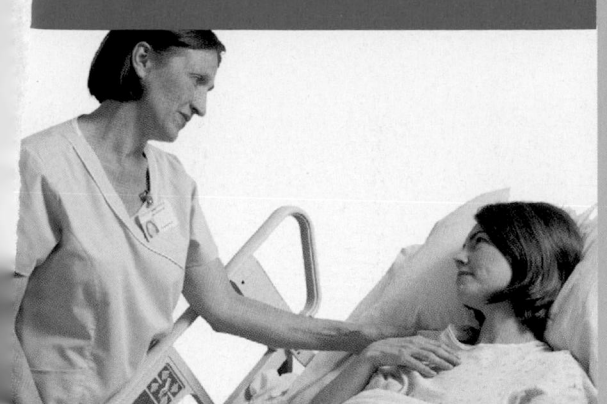

TWELFTH EDITION

VOLUME 2

BRUNNER & SUDDARTH'S
Textbook of
Medical-Surgical
Nursing

Suzanne C. Smeltzer, EdD, RN, FAAN
Professor and Director, Center for Nursing Research
Villanova University College of Nursing
Villanova, Pennsylvania

Brenda G. Bare, RN, MSN
Formerly, Associate Administrator/Chief Nurse Executive
Inova Mount Vernon Hospital
Alexandria, Virginia

Janice L. Hinkle, PhD, RN, CNRN
Formerly, Senior Research Fellow, Acute Stroke Programme
Oxford Brookes University and John Radcliffe Hospital
Oxford, United Kingdom

Kerry H. Cheever, PhD, RN
Professor and Chairperson
St. Luke's School of Nursing at Moravian College
Assistant Vice President
St. Luke's Hospital & Health Network
Bethlehem, Pennsylvania

Wolters Kluwer | Lippincott Williams & Wilkins
Health
Philadelphia · Baltimore · New York · London
Buenos Aires · Hong Kong · Sydney · Tokyo

Senior Acquisitions Editor: Hilarie Surrena
Product Director: Renee Gagliardi
Developmental Editors: Martha Cushman/Megan Klim Duttera
Senior Marketing Manager: Jodi Bukowski
Art Director, Design: Joan Wendt
Art Director, Illustration: Brett MacNaughton/Bob Galindo
Manufacturing Coordinator: Karin Duffield
Compositor: Aptara, Inc.

Twelfth Edition

Library of Congress Cataloging-in-Publication Data

Brunner & Suddarth's textbook of medical-surgical nursing. — 12th ed. /
Suzanne C. Smeltzer ... [et al.].
   p. ; cm.
   Includes bibliographical references and index.
   ISBN 978-0-7817-8589-1 (1 volume American ed. : alk. paper) —
ISBN 978-0-7817-8590-7 (2 volume American ed. : alk. paper) —
ISBN 978-1-60831-080-7 (1 volume international ed.) —
ISBN 978-1-60831-088-3 (2 volume international ed.)
   1. Nursing. 2. Surgical nursing. I. Brunner, Lillian Sholtis. II.
Smeltzer, Suzanne C. O'Connell. III. Title: Brunner and Suddarth's
textbook of medical-surgical nursing. IV. Title: Textbook of
medical-surgical nursing.
   [DNLM: 1. Nursing Care. 2. Perioperative Nursing. WY 150 B8972
2010]
   RT41.T46 2010
   617'.0231—dc22

                                                        2009029135

CONTRIBUTORS

Linda L. Altizer, RN, MSN, ONC, FNE
Health Professions Coordinator
Hagerstown Community College
Hagerstown, Maryland

Chapter 66: Assessment of Musculoskeletal Function

Chapter 69: Management of Patients With Musculoskeletal Trauma

Roberta H. Baron, MSN, RN, AOCN
Clinical Nurse Specialist
Memorial Sloan-Kettering Cancer Center
New York, New York

Chapter 48: Assessment and Management of Patients With Breast Disorders

Janice M. Beitz, RN, PhD, CS, CNOR, CWOCN, CRNP
Professor
La Salle University
Philadelphia, Pennsylvania

Chapter 38: Management of Patients With Intestinal and Rectal Disorders

Catherine M. Belt, MSN, RN, AOCN
Cancer Network Administrator
Abramson Cancer Center of the University of Pennsylvania
Philadelphia, Pennsylvania

Chapter 16: Oncology: Nursing Management in Cancer Care

Elizabeth Blunt, PhD, RN, APRN-BC
Coordinator Nurse Practitioner Programs
Villanova University College of Nursing
Villanova, Pennsylvania

Chapter 53: Assessment and Management of Patients With Allergic Disorders

Lisa Bowman, MSN, RN, CRNP, CNRN
Nurse Practitioner, Division of Cerebrovascular Disease and Neurological Critical Care
Thomas Jefferson University Hospital
Philadelphia, Pennsylvania

Chapter 62: Management of Patients With Cerebrovascular Disorders

Jo Ann Brooks, DNS, RN, FCCP, FAAN
Vice President, Quality
Clarian Health
Indianapolis, Indiana

Chapter 23: Management of Patients With Chest and Lower Respiratory Tract Disorders

Chapter 24: Management of Patients With Chronic Pulmonary Disease

Kim Cantwell-Gab, MN, ARNP-BC, CVN, RVT, RDMS
Acute Care and Adult ARNP
SW Washington Medical Center –Thoracic and Vascular Surgery
Vancouver, Washington

Chapter 31: Assessment and Management of Patients With Vascular Disorders and Problems of Peripheral Circulation

Patricia E. Casey, RN, MSN
Director, NCDR Training and Orientation
American College of Cardiology
Washington, District of Columbia

Chapter 27: Management of Patients With Dysrhythmias and Conduction Problems

Jill Cash, RN, MSN, APRN, CNP
Family Nurse Practitioner
Logan Primary Care
West Frankfort, Illinois

Chapter 59: Assessment and Management of Patients With Hearing and Balance Disorders

Kerry H. Cheever, PhD, RN
Professor and Chairperson
St. Luke's School of Nursing at Moravian College
Assistant Vice President
St. Luke's Hospital & Health Network
Bethlehem, Pennsylvania

Chapter 68: Management of Patients with Musculoskeletal Disorders

Linda Carman Copel, PhD, RN, PHMCNS, BC, CNE, FAPA
Professor
Villanova University
Villanova, Pennsylvania

Chapter 4: Health Education and Health Promotion

Chapter 6: Homeostasis, Stress, and Adaptation

Chapter 7: Individual and Family Considerations Related to Illness

Susanna Garner Cunningham, PhD, BSN, MA, FAAN, FAHA
Professor
University of Washington
Seattle, Washington

Chapter 32: Assessment and Management of Patients With Hypertension

Elizabeth Petit de Mange, PhD, MSN, NP-C, RN
Assistant Professor
Villanova University College of Nursing
Villanova, Pennsylvania

Chapter 42: Assessment and Management of Patients With Endocrine Disorders

Susan K. Dempsey-Walls, MN, RN, AOCNS, ACHPN
Oncology Clinical Nurse Specialist
Orlando Health/M. D. Anderson Cancer Center Orlando
Orlando, Florida

Chapter 49: Assessment and Management of Problems Related to Male
            Reproductive Processes

Nancy Donegan, RN, BSN, MPH
Director, Infection Control
Washington Hospital Center
Washington, District of Columbia

Chapter 70: Management of Patients With Infectious Diseases

Diane K. Dressler, MSN, RN, CCRN
Clinical Assistant Professor
Marquette University College of Nursing
Milwaukee, Wisconsin

Chapter 28: Management of Patients With Coronary Vascular Disorders

Chapter 30: Management of Patients With Complications from
            Heart Disease

Phyllis Dubendorf, RN, MSN, CRNP, CNRN
Clinical Nurse Specialist
Hospital of the University of Pennsylvania
Philadelphia, Pennsylvania

Chapter 61: Management of Patients With Neurologic Dysfunction

Susan M. Fallone, MS, RN, CNN
Clinical Nurse Specialist, Adult and Pediatric Dialysis
Albany Medical Center
Albany, New York

Chapter 43: Assessment of Renal and Urinary Tract Function

Jacqueline D. K. Fenicle, RN, MSN
Director of Patient Care Services
Regional Burn Center and Burn Recovery
Lehigh Valley Health Network
Allentown, Pennsylvania

Chapter 57: Management of Patients With Burn Injury

Eleanor R. Fitzpatrick, RN, BSN, MSN, CCRN
Clinical Nurse Specialist
Thomas Jefferson University Hospital
Philadelphia, Pennsylvania

Chapter 39: Assessment and Management of Patients
            With Hepatic Disorders

Chapter 40: Assessment and Management of Patients
            With Biliary Disorders

Kathleen Kelleher Furniss, RNC, MSN, WHNP-BC, DMH
Coordinator, Women's Imaging and Women's Health NP
Mountainside Hospital and Drew University
Montclair, New Jersey

Chapter 46: Assessment and Management of Female
            Physiologic Processes

Chapter 47: Management of Patients With Female
            Reproductive Disorders

Theresa Lynn Green, PhD, MScHRM, BScN, RN
Assistant Professor
University of Calgary
Calgary, Alberta

Chapter 11: Principles and Practices of Rehabilitation

Margaret J. Griffiths, MSN, RN, CNE
Assistant Dean, Curricular Initiatives
University of Pennsylvania School of Nursing
Philadelphia, Pennsylvania

Chapter 50: Assessment of Immune Function

Chapter 51: Management of Patients With Immunodeficiency

Janice L. Hinkle, PhD, RN, CNRN
Formerly, Senior Research Fellow, Acute Stroke Programme
Oxford Brookes University and John Radcliffe Hospital
Oxford, United Kingdom

Chapter 5: Adult Health and Nutritional Assessment

Chapter 54: Assessment and Management of Patients With Rheumatic
            Disorders

Chapter 64: Management of Patients With Neurologic Infections,
            Autoimmune Disorders, and Neuropathies

Chapter 65: Management of Patients With Oncologic or Degenerative
            Neurologic Disorders

Joyce Young Johnson, RN, MN, PhD
Dean, College of Sciences and Health Professions
    Department of Nursing
Albany State University
Albany, Georgia

Chapter 1: Health Care Delivery and Nursing Practice

Chapter 2: Community-Based Nursing Practice

Chapter 3: Critical Thinking, Ethical Decision Making, and
           the Nursing Process

Chapter 8: Perspectives in Transcultural Nursing

Tamara M. Kear, PhD, MSN, RN, CNN
Assistant Professor
Gwynedd-Mercy College
Gwynedd Valley, Pennsylvania

Chapter 45: Management of Patients With Urinary Disorders

Elizabeth K. Keech, PhD, MA, BSN
Assistant Professor
Villanova University College of Nursing
Villanova University
Villanova, Pennsylvania

Chapter 12: Health Care of the Older Adult

H. Lynne Kennedy, MSN, RN, RNFA, CNOR, CLNC,
    Alumnus CCRN
RNFA, OR Fellowship Instructor, CEU/CME Seminar
    Planner/Instructor
Inova Fair Oaks Hospital
Fairfax, Virginia

Chapter 18: Preoperative Nursing Management

Chapter 19: Intraoperative Nursing Management

Chapter 20: Postoperative Nursing Management

Mary Beth Flynn Makic, PhD, RN, CNS, CCNS, CCRN
Research Nurse Scientist
Critical Care and Assistant Professor
University of Colorado Hospital
University of Colorado Denver–College of Nursing
Aurora, Colorado
Chapter 15: Shock and Multiple Organ Disfunction Syndrome

Barbara J. Maschak-Carey, MSN, RN, CDE
Diabetes Clinical Nurse Specialist
Program Coordinator, Look AHEAD Study
University of Pennsylvania
Philadelphia, Pennsylvania
Chapter 41: Assessment and Management of Patients With Diabetes Mellitus

Agnes Masny, MSN, RN, MPH, CRNP
Nurse Practitioner
Fox Chase Cancer Center
Philadelphia, Pennsylvania
Chapter 9: Genetics and Genomics Perspectives in Nursing

Phyllis J. Mason, MS, ANP-BC
Instructor
The Johns Hopkins University School of Nursing
Baltimore, Maryland
Chapter 34: Assessment of Digestive and Gastrointestinal Function
Chapter 37: Management of Patients With Gastric and Duodenal Disorders

Martha Mulvey, MSN, RN, ANP-BC, ACNS-BC
ANP Neurosciences Epilepsy Program Adult and Pediatrics
The University Hospital
Newark, New Jersey
Chapter 14: Fluid and Electrolytes: Balance and Disturbance

Victoria B. Navarro, MAS, MSN, RN
Director of Nursing
The Wilmer Eye Institute at Johns Hopkins
Baltimore, Maryland
Chapter 58: Assessment and Management of Patients With Eye and Vision Disorders

Donna Nayduch, MSN, RN, ACNP
Trauma Consultant
K-Force Consulting
Tampa, Florida
Chapter 71: Emergency Nursing
Chapter 72: Terrorism, Mass Casualty, and Disaster Nursing

Kathleen M. Nokes, PhD, RN, FAAN
Professor and Director of the Graduate Nursing Program
Hunter College, CUNY Hunter College School of Nursing
New York, New York
Chapter 52: Management of Patients With HIV Infection and AIDS

Janet A. Parkosewich, DNSc, RN, CCRN, FAHA
Interim Nurse Researcher
Yale New Haven Hospital
New Haven, Connecticut
Chapter 26: Assessment of Cardiovascular Function

M. Miki Patterson, PhD, PNP, ONP
Visiting Professor
University of Massachusetts Lowell
Lowell, Massachusetts
Chapter 67: Musculoskeletal Care Modalities

Jana L. Perun, MS, ARNP, AOCNP
Advanced Registered Nurse Practitioner
Cancer Institute of Florida
Altamonte Springs, Florida
Chapter 22: Management of Patients With Upper Respiratory Tract Disorders

Kimberly L. Quinn, MSN, RN, ACNP, ANP, CCRN, ANCP-C
Nurse Practitioner for Thoracic Surgery
Union Memorial Hospital
Baltimore, Maryland
Chapter 35: Management of Patients With Oral and Esophageal Disorders

JoAnne Reifsnyder, PhD, ACHPN
Assistant Professor and Program Director
Chronic Care Management
Jefferson School of Population Health
Thomas Jefferson University
Philadelphia, Pennsylvania
Chapter 17: End-of-Life Care

Judith Reishtein, PhD, RN
Assistant Professor
College of Nursing & Health Professions
Drexel University
Philadelphia, Pennsylvania
Chapter 21: Assessment of Respiratory Function
Chapter 25: Respiratory Care Modalities

Catherine Stewart Sackett, BS, CRNP
Nurse Practitioner
Wilmer Eye Institute at Johns Hopkins
Medstar Research Institute
Baltimore, Maryland
Chapter 58: Assessment and Management of Patients With Eye and Vision Disorders

Linda Schakenbach, MSN, RN, CNS, CCRN, CWCN, ACNS-BC
Clinical Nurse Specialist
Medical Cardiac Nursing
Inova Fairfax Hospital
Inova Heart and Vascular Institute
Falls Church, Virginia
Chapter 29: Management of Patients With Structural, Infectious, and Inflammatory Cardiac Disorders

Suzanne C. Smeltzer, EdD, RN, FAAN
Professor and Director, Center for Nursing Research
Villanova University College of Nursing
Villanova, Pennsylvania
Chapter 10: Chronic Illness and Disability

Karen A. Steffen-Albert, MSN, RN, CCRN, CNRN
Clinical Nurse Specialist, Nursing Research & Quality
Thomas Jefferson University Hospital
Philadelphia, Pennsylvania
Chapter 63: Management of Patients With Neurologic Trauma

Cindy Stern, MSN, RN, CCRP
Cancer Network Administrator
Abramson Cancer Center of the University of
    Pennsylvania Health System
Philadelphia, Pennsylvania
Chapter 16: Oncology: Nursing Management in Cancer Care

Caroline Steward, RN, MSN, APN-C, CCRN, CNN
Nurse Educator Fresenius Medical Care North America
Northern Region Eastern Division
Ewing, New Jersey
Chapter 44: Management of Patients With Renal Disorders

Christina Stewart-Amidei, RN, MSN, CNRN, CCRN
Instructor
University of Central Florida
Orlando, Florida
Chapter 60: Assessment of Neurologic Function

Christine Tea, MSN, RN, NEA-BC, CBN
Service Line Director
Inova Fair Oaks Hospital
Fairfax, Virginia
Chapter 18: Preoperative Nursing Management
Chapter 19: Intraoperative Nursing Management
Chapter 20: Postoperative Nursing Management

Jean Smith Temple, DNS, MSN, BSN
Associate Dean & Associate Professor
Valdosta State University College of Nursing
Valdosta, Georgia
Chapter 1: Health Care Delivery and Nursing Practice
Chapter 2: Community-Based Nursing Practice
Chapter 3: Critical Thinking, Ethical Decision Making, and
    the Nursing Process
Chapter 8: Perspectives in Transcultural Nursing

Mary L. Thomas, MS, RN, AOCN
Hematology Clinical Nurse Specialist
VA Palo Alto Health Care System
Palo Alto, California
Chapter 33: Assessment and Management of Patients With
    Hematologic Disorders

Renay D. Tyler, MSN, RN, ACNP, CNSN
Acute Care Nurse Practitioner
The Parenteral–Enteral Support Service
The Johns Hopkins Hospital
Baltimore, Maryland
Chapter 36: Gastrointestinal Intubation and Special
    Nutritional Modalities

Joyce S. Willens, PhD, RN, BC
Assistant Professor
Villanova University College of Nursing
Villanova, Pennsylvania
Chapter 13: Pain Management

Iris Woodard, BSN, RN-CS, ANP
Nurse Practitioner
Kaiser Permanente
Rockville, Maryland
Chapter 55: Assessment of Integumentary Function
Chapter 56: Management of Patients With Dermatologic Problems

Acknowledgments

The authors gratefully acknowledge the contributions and expertise of Dale Halsey Lea, MS, RN, MPH, FAAN.

PREFACE

The first edition of *Brunner & Suddarth's Textbook of Medical-Surgical Nursing* was published in 1964 under the leadership of Lillian Sholtis Brunner and Doris Smith Suddarth. Lillian and Doris pioneered a medical-surgical nursing textbook that has become a classic. Medical-surgical nursing has come a long way since 1964 but continues to be strongly influenced by the expansion of science, medicine, surgery, and technology, as well as a myriad of social, cultural, economic, and environmental changes throughout the world. Nurses must be particularly skilled in critical thinking and clinical decision-making as well as in consulting and collaborating with other members of the multidisciplinary health care team.

Along with the challenges that today's nurses confront, there are many opportunities to provide skilled, compassionate nursing care in a variety of health care settings, for patients in the various stages of illness, and for patients across the age continuum. At the same time, there are significant opportunities for fostering health promotion activities for individuals and groups; this is an integral part of providing nursing care.

Continuing the tradition of Lillian's and Doris's first edition, this 12th edition of *Brunner & Suddarth's Textbook of Medical-Surgical Nursing* is designed to assist nurses in preparing for their roles and responsibilities within the complex health care delivery system. A goal of the textbook is to provide balanced attention to the art and science of adult medical-surgical nursing. The textbook focuses on physiologic, pathophysiologic, and psychosocial concepts as they relate to nursing care, and emphasis is placed on integrating a variety of concepts from other disciplines such as nutrition, pharmacology, and gerontology. Content relative to health care needs of people with disabilities, nursing research findings, ethical considerations, and evidence-based practice has been expanded to provide opportunities for the nurse to refine clinical decision-making skills.

Organization

Brunner & Suddarth's Textbook of Medical-Surgical Nursing, 12th edition, is organized into 16 units. Units 1 through 4 cover core concepts related to medical-surgical nursing practice. Units 5 through 16 discuss adult health conditions that are treated medically or surgically. Each unit covering adult health conditions is structured in the following way, to facilitate understanding:

- The first chapter in the unit covers assessment and includes a review of normal anatomy and physiology of the body system being discussed.
- The subsequent chapters in the unit cover management of specific disorders. Pathophysiology, clinical manifestations, assessment and diagnostic findings, medical management, and nursing management are presented. Special "Nursing Process" sections, provided for selected conditions, clarify and expand on the nurse's role in caring for patients with these conditions.

Features

Practice-Oriented Features

Nurses assume many different roles when caring for patients. Many of the features in this textbook have been developed to help nurses fulfill these varied roles.

The Nurse as Practitioner

One of the central roles of the nurse is to provide holistic care to patients and their families, both independently and through collaboration with other health care professionals. Many features in *Brunner & Suddarth's Textbook of Medical-Surgical Nursing* are designed to assist students with clinical practice.

Nursing Process sections. The nursing process is the basis for all nursing practice. Special sections throughout the text, organized according to the nursing process framework, clarify the nurse's responsibilities in caring for patients with selected disorders.

Plans of Nursing Care. These plans, provided for selected disorders, illustrate how the nursing process is applied to meet the person's health care and nursing needs.

Applying Concepts from NANDA, NIC, and NOC. Each unit begins with a case study and a chart presenting examples of NANDA, NIC, and NOC terminologies related to the case study. Concept maps, which provide a visual representation of the NANDA, NIC, and NOC chart for each case study, are found on the accompanying Web site thePoint to this book at thepoint.lww.com/Smeltzer12e. This feature introduces the student to the NIC and NOC language and classifications and brings them to life in graphic form.

Assessment charts. These charts help to focus the student's attention on data that should be collected as part of the assessment step of the nursing process.

Risk Factor charts. These charts draw the student's attention to factors that can impair health.

Guidelines charts. These charts review key nursing interventions, and the rationales for those interventions, for specific patient care situations.

Pharmacology charts and tables. Pharmacology charts and tables remind the student of important considerations relative to administering medications and monitoring drug therapy.

Nursing Alerts. These special sections offer brief tips for clinical practice and red-flag warnings to help students avoid common mistakes.

Critical Care. These special sections highlight nursing process considerations for the critically ill patient.

Gerontologic Considerations. In the United States, older adults comprise the fastest-growing segment of the population. This icon is applied to headings, charts, and tables as appropriate to highlight information that pertains specifically to the care of the older adult patient.

Genetics in Nursing Practice charts. These charts summarize and highlight the role that genetics play in many disorders.

Physiology/Pathophysiology figures. These illustrations and algorithms help students to understand normal physiologic and pathophysiologic processes.

The Nurse as Educator

Health education is a primary responsibility of the nursing profession. Nursing care is directed toward promoting, maintaining, and restoring health; preventing illness; and helping patients and families adapt to the residual effects of illness. Teaching, in the form of patient education and health promotion, is central to all of these nursing activities.

Patient Education charts. These charts help the nurse to prepare the patient and family for procedures, assist them with understanding the patient's condition, and explain to them how to provide for self-care after discharge from the health care facility.

Home Care checklists. These checklists review points that should be covered as part of patient education prior to discharge from the health care facility.

Health Promotion charts. These charts review important points that the nurse should discuss with the patient to prevent common health problems from developing.

The Nurse as Patient Advocate

Nurses advocate for patients by protecting their rights (including the right to health care) and assisting patients and their families to make informed decisions about health care.

Ethics and Related Issues charts. These charts present a scenario, a description of potential ethical dilemmas that could arise as a result of the scenario, and a list of questions about the scenario to stimulate thought and discussion.

The Nurse as Researcher

Nurses identify potential research problems and questions to increase nursing knowledge and improve patient care. Use and evaluation of research findings in nursing practice are essential to further the science of nursing.

Nursing Research Profiles. These charts identify the implications and applications of nursing research findings for nursing practice.

EBP *Evidence-Based Practice (EBP) questions.* This icon appears next to critical thinking exercises that encourage the student to think about the evidence base for specific nursing interventions. A journals supplement offers students free online access to over 70 journal articles that relate to the evidence-based practice questions in the text.

Pedagogical Features

Learning Objectives. Each chapter begins with a list of learning objectives. These give the student an overview of the chapter and help to focus his or her reading.

Glossaries. Glossaries provided at the beginning of each chapter let the student review vocabulary words before reading the chapter, and also serve as a useful reference tool while reading.

Critical Thinking Exercises. These questions, which appear at the end of each chapter, foster critical thinking by challenging the student to apply textbook knowledge to clinical scenarios.

References and Selected Readings. A list of current references cited is given at the end of each chapter.

Resources. A resource list at the end of each chapter directs the reader to sources of additional information, Web sites, agencies, and patient education materials.

A Comprehensive Package for Teaching and Learning

To further facilitate teaching and learning, a carefully designed ancillary package is available. In addition to the usual print resources, we are pleased to present multimedia tools that have been developed in conjunction with the text.

Resources for Students

Interactive DVD-ROM. Packaged with the textbook at no additional charge, this DVD helps students test their knowledge and enhance their understanding of medical-surgical nursing. This DVD includes:
- More than 700 study questions organized by unit
- 3,500 NCLEX-style cross-disciplinary questions
- Concepts in Action™ Animations
- Nursing in Action™ Videos
- Clinical Simulations
- Spanish-English Audioglossary
- Drug Monographs
- Other Learning Tools

Study Guide to Accompany Smeltzer, Bare, Hinkle & Cheever: Brunner & Suddarth's Textbook of Medical-Surgical Nursing, 12th edition. Available at student bookstores or at www.LWW.com, this study guide presents a variety of exercises to reinforce the textbook content and enhance learning.

Handbook to Accompany Smeltzer, Bare, Hinkle & Cheever: Brunner & Suddarth's Textbook of Medical-Surgical Nursing, 12th edition. Available at student bookstores or at www.LWW.com, this clinical reference presents need-to-know information on nearly 200 commonly encountered disorders in an easy-to-use alphabetized outline format.

Resources for Instructors

Instructor's Resource DVD-ROM. The instructor's resource DVD contains the following items:
- A thoroughly revised and augmented test generator, containing more than 2,000 NCLEX-style questions
- Sample syllabi for one-, two-, and three-semester courses
- Strategies for effective teaching
- PowerPoint™ lectures, guided lecture notes, and pre-lecture quizzes
- An image bank
- Discussion topics and assignments

Resources for Students and Instructors

ThePoint* (thepoint.lww.com) Students and instructors can visit thePoint to access supplemental multimedia resources to enhance their learning.

It is with pleasure that we introduce these resources—the textbook and the ancillary package—to you. One of our primary goals in creating these resources has been to help nurses and nursing students provide quality care to patients and families across health care settings and in the home. We hope that we have succeeded in that goal, and we welcome feedback from our readers.

Suzanne C. O'Connell Smeltzer, EdD, RN, FAAN

Brenda G. Bare, RN, MSN

Janice L. Hinkle, PhD, RN, CNRN

Kerry H. Cheever, PhD, RN

*thePoint is a trademark of Wolters Kluwer Health.

Earnest Ruth Agnew, RN, MSN
Nursing Instructor/Simulation Lab Coordinator
Itawamba Community College
Fulton, Mississippi

Rita Amerio, PhD(c), RN
Undergraduate Director, College of Nursing and
    Health Professions
Lewis University
Romeoville, Illinois

Linda Barkoozis, RN, MSN
Professor of Nursing
College of DuPage
Glen Ellyn, Illinois

Joanna G. Barnes, MSN, RN
ADN Program Coordinator
Grayson County College
Denison, Texas

Carol A. Berube, RN, MSN
Instructor
Brockton Hospital of Nursing
Brockton, Massachusetts

Dana M. Botz, MSN, RN
Faculty
North Hennepin Community College
Brooklyn Park, Minnesota

Sharon McFadden Bradley, MSN, RN, CNL
Clinical Assistant Professor
Coordinator for Curriculum and Evaluation
University of Florida
Gainesville, Florida

Jo Ellen Branstetter, RN, MS, MS (N), PhD
Professor
Cox College
Springfield, Missouri

Janet Witucki Brown, PhD, RN, CNE
Associate Professor
The University of Tennessee, Knoxville
Knoxville, Tennessee

Julia C. Burgett, MSN, RN, CNE, CNRN
Associate Professor
St. Mary's/Marshall University
Huntington, West Virginia

Patricia Burkard, RNC, MSN
Professor
Moorpark College
Moorpark, California

Janet E. Burton, MSN, RN, CMSRN
Clinical Nurse Specialist/Clinical Instructor
Columbus Regional Hospital
Columbus, Indiana

Patricia W. Campbell, RN, MSN
Faculty
Carolinas College of Health Sciences
Charlotte, North Carolina

Marilyn V. Clithero, RN, MSN
Assistant Professor
Cox College
Springfield, Missouri

Johnnie Sue Cooper, MSN, RN, FNP-BC
Nursing Instructor
Mississippi University for Women
Columbus, Mississippi

Marianne Craven, PhD(c), RN
Professor
Utah Valley University
Orem, Utah

Deborah L. Dalrymple, RN, MSN, CRNI
Professor
Montgomery County Community College
Blue Bell, Pennsylvania

Martha L. Davis, MSN, RN
Associate Degree Nursing Instructor
Itawamba Community College
Fulton, Mississippi

Jane F. deLeon, PhD, RN
Assistant Professor
San Francisco State University
San Francisco, California

David J. Derrico, RN, MSN
Assistant Clinical Professor
University of Florida
Gainesville, Florida

Carol M. Diehl, MSN, MSED, RN
Simulation Coordinator
The Reading Hospital School of Health Sciences
Reading, Pennsylvania

Larinda Dixon, RN, MSN, EdD
Professor
College of DuPage
Glen Ellyn, Illinois

Denise R. Doliveira, RN, MSN
Associate Professor
Community College of Allegheny County, Boyce Campus
Pittsburgh, Pennsylvania

Cynthia L. Donell, MSN, RN, CNE
Campus Director of Nursing
Harrisburg Area Community College, York Campus
York, Pennsylvania

Sandra K. Eggenberger, PhD, RN
Professor
Minnesota State University
Mankato, Minnesota

Cynthia L. Fenske, MS, RN
Lecturer IV
University of Michigan
Ann Arbor, Michigan

Dilyss Gallyot, RN, MS, CCRN
Associate Professor
College of DuPage
Glen Ellyn, Illinois

Theresa A. Glanville, RN, MS, CNE
Professor
Springfield Technical Community College
Springfield, Massachusetts

Cornelia Gordon, RN, BSN, BA, MA
Nursing Instructor
McLennan Community College
Waco, Texas

Kathy Gray-Siracusa, PhD, RN, MBA, CCRN, NEA-BC
Assistant Professor
Villanova University College of Nursing
Villanova, Pennsylvania

Kim Green, RN, MSN
Assistant Professor
Western Kentucky University
Bowling Green, Kentucky

Jacqueline Guhde, MSN, RN, CNS
Assistant Professor
The University of Akron
Akron, Ohio

Karen Toby Haghenbeck, PhD, FNP-BC,
RN-BC, CCRN
Assistant Professor
Pace University
Pleasantville, New York

Mary E. Hanson-Zalot, MSN, RN
Assistant Dean, ASN-BSN
Thomas Jefferson University
Philadelphia, Pennsylvania

Nancy J. Harrer, RN, MS
Assistant Professor
Community College of Baltimore County
Catonsville, Maryland

Kathleen Hayes, RN, MSEd, MSN
Professor
Norwalk Community College
Norwalk, Connecticut

Bonnie Heintzelman, MSN, RN, CMSRN
Instructor
Thomas Jefferson University
Philadelphia, Pennsylvania

Pam Henderson, MSN, RN
Executive Director ADN/PN Programs
University of Arkansas, Fort Smith
Fort Smith, Arkansas

Kevin D. Hite, RN, MSN
Assistant Professor
Fairmont State University
Fairmont, West Virginia

Wanda K. Hoerning, RN, MA, NP-C
Adjunct Instructor
College of Staten Island and Manatee Community College
Staten Island, New York and Bradenton, Florida

Janice J. Hoffman, PhD, RN, CCRN
Assistant Professor and Vice Chair
University of Maryland
Baltimore, Maryland

Jane Hook, RN, MN
Lecturer
California State University, Los Angeles
Los Angeles, California

Connie Houser, MS, RNC-OB, CNE
Nursing Instructor
Central Carolina Technical College
Manning, South Carolina

Norlyn B. Hyde, RN, C, MSN, CNS
Professor
Louisiana Tech University
Ruston, Louisiana

Kathy J. Keister, PhD, RN, CNE
Assistant Professor
Wright State University
Dayton, Ohio

Patricia A. Kent, MS, ACNP-BC
Clinical Assistant Professor
University of Massachusetts Amherst School of Nursing
Amherst, Massachusetts

Penny Y. Kessler, DNS(c), RN
Clinical Assistant Professor
University of Minnesota City
Minneapolis, Minnesota

Deborah R. Klinger, RN, MSN, MBA
Associate Professor
Manatee Community College
Bradenton, Florida

Catherine Lein, MS, FNP-BC
Assistant Professor
MSU College of Nursing
East Lansing, Michigan

Linda C. Lott, RN, MSN
AD Nursing Instructor
Itawamba Community College
Fulton, Mississippi

Tamar Jones Lucas, BSN, MSN, RN, BC
ADN Instructor
Itawamba Community College
Fulton, Mississippi

Billie A. Lynes, FNP, MSN
Professor/Gynocologic Oncology Nurse Practitioner
Mt. San Antonio College
Walnut, California

Shirley B. MacNeill, MSN, RN
ADN Nursing Instructor
Lamar State College, Port Arthur
Porth Arthur, Texas

Phyllis Magaletto, MS, RN, BC
Instructor
Cochran School of Nursing
Yonkers, New York

Gina Maiocco, PhD, RN, CCRN, CCNS
Assistant Professor
Coordinator BS/BA to BSN Program
West Virginia University
Morgantown, West Virginia

Andrea R. Mann, MSN, RN
Instructor, Third Level Chair at Frankford
Instructor Pharmacology at Penn State
Frankford Hospital School of Nursing
Penn State University
Philadelphia, Pennsylvania

Sharon McDonald, MSN, RN
Nursing Instructor
University of Southern Mississippi
Hattiesburg, Mississippi

Nancy Miller, MS, RN
Faculty
Minneapolis Community and Technical College
Minneapolis, Minnesota

Ildiko E. Monahan, MS, RN, ANP
Nurse Educator
St. Elizabeth College of Nursing
Utica, New York

Suzie Morrow, MSN, RN, CNE
Associate Professor
Southwest Baptist University
Springfield, Missouri

Mary Ellen Moyer-Hutcherson, RN, MSN
Professor
Florida Community College
Jacksonville, Florida

Janice A. Neil, RN, PhD
Associate Professor
East Carolina University
Greenville, North Carolina

Pamela S. Newton, RN, BSN
Traveling Nurse
Home Care RN Case Manager IV Team
Pathways Home Health and Hospice
Sunnyvale, California

Rebecca Otten, RN, MSN, EdD
Assistant Professor
California State University Fullerton
Fullerton, California

Verna C. Pangman, RN, MEd, MN
Senior Instructor
University of Manitoba
Winnipeg, Manitoba

Susan R. Parslow, RN, PhD
Associate Professor
Boise State University
Boise, Idaho

Linda Peake, MS, RN, C, CNE
Professor, Curriculum Coordinator
St. Mary's/Marshall University Cooperative and Program
Huntington, West Virginia

Lisa Peden, RN, MSN
Associate Professor
Dalton State College
Dalton, Georgia

Beverly Raway, PhD, RN
Assistant Professor
The College of St. Scholastica
Duluth, Minnesota

Marisue Rayno, RN, MSN, EdD(c)
Faculty
Luzerne County Community College
Nanticoke, Pennsylvania

Kathleen T. Rine, MSN, RN, OCN
Instructor
School of Nursing
Thomas Jefferson University
Philadelphia, Pennsylvania

Kathy Rodger, RN, BSN, MN
Faculty
Nursing Education Program of Saskatchewan (NEPS)
SIAST Wascana Campus
Regina, Saskatchewan

Donna Russo, RN, MSN, CCRN, CNE
Nursing Instructor
Frankford Hospital School of Nursing
Philadelphia, Pennsylvania

Lisa A. Streeter, MSRN, CNE
Nursing Instructor
St. Elizabeth College of Nursing
Utica, New York

Wendy J. Waldspurger Robb, PhD, RN, CNE
Assistant Professor
Director of the Graduate Nursing Program
Cedar Crest College
Allentown, Pennsylvania

Kristen J. Rogers, MSN, CNE, RN
Director, Service Excellence
The Washington Hospital
Washington, Pennsylvania

Tanya Lynn Rogers, APRN, BC, MSN
Associate Professor
Fairmont State University
Fairmont, West Virginia

Judith L. Samsel, RN, MSN
Professor/Chairperson, Nursing Department
Broome Community College
Binghamton, New York

Mary Ellen Santucci, PhD, RN
Assistant Professor
Widener University
Chester, Pennsylvania

Jo-Ann V. Sawatzky, RN, PhD
Associate Professor
University of Manitoba
Winnipeg, Manitoba

Ruth L. Schaffler, PhD, ARNP
Assistant Professor
Pacific Lutheran University
Tacoma, Washington

Donald G. Smith, Jr, MA, PhD, RN, ACRN
Assistant Professor
Hunter College, CUNY
New York, New York

Deborah Steele, PhD, RN, LMFT
Assistant Professor
California State University, Fresno
Fresno, California

Nancy Steffen, RN, MSN
Instructor
Century College
White Bear Lake, Minnesota

Marie H. Thomas, PhD, RN
Instructor
Forsyth Technical Community College
Winston-Salem, North Carolina

Linda Turchin, RN, MSN, CNE
Assistant Professor
Fairmont State University
Fairmont, West Virginia

Carol A. Velas, MSN, RN
Assistant Coordinator, Health Sciences
Associate Professor of Nursing
Moorpark College
Moorpark, California

Mary Walden, RN, MSN, DNP(c), CWOCN
Faculty
Itawamba Community College
Fulton, Mississippi

Terri L. Walker, MSN, RN
Professor
Oklahoma City Community College
Oklahoma City, Oklahoma

Mary Welhaven, PhD, RN
Professor
Winona State University, Rochester
Rochester, Minnesota

Stuart L. Whitney, EdD, RN, CNS
Clinical Associate Professor
University of Vermont
Burlington, Vermont

Donna Williams, RN, MSN, DNP(c)
Faculty
Itawamba Community College
Fulton, Mississippi

Emily Ray Wilson, RN, MSN, MA, AOCN
Instructor and Course Coordinator
Michigan State University
East Lansing, Michigan

Debra Wilson, MSN, FNP
Assistant Professor
California State University, Bakersfield
Bakersfield, California

Thomas Worms, MSN, RN
Professor
Truman College
Chicago, Illinois

Rebecca Yarnell, RN, MSN
Associate Professor
Roane State Community College
Harriman, Tennessee

Jean Yockey, MSN, FNP-BC, CNE
Associate Professor
University of South Dakota
Vermillion, South Dakota

CONTENTS

unit 3
Concepts and Challenges in Patient Management   228

unit 15

Musculoskeletal Function 2006

Metabolic and Endocrine Function

Case Study • Applying Concepts From NANDA, NIC, and NOC

A Patient With Complications of Diabetes

Mr. Johansen is a 58-year-old man with type 2 diabetes, peripheral vascular disease, hyperlipidemia, and peripheral neuropathy. He is also 50 lb over his ideal body weight. He takes an oral antidiabetic agent twice daily and lovastatin for elevated cholesterol levels. Mr. Johansen comes to the clinic for treatment of an unrelated respiratory infection. While there, he tells the nurse that he has numbness and tingling of his feet and has burning pain in his legs if he stands for long periods of time. The nurse assesses his feet and notes decreased sensory function in both feet. Mr. Johansen states that he has not seen his doctor for more than 1 year and only comes to the clinic if he feels sick.

Visit thePoint to view a concept map that illustrates the relationships that exist between the nursing diagnoses, interventions, and outcomes for the patient's clinical problems.

Nursing Classifications and Languages

NANDA NURSING DIAGNOSES	NIC NURSING INTERVENTIONS	NOC NURSING OUTCOMES
		Return to functional baseline status, stabilization of, or improvement in:
INEFFECTIVE TISSUE PERFUSION (ALL TYPES)—Decrease in oxygen resulting in the failure to nourish tissues at the capillary level	**CIRCULATORY CARE: ARTERIAL INSUFFICIENCY**—Promotion of arterial circulation	**CIRCULATION STATUS**—Extent to which blood flows unobstructed, unidirectionally, and at an appropriate pressure through large vessels of the systemic and pulmonary circuits
DISTURBED TACTILE SENSORY PERCEPTION—Change in the amount or patterning of incoming stimuli accompanied by a diminished, exaggerated, distorted, or impaired response to such stimuli	**CIRCULATORY PRECAUTIONS**—Protection of localized area with limited perfusion	**SENSORY FUNCTION: CUTANEOUS**—Extent to which stimulation of the skin is correctly sensed
INEFFECTIVE THERAPEUTIC REGIMEN MANAGEMENT—Pattern of regulating and integrating into daily living a program for treatment of illness and the sequelae of illness that is unsatisfactory for meeting specific health goals	**TEACHING: FOOT CARE**—Preparing an at-risk patient and/or a significant other to provide preventive foot care	**TISSUE INTEGRITY: SKIN AND MUCOUS MEMBRANES**—Structural intactness and normal physiologic function of skin and mucous membranes
	SKIN SURVEILLANCE—Collection and analysis of patient data to maintain skin and mucous membrane integrity	**KNOWLEDGE: DIABETES MANAGEMENT**—Extent of understanding conveyed about diabetes mellitus and its control
	TEACHING: INDIVIDUAL—Planning, implementation, and evaluation of a teaching program designed to address a patient's particular needs	

Bulechek, G. M., Butcher, H. K., & Dochterman, J. M. (2008). *Nursing interventions classification (NIC)* (5th ed.). St. Louis: Mosby.

Johnson, M., Bulechek, G., Butcher, H. K., et al. (2006). *NANDA, NOC, and NIC linkages* (2nd ed.). St. Louis: Mosby.

Moorhead, S., Johnson, M., Mass, M. L., et al. (2008). *Nursing outcomes classification (NOC)* (4th ed.). St. Louis: Mosby.

NANDA International. (2007). *Nursing diagnoses: Definitions & classification 2007–2008*. Philadelphia: North American Nursing Diagnosis Association.

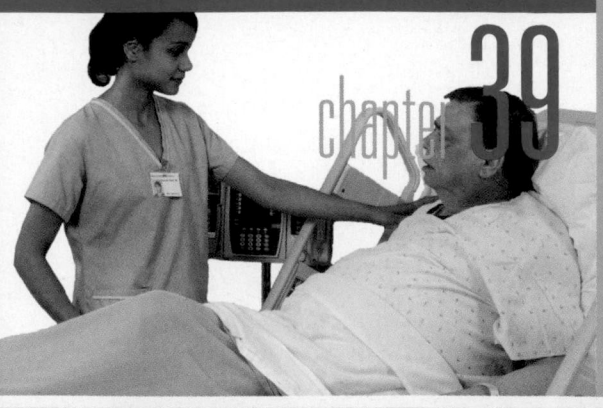

Chapter 39

Assessment and Management of Patients With Hepatic Disorders

LEARNING OBJECTIVES

On completion of this chapter, the learner will be able to:

1 Identify the metabolic functions of the liver and the alterations in these functions that occur with liver disease.

2 Explain liver function tests and the clinical manifestations of liver dysfunction in relation to pathophysiologic alterations of the liver.

3 Relate jaundice, portal hypertension, ascites, varices, nutritional deficiencies, and hepatic coma to pathophysiologic alterations of the liver.

4 Describe the medical, surgical, and nursing management of patients with esophageal varices.

5 Compare the various types of hepatitis and their causes, prevention, clinical manifestations, management, prognosis, and home health care needs.

6 Use the nursing process as a framework for care of the patient with cirrhosis of the liver.

7 Compare the nonsurgical and surgical management of patients with cancer of the liver.

8 Describe the postoperative nursing care of the patient undergoing liver transplantation.

GLOSSARY

asterixis: involuntary flapping movements of the hands associated with metabolic liver dysfunction

balloon tamponade: use of balloons placed within the esophagus and proximal portion of the stomach and inflated to compress bleeding vessels (esophageal and gastric varices)

Budd-Chiari syndrome: hepatic vein thrombosis resulting in non-cirrhotic portal hypertension

cirrhosis: a chronic liver disease characterized by fibrotic changes and the formation of dense connective tissue within the liver, subsequent degenerative changes, and loss of functioning cells

constructional apraxia: inability to draw figures in two or three dimensions

fetor hepaticus: sweet, slightly fecal odor to the breath, presumed to be of intestinal origin; prevalent with the extensive collateral portal circulation in chronic liver disease

fulminant hepatic failure: sudden, severe onset of acute liver failure that occurs within 8 weeks after the first symptoms of jaundice

hepatic encephalopathy: central nervous system dysfunction resulting from liver disease; frequently associated with elevated ammonia levels that produce changes in mental status, altered level of consciousness, and coma

orthotopic liver transplantation (OLT): grafting of a donor liver into the normal anatomic location, with removal of the diseased native liver

portal hypertension: elevated pressure in the portal circulation resulting from obstruction of venous flow into and through the liver

sclerotherapy: the injection of substances into or around esophagogastric varices to cause constriction, thickening, and hardening of the vessel and thus to stop bleeding

variceal banding: procedure that involves the endoscopic placement of a rubber band–like device over esophageal varices to ligate the area and stop bleeding

xenograft: transplantation of organs from one species to another

Liver function is complex, and liver dysfunction affects all body systems. For this reason, the nurse must understand how the liver functions and must have expert clinical assessment and management skills to care for patients undergoing complex diagnostic and treatment procedures. The nurse also must understand technologic advances in the management of liver disorders. Liver disorders are common and may result from a virus, exposure to toxic substances such as alcohol, or tumors.

ASSESSMENT OF THE LIVER

Anatomic and Physiologic Overview

The liver, the largest gland of the body, can be considered a chemical factory that manufactures, stores, alters, and excretes a large number of substances involved in metabolism. The location of the liver is essential in this function because it receives nutrient-rich blood directly from the gastrointestinal (GI) tract and then either stores or transforms these nutrients into chemicals that are used elsewhere in the body for metabolic needs. The liver is especially important in the regulation of glucose and protein metabolism. The liver manufactures and secretes bile, which has a major role in the digestion and absorption of fats in the GI tract. The liver removes waste products from the bloodstream and secretes them into the bile. The bile produced by the liver is stored temporarily in the gallbladder until it is needed for digestion, at which time the gallbladder empties and bile enters the intestine (Fig. 39-1).

Anatomy of the Liver

The liver is a large, highly vascular organ located behind the ribs in the upper right portion of the abdominal cavity. It weighs between 1200 and 1500 g and is divided into four lobes. A thin layer of connective tissue surrounds each lobe, extending into the lobe itself and dividing the liver mass into small, functional units called lobules (Rodes, Benhamou, Blei, et al., 2007).

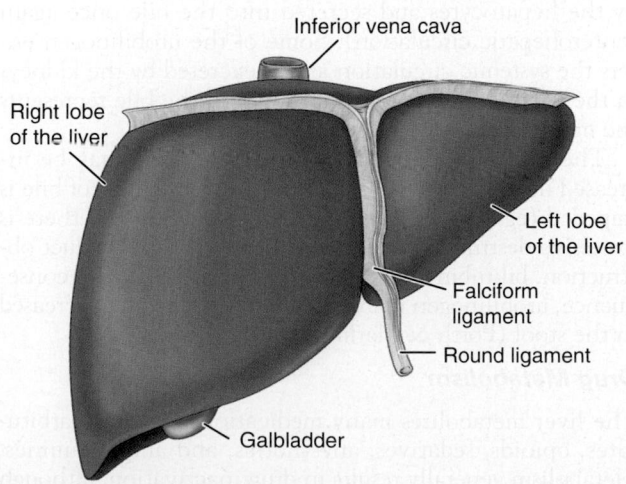

Figure 39-1 The liver and biliary system.

Labels: Inferior vena cava; Right lobe of the liver; Left lobe of the liver; Falciform ligament; Round ligament; Galbladder

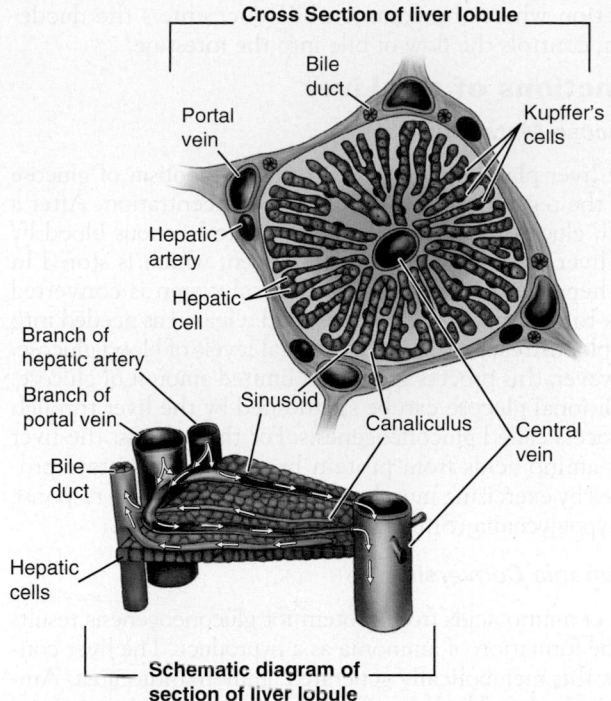

Figure 39-2 A section of liver lobule showing the location of hepatic veins, hepatic cells, liver sinusoids, and branches of the portal vein and hepatic artery.

Labels: Cross Section of liver lobule; Bile duct; Portal vein; Kupffer's cells; Hepatic artery; Hepatic cell; Branch of hepatic artery; Branch of portal vein; Sinusoid; Canaliculus; Bile duct; Central vein; Hepatic cells; Schematic diagram of section of liver lobule

The circulation of the blood into and out of the liver is of major importance to liver function. The blood that perfuses the liver comes from two sources. Approximately 80% of the blood supply comes from the portal vein, which drains the GI tract and is rich in nutrients but lacks oxygen. The remainder of the blood supply enters by way of the hepatic artery and is rich in oxygen. Terminal branches of these two blood vessels join to form common capillary beds, which constitute the sinusoids of the liver (Fig. 39-2). Thus, a mixture of venous and arterial blood bathes the liver cells (hepatocytes). The sinusoids empty into venules that occupy the center of each liver lobule and are called the central veins. The central veins join to form the hepatic vein, which constitutes the venous drainage from the liver and empties into the inferior vena cava, close to the diaphragm (Rodes, et al., 2007).

In addition to hepatocytes, phagocytic cells belonging to the reticuloendothelial system are present in the liver. Other organs that contain reticuloendothelial cells are the spleen, bone marrow, lymph nodes, and lungs. In the liver, these cells are called Kupffer cells. As the most common phagocyte in the human body, their main function is to engulf particulate matter (eg, bacteria) that enters the liver through the portal blood.

The smallest bile ducts, called canaliculi, are located between the lobules of the liver. The canaliculi receive secretions from the hepatocytes and carry them to larger bile ducts, which eventually form the hepatic duct. The hepatic duct from the liver and the cystic duct from the gallbladder join to form the common bile duct, which empties into the small intestine. The sphincter of Oddi, located at the junction where the common bile duct enters the duodenum, controls the flow of bile into the intestine.

Functions of the Liver

Glucose Metabolism

The liver plays a major role in the metabolism of glucose and the regulation of blood glucose concentration. After a meal, glucose is taken up from the portal venous blood by the liver and converted into glycogen, which is stored in the hepatocytes. Subsequently, the glycogen is converted back to glucose (glycogenolysis) and released as needed into the bloodstream to maintain normal levels of blood glucose. However, this process provides a limited amount of glucose. Additional glucose can be synthesized by the liver through a process called gluconeogenesis. For this process, the liver uses amino acids from protein breakdown or lactate produced by exercising muscles. This process occurs in response to hypoglycemia (Shils, Shike, Ross, et al., 2006).

Ammonia Conversion

Use of amino acids from protein for gluconeogenesis results in the formation of ammonia as a byproduct. The liver converts this metabolically generated ammonia into urea. Ammonia produced by bacteria in the intestines is also removed from portal blood for urea synthesis. In this way, the liver converts ammonia, a potential toxin, into urea, a compound that is excreted in the urine (Porth & Matfin, 2009).

Protein Metabolism

The liver also plays an important role in protein metabolism. It synthesizes almost all of the plasma proteins (except gamma-globulin), including albumin, alpha-globulins and beta-globulins, blood clotting factors, specific transport proteins, and most of the plasma lipoproteins. Vitamin K is required by the liver for synthesis of prothrombin and some of the other clotting factors. Amino acids are used by the liver for protein synthesis (Porth & Matfin, 2009).

Fat Metabolism

The liver is also active in fat metabolism. Fatty acids can be broken down for the production of energy and ketone bodies (acetoacetic acid, beta-hydroxybutyric acid, and acetone). Ketone bodies are small compounds that can enter the bloodstream and provide a source of energy for muscles and other tissues. Breakdown of fatty acids into ketone bodies occurs primarily when the availability of glucose for metabolism is limited, as in starvation or in uncontrolled diabetes. Fatty acids and their metabolic products are also used for the synthesis of cholesterol, lecithin, lipoproteins, and other complex lipids (Porth & Matfin, 2009).

In some conditions, lipids may accumulate in the hepatocytes, resulting in the abnormal condition called fatty liver.

Vitamin and Iron Storage

Vitamins A, B, and D and several of the B-complex vitamins are stored in large amounts in the liver. Certain substances, such as iron and copper, are also stored in the liver. Because the liver is rich in these substances, liver extracts have been used for therapy for more than a century for a wide range of nutritional disorders; however, the U.S. Food and Drug Administration (FDA) has urged caution regarding the use of any animal organ extract because of possible risk of exposure to pathogenic organisms.

Bile Formation

Bile is continuously formed by the hepatocytes and collected in the canaliculi and bile ducts. It is composed mainly of water and electrolytes such as sodium, potassium, calcium, chloride, and bicarbonate, and it also contains significant amounts of lecithin, fatty acids, cholesterol, bilirubin, and bile salts. Bile is collected and stored in the gallbladder and is emptied into the intestine when needed for digestion. The functions of bile are excretory, as in the excretion of bilirubin; bile also serves as an aid to digestion through the emulsification of fats by bile salts.

Bile salts are synthesized by the hepatocytes from cholesterol. After conjugation or binding with amino acids (taurine and glycine), bile salts are excreted into the bile. The bile salts, together with cholesterol and lecithin, are required for emulsification of fats in the intestine, which is necessary for efficient digestion and absorption. Bile salts are then reabsorbed, primarily in the distal ileum, into portal blood for return to the liver and are again excreted into the bile. This pathway from hepatocytes to bile to intestine and back to the hepatocytes is called the enterohepatic circulation. Because of the enterohepatic circulation, only a small fraction of the bile salts that enter the intestine are excreted in the feces. This decreases the need for active synthesis of bile salts by the liver cells (Porth & Matfin, 2009).

Bilirubin Excretion

Bilirubin is a pigment derived from the breakdown of hemoglobin by cells of the reticuloendothelial system, including the Kupffer cells of the liver. Hepatocytes remove bilirubin from the blood and chemically modify it through conjugation to glucuronic acid, which makes the bilirubin more soluble in aqueous solutions. The conjugated bilirubin is secreted by the hepatocytes into the adjacent bile canaliculi and is eventually carried in the bile into the duodenum.

In the small intestine, bilirubin is converted into urobilinogen, which is partially excreted in the feces and partially absorbed through the intestinal mucosa into the portal blood. Much of this reabsorbed urobilinogen is removed by the hepatocytes and secreted into the bile once again (enterohepatic circulation). Some of the urobilinogen enters the systemic circulation and is excreted by the kidneys in the urine. Elimination of bilirubin in the bile represents the major route of its excretion.

The bilirubin concentration in the blood may be increased in the presence of liver disease, if the flow of bile is impeded (eg, by gallstones in the bile ducts), or if there is excessive destruction of red blood cells. With bile duct obstruction, bilirubin does not enter the intestine; as a consequence, urobilinogen is absent from the urine and decreased in the stool (Porth & Matfin, 2009).

Drug Metabolism

The liver metabolizes many medications, such as barbiturates, opioids, sedatives, anesthetics, and amphetamines. Metabolism generally results in drug inactivation, although activation may also occur. One of the important pathways for medication metabolism involves conjugation (binding) of the medication with a variety of compounds, such as glucuronic acid or acetic acid, to form more soluble substances. These substances may be excreted in the feces or urine, similar to bilirubin excretion. Bioavailability is the fraction of the administered medication that actually reaches the systemic circulation. The bioavailability of an oral medication (absorbed from the GI tract) can be decreased if the medication is metabolized to a great extent by the liver before it reaches the systemic circulation; this is known as first-pass effect. Some medications have such a large first-pass effect that their use is essentially limited to the parenteral route, or oral doses must be substantially larger than parenteral doses to achieve the same effect.

 ### Gerontologic Considerations

Chart 39-1 summarizes age-related changes in the liver. In the elderly, the most common change in the liver is a decrease in size and weight, accompanied by a decrease in total hepatic blood flow. However, in general, these decreases are proportional to the decreases in body size and weight seen in normal aging. Results of liver function tests do not normally change in the elderly; abnormal results in elderly patients indicate abnormal liver function and are not a result of the aging process itself.

Metabolism of medications by the liver decreases in the elderly, but such changes are usually accompanied by changes in intestinal absorption, renal excretion, and altered body distribution of some medications secondary to changes in fat deposition. These alterations necessitate careful medication administration and monitoring; if appropriate, reduced dosages may be needed to prevent medication toxicity.

Assessment

Health History

If liver function test results are abnormal, the patient is evaluated for liver disease. In such cases, the health history focuses on previous exposure of the patient to hepatotoxic

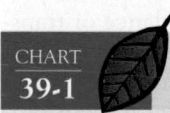

CHART 39-1 *Age-Related Changes of the Hepatobiliary System*

- Steady decrease in size and weight of the liver, particularly in women
- Decrease in blood flow
- Decrease in replacement/repair of liver cells after injury
- Reduced drug metabolism
- Slow clearance of hepatitis B surface antigen
- More rapid progression of hepatitis C infection and lower response rate to therapy
- Decline in drug clearance capability
- Increased prevalence of gallstones due to the increase in cholesterol secretion in bile
- Decreased gallbladder contraction after a meal
- Atypical clinical presentation of biliary disease
- More severe complications of biliary tract disease

substances or infectious agents. The patient's occupational, recreational, and travel history may assist in identifying exposure to hepatotoxins (eg, industrial chemicals, other toxins). The patient's history of alcohol and drug use, including but not limited to the use of intravenous (IV) or injection drugs, provides additional information about exposure to toxins and infectious agents. Many medications (including acetaminophen [Tylenol], ketoconazole [Nizoral], and valproic acid [Depakene]) are responsible for hepatic dysfunction and disease. A thorough medication history should address all current and past prescription medications, over-the-counter medications, herbal remedies, and dietary supplements.

Lifestyle behaviors that increase the risk for exposure to infectious agents are identified. IV or injection drug use, sexual practices, and foreign travel are all potential risk factors for liver disease. The amount and type of alcohol consumption are identified using screening tools (questionnaires) that have been developed for this purpose (see Chapter 5). Men who consume 60 to 80 g/day of alcohol (approximately four glasses of beer, wine, or mixed drinks) and women whose alcohol intake is 40 to 60 g/day are considered at high risk for cirrhosis.

The history also includes an evaluation of the patient's past medical history to identify risk factors for the development of liver disease. Current and past medical conditions, including those of a psychological or psychiatric nature, are identified. The family history includes questions about familial liver disorders that may have their origin in alcohol abuse or gallstone disease, as well as other familial or genetic diseases, such as hemochromatosis, Wilson's disease, or alpha$_1$-antitrypsin disease (see Chart 42-1).

The history also addresses symptoms that suggest liver disease. Symptoms that may have their origin in liver disease but are not specific to hepatic dysfunction include jaundice, malaise, weakness, fatigue, pruritus, abdominal pain, fever, anorexia, weight gain, edema, increasing abdominal girth, hematemesis, melena, hematochezia (passage of bloody stools), easy bruising, changes in mental acuity, personality changes, sleep disturbances, and decreased libido in men and secondary amenorrhea in women.

Physical Assessment

The nurse assesses the patient for physical signs that may occur with liver dysfunction, including the pallor often seen with chronic illness and jaundice. The skin, mucosa, and sclerae are inspected for jaundice, and the extremities are assessed for muscle atrophy, edema, and skin excoriation secondary to scratching. The nurse observes the skin for petechiae or ecchymotic areas (bruises), spider angiomas, and palmar erythema. The male patient is assessed for unilateral or bilateral gynecomastia and testicular atrophy due to hormonal changes. The patient's cognitive status (recall, memory, abstract thinking) and neurologic status are assessed. The nurse observes for general tremor, asterixis, weakness, and slurred speech. These symptoms are discussed later.

The nurse assesses for the presence of an abdominal fluid wave (discussed later). The abdomen is palpated to assess liver size and to detect any tenderness over the liver. The liver may be palpable in the right upper quadrant. A palpable liver presents as a firm, sharp ridge with a smooth surface

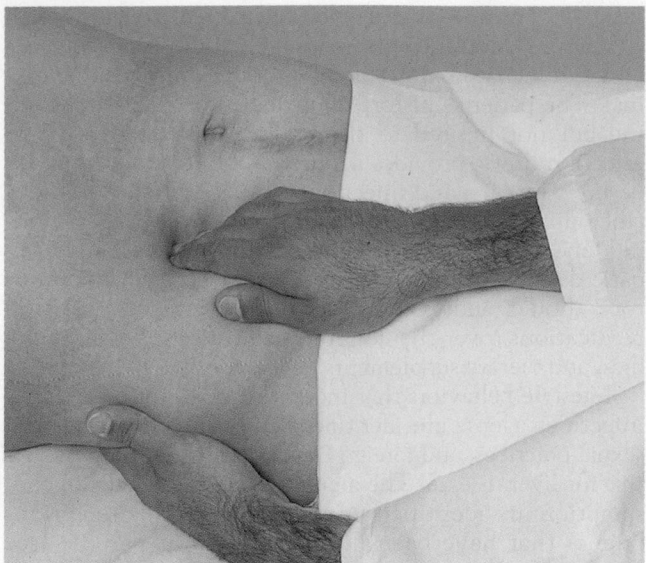

Figure 39-3 Technique for palpating the liver. The examiner places one hand under the right lower rib cage and presses downward with light pressure with the other hand.

(Fig. 39-3). The nurse estimates the size of the liver by percussing its upper and lower borders. If the liver is not palpable but tenderness is suspected, tapping the lower right thorax briskly may elicit tenderness. For comparison, the nurse then performs a similar maneuver on the left lower thorax (Bickley, 2007).

If the liver is palpable, the examiner notes and records its size, its consistency, any tenderness, and whether its outline is regular or irregular. If the liver is enlarged, the degree to which it descends below the right costal margin is recorded to provide some indication of its size. The examiner determines whether the liver's edge is sharp and smooth or blunt and whether the enlarged liver is nodular or smooth. The liver of a patient with cirrhosis is small and hard; whereas the liver of a patient with acute hepatitis is soft, and the hand easily moves the edge.

Tenderness of the liver indicates recent acute enlargement with consequent stretching of the liver capsule. The absence of tenderness may imply that the enlargement is of long-standing duration. The liver of a patient with viral hepatitis is tender; whereas that of a patient with alcoholic hepatitis is not. Enlargement of the liver is an abnormal finding that requires evaluation (Bickley, 2007).

Diagnostic Evaluation

Liver Function Tests

More than 70% of the parenchyma of the liver may be damaged before liver function test results become abnormal. Function is generally measured in terms of serum enzyme activity (ie, serum aminotransferases, alkaline phosphatase, lactic dehydrogenase) and serum concentrations of proteins (albumin and globulins), bilirubin, ammonia, clotting factors, and lipids. Several of these tests may be helpful for as-

sessing patients with liver disease. However, the nature and extent of hepatic dysfunction cannot be determined by these tests alone, because other disorders can affect test results.

Serum aminotransferases (previously called transaminases) are sensitive indicators of injury to the liver cells and are useful in detecting acute liver disease such as hepatitis. Alanine aminotransferase (ALT), aspartate aminotransferase (AST), and gamma-glutamyl transferase (GGT) (also called G-glutamyl transpeptidase) are the most frequently used tests of liver damage. ALT levels increase primarily in liver disorders and may be used to monitor the course of hepatitis or cirrhosis or the effects of treatments that may be toxic to the liver. AST is present in tissues that have high metabolic activity; therefore, the level may be increased if there is damage to or death of tissues of organs such as the heart, liver, skeletal muscle, and kidney. Although not specific to liver disease, levels of AST may be increased in cirrhosis, hepatitis, and liver cancer. Increased GGT levels are associated with cholestasis but can also be due to alcoholic liver disease. Although the kidney has the highest level of the enzyme, the liver is considered the source of normal serum activity. The test determines liver cell dysfunction and is a sensitive indicator of cholestasis. Its main value in liver disease is confirming the hepatic origin of an elevated alkaline phosphatase level. Common liver function tests are summarized in Table 39-1.

Liver Biopsy

Liver biopsy is the removal of a small amount of liver tissue, usually through needle aspiration. It permits examination of liver cells. The most common indication is to evaluate diffuse disorders of the parenchyma and to diagnose space-occupying lesions. Liver biopsy is especially useful when clinical findings and laboratory tests are not diagnostic. Bleeding and bile peritonitis after liver biopsy are the major complications; therefore, coagulation studies are obtained, their values are noted, and abnormal results are treated before liver biopsy is performed. Other techniques for liver biopsy are preferred if ascites or coagulation abnormalities exist. A liver biopsy can be performed percutaneously with ultrasound guidance or transvenously through the right internal jugular vein to right hepatic vein under fluoroscopic control. Liver biopsy can also be performed laparoscopically. Nursing responsibilities related to percutaneous liver biopsy are summarized in Chart 39-2.

Other Diagnostic Tests

Ultrasonography, computed tomography (CT), and magnetic resonance imaging (MRI) are used to identify normal structures and abnormalities of the liver and biliary tree. A radioisotope liver scan may be performed to assess liver size and hepatic blood flow and obstruction.

Laparoscopy (insertion of a fiberoptic endoscope through a small abdominal incision) is used to examine the liver and other pelvic structures. It is also used to perform guided liver biopsy, to determine the cause of ascites, and to diagnose and stage tumors of the liver and other abdominal organs.

Table 39-1	COMMON LABORATORY TESTS TO ASSESS LIVER FUNCTION	
Test	**Normal**	**Clinical Functions**
Pigment Studies		
Serum bilirubin, direct	0–0.3 mg/dL (0–5.1 μmol/L)	These studies measure the ability of the liver to
Serum bilirubin, total	0–0.9 mg/dL (1.7–20.5 μmol/L)	conjugate and excrete bilirubin. Results are
Urine bilirubin	0(0)	abnormal in liver and biliary tract disease and are
Urine urobilinogen	(Urine urobilinogen) 0.05–2.5 mg/24 h (0.5–4.0	associated with jaundice clinically.
Fecal urobilinogen (infrequently	Ehrlich U/24 h)	
used)	(Fecal urobilinogen) 50–300 mg/24 h (100–400	
	Ehrlich U/100 g)	
Protein Studies		
Total serum protein	7.0–7.5 g/dL (70–75 g/L)	Proteins are manufactured by the liver. Their levels
Serum albumin	4.0–5.5 g/dL (40–55 g/L)	may be affected in a variety of liver impairments:
Serum globulin	1.7–3.3 g/dL (17–33 g/L)	albumin is affected in cirrhosis, chronic hepatitis,
Serum protein electrophoresis		edema and ascites, globulins are affected in cirrhosis,
Albumin	4.0–5.5 g/dL (40–55 g/L)	liver disease, chronic obstructive jaundice, and
α_1-Globulin	0.15–0.25 g/dL (1.5–2.5 g/L)	viral hepatitis.
α_2-Globulin	0.43–0.75 g/dL (4.3–7.5 g/L)	
β-Globulin	0.5–1.0 g/dL (5–10 g/L)	
γ-Globulin	0.6–1.3 g/dL (6–13 g/L)	
Albumin/globulin (A/G) ratio	A > G or 1.5:1–2.5:1	A/G ratio is reversed in chronic liver disease (decreased albumin and increased globulin).
Prothrombin Time	100% or 12–16 seconds	Prothrombin time may be prolonged in liver disease. It will not return to normal with vitamin K in severe liver cell damage.
Serum Alkaline Phosphatase	Varies with method: 2–5 Bodansky units 30–50 U/L at 34°C (17–142 U/L at 30°C) (20–90 U/L at 30°C)	Serum alkaline phosphatase is manufactured in bones, liver, kidneys, and intestine and excreted through biliary tract. In the absence of bone disease, it is a sensitive measure of biliary tract obstruction.
Serum Aminotransferase Studies		
AST	10–40 units (4.8–19 U/L)	The studies are based on release of enzymes from
ALT	5–35 units (2.4–17 U/L)	damaged liver cells. These enzymes are elevated in liver cell damage.
GGT, GGTP	10–48 IU/L	Elevated in alcohol abuse. Marker for biliary
LDH	100–200 units (100–225 U/L)	cholestasis.
Ammonia (plasma)	15–45 μg/dL (11–32 μmol/L)	Liver converts ammonia to urea. Ammonia level rises in liver failure
Cholesterol		
Ester	60% of total (fraction of total cholesterol: 0.60)	Cholesterol levels are elevated in biliary obstruction
HDL (high-density lipoprotein)	HDL Male: 35–70 mg/dL, Female: 35–85 mg/dL	and decreased in parenchymal liver disease.
LDL (low-density lipoprotein)	LDL <130 μg/dL	

MANIFESTATIONS OF HEPATIC DYSFUNCTION

Hepatic dysfunction results from damage to the liver's parenchymal cells, directly from primary liver diseases, or indirectly from either obstruction of bile flow or derangements of hepatic circulation. Liver dysfunction may be acute or chronic; the latter is far more common.

Chronic liver disease, including cirrhosis, is the 12th-leading cause of death in the United States among young and middle-aged adults (Mathews, McGuire & Estrada, 2006). At least 40% of those deaths are associated with alcohol use. The rate of chronic liver disease for men is twice that for women, and chronic liver disease is more common in Asian and African countries than it is in Europe and the United States. Compensated cirrhosis, in which the damaged liver is still able to perform normal functions, often goes undetected for extended periods, and as many as 1% of people may have subclinical cirrhosis (Schuppan & Afdhal, 2008).

Disease processes that lead to hepatocellular dysfunction may be caused by infectious agents such as bacteria and viruses and by anoxia, metabolic disorders, toxins and medications, nutritional deficiencies, and hypersensitivity states. The most common cause of parenchymal damage is malnutrition, especially that related to alcoholism.

The parenchymal cells respond to most noxious agents by replacing glycogen with lipids, producing fatty infiltration with or without cell death or necrosis. This is commonly associated with inflammatory cell infiltration and growth of fibrous tissue. Cell regeneration can occur if the disease process is not too toxic to the cells. The result of chronic parenchymal disease is the shrunken, fibrotic liver seen in cirrhosis.

Among the most common and significant manifestations of liver disease are jaundice, portal hypertension, ascites and varices, nutritional deficiencies (resulting from the inability of damaged liver cells to metabolize certain vitamins), and hepatic encephalopathy or coma. The consequences of

CHART
39-2 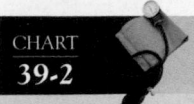 *Guidelines for Assisting With Percutaneous Liver Biopsy*

Equipment

- Liver biopsy tray (contains needles, scalpel, specimen tubes, etc.)
- Sterile gloves
- Antiseptic solution
- Local anesthetic
- Sterile dressing
- Sphygmomanometer to monitor BP

Implementation

Nursing Interventions

Preprocedure

1. Ascertain that results of coagulation tests (prothrombin time, partial thromboplastin time, and platelet count) are available and that compatible donor blood is available.
2. Check for signed consent; confirm that informed consent has been provided.
3. Measure and record the patient's pulse, respirations, and blood pressure immediately before biopsy.
4. Describe to the patient in advance: steps of the procedure; sensations expected; after-effects anticipated; restrictions of activity and monitoring procedures to follow.

During Procedure

1. Support the patient during the procedure.

2. Expose the right side of the patient's upper abdomen (right hypochondriac).
3. Instruct the patient to inhale and exhale deeply several times, finally to exhale, and to hold breath at the end of expiration. The physician promptly introduces the biopsy needle by way of the transthoracic (intercostal) or transabdominal (subcostal) route, penetrates the liver, aspirates, and withdraws.
4. Instruct the patient to resume breathing.

Rationale

1. Many patients with liver disease have clotting defects and are at risk for bleeding.

2. Ensures that the patient consents to this invasive procedure.
3. Prebiopsy values provide a basis on which to compare the patient's vital signs and evaluate status after the procedure.
4. Explanations allay fears and ensure cooperation.

1. Encouragement and support of the nurse enhance comfort and promote a sense of security.
2. The skin at the site of penetration will be cleansed and a local anesthetic will be infiltrated.
3. Holding the breath immobilizes the chest wall and the diaphragm; penetration of the diaphragm thereby is avoided, and the risk of lacerating the liver is minimized.

4. The patient often continues holding his or her breath because of anxiety.

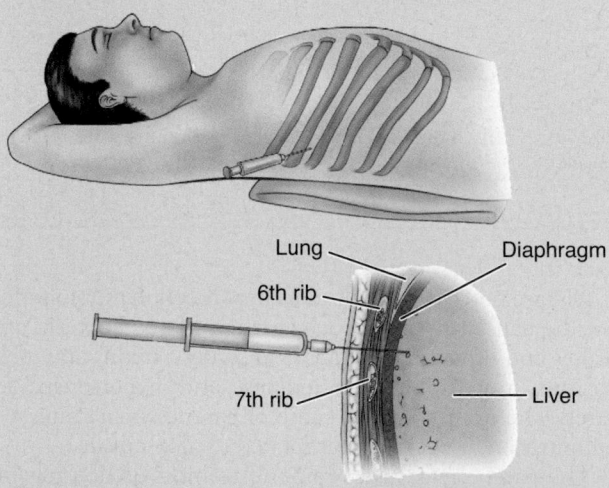

Lung — Diaphragm
6th rib
7th rib — Liver

Postprocedure

1. Immediately after the biopsy, assist the patient to turn on to the right side; place a pillow under the costal margin, and caution the patient to remain in this position, recumbent and immobile, for several hours. Instruct the patient to avoid coughing or straining.
2. Measure and record the patient's pulse, respiratory rate, and blood pressure at 10- to 15-minute intervals for the first hour, then every 30 minutes for the next 1 to 2 hours or until the patient's condition stabilizes.
3. If the patient is discharged after the procedure, instruct the patient to avoid heavy lifting and strenuous activity for 1 week.

1. In this position, the liver capsule at the site of penetration is compressed against the chest wall, and the escape of blood or bile through the perforation is prevented.

2. Changes in vital signs may indicate bleeding, severe hemorrhage, or bile peritonitis, the most frequent complications of liver biopsy.

3. Activity restriction reduces the risk of bleeding at the biopsy puncture site.

liver disease are numerous and varied. Their ultimate effects are often incapacitating or life-threatening, and their presence is ominous. Treatment often is difficult.

Jaundice

When the bilirubin concentration in the blood is abnormally elevated, all the body tissues, including the sclerae and the skin, become tinged yellow or greenish-yellow, a condition called jaundice. Jaundice becomes clinically evident when the serum bilirubin level exceeds 2.5 mg/dL (43 fmol/L). Increased serum bilirubin levels and jaundice may result from impairment of hepatic uptake, conjugation of bilirubin, or excretion of bilirubin into the biliary system. There are several types of jaundice: hemolytic, hepatocellular, and obstructive jaundice, and jaundice due to hereditary hyperbilirubinemia. Hepatocellular and obstructive jaundice are the two types commonly associated with liver disease.

Hemolytic Jaundice

Hemolytic jaundice is the result of an increased destruction of the red blood cells, the effect of which is to flood the plasma with bilirubin so rapidly that the liver, although functioning normally, cannot excrete the bilirubin as quickly as it is formed. This type of jaundice is encountered in patients with hemolytic transfusion reactions and other hemolytic disorders. In these patients, the bilirubin in the blood is predominantly unconjugated or free. Fecal and urine urobilinogen levels are increased, but the urine is free of bilirubin. Patients with this type of jaundice, unless their hyperbilirubinemia is extreme, do not experience symptoms or complications as a result of the jaundice per se. However, prolonged jaundice, even if mild, predisposes to the formation of pigment stones in the gallbladder, and extremely severe jaundice (levels of free bilirubin exceeding 20 to 25 mg/dL) poses a risk for brainstem damage.

Hepatocellular Jaundice

Hepatocellular jaundice is caused by the inability of damaged liver cells to clear normal amounts of bilirubin from the blood. The cellular damage may be caused by hepatitis viruses, other viruses that affect the liver (eg, yellow fever virus, Epstein-Barr virus), medications or chemical toxins (eg, carbon tetrachloride, chloroform, phosphorus, arsenicals, certain medications), or alcohol. Cirrhosis of the liver is a form of hepatocellular disease that may produce jaundice. It is usually associated with excessive alcohol intake, but it may also be a late result of liver cell necrosis caused by viral infection. In prolonged obstructive jaundice, cell damage eventually develops, so that both types of jaundice (ie, obstructive and hepatocellular jaundice) appear together.

Patients with hepatocellular jaundice may be mildly or severely ill, with lack of appetite, nausea, malaise, fatigue, weakness, and possible weight loss. In some cases of hepatocellular disease, jaundice may not be obvious. The serum bilirubin concentration and the urine urobilinogen level may be elevated. In addition, AST and ALT levels may be increased, indicating cellular necrosis. The patient may report headache, chills, and fever if the cause is infectious.

Depending on the cause and extent of the liver cell damage, hepatocellular jaundice may be completely reversible.

Obstructive Jaundice

Obstructive jaundice resulting from extrahepatic obstruction may be caused by occlusion of the bile duct from a gallstone, an inflammatory process, a tumor, or pressure from an enlarged organ (eg, liver, gallbladder). The obstruction may also involve the small bile ducts within the liver (ie, intrahepatic obstruction); this may be caused, for example, by pressure on these channels from inflammatory swelling of the liver or by an inflammatory exudate within the ducts themselves. Intrahepatic obstruction resulting from stasis and inspissation (thickening) of bile within the canaliculi may occur after the ingestion of certain medications, which are referred to as cholestatic agents. These agents include phenothiazines, antithyroid medications, sulfonylureas, tricyclic antidepressant agents, nitrofurantoin, androgens and estrogens, propylthiouracil, amoxicillin-clavulanic acid, and erythromycin estolate.

Regardless of whether the obstruction is intrahepatic or extrahepatic, and regardless of its cause, bile cannot flow normally into the intestine and becomes backed up into the liver substance. It is then reabsorbed into the blood and carried throughout the entire body, staining the skin, mucous membranes, and sclerae. It is excreted in the urine, which becomes deep orange and foamy. Because of the decreased amount of bile in the intestinal tract, the stools become light or clay-colored. The skin may itch intensely, requiring repeated soothing baths. Dyspepsia and intolerance to fatty foods may develop because of impaired fat digestion in the absence of intestinal bile. In general, AST, ALT, and GGT levels rise only moderately, but bilirubin and alkaline phosphatase levels are elevated.

Hereditary Hyperbilirubinemia

Increased serum bilirubin levels (hyperbilirubinemia), resulting from any of several inherited disorders, can also produce jaundice. Gilbert's syndrome is a familial disorder characterized by an increased level of unconjugated bilirubin that causes jaundice. Although serum bilirubin levels are increased, liver histology and liver function test results are normal, and there is no hemolysis. This syndrome affects 3% to 8% of the population, predominantly males (Hauser, Pardi & Poterucha, 2006).

Other conditions that are probably caused by inborn errors of biliary metabolism include Dubin-Johnson syndrome (chronic idiopathic jaundice, with pigment in the liver) and Rotor's syndrome (chronic familial conjugated hyperbilirubinemia, without pigment in the liver); the "benign" cholestatic jaundice of pregnancy, with retention of conjugated bilirubin, probably secondary to unusual sensitivity to the hormones of pregnancy; and benign recurrent intrahepatic cholestasis.

Portal Hypertension

Portal hypotension is the increased pressure throughout the portal venous system that results from obstruction of blood flow through the damaged liver. Commonly associated with hepatic cirrhosis, it can also occur with non-cirrhotic liver disease. Although splenomegaly (enlarged spleen) with possible hypersplenism is a common manifestation of portal hypertension, the two major consequences of portal hypertension are ascites and varices.

Ascites

Pathophysiology

The mechanisms responsible for the development of ascites are not completely understood. Portal hypertension and the resulting increase in capillary pressure and obstruction of venous blood flow through the damaged liver are contributing factors. The vasodilation that occurs in the splanchnic circulation (the arterial supply and venous drainage of the GI system from the distal esophagus to the midrectum including the liver and spleen) is also a suspected causative factor. The failure of the liver to metabolize aldosterone increases sodium and water retention by the kidney. Sodium and water retention, increased intravascular fluid volume, increased lymphatic flow, and decreased synthesis of albumin by the damaged liver all contribute to the movement of fluid from the vascular system into the peritoneal space. The process becomes self-perpetuating; loss of fluid into the peritoneal space causes further sodium and water retention by the kidney in an effort to maintain the vascular fluid volume.

As a result of liver damage, large amounts of albumin-rich fluid, 15 L or more, may accumulate in the peritoneal cavity as ascites. (Ascites may also occur with disorders such as cancer, kidney disease, and heart failure.) With the movement of albumin from the serum to the peritoneal cavity, the osmotic pressure of the serum decreases. This, combined with increased portal pressure, results in movement of fluid into the peritoneal cavity (Fig. 39-4).

Clinical Manifestations

Increased abdominal girth and rapid weight gain are common presenting symptoms of ascites. The patient may be short of breath and uncomfortable from the enlarged abdomen, and striae and distended veins may be visible over the abdominal wall. Umbilical hernias also occur frequently in those patients with cirrhosis. Fluid and electrolyte imbalances are common.

Assessment and Diagnostic Findings

The presence and extent of ascites are assessed by percussion of the abdomen. When fluid has accumulated in the peritoneal cavity, the flanks bulge when the patient assumes a supine position. The presence of fluid can be confirmed either by percussing for shifting dullness or by detecting a fluid wave (Fig. 39-5). A fluid wave is likely to be found only if a large amount of fluid is present. Daily measurement and recording of abdominal girth and body weight are essential to assess the progression of ascites and its response to treatment.

Medical Management

Dietary Modification

The goal of treatment for the patient with ascites is a negative sodium balance to reduce fluid retention. Table salt,

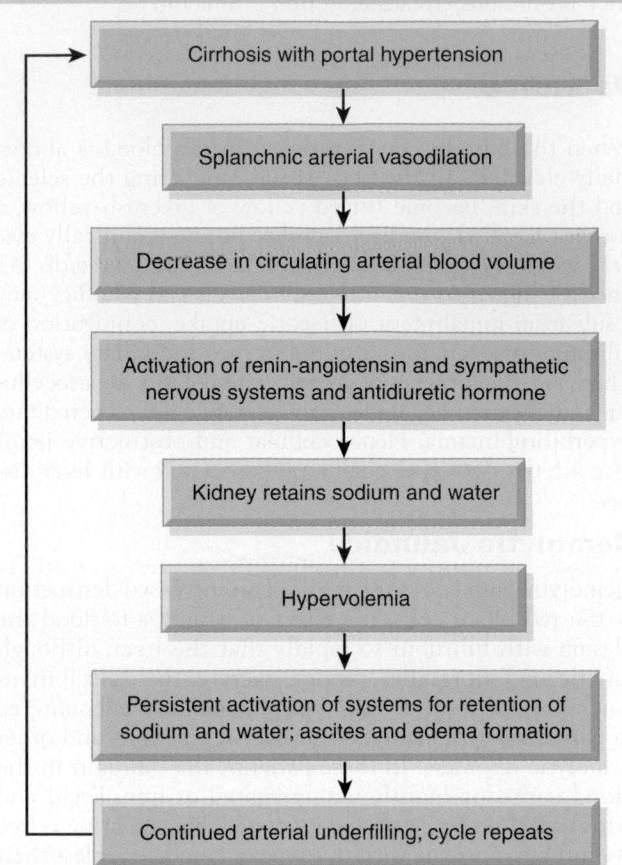

Physiology ■■■ Pathophysiology

Cirrhosis with portal hypertension

↓

Splanchnic arterial vasodilation

↓

Decrease in circulating arterial blood volume

↓

Activation of renin-angiotensin and sympathetic nervous systems and antidiuretic hormone

↓

Kidney retains sodium and water

↓

Hypervolemia

↓

Persistent activation of systems for retention of sodium and water; ascites and edema formation

↓

Continued arterial underfilling; cycle repeats

Figure 39-4 Pathogenesis of ascites (arterial vasodilation theory).

salty foods, salted butter and margarine, and all ordinary canned and frozen foods that are not specifically prepared for low-sodium (2-g sodium) diets should be avoided. It may take 2 to 3 months for the patient's taste buds to adjust to unsalted foods. In the meantime, the taste of unsalted foods can be improved by using salt substitutes such as lemon juice, oregano, and thyme. Commercial salt substitutes need to be approved by the physician, because those that contain ammonia could precipitate hepatic coma. Most salt substitutes contain potassium and should be avoided if the patient has impaired renal function. The patient should make liberal use of powdered, low-sodium milk and milk products. If fluid accumulation is not controlled with this regimen, the daily sodium allowance may be reduced further to 500 mg, and diuretics may be administered.

Dietary control of ascites via strict sodium restriction is difficult to achieve at home. The likelihood that the patient will follow even a 2-g sodium diet increases if the patient and the person preparing meals understand the rationale for the diet and receive periodic guidance about selecting and preparing appropriate foods. Approximately 10% of patients with ascites respond to these measures alone. Nonresponders and those who find sodium restriction difficult require diuretic therapy.

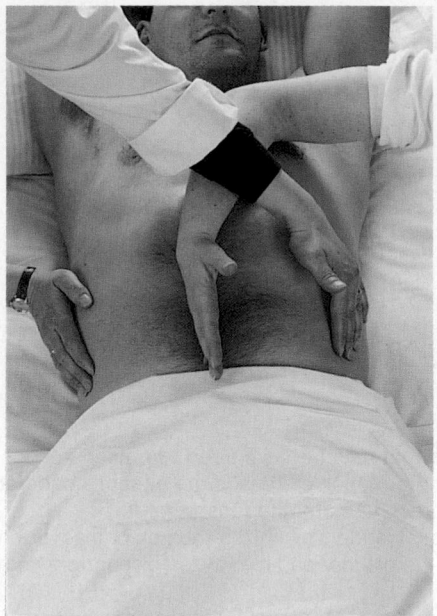

Figure 39-5 Assessing for abdominal fluid wave. The examiner places the hands along the sides of the patient's flanks, then strikes one flank sharply, detecting any fluid wave with the other hand. An assistant's hand is placed (ulnar side down) along the patient's midline to prevent the fluid wave from being transmitted through the tissues of the abdominal wall.

Diuretics

Use of diuretics along with sodium restriction is successful in 90% of patients with ascites. Spironolactone (Aldactone), an aldosterone-blocking agent, is most often the first-line therapy in patients with ascites from cirrhosis. When used with other diuretics, spironolactone helps prevent potassium loss. Oral diuretics such as furosemide (Lasix) may be added but should be used cautiously, because long-term use may induce severe sodium depletion (hyponatremia).

Ammonium chloride and acetazolamide (Diamox) are contraindicated because of the possibility of precipitating hepatic coma. Daily weight loss should not exceed 1 to 2 kg (2.2 to 4.4 lb) in patients with ascites and peripheral edema or 0.5 to 0.75 kg (1.1 to 1.65 lb) in patients without edema. Fluid restriction is not attempted unless the serum sodium concentration is very low.

Possible complications of diuretic therapy include fluid and electrolyte disturbances (including hypovolemia, hypokalemia, hyponatremia, and hypochloremic alkalosis) and encephalopathy. Encephalopathy may be precipitated by dehydration and hypovolemia. In addition, when potassium stores are depleted, the amount of ammonia in the systemic circulation increases, which may cause impaired cerebral functioning and encephalopathy.

Bed Rest

In patients with ascites, an upright posture is associated with activation of the renin–angiotensin–aldosterone system and sympathetic nervous system (Porth & Matfin, 2009). This causes reduced renal glomerular filtration and sodium excretion and a decreased response to loop diuret-

ics. Therefore, bed rest may be a useful therapy, especially for patients whose condition is refractory to diuretics.

Paracentesis

Paracentesis is the removal of fluid (ascites) from the peritoneal cavity through a puncture or a small surgical incision through the abdominal wall under sterile conditions. Ultrasound guidance may be indicated in some patients who are at high risk for bleeding because of an abnormal coagulation profile and in those who have had previous abdominal surgery and may have adhesions. Paracentesis was once considered a routine form of treatment for ascites. However, it is now performed primarily for diagnostic examination of ascitic fluid; for treatment of massive ascites that is resistant to nutritional and diuretic therapy and that is causing severe problems to the patient; and as a prelude to diagnostic imaging studies, peritoneal dialysis, or surgery. A sample of the ascitic fluid may be sent to the laboratory for cell count, albumin and total protein levels, culture, and other tests.

Large-volume (5 to 6 L) paracentesis has been shown to be a safe method for treating patients with severe ascites. This technique, in combination with the IV infusion of salt-poor albumin or other colloid, has become a standard management strategy yielding an immediate effect. Refractive, massive ascites is unresponsive to multiple diuretics and sodium restriction for 2 weeks or more and can result in severe sequelae such as respiratory distress, which requires rapid intervention. Albumin infusions help to correct decreases in effective arterial blood volume that lead to sodium retention. Use of this colloid reduces the incidence of postparacentesis circulatory dysfunction with renal dysfunction, hyponatremia, and rapid reaccumulation of ascites associated with decreased effective arterial volume (Hauser, et al., 2006). The beneficial effects of albumin administration on hemodynamic stability and renal functional status may be related to an improvement in cardiac function as well as a decrease in the degree of arterial vasodilation. Although the patient with cirrhosis has a greatly increased extracellular blood volume, the kidney incorrectly senses that the effective volume has decreased. The renin–angiotensin–aldosterone axis is stimulated, and sodium is reabsorbed (Rodes, et al., 2007). In addition, antidiuretic hormone (ADH) secretion increases, which leads to increased retention of free water and sometimes to the development of dilutional hyponatremia. Therapeutic paracentesis provides only temporary removal of fluid; ascites rapidly recurs, necessitating repeated fluid removal. Nursing care of the patient undergoing paracentesis is presented in Chart 39-3.

Transjugular Intrahepatic Portosystemic Shunt

Transjugular intrahepatic portosystemic shunt (TIPS) is a method of treating ascites in which a cannula is threaded into the portal vein by the transjugular route (Fig. 39-6). To reduce portal hypertension, an expandable stent is inserted to serve as an intrahepatic shunt between the portal circulation and the hepatic vein. TIPS is the treatment of choice for refractory ascites. It is extremely effective in decreasing sodium retention, improving the renal response to diuretic therapy, and preventing recurrence of fluid accumulation (Senzolo, Cholongitas, Tibballs, et al., 2006).

CHART 39-3   *Guidelines for Assisting With a Paracentesis*

Equipment

- Paracentesis tray (contains trocar, syringe, needles, drainage tube)
- Sterile gloves
- Antiseptic solution
- Local anesthetic
- Sterile dressing
- Drainage collection bottles, receptacles
- Sphygmomanometer to monitor BP

Implementation

Nursing Interventions	Rationale
Preprocedure	
1. Check for signed consent form.	1. Ensures that patient has agreed to procedure.
2. Prepare the patient by providing the necessary information and instructions and by offering reassurance.	2. Having information increases the patient's understanding of the procedure and the reason for it.
3. Instruct the patient to void.	3. An empty bladder minimizes the risk of inadvertent puncture of the bladder and minimizes discomfort from a full bladder.
4. Gather appropriate sterile equipment and collection receptacles.	4. Sterility of equipment is essential to minimize risk of infection; having equipment available enables the procedure to be performed smoothly.
5. Place the patient in upright position on the edge of the bed or in a chair with feet supported on a stool. Fowler's position should be used by the patient confined to bed.	5. An upright position results in movement of the peritoneal fluid close to the abdominal wall and promotes easier puncture and removal of fluid.
6. Place the sphygmomanometer cuff around patient's arm.	6. This allows the nurse to monitor the patient's blood pressure during procedure.
Procedure	
1. The physician, using aseptic technique, inserts the trocar through a puncture below the umbilicus. The trocar or needle is connected to a drainage tube, the end of which is inserted into a collecting receptacle.	1. Sterile technique minimizes the risk of infection. Bleeding at the puncture site is minimal at this location. The fluid drains by gravity or mild siphon into the container.
2. Help the patient maintain position throughout the procedure.	2. The patient who is fatigued or weak may have difficulty maintaining an optimal position for drainage of fluid.
3. Measure and record blood pressure at frequent intervals throughout the procedure.	3. Decreased blood pressure may occur with vascular collapse, which can result from removal of the fluid from the peritoneal cavity and fluid shifts.
4. Monitor the patient closely for signs of vascular collapse: pallor, increased pulse rate, or decreased blood pressure.	4. Vascular collapse (hypovolemia) may occur as fluid moves from the vascular system to replace fluid drained from peritoneal cavity.

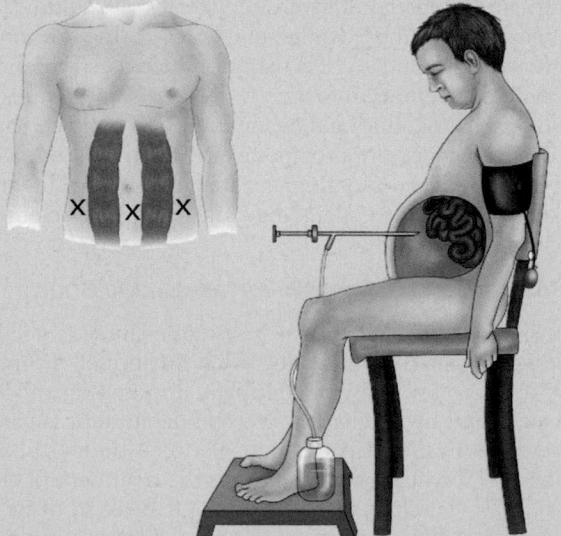

Figure on left shows possible sites for insertion of trocar.

Continued

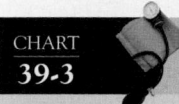

CHART 39-3

Guidelines for Assisting With a Paracentesis (Continued)

Nursing Action	Rationale
Postprocedure	
1. Return the patient to bed or to a comfortable sitting position.	1. The weak or fatigued patient may have difficulty resuming a comfortable position without assistance.
2. Measure, describe, and record the fluid collected.	2. The volume of fluid removed may range from small to very large, and its removal may affect fluid and vascular status; volume should be included in input and output records. The characteristics of the fluid (clear vs. cloudy, red vs. colorless) may be helpful in diagnostic evaluation.
3. Label samples of fluid and send to laboratory.	3. Peritoneal fluid is analyzed as part of the diagnostic workup.
4. Monitor vital signs every 15 min for 1 h, every 30 min for 2 h, every hour for 2 h, and then every 4 h.	4. Vital signs (blood pressure, pulse rate) may change as fluid shifts occur after removal of fluid, especially if a large volume of fluid has been removed.
5. Measure the patient's temperature.	5. An elevated temperature is a sign of infection and should be reported to the patient's physician.
6. Assess for hypovolemia, electrolyte shifts, changes in mental status, and encephalopathy.	6. Changes in fluid and electrolyte states and mental and cognitive status may occur with removal of fluid and fluid shifts, and should be reported.
7. When taking vital signs, check puncture site for leakage or bleeding.	7. Leakage of fluid may occur because of changes in abdominal pressure and may contribute to further loss of fluid if undetected. Leakage suggests a possible site for infection, and bleeding may occur in patients with altered clotting secondary to liver disease.
8. Provide patient teaching regarding need to monitor for bleeding or excessive drainage from puncture site, importance of avoiding heavy lifting or straining, the need to change position slowly, and frequency of monitoring for fever.	8. The patient (or family members) needs to monitor the puncture site for bleeding and excessive drainage if the patient is discharged home after the procedure. Heavy lifting or straining is avoided to enable the puncture site to close. Slow changes in position are recommended because of the risk of hypovolemia related to fluid removal. Monitoring for fever is needed to detect infection.

Because the development of ascites in patients with cirrhosis is associated with a 50% mortality rate, any patient who is considered a candidate for liver transplantation should be referred for TIPS.

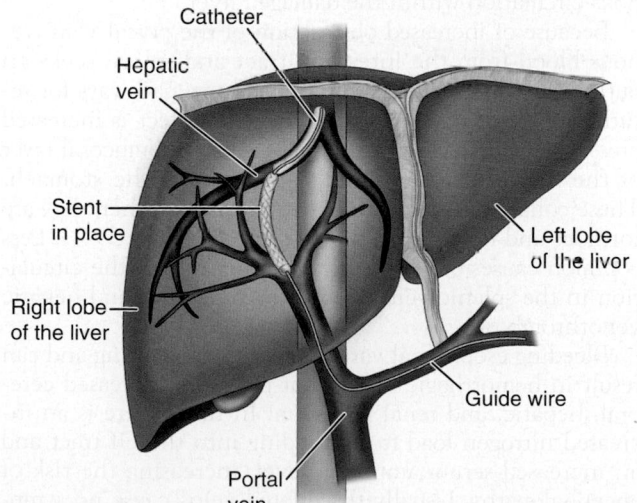

Figure 39-6 Transjugular intrahepatic portosystemic shunt (TIPS). A stent is inserted via catheter to the portal vein to divert blood flow and reduce portal hypertension.

Labels in figure:
Catheter
Hepatic vein
Stent in place
Right lobe of the liver
Left lobe of the liver
Guide wire
Portal vein

Other Methods of Treatment

Ascites can also be treated by the insertion of a peritoneovenous shunt to redirect ascitic fluid from the peritoneal cavity into the systemic circulation. However, this procedure is used only for patients who are not candidates for liver transplantation because of the high complication rate and high incidence of shunt failure.

Nursing Management

If a patient with ascites from liver dysfunction is hospitalized, nursing measures include assessment and documentation of intake and output, abdominal girth, and daily weight to assess fluid status. The nurse monitors serum ammonia and electrolyte levels to assess electrolyte balance, response to therapy, and indicators of encephalopathy.

Promoting Home and Community-Based Care

Teaching Patients Self-Care

The patient treated for ascites is likely to be discharged with some ascites still present. Before hospital discharge, the nurse teaches the patient and family about the treatment plan, including the need to avoid all alcohol intake, adhere to a low-sodium diet, take medications as prescribed, and check with the physician before taking any new medications (Chart 39-4). Additional patient and family teaching

CHART
39-4

HOME CARE CHECKLIST
Management of Ascites

At the completion of the home care instruction, the patient or caregiver will be able to:	PATIENT	CAREGIVER
• Make appropriate dietary choices consistent with dietary prescription and recommendations.	✔	✔
• State the importance of weighing self daily and keeping a daily record of weight.	✔	✔
• Maintain record of daily weight and identify daily weight-loss goals.	✔	✔
• List weight changes (loss or gain) that should be reported to the primary health care provider.	✔	✔
• Explain the rationale for monitoring and recording daily intake and output.	✔	✔
• Identify changes in output that should be reported to primary health care provider (eg, decreasing urine output).	✔	✔
• Identify rationale for fluid restrictions (if needed), and comply with fluid restriction.	✔	✔
• Discuss importance of avoiding nonsteroidal anti-inflammatory agents, medications (eg, cough mixtures) containing alcohol, antibiotics, or antacids containing salt.	✔	✔
• Describe effects, side effects, and monitoring parameters for diuretic therapy.	✔	✔
• Identify need to stop all alcohol intake as critical to well-being.	✔	✔
• Explain how to contact Alcoholics Anonymous or alcohol counselors in related organizations.	✔	✔
• Demonstrate how to care for skin, alleviate pressure over bony prominences by turning when in bed or chair, and decrease edema by position changes.	✔	✔
• Identify early signs and symptoms of complications (encephalopathy, spontaneous bacterial peritonitis, dehydration, electrolyte abnormalities, azotemia).	✔	✔

addresses skin care and the need to weigh the patient daily and to watch for and report signs and symptoms of complications.

Continuing Care

A referral for home care may be warranted, especially if the patient lives alone or cannot provide self-care. The home visit enables the nurse to assess changes in the patient's condition and weight, abdominal girth, skin, and cognitive and emotional status. The home care nurse assesses the home environment and the availability of resources needed to adhere to the treatment plan (eg, a scale to obtain daily weights, facilities to prepare and store appropriate foods, resources to purchase needed medications). It is important to assess the patient's adherence to the treatment plan and the ability to buy, prepare, and eat appropriate foods. The nurse reinforces previous teaching and emphasizes the need for regular follow-up and the importance of keeping scheduled health care appointments.

Esophageal Varices

Esophageal varices develop in the majority of patients with cirrhosis. Varices are varicosities that develop from elevated pressure in the veins that drain into the portal system. They are prone to rupture and often are the source of massive hemorrhages from the upper GI tract and the rectum. In addition, blood clotting abnormalities, often seen in patients with severe liver disease, increase the likelihood of bleeding and significant blood loss.

Once esophageal varices form, they increase in size and eventually bleed (Albillos, 2007); in cirrhosis, they are the most significant source of bleeding. The first bleeding episode has a mortality rate of 30% to 50% and is one of the major causes of death in patients with cirrhosis. The mortality rate increases with each subsequent bleeding episode (Kravetz, 2007).

Pathophysiology

Esophageal varices are dilated, tortuous veins that are usually found in the submucosa of the lower esophagus but may develop higher in the esophagus or extend into the stomach. This condition is almost always caused by portal hypertension, which results from obstruction of the portal venous circulation within the damaged liver.

Because of increased obstruction of the portal vein, venous blood from the intestinal tract and spleen seeks an outlet through collateral circulation (new pathways for return of blood to the right atrium). The effect is increased pressure, particularly in the vessels in the submucosal layer of the lower esophagus and upper part of the stomach. These collateral vessels are not very elastic; rather, they are tortuous and fragile, and they bleed easily (Fig. 39-7). Less common causes of varices are abnormalities of the circulation in the splenic vein or superior vena cava and hepatic venothrombosis.

Bleeding esophageal varices are life-threatening and can result in hemorrhagic shock that produces decreased cerebral, hepatic, and renal perfusion. In turn, there is an increased nitrogen load from bleeding into the GI tract and an increased serum ammonia level, increasing the risk of encephalopathy. Usually the dilated veins cause no symptoms. However, if the portal pressure increases sharply and the mucosa or supporting structures become thin, massive hemorrhaging occurs.

Physiology ■■■ Pathophysiology

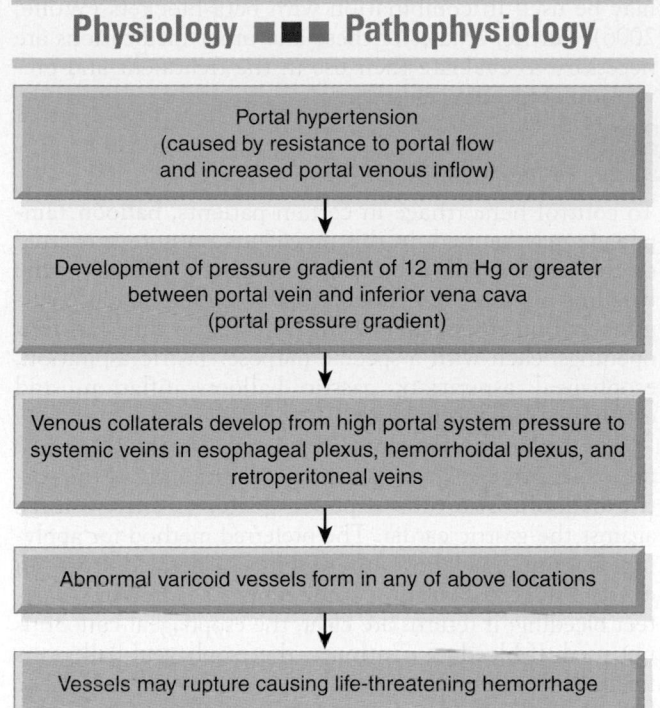

Portal hypertension
(caused by resistance to portal flow
and increased portal venous inflow)

↓

Development of pressure gradient of 12 mm Hg or greater
between portal vein and inferior vena cava
(portal pressure gradient)

↓

Venous collaterals develop from high portal system pressure to
systemic veins in esophageal plexus, hemorrhoidal plexus, and
retroperitoneal veins

↓

Abnormal varicoid vessels form in any of above locations

↓

Vessels may rupture causing life-threatening hemorrhage

Figure 39-7 Pathogenesis of bleeding esophageal varices.

Factors that contribute to hemorrhage are muscular exertion from lifting heavy objects; straining at stool; sneezing, coughing, or vomiting; esophagitis; irritation of vessels by poorly chewed foods or irritating fluids; and reflux of stomach contents (especially alcohol). Salicylates and any medication that erodes the esophageal mucosa or interferes with cell replication also may contribute to bleeding.

Clinical Manifestations

The patient with bleeding esophageal varices may present with hematemesis, melena, or general deterioration in mental or physical status and often has a history of alcohol abuse. Signs and symptoms of shock (cool clammy skin, hypotension, tachycardia) may be present.

Assessment and Diagnostic Findings

Endoscopy is used to identify the bleeding site, along with barium swallow, ultrasonography, CT, and angiography. Because the incidence of varices is 50% in patients with cirrhosis, it is recommended that these patients undergo screening endoscopy every 2 years in an effort to identify and treat large varices, which are the ones most likely to bleed (Wolfe, 2006).

Endoscopy

Immediate endoscopy (see Chapter 34) is indicated to identify the cause and the site of bleeding; at least 30% of patients with suspected bleeding from esophageal varices are actually bleeding from another source (gastritis, ulcer). Nursing support is essential during this often stressful experience. Careful monitoring can detect early signs of cardiac dysrhythmias, perforation, and hemorrhage.

After the examination, fluids are not given until the patient's gag reflex returns. Lozenges and gargles may be used to relieve throat discomfort if the patient's physical condition and mental status permit. If the patient is actively bleeding, oral intake will not be permitted, and the patient will be prepared for further diagnostic and therapeutic procedures.

Portal Hypertension Measurements

Portal hypertension may be suspected if dilated abdominal veins and hemorrhoids are detected. A palpable enlarged spleen (splenomegaly) and ascites may also be present. Portal venous pressure can be measured directly or indirectly. Indirect measurement of the hepatic vein pressure gradient is the most common procedure. The measurement requires insertion of a catheter with a balloon into the antecubital or femoral vein. The catheter is advanced under fluoroscopy to a hepatic vein. Fluid is infused once the catheter is in position to inflate the balloon. A "wedged" pressure (similar to pulmonary artery wedge pressure) is obtained by occluding the blood flow in the blood vessel; pressure in the unoccluded vessel is also measured. Although the values obtained may underestimate portal pressure, this measurement may be taken several times to evaluate the results of therapy.

Direct measurement of portal vein pressure can be obtained by several methods. During laparotomy, a needle may be introduced into the spleen; a manometer reading of more than 20 mL saline is abnormal. Another direct measurement requires insertion of a catheter into the portal vein or one of its branches. Endoscopic measurement of pressure within varices is used only in conjunction with endoscopic sclerotherapy.

Laboratory Tests

Laboratory tests may include various liver function tests, such as serum aminotransferases, bilirubin, alkaline phosphatase, and serum proteins. Splenoportography, which involves serial or segmental x-rays, is used to detect extensive collateral circulation in esophageal vessels, which would indicate varices. Other tests are hepatoportography and celiac angiography. These are usually performed in the operating room or x-ray department.

Medical Management

Bleeding from esophageal varices is an emergency that can quickly lead to hemorrhagic shock. The patient is critically ill, requiring aggressive medical care and expert nursing care, and is usually transferred to the intensive care unit (ICU) for close monitoring and management. See Chapter 15 for a discussion of care of the patient in shock.

The extent of bleeding is evaluated, and vital signs are monitored continuously if hematemesis and melena are present. Signs of potential hypovolemia are noted, such as cold clammy skin, tachycardia, a drop in blood pressure, decreased urine output, restlessness, and weak peripheral pulses. The volume of circulating blood is estimated and monitored with a central venous catheter or pulmonary artery catheter. Blood pressure is monitored via an arterial catheter. Oxygen is administered to prevent hypoxia and to maintain adequate blood oxygenation.

Because patients with bleeding esophageal varices have intravascular volume depletion and are subject to electrolyte imbalance, IV fluids with electrolytes and volume expanders are provided to restore fluid volume and replace electrolytes. Transfusion of blood components also may be required.

Caution must be taken with volume resuscitation so that overhydration does not occur, because this would raise portal pressure and increase bleeding. An indwelling urinary catheter is usually inserted to permit frequent monitoring of urine output.

Although a variety of pharmacologic, endoscopic, and surgical approaches are used to treat bleeding esophageal varices, none is ideal, and most are associated with considerable risk to the patient. Nonsurgical treatment of bleeding esophageal varices is preferable because of the high mortality rate of emergency surgery to control bleeding esophageal varices and because of the poor physical condition that is typical of the patient with severe liver dysfunction.

Pharmacologic Therapy

In an actively bleeding patient, medications are administered initially because they can be obtained and administered quicker than other therapies. Vasopressin (Pitressin) may be the initial mode of therapy in urgent situations because it produces constriction of the splanchnic arterial bed and decreases portal pressure. As previously described, splanchnic circulation comprises the arterial blood supply and venous drainage of the entire GI tract from the distal esophagus to the midrectum, including the liver. Vasopressin constricts distal esophageal and proximal gastric veins, thus reducing the inflow into the portal system and therefore the portal pressure. Vital signs and the presence or absence of blood in the gastric aspirate indicate the effectiveness of vasopressin. Monitoring of fluid intake and output and electrolyte levels is necessary because hyponatremia may develop and vasopressin may have an antidiuretic effect.

Coronary artery disease is a contraindication to the use of vasopressin because coronary vasoconstriction is a side effect that may precipitate myocardial infarction. The combination of vasopressin with nitroglycerin (administered by the IV, sublingual, or transdermal route) has been effective in reducing or preventing the side effects (constriction of coronary vessels and angina) caused by vasopressin alone. Side effects include myocardial and extremity ischemia as well as cardiac dysrhythmias; therefore, vasopressin is used only in urgent situations (Floch, 2005; Wolfe, 2006).

Somatostatin and octreotide (Sandostatin) have been reported to be effective in decreasing bleeding from esophageal varices, and they lack the vasoconstrictive effects of vasopressin. These medications cause selective splanchnic vasoconstriction and are used mainly in the management of active hemorrhage. Propranolol (Inderal) and nadolol (Corgard), beta-blocking agents that decrease portal pressure, are the most common medications used both to prevent a first bleeding episode in patients with known varices and to prevent rebleeding (Wolfe, 2006). Beta-blockers should not be used in acute variceal hemorrhage, but they are effective prophylaxis against such an episode. Nitrates such as isosorbide (Isordil) lower portal pressure by venodilation and decreased cardiac output and

may be used in combination with beta-blockers (Wolfe, 2006). Further studies of these and other medications are necessary to evaluate their use in the treatment and prevention of bleeding episodes.

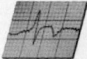 ### Balloon Tamponade

To control hemorrhage in certain patients, **balloon tamponade** may be used. In this procedure, pressure is exerted on the cardia (upper orifice of the stomach) and against the bleeding varices by a double-balloon tamponade (Sengstaken-Blakemore tube) (Fig. 39-8). The tube has four openings, each with a specific purpose: gastric aspiration, esophageal aspiration, gastric balloon inflation, and esophageal balloon inflation.

The balloon in the stomach is inflated with 100 to 200 mL of air. An x-ray confirms proper positioning of the gastric balloon. The tube is pulled gently to exert a force against the gastric cardia. The preferred method for applying traction may be with weights suspended from an overbed trapeze. Irrigation of the tubing is performed to detect bleeding; if returns are clear, the esophageal balloon is not used. If bleeding continues, the esophageal balloon is inflated. The desired pressure in the esophageal and gastric balloons is 25 to 40 mm Hg, as measured by the manometer. On inflation of the esophageal balloon, there is a possibility of injury or rupture of the esophagus, so constant nursing surveillance is necessary.

Gastric suction is provided by connecting the gastric catheter outlet to low suction (80 to 100 mm Hg). The tubing is irrigated hourly, and the color of the drainage indicates whether bleeding has been controlled. Room-temperature lavage or irrigation may be used in the gastric balloon. The pressure within the esophageal balloon is measured and recorded every 2 to 4 hours via the manometer to detect underinflation (which can allow bleeding to continue) or prevent overinflation (which can cause esophageal injury). When it appears that bleeding has stopped, the balloons are deflated carefully and sequentially. The esophageal balloon is deflated first, and the patient is monitored for recurrent bleeding. After several hours without bleeding, the gastric balloon can be deflated safely. If there is still no bleeding, the tamponade tube is removed. The therapy is used for as short a time as possible to control bleeding while emergency treatment is completed and definitive therapies are instituted (no longer than 24 hours).

Although balloon tamponade has been fairly successful, there are some inherent dangers. Displacement of the tube and the inflated balloon into the oropharynx can cause life-threatening obstruction of the airway and asphyxiation. This may occur if the patient pulls on the tube because of confusion or discomfort. It may also result from rupture of the gastric balloon, which causes the esophageal balloon to move into the oropharynx. Sudden rupture of the balloon causes airway obstruction and aspiration of gastric contents into the lungs. Therefore, the tube must be tested before insertion to minimize this risk by ensuring that the balloons can attain and maintain inflation. Aspiration of blood and secretions into the lungs is frequently associated with balloon tamponade, especially in the stuporous or comatose patient. Endotracheal intubation before insertion of the

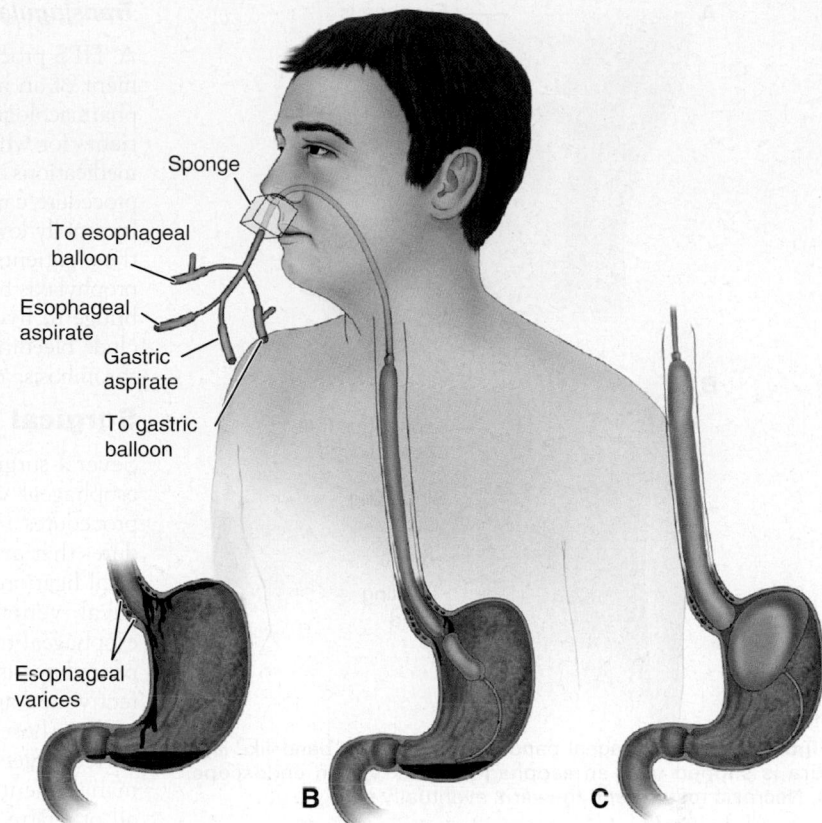

Figure 39-8 Balloon tamponade to treat esophageal varices. **A,** Dilated, bleeding esophageal veins (varices) of the lower esophagus. **B,** A four-lumen esophageal tamponade tube with balloons (uninflated) in place. **C,** Compression of bleeding esophageal varices by inflated esophageal and gastric balloons. The gastric and esophageal outlets permit the nurse to aspirate secretions.

tube protects the airway and minimizes the risk of aspiration. Ulceration and necrosis of the nose, the mucosa of the stomach, or the esophagus may occur if the tube is left in place too long, inflated too long, or inflated at too high a pressure.

 NURSING ALERT

The patient being treated with balloon tamponade must remain under close observation in the ICU because of the risk of serious complications. The patient must be monitored closely and continuously. Precautions must be taken to ensure that the patient does not pull on or inadvertently displace the tube.

Nursing measures include frequent mouth and nasal care. For secretions that accumulate in the mouth, tissues should be within easy reach of the patient. Oral suction may be necessary to remove oral secretions.

The patient with esophageal hemorrhage is usually extremely anxious and frightened. Knowing that the nurse is nearby and ready to respond immediately can help alleviate some of this anxiety. Tube insertion is uncomfortable and never pleasant. Careful explanation during the procedure and while the tube is in place may be reassuring to the patient. Sedation may be prescribed.

Although balloon tamponade stops the bleeding in 90% of patients, bleeding recurs in 60% to 70%, necessitating other treatment modalities, such as sclerotherapy or banding (Wolfe, 2006). Once the balloons are deflated or the tube is removed, the patient must be assessed frequently because of the high risk of recurrent bleeding.

Endoscopic Therapies

In endoscopic **sclerotherapy** (Fig. 39-9), also referred to as injection sclerotherapy, a sclerosing agent is injected through a fiberoptic endoscope into the bleeding esophageal varices to promote thrombosis and eventual sclerosis. The procedure has been used successfully to treat acute GI hemorrhage but is not recommended for prevention of first and subsequent variceal bleeding episodes (Albillos, 2007; Wolfe, 2006).

After treatment for acute hemorrhage, the patient must be observed for bleeding, perforation of the esophagus, aspiration pneumonia, and esophageal stricture. Antacids, histamine-2 antagonists such as cimetidine (Tagamet), or

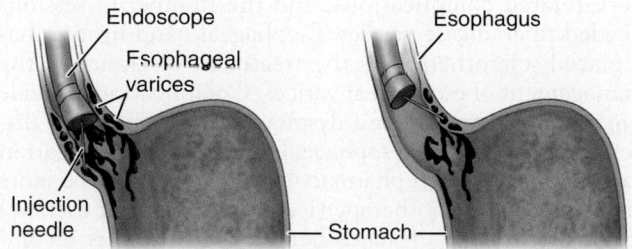

Figure 39-9 Endoscopic or injection sclerotherapy. Injection of sclerosing agent into esophageal varices through an endoscope promotes thrombosis and eventual sclerosis, thereby obliterating the varices.

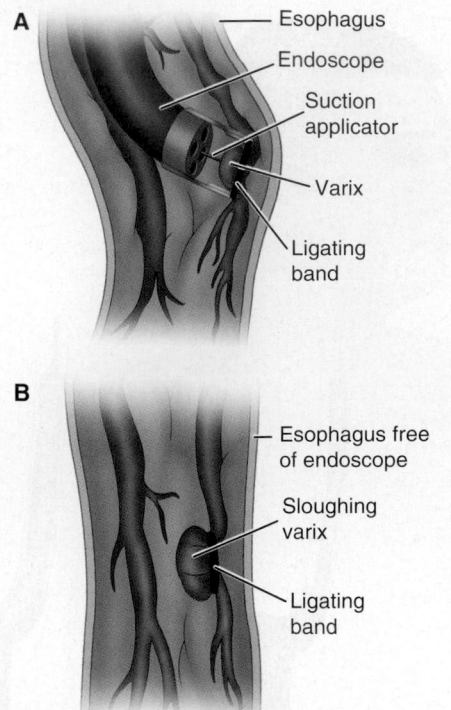

A
- Esophagus
- Endoscope
- Suction applicator
- Varix
- Ligating band

B
- Esophagus free of endoscope
- Sloughing varix
- Ligating band

Figure 39-10 Esophageal banding. **A,** A rubber band–like ligature is slipped over an esophageal varix via an endoscope. **B,** Necrosis results, and the varix eventually sloughs off.

proton pump inhibitors such as pantoprazole (Protonix) may be administered after the procedure to counteract the chemical effects of the sclerosing agent on the esophagus and the acid reflux associated with the therapy.

Esophageal Banding Therapy (Variceal Band Ligation)

In **variceal banding** (Fig. 39-10), also referred to as esophageal variceal ligation (EVL), a modified endoscope loaded with an elastic rubber band is passed through an overtube directly onto the varix (or varices) to be banded. After the bleeding varix is suctioned into the tip of the endoscope, the rubber band is slipped over the tissue, causing necrosis, ulceration, and eventual sloughing of the varix.

Variceal banding is comparable to endoscopic sclerotherapy in its effectiveness in controlling acute bleeding. Compared with sclerotherapy, variceal banding also significantly reduces the rebleeding rate, mortality, procedure-related complications, and the number of sessions needed to eradicate varices. Esophageal band ligation has replaced sclerotherapy as the treatment of choice in the management of esophageal varices. Complications include superficial ulceration and dysphagia, transient chest discomfort, and, rarely, esophageal strictures. Band ligation in combination with pharmacologic therapy may be more effective than monotherapy (ie, a single mode of therapy) in the treatment of acute hemorrhage. EVL is recommended for patients who have experienced variceal bleeding while receiving beta-blocker therapy and for those who cannot tolerate beta-blocking agents (Albillos, 2007).

Transjugular Intrahepatic Portosystemic Shunting

A TIPS procedure (see Fig. 39-6) is indicated for the treatment of an acute episode of variceal bleeding refractory to pharmacologic or endoscopic therapy. In 10% to 20% of patients for whom urgent band ligation or sclerotherapy and medications are not successful in eradicating bleeding, a TIPS procedure can effectively control acute variceal hemorrhage by rapidly lowering portal pressure. TIPS is also indicated for those patients who rebleed after pharmacologic or endoscopic prophylaxis has failed. In addition, this technique is used as a bridge to liver transplantation. Potential complications include bleeding, sepsis, heart failure, organ perforation, shunt thrombosis, and progressive liver failure (Wolfe, 2006).

Surgical Management

Several surgical procedures have been developed to treat esophageal varices and to minimize rebleeding, but these procedures are often accompanied by significant risk. Procedures that may be used for esophageal varices are direct surgical ligation of varices; splenorenal, mesocaval, and portacaval venous shunts to relieve portal pressure; and esophageal transection with devascularization. Use of these procedures is controversial, and studies regarding their effectiveness and outcomes continue. What is known thus far is that these procedures are very effective in controlling variceal bleeding. They may be considered as second-line management (rescue therapy) for those patients for whom all other treatments have failed, those who are not candidates for liver transplantation, and those who require a bridge to transplantation. There is a high incidence of encephalopathy after the surgical shunting procedures, and morbidity and mortality statistics remain high (Rodes, et al., 2007). The TIPS procedure has largely replaced the use of surgical decompressive shunts and ligation procedures.

Surgical Bypass Procedures

Surgical decompression of the portal circulation can prevent variceal bleeding if the shunt remains patent (Rodes, et al., 2007). One of the various surgical shunting procedures (Fig. 39-11) is the distal splenorenal shunt, which is made between the splenic vein and the left renal vein after splenectomy. A mesocaval shunt is created by anastomosing the superior mesenteric vein to the proximal end of the vena cava or to the side of the vena cava using grafting material. The goal of distal splenorenal and mesocaval shunts is to decrease portal pressure by draining only a portion of venous blood from the portal bed; therefore, they are considered selective shunts. The liver continues to receive some portal flow, and the incidence of encephalopathy may be reduced. Portacaval shunts are considered nonselective shunts because they divert all portal flow to the vena cava via end-to-side or side-to-side approaches.

These procedures are extensive and are not always successful because of secondary thrombosis in the veins used for the shunt and because of complications (eg, encephalopathy, accelerated liver failure). The effectiveness of these procedures has been studied extensively. All shunt procedures are equally effective in preventing recurrent variceal bleeding but may cause further impairment of liver function and encephalopathy. Partial portacaval shunts with interposition grafts are as effective as other shunts but

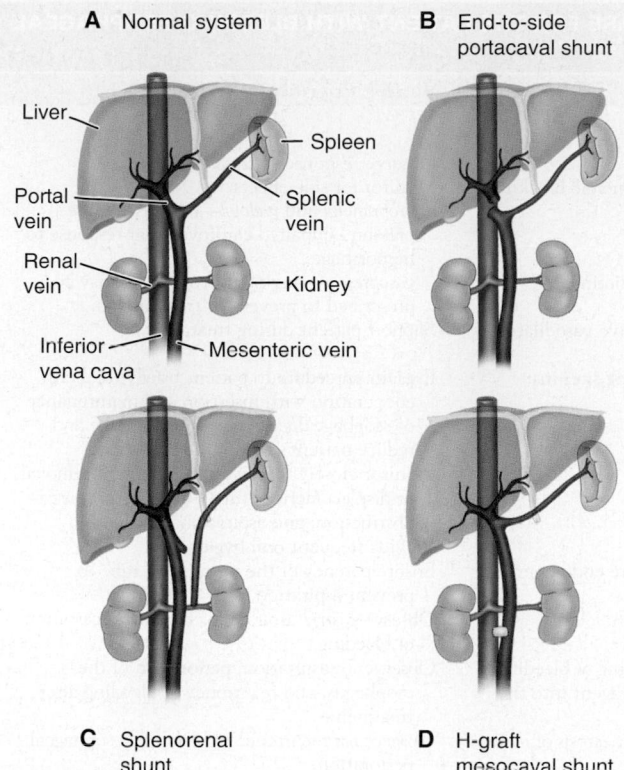

A Normal system

Liver
Spleen
Portal vein
Splenic vein
Renal vein
Kidney
Inferior vena cava
Mesenteric vein

B End-to-side portacaval shunt

C Splenorenal shunt

D H-graft mesocaval shunt

Figure 39-11 Portal systemic shunts. **A,** Normal portal system. **B–D,** Examples of portal shunts to reduce portal pressure.

are associated with a lower rate of encephalopathy (Rodes, et al., 2007). The severity of the disease (by a classification such as the Child-Pugh system, discussed later) and the potential for future liver transplantation guide the treatment decision. If the cause of portal hypertension is the rare Budd-Chiari syndrome or other venous obstructive disease, a portacaval or a mesoatrial shunt may be performed (see Fig. 39-11). The mesoatrial shunt is required when the infrahepatic vena cava is thrombosed and must be bypassed.

Devascularization and Transection

Devascularization and staple-gun transection procedures to separate the bleeding site from the high-pressure portal system have been used in the emergency management of variceal bleeding. The lower end of the esophagus is reached through a small gastrostomy incision; a staple gun permits anastomosis of the transected ends of the esophagus. Rebleeding is a risk, and the outcomes of these procedures vary among patient populations.

> ### ▶ NURSING ALERT
>
> **Postoperative care is similar to that for any abdominal surgery, but the risk of complications (hypovolemic or hemorrhagic shock, hepatic encephalopathy, electrolyte imbalance, metabolic and respiratory alkalosis, alcohol withdrawal syndrome, and seizures) is high. The surgical procedures do not alter the course of the progressive liver disease, and bleeding may recur as new collateral vessels develop.**

Nursing Management

Overall nursing assessment includes monitoring the patient's physical condition and evaluating emotional responses and cognitive status. The nurse monitors and records vital signs and assesses the patient's nutritional and neurologic status. This assessment assists in identifying hepatic encephalopathy, which may result from the breakdown of blood in the GI tract with a rising serum ammonia level. Manifestations range from drowsiness and confusion to profound coma.

If complete rest of the esophagus is indicated because of bleeding, parenteral nutrition is initiated. Gastric suction usually is initiated to keep the stomach as empty as possible and to prevent straining and vomiting. The patient often complains of severe thirst, which may be relieved by frequent oral hygiene and moist sponges to the lips. The nurse closely monitors the blood pressure. Vitamin K therapy and multiple blood transfusions often are indicated because of blood loss. A quiet environment and calm reassurance may help to relieve the patient's anxiety and reduce agitation.

Bleeding anywhere in the body is anxiety provoking, resulting in a crisis for the patient and family. If the patient has been a heavy user of alcohol, delirium secondary to alcohol withdrawal can complicate the situation. The nurse provides support and explanations about medical and nursing interventions. Close monitoring of the patient helps in detecting and managing complications. Management modalities and nursing care of the patient with bleeding esophageal varices are summarized in Table 39-2.

Hepatic Encephalopathy and Coma

Hepatic encephalopathy, or portosystemic encephalopathy (PSE), is a life-threatening complication of liver disease that occurs with profound liver failure. Patients with this condition have no overt signs of the illness but do have abnormalities on neuropsychologic testing (Hauser, et al., 2006). Hepatic encephalopathy is the neuropsychiatric manifestation of hepatic failure associated with portal hypertension and the shunting of blood from the portal venous system into the systemic circulation (Hauser, et al., 2006). This reversible metabolic form of encephalopathy can improve with recovery of liver function. The onset is often insidious and subtle, and initially the disease is termed subclinical or minimal hepatic encephalopathy.

Table 39-3 presents the stages of hepatic encephalopathy, common signs and symptoms, and potential nursing diagnoses for each stage.

Pathophysiology

Despite the frequency with which hepatic encephalopathy occurs, the precise pathophysiology is not fully defined (Feldman, Friedman & Brandt, 2006). Two major alterations underlie its development in acute and chronic liver disease. First, hepatic insufficiency may result in encephalopathy because of the inability of the liver to detoxify toxic byproducts of metabolism. Second, portal-systemic shunting, in which collateral vessels develop as a result of portal hypertension, allows elements of the portal blood

Table 39-2 MANAGEMENT MODALITIES AND NURSING CARE FOR THE PATIENT WITH BLEEDING ESOPHAGEAL VARICES

Treatment Modality*	Action	Nursing Priorities
Nonsurgical Modalities		
Pharmacologic agents		Observe response to therapy.
Propranolol (Inderal)/nadolol (Corgard)	Reduces portal pressure by β-adrenergic blocking action.	Monitor for side effects: *propranolol* and *nadolol*—decreased pulse pressure, impaired cardiovascular response to hemorrhage.
Vasopressin (Pitressin)	Reduces portal pressure by constricting splanchnic arteries.	*vasopressin*—angina; nitroglycerin may be prescribed to prevent or treat angina.
Somatostatin/octreotide (Sandostatin)	Reduces portal pressure by selective vasodilation of portal system.	Support patient during treatment.
Balloon tamponade	Exerts pressure directly to bleeding sites in esophagus and stomach.	Explain procedure to patient briefly to obtain cooperation with insertion and maintenance of esophageal/gastric tamponade tube and reduce patient's fear of the procedure. Monitor closely to prevent inadvertent removal or displacement of tube, subsequent airway obstruction, and aspiration. Provide frequent oral hygiene.
Room-temperature saline lavage	Clears blood and secretions before endoscopy and other procedures.	Ensure patency of the nasogastric tube to prevent aspiration. Observe gastric aspirate for blood and cessation of bleeding.
Injection sclerotherapy	Promotes thrombosis and sclerosing of bleeding sites by injection of sclerosing agent into the esophageal varices.	Observe for aspiration, perforation of the esophagus, and recurrence of bleeding after treatment.
Variceal banding	Provides thrombosis and mucosal necrosis of bleeding sites by band ligation.	Observe for recurrence of bleeding, esophageal perforation.
Transjugular intrahepatic portosystemic shunt (TIPS)	Reduces portal pressure by creating a shunt within the liver between the portal and systemic venous systems.	Observe for rebleeding and signs of infection.
Surgical Modalities		
Portal-systemic shunt	Reduces portal hypertension by diverting blood flow away from obstructed portal system.	Observe for development of portal-systemic encephalopathy (altered mental status, neurologic dysfunction), hepatic failure, and rebleeding. Requires intensive, expert nursing care for prolonged period.
Surgical ligation of varices	Ties off blood vessels at the site of bleeding.	Observe for rebleeding.
Esophageal transection and devascularization	Separates bleeding site from portal system.	Observe for rebleeding. Provide postthoracotomy care.

*Several modalities may be used concurrently or in sequence.

(laden with potentially toxic substances usually extracted by the liver) to enter the systemic circulation (Rodes, et al., 2007). Ammonia is considered the major etiologic factor in the development of encephalopathy. It enters the brain and excites peripheral benzodiazepine-type receptors on astrocyte cells, thus increasing neurosteroid synthesis; this then stimulates gamma-aminobutyric acid (GABA) neurotransmission. GABA causes depression of the central nervous system (Hauser, et al., 2007). Ammonia inhibits neurotransmission and synaptic regulation (Onion, 2006), producing

Table 39-3 STAGES OF HEPATIC ENCEPHALOPATHY AND POSSIBLE NURSING DIAGNOSES*

Stage	Clinical Symptoms	Clinical Signs and EEG Changes	Selected Potential Nursing Diagnoses
1	Normal level of consciousness with periods of lethargy and euphoria; reversal of day–night sleep patterns	Asterixis; impaired writing and ability to draw line figures. Normal EEG.	Activity intolerance Self-care deficit Disturbed sleep pattern
2	Increased drowsiness; disorientation; inappropriate behavior; mood swings; agitation	Asterixis; fetor hepaticus. Abnormal EEG with generalized slowing.	Impaired social interaction Ineffective role performance Risk for injury
3	Stuporous; difficult to rouse; sleeps most of time; marked confusion; incoherent speech	Asterixis; increased deep tendon reflexes; rigidity of extremities. EEG markedly abnormal.	Imbalanced nutrition Impaired mobility Impaired verbal communication
4	Comatose; may not respond to painful stimuli	Absence of asterixis; absence of deep tendon reflexes; flaccidity of extremities. EEG markedly abnormal.	Risk for aspiration Impaired gas exchange Impaired tissue integrity Disturbed sensory perception

*Nursing diagnoses are likely to progress, so that most nursing diagnoses present at earlier stages will occur during later stages as well.

sleep and behavior patterns associated with hepatic encephalopathy.

Circumstances that increase serum ammonia levels tend to aggravate or precipitate hepatic encephalopathy. The largest source of ammonia is the enzymatic and bacterial digestion of dietary and blood proteins in the GI tract. Ammonia from these sources increases as a result of GI bleeding (ie, bleeding esophageal varices, chronic GI bleeding), a high-protein diet, bacterial infection, or uremia. The ingestion of ammonium salts also increases the blood ammonia level. In the presence of alkalosis or hypokalemia, increased amounts of ammonia are absorbed from the GI tract and from the renal tubular fluid. Conversely, serum ammonia is decreased by elimination of protein from the diet and by the administration of antibiotic agents, such as neomycin sulfate (Mycifradin, Neo-fradin), which reduce the number of intestinal bacteria capable of converting urea to ammonia (Dudek, 2006).

Other factors unrelated to increased serum ammonia levels that can cause hepatic encephalopathy in susceptible patients include excessive diuresis, dehydration, infections, surgery, fever, and some medications (sedatives, tranquilizers, analgesics, and diuretics that cause potassium loss). Additional causes include elevated levels of serum manganese (Hauser, et al., 2006), as well as changes in the types of circulating amino acids, mercaptans, and levels of dopamine and other neurotransmitters in the central nervous system (Feldman, et al., 2006). Mercaptans are toxic metabolites of sulfur-containing compounds that are excreted by the liver under normal conditions. Mercaptans and these other so-called "false" neurotransmitters may be generated from an intestinal source or from metabolism of protein by the liver and, with defective hepatic clearance, may precipitate encephalopathy.

Clinical Manifestations

The earliest symptoms of hepatic encephalopathy include minor mental changes and motor disturbances. The patient appears slightly confused and unkempt and has alterations in mood and sleep patterns. The patient tends to sleep during the day and has restlessness and insomnia at night. As hepatic encephalopathy progresses, the patient may become difficult to awaken and completely disoriented with respect to time and place. With further progression, the patient lapses into frank coma and may have seizures.

Asterixis (flapping tremor of the hands) may be seen in stage II encephalopathy (Fig. 39-12). Simple tasks, such as handwriting, become difficult. A handwriting or drawing sample (eg, star figure), taken daily, may provide graphic evidence of progression or reversal of hepatic encephalopathy. Inability to reproduce a simple figure (Fig. 39-13) is referred to as **constructional apraxia.** In the early stages of hepatic encephalopathy, the deep tendon reflexes are hyperactive; with worsening of the encephalopathy, these reflexes disappear and the extremities may become flaccid.

Occasionally, **fetor hepaticus,** a sweet, slightly fecal odor to the breath that is presumed to be of intestinal origin, may be noticed. The odor has also been described as similar to that of freshly mowed grass, acetone, or old wine. Fetor hepaticus is prevalent with extensive collateral portal circulation in chronic liver disease.

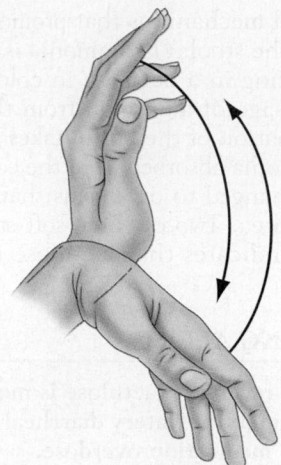

Figure 39-12 Asterixis or "liver flap" may occur in hepatic encephalopathy. The patient is asked to hold the arm out with the hand held upward (dorsiflexed). Within a few seconds, the hand falls forward involuntarily and then quickly returns to the dorsiflexed position.

Assessment and Diagnostic Findings

The electroencephalogram (EEG) shows generalized slowing, an increase in the amplitude of brain waves, and characteristic triphasic waves. The survival rate after a first episode of overt hepatic encephalopathy in patients with cirrhosis is approximately 40% at 1 year. Patients should be referred for liver transplantation after this initial episode (Hauser, et al., 2006).

Medical Management

Medical management of hepatic encephalopathy focuses on identifying and eliminating the precipitating cause if possible, initiating ammonia-lowering therapy, minimizing potential medical complications of cirrhosis and depressed consciousness, and reversing the underlying liver disease, if possible. Correction of the possible reasons for the deterioration such as bleeding, electrolyte abnormalities, sedation, or azotemia is essential (Feldman, et al., 2006). Lactulose (Cephulac) is administered to reduce serum ammonia levels.

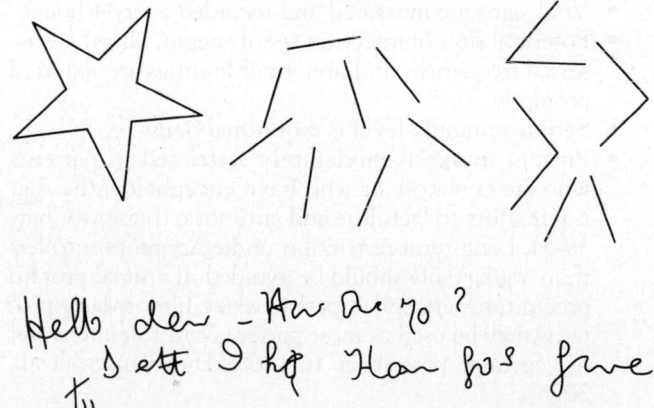

Figure 39-13 Effects of constructional apraxia. Deterioration of handwriting and inability to draw a simple star figure occurs with progressive hepatic encephalopathy. (With permission from Sherlock, S. & Dooley, J. (2002). *Diseases of the liver and biliary system* (11th ed.). Oxford, UK: Blackwell Scientific Ltd.)

It acts by several mechanisms that promote the excretion of ammonia in the stool: (1) ammonia is kept in the ionized state, resulting in a decrease in colon pH, reversing the normal passage of ammonia from the colon to the blood; (2) evacuation of the bowel takes place, which decreases the ammonia absorbed from the colon; and (3) the fecal flora are changed to organisms that do not produce ammonia from urea. Two or three soft stools per day are desirable; this indicates that lactulose is performing as intended.

> ◢ **NURSING ALERT**
>
> **The patient receiving lactulose is monitored closely for the development of watery diarrheal stools, because they indicate a medication overdose.**

Possible side effects of lactulose include intestinal bloating and cramps, which usually disappear within a week. To mask the sweet taste, which some patients dislike, it can be diluted with fruit juice. The patient is closely monitored for hypokalemia and dehydration. Other laxatives are not prescribed during lactulose administration because their effects disturb dosage regulation. Lactulose may be administered by nasogastric tube or enema for patients who are comatose or for those in whom oral administration is contraindicated or impossible.

Other aspects of management include IV administration of glucose to minimize protein breakdown, administration of vitamins to correct deficiencies, and correction of electrolyte imbalances (especially potassium). Antibiotics may also be added to the treatment regimen. Neomycin, metronidazole (Flagyl), and rifaximin (Xifaxan) have been used to reduce levels of ammonia-forming bacteria in the colon. However, no benefit has been shown for long-term treatment with these antibiotics (Hauser, et al., 2006). Additional principles of management of hepatic encephalopathy include the following:

- Neurologic status is assessed frequently.
- Mental status is monitored by keeping a daily record of handwriting and arithmetic performance.
- Fluid intake and output and body weight are recorded each day.
- Vital signs are measured and recorded every 4 hours.
- Potential sites of infection (peritoneum, lungs) are assessed frequently, and abnormal findings are reported promptly.
- Serum ammonia level is monitored daily.
- Protein intake is moderately restricted in patients who are comatose or who have encephalopathy that is refractory to lactulose and antibiotic therapy (Chart 39-5). Long-term restriction of dietary protein to less than 1 g/kg daily should be avoided. If animal protein precipitates encephalopathy, vegetable or dairy proteins may be used as most patients can tolerate a diet of vegetable protein up to 120 g/day (Hauser, et al., 2006).
- Patients and families are advised about foods that are high in protein (eg, meat, eggs), which may need to be eliminated from the diet for the short term to reduce production of ammonia.

Chart 39-5 • *Nutritional Management of Hepatic Encephalopathy*

- Prevent the formation and absorption of toxins, principally ammonia, from the intestine.
- Keep daily protein intake between 1.0 and 1.5 g/kg, depending on the degree of decompensation.
- Avoid protein restriction if possible, even in those with encephalopathy. If necessary, implement temporary restriction of 0.5 to 0.8 g/kg.
- For patients who are truly protein-intolerant, provide additional nitrogen in the form of an amino acid supplement. Use of branched-chain amino acids is still controversial.
- Provide small, frequent meals and an evening snack of complex carbohydrates to avoid protein loading.
- Substitute vegetable protein for animal protein in as high a percentage as possible.

- Enteral feeding is provided for patients whose encephalopathic state persists.
- Reduction in the absorption of ammonia from the GI tract is accomplished by the use of gastric suction, enemas, or oral antibiotics.
- Electrolyte status is monitored and corrected if abnormal.
- Sedatives, tranquilizers, and analgesic medications are discontinued.
- Benzodiazepine antagonists such as flumazenil (Romazicon) may be administered to improve encephalopathy, whether or not the patient has previously taken benzodiazepines. This action may have short-term efficacy because patients with hepatic encephalopathy have an increased concentration of benzodiazepine receptors.

Nursing Management

The nurse is responsible for maintaining a safe environment to prevent injury, bleeding, and infection. The nurse administers the prescribed treatments and monitors the patient for the numerous potential complications. The potential for respiratory compromise is great given the patient's depressed neurological status. The nurse encourages deep breathing and position changes to prevent the development of atelectasis, pneumonia, and other respiratory complications. Despite aggressive pulmonary care, patients may develop respiratory compromise. They may require intubation and mechanical ventilation to protect the airway, and they are frequently admitted to the ICU.

The nurse communicates with the patient's family to inform them about the patient's status and supports them by explaining the procedures and treatments that are part of the patient's care. If the patient recovers from hepatic encephalopathy and coma, rehabilitation is likely to be prolonged. Therefore, the patient and family will require assistance to understand the causes of this severe complication and to recognize that it may recur.

Promoting Home and Community-Based Care

Teaching Patients Self-Care

If the patient has recovered from hepatic encephalopathy and is to be discharged home, the nurse instructs the family to watch for subtle signs of recurrent encephalopathy. In the acute phase of hepatic encephalopathy, dietary protein may be reduced for a brief period to 0.8 to 1.0 g/kg per day. During recovery and in the home situation, it is important to instruct the patient in maintenance of a moderate-protein, high-calorie diet. Protein may then be added in 10-g increments every 3 to 5 days if mental status is improving. Any relapse (worsening neurologic assessment) is treated by returning protein intake to the previous level. The limits of tolerance are usually 1.0 to 1.5 g/kg per day. Continued use of lactulose in the home environment is not uncommon, and the patient and family should closely monitor its efficacy and side effects. They should also be cautioned that constipation can precipitate encephalopathy and should be prevented through the prescribed use of lactulose, which is crucial in preventing constipation. Use of vegetable rather than animal protein may be indicated in patients whose total daily protein tolerance is less than 1 g/kg. Vegetable protein intake may result in improved nitrogen balance without precipitating or advancing hepatic encephalopathy (Feldman, et al., 2006).

Continuing Care

Referral for home care is warranted for the patient who returns home after recovery from hepatic encephalopathy. The home care nurse assesses the patient's physical and mental status and collaborates closely with the physician. The home visit also provides an opportunity for the nurse to assess the home environment and the ability of the patient and family to monitor signs and symptoms and to follow the treatment regimen. It is important to evaluate the patient's fluid volume status and be alert for changes indicative of hypovolemia due to decreased intake and for decreased urine output associated with hepatorenal syndrome. Monitoring of laboratory values continues to be important, and the home care nurse must obtain physician orders to correct abnormalities, especially electrolyte imbalances, which also can worsen encephalopathy.

The safety of the home environment is also assessed closely to identify areas of risk for falls and other injuries. Home care visits are especially important if the patient lives alone because encephalopathy may affect the patient's ability to remember or follow the treatment regimen. The nurse reinforces previous teaching and reminds the patient and family about the importance of dietary restrictions, close monitoring, and follow-up. In addition, the nurse must observe the patient for subtle behavior changes of worsening hepatic encephalopathy. Patients with all types and stages of hepatic encephalopathy should have periodic neurological evaluations to determine their cognitive function so that they do not engage in potentially harmful activities. Even subtle neuropsychiatric abnormalities may preclude patients from driving, operating machinery, or participating in other activities that require psychomotor coordination.

Patients and families may need additional support during those times that the patient exhibits mood disturbances and sleep disorders. Patients should be as active as possible during the day and develop a normal sleep–wake pattern. Sedating medications should be avoided because they may precipitate encephalopathy. Patients and families may require assistance in developing plans to cope with changes in mood and mental status changes. This plan should identify support persons to attend to the patient in the home situation if needed. Social workers and case managers may make appropriate referrals for assistance with physical and psychosocial support and care. Referrals to other experts such as psychologists, psychiatric liaison nurses, case managers, social workers, or therapists may assist family members with coping. Spiritual advisors may also provide another outlet for communication and guidance. If alcohol played a role in the development of the liver disease and encephalopathy, referral to Alcoholics Anonymous or Al-Anon may provide needed support and education.

Other Manifestations of Hepatic Dysfunction

Edema and Bleeding

Many patients with liver dysfunction develop generalized edema caused by hypoalbuminemia due to decreased hepatic production of albumin. The production of blood clotting factors by the liver is also reduced, leading to an increased incidence of bruising, epistaxis, bleeding from wounds, and, as described previously, GI bleeding.

Vitamin Deficiency

Decreased production of several clotting factors may be partially due to deficient absorption of vitamin K from the GI tract. This probably is caused by the inability of liver cells to use vitamin K to make prothrombin. Absorption of the other fat-soluble vitamins (vitamins A, D, and E) as well as dietary fats may also be impaired because of decreased secretion of bile salts into the intestine.

Another group of problems common to patients with severe chronic liver dysfunction results from inadequate intake of sufficient vitamins. These include the following:

- Vitamin A deficiency, resulting in night blindness and eye and skin changes
- Thiamine deficiency, leading to beriberi, polyneuritis, and Wernicke-Korsakoff psychosis
- Riboflavin deficiency, resulting in characteristic skin and mucous membrane lesions
- Pyridoxine deficiency, resulting in skin and mucous membrane lesions and neurologic changes
- Vitamin C deficiency, resulting in the hemorrhagic lesions of scurvy
- Vitamin K deficiency, resulting in hypoprothrombinemia, characterized by spontaneous bleeding and ecchymoses
- Folic acid deficiency, resulting in macrocytic anemia

Because of these avitaminoses, the diet of every patient with chronic liver disease (especially if alcohol related) is supplemented with vitamins A, B complex, C, K, and folic acid.

Metabolic Abnormalities

Abnormalities of glucose metabolism also occur; the blood glucose level may be abnormally high shortly after a meal (a diabetic-type glucose tolerance test result), but hypoglycemia may occur during fasting because of decreased hepatic glycogen reserves and decreased gluconeogenesis. Medications must be used cautiously and in reduced dosages because the ability to metabolize medications is decreased in the patient with liver failure.

Many endocrine abnormalities also occur with liver dysfunction because the liver cannot properly metabolize hormones, including androgens and sex hormones. Failure of the damaged liver to inactivate estrogens normally can cause gynecomastia, amenorrhea, testicular atrophy, loss of pubic hair in the male, menstrual irregularities in the female, and other disturbances of sexual function and sex characteristics.

Pruritus and Other Skin Changes

Patients with liver dysfunction resulting from biliary obstruction commonly develop severe pruritus due to retention of bile salts. Patients may develop vascular (or arterial) spider angiomas (Fig. 39-14) on the skin, usually above the waistline. These are numerous small vessels resembling a spider's legs. They are most often associated with cirrhosis, especially in alcoholic liver disease. Patients may also develop reddened palms ("liver palms" or palmar erythema).

VIRAL HEPATITIS

Viral hepatitis is a systemic, viral infection in which necrosis and inflammation of liver cells produce a characteristic cluster of clinical, biochemical, and cellular changes. To

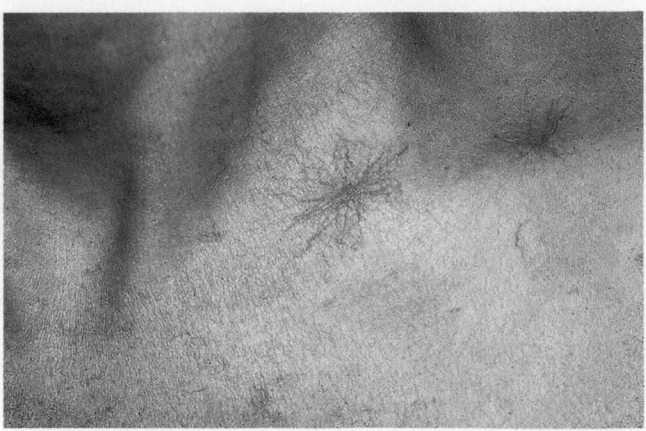

Figure 39-14 Spider angioma. This vascular (arterial) spider appears on the skin. Beneath the elevated center and radiating branches, the blood vessels are looped and tortuous.

date, five definitive types of viral hepatitis have been identified: hepatitis A, B, C, D, and E. Hepatitis A and E are similar in mode of transmission (fecal–oral route), whereas hepatitis B, C, and D share many other characteristics. Terms associated with viral hepatitis are listed in Chart 39-6.

Hepatitis is easily transmitted and causes high morbidity and prolonged loss of time from school or employment. Acute viral hepatitis affects 0.5% to 1% of people in the

Chart 39-6 • *Hepatitis Terms and Abbreviations*

Hepatitis A	
HAV	Hepatitis A virus; etiologic agent of hepatitis A (formerly infectious hepatitis)
Anti-HAV	Antibody to hepatitis A virus; appears in serum soon after onset of symptoms; disappears after 3–12 mo
IgM anti-HAV	IgM antibody to HAV; indicates recent infection with HAV; positive up to 6 mo after infection
Hepatitis B	
HBV	Hepatitis B virus; etiologic agent of hepatitis B (formerly serum hepatitis)
HBsAG	Hepatitis B surface antigen (Australian antigen); indicates acute or chronic hepatitis B or carrier state; indicates infectious state
Anti-HBs	Antibody to hepatitis B surface antigen; indicates prior exposure and immunity to hepatitis; may indicate passive antibody from HBIG or immune response from hepatitis B vaccine
HBeAg	Hepatitis B e-antigen; present in serum early in course; indicates highly infectious stage of hepatitis B; persistence in serum indicates progression to chronic hepatitis
Anti-HBe	Antibody to hepatitis B e-antigen; suggests low titer of HBV
HBcAg	Hepatitis B core antigen; found in liver cells; not easily detected in serum
Anti-HBc	Antibody to hepatitis B core antigen; most sensitive indicator of hepatitis B; appears late in the acute phase of the disease; indicates infection of HBV at some time in the past
IgM anti-HBc	IgM antibody to HBcAg; present for up to 6 mo after HBV infection
Hepatitis C	
HCV	Hepatitis C virus (formerly non-A, non-B virus); may be more than one virus
Hepatitis D	
HDV	Hepatitis D virus (delta agent); etiologic agent to hepatitis D; HBV required for replication
HDAg	Hepatitis delta antigen; detectable in early acute HDV infection
Anti-HDV	Antibody to HDV; indicates past or present infection with HDV
Hepatitis E	
HEV	Hepatitis E virus; etiologic agent of hepatitis E
Hepatitis G	
HGV	Hepatitis G virus; also known as GB virus C or GB-C

Table 39-4   COMPARISON OF MAJOR FORMS OF VIRAL HEPATITIS

	Hepatitis A	Hepatitis B	Hepatitis C	Hepatitis D	Hepatitis E
Previous names	Infectious hepatitis	Serum hepatitis	Non-A, non-B hepatitis		
Epidemiology					
Cause	Hepatitis A virus (HAV)	Hepatitis B virus (HBV)	Hepatitis C virus (HCV)	Hepatitis D virus (HDV)	Hepatitis E virus (HEV)
Mode of transmission	Fecal–oral route; poor sanitation. Person-to-person contact. Waterborne; foodborne. Transmission possible with oral–anal contact during sex.	Parenterally; by intimate contact with carriers or those with acute disease; sexual and oral–oral contact. Perinatal transmission from mothers to infants. An important occupational hazard for health care personnel.	Transfusion of blood and blood products; exposure to contaminated blood through equipment or drug paraphernalia. Transmission possible with sex with infected partner; risk increased with STD.	Same as HBV. HBV surface antigen necessary for replication; pattern similar to that of hepatitis B.	Fecal–oral route; person to person contact may be possible, although risk appears low
Incubation (days)	15–50 days	28–160 days	15–160 days	21–140 days	15–65 days
Immunity	Average: 30 days Homologous	Average: 70–80 days Homologous	Average: 50 days Second attack may indicate weak immunity or infection with another agent.	Average: 35 days Homologous	Average: 42 days Unknown
Nature of Illness					
Signs and symptoms	May occur with or without symptoms; flulike illness *Preicteric phase:* Headache, malaise, fatigue, anorexia, fever *Icteric phase:* Dark urine, jaundice of sclera and skin, tender liver	May occur without symptoms May develop arthralgias, rash	Similar to HBV; less severe and anicteric	Similar to HBV	Similar to HAV. Very severe in pregnant women.
Outcome	Usually mild with recovery. Fatality rate: <1%. No carrier state or increased risk of chronic hepatitis, cirrhosis, or hepatic cancer.	May be severe. Fatality rate: 1–10%. Carrier state possible. Increased risk of chronic hepatitis, cirrhosis, and hepatic cancer.	Frequent occurrence of chronic carrier state and chronic liver disease. Increased risk of hepatic cancer.	Similar to HBV but greater likelihood of carrier state, chronic active hepatitis, and cirrhosis	Similar to HAV except very severe in pregnant women

United States each year. Hepatitis A is responsible for 37% of all cases, and hepatitis B is the offending agent in 18% of cases. The occurrence rate has been decreasing steadily since 1990, largely because of the use of hepatitis A and B vaccines as well as public health education regarding high-risk behaviors (Goldman & Ausiello, 2008). It is estimated that 60% to 90% of viral hepatitis cases go unreported. The occurrence of subclinical cases, failure to recognize mild cases, and misdiagnosis are thought to contribute to the underreporting. Table 39-4 compares the major forms of viral hepatitis.

Hepatitis A Virus

Hepatitis A virus (HAV) accounts for 20% to 25% of cases of clinical hepatitis in the United States and other developed countries (Rodes, et al., 2007). Hepatitis A, formerly called infectious hepatitis, is caused by an RNA virus of the Enterovirus family. In the United States, the disease is seen mainly in the adult population. Fewer than 25% of children have antibodies to HAV. This form of hepatitis is transmitted primarily through the fecal–oral route, by the ingestion of food or liquids infected by the virus. It is more prevalent in countries with overcrowding and poor sanitation. The virus has been found in the stool of infected patients before the onset of symptoms and during the first few days of illness.

Typically, a child or a young adult acquires the infection at school through poor hygiene, hand-to-mouth contact, or close contact during play. The virus is carried home, where haphazard sanitary habits spread it through the family. An infected food handler can spread the disease, and people can contract it by consuming water or shellfish from sewage-contaminated waters. Outbreaks have occurred in day care centers and institutions as a result of poor hygiene among people with developmental disabilities. Hepatitis A can be transmitted during sexual activity; this is more likely with oral–anal contact or anal intercourse and with multiple sex partners (Rodes, et al., 2007). It is rarely, if ever, transmitted by blood transfusions.

The incubation period is estimated to be between 2 to 6 weeks, with a mean of approximately 4 weeks (Rodes, et al., 2007). The illness may be prolonged, lasting 4 to 8 weeks. It usually lasts longer and is more severe in those older than 40 years of age. Most patients recover from hepatitis A; it rarely progresses to acute liver necrosis or fulminant hepatitis resulting in cirrhosis of the liver or death. The mortality rate of hepatitis A is approximately 0.5% for those younger than 40 years of age and 1% to 2% for older people. In patients with underlying chronic liver disease, morbidity and mortality are increased in the presence of an acute hepatitis A infection. No carrier state exists, and no chronic hepatitis is associated with hepatitis A. The virus is present only briefly in the serum; by the time jaundice occurs, the patient is likely to be noninfectious. Although hepatitis A confers immunity against itself, the person may contract other forms of hepatitis.

Clinical Manifestations

Many patients are anicteric (without jaundice) and symptomless. When symptoms appear, they resemble those of a mild, flulike upper respiratory tract infection, with low-grade fever. Anorexia, an early symptom, is often severe. It is thought to result from release of a toxin by the damaged liver or from failure of the damaged liver cells to detoxify an abnormal product. Later, jaundice and dark urine may become apparent. Indigestion is present in varying degrees, marked by vague epigastric distress, nausea, heartburn, and flatulence. The patient may also develop a strong aversion to the taste of cigarettes or the presence of cigarette smoke and other strong odors. These symptoms tend to clear as soon as the jaundice reaches its peak, perhaps 10 days after its initial appearance. Symptoms may be mild in children; in adults, they may be more severe and the course of the disease prolonged.

Assessment and Diagnostic Findings

The liver and spleen are often moderately enlarged for a few days after onset; other than jaundice, there are few other physical signs. Hepatitis A antigen may be found in the stool 7 to 10 days before illness and for 2 to 3 weeks after symptoms appear. HAV antibodies are detectable in the serum, but usually not until symptoms appear. Analysis of subclasses of immunoglobulins can help determine whether the antibody represents acute or past infection.

Prevention

A number of strategies exist to prevent transmission of HAV. Patients and their families are encouraged to follow general precautions that can prevent transmission of the virus. Scrupulous handwashing, safe water supplies, and proper control of sewage disposal are just a few of these prevention strategies.

Effective (95% to 100% after two to three doses) and safe HAV vaccines include Havrix and Vaqta (Goldman &

Ausiello, 2008; Rodes, et al., 2007). It is recommended that the two-dose vaccine be given to adults 18 years of age or older, with the second dose given 6 to 12 months after the first. Protection against hepatitis A develops within several weeks after the first dose of the vaccine. Children and adolescents 2 to 18 years of age receive three doses; the second dose is given 1 month after the first, and the third dose is given 6 to 12 months later. Hepatitis A routine immunization of young children has proved effective in reducing disease incidence and maintaining very low incidence levels among vaccine recipients and across all age groups in many settings (Goldman & Ausiello, 2008; Rodes, et al., 2007). Hepatitis A vaccine is recommended for people traveling to locations where sanitation and hygiene are unsatisfactory. Vaccination is also recommended for those from high-risk groups, such as homosexual men, IV or injection drug users, staff of day care centers, and health care personnel (Hauser, et al., 2006; Rodes, et al., 2007; Wolfe, 2006). The vaccine has also been used to interrupt community-wide outbreaks. As with other vaccinations, precautions must be taken to ensure prevention, detection, and treatment of hypersensitivity reactions to the vaccine.

For people who have not been previously vaccinated, hepatitis A can be prevented by intramuscular administration of globulin during the incubation period, if given within 2 weeks of exposure. This bolsters the person's antibody production and provides 6 to 8 weeks of passive immunity. Immune globulin may suppress overt symptoms of the disease; the resulting subclinical case of hepatitis A would produce immunity to subsequent episodes of the virus.

Immune globulin is also recommended for household members and sexual contacts of people with hepatitis A. Susceptible people in the same household as the patient are usually also infected by the time the diagnosis is made and should receive immune globulin. Institutional contacts of patients with hepatitis A should also receive postexposure prophylaxis with immune globulin. Prophylaxis is not necessary for casual contacts of an infected person, such as classmates, coworkers, or hospital employees (Rodes, et al., 2007). Although they are rare, systemic reactions to immune globulin do occur. Caution is required when anyone who has previously had angioedema, hives, or other allergic reactions is treated with any human immune globulin. Epinephrine should be available in case of systemic, anaphylactic reaction.

Preexposure prophylaxis is recommended for those traveling to developing countries or settings with poor or uncertain sanitation conditions who do not have sufficient time to acquire protection by administration of hepatitis A vaccine (Rodes, et al., 2007). Community interventions for preventing hepatitis A are outlined in Chart 39-7.

Medical Management

Bed rest during the acute stage and a diet that is both acceptable to the patient and nutritious are part of the treatment and nursing care. During the period of anorexia, the patient should receive frequent small feedings, supplemented if necessary by IV fluids with glucose. Because the patient often has an aversion to food, gentle persistence and creativity may be required to stimulate appetite. Optimal

HEALTH PROMOTION
Prevention of Hepatitis

CHART
39-7

- Encourage proper community and home sanitation.
- Encourage conscientious individual hygiene.
- Instruct patients regarding safe practices for preparing and dispensing food.
- Support effective health supervision of schools, dormitories, extended care facilities, barracks, and camps.
- Promote community health education programs.
- Facilitate mandatory reporting of viral hepatitis to local health departments.
- Recommend vaccination for all children 1 year of age and older.
- Recommend vaccination for travelers to developing countries, illegal drug users (injection and noninjection drug users), men who have sex with men, and people with chronic liver disease, and recipients (eg, hemophiliacs) of pooled plasma products.
- Promote vaccination to interrupt community-wide outbreaks.

food and fluid levels are necessary to counteract weight loss and to speed recovery. Even before the icteric phase, however, many patients recover their appetites (Chart 39-8).

The patient's sense of well-being and laboratory test results are generally appropriate guides to bed rest and restriction of physical activity. Gradual but progressive ambulation seems to hasten recovery, provided the patient rests after activity and does not participate in activities to the point of fatigue.

Nursing Management

Management usually occurs in the home unless symptoms are severe. Therefore, the nurse assists the patient and family in coping with the temporary disability and fatigue that are common in hepatitis and instructs them to seek additional health care if the symptoms persist or worsen. The patient and family also need specific guidelines about diet, rest, follow-up blood work, and the importance of avoiding alcohol, as well as sanitation and hygiene measures (particularly handwashing) to prevent spread of the disease to other family members.

Chart 39-8 • *Dietary Management of Viral or Drug-Related Hepatitis*

- Recommend small, frequent meals.
- Provide intake of 2000 to 3000 kcal/d during acute illness.
- Although early studies indicate that a high-protein, high-calorie diet may be beneficial, advise patient not to force food and to restrict fat intake.
- Carefully monitor fluid balance.
- If anorexia and nausea and vomiting persist, enteral feedings may be necessary.
- Instruct patient to abstain from alcohol during acute illness and for at least 6 mo after recovery.
- Advise patient to avoid substances (medications, herbs, illicit drugs, and toxins) that may affect liver function.

Specific teaching to patients and families about reducing the risk of contracting hepatitis A includes good personal hygiene, stressing careful handwashing (after bowel movements and before eating) and environmental sanitation (safe food and water supply, effective sewage disposal).

⚑ **NURSING ALERT**

A combined hepatitis A and B vaccine (Twinrix) is available for vaccination of people 18 years of age and older with indications for both hepatitis A and B vaccination. Vaccination consists of three doses, given on the same schedule as that used for single-antigen hepatitis B vaccine.

Hepatitis B Virus

Unlike HAV, the hepatitis B virus (HBV) is transmitted primarily through blood (percutaneous and permucosal routes). HBV can be found in blood, saliva, semen, and vaginal secretions and can be transmitted through mucous membranes and breaks in the skin. HBV is also transferred from carrier mothers to their infants, especially in areas with a high incidence (eg, Southeast Asia). The infection usually is not transmitted via the umbilical vein but from the mother at the time of birth and during close contact afterward.

HBV has a long incubation period. It replicates in the liver and remains in the serum for relatively long periods, allowing transmission of the virus. Risk factors for HBV infection are summarized in Chart 39-9. Screening of blood donors has greatly reduced the occurrence of hepatitis B after blood transfusion.

Most people (more than 90%) who contract HBV infection develop antibodies and recover spontaneously in 6 months. The mortality rate from hepatitis B has been reported to be as high as 10%. Another 10% of patients who have hepatitis B progress to a carrier state or develop chronic hepatitis with persistent HBV infection and hepatocellular

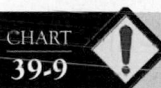

CHART
39-9

Risk Factors for Hepatitis B

- Frequent exposure to blood, blood products, or other body fluids
- Health care workers: hemodialysis staff, oncology and chemotherapy nurses, personnel at risk for needlesticks, operating room staff, respiratory therapists, surgeons, dentists
- Hemodialysis
- Male homosexual and bisexual activity
- IV/injection drug use
- Close contact with carrier of HBV
- Travel to or residence in area with uncertain sanitary conditions
- Multiple sexual partners
- Recent history of sexually transmitted disease
- Receipt of blood or blood products (eg, clotting factor concentrate)

injury and inflammation. It remains a major worldwide cause of cirrhosis and hepatocellular carcinoma.

The elderly patient who contracts hepatitis B has a serious risk of severe liver cell necrosis or fulminant hepatic failure, particularly if other illnesses are present. Because the patient is seriously ill and the prognosis is poor, efforts should be undertaken to eliminate other factors (eg, medications, alcohol) that may affect liver function.

The immune system is altered in the aged. A less responsive immune system may be responsible for the increased incidence and severity of hepatitis B among elderly people and the increased incidence of liver abscesses secondary to decreased phagocytosis by the Kupffer cells. With the advent of hepatitis B vaccine as the standard for prevention, the incidence of hepatic diseases may decrease in the future.

Clinical Manifestations

Clinically, the disease closely resembles hepatitis A, but the incubation period is much longer (1 to 6 months). Signs and symptoms of hepatitis B may be insidious and variable. Fever and respiratory symptoms are rare; some patients have arthralgias and rashes. The patient may have loss of appetite, dyspepsia, abdominal pain, generalized aching, malaise, and weakness. Jaundice may or may not be evident. If jaundice occurs, light-colored stools and dark urine accompany it. The liver may be tender and enlarged to 12 to 14 cm vertically. The spleen is enlarged and palpable in a few patients; the posterior cervical lymph nodes may also be enlarged. Subclinical episodes also occur frequently.

Assessment and Diagnostic Findings

HBV is a DNA virus composed of the following antigenic particles:

- HBcAg—hepatitis B core antigen (antigenic material in an inner core)
- HBsAg—hepatitis B surface antigen (antigenic material on the viral surface, a marker of active replication and infection)
- HBeAg—an independent protein circulating in the blood
- HBxAg—gene product of X gene of HBV DNA

Each antigen elicits its specific antibody and is a marker for different stages of the disease process:

- anti-HBc—antibody to core antigen of HBV; persists during the acute phase of illness; may indicate continuing HBV in the liver
- anti-HBs—antibody to surface determinants on HBV; detected during late convalescence; usually indicates recovery and development of immunity
- anti-HBe—antibody to hepatitis B e-antigen; usually signifies reduced infectivity
- anti-HBxAg—antibody to the hepatitis B x-antigen; may indicate ongoing replication of HBV

HBsAg appears in the circulation in 80% to 90% of infected patients 1 to 10 weeks after exposure to HBV and 2 to 8 weeks before the onset of symptoms or an increase in transferase levels. Patients with HBsAg that persists for 6 months or longer after acute infection are considered to be HBsAg carriers (Rodes, et al., 2007). HBeAg is the next antigen of HBV to appear in the serum. It usually appears within 1 week of the appearance of HBsAg but before

changes in aminotransferase levels; it disappears from the serum within 2 weeks. HBV DNA, detected by polymerase chain reaction testing, appears in the serum at about the same time as HBeAg. HBcAg is not always detected in the serum in HBV infection.

About 15% of American adults are positive for anti-HBs, which indicates that they have had hepatitis B. Anti-HBs may be positive in as many as two thirds of IV or injection drug users. Prevaccination screening for anti-HBs is not recommended except for high-risk adults who may have already been exposed to the disease.

Prevention

Preventing Transmission

Continued screening of blood donors for the presence of hepatitis B antigens further decreases the risk of transmission by blood transfusion. The use of disposable syringes, needles, and lancets and the introduction of needleless IV administration systems have reduced the risk of spreading this infection from one patient to another or to health care personnel during the collection of blood samples or the administration of parenteral therapy. Good personal hygiene is fundamental to infection control. In the clinical laboratory, work areas should be disinfected daily. Gloves are worn when handling all blood and body fluids, as well as HBAg-positive specimens, or when there is potential exposure to blood (eg, blood drawing) or to patients' secretions. Eating and smoking are prohibited in the laboratory and in other areas exposed to secretions, blood, or blood products. Patient education regarding the nature of the disease, its infectiousness, and prognosis is a critical factor in preventing transmission and protecting contacts.

Active Immunization: Hepatitis B Vaccine

Active immunization is recommended for people who are at high risk for hepatitis B (eg, health care personnel, hemodialysis patients). In addition, people with hepatitis C and other chronic liver diseases should receive the vaccine. A yeast-recombinant hepatitis B vaccine (Recombivax HB) is used to provide active immunity and has shown rates of protection greater than 90% in healthy people (Rodes, et al., 2007). Although antibody levels may become low or undetectable, immunologic memory may remain intact for at least 5 to 10 years. Measurable levels of antibodies may not be essential for protection. In general, in those with normal immune systems, booster doses are not required, and no data support the use of booster doses of hepatitis B vaccine among immunocompetent people who have responded to the vaccination series. However, booster doses are recommended for people who are immunocompromised (Rodes, et al., 2007). Additional information is required to determine if booster injections are needed for adults 15 years or more after initial vaccination as well as those at high risk for HBV infection.

A hepatitis B vaccine prepared from plasma of humans chronically infected with HBV is used only rarely in patients who are immunodeficient or allergic to recombinant yeast-derived vaccines.

Both forms of the hepatitis B vaccine are administered intramuscularly in three doses; the second and third doses are given 1 and 6 months, respectively, after the first dose. The third dose is very important in producing prolonged immunity. Hepatitis B vaccination should be administered to adults in the deltoid muscle. Antibody response may be measured by anti-HBs levels 1 to 3 months after completion of the basic course of vaccine, but this testing is not routine and is not currently recommended. People who do not respond may benefit from one to three additional doses (Rodes, et al., 2007).

People who are at high risk, including nurses and other health care personnel exposed to blood or blood products, should receive active immunization. Health care workers who have had frequent contact with blood are screened for anti-HBs to determine whether immunity is already present from previous exposure. The vaccine produces active immunity to HBV in 90% of healthy people (Rodes, et al., 2007). It does not provide protection to those already exposed to HBV, and it provides no protection against other types of viral hepatitis. Side effects of immunization are infrequent; soreness and redness at the injection site are the most common complaints.

Because hepatitis B infection is frequently transmitted sexually, hepatitis B vaccination is recommended for all unvaccinated people being evaluated for a sexually transmitted disease (STD). It is also recommended for those with a history of an STD, people with multiple sex partners, people who have sex with IV or injection drug users, and sexually active men who have sex with other men (Goldman & Ausiello, 2008).

Universal childhood vaccination for hepatitis B prevention has been instituted in the United States, and universal vaccination of all infants is encouraged. Catch-up vaccination is recommended for all children and prepubertal adolescents up to the age of 19 years who have not been previously immunized (Feldman, et al., 2006). Development of chronic carrier states has not been reported in adult responders to the vaccine.

Passive Immunity: Hepatitis B Immune Globulin

Hepatitis B immune globulin (HBIG) provides passive immunity to hepatitis B and is indicated for people exposed to HBV who have never had hepatitis B and have never received hepatitis B vaccine. Specific indications for postexposure vaccine with HBIG include (1) inadvertent exposure to HBAg-positive blood through percutaneous (needlestick) or transmucosal (splashes in contact with mucous membrane) routes, (2) sexual contact with people positive for HBAg, and (3) perinatal exposure (infants born to HBV-infected mothers should receive HBIG within 12 hours after delivery). HBIG is prepared from plasma selected for high titers of anti-HBs. Prompt immunization with HBIG (within hours to a few days after exposure to hepatitis B) increases the likelihood of protection. Both active and passive immunization are recommended for people who have been exposed to hepatitis B through sexual contact or through the percutaneous or transmucosal routes. If HBIG and hepatitis B vaccine are administered at the same time, separate sites and separate syringes should be used. There has been no evidence that human immunodeficiency virus (HIV) infection can be transmitted by HBIG (Wolfe, 2006).

Medical Management

The goals of treatment are to minimize infectivity and liver inflammation and decrease symptoms. Of all the agents that have been used to treat chronic type B viral hepatitis, alpha-interferon as the single modality of therapy that offers the most promise. A regimen of 5 million units daily or 10 million units three times weekly for 16 to 24 weeks results in remission of disease in approximately one third of patients (Wolfe, 2006). A prolonged course of treatment may also have additional benefits and is currently under study. Interferon must be administered by injection and has significant side effects, including fever, chills, anorexia, nausea, myalgias, and fatigue. Delayed side effects are more serious and may necessitate dosage reduction or discontinuation. These include bone marrow suppression, thyroid dysfunction, alopecia, and bacterial infections. Several recombinant forms of alpha-interferon are also available, including the pegylated form (Pegasys), with once-weekly dosing (Wolfe, 2006).

Two antiviral agents, lamivudine (Epivir) and adefovir (Hepsera), oral nucleoside analogs, have been approved for use in chronic hepatitis B in the United States. Studies have revealed improved seroconversion rates, loss of detectable virus, improved liver function, and reduced progression to cirrhosis with lamivudine. It can be used for patients with decompensated cirrhosis who are awaiting liver transplantation (Rodes, et al., 2007). Adefovir may be effective in people who are resistant to lamivudine.

Bed rest may be recommended, regardless of other treatment, until the symptoms of hepatitis have subsided. Activities are restricted until the hepatic enlargement and levels of serum bilirubin and liver enzymes have decreased. Gradually increased activity is then allowed.

Adequate nutrition should be maintained. Proteins are restricted if symptoms indicate that the liver's ability to metabolize protein byproducts is impaired. Measures to control the dyspeptic symptoms and general malaise include the use of antacids and antiemetics, but all medications should be avoided if vomiting occurs. If vomiting persists, the patient may require hospitalization and fluid therapy. Because of the mode of transmission, the patient is evaluated for other bloodborne diseases (eg, HIV infection).

Nursing Management

Convalescence may be prolonged, with complete symptomatic recovery sometimes requiring 3 to 4 months or longer. During this stage, gradual resumption of physical activity is encouraged after the jaundice has resolved.

The nurse identifies psychosocial issues and concerns, particularly the effects of separation from family and friends if the patient is hospitalized during the acute and infective stages. Even if not hospitalized, the patient will be unable to work and must avoid sexual contact. Planning is required to minimize social isolation. Planning that includes the family helps to reduce their fears and anxieties about the spread of the disease.

Promoting Home and Community-Based Care

Teaching Patients Self-Care

Because of the prolonged period of convalescence, the patient and family must be prepared for home care. Provision for adequate rest and nutrition must be ensured. The nurse informs family members and friends who have had intimate contact with the patient about the risks of contracting hepatitis B and makes arrangements for them to receive hepatitis B vaccine or hepatitis B immune globulin as prescribed. Those at risk must be made aware of the early signs of hepatitis B and of ways to reduce risk by avoiding all modes of transmission. Patients with all forms of hepatitis should avoid drinking alcohol and eating raw shellfish.

Continuing Care

Follow-up visits by a home care nurse may be needed to assess the patient's progress and answer family members' questions about disease transmission. During a home visit, the nurse assesses the patient's physical and psychological status and confirms that the patient and family understand the importance of adequate rest and nutrition. The nurse also reinforces previous instructions. Because of the risk of transmission through sexual intercourse, strategies to prevent exchange of body fluids are recommended, such as abstinence or the use of condoms. The nurse emphasizes the importance of keeping follow-up appointments and participating in other health promotion activities and recommended health screenings.

Hepatitis C Virus

A significant proportion of cases of viral hepatitis are neither hepatitis A, hepatitis B, nor hepatitis D, and are classified as hepatitis C. Whereas blood transfusions and sexual contact once accounted for most cases of hepatitis C in the United States, other parenteral means, such as sharing of contaminated needles by IV or injection drug users and unintentional needlesticks and other injuries in health care workers now account for a significant number of cases. Approximately 35,000 new cases of hepatitis C are reported in the United States each year. About 4 million people (1.8% of the U.S. population) have been infected with the hepatitis C virus (HCV), making it the most common chronic bloodborne infection nationally. A fourfold increase in the number of adults diagnosed with HCV infection is projected from 1990 to 2015. The highest prevalence of hepatitis C is in adults 40 to 59 years of age, and in this age group its prevalence is highest among African Americans. There are 10,000 to 12,000 deaths each year in the United States due to hepatitis C, and it has been suggested that deaths from this cause are underestimated. HCV is the underlying cause of about one third of cases of hepatocellular carcinoma, and it is the most common reason for liver transplantation (Wolfe, 2006).

People who are at particular risk for hepatitis C include IV or injection drug users, sexually active people with multiple partners, patients receiving frequent transfusions, those who require large volumes of blood, and health care personnel (Chart 39-10). The incubation period is variable and may range from 15 to 160 days. The clinical course of acute hepatitis C is similar to that of hepatitis B; symptoms are usually mild. However, a chronic carrier state occurs frequently, and there is an increased risk of chronic liver dis-

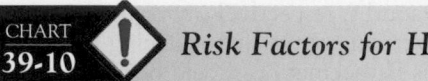

CHART 39-10 — Risk Factors for Hepatitis C

- Recipient of blood products or organ transplant before 1992 or clotting factor concentrates before 1987
- Health care and public safety workers after needlestick injuries or mucosal exposure to blood
- Children born to women infected with hepatitis C virus
- Past/current illicit IV/injection drug use
- Past treatment with chronic hemodialysis
- Multiple sex partners, history of sexually transmitted disease, unprotected sex

ease, including cirrhosis or liver cancer, after hepatitis C. Small amounts of alcohol taken regularly appear to cause progression of the disease. Therefore, alcohol and medications that may affect the liver should be avoided.

There is no benefit from rest, diet, or vitamin supplements. Studies have demonstrated that a combination of two antiviral agents, interferon (Intron-A) and ribavirin (Rebetol), is effective in producing improvement in patients with hepatitis C and in treating relapses. Some patients experience complete remission with combination therapy (Hauser, et al., 2006). Hemolytic anemia, the most frequent side effect, may be severe enough to require discontinuation of treatment. Ribavirin must be used with caution in women of childbearing age. The molecule polyethylene glycol moiety (PEG) is added to the interferon to keep it in the body longer without reducing its efficacy; this extends the dosing interval to once a week. Pegylated interferon (Pegasys) is now available, and some studies have shown it to have a somewhat improved virologic response rate compared with interferon (Hauser, et al., 2006; Wolfe, 2006).

Screening of blood has reduced the incidence of hepatitis C associated with blood transfusion, and public health programs are helping to reduce the number of cases associated with shared needles in IV or injection drug use.

Hepatitis D Virus

Hepatitis D virus (delta agent) infection occurs in some cases of hepatitis B. Because the virus requires hepatitis B surface antigen for its replication, only people with hepatitis B are at risk for hepatitis D. Anti-delta antibodies in the presence of HBAg on testing confirm the diagnosis. Hepatitis D is common among IV or injection drug users, hemodialysis patients, and recipients of multiple blood transfusions. Sexual contact with those with hepatitis B is considered to be an important mode of transmission of hepatitis B and D. The incubation period varies between 30 and 150 days (Goldman & Ausiello, 2008).

The symptoms of hepatitis D are similar to those of hepatitis B, except that patients are more likely to develop fulminant hepatitis and to progress to chronic active hepatitis and cirrhosis. Treatment is similar to that of other forms of hepatitis; interferon as a specific treatment for hepatitis D is under investigation.

Hepatitis E Virus

It is believed that hepatitis E virus (HEV) is transmitted by the fecal–oral route, principally through contaminated water in areas with poor sanitation. The incubation period is variable, estimated to range between 15 and 65 days. In general, hepatitis E resembles hepatitis A. It has a self-limited course with an abrupt onset. Jaundice is almost always present. Chronic forms do not develop.

Avoiding contact with the virus through good hygiene, including handwashing, is the major method of prevention of hepatitis E. The effectiveness of immune globulin in protecting against hepatitis E virus is uncertain.

Hepatitis G Virus and GB Virus-C

It has long been believed that there is another non-A–E agent causing hepatitis in humans. The incubation period for posttransfusion hepatitis is 14 to 145 days, too long for hepatitis B or C. In the United States, about 5% of chronic liver disease remains cryptogenic (ie, does not appear to be autoimmune or viral in origin), and 50% of these patients have received blood transfusions before developing disease. Therefore, another form of hepatitis, called hepatitis G virus (HGV) or GB virus-C (GBV-C) has been described; these are thought to be two different isolates of the same virus. Autoantibodies are absent.

The clinical significance of this virus remains uncertain. Risk factors are similar to those for hepatitis C. There is no clear relationship between HGV/GBV-C infection and progressive liver disease. Persistent infection does occur but does not affect the clinical course.

NONVIRAL HEPATITIS

Certain chemicals have toxic effects on the liver and produce acute liver cell necrosis or toxic hepatitis when inhaled, injected parenterally, or are taken by mouth. The chemicals most commonly implicated in this disease are carbon tetrachloride, phosphorus, chloroform, and gold compounds. These substances are true hepatotoxins. Many medications can induce hepatitis but are only sensitizing rather than toxic. Drug-induced hepatitis is similar to acute viral hepatitis, but parenchymal destruction tends to be more extensive. Medications that can lead to hepatitis include isoniazid (Nydrazid), halothane (Fluothane), acetaminophen, methyldopa (Aldomet), and certain antibiotics, antimetabolites, and anesthetic agents.

Toxic Hepatitis

At the onset of disease, toxic hepatitis resembles viral hepatitis. Obtaining a history of exposure to hepatotoxic chemicals, medications, botanical agents, or other toxic agents assists in early treatment and removal of the causative agent. Anorexia, nausea, and vomiting are the usual symptoms; jaundice and hepatomegaly are noted on physical assessment. Symptoms are more intense for the more severely toxic patient.

Recovery from acute toxic hepatitis is rapid if the hepatotoxin is identified early and removed or if exposure to the agent has been limited. Recovery is unlikely if there is a prolonged period between exposure and onset of symptoms. There are no effective antidotes. The fever rises; the patient becomes toxic and prostrated. Vomiting may be persistent, with the emesis containing blood. Clotting abnormalities may be severe, and hemorrhages may appear under the skin. The severe GI symptoms may lead to vascular collapse. Delirium, coma, and seizures develop, and within a few days the patient may die of fulminant hepatic failure (discussed later) unless he or she receives a liver transplant.

Short of liver transplantation, few treatment options are available. Therapy is directed toward restoring and maintaining fluid and electrolyte balance, blood replacement, and comfort and supportive measures. A few patients recover from acute toxic hepatitis only to develop chronic liver disease. If the liver heals, there may be scarring, followed by postnecrotic cirrhosis.

Drug-Induced Hepatitis

Drug-induced liver disease is the most common cause of acute liver failure, accounting for more than 50% of all cases in the United States (Wolfe, 2006). Manifestations of sensitivity to a medication may occur on the first day of its use or not until several months later. Usually, the onset is abrupt, with chills, fever, rash, pruritus, arthralgia, anorexia, and nausea. Later, there may be jaundice, dark urine, and an enlarged and tender liver. After the offending medication is withdrawn, symptoms may gradually subside. However, reactions can be severe, or even fatal, even if the medication is stopped. If fever, rash, or pruritus occurs from any medication, its use should be stopped immediately.

Although any medication can affect liver function, use of acetaminophen (found in many over-the-counter medications used to treat fever and pain) has been identified as the leading cause of acute liver failure (Wolfe, 2006). Other mechanisms commonly associated with liver injury include many anesthetic agents, medications used to treat rheumatic and musculoskeletal disease, antidepressants, psychotropic medications, anticonvulsants, and antituberculosis agents.

A short course of high-dose corticosteroids may be used in patients with severe hypersensitivity reactions, although its efficacy is uncertain. Liver transplantation is an option for drug-induced hepatitis, but outcomes may not be as successful as with other causes of liver failure.

FULMINANT HEPATIC FAILURE

Fulminant hepatic failure is the clinical syndrome of sudden and severely impaired liver function in a previously healthy person. According to the original and generally accepted definition, fulminant hepatic failure develops within 8 weeks after the first symptoms of jaundice (Hauser, et al., 2006). Patterns of the progression from jaundice to encephalopathy have been identified and have led to proposals of time-based classifications. However, no agreement as to these classifications has been reached. Three categories are frequently cited: hyperacute, acute, and subacute liver failure. In hyperacute liver failure, the duration of jaundice before the onset of encephalopathy is 0 to 7 days; in acute liver failure, it is 8 to 28 days; and in subacute liver failure, it is 28 to 72 days. The prognosis for fulminant hepatic failure is much worse than for chronic liver failure. However, in fulminant failure, the hepatic lesion is potentially reversible, and survival rates are approximately 20% to 50%, depending greatly on the cause of liver failure. Those who do not survive die of massive hepatocellular injury and necrosis (Wolfe, 2006).

Viral hepatitis is a common cause of fulminant hepatic failure; other causes include toxic medications (eg, acetaminophen) and chemicals (eg, carbon tetrachloride), metabolic disturbances (eg, Wilson's disease, a hereditary syndrome with deposition of copper in the liver), and structural changes (eg, Budd-Chiari syndrome, an obstruction to outflow in major hepatic veins).

Jaundice and profound anorexia may be the initial reasons the patient seeks health care. Fulminant hepatic failure is often accompanied by coagulation defects, renal failure and electrolyte disturbances, cardiovascular abnormalities, infection, hypoglycemia, encephalopathy, and cerebral edema.

The key to optimized treatment is rapid recognition of acute liver failure and intensive intervention. Supporting the patient in the ICU and assessing the indications for and feasibility of liver transplantation are hallmarks of management of this population. The use of antidotes for certain conditions may be indicated such as N-acetylcysteine for acetaminophen toxicity and penicillin for mushroom poisoning. Treatment modalities may include plasma exchanges (plasmapheresis) to correct coagulopathy and to stabilize the patient awaiting liver transplantation and prostaglandin therapy to enhance hepatic blood flow; however, more clinical trials are needed to determine the effects or outcomes of these treatments. Hepatocytes within synthetic fiber columns have been tested as liver support systems (liver assist devices) to provide a bridge to transplantation.

Research into interventions for acute liver failure has begun to focus on techniques that combine the efficacy of a whole liver with the convenience and biocompatibility of hemodialysis. The acronyms ELAD (extracorporeal liver assist devices) and BAL (bioartificial liver) have been used to describe these hybrid devices. These short-term devices, which remain experimental, may help patients survive until transplantation is possible. The BAL device exposes separated plasma to a cartridge containing porcine liver cells after the plasma has flowed through a charcoal column that removes substances toxic to hepatocytes. The ELAD exposes whole blood to cartridges containing human hepatoblastoma cells, resulting in removal of toxic substances. In the near future, similar extracorporeal circuits using **xenografts** may be studied as a bridge to liver transplantation. These approaches appear promising and have had success in animal studies. In human clinical application, the use of various BAL systems has resulted in improved neurologic and biochemical parameters. Adding albumin to the dialysate is effective in removing protein-bound toxins and is potentially useful in unstable patients with fulminant liver failure (Rodes, et al., 2007). To fully determine the

clinical applicability of such systems on outcomes and survival rates, controlled, randomized clinical trials in large patient groups are required.

In patients who have fulminant liver failure with stage 4 encephalopathy, there is a high risk of cerebral edema, a life-threatening complication. The cause is not fully understood, although disruption of the blood–brain barrier and plasma leakage into the cerebrospinal fluid may be one cause. An increase in the intracellular osmolarity within cerebral astrocyte cells, possibly related to increased sodium and glutamine in these cells, may be another (Rodes, et al., 2007). These patients require intracranial pressure monitoring. Measures to promote adequate cerebral perfusion include careful fluid balance and hemodynamic assessments, a quiet environment, and diuresis with mannitol (Osmitrol), an osmotic diuretic.

Use of barbiturate anesthesia or pharmacologic paralysis and sedation is indicated to prevent surges in intracranial pressure related to agitation. Other support measures include monitoring for and treating hypoglycemia, coagulopathies, and infection. Despite these treatment modalities, the mortality rate remains high. Consequently, liver transplantation (discussed later) has become the treatment of choice for fulminant hepatic failure.

HEPATIC CIRRHOSIS

Cirrhosis is a chronic disease characterized by replacement of normal liver tissue with diffuse fibrosis that disrupts the structure and function of the liver. There are three types of cirrhosis or scarring of the liver:

- Alcoholic cirrhosis, in which the scar tissue characteristically surrounds the portal areas. This is most frequently caused by chronic alcoholism and is the most common type of cirrhosis.
- Postnecrotic cirrhosis, in which there are broad bands of scar tissue. This is a late result of a previous bout of acute viral hepatitis.
- Biliary cirrhosis, in which scarring occurs in the liver around the bile ducts. This type of cirrhosis usually results from chronic biliary obstruction and infection (cholangitis); it is much less common than the other two types.

The portion of the liver chiefly involved in cirrhosis consists of the portal and the periportal spaces, where the bile canaliculi of each lobule communicate to form the liver bile ducts. These areas become the sites of inflammation, and the bile ducts become occluded with inspissated (thickened) bile and pus. The liver attempts to form new bile channels; hence, there is an overgrowth of tissue made up largely of disconnected, newly formed bile ducts and surrounded by scar tissue.

Pathophysiology

Although several factors have been implicated in the etiology of cirrhosis, alcohol consumption is considered the major causative factor. Cirrhosis occurs with greatest frequency among people with alcoholism. Although nutritional deficiency with reduced protein intake contributes to liver destruction in cirrhosis, excessive alcohol intake is the major causative factor in fatty liver and its consequences. However, cirrhosis has also occurred in people who do not consume alcohol and in those who consume a normal diet and have a high alcohol intake.

Some people appear to be more susceptible than others to this disease, whether or not they have alcoholism or are malnourished. Other factors may play a role, including exposure to certain chemicals (carbon tetrachloride, chlorinated naphthalene, arsenic, or phosphorus) or infectious schistosomiasis. Twice as many men as women are affected, although, for unknown reasons, women are at greater risk for development of alcohol-induced liver disease. Most patients are between 40 and 60 years of age. Each year more than 27,000 people die of chronic liver diseases and cirrhosis in the United States (Rodes, et al., 2007).

Alcoholic cirrhosis is characterized by episodes of necrosis involving the liver cells, which sometimes occur repeatedly throughout the course of the disease. The destroyed liver cells are gradually replaced by scar tissue. Eventually, the amount of scar tissue exceeds that of the functioning liver tissue. Islands of residual normal tissue and regenerating liver tissue may project from the constricted areas, giving the cirrhotic liver its characteristic hobnail appearance. The disease usually has an insidious onset and a protracted course, occasionally proceeding over a period of 30 or more years.

The prognoses for different forms of cirrhosis caused by various liver diseases have been investigated in several studies. Of the many prognostic indicators, the Child-Pugh classification seems most useful in predicting the outcome of patients with liver disease (Table 39-5). It is also used in choosing management approaches.

Clinical Manifestations

Signs and symptoms of cirrhosis increase in severity as the disease progresses. Their severity is used to categorize the disorder as compensated or decompensated cirrhosis (Chart 39-11). Compensated cirrhosis, with its less severe, often vague symptoms, may be discovered secondarily at a routine physical examination. The hallmarks of decompensated cirrhosis result from failure of the liver to synthesize proteins, clotting factors, and other substances and manifestations of portal hypertension (see earlier sections of this chapter for

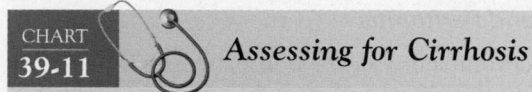

CHART 39-11   *Assessing for Cirrhosis*

Be alert for the following signs and symptoms:

Compensated
- Intermittent mild fever
- Vascular spiders
- Palmar erythema (reddened palms)
- Unexplained epistaxis
- Ankle edema
- Vague morning indigestion
- Flatulent dyspepsia
- Abdominal pain
- Firm, enlarged liver
- Splenomegaly

Decompensated
- Ascites
- Jaundice
- Weakness
- Muscle wasting
- Weight loss
- Continuous mild fever
- Clubbing of fingers
- Purpura (due to decreased platelet count)
- Spontaneous bruising
- Epistaxis
- Hypotension
- Sparse body hair
- White nails
- Gonadal atrophy

clinical manifestations and management of portal hypertension, ascites, varices, and hepatic encephalopathy).

Liver Enlargement

Early in the course of cirrhosis, the liver tends to be large, and the cells are loaded with fat. The liver is firm and has a sharp edge that is noticeable on palpation. Abdominal pain may be present because of recent, rapid enlargement of the liver, which produces tension on the fibrous covering of the liver (Glisson's capsule). Later in the disease, the liver decreases in size as scar tissue contracts the liver tissue. The liver edge, if palpable, is nodular.

Portal Obstruction and Ascites

Portal obstruction and ascites, late manifestations of cirrhosis, are caused partly by chronic failure of liver function and partly by obstruction of the portal circulation. Almost all of the blood from the digestive organs is collected in the portal veins and carried to the liver. Because a cirrhotic liver does not allow free blood passage, blood backs up into the spleen and the GI tract, and these organs become the seat of chronic passive congestion; that is, they are stagnant with blood and therefore cannot function properly. Indigestion and altered bowel function result. Fluid rich in protein may accumulate in the peritoneal cavity, producing ascites. This can be detected through percussion for shifting dullness or a fluid wave (see Fig. 39-5).

Table 39-5   MODIFIED CHILD-PUGH CLASSIFICATION OF THE SEVERITY OF LIVER DISEASE*

Parameter	Points Assigned		
	1	2	3
Ascites	Absent	Slight	Moderate
Bilirubin (mg/dL)	≤ 2	2–3	> 3
Albumin (g/dL)	> 3.5	2.8–3.5	< 2.8
Prothrombin time (seconds over control)	1–3	4–6	> 6
Encephalopathy	None	Grade 1–2	Grade 3–4

*Total score of 1–6, grade A; 7–9, grade B; 10–15, grade C.
Schiff, E. R., Somell, M. F. & Maddrey, W. C. (Eds.) (2006). *Schiff's diseases of the liver* (10th ed.). Philadelphia: Lippincott Williams & Wilkins.

Infection and Peritonitis

Bacterial peritonitis may develop in patients with cirrhosis and ascites in the absence of an intra-abdominal source of infection or an abscess. This condition is referred to as spontaneous bacterial peritonitis (SBP). Bacteremia due to translocation of intestinal flora is believed to be the most likely route of infection. Clinical signs may be absent, necessitating paracentesis for diagnosis. Antibiotic therapy is effective in the treatment and prevention of recurrent episodes of SBP. The most severe complication of SBP is hepatorenal syndrome, a form of renal failure unresponsive to administration of fluid or diuretics. This type of renal failure is characterized by a lack of pathologic changes in the kidney; there is no evidence of dehydration or obstruction of the urinary tract or any other renal disorder.

Gastrointestinal Varices

The obstruction to blood flow through the liver caused by fibrotic changes also results in the formation of collateral blood vessels in the GI system and shunting of blood from the portal vessels into blood vessels with lower pressures. As a result, the patient with cirrhosis often has prominent, distended abdominal blood vessels, which are visible on abdominal inspection (caput medusae) and distended blood vessels throughout the GI tract. The esophagus, stomach, and lower rectum are common sites of collateral blood vessels. These distended blood vessels form varices or hemorrhoids, depending on their location (see Fig. 39-6).

Because these vessels were not intended to carry the high pressure and volume of blood imposed by cirrhosis, they may rupture and bleed. Therefore, assessment must include observation for occult and frank bleeding from the GI tract.

Edema

Another late symptom of cirrhosis is edema, which is attributed to chronic liver failure. A reduced plasma albumin concentration predisposes the patient to the formation of edema. Although edema is generalized, it often affects the lower extremities, the upper extremities, and the presacral area. Facial edema is not typical. Overproduction of aldosterone occurs, causing sodium and water retention and potassium excretion.

Vitamin Deficiency and Anemia

Because of inadequate formation, use, and storage of certain vitamins (notably vitamins A, C, and K), signs of deficiency are common, particularly hemorrhagic phenomena associated with vitamin K deficiency. Chronic gastritis and impaired GI function, together with inadequate dietary intake and impaired liver function, account for the anemia that is often associated with cirrhosis. The patient's anemia, poor nutritional status, and poor state of health result in severe fatigue, which interferes with the ability to carry out routine activities of daily living (ADLs).

Mental Deterioration

Additional clinical manifestations include deterioration of mental and cognitive function with impending hepatic encephalopathy and hepatic coma, as previously described. Neurologic assessment is indicated, including assessment of the patient's general behavior, cognitive abilities, orientation to time and place, and speech patterns.

Assessment and Diagnostic Findings

The extent of liver disease and the type of treatment are determined after review of the laboratory findings. The functions of the liver are complex, and many diagnostic tests provide information about liver function (see Table 39-1). The patient needs to know why these tests are being performed and how to cooperate.

In severe parenchymal liver dysfunction, the serum albumin level tends to decrease, and the serum globulin level rises. Enzyme tests indicate liver cell damage: serum alkaline phosphatase, AST, ALT, and GGT levels increase, and the serum cholinesterase level may decrease. Bilirubin tests are performed to measure bile excretion or retention; increased levels of bilirubin can occur with cirrhosis and other liver disorders. Prothrombin time is prolonged.

Ultrasound scanning is used to measure the difference in density of parenchymal cells and scar tissue. CT, MRI, and radioisotope liver scans give information about liver size and hepatic blood flow and obstruction. Diagnosis is confirmed by liver biopsy. Arterial blood gas analysis may reveal a ventilation–perfusion imbalance and hypoxia.

Medical Management

The management of the patient with cirrhosis is usually based on the presenting symptoms. For example, antacids or histamine-2 (H$_2$) antagonists are prescribed to decrease gastric distress and minimize the possibility of GI bleeding. Vitamins and nutritional supplements promote healing of damaged liver cells and improve the patient's general nutritional status. Potassium-sparing diuretics such as spironolactone or triamterene (Dyrenium) may be indicated to decrease ascites, if present; these diuretics are preferred because they minimize the fluid and electrolyte changes commonly seen with other agents. An adequate diet and avoidance of alcohol are essential. Although the fibrosis of the cirrhotic liver cannot be reversed, its progression may be halted or slowed by such measures.

Preliminary studies indicate that colchicine, an anti-inflammatory agent used to treat the symptoms of gout, may increase survival time in patients with mild to moderate cirrhosis. Many medications have been shown to possess antifibrotic activity for the treatment of cirrhosis. Some of these medications include angiotensin system inhibitors, statins, diuretics, immunosuppressants, and glitazones. These medications have reasonable safety profiles, but their long-term safety and efficacy in patients with cirrhosis has yet to be demonstrated (Schuppan & Afdhal, 2008).

Many patients who have end-stage liver disease (ESLD) with cirrhosis use the herb milk thistle (Silybum marianum) to treat jaundice and other symptoms. This herb has been used for centuries because of its healing and regenerative properties for liver disease. Silymarin from milk thistle has anti-inflammatory and antioxidant properties that may have beneficial effects, especially in hepatitis. The natural compound, SAM-e (s-adenosylmethionine), may improve outcomes in liver disease by improving liver function, possibly through enhancing antioxidant function. Primary biliary cirrhosis has been treated with ursodeoxycholic acid (Actigall, URSO) to improve liver function.

Nursing Management

Nursing management for the patient with cirrhosis of the liver is described in detail in the Plan of Nursing Care for the Patient with Impaired Liver Function (Chart 39-12). Nursing interventions are directed toward promoting patient's rest, improving nutritional status, providing skin care, reducing risk of injury, and monitoring and managing potential complications.

Promoting Rest

The patient with cirrhosis requires rest and other supportive measures to permit the liver to reestablish its functional ability. If the patient is hospitalized, weight and fluid intake and output are measured and recorded daily. The nurse adjusts the patient's position in bed for maximal respiratory efficiency, which is especially important if ascites is marked, because it interferes with adequate thoracic excursion. Oxygen therapy may be required in liver failure to oxygenate the damaged cells and prevent further cell destruction.

Rest reduces the demands on the liver and increases the liver's blood supply. Because the patient is susceptible to the hazards of immobility, efforts to prevent respiratory, circulatory, and vascular disturbances are initiated. These measures may help prevent such problems as pneumonia, thrombophlebitis, and pressure ulcers. After nutritional status improves and strength increases, the nurse encourages the patient to increase activity gradually. Activity and mild exercise, as well as rest, are planned.

Improving Nutritional Status

The patient with cirrhosis without ascites, edema, or signs of impending hepatic coma should receive a nutritious, high-protein diet, if tolerated, supplemented by vitamins of the B complex, as well as A, C, and K. The nurse encourages the patient to eat. If ascites is present, small, frequent meals may be better tolerated than three large meals because of the abdominal pressure exerted by ascites. Patient preferences are considered. Patients with prolonged or severe anorexia and those who are vomiting or eating poorly for any reason may receive nutrients by the enteral or parenteral route.

Patients with fatty stools (steatorrhea) should receive water-soluble forms of fat-soluble vitamins A, D, and E (Aquasol A, D, and E). Folic acid and iron are prescribed to prevent anemia. If the patient shows signs of impending or advancing coma, the amount of protein in the diet is decreased temporarily. Protein is restricted if encephalopathy develops. Incorporating vegetable protein to meet protein needs may decrease the risk for encephalopathy. Sodium restriction is also indicated to prevent ascites.

Providing Skin Care

Providing careful skin care is important because of subcutaneous edema, the patient's immobility, jaundice, and increased susceptibility to skin breakdown and infection. Frequent changes in position are necessary to prevent pressure ulcers. Irritating soaps and the use of adhesive tape are avoided to prevent trauma to the skin. Lotion may be soothing to irritated skin; the nurse takes measures to minimize scratching by the patient.

Reducing Risk of Injury

The nurse protects the patient with cirrhosis from falls and other injuries. The side rails should be in place and padded with blankets or other materials in case the patient becomes agitated or restless. To minimize agitation, the nurse orients the patient to time and place and explains all procedures. The nurse instructs the patient to ask for assistance to get out of bed. The nurse carefully evaluates any injury because of the possibility of internal bleeding.

Because of the risk for bleeding from abnormal clotting, the patient should use an electric razor rather than a safety razor. A soft-bristled toothbrush helps minimize bleeding gums, and pressure applied to all venipuncture sites helps minimize bleeding.

Monitoring and Managing Potential Complications

A major role of the nurse is monitoring of the patient with cirrhosis for complications.

Bleeding and Hemorrhage

The patient is at increased risk for bleeding and hemorrhage because of decreased production of prothrombin and decreased ability of the diseased liver to synthesize the necessary substances for blood coagulation. This was discussed earlier in the section on esophageal varices.

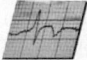 **Hepatic Encephalopathy**

As previously described, hepatic encephalopathy and coma, complications of cirrhosis, may manifest as deteriorating mental status and dementia or as physical signs such as abnormal voluntary and involuntary movements. Hepatic encephalopathy was discussed earlier in the chapter in detail and in Chart 39-12.

Monitoring is an essential nursing function to identify early deterioration in mental status. The nurse monitors the patient's mental status closely and reports changes so that treatment of encephalopathy can be initiated promptly. An extensive neurologic evaluation is key to identify progression through the four stages of encephalopathy.

Each advancing stage demands more intensive nursing interventions aimed at providing for patient safety and prevention and early identification of life-threatening complications such as respiratory failure and cerebral edema, which would necessitate interventions in an ICU. Because electrolyte disturbances can contribute to encephalopathy, serum electrolyte levels are carefully monitored and corrected if abnormal. Oxygen is administered if oxygen desaturation occurs. The nurse monitors for fever or abdominal pain, which may signal the onset of bacterial peritonitis or other infection (see earlier discussion of hepatic encephalopathy).

Fluid Volume Excess

Patients with advanced chronic liver disease develop cardiovascular abnormalities. These occur due to an increased cardiac output and decreased peripheral vascular resistance, possibly resulting from the release of vasodilators.

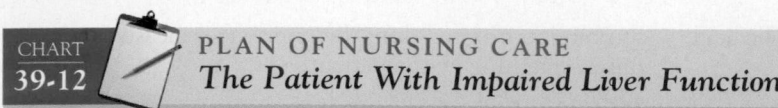

CHART
39-12

PLAN OF NURSING CARE
The Patient With Impaired Liver Function

NURSING DIAGNOSIS: Activity intolerance related to fatigue, lethargy, and malaise
GOAL: Patient reports decrease in fatigue and reports increased ability to participate in activities

Nursing Interventions	Rationale	Expected Outcomes
1. Assess level of activity tolerance and degree of fatigue, lethargy, and malaise when performing routine activities of daily living.	1. Provides baseline for further assessment and criteria for assessment of effectiveness of interventions.	• Exhibits increased interest in activities and events.
2. Assist with activities and hygiene when fatigued.	2. Promotes exercise and hygiene within patient's level of tolerance.	• Participates in activities and gradually increases exercise within physical limits.
3. Encourage rest when fatigued or when abdominal pain or discomfort occurs.	3. Conserves energy and protects the liver.	• Reports increased strength and well-being. • Reports absence of abdominal pain and discomfort.
4. Assist with selection and pacing of desired activities and exercise.	4. Stimulates patient's interest in selected activities.	• Plans activities to allow ample periods of rest.
5. Provide diet high in carbohydrates with protein intake consistent with liver function.	5. Provides calories for energy and protein for healing.	• Takes vitamins as prescribed.
6. Administer supplemental vitamins (A, B complex, C, and K).	6. Provides additional nutrients.	

NURSING DIAGNOSIS: Imbalanced nutrition: less than body requirements, related to abdominal distention and discomfort and anorexia
GOAL: Positive nitrogen balance, no further loss of muscle mass; meets nutritional requirements

Nursing Interventions	Rationale	Expected Outcomes
1. Assess dietary intake and nutritional status through diet history and diary, daily weight measurements, and laboratory data.	1. Identifies deficits in nutritional intake and adequacy of nutritional state.	• Exhibits improved nutritional status by increased weight (without fluid retention) and improved laboratory data. • States rationale for dietary modifications.
2. Provide diet high in carbohydrates with protein intake consistent with liver function.	2. Provides calories for energy, sparing protein for healing.	• Identifies foods high in carbohydrates and within protein requirements (moderate to high protein in cirrhosis and hepatitis, low protein in hepatic failure).
3. Assist patient in identifying low-sodium foods.	3. Reduces edema and ascites formation.	• Reports improved appetite.
4. Elevate the head of the bed during meals.	4. Reduces discomfort from abdominal distention and decreases sense of fullness produced by pressure of abdominal contents and ascites on the stomach.	• Participates in oral hygiene measures. • Reports increased appetite; identifies rationale for smaller, frequent meals.
5. Provide oral hygiene before meals and pleasant environment for meals at meal time.	5. Promotes positive environment and increased appetite; reduces unpleasant taste.	• Demonstrates intake of high-calorie diet; adheres to protein restriction. • Identifies foods and fluids that are nutritious and permitted on diet.
6. Offer smaller, more frequent meals (6 per day).	6. Decreases feeling of fullness, bloating.	• Gains weight without increased edema or ascites formation.
7. Encourage patient to eat meals and supplementary feedings.	7. Encouragement is essential for the patient with anorexia and gastrointestinal discomfort.	• Reports increased appetite and well-being.
8. Provide attractive meals and an aesthetically pleasing setting at meal time.	8. Promotes appetite and sense of well-being.	• Excludes alcohol from diet. • Takes medications for gastrointestinal disorders as prescribed.
9. Eliminate alcohol.	9. Eliminates "empty calories" and further damage from alcohol.	• Reports normal gastrointestinal function with regular bowel function.
10. Apply an ice collar for nausea.	10. May reduce incidence of nausea.	
11. Administer medications prescribed for nausea, vomiting, diarrhea, or constipation.	11. Reduces gastrointestinal symptoms and discomforts that decrease the appetite and interest in food.	
12. Encourage increased fluid intake and exercise if the patient reports constipation.	12. Promotes normal bowel pattern and reduces abdominal discomfort and distention.	

Continued

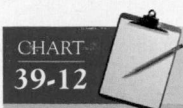

CHART
39-12

PLAN OF NURSING CARE
The Patient With Impaired Liver Function (*Continued*)

NURSING DIAGNOSIS: Impaired skin integrity related to pruritus from jaundice and edema
GOAL: Decrease potential for pressure ulcer development; breaks in skin integrity

Nursing Interventions	Rationale	Expected Outcomes
1. Assess degree of discomfort related to pruritus and edema.	1. Assists in determining appropriate interventions.	• Exhibits intact skin without redness, excoriation, or breakdown.
2. Note and record degree of jaundice and extent of edema.	2. Provides baseline for detecting changes and evaluating effectiveness of interventions.	• Reports relief from pruritus. • Exhibits no skin excoriation from scratching.
3. Keep patient's fingernails short and smooth.	3. Prevents skin excoriation and infection from scratching.	• Uses nondrying soaps and lotions. States rationale for use of nondrying soaps and lotions.
4. Provide frequent skin care; avoid use of soaps and alcohol-based lotions.	4. Removes waste products from skin while preventing dryness of skin.	• Turns self periodically. Exhibits reduced edema of dependent parts of the body.
5. Massage every 2 h with emollients; turn every 2 h.	5. Promotes mobilization of edema.	• Exhibits no areas of skin breakdown.
6. Initiate use of alternating-pressure mattress or low air loss bed.	6. Minimizes prolonged pressure on bony prominences susceptible to breakdown.	• Exhibits decreased edema; normal skin turgor.
7. Recommend avoiding use of harsh detergents.	7. May decrease skin irritation and need for scratching.	
8. Assess skin integrity every 4–8 h. Instruct patient and family in this activity.	8. Edematous skin and tissue have compromised nutrient supply and are vulnerable to pressure and trauma.	
9. Restrict sodium as prescribed.	9. Minimizes edema formation.	
10. Perform range of motion exercises every 4 h, elevate edematous extremities whenever possible.	10. Promotes mobilization of edema.	

NURSING DIAGNOSIS: High risk for injury related to altered clotting mechanisms and altered level of consciousness
GOAL: Reduced risk of injury

Nursing Interventions	Rationale	Expected Outcomes
1. Assess level of consciousness and cognitive level.	1. Assists in determining patient's ability to protect self and comply with required self-protective actions; may detect deterioration of hepatic function.	• Is oriented to time, place, and person. • Exhibits no hallucinations, and demonstrates no efforts to get up unassisted or to leave hospital.
2. Provide safe environment (pad side rails, remove obstacles in room, prevent falls).	2. Minimizes falls and injury if falls occur.	• Exhibits no ecchymoses (bruises), cuts, or hematoma.
3. Provide frequent surveillance to orient patient and avoid use of restraints.	3. Protects patient from harm while stimulating and orienting patient; use of restraints may disturb patient further.	• Uses electric razor rather than sharp-edged razor. • Exhibits absence of frank bleeding from gastrointestinal tract.
4. Replace sharp objects (razors) with safer items.	4. Avoids cuts and bleeding.	• Exhibits absence of restlessness, epigastric fullness, and other indicators of hemorrhage and shock.
5. Observe each stool for color, consistency, and amount.	5. Permits detection of bleeding in gastrointestinal tract.	• Exhibits negative results of test for occult gastrointestinal bleeding.
6. Be alert for symptoms of anxiety, epigastric fullness, weakness, and restlessness.	6. May indicate early signs of bleeding and shock.	• Is free of ecchymotic areas or hematoma formation. • Exhibits normal vital signs.
7. Test each stool and emesis for occult blood.	7. Detects early evidence of bleeding.	• Maintains rest and remains quiet if active bleeding occurs.
8. Observe for hemorrhagic manifestations: ecchymosis, epistaxis, petechiae, and bleeding gums.	8. Indicates altered clotting mechanisms.	• Identifies rationale for blood transfusions and measures to treat bleeding.
9. Record vital signs at frequent intervals, depending on patient acuity (every 1–4 h).	9. Provides baseline and evidence of hypovolemia, and hemorrhagic shock.	• Uses measures to prevent trauma (eg, uses soft toothbrush, blows nose gently, avoids bumps and falls, avoids straining during defecation). • Experiences no side effects of medications.

Continued on following page

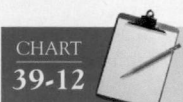

CHART
39-12

PLAN OF NURSING CARE
The Patient With Impaired Liver Function (Continued)

Nursing Interventions	Rationale	Expected Outcomes
10. Keep patient quiet and limit activity.	10. Minimizes risk of bleeding and straining.	• Takes all medications as prescribed.
11. Assist physician in passage of tube for esophageal balloon tamponade, if its insertion is indicated.	11. Promotes nontraumatic insertion of tube in anxious and combative patient for immediate treatment of bleeding.	• Identifies rationale for precautions with use of all medications. • Cooperates with treatment modalities.
12. Observe during blood transfusions.	12. Permits detection of transfusion reactions (risk is increased with multiple blood transfusions needed for active bleeding from esophageal varices).	
13. Measure and record nature, time, and amount of vomitus.	13. Assists in evaluating extent of bleeding and blood loss.	
14. Maintain patient in fasting state, if indicated.	14. Reduces risk of aspiration of gastric contents and minimizes risk of further trauma to esophagus and stomach by preventing vomiting.	
15. Administer vitamin K as prescribed.	15. Promotes clotting by providing fat-soluble vitamin necessary for clotting.	
16. Remain with patient during episodes of bleeding.	16. Reassures anxious patient and permits monitoring and detection of further needs of the patient.	
17. Offer cold liquids by mouth when bleeding stops (if prescribed).	17. Minimizes risk of further bleeding by promoting vasoconstriction of esophageal and gastric blood vessels.	
18. Institute measures to prevent trauma: a. Maintain safe environment.	18. Promotes safety of patient a. Minimizes risk of trauma and bleeding by avoiding falls and cuts, etc.	
b. Encourage *gentle* blowing of nose.	b. Reduces risk of nosebleed (epistaxis) secondary to trauma and decreased clotting.	
c. Provide soft toothbrush and avoid use of toothpicks.	c. Prevents trauma to oral mucosa while promoting good oral hygiene.	
d. Encourage intake of foods with high content of vitamin C. e. Apply cold compresses where indicated. f. Record location of bleeding sites.	d. Promotes healing. e. Minimizes bleeding into tissues by promoting local vasoconstriction. f. Permits detection of new bleeding sites and monitoring of previous sites of bleeding.	
g. Use small-gauge needles for injections.	g. Minimizes oozing and blood loss from repeated injections.	
19. Administer medications carefully; monitor for side effects.	19. Reduces risk of side effects secondary to damaged liver's inability to detoxify (metabolize) medications normally.	

NURSING DIAGNOSIS: Disturbed body image related to changes in appearance, sexual dysfunction, and role function
GOAL: Patient verbalizes feelings consistent with improvement of body image and self-esteem

Nursing Interventions	Rationale	Expected Outcomes
1. Assess changes in appearance and the meaning these changes have for patient and family.	1. Provides information for assessing impact of changes in appearance, sexual function, and role on the patient and family.	• Verbalizes concerns related to changes in appearance, life, and lifestyle.

Continued

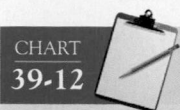

CHART 39-12

PLAN OF NURSING CARE
The Patient With Impaired Liver Function (Continued)

Nursing Interventions	Rationale	Expected Outcomes
2. Encourage patient to verbalize reactions and feelings about these changes. 3. Assess patient's and family's previous coping strategies. 4. Assist and encourage patient to maximize appearance (such as strategies to limit the appearance of jaundice and ascites through careful selection of colors and type of clothing) and explore alternatives to previous sexual and role functions. 5. Assist patient in identifying short-term goals. 6. Encourage and assist patient in decision making about care. 7. Identify with patient resources to provide additional support (counselor, spiritual advisor). 8. Assist patient in identifying previous practices that may have been harmful to self (alcohol and drug abuse). Involve patient in goal-setting and provide positive feedback for accomplishments.	2. Enables patient to identify and express concerns; encourages patient and significant others to share these concerns. 3. Permits encouragement of those coping strategies that are familiar to patient and have been effective in the past. 4. Encourages patient to continue safe roles and functions while encouraging exploration of alternatives. 5. Accomplishing these goals serves as positive reinforcement and increases self-esteem. 6. Promotes patient's control of life and improves sense of well-being and self-esteem. 7. Assists patient in identifying resources and accepting assistance from others when indicated. 8. Recognition and acknowledgment of the harmful effects of these practices are necessary for identifying a healthier lifestyle.	• Shares concerns with significant others. • Identifies past coping strategies that have been effective. • Uses past effective coping strategies to deal with changes in appearance, life, and lifestyle. • Maintains good grooming and hygiene. • Identifies short-term goals and strategies to achieve them. • Takes an active role in decision making about self and care. • Identifies resources that are not harmful. • Verbalizes that some of previous lifestyle practices have been harmful. • Uses healthy expressions of frustration, anger, anxiety.

NURSING DIAGNOSIS: Chronic pain and discomfort related to enlarged tender liver and ascites
GOAL: Increased level of comfort

Nursing Interventions	Rationale	Expected Outcomes
1. Maintain bed rest when patient experiences abdominal discomfort. 2. Administer antispasmodic and analgesic agents as prescribed. 3. Observe, record, and report presence and character of pain and discomfort. 4. Reduce sodium and fluid intake if prescribed. 5. Prepare patient and assist with paracentesis. 6. Encourage the use of distracting activities such as music, reading or meditation.	1. Reduces metabolic demands and protects the liver. 2. Reduces irritability of the gastrointestinal tract and decreases abdominal pain and discomfort. 3. Provides baseline to detect further deterioration of status and to evaluate interventions. 4. Minimizes further formation of ascites. 5. Removal of ascites fluid may decrease abdominal discomfort. 6. Distraction may limit the perception of pain.	• Reports pain and discomfort if present. • Maintains bed rest and decreases activity in presence of pain. • Takes antispasmodic and analgesics as indicated and as prescribed. • Reports decreased pain and abdominal discomfort. • Reduces sodium and fluid intake to prescribed levels if indicated to treat ascites. • Exhibits decreased abdominal girth and appropriate weight changes. • Reports decreased discomfort after paracentesis.

NURSING DIAGNOSIS: Fluid volume excess related to ascites and edema formation
GOAL: Restoration of normal fluid volume

Nursing Interventions	Rationale	Expected Outcomes
1. Restrict sodium and fluid intake if prescribed. 2. Administer diuretics, potassium, and protein supplements as prescribed.	1. Minimizes formation of ascites and edema. 2. Promotes excretion of fluid through the kidneys and maintenance of normal fluid and electrolyte balance.	• Consumes diet low in sodium and within prescribed fluid restriction. • Takes diuretics, potassium, and protein supplements as indicated without experiencing side effects.

Continued on following page

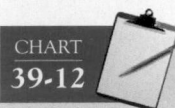

CHART 39-12

PLAN OF NURSING CARE
The Patient With Impaired Liver Function (Continued)

Nursing Interventions	Rationale	Expected Outcomes
3. Record intake and output every 1 to 8 h depending on response to interventions and on patient acuity.	3. Indicates effectiveness of treatment and adequacy of fluid intake.	• Exhibits increased urine output.
4. Measure and record abdominal girth and weight daily.	4. Monitors changes in ascites formation and fluid accumulation.	• Exhibits decreasing abdominal girth.
5. Explain rationale for sodium and fluid restriction.	5. Promotes patient's understanding of restriction and cooperation with it.	• Exhibits no rapid increase in weight.
6. Prepare patient and assist with paracentesis.	6. Paracentesis will temporarily decrease amount of ascites present.	• Identifies rationale for sodium and fluid restriction.
		• Shows a decrease in ascites with decreased weight.

NURSING DIAGNOSIS: Disturbed thought processes and potential for mental deterioration related to abnormal liver function and increased serum ammonia level

GOAL: Improved mental status; safety maintained; ability to cope with cognitive and behavioral changes

Nursing Interventions	Rationale	Expected Outcomes
1. Restrict dietary protein as prescribed for transient period.	1. Reduces source of ammonia (protein foods).	• Adheres to protein restriction.
2. Give frequent, small feedings of carbohydrates.	2. Promotes consumption of adequate carbohydrates for energy requirements and spares protein from breakdown for energy.	• Demonstrates an interest in events and activities in environment.
3. Protect from infection.	3. Minimizes risk for further increase in metabolic requirements.	• Demonstrates normal attention span.
4. Keep environment warm and draft-free.	4. Minimizes shivering, which would increase metabolic requirements.	• Follows and participates in conversation appropriately.
5. Pad the side rails of the bed.	5. Provides protection for the patient should hepatic coma and seizure activity occur.	• Is oriented to person, place, and time.
6. Limit visitors.	6. Minimizes patient's activity and metabolic requirements.	• Remains in bed when indicated.
7. Provide careful nursing surveillance to ensure patient's safety.	7. Provides close monitoring of new symptoms and minimizes trauma to the confused patient.	• Reports no urinary or fecal incontinence.
8. Avoid opioids and barbiturates.	8. Prevents masking of symptoms of hepatic coma and prevents drug overdose secondary to reduced ability of the damaged liver to metabolize opioids and barbiturates. Prevents respiratory depression.	• Experiences no seizures.
		• No neurological or respiratory depression.
9. Awaken at intervals (every 2–4 h) to assess cognitive status.	9. Provides stimulation to the patient and opportunity for observing the patient's level of consciousness.	• Develops no cognitive impairments but if they develop they are quickly identified and treated enhancing the potential of recovery.
10. Identify subtle changes in behavior or sleep–wake pattern (consistent staff caring for the patient enhances this assessment as they become familiar with patient's baseline).	10/11. These changes may herald worsening of encephalopathy which requires rapid intervention including medication.	• Patient and family describe adequate feelings of coping and lowered anxiety. They demonstrate ability to listen and to make decisions as able.
11. Assess handwriting or drawing skill daily as indication of cognitive ability.		• Patient and family communicate their feelings and their needs in a secure and caring environment.
12. Encourage patient and family to participate in therapeutic strategies to enhance coping with episodes of mental deterioration.	12. Promoting activities such as listening to music, relaxation techniques or preillness coping strategies can reduce anxiety.	
13. Encourage patient and family to discuss feeling of fear, powerlessness or emotional distress related to patient's mental deterioration.	13. Actively listening demonstrates caring and concern.	

Continued

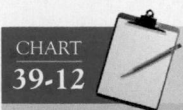

CHART 39-12

PLAN OF NURSING CARE
The Patient With Impaired Liver Function (Continued)

NURSING DIAGNOSIS: Risk for imbalanced body temperature: hyperthermia related to inflammatory process of cirrhosis or hepatitis
GOAL: Maintenance of normal body temperature, free from infection

Nursing Interventions	Rationale	Expected Outcomes
1. Record temperature regularly (every 4 h).	1. Provides baseline to detect fever and to evaluate interventions.	• Exhibits normal temperature and reports absence of chills or sweating.
2. Encourage fluid intake.	2. Corrects fluid loss from perspiration and fever and increases patient's level of comfort.	• Demonstrates adequate intake of fluids.
3. Apply cool sponges or ice bag for elevated temperature.	3. Promotes reduction of fever and increases patient's comfort.	• Exhibits no evidence of local or systemic infection.
4. Administer antibiotics as prescribed.	4. Ensures appropriate serum concentration of antibiotics to treat infection.	• Develops no nosocomial infections related to invasive procedures/lines.
5. Avoid exposure to infections.	5. Minimizes risk of further infection and further increases in body temperature and metabolic rate.	
6. Keep patient at rest while temperature is elevated.	6. Reduces metabolic rate.	
7. Assess for abdominal pain, tenderness.	7. May occur with bacterial peritonitis.	
8. Use sterile technique for all invasive procedures.	8. Many evidence-based practice guidelines (for example central venous catheter care) recommend the use of sterile technique to prevent nosocomial infections.	

NURSING DIAGNOSIS: Ineffective breathing pattern related to ascites and restriction of thoracic excursion secondary to ascites, abdominal distention, and fluid in the thoracic cavity
GOAL: Improved respiratory status

Nursing Interventions	Rationale	Expected Outcomes
1. Elevate head of bed to at least 30 degrees.	1. Reduces abdominal pressure on the diaphragm and permits fuller thoracic excursion and lung expansion.	• Experiences improved respiratory status.
2. Conserve patient's strength by providing rest periods and assisting with activities.	2. Reduces metabolic and oxygen requirements.	• Reports decreased shortness of breath.
3. Change position every 2 h.	3. Promotes expansion and oxygenation of all areas of the lungs.	• Reports increased strength and sense of well-being.
4. Assist with paracentesis or thoracentesis.	4. Paracentesis and thoracentesis (performed to remove fluid from the abdominal and thoracic cavities, respectively) may be frightening to the patient.	• Exhibits normal respiratory rate (12–18/min) with no adventitious sounds.
a. Explain procedure and its purpose to patient.	a. Helps obtain patient's cooperation with procedures.	• Exhibits full thoracic excursion without shallow respirations.
b. Have patient void before paracentesis.	b. Prevents inadvertent bladder injury.	• Exhibits normal arterial blood gases.
c. Support and maintain position during procedure.	c. Prevents inadvertent organ or tissue injury.	• Exhibits adequate oxygen saturation by pulse oximetry.
d. Record both the amount and the character of fluid aspirated.	d. Provides record of fluid removed and indication of severity of limitation of lung expansion by fluid.	• Experiences absence of confusion or cyanosis.
e. Observe for evidence of coughing, increasing dyspnea, or pulse rate.	e. Indicates irritation of the pleural space and evidence of pneumothorax or hemothorax.	

Continued on following page

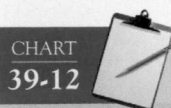

PLAN OF NURSING CARE
The Patient With Impaired Liver Function (Continued)

CHART
39-12

COLLABORATIVE PROBLEM: Gastrointestinal bleeding and hemorrhage
GOAL: Absence of episodes of gastrointestinal bleeding and hemorrhage

Nursing Interventions	Rationale	Expected Outcomes

1. Assess patient for evidence of gastrointestinal bleeding or hemorrhage. If bleeding does occur:
  a. Monitor vital signs (blood pressure, pulse, respiratory rate) every 4 h or more frequently, depending on acuity.
  b. Assess skin temperature, level of consciousness every 4 h or more frequently, depending on acuity.
  c. Monitor gastrointestinal secretions and output (emesis, stool for occult or obvious bleeding). Test emesis for blood once per shift and with any color change. Hematest each stool.
  d. Monitor hematocrit and hemoglobin for trends and changes.
	1. Allows early detection of signs and symptoms of bleeding and hemorrhage.	• Experiences no episodes of bleeding and hemorrhage.
		• Vital signs are within acceptable range for patient.
		• No evidence of bleeding from gastrointestinal tract.
		• Hematocrit and hemoglobin levels within acceptable limits.
		• Turns and moves without straining and increasing intra-abdominal pressure.
		• No straining with bowel movements.
		• No further bleeding episodes if aggressive treatment of bleeding and hemorrhage was needed.
		• Patient and family state rationale for treatments.
		• Patient and family identify supports available to them.
		• Patient and family describe signs and symptoms of a recurrent bleeding episode and identify needed action.

2. Avoid activities that increase intra-abdominal pressure (straining, turning).
  a. Avoid coughing/sneezing.
  b. Assist patient to turn.
  c. Keep all needed items within easy reach.
  d. Use measures to prevent constipation such as adequate fluid intake; stool softeners.
  e. Ensure small meals.
	2. Minimizes increases in intra-abdominal pressure that could lead to rupture and bleeding of esophageal or gastric varices.	

3. Have equipment (Blakemore tube, medications, IV fluids) available if indicated.	3. Equipment, medications, and supplies will be readily available if patient experiences bleeding from ruptured esophageal or gastric varices.	
4. Assist with procedures and therapy needed to treat gastrointestinal bleeding and hemorrhage.	4. Gastrointestinal bleeding and hemorrhage require emergency measures (eg, insertion of Blakemore tube, administration of fluids and medications).	
5. Monitor respiratory status every hour and minimize risk of respiratory complications if balloon tamponade is needed.	5. The patient is at high risk for respiratory complications, including asphyxiation if gastric balloon of tamponade tube ruptures or migrates upward.	
6. Prepare patient physically and psychologically for other treatment modalities if needed.	6. The patient who experiences hemorrhage is very anxious and fearful; minimizing anxiety assists in control of hemorrhage.	
7. Monitor patient for recurrence of bleeding and hemorrhage.	7. Risk of rebleeding is high with all treatment modalities used to halt gastrointestinal bleeding.	
8. Keep family informed of patient's status.	8. Family members are likely to be anxious about the patient's status; providing information will reduce their anxiety level and promote more effective coping.	
9. Once recovered from bleeding episode, provide patient and family with information regarding signs and symptoms of gastrointestinal bleeding.	9. Risk of rebleeding is high. Subtle signs may be more quickly identified.	

Continued

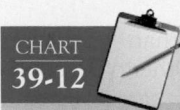

CHART
39-12

PLAN OF NURSING CARE
The Patient With Impaired Liver Function (Continued)

COLLABORATIVE PROBLEM: Hepatic encephalopathy
GOAL: Absence of changes in cognitive status and of injury

Nursing Interventions	Rationale	Expected Outcomes

1. Assess cognitive status every 4–8 h:
  a. Assess patient's orientation to person, place, and time.
  b. Monitor patient's level of activity, restlessness, and agitation. Assess for presence of flapping hand tremors (asterixis).
  c. Obtain and record daily sample of patient's handwriting or ability to construct a simple figure (eg, star).
  d. Assess neurologic signs (deep tendon reflexes, ability to follow instructions).
	1. Data will provide baseline of patient's cognitive status and enable detection of changes.	• Remains awake, alert, and aware of surroundings.
		• Is oriented to time, place, and person.
		• Exhibits no restlessness or agitation.
		• Record of handwriting demonstrates no deterioration in cognitive function.
		• States rationale for treatment used to prevent or treat hepatic encephalopathy.
		• Demonstrates stable serum ammonia level within acceptable limits.
		• Consumes adequate caloric intake and adheres to protein restriction.
		• Takes medications as prescribed.
		• Breath sounds are normal without adventitious sounds.
		• Skin and tissue intact without evidence of pressure or breaks in integrity.
		• Verbalizes understanding of need for treatments and procedures to promote recovery.

2. Monitor medications to prevent administration of those that may precipitate hepatic encephalopathy (sedatives, hypnotics, analgesics).	2. Medications are a common precipitating factor in development of hepatic encephalopathy in patients at risk.	
3. Monitor laboratory data, especially serum ammonia level.	3. Increases in serum ammonia level are associated with hepatic encephalopathy and coma.	
4. Notify physician of even subtle changes in patient's neurologic assessment, cognitive function, sleep pattern, or mood.	4. Allows early initiation of treatment of hepatic encephalopathy and prevention of hepatic coma.	
5. Limit sources of protein from diet if indicated.	5. Reduces breakdown and conversion of protein to ammonia.	
6. Administer medications prescribed to reduce serum ammonia level (eg, lactulose, antibiotics, glucose, benzodiazepine antagonist [Flumazenil] if indicated).	6. Reduces serum ammonia level.	
7. Assess respiratory status and initiate measures to prevent complications.	7. The patient who develops hepatic coma is at risk for respiratory complications (ie, pneumonia, atelectasis, infection).	
8. Protect patient's skin and tissue from pressure and breakdown.	8. The patient in coma is at risk for skin breakdown and pressure ulcer formation.	
9. Provide support and active listening for patient and family as patient's mental status deteriorates.	9. The patient with hepatic encephalopathy can experience episodes of mental deterioration due to liver failure. This can produce feelings of fear and anxiety.	

A hyperdynamic circulatory state develops in patients with cirrhosis, and plasma volume increases. This increase in circulating plasma volume is probably multifactorial, but some studies have implicated excess production of nitrous oxide, like that seen in sepsis, as one causative factor (Rodes, et al., 2007). The greater the degree of hepatic decompensation, the more severe the hyperdynamic state. Close assessment of cardiovascular and respiratory status is of key importance for the care of patients with this disorder. Pulmonary compromise, which is always a potential complication of ESLD because of plasma volume excess, makes prevention of pulmonary complications an important role for the nurse. Administering diuretics, implementing fluid restrictions, and enhancing patient positioning can optimize pulmonary function. Fluid retention may be noted in the development of ascites, lower extremity swelling, and dyspnea. Monitoring of intake and output, daily weight changes, changes in abdominal girth, and edema formation is part of nursing assessment in the hospital or in the home setting. Patients are also monitored for nocturia and, later, for oliguria, because these states indicate increasing severity of liver dysfunction (Rodes, et al., 2007).

Promoting Home and Community-Based Care

Teaching Patients Self-Care

During the hospital stay, the nurse and other health care providers prepare the patient with cirrhosis for discharge, focusing on dietary instruction. Of greatest importance is the exclusion of alcohol from the diet. The patient may need referral to Alcoholics Anonymous, psychiatric care, or counseling or may benefit from support from a spiritual advisor. The patient should also avoid the consumption of raw shellfish.

Sodium restriction will continue for a considerable time, if not permanently. The patient will require written instructions, teaching, reinforcement, and support from the staff as well as family members.

Successful treatment depends on convincing the patient of the need to adhere completely to the therapeutic plan. This includes rest, lifestyle changes, adequate dietary intake, and the elimination of alcohol. The nurse also instructs the patient and family about symptoms of impending encephalopathy, possible bleeding tendencies, and susceptibility to infection.

Recovery is neither rapid nor easy; there are frequent setbacks and apparent lack of improvement. Many patients find it difficult to refrain from using alcohol for comfort or escape. The nurse has a significant role in offering support and encouragement to the patient and in providing positive feedback when the patient experiences success.

Continuing Care

Referral for home care may assist the patient in dealing with the transition from hospital to home. The use of alcohol may have been an important part of normal home and social life in the past. The home care nurse assesses the patient's progress at home and the manner in which the patient and family are coping with the elimination of alcohol and the dietary restrictions. The nurse also reinforces previous teaching and answers questions that may not have occurred to the patient or family until the patient is back home and trying to establish new patterns of eating, drinking, and lifestyle.

CANCER OF THE LIVER

Hepatic tumors may be malignant or benign. Benign liver tumors were uncommon until oral contraceptives were in widespread use. Now benign liver tumors occur most frequently in women in their reproductive years who are taking oral contraceptives.

Primary Liver Tumors

Few cancers originate in the liver. Primary liver tumors usually are associated with chronic liver disease, hepatitis B and C infections, and cirrhosis. Hepatocellular carcinoma (HCC) is the most common type of primary liver cancer, with more than half a million cases diagnosed each year on a worldwide basis. HCC is the third leading cause of cancer-related mortality worldwide. It is rare in the United States and Northern Europe, accounting for less than 5 cases per 100,000 inhabitants (Rodes, et al., 2007). Other types of primary liver cancer include cholangiocellular carcinoma and combined hepatocellular and cholangiocellular carcinoma. HCC is usually nonresectable because of rapid growth and metastasis. If found early, resection of primary liver cancer may be possible, but early detection is unlikely.

Cirrhosis, chronic infection with hepatitis B and C, and exposure to certain chemical toxins (eg, vinyl chloride, arsenic) have been implicated as causes of HCC. Cigarette smoking has also been identified as a risk factor, especially when combined with alcohol use. Some evidence suggests that aflatoxin, a metabolite of the fungus *Aspergillus flavus*, may be a risk factor for HCC. This is especially true in areas where HCC is endemic (ie, Asia and Africa). Aflatoxin and other similar toxic molds can contaminate food such as ground nuts and grains and may act as co-carcinogens with hepatitis B. The risk of contamination is greatest when these foods are stored unrefrigerated in tropical or subtropical climates.

Liver Metastases

Metastases from other primary sites, particularly the digestive system, breast, and lung, are found in the liver 2.5 times more frequently than tumors due to primary liver cancers (Rodes, et al., 2007). Malignant tumors are likely to reach the liver eventually, by way of the portal system or lymphatic channels, or by direct extension from an abdominal tumor. Moreover, the liver apparently is an ideal place for these malignant cells to thrive. Often the first evidence of cancer in an abdominal organ is the appearance of liver metastases; unless exploratory surgery or an autopsy is performed, the primary tumor may never be identified.

Clinical Manifestations

The early manifestations of malignancy of the liver include pain—a continuous dull ache in the right upper quadrant, epigastrium, or back. Weight loss, loss of strength, anorexia, and anemia may also occur. The liver may be enlarged and irregular on palpation. Jaundice is present only if the larger bile ducts are occluded by the pressure of malignant nodules in the hilum of the liver. Ascites develops if such nodules obstruct the portal veins or if tumor tissue is seeded in the peritoneal cavity.

Assessment and Diagnostic Findings

The diagnosis of liver cancer is based on clinical signs and symptoms, the history and physical examination, and the results of laboratory and x-ray studies. Increased serum levels of bilirubin, alkaline phosphatase, AST, GGT, and lactic dehydrogenase may occur. Leukocytosis (increased white blood cells), erythrocytosis (increased red blood cells), hypercalcemia, hypoglycemia, and hypocholesterolemia may also be seen on laboratory assessment.

The serum level of alpha-fetoprotein (AFP), which serves as a tumor marker, is elevated in 30% to 40% of patients with primary liver cancer. The level of carcinoembryonic antigen (CEA), a marker of advanced cancer of the digestive tract, may be elevated. These two markers together are useful to distinguish between metastatic liver disease and primary liver cancer.

Many patients have metastases from the primary liver tumor to other sites by the time the diagnosis is made; metastases occur primarily to the lung but may also occur to regional lymph nodes, adrenals, bone, kidneys, heart, pancreas, or stomach.

X-rays, liver scans, CT scans, ultrasound studies, MRI, arteriography, and laparoscopy may be part of the diagnostic workup and may be performed to determine the extent of the cancer. Positive emission tomograms (PET) scans are used to evaluate a wide range of metastatic tumors of the liver.

Confirmation of a tumor's histology can be made by biopsy under imaging guidance (CT scan or ultrasound) or laparoscopically. Local or systemic dissemination of the tumor by needle biopsy or fine-needle biopsy can occur but is rare. Some clinicians believe that these procedures should not be performed if the tumor is thought to be resectable; rather, primary HCC diagnosis should be confirmed by frozen section at the time of laparotomy in those patients with resectable lesions detected by imaging studies.

Medical Management

Although surgical resection of the liver tumor is possible in some patients, the underlying cirrhosis is so prevalent in cancer of the liver that it increases the risks associated with surgery. Radiation therapy and chemotherapy have been used to treat cancer of the liver with varying degrees of success. Although these therapies may prolong survival and improve quality of life by reducing pain and discomfort, their major effect is palliative.

Radiation Therapy

The use of external beam radiation for the treatment of liver tumors has been limited by the radiosensitivity of normal hepatocytes and the risk of destruction of normal liver parenchyma. More effective methods of delivering radiation to tumors of the liver include (1) IV or intra-arterial injection of antibodies tagged with radioactive isotopes that specifically attack tumor-associated antigens and (2) percutaneous placement of a high-intensity source for interstitial radiation therapy (delivery of radiation directly to the tumor cells). Internal radiotherapy can result in reduction in tumor size, but its effect on survival is yet to be determined.

Chemotherapy

Typically, studies of patients with advanced cases of liver cancer have shown that the use of systemic chemotherapeutic agents leads to poor outcomes. There is no evidence to support a standard systemic chemotherapy and, in the United States, there is no approved systemic treatment for HCC (Wolfe, 2006). However, systemic chemotherapy may be used to treat metastatic liver lesions. Embolization of tumor vessels with chemotherapy (a process known as transarterial chemoembolization [TACE]) produces anoxic necrosis with high concentrations of trapped chemotherapeutic agents. This therapy has begun to show some promising results. An implantable pump has been used to deliver a high concentration of chemotherapy by constant infusion to the liver through the hepatic artery in cases of metastatic disease. This method has shown a moderate response rate, (Rodes, et al., 2007).

Percutaneous Biliary Drainage

Percutaneous biliary or transhepatic drainage is used to bypass biliary ducts obstructed by liver, pancreatic, or bile duct tumors in patients who have inoperable tumors or are considered poor surgical risks. Under fluoroscopy, a catheter is inserted through the abdominal wall and past the obstruction into the duodenum. Such procedures are used to reestablish biliary drainage, relieve pressure and pain from the buildup of bile behind the obstruction, and decrease pruritus and jaundice. As a result, the patient is made more comfortable and quality of life and survival are improved.

For several days after its insertion, the catheter is opened to external drainage. The bile is observed closely for amount, color, and presence of blood and debris. Complications of percutaneous biliary drainage include sepsis, leakage of bile, hemorrhage, and reobstruction of the biliary system by debris in the catheter or by encroaching tumor. Therefore, the patient is observed for fever and chills, bile drainage around the catheter, changes in vital signs, and evidence of biliary obstruction, including increased pain or pressure, pruritus, and recurrence of jaundice.

Other Nonsurgical Treatments

Laser hyperthermia has been used to treat hepatic metastases. Heat has been directed to tumors through several methods to cause necrosis of the tumor cells while sparing normal tissue. In radiofrequency thermal ablation, a needle electrode is inserted into the liver tumor under imaging guidance. Radiofrequency energy passes through to the noninsulated needle tip, causing heat and tumor cell death from coagulation necrosis.

Immunotherapy is another treatment modality under investigation. In this therapy, lymphocytes with antitumor reactivity are administered to the patient with hepatic cancer. Tumor regression has been demonstrated in patients with metastatic cancer for whom standard treatment has failed.

Transcatheter arterial embolization interrupts the arterial blood flow to small tumors by injecting small particulate embolic or chemotherapeutic agents (as previously described) into the artery supplying the tumor. As a result, ischemia and necrosis of the tumor occur.

For multiple small lesions, ultrasound-guided injection of alcohol promotes dehydration of tumor cells and tumor necrosis (Rodes, et al., 2007; Wolfe, 2006).

Surgical Management

Surgical resection is the treatment of choice when HCC is confined to one lobe of the liver and the function of the remaining liver is considered adequate for postoperative recovery. In the case of metastasis, hepatic resection can be performed if the primary site can be completely excised and the metastasis is limited. However, metastases to the liver are rarely limited or solitary. Capitalizing on the regenerative capacity of the liver cells, some surgeons have successfully removed 90% of the liver. However, the presence of cirrhosis limits the ability of the liver to regenerate. Staging of liver tumors aids in predicting the likelihood of surgical cure.

In preparation for surgery, the patient's nutritional, fluid, and general physical status are assessed, and efforts are undertaken to ensure the best physical condition possible. Extensive diagnostic studies may be performed. Specific studies may include liver scan, liver biopsy, cholangiography, selective hepatic angiography, percutaneous needle biopsy, peritoneoscopy, laparoscopy, ultrasound, CT scan, PET scan, MRI, and blood tests, particularly determinations of serum alkaline phosphatase, AST, and GGT and its isoenzymes.

Lobectomy

Removal of a lobe of the liver is the most common surgical procedure for excising a liver tumor. If it is necessary to restrict blood flow from the hepatic artery and portal vein for longer than 15 minutes, it is likely that hypothermia will be used. For a right-liver lobectomy or an extended right lobectomy (including the medial left lobe), a thoracoabdominal incision is used. An extensive abdominal incision is made for a left lobectomy.

Local Ablation

In patients who are not candidates for resection or transplantation, ablation of HCC may be accomplished by chemicals such as ethanol or by physical means such as radiofrequency ablation or microwave coagulation. These techniques may be performed under ultrasound or CT guidance laparoscopically or percutaneously. Radiofrequency ablation is becoming a standard mode of treatment; a tumor up to 5 cm in size can be destroyed in one session. The most common complications following ablation are local pain or bleeding. Serious complications are rare (Wolfe, 2006).

Immunotherapy with interferon has been under study as an adjuvant after liver resection or ablation of HCC. When patients have developed HCC related to hepatitis B or C, interferon may prevent recurrence of the lesion (Clavien, 2007; Rodes, et al., 2007).

Liver Transplantation

Removing the liver and replacing it with a healthy donor organ is another way to treat liver cancer. Studies have shown decreased recurrence rates of the primary liver malignancy after transplantation, with improvement in 5-year survival rates to consistently greater than 70% (Rodes, et al., 2007; Wolfe, 2006). Metastasis and recurrence may be enhanced by the immunosuppressive therapy that is needed to prevent rejection of the transplanted liver. In patients with small (less than 5 cm), single lesions, liver transplantation has been shown to be beneficial, but its use is limited by organ shortages. The increasing use of living donor transplantation may improve this situation and decrease the waiting time and tumor proliferation that is characteristic of patients with liver cancer (see later discussion).

Nursing Management

For the surgical patient, support, explanation, and encouragement are provided to help the patient prepare psychologically for the surgery. After surgery, potential problems related to cardiopulmonary involvement may include vascular complications and respiratory and liver dysfunction. Metabolic abnormalities require careful attention. A constant infusion of 10% glucose may be required in the first 48 hours to prevent a precipitous fall in the blood glucose level that results from decreased gluconeogenesis. Because extensive blood loss may occur as well, the patient receives infusions of blood and IV fluids. The patient requires constant, close monitoring and care for the first 2 or 3 days, similar to postsurgical abdominal and thoracic nursing care.

If the patient is to receive chemotherapy or radiation therapy in an effort to relieve symptoms, he or she may be discharged home while still receiving one or both of these therapies. The patient may also go home with a biliary drainage system or hepatic artery catheter in place. In most cases, the hepatic artery catheter has been inserted surgically and has a prefilled infusion pump that delivers a continuous chemotherapeutic dose until completed. An hepatic artery port may also be inserted to provide access for intermittent chemotherapy infusion. This port dwells under the skin, but, because it provides direct arterial access, it is not used for continuous infusion therapy in the home environment; the access line is discontinued once the chemotherapeutic agent has infused. The patient and family require teaching about care of the biliary catheter and the effects and side effects of hepatic artery chemotherapy. This teaching is necessary because of participation of the patient and family in patient care in the home setting.

Promoting Home and Community-Based Care

Teaching Patients Self-Care

The nurse instructs the patient to recognize and report the potential complications and side effects of the chemotherapy and the desirable and undesirable effects of the specific chemotherapy regimen. The nurse also emphasizes the importance of follow-up visits to assess the patient and the tumor's response to chemotherapy and radiation therapy. In addition, if the patient is receiving chemotherapy on an outpatient basis, the nurse explains the patient's and family's role in managing the chemotherapy infusion and in assessing the infusion or insertion site. The nurse encourages the patient to resume routine activities as soon as possible, while cautioning about activities that may damage the infusion pump or site.

The family of as well as the patient at home with a biliary drainage system in place typically fear that the catheter will become dislodged. Reassurance and instruction can help reduce their fear that the catheter will fall out easily. The patient and family also require instruction on catheter care. The family and the patient need to learn how to keep the catheter site clean and dry and how to assess the catheter and its insertion site. Irrigation of the catheter with sterile normal saline solution or water may be prescribed to keep the catheter patent and free of debris. The patient and caregivers are taught proper technique to avoid introducing bacteria into the biliary system or catheter during irrigation. They are instructed not to aspirate or draw back on the syringe during irrigation, to prevent entry of irritating duodenal contents into the biliary tree or catheter. The patient and caregivers are also instructed about the signs of complications and are encouraged to notify the nurse or physician if problems or questions arise.

Patients with implantable ports are instructed about the chemotherapy regimen, types of medications, effects and side effects that may occur, and appropriate management strategies if problems occur. If a hepatic artery port is inserted for intermittent chemotherapy, patients and their families are provided the same educational content. Such a port has an internal one-way valve; therefore, it is not aspirated for a blood return before the infusion is initiated. The patient is instructed to assess the port site between infusions and to note and report any sign of infection or inflammation.

Continuing Care

In many cases, referral for home care enables the patient with liver cancer to be at home in a familiar environment with family and friends. Because of the poor prognosis associated with liver cancer, the home care nurse serves a vital role in assisting the patient and family to cope with the symptoms that may occur and the prognosis. The home care nurse assesses the patient's physical and psychological status, adequacy of pain relief, nutritional status, and presence of symptoms indicating complications of treatment or progression of disease. During home visits, the nurse assesses the function of the chemotherapy pump, the infusion site, and the biliary drainage system, if indicated. The nurse collaborates with the other members of the health care team, the patient, and the family to ensure effective pain management and to manage potential problems, which include weakness, pruritus, inadequate dietary intake, jaundice, and symptoms associated with metastasis to other sites. The home care nurse also assists the patient and family in making decisions about hospice care and assists with initiation of referrals. The patient is encouraged to discuss preferences for end-of-life care with family members and health care providers (see Chapter 17).

Liver Transplantation

Liver transplantation is used to treat life-threatening ESLD for which no other form of treatment is available. The transplantation procedure involves total removal of the diseased liver and replacement with a healthy liver in the same anatomic location (**orthotopic liver transplantation [OLT]**). Removal of the liver creates a space for the new liver and permits anatomic reconstruction of the hepatic vasculature and biliary tract as close to normal as possible.

The success of liver transplantation depends on successful immunosuppression. Immunosuppressants currently used include cyclosporine (Neoral), tacrolimus (Prograf), corticosteroids, azathioprine (Imuran), mycophenolate mofetil (CellCept), OKT3 (a monoclonal antibody), sirolimus (formerly known as rapamycin [Rapamune]), anti-thymocyte globulin (Thymoglobulin), basiliximab (Simulect), and daclizumab (Zenapax). There is no one, accepted, optimal immunosuppressive regimen. Most centers have developed their own therapeutic practices, largely based on experience. Few large-scale trials have been undertaken and even if they reach established endpoints, many experts agree that newer agents will be developed, making findings less useful (Rodes, et al., 2007).

Despite the success of immunosuppression in reducing the incidence of rejection of transplanted organs, liver transplantation is not routine and may be accompanied by complications related to the lengthy surgical procedure, immunosuppressive therapy, infection, and the technical difficulties encountered in reconstructing the blood vessels and biliary tract. Long-standing systemic problems resulting from the primary liver disease may complicate the preoperative and postoperative course. Previous surgery of the abdomen, including procedures to treat complications of advanced liver disease (ie, shunt procedures used to treat portal hypertension and esophageal varices) increase the complexity of the transplantation procedure.

The indications for liver transplantation are not as limited today as they were when the procedure was first introduced because of advances in immunosuppressive therapy, improvements in biliary tract reconstruction, and, in some cases, the use of venovenous bypass. General indications for liver transplantation include irreversible advanced chronic liver disease, fulminant hepatic failure, metabolic liver diseases, and some hepatic malignancies. Examples of disorders that are indications for liver transplantation include hepatocellular liver diseases (eg, viral hepatitis, drug-induced or alcohol-induced liver disease, Wilson's disease) and cholestatic diseases (primary biliary cirrhosis, sclerosing cholangitis, and biliary atresia).

The patient being considered for liver transplantation frequently has many systemic problems that influence preoperative and postoperative care. Because transplantation is more difficult if the patient has developed severe GI bleeding and hepatic coma, efforts are made to perform the procedure before the disease progresses to this stage. The patient must undergo a thorough evaluation of hepatic reserve and general health. Part of this evaluation includes classification of the degree of medical need, an objective determination known as the Model of End-Stage Liver Disease (MELD) classification, which stratifies the level of illness of those awaiting a liver transplant. The MELD score is derived from a complex formula incorporating bilirubin levels, prothrombin time (reported as international normalized ratio [INR]), creatinine, and the cause of the liver disease (ie, cholestatic, alcoholic, or other). This system has replaced the Child-Pugh classification and other related scoring systems for prioritizing patients on the liver transplantation list (Rodes, et al., 2007; Wolfe, 2006). Although the Child-Pugh score classifies the severity of liver disease and stratifies patients into levels for varied treatment regimens, the MELD score is an indicator of short-term mortality for those with ESLD. Organs are allocated using the MELD score in an effort to provide transplants to the most severely ill patients.

Because liver transplantation is now an established therapeutic modality, rather than an experimental procedure, the number of liver transplantation centers is increasing. Patients requiring transplantation are often referred from distant hospitals to these centers. To prepare the patient and family for liver transplantation, nurses in all settings must understand the processes and procedures of liver transplantation.

Many ethical issues arise concerning liver transplantation, particularly concerning the allocation of organs. The way in which some persons contracted liver disease (eg, alcohol use; hepatitis) leads others to question allocation of organs to them, and some believe that preference should be given to people who need liver transplants but do not have a history of socially unacceptable behavior. Even more controversy exists when a patient requires a second transplant operation because of a return to alcohol or drug use or failure to follow immunosuppressive regimens (Chart 39-13). These are difficult issues with no easy solutions. Transplant recipients must go through a rigorous selection and preparation process that includes counseling and education to aid them in making critical choices for their improved health. Nurses and other health care providers need to be aware of and confront their own biases and work toward improved understanding and acceptance.

Surgical Procedure

During the procedure, the donor liver is freed from other structures, the bile is flushed from the gallbladder to prevent damage to the walls of the biliary tract, and the liver is perfused with a preservative and cooled. Before the donor liver is placed in the recipient, it is flushed with cold lactated Ringer's solution to remove potassium and air bubbles. The presence of portal hypertension increases the difficulty of the procedure.

To minimize this problem, many centers use venovenous bypass, which decompresses the venous system below the diaphragm by temporarily shunting blood to the superior vena cava via the axillary vein (Bayless & Diehl, 2005).

Anastomoses (connections) of the blood vessels and bile duct are performed between the donor liver and the recipient liver. There are two types of biliary anastomoses. Biliary reconstruction is performed with an end-to-end anastomosis of the donor and recipient common bile ducts; a stented T-tube may be inserted for external drainage of bile. In patients with biliary disease such as primary sclerosing cholangitis or if the recipient's bile duct is not suitable for anastomosis for other reasons, a biliary-enteric end-to-side anastomosis with a 40 to 50 cm Roux-en-Y loop of jejunum is created for biliary drainage (known as a Roux-en-Y procedure) (Fig. 39-15A); in this case, bile drainage is internal, and a T-tube is not inserted (Rodes, et al., 2007). Figure 39-15B and C illustrates the final appearance of the grafted liver and final closure and drain placement.

Several additional techniques have been developed to expand the donor pool for liver transplantation. In a split liver transplant, a single organ is used to provide grafts for two individuals with ESLD, with the smaller patient receiving the smaller left lobe. This procedure has resulted in a higher complication rate and lower survival rate than traditional liver transplantation. Auxiliary liver transplantation has been used in adults with fulminant hepatic failure until the patient's own liver recovers function. This procedure incorporates removal of a segment of diseased liver and implantation of a reduced-size graft. Living donor transplantation is being increasingly performed from adult to adult using full right lobes, although it is controversial because it is a major surgical procedure for the donor, and some donor deaths have occurred. The results thus far have indicated that this procedure is most successful when donor and recipient are appropriately selected using careful screening criteria (Rodes, et al., 2007).

Liver transplantation is a long surgical procedure, partly because the patient with liver failure often has portal hypertension, requiring ligation of many venous collateral vessels. Blood loss during the surgical procedure may be extensive. If the patient has adhesions from previous abdominal surgery, lysis of adhesions is often necessary. If a shunt procedure was performed previously, it must be surgically reversed to permit adequate portal venous blood supply to the new liver. During the lengthy surgery, it is important to provide regular updates to the family about the progress of the operation and the patient's status.

Complications

The postoperative complication rate is high, primarily because of technical complications or infection. Immediate postoperative complications may include bleeding, infection, and rejection. Disruption, infection, obstruction of the biliary anastomosis, and impaired biliary drainage may occur. Vascular thrombosis and stenosis are other potential complications.

Bleeding

Bleeding is common in the postoperative period and may result from coagulopathy, portal hypertension, and fibrinolysis caused by ischemic injury to the donor liver. Hypotension

---

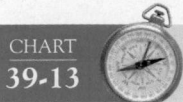

CHART 39-13 *Ethics and Related Issues*

What Ethical Principles Apply When a Candidate for a Second Liver Transplantation Continues His Drug Use?

Situation

A 34-year-old man received a liver transplant a year ago for end-stage liver disease due to hepatitis C (with a history of IV or injection use) and alcoholic liver disease. He experienced a difficult postoperative course with many complications. His liver function has now deteriorated to the point that he is listed to receive a second organ. He is in the hospital, where he is quite ill and in pain. Although he denies further use of alcohol and drug use following his first liver transplant, several bottles of opioids and sedatives are found in his bedside table.

What ethical implications exist in this case? What actions should be taken by the transplant team? What should the nurse document concerning this situation? What factors should be considered when deciding how to proceed in this case?

Dilemma

This patient has already received one liver transplant, and he will not survive unless he receives a another one. He is on the list for a second transplant. Because of the limited availability of livers for transplantation and the fact that there is a strong likelihood of his continued use of drugs, questions have been raised about the appropriateness of a second transplant.

Discussion

1. What ethical principles are involved in this situation?
2. What are the competing issues in this case that must be considered in this man's case?
3. How does the nurse respond if the patient asks about the likelihood of his receiving a second liver transplant?

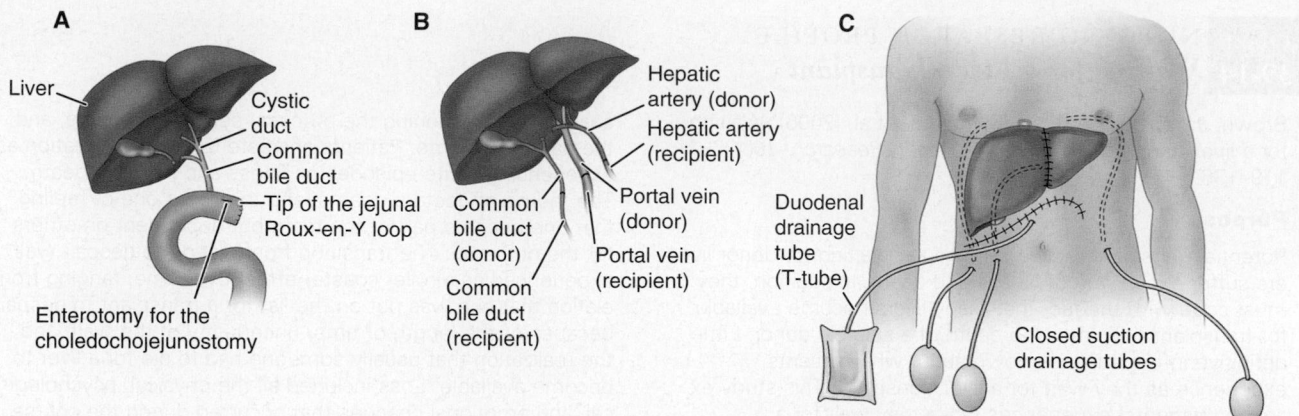

Figure 39-15 A, Some transplant recipients have diseases or conditions that cause their bile ducts to be unusable for anastomosis to the donor liver bile duct. In this case, a loop of jejunum is used as a bridge from the donor liver bile duct to the recipient's small bowel for biliary continuity and drainage. This procedure is termed a Roux-en-Y hepaticojejunostomy. **B,** Final appearance of implanted liver graft with an end-to-end biliary anastomosis. **C,** Final closure and drain placement after liver transplantation with an end-to-end biliary anastomosis and T-tube placement.

may occur in this phase, secondary to blood loss. Administration of platelets, fresh-frozen plasma, or other blood products may be necessary. Hypertension is more common, although its cause is uncertain. Blood pressure elevation that is significant or sustained is treated.

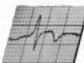

Infection

Infection is the leading cause of death after liver transplantation. Pulmonary and fungal infections are common; susceptibility to infection is increased by the immunosuppressive therapy that is needed to prevent rejection (Rodes, et al., 2007). Therefore, precautions must be taken to prevent healthcare–associated infections. The nurse uses strict asepsis when manipulating central venous catheters, arterial lines, and urine, bile, and other drainage systems; obtaining specimens; and changing dressings. Meticulous hand hygiene is crucial. In the ICU, the nurse uses evidence-based practice guidelines in the care of the postoperative liver transplant patient. Some of these care guidelines include prevention of sepsis and its rapid treatment, prevention of ventilator-associated pneumonia (VAP), and prevention of catheter-related bloodstream infections (American Thoracic Society, 2005).

Rejection

Rejection is a primary concern. A transplanted liver is perceived by the immune system as a foreign antigen. This triggers an immune response, leading to the activation of T lymphocytes that attack and destroy the transplanted liver. Immunosuppressive agents are used as long-term therapy to prevent this response and rejection of the transplanted liver. These agents inhibit the activation of immunocompetent T lymphocytes to prevent the production of effector T cells.

Although the 1- and 5-year survival rates have increased dramatically with the use of new immunosuppressive therapies, these advances are not without major side effects. A major side effect of cyclosporine, which was widely used in

transplantation, is nephrotoxicity; this problem seems to be dose related. Cyclosporine-related side effects have caused many centers to use tacrolimus as first-line therapy because of its efficacy and lower side-effect profile.

Corticosteroids, azathioprine, mycophenolate mofetil, sirolimus (formerly known as rapamycin) anti-thymocyte globulin, basiliximab, daclizumab, and muromonab-CD3 (OKT3) are also used in various regimens of immunosuppression. These agents may be used as the initial therapy to prevent rejection or used later to treat rejection. Liver biopsy and ultrasound may be required to evaluate suspected episodes of rejection.

Retransplantation is usually attempted if the transplanted liver fails, but the success rate of retransplantation does not approach that of initial transplantation.

Nursing Management

The patient considering transplantation, together with the family, must make difficult choices about treatment, use of financial resources, and relocation to another area to be closer to the medical center. They must also be aware of the risks and benefits of the procedure and its consequences. In addition, they must also cope with the patient's long-standing health problems and any social and family problems associated with behaviors that may have caused the patient's liver failure. As a result, considerable emotional stress occurs while the patient and family consider liver transplantation and wait for an available liver (Chart 39-14). The nurse must be aware of these issues and attuned to the emotional and psychological status of the patient and family. Referral to a psychiatric liaison nurse, psychologist, psychiatrist, or spiritual advisor may help them cope with the stressors associated with ESLD and liver transplantation.

If the patient and family are considering undergoing a live donor liver transplant, they are subject to additional stressors. Both the patient and the potential donor must undergo a thorough and exhaustive physical and psychological workup to ensure that all involved parties are physically and emotionally prepared. Often, but not always, the donor

---

CHART 39-14	NURSING RESEARCH PROFILE
	Waiting for a Liver Transplant

Brown, J., Sorrell, J. H., McClaren, J., et al. (2006). Waiting for a liver transplant. *Qualitative Health Research, 16*(1), 119–136.

Purpose

Potential transplant recipients who are waiting for donor livers suffer a high rate of illness and death. In addition, they must cope with the fact that many livers become available for transplant only after the death of a suitable donor. Little definitive information is known about what patients experience as they wait for a liver transplant. This study examined patients' experiences while they wait for a transplant.

Design

Researchers used a phenomenological approach to examine the experience of patients with end-stage liver disease (ESLD) waiting for a transplant. They conducted nine interviews with six patients with ESLD during their wait for a liver transplant. Interviews with six participants were open ended, with three participants having follow-up interviews. The interviews focused on what it was like for patients with ESLD to be on the waiting list for a liver transplant and their experiences during the period of waiting. Researchers performed a qualitative analysis of transcriptions of the interviews to extract statements and ultimately themes that described the experience of waiting for a liver transplant. They identified and verified themes through review of the literature, member checks, and peer review of the data analysis process.

Findings

Eight themes that described the experience of waiting for a liver transplant emerged from the data analysis: transformation; doctors, teams, and trust; transition from elation to de-

spair; loss; questioning the process; searching; coping; and the paradox of time. Patients characterized transformation as experiencing acute episodes of illness and possible death. The theme of doctors, teams, and trust was one of feeling that one became part of the team but dependent on others for the outcome. The transition from elation to despair was experienced as a roller coaster effect over time, ranging from elation that one was put on the list for a transplant to despair because of the length of time, uncertainty of the wait, and the realization that usually someone had to die for a liver to become available. Loss included all the physical, psychological, and emotional changes that occurred during the course of illness and waiting for a transplant. Questioning the process reflected the ambivalence and doubt that were experienced by people as they questioned the wisdom of having a transplant. Searching referred to patients' developing theories about their experiences and the personal search for meaning given their predicament. Coping referred to strategies patients used to grapple with their situation; strategies included denial and patience. Lastly, the paradox of time referred to patients' views of life before and after transplantation and the effect of waiting on their perception of time.

Nursing Implications

The impact on patients of being placed on a wait list for liver transplant needs to be considered by those providing care. The lack of control and the losses experienced by patients waiting for a liver transplant need to be acknowledged and addressed during care by allowing patients to have as much control over their lives as possible. Providing patients with an opportunity to verbalize their fears and concerns about their situation and their future may be helpful in reducing some of the patients' sense of uncertainty and sense of ambivalence about waiting and their uncertain future.

---

is a close family member. Coercion must be excluded as influencing the decision to donate a portion of one's liver to another. The potential donor must be aware of the risks associated with the procedure.

If the patient and family believe that liver transplantation may be appropriate, the nurse, surgeon, hepatologist, and other health care team members provide the patient and family with full explanations about the procedure, the chances of success, and the risks, including the side effects of long-term immunosuppression. The need for close follow-up and lifelong compliance with the therapeutic regimen, including immunosuppression, is emphasized to the patient and family.

Preoperative Nursing Interventions

Once the patient has been accepted as a candidate, he or she is placed on a waiting list at the transplant center, and patient information is entered into the United Network for Organ Sharing (UNOS) computer system. The UNOS system uses the MELD score to determine organ allocation priorities so that the patient with the highest MELD score will receive the first available organ. Candidates may be matched with appropriate organs as they become available.

MELD scores provide the necessary information regarding medical need.

Except in the case of segmental liver transplantation from a living donor, a liver becomes available for transplantation only with the death of another person, usually someone who had been healthy except for severe brain injury and brain death. Therefore, the patient and family undergo a stressful waiting period, and the nurse is often their major source of support. The patient must be accessible at all times in case an appropriate liver becomes available. During this time, liver function may deteriorate further, and the patient may experience other complications from the primary liver disease. Because of the shortage of donor organs, many patients die awaiting transplantation.

Malnutrition, massive ascites, and fluid and electrolyte disturbances are treated before surgery to increase the likelihood of a successful outcome. If the patient's liver dysfunction has a very rapid onset, as in fulminant hepatic failure, there is little time or opportunity for the patient to consider and weigh options and their consequences; often this patient is in a coma, and the decision to proceed with transplantation is made by the family.

The nurse coordinator is an integral member of the transplant team and plays an important role in preparing the patient for liver transplantation. The nurse serves as an advocate for the patient and family and assumes the important role of liaison between the patient and the other members of the transplant team. The nurse also serves as a resource to other nurses and health care team members involved in evaluating and caring for the patient.

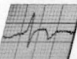

Postoperative Nursing Interventions

The patient is maintained in an environment as free from bacteria, viruses, and fungi as possible, because immunosuppressive medications reduce the body's natural defenses. In the immediate postoperative period, cardiovascular, pulmonary, renal, neurologic, and metabolic functions are monitored continuously. Mean arterial and pulmonary artery pressures are also monitored continuously. Cardiac output, central venous pressure, pulmonary capillary wedge pressure, arterial and mixed venous blood gases, oxygen saturation, oxygen demand and delivery, urine output, heart rate, and blood pressure are used to evaluate the patient's hemodynamic status and intravascular fluid volume. Liver function tests, electrolyte levels, the coagulation profile, chest x-ray, electrocardiogram, and fluid output (including urine, bile from the T-tube, and drainage from Jackson-Pratt tubes) are monitored closely. Because the liver is responsible for the storage of glycogen and the synthesis of protein and clotting factors, these substances need to be monitored and replaced in the immediate postoperative period.

There is a high risk of atelectasis and an altered ventilation–perfusion ratio caused by insult to the diaphragm during the surgical procedure, prolonged anesthesia, immobility, and postoperative pain. The patient will have an endotracheal tube in place and will require mechanical ventilation during the initial postoperative period. Suctioning is performed as required, and sterile humidification is provided. Evidence-based practice guidelines are implemented to prevent the development of VAP in the postoperative liver transplant recipient (American Thoracic Society, 2005). Actions such as keeping the head of the bed elevated at least 30 degrees and performing frequent oral suctioning and cleansing are effective in preventing VAP.

As the patient's condition stabilizes, efforts are made to promote recovery from the trauma of this complex surgery. After removal of the endotracheal tube, the nurse encourages the patient to use an incentive spirometer to decrease the risk of atelectasis. Following extubation, the patient is assisted to get out of bed, to ambulate as tolerated, and to participate in self-care to prevent the complications associated with immobility. Close monitoring for signs and symptoms of liver dysfunction and rejection continue throughout the hospital stay. Plans are made for close follow-up after discharge as well. Teaching is initiated during the preoperative period and continues after surgery.

Promoting Home and Community-Based Care

Teaching Patients Self-Care

Teaching the patient and family about long-term measures to promote health is crucial for the success of transplanta-

tion and is an important role of the nurse. The patient and family must understand why they need to adhere closely to the therapeutic regimen, with special emphasis on the methods of administration, rationale, and side effects of the prescribed immunosuppressive agents. The nurse provides written as well as verbal instructions about how and when to take the medications. To avoid running out of medication or skipping a dose, the patient must make sure that an adequate supply of medication is available. Instructions are also provided about the signs and symptoms that indicate problems necessitating consultation with the transplant team. The patient with a T-tube in place must be taught how to manage the tube, drainage, and skin care.

Continuing Care

The nurse emphasizes the importance of follow-up blood tests and appointments with the transplant team. Trough blood levels of immunosuppressive agents are obtained, along with other blood tests that assess the function of the liver and kidneys. During the first months, the patient is likely to require blood tests two or three times a week. As the patient's condition stabilizes, blood studies and visits to the transplant team are less frequent. The importance of routine ophthalmologic examinations is emphasized because of the increased incidence of cataracts and glaucoma associated with the long-term corticosteroid therapy used with transplantation. Regular oral hygiene and follow-up dental care, with administration of prophylactic antibiotics before dental examinations and treatments, are recommended because of the immunosuppression.

The nurse reminds the patient that preventing rejection and infection is essential and increases the chances for survival and a more normal life than before transplantation. Many patients have lived successful and productive lives after receiving a liver transplant. In fact, pregnancy can be considered 1 year after transplantation. Although successful outcomes have been reported, these pregnancies are considered high risk for both mother and infant. Transplant recipients should be advised about birth control. The 1-year waiting period allows time to establish good health, stable liver function, and lower maintenance levels of immunosuppressive therapy (Rodes, et al., 2007).

Liver Abscesses

Two categories of liver abscess have been identified: amebic and pyogenic. Amebic liver abscesses are most commonly caused by *Entamoeba histolytica*. Most amebic liver abscesses occur in the developing countries of the tropics and subtropics because of poor sanitation and hygiene. Pyogenic liver abscesses are much less common, but they are more common in developed countries than the amebic type.

Pathophysiology

Whenever an infection develops anywhere along the biliary or GI tract, infecting organisms may reach the liver through the biliary system, portal venous system, or hepatic arterial or lymphatic system. Most bacteria are destroyed promptly, but occasionally some gain a foothold. The bacterial toxins destroy the neighboring liver cells, and the resulting necrotic tissue serves as a protective wall for the organisms.

Meanwhile, leukocytes migrate into the infected area. The result is an abscess cavity full of a liquid containing living and dead leukocytes, liquefied liver cells, and bacteria. Pyogenic abscesses of this type may be either single or multiple and small. Examples of causes of pyogenic liver abscess include cholangitis (usually related to benign or malignant obstruction of the biliary tree) and abdominal trauma.

Clinical Manifestations

The clinical picture is one of sepsis with few or no localizing signs. Fever with chills and diaphoresis, malaise, anorexia, nausea, vomiting, and weight loss may occur. The patient may complain of dull abdominal pain and tenderness in the right upper quadrant of the abdomen. Hepatomegaly, jaundice, anemia, and pleural effusion may develop. Sepsis and shock may be severe and life-threatening. In the past, the mortality rate was 100% because of the vague clinical symptoms, inadequate diagnostic tools, and inadequate surgical drainage of the abscess. With the aid of ultrasound, CT, MRI, and liver scans, early diagnosis and surgical drainage of abscesses have greatly reduced the mortality rate.

Assessment and Diagnostic Findings

Although blood cultures are obtained, the organism may not be identified. Aspiration of the liver abscess, guided by ultrasound, CT, or MRI, may be performed to assist in diagnosis and to obtain cultures of the organism. Percutaneous drainage of pyogenic abscesses is carried out to evacuate the abscess material and promote healing. A catheter may be left in place for continuous drainage; the patient must be instructed about its management.

Medical Management

Treatment includes IV antibiotic therapy; the specific antibiotic used in treatment depends on the organism identified. Continuous supportive care is indicated because of the serious condition of the patient. Open surgical drainage may be required if antibiotic therapy and percutaneous drainage are ineffective.

Nursing Management

Although the manifestations of liver abscess vary with the type of abscess, most patients appear acutely ill. Others appear to be chronically ill and debilitated. The nursing management depends on the patient's physical status and the medical management that is indicated. For patients who undergo evacuation and drainage of an abscess, monitoring of the drainage and skin care are imperative. Strategies must be implemented to contain the drainage and to protect the patient from other sources of infection. Vital signs are monitored to detect changes in the patient's physical status. Deterioration in vital signs or the onset of new symptoms such as increasing pain, which may indicate rupture or extension of the abscess, is reported promptly. The nurse administers IV antibiotic therapy as prescribed. The white blood cell count and other laboratory test results are monitored closely for changes consistent with worsening infection. The nurse prepares the patient for discharge by providing instruction about symptom management, signs and symptoms that should be reported to the physician, management of drainage, and the importance of taking antibiotics as prescribed.

CRITICAL THINKING EXERCISES

1 A 56-year-old professor and consultant has just received unexpected notice that she must travel to Nicaragua for a conference in 2 days. What prophylactic measures to reduce her risk of contracting hepatitis A are available before she leaves for her trip? What signs and symptoms are important for her to watch for and to report to her health care provider? What modifications, if any, should be implemented for her close household contacts? If this woman had 6 months to prepare for her trip, how would the answers to these questions be different?

2 A 36-year-old African man came to the United States from Botswana 3 years ago to live with relatives. He is being treated for end-stage liver disease (ESLD) with cirrhosis related to hepatitis B and is undergoing evaluation for liver transplantation. The sequelae of ESLD that he is experiencing include encephalopathy and ascites. What would you anticipate this patient's treatment regimen to include? What medications would be most appropriate for him? What would you include in your cultural assessment when you develop a preoperative teaching plan for this patient? What alternative therapies might be used preoperatively? Once the patient receives a liver transplant, what medications would you expect to be prescribed for him in addition to an immunosuppressant regimen?

3 A 68-year-old man is admitted to the hospital with a diagnosis of bleeding esophageal varices. Describe the monitoring you would initiate. What possible management strategies to prevent bleeding and to treat active bleeding of the esophageal varices would you anticipate? What are the nursing implications for each of these strategies? How would medical management and nursing care be modified if the patient had chronic obstructive pulmonary disease in addition to esophageal varices? How would you explain treatment strategies to the patient and his family if one or more of them had hearing impairment?

4 A 26-year-old man is transferred to your transplant center with the diagnosis of end-stage liver disease with a severe coagulopathy and encephalopathy. He presents with extreme jaundice, multiple bruises, and severe confusion and agitation. In addition, he is trying to climb out of bed and strike family members and hospital personnel. The cause of his liver failure is hepatitis C from intravenous (IV) or injection drug use along with alcohol abuse. The referring institution had indicated that the man had not used drugs or alcohol for more than 6 months. On obtaining a detailed history from the patient's mother and sister, the nurse and physician learn that his family had seen him use IV or injection drugs only 2 weeks prior to admission. What are the nursing priorities in the care of this patient? What measures would you institute to ensure patient safety? What medications are likely to be used to improve the patient's mental status? Is the patient an appropriate candidate for a liver transplant? If the patient does not receive a liver transplant, what is the likely outcome?

EBP   **5**   A 19-year-old college student with fulminant liver failure is hospitalized with hepatic coma related to an acetaminophen overdose. She is in the intensive care unit, intubated and on a ventilator. A pulmonary artery catheter has been placed as well as an arterial line and indwelling urinary catheter. She has also had a device placed to monitor and treat intracranial hypertension. What factors place her at high risk for infection? What particular types of infection are most likely? What evidence-based practice guidelines are you most likely to institute to prevent sepsis in this patient? What criteria will you use to determine the strength of the evidence? On receiving a liver transplant, what other risk factors for infection will she have?

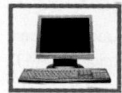 The Smeltzer suite offers these additional resources to enhance learning and facilitate understanding of this chapter:

• thePoint on line resource, thepoint.lww.com/Smeltzer12E
• Student CD-ROM included with the book
• *Study Guide to Accompany Brunner & Suddarth's Textbook of Medical-Surgical Nursing*
• *Handbook for Brunner & Suddarth's Textbook of Medical-Surgical Nursing*

REFERENCES AND SELECTED READINGS

Asterisk indicates nursing research.

Books

Ajani, J. A., Curley, S. A., Janjan, N. A. et al. (Eds.). (2005). *Gastrointestinal cancer.* New York: Springer Science.
American Cancer Society. (2008). *Cancer facts and figures.* Atlanta: Author.
Bayless, T. M. & Diehl, A. M. (Eds.). (2005). *Advanced therapy in gastroenterology and liver disease.* Hamilton, Ontario: B. C. Decker.
Bergin, J. D. (2008). *Medicine recall.* Philadelphia: Wolters Kluwer Health/Lippincott Williams & Wilkins.
Bickley, L. S. (2007). *Bates' guide to physical examination and history taking* (9th ed.). Philadelphia: Lippincott Williams & Wilkins.
Boyer, T. D., Wright, T. L. & Manns, M. P. (Eds.). (2006). *Zakim & Boyer's hepatology: Textbook of liver disease* (5th ed.). Philadelphia: Saunders Elsevier.
Dudek, S. G. (2006). *Nutrition essentials for nursing practice* (5th ed.). Philadelphia: Lippincott Williams & Wilkins.
Feldman, M., Friedman, L. S. & Brandt, L. J. (Eds.) (2006). *Sleisenger and Fordtran's gastrointestinal and liver disease: Pathophysiology, diagnosis, and management.* Philadelphia: Saunders.
Floch, M. H. (Ed.). (2005). *Netter's gastroenterology.* Carlstadt, NJ: Icon Learning Systems.
Forbes, A. (2005). *Atlas of clinical gastroenterology.* Edinburgh; New York: Elsevier Mosby.
Goldman, L. & Ausiello, D. (2008). *Cecil Medicine* (23rd ed.). Philadelphia: Saunders Elsevier.
Hauser, S. C., Pardi, D. S. & Poterucha, J. J. (Eds.). (2006). *Mayo Clinic gastroenterology and hepatology board review* (2nd ed.). Rochester, MN: Mayo Foundation for Medical Education and Research.
Maingot, R. (2007). *Maingot's abdominal operations.* New York: McGraw-Hill.
Onion, D. K. (Ed.). (2006). *The little black book of gastroenterology* (2nd ed.). Sudbury, MA: Jones and Bartlett.

Porth, C. M. & Matfin, G. (2009). *Pathophysiology: Concepts of altered health states* (8th ed.). Philadelphia: Lippincott Williams & Wilkins.
Rodes, J., Benhamou, J. P., Blei, A. T., et al. (Eds.). (2007). *Textbook of hepatology: From basic science to clinical practice* (3rd ed.). Malden, MA: Blackwell.
Schiff, E. R., Sorrell, M. F. & Maddrey, L. C. (Eds.). (2006). *Schiff's diseases of the liver* (10th ed.). Philadelphia: Lippincott Williams & Wilkins.
Shils, M. E., Shike, M., Ross, A. C., et al. (Eds.). (2006). *Modern nutrition in health and disease* (10th ed.). Philadelphia: Lippincott Williams & Wilkins.
Tierney, L. M., McPhee, S. J. & Papadakis, M. A. (2007). *Current medical diagnosis and treatment* (46th ed.). New York: Lange Medical Books/McGraw-Hill.
Weinstein, W. M., Hawkey, J. & Bosch, J. (2005). *Clinical gastroenterology and hepatology.* Edinburgh: Elsevier Mosby.
Wolfe, M. M. (Ed.). (2006). *Therapy of digestive disorders* (2nd ed.). Philadelphia: Saunders Elsevier.
Yamada, T. (2005). *Handbook of gastroenterology.* Philadelphia: Lippincott Williams & Wilkins.

Journals and Electronic Documents

General

American Thoracic Society. (2005). Guidelines for the management of adults with hospital-acquired, ventilator-associated, and healthcare-associated pneumonia. *American Journal of Respiratory and Critical Care Medicine, 171*(4), 388–416.
Clark, J. M. (2006). The epidemiology of nonalcoholic fatty liver disease in adults. *Journal of Clinical Gastroenterology, 40*(3 Suppl 1), S5–S 10.
Czaja, A. J. (2007). Autoimmune liver disease. *Current Opinion in Gastroenterology, 23*(3), 255–262.
Freeman, R. B. (2008). Model for end-stage liver disease (MELD) for liver allocation: A 5 year score card. *Hepatology, 47*(3), 1052–1057.
Hankins, J. (2007). The role of albumin in fluid balance. *Nursing, 37*(12), 14–15.
Kaplan, M. M. & Gershwin, M. E. (2005). Primary biliary cirrhosis. *New England Journal of Medicine, 353*(12), 1261–1273.
Khanna, S. & Gopalan, S. (2007). Role of branched-chain amino acids in liver disease: The evidence for and against. *Current Opinion in Clinical Nutrition and Metabolic Care, 10*(3), 297–303.
Kotronen, A. & Yki-Jarvinen, H. (2008). Fatty liver: A novel component of the metabolic syndrome. *Arteriosclerosis, Thrombosis and Vascular Biology, 28*(1), 27–38.
Reuben, A. (2007). Alcohol and the liver. *Current Opinion in Gastroenterology, 23*(3), 283–291.
Sakka, S. G. (2007). Assessing liver function. *Current Opinion in Critical Care, 13*(2), 207–214.
Senzolo, M., Cholongitas, E., Tibballs, J., et al. (2006). Transjugular intrahepatic portosystemic shunt in the management of ascites and hepatorenal syndrome. *European Journal of Gastroenterology & Hepatology, 18*(11), 1143–1150.
Stadlbauer, V. & Jalan, R. (2007). Acute liver failure: Liver support therapies. *Current Opinion in Critical Care, 13*(2), 215–221.
Sublett, L. (2007). Deconstructing nonalcoholic fatty liver disease. *Nurse Practitioner, 32*(8), 12–17.
Udayakumar, N., Subramaniam, K., Umashandar, L., et al. (2007). Predictors of mortality in hepatic encephalopathy in acute and chronic liver disease: A preliminary observation. *Journal of Clinical Gastroenterology, 41*(10), 922–926.

Cirrhosis and Esophageal Varices

Abraides, J. G. & Bosch, J. (2007). The treatment of acute variceal bleeding. *Journal of Clinical Gastroenterology, 41*(Suppl 3), S312–S317.
Albillos, A. (2007). Preventing first variceal hemorrhage in cirrhosis. *Journal of Clinical Gastroenterology, 41*(Suppl 3), S305–S311.
Blei, A. T. (2007). Portal hypertension and its complications. *Current Opinion in Gastroenterology, 23*(3), 275–282.
Colombato, L. (2007). The role of transjugular intrahepatic portosystemic shunt (TIPS) in the management of portal hypertension. *Journal of Clinical Gastroenterology, 41*(Suppl 3), S344–S351.
De Franchis, R. & Dell'Era, A. (2007). Diagnosis and therapy of esophageal vascular disorders. *Current Opinion in Gastroenterology, 23*(4), 422–427.
dePaulo, G. A., Ardengh, J. C., Nakao, F. S., et al. (2006). Treatment of esophageal varices: A randomized controlled trial comparing endoscopic sclerotherapy and EUS-guided sclerotherapy of esophageal collateral veins. *Gastrointestinal Endoscopy, 63*(3), 396–402.
Everson, G. T. (2005). Management of cirrhosis due to chronic hepatitis C. *Journal of Hepatology, 42*(Suppl), S65–S74.

Garcia-Tsao, G. (2006). Portal hypertension. *Current Opinion in Gastroenterology, 22*(3), 254–262.

Kravetz, D. (2007). Prevention of recurrent esophageal variceal hemorrhage: Review and current recommendations. *Journal of Clinical Gastroenterology, 41*(Suppl 3), S318–S322.

Lazaridis, K. N. & Talwalkar, J. A. (2007). Clinical epidemiology of primary biliary cirrhosis: Incidence, prevalence, and impact of therapy. *Journal of Clinical Gastroenterology, 41*(5), 494–500.

Longacre, A. V. & Garcia-Tsao, G. (2006). A commonsense approach to esophageal varices. *Clinics in Liver Disease, 10*(3), 613–625.

Mathews, R. E., McGuire, B. M. & Estrada, C. A. (2006). Outpatient management of cirrhosis: A narrative review. *Southern Medical Journal, 99*(6), 600–606.

Saab, S., Nieto, J. M., Lewis, S. K., et al. (2006). TIPS versus paracentesis for cirrhotic patients with refractory ascites. *Cochrane Database System Review,* (4), CD004889.

Schuppan, D. & Afdhal, N. H. (2008). Liver cirrhosis. *Lancet, 371*(9615), 838–851.

Spiegel, B. M. R., Esrailian, E. & Eisen, G. (2007). The budget impact of endoscopic screening for esophageal varices in cirrhosis. *Gastrointestinal Endoscopy, 66*(4), 679–692.

Talwalkar, J. A. (2006). Cost-effectiveness of treating esophageal varices. *Clinics in Liver Disease, 10*(3), 679–689.

Tripathi, D., Graham, C. & Hayes, P. C. (2007). Variceal band ligation versus beta-blockers for primary prevention of variceal bleeding: a meta analysis. *European Journal of Gastroenterology & Hepatology, 19*(10), 835–845.

Zaman, A. (2006). Portal hypertension-related bleeding: Management of difficult cases. *Clinics in Liver Disease, 10*(2), 353–370.

Hepatitis

American Academy of Pediatrics Committee on Infectious Diseases. (2007). Hepatitis A vaccine recommendations. *Pediatrics, 120*(1), 189–199.

Blaine, H. F., Bell, B., Levy-Bruhl, D., et al. (2007). Hepatitis A and B vaccination and public health. *Journal of Viral Hepatitis, 14*(Suppl 1), 1–5.

Caccamo, L., Agnelli, F. & Reggiani, P., et al. (2007). Role of lamivudine in the posttransplant prophylaxis of chronic hepatitis B virus and hepatitis delta virus coinfection. *Transplantation, 83*(10), 1341–1344.

Craig, A. S., Watson, B., Zink, T. K., et al. (2007). Hepatitis A outbreak activity in the United States: Responding to a vaccine-preventable disease. *American Journal of the Medical Sciences, 334*(3), 180–183.

Giovanna, F., Bortolotti, F. & Francesco, D. (2008). Natural history of chronic hepatitis B: Special emphasis on disease progression and prognostic factors. *Journal of Hepatology, 48*(2), 335–352.

*Hamilton, H. E., Gordon, C., Nelson, M., et al. (2006). Physicians, nonphysician healthcare providers, and patients communicating in hepatitis C: An in-office sociolinguistic study. *Gastroenterology Nursing, 29*(5), 364–370.

National Institutes of Health. (2002). Consensus statement on management of hepatitis C. *NIH Consensus and State-of-the-Science Statements, 19*(3), 1–46.

Page-Shafer, K., Hahn, J. A. & Lum, P. J. (2007). Preventing hepatitis C virus infection in injection drug users: Risk reduction is not enough. *AIDS, 21*(14), 1967–1969.

Sanyal, A. J., Fontana, R. J. & DeBisceglie, A. M. (2006). The prevalence and risk factors associated with esophageal varices in subjects with hepatitis C and advanced fibrosis. *Gastrointestinal Endoscopy, 64*(6), 855–864.

*Sheppard, K. & Hubbert, A. (2006). The patient experience of treatment for hepatitis C. *Gastroenterology Nursing, 29*(4), 309–315.

*Stringer, M., Ratcliffe, S. J. & Gross, R. (2006). Acceptance of hepatitis B vaccination by pregnant adolescents. *MCN: The American Journal of Maternal/Child Nursing, 31*(1), 54–60.

Tan, J. & Lok, A. S. F. (2007). Update on viral hepatitis: 2006. *Current Opinion in Gastroenterology, 23*(3), 263–267.

Victor, J. C., Monto, A. S., Surdian, T. Y., et al. (2007). Hepatitis A vaccine versus immune globulin for postexposure prophylaxis. *New England Journal of Medicine, 357*(17), 1685–1694.

Wasley, A., Grytdal, S. & Gallagher, K. (2008). Surveillance for acute viral hepatitis—United States, 2006. *Morbidity & Mortality Weekly Report, 57*(SS02), 1–24.

Wasley, A., Samandari, T. & Bell, B. P. (2005). Incidence of hepatitis A in the United States in the era of vaccination. *Journal of American Medical Association, 294*(2), 194–201.

*Zucker, D. (2006a). A case of health disparity: Treatment issues in women with hepatitis C. *Gastroenterology Nursing, 29*(2), 137–141.

*Zucker, D. (2006b). Hepatitis C prevention in a county correctional facility. *Gastroenterology Nursing, 29*(2), 173.

Liver Cancer

Abdalla, E. K., Denys, A., Hasegawa, K., et al. (2008). Treatment of large and advanced hepatocellular carcinoma. *Annals of Surgical Oncology, 15*(4), 979–985.

Clavien, P. A. (2007). Interferon: The magic bullet to prevent hepatocellular recurrence after resection? *Annals of Surgery, 245*(6), 843–845.

Kallwitz, E. R. & Cotler, S. J. (2007). Screening for hepatocellular carcinoma in clinical practice: Miles to go before we sleep. *Journal of Clinical Gastroenterology, 41*(8), 729–730.

Krishnan, S., Dawson, L. A., Seong, J., et al. (2008). Radiotherapy for hepatocellular carcinoma: An overview. *Annals of Surgical Oncology, 15*(4), 1015–1024.

Kulik, L. M. (2007). Advancements in hepatocellular carcinoma. *Current Opinion in Gastroenterology, 23*(3), 268–274.

Kulik, L. M., Mulcahy, M. F., Omary, R. A., et al. (2007). Emerging approaches in hepatocellular carcinoma. *Journal of Clinical Gastroenterology, 41*(9), 839–854.

La Vecchia, C. (2007). Alcohol and liver cancer. *European Journal of Cancer Prevention, 16*(6), 495–497.

Lo, C. M., Liu, C. L., Chan, S. C., et al. (2007). A randomized, controlled trial of postoperative adjuvant interferon therapy after resection of hepatocellular carcinoma. *Annals of Surgery, 245*(6), 831–842.

Mocherla, B., Jongho, K., Roayale, S., et al. (2007). FDG PET/CT imaging to rule out extrahepatic metastases before liver transplantation. *Clinical Nuclear Medicine, 32*(12), 947–948.

Raoul, J. L. (2008). Natural history of hepatocellular carcinoma and current treatment options. *Seminars in Nuclear Medicine, 38*(2), S13–S18.

Takayama, T., Makuuchi, M., Kojiro, M., et al. (2008). Early hepatocellular carcinoma: Pathology, imaging and therapy. *Annals of Surgical Oncology, 15*(4), 972–978.

Thomas, M. B., O'Beirne, J. P., Furuse, J., et al. (2008). Systemic therapy for hepatocellular carcinoma: Cytotoxic chemotherapy, targeted therapy and immunotherapy. *Annals of Surgical Oncology, 15*(4), 1008–1014.

Liver Transplantation

Aranda-Michel, J., Dickson, R. C., Bonatti, H., et al. (2008). Patient selection for liver transplant: 1-year experience with 555 patients at a single center. *Mayo Clinic Proceedings, 83*(2), 165–168.

*Brown, J., Sorrell, J. H., McClaren, J., et al. (2006). Waiting for a liver transplant. *Qualitative Health Research, 16*(1), 199–136.

Dew, M. A., DiMartini, A. F., Steel, J., et al. (2008). Meta-analysis of risk for relapse to substance use after transplantation of the liver or other solid organ. *Liver Transplantation, 14*(2), 159–172.

Herrero, J. L., Pardo, F., Alegre, F., et al. (2008). Outcome of liver transplantation in older recipients. *Archives of Surgery, 143*(3), 313.

Karasu, Z., Akyildiz, M., Kilic, M., et al. (2007). Living donor liver transplantation for hepatitis B cirrhosis. *Journal of Gastroenterology & Hepatology, 22*(12), 2142–2149.

Mazzaferro, V., Chun, Y. S., Poon, R. T., et al. (2008). Liver transplantation for hepatocellular carcinoma. *Annals of Surgical Oncology, 15*(4), 1001–1007.

Said, A., Einstein, M. & Lucey, M. R. (2007). Liver transplantation: 2007. *Current Opinion in Gastroenterology, 23*(3), 292–298.

Stickel, F., Inderbitzin, D. & Candinas, D. (2008). Role of nutrition in liver transplantation for end-stage chronic liver disease. *Nutrition Reviews, 66*(1), 47–54.

Tome, S., Said, A. & Lucey, M. R. (2008). Addictive behavior after solid organ transplantation: What do we know already and what do we need to know? *Liver Transplantation, 14*(2), 262.

Yilmaz, N., Shiffman, M. L., Todd, S. R., et al. (2008). Prophylaxis against recurrence of hepatitis B virus after liver transplantation: A retrospective analysis spanning 20 years. *Liver International, 28*(10), 72–78.

RESOURCES

Al-Anon Family Group Headquarters, www.al-anon.alateen.org
Alcoholics Anonymous World Services, http://aa.org
American Association for the Study of Liver Diseases, www.aasld.org
American College of Gastroenterology, www.acg.gi.org
American Liver Foundation, www.liverfoundation.org
Hepatitis Foundation International, www.hepfi.org
National Council on Alcoholism and Drug Dependence, www.ncadd.org
National Digestive Diseases Information Clearing House, www.niddk.nih.gov
National Institute on Alcohol Abuse and Alcoholism, www.niaaa.nih.gov
United Network for Organ Sharing, www.unos.org

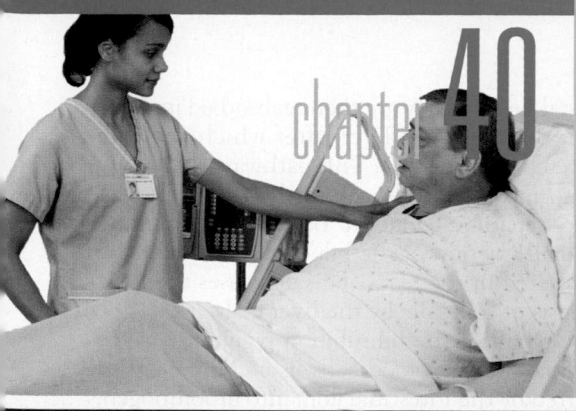

chapter 40

Assessment and Management of Patients With Biliary Disorders

LEARNING OBJECTIVES

On completion of this chapter, the learner will be able to:

1 Compare approaches to management of cholelithiasis.

2 Use the nursing process as a framework for care of patients with cholelithiasis and those undergoing laparoscopic or open cholecystectomy.

3 Differentiate between acute and chronic pancreatitis.

4 Describe nursing management of patients with acute pancreatitis.

5 Describe the nutritional and metabolic effects of surgical treatment of tumors of the pancreas.

GLOSSARY

amylase: pancreatic enzyme; aids in the digestion of carbohydrates

cholecystectomy: removal of the gallbladder

cholecystitis: inflammation of the gallbladder

cholecystojejunostomy: anastomosis of the jejunum to the gallbladder to divert bile flow

cholecystokinin-pancreozymin (CCK-PZ): hormone; major stimulus for digestive enzyme secretion; stimulates contraction of the gallbladder

cholecystostomy: opening and drainage of the gallbladder

choledochojejunostomy: anastomosis of common duct to jejunum

choledocholithiasis: stones in the common duct

choledocholithotomy: incision of common bile duct for removal of stones

choledochostomy: opening into the common duct

cholelithiasis: calculi in the gallbladder

GLOSSARY *(Continued)*

dissolution therapy: use of medications to break up/dissolve gallstones

endocrine: secreting internally; hormonal secretion of a ductless gland

endoscopic retrograde cholangiopancreatography (ERCP): an endoscopic procedure using fiberoptic technology to visualize the biliary system

exocrine: secreting externally; hormonal secretion from excretory ducts

laparoscopic cholecystectomy: removal of gallbladder through an endoscopic procedure

lipase: pancreatic enzyme; aids in the digestion of fats

llthotripsy: disintegration of gallstones by shock waves

pancreaticojejunostomy: joining of the pancreatic duct to the jejunum by side-to-side anastomosis; allows drainage of the pancreatic secretions into the jejunum

pancreatitis: inflammation of the pancreas; may be acute or chronic

secretin: hormone responsible for stimulating secretion of pancreatic juice; also used as an aid in diagnosing pancreatic exocrine disease and in obtaining desquamated pancreatic cells for cytologic examination

steatorrhea: frothy, foul-smelling stools with a high fat content; results from impaired digestion of proteins and fats due to a lack of pancreatic juice in the intestine

trypsin: pancreatic enzyme; aids in digestion of proteins

wound-ostomy-continence (WOC) nurse: nurse specially educated in appropriate skin, wound, ostomy, and continence care; often referred to as wound-care specialist or enterostomal therapist

Zollinger-Ellison tumor: hypersecretion of gastric acid that produces peptic ulcers as a result of a non–beta-cell tumor of the pancreatic islets

Disorders of the biliary tract and pancreas are common and include gallbladder stones and pancreatic dysfunction. An understanding of the structure and function of the biliary tract and pancreas is essential, along with an understanding of how biliary tract disorders are closely linked with liver disease. Patients with acute or chronic biliary tract or pancreatic disease require care from nurses who are knowledgeable about the diagnostic procedures and interventions that are used in the management of gallbladder and pancreatic disorders.

ANATOMIC AND PHYSIOLOGIC OVERVIEW

The Gallbladder

The gallbladder, a pear-shaped, hollow, saclike organ, 7.5 to 10 cm (3 to 4 in) long, lies in a shallow depression on the inferior surface of the liver, to which it is attached by loose connective tissue. The capacity of the gallbladder is 30 to 50 mL of bile. Its wall is composed largely of smooth muscle. The gallbladder is connected to the common bile duct by the cystic duct (Fig. 40-1).

The gallbladder functions as a storage depot for bile. Between meals, when the sphincter of Oddi is closed, bile produced by the hepatocytes enters the gallbladder. During storage, a large portion of the water in bile is absorbed through the walls of the gallbladder, so that bile in the gallbladder is five to 10 times more concentrated than that originally secreted by the liver. When food enters the duodenum, the gallbladder contracts and the sphincter of Oddi (located at the junction of the common bile duct with the duodenum) relaxes. Relaxation of this sphincter allows the bile to enter the intestine. This response is mediated by secretion of the hormone **cholecystokinin-pancreozymin (CCK-PZ)** from the intestinal wall. Bile is composed of water and electrolytes (sodium, potassium, calcium, chloride, and bicarbonate) along with significant amounts of lecithin, fatty acids, cholesterol, bilirubin, and bile salts. The bile salts, together with cholesterol, assist in emulsification of fats in the distal ileum. They are then reabsorbed into the portal blood for return to the liver, after which they are once again excreted into the bile. This pathway from hepatocytes to bile to intestine and back to the hepatocytes is called the enterohepatic circulation. Because of this circulation, only a small fraction of the bile salts that enter the intestine are excreted in the feces. This decreases the need for active synthesis of bile salts by the liver cells.

Approximately half of the bilirubin, a pigment derived from the breakdown of red blood cells, is a component of bile. It is converted by the intestinal flora into urobilinogen, a highly soluble substance. Urobilinogen is either excreted in the feces or returned to the portal circulation, where it is reexcreted into the bile. About 5% is normally absorbed into the general circulation and then excreted by the kidneys (Porth & Matfin, 2009).

If the flow of bile is impeded (eg, by gallstones in the bile ducts), bilirubin does not enter the intestine. As a result, blood levels of bilirubin increase. This causes increased renal excretion of urobilinogen, which results from conversion of bilirubin in the small intestine, and decreased excretion in the stool. These changes produce many of the signs and symptoms seen in gallbladder disorders.

The Pancreas

The pancreas, located in the upper abdomen, has **endocrine** as well as **exocrine** functions (see Fig. 40-1). The exocrine functions include secretion of pancreatic enzymes into the gastrointestinal (GI) tract through the pancreatic duct. The endocrine functions include secretion of insulin, glucagon, and somatostatin directly into the bloodstream.

The Exocrine Pancreas

The secretions of the exocrine portion of the pancreas are collected in the pancreatic duct, which joins the common bile duct and enters the duodenum at the ampulla of Vater. Surrounding the ampulla is the sphincter of Oddi, which partially controls the rate at which secretions from the pancreas and the gallbladder enter the duodenum.

The secretions of the exocrine pancreas are digestive enzymes high in protein content and an electrolyte-rich fluid. The secretions, which are very alkaline because of their high concentration of sodium bicarbonate, are capable of neutralizing the highly acid gastric juice that enters the duodenum. The enzyme secretions include **amylase,** which aids in the digestion of carbohydrates; **trypsin,** which aids in the digestion of proteins; and **lipase,** which aids in the digestion of fats. Other enzymes that promote the breakdown of more complex foodstuffs are also secreted.

Hormones originating in the GI tract stimulate the secretion of these exocrine pancreatic juices. The hormone **secretin** is the major stimulus for increased bicarbonate secretion from the pancreas, and the major stimulus for digestive enzyme secretion is the hormone CCK-PZ. The vagus nerve also influences exocrine pancreatic secretion.

The Endocrine Pancreas

The islets of Langerhans, the endocrine part of the pancreas, are collections of cells embedded in the pancreatic tissue. They are composed of alpha, beta, and delta cells. The hormone produced by the beta cells is called insulin;

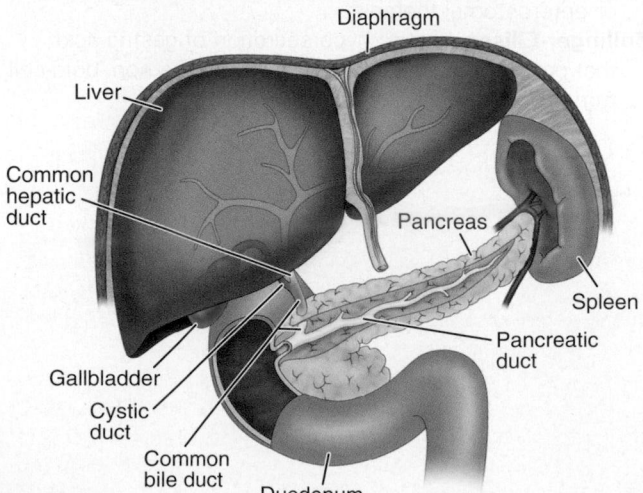

Figure 40-1 The liver, biliary system, and pancreas.

the alpha cells secrete glucagon, and the delta cells secrete somatostatin.

Insulin

A major action of insulin is to lower blood glucose by permitting entry of glucose into the cells of the liver, muscle, and other tissues, where it is either stored as glycogen or used for energy. Insulin also promotes the storage of fat in adipose tissue and the synthesis of proteins in various body tissues. In the absence of insulin, glucose cannot enter the cells and is excreted in the urine. This condition, called diabetes mellitus, can be diagnosed by high levels of glucose in the blood. In diabetes mellitus, stored fats and protein are used for energy instead of glucose, causing loss of body mass. (Diabetes mellitus is discussed in detail in Chapter 41.) The level of glucose in the blood normally regulates the rate of insulin secretion from the pancreas.

Glucagon

The effect of glucagon (opposite to that of insulin) is chiefly to raise the blood glucose by converting glycogen to glucose in the liver. Glucagon is secreted by the pancreas in response to a decrease in the level of blood glucose.

Somatostatin

Somatostatin exerts a hypoglycemic effect by interfering with release of growth hormone from the pituitary and glucagon from the pancreas, both of which tend to raise blood glucose levels.

Endocrine Control of Carbohydrate Metabolism

Glucose required for energy is derived by metabolism of ingested carbohydrates and also from proteins by the process of gluconeogenesis. Glucose can be stored temporarily in the form of glycogen in the liver, muscles, and other tissues. The endocrine system controls the level of blood glucose by regulating the rate at which glucose is synthesized, stored, and moved to and from the bloodstream. Through the action of hormones, blood glucose is normally maintained at less than 100 mg/dL (5.5 mmol/L). Insulin is the primary hormone that lowers the blood glucose level. Hormones that raise the blood glucose level are glucagon, epinephrine, adrenocorticosteroids, growth hormone, and thyroid hormone.

The endocrine and exocrine functions of the pancreas are interrelated. The major exocrine function is to facilitate digestion through secretion of enzymes into the proximal duodenum. Secretin and CCK-PZ are hormones from the GI tract that aid in the digestion of food substances by controlling the secretions of the pancreas. Neural factors also influence pancreatic enzyme secretion. Considerable dysfunction of the pancreas must occur before enzyme secretion decreases and protein and fat digestion becomes impaired. Pancreatic enzyme secretion is normally 1500 to 2500 mL/day.

 ### Gerontologic Considerations

There is little change in the size of the pancreas with age. However, there is an increase in fibrous material and some fatty deposition in the normal pancreas in people older than 70 years of age. Some localized arteriosclerotic changes occur with age. There is also a decreased rate of pancreatic secretion (decreased lipase, amylase, and trypsin) and decreased bicarbonate output in older people. Some impairment of normal fat absorption occurs with increasing age, possibly because of delayed gastric emptying and pancreatic insufficiency. Decreased calcium absorption may also occur. These changes require care in interpreting diagnostic test results in the normal elderly patient and in providing dietary counseling.

DISORDERS OF THE GALLBLADDER

Several disorders affect the biliary system and interfere with normal drainage of bile into the duodenum. These disorders include inflammation of the biliary system and carcinoma that obstructs the biliary tree. Gallbladder disease with gallstones is the most common disorder of the biliary system. Although not all occurrences of gallbladder inflammation (**cholecystitis**) are related to gallstones (**cholelithiasis**), more than 90% of patients with acute cholecystitis have gallstones. However, most of the 15 million Americans with gallstones have no pain and are unaware of the presence of stones.

Cholecystitis

Cholecystitis, acute inflammation of the gallbladder, causes pain, tenderness, and rigidity of the upper right abdomen that may radiate to the midsternal area or right shoulder and is associated with nausea, vomiting, and the usual signs of an acute inflammation. An empyema of the gallbladder develops if the gallbladder becomes filled with purulent fluid (pus).

Calculous cholecystitis is the cause of more than 90% of cases of acute cholecystitis (Feldman, Friedman & Brandt, 2006). In calculous cholecystitis, a gallbladder stone obstructs bile outflow. Bile remaining in the gallbladder initiates a chemical reaction; autolysis and edema occur; and the blood vessels in the gallbladder are compressed, compromising its vascular supply. Gangrene of the gallbladder with perforation may result. Bacteria play a minor role in acute cholecystitis; however, secondary infection of bile occurs in approximately 50% of cases. The organisms involved are generally enteric (normally live in the GI tract) and include *Escherichia coli*, *Klebsiella* species, and *Streptococcus*. Bacterial contamination is not believed to stimulate the actual onset of acute cholecystitis (Feldman, et al., 2006).

Acalculous cholecystitis describes acute gallbladder inflammation in the absence of obstruction by gallstones. Acalculous cholecystitis occurs after major surgical procedures, severe trauma, or burns. Other factors associated with this type of cholecystitis include torsion, cystic duct obstruction, primary bacterial infections of the gallbladder, and multiple blood transfusions. It is speculated that acalculous cholecystitis is caused by alterations in fluids and electrolytes and alterations in regional blood flow in the visceral circulation. Bile stasis (lack of gallbladder contraction) and increased viscosity of the bile are also thought to play a role.

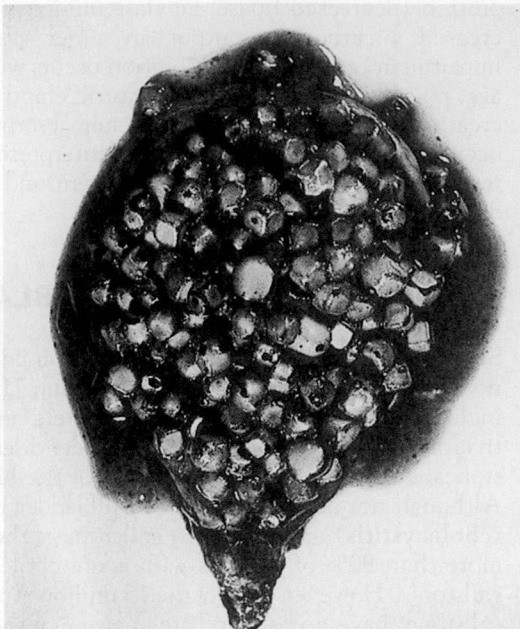
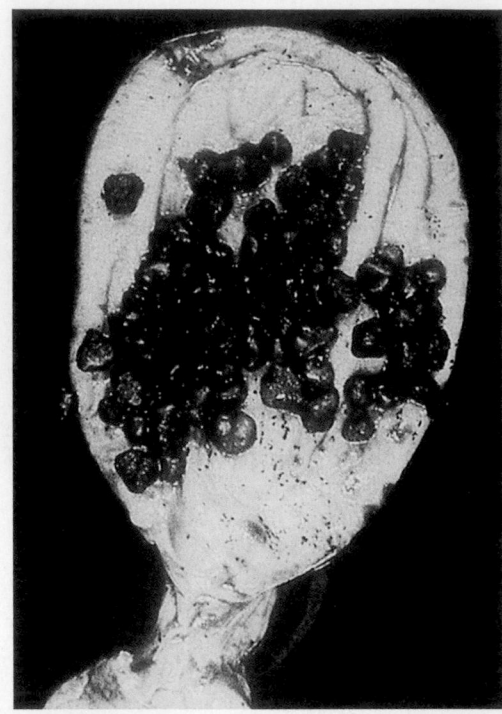

Figure 40-2 Examples of cholesterol gallstones (*left*) made up of a coalescence of multiple small stones and pigment gallstones (*right*) composed of calcium bilirubinate. From Rubin, E. & Farber, J. L. (2005). *Pathology* (4th ed.). Philadelphia: Lippincott Williams & Wilkins.

The occurrence of acalculous cholecystitis with major surgical procedures or trauma makes its diagnosis difficult.

Cholelithiasis

Calculi, or gallstones, usually form in the gallbladder from the solid constituents of bile; they vary greatly in size, shape, and composition (Fig. 40-2). They are uncommon in children and young adults but become more prevalent with increasing age, affecting 30% to 40% of people by the age of 80 years.

Pathophysiology

There are two major types of gallstones: those composed predominantly of pigment and those composed primarily of cholesterol. Pigment stones probably form when unconjugated pigments in the bile precipitate to form stones; these stones account for about 10% to 25% of cases in the United States (Feldman, et al., 2006). The risk of developing such stones is increased in patients with cirrhosis, hemolysis, and infections of the biliary tract. Pigment stones cannot be dissolved and must be removed surgically.

Cholesterol stones account for most of the remaining 75% of cases of gallbladder disease in the United States. Cholesterol, a normal constituent of bile, is insoluble in water. Its solubility depends on bile acids and lecithin (phospholipids) in bile. In gallstone-prone patients, there is decreased bile acid synthesis and increased cholesterol synthesis in the liver, resulting in bile supersaturated with cholesterol, which precipitates out of the bile to form stones. The cholesterol-saturated bile predisposes to the formation of gallstones and acts as an irritant that produces inflammatory changes in the gallbladder.

Two to three times more women than men develop cholesterol stones and gallbladder disease; affected women are usually older than 40 years of age, multiparous, and obese. Stone formation is more frequent in people who use oral contraceptives, estrogens, or clofibrate; these medications are known to increase biliary cholesterol saturation. The incidence of stone formation increases with age as a result of increased hepatic secretion of cholesterol and decreased bile acid synthesis. In addition, there is an increased risk because of malabsorption of bile salts in patients with GI disease or T-tube fistula and in those who have undergone ileal resection or bypass. The incidence is also greater in people with diabetes (Chart 40-1).

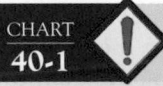 **CHART 40-1** ! *Risk Factors for Cholelithiasis*

- Obesity
- Women, especially those who have had multiple pregnancies or who are of Native American or U.S. Southwestern Hispanic ethnicity
- Frequent changes in weight
- Rapid weight loss (leads to rapid development of gallstones and high risk of symptomatic disease)
- Treatment with high-dose estrogen (eg, in prostate cancer)
- Low-dose estrogen therapy–a small increase in the risk of gallstones
- Ileal resection or disease
- Cystic fibrosis
- Diabetes mellitus

Clinical Manifestations

Gallstones may be silent, producing no pain and only mild GI symptoms. Such stones may be detected incidentally during surgery or evaluation for unrelated problems.

The patient with gallbladder disease resulting from gallstones may develop two types of symptoms: those due to disease of the gallbladder itself and those due to obstruction of the bile passages by a gallstone. The symptoms may be acute or chronic. Epigastric distress, such as fullness, abdominal distention, and vague pain in the right upper quadrant of the abdomen, may occur. This distress may follow a meal rich in fried or fatty foods.

Pain and Biliary Colic

If a gallstone obstructs the cystic duct, the gallbladder becomes distended, inflamed, and eventually infected (acute cholecystitis). The patient develops a fever and may have a palpable abdominal mass. The patient may have biliary colic with excruciating upper right abdominal pain that radiates to the back or right shoulder. Biliary colic is usually associated with nausea and vomiting, and it is noticeable several hours after a heavy meal. The patient moves about restlessly, unable to find a comfortable position. In some patients, the pain is constant rather than colicky.

Such a bout of biliary colic is caused by contraction of the gallbladder, which cannot release bile because of obstruction by the stone. When distended, the fundus of the gallbladder comes in contact with the abdominal wall in the region of the right ninth and tenth costal cartilages. This produces marked tenderness in the right upper quadrant on deep inspiration and prevents full inspiratory excursion.

The pain of acute cholecystitis may be so severe that analgesics are required. The use of morphine has traditionally been avoided because of concern that it could cause spasm of the sphincter of Oddi, and meperidine (Demerol) has been used instead. This is controversial, because morphine is the preferred analgesic agent for management of acute pain, and some metabolites of meperidine are toxic to the central nervous system (CNS). Furthermore, all opioids stimulate the sphincter of Oddi to some degree (Porth & Matfin, 2009).

If the gallstone is dislodged and no longer obstructs the cystic duct, the gallbladder drains and the inflammatory process subsides after a relatively short time. If the gallstone continues to obstruct the duct, abscess, necrosis, and perforation with generalized peritonitis may result.

Jaundice

Jaundice occurs in a few patients with gallbladder disease, usually with obstruction of the common bile duct. The bile, which is no longer carried to the duodenum, is absorbed by the blood and gives the skin and mucous membranes a yellow color. This is frequently accompanied by marked pruritus (itching) of the skin.

Changes in Urine and Stool Color

The excretion of the bile pigments by the kidneys gives the urine a very dark color. The feces, no longer colored with bile pigments, are grayish, like putty, or clay-colored.

Vitamin Deficiency

Obstruction of bile flow interferes with absorption of the fat-soluble vitamins A, D, E, and K. Patients may exhibit deficiencies of these vitamins if biliary obstruction has been prolonged. For example, a patient may have bleeding caused by vitamin K deficiency (vitamin K is necessary for normal blood clotting).

Assessment and Diagnostic Findings

Table 40-1 identifies various procedures and their diagnostic uses.

Abdominal X-Ray

If gallbladder disease is suspected, an abdominal x-ray may be obtained to exclude other causes of symptoms. However, only 15% to 20% of gallstones are calcified sufficiently to be visible on such x-ray studies.

Ultrasonography

Ultrasonography has replaced cholecystography (discussed later) as the diagnostic procedure of choice because it is rapid and accurate and can be used in patients with liver dysfunction and jaundice. It does not expose patients to ionizing radiation. The procedure is most accurate if the patient fasts overnight so that the gallbladder is distended. Ultrasonography can detect calculi in the gallbladder or a dilated common bile duct with 95% accuracy.

Table 40-1	STUDIES USED IN THE DIAGNOSIS OF BILIARY TRACT AND PANCREATIC DISEASE
Studies	**Diagnostic Uses**
Cholecystogram, cholangiogram	To visualize gallbladder and bile duct
Celiac axis arteriography	To visualize liver and pancreas
Laparoscopy	To visualize anterior surface of liver, gallbladder, and mesentery through a trocar
Ultrasonography	To show size of abdominal organs and presence of masses
Helical computed tomography (CT scans) and magnetic resonance imaging (MRI)	To detect neoplasms; diagnose cysts, pseudocysts, abscess, and hematomas
Endoscopic retrograde cholangiopancreatography (ERCP)	To visualize biliary structures and pancreas via endoscopy
Endoscopic ultrasound (EUS)	To identify small tumors and to facilitate fine-needle aspiration biopsy of tumors or lymph nodes for diagnosis
Serum alkaline phosphatase	In absence of bone disease, to measure biliary tract obstruction
Gamma-glutamyl (GGT), gamma-glutamyl trans-peptidase (GGTP), lactate dehydrogenase (LDH)	Markers for biliary stasis; also elevated in alcohol abuse
Cholesterol levels	Elevated in biliary obstruction; decreased in parenchymal liver disease

Radionuclide Imaging or Cholescintigraphy

Cholescintigraphy is used successfully in the diagnosis of acute cholecystitis or blockage of a bile duct. In this procedure, a radioactive agent is administered intravenously. It is taken up by the hepatocytes and excreted rapidly through the biliary tract. The biliary tract is then scanned, and images of the gallbladder and biliary tract are obtained. This test is more expensive than ultrasonography, takes longer to perform, exposes the patient to radiation, and cannot detect gallstones. It is often used when ultrasonography is not conclusive.

Cholecystography

Although cholecystography has been replaced by ultrasonography as the test of choice, it is still used if ultrasound equipment is not available or if the ultrasound results are inconclusive. Oral cholangiography may be performed to detect gallstones and to assess the ability of the gallbladder to fill, concentrate its contents, contract, and empty. If the patient is not allergic to iodine or seafood, an iodide-containing contrast agent that is excreted by the liver and concentrated in the gallbladder is administered 10 to 12 hours before the x-ray study. The normal gallbladder fills with this radiopaque substance. If gallstones are present, they appear as shadows on the x-ray film.

Oral cholecystography is likely to continue to be used as part of the evaluation of the few patients who have been treated with gallstone **dissolution therapy** or lithotripsy.

Endoscopic Retrograde Cholangiopancreatography

Endoscopic retrograde cholangiopancreatography (ERCP) permits direct visualization of structures that previously could be seen only during laparotomy. The examination of the hepatobiliary system is carried out via a side-viewing flexible fiberoptic endoscope inserted through the esophagus to the descending duodenum (Fig. 40-3). Multiple position changes are required to pass the endoscope during the procedure, beginning in the left semiprone position.

Fluoroscopy and multiple x-rays are used during ERCP to evaluate the presence and location of ductal stones. Careful insertion of a catheter through the endoscope into the common bile duct is the most important step in sphincterotomy (division of the muscles of the biliary sphincter) for gallstone extraction via this technique (see later discussion).

Nursing Implications

The procedure requires a cooperative patient to permit insertion of the endoscope without damage to the GI tract structures, including the biliary tree. Before the procedure, the patient is given an explanation of the procedure and his or her role in it. The patient takes nothing by mouth for several hours before the procedure. Moderate sedation is used, and the sedated patient must be monitored closely. It may be necessary to administer medications, such as glucagon or anticholinergics, to make cannulation easier by decreasing duodenal peristalsis. The nurse observes closely for signs of respiratory and central nervous system depression, hypotension, oversedation, and vomiting (if glucagon is administered). During ERCP, the nurse monitors intravenous (IV) fluids, administers medications, and positions the patient.

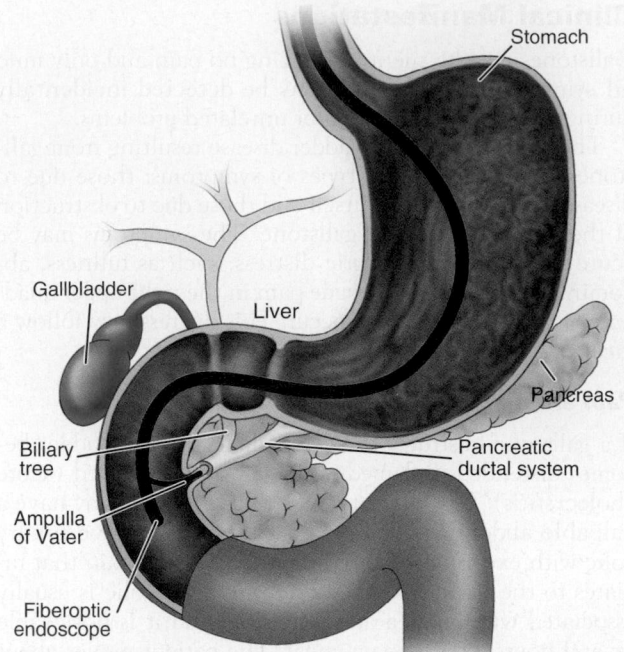

Figure 40-3 Endoscopic retrograde cholangiopancreatography (ERCP). A fiberoptic duodenoscope, with side-viewing apparatus, is inserted into the duodenum. The ampulla of Vater is catheterized, and the biliary tree is injected with contrast agent. The pancreatic ductal system is also assessed, if indicated. This procedure is of special value in visualizing neoplasms of the ampulla area and extracting a biopsy specimen.

After the procedure, the nurse monitors the patient's condition, observing vital signs and monitoring for signs of perforation or infection. The nurse also monitors the patient for side effects of any medications received during the procedure and for return of the gag and cough reflexes after the use of local anesthetics.

Percutaneous Transhepatic Cholangiography

Percutaneous transhepatic cholangiography involves the injection of dye directly into the biliary tract. Because of the relatively large concentration of dye that is introduced into the biliary system, including the hepatic ducts within the liver, the entire length of the common bile duct, the cystic duct, and the gallbladder is outlined clearly.

This procedure can be carried out even in the presence of liver dysfunction and jaundice. It is useful for (1) distinguishing jaundice caused by liver disease (hepatocellular jaundice) from that caused by biliary obstruction, (2) investigating the GI symptoms of a patient whose gallbladder has been removed, (3) locating stones within the bile ducts, and (4) diagnosing cancer involving the biliary system.

This sterile procedure is performed under moderate sedation on a patient who has been fasting; the patient receives local anesthesia and moderate sedation. Coagulation parameters and platelet count should be normal to minimize the risk of bleeding. Broad-spectrum antibiotics are administered during the procedure because of the high prevalence of bacterial colonization from obstructed biliary systems. After infiltration with a local anesthetic agent has occurred, a flexible needle is inserted into the liver from the right side in the midclavicular line immediately beneath the right costal margin. Successful entry of a duct is noted when bile is aspirated or on injection of a contrast agent. Ultrasound can be used to guide puncture of the duct. Bile is aspirated and samples are sent for bacteriology and cytology. A water-soluble contrast agent is injected to fill the biliary system. The fluoroscopy table is tilted and the patient is repositioned to allow x-rays to be taken in multiple projections. Delayed x-ray views can identify abnormalities of more distant ducts and determine the length of a stricture or multiple strictures. Before the needle is removed, as much dye and bile as possible are aspirated to forestall subsequent leakage into the needle tract and eventually into the peritoneal cavity, thus minimizing the risk of bile peritonitis.

▶ NURSING ALERT

Although the complication rate after this procedure is low, the nurse must closely observe the patient for symptoms of bleeding, peritonitis, and septicemia. The nurse assesses the patient for pain and indications of these complications and reports them promptly to the physician. Antibiotic agents are often prescribed to minimize the risk of sepsis and septic shock.

Medical Management

The major objectives of medical therapy are to reduce the incidence of acute episodes of gallbladder pain and cholecystitis by supportive and dietary management and, if possible, to remove the cause of cholecystitis by pharmacologic therapy, endoscopic procedures, or surgical intervention. Although nonsurgical approaches eliminate risks associated with surgery, these approaches are associated with persistent symptoms or recurrent stone formation. Most of the nonsurgical approaches, including lithotripsy and dissolution of gallstones, provide only temporary solutions to gallstone problems and are infrequently used in the United States. In some instances, other treatment approaches may be indicated; these are described later.

Removal of the gallbladder (**cholecystectomy**) through traditional surgical approaches was the standard treatment for more than 100 years. It has largely been replaced by **laparoscopic cholecystectomy** (removal of the gallbladder through a small incision through the umbilicus). As a result, surgical risks have decreased, along with the length of hospital stay and the long recovery period required after standard surgical cholecystectomy. In relatively rare instances, a standard surgical procedure may be necessary.

Nutritional and Supportive Therapy

Approximately 80% of the patients with acute gallbladder inflammation achieve remission with rest, IV fluids, nasogastric suction, analgesia, and antibiotic agents. Unless the patient's condition deteriorates, surgical intervention is delayed just until the acute symptoms subside (usually within a few days). At this time, the patient should undergo a laparoscopic cholecystectomy (Goldman & Ausiello, 2008).

The diet required immediately after an episode is usually limited to low-fat liquids. These can include powdered supplements high in protein and carbohydrate stirred into skim milk. Cooked fruits, rice or tapioca, lean meats, mashed potatoes, non–gas-forming vegetables, bread, coffee, or tea may be added as tolerated. The patient should avoid eggs, cream, pork, fried foods, cheese, rich dressings, gas-forming vegetables, and alcohol. It is important to remind the patient that fatty foods may induce an episode of cholecystitis. Dietary management may be the major mode of therapy in patients who have had only dietary intolerance to fatty foods and vague GI symptoms (Dudek, 2006).

Pharmacologic Therapy

Ursodeoxycholic acid (UDCA [URSO, Actigall]) and chenodeoxycholic acid (chenodiol or CDCA [Chenix]) have been used to dissolve small, radiolucent gallstones composed primarily of cholesterol. UDCA has fewer side effects than chenodiol and can be administered in smaller doses to achieve the same effect. It acts by inhibiting the synthesis and secretion of cholesterol, thereby desaturating bile. Treatment with UDCA can reduce the size of existing stones, dissolve small stones, and prevent new stones from forming. Six to 12 months of therapy are required in many patients to dissolve stones, and monitoring of the patient for recurrence of symptoms or the occurrence of side effects (eg, GI symptoms, pruritus, headache) is required during this time. The effective dose of medication depends on body weight. This method of treatment is generally indicated for patients who refuse surgery or for whom surgery is considered too risky.

Patients with significant, frequent symptoms; cystic duct occlusion; or pigment stones are not candidates for therapy with UDCA. Laparoscopic or open cholecystectomy is more appropriate for symptomatic patients with acceptable operative risk.

Nonsurgical Removal of Gallstones

Dissolving Gallstones

Several methods have been used to dissolve gallstones by infusion of a solvent (mono-octanoin or methyl tertiary butyl ether [MTBE]) into the gallbladder. The solvent can be infused through the following routes: through a tube or catheter inserted percutaneously directly into the gallbladder; through a tube or drain inserted through a T-tube tract to dissolve stones not removed at the time of surgery; endoscopically with ERCP; or via a transnasal biliary catheter.

In the latter procedure, the catheter is introduced through the mouth and inserted into the common bile duct. The upper end of the tube is then rerouted from the mouth to the nose and left in place. This enables the patient to eat and drink normally while passage of stones is monitored or chemical solvents are infused to dissolve the stones. This method of dissolution of stones is not widely used.

Stone Removal by Instrumentation

Several nonsurgical methods are used to remove stones that were not removed at the time of cholecystectomy or have become lodged in the common bile duct (Fig. 40-4A,B). A catheter and instrument with a basket attached are threaded through the T-tube tract or fistula formed at the time of T-tube insertion; the basket is used to retrieve and remove the stones lodged in the common bile duct.

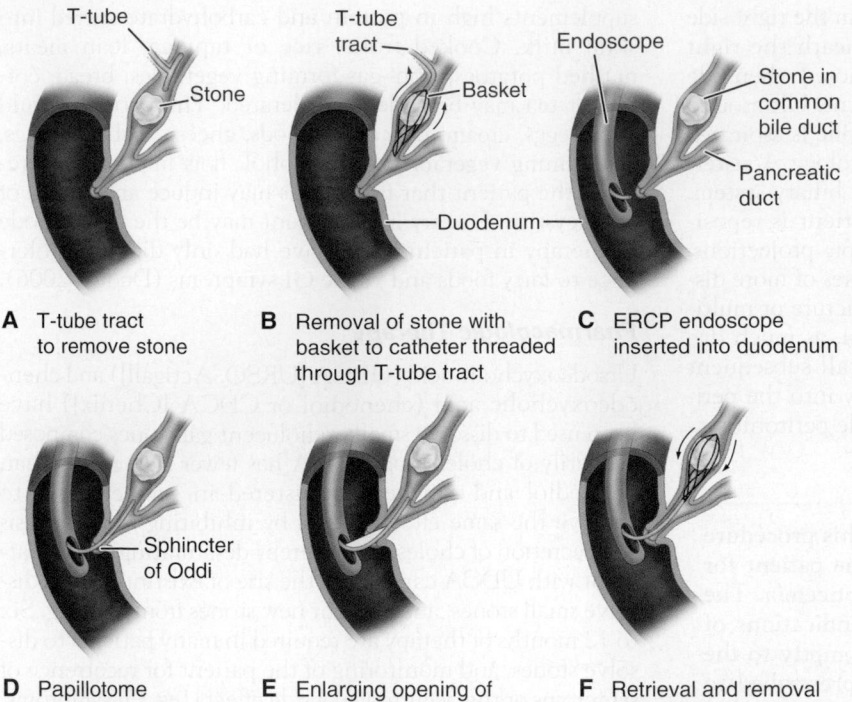

A T-tube tract to remove stone

B Removal of stone with basket to catheter threaded through T-tube tract

C ERCP endoscope inserted into duodenum

D Papillotome inserted into common bile duct

E Enlarging opening of sphincter of Oddi

F Retrieval and removal of stone with basket inserted through endoscope

Figure 40-4 Nonsurgical techniques for removing gallstones.

A second procedure involves the use of the ERCP endoscope (Fig. 40-4C). After the endoscope is inserted, a cutting instrument is passed through the endoscope into the ampulla of Vater of the common bile duct. It may be used to cut the submucosal fibers, or papilla, of the sphincter of Oddi, enlarging the opening, which may allow the lodged stones to pass spontaneously into the duodenum. Another instrument with a small basket or balloon at its tip may be inserted through the endoscope to retrieve the stones (Fig. 40-4D–F). The patient is observed closely for bleeding, perforation, and the development of pancreatitis or sepsis.

The ERCP procedure is particularly useful in diagnosis and treatment of patients who have symptoms after biliary tract surgery, patients with intact gallbladders, and patients for whom surgery is particularly hazardous.

Intracorporeal Lithotripsy

Stones in the gallbladder or common bile duct may be fragmented by means of laser pulse technology. A laser pulse is directed under fluoroscopic guidance with the use of devices that can distinguish between stones and tissue. The laser pulse produces rapid expansion and disintegration of plasma on the stone surface, resulting in a mechanical shock wave. Electrohydraulic lithotripsy uses a probe with two electrodes that deliver electric sparks in rapid pulses, creating expansion of the liquid environment surrounding the gallstones. This results in pressure waves that cause stones to fragment. This technique can be used percutaneously with a basket or balloon catheter system or by direct visualization through an endoscope. Repeated procedures may be necessary because of stone size, local anatomy, bleeding, or technical difficulty. A nasobiliary tube can be inserted to allow

for biliary decompression and to prevent stone impaction in the common bile duct. This approach allows time for improvement in the patient's clinical condition until gallstones are cleared endoscopically, percutaneously, or surgically.

Extracorporeal Shock Wave Lithotripsy

Extracorporeal shock wave therapy (lithotripsy or ESWL) has been used for nonsurgical fragmentation of gallstones. **Lithotripsy,** a noninvasive procedure, uses repeated shock waves directed at the gallstones in the gallbladder or common bile duct to fragment the stones. The waves are transmitted to the body through a fluid-filled bag or by immersing the patient in a water bath. After the stones are gradually broken up, the stone fragments can be spontaneously passed from the gallbladder or common bile duct, removed by endoscopy, or dissolved with oral bile acid or solvents. Because the procedure requires no incision and no hospitalization, patients are usually treated as outpatients, but usually several sessions are necessary. This procedure has largely been replaced by laparoscopic cholecystectomy. ESWL is used in some centers for a small percentage of suitable patients (those with common bile duct stones who may not be surgical candidates), sometimes in combination with dissolution therapy.

Surgical Management

Surgical treatment of gallbladder disease and gallstones is carried out to relieve persistent symptoms, to remove the cause of biliary colic, and to treat acute cholecystitis. Surgery may be delayed until the patient's symptoms have subsided, or it may be performed as an emergency procedure, if necessitated by the patient's condition.

Preoperative Measures

Chest x-ray, electrocardiogram (ECG), and liver function tests may be performed in addition to x-ray studies of the gallbladder. Vitamin K may be administered if the prothrombin level is low. Nutritional requirements are considered, and, if the nutritional status is suboptimal, it may be necessary to provide IV glucose with protein supplements to aid wound healing and help prevent liver damage.

Preparation for gallbladder surgery is similar to that for any upper abdominal laparotomy or laparoscopy. Instructions and explanations are given before surgery with regard to turning and deep breathing. Postoperative pneumonia and atelectasis can be avoided by deep-breathing exercises and frequent turning. The patient should be informed that drainage tubes and a nasogastric tube and suction might be required during the immediate postoperative period if an open cholecystectomy is performed.

Laparoscopic Cholecystectomy

Laparoscopic cholecystectomy (Fig. 40-5) has dramatically changed the approach to the management of cholecystitis. It has become the new standard for therapy of symptomatic gallstones. Approximately 700,000 patients in the United States require surgery each year for removal of the gallbladder, and 80% to 90% of them are candidates for laparoscopic cholecystectomy (Feldman, et al., 2006). If the common bile duct is thought to be obstructed by a gallstone, an ERCP with sphincterotomy may be performed to explore the duct before laparoscopy.

Before the procedure, the patient is informed that an open abdominal procedure may be necessary, and general anesthesia is administered. Laparoscopic cholecystectomy is performed through a small incision or puncture made through the abdominal wall at the umbilicus. The abdominal cavity is insufflated with carbon dioxide (pneumoperitoneum) to assist in inserting the laparoscope and to aid in visualizing the abdominal structures. The fiberoptic scope is inserted through the small umbilical incision. Several additional punctures or small incisions are made in the abdominal wall to introduce other surgical instruments into the operative field. A camera attached to the laparoscope permits the surgeon to view the intra-abdominal field and biliary system on a television monitor. After the cystic duct is dissected, the common bile duct can be visualized by ultrasound or cholangiography to evaluate the anatomy and identify stones. The cystic artery is dissected free and clipped. The gallbladder is separated from the hepatic bed and removed from the abdominal cavity after bile and small stones are aspirated. Stone forceps also can be used to remove or crush larger stones.

With the laparoscopic procedure, the patient does not experience the paralytic ileus that occurs with open abdominal surgery and has less postoperative abdominal pain. The patient is often discharged from the hospital on the same day of surgery or within 1 or 2 days and resumes full activity and employment within 1 week after the surgery.

Conversion to a traditional abdominal surgical procedure may be necessary if problems are encountered during the laparoscopic procedure; this occurs in 2.2% of cases in the United States and 3.6% to 8.2% of cases internationally. Conversion to an open procedure occurs if there is inflammation in and around the gallbladder, making safe dissection of the porta hepatis difficult (Feldman, et al., 2006).

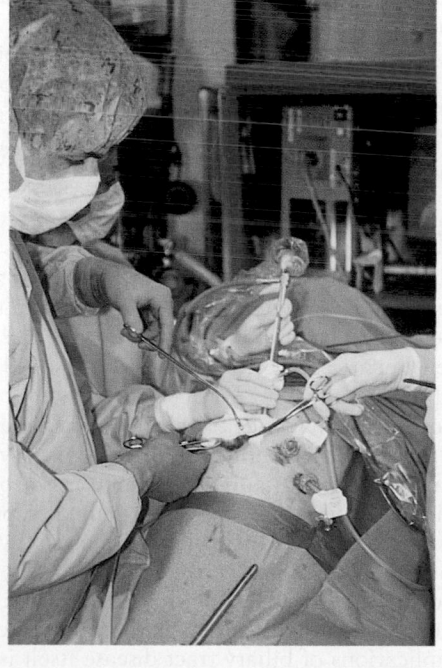
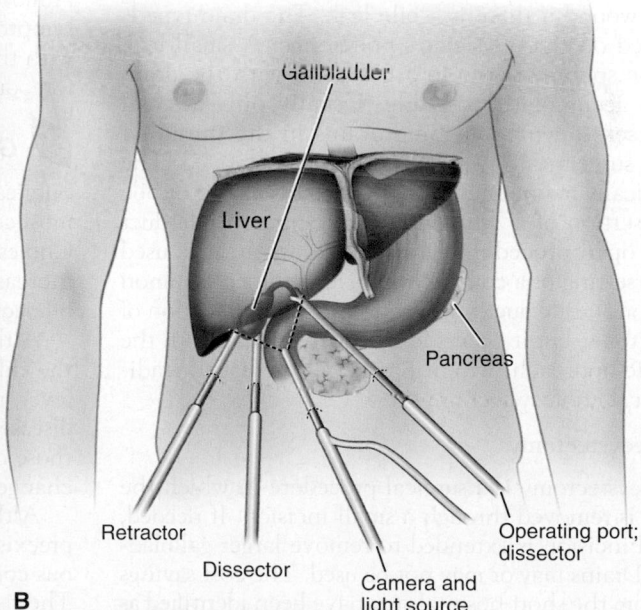

Figure 40-5 **A,** In laparoscopic cholecystectomy, the surgeon makes four small incisions (less than one half inch each) in the abdomen **(B)** and inserts a laparoscope with a miniature camera through the umbilical incision. The camera apparatus displays the gallbladder and adjacent tissues on a screen, allowing the surgeon to visualize the sections of the organ for removal.

(The porta hepatis is the fissure of the liver where the portal vein and the hepatic artery enter and the hepatic ducts exit the liver.) Careful screening of patients and identification of those at low risk for complications limit the frequency of conversion to an open abdominal procedure. However, with increasing use of laparoscopic procedures, the number of such conversions may increase.

The most serious complication after laparoscopic cholecystectomy is a bile duct injury, which may be identified and corrected at the time of the procedure. Patients with a postoperative bile leak may not develop symptoms until several days after the procedure, and some have an even more prolonged period before injury to the bile duct becomes apparent (Massoumi, Kiyici & Hertan, 2007). A bile leak may result in fluid collections, which can usually be managed by endoscopic stent placement. Bile peritonitis, a rare complication, may result in serious illness or death.

Because of the short hospital stay with uncomplicated laparoscopic cholecystectomies, it is important to provide written and verbal instructions about managing postoperative pain and reporting signs and symptoms of intra-abdominal complications, including loss of appetite, vomiting, pain, distention of the abdomen, and temperature elevation. Although recovery from laparoscopic cholecystectomy is rapid, patients are drowsy afterward. The patient must have assistance at home during the first 24 to 48 hours. If pain occurs in the right shoulder or scapular area (from migration of the carbon dioxide used to insufflate the abdominal cavity during the procedure), the nurse may recommend a heating pad for 15 to 20 minutes hourly.

Cholecystectomy

In cholecystectomy, the gallbladder is removed through an abdominal incision (usually right subcostal) after the cystic duct and artery are ligated. The procedure is performed for acute and chronic cholecystitis. In some patients, a drain is placed close to the gallbladder bed and brought out through a puncture wound if there is a bile leak. The drain type is chosen based on the physician's preference. A small leak should close spontaneously in a few days, with the drain preventing accumulation of bile. Usually only a small amount of serosanguineous fluid drains in the initial 24 hours after surgery; afterward, the drain is removed. The drain is typically maintained if there is excess oozing or bile leakage. Insertion of a T-tube into the common bile duct during the open procedure is now uncommon; it is used only in the setting of a complication (ie, retained common bile duct stone). Bile duct injury is a serious complication of cholecystectomy, but it occurs less frequently than with the laparoscopic approach, which has largely replaced traditional surgical cholecystectomy.

Mini-Cholecystectomy

Mini-cholecystectomy is a surgical procedure in which the gallbladder is removed through a small incision. If needed, the surgical incision is extended to remove larger gallbladder stones. Drains may or may not be used. The cost savings resulting from the short hospital stay have been identified as a major reason for pursuing this type of procedure. The procedure is controversial because it limits exposure to all the involved biliary structures.

Choledochostomy

Choledochostomy is reserved for the patient with acute cholecystitis who may be too ill to undergo a surgical procedure. It involves making an incision in the common duct, usually for removal of stones (choledochostomy). After the stones have been evacuated, a tube is usually inserted into the duct for drainage of bile until edema subsides. This tube is connected to gravity drainage tubing; the patient is monitored closely, and a laparoscopic cholecystectomy is planned for a future date after acute inflammation has resolved.

Surgical Cholecystostomy

Cholecystostomy is performed when the patient's condition precludes more extensive surgery or when an acute inflammatory reaction is severe. The gallbladder is surgically opened, stones and the bile or the purulent drainage are removed, and a drainage tube is secured with a purse-string suture. The drainage tube is connected to a drainage system to prevent bile from leaking around the tube or escaping into the peritoneal cavity. After recovery from the acute episode, the patient may return for subsequent laparoscopic cholecystectomy. Despite its lower risk, surgical cholecystostomy has a high mortality rate (reported to be as high as 20% to 30%) because of the underlying disease process.

Percutaneous Cholecystostomy

Percutaneous cholecystostomy has been used in the treatment and diagnosis of acute cholecystitis in patients who are poor risks for any surgical procedure or for general anesthesia. These may include patients with sepsis or severe cardiac, renal, pulmonary, or liver failure. Under local anesthesia, a fine needle is inserted through the abdominal wall and liver edge into the gallbladder under the guidance of ultrasound or computed tomography (CT). Bile is aspirated to ensure adequate placement of the needle, and a catheter is inserted into the gallbladder to decompress the biliary tract. Almost immediate relief of pain and resolution of signs and symptoms of sepsis and cholecystitis have been reported with this procedure. Antibiotic agents are administered before, during, and after the procedure.

 Gerontologic Considerations

Surgical intervention for disease of the biliary tract is the most common operative procedure performed in the elderly. Cholesterol saturation of bile increases with age because of increased hepatic secretion of cholesterol and decreased bile acid synthesis.

Although the incidence of gallstones increases with age, the elderly patient may not exhibit the typical symptoms of fever, pain, chills, and jaundice. Symptoms of biliary tract disease in the elderly may be accompanied or preceded by those of septic shock, which include oliguria, hypotension, changes in mental status, tachycardia, and tachypnea.

Although surgery in the elderly presents a risk because of preexisting associated diseases, the mortality rate from serious complications of biliary tract disease itself is also high. The risk of death and complications is increased in the elderly patient who undergoes emergency surgery for life-threatening disease of the biliary tract. Despite chronic illness in many elderly patients, elective cholecystectomy is usually well tolerated and can be carried out with low risk if expert assessment and care are provided before, during, and after the surgical procedure.

Because of recent changes in reimbursement for health care expenses, there has been a decrease in the number of elective surgical procedures performed, including cholecystectomies. As a result, patients requiring the procedure are seen in later stages of disease. At the same time, patients undergoing surgery are increasingly older than 60 years of age and may have complicated acute cholecystitis. The higher risk of complications and shorter hospital stay make it essential that older patients and their family members receive specific information about signs and symptoms of complications and measures to prevent them.

NURSING PROCESS

THE PATIENT UNDERGOING SURGERY FOR GALLBLADDER DISEASE

Assessment

The patient who is to undergo surgical treatment of gallbladder disease is often admitted to the hospital or same-day surgery unit on the morning of surgery. Preadmission testing is often completed a week or longer before admission. At that time, the nurse instructs the patient about the need to avoid smoking, to enhance pulmonary recovery postoperatively, and to avoid respiratory complications. It also is important to instruct the patient to avoid the use of aspirin and other agents (over-the-counter medications and herbal remedies) that can alter coagulation and other biochemical processes.

Assessment should focus on the patient's respiratory status. If a traditional surgical approach is planned, the high abdominal incision required during surgery may interfere with full respiratory excursion. The nurse notes a history of smoking, previous respiratory problems, shallow respirations, a persistent or ineffective cough, and the presence of adventitious breath sounds. Nutritional status is evaluated through a dietary history and a general examination performed at the time of preadmission testing. The nurse also reviews previously obtained laboratory results to obtain information about the patient's nutritional status.

Diagnosis

Nursing Diagnoses

Based on all the assessment data, the major postoperative nursing diagnoses for the patient undergoing surgery for gallbladder disease may include the following:

- Acute pain and discomfort related to surgical incision
- Impaired gas exchange related to the high abdominal surgical incision (if traditional surgical cholecystectomy was performed)
- Impaired skin integrity related to altered biliary drainage after surgical intervention (if a T-tube was inserted because of retained stones in the common bile duct or another drainage device was employed)
- Imbalanced nutrition, less than body requirements, related to inadequate bile secretion

- Deficient knowledge about self-care activities related to incision care, dietary modifications (if needed), medications, and reportable signs or symptoms (eg, fever, bleeding, vomiting)

Collaborative Problems/Potential Complications

Based on assessment data, potential complications may include the following:

- Bleeding
- GI symptoms (may be related to biliary leak or injury to the bowel)

Planning and Goals

The goals for the patient include relief of pain, adequate ventilation, intact skin and improved biliary drainage, optimal nutritional intake, absence of complications, and understanding of self-care routines.

Postoperative Nursing Interventions

After recovery from anesthesia, the patient is placed in the low Fowler's position. Fluids may be administered intravenously, and nasogastric suction (a nasogastric tube was probably inserted immediately before surgery for a nonlaparoscopic procedure) may be instituted to relieve abdominal distention. Water and other fluids are administered within hours after laparoscopic procedures. A soft diet is started after bowel sounds return, which is usually the next day if the laparoscopic approach is used.

Relieving Pain

The location of the subcostal incision in nonlaparoscopic gallbladder surgery often causes the patient to avoid turning and moving, to splint the affected site, and to take shallow breaths to prevent pain. Because full expansion of the lungs and gradually increased activity are necessary to prevent postoperative complications, the nurse administers analgesic agents as prescribed to relieve the pain and to promote well-being in addition to helping the patient turn, cough, breathe deeply, and ambulate as indicated. Use of a pillow or binder over the incision may reduce pain during these maneuvers.

Improving Respiratory Status

Patients undergoing biliary tract surgery are especially prone to pulmonary complications, as are all patients with upper abdominal incisions. Therefore, the nurse reminds the patient to take deep breaths and cough every hour to expand the lungs fully and prevent atelectasis. The early and consistent use of incentive spirometry also helps improve respiratory function. Early ambulation prevents pulmonary complications as well as other complications, such as thrombophlebitis. Pulmonary complications are more likely to occur in elderly patients, obese patients, and those with preexisting pulmonary disease.

Maintaining Skin Integrity and Promoting Biliary Drainage

In patients who have undergone a cholecystostomy or choledochostomy, the drainage tube must be connected immediately to a drainage receptacle. The nurse should fasten the tubing to the dressings or to the patient's gown, with enough leeway for the patient to move without dislodging or kinking the tube. Because a drainage system remains attached when the patient is ambulating, the drainage bag may be placed in a bathrobe pocket or fastened so that it is below the waist or common duct level. If a Penrose drain is used, the nurse changes the dressings as required.

After these surgical procedures, the patient is observed for indications of infection, leakage of bile into the peritoneal cavity, and obstruction of bile drainage. If bile is not draining properly, an obstruction is probably causing bile to be forced back into the liver and bloodstream. Because jaundice may result, the nurse should assess the color of the sclerae. The nurse should note and report right upper quadrant abdominal pain, nausea and vomiting, bile drainage around any drainage tube, clay-colored stools, and a change in vital signs.

Bile may continue to drain from the drainage tract in considerable quantities for some time, necessitating frequent changes of the outer dressings and protection of the skin from irritation (bile is corrosive to the skin).

To prevent total loss of bile, the physician may want the drainage tube or collection receptacle elevated above the level of the abdomen so that the bile drains externally only if pressure develops in the duct system. Every 24 hours, the nurse measures the bile collected and records the amount, color, and character of the drainage. After several days of drainage, the tube may be clamped for 1 hour before and after each meal to deliver bile to the duodenum to aid in digestion. Within 7 to 14 days, the drainage tube is removed. The patient who goes home with a drainage tube in place requires instruction and reassurance about the function and care of the tube.

In all patients with biliary drainage, the nurse (or the patient, if at home) observes the color of stools daily. Urine and stool specimens may be sent to the laboratory for examination for bile pigments. In this way, it is possible to determine whether the bile pigment is disappearing from the blood and is draining again into the duodenum. Maintaining a careful record of fluid intake and output is important.

Improving Nutritional Status

The nurse encourages the patient to eat a diet that is low in fats and high in carbohydrates and proteins immediately after surgery. At the time of hospital discharge, there are usually no special dietary instructions other than to maintain a nutritious diet and avoid excessive fats. Fat restriction usually is lifted in 4 to 6 weeks, when the biliary ducts dilate to accommodate the volume of bile once held by the gallbladder and when the ampulla of Vater again functions effectively. After this time, when the patient eats fat, adequate bile will be released into the GI tract to emulsify the fats and allow their digestion. This is in contrast to the condition before surgery, when fats may not have been digested completely or adequately and flatulence may have occurred. One purpose of gallbladder surgery is to allow a normal diet.

Monitoring and Managing Potential Complications

Bleeding may occur as a result of inadvertent puncture or injury to a major blood vessel. Postoperatively, the nurse closely monitors vital signs and inspects the surgical incisions and any drains for bleeding. The nurse also assesses the patient for increased tenderness and rigidity of the abdomen. If these signs and symptoms occur, they are reported to the

surgeon. The nurse instructs the patient and family to report any change in the color of stools, because this may indicate complications. GI symptoms, although not common, may occur with manipulation of the intestines during surgery.

After laparoscopic cholecystectomy, the nurse assesses the patient for anorexia, vomiting, pain, abdominal distension, and temperature elevation. These may indicate infection or disruption of the GI tract and should be reported to the surgeon promptly. Because the patient is discharged soon after laparoscopic surgery, the patient and family are instructed verbally and in writing about the importance of reporting these symptoms promptly.

Promoting Home and Community-Based Care

TEACHING PATIENTS SELF-CARE. The nurse instructs the patient about the medications that are prescribed (vitamins, anticholinergics, and antispasmodics) and their actions. It also is important to inform the patient and family about symptoms that should be reported to the physician, including jaundice, dark urine, pale-colored stools, pruritus, and signs of inflammation and infection, such as pain or fever.

Some patients report one to three bowel movements a day, which is a result of a continual trickle of bile through the choledochoduodenal junction after cholecystectomy. Usually, such frequency diminishes over a period of a few weeks to several months.

If a patient is discharged from the hospital with a drainage tube still in place, the patient and family need instructions about its management. The nurse instructs them in proper care of the drainage tube and the importance of reporting promptly any changes in the amount or characteristics of drainage. Assistance in securing the appropriate dressings reduces the patient's anxiety about going home with the drain or tube still in place. See Chart 40-2 for additional details.

CONTINUING CARE. With sufficient support at home, most patients recover quickly from a cholecystectomy. However, elderly or frail patients and those who live alone may require a referral for home care. During home visits, the nurse assesses the patient's physical status, especially wound healing, and progress toward recovery. Assessing the patient for adequacy of pain relief and pulmonary exercises is also important. If the patient has a drainage system in place, the nurse assesses it for patency and appropriate management by the patient and family. Assessing for signs of infection and teaching the patient about the signs and symptoms of infection are also important nursing interventions. The patient's understanding of the therapeutic regimen (medications, gradual return to normal activities) is assessed, and previous teaching is reinforced. The nurse emphasizes the importance of keeping follow-up appointments and reminds the patient and family of the importance of participating in health promotion activities and recommended health screening.

Evaluation

Expected Patient Outcomes

Expected patient outcomes may include the following:

1. Reports decrease in pain
   a. Splints abdominal incision to decrease pain

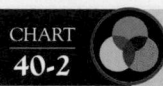

CHART 40-2

PATIENT EDUCATION
Managing Self-Care After Laparoscopic Cholecystectomy

Resuming Activity

- Begin light exercise (walking) immediately.
- Take a shower or bath after 1 or 2 days.
- Drive a car after 3 or 4 days.
- Avoid lifting objects exceeding 5 pounds after surgery, usually for 1 week.
- Resume sexual activity when desired.

Caring for the Wound

- Check puncture site daily for signs of infection.
- Wash puncture site with mild soap and water.
- Allow special adhesive strips on the puncture site to fall off. Do not pull them off.

Resuming Eating

- Resume your normal diet.
- If you had fat intolerance before surgery, gradually add fat back into your diet in small increments.

Managing Pain

- You may experience pain or discomfort in your right shoulder from the gas used to inflate your abdominal area during surgery. Sitting upright in bed or a chair, walking, or use of a heating pad may ease the discomfort.
- Take analgesics as needed and as prescribed. Report to surgeon if pain is unrelieved even with analgesic use.

Managing Follow-Up Care

- Make an appointment with your surgeon for 7 to 10 days after discharge.
- Call your surgeon if you experience any signs or symptoms of infection at or around the puncture site: redness, tenderness, swelling, heat, or drainage.
- Call your surgeon if you experience a fever of 37.7°C (100°F) or more for 2 consecutive days.
- Call your surgeon if you develop nausea, vomiting, or abdominal pain.

---

b. Avoids foods that cause pain

c. Uses postoperative analgesia as prescribed

2. Demonstrates appropriate respiratory function

a. Achieves full respiratory excursion, with deep inspiration and expiration

b. Coughs effectively, using pillow to splint abdominal incision

c. Uses postoperative analgesia as prescribed

d. Exercises as prescribed (eg, turns, ambulates)

3. Exhibits normal skin integrity around biliary drainage site (if applicable)

a. Is free of fever, abdominal pain, change in vital signs, and presence of bile, foul-smelling drainage, or pus around drainage tube

b. Demonstrates correct management of drainage tube (if applicable)

c. Identifies signs and symptoms of biliary obstruction to be noted and reported

d. Has serum bilirubin level within normal range

4. Obtains relief from dietary intolerance

a. Maintains adequate dietary intake and avoids foods that cause gastrointestinal symptoms

b. Reports decreased or absent nausea, vomiting, diarrhea, flatulence, and abdominal discomfort

5. Absence of complications

a. Has normal vital signs (blood pressure, pulse, respiratory rate and pattern, and temperature)

b. Reports absence of bleeding from GI tract and from biliary drainage tube or catheter (if present) and no evidence of bleeding in stool

c. Reports return of appetite and no evidence of vomiting, abdominal distention, or pain

d. Lists symptoms that should be reported to surgeon promptly and demonstrates an understanding of self-care, including wound care

DISORDERS OF THE PANCREAS

Pancreatitis (inflammation of the pancreas) is a serious disorder. The most basic classification system used to describe or categorize the various stages and forms of pancreatitis divides the disorder into acute and chronic forms. Acute pancreatitis can be a medical emergency associated with a high risk of life-threatening complications and mortality, whereas chronic pancreatitis often goes undetected until 80% to 90% of the exocrine and endocrine tissue is destroyed. Acute pancreatitis does not usually lead to chronic pancreatitis unless complications develop. However, chronic pancreatitis can be characterized by acute episodes.

Although the mechanisms causing pancreatic inflammation are unknown, pancreatitis is commonly described as autodigestion of the pancreas. It is believed that the pancreatic duct becomes temporarily obstructed, accompanied by hypersecretion of the exocrine enzymes of the pancreas. These enzymes enter the bile duct, where they are activated and, together with bile, back up (reflux) into the pancreatic duct, causing pancreatitis.

Acute Pancreatitis

Acute pancreatitis ranges from a mild, self-limited disorder to a severe, rapidly fatal disease that does not respond to any treatment. Approximately 185,000 cases of acute pancreatitis occur in the United States each year, of which 150,000 are the result of cholelithiasis or sustained alcohol abuse (Zinner & Ashley, 2007). Mild acute pancreatitis is characterized by edema and inflammation confined to the pancreas. Minimal organ dysfunction is present, and return to normal function usually occurs within 6 months. Although this is considered the milder form of pancreatitis, the patient is acutely ill and at risk for hypovolemic shock, fluid and electrolyte disturbances, and sepsis. A more widespread and complete enzymatic digestion of the gland characterizes severe acute pancreatitis. Enzymes damage the local blood vessels, and bleeding and thrombosis can occur. The tissue may become necrotic, with damage extending into the retroperitoneal tissues. Local complications include pancreatic cysts or abscesses and acute fluid collections in or near the pancreas. Patients who develop systemic complications with organ failure, such as pulmonary insufficiency with hypoxia, shock, renal failure, and GI bleeding, are also characterized as having severe acute pancreatitis.

 ## Gerontologic Considerations

Acute pancreatitis affects people of all ages, but the mortality rate associated with acute pancreatitis increases with advancing age. In addition, the pattern of complications changes with age. Younger patients tend to develop local complications; the incidence of multiple organ failure increases with age, possibly as a result of progressive decreases in physiologic function of major organs with increasing age. Close monitoring of major organ function (ie, lungs, kidneys) is essential, and aggressive treatment is necessary to reduce mortality from acute pancreatitis in the elderly.

Pathophysiology

Self-digestion of the pancreas by its own proteolytic enzymes, principally trypsin, causes acute pancreatitis. Eighty percent of patients with acute pancreatitis have biliary tract disease or a history of long-term alcohol abuse. These patients usually have had undiagnosed chronic pancreatitis before their first episode of acute pancreatitis. Gallstones enter the common bile duct and lodge at the ampulla of Vater, obstructing the flow of pancreatic juice or causing a reflux of bile from the common bile duct into the pancreatic duct, thus activating the powerful enzymes within the pancreas. Normally, these remain in an inactive form until the pancreatic secretions reach the lumen of the duodenum. Activation of the enzymes can lead to vasodilation, increased vascular permeability, necrosis, erosion, and hemorrhage (Zinner & Ashley, 2007).

Other less common causes of pancreatitis include bacterial or viral infection, with pancreatitis occasionally developing as a complication of mumps virus. Spasm and edema of the ampulla of Vater, caused by duodenitis, can probably produce pancreatitis. Blunt abdominal trauma, peptic ulcer disease, ischemic vascular disease, hyperlipidemia, hypercalcemia, and the use of corticosteroids, thiazide diuretics, oral contraceptives, and other medications have also been associated with an increased incidence of pancreatitis. Acute pancreatitis may develop after surgery on or near the pancreas or after instrumentation of the pancreatic duct. Acute idiopathic pancreatitis accounts for up to 10% of the cases of acute pancreatitis. Some experts postulate that these cases may be related to occult microlithiasis (small stones in the bile) (Zinner & Ashley, 2007). In addition, there is a small incidence of hereditary pancreatitis.

The overall mortality rate of patients with acute pancreatitis is high (2% to 10%) because of shock, anoxia, hypotension, or fluid and electrolyte imbalances. This mortal-

Chart 40-3 • *Criteria for Predicting Severity of Pancreatitis**

Criteria on Admission to Hospital

Age >55 years
WBC >16,000 mm³
Serum glucose >200 mg/dL (>11.1 mmol/L)
Serum LDH >350 IU/L (>350 U/L)
AST >250 U/mL (120 U/L)

Criteria Within 48 Hours of Hospital Admission

Fall in hematocrit >10% (>0.10)
BUN increase >5 mg/dL (>1.7 mmol/L)
Serum calcium <8 mg/dL (<2.0 mmol/L)
Base deficit >4 mEq/L (>4 mmol/L)
Fluid retention or sequestration >6 L
PO_2 <60 mm Hg

Two or fewer signs, 1% mortality; 3 or 4 signs, 15% mortality; 5 or 6 signs, 40% mortality; >6 signs, 100% mortality.
*Note: The more risk factors a patient has, the greater the severity and likelihood of complications or death.

ity rate may also be related to the 10% to 30% of patients with severe acute disease characterized by pancreatic and peripancreatic necrosis (Zinner & Ashley, 2007). Attacks of acute pancreatitis may result in complete recovery, may recur without permanent damage, or may progress to chronic pancreatitis. The patient who is admitted to the hospital with a diagnosis of pancreatitis is acutely ill and needs expert nursing and medical care.

The severity of acute alcoholic pancreatitis and its outcomes can be predicted based on clinical and laboratory data (Chart 40-3).

Clinical Manifestations

Severe abdominal pain is the major symptom of pancreatitis that causes the patient to seek medical care. Abdominal pain and tenderness and back pain result from irritation and edema of the inflamed pancreas. Increased tension on the pancreatic capsule and obstruction of the pancreatic ducts also contribute to the pain. Typically, the pain occurs in the midepigastrium. Pain is frequently acute in onset, occurring 24 to 48 hours after a very heavy meal or alcohol ingestion, and it may be diffuse and difficult to localize. It is generally more severe after meals and is unrelieved by antacids. Pain may be accompanied by abdominal distention; a poorly defined, palpable abdominal mass; decreased peristalsis; and vomiting that fails to relieve the pain or nausea.

The patient appears acutely ill. Abdominal guarding is present. A rigid or boardlike abdomen may develop and is generally an ominous sign, usually indicating peritonitis. Ecchymosis (bruising) in the flank or around the umbilicus may indicate severe pancreatitis. Nausea and vomiting are common in acute pancreatitis. The emesis is usually gastric in origin but may also be bile stained. Fever, jaundice, mental confusion, and agitation may also occur.

Hypotension is typical and reflects hypovolemia and shock caused by the loss of large amounts of protein-rich fluid into the tissues and peritoneal cavity. In addition to hypotension, the patient may develop tachycardia, cyanosis, and cold, clammy skin. Acute renal failure is common.

Respiratory distress and hypoxia are common, and the patient may develop diffuse pulmonary infiltrates, dyspnea, tachypnea, and abnormal blood gas values. Myocardial depression, hypocalcemia, hyperglycemia, and disseminated intravascular coagulation may also occur with acute pancreatitis.

Assessment and Diagnostic Findings

The diagnosis of acute pancreatitis is based on a history of abdominal pain, the presence of known risk factors, physical examination findings, and diagnostic findings. Serum amylase and lipase levels are used in making the diagnosis of acute pancreatitis, although their elevation can be attributed to many other causes (Feldman, et al., 2006). In most cases, serum amylase and lipase levels are elevated within 24 hours of the onset of the symptoms. Serum amylase usually returns to normal within 48 to 72 hours, but serum lipase levels may remain elevated for a longer period, often days longer than amylase. Urinary amylase levels also become elevated and remain elevated longer than serum amylase levels. The white blood cell count is usually elevated; hypocalcemia is present in many patients and correlates well with the severity of pancreatitis. Transient hyperglycemia and glucosuria and elevated serum bilirubin levels occur in some patients with acute pancreatitis.

X-ray studies of the abdomen and chest may be obtained to differentiate pancreatitis from other disorders that can cause similar symptoms and to detect pleural effusions. Ultrasound and contrast-enhanced CT scans are used to identify an increase in the diameter of the pancreas and to detect pancreatic cysts, abscesses, or pseudocysts.

Hematocrit and hemoglobin levels are used to monitor the patient for bleeding. Peritoneal fluid, obtained through paracentesis or peritoneal lavage, may contain increased levels of pancreatic enzymes. ERCP is rarely used in the diagnostic evaluation of acute pancreatitis, because the patient is acutely ill; however, it may be valuable in the treatment of gallstone pancreatitis.

Medical Management

Management of acute pancreatitis is directed toward relieving symptoms and preventing or treating complications. All oral intake is withheld to inhibit stimulation of the pancreas and its secretion of enzymes. Parenteral nutrition plays an important role in the nutritional support of patients with severe acute pancreatitis, particularly in those who are debilitated and those with a prolonged paralytic ileus (more than 48 to 72 hours) (Zinner & Ashley, 2007). Ongoing research has shown positive outcomes with the use of enteral feedings. The current recommendation is that, whenever possible, the enteral route should be used to meet nutritional needs in patients with pancreatitis. This strategy also has been found to prevent infectious complications, safely and cost effectively (DiMagno & DiMagno, 2007; Zinner & Ashley, 2007). Enteral feedings should be started early in the course of acute pancreatitis. Patients who do not tolerate enteral feeding require parenteral nutrition. Nasogastric suction may be used to relieve nausea and vomiting and to decrease painful abdominal distention and paralytic ileus. Research data do not support the routine use of nasogastric tubes to remove gastric secretions in an effort to limit pancreatic secretion. Histamine-2 (H_2) antagonists such as cimetidine (Tagamet) and ranitidine (Zantac) may be prescribed to decrease pancreatic activity by inhibiting secretion of gastric acid. Proton pump inhibitors such as pantoprazole (Protonix) may be used for patients who do not tolerate H_2 antagonists or for whom this therapy is ineffective.

Pain Management

Adequate administration of analgesia is essential during the course of acute pancreatitis to provide sufficient pain relief and to minimize restlessness, which may stimulate pancreatic secretion further. Pain relief may require parenteral opioids such as morphine, fentanyl (Sublimaze), or hydromorphone (Dilaudid) (Hauser, Pardi & Poterucha, 2006). The use of morphine was avoided in the past because of concern that it could cause painful spasms of the sphincter of Oddi and worsen pancreatitis; however, all opioids stimulate this sphincter to some degree. There is no clinical evidence to support the use of meperidine for pain relief in pancreatitis, and, in fact, accumulation of its metabolites can cause CNS irritability and possibly seizures. The current recommendation for pain management is the use of opioids, with assessment for their effectiveness and altering therapy if pain is not controlled or increased (Wolfe, Davis, Farraye, et al., 2006). More research is needed to identify the best option for pain management in the patient with acute pancreatitis (Hauser, et al., 2006). Antiemetic agents may be prescribed to prevent vomiting.

Intensive Care

Correction of fluid and blood loss and low albumin levels is necessary to maintain fluid volume and prevent renal failure. The patient is usually acutely ill and is monitored in the intensive care unit, where hemodynamic monitoring and arterial blood gas monitoring are initiated. Antibiotic agents may be prescribed if infection is present. The role of prophylactic antibiotics is controversial and still under study. Insulin may be required if hyperglycemia occurs. Intensive insulin therapy (continuous infusion) in the critically ill patient has undergone much study and has shown promise in terms of positive patient outcomes when compared with intermittent insulin dosing. Glycemic control with normal or near normal blood glucose levels improves patient outcomes.

Respiratory Care

Aggressive respiratory care is indicated because of the high risk of elevation of the diaphragm, pulmonary infiltrates and effusion, and atelectasis. Hypoxemia occurs in a significant number of patients with acute pancreatitis, even with normal x-ray findings. Respiratory care may range from close monitoring of arterial blood gases to use of humidified oxygen to intubation and mechanical ventilation (see Chapter 25 for further discussion).

Biliary Drainage

Placement of biliary drains (for external drainage) and stents (indwelling tubes) in the pancreatic duct through endoscopy has been performed to reestablish drainage of the

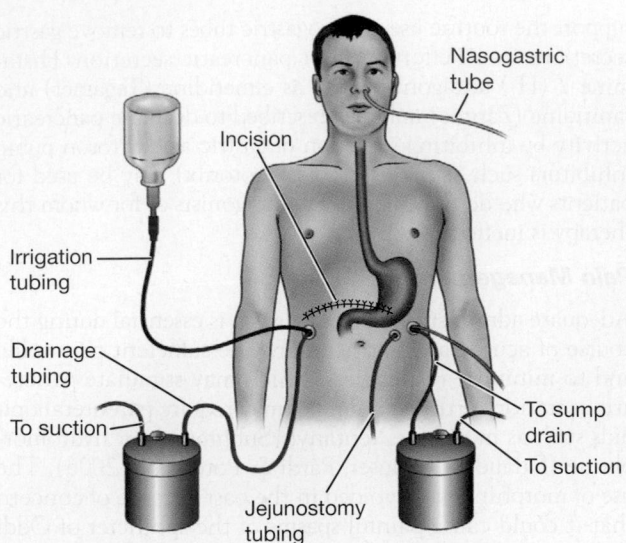

Figure 40-6 Multiple sump tubes are used after pancreatic surgery. Triple-lumen tubes consist of ports that provide tubing for irrigation, air venting, and drainage.

pancreas. This has resulted in decreased pain and increased weight gain.

Surgical Intervention

Although surgery is often risky because the acutely ill patient is a poor surgical risk, it may be performed to assist in the diagnosis of pancreatitis (diagnostic laparotomy), to establish pancreatic drainage, or to resect or débride a necrotic pancreas. The patient who undergoes pancreatic surgery may have multiple drains in place postoperatively, as well as a surgical incision that is left open for irrigation and repacking every 2 to 3 days to remove necrotic debris (Fig. 40-6).

Postacute Management

Antacids may be used after acute pancreatitis begins to resolve. Oral feedings that are low in fat and protein are initiated gradually. Caffeine and alcohol are eliminated from the diet. If the episode of pancreatitis occurred during treatment with thiazide diuretics, corticosteroids, or oral contraceptives, these medications are discontinued. Follow-up may include ultrasound, x-ray studies, or ERCP to determine whether the pancreatitis is resolving and to assess for abscesses and pseudocysts. ERCP may also be used to identify the cause of acute pancreatitis if it is in question and for endoscopic sphincterotomy and removal of gallstones from the common bile duct.

Nursing Management

Relieving Pain and Discomfort

Because the pathologic process responsible for pain is autodigestion of the pancreas, the objectives of therapy are to relieve pain and decrease secretion of pancreatic enzymes. The pain of acute pancreatitis is often very severe, necessitating the liberal use of analgesics. The current recommendation for pain management in this population is parenteral opioids, including morphine, hydromorphone, or fentanyl

via patient-controlled analgesia or bolus (Hauser, et al., 2006; Wolfe, et al., 2006). In critically ill patients, a continuous infusion may be needed. Because most opioids stimulate spasm of the sphincter of Oddi to some degree, consensus has not been reached on the most effective agent. Ensuring patient comfort, regardless of the opioid prescribed, is the most essential aspect of care. The nurse frequently assesses the pain and the effectiveness of the pharmacologic (and nonpharmacologic) interventions. Changes may be needed in the regimen for pain management based on the achievement of pain control. Pain assessment tools (see Chapter 13) are available for the nurse to ensure an accurate rating of pain. Nonpharmacologic interventions such as proper positioning, music, distraction, and imagery may be effective in reducing pain when used along with medications.

In addition, oral feedings are withheld to decrease the secretion of secretin. Parenteral fluids and electrolytes are prescribed to restore and maintain fluid balance. Nasogastric suction may be used to relieve nausea and vomiting or to treat abdominal distention and paralytic ileus. The nurse provides frequent oral hygiene and care to decrease discomfort from the nasogastric tube and relieve dryness of the mouth.

The acutely ill patient is maintained on bed rest to decrease the metabolic rate and reduce the secretion of pancreatic and gastric enzymes. If the patient experiences increasing severity of pain, the nurse reports this to the physician because the patient may be experiencing hemorrhage of the pancreas or the dose of analgesic may be inadequate.

The patient with acute pancreatitis often has a clouded sensorium because of severe pain, fluid and electrolyte disturbances, and hypoxia. Therefore, the nurse provides frequent and repeated but simple explanations about the need for withholding fluids, maintenance of gastric suction, and bed rest.

Improving Breathing Pattern

The nurse maintains the patient in a semi-Fowler's position to decrease pressure on the diaphragm by a distended abdomen and to increase respiratory expansion. Frequent changes of position are necessary to prevent atelectasis and pooling of respiratory secretions. Pulmonary assessment, including monitoring of pulse oximetry or arterial blood gases, is essential to detect changes in respiratory status so that early treatment can be initiated. The nurse instructs the patient in techniques of coughing and deep breathing and in the use of incentive spirometry to improve respiratory function and assists the patient to perform these activities every hour.

Improving Nutritional Status

Oral food or fluid intake is not permitted. However, it is important to assess the patient's nutritional status and to note factors that alter the patient's nutritional requirements (eg, temperature elevation, surgery, drainage). Laboratory test results and daily weights are useful to monitor the nutritional status.

Enteral or parenteral nutrition may be prescribed. In addition to administering enteral or parenteral nutrition, the nurse monitors serum glucose levels every 4 to 6 hours. As the acute symptoms subside, oral feedings are gradually reintroduced.

Between acute attacks, the patient receives a diet that is high in carbohydrates and low in fats and proteins. The patient should avoid heavy meals and alcoholic beverages.

Maintaining Skin Integrity

The patient is at risk for skin breakdown because of poor nutritional status, enforced bed rest, and restlessness, which may result in pressure ulcers and breaks in tissue integrity. In addition, the patient who has undergone surgery may have multiple drains or an open surgical incision and is at risk for skin breakdown and infection. The nurse carefully assesses the wound, drainage sites, and skin for signs of infection, inflammation, and breakdown. The nurse carries out wound care as prescribed and takes precautions to protect intact skin from contact with drainage. Consultation with a **wound-ostomy-continence (WOC) nurse** (formerly referred to as a wound care specialist or enterostomal therapist) is often helpful in identifying appropriate skin care devices and protocols. It is important to turn the patient every 2 hours; use of specialty beds may be indicated to prevent skin breakdown.

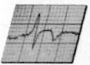

Monitoring and Managing Potential Complications

Fluid and electrolyte disturbances are common complications because of nausea, vomiting, movement of fluid from the vascular compartment to the peritoneal cavity, diaphoresis, fever, and the use of gastric suction. The nurse assesses the patient's fluid and electrolyte status by noting skin turgor and moistness of mucous membranes. The nurse weighs the patient daily and carefully measures fluid intake and output, including urine output, nasogastric secretions, and diarrhea. In addition, it is important to assess for other factors that may affect fluid and electrolyte status, including increased body temperature and wound drainage. The nurse assesses the patient for ascites and measures abdominal girth daily if ascites is suspected.

Fluids are administered intravenously and may be accompanied by infusion of blood or blood products to maintain the blood volume and to prevent or treat hypovolemic shock. It is important to keep emergency medications readily available because of the risk of circulatory collapse and shock. The nurse promptly reports decreased blood pressure and reduced urine output, which indicate hypovolemia and shock or renal failure. Low serum calcium and magnesium levels may occur and require prompt treatment.

Pancreatic necrosis is a major cause of morbidity and mortality in patients with acute pancreatitis because of resulting hemorrhage, septic shock, and multiple organ failure. The patient may undergo diagnostic procedures for confirmation of pancreatic necrosis, for surgical débridement, or for insertion of multiple drains. The patient with pancreatic necrosis is usually critically ill and requires expert medical and nursing management, including hemodynamic monitoring in the intensive care unit.

In addition to carefully monitoring vital signs and other signs and symptoms, the nurse is responsible for administering prescribed fluids, medications, and blood products; assisting with supportive management, such as use of a ventilator; preventing additional complications; and providing physical and psychological care.

Shock and multiple organ failure may occur with acute pancreatitis. Hypovolemic shock may occur as a result of hypovolemia and sequestering of fluid in the peritoneal cavity. Hemorrhagic shock may occur with hemorrhagic pancreatitis. Septic shock may occur with bacterial infection of the pancreas. Cardiac dysfunction may occur as a result of fluid and electrolyte disturbances, acid–base imbalances, and release of toxic substances into the circulation.

The nurse closely monitors the patient for early signs of neurologic, cardiovascular, renal, and respiratory dysfunction. The nurse must be prepared to respond quickly to rapid changes in the patient's status, treatments, and therapies. In addition, it is important to inform the family about the status and progress of the patient and to allow them to spend time with the patient. (Management of shock is discussed in detail in Chapter 15.)

Promoting Home and Community-Based Care

Teaching Patients Self-Care

The patient who has survived an episode of acute pancreatitis has been acutely ill. A prolonged period is needed to regain strength and return to the previous level of activity. The patient is often still weak and debilitated for weeks or months after an acute episode of pancreatitis. Because of the severity of the acute illness, the patient may not recall many of the explanations and instructions given during the acute phase. Teaching often needs to be repeated and reinforced. The nurse instructs the patient about the factors implicated in the onset of acute pancreatitis and about the need to avoid high-fat foods, heavy meals, and alcohol. It is important to give the patient and family verbal and written instructions about signs and symptoms of acute pancreatitis and possible complications that should be reported promptly to the physician.

If acute pancreatitis is a result of biliary tract disease, such as gallstones and gallbladder disease, additional explanations are needed about required dietary modifications. If the pancreatitis is a result of alcohol abuse, the nurse reinforces the need to avoid all alcohol.

Continuing Care

A referral for home care is often indicated. This enables the nurse to assess the patient's physical and psychological status and adherence to the therapeutic regimen. The nurse also assesses the home situation and reinforces instructions about fluid and nutrition intake and avoidance of alcohol. After the acute attack has subsided, some patients may be inclined to return to their previous drinking habits. The nurse provides specific information about resources and support groups that may be of assistance in avoiding alcohol in the future. Referral to Alcoholics Anonymous or other appropriate support groups is essential. See the accompanying plan of nursing care in Chart 40-4 for the patient with acute pancreatitis.

Chronic Pancreatitis

Chronic pancreatitis is an inflammatory disorder characterized by progressive destruction of the pancreas. As cells are replaced by fibrous tissue with repeated attacks of pancreatitis,

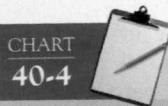

PLAN OF NURSING CARE
Care of the Patient With Acute Pancreatitis

CHART 40-4

NURSING DIAGNOSIS: Acute pain and discomfort related to edema, distention of the pancreas, and peritoneal irritation
GOAL: Relief of pain and discomfort

Nursing Interventions	Rationale	Expected Outcomes
1. Administer morphine, fentanyl, or hydromorphone frequently, as prescribed, to achieve level of pain acceptable to patient based on patient's level of pain and discomfort.	1. Morphine, fentanyl, and hydromorphone act by depressing the central nervous system and thereby increasing the patient's pain threshold. Meperidine (Demerol) is avoided because it has failed acute pain studies and it possesses toxic metabolites.	• Reports relief of pain. • Moves and turns without increasing pain and discomfort. • Rests comfortably and sleeps for increasing periods. • Reports less frequent episodes of pain, discomfort, and cramping. • Experiences enhanced pain relief. • Reports increased feelings of well-being and security with the health care team.
2. Using a pain scale, assess pain level before and after administration of analgesic.	2. Assessment and control of pain are important because restlessness increases body metabolism, which stimulates the secretion of pancreatic and gastric enzymes.	
3. Report unrelieved pain or increasing intensity of pain.	3. Pain may increase pancreatic enzymes and may also indicate pancreatic hemorrhage.	
4. Assist the patient to assume positions of comfort; turn and reposition every 2 hours.	4. Frequent turning relieves pressure and assists in preventing pulmonary and vascular complications.	
5. Use nonpharmacologic interventions for relieving pain (eg, relaxation, focused breathing, diversion).	5. Use of nonpharmacologic methods will enhance the effects of analgesics. Gate control theory suggests that cutaneous stimulation closes the pain pathways.	
6. Listen to patient's expression of pain experience.	6. Demonstration of caring can help to decrease anxiety.	

NURSING DIAGNOSIS: Acute pain and discomfort related to excess stimulation of pancreatic secretions
GOAL: Relief of pain related to stimulation of the pancreas

Nursing Interventions	Rationale	Expected Outcomes
1. Administer anticholinergic medications as prescribed.	1. Anticholinergic medications reduce gastric and pancreatic secretion.	• Reports relief of pain, discomfort, and abdominal cramping. • Consumes no fluid and food during acute phase. • Maintains bed rest. • Identifies rationale for fluid and dietary restrictions and use of nasogastric drainage. • Cooperates with insertion of nasogastric tube and suction.
2. Withhold oral intake.	2. Pancreatic secretion is increased by food and fluid intake.	
3. Maintain the patient on bed rest.	3. Bed rest decreases body metabolism and thus reduces pancreatic and gastric secretions.	

4. Maintain continuous nasogastric drainage if paralytic ileus or nausea and vomiting, abdominal distention are present.
  a. Measure gastric secretions at specified intervals.
  b. Observe and record color and viscosity of gastric secretions.
  c. Ensure that the nasogastric tube is patent to permit free drainage.
	4. Nasogastric suction relieves nausea, vomiting, and abdominal distention. Decompression of the intestines (if intestinal intubation is used) also assists in relieving respiratory distress.	

NURSING DIAGNOSIS: Discomfort related to nasogastric tube
GOAL: Relief of discomfort associated with nasogastric intubation used to treat ileus, vomiting, distention

Nursing Interventions	Rationale	Expected Outcomes
1. Use water-soluble lubricant around external nares.	1. Prevents irritation of nares.	• Exhibits intact skin and tissue of nares at site of nasogastric tube insertion. • Reports no pain or irritation of nares or oropharynx.
2. Turn patient at intervals; avoid pressure or tension on nasogastric tube.	2. Relieves pressure of tube on esophageal and gastric mucosa.	

Continued

CHART 40-4

PLAN OF NURSING CARE
Care of the Patient With Acute Pancreatitis (Continued)

Nursing Interventions	Rationale	Expected Outcomes
3. Provide oral hygiene and gargling solutions without alcohol. 4. Explain rationale for use of nasogastric drainage	3. Relieves dryness and irritation of oropharynx. 4. Assists patient to cooperate with the drainage, nasogastric tube, and suction.	• Exhibits moist, clean mucous membranes of mouth and nasopharynx. • States that thirst is relieved by oral hygiene. • Identifies rationale for nasogastric tube and suction.

NURSING DIAGNOSIS: Imbalanced nutrition: less than body requirements related to inadequate dietary intake, impaired pancreatic secretions, increased nutritional needs secondary to acute illness, and increased body temperature
GOAL: Improvement in nutritional status

Nursing Interventions	Rationale	Expected Outcomes
1. Assess current nutritional status and increased metabolic requirements. 2. Monitor serum glucose levels and administer insulin as prescribed. 3. Administer intravenous fluid and electrolytes, enteral or parenteral nutrition as prescribed. 4. Provide high-carbohydrate, low-protein, low-fat diet when tolerated. 5. Instruct patient to eliminate alcohol and refer to Alcoholics Anonymous if indicated. 6. Counsel patient to avoid excessive use of coffee and spicy foods. 7. Monitor daily weights.	1. Alteration in pancreatic secretions interferes with normal digestive processes. Acute illness, infection, and fever increase metabolic needs. 2. Impairment of endocrine function of the pancreas leads to increased serum glucose levels. 3. Parenteral administration of fluids and electrolytes, and enteral or parenteral nutrients are essential to provide fluids, calories, electrolytes, and nutrients when oral intake is prohibited. 4. These foods increase caloric intake without stimulating pancreatic secretions beyond the ability of the pancreas to respond. 5. Alcohol intake produces further damage to pancreas and precipitates attacks of acute pancreatitis. 6. Coffee and spicy foods increase pancreatic and gastric secretions. 7. This provides a baseline and a means to measure weight gain or weight loss.	• Maintains normal body weight. • Demonstrates no additional weight loss. • Maintains normal serum glucose levels. • Reports decreasing episodes of vomiting and diarrhea. • Reports return of normal stool characteristics and bowel pattern. • Consumes foods high in carbohydrates, low in fat and protein. • Explains rationale for high-carbohydrate, low-fat, low-protein diet. • Eliminates alcohol from diet. • Explains rationale for limiting coffee intake and avoiding spicy foods. • Participates in Alcoholics Anonymous or other counseling approach. • Returns to and maintains desirable weight.

NURSING DIAGNOSIS: Ineffective breathing pattern related to splinting from severe pain, pulmonary infiltrates, pleural effusion, and atelectasis
GOAL: Improvement in respiratory function

Nursing Interventions	Rationale	Expected Outcomes
1. Assess respiratory status (rate, pattern, breath sounds), pulse oximetry, and arterial blood gases. 2. Maintain semi-Fowler's position. 3. Instruct and encourage patient to take deep breaths and to cough every hour. 4. Assist patient to turn and change position every 2 hours.	1. Acute pancreatitis produces retroperitoneal edema, elevation of the diaphragm, pleural effusion, and inadequate lung ventilation. Intra-abdominal infection and labored breathing increase the body's metabolic demands, which further decreases pulmonary reserve and leads to respiratory failure. 2. Decreases pressure on diaphragm and allows greater lung expansion. 3. Taking deep breaths and coughing will clear the airways and reduce atelectasis. 4. Changing position frequently assists aeration and drainage of all lobes of the lungs.	• Demonstrates normal respiratory rate and pattern and full lung expansion. • Demonstrates normal breath sounds and absence of adventitious breath sounds. • Demonstrates normal arterial blood gases and pulse oximetry. • Maintains semi-Fowler's position when in bed. • Changes position in bed frequently. • Coughs and takes deep breaths at least every hour. • Demonstrates normal body temperature. • Exhibits no signs or symptoms of respiratory infection or impairment. • Is alert and responsive to environment.

Continued on following page

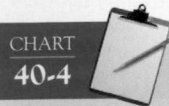

CHART
40-4

PLAN OF NURSING CARE
Care of the Patient With Acute Pancreatitis (Continued)

Nursing Interventions	Rationale	Expected Outcomes

5. Reduce the excessive metabolism of the body.
  a. Administer antibiotics as prescribed.
  b. Place patient in an air-conditioned room.
  c. Administer nasal oxygen as required for hypoxia.
  d. Use a hypothermia blanket if necessary.
	5. Pancreatitis produces a severe peritoneal and retroperitoneal reaction that causes fever, tachycardia, and accelerated respirations. Placing the patient in an air-conditioned room and supporting the patient with oxygen therapy decrease the workload of the respiratory system and the tissue utilization of oxygen. Reduction of fever and pulse rate decreases the metabolic demands on the body.	

COLLABORATIVE PROBLEM: Fluid and electrolyte disturbances, hypovolemia, shock
GOAL: Improvement in fluid and electrolyte status, prevention of hypovolemia and shock

Nursing Interventions	Rationale	Expected Outcomes
1. Assess fluid and electrolyte status (skin turgor, mucous membranes, urine output, vital signs, hemodynamic parameters).	1. The amount and type of fluid and electrolyte replacement are determined by the status of the blood pressure, the laboratory evaluations of serum electrolyte and blood urea nitrogen levels, the urinary volume, and the assessment of the patient's condition.	• Exhibits moist mucous membranes and normal skin turgor. • Exhibits normal blood pressure without evidence of postural (orthostatic) hypotension. • Excretes adequate urine volume. • Exhibits normal, not excessive, thirst. • Maintains normal pulse and respiratory rate.

2. Assess sources of fluid and electrolyte loss (vomiting, diarrhea, nasogastric drainage, excessive diaphoresis).
3. Combat shock if present.
  a. Administer corticosteroids as prescribed if patient does not respond to conventional treatment.
  b. Evaluate the amount of urinary output. Attempt to maintain this at 50 mL/h.
	2. Electrolyte losses occur from nasogastric suctioning, severe diaphoresis, emesis, and as a result of the patient's being in a fasting state.
	3. Extensive acute pancreatitis may cause peripheral vascular collapse and shock. Blood and plasma may be lost into the abdominal cavity, and, therefore, there is a decreased blood and plasma volume. The toxins from the bacteria of a necrotic pancreas may cause shock.
		• Remains alert and responsive.
		• Exhibits normal arterial pressures and blood gases.
		• Exhibits normal electrolyte levels.
		• Exhibits no signs or symptoms of calcium deficit (eg, tetany, carpopedal spasm).

4. Administer blood products, fluids, and electrolytes (sodium, potassium, chloride) as prescribed. 5. Administer plasma and blood products as prescribed.	4. Patients with hemorrhagic pancreatitis lose large amounts of blood and plasma, which decreases effective circulation and blood volume. 5. Replacement with blood, plasma or albumin assists in ensuring effective circulating blood volume.	• Exhibits no additional losses of fluids and electrolytes through vomiting, diarrhea, or diaphoresis. • Reports stabilization of weight. • Demonstrates no increase in abdominal girth.
6. Keep a supply of intravenous calcium gluconate readily available.	6. Calcium may be prescribed to prevent or treat tetany, which may result from calcium losses into retroperitoneal (peripancreatic) exudate.	• Demonstrates no fluid wave on palpation of the abdomen. • Demonstrates stable organ function without manifestations of failure.

7. Assess abdomen for ascites formation:
  a. Measure abdominal girth daily.
  b. Weigh patient daily.
  c. Palpate abdomen for fluid wave.
8. Monitor for manifestations of multiple organ failure: neurologic, cardiovascular, renal, and respiratory dysfunction.
	7. During acute pancreatitis, plasma may be lost into the abdominal cavity, which diminishes the blood volume.
	
	8. All body systems may fail if pancreatitis is severe and treatment is ineffective.	

pressure within the pancreas increases. The result is obstruction of the pancreatic and common bile ducts and the duodenum. Additionally, there is atrophy of the epithelium of the ducts, inflammation, and destruction of the secreting cells of the pancreas.

Alcohol consumption in Western societies and malnutrition worldwide are the major causes of chronic pancreatitis. The median age of patients diagnosed with chronic pancreatitis is 37 to 40 years. Frequently, at that age, patients already report a long history of alcohol abuse. Excessive and prolonged consumption of alcohol accounts for approximately 70% to 80% of all cases of chronic pancreatitis (Zinner & Ashley, 2007). The incidence of pancreatitis is 50 times greater in people with alcoholism than in those who do not abuse alcohol. Long-term alcohol consumption causes hypersecretion of protein in pancreatic secretions, resulting in protein plugs and calculi within the pancreatic ducts. Alcohol also has a direct toxic effect on the cells of the pancreas. Damage to these cells is more likely to occur and to be more severe in patients whose diets are poor in protein content and either very high or very low in fat.

Smoking is another factor in the development of chronic pancreatitis. Because heavy drinkers usually smoke, it is difficult to separate the effects of the alcohol abuse and smoking (Lankisch, 2007).

Clinical Manifestations

Chronic pancreatitis is characterized by recurring attacks of severe upper abdominal and back pain, accompanied by vomiting. Attacks are often so painful that opioids, even in large doses, do not provide relief. The risk of opioid dependence is increased in pancreatitis because of the chronic nature and severity of the pain. As the disease progresses, recurring attacks of pain are more severe, more frequent, and of longer duration. Some patients experience continuous severe pain, and others have dull, nagging constant pain. Periods of well-being sometimes follow the episodes of pain (Wolfe, et al., 2006). In fact, in some patients, chronic pancreatitis is painless. The natural history of abdominal pain (character, timing, severity) is variable, and many studies have documented a decrease in pain ("burnout") over time in a majority of patients (Dominguez-Muñoz & Malfertheiner, 2005).

Weight loss is a major problem in chronic pancreatitis: More than 80% of patients experience significant weight loss, which is usually caused by decreased dietary intake secondary to anorexia or fear that eating will precipitate another attack (Wolfe, et al., 2006). Malabsorption occurs late in the disease, when as little as 10% of pancreatic function remains (Dominguez-Muñoz & Malfertheiner, 2005). As a result, digestion, especially of proteins and fats, is impaired. The stools become frequent, frothy, and foul-smelling because of impaired fat digestion, which results in stools with a high fat content. This is referred to as **steatorrhea.** As the disease progresses, calcification of the gland may occur, and calcium stones may form within the ducts.

Assessment and Diagnostic Findings

ERCP is the most useful study in the diagnosis of chronic pancreatitis. It provides details about the anatomy of the pancreas and the pancreatic and biliary ducts. It is also helpful in obtaining tissue for analysis and differentiating pancreatitis from other conditions, such as carcinoma. Various imaging procedures, including magnetic resonance imaging (MRI), CT scans, and ultrasound, are used in the diagnostic evaluation of patients with suspected pancreatic disorders. A CT scan or ultrasound study is also helpful to detect pancreatic cysts.

A glucose tolerance test evaluates pancreatic islet cell function and provides necessary information for making decisions about surgical resection of the pancreas. An abnormal glucose tolerance test may indicate the presence of diabetes associated with pancreatitis. Acute exacerbations of chronic pancreatitis may result in increased serum amylase levels. Steatorrhea is best confirmed by laboratory analysis of fecal fat content (Dominguez-Muñoz & Malfertheiner, 2005).

Medical Management

The management of chronic pancreatitis depends on its probable cause in each patient. Treatment is directed toward preventing and managing acute attacks, relieving pain and discomfort, and managing exocrine and endocrine insufficiency of pancreatitis.

Nonsurgical Management

Nonsurgical approaches may be indicated for the patient who refuses surgery, who is a poor surgical risk, or whose disease and symptoms do not warrant surgical intervention. Endoscopy to remove pancreatic duct stones, correct strictures, and drain cysts may be effective in selected patients to manage pain and relieve obstruction (Zinner & Ashley, 2007).

Management of abdominal pain and discomfort is similar to that of acute pancreatitis; however, the focus is usually on the use of nonopioid methods to manage pain. Antioxidants that may relieve pain and improve reported quality of life are being studied (Kirk, White, McKie, et al., 2006). Researchers have proposed that yoga may be an effective nonpharmacologic method for pain reduction and for relief of other coexisting symptoms of chronic pancreatitis (Sareen & Kumari, 2006). Persistent, unrelieved pain is often the most difficult aspect of management (Zinner & Ashley, 2007). The physician, nurse, and dietitian emphasize to the patient and family the importance of avoiding alcohol and foods that have produced abdominal pain and discomfort in the past. The health care team stresses to the patient that no other treatment is likely to relieve pain if the patient continues to consume alcohol.

Diabetes mellitus resulting from dysfunction of the pancreatic islet cells is treated with diet, insulin, or oral antidiabetic agents. The hazard of severe hypoglycemia with alcohol consumption is stressed to the patient and family. Pancreatic enzyme replacement is indicated for the patient with malabsorption and steatorrhea.

Surgical Management

Chronic pancreatitis is not often managed by surgery. However, surgery may be indicated to relieve persistent abdominal pain and discomfort, restore drainage of pancreatic secretions, and reduce the frequency of acute attacks of pancreatitis and hospitalization (Zinner & Ashley, 2007).

The type of surgery performed depends on the anatomic and functional abnormalities of the pancreas, including the location of disease within the pancreas, the presence of diabetes, exocrine insufficiency, biliary stenosis, and pseudocysts of the pancreas. Other considerations for surgery selection include the patient's likelihood for continued use of alcohol and the likelihood that the patient will be able to manage the endocrine or exocrine changes that are expected after surgery.

Pancreaticojejunostomy (also referred to as Roux-en-Y), with a side-to-side anastomosis or joining of the pancreatic duct to the jejunum, allows drainage of the pancreatic secretions into the jejunum. Pain relief occurs within 6 months in more than 85% of the patients who undergo this procedure, but pain returns in a substantial number of patients as the disease progresses (Zinner & Ashley, 2007).

Other surgical procedures may be performed for different degrees and types of underlying disorders. These procedures include revision of the sphincter of the ampulla of Vater, internal drainage of a pancreatic cyst into the stomach (see later discussion), insertion of a stent, and wide resection or removal of the pancreas. A Whipple resection (pancreaticoduodenectomy) can be carried out to relieve the pain of chronic pancreatitis. In an effort to provide permanent pain relief and avoid endocrine and exocrine insufficiency that ensue with major resections of the pancreas, surgeons have designed new procedures that combine limited resection of the head of the pancreas with a pancreaticojejunostomy. These procedures, known as the Beger or Frey operations, remove most of the head of the pancreas except for a shell of pancreatic tissue posteriorly (Bayless & Diehl, 2005; Zinner & Ashley, 2007).

When chronic pancreatitis develops as a result of gallbladder disease, surgery is performed to explore the common duct and remove the stones; usually, the gallbladder is removed at the same time. In addition, an attempt is made to improve the drainage of the common bile duct and the pancreatic duct by dividing the sphincter of Oddi, a muscle that is located at the ampulla of Vater (this surgical procedure is known as a sphincterotomy). A T-tube usually is placed in the common bile duct, requiring a drainage system to collect the bile postoperatively. Nursing care after such surgery is similar to that indicated after other biliary tract surgery.

Approximately two thirds of all patients with chronic pancreatitis can be managed with endoscopic or laparoscopic intervention (Wolfe, et al., 2006). Endoscopic and laparoscopic procedures such as distal pancreatectomy, longitudinal decompression of the pancreatic duct, nerve denervation, and stenting have been performed in patients with jaundice or recurrent inflammation and are being refined. Minimally invasive procedures to treat chronic pancreatitis may prove to be successful adjuncts in the management of this complex disorder (Beger & Bettina, 2007; Wolfe, et al., 2006).

Patients who undergo surgery for chronic pancreatitis may experience weight gain and improved nutritional status; this may result from reduction in pain associated with eating rather than from correction of malabsorption. However, morbidity and mortality after these surgical procedures are high because of the poor physical condition of the patient before surgery and the concomitant presence of cirrhosis. Even after undergoing these surgical procedures, the patient is likely to continue to have pain and impaired digestion secondary to pancreatitis, unless alcohol is avoided completely.

Pancreatic Cysts

As a result of the local necrosis that occurs at the time of acute pancreatitis, collections of fluid may form close to the pancreas. These fluid collections become walled off by fibrous tissue and are called pancreatic pseudocysts. They are the most common type of pancreatic cyst. Less common cysts occur as a result of congenital anomalies or secondary to chronic pancreatitis or trauma to the pancreas.

Diagnosis of pancreatic cysts and pseudocysts is made by ultrasound, CT scan, and ERCP. ERCP may be used to define the anatomy of the pancreas and evaluate the patency of pancreatic drainage. Pancreatic pseudocysts may be of considerable size. When pancreatic pseudocysts enlarge, they impinge on and displace the adjacent stomach or the colon because of the location of pseudocysts behind the posterior peritoneum. Eventually, through pressure or secondary infection, they produce symptoms and require drainage.

Drainage into the GI tract or through the skin and abdominal wall may be established. In the latter instance, the drainage is likely to be profuse and destructive to tissue because of the enzyme contents. Hence, steps (including application of skin ointment) must be taken to protect the skin near the drainage site from excoriation. A suction apparatus may be used to continuously aspirate digestive secretions from the drainage tract so that skin contact with the digestive enzymes is avoided. Expert nursing attention is required to ensure that the suction tube does not become dislodged and suction is not interrupted. Consultation with a WOC nurse is indicated to identify appropriate strategies for maintaining drainage and protecting the skin.

Cancer of the Pancreas

Pancreatic cancer is the fourth leading cause of cancer death in men in the United States and the fifth leading cause of cancer death in women. It is very rare before the age of 45 years, and the majority of patients present in or beyond the sixth decade of life (Feldman, et al., 2006; Zinner & Ashley, 2007). The incidence of pancreatic cancer increases with age, peaking in the seventh and eighth decades for both men and women (American Cancer Society, 2009). The frequency of pancreatic cancer has decreased slightly over the past 25 years among non-Caucasian men. There is a slight male preponderance, and in the United States, incidence is highest in African American males (Zinner & Ashley, 2007). Cigarette smoking, exposure to industrial chemicals or toxins in the environment, and a diet high in fat, meat, or both are associated with pancreatic cancer, although their roles are not completely clear. The risk of pancreatic cancer increases as the extent of cigarette smoking increases. Diabetes mellitus, chronic pancreatitis, and hereditary pancreatitis are also associated with pancreatic cancer. The pancreas can also be the site of metastasis from other tumors.

Cancer may develop in the head, body, or tail of the pancreas; clinical manifestations vary depending on the site and whether functioning insulin-secreting pancreatic islet cells are involved. Approximately 70% of pancreatic cancers originate in the head of the pancreas and give rise to a distinctive clinical picture (Zinner & Ashley, 2007). Functioning islet cell tumors, whether benign (adenoma) or malignant (carcinoma), are responsible for the syndrome of hyperinsulinism. The symptoms are typically nonspecific, and patients usually do not seek medical attention until late in the disease. Only about 7% of cases are diagnosed in early stages; 80% to 85% of patients have advanced, unresectable tumor when first detected. As a result, pancreatic carcinoma has only a 5% survival rate at 5 years regardless of the stage of disease at diagnosis or treatment (American Cancer Society, 2009).

Clinical Manifestations

Pain, jaundice, or both are present in more than 80% of patients and, along with weight loss, are considered classic signs of pancreatic carcinoma (Hauser, et al., 2006). However, they often do not appear until the disease is far advanced. Other signs include rapid, profound, and progressive weight loss as well as vague upper or midabdominal pain or discomfort that is unrelated to any GI function and is often difficult to describe. Such discomfort radiates as a boring pain in the midback and is unrelated to posture or activity. It is often progressive and severe, requiring the use of opioids. It is often more severe at night and is accentuated when lying supine. Relief may be obtained by sitting up and leaning forward.

Malignant cells from pancreatic cancer are often shed into the peritoneal cavity, increasing the likelihood of metastasis. The formation of ascites is common. An important sign, if it is present, is the onset of symptoms of insulin deficiency: glucosuria, hyperglycemia, and abnormal glucose tolerance. Therefore, diabetes may be an early sign of carcinoma of the pancreas. Meals often aggravate epigastric pain, which usually occurs before the appearance of jaundice and pruritus.

Assessment and Diagnostic Findings

Spiral (helical) CT is more than 85% to 90% accurate in the diagnosis and staging of pancreatic cancer and is currently the most useful preoperative imaging technique. MRI may also be used. ERCP is also used in the diagnosis of pancreatic carcinoma. Endoscopic ultrasound (EUS) is useful in identifying small tumors and in performing fine-needle aspiration biopsy of the primary tumor or lymph nodes (Hauser, et al., 2006). Cells obtained during ERCP are sent to the laboratory for analysis. GI x-ray findings may demonstrate deformities in adjacent organs caused by the impinging pancreatic mass.

A histologic diagnosis is not usually required in patients who are candidates for surgery. The tissue diagnosis is made at the time of the surgical procedure. Percutaneous fine-needle aspiration biopsy of the pancreas, which is used to diagnose pancreatic tumors, is also used to confirm the diagnosis in patients whose tumors are not resectable so that

a palliative plan of care can be determined. This may eliminate the stress and postoperative pain of ineffective surgery. In this procedure, a needle is inserted through the anterior abdominal wall into the pancreatic mass, guided by CT, ultrasound, ERCP, or other imaging techniques. The aspirated material is examined for malignant cells. Although percutaneous biopsy is a valuable diagnostic tool, it has some potential drawbacks: a false-negative result if small tumors are missed and the risk of seeding of cancer cells along the needle track. Low-dose radiation to the site may be used before the biopsy to reduce this risk.

Percutaneous transhepatic cholangiography is another procedure that may be performed to identify obstructions of the biliary tract by a pancreatic tumor. Several tumor markers (eg, cancer antigen [CA] 19-9, carcinoembryonic antigen [CEA], DU-PAN-2) may be used in the diagnostic workup, but they are nonspecific for pancreatic carcinoma. These tumor markers are useful as indicators of disease progression.

Angiography, CT scans, and laparoscopy may be performed to determine whether the tumor can be removed surgically. Intraoperative ultrasonography has been used to determine whether there is metastatic disease to other organs.

Medical Management

If the tumor is resectable and localized (typically tumors in the head of the pancreas), the surgical procedure to remove it is usually extensive (see later discussion). However, total excision of the lesion often is not possible for two reasons: (1) extensive growth of tumor before diagnosis and (2) probable widespread metastases (especially to the liver, lungs, and bones). More often, treatment is limited to palliative measures.

Although pancreatic tumors may be resistant to standard radiation therapy, the patient may be treated with radiation and chemotherapy (5-fluorouracil [5-FU, Adrucil], leucovorin [Wellcovorin], and gemcitabine [Gemzar]). Currently, gemcitabine is the standard of care for patients with metastatic pancreatic cancer (Feldman, et al., 2006). At present, newer biologic agents, including farnesyl transferase inhibitors and monoclonal antibodies, are under study for the treatment of metastatic pancreatic cancer (Feldman, et al., 2006; Zinner & Ashley, 2007). If the patient undergoes surgery, intraoperative radiation therapy (IORT) may be used to deliver a high dose of radiation to the tumor with minimal injury to other tissues; this may also be helpful in relief of pain. Interstitial implantation of radioactive sources has also been used, although the rate of complications is high. A large biliary stent inserted percutaneously or by endoscopy may be used to relieve jaundice.

Nursing Management

Pain management and attention to nutritional requirements are important nursing measures that improve the level of patient comfort. Skin care and nursing measures are directed toward relief of pain and discomfort associated with jaundice, anorexia, and profound weight loss. Specialty mattresses are beneficial and protect bony prominences from pressure. Pain associated with pancreatic cancer may be severe and may require liberal use of opioids;

patient-controlled analgesia should be considered for the patient with severe, escalating pain.

Because of the poor prognosis and likelihood of short survival, end-of-life preferences are discussed and honored. If appropriate, the nurse refers the patient to hospice care. (See Chapters 16 and 17 for care of the patient with cancer and end-of-life care, respectively.)

Promoting Home and Community-Based Care

Teaching Patients Self-Care

The specific teaching for the patient and family varies with the stage of disease and the treatment choices made by the patient. If the patient elects to receive chemotherapy, the nurse focuses teaching on prevention of side effects and complications of the agents used. If surgery is performed to relieve obstruction and establish biliary drainage, teaching addresses management of the drainage system and monitoring for complications. The nurse instructs the family about changes in the patient's status that should be reported to the physician.

Continuing Care

A referral for home care is indicated to help the patient and family deal with the physical problems and discomforts associated with pancreatic cancer and the psychological impact of the disease. The home care nurse assesses the patient's physical status, fluid and nutritional status, skin integrity, and the adequacy of pain management. The nurse teaches the patient and family strategies to prevent skin breakdown and relieve pain, pruritus, and anorexia. It is important to discuss and arrange palliative care (hospice services) in an effort to relieve patient discomfort, assist with care, and comply with the patient's end-of-life decisions and wishes.

Tumors of the Head of the Pancreas

Sixty percent to 80% of pancreatic tumors occur in the head of the pancreas (Zinner & Ashley, 2007). Tumors in this region of the pancreas obstruct the common bile duct where the duct passes through the head of the pancreas to join the pancreatic duct and empty at the ampulla of Vater into the duodenum. The tumors producing the obstruction may arise from the pancreas, the common bile duct, or the ampulla of Vater.

Clinical Manifestations

The obstructed flow of bile produces jaundice, clay-colored stools, and dark urine. Malabsorption of nutrients and fat-soluble vitamins may result if the tumor obstructs the entry of bile to the GI tract. Abdominal discomfort or pain and pruritus may be noted, along with anorexia, weight loss, and malaise. If these signs and symptoms are present, cancer of the head of the pancreas is suspected.

The jaundice of this disease must be differentiated from that due to a biliary obstruction caused by a gallstone in the common duct. Jaundice caused by a gallstone is usually intermittent and appears typically in obese patients, who are most often women, and who have had previous symptoms of gallbladder disease.

Assessment and Diagnostic Findings

Diagnostic studies may include duodenography, angiography by hepatic or celiac artery catheterization, pancreatic scanning, percutaneous transhepatic cholangiography, ERCP, and percutaneous needle biopsy of the pancreas. Results of a biopsy of the pancreas may aid in the diagnosis.

Medical Management

Before extensive surgery can be performed, a fairly long period of preparation is often necessary, because the patient's nutritional status and physical condition are often quite compromised. Various liver and pancreatic function studies are performed. A diet high in protein along with pancreatic enzymes is often prescribed. Preoperative preparation includes adequate hydration, correction of prothrombin deficiency with vitamin K, and treatment of anemia to minimize postoperative complications. Parenteral nutrition and blood component therapy are frequently required.

A biliary-enteric shunt may be performed to relieve the jaundice and, perhaps, to provide time for a thorough diagnostic evaluation. Total pancreatectomy (removal of the pancreas) may be performed if there is no evidence of direct extension of the tumor to adjacent tissues or regional lymph nodes. A pancreaticoduodenectomy (Whipple's procedure or resection) is used for potentially resectable cancer of the head of the pancreas (Fig. 40-7). This procedure involves removal of the gallbladder, a portion of the stomach, duodenum, proximal jejunum, head of the pancreas, and distal common bile duct. Reconstruction involves anastomosis of the remaining pancreas and stomach to the jejunum (Hauser, et al., 2006). The result is removal of the tumor, allowing flow of bile into the jejunum. If the tumor cannot be excised, the jaundice may be relieved by diverting the bile flow into the jejunum by anastomosing the jejunum to the gallbladder, a procedure known as **cholecystojejunostomy.**

The postoperative management of patients who have undergone a pancreatectomy or a pancreaticoduodenectomy is similar to the management of patients after extensive gastrointestinal or biliary surgery. The patient's physical status is often suboptimal, increasing the risk of postoperative complications. Hemorrhage, vascular collapse, and hepatorenal failure remain the major postoperative complications. The mortality rate associated with these procedures has decreased because of advances in nutritional support and improved surgical techniques. A nasogastric tube with suction and parenteral nutrition allow the GI tract to rest while promoting adequate nutrition.

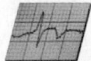

Nursing Management

Preoperatively and postoperatively, nursing care is directed toward promoting patient comfort, preventing complications, and assisting the patient to return to and maintain as normal and comfortable a life as possible. The nurse closely monitors the patient in the intensive care unit after surgery; in the immediate postoperative period, multiple IV and arterial lines are used for fluid and blood replacement and hemodynamic monitoring, and a mechanical ventilator may be used. It is important to note and report changes in vital

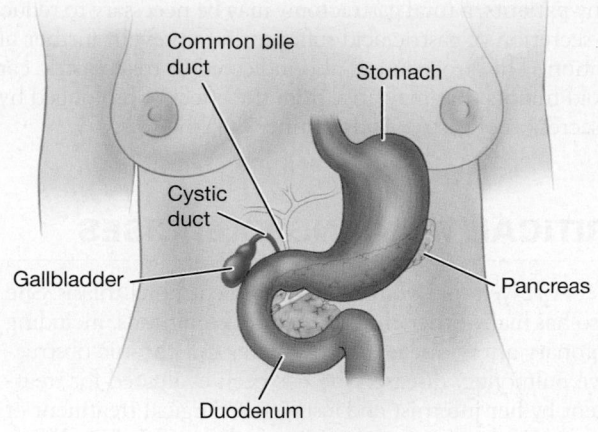

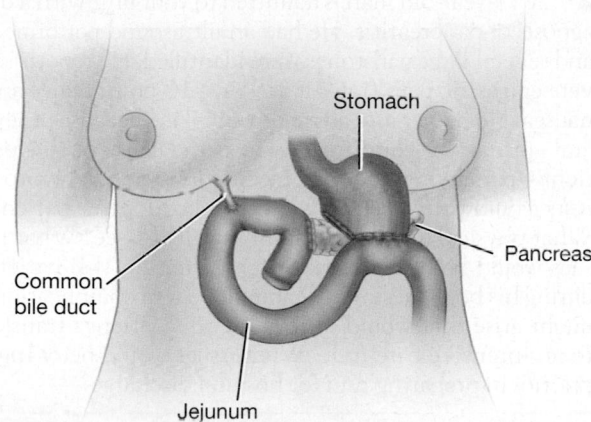

Figure 40-7 Pancreatoduodenectomy (Whipple's procedure or resection). End result of resection of carcinoma of the head of the pancreas or the ampulla of Vater. The common duct is sutured to the side of the jejunum (choledochojejunostomy), and the remaining portion of the pancreas and the end of the stomach are sutured to the side of the jejunum.

signs, arterial blood gases and pressures, pulse oximetry, laboratory values, and urine output. The nurse must also consider the patient's compromised nutritional status and risk of bleeding. Depending on the type of surgical procedure performed, malabsorption syndrome and diabetes mellitus are likely; the nurse must address these issues during acute and long-term patient care.

Although the patient's physiologic status is the focus of the health care team in the immediate postoperative period, the patient's psychological and emotional states must be considered, along with that of the family. The patient has undergone a major high-risk surgery and is critically ill; anxiety and depression may affect recovery. The immediate and long-term outcomes of this extensive surgical resection are uncertain, and the patient and family require emotional support and understanding in the critical and stressful preoperative and postoperative periods.

Promoting Home and Community-Based Care

Teaching Patients Self-Care

The patient who has undergone this extensive surgery requires careful and thorough preparation for self-care at home. The nurse instructs the patient and family about the need for modifications in the diet because of malabsorption and hyperglycemia resulting from the surgery. It is important to instruct the patient and family about the continuing need for pancreatic enzyme replacement, a low-fat diet, and vitamin supplementation.

The nurse teaches the patient and family strategies to relieve pain and discomfort, along with strategies to manage drains, if present, and to care for the surgical incision. The patient and family members may require instruction about use of patient-controlled analgesia, parenteral nutrition, wound care, skin care, and management of drainage. It is important to describe, verbally and in writing, the signs and symptoms of complications and to teach the patient and family about indicators of complications that should be reported promptly.

Discharge of the patient to a long-term care or rehabilitation facility may be warranted after surgery as extensive as pancreatectomy or pancreaticoduodenectomy, particularly if the patient's preoperative status was not optimal. Information about the teaching that has been provided is shared with the long-term care staff so that instructions can be clarified and reinforced. During the recovery or long-term phase of care, the patient and family receive further instructions about self-care in the home.

Continuing Care

A referral for home care may be indicated when the patient returns home. The home care nurse assesses the patient's physical and psychological status and the ability of the patient and family to manage needed care. The home care nurse provides needed physical care and monitors the adequacy of pain management. In addition, it is important to assess the patient's nutritional status and monitor the use of enteral or parenteral nutrition, if used. The nurse discusses the use of hospice services with the patient and family and makes a referral if indicated.

Pancreatic Islet Tumors

The pancreas contains the islets (islands) of Langerhans, small nests of cells that secrete hormones directly into the bloodstream and therefore are part of the endocrine system. The hormone insulin is essential for the metabolism of glucose. Diabetes mellitus (see Chapter 41) is the result of deficient insulin secretion. At least two types of tumors of the pancreatic islet cells are known: those that secrete insulin (insulinoma) and those in which insulin secretion is not increased (nonfunctioning islet cell cancer). Insulinomas produce hypersecretion of insulin and cause an excessive rate of glucose metabolism. The resulting hypoglycemia may produce symptoms of weakness, mental confusion, and seizures. These symptoms may be relieved almost immediately by oral or IV administration of glucose. The 5-hour glucose tolerance test is helpful to diagnose insulinoma and to distinguish this diagnosis from other causes of hypoglycemia.

Surgical Management

If a tumor of the islet cells has been diagnosed, surgical treatment with removal of the tumor is usually recommended (Zinner & Ashley, 2007). The tumors may be benign adenomas or they may be malignant. Complete removal usually results in almost immediate relief of symptoms. In some patients, symptoms may be produced by simple hypertrophy of this tissue rather than a tumor of the islet cells. In such cases, a partial pancreatectomy (removal of the tail and part of the body of the pancreas) is performed.

Nursing Management

In preparing the patient for surgery, the nurse must be alert for symptoms of hypoglycemia and be ready to administer glucose as prescribed if symptoms occur. Postoperatively, the nursing management is the same as after other upper abdominal surgical procedures, with special emphasis on monitoring serum glucose levels. Patient teaching is determined by the extent of surgery and alterations in pancreatic function.

Hyperinsulinism

Hyperinsulinism is caused by overproduction of insulin by the pancreatic islets. Symptoms resemble those of excessive doses of insulin and are attributable to the same mechanism: an abnormal reduction in blood glucose levels. Clinically it is characterized by episodes during which the patient experiences unusual hunger, nervousness, sweating, headache, and faintness; in severe cases, seizures and episodes of unconsciousness may occur. The findings at the time of surgery or at autopsy may indicate hyperplasia (overgrowth) of the islets of Langerhans or a benign or malignant tumor involving the islets that is capable of producing large amounts of insulin (see preceding discussion). Occasionally, tumors of nonpancreatic origin produce an insulin-like material that can cause severe hypoglycemia and may be responsible for seizures coinciding with blood glucose levels that are too low to sustain normal brain function (ie, lower than 30 mg/dL [1.6 mmol/L]).

All the symptoms that accompany spontaneous hypoglycemia are relieved by the oral or parenteral administration of glucose. Surgical removal of the hyperplastic or neoplastic tissue from the pancreas is the only successful method of treatment. About 15% of patients with spontaneous or functional hypoglycemia eventually develop diabetes mellitus.

Ulcerogenic Tumors

Some tumors of the islets of Langerhans are associated with hypersecretion of gastric acid that produces ulcers in the stomach, duodenum, and jejunum. This is referred to as **Zollinger-Ellison syndrome.** The hypersecretion is so excessive that even after partial gastric resection enough acid is produced to cause further ulceration. If a marked tendency to develop gastric and duodenal ulcers is noted, an ulcerogenic tumor of the islets of Langerhans is considered.

These tumors, which may be benign or malignant, are treated by excision, if possible. Frequently, however, removal is not possible because of extension beyond the pancreas. In many patients, a total gastrectomy may be necessary to reduce the secretion of gastric acid sufficiently to prevent further ulceration. This procedure is also indicated to treat gastric carcinoid tumors that may arise from the effect of prolonged hypersecretion of gastric acids (Zinner & Ashley, 2007).

CRITICAL THINKING EXERCISES

1 A 72-year-old woman has confirmed cholelithiasis. She also has many other chronic medical conditions, including coronary artery disease, heart failure, and chronic obstructive pulmonary disease. She has been evaluated for treatment by her internist and a surgeon. Surgical treatment of her cholelithiasis is inappropriate for her at this time. What options exist for this patient? How would you educate and prepare her for nonsurgical interventions? What will her likely outcome be with this treatment approach? What are possible adverse effects of nonsurgical treatment?

2 A 44-year-old man is admitted to your unit with a diagnosis of pancreatitis. He had an ultrasound performed, and several large gallstones were identified. He reports severe epigastric pain (rates it at 9 on a 10-point scale) and nausea. He has a nasogastric tube in place because of several episodes of vomiting. What is the cause of this patient's pancreatitis? What medications and laboratory tests would you expect to see prescribed for this patient? What physical assessment findings will you see? What issues would be of high priority in caring for this patient during his hospital stay? What multisystem complications might arise that would necessitate this patient's transfer to an intensive care unit? What issues would be of high priority in preparing him for hospital discharge?

EBP **3** A 68-year-old woman has undergone a Whipple procedure. For what immediate postoperative complications must you be alert? What assessment strategies are used to monitor for the development of complications? Describe two evidence-based preventive interventions for postoperative care. What type of nutritional interventions might you expect? What education is needed prior to the patient's hospital discharge? What follow-up will be necessary?

EBP **4** A 35-year-old woman is scheduled for a laparoscopic cholecystectomy. She is being discharged on the day of surgery. What information should you collect regarding the patient's home situation before she is discharged? What information should you provide about expectations for postoperative pain and other complications, and what instructions should you provide to the patient about pharmacologic and nonpharmacologic pain management strategies? What is the evidence base for the pain management strategies you provide, and what is the strength of that evidence?

5 Compare and contrast the nursing care of a 46-year-old patient with a diagnosis of acute pancreatitis with that of a 64-year-old patient with a diagnosis of chronic pancreatitis. Explain the rationale for differences in care for patients with these two diagnoses.

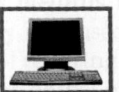
The Smeltzer suite offers these additional resources to enhance learning and facilitate understanding of this chapter:

- thePoint on line resource, thepoint.lww.com/Smeltzer12E
- Student CD-ROM included with the book
- *Study Guide to Accompany Brunner & Suddarth's Textbook of Medical-Surgical Nursing*
- *Handbook for Brunner & Suddarth's Textbook of Medical-Surgical Nursing*

REFERENCES AND SELECTED READINGS

Books

Ajani, J. A., Curley, S. A., Janjan, N. A., et al. (2005). *Gastrointestinal cancer.* New York: Springer Science.

Bayless, T. M. & Diehl, A. M. (Eds.). (2005). *Advanced therapy in gastroenterology and liver disease* (5th ed.). Hamilton: B.C. Decker, Inc.

Bergin, J. D. (2008). *Advanced medicine recall.* Philadelphia: Wolters Kluwer Health/Lippincott Williams & Wilkins.

Corry, R. J. (2007). *Pancreatitis.* New York: Informa Healthcare.

Dominguez-Muñoz, J. E. & Malfertheiner, P. (Ed.). (2005). *Clinical pancreatology for practising gastroenterologists and surgeons.* Malden, MA: Blackwell.

Dudek, S. (2006). *Nutrition essentials for nursing practice.* Philadelphia: Lippincott Williams & Wilkins.

Feldman, M., Friedman, L. S. & Brandt, L. J. (Eds.). (2006). *Sleisenger and Fordtran's gastrointestinal and liver disease: Pathophysiology, diagnosis, and management.* Philadelphia: Saunders.

Floch, M. H., Floch, N. R. & Kowdley, K. V. (Eds.). (2005). *Netter's gastroenterology.* Carlstadt, NJ: Icon Learning Systems.

Forbes, A. (2005). *Atlas of clinical gastroenterology.* Edinburgh; New York: Elsevier Mosby.

Forsmark, C. E. (2005). *Pancreatitis and its complications.* Totowa, NJ: Humana Press. Science.

Goldman, L. & Ausiello, D. A. (2008). *Cecil medicine* (23rd ed.). Philadelphia: Saunders Elsevier.

Hauser, S. C., Pardi, D. S. & Poterucha, J. J. (Eds.). (2006). *Mayo Clinic gastroenterology and hepatology board review* (2nd ed.). Rochester, MN: Mayo Foundation for Medical Education and Research.

Porth, C. M. & Matfin, G. (2009). *Pathophysiology: Concepts of altered health states* (8th ed.). Philadelphia: Lippincott Williams & Wilkins.

Shils, M. E., Shike, M., Ross, A. C., et al. (Eds.). (2006). *Modern nutrition in health and disease* (10th ed.). Philadelphia: Lippincott Williams & Wilkins.

Su, G. H. (Ed.). (2005). *Pancreatic cancer: Methods and protocols.* Totowa, NJ: Humana Press.

Tierney, L. M., McPhee, S. J. & Papadakis, M. A. (2008). *Current medical diagnosis and treatment* (47th ed.). New York: McGraw-Hill.

Weinstein, W. M., Hawkey, J. & Bosch, J. (2005). *Clinical gastroenterology and hepatology.* Edinburgh: Elsevier Mosby.

Wolfe, M. M., Davis, G., Farraye, F., et al. (Eds.). (2006). *Therapy of digestive disorders* (2nd ed.). Philadelphia: Saunders Elsevier.

Yamada, T. (2005). *Handbook of gastroenterology.* Philadelphia: Lippincott Williams & Wilkins.

Zinner, M. J. & Ashley, S.W. (Eds.). (2007). *Maingot's abdominal operations* (11th ed.). New York: McGraw-Hill.

Journals and Electronic Documents

Gallbladder Disease

Al-azawi, D., Mc Mahon, D. & Rajpal, P. K. (2007). The diagnosis of acute cholecystitis in patients undergoing early laparoscopic cholecystectomy in a community hospital. *Surgical Laparoscopy, Endoscopy and Percutaneous Techniques, 17*(1), 19–21.

Baltimore, J. J. & Davidson, J. (2007). Caring for a patient with acute cholecystitis. *Nursing 2008, 37*(3), 64hn1–64hn4.

Kanamaru, T., Sakata, K., Nakamura, Y., et al. (2007). Laparoscopic choledochotomy in management of choledocholithiasis. *Surgical Laparoscopy, Endoscopy and Percutaneous Techniques, 17*(4), 262–266.

Massoumi, H., Kiyici, N. & Hertan, H. (2007). Bile leak after laparoscopic cholecystectomy. *Journal of Clinical Gastroenterology, 41*(3), 301–305.

Shamiyeh, A., Danis, J., Wayand, W., et al. (2007). A 14-year analysis of laparoscopic cholecystectomy: Conversion-when and why? *Surgical Laparoscopy, Endoscopy & Percutaneous Techniques, 17*(4), 271–276.

Tsujino, T., Sugita, R., Yoshida, H., et al. (2007). Risk factors for acute suppurative cholangitis caused by bile duct stones. *European Journal of Gastroenterology and Hepatology, 19*(7), 585–588.

Tsushimi, T., Matsui, N., Takemoto, Y., et al. (2007). Early laparoscopic cholecystectomy for acute gangrenous cholecystitis. *Surgical Laparoscopy, Endoscopy and Percutaneous Technique, 17*(1), 14–18.

Tuveri, M. & Tuveri, A. (2007). Laparoscopic cholecystectomy: Complications and conversions with the 3-trocar technique: A 10-year review. *Surgical Laparoscopy, Endoscopy and Percutaneous Techniques, 17*(5), 380–384.

Pancreatic Disorders

American Academy of Family Physicians. (2007). Chronic pancreatitis: What you should know. *American Family Physician, 76*(11), 1693–1694.

American Cancer Society. (2008). *Cancer facts and figures 2009.* Atlanta: Author.

Beger, H. G. & Bettina, M. (2007). New advances in pancreatic surgery. *Current Opinion in Gastroenterology, 23*(5), 522–534.

Behrman, S. W. & Fowler, E. S. (2007). Pathophysiology of chronic pancreatitis. *Surgical Clinics of North America, 87*(6), 1309–1324.

Ben-Menachem, T. (2007). Risk factors for cholangiocarcinoma. *European Journal of Gastroenterology and Hepatology, 19*(8), 615–617.

Criddle, D. N., McLaughlin, E., Murphy, J. A., et al. (2007). The pancreas misled: Signals to pancreatitis. *Pancreatology, 7*(5–6), 436–446.

DiMagno, M. J. & DiMagno, E. (2007). New advances in acute pancreatitis. *Current Opinion in Gastroenterology, 23*(5), 494–501.

Grote, T. & Logsdon, C. D. (2007). Progress on molecular markers of pancreatic cancer. *Current Opinion in Gastroenterology, 23*(5), 508–514.

Holcomb, S. S. (2007). Stopping the destruction of acute pancreatitis. *Nursing, 37*(6), 42–47.

Kirk, G. R., White, J. S., McKie, L., et al. (2006). Combined antioxidant therapy reduces pain and improves quality of life in chronic pancreatitis. *Journal of Gastrointestinal Surgery, 10*(4), 499–503.

Kocher, H. M. (2008). Chronic pancreatitis. *American Family Physician, 77*(5), 661–662.

Lankisch, P. G. (2007). Chronic pancreatitis. *Current Opinion in Gastroenterology, 23*(5), 502–507.

Lee, J. K. & Enns, R. (2007). Review of Idiopathic pancreatitis. *World Journal of Gastroenterology, 13*(47), 6296–6313.

Nair, R. J., Lawler, L. & Miller, M. R. (2007). Chronic pancreatitis. *American Family Physician, 76*(11), 1693–1694.

National Pancreas Foundation. (2007). Pancreatic disorders: State of the science and future directions. *Pancreas, 35*(3), 276–280.

Pausawasdi, N. & Scheiman, J. (2007). Endoscopic evaluation and palliation of pancreatic adenocarcinoma. *Current Opinion in Gastroenterology, 23*(5), 515–521.

Petrov, M. S., van Santvoort, H. C., Besselink, M. G., et al. (2008). Early endoscopic retrograde cholangiopancreatography versus conservative management in acute biliary pancreatitis without cholangitis: A meta-analysis of randomized trials. *Annals of Surgery, 247*(2), 250–257.

Plate, J. M. (2007). Current immunotherapeutic strategies in pancreatic cancer. *Surgical Oncology Clinics of North America, 16*(4), 919–943.

Ranson, J. H. Rifkind, K. M. Roses, D. F., et al. (1974). Prognostic signs and the role of operative management in acute pancreatitis. *Surgery, Gynecology, & Obstetrics, 139*(1), 69–81.

Rodriguez, J. R., Razo, A. O., Targarona, J., et al. (2008). Debridement and closed packing for sterile or infected necrotizing pancreatitis: Insights into indications and outcomes in 167 patients. *Annals of Surgery, 247*(2), 294–299.

Sareen, S. & Kumari, V. (2006). Yoga for rehabilitation in chronic pancreatitis. *Gut, 55*(3), 1051.

Takai, S., Satoi, S., Yanagimoto, H., et al. (2008). Neoadjuvant chemoradiation in patients with potentially resectable pancreatic cancer. *Pancreas, 36*(1), 26–32.

Vitale, G. C. (2007). Early management of acute gallstone pancreatitis. *Annals of Surgery, 245*(1), 18–19.

Yekebas, E. F., Bogoevski, D., Cataldegirmen, G., et al. (2008). En bloc resection for locally advanced pancreatic malignancies infiltrating major blood vessels: Perioperative outcome and long-term survival. *Annals of Surgery, 247*(2), 300–309.

RESOURCES

American Gastroenterological Association, www.gastro.org

National Digestive Diseases Information Clearing House, www.niddk.nih.gov

National Endocrine Society, www.endo-society.org

National Pancreas Foundation, www.pancreasfoundation.org

Table 41-1	CLASSIFICATION OF DIABETES MELLITUS AND RELATED GLUCOSE INTOLERANCES
Current Classification	**Clinical Characteristics and Clinical Implications**
Type 1 (5–10% of all diabetes) (Previously classified as juvenile-onset diabetes, juvenile-onset diabetes, ketosis-prone diabetes, brittle diabetes, and insulin-dependent diabetes mellitus [IDDM])	Onset any age, but usually young (<30 y) Usually thin at diagnosis; recent weight loss Etiology includes genetic, immunologic, and environmental factors (eg, virus) Often have islet cell antibodies Often have antibodies to insulin even before insulin treatment Little or no endogenous insulin Need insulin to preserve life Ketosis prone when insulin absent Acute complication of hyperglycemia: diabetic ketoacidosis
Type 2 (90–95% of all diabetes: obese—80% of type 2; nonobese—20% of type 2) (Previously classified as adult-onset diabetes, maturity-onset diabetes, ketosis-resistant diabetes, stable diabetes, and non–insulin-dependent diabetes [NIDDM])	Onset any age, usually over 30 y Usually obese at diagnosis Causes include obesity, heredity, and environmental factors No islet cell antibodies Decrease in endogenous insulin, or increased with insulin resistance Most patients can control blood glucose through weight loss if obese Oral antidiabetic agents may improve blood glucose levels if dietary modification and exercise are unsuccessful May need insulin on a short-term or long-term basis to prevent hyperglycemia Ketosis uncommon, except in stress or infection Acute complication: hyperglycemic hyperosmolar nonketotic syndrome
Diabetes mellitus associated with other conditions or syndromes (Previously classified as secondary diabetes)	Accompanied by conditions known or suspected to cause the disease: pancreatic diseases, hormonal abnormalities, medications such as corticosteroids and estrogen-containing preparations Depending on the ability of the pancreas to produce insulin, the patient may require treatment with oral antidiabetic agents or insulin
Gestational diabetes	Onset during pregnancy, usually in the second or third trimester Due to hormones secreted by the placenta, which inhibit the action of insulin Above-normal risk for perinatal complications, especially macrosomia (abnormally large babies) Treated with diet and, if needed, insulin to strictly maintain normal blood glucose levels Occurs in about 2–5% of all pregnancies Glucose intolerance transitory but may recur: • In subsequent pregnancies • 30–40% will develop overt diabetes (usually type 2) within 10 years (especially if obese) Risk factors include obesity, age older than 30 years, family history of diabetes, previous large babies (>9 lb) Screening tests (glucose challenge test) should be performed on all pregnant women between 24- and 28-weeks gestation Should be screened for diabetes periodically
Prediabetes (Previously classified as previous abnormality of glucose tolerance [PrevAGT])	Previous history of hyperglycemia (eg, during pregnancy or illness) Current normal glucose metabolism Impaired glucose tolerance or impaired fasting glucose screening after age 40 years if there is a family history of diabetes or if symptomatic Encourage ideal body weight, because loss of 10–15 lb may improve glycemic control

and the glucagon together maintain a constant level of glucose in the blood by stimulating the release of glucose from the liver.

Initially, the liver produces glucose through the breakdown of glycogen (glycogenolysis). After 8 to 12 hours without food, the liver forms glucose from the breakdown of noncarbohydrate substances, including amino acids (gluconeogenesis).

Type 1 Diabetes

Type 1 diabetes affects approximately 5% to 10% of people with the disease; it is characterized by an acute onset, usually before 30 years of age (CDC, 2008). Type 1 diabetes is characterized by destruction of the pancreatic beta cells. Combined genetic, immunologic, and possibly environmental (eg, viral) factors are thought to contribute to beta-cell destruction. Although the events that lead to beta-cell destruction are not fully understood, it is generally accepted that a genetic susceptibility is a common underlying factor

in the development of type 1 diabetes. People do not inherit type 1 diabetes itself but rather a genetic predisposition, or tendency, toward development of type 1 diabetes. This genetic tendency has been found in people with certain human leukocyte antigen (HLA) types. There is also evidence of an autoimmune response in type 1 diabetes. This is an abnormal response in which antibodies are directed against normal tissues of the body, responding to these tissues as if they were foreign. Autoantibodies against islet cells and against endogenous (internal) insulin have been detected in people at the time of diagnosis and even several years before the development of clinical signs of type 1 diabetes. In addition to genetic and immunologic components, environmental factors, such as viruses or toxins, that may initiate destruction of the beta cell are being investigated.

Regardless of the specific cause, the destruction of the beta cells results in decreased insulin production, unchecked glucose production by the liver, and fasting hyperglycemia. In addition, glucose derived from food cannot be stored in the liver but instead remains in the bloodstream and contributes to postprandial (after meals) hyperglycemia. If the concentration of glucose in the blood exceeds the renal threshold for glucose, usually 180 to 200 mg/dL (9.9 to 11.1 mmol/L), the kidneys may not reabsorb all of the filtered glucose; the glucose then appears in the urine (glycosuria). When excess glucose is excreted in the urine, it is accompanied by excessive loss of fluids and electrolytes. This is called osmotic diuresis.

Because insulin normally inhibits glycogenolysis (break-down of stored glucose) and gluconeogenesis (production of new glucose from amino acids and other substrates), these processes occur in an unrestrained fashion in people with insulin deficiency and contribute further to hyperglycemia. In addition, fat breakdown occurs, resulting in an increased production of **ketone** bodies, which are the byproducts of fat breakdown.

 NURSING ALERT

Ketone bodies are acids that disturb the acid–base balance of the body when they accumulate in excessive amounts. The resulting **diabetic ketoacidosis (DKA)** may cause signs and symptoms such as abdominal pain, nausea, vomiting, hyperventilation, a fruity breath odor, and, if left untreated, altered level of consciousness, coma, and death. Initiation of insulin treatment, along with fluid and electrolytes as needed, is essential to treat hyperglycemia and DKA and rapidly improves the metabolic abnormalities.

Type 2 Diabetes

Type 2 diabetes affects approximately 90% to 95% of people with the disease (CDC, 2008). It occurs more commonly among people who are older than 30 years of age and obese (National Institute of Diabetes and Digestive and Kidney Diseases [NIDDK], 2005), although its incidence is rapidly increasing in younger people because of the growing epidemic of obesity in children, adolescents, and young adults (CDC, 2008). The two main problems related to insulin in type 2 diabetes are insulin resistance and impaired insulin secretion. Insulin resistance refers to a decreased tissue sensitivity to insulin. Normally, insulin binds to special receptors on cell surfaces and initiates a series of reactions involved in glucose metabolism. In type 2 diabetes, these intracellular reactions are diminished, making insulin less effective at stimulating glucose uptake by the tissues and at regulating glucose release by the liver (Fig. 41-1). The exact mechanisms that lead to insulin resistance and impaired insulin secretion in type 2 diabetes are unknown, although genetic factors are thought to play a role.

To overcome insulin resistance and to prevent the buildup of glucose in the blood, increased amounts of insulin must be secreted to maintain the glucose level at a normal or slightly elevated level. This is called metabolic syndrome, which includes hypertension, hypercholesterolemia, and abdominal obesity. However, if the

Physiology ■■■ Pathophysiology

Figure 41-1 Pathogenesis of type 2 diabetes.

beta cells cannot keep up with the increased demand for insulin, the glucose level rises and type 2 diabetes develops.

Despite the impaired insulin secretion that is characteristic of type 2 diabetes, there is enough insulin present to prevent the breakdown of fat and the accompanying production of ketone bodies. Therefore, DKA does not typically occur in type 2 diabetes. However, uncontrolled type 2 diabetes may lead to another acute problem—hyperglycemic hyperosmolar nonketotic syndrome (see later discussion).

Because type 2 diabetes is associated with a slow, progressive glucose intolerance, its onset may go undetected for many years. If the patient experiences symptoms, they are frequently mild and may include fatigue, irritability, polyuria, polydipsia, poorly healing skin wounds, vaginal infections, or blurred vision (if glucose levels are very high).

For most patients (approximately 75%), type 2 diabetes is detected incidentally (eg, when routine laboratory tests or ophthalmoscopic examinations are performed). One consequence of undetected diabetes is that long-term diabetes complications (eg, eye disease, peripheral neuropathy, peripheral vascular disease) may have developed before the actual diagnosis of diabetes is made (ADA, 2009a), signifying that the blood glucose has been elevated for a time before diagnosis.

Gestational Diabetes

Gestational diabetes mellitus (GDM) is any degree of glucose intolerance with its onset during pregnancy. Hyperglycemia develops during pregnancy because of the secretion of placental hormones, which causes insulin resistance. Gestational diabetes occurs in as many as 14% of pregnant women and increases their risk for hypertensive disorders during pregnancy (ADA, 2009a).

Women who are considered to be at high risk for GDM and who should be screened by blood glucose testing at their first prenatal visit are those with marked obesity, a personal history of GDM, glycosuria, or a strong family history of diabetes. High-risk ethnic groups include Hispanic Americans, Native Americans, Asian Americans, African Americans, and Pacific Islanders. If these high-risk women do not have GDM at initial screening, they should be retested between 24 and 28 weeks of gestation. All women of average risk should be tested at 24 to 28 weeks of gestation. Testing is not specifically recommended for women identified as being at low risk. Low-risk women are those who meet all of the following criteria: age younger than 25 years, normal weight before pregnancy, member of an ethnic group with low prevalence of GDM, no history of abnormal glucose tolerance, no known history of diabetes in first-degree relatives, and no history of poor obstetric outcome (ADA, 2009a). Women considered to be at high risk or average risk should have either an oral glucose tolerance test (OGTT) or a glucose challenge test (GCT) followed by OGTT in women who exceed the glucose threshold value of 140 mg/dL (7.8 mmol/L) (ADA, 2009a).

Initial management includes dietary modification and blood glucose monitoring. If hyperglycemia persists, insulin is prescribed. Goals for blood glucose levels during pregnancy are 105 mg/dL (5.8 mmol/L) or less before meals and 130 mg/dL (7.2 mmol/L) or less 2 hours after meals (ADA, 2009a).

After delivery, blood glucose levels in women with GDM usually return to normal. However, many women who have had GDM develop type 2 diabetes later in life. For this reason, a woman who has had GDM should be counseled to maintain her ideal body weight and to exercise regularly to reduce her risk for type 2 diabetes (Kitzmiller, Dang-Kilduff & Taslimi, 2007).

Prevention

In 2002 the Diabetes Prevention Program Research Group reported that type 2 diabetes can be prevented with appropriate changes in lifestyle. Persons at high risk for type 2 diabetes (BMI 24 or greater, fasting and postprandial plasma glucose levels elevated but not to levels diagnostic of diabetes) received either standard lifestyle recommendations plus metformin, standard lifestyle recommendations plus placebo, or an intensive program of lifestyle modifications. The 16-lesson curriculum of the intensive program of lifestyle modifications focused on weight reduction of greater than 7% of initial body weight and physical activity of moderate intensity. It also included behavior modification strategies designed to help patients achieve the goals of weight reduction and participation in exercise. The lifestyle intervention group had a 58% lower incidence of diabetes and the metformin group had a 31% lower incidence of diabetes compared to the placebo group. These findings were found in both genders and all racial and ethnic groups. These findings demonstrate that type 2 diabetes can be prevented or delayed in persons at high risk for the disease.

Clinical Manifestations

Clinical manifestations depend on the patient's level of hyperglycemia. Classic clinical manifestations of all types of diabetes include the "three Ps": polyuria, polydipsia, and polyphagia. Polyuria (increased urination) and polydipsia (increased thirst) occur as a result of the excess loss of fluid associated with osmotic diuresis. Patients also experience polyphagia (increased appetite) that results from the catabolic state induced by insulin deficiency and the breakdown of proteins and fats. Other symptoms include fatigue and weakness, sudden vision changes, tingling or numbness in hands or feet, dry skin, skin lesions or wounds that are slow to heal, and recurrent infections. The onset of type 1 diabetes may also be associated with sudden weight loss or nausea, vomiting, or abdominal pains, if DKA has developed.

Assessment and Diagnostic Findings

An abnormally high blood glucose level is the basic criterion for the diagnosis of diabetes. **Fasting plasma glucose (FPG),** random plasma glucose, and glucose level 2 hours after receiving glucose (2-hour postload) may be used. The OGTT and the intravenous (IV) glucose tolerance test are no longer recommended for routine clinical use. See Chart 41-2 for the ADA's diagnostic criteria for diabetes mellitus (ADA, 2009a).

In addition to the assessment and diagnostic evaluation performed to diagnose diabetes, ongoing specialized assessment of patients with known diabetes and evaluation for complications in patients with newly diagnosed diabetes are important components of care. Parameters that should be regularly assessed are discussed in Chart 41-3.

Chart 41-2 • *Criteria for the Diagnosis of Diabetes Mellitus*

1. Symptoms of diabetes plus casual plasma glucose concentration equal to or greater than 200 mg/dL (11.1 mmol/L). Casual is defined as any time of day without regard to time since last meal. The classic symptoms of diabetes include polyuria, polydipsia, and unexplained weight loss.

or

2. Fasting plasma glucose greater than or equal to 126 mg/dL (7.0 mmol/L). Fasting is defined as no caloric intake for at least 8 hours.

or

3. Two-hour postload glucose equal to or greater than 200 mg/dL (11.1 mmol/L) during an oral glucose tolerance test. The test should be performed as described by the World Health Organization, using a glucose load containing the equivalent of 75 g anhydrous glucose dissolved in water.

In the absence of unequivocal hyperglycemia with acute metabolic decompensation, these criteria should be confirmed by repeat testing on a different day. The third measure is not recommended for routine clinical use.

Used with permission of American Diabetes Association. (2009a). Report of the Expert Committee on the Diagnosis and Classification of Diabetes Mellitus, *Diabetes Care, 32*(Suppl. 1), S62–S67.

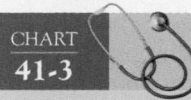

CHART 41-3 *Assessing the Patient With Diabetes*

History

- Symptoms related to the diagnosis of diabetes:
  Symptoms of hyperglycemia
  Symptoms of hypoglycemia
    Frequency, timing, severity, and resolution
- Results of blood glucose monitoring
- Status, symptoms, and management of chronic complications of diabetes:
    Eye; kidney; nerve; genitourinary and sexual, bladder, and gastrointestinal
    Cardiac; peripheral vascular; foot complications associated with diabetes
- Adherence to/ability to follow prescribed dietary management plan
- Adherence to prescribed exercise regimen
- Adherence to/ability to follow prescribed pharmacologic treatment (insulin or oral antidiabetic agents)
- Use of tobacco, alcohol, and prescribed and over-the-counter medications/drugs
- Lifestyle, cultural, psychosocial, and economic factors that may affect diabetes treatment
- Effects of diabetes or its complications on functional status (eg, mobility, vision)

Physical Examination

- Blood pressure (sitting and standing to detect orthostatic changes)

- Body mass index (height and weight)
- Fundoscopic examination and visual acuity
- Foot examination (lesions, signs of infection, pulses)
- Skin examination (lesions and insulin-injection sites)
- Neurologic examination
  Vibratory and sensory examination using monofilament
  Deep tendon reflexes
- Oral examination

Laboratory Examination

- $HgbA_{1C}$ (A1C)
- Fasting lipid profile
- Test for microalbuminuria
- Serum creatinine level
- Urinalysis
- Electrocardiogram

Need for Referrals

- Ophthalmology
- Podiatry
- Dietitian
- Diabetes educator
- Others if indicated

Gerontologic Considerations

Elevated blood glucose levels appear to be age related and occur in both men and women throughout the world. Elevated blood glucose levels commonly appear in the fifth decade of life and increase in frequency with advancing age. Approximately 10% to 30% of elderly people have age-related hyperglycemia, not counting those with overt diabetes. What causes age-related changes in carbohydrate metabolism is not known. Possibilities include poor diet, physical inactivity, a decrease in the lean body mass in which ingested carbohydrate may be stored, altered insulin secretion, and increase in fat tissue, which increases insulin resistance (ADA, 2009b).

Medical Management

The main goal of diabetes treatment is to normalize insulin activity and blood glucose levels to reduce the development of vascular and neuropathic complications. The Diabetes Control and Complications Trial (DCCT), a 10-year prospective clinical trial conducted from 1983 to 1993, demonstrated the importance of achieving blood glucose control in the normal, nondiabetic range. This landmark trial demonstrated that intensive glucose control dramatically reduced the development and progression of complications such as **retinopathy, nephropathy,** and **neuropathy.** Intensive treatment is defined as three or four insulin injections per day or **continuous subcutaneous insulin infusion, insulin pump** therapy plus frequent blood glucose

monitoring and weekly contacts with diabetes educators. The American Diabetes Association now recommends that all patients with diabetes strive for glucose control to reduce their risk of complications (ADA, 2009b).

Intensive therapy must be initiated with caution and must be accompanied by thorough education of the patient and family and by responsible behavior of the patient. Careful screening of patients is a key step in initiating intensive therapy.

A study conducted in the United Kingdom demonstrated a decrease in complications among patients with type 2 diabetes receiving intensive therapy compared to those receiving conventional therapy (United Kingdom Prospective Diabetes Study Group [UKPDS], 1998; see also ADA, 2009b).

The results of the DCCT and UKPDS have been supported by follow-up studies, including the Epidemiology of Diabetes Interventions and Complications (EDIC) study (Nathan, Cleary, Backlund, et al., 2005). Therefore, the therapeutic goal for diabetes management is to achieve normal blood glucose levels (euglycemia) without hypoglycemia while maintaining a high quality of life. Diabetes management has five components: nutritional therapy, exercise, monitoring, pharmacologic therapy, and education. Diabetes management involves constant assessment and modification of the treatment plan by health professionals and daily adjustments in therapy by the patient. Although the health care team directs the treatment, it is the individual patient who must manage the complex therapeutic regimen. For this reason, patient and family education is an essential component of diabetes treatment and is as important as all other components of the regimen.

Nutritional Therapy

Nutrition, meal planning, and weight control are the foundation of diabetes management. The most important objectives in the dietary and nutritional management of diabetes are control of total caloric intake to attain or maintain a reasonable body weight, control of blood glucose levels, and normalization of lipids and blood pressure to prevent heart disease. Success in this area alone is often associated with reversal of hyperglycemia in type 2 diabetes. However, achieving these goals is not always easy. Because **medical nutrition therapy** (MNT, nutritional management) of diabetes is complex, a registered dietitian who understands diabetes management has the major responsibility for designing and teaching this aspect of the therapeutic plan. Nurses and all other members of the health care team must be knowledgeable about nutritional therapy and supportive of patients who need to implement nutritional and lifestyle changes. Nutritional management of diabetes includes the following goals (ADA, 2008b).

1. To achieve and maintain
   • Blood glucose levels in the normal range or as close to normal as is safely possible
   • A lipid and lipoprotein profile that reduces the risk for vascular disease
   • Blood pressure levels in the normal range or as close to normal as is safely possible
2. To prevent, or at least slow, the rate of development of the chronic complications of diabetes by modifying nutrient intake and lifestyle
3. To address individual nutrition needs, taking into account personal and cultural preferences and willingness to change
4. To maintain the pleasure of eating by only limiting food choices when indicated by scientific evidence.

For obese patients with diabetes (especially those with type 2 diabetes), weight loss is the key to treatment. (It is also a major factor in preventing diabetes.) In general, overweight is considered to be a body mass index (BMI) of 25 to 29; obesity is defined as 20% above ideal body weight or a BMI equal to or greater than 30 (National Institutes of Health, 2000). BMI is a weight-to-height ratio calculated by dividing body weight (in kilograms) by the square of the height (in meters). Calculation of BMI is discussed in Chapter 5. Obese patients who have type 2 diabetes and who require insulin or oral agents to control blood glucose levels may be able to reduce or eliminate the need for medication through weight loss. A weight loss as small as 5% to 10% of total weight may significantly improve blood glucose levels (ADA, 2009b). For obese patients with diabetes who do not take insulin or sulfonylureas, consistent meal content or timing is important but not as critical. Rather, decreasing the overall caloric intake assumes more importance. However, meals should not be skipped. Pacing food intake throughout the day places more manageable demands on the pancreas.

Consistently following a meal plan is one of the most challenging aspects of diabetes management. It may be more realistic to restrict calories only moderately. For patients who have lost weight, maintaining the weight loss may be difficult. To help these patients incorporate new dietary habits into their lifestyles, diet education, behavioral therapy, group support, and ongoing nutrition counseling are encouraged.

Meal Planning and Related Teaching

The meal plan must consider the patient's food preferences, lifestyle, usual eating times, and ethnic and cultural background. For patients who require insulin to help control blood glucose levels, maintaining as much consistency as possible in the amount of calories and carbohydrates ingested at each meal is essential. In addition, consistency in the approximate time intervals between meals, with the addition of snacks if necessary, helps prevent hypoglycemic reactions and maintain overall blood glucose control. For patients who can master the insulin-to-carbohydrate calculations, lifestyle can be more flexible and diabetes control more predictable. For those using intensive insulin therapy, there may be greater flexibility in the timing and content of meals by allowing adjustments in insulin dosage for changes in eating and exercise habits. Advances in insulin management (new insulin analogues, insulin algorithms, insulin pumps) permit greater flexibility of schedules than was previously possible. This contrasts with the older concept of maintaining a constant dose of insulin, which required strict scheduling of meals to match the actions and duration of the insulin.

The first step in preparing a meal plan is a thorough review of the patient's diet history to identify his or her eating habits and lifestyle. This includes a thorough assessment of the patient's need for weight loss, gain, or maintenance. In most instances, people with type 2 diabetes require weight reduction.

In teaching about meal planning, clinical dietitians use various educational tools, materials, and approaches. Initial education addresses the importance of consistent eating habits, the relationship of food and insulin, and the provision of an individualized meal plan. In-depth follow-up education then focuses on management skills, such as eating at restaurants, reading food labels, and adjusting the meal plan for exercise, illness, and special occasions. The nurse plays an important role in communicating pertinent information to the dietitian and reinforcing the patient's understanding.

Certain aspects of meal planning, such as the food exchange system, may be difficult to learn. This may be related to limitations in the patient's intellectual level or to emotional issues, such as difficulty accepting the diagnosis of diabetes or feelings of deprivation and undue restriction in eating. In any case, it helps to emphasize that using the exchange system (or any food classification system) provides a new way of thinking about food rather than a new way of eating. It is also important to simplify information as much as possible and to provide opportunities for the patient to practice and repeat activities and information.

Caloric Requirements.
Calorie-controlled diets are planned by first calculating a person's energy needs and caloric requirements based on age, gender, height, and weight. An activity element is then factored in to provide

the actual number of calories required for weight maintenance. To promote a 1- to 2-pound weight loss per week, 500 to 1000 calories are subtracted from the daily total. The calories are distributed into carbohydrates, proteins, and fats, and a meal plan is then developed, taking into account the patient's lifestyle and food preferences.

In contrast to the priority for the obese person with type 2 diabetes, the priority for a young patient with type 1 diabetes should be a diet with enough calories to maintain normal growth and development. Some patients may be underweight at the onset of type 1 diabetes because of rapid weight loss from severe hyperglycemia. The goal initially may be to provide a higher-calorie diet to regain lost weight and blood glucose control.

Caloric Distribution. A meal plan for diabetes focuses on the percentages of calories that come from carbohydrates, proteins, and fats.

Carbohydrates. The caloric distribution currently recommended is higher in carbohydrates than in fat and protein. In general, carbohydrate foods have the greatest effect on blood glucose levels because they are more quickly digested than other foods and are converted into glucose rapidly. However, research into the appropriateness of a higher-carbohydrate diet in patients with decreased glucose tolerance is ongoing, and recommendations may change accordingly. Currently, the ADA and the American Dietetic Association recommend that for all levels of caloric intake, 50% to 60% of calories should be derived from carbohydrates, 20% to 30% from fat, and the remaining 10% to 20% from protein. The majority of the selections for carbohydrates should come from whole grains. These recommendations are also consistent with those of the American Heart Association and American Cancer Society.

Carbohydrates consist of sugars (eg, sucrose) and starches (eg, rice, pasta, bread). Low glycemic index diets (described later) may reduce postprandial glucose levels. Therefore, the nutrition guidelines recommend that all carbohydrates should be eaten in moderation to avoid high postprandial blood glucose levels (ADA, 2008b).

Foods high in carbohydrates, such as sucrose (concentrated sweets), are not totally eliminated from the diet but should be eaten in moderation (up to 10% of total calories), because they are typically high in fat and lack vitamins, minerals, and fiber.

Fats. The recommendations regarding fat content of the diabetic diet include both reducing the total percentage of calories from fat sources to less than 30% of total calories and limiting the amount of saturated fats to 10% of total calories. Additional recommendations include limiting the total intake of dietary cholesterol to less than 300 mg/day. This approach may help reduce risk factors such as increased serum cholesterol levels, which are associated with the development of coronary artery disease, the leading cause of death and disability among people with diabetes (ADA, 2008c).

Protein. The meal plan may include the use of some nonanimal sources of protein (eg, legumes, whole grains), to help reduce saturated fat and cholesterol intake. In addition, the amount of protein intake may be reduced in patients with early signs of renal disease.

Fiber. Increased fiber in the diet may improve blood glucose levels, decrease the need for exogenous insulin, and lower total cholesterol and low-density lipoprotein levels in the blood (ADA, 2008b).

There are two types of dietary fibers: soluble and insoluble. Soluble fiber—in foods such as legumes, oats, and some fruits—plays more of a role in lowering blood glucose and lipid levels than does insoluble fiber, although the clinical significance of this effect is probably small (ADA, 2008b). Soluble fiber slows stomach emptying and the movement of food through the upper digestive tract. The potential glucose-lowering effect of fiber may be caused by the slower rate of glucose absorption from foods that contain soluble fiber. Insoluble fiber is found in whole-grain breads and cereals and in some vegetables. This type of fiber along with soluble fiber increases satiety, which is helpful for weight loss. At least 25 g of fiber should be ingested daily.

One risk involved in suddenly increasing fiber intake is that it may require adjusting the dosage of insulin or oral agents to prevent hypoglycemia. Other problems may include abdominal fullness, nausea, diarrhea, increased flatulence, and constipation if fluid intake is inadequate. If fiber is added to or increased in the meal plan, it should be done gradually and in consultation with a dietitian. The exchange lists (ADA, 2008b) serve as an excellent guide for increasing fiber intake. Fiber-rich food choices within the vegetable, fruit, and starch/bread exchanges are highlighted in the lists.

Food Classification Systems. To teach diet principles and to help in meal planning, several systems have been developed in which foods are organized into groups with common characteristics, such as number of calories, composition of foods (ie, amount of protein, fat, or carbohydrate in the food), or effect on blood glucose levels. Several of these are listed here.

Exchange Lists. A commonly used tool for nutritional management is the exchange lists for meal planning (ADA, 2008b). There are six main exchange lists: bread/starch, vegetable, milk, meat, fruit, and fat. Foods within one group (in the portion amounts specified) contain equal numbers of calories and are approximately equal in grams of protein, fat, and carbohydrate. Meal plans can be based on a recommended number of choices from each exchange list. Foods on one list may be interchanged with one another, allowing for variety while maintaining as much consistency as possible in the nutrient content of foods eaten. Table 41-2 presents three sample lunch menus that are interchangeable in terms of carbohydrate, protein, and fat content.

Exchange list information on combination foods such as pizza, chili, and casseroles, as well as convenience foods, desserts, snack foods, and fast foods, is available from the American Diabetes Association (see Resources). Some food manufacturers and restaurants publish exchange lists that describe their products.

Nutrition Labels. Food manufacturers are required to have the nutrition content of foods listed on package labels, and reading food labels is an important skill for patients to learn and use when food shopping. The label includes information about how many grams of carbohydrate are in a serving

Table 41-2	SELECTED SAMPLE MENUS FROM EXCHANGE LISTS		
Exchanges	**Sample Lunch #1**	**Sample Lunch #2**	**Sample Lunch #3**
2 starch	2 slices bread	Hamburger bun	1 cup cooked pasta
3 meat	2 oz sliced turkey and 1 oz lowfat cheese	3 oz lean beef patty	3 oz boiled shrimp
1 vegetable	Lettuce, tomato, onion	Green salad	½ cup plum tomatoes
1 fat	1 tsp mayonnaise	1 tbsp salad dressing	1 tsp olive oil
1 fruit	1 medium apple	1¼ cup watermelon	1¼ cup fresh strawberries
"Free" items (optional)	Unsweetened iced tea	Diet soda	Ice water with lemon
	Mustard, pickle, hot pepper	1 tbsp catsup, pickle, onions	Garlic, basil

of food. This information can be used to determine how much medication is needed. For example, a patient who takes premeal insulin may use the algorithm, 1 unit of insulin for 15 g of carbohydrate. Patients can also be taught to have a "carbohydrate budget" per meal (eg, 45 to 60 g).

Carbohydrate counting is a nutritional tool used for blood glucose management because carbohydrates are the main nutrients in food that influence blood glucose levels. This method provides flexibility in food choices, can be less complicated to understand than the diabetic food exchange list, and allows more accurate management with multiple daily injections (insulin before each meal). However, if carbohydrate counting is not used with other meal-planning techniques, weight gain can result. A variety of methods are used to count carbohydrates. When developing a diabetic meal plan using carbohydrate counting, all food sources should be considered.

Once digested, 100% of carbohydrates are converted to glucose. Approximately 50% of protein foods (meat, fish, and poultry) are also converted to glucose, but this has minimal effect on blood glucose levels.

Carbohydrate counting consists of counting grams of carbohydrates. If target goals are not reached by counting carbohydrates alone, protein is factored into the calculations. This is especially true if the meal consists only of meat, fish, and nonstarchy vegetables.

Although carbohydrate counting is now commonly used for blood glucose management with type 1 and type 2 diabetes, it is not a perfect system. All carbohydrates affect the blood glucose level to different degrees, regardless of equivalent serving size. When carbohydrate counting is used, reading labels on food items is the key to success. Knowing what the "carbohydrate budget" for the meal is and knowing how many grams of carbohydrate are in a serving of a food, the patient can calculate the amount in one serving.

Healthy Food Choices. An alternative to counting grams of carbohydrate is measuring servings or choices. This method is used more often by people with type 2 diabetes. It is similar to the food exchange list and emphasizes portion control of total servings of carbohydrate at meals and snacks. One carbohydrate serving is equivalent to 15 g of carbohydrate. Examples of one serving are an apple 2 inches in diameter and one slice of bread. Vegetables and meat are counted as one third of a carbohydrate serving. This system works well for those who have difficulty with the other complicated systems.

Food Guide Pyramid. The Food Guide Pyramid (ie, MyPyramid) is another tool used to develop meal plans. It is commonly used for patients with type 2 diabetes who have a difficult time following a calorie-controlled diet. The 2005 food pyramid consists of the following food groups: (1) grains, (2) vegetables, (3) fruits, (4) milk and other dairy products, and (5) meats and beans. Oils and other high-fat foods comprise another food group on the pyramid (see Chapter 5). Foods (starches, fruits, and vegetables) that are lowest in calories and fat and highest in fiber should make up the basis of the diet. For those with diabetes, as well as for the general population, 50% to 60% of the daily caloric intake should be from these three groups. Foods higher in fat (particularly saturated fat) should account for a smaller percentage of the daily caloric intake. Fats, oils, and sweets should be used sparingly to obtain weight and blood glucose control and to reduce the risk for cardiovascular disease. Reliance on the MyPyramid may result in fluctuations in blood glucose levels, however, because high-carbohydrate foods may be grouped with low-carbohydrate foods. The pyramid is appropriately used only as a first-step teaching tool for patients who are learning how to control food portions and how to identify which foods contain carbohydrate, protein, and fat.

Glycemic Index. One of the main goals of diet therapy in diabetes is to avoid sharp, rapid increases in blood glucose levels after food is eaten. The term glycemic index is used to describe how much a given food increases the blood glucose level compared with an equivalent amount of glucose. The effects of use of the glycemic index on blood glucose levels and on long-term patient outcomes are unclear, but it may be beneficial (ADA, 2008b). Although more research is necessary, the following guidelines may be helpful when making dietary recommendations:

- Combining starchy foods with protein-containing and fat-containing foods tends to slow their absorption and lower the glycemic response.
- In general, eating foods that are raw and whole results in a lower glycemic response than eating chopped, puréed, or cooked foods.
- Eating whole fruit instead of drinking juice decreases the glycemic response, because fiber in the fruit slows absorption.
- Adding foods with sugars to the diet may result in a lower glycemic response if these foods are eaten with foods that are more slowly absorbed.

Patients can create their own glycemic index by monitoring their blood glucose level after ingestion of a particular food. This can help improve blood glucose control through individualized manipulation of the diet. Many patients who use frequent monitoring of blood glucose levels can use this information to adjust their insulin doses in accordance with variations in food intake.

Other Dietary Concerns

Alcohol Consumption. Patients with diabetes do not need to give up alcoholic beverages entirely, but they and health care professionals must be aware of the potential adverse effects of alcohol specific to diabetes. Alcohol is absorbed before other nutrients and does not require insulin for absorption. Large amounts can be converted to fats, increasing the risk for DKA. In general, the same precautions regarding the use of alcohol by people without diabetes should be applied to patients with diabetes. Moderation is recommended. A major danger of alcohol consumption by the patient with diabetes is hypoglycemia, especially for patients who take insulin or insulin secretagogues (medications that increase the secretion of insulin by the pancreas). Alcohol may decrease the normal physiologic reactions in the body that produce glucose (gluconeogenesis). Therefore, if a patient with diabetes consumes alcohol on an empty stomach, there is an increased likelihood of hypoglycemia. In addition, excessive alcohol intake may impair the patient's ability to recognize and treat hypoglycemia or to follow a prescribed meal plan to prevent hypoglycemia. To reduce the risk of hypoglycemia, the patient should be cautioned to consume food along with the alcohol; however, carbohydrate consumed with alcohol may raise blood glucose (ADA, 2008b).

Alcohol consumption may lead to excessive weight gain (from the high caloric content of alcohol), hyperlipidemia, and elevated glucose levels (especially with mixed drinks and liqueurs). Patient teaching regarding alcohol intake must emphasize moderation in the amount of alcohol consumed. Moderate intake is considered to be one alcoholic beverage per day for women and two per day for men. Lower-calorie or less sweet drinks (eg, light beer, dry wine) and food intake along with alcohol consumption are advised. Especially for patients with type 2 diabetes who wish to control their weight, it is important to incorporate the calories from alcohol into the overall meal plan.

Sweeteners. Use of artificial sweeteners is acceptable, especially if it assists in overall dietary adherence. Moderation in the amount of sweetener used is encouraged to avoid potential adverse effects. There are two main types of sweeteners: nutritive and nonnutritive. The nutritive sweeteners contain calories, and the nonnutritive sweeteners have few or no calories in the amounts normally used.

Nutritive sweeteners include fructose (fruit sugar), sorbitol, and xylitol, all of which provide calories in amounts similar to those in sucrose (table sugar). They cause less elevation in blood sugar levels than sucrose does and are often used in "sugar-free" foods. Sweeteners containing sorbitol may have a laxative effect.

Nonnutritive sweeteners have minimal or no calories. They are used in food products and are also available for table use. They produce minimal or no elevation in blood glucose levels and have been approved by the U.S. Food and Drug Administration (FDA) as safe for people with diabetes. Nonnutritive sweeteners include saccharin, aspartame (NutraSweet), acesulfame-K (Sunnette), and sucralose (Splenda) (ADA, 2009b).

Misleading Food Labels. Foods labeled "sugarless" or "sugar-free" may still provide calories equal to those of the equivalent sugar-containing products if they are made with nutritive sweeteners. Therefore, these foods should not be considered "free" foods to be eaten in unlimited quantity, because they can elevate blood glucose levels. Foods labeled "dietetic" are not necessarily reduced-calorie foods. Patients are advised that foods labeled "dietetic" may still contain significant amounts of sugar or fat.

It is important that patients read the labels of "health foods"—especially snacks—because they often contain carbohydrates (eg, honey, brown sugar, corn syrup) and saturated vegetable fats (eg, coconut or palm oil), hydrogenated vegetable fats, or animal fats, which may be contraindicated in people with elevated blood lipid levels.

Exercise

Exercise is extremely important in diabetes management because of its effects on lowering blood glucose and reducing cardiovascular risk factors. Exercise lowers blood glucose levels by increasing the uptake of glucose by body muscles and by improving insulin utilization. It also improves circulation and muscle tone. Resistance (strength) training, such as weight lifting, can increase lean muscle mass, thereby increasing the resting metabolic rate. These effects are useful in diabetes in relation to losing weight, easing stress, and maintaining a feeling of well-being. Exercise also alters blood lipid concentrations, increasing levels of high-density lipoproteins and decreasing total cholesterol and triglyceride levels. This is especially important for people with diabetes because of their increased risk of cardiovascular disease (Nathan, et al., 2005).

Exercise Recommendations

Ideally, a person with diabetes should exercise at the same time (preferably when blood glucose levels are at their peak) and in the same amount each day. Regular daily exercise, rather than sporadic exercise, should be encouraged. Exercise recommendations must be altered as necessary for patients with diabetic complications such as retinopathy, autonomic neuropathy, sensorimotor neuropathy, and cardiovascular disease (ADA, 2009b). Increased blood pressure associated with exercise may aggravate diabetic retinopathy and increase the risk of a hemorrhage into the vitreous or retina. Patients with ischemic heart disease risk triggering angina or a myocardial infarction, which may be silent. Avoiding trauma to the lower extremities is especially important in patients with numbness related to neuropathy.

In general, a slow, gradual increase in the exercise period is encouraged. For many patients, walking is a safe and beneficial form of exercise that requires no special equipment (except for proper shoes) and can be performed anywhere. People with diabetes should discuss an exercise program with their health care providers and undergo a careful medical evaluation with appropriate diagnostic studies before beginning program (ADA, 2009b).

For patients who are older than 30 years and who have two or more risk factors for heart disease, an exercise stress test is recommended. Risk factors for heart disease include hypertension, obesity, high cholesterol levels, abnormal resting electrocardiogram (ECG), sedentary lifestyle, smoking, male gender, and a family history of heart disease. An abnormal stress test may indicate cardiac ischemia. Typically, an abnormal stress test is followed up with a cardiac catheterization and, in some cases, with an intervention such as angioplasty, stent replacement, or cardiac surgery.

Exercise Precautions

Patients who have blood glucose levels exceeding 250 mg/dL (14 mmol/L) and who have ketones in their urine should not begin exercising until the urine test results are negative for ketones and the blood glucose level is closer to normal. Exercising with elevated blood glucose levels increases the secretion of glucagon, growth hormone, and catecholamines. The liver then releases more glucose, and the result is an increase in the blood glucose level (ADA, 2009b).

The physiologic decrease in circulating insulin that normally occurs with exercise cannot occur in patients treated with insulin. Initially, patients who require insulin should be taught to eat a 15-g carbohydrate snack (a fruit exchange) or a snack of complex carbohydrates with a protein before engaging in moderate exercise to prevent unexpected hypoglycemia. The exact amount of food needed varies from person to person and should be determined by blood glucose monitoring.

Another potential concern for patients who take insulin is hypoglycemia that occurs many hours after exercise. To avoid postexercise hypoglycemia, especially after strenuous or prolonged exercise, the patient may need to eat a snack at the end of the exercise session and at bedtime and monitor the blood glucose level more frequently. Patients who are capable, knowledgeable, and responsible can learn to adjust their own insulin doses by working closely with a diabetes educator. Others need specific instructions on what to do when they exercise.

Patients taking insulin and participating in extended periods of exercise should test their blood glucose levels before, during, and after the exercise period, and they should snack on carbohydrates as needed to maintain blood glucose levels (ADA, 2006a). Other participants or observers should be aware that the person exercising has diabetes, and they should know what assistance to give if severe hypoglycemia occurs.

In obese people with type 2 diabetes, exercise in addition to dietary management both improves glucose metabolism and enhances loss of body fat. Exercise coupled with weight loss improves insulin sensitivity and may decrease the need for insulin or oral antidiabetic agents (ADA, 2006a). Eventually, the patient's glucose tolerance may return to normal. Patients with type 2 diabetes who are not taking insulin or an oral agent may not need extra food before exercise.

General precautions for exercise in diabetes are presented in Chart 41-4.

 Gerontologic Considerations

Physical activity that is consistent and realistic is beneficial to elderly people with diabetes. Physical fitness in the elderly population with diabetes may lead to improved

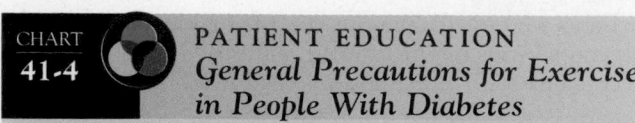

CHART 41-4

PATIENT EDUCATION
General Precautions for Exercise in People With Diabetes

- Use proper footwear and, if appropriate, other protective equipment.
- Avoid exercise in extreme heat or cold.
- Inspect feet daily after exercise.
- Avoid exercise during periods of poor metabolic control.

glycemic control, decreased risk for chronic vascular disease, and an improved quality of life (ADA, 2006a). Advantages of exercise in this population include a decrease in hyperglycemia, a general sense of well-being, and better use of ingested calories, resulting in weight reduction. Because there is an increased incidence of cardiovascular problems in the elderly, a physical examination and exercise stress test may be warranted before an exercise program is initiated. A pattern of gradual, consistent exercise, including resistance exercise, should be planned that does not exceed the patient's physical capacity. Physical impairment due to other chronic diseases must also be considered. In some cases, a physical therapy evaluation may be indicated, with the goal of determining exercises specific to the patient's needs and abilities. Tools such as the "Armchair Fitness" video may be helpful. For more information about age-related changes that affect diabetes management, see Chart 41-5.

Monitoring Glucose Levels and Ketones

Blood glucose monitoring is a cornerstone of diabetes management, and **self-monitoring of blood glucose (SMBG)** levels has dramatically altered diabetes care.

Self-Monitoring of Blood Glucose

Using frequent SMBG and learning how to respond to the results enable people with diabetes to adjust their treatment regimen to obtain optimal blood glucose control. This allows for detection and prevention of hypoglycemia and hyperglycemia and plays a crucial role in normalizing blood glucose levels, which in turn may reduce the risk of long-term diabetic complications.

Various methods for SMBG are available. Most involve obtaining a drop of blood from the fingertip, applying the blood to a special reagent strip, and allowing the blood to stay on the strip for the amount of time specified by the manufacturer (usually 5 to 30 seconds). The meter gives a digital readout of the blood glucose value. The meters available for SMBG offer various features and benefits such as monthly averages, tracking of events like exercise and food consumption, and downloading capacity. Some meters are biosensors that can use blood obtained from alternative test sites, such as the forearm. They have a special lancing device that is useful for patients who have painful fingertips or experience pain with fingersticks.

Because laboratory methods measure plasma glucose, most blood glucose monitors approved for patients' use in the home and some test strips calibrate blood glucose readings to plasma values. Plasma glucose values are 10% to 15% higher than whole blood glucose values, and it is

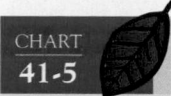

CHART
41-5

GERONTOLOGIC CONSIDERATIONS
Age-Related Changes That May Affect Diabetes and Its Management

Sensory Changes

Decreased vision
Decreased smell
Taste changes
Decreased proprioception
Diminished thirst

Gastrointestinal Changes

Dental problems
Appetite changes
Delayed gastric emptying
Decreased bowel motility

Activity/exercise Pattern Changes

More sedentary

Renal Function Changes

Decreased function
Decreased drug clearance

Affective/cognitive Changes

Medications/meals omitted or taken erratically

Socioeconomic Factors

Fad diets
Loneliness/living alone
Lack of money/lack of support system

Chronic Diseases

Hypertension
Arthritis
Neoplasms
Acute/chronic infections

Potential Drug Interactions

Use of another person's medications
Consulting multiple physicians for different illnesses
Alcohol use/abuse

---

crucial for patients with diabetes to know whether their monitor and strips provide whole blood or plasma results.

Methods for SMBG must match the skill level of patients. Factors affecting SMBG performance include visual acuity, fine motor coordination, cognitive ability, comfort with technology and willingness to use it, and cost. Some meters can be used by patients with visual impairments that have audio components to assist in performing the test and obtaining the result. In addition, meters are available to check both blood glucose and blood ketone levels by those who are particularly susceptible to DKA. Most insurance companies cover some or all of the costs of meters and strips.

A potential hazard of all methods of SMBG is that the patient may obtain and report erroneous blood glucose values as a result of using incorrect techniques. Some common sources of error include improper application of blood (eg, drop too small), damage to the reagent strips caused by heat or humidity, use of outdated strips, and improper meter cleaning and maintenance.

Nurses play an important role in providing initial teaching about SMBG techniques. Equally important is evaluating the techniques of patients who are experienced in self-monitoring. Every 6 to 12 months, patients should conduct a comparison of their meter result with a simultaneous laboratory-measured blood glucose level in their physician's office and have their technique observed. The accuracy of the meter and strips can also be assessed with control solutions specific to that meter whenever a new vial of strips is used and whenever the validity of the reading is in doubt.

Candidates for Self-Monitoring of Blood Glucose. SMBG is a useful tool for managing self-care for everyone with diabetes. It is a key component of treatment for any intensive insulin therapy regimen (ie, two to four injections per day or use of an insulin pump) and for diabetes management during pregnancy. It is also recommended for patients with the following conditions:

- Unstable diabetes (severe swings from very high to very low blood glucose levels within a 24-hour day)
- A tendency to develop severe ketosis or hypoglycemia
- Hypoglycemia without warning symptoms

For patients not taking insulin, SMBG is helpful for monitoring the effectiveness of exercise, diet, and oral antidiabetic agents. It can also help motivate patients to continue with treatment. For patients with type 2 diabetes, SMBG is recommended during periods of suspected hyperglycemia (eg, illness) or hypoglycemia (eg, unusual increased activity levels) and when the medication or dosage of medication is modified (ADA, 2009b).

Frequency of Self-Monitoring of Blood Glucose. For most patients who require insulin, SMBG is recommended two to four times daily (usually before meals and at bedtime). For patients who take insulin before each meal, SMBG is required at least three times daily before meals to determine each dose (ADA, 2009b). Those not receiving insulin may be instructed to assess their blood glucose levels at least two or three times per week, including a 2-hour postprandial test. For all patients, testing is recommended whenever hypoglycemia or hyperglycemia is suspected, with changes in medications, activity, or diet, and with stress or illness.

Responding to Self-Monitoring of Blood Glucose Results. Patients are asked to keep a record or logbook of blood glucose levels so that they can detect patterns. Testing is done at the peak action time of the medication to evaluate the need for dosage adjustments. To evaluate basal insulin and determine bolus insulin doses, testing is performed before meals. To determine bolus doses of regular or rapid-acting insulin (lispro [Humalog], aspart [Novolog], or glulisine [Apidra]), testing is done 2 hours after meals. Patients with type 2 diabetes are encouraged to test daily before and 2 hours after the largest meal of the day until stabilized. Thereafter, testing should be done periodically before and after meals. Patients who take insulin at bedtime or who use an insulin infusion pump should also test at 3 AM once a week to document that the blood glucose level is not decreasing during the night. If the patient is unwilling or cannot afford to test frequently, then once or twice a day may be sufficient if the time of testing is varied (eg, before breakfast one day and before lunch the next day).

A tendency to discontinue SMBG is more likely to occur if the patient does not receive instruction about using the results to alter the treatment regimen, if positive reinforcement is not given, and if costs of testing increase. At the very least, the patient should be given parameters for contacting the physician. Patients using intensive insulin therapy regimens may be instructed in the use of algorithms (rules or decision trees) for changing the insulin doses based on patterns of values greater or less than the target range and the amount of carbohydrate to be consumed. Baseline patterns should be established by SMBG for 1 to 2 weeks.

Using a Continuous Glucose Monitoring System

A **continuous glucose monitoring system (CGMS)** can be used to continuously monitor blood glucose levels (Fig. 41-2). A sensor attached to an infusion set, which is similar to an insulin pump infusion set, is inserted subcutaneously in the abdomen and connected to the device worn on a belt. After 72 hours, the data from the device are downloaded, and blood glucose readings are analyzed. Although the CGMS cannot be used for making decisions about specific insulin doses, it can be used to determine whether treatment is adequate over a 24-hour period. This device will be refined in the future so that it can be used by patients to make daily treatment decisions.

Testing for Glycated Hemoglobin

Glycated hemoglobin (also referred to as **glycosylated hemoglobin, HgbA$_{1C}$, or A1C**) is a blood test that reflects average blood glucose levels over a period of approximately

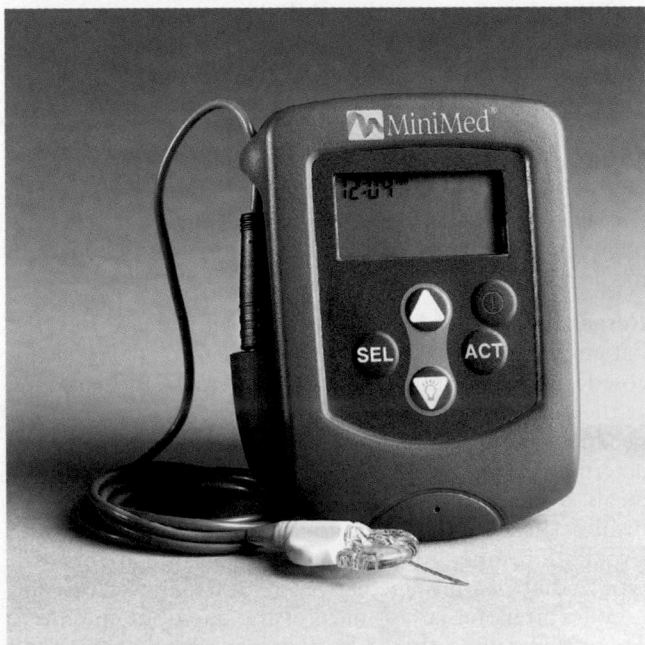

Figure 41-2 MiniMed CGMS System Gold Continuous Glucose Monitoring System. (Courtesy of Medtronic Diabetes.)

2 to 3 months (ADA, 2009b). When blood glucose levels are elevated, glucose molecules attach to hemoglobin in red blood cells. The longer the amount of glucose in the blood remains above normal, the more glucose binds to hemoglobin and the higher the glycated hemoglobin level becomes. This complex (hemoglobin attached to the glucose) is permanent and lasts for the life of an individual red blood cell, approximately 120 days. If near-normal blood glucose levels are maintained, with only occasional increases, the overall value will not be greatly elevated. However, if the blood glucose values are consistently high, then the test result is also elevated. If the patient reports mostly normal SMBG results but the glycated hemoglobin is high, there may be errors in the methods used for glucose monitoring, errors in recording results, or frequent elevations in glucose levels at times during the day when the patient is not usually monitoring blood sugar levels. Normal values typically range from 4% to 6% and indicate consistently near-normal blood glucose concentrations. The target range for people with diabetes is less than 7% (ADA, 2009b).

Testing for Ketones

Ketones (or ketone bodies) are byproducts of fat breakdown, and they accumulate in the blood and urine. Ketones in the urine signal that there is a deficiency of insulin and control of type 1 diabetes is deteriorating. The risk of DKA is high. When there is almost no effective insulin available, the body starts to break down stored fat for energy. Urine testing is the most common method used for self-testing of ketone bodies by patients. A meter that enables testing of blood for ketones is available.

Most commonly, the patient uses a urine dipstick (Ketostix or Chemstrip uK) to detect ketonuria. The reagent pad on the strip turns purple when ketones are present. (One of the ketone bodies is called acetone, and this term is frequently used interchangeably with the term ketones.) Other strips are available for measuring both urine glucose and ketones (Keto-Diastix or Chemstrip uGK). Large amounts of ketones may depress the color response of the glucose test area.

Urine ketone testing should be performed whenever patients with type 1 diabetes have glycosuria or persistently elevated blood glucose levels (more than 240 mg/dL or 13.2 mmol/L for two testing periods in a row) and during illness, in pregnancy with preexisting diabetes, and in gestational diabetes (ADA, 2009b).

Pharmacologic Therapy

As previously stated, insulin is secreted by the beta cells of the islets of Langerhans and works to lower the blood glucose level after meals by facilitating the uptake and utilization of glucose by muscle, fat, and liver cells. In the absence of adequate insulin, pharmacologic therapy is essential.

Insulin Therapy

In type 1 diabetes, exogenous insulin must be administered for life because the body loses the ability to produce insulin. In type 2 diabetes, insulin may be necessary on a long-term basis to control glucose levels if meal planning and oral agents are ineffective. In addition, some patients in whom type 2 diabetes is usually controlled by meal planning alone or by meal planning and an oral antidiabetic agent may require insulin temporarily during illness, infection, pregnancy, surgery, or some other stressful event. In many cases, insulin injections are administered two or more times daily to control the blood glucose level. Because the insulin dose required by the individual patient is determined by the level of glucose in the blood, accurate monitoring of blood glucose levels is essential; thus, SMBG is a cornerstone of insulin therapy.

Preparations. A number of insulin preparations are available. They vary according to three main characteristics: time course of action, species (source), and manufacturer.

Time Course of Action. Insulins may be grouped into several categories based on the onset, peak, and duration of action (Table 41-3). Human insulin preparations have a shorter duration of action than insulin from animal sources because the presence of animal proteins triggers an immune response that results in the binding of animal insulin, which slows its availability.

Rapid-acting insulins produce a more rapid effect that is of shorter duration than regular insulin. Because of their rapid onset, the patient should be instructed to eat no more than 5 to 15 minutes after injection. Because of the short duration of action of these insulin analogues, patients with type 1 diabetes and some patients with type 2 or gestational diabetes also require a long-acting insulin (basal insulin) to maintain glucose control. Basal insulin is necessary to maintain blood glucose levels irrespective of meals. A constant level of insulin is required at all times. Intermediate-acting insulins function as basal insulins but may have to be split into two injections to achieve 24-hour coverage.

Short-acting insulins are called regular insulin (marked R on the bottle). Regular insulin is a clear solution and is usually administered 20 to 30 minutes before a meal, either alone or in combination with a longer-acting insulin. Regular insulin is the only insulin approved for IV use.

Intermediate-acting insulins are called NPH insulin (neutral protamine Hagedorn) or Lente insulin. Intermediate-acting insulins, which are similar in their time course of action, appear white and cloudy. If NPH or Lente insulin is taken alone, it is not crucial that it be taken 30 minutes before the meal. However, it is important that patients eat some food around the time of the onset and peak of these insulins.

"Peakless" basal or very long-acting insulins are approved by the FDA for use as a basal insulin—that is, the insulin is absorbed very slowly over 24 hours and can be given once a day. Because the insulin is in a suspension with a pH of 4, it cannot be mixed with other insulins because this would cause precipitation. It was originally approved to be given once a day at bedtime; however, it has now been approved to be given once a day at any time of the day but must be given at the same time each day to prevent overlap of action. Many patients fall asleep, forgetting to take their bedtime insulin or may be wary of taking insulin before going to sleep. Having these patients take their insulin in the morning ensures that the dose is taken.

> ### NURSING ALERT
>
> When administering insulin, it is very important to read the label carefully and to be sure that the correct type of insulin is administered. It is also important to avoid mistaking Lantus insulin for Lente insulin and vice versa.

The nurse should emphasize which meals and snacks—are being "covered" by which insulin doses. In general, the rapid-acting and short-acting insulins are expected to cover the increase in glucose levels after meals, immediately after the injection; the intermediate-acting insulins are expected to cover subsequent meals; and the long-acting insulins provide a relatively constant level of insulin and act as a basal insulin.

Species (Source). In the past, all insulins were obtained from beef (cow) and pork (pig) pancreases. Human insulins are now widely available. They are produced by recombinant

Table 41-3	**CATEGORIES OF INSULIN**				
Time Course	**Agent**	**Onset**	**Peak**	**Duration**	**Indications**
Rapid-acting	Lispro (Humalog)	10–15 min	1 h	2–4 h	Used for rapid reduction of glucose
	Aspart (Novolog)	5–15 min	40–50 min	2–4 h	level, to treat postprandial
	Glulisine (Apidra)	5–15 min	30–60 min	2 h	hyperglycemia, and/or to prevent nocturnal hypoglycemia
Short-acting	Regular (Humalog R, Novolin R, Iletin II Regular)	½–1 h	2–3 h	4–6 h	Usually administered 20–30 min before a meal; may be taken alone or in combination with longer-acting insulin
Intermediate-acting	NPH (neutral protamine Hagedorn)	2–4 h	4–12 h	16–20 h	Usually taken after food
	(Humulin N, Iletin II Lente, Iletin II NPH, Novolin L [Lente], Novolin N [NPH])	3–4 h	4–12 h	16–20 h	
Very long-acting	Glargine (Lantus) Detemir (Levemir)	1 h	Continuous (no peak)	24 h	Used for basal dose

DNA technology and have largely replaced insulin from animal sources. These insulins are preferable to animal source insulins because they are not antigenic and do not depend on sufficient animal sources. Human insulin preparations have a shorter duration of action than insulin from animal sources because the presence of animal proteins triggers an immune response that results in the binding of animal insulin, which slows its availability.

Insulin Regimens. Insulin regimens vary from one to four injections per day. Usually there is a combination of a short-acting insulin and a longer-acting insulin. The normally functioning pancreas continuously secretes small amounts of insulin during the day and night. In addition, whenever blood glucose increases after ingestion of food, there is a rapid burst of insulin secretion in proportion to the glucose-raising effect of the food. The goal of all but the simplest, one-injection insulin regimens is to mimic this normal pattern of insulin secretion in response to food intake and activity patterns. Table 41-4 describes several insulin regimens and the advantages and disadvantages of each.

There are two general approaches to insulin therapy: conventional and intensive (described in detail below). The patient can learn to use SMBG results and carbohydrate counting to vary the insulin doses. This allows more flexibility in timing and content of meals and exercise periods. However, complex insulin regimens require a strong level of commitment, intensive education, and close follow-up by the health care team.

The patient should be very involved in the decision regarding which insulin regimen to use. The patient should compare the potential benefits of different regimens with the potential costs (eg, time involved, number of injections or fingersticks for glucose testing, amount of record keeping). There are no set guidelines as to which insulin regimen should be used for which patient. It must not be assumed that elderly patients should automatically be given a simplified regimen. Likewise, it must not be assumed that all people want to be involved in a complex treatment regimen. The nurse plays an important role in educating the patient about the various approaches to insulin therapy. The nurse should refer the patient to a diabetes specialist or a diabetes education center, if available, for further training and education in the insulin treatment regimens.

Conventional Regimen. One approach is to simplify the insulin regimen as much as possible, with the aim of avoiding the acute complications of diabetes (hypoglycemia and symptomatic hyperglycemia). With this type of simplified regimen (eg, one or more injections of a mixture of short-acting and intermediate-acting insulins per day), the patient should not vary meal patterns and activity levels. The simplified regimen would be appropriate for the terminally ill, the frail elderly with limited self-care abilities, or patients who are completely unwilling or unable to engage in the self-management activities that are part of a more complex insulin regimen.

Intensive Regimen. The second approach is to use a more complex insulin regimen to achieve as much control over blood glucose levels as is safe and practical. A more complex insulin regimen allows the patient more flexibility to change the insulin doses from day to day in accordance with changes in eating and activity patterns, with stress and illness, and as needed for variations in the prevailing glucose level.

Although the DCCT Research Group (1993) found that intensive treatment (three or four injections of insulin per day) reduced the risk of complications, not all people with diabetes are candidates for very tight control of blood glucose. The DCCT also found that the risk of severe hypoglycemia was increased threefold in patients receiving intensive treatment (ADA, 2009b). Patients who have received a kidney transplant because of nephropathy and chronic renal failure should follow an intensive insulin regimen to preserve function of the new kidney.

Those who are not candidates include those with:
- Nervous system disorders rendering them unaware of hypoglycemic episodes (eg, those with autonomic neuropathy)
- Recurring severe hypoglycemia
- Irreversible diabetic complications, such as blindness or end-stage renal disease
- Cerebrovascular or cardiovascular disease
- Ineffective self-care skills

Complications of Insulin Therapy

Local Allergic Reactions. A local allergic reaction (redness, swelling, tenderness, and induration or a 2- to 4-cm wheal) may appear at the injection site 1 to 2 hours after the insulin administration. These reactions, which usually occur during the beginning stages of therapy and disappear with continued use of insulin, are becoming rare because of the increased use of human insulins. The physician may prescribe an antihistamine to be taken 1 hour before the injection if such a local reaction occurs.

Systemic Allergic Reactions. Systemic allergic reactions to insulin are rare. When they do occur, there is an immediate local skin reaction that gradually spreads into generalized urticaria (hives). These rare reactions are occasionally associated with generalized edema or anaphylaxis. The treatment is desensitization, with small doses of insulin administered in gradually increasing amounts using a desensitization kit.

Insulin Lipodystrophy. Lipodystrophy refers to a localized reaction, in the form of either lipoatrophy or lipohypertrophy, occurring at the site of insulin injections. Lipoatrophy is loss of subcutaneous fat; it appears as slight dimpling or more serious pitting of subcutaneous fat. The use of human insulin has almost eliminated this disfiguring complication.

Lipohypertrophy, the development of fibrofatty masses at the injection site, is caused by the repeated use of an injection site. If insulin is injected into scarred areas, absorption may be delayed. This is one reason that rotation of injection sites is so important. Patients should avoid injecting insulin into these areas until the hypertrophy disappears.

Resistance to Injected Insulin. Most patients have some degree of insulin resistance at one time or another. This may occur for various reasons, the most common being obesity, which can be overcome by weight loss. Clinical insulin resistance has been defined as a daily insulin requirement of

Table 41-4 INSULIN REGIMENS

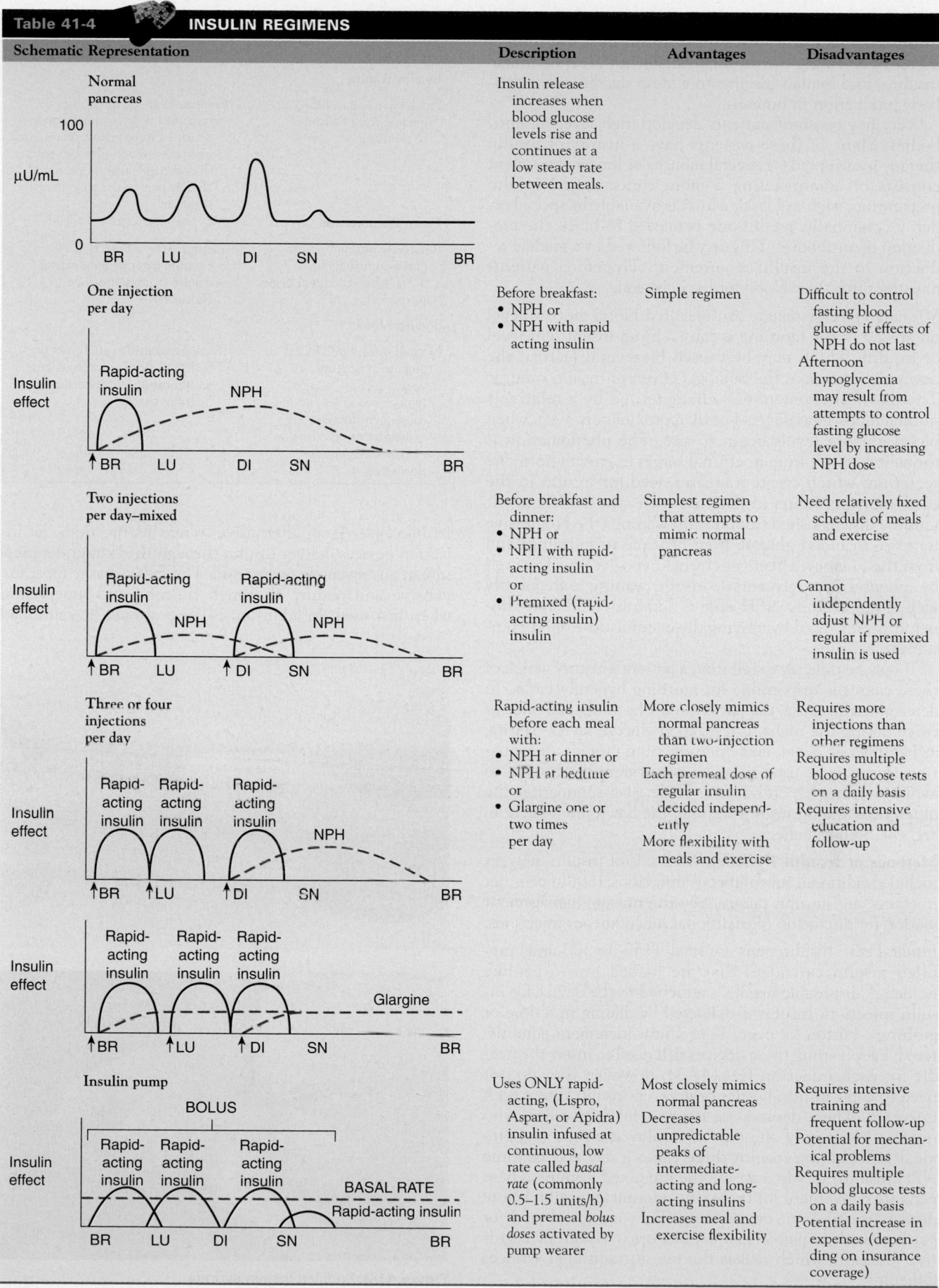

Schematic Representation	Description	Advantages	Disadvantages
Normal pancreas	Insulin release increases when blood glucose levels rise and continues at a low steady rate between meals.		
One injection per day	Before breakfast: • NPH or • NPH with rapid acting insulin	Simple regimen	Difficult to control fasting blood glucose if effects of NPH do not last Afternoon hypoglycemia may result from attempts to control fasting glucose level by increasing NPH dose
Two injections per day—mixed	Before breakfast and dinner: • NPH or • NPH with rapid-acting insulin or • Premixed (rapid-acting insulin) insulin	Simplest regimen that attempts to mimic normal pancreas	Need relatively fixed schedule of meals and exercise Cannot independently adjust NPH or regular if premixed insulin is used
Three or four injections per day	Rapid-acting insulin before each meal with: • NPH at dinner or • NPH at bedtime or • Glargine one or two times per day	More closely mimics normal pancreas than two-injection regimen Each premeal dose of regular insulin decided independently More flexibility with meals and exercise	Requires more injections than other regimens Requires multiple blood glucose tests on a daily basis Requires intensive education and follow-up
Insulin pump	Uses ONLY rapid-acting, (Lispro, Aspart, or Apidra) insulin infused at continuous, low rate called *basal rate* (commonly 0.5–1.5 units/h) and premeal *bolus doses* activated by pump wearer	Most closely mimics normal pancreas Decreases unpredictable peaks of intermediate-acting and long-acting insulins Increases meal and exercise flexibility	Requires intensive training and frequent follow-up Potential for mechanical problems Requires multiple blood glucose tests on a daily basis Potential increase in expenses (depending on insurance coverage)

BR, breakfast; LU, lunch; DI, dinner; SN, snack; REG, regular; ↑ indicates insulin injections.
Rapid acting insulin; lispro, aspart, or glulisine [Apidra]

200 units or more. In most patients with diabetes who take insulin, immune antibodies develop and bind the insulin, thereby decreasing the insulin available for use. All animal insulins, and human insulins to a lesser degree, cause antibody production in humans.

Very few resistant patients develop high levels of antibodies. Many of these patients have a history of insulin therapy interrupted for several months or longer. Treatment consists of administering a more concentrated insulin preparation, such as U500, which is available by special order. Occasionally, prednisone is needed to block the production of antibodies. This may be followed by a gradual reduction in the insulin requirement. Therefore, patients must monitor their blood for hypoglycemia.

Morning Hyperglycemia. An elevated blood glucose level on arising in the morning is caused by an insufficient level of insulin, which may be caused by several factors: the dawn phenomenon, the Somogyi effect, or insulin waning. The dawn phenomenon is characterized by a relatively normal blood glucose level until approximately 3 AM, when blood glucose levels begin to rise. The phenomenon is thought to result from nocturnal surges in growth hormone secretion, which create a greater need for insulin in the early morning hours in patients with type 1 diabetes. It must be distinguished from insulin waning (the progressive increase in blood glucose from bedtime to morning) and from the Somogyi effect (nocturnal hypoglycemia followed by rebound hyperglycemia). Insulin waning is frequently seen if the evening NPH dose is administered before dinner; it is prevented by moving the evening dose of NPH insulin to bedtime.

It may be difficult to tell from a patient's history which of these causes is responsible for morning hyperglycemia. To determine the cause, the patient must be awakened once or twice during the night to test blood glucose levels. Testing at bedtime, at 3 AM, and on awakening provides information that can be used to make adjustments in insulin to avoid morning hyperglycemia. Table 41-5 summarizes the differences among insulin waning, the dawn phenomenon, and the Somogyi effect.

Methods of Insulin Delivery. Methods of insulin delivery include traditional subcutaneous injections, insulin pens, jet injectors, and insulin pumps. See the nursing management section for discussion of traditional subcutaneous injections.

Insulin Pens. Insulin pens use small (150- to 300-unit) prefilled insulin cartridges that are loaded into a penlike holder. A disposable needle is attached to the device for insulin injection. Insulin is delivered by dialing in a dose or pushing a button for every 1- or 2-unit increment administered. People using these devices still need to insert the needle for each injection (Fig. 41-3); however, they do not need to carry insulin bottles or draw up insulin before each injection. These devices are most useful for patients who need to inject only one type of insulin at a time (eg, premeal rapid-acting insulin three times a day and bedtime NPH insulin) or who can use the premixed insulins. These pens are convenient for those who administer insulin before dinner if eating out or traveling. They are also useful for patients with impaired manual dexterity, vision, or cognitive function, which makes the use of traditional syringes difficult.

Table 41-5	**CAUSES OF MORNING HYPERGLYCEMIA**
Characteristic	**Treatment**
Insulin Waning	
Progressive rise in blood glucose from bedtime to morning	Increase evening (predinner or bedtime) dose of intermediate-acting or long-acting insulin, or institute a dose of insulin before the evening meal if one is not already part of the treatment regimen.
Dawn Phenomenon	
Relatively normal blood glucose until about 3 AM, when the level begins to rise	Change time of injection of evening intermediate-acting insulin from dinnertime to bedtime.
Somogyi Effect	
Normal or elevated blood glucose at bedtime, a decrease at 2–3 AM to hypoglycemic levels, and a subsequent increase caused by the production of counterregulatory hormones	Decrease evening (predinner or bedtime) dose of intermediate-acting insulin, or increase bedtime snack.

Jet Injectors. As an alternative to needle injections, jet injection devices deliver insulin through the skin under pressure in an extremely fine stream. These devices are more expensive and require thorough training and supervision when first used. In addition, patients should be cautioned

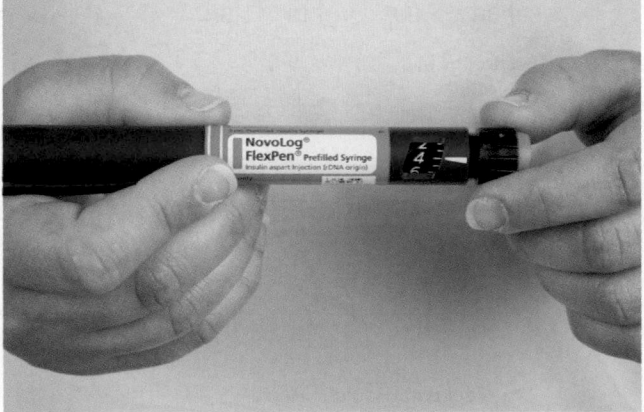

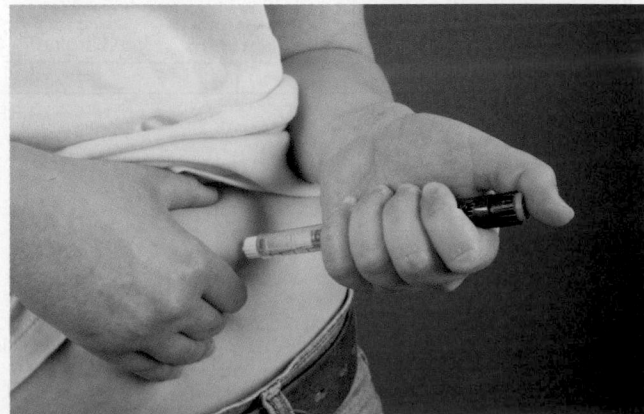

Figure 41-3 Prefilled insulin syringe.

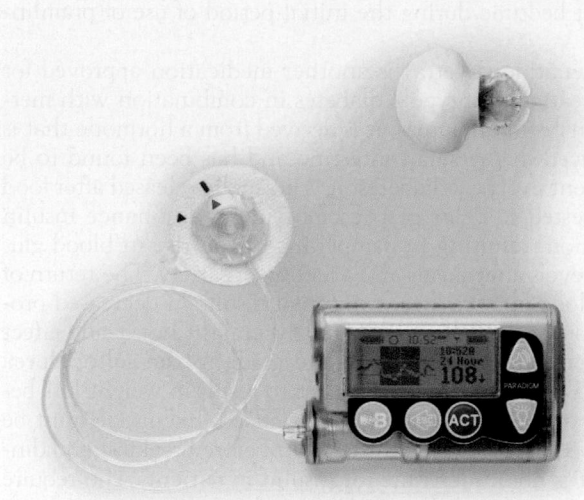

Figure 41-4 MiniMed Paradigm real-time insulin pump and continuous glucose monitoring system. (Courtesy of Medtronic Diabetes.)

that absorption rates, peak insulin activity, and insulin levels may be different when changing to a jet injector. (Insulin administered by jet injector is usually absorbed faster.) Use of jet injectors has been associated with bruising in some patients.

Insulin Pumps. Continuous subcutaneous insulin infusion involves the use of small, externally worn devices (insulin pumps) that closely mimic the functioning of the normal pancreas (ADA, 2009b). Insulin pumps contain a 3-mL syringe attached to a long (24- to 42-in), thin, narrow-lumen tube with a needle or Teflon catheter attached to the end (Fig. 41-4). The patient inserts the needle or catheter into subcutaneous tissue (usually on the abdomen) and secures it with tape or a transparent dressing. The needle or catheter is changed at least every 3 days. The pump is then worn either on a belt or in a pocket. Some women keep the pump tucked into the front or side of the bra or wear it on a garter belt on the thigh.

When an insulin pump is used, insulin is delivered by subcutaneous infusion at a basal rate (eg, 0.5 to 2.0 units/h). When a meal is consumed, the patient calculates a dose of insulin to metabolize the meal by counting the total amount of carbohydrate for the meal using a predetermined insulin-to-carbohydrate ratio; for example, a ratio of 1 unit of insulin for every 15 g of carbohydrate would require 3 units for a meal with 45 g of carbohydrate. This allows flexibility of meal timing and content.

Possible disadvantages of insulin pumps are unexpected disruptions in the flow of insulin from the pump that may occur if the tubing or needle becomes occluded, if the supply of insulin runs out, or if the battery is depleted, increasing the risk of DKA. Effective teaching to produce knowledgeable patients minimizes this risk. Another disadvantage is the potential for infection at needle insertion sites. Hypoglycemia may occur with insulin pump therapy; however, this is usually related to the lowered blood glucose levels many patients achieve rather than to a specific problem with the pump itself. The tight diabetes control associated with use of an insulin pump may increase the incidence of hypoglycemia unawareness because of the very gradual decline in serum glucose level, from more than 70 mg/dL (3.9 mmol/L) to less than 60 mg/dL (3.3 mmol/L).

Some patients find that wearing the pump for 24 hours each day is inconvenient. However, the pump can easily be disconnected, per patient preference, for limited periods, such as for showering, exercise, or sexual activity.

Candidates for the insulin pump must be willing to assess their blood glucose level several times daily. In addition, they must be psychologically stable and open about having diabetes, because the insulin pump is often a visible sign to others and a constant reminder to patients that they have diabetes. Most important, patients using insulin pumps must have extensive education in the use of the pump and in self-management of blood glucose and insulin doses. They must work closely with a team of health care professionals who are experienced in insulin pump therapy—specifically, a diabetologist/endocrinologist, a dietitian, and a certified diabetes educator.

The most common risk of insulin pump therapy is ketoacidosis, which can occur if there is an occlusion in the infusion set or tubing. Because only rapid-acting insulin is used in the pump, any interruption in the flow of insulin may rapidly cause the patient to be without insulin. The patient should be taught to administer insulin by manual injection if an insulin interruption is suspected (eg, no response in blood glucose level after a meal bolus).

Many insurance companies cover the cost of pump therapy. If not, the extra expense of the pump and associated supplies may be a deterrent for some patients. Medicare covers insulin pump therapy for patients with type 1 diabetes.

Insulin pumps have been used in patients with type 2 diabetes whose beta-cell function has diminished and who require insulin. Patients with a hectic lifestyle often do well with an insulin pump. There is no risk of DKA when there is an interruption of the flow of insulin in people with type 2 diabetes wearing an insulin pump.

Future Insulin Delivery. Research into mechanical delivery of insulin has involved implantable insulin pumps that can be externally programmed according to blood glucose test results. Clinical trials with these devices are continuing. In addition, there is research into the development of implantable devices that both measure the blood glucose level and deliver insulin as needed. Methods of administering insulin by the oral route (oral spray or capsule) and skin patch are undergoing intensive study.

Transplantation of Pancreatic Cells. Transplantation of the whole pancreas or a segment of the pancreas is being performed on a limited population (mostly patients with diabetes who are receiving a kidney transplantation simultaneously). One main issue is weighing the risks of antirejection medications against the advantages of pancreas transplantation. Implantation of insulin-producing pancreatic islet cells is another approach under investigation. This latter approach involves a less extensive surgical procedure and a potentially lower incidence of immunogenic problems (ADA, 2006b). However, thus far, independence from exogenous insulin has been limited to 2 years after transplantation of islet cells. Results of recent studies of patients with

islet cell transplants using less toxic antirejection drugs have shown some promise (NIDDK, 2007).

Oral Antidiabetic Agents

Oral antidiabetic agents may be effective for patients who have type 2 diabetes that cannot be treated effectively with MNT and exercise alone. In the United States, oral antidiabetic agents include first-generation and second-generation **sulfonylureas,** biguanides, alpha-glucosidase inhibitors, non-sulfonylurea insulin secretogogues (meglitinides and phenylalanine derivatives), **thiazolidinediones** (glitazones), and dipeptide-peptidase-4 (DPP-4) inhibitors (Table 41-6). Sulfonylureas and meglitinides are considered insulin secretagogues because their action increases the secretion of insulin by the pancreatic beta cells.

Patients must understand that oral agents are prescribed as an addition to (not as a substitute for) other treatment modalities, such as MNT and exercise. Use of oral antidiabetic medications may need to be halted temporarily and insulin prescribed if hyperglycemia develops that is attributable to infection, trauma, or surgery.

In time, oral antidiabetic agents may no longer be effective in controlling diabetes because of decline in function of beta cells. In such cases, the patient is treated with insulin. Approximately half of all patients who initially use oral antidiabetic agents eventually require insulin. This is referred to as a secondary failure. Primary failure occurs when the blood glucose level remains high 1 month after initial medication use.

Because mechanisms of action vary (Fig. 41-5), effects may be enhanced with the use of multidose, multiple medications. Use of multiple medications with different mechanisms of action is very common today. A combination of oral agents with insulin, usually glargine at bedtime, has also been used frequently as a treatment for some patients with type 2 diabetes.

Other Pharmacologic Therapy

Two new medications became available in 2005 for use in the pharmacologic management of diabetes. Both are injectable medications; neither is a substitute for insulin if insulin is required to control diabetes.

Pramlintide (Symlin), a synthetic analogue of human amylin, a hormone that is secreted by the beta cells of the pancreas, has recently been approved for treatment of both type 1 and type 2 diabetes. It is used to control hyperglycemia in adults who have not achieved acceptable levels of glucose control despite the use of insulin at mealtimes. It is used with insulin, not in place of insulin. Although pramlintide is not yet widely used, it is anticipated that it will be useful to minimize fluctuations in daily glucose levels and provide better glucose control. Risks associated with pramlintide include hypoglycemia; therefore, a source of glucose must be available if hypoglycemia occurs. Pramlintide must be injected into the abdomen or thigh because of variable absorption rates if it is injected into the arm. It should not be injected close to an insulin injection site. Caution must be exercised in preparing and administering pramlintide to avoid errors in dosing. Patients are instructed to monitor their blood glucose level before each meal, 2 hours afterward, and at bedtime during the initial period of use of pramlintide.

Exenatide (Byetta) is another medication approved for the treatment of type 2 diabetes in combination with metformin or sulfonylureas. It is derived from a hormone that is produced in the small intestine and has been found to be deficient in type 2 diabetes. It is normally released after food is ingested to delay gastric emptying and enhance insulin secretion, resulting in dampening of the rise in blood glucose levels after meals and a feeling of satiety. The return of the blood glucose level to normal results in decreased production of the hormone. Hypoglycemia is not a side effect of exenatide if adjustments are made in the sulfonylurea dose. Exenatide has been shown to result in weight loss because of the increased satiety produced. Exenatide must be injected twice a day within 1 hour before breakfast and dinner. It is not a substitute for insulin in patients who require insulin to control their diabetes.

Nursing Management

Nursing management of patients with diabetes can involve treatment of a wide variety of physiologic disorders, depending on the patient's health status and whether the patient is newly diagnosed or seeking care for an unrelated health problem. Nursing management of patients with DKA and hyperglycemic hyperosmolar nonketotic syndrome and of those with diabetes as a secondary diagnosis is discussed in subsequent sections of this chapter.

Because all patients with diabetes must master the concepts and skills necessary for long-term management and avoidance of potential complications of diabetes, a solid educational foundation is necessary for competent self-care and is an ongoing focus of nursing care.

Providing Patient Education

Diabetes mellitus is a chronic illness that requires a lifetime of special self-management behaviors. Because MNT, physical activity, and physical and emotional stress affect diabetic control, patients must learn to balance a multitude of factors.

Developing a Diabetic Teaching Plan

Changes in the health care system as a whole have had a major impact on diabetes education and training. Patients with new-onset type 1 diabetes are hospitalized for much shorter periods or may be managed completely on an outpatient basis. Patients with new-onset type 2 diabetes are rarely hospitalized for initial care. There has been a proliferation of outpatient diabetes education and training programs, with increasing support of third-party reimbursement. All encounters with patients with diabetes are opportunities for reinforcement of self-management skills, regardless of the setting.

Many hospitals employ nurses who specialize in diabetes education and management and who are certified by the National Certification Board of Diabetes Educators as Certified Diabetes Educators (CDEs). However, because of the large number of patients with diabetes who are admitted to every unit of a hospital for reasons other than diabetes or its complications, staff nurses play a vital role in identifying patients with diabetes, assessing self-care skills, providing

Table 41-6   **ORAL ANTIDIABETIC AGENTS**

Generic (Trade) Name	Action/Indications	Side Effects	Implications
First-Generation Sulfonylureas Acetohexamide (Dymelor) Chlorpropamide (Diabinese) Tolazamide (Tolinase) Tolbutamide (Orinase)	Used infrequently in U.S. today Used in type 2 diabetes to control blood glucose levels Stimulate beta cells of the pancreas to secrete insulin; may improve binding between insulin and insulin receptors or increase the number of insulin receptors	Hypoglycemia Mild GI symptoms Weight gain Drug–drug interactions (NSAIDs, warfarin, sulfonamides) Sulfa allergy Skin reactions	Monitor patient for hypoglycemia Monitor blood glucose and urine ketone levels to assess effectiveness of therapy Patients at high risk for hypoglycemia: advanced age, renal insufficiency When taken with beta-adrenergic blocking agents may mask usual warning signs and symptoms of hypoglycemia Instruct patients to avoid use of alcohol Check for interactions with other medications
Second-Generation Sulfonylureas Glipizide (Glucotrol, Glucotrol XL) Glyburide (Micronase, Glynase, Dia-Beta) Glimepiride (Amaryl)	Stimulate beta cells of the pancreas to secrete insulin; may improve binding between insulin and insulin receptors or increase the number of insulin receptors Used in type 2 diabetes to control blood glucose levels Have more potent effects than first-generation sulfonylureas May be used in combination with metformin or insulin to improve glucose control	Hypoglycemia Mild GI symptoms Weight gain Drug–drug interactions (NSAIDs, warfarin, sulfonamides) Sulfa allergy	Monitor patient for hypoglycemia Monitor blood glucose and urine ketone levels to assess effectiveness of therapy Patients at high risk for hypoglycemia: advanced age, renal insufficiency When taken with beta-adrenergic blocking agents, may mask usual warning signs and symptoms of hypoglycemia Instruct patients to avoid use of alcohol
Biguanides Metformin (Glucophage, Glucophage XL, Fortamet) Metformin with glyburide (Glucovance)	Inhibit production of glucose by the liver Increase body tissues' sensitivity to insulin Decrease hepatic synthesis of cholesterol Used in type 2 diabetes to control blood glucose levels	Lactic acidosis Hypoglycemia if metformin is used in combination with insulin or other antidiabetic agents Drug–drug interaction GI disturbances Contraindicated in patients with impaired renal or liver function, respiratory insufficiency, severe infection, or alcohol abuse	Monitor for lactic acidosis and hypoglycemia Monitor renal function Patients taking metformin are at increased risk of acute renal failure and lactic acidosis with use of iodinated contrast material for diagnostic studies; metformin should be stopped 48 h prior to and for 48 h after use of contrast agent or until renal function is evaluated and normal Check for interactions with other medications
Alpha-Glucosidase Inhibitors Acarbose (Precose) Miglitol (Glyset)	Delay absorption of complex carbohydrates in the intestine and slow entry of glucose into systemic circulation Do not increase insulin secretion Used in type 2 diabetes to control blood glucose levels Can be used alone or in combination with sulfonylureas, metformin, or insulin to improve glucose control	Hypoglycemia (risk increased if used with insulin or other antidiabetic agents) GI side effects (abdominal discomfort or distention, diarrhea, flatulence) Drug–drug interactions	Must be taken with first bite of food to be effective Monitor for GI side effects (diarrhea, abdominal distention) Monitor for blood glucose levels to assess effectiveness of therapy Monitor liver function studies every 3 mo for 1 y, then periodically Contraindicated in patients with GI or renal dysfunction, or cirrhosis **Alert: Hypoglycemia must be treated with glucose, not sucrose**

Continued on following page

Table 41-6		ORAL ANTIDIABETIC AGENTS (Continued)	
Generic (Trade) Name	Action/Indications	Side Effects	Implications
Non-Sulfonylurea Insulin Secretagogues			
Repaglinide (Prandin) categorized as a meglitinide Nateglinide (Starlix) categorized as a D-phenylalanine derivative	Stimulate pancreas to secrete insulin Used in type 2 diabetes to control blood glucose levels Can be used alone or in combination with metformin or thiazolidinediones to improve glucose control	Hypoglycemia/weight gain less likely than sulfonylureas Drug–drug interactions (with ketoconazole, fluconazole, erythromycin, rifampin, isoniazid)	Monitor blood glucose levels to assess effectiveness of therapy Has rapid action and short half-life Should be taken only if able to eat a meal immediately Teach patients symptoms of hypoglycemia Monitor patients with impaired liver function and renal impairment Has no effect on plasma lipids Is taken before each meal Check for interactions with other medications
Thiazolidinediones (or glitazones)			
Pioglitazone (Actos) Rosiglitazone (Avandia)	Sensitize body tissue to insulin; stimulate insulin receptor sites to lower blood glucose and improve action of insulin May be used alone or in combination with sulfonylurea, metformin, or insulin	Hypoglycemia (risk increased with use of insulin or other antidiabetic agents) Anemia Weight gain, edema Decrease effectiveness of oral contraceptives Possible liver dysfunction Drug–drug interactions Hyperlipidemia (has variable effect on lipids; pioglitazone may be preferred choice in patients with lipid abnormalities) Impaired platelet function	Monitor blood glucose levels to assess effectiveness of therapy Monitor liver function tests Arrange dietary teaching to establish weight control program Instruct patient taking oral contraceptives about increased risk of pregnancy
Dipeptidyl Peptidase-4 (DPP-4) Inhibitor			
Sitagliptin (Januvia) Vildagliptin (Galvus)	Increase and prolongs the action of incretin, a hormone that increases insulin release and decreases glucagon levels, with the result of improved glucose control	Upper respiratory infection Stuffy or runny nose and sore throat Headache Stomach discomfort and diarrhea Hypoglycemia, if used with sulfonylurea	Usually administered once a day Used alone or with other oral antidiabetic agents Instruct patient about signs and symptoms of hypoglycemia and other adverse effects to report Monitor renal function

basic education, reinforcing the teaching provided by the specialist, and referring patients for follow-up care after discharge. Diabetes patient education programs that have been peer-reviewed by the ADA as meeting National Standards for Diabetes Education can be reimbursed for education.

Organizing Information. There are various strategies for organizing and prioritizing the vast amount of information that must be taught to patients with diabetes. In addition, many hospitals and outpatient diabetes centers have devised written guidelines, care plans, and documentation forms (often based on ADA guidelines) that may be used to document and evaluate teaching. One approach is to organize education using the seven tips for managing diabetes identified and developed by the American Association of Diabetes Educators (AADE, 2005): healthy eating, being active, monitoring, taking medication, problem solving, healthy coping, and reducing risks. The AADE can be contacted for additional information about assessment and documentation of outcomes of this approach to teaching.

Another general approach is to organize information and skills into two main types: basic, initial, or "survival" skills and information, and in-depth (advanced) or continuing education.

Teaching Survival Skills. Survival skills must be taught to all patients with newly diagnosed type 1 or type 2 diabetes and all patients receiving insulin for the first time. This basic information is literally what patients must know to survive (eg, to avoid severe hypoglycemic or acute hyperglycemic complications after discharge). An outline of survival information includes the following:

1. Simple pathophysiology
   a. Basic definition of diabetes (having a high blood glucose level)
   b. Normal blood glucose ranges and target blood glucose levels
   c. Effect of insulin and exercise (decrease glucose)
   d. Effect of food and stress, including illness and infections (increase glucose)
   e. Basic treatment approaches

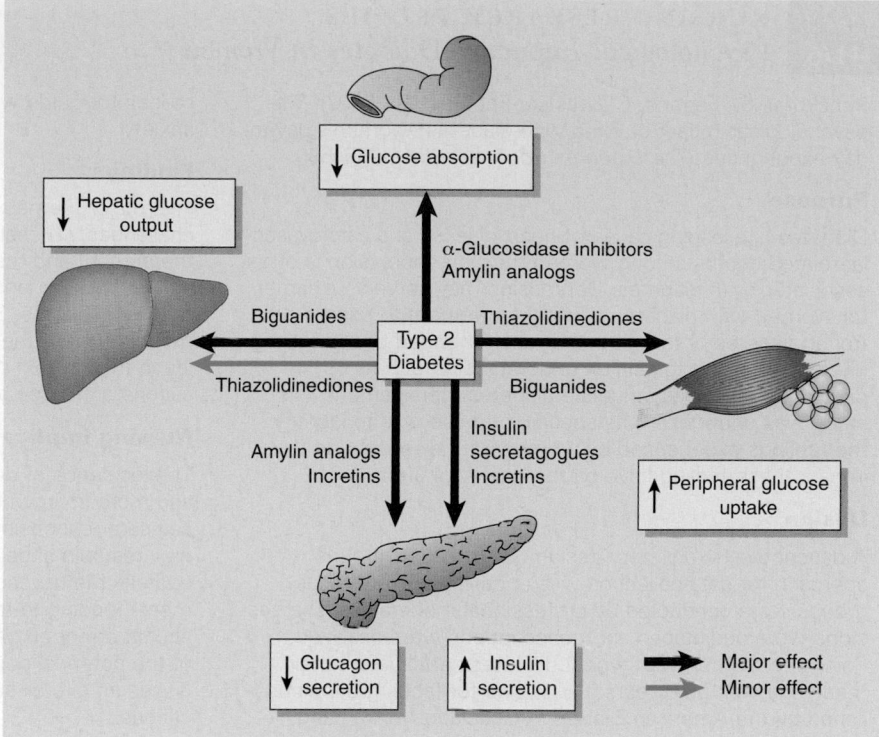

Figure 41-5 Action sites of hypoglycemic agents and mechanisms of lowering blood glucose in type 2 diabetes. The incretins are the dipeptidyl peptidase-4 (DPP-4) inhibitors and glucagon-like peptide-1 (GLP-1) agonists.

2. Treatment modalities
   a. Administration of insulin and oral antidiabetes medications
   b. Meal planning (food groups, timing of meals)
   c. Monitoring of blood glucose and urine ketones
3. Recognition, treatment, and prevention of acute complications
   a. Hypoglycemia
   b. Hyperglycemia
4. Pragmatic information
   a. Where to buy and store insulin, syringes, and glucose monitoring supplies
   b. When and how to contact the physician

For patients with newly diagnosed type 2 diabetes, emphasis is initially placed on meal planning and exercise. Those who are starting to take oral sulfonylureas or insulin secretagogues need to know about detecting, preventing, and treating hypoglycemia. If diabetes has gone undetected for many years, the patient may already be experiencing some chronic diabetic complications. Therefore, for some patients with newly diagnosed type 2 diabetes, basic diabetes teaching must include information on preventive skills, such as foot care and eye care (eg, planning yearly or more frequent complete [dilated eye] examinations by an ophthalmologist, understanding that retinopathy is largely asymptomatic until advanced stages).

Patients also need to realize that once they master the basic skills and information, further diabetes education must be pursued. Acquiring in-depth and advanced diabetes knowledge occurs throughout the patient's lifetime, both formally through programs of continuing education and informally through experience and sharing of information with other people with diabetes.

Planning In-Depth and Continuing Education. This education involves teaching more detailed information related to survival skills (eg, learning to vary food choices and insulin, preparing for travel) as well as learning preventive measures for avoiding long-term diabetic complications. Preventive measures include foot care, eye care, general hygiene (eg, skin care and oral hygiene), and risk factor management (eg, blood pressure control and blood glucose normalization).

More advanced continuing education may include alternative methods for insulin delivery, such as the insulin pump, and algorithms or rules for evaluating and adjusting insulin doses. The degree of advanced diabetes education to be provided depends on the patient's interest and ability. However, learning preventive measures (especially foot care and eye care) is mandatory for early detection and treatment to reduce the occurrence of amputations and blindness in patients with diabetes.

Assessing Readiness to Learn

Before initiating diabetes education, the nurse assesses the patient's (and family's) readiness to learn. When patients are first diagnosed with diabetes (or first told of their need for insulin), they often go through various stages of the grieving process. These stages may include shock and denial, anger, depression, negotiation, and acceptance. The amount of time it takes for the patient and family members to work through the grieving process varies from patient to patient. They may experience helplessness, guilt, altered body image, loss of self-esteem, and concern about the future. The nurse must assess the patient's coping strategies and reassure the patient and family that feelings of depression and shock are normal (Chart 41-6).

Asking the patient and family about their major concerns or fears is an important way to learn about any

---

<table>
<tr><td>CHART
41-6</td><td>NURSING RESEARCH PROFILE
Psychological Impact of Diabetes in Women</td></tr>
</table>

Penckofer, S., Ferrans, C. & Velsor-Friedrich, B. (2007). The psychological impact of living with diabetes: Women's day-to-day experiences. *The Diabetes Educator, 33*(4), 680–690.

Purpose

Diabetes is a leading cause of heart disease and cardiovascular-related deaths among women; further, depression is often associated with diabetes. Depression may serve as a barrier for women with diabetes to obtain treatment to ensure control of diabetes or to follow the recommended treatment regimen. In an effort to gain an understanding of how psychological issues influence diabetes management, this study was undertaken. Its specific purpose was to identify the feelings experienced by women with diabetes and the impact these feeling have on the quality of life.

Design

A descriptive, exploratory design using a focus groups approach for data collection was undertaken. Four focus groups were conducted by professional moderators. The sessions were audiotaped and transcriptions were analyzed. Forty-one women with type 2 diabetes participated; their mean age was 55.6 years. Guidelines for focus groups published by the American Diabetes Association were used. A moderator guide was used to explore depression, anger, and anxiety.

Findings

Five major themes were identified: (1) struggling with health challenges, (2) challenges in relationships, (3) worrying about the present and the future, (4) multiple responsibilities for self and others, and (5) choosing to take a break from caring for their diabetes. Struggling with health situations was the most prevalent theme. The difficulty of carrying on a normal life in the context of experiencing hypoglycemia and complications promoted angry feelings.

Nursing Implications

The incidence of depression is high in people with diabetes and more so in women than in men. The burden to take on self-care responsibilities while being responsible for others may result in anger. The findings support the need to address the psychological impact of having diabetes on treatment. Tending to the psychological component of diabetes and its effect on patients and families is important because of the potential negative effect of unresolved psychological issues on overall health and prevention of long-term complications.

---

misinformation that may be contributing to anxiety. Some common misconceptions regarding diabetes and its treatment are listed in Table 41-7. Simple, direct information should be provided to dispel misconceptions. More information can be provided once the patient masters survival skills.

Nurses whose patients are in the hospital rarely have the luxury of waiting until the patient feels ready to learn; short hospital stays necessitate initiation of survival skill education as early as possible. This gives the patient the opportunity to practice skills with supervision by the nurse before discharge. Follow-up by home health nurses is often necessary for reinforcement of survival skills.

The nurse evaluates the patient's social situation for factors that may influence the diabetes treatment and education plan, such as

- Low literacy level (may be evaluated while assessing for visual deficits by having the patient read from teaching materials)
- Limited financial resources or lack of health insurance
- Presence or absence of family support
- Typical daily schedule (the patient is asked about timing and number of usual daily meals, work and exercise schedule, plans for travel)
- Neurologic deficits caused by stroke, other neurologic disorders, or other disabling conditions, obtained from the patient's health history and physical assessment (the patient is assessed for aphasia or decreased ability to follow simple commands)

Teaching Experienced Patients

Nurses should continue to assess the skills and self-care behaviors of patients who have had diabetes for many years,

because it is estimated that as many as 50% of patients make errors in self-care. Assessment of these patients must include direct observation of skills, not just the patient's self-report of self-care behaviors. In addition, these patients must be fully aware of preventive measures related to foot care, eye care, and risk factor management. Those experiencing long-term diabetic complications for the first time may go through the grieving process again. Some patients may have a renewed interest in diabetes self-care in the hope of delaying further complications. Others may be overwhelmed by feelings of guilt and depression. The patient is encouraged to discuss feelings and fears related to complications. Meanwhile, the nurse provides appropriate information regarding diabetic complications.

Determining Teaching Methods

Maintaining flexibility with regard to teaching approaches is important. Teaching skills and information in a logical sequence is not always the most helpful method for patients. For example, many patients fear self-injection. Before they learn how to prepare, purchase, store, and mix insulins, they should be taught to insert the needle and inject insulin (or practice with saline solution).

Various tools can be used to complement teaching. Many of the companies that manufacture products for diabetes self-care also provide booklets and videotapes to assist in patient teaching. Teaching/educational materials are also available from the AADE and the ADA. It is important to use a variety of written handouts that match the patient's learning needs (including different languages, low-literacy information, large print) and reading level and to ensure that these materials are technically accurate. Patients can continue learning about diabetes care by participating in

Table 41-7 MISCONCEPTIONS RELATED TO INSULIN TREATMENT

Misconception	Response
Once insulin injections are started (for treatment of type 2 diabetes), they can never be discontinued	During periods of acute stress (eg, illness, infection, surgery) or when receiving certain medications that cause elevations in blood glucose, some patients with type 2 diabetes require insulin. If the diabetes had previously been well controlled with diet alone or diet with oral antidiabetic agents, the patient should be able to resume previous methods for control of diabetes after the stress is resolved. In addition, insulin is sometimes used to control blood glucose levels in obese type 2 diabetic patients who have been unsuccessful at weight loss. If the patient can lose weight after insulin therapy is initiated, the insulin doses may be tapered and the patient may be able to switch to diet and exercise alone or with oral antidiabetic agents for control of blood glucose. (For patients with type 1 diabetes, insulin is needed on an ongoing basis. For thin patients with type 2 diabetes, once insulin has to be started, it is usually required permanently.)
If increasing doses of insulin are needed to control the blood glucose, the diabetes must be getting "worse"	Explain to the patient that unlike other medications that are given in standard doses, there is not a standard dose of insulin that is effective for all patients. Rather, the dose must be adjusted according to blood glucose test results. If the initial insulin dose prescribed for the patient does not adequately decrease the glucose level, the patient may assume that he or she has a "bad" case of diabetes or that the diabetes is getting worse. It is important to instruct patients that many different factors may affect the ability of insulin to lower the glucose, including obesity, puberty, pregnancy, illness, and certain medications. In addition, to avoid hypoglycemia, physicians frequently initiate insulin therapy with smaller dosages than will eventually be needed. The doses are then increased in small increments until blood glucose levels are in the desired range.
Insulin causes blindness (or other diabetic complications)	If the patient has a diabetic acquaintance in whom the initiation of insulin therapy happened to coincide with the onset of diabetic complications, the patient may view insulin as the cause of complications such as blindness or amputation. In these situations, the acquaintance probably had type 2 diabetes that was no longer controllable with diet and oral hypoglycemic agents. It must be explained to the patient that factors such as elevated blood glucose (and not insulin therapy) contribute to some of the diabetic complications. Further, emphasize that insulin is a natural hormone that is present in every person's body, helps control blood glucose levels, and definitely does *not* cause long-term complications of diabetes.
Insulin must be injected directly into the vein	When patients first learn that one area used for insulin injections is on the arm, they may envision inserting the needle directly into a vein in the antecubital area, as in blood withdrawal. The patient must be reassured that insulin is injected into the fat tissue on the *back* of the arm (or on the abdomen, thigh, or hip) and that the needle is much shorter than that used for venipuncture.
There is extreme danger in injecting insulin if there are any air bubbles in the syringe	Patients may have a fear of dying if air bubbles are injected with a syringe. (This may be related to the misconception that insulin is injected directly into the vein.) Reassure patients that the main danger in having air bubbles in the insulin syringe is that the amount of insulin being injected is less than the required dose. It is often difficult to remove every small "champagne" bubble from the syringe. Thus, patients should be reassured that injection of insulin when these bubbles are present does not cause any harm.
Insulin always causes people to have bad (hypoglycemic) reactions	First, make sure that patients are aware that low blood sugar reactions are often related to an imbalance with the insulin, food, and activity and can often be avoided. Thus, before starting on insulin, patients should discuss their usual schedule of meals and activities as well as the content of meals with the health care team. Make sure that patients are aware that various different insulins and insulin schedules can be used to try to allow patients to maintain some of their usual lifestyle habits. Reassure patients that avoiding hypoglycemic reactions is a high priority for the diabetes team. In addition, tell patients of the importance of reporting any hypoglycemic reactions to the health care team immediately so that early adjustments can be made in the insulin dosage. Focus early insulin education on treatment and prevention of hypoglycemia.
People who take insulin must travel only where there is a refrigerator to store the insulin	Insulin bottles in use may be kept at room temperature. Therefore, for most business trips or vacations, keeping the insulin in a purse or briefcase (or special diabetes supply case) is acceptable. If a prolonged trip is planned (more than 2 to 3 months), patients may want to consult the pharmacist or insulin manufacturer for suggestions. Most importantly, emphasize with patients that taking insulin should never deter them from pursuing activities they enjoy.

Pearce, M. A., Rosenberg, C. S. & Davidson, M. B. (2003). Patient education. In Davidson, M. B. (Ed.). *Diabetes mellitus: Diagnosis and treatment* (4th ed.). New York: Churchill Livingstone. Reprinted with permission from Elsevier Science.

activities sponsored by local hospitals and diabetes organizations. In addition, magazines and Web sites with information on diabetes management are available (see Resources).

Teaching Patients to Self-Administer Insulin

Insulin injections are self-administered into the subcutaneous tissue with the use of special insulin syringes. Basic information includes explanations of the equipment, insulins, and syringes and how to mix insulin.

Storing Insulin. Whether insulin is the short-acting or the long-acting preparation, vials not in use, including spare vials, should be refrigerated. Extremes of temperature should be avoided; insulin should not be allowed to freeze and should not be kept in direct sunlight or in a hot car. The insulin vial in use should be kept at room temperature to reduce local irritation at the injection site, which may occur if cold insulin is injected. If a vial of insulin will be used up within 1 month, it may be kept at room temperature. The patient should be instructed to always have a spare vial of the type or types of insulin he or she uses (ADA, 2004). Cloudy insulins should be thoroughly mixed by gently inverting the vial or rolling it between the hands before drawing the solution into a syringe or a pen.

Bottles of intermediate-acting insulin should also be inspected for flocculation, which is a frosted, whitish coating inside the bottle. This occurs most commonly with human insulins that are exposed to extremes of temperature. If a frosted, adherent coating is present, some of the insulin is bound, and it should not be used.

Selecting Syringes. Syringes must be matched with the insulin concentration (eg, U-100). Currently, three sizes of U-100 insulin syringes are available:

- 1-mL syringes that hold 100 units
- 0.5-mL syringes that hold 50 units
- 0.3-mL syringes that hold 30 units

The concentration of insulin used in the United States is U-100; that is, there are 100 units per milliliter (or cubic centimeter). Small syringes allow patients who require small amounts of insulin to measure and draw up the amount of insulin accurately. Patients who require large amounts of insulin use larger syringes. There is a U-500 (500 units/mL) concentration of insulin available by special order for patients who have severe insulin resistance and require massive doses of insulin.

Most insulin syringes have a disposable 27- to 29-gauge needle that is approximately 0.5 inch long. The smaller syringes are marked in 1-unit increments and may be easier to use for patients with visual deficits and those taking very small doses of insulin. The 1-mL syringes are marked in 1- and 2-unit increments. A small disposable insulin needle (31 gauge, 8 mm long) is available for very thin patients and children.

Mixing Insulins. When rapid-acting or short-acting insulins are to be given simultaneously with longer-acting insulins, they are usually mixed together in the same syringe; the longer-acting insulins must be mixed thoroughly before drawing into the syringe. The most important issue is that patients be consistent in how they prepare their insulin injections from day to day.

There are varying opinions regarding which type of insulin (short-acting or longer-acting) should be drawn up into the syringe first when they are going to be mixed, but the ADA recommends that the regular insulin be drawn up first. Again, the most important issues are (1) that patients be consistent in technique, so as not to draw up the wrong dose in error or the wrong type of insulin, and (2) that patients not inject one type of insulin into the bottle containing a different type of insulin (ADA, 2004). Injecting cloudy insulin into a vial of clear insulin contaminates the entire vial of clear insulin and alters its action.

For patients who have difficulty mixing insulins, several options are available: they may use a premixed insulin, they may have prefilled syringes prepared (see Fig. 41-3), or they may take 2 injections. Premixed insulins are available in several different ratios of NPH insulin to regular insulin. The ratio of 70/30 (70% NPH and 30% regular insulin in one bottle) is most common; this combination is available as Novolin 70/30 (Novo-Nordisk) and Humulin 70/30 (Lilly). Combinations with a ratio of 75% NPL (neutral protamine lispro) and 25% insulin lispro are also available (ADA, 2004). NPL is used only in the mix with Humalog; its action is the same as NPH. The appropriate initial dosage of premixed insulin must be calculated so that the ratio of NPH to regular insulin most closely approximates the separate doses needed.

For patients who can inject insulin but who have difficulty drawing up a single or mixed dose, syringes may be prefilled with the help of home care nurses or family and friends. A 3-week supply of insulin syringes may be prepared and kept in the refrigerator. The prefilled syringes should be stored with the needle in an upright position to avoid clogging of the needle (ADA, 2004); they should be mixed thoroughly before the insulin is injected.

Withdrawing Insulin. Most (if not all) of the printed materials available on insulin dose preparation instruct patients to inject air into the bottle of insulin equivalent to the number of units of insulin to be withdrawn. The rationale for this is to prevent the formation of a vacuum inside the bottle, which would make it difficult to withdraw the proper amount of insulin.

Selecting and Rotating the Injection Site. The four main areas for injection are the abdomen, upper arms (posterior surface), thighs (anterior surface), and hips (Fig. 41-6). Insulin is absorbed faster in some areas of the body than others. The speed of absorption is greatest in the abdomen and decreases progressively in the arm, thigh, and hip, respectively.

Systematic rotation of injection sites within an anatomic area is recommended to prevent localized changes in fatty tissue (lipodystrophy). In addition, to promote consistency in insulin absorption, the patient should be encouraged to use all available injection sites within one area rather than randomly rotating sites from area to area (ADA, 2004). For example, some patients almost exclusively use the abdominal area, administering each injection 0.5 to 1 inch away from the previous injection. Another approach to rotation is always to use the same area at the same time of day. For example, patients may inject morning doses into the abdomen and evening doses into the arms or legs.

A few general principles apply to all rotation patterns. First, the patient should try not to use the same site more than once in 2 to 3 weeks. In addition, if the patient is planning to exercise, insulin should not be injected into

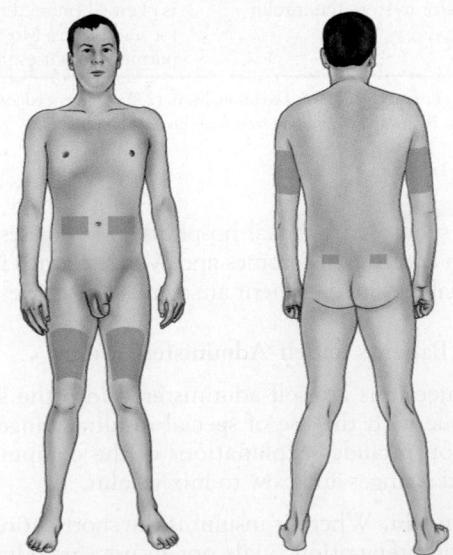

Figure 41-6 Suggested areas for insulin injection.

the limb that will be exercised because this will cause the drug to be absorbed faster, which may result in hypoglycemia.

In the past, patients were taught to rotate injections from one area to the next (eg, injecting once in the right arm, then once in the right abdomen, then once in the right thigh). Patients who still use this system must be taught to avoid repeated injections into the same site within an area. However, as previously stated, it is preferable for patients to use the same anatomic area at the same time of day consistently; this reduces day-to-day variation in blood glucose levels caused by different absorption rates.

Preparing the Skin. Use of alcohol to cleanse the skin is not recommended, but patients who have learned this technique often continue to use it. They should be cautioned to allow the skin to dry after cleansing with alcohol. If the skin is not allowed to dry before the injection, the alcohol may be carried into the tissues, resulting in a localized reddened area and a burning sensation.

Inserting the Needle. There are varying approaches to inserting the needle for insulin injections. The correct technique is based on the need for the insulin to be injected into the subcutaneous tissue (Chart 41-7). Injection that is too deep (eg, intramuscular) or too shallow may affect the rate of absorption of the insulin. For a normal or overweight person, a 90-degree angle is the best insertion angle. Aspiration (inserting the needle and then pulling back on the plunger to assess for blood being drawn into the syringe) is generally not recommended with self-injection of insulin. Many patients who have been using insulin for an extended

---

CHART 41-7 PATIENT EDUCATION
Self-Injection of Insulin

1. With one hand, stabilize the skin by spreading it or pinching up a large area.

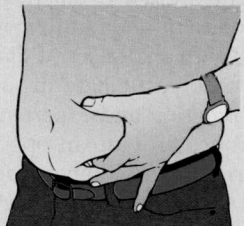

Pinching the skin

2. Pick up syringe with the other hand and hold it as you would a pencil. Insert needle straight into the skin.*

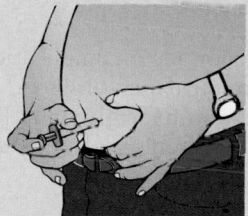

Inserting the needle into the skin

3. To inject the insulin, push the plunger all the way in.

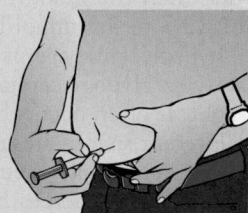

Injecting the insulin

4. Pull needle straight out of skin. Press cotton ball over injection site for several seconds.

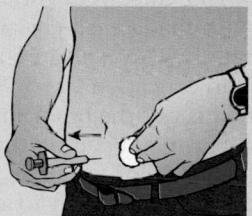

Removing the needle and holding cotton ball over site

5. Use disposable syringe *only once* and discard into hard plastic container (with a tight-fitting top) such as an empty bleach or detergent container.† Follow state regulations for disposal of syringes and needles.

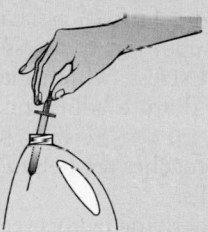

Disposing of syringe

*Some patients may be taught to insert the needle at a 45-degree angle.
†Although some studies suggest that reusing disposable syringes may be safe, it is recommended that this be done only in the absence of poor personal hygiene, an acute concurrent illness, open wounds on the hands, or decreased resistance to infection.

period have eliminated this step from their insulin injection routine with no apparent adverse effects.

Disposing of Syringes and Needles. Insulin syringes and pens, needles, and lancets should be disposed of according to local regulations. If community disposal programs are unavailable, used sharps should be placed in a puncture-resistant container. The patient should contact local trash authorities for instructions about proper disposal of filled containers, which should not be mixed with containers to be recycled.

Promoting Home and Community-Based Care

Promoting Self-Care

If problems exist with glucose control or with the development of preventable complications, it is the nurse's responsibility to assess the reasons for the patient's ineffective management of the treatment regimen. It should not be assumed that problems with diabetes management are related to the patient's willful decision to ignore self-management. The patient may have forgotten or never learned certain information. The problem may be correctable simply through providing complete information and ensuring that the patient understands the information. The focus of diabetes education should be patient empowerment. Patient education should address behavior change, self-efficacy, and health beliefs. Chart 41-8 details how to evaluate the effectiveness of self-injection of insulin education.

If knowledge deficit is not the problem, certain physical or emotional factors may be impairing the patient's ability to perform self-care skills. For example, decreased visual acuity may impair the patient's ability to administer insulin accurately, measure the blood glucose level, or inspect the skin and feet. In addition, decreased joint mobility (especially in the elderly) or preexisting disability may impair the patient's ability to inspect the bottom of the feet. Denial of the diagnosis or depression may impair the patient's ability to carry out multiple daily self-care measures. The patient whose family, personal, or work problems may be of higher priority may benefit from assistance in establishing priorities. It is also important to assess the patient for infection or emotional stress, which may lead to elevated blood glucose levels despite adherence to the treatment regimen.

The following approaches are helpful for promoting self-care management skills:

- Address any underlying factors (eg, knowledge deficit, self-care deficit, illness) that may affect diabetic control.
- Simplify the treatment regimen if it is too difficult for the patient to follow.
- Adjust the treatment regimen to meet patient requests (eg, adjust diet or insulin schedule to allow increased flexibility in meal content or timing).
- Establish a specific plan or contract with each patient with simple, measurable goals.
- Provide positive reinforcement of self-care behaviors performed instead of focusing on behaviors that were neglected (eg, positively reinforce blood glucose tests that were performed instead of focusing on the number of missed tests).

- Help the patient identify personal motivating factors rather than focusing on wanting to please physicians or nurses.
- Encourage the patient to pursue life goals and interests, and discourage an undue focus on diabetes.

Continuing Care

The degree to which patients interact with health care providers to obtain ongoing care depends on many factors. Age, socioeconomic level, existing complications, type of diabetes, and comorbid conditions all may dictate the frequency of follow-up visits. Many patients with diabetes are seen by home health nurses for diabetes education, wound care, insulin preparation, or assistance with glucose monitoring. Even patients who achieve excellent glucose control and have no complications can expect to see their primary health care provider at least twice a year for ongoing evaluation and should receive routine nutrition updates. In addition, the nurse should remind the patient to participate in recommended health promotion activities (eg, immunizations) and age-appropriate health screenings (eg, pelvic examinations, mammograms).

In addition, participation in support groups is encouraged for patients who have had diabetes for many years as well as for those who are newly diagnosed. Such participation may help the patient and family cope with changes in lifestyle that occur with the onset of diabetes and its complications. People who participate in support groups often share valuable information and experiences and learn from others. Support groups provide an opportunity for discussion of strategies to deal with diabetes and its management and to clarify and verify information with nurses or other health care professionals. Participation in support groups may also promote healthy activities.

ACUTE COMPLICATIONS OF DIABETES

There are three major acute complications of diabetes related to short-term imbalances in blood glucose levels: hypoglycemia, DKA, and hyperglycemic hyperosmolar nonketotic syndrome, which is also called hyperglycemic hyperosmolar syndrome or state.

Hypoglycemia (Insulin Reactions)

Hypoglycemia occurs when the blood glucose falls to less than 50 to 60 mg/dL (2.7 to 3.3 mmol/L), because of too much insulin or oral hypoglycemic agents, too little food, or excessive physical activity. Hypoglycemia may occur at any time of the day or night. It often occurs before meals, especially if meals are delayed or snacks are omitted. For example, midmorning hypoglycemia may occur when the morning regular insulin is peaking, whereas hypoglycemia that occurs in the late afternoon coincides with the peak of the morning NPH or Lente insulin. Middle-of-the-night hypoglycemia may occur because of peaking evening or predinner NPH or Lente insulins, especially in patients who have not eaten a bedtime snack.

Chart 41-8 • *Outcome Criteria for Determining Effectiveness of Self-Injection of Insulin Education*

Equipment

Insulin

1. Identifies information on label of insulin bottle:
   - Type (eg, NPH, regular, 70/30)
   - Species (human, biosynthetic, pork)
   - Manufacturer (Lilly, Novo Nordisk)
   - Concentration (eg, U-100)
   - Expiration date
2. Checks appearance of insulin:
   - Clear or milky white
   - Checks for flocculation (clumping, frosted appearance)
3. Identifies where to purchase and store insulin:
   - Indicates approximately how long bottle will last (1,000 units per bottle U-100 insulin)
   - Indicates how long opened bottles can be used

Syringes

1. Identifies concentration (U-100) marking on syringe
2. Identifies size of syringe (eg, 100-unit, 50-unit, 30-unit)
3. Describes appropriate disposal of used syringe

Preparation and Administration of Insulin Injection

1. Draws up correct amount and type of insulin
2. Properly mixes two insulins if necessary
3. Inserts needle and injects insulin
4. Describes site rotation:
   - Demonstrates injection with all anatomic areas to be used
   - Describes pattern for rotation, such as using abdomen only or using certain areas at the same time of day
   - Describes system for remembering site locations, such as horizontal pattern across the abdomen as if drawing a dotted line

Knowledge of Insulin Action

1. Lists prescription:
   - Type and dosage of insulin
   - Timing of insulin injections
2. Describes approximate time course of insulin action:
   - Identifies longing and short-acting insulins by name
   - States approximate time delay until onset of insulin action
   - Identifies need to delay food until 5 to 15 min after injection of rapid-acting insulin (lispro, aspart, glulisine [Apidra])
   - Knows that longer time delays are safe when blood glucose level is high, and time delays may need to be shortened when blood glucose level is low

Incorporation of Insulin Injections Into Daily Schedule

1. Recites proper order of premeal diabetes activities:
   - May use mnemonic device such as the word "tie," which helps the patient remember the order of activities ("t" = test [blood glucose], "i" = insulin injection, "e" = eat)
   - Describes daily schedule, such as test, insulin, eat before breakfast and dinner; test and eat, before lunch and bedtime
2. Describes information regarding hypoglycemia:
   - Symptoms: shakiness, sweating, nervousness, hunger, weakness
   - Causes: too much insulin, too much exercise, not enough food
   - Treatment: 15 g concentrated carbohydrate, such as two or three glucose tablets, 1 tube glucose gel, 0.5 cup juice
   - After initial treatment, follow with snack including starch and protein, such as cheese and crackers, milk and crackers, half sandwich
3. Describes information regarding prevention of hypoglycemia:
   - Avoids delays in meal timing
   - Eats a meal or snack approximately every 4 to 5 h (while awake)
   - Does not skip meals
   - Increases food intake before exercise if blood glucose level is <100 mg/dL
   - Checks blood glucose regularly
   - Identifies safe modification of insulin doses consistent with management plan
   - Carries a form of fast-acting sugar at all times
   - Wears a medical identification bracelet
   - Teaches family, friends, coworkers about signs and treatment of hypoglycemia
   - Has family, roommates, traveling companions learn to use injectable glucagon for severe hypoglycemic reactions
4. Maintains regular follow-up for evaluation of diabetes control:
   - Keeps written record of blood glucose, insulin doses, hypoglycemic reactions, variations in diet
   - Keeps all appointments with health professionals
   - Sees health care provider regularly (usually two to four times per year)
   - States how to contact health care provider in case of emergency
   - States when to call health care provider to report variations in blood glucose levels

 Gerontologic Considerations

In elderly patients with diabetes, hypoglycemia is a particular concern for many reasons:
- Elderly people frequently live alone and may not recognize the symptoms of hypoglycemia.
- With decreasing renal function, it takes longer for oral hypoglycemic agents to be excreted by the kidneys.
- Skipping meals may occur because of decreased appetite or financial limitations.

- Decreased visual acuity may lead to errors in insulin administration.

Clinical Manifestations

The clinical manifestations of hypoglycemia may be grouped into two categories: adrenergic symptoms and central nervous system (CNS) symptoms.

In mild hypoglycemia, as the blood glucose level falls, the sympathetic nervous system is stimulated, resulting in a surge of epinephrine and norepinephrine. This causes symptoms such as sweating, tremor, tachycardia, palpitation, nervousness, and hunger.

In moderate hypoglycemia, the drop in blood glucose level deprives the brain cells of needed fuel for functioning. Signs of impaired function of the CNS may include inability to concentrate, headache, lightheadedness, confusion, memory lapses, numbness of the lips and tongue, slurred speech, impaired coordination, emotional changes, irrational or combative behavior, double vision, and drowsiness. Any combination of these symptoms (in addition to adrenergic symptoms) may occur with moderate hypoglycemia.

In severe hypoglycemia, CNS function is so impaired that the patient needs the assistance of another person for treatment of hypoglycemia. Symptoms may include disoriented behavior, seizures, difficulty arousing from sleep, or loss of consciousness.

Assessment and Diagnostic Findings

Symptoms of hypoglycemia may occur suddenly and vary considerably from person to person. To some degree, this may be related to the actual level to which the blood glucose falls or to the rate at which it falls. For example, patients who usually have a blood glucose level in the hyperglycemic range (eg, 200 mg/dL or greater) may feel hypoglycemic (adrenergic) symptoms when their blood glucose falls rapidly to 120 mg/dL (6.6 mmol/L) or less. Conversely, patients who frequently have a glucose level in the low range of normal (eg, 80 to 100 mg/dL) may be asymptomatic when the blood glucose falls slowly to less than 50 mg/dL (2.7 mmol/L).

Decreased hormonal (adrenergic) response to hypoglycemia may also contribute to lack of symptoms of hypoglycemia. This occurs in some patients who have had diabetes for many years. It may be related to autonomic neuropathy, a chronic diabetic complication (see later discussion). As the blood glucose level falls, the normal surge in adrenalin does not occur, and the usual adrenergic symptoms, such as sweating and shakiness, do not take place. The hypoglycemia may not be detected until moderate or severe CNS impairment occurs. Affected patients must perform SMBG on a frequent regular basis, especially before driving or engaging in other potentially dangerous activities.

Management

Treating with Carbohydrates

Immediate treatment must be given when hypoglycemia occurs. The usual recommendation is for 15 g of a fast-acting concentrated source of carbohydrate such as the following, given orally:

- Three or four commercially prepared glucose tablets
- 4 to 6 oz of fruit juice or regular soda
- 6 to 10 hard candies
- 2 to 3 teaspoons of sugar or honey

It is not necessary to add sugar to juice, even if it is labeled as unsweetened juice: the fruit sugar in juice contains enough carbohydrate to raise the blood glucose level. Adding table sugar to juice may cause a sharp increase in the blood glucose level, and patients may experience hyperglycemia for hours after treatment.

The blood glucose level should be retested in 15 minutes and retreated if it is less than 70 to 75 mg/dL (3.8 to 4 mmol/L). If the symptoms persist for longer than 10 to 15 minutes after initial treatment, the treatment is repeated even if blood glucose testing is not possible. Once the symptoms resolve, a snack containing protein and starch (eg, milk or cheese and crackers) is recommended unless the patient plans to eat a regular meal or snack within 30 to 60 minutes.

Initiating Emergency Measures

In emergency situations, for adults who are unconscious and cannot swallow, an injection of glucagon 1 mg can be administered either subcutaneously or intramuscularly. Glucagon is a hormone produced by the alpha cells of the pancreas that stimulates the liver to breakdown glycogen, the stored glucose. Injectable glucagon is packaged as a powder in 1-mg vials and must be mixed with a diluent immediately before being injected. After injection of glucagon, the patient may take as long as 20 minutes to regain consciousness. A concentrated source of carbohydrate followed by a snack should be given to the patient on awakening to prevent recurrence of hypoglycemia (because the duration of the action of 1 mg of glucagon is brief—its onset is 8 to 10 minutes, and its action lasts 12 to 27 minutes) and to replenish liver stores of glucose. Some patients experience nausea after the administration of glucagon. If this occurs, the patient should be turned to the side to prevent aspiration in case the patient vomits.

Glucagon is sold by prescription only and should be part of the emergency supplies available to patients with diabetes who require insulin. Family members, friends, neighbors, and coworkers should be instructed in the use of glucagon, especially for patients who have little or no warning of hypoglycemic episodes. Patients should be instructed to notify their physician after severe hypoglycemia has occurred and been treated.

In hospitals and emergency departments, for patients who are unconscious or cannot swallow, 25 to 50 mL of 50% dextrose in water ($D_{50}W$) may be administered IV. The effect is usually seen within minutes. The patient may complain of a headache and of pain at the injection site. Assuring patency of the IV line used for injection of 50% dextrose is essential because hypertonic solutions such as 50% dextrose are very irritating to veins.

Providing Patient Education

Hypoglycemia is prevented by a consistent pattern of eating, administering insulin, and exercising. Between-meal and bedtime snacks may be needed to counteract the maximum insulin effect. In general, the patient should cover the time of peak activity of insulin by eating a snack and by taking additional food when physical activity is increased. Routine blood glucose tests are performed so that changing insulin requirements may be anticipated and the dosage adjusted. Because unexpected hypoglycemia can occur, all patients treated with insulin should wear an identification bracelet or tag stating that they have diabetes.

Patients and family members must be instructed to recognize the symptoms of hypoglycemia. Family members in particular must be made aware that any subtle (but unusual) change in behavior may be an indication of hypoglycemia. They should be taught to encourage and even insist that the person with diabetes assess blood glucose levels if hypoglycemia is suspected. When some patients are hypoglycemic, they become very resistant to testing or eating and become angry at family members who are trying to treat the hypoglycemia. Family members must be taught to persevere and to understand that the hypoglycemia can cause irrational behavior.

Autonomic neuropathy or beta-blockers such as propranolol (Inderal) to treat hypertension or cardiac dysrhythmias may mask the typical symptoms of hypoglycemia. It is very important that these patients perform blood glucose tests on a frequent and regular basis. Patients who have type 2 diabetes and who take oral sulfonylurea agents may also develop hypoglycemia, which can be prolonged and severe; this is a particular risk for elderly patients.

It is important that patients with diabetes, especially those receiving insulin, learn to carry some form of simple sugar with them at all times (ADA, 2008b). There are many different commercially prepared glucose tablets and gels that the patient may find convenient to carry. If the patient has a hypoglycemic reaction and does not have any of the recommended emergency foods available, he or she should eat any available food (preferably a carbohydrate food).

Patients are advised to refrain from eating high-calorie, high-fat dessert foods (eg, cookies, cakes, doughnuts, ice cream) to treat hypoglycemia because their high fat content may slow the absorption of the glucose and resolution of the hypoglycemic symptoms. The patient may subsequently eat more of the foods when symptoms do not resolve rapidly, which may cause very high blood glucose levels for several hours and may contribute to weight gain.

Patients who feel unduly restricted by their meal plan may view hypoglycemic episodes as a time to reward themselves with desserts. It may be more prudent to teach these patients to incorporate occasional desserts into the meal plan. This may make it easier for them to limit their treatment of hypoglycemic episodes to simple (low-calorie) carbohydrates such as juice or glucose tablets.

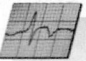

Diabetic Ketoacidosis

DKA is caused by an absence or markedly inadequate amount of insulin. This deficit in available insulin results in disorders in the metabolism of carbohydrate, protein, and fat. The three main clinical features of DKA are
- Hyperglycemia
- Dehydration and electrolyte loss
- Acidosis

Pathophysiology

Without insulin, the amount of glucose entering the cells is reduced, and production and release of glucose by the liver (gluconeogenesis) is increased, leading to hyperglycemia (Fig. 41-7). In an attempt to rid the body of the excess glucose, the kidneys excrete the glucose along with water and electrolytes (eg, sodium, potassium). This osmotic diuresis, which is characterized by excessive urination (polyuria),

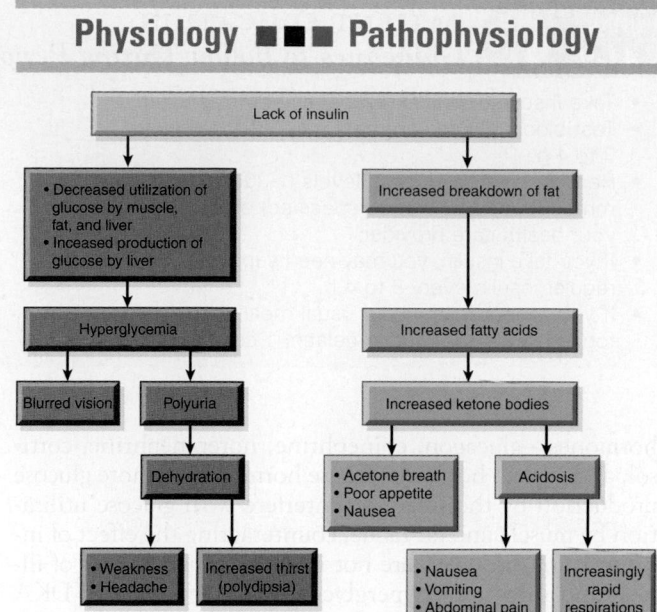

Figure 41-7 Abnormal metabolism that causes signs and symptoms of diabetic ketoacidosis. (Redrawn from Pearce, M. A., Rosenberg, C. S. & Davidson, M. D. (2003). Patient education. In Davidson, M. B. (Ed.). *Diabetes mellitus: Diagnosis and treatment.* New York: Churchill Livingstone.)

leads to dehydration and marked electrolyte loss. Patients with severe DKA may lose up to 6.5 L of water and up to 400 to 500 mEq each of sodium, potassium, and chloride over a 24-hour period.

Another effect of insulin deficiency or deficit is the breakdown of fat (lipolysis) into free fatty acids and glycerol. The free fatty acids are converted into ketone bodies by the liver. Ketone bodies are acids; their accumulation in the circulation due to lack of insulin leads to metabolic acidosis.

Three main causes of DKA are decreased or missed dose of insulin, illness or infection, and undiagnosed and untreated diabetes (DKA may be the initial manifestation of diabetes). An insulin deficit may result from an insufficient dosage of insulin prescribed or from insufficient insulin being administered by the patient. Errors in insulin dosage may be made by patients who are ill and who assume that if they are eating less or if they are vomiting, they must decrease their insulin doses. (Because illness, especially infections, can cause increased blood glucose levels, the patient does not need to decrease the insulin dose to compensate for decreased food intake when ill and may even need to increase the insulin dose.)

Other potential causes of decreased insulin include patient error in drawing up or injecting insulin (especially in patients with visual impairments), intentional skipping of insulin doses (especially in adolescents with diabetes who are having difficulty coping with diabetes or other aspects of their lives), or equipment problems (eg, occlusion of insulin pump tubing). Illness and infections are associated with insulin resistance. In response to physical (and emotional) stressors, there is an increase in the level of "stress"

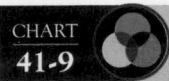

CHART 41-9

PATIENT EDUCATION
Guidelines to Follow During Periods of Illness ("Sick Day Rules")

- Take insulin or oral antidiabetic agents as usual.
- Test blood glucose and test urine ketones every 3 to 4 h.
- Report elevated glucose levels (>300 mg/dL [16.6 mmol/L] or as otherwise specified) or urine ketones to your health care provider.
- If you take insulin, you may need supplemental doses of regular insulin every 3 to 4 h.
- If you cannot follow your usual meal plan, substitute soft foods (eg, ⅓ cup regular gelatin, 1 cup cream soup, ½ cup custard, 3 squares graham crackers) six to eight times per day.
- If vomiting, diarrhea, or fever persists, take liquids (eg, ½ cup regular cola or orange juice, ½ cup broth, 1 cup Gatorade) every ½ to 1 hour to prevent dehydration and to provide calories.
- Report nausea, vomiting, and diarrhea to your health care provider, because extreme fluid loss may be dangerous.
- If you are unable to retain oral fluids, you may require hospitalization to avoid diabetic ketoacidosis and possibly coma.

hormones—glucagon, epinephrine, norepinephrine, cortisol, and growth hormone. These hormones promote glucose production by the liver and interfere with glucose utilization by muscle and fat tissue, counteracting the effect of insulin. If insulin levels are not increased during times of illness and infection, hyperglycemia may progress to DKA (ADA, 2006c).

Prevention

For prevention of DKA related to illness, "sick day" rules for managing their diabetes when ill (Chart 41-9) should be reviewed. The most important concept in this is to never eliminate insulin doses when nausea and vomiting occur. Instead, the patient should take the usual insulin dose (or previously prescribed special "sick day" doses) and then attempt to consume frequent small portions of carbohydrates (including foods usually avoided, such as juices, regular sodas, and gelatin). Drinking fluids every hour is important to prevent dehydration. Blood glucose and urine ketones must be assessed every 3 to 4 hours.

If the patient cannot take fluids without vomiting, or if elevated glucose or ketone levels persist, the physician must be contacted. Patients are taught to have foods available for use on sick days. In addition, a supply of urine test strips (for ketone testing) and blood glucose test strips should be available. The patient must know how to contact his or her physician 24 hours a day. These materials should be assembled in a "sick day" kit.

After the acute phase of DKA has resolved, the nurse should assess for underlying causes of DKA. If there are psychological reasons for the patient's deliberately missing insulin doses, the patient and family may be referred for evaluation and counseling or therapy.

Clinical Manifestations

The hyperglycemia of DKA leads to polyuria and polydipsia (increased thirst). In addition, the patient may experience blurred vision, weakness, and headache. Patients with marked intravascular volume depletion may have orthostatic hypotension (drop in systolic blood pressure of 20 mm Hg or more on changing from a reclining to a standing position). Volume depletion may also lead to frank hypotension with a weak, rapid pulse.

The ketosis and acidosis of DKA lead to gastrointestinal symptoms such as anorexia, nausea, vomiting, and abdominal pain. The abdominal pain and physical findings on examination can be so severe that they resemble an acute abdominal disorder that requires surgery. The patient may have acetone breath (a fruity odor), which occurs with elevated ketone levels. In addition, hyperventilation (with very deep, but not labored, respirations) may occur. These Kussmaul respirations represent the body's attempt to decrease the acidosis, counteracting the effect of the ketone buildup. In addition, mental status in DKA varies widely. The patient may be alert, lethargic, or comatose.

Assessment and Diagnostic Findings

Blood glucose levels may vary between 300 and 800 mg/dL (16.6 to 44.4 mmol/L). Some patients have lower glucose values, and others have values of 1000 mg/dL (55.5 mmol/L) or higher (usually depending on the degree of dehydration). The severity of DKA is not necessarily related to the blood glucose level. Evidence of ketoacidosis is reflected in low serum bicarbonate (0 to 15 mEq/L) and low pH (6.8 to 7.3) values. A low partial pressure of carbon dioxide (PCO_2; 10 to 30 mm Hg) reflects respiratory compensation (Kussmaul respirations) for the metabolic acidosis. Accumulation of ketone bodies (which precipitates the acidosis) is reflected in blood and urine ketone measurements.

Sodium and potassium concentrations may be low, normal, or high, depending on the amount of water loss (dehydration). Despite the plasma concentration, there has been a marked total body depletion of these (and other) electrolytes and they will need to be replaced.

Increased levels of creatinine, blood urea nitrogen (BUN), and hematocrit may also be seen with dehydration. After rehydration, continued elevation in the serum creatinine and BUN levels suggests underlying renal insufficiency.

Management

In addition to treating hyperglycemia, management of DKA is aimed at correcting dehydration, electrolyte loss, and acidosis.

Rehydration

In dehydrated patients, rehydration is important for maintaining tissue perfusion. In addition, fluid replacement enhances the excretion of excessive glucose by the kidneys. The patient may need as much as 6 to 10 L of IV fluid to replace fluid losses caused by polyuria, hyperventilation, diarrhea, and vomiting.

Initially, 0.9% sodium chloride (normal saline) solution is administered at a rapid rate, usually 0.5 to 1 L/h for 2 to 3 hours. Half-strength normal saline (0.45%) solution (also known as hypotonic saline solution) may be used for patients with hypertension or hypernatremia and those at risk for heart failure. After the first few hours, half-strength normal saline solution is the fluid of choice for continued rehydration, provided the blood pressure is stable and the sodium level is not low. Moderate to high rates of infusion (200 to 500 mL/h) may be needed for several more hours. When the blood glucose level reaches 300 mg/dL (16.6 mmol/L) or less, the IV solution may be changed to dextrose 5% in water (D$_5$W) to prevent a precipitous decline in the blood glucose level (Fowler, 2009).

Monitoring of fluid volume status involves frequent measurements of vital signs (including monitoring for orthostatic changes in blood pressure and heart rate), lung assessment, and monitoring of intake and output. Initial urine output lags behind IV fluid intake as dehydration is corrected. Plasma expanders may be necessary to correct severe hypotension that does not respond to IV fluid treatment. Monitoring for signs of fluid overload is especially important for patients who are older, have renal impairment, or are at risk for heart failure.

Restoring Electrolytes

The major electrolyte of concern during treatment of DKA is potassium. Although the initial plasma concentration of potassium may be low, normal, or even high, there is a major loss of potassium from body stores and an intracellular-to-extracellular shift of potassium. Furthermore, the serum level of potassium decreases as potassium reenters the cells during the course of treatment of DKA; therefore, the serum potassium level must be monitored frequently. Some of the factors related to treating DKA that reduce the serum potassium concentration include rehydration, which leads to increased plasma volume and subsequent decreases in the concentration of serum potassium. Rehydration also leads to increased urinary excretion of potassium. Insulin administration enhances the movement of potassium from the extracellular fluid into the cells.

Cautious but timely potassium replacement is vital to avoid dysrhythmias that may occur with hypokalemia. As much as 40 mEq/h may be needed for several hours. Because extracellular potassium levels decrease during DKA treatment, potassium must be infused even if the plasma potassium level is normal.

Frequent (every 2 to 4 hours initially) ECGs and laboratory measurements of potassium are necessary during the first 8 hours of treatment. Potassium replacement is withheld only if hyperkalemia is present or if the patient is not urinating.

 NURSING ALERT

Because a patient's serum potassium level may drop quickly as a result of rehydration and insulin treatment, potassium replacement must begin once potassium levels drop to normal.

Reversing Acidosis

Ketone bodies (acids) accumulate as a result of fat breakdown. The acidosis that occurs in DKA is reversed with insulin, which inhibits fat breakdown, thereby stopping acid buildup. Insulin is usually infused intravenously at a slow, continuous rate (eg, 5 units/h). Hourly blood glucose values must be measured. IV fluid solutions with higher concentrations of glucose, such as normal saline (NS) solution (eg, D$_5$NS, D$_5$·45NS), are administered when blood glucose levels reach 250 to 300 mg/dL (13.8 to 16.6 mmol/L) to avoid too rapid a drop in the blood glucose level (ie, hypoglycemia) during treatment.

Regular insulin, the only type of insulin approved for IV use, may be added to IV solutions. The nurse must convert hourly rates of insulin infusion (frequently prescribed as units per hour) to IV drip rates. For example, if 100 units of regular insulin are mixed into 500 mL of 0.9% NS, then 1 unit of insulin equals 5 mL; therefore, an initial insulin infusion rate of 5 units/h would equal 25 mL/h. The insulin is often infused separately from the rehydration solutions to allow frequent changes in the rate and content of the latter.

Insulin must be infused continuously until subcutaneous administration of insulin can be resumed. Any interruption in administration may result in the reaccumulation of ketone bodies and worsening acidosis. Even if blood glucose levels are decreasing and returning to normal, the insulin drip must not be stopped until subcutaneous insulin therapy has been started. Rather, the rate or concentration of the dextrose infusion should be increased. Blood glucose levels are usually corrected before the acidosis is corrected. Therefore, IV insulin may be continued for 12 to 24 hours, until the serum bicarbonate level increases (to at least 15 to 18 mEq/L) and until the patient can eat. In general, bicarbonate infusion to correct severe acidosis is avoided during treatment of DKA because it precipitates further, sudden (and potentially fatal) decreases in serum potassium levels. Continuous insulin infusion is usually sufficient for reversal of DKA (ADA, 2006c).

 NURSING ALERT

When mixing the insulin drip, it is important to flush the insulin solution through the entire IV infusion set and to discard the first 50 mL of fluid. Insulin molecules adhere to the inner surface of IV infusion sets; therefore, the initial fluid may contain a decreased concentration of insulin.

Hyperglycemic Hyperosmolar Nonketotic Syndrome

Hyperglycemic hyperosmolar nonketotic syndrome (HHNS) is a serious condition in which hyperosmolarity and hyperglycemia predominate, with alterations of the sensorium (sense of awareness). At the same time, ketosis is usually minimal or absent. The basic biochemical defect is lack of effective insulin (ie, insulin resistance). Persistent hyperglycemia causes osmotic diuresis, which results in losses of water and electrolytes. To maintain osmotic equilibrium, water shifts from the intracellular fluid space to the

Table 41-8 COMPARISON OF DIABETIC KETOACIDOSIS (DKA) AND HYPERGLYCEMIC HYPEROSMOLAR NONKETOTIC SYNDROME (HHNS)

Characteristics	DKA	HHNS
Patients most commonly affected	Can occur in type 1 or type 2 diabetes; more common in type 1 diabetes	Can occur in type 1 or type 2 diabetes; more common in type 2 diabetes, especially elderly patients with type 2 diabetes
Precipitating event	Omission of insulin; physiologic stress (infection, surgery, CVA, MI)	Physiologic stress (infection, surgery, CVA, MI)
Onset	Rapid (<24 h)	Slower (over several days)
Blood glucose levels	Usually >250 mg/dL (>13.9 mmol/L)	Usually >600 mg/dL (>33.3 mmol/L)
Arterial pH level	<7.3	Normal
Serum and urine ketones	Present	Absent
Serum osmolality	300–350 mOsm/L	>350 mOsm/L
Plasma bicarbonate level	<15 mEq/L	Normal
BUN and creatinine levels	Elevated	Elevated
Mortality rate	<5%	10–40%

BUN, blood urea nitrogen; CVA, cerebrovascular accident; MI, myocardial infarction.

extracellular fluid space. With glycosuria and dehydration, hypernatremia and increased osmolarity occur. Table 41-8 compares DKA and HHNS.

HHNS occurs most often in older people (50 to 70 years of age) who have no known history of diabetes or who have type 2 diabetes. HHNS often can be traced to a precipitating event such as an acute illness (eg, pneumonia, cerebrovascular accident [CVA]), medications that exacerbate hyperglycemia (eg, thiazides), or treatments such as dialysis. The history includes days to weeks of polyuria with adequate fluid intake. What distinguishes HHNS from DKA is that ketosis and acidosis generally do not occur in HHNS, partly because of differences in insulin levels. In DKA, no insulin is present, and this promotes the breakdown of stored glucose, protein, and fat, which leads to the production of ketone bodies and ketoacidosis. In HHNS, the insulin level is too low to prevent hyperglycemia (and subsequent osmotic diuresis), but it is high enough to prevent fat breakdown. Patients with HHNS do not have the ketosis-related gastrointestinal symptoms that lead them to seek medical attention. Instead, they may tolerate polyuria and polydipsia until neurologic changes or an underlying illness (or family members or others) prompts them to seek treatment. Because of possible delays in therapy, hyperglycemia, dehydration, and hyperosmolarity may be more severe in HHNS.

Clinical Manifestations

The clinical picture of HHNS is one of hypotension, profound dehydration (dry mucous membranes, poor skin turgor), tachycardia, and variable neurologic signs (eg, alteration of sensorium, seizures, hemiparesis). The mortality rate ranges from 10% to 40%, usually related to an underlying illness, the vulnerability of the elderly patient, and the severity of HHNS.

Assessment and Diagnostic Findings

Diagnostic assessment includes a range of laboratory tests, including blood glucose, electrolytes, BUN, complete blood count, serum osmolality, and arterial blood gas analysis. The blood glucose level is usually 600 to 1200 mg/dL, and the osmolality exceeds 350 mOsm/kg. Electrolyte and

BUN levels are consistent with the clinical picture of severe dehydration. Mental status changes, focal neurologic deficits, and hallucinations are common secondary to the cerebral dehydration that results from extreme hyperosmolality. Postural hypotension accompanies the dehydration.

Management

The overall approach to the treatment of HHNS is similar to that of DKA: fluid replacement, correction of electrolyte imbalances, and insulin administration. Because patients with HHNS are typically older, close monitoring of volume and electrolyte status is important for prevention of fluid overload, heart failure, and cardiac dysrhythmias. Fluid treatment is started with 0.9% or 0.45% NS, depending on the patient's sodium level and the severity of volume depletion. Central venous or hemodynamic pressure monitoring guides fluid replacement. Potassium is added to IV fluids when urinary output is adequate and is guided by continuous ECG monitoring and frequent laboratory determinations of potassium.

Extremely elevated blood glucose concentrations decrease as the patient is rehydrated. Insulin plays a less important role in the treatment of HHNS because it is not needed for reversal of acidosis, as in DKA. Nevertheless, insulin is usually administered at a continuous low rate to treat hyperglycemia, and replacement IV fluids with dextrose are administered (as in DKA) after the glucose level has decreased to the range of 250 to 300 mg/dL (13.8 to 16.6 mmol/L) (ADA, 2008d; Fowler, 2009).

Other therapeutic modalities are determined by the underlying illness and the results of continuing clinical and laboratory evaluation. It may take 3 to 5 days for neurologic symptoms to clear, and treatment of HHNS usually continues well after metabolic abnormalities have resolved. After recovery from HHNS, many patients can control their diabetes with MNT alone or with MNT and oral antidiabetic medications. Insulin may not be needed once the acute hyperglycemic complication is resolved. Frequent SBGM is important in prevention of recurrence of HHNS.

NURSING PROCESS

THE PATIENT WITH DIABETIC KETOACIDOSIS OR HYPERGLYCEMIC HYPEROSMOLAR NONKETOTIC SYNDROME

Assessment

For the patient with DKA, the nurse monitors the ECG for dysrhythmias indicating abnormal potassium levels. Vital signs (especially blood pressure and pulse), arterial blood gases, breath sounds, and mental status are assessed every hour and recorded on a flow sheet. Neurologic status checks are included as part of the hourly assessment as cerebral edema can be a severe and sometimes fatal outcome.

For the patient with HHNS, the nurse assesses vital signs, fluid status, and laboratory values. Fluid status and urine output are closely monitored because of the high risk of renal failure secondary to severe dehydration. Because HHNS tends to occur in older patients, the physiologic changes that occur with aging should be considered. Careful assessment of cardiovascular, pulmonary, and renal function throughout the acute and recovery phases of HHNS is important.

Diagnosis

Nursing Diagnoses

Based on the assessment data, major nursing diagnoses may include the following:

- Risk for fluid volume deficit related to polyuria and dehydration
- Fluid and electrolyte imbalance related to fluid loss or shifts
- Deficient knowledge about diabetes self-care skills or information
- Anxiety related to loss of control, fear of inability to manage diabetes, misinformation related to diabetes, fear of diabetes complications

Collaborative Problems/Potential Complications

Based on assessment data, potential complications may include the following:

- Fluid overload, pulmonary edema, and heart failure
- Hypokalemia
- Hyperglycemia and ketoacidosis
- Hypoglycemia
- Cerebral edema

Planning and Goals

The major goals for the patient may include maintenance of fluid and electrolyte balance, optimal control of blood glucose levels, ability to perform diabetes survival skills and self-care activities, and absence of complications.

Nursing Interventions

Maintaining Fluid and Electrolyte Balance

Intake and output are measured. IV fluids and electrolytes are administered as prescribed, and oral fluid intake is encouraged when it is permitted. Laboratory values of serum electrolytes (especially sodium and potassium) are monitored. Vital signs are monitored hourly for signs of dehydration (tachycardia, orthostatic hypotension) along with assessment of breath sounds, level of consciousness, presence of edema, and cardiac status (ECG rhythm strips).

Increasing Knowledge About Diabetes Management

The development of DKA or HHNS suggests the need for the nurse to carefully assess the patient's understanding of and adherence to the diabetes management plan. Further, factors that may have led to the development of DKA or HHNS are explored with the patient and family. If the patient's blood glucose monitoring, dietary intake, use of antidiabetes (insulin or oral agents) medications, and exercise patterns differ from those identified in the diabetes management plan, their relationship to the development of DKS or HHNS is discussed, along with early manifestations of DKA or HHNS. If other factors, such as trauma, illness, surgery, or stress, are implicated, appropriate strategies to respond to these and similar situations in the future are described so that the patient can respond in the future without developing life-threatening complications. It may be necessary to reteach survival skills to patients who may not be able to recall them. If the patient has omitted insulin or oral antidiabetes agents that have been prescribed, it is important to explore the reasons for doing so and address those issues to prevent future recurrence and readmissions for treatment of these complications.

If the patient has not previously been diagnosed with diabetes, the opportunity is used to teach the patient about the need for maintaining blood glucose at a normal level and learning about diabetes management and survival skills.

Monitoring and Managing Potential Complications

FLUID OVERLOAD. Fluid overload can occur because of the administration of a large volume of fluid at a rapid rate, which is often required to treat patients with DKA or HHNS. This risk is increased in elderly patients and in those with preexisting cardiac or renal disease. To avoid fluid overload and resulting heart failure and pulmonary edema, the nurse monitors the patient closely during treatment by measuring vital signs and intake and output at frequent intervals. Central venous pressure monitoring and hemodynamic monitoring may be initiated to provide additional measures of fluid status. Physical examination focuses on assessment of cardiac rate and rhythm, breath sounds, venous distention, skin turgor, and urine output. The nurse monitors fluid intake and keeps careful records of IV and other fluid intake, along with urine output measurements.

HYPOKALEMIA. As previously described, hypokalemia is a potential complication during the treatment of DKA as potassium is lost from body stores. Low serum potassium levels may result from rehydration, increased urinary excretion of potassium, and movement of potassium from the extracellular fluid into the cells with insulin administration.

Prevention of hypokalemia includes cautious replacement of potassium; however, before its administration, it is important to ensure that a patient's kidneys are functioning. Because of the adverse effects of hypokalemia on cardiac function, monitoring of the cardiac rate, cardiac rhythm, ECG, and serum potassium levels is essential.

CEREBRAL EDEMA. Although the cause of cerebral edema is unknown, rapid correction of hyperglycemia, resulting in fluid shifts, is thought to be the cause. Cerebral edema, which occurs more often in children than in adults, can be prevented by gradual reduction in the blood glucose level (ADA, 2006c). An hourly flow sheet is used to enable close monitoring of the blood glucose level, serum electrolyte levels, urine output, mental status, and neurologic signs. Precautions are taken to minimize activities that could increase intracranial pressure.

Teaching Patients Self-Care

The patient is taught survival skills, including treatment modalities (diet, insulin administration, monitoring of blood glucose, and, for type 1 diabetes, monitoring of urine ketones); recognition, treatment, and prevention of DKA and HHNS. Teaching addresses those factors leading to DKA or HHNS. Follow-up education is arranged with a home care nurse and dietitian or an outpatient diabetes education center. This is particularly important for patients who have experienced DKA or HHNS because of the need to address factors that led to its occurrence. The importance of self-monitoring and of monitoring and follow-up by primary health care providers is reinforced, and the patient is reminded about the importance of keeping follow-up appointments.

Evaluation

Expected Outcomes

1. Achieves fluid and electrolyte balance
   a. Demonstrates intake and output balance
   b. Exhibits electrolyte values within normal limits
   c. Exhibits vital signs that remain stable, with resolution of orthostatic hypotension and tachycardia
2. Demonstrates knowledge about DKA and HHNS
   a. Identifies factors leading to DKA and HHNS
   b. Describes signs and symptoms of DKA and HHNS
   c. Describes short-term and long-term consequences of DKA and HHNS
   d. Identifies strategies to prevent the development of DKA and HHNS
   e. States when contact with health care provider is needed to treat early signs of DKS and HHNS
3. Absence of complications
   a. Exhibits normal cardiac rate and rhythm and normal breath sounds
   b. Exhibits no jugular venous distention
   c. Exhibits blood glucose and urine ketone levels within target range
   d. Exhibits no manifestations of hypoglycemia or hyperglycemia
   e. Shows improved mental status without signs of cerebral edema

LONG-TERM COMPLICATIONS OF DIABETES

There has been a steady decline in the number of deaths attributable to ketoacidosis and infection in patients with diabetes but an alarming increase in the number of deaths from cardiovascular and renal complications. Long-term complications, which are becoming more common as more people live longer with diabetes, can affect almost every organ system of the body and are a major cause of disability. The general categories of long-term diabetic complications are macrovascular disease, microvascular disease, and neuropathy.

The specific causes and pathogenesis of each type of complication are still being investigated. However, it appears that increased levels of blood glucose may play a role in neuropathic disease, microvascular complications, and risk factors contributing to macrovascular complications. Hypertension may also be a major contributing factor, especially in macrovascular and microvascular diseases.

Long-term complications are seen in both type 1 and type 2 diabetes but usually do not occur within the first 5 to 10 years after diagnosis. However, evidence of these complications may be present at the time of diagnosis of type 2 diabetes, because patients may have had undiagnosed diabetes for many years. Renal (microvascular) disease is more prevalent in patients with type 1 diabetes, and cardiovascular (macrovascular) complications are more prevalent in older patients with type 2 diabetes.

Macrovascular Complications

Diabetic macrovascular complications result from changes in the medium to large blood vessels. Blood vessel walls thicken, sclerose, and become occluded by plaque that adheres to the vessel walls. Eventually, blood flow is blocked. These atherosclerotic changes tend to occur more often and at an earlier age in patients with diabetes. Coronary artery disease, cerebrovascular disease, and peripheral vascular disease are the three main types of macrovascular complications that occur frequently in the diabetic population.

Myocardial infarction (MI) is twice as common in men with diabetes and three times as common in women with diabetes, compared to people without diabetes. There is also an increased risk for complications resulting from MI and an increased likelihood of a second MI. Coronary artery disease may account for 50% to 60% of all deaths among patients with diabetes. The typical ischemic symptoms may be absent in patients with diabetes. Therefore, the patient may not experience the early warning signs of decreased coronary blood flow and may have "silent" MIs, which may be discovered only as changes on the ECG. However, ECG changes may not be apparent. This lack of ischemic symptoms may be secondary to autonomic neuropathy (see later discussion). Cardiac disease is discussed in detail in Chapter 28.

Cerebral blood vessels are similarly affected by accelerated atherosclerosis. Occlusive changes or the formation of an embolus elsewhere in the vasculature that lodges in a cerebral blood vessel can lead to transient ischemic attacks and strokes. People with diabetes have twice the risk of developing cerebrovascular disease, and an increased risk of death from CVA. In addition, recovery from a stroke may be impaired in patients who have elevated blood glucose levels at the time of and immediately after a stroke. Because symptoms of CVA may be similar to symptoms of acute diabetic complications (HHNS or hypoglycemia), it is very important to assess the blood glucose level (and treat abnormal levels) rapidly in patients with these symptoms, so that testing and treatment of CVA (stroke) can be initiated promptly if indicated.

Atherosclerotic changes in the large blood vessels of the lower extremities are responsible for the increased incidence (two to three times higher than in nondiabetic people) of occlusive peripheral arterial disease in patients with diabetes. Signs and symptoms of peripheral vascular disease include diminished peripheral pulses and intermittent claudication (pain in the buttock, thigh, or calf during walking). The severe form of arterial occlusive disease in the lower extremities is largely responsible for the increased incidence of gangrene and subsequent amputation in patients with diabetes. Neuropathy and impairments in wound healing also play a role in diabetic foot disease (see later discussion).

Role of Diabetes in Macrovascular Diseases

Researchers continue to investigate the relationship between diabetes and macrovascular diseases. The main feature unique to diabetes is elevated blood glucose; however, a direct link has not been found between hyperglycemia and atherosclerosis. Although it may be tempting to attribute the increased prevalence of macrovascular diseases to the increased prevalence of certain risk factors (eg, obesity, increased triglyceride levels, hypertension) in patients with diabetes, there is a higher-than-expected rate of macrovascular diseases among patients with diabetes compared with patients without diabetes who have the same risk factors (ADA, 2009b). Therefore, diabetes itself is seen as an independent risk factor for accelerated atherosclerosis. Other potential factors that may play a role in diabetes-related atherosclerosis include platelet and clotting factor abnormalities, decreased flexibility of red blood cells, decreased oxygen release, changes in the arterial wall related to hyperglycemia, and possibly hyperinsulinemia.

Management

The focus of management is aggressive modification and reduction of risk factors. This involves prevention and treatment of the commonly accepted risk factors for atherosclerosis. MNT and exercise are important in managing obesity, hypertension, and hyperlipidemia. In addition, the use of medications to control hypertension and hyperlipidemia is indicated. Smoking cessation is essential. Control of blood glucose levels may reduce triglyceride concentrations and can significantly reduce the incidence of complications.

When macrovascular complications do occur, patients may require increased amounts of insulin or may need to switch from oral antidiabetic agents to insulin during illnesses.

Microvascular Complications

Diabetic microvascular disease (or microangiopathy) is characterized by capillary basement membrane thickening. The basement membrane surrounds the endothelial cells of the capillary. Researchers believe that increased blood glucose levels react through a series of biochemical responses to thicken the basement membrane to several times its normal thickness. Two areas affected by these changes are the retina and the kidneys.

DIABETIC RETINOPATHY

Diabetic retinopathy is the leading cause of blindness among people between 20 and 74 years of age in the United States; it occurs in both type 1 and type 2 diabetes (ADA, 2009b; CDC, 2008).

People with diabetes are subject to many visual complications (Table 41-9). The eye pathology referred to as diabetic retinopathy is caused by changes in the small blood vessels in the retina, the area of the eye that receives images and sends information about the images to the brain (Fig. 41-8). The retina is richly supplied with blood vessels of all

Table 41-9	OCULAR COMPLICATIONS OF DIABETES
Eye Disorder	**Characteristics**
Retinopathy	Deterioration of the small blood vessels that nourish the retina.
Background	Early stage, asymptomatic retinopathy. Blood vessels within the retina develop microaneurysms that leak fluid, causing swelling and forming deposits (exudates). In some cases, macular edema causes distorted vision.
Preproliferative	Represents increased destruction of retinal blood vessels.
Proliferative	Abnormal growth of new blood vessels on the retina. New vessels rupture, bleeding into the vitreous and blocking light. Ruptured blood vessels in the vitreous form scar tissue, which can pull on and detach the retina.
Cataracts	Opacity of the lens of the eye; cataracts occur at an earlier age in patients with diabetes.
Lens Changes	The lens of the eye can swell when blood glucose levels are elevated. For some patients, visual changes related to lens swelling may be the first symptoms of diabetes. It may take up to 2 months of improved blood glucose control before hyperglycemic swelling subsides and vision stabilizes. Therefore, patients are advised not to change eyeglass prescriptions during the 2 months after discovery of hyperglycemia.
Extraocular Muscle Palsy	This may occur as a result of diabetic neuropathy. The involvement of various cranial nerves responsible for ocular movements may lead to double vision. This usually resolves spontaneously.
Glaucoma	Results from occlusion of the outflow channels by new blood vessels. Glaucoma may occur with slightly higher frequency in the diabetic population.

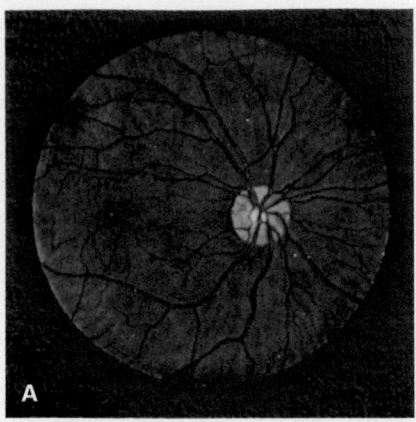
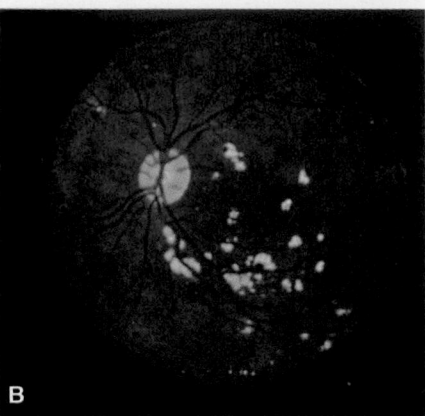

Figure 41-8 Diabetic retinopathy. **A,** In the fundus photograph of a normal eye, the light circular area over which a number of blood vessels converge is the optic disk, where the optic nerve meets the back of the eye. **B,** The fundus photograph of a patient with diabetic retinopathy shows characteristic waxy-looking retinal lesions, microaneurysms of the vessels, and hemorrhages. (Courtesy of American Optometric Association.)

kinds: small arteries and veins, arterioles, venules, and capillaries. Retinopathy has three main stages: nonproliferative (background), preproliferative, and proliferative.

Almost all patients with type 1 diabetes and more than 60% of patients with type 2 diabetes have some degree of retinopathy after 20 years (ADA, 2009b). Changes in the microvasculature include microaneurysms, intraretinal hemorrhage, hard exudates, and focal capillary closure. Although most patients do not develop visual impairment, it can be devastating if it occurs. A complication of nonproliferative retinopathy, macular edema, occurs in approximately 10% of people with type 1 or type 2 diabetes and may lead to visual distortion and loss of central vision (ADA, 2008e).

An advanced form of background retinopathy, preproliferative retinopathy, is considered to be a precursor to the more serious proliferative retinopathy. In preproliferative retinopathy, there are more widespread vascular changes and loss of nerve fibers. Epidemiologic evidence suggests that 10% to 50% of patients with preproliferative retinopathy will develop proliferative retinopathy within a short time (possibly as little as 1 year). As with background retinopathy, if visual changes occur during the preproliferative stage, they are usually caused by macular edema.

Proliferative retinopathy represents the greatest threat to vision and is characterized by the proliferation of new blood vessels growing from the retina into the vitreous. These new vessels are prone to bleeding. The visual loss associated with proliferative retinopathy is caused by this vitreous hemorrhage, retinal detachment, or both. The vitreous is normally clear, allowing light to be transmitted to the retina. When there is a hemorrhage, the vitreous becomes clouded and cannot transmit light, resulting in loss of vision. Another consequence of vitreous hemorrhage is that resorption of the blood in the vitreous leads to the formation of fibrous scar tissue. This scar tissue may place traction on the retina, resulting in retinal detachment and subsequent visual loss.

Clinical Manifestations

Retinopathy is a painless process. In nonproliferative and preproliferative retinopathy, blurry vision secondary to macular edema occurs in some patients, although many patients are asymptomatic. Even patients with a significant degree of proliferative retinopathy and some hemorrhaging may not experience major visual changes. However, symptoms indicative of hemorrhaging include floaters or cobwebs in the visual field, sudden visual changes including spotty or hazy vision, or complete loss of vision.

Assessment and Diagnostic Findings

Diagnosis is by direct visualization of the retina through dilated pupils with an ophthalmoscope or with a technique known as fluorescein angiography. Fluorescein angiography can document the type and activity of the retinopathy. Dye is injected into an arm vein and is carried to various parts of the body through the blood, but especially through the vessels of the retina of the eye. This technique allows an ophthalmologist, using special instruments, to see the retinal vessels in bright detail and gives useful information that cannot be obtained with just an ophthalmoscope.

Side effects of this diagnostic procedure may include nausea during the dye injection; yellowish, fluorescent discoloration of the skin and urine lasting 12 to 24 hours; and occasionally allergic reactions, usually manifested by hives or itching. However, the diagnostic procedure is generally safe.

Medical Management

The first focus of management of retinopathy is on primary and secondary prevention. The DCCT study (1993) demonstrated that in patients without preexisting retinopathy, maintenance of blood glucose to a normal or near-normal level in type 1 diabetes through intensive insulin therapy and patient education decreased the risk of retinopathy by 76%, compared with conventional therapy. The progression of retinopathy was decreased by 54% in patients with very mild to moderate nonproliferative retinopathy at the time of initiation of treatment. Similarly, the UKPDS study (1998) demonstrated that better control of blood glucose levels in patients with type 2 diabetes led to reduced risk of retinopathy.

Other strategies that may slow the progression of diabetic retinopathy include control of hypertension, control of blood glucose, and cessation of smoking.

For advanced cases of diabetic retinopathy, the main treatment is argon laser photocoagulation. The laser treatment destroys leaking blood vessels and areas of neovascularization. For patients who are at increased risk for hemorrhage, panretinal photocoagulation may significantly reduce the rate of progression to blindness. Panretinal photocoagulation involves the systematic application of multiple (more than 1000) laser burns throughout the retina (except in the macular region). This stops the widespread growth of new vessels and hemorrhaging of damaged vessels. The role of "mild" panretinal photocoagulation (with only one-third to one-half as many laser burns) in the early stages of proliferative retinopathy or in patients with preproliferative changes is being investigated. For patients with macular edema, focal photocoagulation is used to apply smaller laser burns to specific areas of microaneurysms in the macular region. This may reduce the rate of visual loss from macular edema by 50% (ADA, 2008e).

Photocoagulation treatments are usually performed on an outpatient basis, and most patients can return to their usual activities by the next day. Limitations may be placed on activities involving weight bearing or bearing down. In most cases, the treatment does not cause intense pain, although patients may report varying degrees of discomfort. Usually an anesthetic eye drop is all that is needed during the treatment. A few patients may experience slight visual loss, loss of peripheral vision, or impairments in adaptation to the dark. However, the risk of slight visual changes from the laser treatment itself is much less than the potential for loss of vision from progression of retinopathy.

A major hemorrhage into the vitreous may occur, with the vitreous fluid becoming mixed with blood, preventing light from passing through the eye; this can cause blindness. A vitrectomy is a surgical procedure in which vitreous humor filled with blood or fibrous tissue is removed with a special drill-like instrument and replaced with saline or another liquid. A vitrectomy is performed for patients who already have visual loss and in whom the vitreous hemorrhage has not cleared on its own after 6 months. The purpose is to restore useful vision; recovery to near-normal vision is not usually expected.

Nursing Management

Nursing management of patients with diabetic retinopathy or other eye disorders involves implementing the individual plan of care and providing patient education. Education focuses on prevention through regular ophthalmologic examinations and blood glucose control and self-management of eye care regimens. The effectiveness of early diagnosis and prompt treatment is emphasized in teaching the patient and family. If vision loss occurs, nursing care must also address the patient's adjustment to impaired vision and use of adaptive devices for diabetes self-care as well as activities of daily living. Nursing care for patients with low vision or loss of vision is discussed in detail in Chapter 58.

Promoting Home and Community-Based Care

Teaching Patients Self-Care

Because the course of the retinopathy may be long and stressful, patient teaching is essential. In teaching and counseling patients, it is important to stress the following:

- Retinopathy may appear after many years of diabetes, and its appearance does not necessarily mean that the diabetes is on a downhill course.
- The odds for maintaining vision are in the patient's favor, especially with adequate control of glucose levels and blood pressure.
- Frequent eye examinations allow for the detection and prompt treatment of retinopathy.

A patient's response to vision loss depends on personality, self-concept, and coping mechanisms. Acceptance of blindness occurs in stages; some patients may learn to accept blindness in a rather short period, and others may never do so. An important issue in teaching patients is that several complications of diabetes occur simultaneously. For example, a patient who is blind due to diabetic retinopathy may also have peripheral neuropathy and may experience impairment of manual dexterity and tactile sensation. To prevent further losses, glycemic control remains a priority.

Continuing Care

The importance of careful diabetes management is emphasized as one means of slowing the progression of visual changes. The patient is reminded of the need to see an ophthalmologist regularly. If eye changes are progressive and unrelenting, the patient should be prepared for inevitable blindness. Therefore, consideration is given to making referrals for teaching the patient Braille and for training him or her with guide (ie, service) dogs. Referral to state agencies should be made to ensure that the patient receives services for the blind. Family members are also taught how to assist the patient to remain as independent as possible despite decreasing visual acuity.

Referral for home care may be indicated for some patients, particularly those who live alone, those who are not coping well, and those who have other health problems or complications of diabetes that may interfere with their ability to perform self-care. During home visits, the nurse can assess the patient's home environment and his or her ability to manage diabetes despite visual impairments. Medical management and nursing care of patients with visual disturbances are discussed in detail in Chapter 58.

NEPHROPATHY

Nephropathy, or renal disease secondary to diabetic microvascular changes in the kidney, is a common complication of diabetes (ADA, 2008f, 2009b). In the United States each year, people with diabetes account for almost 50% of new cases of end-stage renal disease (ESRD) and about 25% of those require dialysis or transplantation. About 20% to 30% of people with type 1 or type 2 diabetes develop nephropathy, but fewer of those with type 2 diabetes progress to ESRD. Native American, Latino, African American, Asian American, and Pacific Island people with type 2 diabetes are at greater risk for ESRD than non-Latino whites (ADA, 2009b).

Patients with type 1 diabetes frequently show initial signs of renal disease after 10 to 15 years; patients with type 2 diabetes develop renal disease within 10 years after the diagnosis of diabetes. Many patients with type 2 diabetes have had diabetes for many years before the diabetes is diagnosed and treated. Therefore, they may have evidence of nephropathy at the time of diagnosis (ADA, 2008f). If blood glucose levels are elevated consistently for a significant period of time, the kidney's filtration mechanism is stressed, allowing blood proteins to leak into the urine. As a result, the pressure in the blood vessels of the kidney increases. It is thought that this elevated pressure serves as the stimulus for the development of nephropathy. Various medications and diets are being tested to prevent these complications.

The DCCT (1993) results showed that intensive treatment of type 1 diabetes with a goal of achieving a hemoglobin A_{1C} level as close to the nondiabetic range as possible reduced the occurrence of early signs of nephropathy. Similarly, the UKPDS study (1998) demonstrated a reduced incidence of overt nephropathy in patients with type 2 diabetes who controlled their blood glucose levels.

Clinical Manifestations

Most of the signs and symptoms of renal dysfunction in patients with diabetes are similar to those seen in patients without diabetes (see Chapter 44). In addition, as renal failure progresses, the catabolism (breakdown) of both exogenous and endogenous insulin decreases, and frequent hypoglycemic episodes may result. Insulin needs change as a result of changes in the catabolism of insulin, changes in diet related to the treatment of nephropathy, and changes in insulin clearance that occur with decreased renal function. The stress of renal disease affects self-esteem, family relationships, marital relations, and virtually all aspects of daily life. As renal function decreases, patients commonly have multiple-system failure (eg, declining visual acuity, impotence, foot ulcerations, heart failure, nocturnal diarrhea).

Assessment and Diagnostic Findings

Albumin is one of the most important blood proteins that leaks into the urine. Although small amounts may leak undetected for years, its leakage into the urine is among the earliest signs that can be detected. Clinical nephropathy eventually develops in more than 85% of people with microalbuminuria but in fewer than 5% of people without microalbuminuria. The urine should be checked annually for the presence of microalbumin. If the microalbuminuria exceeds 30 mg/24 hours on two consecutive random urine tests, a 24-hour urine sample should be obtained and tested. If results are positive, treatment is indicated (see later discussion).

In addition, tests for serum creatinine and BUN levels should be conducted annually. Diagnostic testing for cardiac or other systemic disorders may also be required with progression of other complications, and caution is indicated if contrast agents are used with these tests. Contrast agents and dyes used for some diagnostic tests may not be easily cleared by the damaged kidney, and the potential benefits of these diagnostic tests must be weighed against their potential risks.

Hypertension often develops in patients (with and without diabetes) who are in the early stages of renal disease. However, hypertension occurs in as many as 50% of all people with diabetes (for unknown reasons). Therefore, this symptom may or may not be due to renal disease; other diagnostic criteria must also be present.

Management

In addition to achieving and maintaining near-normal blood glucose levels, management for all patients with diabetes should include careful attention to the following:

- Control of hypertension (the use of angiotensin-converting enzyme [ACE] inhibitors, such as captopril [Capoten]), because control of hypertension may also decrease or delay the onset of early proteinuria
- Prevention or vigorous treatment of urinary tract infections
- Avoidance of nephrotoxic substances (eg, antibiotics, other selected medications)
- Adjustment of medications as renal function changes
- Low-sodium diet
- Low-protein diet

If the patient has already developed microalbuminuria and its level exceeds 30 mg/24 hours on two consecutive tests, an ACE inhibitor should be prescribed. ACE inhibitors lower blood pressure and reduce microalbuminuria, thereby protecting the kidney. Alternatively, angiotensin-receptor blocking (ARB) agents may be prescribed. This preventive strategy should be part of the standard of care for all people with diabetes. Carefully designed low-protein diets also appear to reverse early leakage of small amounts of protein from the kidney.

In chronic or end-stage renal failure, two types of treatment are available: dialysis (hemodialysis or peritoneal dialysis) and transplantation from a relative or a cadaver. Hemodialysis for patients with diabetes is similar to that for patients without the disease (see Chapter 44). Because hemodialysis creates additional stress on patients with cardiovascular disease, it may not be appropriate for some patients.

Continuous ambulatory peritoneal dialysis is being used by an increasing number of patients with diabetes, mainly because of the independence it allows. In addition, insulin can be mixed into the dialysate, which may result in better blood glucose control and end the need for insulin injections. In some cases, they may require higher doses of insulin because the dialysate contains glucose. Major risks of peritoneal dialysis are infection and peritonitis. The mortality rate for patients with diabetes undergoing dialysis is higher than that for patients without diabetes undergoing dialysis and is closely related to the severity of cardiovascular problems.

Renal disease is frequently accompanied by advancing retinopathy that may require laser treatments and surgery. Severe hypertension also worsens eye disease because of the additional stress it places on the blood vessels. Patients being treated with hemodialysis who require eye surgery may be changed to peritoneal dialysis and have their hypertension aggressively controlled for several weeks before surgery to prevent bleeding and damage to the retina. The rationale for this change is that hemodialysis requires anticoagulants that can increase the risk of bleeding after the surgery, and peritoneal dialysis minimizes pressure changes in the eyes.

The success rate for kidney transplantation in patients with diabetes has improved. In medical centers performing large numbers of transplantations, the chances are 75% to 80% that the transplanted kidney will continue to function in patients with diabetes for at least 5 years. Like the original kidneys, transplanted kidneys can eventually be damaged if blood glucose levels are consistently high after the transplantation. Therefore, monitoring blood glucose levels frequently and adjusting insulin levels in patients with diabetes are essential for long-term success of kidney transplantation.

Diabetic Neuropathies

Diabetic neuropathy refers to a group of diseases that affect all types of nerves, including peripheral (sensorimotor), autonomic, and spinal nerves. The disorders appear to be clinically diverse and depend on the location of the affected nerve cells. The prevalence increases with the age of the patient and the duration of the disease and may be as high as 50% in patients who have had diabetes for 25 years (NIDDK, 2008a).

The etiology of neuropathy may involve elevated blood glucose levels over a period of years. The DCCT results (1993) showed that control of blood glucose levels to normal or near-normal levels decreased the incidence of neuropathy by 60%. The pathogenesis of neuropathy may be attributed to either a vascular or metabolic mechanism or both. Capillary basement membrane thickening and capillary closure may be present. In addition, there may be demyelinization of the nerves, which is thought to be related to hyperglycemia. Nerve conduction is disrupted when there are aberrations of the myelin sheaths.

The two most common types of diabetic neuropathy are sensorimotor polyneuropathy and autonomic neuropathy. Sensorimotor polyneuropathy is also called peripheral neuropathy. Cranial mononeuropathies—those affecting the oculomotor nerve—also occur in diabetes, especially in the elderly.

Peripheral Neuropathy

Peripheral neuropathy most commonly affects the distal portions of the nerves, especially the nerves of the lower extremities; it affects both sides of the body symmetrically and may spread in a proximal direction.

Clinical Manifestations

Although approximately half of patients with diabetic neuropathy do not have symptoms, initial symptoms may include paresthesias (prickling, tingling, or heightened sensation) and burning sensations (especially at night). As the neuropathy progresses, the feet become numb. In addition, a decrease in proprioception (awareness of posture and movement of the body and of position and weight of objects in relation to the body) and a decreased sensation of light touch may lead to an unsteady gait. Decreased sensations of pain and temperature place patients with neuropathy at increased risk for injury and undetected foot infections. Deformities of the foot may also occur; neuropathy-related joint changes produce Charcot joints. These joint deformities result from the abnormal weight distribution on joints resulting from lack of proprioception.

On physical examination, a decrease in deep tendon reflexes and vibratory sensation is found. For patients who have few or no symptoms of neuropathy, these physical findings may be the only indication of neuropathic changes. For patients with signs or symptoms of neuropathy, it is important to rule out other possible causes, including alcohol-induced and vitamin-deficiency neuropathies.

Management

The results of the DCCT study (1993) demonstrated that intensive insulin therapy and control of blood glucose levels delay the onset and slow the progression of neuropathy. Pain, particularly of the lower extremities, is a disturbing symptom in some people with neuropathy secondary to diabetes. In some cases, neuropathic pain spontaneously resolves within 6 months; for others, pain persists for many years. Various approaches to pain management can be tried. These include analgesics (preferably nonopioid); tricyclic antidepressants; antiseizure medications (phenytoin [Dilantin], carbamazepine [Tegretol], or gabapentin [Neurontin]); mexiletine (Mexitil, an antiarrhythmic); and transcutaneous electrical nerve stimulation (TENS).

Duloxetine (Cymbalta), an antidepressant medication, has been approved for treatment of peripheral diabetic neuropathy.

Autonomic Neuropathies

Neuropathy of the autonomic nervous system results in a broad range of dysfunctions affecting almost every organ system of the body (NIDDK, 2008a).

Clinical Manifestations

Three manifestations of autonomic neuropathy are related to the cardiac, gastrointestinal, and renal systems. Cardiovascular symptoms range from a fixed, slightly tachycardic heart rate and orthostatic hypotension to silent, or painless, myocardial ischemia and infarction. Delayed gastric emptying may occur with the typical gastrointestinal symptoms of early satiety, bloating, nausea, and vomiting. "Diabetic" constipation or diarrhea (especially nocturnal diarrhea) may occur as a result. In addition, there may be unexplained wide swings in blood glucose levels related to inconsistent absorption of the glucose from ingested foods secondary to the inconsistent gastric emptying.

Urinary retention, a decreased sensation of bladder fullness, and other urinary symptoms of neurogenic bladder result from autonomic neuropathy. The patient with a neurogenic bladder is predisposed to development of urinary tract infections because of the inability to empty the bladder completely. This is especially true of patients with poorly controlled diabetes because hyperglycemia impairs resistance to infection.

Hypoglycemic Unawareness

Autonomic neuropathy that affects the adrenal medulla is responsible for diminished or absent adrenergic symptoms of hypoglycemia. Patients may report that they no longer feel the typical shakiness, sweating, nervousness, and palpitations associated with hypoglycemia. Frequent blood glucose monitoring is recommended for these patients. Their inability to detect and treat these warning signs of hypoglycemia puts them at risk for development of dangerously low blood glucose levels. Therefore, their goals for blood glucose levels may need to be adjusted to reduce the risk for hypoglycemia. Patients and families need to be taught to recognize subtle and atypical symptoms of hypoglycemia, such as numbness around the mouth and impaired ability to concentrate.

Sudomotor Neuropathy

The neuropathic condition called sudomotor neuropathy refers to a decrease or absence of sweating (anhidrosis) of the extremities, with a compensatory increase in upper body sweating. Dryness of the feet increases the risk for the development of foot ulcers.

Sexual Dysfunction

Sexual dysfunction, especially erectile dysfunction in men, is a complication of diabetes. The effects of autonomic neuropathy on female sexual functioning are not well documented. Reduced vaginal lubrication has been mentioned as a possible neuropathic effect. Other possible changes in sexual function in women with diabetes include decreased libido and lack of orgasm. Vaginal infection, which increases in incidence in women with diabetes, may be associated with decreased lubrication and vaginal pruritus (itching) and tenderness. Urinary tract infections and vaginitis may also affect sexual function.

Impotence (inability of the penis to become rigid and sustain an erection adequate for penetration) occurs with greater frequency in men with diabetes than in other men of the same age. Some men with autonomic neuropathy have normal erectile function and can experience orgasm but do not ejaculate normally. Retrograde ejaculation occurs; seminal fluid is propelled backward through the posterior urethra and into the urinary bladder. Examination of the urine confirms the diagnosis because of the large number of active sperm present. Fertility counseling may be necessary for couples attempting conception.

Diabetic neuropathy is not the only cause of impotence in men with diabetes. Medications such as antihypertensive agents, psychological factors, and other medical conditions (eg, vascular insufficiency) that may affect other men also play a role in impotence in men with diabetes (see Chapter 49).

Management

Management strategies for autonomic neuropathy focus on alleviating symptoms and on modification and management of risk factors. The prognosis for painless cardiac ischemia is poor. However, detection is important so that education about avoiding strenuous exercise can be provided. Orthostatic hypotension may respond to a diet high in sodium, discontinuation of medications that impede autonomic nervous system responses, use of sympathomimetics and other agents (eg, caffeine) that stimulate an autonomic response, mineralocorticoid therapy, and use of lower-body elastic garments that maximize venous return and prevent pooling of blood in the extremities.

Treatment of delayed gastric emptying includes a low-fat diet, frequent small meals, frequent blood glucose monitoring, and use of agents that increase gastric motility (eg, metoclopramide [Reglan], bethanechol [Myotonachol]). Treatment of diabetic diarrhea may include bulk-forming laxatives or antidiarrheal agents. Constipation is treated with a high-fiber diet and adequate hydration; medications, laxatives, and enemas may be necessary if consti-

pation is severe. Management of sexual dysfunction in women and men is discussed in Chapters 47 and 49, respectively.

Treatment of sudomotor dysfunction focuses on education about skin care and heat intolerance.

Foot and Leg Problems

Between 50% and 75% of lower extremity amputations are performed on people with diabetes. More than 50% of these amputations are thought to be preventable, provided patients are taught foot care measures and practice them on a daily basis (ADA, 2009b). Complications of diabetes that contribute to the increased risk of foot problems and infections include the following:

- Neuropathy: Sensory neuropathy leads to loss of pain and pressure sensation, and autonomic neuropathy leads to increased dryness and fissuring of the skin (secondary to decreased sweating). Motor neuropathy results in muscular atrophy, which may lead to changes in the shape of the foot.
- Peripheral vascular disease: Poor circulation of the lower extremities contributes to poor wound healing and the development of gangrene.
- Immunocompromise: Hyperglycemia impairs the ability of specialized leukocytes to destroy bacteria. Therefore, in poorly controlled diabetes, there is a lowered resistance to certain infections.

The typical sequence of events in the development of a diabetic foot ulcer begins with a soft tissue injury of the foot, formation of a fissure between the toes or in an area of dry skin, or formation of a callus (Fig. 41-9). Patients with an insensitive foot do not feel injuries, which may be thermal (eg, from using heating pads, walking barefoot on hot concrete, testing bath water with the foot), chemical (eg, burning the foot while using caustic agents on calluses, corns, or bunions), or traumatic (eg, injuring skin while cutting nails, walking with an undetected foreign object in the shoe, or wearing ill-fitting shoes and socks).

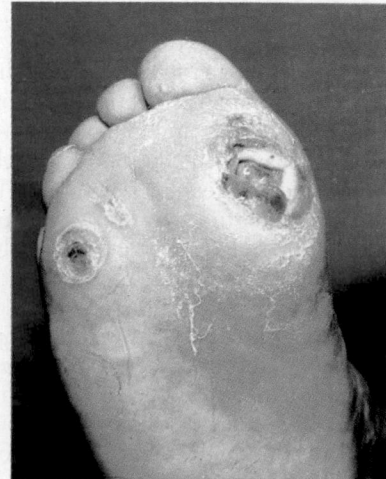

Figure 41-9 Neuropathic ulcers occur on pressure points in areas with diminished sensation in diabetic polyneuropathy. Because pain is absent, the ulcer may go unnoticed.

If the patient is not in the habit of thoroughly inspecting both feet on a daily basis, the injury or fissure may go unnoticed until a serious infection has developed. Drainage, swelling, redness of the leg (from cellulitis), or gangrene may be the first sign of foot problems that the patient notices. Treatment of foot ulcers involves bed rest, antibiotics, and débridement. In addition, controlling glucose levels, which tend to increase when infections occur, is important for promoting wound healing. When peripheral vascular disease is present, foot ulcers may not heal because of the decreased ability of oxygen, nutrients, and antibiotics to reach the injured tissue. Amputation may be necessary to prevent the spread of infection, particularly if it involves the bone (osteomyelitis).

Foot assessment and foot care instructions are most important when caring for patients who are at high risk for foot infections. Some of the high-risk characteristics include:

- Duration of diabetes more than 10 years
- Age older than 40 years
- History of smoking
- Decreased peripheral pulses
- Decreased sensation
- Anatomic deformities or pressure areas (eg, bunions, calluses, hammer toes)
- History of previous foot ulcers or amputation

Management

Teaching proper foot care is a nursing intervention that can prevent costly and painful complications that result in disability (Chart 41-10). Preventive foot care begins with careful daily assessment of the feet, which should be inspected on a daily basis for any redness, blisters, fissures, calluses, ulcerations, changes in skin temperature, or development of foot deformities (hammer toes, bunions). Visual impairment or decreased joint mobility (especially in the elderly) requires use of a mirror to inspect the bottoms of both feet or the help of a family member in foot inspection. The interior surfaces of shoes should also be inspected for any rough spots or foreign objects (NIDDK, 2008b).

In addition to the daily visual and manual inspection of the feet, the feet should be examined during every health care visit or at least once per year (more often if there is an increase in risk) by a podiatrist, physician, or nurse (ADA, 2009b). All patients should be assessed for neuropathy and undergo evaluation of neurologic status by an experienced examiner using a monofilament device (Fig. 41-10). Pressure areas, such as calluses, or thick toenails should be treated by a podiatrist in addition to routine trimming of nails.

Additional aspects of preventive foot care that are taught to patients and families include the following:

- Properly bathing, drying, and lubricating the feet, taking care not to allow moisture (water or lotion) to accumulate between the toes
- Wearing closed-toed shoes that fit well. A podiatrist can provide the patient with inserts (orthotics) to remove pressure from pressure points on the foot. New shoes should be broken in slowly (ie, worn for 1 to 2 hours initially, with gradual increases in the length of

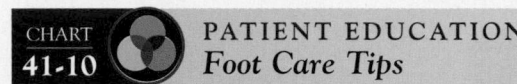

CHART 41-10 **PATIENT EDUCATION**
Foot Care Tips

1. Take care of your diabetes.
   - Work with your health care team to keep your blood glucose level within a normal range.
2. Inspect your feet every day.
   - Look at your bare feet every day for cuts, blisters, red spots, and swelling.
   - Use a mirror to check the bottoms of your feet or ask a family member for help if you have trouble seeing.
   - Check for changes in temperature.
3. Wash your feet every day.
   - Wash your feet in warm, not hot, water.
   - Dry your feet well. Be sure to dry between the toes.
   - Do not soak your feet.
   - Do not check water temperature with your feet; use a thermometer or elbow.
4. Keep the skin soft and smooth.
   - Rub a thin coat of skin lotion over the tops and bottoms of your feet, but not between your toes.
5. Smooth corns and calluses gently.
   - Use a pumice stone to smooth corns and calluses.
6. Trim your toenails each week or when needed.
   - Trim your toenails straight across and file the edges with an emery board or nail file.
7. Wear shoes and socks at all times.
   - Never walk barefoot.
   - Wear comfortable shoes that fit well and protect your feet.
   - Feel inside your shoes before putting them on each time to make sure the lining is smooth and there are no objects inside.
8. Protect your feet from hot and cold.
   - Wear shoes at the beach or on hot pavement.
   - Wear socks at night if your feet get cold.
9. Keep the blood flowing to your feet.
   - Put your feet up when sitting.
   - Wiggle your toes and move your ankles up and down for 5 minutes, 2 or 3 times a day.
   - Do not cross your legs for long periods of time.
   - Do not smoke.
10. Check with your health care provider.
    - Have your health care provider check your bare feet and find out whether you are likely to have serious foot problems. Remember that you may not feel the pain of an injury.
    - Call your health care provider right away if a cut, sore, blister, or bruise on your foot does not begin to heal after one day.
    - Follow your health care provider's advice about foot care.
    - Do not self-medicate or use home remedies or over-the-counter agents to treat foot problems.

time worn) to avoid blister formation. Patients with bony deformities may need custom-made shoes with extra width or depth. High-risk behaviors, such as walking barefoot, using heating pads on the feet, wearing open-toed shoes, soaking the feet, and shaving calluses, should be avoided.
- Trimming toenails straight across and filing sharp corners to follow the contour of the toe. If the patient has

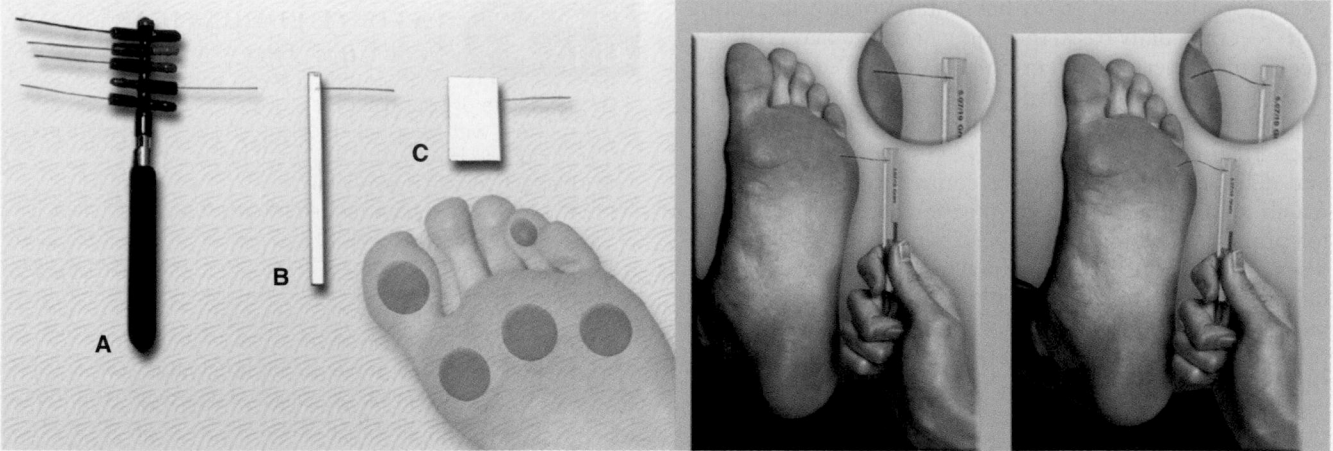

Figure 41-10 The monofilament test is used to assess the sensory threshold in patients with diabetes. The test instrument—a monofilament—is gently applied to about five pressure points on the foot (as shown in image on *left*). **A,** Example of a monofilament used for advanced quantitative assessment. **B,** Semmes-Weinstein monofilament used by clinicians. **C,** Disposable monofilament used by patients. The examiner applies the monofilament to the test area to determine whether the patient feels the device. (Adapted with permission from Cameron, B. L. (2002). Making diabetes management routine. *American Journal of Nursing, 102*(2), 26–32.)

visual deficits, is unable to reach the feet because of disability, or has thickened toenails, a podiatrist should cut the nails.
- Reducing risk factors, such as smoking and elevated blood lipids, that contribute to peripheral vascular disease.
- Avoiding home remedies, over-the-counter agents, and self-medicating to treat foot problems.

Blood glucose control is important for avoiding decreased resistance to infections and for preventing diabetic neuropathy.

SPECIAL ISSUES IN DIABETES CARE

Patients With Diabetes Who Are Undergoing Surgery

During periods of physiologic stress, such as surgery, blood glucose levels tend to increase, because levels of stress hormones (epinephrine, norepinephrine, glucagon, cortisol, and growth hormone) increase. If hyperglycemia is not controlled during surgery, the resulting osmotic diuresis may lead to excessive loss of fluids and electrolytes. Patients with type 1 diabetes also risk developing ketoacidosis during periods of stress.

Hypoglycemia is also a concern in patients with diabetes who are undergoing surgery. For example, this is a special concern during the preoperative period if surgery is delayed beyond the morning in a patient who received a morning injection of intermediate-acting insulin.

There are various approaches to managing glucose control during the perioperative period. Frequent blood glucose monitoring is essential throughout the preoperative and postoperative periods, regardless of the method used for glucose control. Examples of these approaches are described in Chart 41-11. The use of IV insulin and dextrose has become widespread with the increased availability of meters for intraoperative glucose monitoring.

During the postoperative period, patients with diabetes must also be closely monitored for cardiovascular complications because of the increased prevalence of atherosclerosis, wound infections, and skin breakdown (especially in patients with decreased sensation in the extremities due to neuropathy). Maintaining adequate nutrition and blood glucose control promote wound healing.

Management of Hospitalized Patients With Diabetes

At any one time, 10% to 20% of hospitalized general medical-surgical patients have diabetes. This number may increase as elderly patients make up an increasing proportion of the hospitalized population. Often diabetes is not the primary medical diagnosis, yet problems with control of diabetes frequently result from changes in the patient's normal routine or from surgery or illness. During the course of treatment for the primary medical diagnosis, blood glucose control may worsen. In addition, the only opportunity for some patients with diabetes to update their knowledge about diabetes self-care and prevention of complications may be during hospitalization. It is important for nurses caring for patients with diabetes to focus attention on the diabetes as well as the primary health issue. Control of blood glucose levels is important because hyperglycemia impairs resistance to certain infections and impedes wound healing.

Self-Care Issues

For patients who are actively involved in diabetes self-management (especially insulin dose adjustment), relinquishing control over meal timing, insulin timing, and insulin dosage can be particularly difficult and anxiety provoking. The patient may fear hypoglycemia and express much concern over possible delays in receiving attention from the nurse if hypoglycemic symptoms occur or may disagree with a planned dose of insulin.

Chart 41-11•*Approaches to Management of Glucose Control During the Perioperative Period*

- Monitor blood glucose levels frequently (every 1 to 2 h).
- For patients taking insulin
  1. The morning of surgery, all subcutaneous insulin doses are withheld, unless the blood glucose level is elevated (eg, >200 mg/dL [11.1 mmol/L]), in which case a small dose of subcutaneous regular insulin may be prescribed. The blood glucose level is controlled during surgery with the IV infusion of regular insulin, which is balanced by an infusion of dextrose. The insulin and dextrose infusion rates are adjusted according to frequent (hourly) capillary glucose determinations. After surgery, the insulin infusion may be continued until the patient can eat. If IV insulin is discontinued, subcutaneous regular insulin may be administered at set intervals (every 4–6 h), or intermediate-acting insulin may be administered every 12 h with supplemental regular insulin as necessary until the patient is eating and the usual pattern of insulin dosing is resumed.
     - Carefully monitor the insulin infusion rate and blood glucose levels in a patient with diabetes who is receiving IV insulin. IV insulin has a much shorter duration of action than subcutaneous insulin. If the infusion is interrupted or discontinued, hyperglycemia will develop rapidly (within 1 h in type 1 diabetes and within a few hours in type 2 diabetes).
     - Ensure that subcutaneous insulin is administered 30 min before the IV insulin infusion is discontinued.

  2. One half to two thirds of the patient's usual morning dose of insulin (either intermediate-acting insulin alone or both short-act and intermediate-acting insulins) is administered subcutaneously in the morning before surgery. The remainder is then administered after surgery.
  3. The patient's usual daily dose of subcutaneous insulin is divided into four equal doses of regular insulin. These are then administered at 6-h intervals. The last two approaches do not provide the control achieved by IV administration of insulin and dextrose.
- Patients with type 2 diabetes who do not usually take insulin may require insulin during the perioperative period to control blood glucose elevations. Patients who are taking metformin may be instructed to discontinue the oral agent 24 to 48 h before surgery, if possible. Some of these patients may resume their usual regimen of diet and oral agent during the recovery period. Other patients (whose diabetes is probably not well controlled with diet and an oral antidiabetic agent before surgery) need to continue with insulin injections after discharge.
- For patients with type 2 diabetes who are undergoing minor surgery but who do not normally take insulin, glucose levels may remain stable provided no dextrose is infused during the surgery. After surgery, these patients may require small doses of regular insulin until the usual diet and oral agent are resumed.

It is important for the nurse to acknowledge the patient's concerns and involve the patient in the plan of care as much as possible. If the patient disagrees with certain aspects of the nursing or medical care related to diabetes, the nurse must communicate this to other members of the health care team. Nurses and other health care providers must pay particular attention to patients who are successful in managing self-care; they should assess these patients' self-care management skills and encourage them to continue if their performance is correct and effective.

Hospitalization of a patient with diabetes should be considered an opportunity to evaluate the patient's self-care skills and to reinforce teaching that might be needed. The nurse observes the patient preparing and injecting the insulin, monitoring blood glucose, and performing foot care. (Simply questioning the patient about these skills without actually observing performance of the skills is not sufficient.) The patient's knowledge about diet can be assessed with the help of a dietitian through direct questioning and review of the patient's menu choices. The patient's understanding about signs and symptoms, treatment, and prevention of hypoglycemia and hyperglycemia is assessed, along with knowledge of risk factors for macrovascular disease, including hypertension, increased lipids, and smoking. In addition, the patient is asked the date of his or her last eye examination (including dilation of the pupils). Teaching about these issues is critical.

Hyperglycemia During Hospitalization

Hyperglycemia may occur in hospitalized patients as a result of the original illness that led to the need for hospitalization. A number of other factors may contribute to hyperglycemia; examples include:

- Changes in the usual treatment regimen (eg, increased food, decreased insulin, decreased activity)
- Medications (eg, corticosteroids such as prednisone, which are used in the treatment of a variety of inflammatory disorders)
- IV dextrose, which may be part of the maintenance fluids or may be used for the administration of antibiotics and other medications, without adequate insulin therapy
- Overly vigorous treatment of hypoglycemia
- Inappropriate withholding of insulin or inappropriate use of "sliding scales"
- Mismatched timing of meals and insulin (eg, postmeal hyperglycemia may occur if short-acting insulin is administered immediately before or even after a meal)

Nursing actions to correct some of these factors are important for avoiding hyperglycemia. Assessment of the patient's usual home routine is important. The nurse should try to approximate as much as possible the home schedule of insulin, meals, and activities. Monitoring blood glucose levels has been identified by the ADA as an additional "vital sign" essential in assessment of patients (ADA, 2009b). The results of blood glucose monitoring provide information needed to obtain orders for extra doses of insulin (at times when insulin is usually taken), an important nursing function. Insulin doses must not be withheld when blood glucose levels are normal.

Short-acting insulin is usually needed to avoid postprandial hyperglycemia (even in patients with normal premeal glucose levels), and NPH insulin does not peak until many hours after the dose is given. IV antibiotics should be mixed

NURSING RESEARCH PROFILE
Hypoglycemia in Hospitalized Patients With Diabetes

Anthony, M. (2007). Treatment of hypoglycemia in hospitalized adults, A descriptive study. *The Diabetes Educator, 33*(4), 709–715.

Purpose

Diabetes mellitus is a primary or secondary reason for over 24 million days spent in the hospital. The goal of achieving normal blood glucose levels is a challenge in hospitalized patients but has the potential to improve patient outcomes. This goal may, however, result in increased risk of hypoglycemia in patients with diabetes who are hospitalized. The purpose of this study was to describe the treatment of hypoglycemia in two Midwestern hospitals to determine patterns and adherence to policies and procedures.

Design

A retrospective chart audit was conducted on 210 patients who had experienced hypoglycemia while hospitalized. The purpose of the audit was to examine adherence to five steps identified in hospital policies and procedures for treatment of hypoglycemia. The five steps were: (1) administer 15 g of carbohydrates, (2) retest blood glucose in 15 minutes, (3) retest in 1 hour, (4) notify the physician, and (5) document the event in the patient's record. A checklist of expected behaviors was derived from the practice manual and used as the evaluation tool.

Findings

A total of 484 episodes of hypoglycemia in 105 patients at two hospitals were analyzed. Hypoglycemia was defined as a blood glucose level of less than 70 mg/dL. Adherence to practice guidelines for treatment of hypoglycemia was low. There was not one case where all five steps were followed. The adherence ranged from 2.1% for the 1-hour retest to a high of 70.9% for documentation.

Nursing Implications

Nursing policy and procedures are put in place to ensure that a standard of care is followed for patient safety. The treatment of hypoglycemia is an important patient safety issue because severe hypoglycemia can threaten the patient's well-being and lead to seizures, coma, or a fall. Following guidelines provides for the treatment of the condition and a return of blood glucose levels to normal without causing hyperglycemia. Although it is possible that all five steps of the guidelines were taken but not documented, if actions are not documented it is assumed that the actions were not taken. The findings indicate that staff education is needed to increase the likelihood that important guidelines are followed to improve patient safety and prevent catastrophic outcomes.

---

in normal saline (if possible) to avoid excess infusion of dextrose (especially in patients who are eating). It is important to avoid overly vigorous treatment of hypoglycemia, which may lead to hyperglycemia.

Hypoglycemia During Hospitalization

Hypoglycemia in hospitalized patients is usually the result of too much insulin or delays in eating (Chart 41-12). Specific examples include:

- Overuse of "sliding scale" regular insulin, particularly as a supplement to regularly scheduled, twice-daily short-acting and intermediate-acting insulins
- Lack of change in insulin dosage when dietary intake is changed (eg, in the patient taking nothing by mouth [NPO])
- Overly vigorous treatment of hyperglycemia (eg, giving too-frequent successive doses of regular insulin before the time of peak insulin activity is reached), resulting in a cumulative effect
- Delayed meal after administration of lispro, aspart, or glulisine [Apidra] insulin (the patient should eat within 5 to 15 minutes after insulin administration)

Treatment of hypoglycemia should be based on the established hospital protocol. If the initial treatment does not increase the glucose level adequately, the same treatment may be repeated after 15 minutes. The nurse must assess the pattern of glucose values and avoid giving doses of insulin that repeatedly lead to hypoglycemia. Successive doses of subcutaneous regular insulin should be administered no more frequently than every 3 to 4 hours. For patients receiving NPH or Lente insulin before breakfast and dinner, the nurse must use caution in administering supplemental doses of regular insulin at lunch and bedtime. Hypoglycemia may occur when two insulins peak at similar times (eg, morning NPH peaks with lunchtime regular insulin and may lead to late-afternoon hypoglycemia; dinnertime NPH peaks with bedtime regular insulin and may lead to nocturnal hypoglycemia). To avoid hypoglycemic reactions caused by delayed food intake, the nurse should arrange for snacks to be given to the patient if meals are going to be delayed because of procedures, physical therapy, or other activities.

Common Alterations in Diet

Dietary modifications commonly prescribed during hospitalization require special consideration for patients who have diabetes (ADA, 2008b).

Nothing by Mouth

For patients who must be NPO in preparation for diagnostic or surgical procedures, the nurse must ensure that the usual insulin dosage has been changed. These changes may include eliminating the rapid-acting insulin and giving a decreased amount (eg, half the usual dose) of intermediate-acting NPH or Lente insulin. Another approach is to use frequent (every 3 to 4 hours) dosing of rapid-acting insulin only. IV dextrose may be administered to provide calories and to avoid hypoglycemia.

Even without food, glucose levels may increase as a result of hepatic glucose production, especially in patients with type 1 diabetes and lean patients with type 2 diabetes. Furthermore, in type 1 diabetes, elimination of the insulin dose may lead to the development of DKA. Therefore, administration of insulin to patients with type 1 diabetes who are NPO is an important nursing action.

For patients with type 2 diabetes who are taking insulin, DKA does not usually develop when insulin doses are eliminated because the patient's pancreas produces some insulin. Therefore, skipping the insulin dose altogether (when the patient is receiving IV dextrose) may be safe; however, close monitoring of blood glucose levels is essential.

For patients who are NPO for extended periods (24 hours), glucose testing and insulin administration should be performed at regular intervals, usually four times per day. Insulin regimens for the patient who is NPO for an extended period may include NPH insulin every 12 hours (with rapid-acting insulin added to the NPH, depending on the results of glucose testing) or rapid-acting insulin only every 4 to 6 hours. These patients should receive dextrose infusions to provide some calories and limit ketosis.

To prevent the problems that result from the need to withhold food, diagnostic tests and procedures and surgery should be scheduled early in the morning if possible.

Clear Liquid Diet

When the diet is advanced to include clear liquids, patients with diabetes receive more simple carbohydrate foods, such as juice and gelatin desserts, than are usually included in the diabetic diet. It is important for hospitalized patients to maintain their nutritional status as much as possible to promote healing. Therefore, the use of reduced-calorie substitutes such as diet soda or diet gelatin desserts would not be appropriate when the only source of calories is clear liquids. Simple carbohydrates, if eaten alone, cause a rapid rise in blood glucose levels; therefore, it is important to try to match peak times of insulin effect with peaks in the blood glucose concentration. If the patient receives insulin at regular intervals while NPO, the scheduled times for glucose tests and insulin injections must match meal times.

Enteral Tube Feedings

Tube feeding formulas contain more simple carbohydrates and less protein and fat than the typical meal plan for diabetes. This results in increased levels of glucose in patients with diabetes who are receiving tube feedings. It is important that insulin doses be administered at regular intervals (eg, NPH every 12 hours or regular insulin every 4 to 6 hours) when continuous tube feedings are administered. If insulin is administered at routine (prebreakfast and predinner) times, hypoglycemia during the day may result (because the patient receives more insulin without more calories); and hyperglycemia may occur during the night if feedings continue but insulin action decreases.

A common cause of hypoglycemia in patients receiving both continuous tube feedings and insulin is inadvertent or purposeful discontinuation of the feeding. The nurse must discuss with the medical team any plans for temporarily discontinuing the tube feeding (eg, when the patient is away from the unit). Planning ahead may allow for alterations to be made in the insulin dose or for administration of IV dextrose. In addition, if problems with the tube feeding develop unexpectedly (eg, the patient pulls out the tube, the tube clogs, the feeding is discontinued when residual gastric contents are found), the nurse must notify the physician, assess blood glucose levels more frequently, and administer IV dextrose if indicated.

Parenteral Nutrition

Patients receiving parenteral nutrition may receive both IV insulin (added to the parenteral nutrition container) and subcutaneous intermediate-acting or short-acting insulins. If the patient is receiving continuous parenteral nutrition, the blood glucose level should be monitored and insulin administered at regular intervals. If the parenteral nutrition is infused over a limited number of hours, subcutaneous insulin should be administered so that peak times of insulin action coincide with times of parenteral nutrition infusion.

Hygiene

Nurses caring for hospitalized patients with diabetes must focus attention on oral hygiene and skin care. Because these patients are at increased risk for periodontal disease, it is important for the nurse to assist the patient with daily dental care. The patient may also require assistance in keeping the skin clean and dry, especially in areas of contact between two skin surfaces (eg, groin, axilla, under the breasts), where chafing and fungal infections tend to occur.

Careful assessment of the skin, especially at pressure points and on the lower extremities, is important. The skin is assessed for dryness, cracks, skin breakdown, and redness. The patient is asked about symptoms of neuropathy, such as tingling and pain or numbness of the feet. Deep tendon reflexes are assessed.

As with any patient confined to bed, nursing care must emphasize the prevention of skin breakdown at pressure points. The heels are particularly susceptible to breakdown because of loss of sensation of pain and pressure associated with sensory neuropathy.

Feet should be cleaned, dried, lubricated with lotion (but not between the toes), and inspected frequently. If the patient is in the supine position, pressure on the heels can be alleviated by elevating the lower legs on a pillow, with the heels positioned over the edge of the pillow. When the patient is seated in a chair, the feet should be positioned so that pressure is not placed on the heels. If the patient has an ulcer on one foot, it is important to provide preventive care to the unaffected foot as well as special care of the affected foot.

As always, every opportunity should be taken to teach the patient about diabetes self-management, including daily oral, skin, and foot care. Female patients should also be instructed about measures for the avoidance of vaginal infections, which occur more frequently when blood glucose levels are elevated. Patients often take their cues from nurses and realize the importance of daily personal hygiene if this is emphasized during their hospitalization.

Stress

Physiologic stress, such as infections and surgery, contributes to hyperglycemia and may precipitate DKA or HHNS. Emotional stress related to hospitalization for any reason can also have a negative impact on diabetic control. An increase in stress hormones leads to an increase in glucose levels, especially if intake of food and insulin remains unchanged. In addition, during periods of emotional stress, people with diabetes may alter their usual pattern of meals, exercise, and medication. This can contribute to hyperglycemia or even hypoglycemia (eg, in the patient taking insulin or oral antidiabetic agents who stops eating in response to stress).

People with diabetes must be made aware of the potential deterioration in diabetic control that can accompany emotional stress. They must be encouraged to follow the diabetes treatment plan as much as possible during times of stress. In addition, learning strategies for minimizing stress and coping with stress when it does occur are important aspects of diabetes education. Healthy coping is one of the seven steps to managing diabetes identified by the AADE (2007).

 Gerontologic Considerations

Because people with diabetes are living longer, both type 1 and type 2 diabetes are being seen more frequently in elderly patients hospitalized for various reasons. Regardless of the type or duration of diabetes, the goals of diabetes treatment may need to be altered when caring for hospitalized elderly patients. The focus is on quality-of-life issues, such as maintaining independent functioning and promoting general well-being.

Some of the barriers to learning and self-care during hospital stays and in preparing patients for discharge include decreased vision, hearing loss, memory deficits, decreased mobility and fine motor coordination, increased tremors, depression and isolation, decreased financial resources, and limitations related to disabilities and other medical disorders. Assessing these barriers is important in planning diabetes treatment and educational activities. Presenting brief, simplified instructions with ample opportunity for practice of skills is important. The use of special devices such as a magnifier for the insulin syringe, an insulin pen, or a mirror for foot inspection is helpful. Frequent evaluation of self-care skills (insulin administration, blood glucose monitoring, foot care, diet planning) is essential, especially in patients with deteriorating vision and memory.

If appropriate, family members may be called on to assist with diabetes survival skills, and referral to community resources may be made. It is preferable to teach the patient or family members to test blood glucose at home; the choice of meter should be tailored to the patient's visual and cognitive status and dexterity.

 NURSING ALERT

Careful monitoring for diabetes complications must not be neglected in elderly patients. Hypoglycemia is especially dangerous, because it may go undetected and result in falls. Dehydration is a concern in patients who have chronically elevated blood glucose levels. Assessment for long-term complications, especially eye and foot problems, is important. Avoiding blindness and amputation through early detection and treatment of retinopathy and foot ulcers may mean the difference between placement in a long-term care facility and continued independent living for the elderly person with diabetes.

Monitoring and Managing Potential Complications

Assessment for hypoglycemia and hyperglycemia involves frequent blood glucose monitoring (usually prescribed before meals and at bedtime) and monitoring for signs and symptoms of hypoglycemia or prolonged hyperglycemia (including DKA or HHNS), as described previously. Inadequate control of blood glucose levels may hinder recovery from the primary health problem. Blood glucose levels are monitored, and insulin is administered as prescribed. It is important for the nurse to ensure that prescribed insulin dosage is modified as needed to compensate for changes in the patient's schedule or eating pattern. Treatment is given for hypoglycemia (with oral glucose) or hyperglycemia (with supplemental regular insulin no more often than every 3 to 4 hours). Blood glucose records are assessed for patterns of hypoglycemia and hyperglycemia at the same time of day, and findings are reported to the physician for modification in insulin orders. In the patient with prolonged elevations in blood glucose, laboratory values and the patient's physical condition are monitored for signs and symptoms of DKA or HHNS.

Promoting Home and Community-Based Case

Teaching Patients Self-Care

Even if the patient has had diabetes for many years, it is important to assess his or her knowledge and adherence to the plan of care. A new plan of care may need to be devised using concepts mentioned earlier. The nurse also reminds the patient and family about the importance of health promotion activities and recommended health screening.

Continuing Care

A patient who is hospitalized may require referral for home care. The home care nurse can use this opportunity to assess the patient's knowledge about diabetes management and the patient's and family's ability to carry out that management. The nurse reinforces the teaching provided in the hospital, clinic, office, or diabetes education center and assesses the home care environment to determine its adequacy for self-care and safety.

CRITICAL THINKING EXERCISES

1 A 35-year-old pregnant woman with type 2 diabetes is admitted to the hospital for an elective Caesarean section. What modifications in her diabetes care are needed before, during, and after her Caesarean section? How would her care differ if she had type 1 diabetes?

EBP **2** A 25-year-old patient is newly diagnosed with type 1 diabetes. His physician has discussed intensive insulin therapy with him, although the patient indicates that he needs more information about the advantages and disadvantages of intensive therapy before he can make a decision about therapy. What is the evidence base for intensive insulin therapy and the strength of that evidence?

How would you present information to him about the advantages and disadvantages of intensive therapy?

3 You are the nurse in a diabetes education center with many patients with type 1 and type 2 diabetes. Identify strategies you would use to provide diabetes education for the following patients: (1) a patient who has managed her diabetes well for 20 years, but has recently been prescribed insulin for the first time, (2) a patient who has cerebral palsy that affects her lower extremities and one hand, (3) a patient who speaks very little English, and (4) a patient who is angry and resentful that he has developed diabetes.

4 You are providing discharge instructions for a 55-year-old executive being discharged from the hospital after carotid endarterectomy and cardiac artery bypass surgery. He indicates that although he has had diabetes for 10 years, he has only "a little diabetes" because until recently he has not required insulin. He is a smoker and travels extensively. Develop a teaching plan for this patient and identify the priorities of teaching for him.

5 A 68-year-old woman who was found at home unresponsive by her neighbors is admitted to the emergency department with possible diabetic ketoacidosis. She is well known to the emergency department personnel because of repeated episodes of hypoglycemia in the past. Compare the pathophysiology and signs and symptoms of diabetic ketoacidosis and hypoglycemia. How would assessment, medical management, and nursing care for these two disorders compare? What would be your priorities for patient teaching once she has recovered from the acute medical problem?

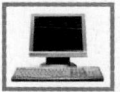

The Smeltzer suite offers these additional resources to enhance learning and facilitate understanding of this chapter:
- thePoint online resource, thepoint.lww.com/Smeltzer12E
- Student CD-ROM included with the book
- *Study Guide to Accompany Brunner & Suddarth's Textbook of Medical-Surgical Nursing*
- *Handbook for Brunner & Suddarth's Textbook of Medical-Surgical Nursing*

REFERENCES AND SELECTED READINGS

*Asterisk indicates nursing research.
**Double asterisk indicates classic reference.

Books

American Nurses Association and American Association of Diabetes Educators. (2003). *Scope and standards of diabetes nursing practice.* Washington, DC: American Nurses Publishing.

Centers for Disease Control and Prevention (CDC). (2008). *National diabetes fact sheet: National estimates on diabetes.* Atlanta: Author.

Davidson, M. B., Harmel., A. P. & Mathur, R. (2004). *Davidson's diabetes mellitus: Diagnosis and treatment* (5th ed.). Philadelphia: Saunders.

National Institute of Diabetes and Digestive and Kidney Diseases (NIDDK). (2005). *National Diabetes Statistics fact sheet: General information and national estimates on diabetes in the United States, 2005.* Bethesda, MD: U.S. Department of Health and Human Services, National Institutes of Health, NIH Publication 06-3892.

National Institute of Diabetes and Digestive and Kidney Diseases (NIDDK). (2007). *Pancreatic islet transplantation.* Bethesda, MD: U.S. Department of Health and Human Services, National Institutes of Health, NIH Publication 07-4693.

National Institute of Diabetes and Digestive and Kidney Diseases (NIDDK). (2008a). *Diabetic neuropathies: The nerve damage of diabetes.* Bethesda, MD: U.S. Department of Health and Human Services, National Institutes of Health, NIH Publication 08-3185.

National Institute of Diabetes and Digestive and Kidney Diseases (NIDDK). (2008b). *Prevent diabetes problems: Keep your feet and skin healthy.* Bethesda, MD: U.S. Department of Health and Human Services, National Institutes of Health, NIH Publication 08-4282.

National Institutes of Health, National Heart, Lung and Blood Institute, North American Association for the Study of Obesity. (2000). *The practical guide: Identification, evaluation and treatment of overweight and obesity in adults.* Bethesda, MD: U.S. Department of Health and Human Services, National Institutes of Health, NIH Publication 00-4084.

Porth, C. M. & Matfin, G. (2009). *Pathophysiology: Concepts of altered health states* (8th ed.). Philadelphia: Lippincott Williams & Wilkins.

U.S. Department of Agriculture. (2005). *Nutrition and your health: Dietary guidelines for Americans.* Washington, DC: U.S. Government Printing Office.

U.S. Department of Health and Human Services. (2005). *Healthy people 2010: Midcourse review.* Washington, DC: U.S. Government Printing Office.

Journals and Electronic Documents

General

American Association of Diabetes Educators (AADE). (2005). The scope of practice, standards of practice, and standards of professional performance for diabetes educators. *Diabetes Educators, 31*(4), 487–513.

American Association of Diabetes Educators (AADE). (2007). AADE position statement: Individualization of diabetes self-management education. *The Diabetes Educator, 33*(1), 45–49.

American Diabetes Association (ADA). (2008a). Economic costs of diabetes in the U.S. in 2007. *Diabetes Care, 31*(3), 1–20.

American Diabetes Association (ADA). (2008b). Third party reimbursement for diabetes care, self-management education, and supplies. *Diabetes Care, 31*(1), S95–S96.

American Diabetes Association (ADA). (2009a). Diagnosis and classification of diabetes mellitus. *Diabetes Care, 32*(Suppl 1), S62–S67.

American Diabetes Association (ADA). (2009b). Standards of medical care in diabetes—2009. (Position statement). *Diabetes Care, 32*(Suppl 1), S13–S61.

Centers for Disease Control and Prevention (CDC). (2008). *National diabetes fact sheet: General information and national estimates on diabetes in the United States, 2007.* Atlanta, GA: U.S. Department of Health and Human Services, Centers for Disease Control and Prevention.

Diabetes Prevention Program Research Group. (2002). Reduction in the incidence of type 2 diabetes with lifestyle intervention or metformin. *New England Journal of Medicine, 346*(6), 393–403.

Fowler, M. (2009). Hyperglycemic crisis in adults: Pathophysiology, presentation, pitfalls, and prevention. *Clinical Diabetes, 27*(1), 19–23.

Funnell, M. M., Brown, T. L., Childs, B. P., et al. (2009). National standards for diabetes self-management education. *Diabetes Care, 32*(Suppl 1), S87–S94.

Geil, P. B. (2008). Choose your foods: Exchange lists for diabetes: The 2008 revision of exchange lists for meal planning. *Diabetes Spectrum, 21*(4), 281–283.

Grandjean, C. & Moran, B. (2007). The impact of diabetes mellitus on female sexual well-being. *Nursing Clinics of North America, 42*(4), 581–592.

Kitzmiller, J. L., Dang-Kilduff, L. & Taslimi, M. M. (2007). Gestational diabetes after delivery: Short-term management and long-term risks. *Diabetes Care, 30*(2), S225–S235.

Nathan, D. M., Buse, J. B., Davidson, M. B., et al. (2009). Medical management of hyperglycemia in type 2 diabetes: A consensus algorithm for the initiation and adjustment of therapy: A consensus statement from the American Diabetes Association and the European Association for the Study of Diabetes. *Diabetes Care, 32*(1), 193–203.

*Penckofer, S., Ferrans, C. & Velsor-Friedrich, B. (2007). The psychological impact of living with diabetes: Women's day-to-day experiences. *The Diabetes Educator, 33*(4), 680–690.

World Health Organization. (2008). Diabetes. Fact sheet no. 312. www.who.int/mediacentre/factsheets/fs312/en/index.html

Complications

American Diabetes Association (ADA). (2008d). Hyperglycemic crisis in diabetes. *Diabetes Care, 31*(Suppl 1), S94–S102.

American Diabetes Association (ADA). (2006c). Hyperglycemic crisis in adults. *Diabetes Care, 29*(12), 2739–2748.

American Diabetes Association (ADA). (2008f). Nephropathy in diabetes. *Diabetes Care, 31*(Suppl 1), S79–S83.

American Diabetes Association (ADA). (2008e). Retinopathy in diabetes. *Diabetes Care, 31*(Suppl 1), S84–S87.

Bloomgarden, Z. T. (2007). Diabetic neuropathy. *Diabetes Care, 30*(4), 1027–1032.

Bloomgarden, Z. T. (2008a). Diabetic nephropathy. *Diabetes Care, 31*(4), 823–827.

Bloomgarden, Z. T. (2008b). Diabetic retinopathy. *Diabetes Care, 31*(5), 1080–1083.

**Diabetes Control and Complications Trial (DCCT) Research Group. (1993). The effect of intensive treatment of diabetes on the development and progression of long-term complications in insulin-dependent diabetes mellitus. *New England Journal of Medicine, 329*(14), 977–986.

Management

American Diabetes Association (ADA). (2004). Insulin administration [position statement]. *Diabetes Care, 27*(1), 106–107.

American Diabetes Association (ADA). (2006a). Physical activity/exercise and type 2 diabetes [consensus statement]. *Diabetes Care, 29*(6), 1433–1438.

American Diabetes Association (ADA). (2006b). Pancreas and islet transplantation in type 1 diabetes [position statement]. *Diabetes Care, 29*(4), 935.

American Diabetes Association (ADA). (2008b). Nutrition recommendations and interventions for diabetes [position statement]. *.Diabetes Care, 31*(Suppl 1), S61–S78.

American Diabetes Association (ADA). (2008c). Lipoprotein management in patients with cardiometabolic risk. Consensus statement from ADA and American College of Cardiology Foundation [consensus statement]. *Diabetes Care, 31*(4), 811–822.

Blonde, L., Klein, E. J., Han, J., et al. (2006). Interim analysis of the effects of exenatide treatment on A1C, weight and cardiovascular risk factors over 82 weeks in 314 overweight patients with type 2 diabetes. *Diabetes, Obesity and Metabolism, 8*(4), 436–447.

Capriotti, T. (2005). Type 2 diabetes epidemic increases use of oral anti-diabetic agents. *MedSurg Nursing, 14*(5), 341–347.

Durso, S. C. (2006). Using clinical guidelines designed for older adults with diabetes mellitus and complex health status. *Journal of the American Medical Association, 295*(6), 1935–1940.

Hirsch, I. B. (2005). Insulin analogues. *New England Journal of Medicine, 352*(2), 174–183.

**Jacobson, A. F. (1999). Saving limbs with Semmes-Weinstein monofilament. *American Journal of Nursing, 99*(2), 76.

Lachance, P. A. & Fisher, M. C. (2005). Reinvention of the food pyramid to promote health. *Advances in Food and Nutrition Research, 49,* 1–39.

Nathan, D. M., Cleary, P. A., Backlund, J-Y. C., et al. (2005). Intensive diabetes treatment and cardiovascular disease in patients with type 1 diabetes. *New England Journal of Medicine, 353*(25), 2643–2653.

Singh, S., Loke, Y. & Furberg, C. (2007). Long-term risk of cardiovascular events with rosiglitazone: A meta-analysis. *Journal of American Medical Association, 298*(10), 1189–1195.

**United Kingdom Prospective Diabetes Study Group (UKPDS). (1998). Intensive blood glucose control with sulfonylureas or insulin compared with conventional treatment and risk of complications with type 2 diabetes. *Lancet, 352*(9131), 837–853.

Webb, K. E. (2006). Use of insulin pumps for diabetes management. *MedSurg Nursing, 15*(2), 61–68, 94.

Pregnancy and Gestational Diabetes

American Diabetes Association (ADA). (2008g). Managing preexisting diabetes for pregnancy: Summary of evidence and consensus recommendations for care. *Diabetes Care, 31*(6), 1060–1079.

Owens, M. D., Kieffer, K. C. & Chowdhury, F. M. (2006). Preconception care and women with or at risk for diabetes: Implications for community intervention. *Maternal and Child Health Journal, 10*(Suppl 1), 137–141.

RESOURCES

American Association of Diabetes Educators, www.aadenet.org/

American Diabetes Association, www.diabetes.org

American Dietetic Association, www.eatright.org

American Foundation for the Blind, www.afb.org

Armchair Fitness Series, CC-M Productions, Inc. 7755 16th Street, NW, District of Columbia, Washington, 20012. http://armchairfitness.stores.yahoo.net/index.html.

Centers for Disease Control and Prevention, www.cdc.gov/diabetes/pubs/factsheet.htm

Juvenile Diabetes Research Foundation International, www.jdrf.org

MedicAlert Foundation International, www.medicalert.org

National Diabetes Information Clearinghouse, www.niddk.nih.gov

National Library Services for the Blind and Physically Handicapped (NLSBPH), www.loc.gov/nls/

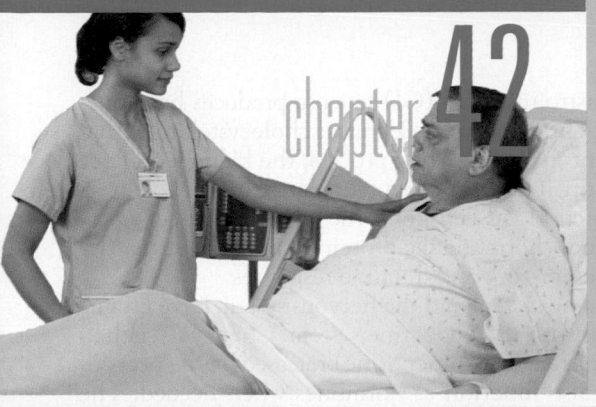

Assessment and Management of Patients With Endocrine Disorders

chapter 42

LEARNING OBJECTIVES

On completion of this chapter, the learner will be able to:

1 Describe the functions of each of the endocrine glands and their hormones.
2 Identify the diagnostic tests used to determine alterations in function of each of the endocrine glands.
3 Compare hypothyroidism and hyperthyroidism: their causes, clinical manifestations, management, and nursing interventions.
4 Develop a plan of nursing care for the patient undergoing thyroidectomy.
5 Compare hyperparathyroidism and hypoparathyroidism: their causes, clinical manifestations, management, and nursing interventions.
6 Compare Addison's disease with Cushing's syndrome: their causes, clinical manifestations, management, and nursing interventions.
7 Describe nursing management of patients with adrenal insufficiency.
8 Use the nursing process as a framework for care of patients with Cushing's syndrome.
9 Identify the teaching needs of patients requiring corticosteroid therapy.

GLOSSARY

acromegaly: disease process resulting from excessive secretion of somatotropin; causes progressive enlargement of peripheral body parts
addisonian crisis: acute adrenocortical insufficiency; characterized by hypotension, cyanosis, fever, nausea/vomiting, and classic signs of shock; precipitated by stress or abrupt withdrawal of therapeutic glucocorticoids
Addison's disease: chronic adrenocortical insufficiency secondary to destruction of the adrenal glands
adrenalectomy: surgical removal of one or both adrenal glands
adrenocorticotropic hormone (ACTH): hormone secreted by the anterior pituitary; essential for growth and development
adrenogenital syndrome: masculinization in women, feminization in men, or premature sexual development in children; result of abnormal secretion of adrenocortical hormones, especially androgens
androgens: hormones secreted by the adrenal cortex; stimulate activity of accessory male sex organs and development of male sex characteristics
basal metabolic rate: chemical reactions occurring when the body is at rest
calcitonin: hormone secreted by the parafollicular cells of the thyroid gland; participates in calcium regulation
Chvostek's sign: spasm of the facial muscles produced by sharply tapping over the facial nerve in front of the parotid gland and anterior to the ear; suggestive of latent tetany in patients with hypocalcemia
corticosteroids: hormones produced by the adrenal cortex or their synthetic equivalents; also referred to as adrenal-cortical hormone and adrenocorticosteroid; consist of glucocorticoids, mineralocorticoids, and androgens
cretinism: stunted body growth and mental development appearing during the first year of life as a result of congenital hypothyroidism
Cushing's syndrome: group of symptoms produced by an excess of free circulating cortisol from the adrenal cortex; characterized by truncal obesity, "moon face," acne, abdominal striae, and hypertension

GLOSSARY *(Continued)*

diabetes insipidus: condition in which abnormally large volumes of dilute urine are excreted as a result of deficient production of vasopressin
dwarfism: generalized limited growth resulting from insufficient secretion of growth hormone during childhood
endocrine: secreting internally; hormonal secretion of a ductless gland
euthyroid: state of normal thyroid hormone production
exocrine: secreting externally; hormonal secretion from excretory ducts
exophthalmos: abnormal protrusion of one or both eyeballs
glucocorticoids: steroid hormones secreted by the adrenal cortex in response to ACTH; produce a rise of liver glycogen and blood glucose
goiter: enlargement of the thyroid gland; usually caused by an iodine-deficient diet
Graves' disease: a form of hyperthyroidism; characterized by a diffuse goiter and exophthalmos
hormones: chemical transmitter substances produced in one organ or part of the body and carried by the bloodstream to other cells or organs on which they have a specific regulatory effect; produced mainly by endocrine glands
hypophysectomy: removal or destruction of all or part of the pituitary gland
mineralocorticoid: steroid of the adrenal cortex
myxedema: severe hypothyroidism characterized by an accumulation of mucopolysaccharides in interstitial tissues, a masklike expression, puffy eyelids, loss of eyebrow hair, thick lips, and a broad tongue
negative feedback: regulating mechanism in which an increase or decrease in the level of a substance decreases or increases the function of the organ producing the substance
oxytocin: hormone secreted by the posterior pituitary; causes myometrial contraction at term and milk release during lactation
pheochromocytoma: chromaffin cell tumor, usually benign, located in the adrenal medulla; characterized by secretion of catecholamines resulting in hypertension, severe headache, profuse sweating, visual blurring, anxiety, and nausea
syndrome of inappropriate antidiuretic hormone (SIADH) secretion: excessive secretion of antidiuretic hormone (ADH) from the pituitary gland despite low serum osmolality level
thyroidectomy: surgical removal of all or part of the thyroid gland
thyroiditis: inflammation of the thyroid gland; may lead to chronic hypothyroidism or may resolve spontaneously
thyroid-stimulating hormone: released from the pituitary gland; causes stimulation of the thyroid, resulting in release of T3 and T4
thyroid storm: severe life-threatening hyperthyroidism precipitated by stress; characterized by high fever, extreme tachycardia, and altered mental state
thyrotoxicosis: condition produced by excessive endogenous or exogenous thyroid hormone
thyroxine (T_4): thyroid hormone; active iodine compound formed and stored in the thyroid; deiodinated in peripheral tissues to form triiodothyronine; maintains body metabolism in a steady state
triiodothyronine (T_3): thyroid hormone; formed and stored in the thyroid; released in smaller quantities, biologically more active and with faster onset of action than T_4; widespread effect on cellular metabolism
Trousseau's sign: carpopedal spasm induced when blood flow to the arm is occluded using a blood pressure cuff or tourniquet, causing ischemia to the distal nerves; suggestive sign for latent tetany in hypocalcemia
vasopressin: ADH secreted by the posterior pituitary; causes contraction of smooth muscle, particularly blood vessels

The endocrine system plays a vital role in growth and development, the metabolism of energy, muscle and adipose tissue distribution, sexual development, fluid and electrolyte balance, and inflammation and immune responses (Porth & Matfin, 2009). This interconnected network of glands is closely linked with the nervous and immune systems regulating the functions of multiple body organs. Disorders of the endocrine system are common and are manifested as hyperfunction and hypofunction.

Nursing interventions are essential in the management of patients with endocrine disorders. This chapter focuses on the anatomy and physiology of the endocrine system; the most common endocrine disorders of the pituitary, thyroid, parathyroid, and adrenal glands; clinical manifestations; diagnostic studies; medical management; and nursing interventions. The unique endocrine and exocrine functions of the pancreas, pancreatic function, and associated pancreatic disorders are discussed in Chapters 40 and 41, and reproductive structures, including the ovaries and testes, are discussed in Chapters 46 and 49.

ASSESSMENT OF THE ENDOCRINE SYSTEM

Anatomic and Physiologic Overview

The **endocrine** system involves the release of chemical substances known as **hormones** to regulate and integrate body functions. Generally, these hormones are produced by the endocrine glands, but some are also produced by other tis-sues. The gastrointestinal (GI) mucosa produces hormones (eg, gastrin, enterogastrone, secretin, cholecystokinin) that are important in the digestive process; the kidneys produce erythropoietin, a hormone that stimulates the bone marrow to produce red blood cells; and the white blood cells produce cytokines (hormonelike proteins) that actively participate in inflammatory and immune responses.

The immune system and the nervous system have unique relationships with the endocrine system. Chemicals such as neurotransmitters (eg, epinephrine) released by the nervous system can also function as hormones when needed. The immune system responds to the introduction of foreign agents by means of chemical messengers (cytokines), which are hormonelike proteins, while it is also subject to regulation by adrenal corticosteroid hormones (Porth & Matfin, 2009).

Glands of the Endocrine System

The endocrine system is composed of several glands: the pituitary, the thyroid gland, parathyroid glands, adrenal glands, pancreatic islets, ovaries, and testes (Fig. 42-1). Unlike the **exocrine** glands, most hormones secreted from endocrine glands are released directly into the bloodstream. Exocrine glands, such as sweat glands, secrete their products through ducts onto epithelial surfaces or into the GI tract.

Function and Regulation of Hormones

Hormones help regulate organ function in concert with the nervous system. This dual regulatory system, in which rapid action by the nervous system is balanced by slower hormonal action, permits precise control of organ functions in

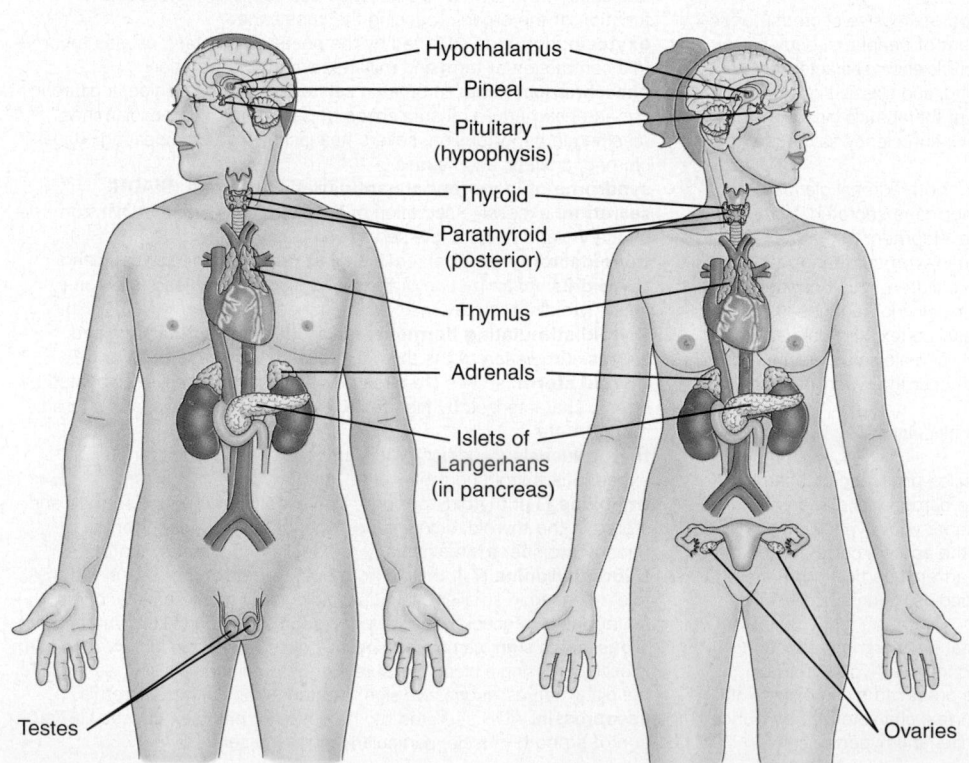

Figure 42-1 Major hormone-secreting glands of the endocrine system.

Hypothalamus
Pineal
Pituitary (hypophysis)
Thyroid
Parathyroid (posterior)
Thymus
Adrenals
Islets of Langerhans (in pancreas)
Testes
Ovaries

Table 42-1   MAJOR ACTION AND SOURCE OF SELECTED HORMONES

Source	Hormone	Major Action

Hypothalamus	Releasing and inhibiting hormones
	  Corticotropin-releasing hormone (CRH)
	  Thyrotropin-releasing hormone (TRH)
	  Growth hormone–releasing hormone (GHRH)
	  Gonadotropin–releasing hormone (GnRH)
		Controls the release of pituitary hormones

	Somatostatin	Inhibits growth hormone and thyroid-stimulating hormone
Anterior pituitary	Growth hormone (GH)	Stimulates growth of bone and muscle, promotes protein synthesis and fat metabolism, decreases carbohydrate metabolism
	Adrenocorticotropic hormone (ACTH)	Stimulates synthesis and secretion of adrenal cortical hormones
	Thyroid-stimulating hormone (TSH)	Stimulates synthesis and secretion of thyroid hormone
	Follicle-stimulating hormone (FSH)	Female: stimulates growth of ovarian follicle, ovulation Male: stimulates sperm production
	Luteinizing hormone (LH)	Female: stimulates development of corpus luteum, release of oocyte, production of estrogen and progesterone Male: stimulates secretion of testosterone, development of interstitial tissue of testes
	Prolactin	Prepares female breast for breast-feeding
Posterior pituitary	Antidiuretic hormone (ADH)	Increases water reabsorption by kidney
	Oxytocin	Stimulates contraction of pregnant uterus, milk ejection from breasts after childbirth
Adrenal cortex	Mineralocorticosteroids, mainly aldosterone	Increase sodium absorption, potassium loss by kidney
	Glucocorticoids, mainly cortisol	Affect metabolism of all nutrients; regulates blood glucose levels, affects growth, has anti-inflammatory action, and decreases effects of stress
	Adrenal androgens, mainly dehydroepiandrosterone (DHEA) and androstenedione	Have minimal intrinsic androgenic activity; they are converted to testosterone and dihydrotestosterone in the periphery
Adrenal medulla	Epinephrine Norepinephrine	Serve as neurotransmitters for the sympathetic nervous system
Thyroid (follicular cells)	Thyroid hormones: triiodothyronine (T_3), thyroxine (T_4)	Increase the metabolic rate; increase protein and bone turnover; increase responsiveness to catecholamines; necessary for fetal and infant growth and development
Thyroid C cells	Calcitonin	Lowers blood calcium and phosphate levels
Parathyroid glands	Parathormone (PTH, parathyroid hormone)	Regulates serum calcium
Pancreatic islet cells	Insulin	Lowers blood glucose by facilitating glucose transport across cell membranes of muscle, liver, and adipose tissue
	Glucagon	Increases blood glucose concentration by stimulation of glycogenolysis and glyconeogenesis
	Somatostatin	Delays intestinal absorption of glucose
Kidney	1,25-Dihydroxyvitamin D	Stimulates calcium absorption from the intestine
	Renin	Activates renin–angiotensin–aldosterone system
	Erythropoietin	Increases red blood cell production
Ovaries	Estrogen	Affects development of female sex organs and secondary sex characteristics
	Progesterone	Influences menstrual cycle; stimulates growth of uterine wall; maintains pregnancy
Testes	Androgens, mainly testosterone	Affect development of male sex organs and secondary sex characteristics; aid in sperm production

Reproduced with permission from Porth, C. M. & Matfin, G. (2009). *Pathophysiology: Concepts of altered health states* (8th ed.). Philadelphia: Lippincott Williams & Wilkins.

response to varied changes within and outside the body. Table 42-1 lists the major hormones, their target tissues, and some of their properties.

The endocrine glands are composed of secretory cells arranged in minute clusters known as acini. No ducts are present, but the glands have a rich blood supply, so the hormones they produce enter the bloodstream rapidly. In the healthy physiologic state, hormone concentration in the bloodstream is maintained at a relatively constant level. **Negative feedback** is the mechanism for regulating hormone concentration in the bloodstream. When the hormone concentration increases, further production of that hormone is inhibited. Conversely, when the hormone concentration decreases, the rate of production of that hormone increases.

Hormones are generally transported in body fluids, and the amount of specific hormones circulating at any given time depends on the body's needs. Hormones are special in that particular ones may affect different tissues in various ways or that several may be necessary for the regulation of a certain body function.

Classification and Action of Hormones

Hormones are classified into four categories according to their structure: (1) amines and amino acids (eg, epinephrine, norepinephrine, and thyroid hormones); (2) peptides, polypeptides, proteins, and glycoproteins (eg, thyrotropin-releasing hormone, follicle-stimulating hormone, and growth hormone); (3) steroids (eg, corticosteroids); and (4) fatty acid derivatives (eg, eicosanoid, retinoids) (Porth &

Matfin, 2009). These different classes of hormones act on the target tissues by different mechanisms.

Hormones can alter the function of the target tissue by interacting with chemical receptors located either on the cell membrane or in the interior of the cell. For example, *peptide and protein hormones* interact with receptor sites on the cell surface, resulting in stimulation of the intracellular enzyme adenyl cyclase. This causes increased production of cyclic 3′,5′-adenosine monophosphate (cyclic AMP). The cyclic AMP inside the cell alters enzyme activity. Thus, cyclic AMP is the "second messenger" that links the peptide hormone at the cell surface to a change in the intracellular environment. Some protein and peptide hormones also act by changing membrane permeability and act within seconds or minutes. The mechanism of action for *amine hormones* is similar to that for peptide hormones.

Steroid hormones, because of their smaller size and higher lipid solubility, penetrate cell membranes and interact with intracellular receptors. The steroid–receptor complex modifies cell metabolism and the formation of messenger ribonucleic acid (mRNA) from deoxyribonucleic acid (DNA). The mRNA then stimulates protein synthesis within the cell. Steroid hormones require several hours to exert their effects, because they exert their action by the modification of protein synthesis.

Although most hormones released by endocrine glands can be transported to distant target sites for action, some hormones and hormonelike substances never enter the bloodstream. Some hormones act locally in the area where they are released; this is called paracrine action (eg, the effect of sex hormones on the ovaries). Others may act on the actual cells from which they were released; this is called autocrine action (eg, the effect of insulin from pancreatic beta cells on those cells) (Porth & Matfin, 2009).

Assessment

Health History

Although specific endocrine disorders are often accompanied by specific clinical symptoms, more general manifestations may also occur. Some common signs and symptoms of endocrine imbalances include changes in energy level, tolerance to heat or cold, weight, fat and fluid distribution, secondary sexual characteristics, sexual dysfunction, memory, concentration, sleep patterns, and mood. The health history should include information regarding (1) the severity of these changes, (2) the length of time the patient has experienced these changes, (3) the way in which these changes have affected the patient's ability to carry out activities of daily living, and (4) the effect of the changes on the patient's self-perception. Specific symptoms of various endocrine disorders are discussed with each disorder. Possible genetics-related issues may also be important (Chart 42-1).

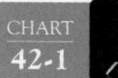

CHART 42-1

GENETICS IN NURSING PRACTICE
Metabolic Disorders

Some examples of metabolic and endocrine disorders influenced by genetic factors include the following:
- Alpha-1 antitrypsin deficiency
- Cystic fibrosis
- Diabetes mellitus type 1 and type 2
- Hereditary hemochromatosis
- Multiple endocrine neoplasia (MEN) type I and type II
- Von Hippel-Lindau syndrome
- Wilson's disease

Nursing Assessments

Family History Assessment
- Assess family history for relatives with early-onset hepatic, pancreatic, or endocrine disease.
- Inquire about family members with diabetes and their ages at onset.
- Assess family history of other related genetic conditions such as cystic fibrosis, alpha-1 antitrypsin deficiency, and hereditary hemochromatosis.

Patient Assessment
- Assess for physical symptoms such as mucosal neuromas, hypertrophied lips, skeletal abnormalities, and marfanoid appearance.
- Assess for signs of arthritis and bronze pigmentation of the skin (hereditary hemochromatosis).

Management Issues Specific to Genetics
- Inquire whether DNA mutation testing has been performed on any affected family member.

- If indicated, refer for further genetic counseling and evaluation so that family members can discuss inheritance, risk to other family members, and availability of genetic testing and gene-based interventions.
- Offer appropriate genetics information and resources.
- Assess patient's understanding of genetics information.
- Provide support to families with newly diagnosed genetics-related metabolic and endocrine conditions.
- Participate in management and coordination of care of patients with genetic conditions and people predisposed to develop or pass on a genetic condition.

Genetics Resources for Nurses and Their Patients on the Web

Genetic Alliance—a directory of support groups for patients and families with genetic conditions, www.geneticalliance.org

Gene Clinics—a listing of common genetics disorders with clinical summaries and genetic counseling and testing information, www.geneclinics.org

National Organization of Rare Disorders—a directory of support groups and information for patients and families with rare genetic disorders, www.rarediseases.org

OMIM: Online Mendelian Inheritance in Man—a complete listing of inherited genetic conditions, www.ncbi.nlm.nih.gov/projects/omim

Physical Assessment

The physical examination should include vital signs, a visual head-to-toe assessment, and tactile examination. Findings should be compared with previous findings if available. Changes in physical characteristics such as appearance of facial hair in women, "moon face," "buffalo hump," exophthalmos, edema, thinning of the skin, obesity of the trunk, thinness of the extremities, increased size of the feet and hands, and edema may signify disorders of the thyroid, adrenal cortex, or pituitary gland. Exophthalmos and other eye symptoms may occur with hyperthyroidism and Graves' disease. Alteration in skin texture is associated with hypofunction and hyperfunction of the thyroid gland. Elevated blood pressure may occur with hyperfunction of the adrenal cortex or tumor of the adrenal medulla. Decreased blood pressure may occur with hypofunction of the adrenal cortex. Behavioral changes such as agitation, nervousness, a flat affect, or a lack of concern about personal appearance may also be present.

Diagnostic Evaluation

A variety of diagnostic studies are used to evaluate the endocrine system. The most common tests are discussed in this section.

Blood tests are used to determine hormone blood levels. Knowing the serum levels of a specific hormone may provide information about whether there is hypofunction or hyperfunction of the endocrine system and the site of dysfunction. Other blood tests are used to detect autoantibodies or to assess the effect of the hormone on other substances (eg, the effect of insulin on blood glucose levels). Radioimmunoassays are radioisotope-labeled antigen tests used to measure the levels of hormones or other substances.

Urine tests may be used to measure the amount of hormones or the end products of hormones excreted by the kidneys. One-time specimens are obtained, or in some disorders 24-hour urine specimens are collected to measure hormones or their metabolites. For example, urinary levels of free catecholamines (norepinephrine, epinephrine, and dopamine) may be measured in patients with suspected tumors of the adrenal medulla (pheochromocytoma). Urine tests have several disadvantages, such as the inability of patients to urinate at scheduled intervals and the effect of some medications or disease states on the test results (Porth & Matfin, 2009).

Stimulation tests can determine how an endocrine gland responds to the administration of stimulating hormones that are normally produced or released by the hypothalamus or pituitary gland. If the endocrine gland responds to this stimulation, the specific disorder may be in the hypothalamus or pituitary. Failure of the endocrine gland to respond to this stimulation helps identify the problem as being in the endocrine gland itself.

Suppression tests may be used to determine whether negative feedback mechanisms that normally control secretion of hormones from the hypothalamus or pituitary gland are intact. They test the effect of administration of an exogenous dose of the hormone on the endogenous secretion of the hormone or on the secretion of stimulation hormones from the hypothalamus or pituitary gland.

Imaging studies include radioactive scanning, magnetic resonance imaging (MRI), computed tomography (CT), ultrasonography, positron emission tomography (PET), and dual-energy x-ray absorptiometry (DEXA).

Genetic screening is increasingly becoming more available. DNA testing is expected to lead to the identification of specific genes associated with endocrine disorders, selective targeting for drug development, and increased understanding of the function of the endocrine system (Porth & Matfin, 2009). Genetic screening is used to determine the presence of a gene mutation that may predispose an individual to a certain condition. The use of genetic screening must be considered carefully by the physician and patient.

THE PITUITARY GLAND

Anatomic and Physiologic Overview

The pituitary gland, or hypophysis, is commonly referred to as the master gland because of the influence it has on secretion of hormones by other endocrine glands (Fig. 42-2) (Porth & Matfin, 2009). The round structure, about 1.27 cm (1/2 inch) in diameter, is located on the inferior aspect of the brain. The pituitary gland is divided into anterior and posterior lobes. It is controlled by the hypothalamus, an adjacent area of the brain that is connected to the pituitary by the pituitary stalk.

Anterior Pituitary

The major hormones of the anterior pituitary gland are follicle-stimulating hormone (FSH), luteinizing hormone (LH), prolactin, **adrenocorticotropic hormone (ACTH), thyroid-stimulating hormone (TSH),** and growth hormone (GH) (also referred to as somatotropin). The secretion of these major hormones is controlled by releasing factors secreted by the hypothalamus. These releasing factors reach the anterior pituitary by way of the bloodstream in a special circulation called the pituitary portal blood system. Other hormones include melanocyte-stimulating hormone and beta-lipotropin; the function of lipotropin is poorly understood.

The hormones released by the anterior pituitary enter the general circulation and are transported to their target organs. The main function of TSH, ACTH, FSH, and LH is the release of hormones from other endocrine glands. Prolactin acts on the breast to stimulate milk production. Hormones that stimulate other organs and tissues are discussed in conjunction with their target organs.

GH is a protein hormone that increases protein synthesis in many tissues, increases the breakdown of fatty acids in adipose tissue, and increases the glucose level in the blood. These actions of GH are essential for normal growth, although other hormones, such as thyroid hormone and insulin, are required as well. Stress, exercise, and low blood glucose levels increase the secretion of GH. The half-life of GH activity in the blood is 20 to 30 minutes; the hormone is largely inactivated in the liver.

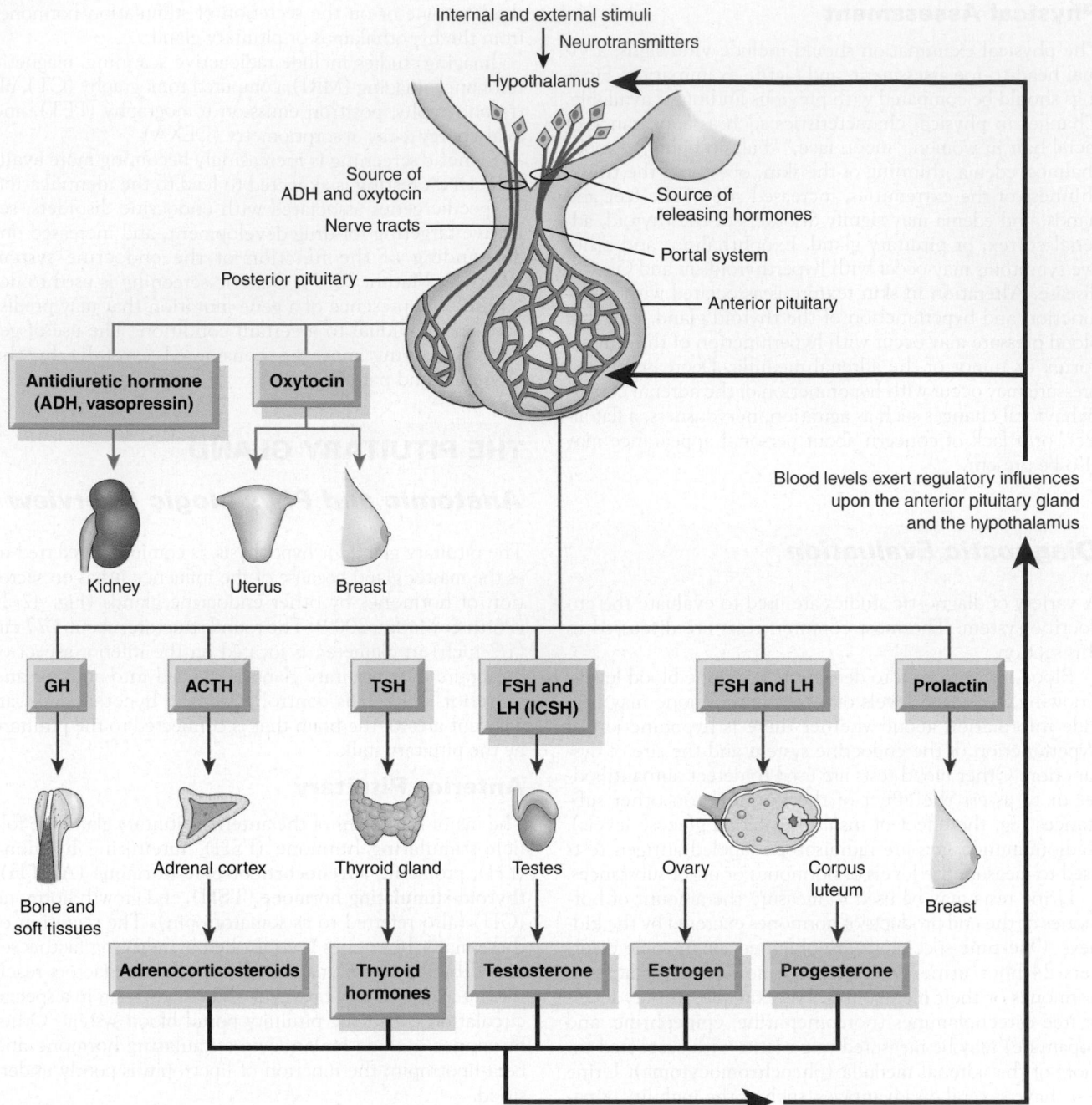

Figure 42-2 The pituitary gland, the relationship of the brain to pituitary action, and the hormones secreted by the anterior and posterior pituitary lobes. ACTH, adrenocorticotropic hormone; ADH, antidiuretic hormone; FSH, follicle-stimulating hormone; GH, growth hormone; ICSH, interstitial cell-stimulating hormone; LH, luteinizing hormone; TSH, thyroid-stimulating hormone.

Posterior Pituitary

The important hormones secreted by the posterior lobe of the pituitary gland are **vasopressin,** also called antidiuretic hormone (ADH), and **oxytocin.** These hormones are synthesized in the hypothalamus and travel from the hypothalamus to the posterior pituitary gland for storage. Vasopressin controls the excretion of water by the kidney; its secretion is stimulated by an increase in the osmolality of the blood or by a decrease in blood pressure. Oxytocin secretion is stimulated during pregnancy and at childbirth. It

facilitates milk ejection during lactation and increases the force of uterine contractions during labor and delivery.

Pathophysiology

Abnormalities of pituitary function are caused by oversecretion or undersecretion of any of the hormones produced or released by the gland. Abnormalities of the anterior and posterior portions of the gland may occur independently.

Hypofunction of the pituitary gland (hypopituitarism) can result from disease of the pituitary gland itself or disease of the hypothalamus; the result is essentially the same. Hypopituitarism can result from radiation therapy to the head and neck area. The total destruction of the pituitary gland by trauma, tumor, or vascular lesion removes all stimuli that are normally received by the thyroid, the gonads, and the adrenal glands. The result is extreme weight loss, emaciation, atrophy of all endocrine glands and organs, hair loss, impotence, amenorrhea, hypometabolism, and hypoglycemia. Coma and death occur if the missing hormones are not replaced.

Anterior Pituitary

Oversecretion (hypersecretion) of the anterior pituitary gland most commonly involves ACTH or GH and results in **Cushing's syndrome** or **acromegaly,** respectively. Acromegaly, an excess of GH in adults, results in bone and soft tissue deformities and enlargement of the viscera without an increase in height. It occurs in approximately 3 cases per 1 million people per year (Melmed, 2006). Oversecretion of GH results in gigantism in children; a person may be 7 or even 8 feet tall. Conversely, insufficient secretion of GH during childhood results in generalized limited growth and **dwarfism** (Porth & Matfin, 2009). Undersecretion (hyposecretion) commonly involves all of the anterior pituitary hormones and is termed *panhypopituitarism*. In this condition, the thyroid gland, the adrenal cortex, and the gonads atrophy (shrink) because of loss of the trophic-stimulating hormones. Hypopituitarism may result from destruction of the anterior lobe of the pituitary gland. Postpartum pituitary necrosis (Sheehan's syndrome) is another uncommon cause of failure of the anterior pituitary. It is more likely to occur in women with severe blood loss, hypovolemia, and hypotension at the time of delivery.

Posterior Pituitary

The most common disorder related to posterior lobe dysfunction is **diabetes insipidus,** a condition in which abnormally large volumes of dilute urine are excreted as a result of deficient production of vasopressin.

Specific Disorders of the Pituitary Gland

PITUITARY TUMORS

Pituitary tumors are usually benign and may be primary or secondary (Porth & Matfin, 2009). Functionality is also important. Functional tumors secrete pituitary hormones, whereas nonfunctional tumors do not. The location and effects of these tumors on hormone production by target organs can have life-threatening effects. Three principal types of pituitary tumors represent an overgrowth of (1) eosinophilic cells, (2) basophilic cells, or (3) chromophobic cells (ie, cells with no affinity for either eosinophilic or basophilic stains).

Clinical Manifestations

Eosinophilic tumors that develop early in life result in gigantism. The affected person may be more than 7 feet tall and large in all proportions, yet so weak and lethargic that he or she can hardly stand. If the disorder begins during adult life, the excessive skeletal growth occurs only in the feet, the hands, the superciliary ridge, the molar eminences, the nose, and the chin, giving rise to the clinical picture called acromegaly. However, enlargement involves all tissues and organs of the body (Melmed, 2006). Many of these patients suffer from severe headaches and visual disturbances because the tumors exert pressure on the optic nerves (Porth & Matfin, 2009). Assessment of central vision and visual fields may reveal loss of color discrimination, diplopia (double vision), or blindness in a portion of a field of vision. Decalcification of the skeleton, muscular weakness, and endocrine disturbances, similar to those occurring in patients with hyperthyroidism, also are associated with this type of tumor.

Basophilic tumors give rise to Cushing's syndrome with features largely attributable to hyperadrenalism, including masculinization and amenorrhea in females, truncal obesity, hypertension, osteoporosis, and polycythemia.

Chromophobic tumors represent 90% of pituitary tumors. These tumors usually produce no hormones but destroy the rest of the pituitary gland, causing hypopituitarism. People with this disease are often obese and somnolent and exhibit fine, scanty hair; dry, soft skin; a pasty complexion; and small bones. They also experience headaches, loss of libido, and visual defects progressing to blindness. Other signs and symptoms include polyuria, polyphagia, a lowering of the **basal metabolic rate,** and a subnormal body temperature.

Assessment and Diagnostic Findings

Diagnostic evaluation requires a careful history and physical examination, including assessment of visual acuity and visual fields. CT and MRI are used to diagnose the presence and extent of pituitary tumors. Serum levels of pituitary hormones may be obtained along with measurements of hormones of target organs (eg, thyroid, adrenal) to assist in diagnosis.

Medical Management

Surgical removal of the pituitary tumor **(hypophysectomy)** through a transsphenoidal approach is the usual treatment. Stereotactic radiation therapy, which requires use of a neurosurgery-type stereotactic frame, may be used to deliver external beam radiation therapy precisely to the pituitary tumor with minimal effect on normal tissue (see Chapter 16). Other treatments include conventional radiation therapy, bromocriptine (Parlodel, a dopamine antagonist), and octreotide (Sandostatin, a synthetic analogue of GH). These medications inhibit the production or release of GH and may bring about marked improvement of symptoms. Octreotide and lanreotide (Somatuline Depot, a somatostatin analogue) may also be used preoperatively to improve the patient's clinical condition and to shrink the tumor (Melmed, 2006).

Surgical Management

Hypophysectomy is the treatment of choice in patients with Cushing's syndrome resulting from excessive production of ACTH by a pituitary tumor. Hypophysectomy may also be performed on occasion as a palliative measure to relieve bone pain secondary to metastasis of malignant lesions of the breast and prostate.

Several approaches are used to remove or destroy the pituitary gland, including surgical removal by transfrontal, subcranial, or oronasal–transsphenoidal approaches; irradiation; and cryosurgery. (The transsphenoidal approach and the nursing management of a patient undergoing cranial surgery are discussed in Chapter 61.) Features or symptoms of acromegaly are unaffected by surgical removal of the tumor.

The absence of the pituitary gland alters the function of many body systems. Menstruation ceases and infertility occurs after total or near-total ablation of the pituitary gland. Replacement therapy with corticosteroids and thyroid hormone is necessary; therefore, patient teaching is imperative (see later discussion).

DIABETES INSIPIDUS

Diabetes insipidus (DI) is a disorder of the posterior lobe of the pituitary gland that is characterized by a deficiency of ADH (vasopressin). Excessive thirst (polydipsia) and large volumes of dilute urine characterize the disorder. It may occur secondary to head trauma, brain tumor, or surgical ablation or irradiation of the pituitary gland. It may also occur with infections of the central nervous system (meningitis, encephalitis, tuberculosis) or with tumors (eg, metastatic disease, lymphoma of the breast or lung). Another cause of DI is failure of the renal tubules to respond to ADH; this nephrogenic form may be related to hypokalemia, hypercalcemia, and a variety of medications (eg, lithium, demeclocycline [Declomycin]).

Clinical Manifestations

Without the action of ADH on the distal nephron of the kidney, an enormous daily output of very dilute, waterlike urine with a specific gravity of 1.001 to 1.005 occurs. The urine contains no abnormal substances such as glucose or albumin. Because of the intense thirst, the patient tends to drink 2 to 20 L of fluid daily and craves cold water. In the hereditary form of DI, the primary symptoms may begin at birth. In adults, the onset of DI may be insidious or abrupt.

The disease cannot be controlled by limiting fluid intake, because the high-volume loss of urine continues even without fluid replacement. Attempts to restrict fluids cause the patient to experience an insatiable craving for fluid and to develop hypernatremia and severe dehydration.

Assessment and Diagnostic Findings

The fluid deprivation test is carried out by withholding fluids for 8 to 12 hours or until 3% to 5% of the body weight is lost. The patient is weighed frequently during the test. Plasma and urine osmolality studies are performed at the beginning and end of the test. The inability to increase the specific gravity and osmolality of the urine is characteristic of DI. The patient continues to excrete large volumes of urine with low specific gravity and experiences weight loss, increasing serum osmolality, and elevated serum sodium levels. The patient's condition needs to be monitored frequently during the test, and the test is terminated if tachycardia, excessive weight loss, or hypotension develops.

Other diagnostic procedures include concurrent measurements of plasma levels of ADH and plasma and urine osmolality as well as a trial of desmopressin (synthetic vasopressin) therapy and intravenous (IV) infusion of hypertonic saline solution. If the diagnosis is confirmed and the cause (eg, head injury) is not obvious, the patient is carefully assessed for tumors that may be causing the disorder.

Medical Management

The objectives of therapy are (1) to replace ADH (which is usually a long-term therapeutic program), (2) to ensure adequate fluid replacement, and (3) to identify and correct the underlying intracranial pathology. Nephrogenic causes require different management approaches.

Pharmacologic Therapy

Desmopressin (DDAVP), a synthetic vasopressin without the vascular effects of natural ADH, is particularly valuable because it has a longer duration of action and fewer adverse effects than other preparations previously used to treat the disease. It is administered intranasally; the patient sprays the solution into the nose through a flexible calibrated plastic tube. One or two administrations daily (ie, every 12 to 24 hours) usually control the symptoms (Tierney, McPhee & Papadakis, 2005). Vasopressin causes vasoconstriction; thus, it must be used cautiously in patients with coronary artery disease.

Intramuscular administration of ADH, vasopressin tannate in oil, is used if the intranasal route is not possible. The medication is administered every 24 to 96 hours. The vial of medication should be warmed or shaken vigorously before administration. The injection is administered in the evening so that maximum results are obtained during sleep. Abdominal cramps are a side effect of this medication. Rotation of injection sites is necessary to prevent lipodystrophy.

Clofibrate (Atromid-S), a hypolipidemic agent, has been found to have an antidiuretic effect on patients with DI who have some residual hypothalamic vasopressin. Chlorpropamide (Diabinese) and thiazide diuretics are also used in mild forms of the disease because they potentiate the action of vasopressin. Hyperglycemia is possible.

If the DI is renal in origin, the previously described treatments are ineffective. Thiazide diuretics, mild salt depletion, and prostaglandin inhibitors (ibuprofen [Advil, Motrin], indomethacin [Indocin], and aspirin) are used to treat the nephrogenic form of DI.

Nursing Management

The nurse must teach the patient and family about follow-up care and emergency measures and provide specific verbal and written instructions, including the actions and side effects of all medications. In addition to demonstrating correct medication administration, the nurse should observe return demonstrations. It is necessary to provide information regarding the signs and symptoms of hyponatremia. Finally, the nurse should advise wearing a medical identification bracelet and carrying medication and information about DI at all times.

SYNDROME OF INAPPROPRIATE ANTIDIURETIC HORMONE SECRETION

The **syndrome of inappropriate antidiuretic hormone (SIADH) secretion** includes excessive ADH secretion from the pituitary gland even in the face of subnormal serum osmolality. Patients cannot excrete a dilute urine, retain fluids, and develop a sodium deficiency known as dilutional hyponatremia. SIADH is often of nonendocrine origin; for instance, the syndrome may occur in patients with bronchogenic carcinoma in which malignant lung cells synthesize and release ADH. SIADH has also occurred in patients with severe pneumonia, pneumothorax, and other disorders of the lungs, as well as malignant tumors that affect other organs (Porth & Matfin, 2009).

Disorders of the central nervous system, such as head injury, brain surgery or tumor, and infection, are thought to produce SIADH by direct stimulation of the pituitary gland. Some medications (eg, vincristine [Oncovin], phenothiazines, tricyclic antidepressants, thiazide diuretics) and nicotine have been implicated in SIADH; they either directly stimulate the pituitary gland or increase the sensitivity of renal tubules to circulating ADH.

Interventions include the elimination of the underlying cause, if possible, and restricting fluid intake. Because retained water is excreted slowly through the kidneys, the extracellular fluid volume contracts and the serum sodium concentration gradually increases toward normal. Diuretics such as furosemide (Lasix) may be used along with fluid restriction if severe hyponatremia is present.

Close monitoring of fluid intake and output, daily weight, urine and blood chemistries, and neurologic status is indicated for the patient at risk for SIADH. Supportive measures and explanations of procedures and treatments assist the patient in managing this disorder.

THE THYROID GLAND

The thyroid gland is a butterfly-shaped organ located in the lower neck, anterior to the trachea (Fig. 42-3). It consists of two lateral lobes connected by an isthmus. The gland is about 5 cm long and 3 cm wide and weighs about 30 g. The blood flow to the thyroid is very high (about 5 mL/min per gram of thyroid tissue), approximately five times the blood flow to the liver. This reflects the high metabolic activity of the thyroid gland. The thyroid gland produces three hormones: **thyroxine (T_4)**, **triiodothyronine (T_3)**, and **calcitonin**.

Anatomic and Physiologic Overview

Various hormones and chemicals are responsible for normal thyroid function. Key among them are thyroid hormone, calcitonin, and iodine.

Thyroid Hormone

T_4 and T_3, which are referred to collectively as thyroid hormone, are two separate hormones produced by the thyroid gland. Both are amino acids that contain iodine molecules bound to the amino acid structure; T_4 contains four iodine atoms in each molecule, and T_3 contains three. These hormones are synthesized and stored bound to proteins in the cells of the thyroid gland until needed for release into the bloodstream. About 75% of bound thyroid hormone is bound to thyroxine-binding globulin (TBG); the remaining bound thyroid hormone is bound to thyroid-binding prealbumin and albumin.

Synthesis of Thyroid Hormone

Iodine is essential to the thyroid gland for synthesis of its hormones. The major use of iodine in the body is by the thyroid, and the major derangement in iodine deficiency is alteration of thyroid function. Iodide is ingested in the diet and absorbed into the blood in the GI tract. The thyroid gland is extremely efficient at taking up iodide from the blood and concentrating it within the cells, where iodide ions are converted to iodine molecules, which react with tyrosine (an amino acid) to form the thyroid hormones.

Regulation of Thyroid Hormone

The secretion of T_3 and T_4 by the thyroid gland is controlled by TSH (also called thyrotropin) from the anterior pituitary gland. TSH controls the rate of thyroid hormone release through a negative feedback mechanism. In turn, the level of thyroid hormone in the blood determines the release of TSH. If the thyroid hormone concentration in the blood decreases, the release of TSH increases, which causes increased output of T_3 and T_4. The term **euthyroid** refers to thyroid hormone production that is within normal limits.

Thyrotropin-releasing hormone (TRH), secreted by the hypothalamus, exerts a modulating influence on the release of TSH from the pituitary. Environmental factors, such as a decrease in temperature, may lead to increased secretion of TRH, resulting in elevated secretion of thyroid hormones. Figure 42-4 shows the hypothalamic–pituitary–thyroid axis, which regulates thyroid hormone production.

Function of Thyroid Hormone

The primary function of thyroid hormone is to control cellular metabolic activity. T_4, a relatively weak hormone, maintains body metabolism in a steady state. T_3 is about five

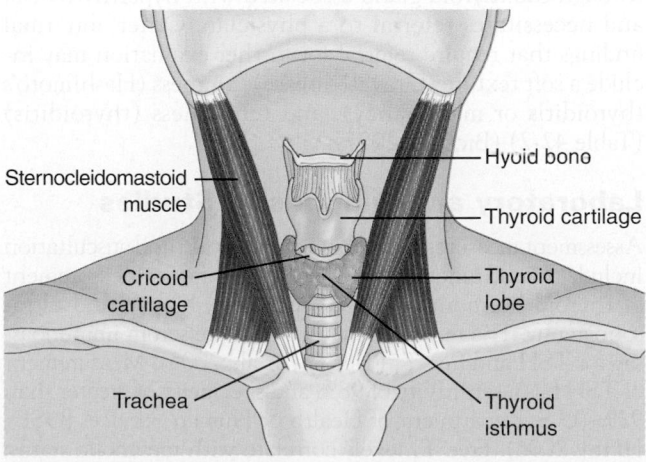

Figure 42-3 The thyroid gland and surrounding structures.

Sternocleidomastoid muscle

Cricoid cartilage

Trachea

Hyoid bone

Thyroid cartilage

Thyroid lobe

Thyroid isthmus

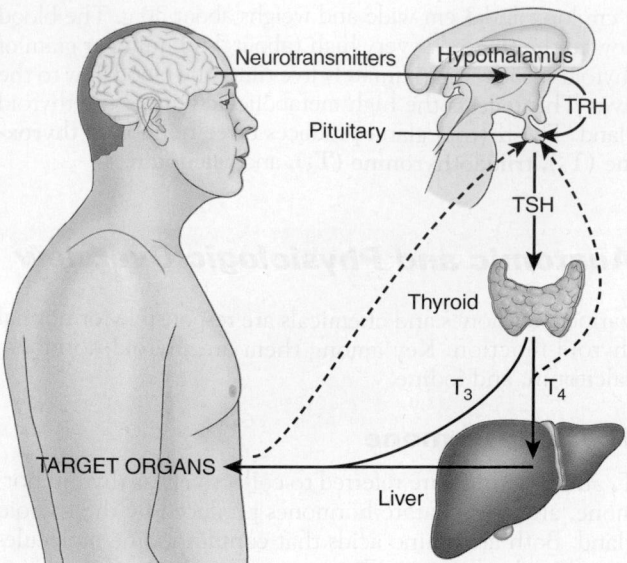

Figure 42-4 The hypothalamic–pituitary–thyroid axis. Thyroid-releasing hormone (TRH) from the hypothalamus stimulates the pituitary gland to secrete thyroid-stimulating hormone (TSH). TSH stimulates the thyroid to produce thyroid hormone (tri-iodothyronine [T_3] and thyroxine [T_4]). High circulating levels of T_3 and T_4 inhibit further TSH secretion and thyroid hormone production through a negative feedback mechanism (*dashed lines*).

times as potent as T_4 and has a more rapid metabolic action. These hormones accelerate metabolic processes by increasing the level of specific enzymes that contribute to oxygen consumption and altering the responsiveness of tissues to other hormones. The thyroid hormones influence cell replication and are important in brain development. Thyroid hormone is also necessary for normal growth. The thyroid hormones, through their widespread effects on cellular metabolism, influence every major organ system.

Calcitonin

Calcitonin, or thyrocalcitonin, is another important hormone secreted by the thyroid gland. It is secreted in response to high plasma levels of calcium, and it reduces the plasma level of calcium by increasing its deposition in bone.

Pathophysiology

Inadequate secretion of thyroid hormone during fetal and neonatal development results in stunted physical and mental growth **(cretinism)** because of general depression of metabolic activity. In adults, hypothyroidism manifests as lethargy, slow mentation, and generalized slowing of body functions.

Oversecretion of thyroid hormones (hyperthyroidism) is manifested by a greatly increased metabolic rate. Many of the other characteristics of hyperthyroidism result from the increased response to circulating catecholamines (epinephrine and norepinephrine). Oversecretion of thyroid hormones is usually associated with an enlarged thyroid gland known as a **goiter.** Goiter also commonly occurs with iodine deficiency. In this latter condition, lack of iodine results in

low levels of circulating thyroid hormones, which causes increased release of TSH; the elevated TSH causes overproduction of thyroglobulin (a precursor of T_3 and T_4) and hypertrophy of the thyroid gland.

Assessment and Diagnostic Findings

Physical Examination

The thyroid gland is inspected and palpated routinely in all patients. Inspection begins with identification of landmarks. The lower neck region between the sternocleidomastoid muscles is inspected for swelling or asymmetry. The patient is instructed to extend the neck slightly and swallow. Thyroid tissue rises normally with swallowing. The thyroid is then palpated for size, shape, consistency, symmetry, and the presence of tenderness (Bickley, 2007).

The clinician may examine the thyroid from an anterior or a posterior position. In the posterior position, both hands encircle the patient's neck. The thumbs rest on the nape of the neck, while the index and middle fingers palpate for the thyroid isthmus and the anterior surfaces of the lateral lobes. When palpable, the isthmus is perceived as firm and of a rubber-band consistency.

The left lobe is examined by positioning the patient so that the neck flexes slightly forward and to the left. The thyroid cartilage is then displaced to the left with the fingers of the right hand. This maneuver displaces the left lobe deep into the sternocleidomastoid muscle, where it can be more easily palpated. The left lobe is then palpated by placing the left thumb deep into the posterior area of the sternocleidomastoid muscle, while the index and middle fingers exert opposite pressure in the anterior portion of the muscle. Having the patient swallow during the maneuver may assist the examiner to locate the thyroid as it ascends in the neck. The procedure is reversed to examine the right lobe. The isthmus is the only portion of the thyroid that is normally palpable. If a patient has a very thin neck, two thin, smooth, nontender lobes may also be palpable.

If palpation discloses an enlarged thyroid gland, both lobes are auscultated using the diaphragm of the stethoscope. Auscultation identifies the localized audible vibration of a bruit. This is indicative of increased blood flow through the thyroid gland associated with hyperthyroidism and necessitates referral to a physician. Other abnormal findings that require referral for further evaluation may include a soft texture (Graves' disease), firmness (Hashimoto's thyroiditis or malignancy), and tenderness (thyroiditis) (Table 42-2) (Bickley, 2007).

Laboratory and Diagnostic Studies

Assessment measures in addition to palpation and auscultation include thyroid function tests, such as laboratory measurement of thyroid hormones, thyroid scanning, biopsy, and ultrasonography. The most widely used tests are serum immunoassay for TSH and free T_4 (Tierney, et al., 2005). Measurement of TSH has a sensitivity of 98% and specificity of greater than 92% (U.S. Department of Health & Human Services [USDHHS], 2006). Free T_4 levels correlate with metabolic status; they are elevated in hyperthyroidism and decreased in

Table 42-2	SUMMARY OF FINDINGS ON PHYSICAL EXAMINATION OF THE THYROID GLAND	
Physical Finding	**Differential Diagnosis**	**Special Features**
Single nodule	Autonomously functioning adenoma	Opposite lobe not palpable
	Adenoma or adenomatous nodule	Rubbery, firm; tenderness suggests recent hemorrhage or infarction
	Cancer	Usually hard; may have associated lymph node enlargement or vocal cord palsy
	Hyperplasia secondary to unilobar agenesis	Opposite lobe not palpable
Multiple nodules	Multinodular goiter	Firm lobes or irregular surface may be misinterpreted as multiple nodules
	Hashimoto's thyroiditis	
Diffuse goiter	Graves' disease	Bruit or thrill; pyramidal lobe
	Hashimoto's thyroiditis	Irregular surface; pyramidal lobe; rubbery or firm; occasionally tender; fibrous variant may be hard
	Thyroid lymphoma	Rapidly growing goiter, particularly in setting of preexisting Hashimoto's thyroiditis
	Multinodular goiter	Nodules may be hidden within gland and may become apparent with thyroid hormone suppression
Tenderness	Subacute thyroiditis	Unilateral or bilateral; tenderness often severe
	Hemorrhagic or infarcted adenoma	Discrete nodule with tenderness
	Hashimoto's thyroiditis	Mild tenderness
	Cancer	Irregular, firm thyroid nodule with chronic tenderness

hypothyroidism. Ultrasound, CT, and MRI may be used to clarify or confirm the results of other diagnostic studies.

Thyroid Tests

Serum Thyroid-Stimulating Hormone

Measurement of the serum TSH concentration is the single best screening test of thyroid function in outpatients because of its high sensitivity. The ability to detect minute changes in serum TSH makes it possible to distinguish subclinical thyroid disease from euthyroid states in patients with low or high normal values. Measurement of TSH is also used for monitoring thyroid hormone replacement therapy and for differentiating between disorders of the thyroid gland itself and disorders of the pituitary or hypothalamus. Current recommendations suggest TSH screening for all adults beginning at 35 years of age and every 5 years thereafter (USDHHS, 2006).

Serum Free T_4

The test most commonly used to confirm an abnormal TSH result is free T_4. It is a direct measurement of free (unbound) thyroxine, the only metabolically active fraction of T_4. The range of free T_4 in serum is normally 0.9 to 1.7 ng/dL (11.5 to 21.8 pmol/L). When measured by the dialysis method, free T_4 is not affected by variations in protein binding and is the procedure of choice for monitoring the changes in T_4 secretion during treatment of hyperthyroidism.

Serum T_3 and T_4

Measurement of total T_3 or T_4 includes protein-bound and free hormone levels that occur in response to TSH secretion. T_4 is 70% bound to TBG; T_3 is bound less firmly. Only 0.03% of T_4 and 0.3% of T_3 are unbound. Serious systemic illnesses, medications (eg, oral contraceptives, corticosteroids, phenytoin, salicylates) and protein wasting as a result of nephrosis or use of androgens may interfere with accurate test results. Normal range for T_4 is 4.5 to 11.5 μg/dL (58.5 to 150 nmol/L). Although serum T_3 and T_4 levels generally increase or decrease together, the T_3 level appears to be a more accurate indicator of hyperthyroidism, which

causes a greater increase in T_3 than in T_4 levels. The normal range for serum T_3 is 70 to 220 ng/dL (1.15 to 3.10 nmol/L).

T_3 Resin Uptake Test

The T_3 resin uptake test is an indirect measure of unsaturated TBG. Its purpose is to determine the amount of thyroid hormone bound to TBG and the number of available binding sites. This provides an index of the amount of thyroid hormone already present in the circulation. Normally, TBG is not fully saturated with thyroid hormone, and additional binding sites are available to combine with radioiodine-labeled T_3 added to the blood specimen. The normal T_3 uptake value is 25% to 35% (relative uptake fraction, 0.25 to 0.35), which indicates that about one third of the available sites of TBG are occupied by thyroid hormone. If the number of free or unoccupied binding sites is low, as in hyperthyroidism, the T_3 uptake is greater than 35% (0.35). If the number of available sites is high, as occurs in hypothyroidism, the test result is less than 25% (0.25).

T_3 uptake is useful in the evaluation of thyroid hormone levels in patients who have received diagnostic or therapeutic doses of iodine. The test results may be altered by the use of estrogens, androgens, salicylates, phenytoin, anticoagulants, or corticosteroids.

Thyroid Antibodies

Autoimmune thyroid diseases include both hypothyroid and hyperthyroid conditions. Results of testing by immunoassay techniques for antithyroid antibodies are positive in chronic autoimmune thyroid disease (90%), Hashimoto's thyroiditis (100%), Graves' disease (80%), and other organ-specific autoimmune diseases, such as lupus erythematosus and rheumatoid arthritis. Antithyroid antibody titers are normally present in 5% to 10% of the population and increase with age.

Radioactive Iodine Uptake

The radioactive iodine uptake test measures the rate of iodine uptake by the thyroid gland. The patient is administered a tracer dose of iodine 123 (^{123}I) or another radionuclide, and a count is made over the thyroid gland with a scintillation counter, which detects and counts the gamma rays released from the breakdown of ^{123}I in the thyroid. It measures the proportion of the administered dose that is present in the thyroid gland at a specific time after its administration. It is a simple test and provides reliable results. It is affected by the patient's intake of iodide or thyroid hormone; therefore, a careful preliminary clinical history is essential in evaluating results. Normal values vary from one geographic region to another and with the intake of iodine. Patients with hyperthyroidism exhibit a high uptake of the ^{123}I (in some patients, as high as 90%), whereas patients with hypothyroidism exhibit a very low uptake.

Fine-Needle Aspiration Biopsy

Use of a small-gauge needle to sample the thyroid tissue for biopsy is a safe and accurate method of detecting malignancy. It is often the initial test for evaluation of thyroid masses. Results are reported as (1) negative (benign), (2) positive (malignant), (3) indeterminate (suspicious), and (4) inadequate (nondiagnostic).

Thyroid Scan, Radioscan, or Scintiscan

In a thyroid scan, a scintillation detector or gamma camera moves back and forth across the area to be studied in a series of parallel tracks, and a visual image is made of the distribution of radioactivity in the area being scanned. Although ^{123}I has been the most commonly used isotope, technetium 99m (^{99m}Tc) pertechnetate, thallium, and americium are also used.

Scans are helpful in determining the location, size, shape, and anatomic function of the thyroid gland, particularly when thyroid tissue is substernal or large. Identifying areas of increased function ("hot" areas) or decreased function ("cold" areas) can assist in diagnosis. Although most areas of decreased function do not represent malignancies, lack of function increases the likelihood of malignancy, particularly if only one nonfunctioning area is present. Scanning of the entire body, to obtain the total body profile, may be carried out in a search for a functioning thyroid metastasis (ie, a lesion that produces thyroid hormones).

Serum Thyroglobulin

Thyroglobulin (Tg) can be measured reliably in the serum by radioimmunoassay. Clinically, it is used to detect persistence or recurrence of thyroid carcinoma.

Nursing Implications

When thyroid tests are scheduled, it is necessary to determine whether the patient has taken medications or agents that contain iodine, because these may alter the test results. Iodine-containing medications include contrast agents and those used to treat thyroid disorders. Less obvious sources of iodine are topical antiseptics, multivitamin preparations, and food supplements frequently found in health food stores; cough syrups; and amiodarone (Cordarone), an antiarrhythmic agent. Other medications that may affect test results are estrogens, salicylates, amphetamines, chemotherapeutic agents, antibiotics, corticosteroids, and mercurial diuretics. The nurse asks the patient about the use of these medications and notes their use on the laboratory requisi-

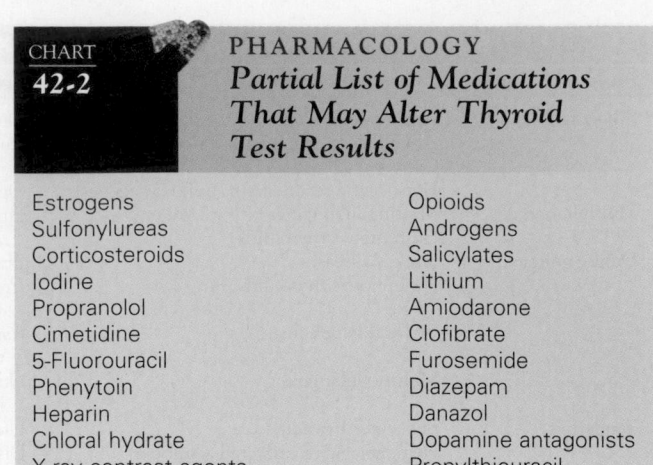

CHART 42-2

PHARMACOLOGY
Partial List of Medications That May Alter Thyroid Test Results

Estrogens	Opioids
Sulfonylureas	Androgens
Corticosteroids	Salicylates
Iodine	Lithium
Propranolol	Amiodarone
Cimetidine	Clofibrate
5-Fluorouracil	Furosemide
Phenytoin	Diazepam
Heparin	Danazol
Chloral hydrate	Dopamine antagonists
X-ray contrast agents	Propylthiouracil

tion. Chart 42-2 gives a partial list of agents that may interfere with accurate testing of thyroid gland function.

Specific Disorders of the Thyroid Gland

HYPOTHYROIDISM

Hypothyroidism results from suboptimal levels of thyroid hormone. Thyroid deficiency can affect all body functions and can range from mild, subclinical forms to **myxedema,** an advanced form. The most common cause of hypothyroidism in adults is autoimmune thyroiditis (Hashimoto's disease), in which the immune system attacks the thyroid gland. Symptoms of hyperthyroidism may later be followed by those of hypothyroidism and myxedema. Hypothyroidism also commonly occurs in patients with previous hyperthyroidism that has been treated with radioiodine or antithyroid medications or thyroidectomy. The condition occurs most frequently in older women. In addition, there is an increased incidence of thyroid cancer in men who have undergone radiation therapy for head and neck cancer. Therefore, testing of thyroid function is recommended for all patients who receive such treatment. Other causes of hypothyroidism are presented in Chart 42-3.

Chart 42-3 • *Causes of Hypothyroidism*

Autoimmune disease (Hashimoto's thyroiditis, post-Graves' disease)
Atrophy of thyroid gland with aging
Therapy for hyperthyroidism
   Radioactive iodine (^{131}I)
   Thyroidectomy
Medications
   Lithium
   Iodine compounds
   Antithyroid medications
Radiation to head and neck for treatment of head and neck cancers, lymphoma
Infiltrative diseases of the thyroid (amyloidosis, scleroderma, lymphoma)
Iodine deficiency and iodine excess

More than 95% of patients with hypothyroidism have primary or thyroidal hypothyroidism, which refers to dysfunction of the thyroid gland itself. If the cause of the thyroid dysfunction is failure of the pituitary gland, the hypothalamus, or both, the hypothyroidism is known as central hypothyroidism. If the cause is entirely a pituitary disorder, it may be referred to as pituitary or secondary hypothyroidism. If the cause is a disorder of the hypothalamus resulting in inadequate secretion of TSH due to decreased stimulation of TRH, it is referred to as hypothalamic or tertiary hypothyroidism. If thyroid deficiency is present at birth, it is referred to as cretinism. In such instances, the mother may also have thyroid deficiency.

The term *myxedema* refers to the accumulation of mucopolysaccharides in subcutaneous and other interstitial tissues. Although myxedema occurs in long-standing hypothyroidism, the term is used appropriately only to describe the extreme symptoms of severe hypothyroidism.

Clinical Manifestations

Extreme fatigue makes it difficult for the person to complete a full day's work or participate in usual activities. Reports of hair loss, brittle nails, and dry skin are common, and numbness and tingling of the fingers may occur. On occasion, the voice may become husky, and the patient may complain of hoarseness. Menstrual disturbances such as menorrhagia or amenorrhea occur, in addition to loss of libido. Hypothyroidism affects women five times more frequently than men and occurs most often between 40 and 70 years of age. The prevalence of the disease increases with increasing age.

Severe hypothyroidism results in a subnormal body temperature and pulse rate. The patient usually begins to gain weight even without an increase in food intake, although he or she may be cachectic. The skin becomes thickened because of an accumulation of mucopolysaccharides in the subcutaneous tissues. The hair thins and falls out, and the face becomes expressionless and masklike. The patient often complains of being cold even in a warm environment.

At first, the patient may be irritable and may complain of fatigue, but as the condition progresses, the emotional responses are subdued. The mental processes become dulled, and the patient appears apathetic. Speech is slow, the tongue enlarges, and the hands and feet increase in size, and deafness may occur. The patient frequently complains of constipation.

Advanced hypothyroidism may produce personality and cognitive changes characteristic of dementia. Inadequate ventilation and sleep apnea can occur with severe hypothyroidism. Pleural effusion, pericardial effusion, and respiratory muscle weakness may also occur.

Severe hypothyroidism is associated with an elevated serum cholesterol level, atherosclerosis, coronary artery disease, and poor left ventricular function. The patient with advanced hypothyroidism is hypothermic and abnormally sensitive to sedatives, opioids, and anesthetic agents, which must be administered with extreme caution.

Patients with unrecognized hypothyroidism who are undergoing surgery are at increased risk for intraoperative hypotension, postoperative heart failure, and altered mental status.

Myxedema coma is a rare life-threatening condition. It is the decompensated state of severe hypothyroidism in which the patient is hypothermic and unconscious (Kwaku & Burman, 2007). This condition may develop with undiagnosed hypothyroidism and may be precipitated by infection or other systemic disease or by use of sedatives or opioid analgesic agents. The condition occurs most often among elderly women in the winter months and appears to be precipitated by cold. However, the disorder can affect any age group.

In myxedema coma, the patient may initially show signs of depression, diminished cognitive status, lethargy, and somnolence (Kwaku & Burman, 2007). Increasing lethargy may progress to stupor. The patient's respiratory drive is depressed, resulting in alveolar hypoventilation, progressive carbon dioxide retention, narcosis, and coma. These symptoms, along with cardiovascular collapse and shock, require aggressive and intensive supportive and hemodynamic therapy if the patient is to survive. Although there has been a decline in mortality rates over the past two decades due to early intervention and improved therapies, the mortality rate (20% to 25%) remains high even with vigorous treatment (Kwaku & Burman, 2007).

NURSING ALERT

In all patients with hypothyroidism, the effects of analgesic agents, sedatives, and anesthetic agents are prolonged; special caution is necessary in administering these agents to elderly patients because of concurrent changes in liver and renal function.

Medical Management

The primary objective in the management of hypothyroidism is to restore a normal metabolic state by replacing the missing hormone.

Pharmacologic Therapy

Synthetic levothyroxine (Synthroid or Levothroid) is the preferred preparation for treating hypothyroidism and suppressing nontoxic goiters. Its dosage is based on the patient's serum TSH concentration. Desiccated thyroid is used infrequently today, because it often results in transient elevated serum concentrations of T_3, with occasional symptoms of hyperthyroidism. If replacement therapy is adequate, the symptoms of myxedema disappear and normal metabolic activity is resumed.

Prevention of Cardiac Dysfunction

Any patient who has had hypothyroidism for a long period is almost certain to have elevated serum cholesterol, atherosclerosis, and coronary artery disease. As long as metabolism is subnormal and the tissues, including the myocardium, require relatively little oxygen, a reduction in blood supply is tolerated without overt symptoms of coronary artery disease. When thyroid hormone is administered, the oxygen demand increases, but oxygen delivery cannot be increased unless, or until, the atherosclerosis improves. This occurs very slowly, if at all. The occurrence of angina is the signal that the oxygen needs of the myocardium exceed its blood supply. Angina or dysrhythmias can occur when thyroid replacement is initiated because thyroid hormones enhance the cardiovascular effects of catecholamines.

NURSING ALERT

The nurse must monitor for myocardial ischemia or infarction, which can occur in response to therapy in patients with severe, long-standing hypothyroidism or myxedema coma. The nurse must also be alert for signs of angina, especially during the early phase of treatment; if detected, it must be reported and treated at once to avoid a fatal myocardial infarction.

Obviously, if angina or dysrhythmias occur, thyroid hormone administration must be discontinued immediately. Later, when it can be resumed safely, it should be prescribed cautiously at a lower dosage and under the close observation of the physician and the nurse.

Prevention of Medication Interactions

Precautions must be taken during the course of therapy because thyroid hormones may interact with other medications. Thyroid hormones may increase blood glucose levels, which may necessitate adjustment in the dosage of insulin or oral antidiabetic agents in patients with diabetes. Thyroid hormones may also increase the pharmacologic effects of digitalis glycosides, anticoagulant agents, and indomethacin (Indocin). Phenytoin (Dilantin) and tricyclic antidepressant agents may increase the effects of thyroid hormone. Bone loss and osteoporosis may also occur with thyroid therapy.

Even in small doses, hypnotic and sedative agents may induce profound somnolence, lasting far longer than anticipated and leading to narcosis (stuporlike condition). Furthermore, they are likely to cause respiratory depression, which can easily be fatal because of decreased respiratory reserve and alveolar hypoventilation. The dose of these medications should be one half or one third of that typically prescribed for patients of similar age and weight with normal thyroid function.

Supportive Therapy

In severe hypothyroidism and myxedema coma, management includes maintaining vital functions. Arterial blood gases may be measured to determine carbon dioxide retention and to guide the use of assisted ventilation to combat hypoventilation. Oxygen saturation levels should be monitored using pulse oximetry. Fluids are administered cautiously because of the danger of water intoxication. Application of external heat (eg, heating pads) is avoided, because it increases oxygen requirements and may lead to vascular collapse. If hypoglycemia is evident, concentrated glucose may be prescribed to provide glucose without precipitating fluid overload. If myxedema has progressed to myxedema coma, thyroid hormone (usually levothyroxine [Synthroid]) is administered intravenously until consciousness is restored. Treatment then continues with oral thyroid hormone therapy. Because of an associated adrenocortical insufficiency, corticosteroid therapy may be necessary.

Nursing Management

Nursing care of the patient with hypothyroidism and myxedema is summarized in the plan of nursing care in Chart 42-4.

NURSING ALERT

Medications are administered to the patient with hypothyroidism with extreme caution because of the potential for altered metabolism and excretion as well as depressed metabolic rate and respiratory status.

Promoting Home and Community-Based Care

Teaching Patients Self-Care

The patient and family require education and support to manage this complex disorder at home. Oral and written instructions should be provided regarding the following:

- Desired actions and side effects of medications
- Correct medication administration
- Importance of continuing to take the medications as prescribed even after symptoms improve
- When to seek medical attention
- Importance of nutrition and diet to promote weight loss and normal bowel patterns
- Importance of periodic follow-up testing

The patient and family should be informed that many of the symptoms observed during the course of the disorder will disappear with effective treatment (Chart 42-5).

Continuing Care

If indicated, a referral is made for home care. The home care nurse monitors the patient's recovery and ability to cope with the recent changes, along with the patient's physical and cognitive status and the patient's and family's understanding of the instructions provided before hospital discharge. The home care nurse documents and reports to the patient's primary health care provider subtle signs and symptoms that may indicate either inadequate or excessive thyroid hormone.

 Gerontologic Considerations

The prevalence of hypothyroidism increases with age, most often among women. The higher prevalence of hypothyroidism among elderly people may be related to alterations in immune function with age and complicated by multiple comorbidities. Screening of TSH levels is recommended for women older than 50 years of age who have one or more symptoms, because they are at high risk for hypothyroidism (USDHHS, 2006). It is estimated that approximately 10% of women 65 years of age and 15% of those older than 75 years of age experience hypothyroidism (Singer, 2006).

Most patients with primary hypothyroidism present with long-standing mild to moderate hypothyroidism. Subclinical disease is common among older women and can be asymptomatic or mistaken for other medical conditions. Subtle symptoms of hypothyroidism, such as fatigue, muscle aches, and mental confusion, may be attributed to the normal aging process by patients, families, and health care

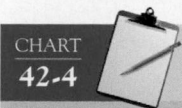

CHART
42-4

PLAN OF NURSING CARE
Care of the Patient With Hypothyroidism

NURSING DIAGNOSIS: Activity intolerance related to fatigue and depressed cognitive process
GOAL: Increased participation in activities and increased independence

Nursing Interventions	Rationale	Expected Outcomes

1. Promote independence in self-care activities.
  a. Space activities to promote rest and exercise as tolerated.
  b. Assist with self-care activities when patient is fatigued.
  c. Provide stimulation through conversation and nonstressful activities.
  d. Monitor patient's response to increasing activities
	1. Encouragement needed in fatigued, often depressed patient
	  a. Encourages activities while allowing time for adequate rest
	  b. Permits patient to participate to the extent possible in self-care activities
	  c. Promotes interest without overly stressing the patient
	  d. Guards against over- and under-exertion by the patient
		• Participates in self-care activities
		• Reports decreased level of fatigue
		• Displays interest and awareness in environment
		• Participates in activities and events in environment
		• Participates in family events and activities
		• Reports no chest pain, increased fatigue, or breathlessness with increased level of activity

NURSING DIAGNOSIS: Risk for imbalanced body temperature
GOAL: Maintenance of normal body temperature

Nursing Interventions	Rationale	Expected Outcomes
1. Provide extra layer of clothing or extra blanket. 2. Avoid and discourage use of external heat source (eg, heating pads, electric or warming blankets). 3. Monitor patient's body temperature and report decreases from patient's baseline value. 4. Protect from exposure to cold and drafts.	1. Minimizes heat loss 2. Reduces risk of peripheral vasodilation and vascular collapse 3. Detects decreased body temperature and onset of myxedema coma 4. Increases patient's level of comfort and decreases further heat loss	• Experiences relief of discomfort and cold intolerance • Maintains baseline body temperature • Reports adequate feeling of warmth and lack of chilling • Uses extra layer of clothing or extra blanket • Explains rationale for avoiding external heat source

NURSING DIAGNOSIS: Constipation related to depressed gastrointestinal function
GOAL: Return of normal bowel function

Nursing Interventions	Rationale	Expected Outcomes
1. Encourage increased fluid intake within limits of fluid restriction. 2. Provide foods high in fiber. 3. Instruct patient about foods with high water content. 4. Monitor bowel function. 5. Encourage increased mobility within patient's exercise tolerance. 6. Encourage patient to use laxatives and enemas sparingly.	1. Promotes passage of soft stools 2. Increases bulk of stools and more frequent bowel movements 3. Provides rationale for patient to increase fluid intake 4. Permits detection of constipation and return to normal bowel pattern 5. Promotes evacuation of the bowel 6. Minimizes patient's dependence on laxatives and enemas and encourages normal pattern of bowel evacuation	• Reports normal bowel function • Identifies and consumes foods high in fiber • Drinks recommended amount of fluid each day • Participates in gradually increasing exercises • Uses laxatives as prescribed and avoids excessive dependence on laxatives and enemas

NURSING DIAGNOSIS: Deficient knowledge about the therapeutic regimen for lifelong thyroid replacement therapy
GOAL: Knowledge and acceptance of the prescribed therapeutic regimen

Nursing Interventions	Rationale	Expected Outcomes
1. Explain rationale for thyroid hormone replacement. 2. Describe desired effects of medication to patient.	1. Provides rationale for patient to use thyroid hormone replacement as prescribed 2. Provides encouragement to patient by identifying improved physical status and well-being that will occur with thyroid hormone therapy and return to a euthyroid state	• Describes therapeutic regimen correctly • Explains rationale for thyroid hormone replacement • Identifies positive outcomes of thyroid hormone replacement

Continued on following page

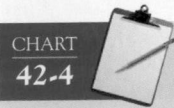

CHART 42-4 PLAN OF NURSING CARE
Care of the Patient With Hypothyroidism (*Continued*)

Nursing Interventions	Rationale	Expected Outcomes
3. Assist patient to develop schedule and checklist to ensure self-administration of thyroid replacement. 4. Describe signs and symptoms of over- and underdose of medication. 5. Explain the necessity for long-term follow-up to patient and family	3. Increases chances that medication will be taken as prescribed 4. Serves as check for patient to determine if therapeutic goals are met 5. Increases likelihood that hypo- or hyperthyroidism will be detected and treated	• Administers medication to self as prescribed • Identifies adverse side effects that should be reported promptly to physician: recurrence of symptoms of hypothyroidism and occurrence of symptoms of hyperthyroidism • Restates need for periodic/long-term follow-up visits to physician

NURSING DIAGNOSIS: Ineffective breathing pattern related to depressed ventilation
GOAL: Improved respiratory status and maintenance of normal breathing pattern

Nursing Interventions	Rationale	Expected Outcomes
1. Monitor respiratory rate, depth, pattern, pulse oximetry, and arterial blood gases. 2. Encourage deep breathing, coughing, and use of incentive spirometry. 3. Administer medications (hypnotics and sedatives) with caution. 4. Maintain patent airway through suction and ventilatory support if indicated (see Chapter 25 for care of patients requiring mechanical ventilation).	1. Identifies patient's baseline to monitor further changes and evaluate effectiveness of interventions 2. Prevents atelectasis and promotes adequate ventilation 3. Patients with hypothyroidism are very susceptible to respiratory depression with use of hypnotics and sedatives. 4. Use of an artificial airway and ventilatory support may be necessary with respiratory depression.	• Shows improved respiratory status and maintenance of normal breathing pattern • Demonstrates normal respiratory rate, depth, and pattern • Takes deep breaths, coughs, and uses incentive spirometry when encouraged • Demonstrates normal breath sounds without adventitious sounds on auscultation • Explains rationale for cautious use of medications • Cooperates with suction procedure and ventilator support when necessary

NURSING DIAGNOSIS: Disturbed thought processes related to depressed metabolism and altered cardiovascular and respiratory status
GOAL: Improved thought processes

Nursing Interventions	Rationale	Expected Outcomes
1. Orient patient to time, place, date, and events around him or her. 2. Provide stimulation through conversation and nonthreatening activities. 3. Explain to patient and family that change in cognitive and mental functioning is a result of disease process. 4. Monitor cognitive and mental processes and response of these to medication and other therapy.	1. Provides reality orientation to patient 2. Provides stimulation within patient's level of tolerance for stress 3. Reassures patient and family about the cause of the cognitive changes and that a positive outcome is possible with appropriate treatment 4. Permits evaluation of the effectiveness of treatment	• Shows improved cognitive functioning • Identifies time, place, date, and events correctly • Responds when stimulated • Responds spontaneously as treatment becomes effective • Interacts spontaneously with family and environment • Explains that change in mental and cognitive processes is a result of disease processes • Takes medications as prescribed to prevent decrease in cognitive processes

COLLABORATIVE PROBLEM: Myxedema and myxedema coma
GOAL: Absence of complications

Nursing Interventions	Rationale	Expected Outcomes

1. Monitor patient for increasing severity of signs and symptoms of hypothyroidism:
  a. Decreased level of consciousness; dementia
  b. Decreased vital signs (blood pressure, respiratory rate, temperature, pulse rate)
  c. Increasing difficulty in awakening or arousing patient
	1. Extreme hypothyroidism may lead to myxedema, myxedema coma, and slowing of all body systems if untreated.	• Exhibits reversal of myxedema and myxedema coma
		• Responds appropriately to questions and surroundings
		• Vital signs return to normal or near-normal ranges
		• Respiratory status improves with adequate spontaneous ventilatory effort

Continued

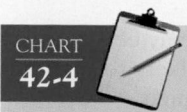

CHART 42-4

PLAN OF NURSING CARE
Care of the Patient With Hypothyroidism (Continued)

Nursing Interventions	Rationale	Expected Outcomes
2. Assist in ventilatory support if respiratory depression and failure occur.	2. Ventilatory support is necessary to maintain adequate oxygenation and maintenance of airway.	• Reports no episodes of angina or other indicators of cardiac insufficiency
3. Administer prescribed medications (eg, thyroxine) with extreme caution.	3. The slow metabolism and atherosclerosis of myxedema may result in angina with administration of thyroxine.	• Experiences minimal or no complications caused by immobility
4. Turn and reposition patient at intervals.	4. Minimizes risks associated with immobility	
5. Avoid use of hypnotic, sedative, and analgesic agents.	5. Altered metabolism of these agents greatly increases the risks of their use in myxedema.	

providers; therefore, these symptoms require close attention (Dominguez, Bevilacqua, DiBella, et al., 2008). In addition, signs and symptoms of hypothyroidism in elderly people are often atypical, and manifestations of hypothyroidism and hyperthyroidism may blur. Patients may have few or no symptoms until dysfunction is severe. Depression, apathy, and decreased mobility or activity may be the major initial symptoms and may be accompanied by significant weight loss. Constipation affects one fourth of elderly patients.

In elderly patients with mild to moderate hypothyroidism, thyroid hormone replacement is individually tailored and must be started with low dosages and increased gradually to prevent serious cardiovascular and neurologic side effects. Angina, for example, may occur with rapid thyroid replacement in the presence of coronary artery disease secondary to the hypothyroid state. Heart failure and tachydysrhythmias may worsen during the transition from the hypothyroid state to the normal metabolic state. Dementia

may become more apparent during early thyroid hormone replacement in elderly patients.

Elderly patients with severe hypothyroidism and atherosclerosis may become confused and agitated if their metabolic rate is increased too quickly. Marked clinical improvement follows the administration of hormone replacement; such medication must be continued for life, even though signs of hypothyroidism disappear within 3 to 12 weeks.

Myxedema and myxedema coma usually occur exclusively in patients older than 50 years of age (Kwaku & Burman, 2007). The high mortality rate of myxedema coma mandates immediate IV administration of high doses of thyroid hormone as well as supportive care.

Elderly patients require periodic follow-up monitoring of serum TSH levels, because poor compliance with therapy may occur or the patient may take the medications erratically. A careful history can identify the need for further teaching about the importance of the medication.

CHART 42-5

HOME CARE CHECKLIST
The Patient With Hypothyroidism (Myxedema)

At the completion of the home care instruction, the patient or caregiver will be able to:	PATIENT	CAREGIVER
• State present and potential effects of hypothyroidism on the body.	✔	✔
• State precipitating factors and interventions for complications (hyperthyroidism, myxedema coma).	✔	✔
• Explain the purpose, dose, route, schedule, side effects, and precautions of prescribed medication (synthetic thyroid hormone).	✔	✔
• State that compliance with medical regimen is lifelong.	✔	✔
• State the need to avoid extreme cold temperature until condition is stable.	✔	✔
• State importance of regular follow-up visits with health care provider.	✔	✔
• Identify dietary strategies to promote weight reduction and prevent constipation (high fiber, low calorie, adequate fluid intake).	✔	✔
• State potential for menstrual irregularities and potential for pregnancy for women.	✔	✔
• State the importance of avoiding infection.	✔	✔
• Identify changes in personality as related to hypothyroidism.	✔	✔
• Identify areas of activity limitations and impact on lifestyle.	✔	✔

HYPERTHYROIDISM

Hyperthyroidism is the second most prevalent endocrine disorder, after diabetes mellitus. **Graves' disease,** the most common type of hyperthyroidism, results from an excessive output of thyroid hormones caused by abnormal stimulation of the thyroid gland by circulating immunoglobulins (Porth & Matfin, 2009). It affects women eight times more frequently than men, with onset usually between the second and fourth decades (Tierney, et al., 2005). The disorder may appear after an emotional shock, stress, or an infection, but the exact significance of these relationships is not understood. Other common causes of hyperthyroidism include thyroiditis and excessive ingestion of thyroid hormone.

Clinical Manifestations

Patients with well-developed hyperthyroidism exhibit a characteristic group of signs and symptoms (sometimes referred to as **thyrotoxicosis**). The presenting symptom is often nervousness. These patients are often emotionally hyperexcitable, irritable, and apprehensive; they cannot sit quietly; they suffer from palpitations; and their pulse is abnormally rapid at rest as well as on exertion. They tolerate heat poorly and perspire unusually freely. The skin is flushed continuously, with a characteristic salmon color, and is likely to be warm, soft, and moist. However, patients may report dry skin and diffuse pruritus. A fine tremor of the hands may be observed. Patients may exhibit ophthalmopathy, such as **exophthalmos** (bulging eyes), which produces a startled facial expression. Despite treatment, these ocular changes are not always reversible. Patients should be informed that smoking has been shown to aggravate ocular changes (Asvold, Bjoro, Nilsen, et al., 2007).

Other manifestations include an increased appetite and dietary intake, progressive weight loss, abnormal muscular fatigability and weakness (difficulty in climbing stairs and rising from a chair), amenorrhea, and changes in bowel function. The pulse rate ranges constantly between 90 and 160 bpm; the systolic, but characteristically not the diastolic, blood pressure is elevated; atrial fibrillation may occur; and cardiac decompensation in the form of heart failure is common, especially in elderly patients. Osteoporosis and fracture are also associated with hyperthyroidism.

Cardiac effects may include sinus tachycardia or dysrhythmias, increased pulse pressure, and palpitations; these changes may be related to increased sensitivity to catecholamines or to changes in neurotransmitter turnover. Myocardial hypertrophy and heart failure may occur if the hyperthyroidism is severe and untreated.

The course of the disease may be mild, characterized by remissions and exacerbations, and terminate with spontaneous recovery in a few months or years. Conversely, it may progress relentlessly, with the untreated person becoming emaciated, intensely nervous, delirious, and even disoriented; eventually, the heart fails.

Symptoms of hyperthyroidism may occur with the release of excessive amounts of thyroid hormone as a result of inflammation after irradiation of the thyroid or destruction of thyroid tissue by tumor. Such symptoms may also occur with excessive administration of thyroid hormone for treatment of hypothyroidism. Long-standing use of thyroid hormone in the absence of close monitoring may be a cause of symptoms of hyperthyroidism. It is also likely to result in premature osteoporosis, particularly in women.

Assessment and Diagnostic Findings

The thyroid gland invariably is enlarged to some extent. It is soft and may pulsate; a thrill often can be palpated, and a bruit is heard over the thyroid arteries. These are signs of greatly increased blood flow through the thyroid gland. In advanced cases, the diagnosis is made on the basis of the symptoms, a decrease in serum TSH, increased free T_4, and an increase in radioactive iodine uptake.

Medical Management

Appropriate treatment of hyperthyroidism depends on the underlying cause and often consists of a combination of therapies, including antithyroid agents, radioactive iodine, and surgery. Treatment of hyperthyroidism is directed toward reducing thyroid hyperactivity to relieve symptoms and preventing complications. Use of radioactive iodine is the most common form of treatment for Graves' disease in North America. Beta-adrenergic blocking agents (eg, propranolol [Inderal]) are used as adjunctive therapy for symptomatic relief, particularly in transient thyroiditis (Cooper, 2005). Surgical removal of most of the thyroid gland is a nonpharmacologic alternative.

No treatment for thyrotoxicosis is without side effects, and all three treatments (radioactive iodine therapy, antithyroid medications, and surgery) share the same complications: relapse or recurrent hyperthyroidism and permanent hypothyroidism. The rate of relapse increases in patients who have had very severe disease, a long history of dysfunction, ocular and cardiac symptoms, large goiter, or relapse after previous treatment. The relapse rate after radioactive iodine therapy depends on the dose used in treatment. Patients receiving a lower dose of radioactive iodine are more likely to require subsequent treatment than those treated with a higher dose. The remission rate achieved with a single dose of radioactive iodine is 80% (Reid & Wheeler, 2005, Brent, 2008).

Pharmacologic Therapy

Two forms of pharmacotherapy are available for treating hyperthyroidism and controlling excessive thyroid activity: (1) use of irradiation by administration of the radioisotope iodine 131 (^{131}I) for destructive effects on the thyroid gland and (2) antithyroid medications that interfere with the synthesis of thyroid hormones and other agents that control manifestations of hyperthyroidism.

Radioactive Iodine Therapy

The goal of radioactive iodine therapy (^{131}I) is to destroy the overactive thyroid cells. Almost all the iodine that enters and is retained in the body becomes concentrated in the thyroid gland. Therefore, the radioactive isotope of iodine is concentrated in the thyroid gland, where it destroys thyroid cells without jeopardizing other radiosensitive tissues. Over a period of several weeks, thyroid cells exposed to the radioactive iodine are destroyed, resulting in reduction of the hyperthyroid state and inevitably hypothyroidism.

Chart 42-6• *Thyroid Storm (Thyrotoxic Crisis, Thyrotoxicosis)*

Thyroid storm (thyrotoxic crisis) is a form of severe hyperthyroidism, usually of abrupt onset. Untreated, it is almost always fatal, but with proper treatment the mortality rate is reduced substantially. The patient with thyroid storm or crisis is critically ill and requires astute observation and aggressive and supportive nursing care during and after the acute stage of illness.

Clinical Manifestations

Thyroid storm is characterized by:

- High fever (hyperpyrexia) above 38.5°C (101.3°F)
- Extreme tachycardia (more than 130 bpm)
- Exaggerated symptoms of hyperthyroidism with disturbances of a major system—for example, gastrointestinal (weight loss, diarrhea, abdominal pain) or cardiovascular (edema, chest pain, dyspnea, palpitations)
- Altered neurologic or mental state, which frequently appears as delirium psychosis, somnolence, or coma

Life-threatening thyroid storm is usually precipitated by stress, such as injury, infection, thyroid and nonthyroid surgery, tooth extraction, insulin reaction, diabetic ketoacidosis, pregnancy, digitalis intoxication, abrupt withdrawal of antithyroid medications, extreme emotional stress, or vigorous palpation of the thyroid. These factors can precipitate thyroid storm in the partially controlled or completely untreated patient with hyperthyroidism. Current methods of diagnosis and treatment for hyperthyroidism have greatly decreased the incidence of thyroid storm, making it uncommon today.

Management

Immediate objectives are reduction of body temperature and heart rate and prevention of vascular collapse. Measures to accomplish these objectives include:

- A hypothermia mattress or blanket, ice packs, a cool environment, hydrocortisone, and acetaminophen (Tylenol). Salicylates (eg, aspirin) are not used because they displace thyroid hormone from binding proteins and worsen the hypermetabolism.
- Humidified oxygen is administered to improve tissue oxygenation and meet the high metabolic demands. Arterial blood gas levels or pulse oximetry may be used to monitor respiratory status.
- Intravenous fluids containing dextrose are administered to replace liver glycogen stores that have been decreased in the hyperthyroid patient.
- PTU or methimazole is administered to impede formation of thyroid hormone and block conversion of T_4 to T_3, the more active form of thyroid hormone.
- Hydrocortisone is prescribed to treat shock or adrenal insufficiency.
- Iodine is administered to decrease output of T_4 from the thyroid gland. For cardiac problems such as atrial fibrillation, dysrhythmias, and heart failure, sympatholytic agents may be administered. Propranolol, combined with digitalis, has been effective in reducing severe cardiac symptoms.

The patient is instructed about what to expect with this tasteless, colorless radioiodine, which may be administered by the radiologist. Typically, a single dose is needed (Reid & Wheeler, 2005). About 95% of patients are cured by one dose of radioactive iodine. The additional 5% require two doses; rarely is a third dose necessary. Use of an ablative dose of radioactive iodine initially causes an acute release of thyroid hormone from the thyroid gland and may cause increased symptoms. The patient is observed for signs of **thyroid storm** (Chart 42-6), a life-threatening condition manifested by cardiac dysrhythmias, fever, and neurologic impairment (Harris, 2007). Propranolol (Inderal) is useful in controlling these symptoms.

After treatment with radioactive iodine, the patient is monitored closely until the euthyroid state is reached. In 3 to 4 weeks, symptoms of hyperthyroidism subside. Close follow-up is required to evaluate thyroid function, because the incidence of hypothyroidism after this form of treatment is very high. Approximately 20% of patients become hypothyroid within 2 years after treatment, and another 3% to 5% of patients each year thereafter (Reid & Wheeler, 2005). Thyroid hormone replacement is necessary; small doses are usually prescribed, with the dose gradually increased over a period of months (up to about 1 year) until the free T_4 and TSH levels stabilize within normal ranges.

Radioactive iodine has been used to treat toxic adenomas, multinodular goiter, and most varieties of thyrotoxicosis (rarely with permanent success). It is preferred for treating patients beyond the childbearing years who have diffuse toxic goiter. Radioactive iodine is contraindicated during pregnancy (because it crosses the placenta) and while breast-feeding (because it is secreted in breast milk) to prevent hypothyroidism in the fetus (Cooper, Doherty, Haugen, et al., 2006). Pregnancy should be postponed for at least 6 months after treatment.

A major advantage of treatment with radioactive iodine is that it avoids many of the side effects associated with antithyroid medications. However, some patients and their families fear medications that are radioactive. For this reason, patients may elect to take antithyroid medications rather than radioactive iodine.

Antithyroid Medications

Antithyroid medications are summarized in Table 42-3. The objective of pharmacotherapy is to inhibit one or more stages in thyroid hormone synthesis or hormone release. Antithyroid agents block the utilization of iodine by interfering with the iodination of tyrosine and the coupling of iodotyrosines in the synthesis of thyroid hormones. This prevents the synthesis of thyroid hormone. Most commonly, propylthiouracil (PTU) or methimazole (Tapazole) is used until the patient is euthyroid (ie, neither hyperthyroid nor hypothyroid). These medications block extrathyroidal conversion of T_4 to T_3.

The therapeutic dose is determined on the basis of clinical criteria, including changes in pulse rate, pulse pressure, body weight, size of the goiter, and results of laboratory studies of thyroid function. Because antithyroid

Table 42-3	PHARMACOLOGIC AGENTS USED TO TREAT HYPERTHYROIDISM	
Agent	**Action**	**Nursing Considerations**
Propylthiouracil (PTU)	Blocks synthesis of hormones (conversion of T_3 to T_4)	Monitor cardiac parameters. Observe for conversion to hypothyroidism. Must be given by mouth. Watch for rash, nausea, vomiting, agranulocytosis, lupus syndrome.
Methimazole	Blocks synthesis of thyroid hormone	More toxic than PTU. Watch for rash and other symptoms as for PTU.
Sodium iodide	Suppresses release of thyroid hormone	Given 1 h after PTU or methimazole. Watch for edema, hemorrhage, gastrointestinal upset.
Potassium iodide	Suppresses release of thyroid hormone	Discontinue for rash. Watch for signs of toxic iodinism.
Saturated solution of potassium iodide (SSKI)	Suppresses release of thyroid hormone	Mix with juice or milk. Give by straw to prevent staining of teeth.
Dexamethasone	Suppresses release of thyroid hormone	Monitor input and output. Monitor glucose. May cause hypertension, nausea, vomiting, anorexia, infection.
Beta-blocker (eg, propranolol)	Beta-adrenergic blocking agent	Monitor cardiac status. Hold for bradycardia or decreased cardiac output. Use with caution in patients with heart failure.

Adapted from Morton, P. G. & Fontaine, D. K. (2009). *Critical care nursing: A holistic approach*. Philadelphia: Lippincott Williams & Wilkins.

medications do not interfere with release or activity of previously formed thyroid hormones, it may take several weeks until relief of symptoms occurs. At that time, the maintenance dose is established, and a gradual withdrawal of the medication over the next several months follows.

Toxic complications of antithyroid medications are relatively uncommon; nevertheless, the importance of periodic follow-up is emphasized, because medication sensitization, fever, rash, urticaria, or even agranulocytosis and thrombocytopenia (decrease in granulocytes and platelets) may develop. With any sign of infection, especially pharyngitis and fever or the occurrence of mouth ulcers, the patient is advised to stop the medication, notify the physician immediately, and undergo hematologic studies. Rash, arthralgias, and fever occur in 1% to 5% of patients (Reid & Wheeler, 2005). Agranulocytosis, the most serious toxic side effect, occurs in approximately 0.5% of patients. Its incidence is higher in patients older than 40 years of age. It usually occurs within the first 3 months but may occur up to 1 year after therapy is started.

Patients taking antithyroid medications are instructed not to use decongestants for nasal stuffiness, because these agents are poorly tolerated. PTU is the treatment of choice during pregnancy. Once the thyrotoxicity is under control, the dose is decreased to prevent fetal hypothyroidism. Antithyroid medications are contraindicated in late pregnancy, because they may produce goiter and cretinism in the fetus (Cooper, 2005).

Another goal of therapy is to reduce the amount of thyroid tissue, with resulting decreased thyroid hormone production. Thyroid hormone is occasionally administered with antithyroid medications to put the thyroid gland at rest. In this approach, hypothyroidism from excess antithyroid medication is avoided, as is stimulation of the thyroid gland by TSH. Levothyroxine sodium (Synthroid) is the most common thyroid hormone preparation used. It takes approximately 10 days of its administration to achieve full effect. Liothyronine sodium (Cytomel) has a more rapid

onset, and its action is of short duration. Antithyroid medications may also be used to normalize thyroid function before radioactive iodine is administered, to suppress symptoms of thyrotoxicosis that may occur with this therapy (Cooper, 2005).

Relapse usually occurs within the first 3 to 6 months after medication is stopped. Thereafter, the rate of recurrence decreases and stabilizes after 1 to 2 years, for an overall recurrence rate of approximately 50% to 60% (Cooper, 2005). Discontinuation of antithyroid medications before therapy is complete usually results in relapse within 6 months. The incidence of relapse with subtotal thyroidectomy is 19% at 18 months; an incidence of hypothyroidism of 25% has been reported at 18 months after surgery. The risk of these complications illustrates the importance of long-term follow-up of patients treated for hyperthyroidism. It is important that the possibility of relapse be discussed so that a treatment strategy will be in place if relapse occurs.

Adjunctive Therapy

Iodine or iodide compounds, once the only therapy available for patients with hyperthyroidism, are no longer used as the sole method of treatment. Such compounds decrease the release of thyroid hormones from the thyroid gland and reduce the vascularity and size of the thyroid. Compounds such as potassium iodide (KI), Lugol's solution, and saturated solution of potassium iodide (SSKI) may be used in combination with antithyroid agents or beta-adrenergic blockers to prepare the patient with hyperthyroidism for surgery. These agents reduce the activity of the thyroid hormone and the vascularity of the thyroid gland, making the surgical procedure safer (Brent, 2008). Solutions of iodine and iodide compounds are more palatable in milk or fruit juice and are administered through a straw to prevent staining of the teeth. These compounds reduce the metabolic rate more rapidly than antithyroid medications do, but their action does not last as long.

NURSING ALERT

Patients receiving iodide medications should be observed for the development of goiter and should be cautioned against use of iodide-containing over-the-counter medications that can increase the response to iodide therapy. Cough medications, expectorants, bronchodilators, and salt substitutes may contain iodide and should be avoided.

Beta-adrenergic blocking agents are important in controlling the sympathetic nervous system effects of hyperthyroidism. For example, propranolol is used to control nervousness, tachycardia, tremor, anxiety, and heat intolerance. The patient continues taking propranolol until the free T_4 is within the normal range and the TSH level approaches normal.

Surgical Management

Surgery to remove thyroid tissue was once the primary method of treating hyperthyroidism. Today, surgery is reserved for special circumstances—for example, in pregnant women who are allergic to antithyroid medications, in patients with large goiters, or in patients who are unable to take antithyroid agents. Surgery for treatment of hyperthyroidism is performed soon after the thyroid function has returned to normal (4 to 6 weeks).

The surgical removal of about five sixths of the thyroid tissue (subtotal thyroidectomy) reliably results in a prolonged remission in most patients with exophthalmic goiter. Its use today is reserved for patients with obstructive symptoms, for pregnant women in the second trimester, and for patients with a need for rapid normalization of thyroid function. Before surgery, PTU is administered until signs of hyperthyroidism have disappeared. A beta-adrenergic blocking agent (eg, propranolol) may be used to reduce the heart rate and other signs and symptoms of hyperthyroidism; however, this does not create a euthyroid state. Iodine (Lugol's solution or KI) may be prescribed in an effort to reduce blood loss; however, the effectiveness of this treatment is unknown. Medications that may prolong clotting (eg, aspirin) are stopped several weeks before surgery to reduce the risk for postoperative bleeding. Patients receiving iodine medication must be monitored for evidence of iodine toxicity (iodism), which requires immediate withdrawal of the medication. Symptoms of iodism include swelling of the buccal mucosa, excessive salivation, coryza, and skin eruptions.

 Gerontologic Considerations

Although hyperthyroidism is much less common in elderly people than hypothyroidism, patients older than 60 years of age account for 10% to 15% of the cases of thyrotoxicosis. They often develop atypical signs and symptoms of endocrine disorders, including thyrotoxicosis. The only presenting manifestations may be anorexia and weight loss, absence of ocular signs, or isolated atrial fibrillation. (New or worsening heart failure or angina is more likely to occur in elderly than in younger patients.) These signs and symptoms may mask the underlying thyroid disease. Elderly patients also tend to have symptoms for longer periods of time and commonly present with vague and nonspecific signs and symptoms, making disorders difficult to detect (Dominguez, et al., 2008). Symptoms such as tachycardia, fatigue, mental confusion, weight loss, change in bowel habits, and depression can be attributed to age and other illnesses that are common in elderly people. In addition, patients may report cardiovascular symptoms and difficulty climbing stairs or rising from a chair because of muscle weakness. Elderly patients may have only a single manifestation (eg, anorexia, weight loss) of thyroid disease.

Spontaneous remission of hyperthyroidism is rare in elderly patients. Measurement of TSH is indicated in elderly patients who have unexplained physical or mental deterioration. The use of radioactive iodine is generally recommended for treatment of thyrotoxicosis in elderly patients unless an enlarged thyroid gland is pressing on the airway. The hypermetabolic state of thyrotoxicosis must be controlled by antithyroid medications before radioactive iodine is administered, because radiation therapy may precipitate thyroid storm by increasing the release of hormone from the thyroid gland. Thyroid storm, if it occurs, has a mortality rate of 10% in elderly patients.

Long-term use of antithyroid medications is not generally recommended for elderly patients because of the increased incidence of side effects, such as granulocytopenia, and the need for frequent monitoring. The dosage of other medications used to treat other chronic illnesses in elderly patients may need to be modified because of the altered rate of metabolism in hyperthyroidism. In addition, antithyroid medications are considered to be less effective in the treatment of toxic nodular goiter, the most common cause of thyrotoxicosis in the elderly.

Use of beta-adrenergic blocking agents (eg, propranolol) may be indicated to decrease the cardiovascular and neurologic signs and symptoms of thyrotoxicosis. These agents must be used with extreme caution in elderly patients to minimize adverse effects on cardiac function that may produce heart failure.

NURSING PROCESS

THE PATIENT WITH HYPERTHYROIDISM

Assessment

The health history and examination focus on symptoms related to accelerated or exaggerated metabolism. These include the patient's and family's reports of irritability and increased emotional reaction and the impact these changes have had on the patient's interactions with family, friends, and coworkers. The history includes other stressors and the patient's ability to cope with stress.

The nurse assesses the patient's nutritional status and the presence of symptoms. Symptoms related to excessive nervous system output and changes in vision and appearance of the eyes are noted. The nurse periodically assesses and monitors the patient's cardiac status, including heart rate, blood pressure, heart sounds, and peripheral pulses.

Because emotional changes are associated with hyperthyroidism, the patient's emotional state and psychological status are evaluated, as well as such symptoms as irritability, anxiety, sleep disturbances, apathy, and lethargy, all of which may occur with hyperthyroidism. The family may also provide information about recent changes in the patient's emotional status.

Diagnosis

Nursing Diagnoses

Based on all the assessment data, the major nursing diagnoses of the patient with hyperthyroidism may include the following:

- Imbalanced nutrition, less than body requirements, related to exaggerated metabolic rate, excessive appetite, and increased GI activity
- Ineffective coping related to irritability, hyperexcitability, apprehension, and emotional instability
- Low self-esteem related to changes in appearance, excessive appetite, and weight loss
- Altered body temperature

Collaborative Problems/Potential Complications

Based on assessment data, potential complications may include the following:

- Thyrotoxicosis or thyroid storm
- Hypothyroidism

Planning and Goals

The goals for the patient may be improved nutritional status, improved coping ability, improved self-esteem, maintenance of normal body temperature, and absence of complications.

Nursing Interventions

Improving Nutritional Status

Hyperthyroidism affects all body systems, including the GI system. The appetite is increased but may be satisfied by several well-balanced meals of small size, even up to six meals a day. Foods and fluids are selected to replace fluid lost through diarrhea and diaphoresis and to control the diarrhea that results from increased peristalsis. Rapid movement of food through the GI tract may result in nutritional imbalance and further weight loss. To reduce diarrhea, highly seasoned foods and stimulants such as coffee, tea, cola, and alcohol are discouraged. High-calorie, high-protein foods are encouraged. A quiet atmosphere during mealtime may aid digestion. Weight and dietary intake are recorded to monitor nutritional status.

Enhancing Coping Measures

The patient with hyperthyroidism needs reassurance that the emotional reactions being experienced are a result of the disorder and that with effective treatment those symptoms will be controlled. Because of the negative effect these symptoms have on family and friends, they too need reassurance that the symptoms are expected to disappear with treatment.

It is important to use a calm, unhurried approach with the patient. Stressful experiences are minimized; therefore, if hospitalized, the patient is not placed in a room with very ill or talkative patients. The environment is kept quiet and uncluttered. Noises, such as loud music, conversation, and equipment alarms, are minimized. The nurse encourages relaxing activities if they do not overstimulate the patient.

If thyroidectomy is planned, the patient needs to know that pharmacologic therapy is necessary to prepare the thyroid gland for surgical treatment. The nurse instructs and reminds the patient to take the medications as prescribed. Because of hyperexcitability and shortened attention span, the patient may require repetition of this information and written instructions.

Improving Self-Esteem

The patient with hyperthyroidism is likely to experience changes in appearance, appetite, and weight. These factors, along with the patient's inability to cope well with family and the illness, may result in loss of self-esteem. The nurse conveys an understanding of the patient's concern about these problems and promotes use of effective coping strategies. The patient and family need to know that these changes are a result of the thyroid dysfunction and are, in fact, out of the patient's control.

If changes in appearance are very disturbing to the patient, mirrors may be covered or removed. In addition, the nurse reminds family members and personnel to avoid bringing these changes to the patient's attention. The nurse explains to the patient and family that most of these changes are expected to disappear with effective treatment.

If the patient experiences ocular changes secondary to hyperthyroidism, eye care and protection may be necessary. The patient may need instructions about instillation of eye drops or ointment prescribed to soothe the eyes and protect the exposed cornea. The patient should also be discouraged from smoking.

The patient may be embarrassed by the need to eat large meals. Therefore, the nurse arranges for the patient to eat alone if desired and avoids commenting on the patient's large dietary intake while making sure that the patient receives sufficient food.

Maintaining Normal Body Temperature

The patient with hyperthyroidism frequently finds a normal room temperature too warm because of an exaggerated metabolic rate and increased heat production. If the patient is hospitalized, the nurse maintains the environment at a cool, comfortable temperature and changes bedding and clothing as needed. Cool baths and cool or cold fluids are encouraged, because they may provide relief.

Monitoring and Managing Potential Complications

The nurse closely monitors the patient with hyperthyroidism for signs and symptoms that may be indicative of thyroid storm. Cardiac and respiratory function are assessed by measuring vital signs and cardiac output, electrocardiographic (ECG) monitoring, arterial blood gases, and pulse oximetry. Assessment continues after treatment is initiated because of the potential effects of treatment on cardiac function. Oxygen is administered to prevent hypoxia, to improve tissue oxygenation, and to meet the high metabolic demands. IV fluids may be necessary to maintain blood glucose levels and to replace lost fluids. Antithyroid medications (PTU or methimazole) may be prescribed to reduce thyroid hormone levels. In addition, propranolol and digitalis may be prescribed to treat cardiac symptoms. If shock develops, treatment strategies must be implemented (see Chapter 15).

Hypothyroidism is likely to occur with any of the treatments used for hyperthyroidism. Therefore, the nurse periodically monitors the patient. Most patients report a greatly improved sense of well-being after treatment of hyperthyroidism, and some fail to continue to take prescribed thyroid replacement therapy. Therefore, part of patient and family teaching is instruction about the importance of continuing therapy indefinitely after discharge and a discussion of the consequences of failing to take medication.

Promoting Home and Community-Based Care

TEACHING PATIENTS SELF-CARE. The nurse teaches the patient with hyperthyroidism how and when to take prescribed medication and provides instruction about the essential role of the medication in the broader therapeutic plan. Because of the hyperexcitability and decreased attention span associated with hyperthyroidism, the nurse provides a written plan for the patient to use at home. The type and amount of information given depend on the patient's stress and anxiety levels. The patient and family members receive verbal and written information about the actions and possible side effects of the medications. The nurse identifies adverse effects that should be reported if they occur (Chart 42-7).

If a total or subtotal thyroidectomy is anticipated, the patient needs information about what to expect. This information is repeated as the time of surgery approaches. The nurse also advises the patient to avoid stressful situations that may precipitate thyroid storm.

CONTINUING CARE. Referral for home care, if indicated, allows the home care nurse to assess the home and family environment and the patient's and family's understanding of the importance of adhering to the therapeutic regimen and the recommended follow-up monitoring. The nurse reinforces to the patient and family the importance of long-term follow-up because of the risk of hypothyroidism after thyroidectomy or treatment with antithyroid medications or radioactive iodine. The nurse also assesses the patient for changes indicating return to normal thyroid function and signs and symptoms of hyperthyroidism and hypothyroidism. Furthermore, the nurse reminds the patient and family about the importance of health promotion activities and recommended health screening.

Evaluation

Expected Patient Outcomes

Expected patient outcomes may include the following:

1. Improves nutritional status
   a. Reports adequate dietary intake and decreased hunger
   b. Identifies high-calorie, high-protein foods; identifies foods to be avoided
   c. Avoids use of alcohol and other stimulants
   d. Stops smoking
   e. Reports decreased episodes of diarrhea
2. Demonstrates effective coping methods in dealing with family, friends, and coworkers
   a. Explains reasons for irritability and emotional instability
   b. Avoids stressful situations, events, and people
   c. Participates in relaxing, nonstressful activities
3. Achieves increased self-esteem
   a. Verbalizes feelings about self and illness
   b. Describes feelings of frustration and loss of control
   c. Describes reasons for increased appetite

CHART 42-7

HOME CARE CHECKLIST
The Patient With Hyperthyroidism

At the completion of the home care instruction, the patient or caregiver will be able to:	PATIENT	CAREGIVER
• State present and potential effects of hyperthyroidism on the body.	✔	✔
• State precipitating factors and interventions for complications (hypothyroidism, thyroid storm).	✔	✔
• State the purpose, dose, route, schedule, side effects, and precautions of prescribed medications (propylthiouracil, radioactive iodine).	✔	✔
• State the need to contact health care provider before taking over-the-counter medications.	✔	✔
• State need for regular follow-up visits with health care provider.	✔	✔
• Identify the need for planned rest periods and methods to improve sleep patterns.	✔	✔
• Identify the need for increased dietary intake until weight stabilizes.	✔	✔
• Identify areas of physical and emotional stress.	✔	✔
• State that emotional lability is part of disease process.	✔	✔
• Describe the potential benefits and risks of surgical intervention or radioactive iodine therapy.	✔	✔
• Identify potential for menstrual irregularities, increased risk for osteoporosis, and potential for pregnancy for women.	✔	✔
• State need to wear medical identification and carry medical information card.	✔	✔
• Identify rationale for smoking cessation and take steps to stop smoking.	✔	

4. Maintains normal body temperature
5. Absence of complications
   a. Has serum thyroid hormone and TSH levels within normal limits
   b. Identifies signs and symptoms of thyroid storm and hypothyroidism
   c. Has vital signs and results of ECG, arterial blood gases, and pulse oximetry within normal limits
   d. States importance of regular follow-up and life-long maintenance of prescribed therapy

THYROIDITIS

Thyroiditis, inflammation of the thyroid gland, can be acute, subacute, or chronic. Each type of thyroiditis is characterized by inflammation, fibrosis, or lymphocytic infiltration of the thyroid gland. Several forms of thyroiditis are characterized by autoimmune damage to the thyroid. The various forms of thyroiditis may cause thyrotoxicosis, hypothyroidism, or both (Bindra & Braunstein, 2006).

Acute Thyroiditis

Acute thyroiditis is a rare disorder caused by infection of the thyroid gland by bacteria, fungi, mycobacteria, or parasites. *Staphylococcus aureus* and other staphylococci are the most common causes. Infection typically causes anterior neck pain and swelling, fever, dysphagia, and dysphonia. Pharyngitis or pharyngeal pain is often present. Examination may reveal warmth, erythema (redness), and tenderness of the thyroid gland. Treatment of acute thyroiditis includes antimicrobial agents and fluid replacement. Surgical incision and drainage may be needed if an abscess is present.

Subacute Thyroiditis

Subacute thyroiditis may be subacute granulomatous thyroiditis (de Quervain's thyroiditis) or painless thyroiditis (silent thyroiditis or subacute lymphocytic thyroiditis). Subacute granulomatous thyroiditis is an inflammatory disorder of the thyroid gland that predominantly affects women between the ages of 40 and 50 years (Bindra & Braunstein, 2006). The condition is usually associated with a viral respiratory infection and has a summer peak incidence that coincides with coxsackievirus groups A and B and echovirus infections. Signs and symptoms include myalgias, pharyngitis, low-grade fever, and fatigue. These progress to a painful swelling in the anterior neck that lasts 1 to 2 months and then disappears spontaneously without residual effect. The thyroid enlarges symmetrically and may be painful. The overlying skin is often reddened and warm. Swallowing may be difficult and uncomfortable. Irritability, nervousness, insomnia, and weight loss—manifestations of hyperthyroidism—are common, and many patients experience chills and fever as well. There is no thrill or bruit found on physical examination of the thyroid gland in hyperthyroidism with subacute thyroiditis. The absence of this sign assists in the differentiation of hyperthyroidism associated with subacute thyroiditis and hyperthyroidism associated with Graves' disease (Bindra & Braunstein, 2006).

Treatment is directed toward control of the inflammation. In general, nonsteroidal anti-inflammatory drugs are used to relieve neck pain. Acetylsalicylic acid (aspirin) is avoided if symptoms of hyperthyroidism occur, because aspirin displaces thyroid hormone from its binding sites and increases the amount of circulating hormone. Beta-blocking agents (eg, propranolol [Inderal]) may be used to control symptoms of hyperthyroidism. Antithyroid agents, which block the synthesis of T_3 and T_4, are not effective because the associated thyrotoxicosis results from the release of stored thyroid hormones rather than from their increased synthesis. In cases that are more severe and do not respond to treatment within 5 weeks, oral corticosteroids may be prescribed to reduce swelling and relieve pain. However, corticosteroids do not usually affect the underlying cause (Bindra & Braunstein, 2006). In some cases, temporary hypothyroidism may develop and may necessitate thyroid hormone therapy. Follow-up monitoring is necessary to document the patient's return to a euthyroid state.

Painless thyroiditis (subacute lymphocytic thyroiditis) often occurs in the postpartum period and is thought to be an autoimmune process. Symptoms of hyperthyroidism or hypothyroidism are possible. Treatment is directed at symptoms, and yearly follow-up is recommended to determine the patient's need for treatment of subsequent hypothyroidism.

Chronic Thyroiditis (Hashimoto's Disease)

Chronic thyroiditis, which occurs most frequently in women between the ages of 30 and 50 years, has been termed Hashimoto's disease, or chronic lymphocytic thyroiditis. In contrast to acute thyroiditis, the chronic forms usually are not accompanied by pain, pressure symptoms, or fever, and thyroid activity usually is normal or low rather than increased. Cell-mediated immunity may play a significant role in the pathogenesis of chronic thyroiditis, and there may be a genetic predisposition to it. Diagnosis is based on the histologic appearance of the inflamed thyroid gland. Patients with Hashimoto's disease should also be evaluated for primary thyroid lymphoma if they present with a rapidly growing nodule, because they are 60 to 80 times more likely to develop this condition than the general population (Bindra & Braunstein, 2006). If untreated, the disease runs a slow, progressive course, leading eventually to hypothyroidism. Indications for treatment include goiter or clinical hypothyroidism.

The objective of treatment is to reduce the size of the thyroid gland and prevent hypothyroidism. Thyroid hormone therapy is prescribed to reduce thyroid activity and the production of thyroglobulin. If hypothyroid symptoms are present, thyroid hormone therapy is prescribed. Surgery may be required if pressure symptoms persist.

THYROID TUMORS

Tumors of the thyroid gland are classified on the basis of being benign or malignant, the presence or absence of associated thyrotoxicosis, and the diffuse or irregular quality of the glandular enlargement. If the enlargement is sufficient to cause a visible swelling in the neck, the tumor is referred to as a goiter.

All grades of goiter are encountered, from those that are barely visible to those producing disfigurement. Some are symmetric and diffuse; others are nodular. Some are accompanied by hyperthyroidism, in which case they are described as toxic; others are associated with a euthyroid state and are called nontoxic goiters.

Endemic (Iodine-Deficient) Goiter

The most common type of goiter, once encountered chiefly in geographic regions where the natural supply of iodine is deficient (eg, the Great Lakes areas of the United States), is the so-called simple or colloid goiter. In addition to being caused by an iodine deficiency, simple goiter may be caused by an intake of large quantities of goitrogenic substances in patients with unusually susceptible glands. These substances include excessive amounts of iodine or lithium, which is used in treating bipolar disorders.

Simple goiter represents a compensatory hypertrophy of the thyroid gland, caused by stimulation by the pituitary gland. The pituitary gland produces thyrotropin or TSH, a hormone that controls the release of thyroid hormone from the thyroid gland. Its production increases if there is subnormal thyroid activity, as when insufficient iodine is available for production of the thyroid hormone. Such goiters usually cause no symptoms, except for the swelling in the neck, which may result in tracheal compression when excessive.

Many goiters of this type recede after the iodine imbalance is corrected. Supplementary iodine, such as SSKI, is prescribed to suppress the pituitary's thyroid-stimulating activity. When surgery is recommended, the risk of postoperative complications is minimized by ensuring a preoperative euthyroid state through treatment with antithyroid medications and iodide to reduce the size and vascularity of the goiter.

Providing children in iodine-poor regions with iodine compounds can prevent simple or endemic goiter. Although the introduction of iodized salt has been the single most effective means of preventing goiter in at-risk populations, the World Health Organization (2007) is exploring alternative strategies to ensure iodine intake because of the health risks associated with excessive salt intake.

Nodular Goiter

Some thyroid glands are nodular because of areas of hyperplasia (overgrowth). No symptoms may arise as a result of this condition, but not uncommonly these nodules slowly increase in size, with some descending into the thorax, where they cause local pressure symptoms. Some nodules become malignant, and some are associated with a hyperthyroid state. Therefore, the patient with many thyroid nodules may eventually require surgery.

Thyroid Cancer

Cancer of the thyroid is much less prevalent than other forms of cancer; however, it accounts for 90% of endocrine malignancies. According to the American Cancer Society (2009), more than 37,000 new cases of thyroid cancer are diagnosed each year, with one fourth of the cases occurring in men and three fourths in women. About 1600 people die annually from this malignancy. There are several types of cancer of the thyroid gland; the type determines the course and prognosis (Table 42-4).

External radiation of the head, neck, or chest in infancy and childhood increases the risk of thyroid carcinoma. The incidence of thyroid cancer appears to increase 5 to 40 years after irradiation. Consequently, people who underwent radiation treatment or were otherwise exposed to radiation as children should consult a physician, request an isotope thyroid scan as part of the evaluation, follow recommended treatment of abnormalities of the gland, and continue with annual checkups (Chart 42-8).

Assessment and Diagnostic Findings

Lesions that are single, hard, and fixed on palpation or associated with cervical lymphadenopathy suggest malignancy. Thyroid function tests may be helpful in evaluating thyroid nodules and masses; however, results are rarely

Table 42-4 TYPES OF THYROID CANCERS

Type of Thyroid Cancer	Incidence (%)	Characteristics
Papillary adenocarcinoma	70	Most common and least aggressive Asymptomatic nodule in a normal gland Starts in childhood or early adult life, remains localized Metastasizes along the lymphatics if untreated More aggressive in the elderly
Follicular adenocarcinoma	15	Appears after 40 y of age Encapsulated; feels elastic or rubbery on palpation Spreads through the bloodstream to bone, liver, and lung Prognosis is not as favorable as for papillary adenocarcinoma
Medullary	5	Appears after 50 y of age Occurs as part of multiple endocrine neoplasia (MEN) Hormone-producing tumor causing endocrine dysfunction symptoms Metastasizes by lymphatics and bloodstream Moderate survival rate
Anaplastic	5	50% of anaplastic thyroid carcinomas occur in patients older than 60 y Hard, irregular mass that grows quickly and spreads by direct invasion to adjacent tissues May be painful and tender Survival for patients with anaplastic cancer is usually less than 6 mo
Thyroid lymphoma	5	Appears after age 40 y May have history of goiter, hoarseness, dyspnea, pain, and pressure Good prognosis

Chart 42-8 • *Radiation-Induced Thyroid Damage and Cancer*

The thyroid gland has a very efficient mechanism to remove iodine from the bloodstream and concentrate or "trap" it for subsequent synthesis of thyroid hormone. The effectiveness of this mechanism to concentrate iodide is reflected in a concentration of iodide 20 to 40 times the concentration of iodide in the plasma.

If milk and other food sources become contaminated with radioactivity as a result of a nuclear detonation or a nuclear power plant incident or mishap, the radioactive iodide would become concentrated in the thyroid gland at a very high concentration and would irradiate the thyroid gland, increasing the risk for thyroid gland cancer. Therefore, in communities exposed to increased radioactivity, attempts have been made to block the uptake of radioactive iodide by flooding or saturating the thyroid gland with nonradioactive iodide.

Administration of potassium iodide (KI) or other iodide preparations as soon as possible after exposure almost completely inhibits thyroid absorption of the radioactive iodide and promotes rapid excretion of any that is absorbed. In 2001, the Food and Drug Administration issued a statement recommending KI administration in advance of exposure to radioactive iodine—that is, when exposure is imminent (Thyroid Carcinoma Task Force, 2001).

conclusive. Needle biopsy of the thyroid gland is used as an outpatient procedure to make a diagnosis of thyroid cancer, to differentiate cancerous thyroid nodules from noncancerous nodules, and to stage the cancer if detected. The procedure is safe and usually requires only a local anesthetic agent. However, patients who undergo the procedure are monitored closely, because cancerous tissues may be missed during the procedure. A second type of aspiration or biopsy uses a large-bore needle rather than the fine needle used in standard biopsy; it may be used when the results of the standard biopsy are inconclusive or with rapidly growing tumors. Additional diagnostic studies include ultrasound, MRI, CT, thyroid scans, radioactive iodine uptake studies, and thyroid suppression tests.

Medical Management

The treatment of choice for thyroid carcinoma is surgical removal. Total or near-total **thyroidectomy** is performed if possible. Modified neck dissection or more extensive radical neck dissection is performed if there is lymph node involvement.

Efforts are made to spare parathyroid tissue to reduce the risk of postoperative hypocalcemia and tetany. After surgery, ablation procedures are carried out with radioactive iodine to eradicate residual thyroid tissue if the tumor is radiosensitive. Radioactive iodine also maximizes the chance of discovering thyroid metastasis at a later date if total-body scans are carried out.

After surgery, thyroid hormone is administered in suppressive doses to lower the levels of TSH to a euthyroid state (Cooper, et al., 2006). If the remaining thyroid tissue is inadequate to produce sufficient thyroid hormone, thyroxine is required permanently.

Several routes are available for administering radiation to the thyroid or tissues of the neck, including oral administration of radioactive iodine and external administration of radiation therapy. The patient who receives external sources of radiation therapy is at risk for mucositis, dryness of the mouth, dysphagia, redness of the skin, anorexia, and fatigue (see Chapter 16). Chemotherapy is infrequently used to treat thyroid cancer.

Patients whose thyroid cancer is detected early and who are appropriately treated usually do very well. Patients who have had papillary cancer, the most common and least aggressive tumor, have a 10-year survival rate greater than 90%. Long-term survival is also common in follicular cancer, a more aggressive form of thyroid cancer (Tierney, et al., 2005). However, continued thyroid hormone therapy and periodic follow-up and diagnostic testing are important to ensure the patient's well-being (Cooper, et al., 2006).

Postoperatively, the patient is instructed to take exogenous thyroid hormone to prevent hypothyroidism. Later follow-up includes clinical assessment for recurrence of nodules or masses in the neck and signs of hoarseness, dysphagia, or dyspnea. Total-body scans are performed 2 to 4 months after surgery to detect residual thyroid tissue or metastatic disease. Thyroid hormones are stopped for about 6 weeks before the tests. Care must be taken to avoid iodine-containing foods and contrast agents. A repeat scan is performed 1 year after the initial surgery. If measurements are stable, a final scan is obtained in 3 to 5 years.

Free T_4, TSH, and serum calcium and phosphorus levels are monitored to determine whether the thyroid hormone supplementation is adequate and to note whether calcium balance is maintained.

Although local and systemic reactions to radiation may occur and may include neutropenia or thrombocytopenia, these complications are rare when radioactive iodine is used. Patients who undergo surgery that is combined with radioactive iodine have a higher survival rate than those who undergo surgery alone. Patient teaching emphasizes the importance of taking prescribed medications and following recommendations for follow-up monitoring. The patient who is undergoing radiation therapy is also instructed in how to assess and manage side effects of treatment.

Nursing Management

Important preoperative goals are to gain the patient's confidence and reduce anxiety. Often, the patient's home life has become tense because of his or her restlessness, irritability, and nervousness secondary to hyperthyroidism. Efforts are necessary to protect the patient from such tension and stress to avoid precipitating thyroid storm. If the patient reports increased stress when with family or friends, suggestions are made to limit contact with them. Quiet and relaxing forms of recreation or occupational therapy may be helpful.

Providing Preoperative Care

The nurse instructs the patient about the importance of eating a diet high in carbohydrates and proteins. A high daily caloric intake is necessary because of the increased metabolic activity and rapid depletion of glycogen reserves. Supplementary vitamins, particularly thiamine and ascorbic acid, may be prescribed. The patient is reminded to avoid tea, coffee, cola, and other stimulants.

The nurse also informs the patient about the purpose of preoperative tests, if they are to be performed, and explains what preoperative preparations to expect. This information should help to reduce the patient's anxiety about the surgery. In addition, special efforts are made to ensure a good night's rest before surgery, although many patients are admitted to the hospital on the day of surgery.

Preoperative teaching includes demonstrating to the patient how to support the neck with the hands after surgery to prevent stress on the incision. This involves raising the elbows and placing the hands behind the neck to provide support and reduce strain and tension on the neck muscles and the surgical incision.

Providing Postoperative Care

The nurse periodically assesses the surgical dressings and reinforces them if necessary. When the patient is in a recumbent position, the nurse observes the sides and the back of the neck as well as the anterior dressing for bleeding. In addition to monitoring the pulse and blood pressure for any indication of internal bleeding, it is important to be alert for complaints of a sensation of pressure or fullness at the incision site. Such symptoms may indicate subcutaneous hemorrhage and hematoma formation and should be reported.

Difficulty in respiration can occur as a result of edema of the glottis, hematoma formation, or injury to the recurrent laryngeal nerve. This complication requires that an airway be inserted. Therefore, a tracheostomy set is kept at the bedside at all times, and the surgeon is summoned at the first indication of respiratory distress. If the respiratory distress is caused by hematoma, surgical evacuation is required.

The intensity of pain is assessed, and analgesic agents are administered as prescribed for pain. The nurse should anticipate apprehension in the patient and should inform the patient that oxygen will assist breathing. When moving and turning the patient, the nurse carefully supports the patient's head and avoids tension on the sutures. The most comfortable position is the semi-Fowler's position, with the head elevated and supported by pillows.

IV fluids are administered during the immediate postoperative period. Water may be given by mouth as soon as nausea subsides. Usually, there is a little difficulty in swallowing; initially, cold fluids and ice may be taken better than other fluids. Often, patients prefer a soft diet to a liquid diet in the immediate postoperative period.

The patient is advised to talk as little as possible to reduce edema to the vocal cords; however, when the patient does speak, any voice changes are noted, which might indicate injury to the recurrent laryngeal nerve, which lies just behind the thyroid next to the trachea. An overbed table is provided for access to frequently used items so the patient avoids turning his or her head. The table can also be used to support a humidifier when vapor-mist inhalations are prescribed for the relief of excessive mucus accumulation.

The patient is usually permitted out of bed as soon as possible and is encouraged to eat foods that are easily swallowed. A high-calorie diet may be prescribed to promote weight gain. Sutures or skin clips are usually removed on the second day. The patient is usually discharged from the hospital on the day of surgery or soon afterward if the postoperative course is uncomplicated.

Monitoring and Managing Potential Complications

Hemorrhage, hematoma formation, edema of the glottis, and injury to the recurrent laryngeal nerve are complications that have been reviewed previously in this chapter. Occasionally in thyroid surgery, the parathyroid glands are injured or removed, producing a disturbance in calcium metabolism. As the blood calcium level falls, hyperirritability of the nerves occurs, with spasms of the hands and feet and muscle twitching (see Chapter 14). This group of symptoms is termed tetany, and the nurse must immediately report its appearance, because laryngospasm, although rare, may occur and obstruct the airway. Tetany of this type is usually treated with IV calcium gluconate. This calcium abnormality is usually temporary after thyroidectomy unless all parathyroid tissue was removed.

Promoting Home and Community-Based Care

The patient is usually discharged within 1 or 2 days. Therefore, the patient and family need to be knowledgeable about the signs and symptoms of the complications that may occur and those that should be reported. Strategies are suggested for managing postoperative pain at home and for increasing humidification. The nurse explains to the patient and family the need for rest, relaxation, and nutrition. The patient is permitted to resume his or her former activities and responsibilities completely once recovered from surgery.

If indicated, a referral to home care is made. The home care nurse assesses the patient's recovery from surgery. The nurse also assesses the surgical incision and reinforces instruction about limiting activities that put strain on the incision and sutures. Family responsibilities and factors relating to the home environment that produce emotional tension have often been implicated as precipitating causes of thyrotoxicosis. A home visit provides an opportunity to evaluate these factors and to suggest ways to improve the home and family environment. The nurse instructs the patients about the importance of follow-up visits to the physician or the clinic for monitoring of thyroid status.

THE PARATHYROID GLANDS

Anatomic and Physiologic Overview

The parathyroid glands (normally four) are situated in the neck and embedded in the posterior aspect of the thyroid gland (Fig. 42-5). Parathormone (parathyroid hormone), the protein hormone produced by the parathyroid glands, regulates calcium and phosphorus metabolism. Increased secretion of parathormone results in increased calcium absorption from the kidney, intestine, and bones, which raises the blood calcium level. Some actions of this hormone are increased by the presence of vitamin D. Parathormone also tends to lower the blood phosphorus level. The serum level of ionized calcium regulates the output of parathormone. Increased serum calcium results in decreased parathormone secretion, creating a negative feedback system.

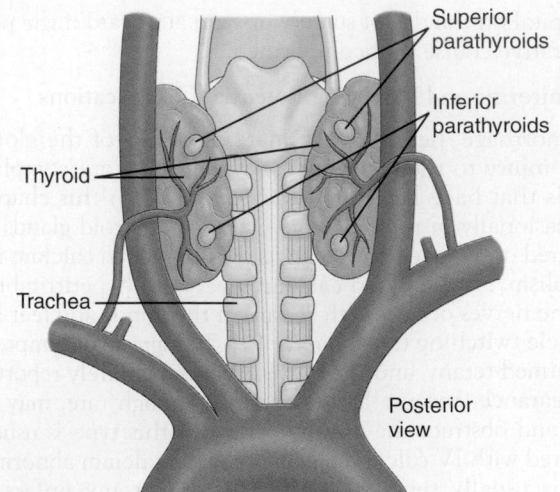

Figure 42-5 The parathyroid glands are located behind the thyroid gland. The parathyroids may be embedded in the thyroid tissue.

Pathophysiology

Excess parathormone can result in markedly increased levels of serum calcium, a potentially life-threatening situation. When the product of serum calcium and serum phosphorus (calcium × phosphorus) rises, calcium phosphate may precipitate in various organs of the body (eg, the kidneys) and cause tissue calcification.

Specific Disorders of the Parathyroid Glands

HYPERPARATHYROIDISM

Hyperparathyroidism, which is caused by overproduction of parathormone by the parathyroid glands, is characterized by bone decalcification and the development of renal calculi (kidney stones) containing calcium.

Primary hyperparathyroidism occurs two to four times more often in women than in men and is most common in people between 60 and 70 years of age. Its incidence is approximately 25 cases per 100,000 (Suliburk & Perrier, 2007). The disorder is rare in children younger than 15 years of age, but its incidence increases 10-fold between the ages of 15 and 65 years. Half of the people diagnosed with hyperparathyroidism do not have symptoms.

Secondary hyperparathyroidism, with manifestations similar to those of primary hyperparathyroidism, occurs in patients who have chronic renal failure and so-called renal rickets as a result of phosphorus retention, increased stimulation of the parathyroid glands, and increased parathormone secretion.

Clinical Manifestations

The patient may have no symptoms or may experience signs and symptoms resulting from involvement of several body systems. Apathy, fatigue, muscle weakness, nausea, vomiting, constipation, hypertension, and cardiac dysrhythmias may occur. All these signs and symptoms are attributable to the increased concentration of calcium in the blood. Psychological effects may vary from irritability and neurosis to psychoses caused by the direct action of calcium on the brain and nervous system. An increase in calcium produces a decrease in the excitation potential of nerve and muscle tissue.

The formation of stones in one or both kidneys, related to the increased urinary excretion of calcium and phosphorus, is one of the important complications of hyperparathyroidism and occurs in 55% of patients with primary hyperparathyroidism. Renal damage results from the precipitation of calcium phosphate in the renal pelvis and parenchyma, which causes renal calculi (kidney stones), obstruction, pyelonephritis, and renal failure.

Musculoskeletal symptoms accompanying hyperparathyroidism may be caused by demineralization of the bones or by bone tumors composed of benign giant cells resulting from overgrowth of osteoclasts. The patient may develop skeletal pain and tenderness, especially of the back and joints; pain on weight bearing; pathologic fractures; deformities; and shortening of body stature. Bone loss attributable to hyperparathyroidism increases the risk of fracture.

The incidence of peptic ulcer and pancreatitis is increased with hyperparathyroidism and may be responsible for many of the GI symptoms that occur.

Assessment and Diagnostic Findings

Primary hyperparathyroidism is diagnosed by persistent elevation of serum calcium levels and an elevated concentration of parathormone. Radioimmunoassays for parathormone are sensitive and differentiate primary hyperparathyroidism from other causes of hypercalcemia in more than 90% of patients with elevated serum calcium levels. An elevated serum calcium level alone is a nonspecific finding, because serum levels may be altered by diet, medications, and renal and bone changes. Bone changes may be detected on x-ray or bone scans in advanced disease. The double-antibody parathyroid hormone test is used to distinguish between primary hyperparathyroidism and malignancy as a cause of hypercalcemia. Ultrasound, MRI, thallium scan, and fine-needle biopsy have been used to evaluate the function of the parathyroids and to localize parathyroid cysts, adenomas, or hyperplasia.

Medical Management

Surgical Management

The recommended treatment for primary hyperparathyroidism is the surgical removal of abnormal parathyroid tissue (parathyroidectomy) (Rodgers, Lew & Solorzano, 2008; Suliburk & Perrier, 2007). In the past, the standard parathyroidectomy involved a bilateral neck exploration under general anesthesia. Today, minimally invasive parathyroidectomy techniques allow for unilateral neck exploration using local anesthesia; these are performed on an outpatient basis. In some cases only the removal of a single diseased gland is necessary, reducing morbidity rates associated with surgery. For asymptomatic patients who have only mildly elevated serum calcium concentrations and normal renal function, surgery may be delayed and the patient monitored closely for worsening of hypercalcemia, bone deterioration, renal impairment, or the development of kidney stones.

Surgery is recommended for asymptomatic patients who meet the following criteria: (1) younger than 50 years of age, (2) unable or unlikely to participate in follow-up care, (3) serum calcium level more than 1.0 mg/dL (0.25 mmol/L) above normal reference range, (4) urinary calcium level greater than 400 mg/day (10 mmol/day), (5) a 30% or greater decrease in renal function, or (6) with complaints of primary hyperparathyroidism, including nephrocalcinosis, osteoporosis, or a severe psychoneurologic disorder (AACE/AAES Task Force on Primary Hyperparathyroidism, 2005).

However, according to several authors, these criteria are too conservative; there is little evidence to support long-term medical management of asymptomatic patients who do not meet these criteria (Rodgers, et al., 2008; Suliburk & Perrier, 2007).

Hydration Therapy

Because kidney involvement is possible, patients with hyperparathyroidism are at risk for renal calculi. Therefore, a daily fluid intake of 2000 mL or more is encouraged to help prevent calculus formation. Cranberry juice is suggested, because it may lower the urinary pH. It can be added to other juices or to ginger ale for variety. Cranberry extract tablets are an alternative to reduce urinary pH. The patient is instructed to report other manifestations of renal calculi, such as abdominal pain and hematuria. Thiazide diuretics are avoided, because they decrease the renal excretion of calcium and further elevate serum calcium levels. Because of the risk of hypercalcemic crisis (see later discussion), the patient is instructed to avoid dehydration and to seek immediate health care if conditions that commonly produce dehydration (eg, vomiting, diarrhea) occur.

Mobility

Mobility of the patient, with walking or use of a rocking chair for those with limited mobility, is encouraged as much as possible, because bones that are subjected to normal stress give up less calcium. Bed rest increases calcium excretion and the risk for renal calculi. Oral phosphates lower the serum calcium level in some patients; long-term use is not recommended because of the risk of ectopic calcium phosphate deposition in soft tissues.

Diet and Medications

Nutritional needs are met, but the patient is advised to avoid a diet with restricted or excess calcium. If the patient has a coexisting peptic ulcer, prescribed antacids and protein feedings are necessary. Because anorexia is common, efforts are made to improve the appetite. Prune juice, stool softeners, and physical activity, along with increased fluid intake, help offset constipation, which is common postoperatively.

Nursing Management

The insidious onset and chronic nature of hyperparathyroidism and its diverse and commonly vague symptoms may result in depression and frustration. The family may have considered the patient's illness to be psychosomatic. An awareness of the course of the disorder and an understanding approach by the nurse may help the patient and family deal with their reactions and feelings.

The nursing management of the patient undergoing parathyroidectomy is essentially the same as that of a patient undergoing thyroidectomy. However, the previously described precautions about airway patency, dehydration, immobility, and diet are particularly important in the patient who is awaiting or recovering from parathyroidectomy. Although not all parathyroid tissue is removed during surgery in an effort to control the calcium–phosphorus balance, the nurse closely monitors the patient to detect symptoms of tetany (which may be an early postoperative complication). Most patients quickly regain function of the remaining parathyroid tissue and experience only mild, transient postoperative hypocalcemia. In patients with significant bone disease or bone changes, a more prolonged period of hypocalcemia should be anticipated. The nurse reminds the patient and family about the importance of follow-up to ensure return of serum calcium levels to normal (Chart 42-9).

Complications: Hypercalcemic Crisis

Acute hypercalcemic crisis can occur with extreme elevation of serum calcium levels. Serum calcium levels greater than 15 mg/dL (3.7 mmol/L) result in neurologic, cardiovascular, and renal symptoms that can be life-threatening. Treatment includes rehydration with large volumes of IV fluids, diuretic agents to promote renal excretion of excess calcium, and phosphate therapy to correct hypophosphatemia and decrease serum calcium levels by promoting calcium deposition in bone and reducing the gastrointestinal absorption of calcium. Cytotoxic agents (eg, mithramycin), calcitonin, and dialysis may be used in emergency situations to decrease serum calcium levels quickly.

 NURSING ALERT

The patient in acute hypercalcemic crisis requires close monitoring for life-threatening complications and prompt treatment to reduce serum calcium levels.

A combination of calcitonin and corticosteroids has been administered in emergencies to reduce the serum calcium level by increasing calcium deposition in bone. Other agents that may be administered to decrease serum calcium levels include bisphosphonates (eg, etidronate [Didronel], pamidronate [Aredia]).

Expert assessment and care are required to minimize complications and reverse the life-threatening hypercalcemia. Medications are administered with care, and attention is given to fluid balance to promote return of normal fluid and electrolyte balance. Supportive measures are necessary for the patient and family. (See Chapters 14 and 16 for further discussion of hypercalcemic crisis.)

HYPOPARATHYROIDISM

The most common cause of hypoparathyroidism is inadequate secretion of parathormone after interruption of the blood supply or surgical removal of parathyroid gland tissue during thyroidectomy, parathyroidectomy, or radical neck dissection. These small glands are easily overlooked and can be removed inadvertently during thyroid surgery. Atrophy

CHART
42-9

HOME CARE CHECKLIST
The Patient With Hyperparathyroidism

At the completion of the home care instruction, the patient or caregiver will be able to:	PATIENT	CAREGIVER
• State present and potential effects of hyperparathyroidism on the body.	✔	✔
• State precipitating factors and interventions for complications.	✔	✔
• State importance of regular follow-up visits with health care provider.	✔	✔
• Describe potential benefits and risks of parathyroidectomy.	✔	✔
• State the purpose, dose, route, schedule, side effects, and precautions of prescribed medications (loop diuretics, phosphate, calcitonin, mithramycin).	✔	✔
• State the need to contact health care provider before taking over-the-counter medication containing calcium.	✔	✔
• State need to take pain medications on a scheduled basis.	✔	✔
• Describe nonpharmacologic methods of pain management.	✔	✔
• Identify safety hazards and methods of injury prevention.	✔	✔
• Identify areas of activity limitations and impact on lifestyle.	✔	✔
• State need for increased fluid intake and diet low in calcium and vitamin D.	✔	✔

of the parathyroid glands of unknown cause is a less common cause of hypoparathyroidism.

Deficiency of parathormone results in increased blood phosphate (hyperphosphatemia) and decreased blood calcium (hypocalcemia) levels. In the absence of parathormone, there is decreased intestinal absorption of dietary calcium and decreased resorption of calcium from bone and through the renal tubules. Decreased renal excretion of phosphate causes hypophosphaturia, and low serum calcium levels result in hypocalciuria.

Clinical Manifestations

Hypocalcemia causes irritability of the neuromuscular system and contributes to the chief symptom of hypoparathyroidism—tetany. Tetany is a general muscle hypertonia, with tremor and spasmodic or uncoordinated contractions occurring with or without efforts to make voluntary movements. Symptoms of latent tetany are numbness, tingling, and cramps in the extremities, and the patient complains of stiffness in the hands and feet. In overt tetany, the signs include bronchospasm, laryngeal spasm, carpopedal spasm (flexion of the elbows and wrists and extension of the carpophalangeal joints and dorsiflexion of the feet), dysphagia, photophobia, cardiac dysrhythmias, and seizures. Other symptoms include anxiety, irritability, depression, and even delirium. ECG changes and hypotension also may occur.

Assessment and Diagnostic Findings

A positive Trousseau's sign or a positive Chvostek's sign suggests latent tetany. **Trousseau's sign** is positive when carpopedal spasm is induced by occluding the blood flow to the arm for 3 minutes with a blood pressure cuff. **Chvostek's sign** is positive when a sharp tapping over the facial nerve just in front of the parotid gland and anterior to the ear causes spasm or twitching of the mouth, nose, and eye (see Chapter 14).

The diagnosis of hypoparathyroidism often is difficult because of the vague symptoms, such as aches and pains. There-

fore, laboratory studies are especially helpful. Tetany develops at serum calcium levels of 5 to 6 mg/dL (1.2 to 1.5 mmol/L) or lower. Serum phosphate levels are increased, and x-rays of bone show increased density. Calcification is detected on x-rays of the subcutaneous or paraspinal basal ganglia of the brain.

Medical Management

The goal of therapy is to increase the serum calcium level to 9 to 10 mg/dL (2.2 to 2.5 mmol/L) and to eliminate the symptoms of hypoparathyroidism and hypocalcemia. When hypocalcemia and tetany occur after a thyroidectomy, the immediate treatment is administration of IV calcium gluconate. If this does not decrease neuromuscular irritability and seizure activity immediately, sedative agents such as pentobarbital may be administered.

Parenteral parathormone can be administered to treat acute hypoparathyroidism with tetany. However, the high incidence of allergic reactions to injections of parathormone limits its use to acute episodes of hypocalcemia. The patient receiving parathormone is monitored closely for allergic reactions and changes in serum calcium levels.

Because of neuromuscular irritability, the patient with hypocalcemia and tetany requires an environment that is free of noise, drafts, bright lights, or sudden movement. Tracheostomy or mechanical ventilation may become necessary, along with bronchodilating medications, if the patient develops respiratory distress.

Therapy for chronic hypoparathyroidism is determined after serum calcium levels are obtained. A diet high in calcium and low in phosphorus is prescribed. Although milk, milk products, and egg yolk are high in calcium, they are restricted because they also contain high levels of phosphorus. Spinach also is avoided because it contains oxalate, which would form insoluble calcium substances. Oral tablets of calcium salts, such as calcium gluconate, may be used to supplement the diet. Aluminum hydroxide gel or aluminum carbonate (Gelusil, Amphojel) also is administered after

CHART
42-10

HOME CARE CHECKLIST
The Patient With Hypoparathyroidism

At the completion of the home care instruction, the patient or caregiver will be able to:	PATIENT	CAREGIVER
• State present and potential effects of hypoparathyroidism on the body.	✔	✔
• State precipitating factors and interventions for complications (seizure, cardiac dysrhythmias, cardiac arrest).	✔	✔
• State necessary actions for seizure activity.		✔
• State importance of regular follow-up visits with health care provider.	✔	✔
• State purpose, dose, route, schedule, side effects, and precautions of prescribed medications (calcium, phosphate binders).	✔	✔
• State need to alternate activity and rest periods.	✔	✔
• Identify areas of activity limitations and impact on lifestyle.	✔	✔
• Identify foods high in calcium and vitamin D, low in phosphorus.	✔	✔

meals to bind phosphate and promote its excretion through the GI tract.

Variable dosages of a vitamin D preparation—dihydrotachysterol (AT 10 or Hytakerol), ergocalciferol (vitamin D), or cholecalciferol (vitamin D)—are usually required and enhance calcium absorption from the GI tract.

Nursing Management

Nursing management of the patient with possible acute hypoparathyroidism includes the following:

- Care of postoperative patients who have undergone thyroidectomy, parathyroidectomy, or radical neck dissection is directed toward detecting early signs of hypocalcemia and anticipating signs of tetany, seizures, and respiratory difficulties.
- Calcium gluconate is kept at the bedside with equipment necessary for emergency IV administration. If the patient requiring administration of calcium gluconate has a cardiac disorder, is subject to dysrhythmias, or is receiving digitalis, the calcium gluconate is administered slowly and cautiously.
- Calcium and digitalis increase systolic contraction and also potentiate each other; this can produce potentially fatal dysrhythmias. Consequently, the cardiac patient requires continuous cardiac monitoring and careful assessment.

An important aspect of nursing care is teaching about medications and diet therapy. The patient needs to know the reason for high calcium and low phosphate intake and the symptoms of hypocalcemia and hypercalcemia; he or she should know to contact the physician immediately if these symptoms occur (Chart 42-10).

THE ADRENAL GLANDS

Anatomic and Physiologic Overview

Each person has two adrenal glands, one attached to the upper portion of each kidney (Porth & Matfin, 2009). Each adrenal gland is, in reality, two endocrine glands with sepa-

rate, independent functions. The adrenal medulla at the center of the gland secretes catecholamines, and the outer portion of the gland, the adrenal cortex, secretes steroid hormones (Fig. 42-6). The secretion of hormones from the adrenal cortex is regulated by the hypothalamic–pituitary–adrenal axis. The hypothalamus secretes corticotropin-releasing hormone (CRH), which stimulates the pituitary gland to secrete ACTH, which in turn stimulates

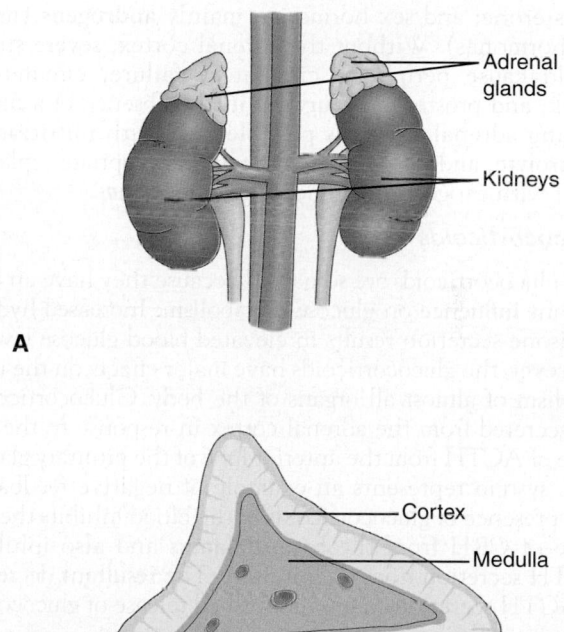

Figure 42-6 **A,** The adrenal glands sit on top of the kidneys. **B,** Each gland is composed of an outer cortex and an inner medulla. Each area secretes specific hormones. The adrenal medulla secretes catecholamines—epinephrine and norepinephrine; the adrenal cortex secretes glucocorticoids, mineralocorticoids, and sex hormones. Adapted from Porth, C. (2006). *Essentials of pathophysiology: Concepts of altered health states* (2nd ed.). Philadelphia: Lippincott Williams & Wilkins.

the adrenal cortex to secrete glucocorticoid hormone (cortisol). Increased levels of the adrenal hormone then inhibit the production or secretion of CRH and ACTH. This system is an example of a negative feedback mechanism.

Adrenal Medulla

The adrenal medulla functions as part of the autonomic nervous system. Stimulation of preganglionic sympathetic nerve fibers, which travel directly to the cells of the adrenal medulla, causes release of the catecholamine hormones epinephrine and norepinephrine. About 90% of the secretion of the human adrenal medulla is epinephrine (also called adrenaline). Catecholamines regulate metabolic pathways to promote catabolism of stored fuels to meet caloric needs from endogenous sources. The major effects of epinephrine release are to prepare to meet a challenge (fight-or-flight response). Secretion of epinephrine causes decreased blood flow to tissues that are not needed in emergency situations, such as the GI tract, and increased blood flow to tissues that are important for effective fight or flight, such as cardiac and skeletal muscle. Catecholamines also induce the release of free fatty acids, increase the basal metabolic rate, and elevate the blood glucose level.

Adrenal Cortex

A functioning adrenal cortex is necessary for life; adrenocortical secretions make it possible for the body to adapt to stress of all kinds. The three types of steroid hormones produced by the adrenal cortex are **glucocorticoids,** the prototype of which is hydrocortisone; **mineralocorticoids,** mainly aldosterone; and sex hormones, mainly **androgens** (male sex hormones). Without the adrenal cortex, severe stress would cause peripheral circulatory failure, circulatory shock, and prostration. Survival in the absence of a functioning adrenal cortex is possible only with nutritional, electrolyte, and fluid replacement and appropriate replacement with exogenous adrenocortical hormones.

Glucocorticoids

The glucocorticoids are so named because they have an important influence on glucose metabolism: Increased hydrocortisone secretion results in elevated blood glucose levels. However, the glucocorticoids have major effects on the metabolism of almost all organs of the body. Glucocorticoids are secreted from the adrenal cortex in response to the release of ACTH from the anterior lobe of the pituitary gland. This system represents an example of negative feedback. The presence of glucocorticoids in the blood inhibits the release of CRH from the hypothalamus and also inhibits ACTH secretion from the pituitary. The resultant decrease in ACTH secretion causes diminished release of glucocorticoids from the adrenal cortex.

Glucocorticoids (in the form of **corticosteroids**) are administered frequently to inhibit the inflammatory response to tissue injury and to suppress allergic manifestations. Their side effects include the development of diabetes mellitus, osteoporosis, peptic ulcer, increased protein breakdown resulting in muscle wasting and poor wound healing, and redistribution of body fat. Large amounts of exogenously administered glucocorticoids in the blood inhibit the release of ACTH and endogenous glucocorticoids. Because

of this, the adrenal cortex can atrophy. If exogenous glucocorticoid administration is discontinued suddenly, adrenal insufficiency results because of the inability of the atrophied cortex to respond adequately.

Mineralocorticoids

Mineralocorticoids exert their major effects on electrolyte metabolism. They act principally on the renal tubular and GI epithelium to cause increased sodium ion absorption in exchange for excretion of potassium or hydrogen ions. ACTH only minimally influences aldosterone secretion. It is primarily secreted in response to the presence of angiotensin II in the bloodstream. Angiotensin II is a substance that elevates the blood pressure by constricting arterioles. Its concentration is increased when renin is released from the kidney in response to decreased perfusion pressure. The resultant increased aldosterone levels promote sodium reabsorption by the kidney and the GI tract, which tends to restore blood pressure to normal. The release of aldosterone is also increased by hyperkalemia. Aldosterone is the primary hormone for the long-term regulation of sodium balance.

Adrenal Sex Hormones (Androgens)

Androgens, the third major type of steroid hormones produced by the adrenal cortex, exert effects similar to those of male sex hormones. The adrenal gland may also secrete small amounts of some estrogens, or female sex hormones. ACTH controls the secretion of adrenal androgens. When secreted in normal amounts, the adrenal androgens probably have little effect, but when secreted in excess, as in certain inborn enzyme deficiencies, masculinization may result. This is termed the **adrenogenital syndrome.**

Specific Disorders of the Adrenal Glands

PHEOCHROMOCYTOMA

Pheochromocytoma is a tumor that is usually benign and originates from the chromaffin cells of the adrenal medulla. In 90% of patients (Porth & Matfin, 2009), the tumor arises in the medulla; in the remaining patients, it occurs in the extra-adrenal chromaffin tissue located in or near the aorta, ovaries, spleen, or other organs. Pheochromocytoma may occur at any age, but its peak incidence is between 40 and 50 years of age affecting men and women equally. Ten percent of the tumors are bilateral, and 10% are malignant. Because of the high incidence of pheochromocytoma in family members of affected people, the patient's family members should be alerted and screened for this tumor. Pheochromocytoma may occur in the familial form as part of multiple endocrine neoplasia type 2; therefore, it should be considered a possibility in patients who have medullary thyroid carcinoma and parathyroid hyperplasia or tumor.

Pheochromocytoma is the cause of high blood pressure in 0.1% of patients with hypertension. Although it is uncommon, it is one form of hypertension that is usually cured by surgery; however, without detection and treatment, it is usually fatal.

Clinical Manifestations

The nature and severity of symptoms of functioning tumors of the adrenal medulla depend on the relative proportions of epinephrine and norepinephrine secretion. The typical triad of symptoms is headache, diaphoresis, and palpitations in the patient with hypertension. Approximately 8% of patients are completely asymptomatic. Hypertension and other cardiovascular disturbances are common. The hypertension may be intermittent or persistent. However, only half of patients with pheochromocytoma have sustained or persistent hypertension. If the hypertension is sustained, it may be difficult to distinguish from other causes of hypertension. Other symptoms may include tremor, headache, flushing, and anxiety. Hyperglycemia may result from conversion of liver and muscle glycogen to glucose due to epinephrine secretion; insulin may be required to maintain normal blood glucose levels.

The clinical picture in the paroxysmal form of pheochromocytoma is usually characterized by acute, unpredictable attacks lasting seconds or several hours. Symptoms usually begin abruptly and subside slowly. During these attacks, the patient is extremely anxious, tremulous, and weak. The patient may experience headache, vertigo, blurring of vision, tinnitus, air hunger, and dyspnea. Other symptoms include polyuria, nausea, vomiting, diarrhea, abdominal pain, and a feeling of impending doom. Palpitations and tachycardia are common (Porth & Matfin, 2009). Blood pressures exceeding 250/150 mm Hg have been recorded. Such blood pressure elevations are life-threatening and can cause severe complications, such as cardiac dysrhythmias, dissecting aneurysm, stroke, and acute renal failure. Postural hypotension (decrease in systolic blood pressure, lightheadedness, dizziness on standing) occurs in 70% of patients with untreated pheochromocytoma.

Assessment and Diagnostic Findings

Pheochromocytoma is suspected if signs of sympathetic nervous system overactivity occur in association with marked elevation of blood pressure. These signs can be associated with the "five H's": hypertension, headache, hyperhidrosis (excessive sweating), hypermetabolism, and hyperglycemia. The presence of these signs is highly predictive of pheochromocytoma. Paroxysmal symptoms of pheochromocytoma commonly develop in the fifth decade of life.

Measurements of urine and plasma levels of catecholamines and metanephrine (MN), a catecholamine metabolite, are the most direct and conclusive tests for overactivity of the adrenal medulla. A new test for detecting pheochromocytoma has recently been developed that measures free MN in plasma by high-pressure liquid chromatography and electrochemical detection. A negative test result virtually excludes pheochromocytoma. However, increased levels of at least one catecholamine or MN can occur in 10% of patients with essential hypertension.

Measurements of catecholamine metabolites (MN and vanillylmandelic acid [VMA]) or free catecholamines have been extensively used in the clinical setting. In most cases, pheochromocytoma can be diagnosed or confirmed based on a properly collected 24-hour urine sample. Levels can be as high as two times the normal limit. A 24-hour specimen of urine is collected for determination of free catecholamines, MN, and VMA; the use of combined tests increases the diagnostic accuracy of testing. A number of medications and foods, such as coffee and tea (including decaffeinated varieties), bananas, chocolate, vanilla, and aspirin, may alter the results of these tests; therefore, careful instructions to avoid restricted items must be given to the patient. Urine collected over a 2- or 3-hour period after an attack of hypertension can be assayed for catecholamine content.

The total plasma catecholamine (epinephrine and norepinephrine) concentration is measured with the patient supine and at rest for 30 minutes. To prevent elevation of catecholamine levels resulting from the stress of venipuncture, a butterfly needle, scalp vein needle, or venous catheter may be inserted 30 minutes before the blood specimen is obtained.

Factors that may elevate catecholamine concentrations must be controlled to obtain valid results; these factors include consumption of coffee or tea (including decaffeinated varieties), use of tobacco, emotional and physical stress, and use of many prescription and over-the-counter medications (eg, amphetamines, nose drops or sprays, decongestant agents, bronchodilators).

Normal plasma values of epinephrine are 100 pg/mL (590 pmol/L); normal values of norepinephrine are generally less than 100 to 550 pg/mL (590 to 3240 pmol/L). Values of epinephrine greater than 400 pg/mL (2180 pmol/L) or norepinephrine values greater than 2000 pg/mL (11,800 pmol/L) are considered diagnostic of pheochromocytoma. Values that fall between normal levels and those diagnostic of pheochromocytoma indicate the need for further testing.

A clonidine suppression test may be performed if the results of plasma and urine tests of catecholamines are inconclusive. Clonidine (Catapres) is a centrally acting anti-adrenergic medication that suppresses the release of neurogenically mediated catecholamines. The suppression test is based on the principle that catecholamine levels are normally increased through the activity of the sympathetic nervous system. In pheochromocytoma, increased catecholamine levels result from the diffusion of excess catecholamines into the circulation, bypassing normal storage and release mechanisms. Therefore, in patients with pheochromocytoma, clonidine does not suppress the release of catecholamines.

Imaging studies, such as CT, MRI, and ultrasonography, may also be carried out to localize the pheochromocytoma and to determine whether more than one tumor is present. Use of ^{131}I-metaiodobenzylguanidine (MIBG) scintigraphy may be required to determine the location of the pheochromocytoma and to detect metastatic sites outside the adrenal gland. MIBG is a specific isotope for catecholamine-producing tissue. It has been helpful in identifying tumors not detected by other tests or procedures. MIBG scintigraphy is a noninvasive, safe procedure that has increased the accuracy of diagnosis of adrenal tumors.

Other diagnostic studies may focus on evaluating the function of other endocrine glands because of the association of pheochromocytoma in some patients with other endocrine tumors.

Medical Management

During an episode or attack of hypertension, tachycardia, anxiety, and the other symptoms of pheochromocytoma, bed rest with the head of the bed elevated is prescribed to promote an orthostatic decrease in blood pressure.

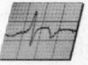

Pharmacologic Therapy

The patient may be moved to the intensive care unit for close monitoring of ECG changes and careful administration of alpha-adrenergic blocking agents (eg, phentolamine [Regitine]) or smooth muscle relaxants (eg, sodium nitroprusside [Nipride]) to lower the blood pressure quickly.

Phenoxybenzamine (Dibenzyline), a long-acting alphablocker, may be used after the blood pressure is stable to prepare the patient for surgery. Calcium channel blockers such as nifedipine (Procardia) are usually well tolerated by patients and have reduced perioperative fluid requirements. They are also useful for prevention of cardiovascular complications, because they prevent catecholamine-induced coronary vasospasm and myocarditis. Beta-adrenergic blocking agents such as propranolol (Inderal) may be used in patients with cardiac dysrhythmias and in those not responsive to alpha-blockers. Alpha-adrenergic and beta-adrenergic blocking agents must be used with caution, because patients with pheochromocytoma may have increased sensitivity to them. Still other medications that may be used preoperatively are catecholamine synthesis inhibitors, such as alpha-methyl-p-tyrosine (metyrosine [Demser]). These are occasionally used if adrenergic blocking agents do not reduce the effects of catecholamines.

Surgical Management

The definitive treatment of pheochromocytoma is surgical removal of the tumor, usually with **adrenalectomy.** Bilateral adrenalectomy may be necessary if tumors are present in both adrenal glands. Patient preparation includes control of blood pressure and blood volumes; usually this is carried out over 4 to 7 days. Nifedipine (Procardia) and nicardipine (Cardene) may be used safely without causing undue hypotension. For episodes of severe hypertension, nifedipine is a fast and effective treatment, because the capsules can be pierced and chewed. The patient needs to be well hydrated before, during, and after surgery to prevent hypotension.

Manipulation of the tumor during surgical excision may cause release of stored epinephrine and norepinephrine, with marked increases in blood pressure and changes in heart rate. Therefore, use of sodium nitroprusside (Nipride) and alpha-adrenergic blocking agents may be required during and after surgery. Exploration of other possible tumor sites is frequently undertaken to ensure removal of all tumor tissue. As a result, the patient is subject to the stress and effects of a long surgical procedure, which may increase the risk of hypertension postoperatively.

Corticosteroid replacement is required if bilateral adrenalectomy has been necessary. Corticosteroids may also be required for the first few days or weeks after removal of a single adrenal gland. IV administration of corticosteroids (methylprednisolone sodium succinate [Solu-Medrol]) may begin on the evening before surgery and continue during the early postoperative period to prevent adrenal insufficiency. Oral preparations of corticosteroids (prednisone) are prescribed after the acute stress of surgery diminishes.

Hypotension and hypoglycemia may occur in the postoperative period because of the sudden withdrawal of excessive amounts of catecholamines. Therefore, careful attention is directed toward monitoring and treating these changes. Blood pressure is expected to return to normal with treatment; however, one third of patients continue to be hypertensive after surgery. This may result if not all pheochromocytoma tissue was removed, if pheochromocytoma recurs, or if the blood vessels were damaged by severe and prolonged hypertension. Several days after surgery, urine and plasma levels of catecholamines and their metabolites are measured to determine whether the surgery was successful.

Nursing Management

The patient who has undergone surgery to treat pheochromocytoma has experienced a stressful preoperative and postoperative course and may remain fearful of repeated attacks. Although it is usually expected that all pheochromocytoma tissue has been removed, there is a possibility that other sites were undetected and that attacks may recur. The patient is monitored for several days in the intensive care unit with special attention given to ECG changes, arterial pressures, fluid and electrolyte balance, and blood glucose levels. Several IV lines are inserted for administration of fluids and medications.

Promoting Home and Community-Based Care

Teaching Patients Self-Care

During the preoperative and postoperative phases of care, the nurse informs the patient about the importance of follow-up monitoring to ensure that pheochromocytoma does not recur undetected. After adrenalectomy, use of corticosteroids may be needed. Therefore, the nurse instructs the patient about their purpose, the medication schedule, and the risks of skipping doses or stopping their administration abruptly.

It is important to teach the patient and family how to measure the patient's blood pressure and when to notify the physician about changes in blood pressure. In addition, the nurse provides verbal and written instructions about the procedure for collecting 24-hour urine specimens to monitor urine catecholamine levels.

Continuing Care

A follow-up visit from a home care nurse may be indicated to assess the patient's postoperative recovery, surgical incision, and compliance with the medication schedule. This may help reinforce previous teaching about management and monitoring. The home care nurse also obtains blood pressure measurements and assists the patient in preventing or dealing with problems that may result from long-term use of corticosteroids.

Because of the risk of recurrence of hypertension, periodic checkups are required, especially in young patients and in those whose families have a history of pheochromocytoma. The patient is scheduled for periodic follow-up appointments to observe for return of normal blood pressure and plasma and urine levels of catecholamines.

ADRENOCORTICAL INSUFFICIENCY (ADDISON'S DISEASE)

Addison's disease, or adrenocortical insufficiency, occurs when adrenal cortex function is inadequate to meet the patient's need for cortical hormones. Autoimmune or idiopathic atrophy of the adrenal glands is responsible for the vast majority of cases. Other causes include surgical removal of both adrenal glands and infection of the adrenal glands. Tuberculosis and histoplasmosis are the most common infections that destroy adrenal gland tissue. Although autoimmune destruction has replaced tuberculosis as the principal cause of Addison's disease, tuberculosis should be considered in the diagnostic workup because of its increasing incidence. Inadequate secretion of ACTH from the pituitary gland also results in adrenal insufficiency because of decreased stimulation of the adrenal cortex.

Therapeutic use of corticosteroids is the most common cause of adrenocortical insufficiency (Porth & Matfin, 2009). Symptoms of adrenocortical insufficiency may also result from the sudden cessation of exogenous adrenocortical hormonal therapy, which suppresses the body's normal response to stress and interferes with normal feedback mechanisms. Treatment with daily administration of corticosteroids for 2 to 4 weeks may suppress function of the adrenal cortex; therefore, adrenal insufficiency should be considered in any patient who has been treated with corticosteroids.

Clinical Manifestations

Addison's disease is characterized by muscle weakness; anorexia; GI symptoms; fatigue; emaciation; dark pigmentation of the mucous membranes and the skin, especially of the knuckles, knees, and elbows; hypotension; and low blood glucose, low serum sodium, and high serum potassium levels. Mental status changes such as depression, emotional lability, apathy, and confusion are present in 60% to 80% of patients. In severe cases, the disturbance of sodium and potassium metabolism may be marked by depletion of sodium and water and severe, chronic dehydration.

With disease progression and acute hypotension, **addisonian crisis** develops. This condition is characterized by cyanosis and the classic signs of circulatory shock: pallor, apprehension, rapid and weak pulse, rapid respirations, and low blood pressure. In addition, the patient may complain of headache, nausea, abdominal pain, and diarrhea and may show signs of confusion and restlessness. Even slight overexertion, exposure to cold, acute infection, or a decrease in salt intake may lead to circulatory collapse, shock, and death if untreated. The stress of surgery or dehydration resulting from preparation for diagnostic tests or surgery may precipitate an addisonian or hypotensive crisis.

Assessment and Diagnostic Findings

Although the clinical manifestations presented appear specific, the onset of Addison's disease usually occurs with nonspecific symptoms. The diagnosis is confirmed by laboratory test results. Combined measurements of early-morning serum cortisol and plasma ACTH are performed to differentiate primary adrenal insufficiency from secondary adrenal insufficiency and from normal adrenal function. Patients with primary insufficiency have a greatly increased plasma ACTH level (more than 22.0 pmol/L) and a serum cortisol concentration lower than the normal range (less than 165 nmol/L) or in the low-normal range. Other laboratory findings include decreased levels of blood glucose (hypoglycemia) and sodium (hyponatremia), an increased serum potassium concentration (hyperkalemia), and an increased white blood cell count (leukocytosis).

The diagnosis is confirmed by low levels of adrenocortical hormones in the blood or urine and decreased serum cortisol levels. If the adrenal cortex is destroyed, baseline values are low, and ACTH administration fails to cause the normal increase in plasma cortisol and urinary 17-hydroxycorticosteroids. If the adrenal gland is normal but not stimulated properly by the pituitary, a normal response to repeated doses of exogenous ACTH is seen, but no response occurs after the administration of metyrapone (Metopirone), which stimulates endogenous ACTH.

Medical Management

Immediate treatment is directed toward combating circulatory shock: restoring blood circulation, administering fluids and corticosteroids, monitoring vital signs, and placing the patient in a recumbent position with the legs elevated. Hydrocortisone (Solu-Cortef) is administered by IV, followed by 5% dextrose in normal saline. Vasopressor amines may be required if hypotension persists.

Antibiotics may be administered if infection has precipitated adrenal crisis in a patient with chronic adrenal insufficiency. In addition, the patient is assessed closely to identify other factors, stressors, or illnesses that led to the acute episode.

Oral intake may be initiated as soon as tolerated. IV fluids are gradually decreased after oral fluid intake is adequate to prevent hypovolemia. If the adrenal gland does not regain function, the patient needs lifelong replacement of corticosteroids and mineralocorticoids to prevent recurrence of adrenal insufficiency. During stressful procedures or significant illnesses, additional supplementary therapy with glucocorticoids is required to prevent addisonian crisis. In addition, the patient may need to supplement dietary intake with added salt during gastrointestinal losses of fluids through vomiting and diarrhea.

Nursing Management

Assessing the Patient

The health history and examination focus on the presence of symptoms of fluid imbalance and on the patient's level of stress. The nurse should monitor the blood pressure and pulse rate as the patient moves from a lying, sitting, and standing position to assess for inadequate fluid volume. A decrease in systolic pressure (20 mm Hg or more) may indicate depletion of fluid volume, especially if accompanied by symptoms. The skin should be assessed for changes in color and turgor, which could indicate chronic adrenal insufficiency and hypovolemia. The patient is assessed for change in weight, muscle weakness, fatigue, and any illness or stress that may have precipitated the acute crisis.

Monitoring and Managing Addisonian Crisis

The patient at risk is monitored for signs and symptoms indicative of addisonian crisis, which can include shock; hypotension; rapid, weak pulse; rapid respiratory rate; pallor; and extreme weakness (see Chapter 15). Physical and psychological stressors such as cold exposure, overexertion, infection, and emotional distress should be avoided.

The patient with addisonian crisis requires immediate treatment with IV administration of fluid, glucose, and electrolytes, especially sodium; replacement of missing steroid hormones; and vasopressors. The nurse anticipates and meets the patient's needs to promote return to a precrisis state.

Restoring Fluid Balance

The nurse encourages the patient to consume foods and fluids that assist in restoring and maintaining fluid and electrolyte balance. Along with the dietitian, the nurse helps the patient select foods high in sodium during GI disturbances and in very hot weather.

The nurse instructs the patient and family to administer hormone replacement as prescribed and to modify the dosage during illness and other stressful situations. Written and verbal instructions are provided about the administration of mineralocorticoid (Florinef) or corticosteroid (prednisone) as prescribed.

Improving Activity Tolerance

Until the patient's condition is stabilized, the nurse takes precautions to avoid unnecessary activity and stress that could precipitate another hypotensive episode. Efforts are made to detect signs of infection or the presence of other stressors. Explaining the rationale for minimizing stress during the acute crisis assists the patient to increase activity gradually.

Promoting Home and Community-Based Care

Teaching Patients Self-Care

Because of the need for lifelong replacement of adrenal cortex hormones to prevent addisonian crises, the patient and family members receive explicit verbal and written instructions about the rationale for replacement therapy and proper dosage. In addition, they are instructed about how to modify the medication dosage and increase salt intake in times of illness, very hot weather, and other stressful situations. The patient also learns how to modify diet and fluid intake to help maintain fluid and electrolyte balance.

The patient and family are frequently prescribed preloaded, single-injection syringes of corticosteroid for use in emergencies. Specific instructions about how and when to use the injection are also provided. It is important to instruct the patient to inform other health care providers, such as dentists, about the use of corticosteroids; to wear a medical alert bracelet; and to carry information at all times about the need for corticosteroids. If the patient with Addison's disease requires surgery, careful administration of fluids and corticosteroids is necessary before, during, and after surgery to prevent addisonian crisis.

The patient and family need to know the signs of excessive or insufficient hormone replacement. The development of edema or weight gain may signify too high a dose of hormone; postural hypotension and weight loss frequently signify too low a dose (Chart 42-11).

CHART 42-11   **HOME CARE CHECKLIST**
The Patient With Adrenal Insufficiency (Addison's Disease)

At the completion of the home care instruction, the patient or caregiver will be able to:	PATIENT	CAREGIVER
• State present and potential effects of adrenal insufficiency on the body.	✔	✔
• State warning signs of adrenal crisis and need for emergency care.	✔	✔
• Explain components of an emergency kit and indications for their use; demonstrate how to use them.	✔	✔
• State strategies for dealing with stress and avoiding adrenal crisis.	✔	✔
• State the purpose, dose, route, schedule, side effects, and precautions of prescribed medications (corticosteroid replacement).	✔	✔
• State that compliance with medical regimen is lifelong.	✔	✔
• State importance of regular follow-up visits with health care provider.	✔	✔
• Recognize the need for dosage adjustment during times of stress.	✔	✔
• State need to wear medical alert identification and carry medical information card.	✔	✔
• State need to notify health care providers about disease before treatment or procedure.	✔	✔
• State need to avoid strenuous activity in hot, humid weather.	✔	✔
• State need for increased fluid intake and salt with excessive perspiration.	✔	✔
• State need for high-carbohydrate, high-protein diet with adequate sodium intake.	✔	✔
• Identify needed activity limitations and impact on lifestyle.	✔	✔

Continuing Care

Although most patients can return to their job and family responsibilities soon after hospital discharge, others cannot do so because of concurrent illnesses or incomplete recovery from the episode of adrenal insufficiency. In these circumstances, a referral for home care enables the home care nurse to assess the patient's recovery, monitor hormone replacement, and evaluate stress in the home. The nurse assesses the patient's and family's knowledge about medication therapy and dietary modifications. A home visit also allows the nurse to assess the patient's plans for follow-up visits to the clinic or physician's office. The nurse reminds the patient and family about the importance of participating in health promotion activities and health screening.

CUSHING'S SYNDROME

Cushing's syndrome results from excessive, rather than deficient, adrenocortical activity (Porth & Matfin, 2009). Cushing's syndrome is commonly caused by use of corticosteroid medications and is infrequently the result of excessive corticosteroid production secondary to hyperplasia of the adrenal cortex. However, overproduction of endogenous corticosteroids may be caused by several mechanisms, including a tumor of the pituitary gland that produces ACTH and stimulates the adrenal cortex to increase its hormone secretion despite production of adequate amounts. Primary hyperplasia of the adrenal glands in the absence of a pituitary tumor is less common. Another less common cause of Cushing's syndrome is the ectopic production of ACTH by malignancies; bronchogenic carcinoma is the most common type. Regardless of the cause, the normal feedback mechanisms that control the function of the adrenal cortex become ineffective, and the usual diurnal pattern of cortisol is lost. The signs and symptoms of Cushing's syndrome are primarily a result of oversecretion of glucocorticoids and androgens (sex hormones), although mineralocorticoid secretion also may be affected (Porth & Matfin, 2009).

Clinical Manifestations

When overproduction of the adrenal cortical hormone occurs, arrest of growth, obesity, and musculoskeletal changes occur along with glucose intolerance. The classic picture of Cushing's syndrome in the adult is that of central-type obesity, with a fatty "buffalo hump" in the neck and supraclavicular areas, a heavy trunk, and relatively thin extremities. The skin is thin, fragile, and easily traumatized; ecchymoses (bruises) and striae develop. The patient complains of weakness and lassitude. Sleep is disturbed because of altered diurnal secretion of cortisol.

Excessive protein catabolism occurs, producing muscle wasting and osteoporosis. Kyphosis, backache, and compression fractures of the vertebrae may result. Retention of sodium and water occurs as a result of increased mineralocorticoid activity, producing hypertension and heart failure.

The patient develops a "moon-faced" appearance and may experience increased oiliness of the skin and acne. There is increased susceptibility to infection. Hyperglycemia or overt diabetes may develop. The patient may also report weight gain, slow healing of minor cuts, and bruises.

Women between the ages of 20 and 40 years are five times more likely than men to develop Cushing's syndrome. In females of all ages, virilization may occur as a result of excess androgens. Virilization is characterized by the appearance of masculine traits and the recession of feminine traits. There is an excessive growth of hair on the face (hirsutism), the breasts atrophy, menses cease, the clitoris enlarges, and the voice deepens. Libido is lost in men and women.

Changes occur in mood and mental activity, and psychosis may develop. Distress and depression are common and are increased by the severity of the physical changes that occur with this syndrome. If Cushing's syndrome is a consequence of pituitary tumor, visual disturbances may occur because of pressure of the growing tumor on the optic chiasm. Chart 42-12 summarizes the changes associated with Cushing's syndrome.

Assessment and Diagnostic Findings

An overnight dexamethasone suppression test is the most widely used and most sensitive screening test for diagnosis of pituitary and adrenal causes of Cushing's syndrome. It can be performed on an outpatient basis. Dexamethasone (1 mg) is administered orally at 11 PM, and a plasma cortisol level is obtained at 8 AM the next morning. Suppression of cortisol to less than 5 mg/dL indicates that the hypothalamic–pituitary–adrenal axis is functioning properly. Stress, obesity, depression, and medications such as antiseizure agents, estrogen (during pregnancy or as oral medications), and rifampin (Rifadin) can falsely elevate cortisol levels. Nighttime salivary cortisol levels show promise in screening for Cushing's syndrome (Gross, Mindea, Pick, et al., 2007).

Indicators of Cushing's syndrome include an increase in serum sodium and blood glucose levels and a decrease in serum potassium, a reduction in the number of blood eosinophils, and disappearance of lymphoid tissue. Measurements of plasma and urinary cortisol levels are obtained. Several blood samples may be collected to determine whether the normal diurnal variation in plasma levels is present; this variation is frequently absent in adrenal dysfunction. If several blood samples are required, they must be collected at the times specified, and the time of collection must be noted on the requisition slip. Other diagnostic studies include a 24-hour urinary free cortisol level and a low-dose dexamethasone suppression test. Low-dose suppression tests are similar to the overnight test but vary in dosage and timing.

Measurement of plasma ACTH by radioimmunoassay is used in conjunction with the high-dose suppression test to distinguish pituitary tumors from ectopic sites of ACTH production as the cause of Cushing's syndrome. Elevation of both ACTH and cortisol indicates pituitary or hypothalamic disease. A low ACTH with a high cortisol level indicates adrenal disease. CT, ultrasound, or MRI may be performed to localize adrenal tissue and detect tumors of the adrenal gland.

Medical Management

If Cushing's syndrome is caused by pituitary tumors rather than tumors of the adrenal cortex, treatment is directed at the pituitary gland. Surgical removal of the tumor by transsphenoidal hypophysectomy (see Chapter 61) is the

Chart 42-12 • *Clinical Manifestations of Cushing's Syndrome*

Ophthalmic	Skeletal
Cataracts	Osteoporosis
Glaucoma	Spontaneous fractures
	Aseptic necrosis of femur
Cardiovascular	Vertebral compression
Hypertension	fractures
Heart failure	**Gastrointestinal**
Endocrine/Metabolic	Peptic ulcer
Truncal obesity	Pancreatitis
Moon face	
Buffalo hump	**Muscular**
Sodium retention	Myopathy
Hypokalemia	Muscle weakness
Metabolic alkalosis	
Hyperglycemia	**Dermatologic**
Menstrual irregularities	Thinning of skin
Impotence	Petechiae
Negative nitrogen	Ecchymoses
balance	Striae
Altered calcium	Acne
metabolism	
Adrenal suppression	**Psychiatric**
	Mood alterations
Immune Function	Psychoses
Decreased inflammatory	
responses	
Impaired wound healing	
Increased susceptibility to	
infections	

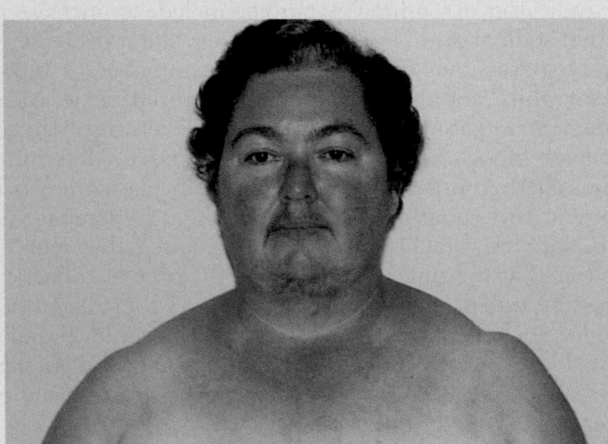

This woman with Cushing's syndrome has several classic signs, including facial hair, buffalo hump, and moon face. From Rubin, E. & Farber, J. L. (2005). *Pathology* (4th ed.). Philadelphia: Lippincott Williams & Wilkins.

treatment of choice and has an 80% success rate. Radiation of the pituitary gland also has been successful, although it may take several months for control of symptoms. Adrenalectomy is the treatment of choice in patients with primary adrenal hypertrophy.

Postoperatively, symptoms of adrenal insufficiency may begin to appear 12 to 48 hours after surgery because of reduction of the high levels of circulating adrenal hormones. Temporary replacement therapy with hydrocortisone may be necessary for several months, until the adrenal glands begin to respond normally to the body's needs. If both adrenal glands have been removed (bilateral adrenalectomy), lifetime replacement of adrenal cortex hormones is necessary.

Adrenal enzyme inhibitors (eg, metyrapone [Metopirone], aminoglutethimide [Cytadren], mitotane [Lysodren], and ketoconazole [Nizoral]) may be used to reduce hyperadrenalism if the syndrome is caused by ectopic ACTH secretion by a tumor that cannot be eradicated. Close monitoring is necessary, because symptoms of inadequate adrenal function may result and side effects of the medications may occur.

If Cushing's syndrome is a result of the administration of corticosteroids, an attempt is made to reduce or taper the medication to the minimum dosage needed to treat the underlying disease process (eg, autoimmune or allergic disease, rejection of a transplanted organ). Frequently, alternate-day therapy decreases the symptoms of Cushing's syndrome and allows recovery of the adrenal glands' responsiveness to ACTH.

NURSING PROCESS

THE PATIENT WITH CUSHING'S SYNDROME

Assessment

The health history and examination focus on the effects on the body of high concentrations of adrenal cortex hormones and on the inability of the adrenal cortex to respond to changes in cortisol and aldosterone levels. The history includes information about the patient's level of activity and ability to carry out routine and self-care activities. The skin is observed and assessed for trauma, infection, breakdown, bruising, and edema. Changes in physical appearance are noted, and the patient's responses to these changes are elicited. The nurse assesses the patient's mental function, including mood, responses to questions, awareness of environment, and level of depression. The family is often a good source of information about gradual changes in the patient's physical appearance as well as emotional status.

Diagnosis

Nursing Diagnoses

Based on all the assessment data, the major nursing diagnoses of the patient with Cushing's syndrome include the following:

- Risk for injury related to weakness
- Risk for infection related to altered protein metabolism and inflammatory response
- Self-care deficit related to weakness, fatigue, muscle wasting, and altered sleep patterns
- Impaired skin integrity related to edema, impaired healing, and thin and fragile skin
- Disturbed body image related to altered physical appearance, impaired sexual functioning, and decreased activity level
- Disturbed thought processes related to mood swings, irritability, and depression

Collaborative Problems/Potential Complications

Potential complications may include the following:

- Addisonian crisis
- Adverse effects of adrenocortical activity

Planning and Goals

The major goals for the patient include decreased risk of injury, decreased risk of infection, increased ability to carry out self-care activities, improved skin integrity, improved body image, improved mental function, and absence of complications.

Nursing Interventions

Decreasing Risk of Injury

Establishing a protective environment helps prevent falls, fractures, and other injuries to bones and soft tissues. The patient who is very weak may require assistance from the nurse in ambulating to avoid falling or bumping into sharp corners of furniture. Foods high in protein, calcium, and vitamin D are recommended to minimize muscle wasting and osteoporosis. Referral to a dietitian may assist the patient in selecting appropriate foods that are also low in sodium and calories.

Decreasing Risk of Infection

The patient should avoid unnecessary exposure to others with infections. The nurse frequently assesses the patient for subtle signs of infection, because the anti-inflammatory effects of corticosteroids may mask the common signs of inflammation and infection.

Preparing the Patient for Surgery

The patient is prepared for adrenalectomy, if indicated, and the postoperative course (see later discussion). If Cushing's syndrome is a result of a pituitary tumor, a transsphenoidal hypophysectomy may be performed (see Chapter 61). Diabetes mellitus and peptic ulcer are common in patients with Cushing's syndrome. Therefore, insulin therapy and medication to treat peptic ulcer are initiated if needed. Before, during, and after surgery, blood glucose monitoring and assessment of stools for blood are carried out to monitor for these complications. If the patient has other symptoms of Cushing's syndrome, these are considered in the preoperative preparation. For example, if the patient has experienced weight gain, special instruction is given about postoperative breathing exercises.

Encouraging Rest and Activity

Although the patient with Cushing's syndrome experiences insomnia, weakness, fatigue, and muscle wasting, the nurse should encourage moderate activity to prevent complications of immobility and promote increased self-esteem. It is important to help the patient plan and space rest periods throughout the day and promote a relaxing, quiet environment for rest and sleep.

Promoting Skin Integrity

Meticulous skin care is necessary to avoid traumatizing the patient's fragile skin. Use of adhesive tape is avoided, because it can irritate the skin and tear the fragile tissue when the tape is removed. The nurse frequently assesses the skin and bony prominences and encourages and assists the patient to change positions frequently to prevent skin breakdown.

Improving Body Image

If treated successfully, the major physical changes associated with Cushing's syndrome disappear in time. The patient may benefit from discussion of the effect the changes have had on his or her self-concept and relationships with others. Weight gain and edema may be modified by a low-carbohydrate, low-sodium diet, and a high protein intake may reduce some of the other bothersome symptoms.

Improving Thought Processes

Explanations to the patient and family members about the cause of emotional instability are important in helping them cope with the mood swings, irritability, and depression that may occur. Psychotic behavior may occur in a few patients and should be reported. The nurse encourages the patient and family members to verbalize their feelings and concerns.

Monitoring and Managing Potential Complications

ADDISONIAN CRISIS. The patient with Cushing's syndrome whose symptoms are treated by withdrawal of corticosteroids, by adrenalectomy, or by removal of a pituitary tumor is at risk for adrenal hypofunction and addisonian crisis. If high levels of circulating adrenal hormones have suppressed the function of the adrenal cortex, atrophy of the adrenal cortex is likely. If the circulating hormone level is decreased rapidly because of surgery or abrupt cessation of corticosteroid agents, manifestations of adrenal hypofunction and addisonian crisis may develop. Therefore, the patient with Cushing's syndrome should be assessed for signs and symptoms of addisonian crisis as previously discussed. If addisonian crisis occurs, the patient is treated for circulatory collapse and shock (see Chapter 15).

ADVERSE EFFECTS OF ADRENOCORTICAL ACTIVITY. The nurse assesses fluid and electrolyte status by monitoring laboratory values and daily weights. Because of the increased risk of glucose intolerance and hyperglycemia, blood glucose monitoring is initiated. The nurse reports elevated blood glucose levels to the physician so that treatment can be prescribed if indicated.

Promoting Home and Community-Based Care

TEACHING PATIENTS SELF-CARE. The patient and family should be informed that acute adrenal insufficiency and underlying symptoms will recur if corticosteroid therapy is stopped abruptly without medical supervision. The patient should be instructed to always have an adequate supply of the corticosteroid medication to avoid running out (see Therapeutic Uses of Corticosteroids).

The nurse stresses the need for dietary modifications to ensure adequate calcium intake without increasing the risks for hypertension, hyperglycemia, and weight gain. The patient and family can be taught to monitor blood pressure, blood glucose levels, and weight. Patients should be advised to wear a medical alert bracelet and to notify other health care providers (eg, dentist) about their condition (Chart 42-13).

CHART 42-13   HOME CARE CHECKLIST
The Patient With Cushing's Syndrome

At the completion of the home care instruction, the patient or caregiver will be able to:	PATIENT	CAREGIVER
• State present and potential effects of Cushing's syndrome on the body.	✔	✔
• Identify signs and symptoms of excessive and insufficient adrenal hormone.	✔	✔
• State the relationship between adrenal hormones, emotional state, and stress.	✔	✔
• Identify methods for managing labile emotions.	✔	✔
• Describe protective skin care measures and use of protective devices and practices.	✔	✔
• State the importance of regular follow-up visits with primary health care provider.	✔	✔
• State the purpose, dose, route, schedule, side effects, and precautions for prescribed medications (adrenocortical inhibitors).	✔	✔
• Identify need to wear medical alert identification and carry medical information card.	✔	✔
• State importance of compliance with medical regimen.	✔	✔
• State the need to contact health care provider before taking over-the-counter medications.	✔	✔
• Identify foods high in potassium and low in sodium, calories, and carbohydrates.	✔	✔
• Identify areas of activity limitations and impact on lifestyle.	✔	✔

CONTINUING CARE. The need for follow-up depends on the origin and duration of the disease and its management. The patient who has been treated by adrenalectomy or removal of a pituitary tumor requires close monitoring to ensure that adrenal function has returned to normal and to ensure adequacy of circulating adrenal hormones. The patient who requires continued corticosteroid therapy is monitored to ensure understanding of the medications and the need for a dosage that treats the underlying disorder while minimizing the side effects. Home care referral may be indicated to ensure a safe environment that minimizes stress and risk of falls and other side effects. The home care nurse assesses the patient's physical and psychological status and reports changes to the physician. The nurse also assesses the patient's understanding of the medication regimen and his or her compliance with the regimen and reinforces previous teaching about the medications and the importance of taking them as prescribed. The nurse emphasizes the importance of regular medical follow-up, the side effects and toxic effects of medications, and the need to wear medical identification with Addison's and Cushing's disease. In addition, the nurse reminds the patient and family about the importance of health promotion activities and recommended health screening, including bone mineral density testing.

Evaluation

Expected Patient Outcomes

Expected patient outcomes may include the following:

1. Decreases risk of injury
   a. Is free of fractures or soft tissue injuries
   b. Is free of ecchymotic areas
2. Decreases risk of infection
   a. Experiences no temperature elevation, redness, pain, or other signs of infection or inflammation
   b. Avoids contact with others who have infections

3. Increases participation in self-care activities
   a. Plans activities and exercises to allow alternating periods of rest and activity
   b. Reports improved well-being
   c. Is free of complications of immobility
4. Attains/maintains skin integrity
   a. Has intact skin, without evidence of breakdown or infection
   b. Exhibits decreased edema in extremities and trunk
   c. Changes position frequently and inspects bony prominences daily
5. Achieves improved body image
   a. Verbalizes feelings about changes in appearance, sexual function, and activity level
   b. States that physical changes are a result of excessive corticosteroids
6. Exhibits improved mental functioning
7. Exhibits absence of complications
   a. Exhibits normal vital signs and weight and is free of symptoms of addisonian crisis
   b. Identifies signs and symptoms of adrenocortical hypofunction that should be reported and measures to take in case of severe illness and stress
   c. Identifies strategies to minimize complications of Cushing's syndrome
   d. Complies with recommendations for follow-up appointments and health screening

PRIMARY ALDOSTERONISM

The principal action of aldosterone is to conserve body sodium. Under the influence of this hormone, the kidneys excrete less sodium and more potassium and hydrogen. Excessive production of aldosterone, which occurs in some patients with functioning tumors of the adrenal gland, causes a distinctive pattern of biochemical changes and a corresponding set of clinical manifestations that are diagnostic of this condition.

Clinical Manifestations

Patients with aldosteronism exhibit a profound decline in the serum levels of potassium (hypokalemia) and hydrogen ions (alkalosis), as demonstrated by an increase in pH and serum bicarbonate concentration. The serum sodium level is normal or elevated, depending on the amount of water reabsorbed with the sodium. Hypertension is the most prominent and almost universal sign of aldosteronism and is present in up to 10% of individuals with hypertension (Mulatero, Dluhy, Giacchetti, et al., 2005).

Hypokalemia is responsible for the variable muscle weakness, cramping, and fatigue in patients with aldosteronism, as well as an inability on the part of the kidneys to acidify or concentrate the urine. Accordingly, the urine volume is excessive, leading to polyuria. Serum, by contrast, becomes abnormally concentrated, contributing to excessive thirst (polydipsia) and arterial hypertension. A secondary increase in blood volume and possible direct effects of aldosterone on nerve receptors, such as the carotid sinus, are other factors that result in hypertension.

Hypokalemic alkalosis may decrease the ionized serum calcium level and predispose the patient to tetany and paresthesias. Trousseau's and Chvostek's signs may be used to assess neuromuscular irritability before overt paresthesia and tetany occur. Glucose intolerance may occur, because hypokalemia interferes with insulin secretion from the pancreas.

Assessment and Diagnostic Findings

In addition to a high or normal serum sodium level and a low serum potassium level, diagnostic studies indicate high serum aldosterone and low serum renin levels. The measurement of the aldosterone excretion rate after salt loading is a useful diagnostic test for primary aldosteronism. The renin–aldosterone stimulation test and bilateral adrenal venous sampling are useful in differentiating the cause of primary aldosteronism. Antihypertensive medication may be discontinued up to 2 weeks before testing.

Medical Management

Treatment of primary aldosteronism usually involves surgical removal of the adrenal tumor through adrenalectomy. Hypokalemia resolves for all patients after surgery, but hypertension may persist. Spironolactone (Aldactone) may be prescribed to control hypertension.

Adrenalectomy is performed through an incision in the flank or the abdomen. In general, the postoperative care resembles that for other abdominal surgery. However, the patient is susceptible to fluctuations in adrenocortical hormones and requires administration of corticosteroids, fluids, and other agents to maintain blood pressure and prevent acute complications. If the adrenalectomy is bilateral, replacement of corticosteroids will be lifelong; if one adrenal gland is removed, replacement therapy may be temporarily necessary because of suppression of the remaining adrenal gland by high levels of adrenal hormones. A normal serum glucose level is maintained with insulin, appropriate IV fluids, and dietary modifications.

Nursing Management

Nursing management in the postoperative period includes frequent assessment of vital signs to detect early signs and symptoms of adrenal insufficiency and crisis or hemorrhage. Explaining all treatments and procedures, providing comfort measures, and providing rest periods can reduce the patient's stress and anxiety level.

Corticosteroid Therapy

Corticosteroids are used extensively for adrenal insufficiency and are also widely used in suppressing inflammation and autoimmune reactions, controlling allergic reactions, and reducing the rejection process in transplantation. Commonly used corticosteroid preparations are listed in Table 42-5. Their anti-inflammatory and antiallergy actions make corticosteroids effective in treating rheumatic or connective tissue diseases, such as rheumatoid arthritis and systemic lupus erythematosus. They are also frequently used in the treatment of asthma, multiple sclerosis, and other autoimmune disorders.

High doses appear to allow patients to tolerate high degrees of stress. Such antistress action may be caused by the ability of corticosteroids to aid circulating vasopressor substances in keeping the blood pressure elevated; other effects, such as maintenance of the serum glucose level, also may keep blood pressure elevated.

Table 42-5	COMMONLY USED CORTICOSTEROID PREPARATIONS
Generic Names	**Trade Names**
Hydrocortisone	Cortisol, Cortef, Hydrocortone, Solu-Cortef
Cortisone	Cortone, Cortate, Cortogen
Dexamethasone	Decadron, Dexameth, Deronil, Delalone, Dexasone, Dexone, Hexadrol
Prednisone	Meticorten, Deltasone, Orasone, Panasol, Novo-prednisone
Prednisolone	Meticortelone, Delta-Cortef, Prelone, Predalone
Methylprednisolone	Medrol, Solu-Medrol, Meprolone
Triamcinolone	Aristocort, Kenacort, Kenalog, Cenocort, Azmacort, Aristospan
Beclomethasone	Beconase, Beclovent, Vanceril, Vancenase, Propaderm
Betamethasone	Celestone, Betameth, Betnesol, Betnelan

Side Effects

Although the synthetic corticosteroids are safer for some patients because of relative freedom from mineralocorticoid activity, most natural and synthetic corticosteroids produce similar kinds of side effects. The dose required for anti-inflammatory and antiallergy effects also produces metabolic effects, pituitary and adrenal gland suppression, and changes in the function of the central nervous system. Therefore, although corticosteroids are highly effective therapeutically, they may also be very dangerous. Dosages of these medications are frequently altered to allow high concentrations when necessary and then tapered in an attempt to avoid undesirable effects. This requires that patients be observed closely for side effects and that the dose be reduced when high doses are no longer required. Suppression of the adrenal cortex may persist up to 1 year after a course of corticosteroids of only 2 weeks' duration.

Therapeutic Uses of Corticosteroids

The dosage of corticosteroids is determined by the nature and chronicity of the illness as well as the patient's other medical conditions. Rheumatoid arthritis, bronchial asthma, and multiple sclerosis are chronic disorders that corticosteroids do not cure; however, these medications may be useful when other measures do not provide adequate control of symptoms. In addition, corticosteroids may be used to treat acute exacerbations of these disorders.

In such situations, the adverse effects of corticosteroids are weighed against the patient's current condition. These medications may be used for a period but then are gradually reduced or tapered as the symptoms subside. The nurse plays an important role in providing encouragement and understanding during times when the patient is experiencing (or is apprehensive about experiencing) recurrence of symptoms while taking smaller doses.

Treatment of Acute Conditions

Acute flare-ups and crises are treated with large doses of corticosteroids. Examples include emergency treatment for bronchial obstruction in status asthmaticus and for septic shock from septicemia caused by gram-negative bacteria. Other measures, such as anti-infective agents or medications, are also used with corticosteroids to treat shock and other major symptoms. At times, corticosteroids are continued past the acute flare-up stage to prevent serious complications.

Ophthalmologic Treatment

Outer eye infections can be treated by topical application of corticosteroid eye drops, because the agents do not cause systemic toxicity. However, long-term application can cause an increase in intraocular pressure, which leads to glaucoma in some patients. In addition, prolonged use of corticosteroids can sometimes lead to cataract formation.

Dermatologic Disorders

Topical administration of corticosteroids in the form of creams, ointments, lotions, and aerosols is especially effective in many dermatologic disorders. It may be more effective in some conditions to use occlusive dressings around the affected part to achieve maximum absorption of the medication. Penetration and absorption are also increased if the medication is applied when the skin is hydrated or moist (eg, immediately after bathing).

Absorption of topical agents varies with body location. For example, absorption is greater through the layers of skin on the scalp, face, and genital area than on the forearm; as a result, use of topical agents on these sites increases the risk of side effects. The availability of over-the-counter topical corticosteroids increases the risk of side effects in patients who are unaware of their potential risks. Excessive use of these agents, especially on large surface areas of inflamed skin, can lead to decreased therapeutic effects and increased side effects.

Dosage

Attempts have been made to determine the best time to administer pharmacologic doses of steroids. If symptoms have been controlled on a 6-hour or 8-hour program, a once-daily or every-other-day schedule may be implemented. In keeping with the natural secretion of cortisol, the best time of day for the total corticosteroid dose is in the early morning, between 7 AM and 8 AM. Large-dose therapy at 8 AM., when the adrenal gland is most active, produces maximal suppression of the gland. A large 8 AM dose is more physiologic because it allows the body to escape effects of the steroids from 4 PM to 6 AM, when serum levels are normally low, hence minimizing cushingoid effects. If symptoms of the disorder being treated are suppressed, alternate-day therapy is helpful in reducing pituitary–adrenal suppression in patients requiring prolonged therapy. Some patients report discomfort associated with symptoms of their primary illness on the second day; therefore, it is important to explain to patients that this regimen is necessary to minimize side effects and suppression of adrenal function.

Tapering

Corticosteroid dosages are reduced gradually (tapered) to allow normal adrenal function to return and to prevent steroid-induced adrenal insufficiency. Up to 1 year or longer after use of corticosteroids, the patient is still at risk for adrenal insufficiency in times of stress. For example, if surgery for any reason is necessary, the patient is likely to require IV corticosteroids during and after surgery to reduce the risk of acute adrenal crisis. Patients receiving corticosteroids must have an adequate supply of medication on hand, so that they do not miss a scheduled dose and increase their risk of adrenal insufficiency. Table 42-6 provides an overview of the effects of corticosteroid therapy and their nursing implications.

Table 42-6	SIDE EFFECTS OF CORTICOSTEROID THERAPY AND IMPLICATIONS FOR NURSING PRACTICE
Side Effects	**Collaborative Interventions**
Cardiovascular Effects Hypertension Thrombophlebitis Thromboembolism Accelerated atherosclerosis	Monitor for elevated blood pressure. Assess for signs and symptoms of deep venous thrombosis: redness, warmth, tenderness, and edema of an extremity. Remind patient to avoid positions and situations that restrict blood flow (eg, crossing legs, prolonged sitting in same position). Encourage foot and leg exercises when recumbent. Encourage low sodium intake. Encourage limited intake of fat.
Immunologic Effects Increased risk of infection and masking of signs of infection	Assess for subtle signs of infection and inflammation. Encourage patient to avoid exposure to others with upper respiratory infection. Monitor patient for fungal infections. Encourage hand washing.
Ophthalmologic Changes Glaucoma Corneal lesions	Encourage frequent eye examinations. Refer patient to ophthalmologist if changes in visual acuity are detected.
Musculoskeletal Effects Muscle wasting Poor wound healing Osteoporosis with vertebral compression fractures, pathologic fractures of long bones, aseptic necrosis of head of the femur	Encourage high protein intake. Encourage high protein intake and vitamin C supplementation. Encourage diet high in calcium and vitamin D or calcium and vitamin D supplementation if indicated. Take measures to avoid falls and other trauma. Use caution in moving and turning patient. Encourage postmenopausal women on corticosteroids to consider bone mineral density testing and treatment, if indicated. Instruct patient to rise slowly from bed or chair to avoid falling due to postural hypotension.
Metabolic Effects Alterations in glucose metabolism Steroid withdrawal syndrome	Monitor blood glucose levels at periodic intervals. Instruct patient about medications, diet, and exercise prescribed to control blood glucose level. Report signs of adrenal insufficiency. Administer corticosteroids and mineralocorticoids as prescribed. Monitor fluid and electrolyte balance. Administer fluids and electrolytes as prescribed. Instruct patient about importance of taking corticosteroids as prescribed without abruptly stopping therapy. Encourage patient to obtain and wear a medical identification bracelet. Advise patient to notify all health care providers (eg, dentist) about need for corticosteroid therapy.
Changes in Appearance Moon face Weight gain Acne	Encourage low-caloric, low-sodium diet. Assure patient that most changes in appearance are temporary and will disappear if and when corticosteroid therapy is no longer necessary.

CRITICAL THINKING EXERCISES

1 A 72-year-old man has been diagnosed with hyperparathyroidism. He is scheduled for a minimally invasive parathyroidectomy in 1 week. How would you explain this disorder to the patient? Describe what he and his family can expect postoperatively. Describe the nursing role preoperatively and postoperatively. Discuss the importance of nutrition and activity as related to this disorder.

2 A 40-year-old woman is seen in the emergency department for severe nausea, vomiting, tachycardia, and agitation. Her eyes appear to bulge. She is diagnosed with severe hyperthyroidism and thyroid storm. What factors could have precipitated her condition? What is the significance of the bulging eyes? What nursing precautions should be taken? How would you explain this condition to the patient, and what information would you provide to the family to assist them in understanding her symptoms? What diagnostic tests are likely to be performed? Describe the treatment for this condition.

EBP **3** A 50-year-old woman of Japanese descent is undergoing testing for thyroid disease because of symptoms of hyperthyroidism. Her physician has suggested that she receive treatment with radioactive iodine (RAI). Information the patient found on the Internet has convinced her that RAI is not safe or necessary to treat her disorder. Her grandparents lived in Nagasaki during World War II, and she recalls stories of horrible effects of the radiation on her grandfather and other relatives. Only her grandmother survived the atomic blast.

If untreated, the patient's condition can lead to serious complications. How would you address this patient's concerns and assist her in making an informed decision about treatment? What sources of information would you use, and how would you evaluate the available evidence about the effectiveness and possible adverse effects of RAI?

4 A 50-year-old woman is recovering from acute adrenal insufficiency. Corticosteroid therapy has been prescribed, and she will be required to take it for the rest of her life. What instructions should you provide regarding precautions to take related to corticosteroid therapy? How can the patient and family prevent a reoccurrence of this disorder?

5 A 24-year-old man is scheduled for diagnostic testing for possible pheochromocytoma. Identify the major signs and symptoms of pheochromocytoma and their cause. If pheochromocytoma is diagnosed and the patient is scheduled for an adrenalectomy, what preoperative and postoperative nursing care would you anticipate? What teaching, if any, would you provide to the patient's family?

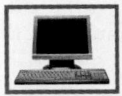

The Smeltzer suite offers these additional resources to enhance learning and facilitate understanding of this chapter:
• thePoint online resource, thepoint.lww.com/Smeltzer12E
• Student CD-ROM included with the book
• *Study Guide to Accompany Brunner & Suddarth's Textbook of Medical-Surgical Nursing*
• *Handbook for Brunner & Suddarth's Textbook of Medical-Surgical Nursing*

REFERENCES AND SELECTED READINGS

Books

American Cancer Society. (2009). *Cancer facts & figures – 2009*. Atlanta, GA: Author.
Bickley, L. S. (2007). *Bates' guide to physical examination and history taking* (9th ed.). Philadelphia: Lippincott Williams & Wilkins.
Ferri, F. (Ed.). (2005). *Ferri clinical advisor: Instant diagnosis and treatment* (5th ed.). Philadelphia: Mosby.
Fink, M. P., Abraham, E., Kochanek, P., et al. (Eds.). (2005). *Textbook of critical care* (5th ed.). Philadelphia: W. B. Saunders.
Morton, P. G., Fontaine, D. K., Hudak, C. M., et al. (2005). *Critical care nursing: A holistic approach* (8th ed.). Philadelphia: Lippincott Williams & Wilkins.
Porth, C. M. (2006). *Essentials of pathophysiology: Concepts for altered health states* (2nd ed.). Philadelphia: Lippincott Williams & Wilkins.
Porth, C. M. & Matfin, G. (2009). *Pathophysiology: Concepts of altered health states* (8th ed.). Philadelphia: Lippincott Williams & Wilkins.
Rakel, R. E. & Bope, E. T. (Eds.). (2008). *Conn's current therapy 2008*. Philadelphia: W. B. Saunders Elsevier.
Singer, P. A. (2006). Hypothyroidism. In R. E. Rakel & E. T. Bope (Eds.), *Conn's current therapy*. Philadelphia: W. B. Saunders Elsevier.
Tierney, L. M., McPhee, S. J. & Papadakis, M. A. (Eds.). (2005). *Current medical diagnosis and treatment*. New York: Lange Medical Books/McGraw-Hill.
Wartofsky, L. & Van Nostrand, D. (2006). *Thyroid cancer: A comprehensive guide to clinical management* (2nd ed.). Towata, NJ: Humana Press.

Journals and Electronic Documents

General

Bauer, D. G. (2005). Review of the endocrine system. *MedSurg Nursing, 14*(5), 335–337.

Pituitary Gland

Carlé, A., Laurberg, P., Pedersen, I. B., et al. (2007). Age modifies the pituitary TSH response to thyroid failure. *Thyroid, 17*(2), 139–144.
Espiritu, J. R. (2008). Aging-related sleep changes. *Clinics in Geriatric Medicine, 24*(1), 1–14.

Growth Hormone Guideline Task Force. (2006). Evaluation and treatment of adult growth hormone deficiency: An Endocrine Society clinical practice guideline. *Journal of Clinical Endocrinology and Metabolism, 91*(5), 1621–1634.
Hanberg, A. (2005). Common disorders of the pituitary gland: Hyposecretion versus hypersecretion. *Journal of Infusion Nursing, 28*(1), 36–44.
Haskal, R. (2007). Current issues for nurse practitioners: Hyponatremia. *Journal of the American Academy of Nurse Practitioners, 19*(11), 563–579.
Hudson, M. J. (2007). Complications of diabetes insipidus: The significance of headache. *Pediatric Nursing, 33*(1), 58–59.
Melmed, S. (2006). Acromegaly. *New England Journal of Medicine, 355*(24), 2558–2575.
Urban, R. J., Harris, P. & Masal, B. (2005). Anterior hypopituitarism following traumatic brain injury. *Brain Injury, 19*(5), 349–358.

Thyroid Gland

Agency for Health and Research Quality. (2006). Studies examine the source of diagnostic errors in thyroid and lung cancers. *Agency for Health and Research Quality Research Activities Newsletter, 312*, 9–10.
Asvold, B. O., Bjoro, T., Nilsen, T. I., et al. (2007). Tobacco smoking and thyroid function. *Archives of Internal Medicine, 167*(13), 1428–1432.
Barrows, F. B., Shockley, W. W., Wright, J. D., et al. (2006). Metastatic medullary thyroid cancer in a pediatric patient with MEN 2B: Emphasis on the need for early recognition of extrathyroidal clinical findings associated with MEN 2B. *Clinical Pediatrics, 45*(5), 463–467.
Bindra, A. & Braunstein, G. D. (2006). Thyroiditis. *American Family Physician, 73*(10), 1769–1773.
Brent, G. A. (2008). Graves' disease. *New England Journal of Medicine, 358*(24), 2594–2605.
Cooper, D. S. (2005). Drug therapy: Antithyroid drugs. *New England Journal of Medicine, 352*(9), 905–917.
Cooper, D. S., Doherty, G. M., Haugen, B. R., et al. (2006). Management guidelines for patients with thyroid nodules and differentiated thyroid cancer. *Thyroid, 16*(2), 109–142.
Dominguez, L. J., Bevilacqua, M., DiBella, G., et al. (2008). Diagnosing and managing thyroid disease in the nursing home. *Journal of the American Medical Directors Association, 9*(1), 9–17.
Franklyn, J. A., Sheppard, M. C. & Maisonneuve, P. (2005). Thyroid function and mortality in patients treated for hypertension. *Journal of the American Medical Association, 294*(1), 71–80.
Harris, C. (2007). Recognizing thyroid storm in the neurologically impaired patient. *American Association of Neuroscience Nursing, 39*(1), 55–57.
Karlsson, F. A. (2006). Endocrine ophthalmopathy and radioiodine therapy. *Acta Onologica, 45*(8), 1046–1050.
Kwaku, M. P. & Burman, K. D. (2007). Myxedema coma. *Journal of Intensive Care Medicine, 22*(4), 224–231.
Nyenwe, E. A. & Dagogo, D. S. (2007). Recognizing iodine deficiency in iodine-replete environments. *New England Journal of Medicine, 357*(12), 1263–1264.
Reid, J. R. & Wheeler, S. F. (2005). Hyperthyroidism: Diagnosis and treatment. *American Family Physician, 72*(4), 623–630.
Rosenthal, M. S. (2006). Patient misconceptions and ethical challenges in radioactive iodine scanning and therapy. *Journal of Nuclear Medicine Technology, 34*(3), 143–150.
Seiberling, K., Dutra, J. C. & Baharamovic, S. (2007). Hypothyroidism following hemithyroidectomy for benign nontoxic thyroid disease. *Ear, Nose, & Throat Journal, 86*(5), 295–299.
Thyroid Carcinoma Task Force (2001). AACE/AAES medical/surgical guidelines for clinical practice: Management of thyroid carcinoma. *Endocrine Practice, 7*(3), 2002–2020.
U.S. Department of Health and Human Services (USDHHS). Agency for Healthcare Research and Quality. (2006). *The guide to clinical preventive services 2006: Recommendations of the U.S. Preventive Services Task Force*. www.ahrq.gov
Warren, E. (2007). Thyroid disease. *Update, 74*(3), 20–25.
World Health Organization. (2007). *Reducing salt intake in populations. Report of a WHO Forum and Technical Meeting 5–7 October 2006, Paris, France*. Geneva, Switzerland: Author.
Zablotska, L. B., Bogdanova, T. I., Ovsly, E. R, et al. (2008). A cohort study of thyroid diseases after the Chernobyl accident: Dose-response analysis of thyroid follicular adenomas detected during first screening in Ukraine (1998–2000). *American Journal of Epidemiology, 167*(3), 305–313.

Parathyroid Glands

AACE/AAES Task Force on Primary Hyperparathyroidism. (2005). The American Association of Clinical Endocrinologists and the American

Association of Endocrine Surgeons position statement on the diagnosis and management of primary hyperparathyroidism. *Endocrine Practice, 11*(1), 49–54.

Conn, C. A., Clark, J., Bumpous, J., et al. (2006). Hypocalcemia after neck exploration for untreated primary hyperparathyroidism. *American Surgeon, 72*(12), 1234–1237.

Norman, J. & Politz, D. (2008). Shingles (varicella zoster) outbreaks in patients with hyperparathyroidism and their relationship to hypercalcemia. *Clinical Infectious Diseases, 46*(9), 1452.

Rodgers, S. E., Lew J. I. & Solorzano, C. C. (2008). Primary hyperparathyroidism. *Current Opinion in Oncology, 20*(1), 52–58.

Shoback, D. (2008). Hypoparathyroidism. *New England Journal of Medicine, 359*(4), 391–403.

Suliburk, J. W. & Perrier, N. D. (2007). Primary hyperparathyroidism. *The Oncologist, 12*, 644–653.

Tomasello, S. (2008). Secondary hyperparathyroidism and chronic kidney disease. *Diabetes Spectrum, 21*(1), 19–25.

Adrenal Glands

Brender, E. (2005). Adrenal insufficiency [JAMA patient page]. *Journal of the American Medical Association, 294*(19), 2528.

Findling, J. W. & Raff, H. (2005). Screening and diagnosis of Cushing's syndrome. *Endocrinology and Metabolism Clinics of North America, 34*(2), 385–402.

Gross, B. A., Mindea, S. A., Pick, A. J., et al. (2007). Diagnostic approach to Cushing disease. *Neurosurgical Focus, 23*(2), E1.

Mulatero, P., Dluhy, R. G., Giacchetti, G., et al. (2005). Diagnosis of primary aldosteronism: From screening to subtype differentiation. *Trends in Endocrinology and Metabolism, 16*(3), 114–119.

National Comprehensive Cancer Network. (2008). NCCN clinical practice guidelines in oncology. *Neuroendocrine Tumors V. 1. 2008.* www.nccn.org

Nieman, L. K., Biller, B. M. K., Findling, J. W., et al. (2008). The Endocrine Society's clinical guidelines: The diagnosis of Cushing's syndrome: An Endocrine Society clinical practice guideline. *Journal of Clinical Endocrinology & Metabolism, 93*(5), 1526–1540.

Rhen, T. & Cidlowski, J. A. (2005). Antiinflammatory action of glucocorticoids: New mechanisms for old drugs. *New England Journal of Medicine, 353*(16), 1711–1723.

Salvatori, R. (2005). Adrenal insufficiency. *Journal of the American Medical Association, 294*(19), 2481–2488.

Young, W. F. (2007). The incidentally discovered adrenal mass. *New England Journal of Medicine, 356*(6), 601–610.

RESOURCES

American Association of Clinical Endocrinologists, www.aace.com
American Thyroid Association, Inc., www.thyroid.org
Cushing's Support and Research Foundation, http://csrf.net
The Endocrine Society, www.endo-society.org
National Adrenal Disease Foundation, www.nadf.us
National Cancer Institute, Cancer Net for Health Professionals, www.nci.nih.gov
The Thyroid Society for Education and Research, www.the-thyroid-society.org

Urinary Tract Function

A Patient With Involuntary Urine Loss During Physical Exertion and Ineffective Bladder Emptying

Mrs. Lopez is a 38-year-old woman with no significant past medical history. She has three children. During her annual physical examination, she tells the women's health nurse practitioner that when she jogs, coughs, or sneezes, she experiences an involuntary loss of small amounts of urine. The patient's urinalysis is normal. On physical examination, the nurse finds that Mrs. Lopez has a moderate cystocele and that her bladder feels mildly distended, although she had just voided to provide a urine sample. The nurse catheterizes Mrs. Lopez to check for postvoid residual urine and obtains 120 mL of clear urine.

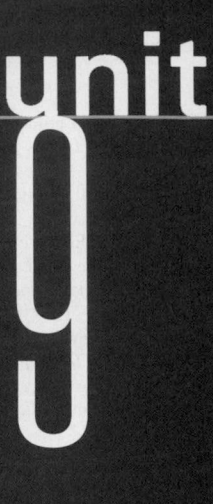

Visit thePoint to view a concept map that illustrates the relationships that exist between the nursing diagnoses, interventions, and outcomes for the patient's clinical problems.

Nursing Classifications and Languages

NANDA NURSING DIAGNOSES	NIC NURSING INTERVENTIONS	NOC NURSING OUTCOMES
		Return to functional baseline status, stabilization of, or improvement in:
STRESS URINARY INCONTINENCE— Loss of less than 50 mL of urine occurring with increased abdominal pressure	**PELVIC MUSCLE EXERCISES—** Strengthening and training the levator ani and urogenital muscles through voluntary, repetitive contraction to decrease stress, urge, or mixed types of urinary incontinence	**SYMPTOM CONTROL—**Personal actions to minimize perceived changes in physical and emotional functioning
URINARY RETENTION—Incomplete emptying of the bladder	**URINARY BLADDER TRAINING—** Improving bladder function for those with urge incontinence by increasing the bladder's ability to hold urine and the patient's ability to suppress urination	**URINARY CONTINENCE—**Control of elimination of urine from the bladder
RISK FOR INFECTION—At increased risk for being invaded by pathogenic organisms	**URINARY CATHETERIZATION: INTERMITTENT—**Regular periodic use of a catheter to empty the bladder **INFECTION PROTECTION—** Prevention and early detection of infection in a patient at risk	**INFECTION SEVERITY—**Severity of infection and associated symptoms

Bulechek, G. M., Butcher, H. K., & Dochterman, J. M. (2008). *Nursing interventions classification (NIC)* (5th ed.). St. Louis: Mosby.
Johnson, M., Bulechek, G., Butcher, H. K., et al. (2006). *NANDA, NOC, and NIC linkages* (2nd ed.). St. Louis: Mosby.
Moorhead, S., Johnson, M., Mass, M. L., et al. (2008). *Nursing outcomes classification (NOC)* (4th ed.). St. Louis: Mosby.
NANDA International. (2007). *Nursing diagnoses: Definitions & classification 2007–2008.* Philadelphia: North American Nursing Diagnosis Association.

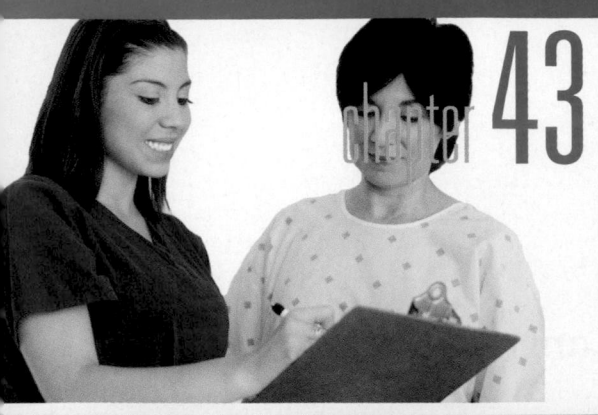

chapter 43

Assessment of Renal and Urinary Tract Function

LEARNING OBJECTIVES

On completion of this chapter, the learner will be able to:

1 Describe the anatomy and physiology of the renal and urinary systems.

2 Discuss the role of the kidneys in regulating fluid and electrolyte balance, acid–base balance, and blood pressure.

3 Describe the diagnostic studies used to determine upper and lower urinary tract function.

4 Identify the assessment parameters used for determining the status of upper and lower urinary tract function.

5 Initiate education and preparation for patients undergoing assessment of the urinary system.

GLOSSARY

aldosterone: hormone synthesized and released by the adrenal cortex; causes the kidneys to reabsorb sodium

antidiuretic hormone: hormone secreted by the posterior pituitary gland; causes the kidneys to reabsorb more water; also called vasopressin

anuria: total urine output less than 50 mL in 24 hours

bacteriuria: bacteria in the urine; bacterial count higher than 100,000 colonies/mL

creatinine: endogenous waste product of muscle energy metabolism

diuresis: increased formation and secretion of urine

dysuria: painful or difficult urination

frequency: voiding more frequently than every 3 hours

glomerular filtration: plasma filtered at the glomerulus into the kidney tubules

glomerulus: tuft of capillaries forming part of the nephron through which filtration occurs

hematuria: red blood cells in the urine

micturition: urination or voiding

nephron: structural and functional unit of the kidney responsible for urine formation

nocturia: awakening at night to urinate

oliguria: total urine output less than 500 mL in 24 hours

proteinuria: protein in the urine

pyuria: white blood cells in the urine

renal clearance: volume of plasma that the kidneys can clear of a specific solute (eg, creatinine); expressed in milliliters per minute

renal glycosuria: recurring or persistent excretion of glucose in the urine

specific gravity: reflects the weight of particles dissolved in the urine; expression of the degree of concentration of the urine

tubular reabsorption: movement of a substance from the kidney tubule into the blood in the peritubular capillaries or vasa recta

tubular secretion: movement of a substance from the blood in the peritubular capillaries or vasa recta into the kidney tubule

urea nitrogen: nitrogenous end product of protein metabolism

Chart 43-1•*Functions of the Kidney*

- Urine formation
- Excretion of waste products
- Regulation of electrolytes
- Regulation of acid–base balance
- Control of water balance
- Control of blood pressure
- Renal clearance
- Regulation of red blood cell production
- Synthesis of vitamin D to active form
- Secretion of prostaglandins
- Regulates calcium and phosphorus balance

Function of the renal and urinary systems is essential to life. The primary purpose of the renal and urinary systems is to maintain the body's state of homeostasis by carefully regulating fluid and electrolytes, removing wastes, and providing other functions (Chart 43-1). Dysfunction of the kidneys and lower urinary tract is common and may occur at any age and with varying degrees of severity. Assessment of upper and lower urinary tract function is part of every health examination and necessitates an understanding of the anatomy and physiology of the urinary system as well as the effects of changes in the system on other physiologic functions.

Anatomic and Physiologic Overview

Anatomy of the Renal and Urinary Tract Systems

The renal and urinary systems include the kidneys, ureters, bladder, and urethra. Urine is formed by the kidney and flows through the other structures to be eliminated from the body.

Kidneys

The kidneys are a pair of bean-shaped, brownish-red structures located retroperitoneally (behind and outside the peritoneal cavity) on the posterior wall of the abdomen—from the 12th thoracic vertebra to the third lumbar vertebra in the adult (Fig. 43-1A). The average adult kidney weighs approximately 113 to 170 g (about 4.5 oz) and is 10 to 12 cm long, 6 cm wide, and 2.5 cm thick (Porth & Matfin, 2009). The right kidney is slightly lower than the left due to the location of the liver.

Externally, the kidneys are well protected by the ribs and by the muscles of the abdomen and back. Internally, fat deposits surround each kidney, providing protection against jarring. The kidneys and surrounding fat are suspended from the abdominal wall by renal fascia made of connective tissue. The fibrous connective tissue, blood vessels, and lymphatics surrounding each kidney are known as the renal capsule. An adrenal gland lies on top of each kidney. The kidneys and adrenals are independent in function, blood supply, and innervation.

The renal parenchyma is divided into two parts: the cortex and the medulla (Fig. 43-1B). The medulla, which is approximately 5 cm wide, is the inner portion of the kidney. It contains the loops of Henle, the vasa recta, and the collecting ducts of the juxtamedullary nephrons. The collecting ducts from both the juxtamedullary and the cortical nephrons connect to the renal pyramids, which are triangular and are situated with the base facing the concave surface of the kidney and the point (papilla) facing the hilum, or pelvis. Each kidney contains approximately 8 to 18 pyramids. The pyramids drain into minor calices, which drain into major calices that open directly into the renal pelvis. The renal pelvis is the beginning of the collecting system and is composed of structures that are designed to collect and transport urine. Once the urine leaves the renal pelvis, the composition or amount of urine does not change.

The cortex, which is approximately 1 cm wide, is located farthest from the center of the kidney and around the

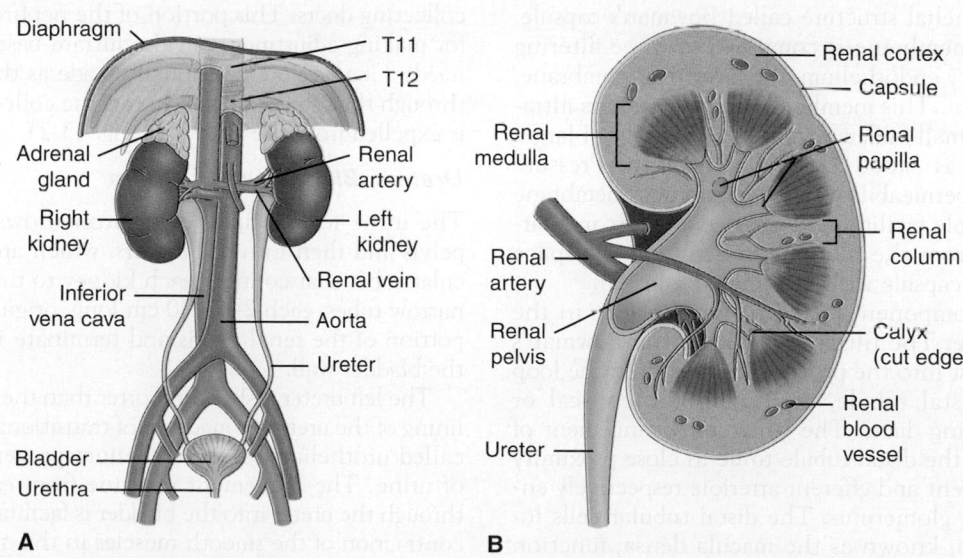

Figure 43-1 **A,** Kidneys, ureters, and bladder. **B,** Internal structure of the kidney. Redrawn from Porth, C. M. & Matfin, G. (2009). *Pathophysiology: Concepts of altered health status* (8th ed.). Philadelphia: Lippincott Williams & Wilkins.

Diaphragm — T11 / T12
Adrenal gland — Renal artery
Right kidney — Left kidney
Inferior vena cava — Renal vein
— Aorta
— Ureter
Bladder
Urethra
A

Renal cortex — Capsule
Renal medulla — Renal papilla
Renal artery — Renal column
Renal pelvis — Calyx (cut edge)
Ureter — Renal blood vessel
B

outermost edges. It contains the **nephrons** (the functional units of the kidney), which are discussed below.

Blood Supply to the Kidneys

The hilum is the concave portion of the kidney through which the renal artery enters and the ureters and renal vein exit. The kidneys receive 20% to 25% of the total cardiac output, which means that all of the body's blood circulates through the kidneys approximately 12 times per hour. The renal artery (arising from the abdominal aorta) divides into smaller and smaller vessels, eventually forming the afferent arterioles. Each afferent arteriole branches to form a **glomerulus,** which is the capillary bed responsible for glomerular filtration. Blood leaves the glomerulus through the efferent arteriole and flows back to the inferior vena cava through a network of capillaries and veins.

Nephrons

Each kidney has 1 million nephrons that are located within the renal parenchyma and are responsible for the initial formation of urine. The large number of nephrons allows for adequate renal function even if the opposite kidney is damaged or becomes nonfunctional. If the total number of functioning nephrons is less then 20% of normal, renal replacement therapy needs to be considered.

There are two types of nephrons. The cortical nephrons, which make up 80% to 85% of the total number, are located in the outermost part of the cortex, and the juxtamedullary nephrons, which make up the remaining 15% to 20%, are located deeper in the cortex. The juxtamedullary nephrons are distinguished by long loops of Henle and are surrounded by long capillary loops called vasa recta that dip into the medulla of the kidney. The length of the tubular component of the nephron is directly related to its ability to concentrate urine.

Nephrons are made up of two basic components: a filtering element composed of an enclosed capillary network (the glomerulus) and the attached tubule (Fig. 43-2). The glomerulus is a unique network of capillaries suspended between the afferent and efferent blood vessels, which are enclosed in an epithelial structure called Bowman's capsule. The glomerular membrane is composed of three filtering layers: the capillary endothelium, the basement membrane, and the epithelium. This membrane normally allows filtration of fluid and small molecules yet limits passage of larger molecules, such as blood cells and albumin. Pressure changes and the permeability of the glomerular membrane of Bowman's capsule facilitate the passage of fluids and various substances from the blood vessels, filling the space within Bowman's capsule with this filtered solution.

The tubular component of the nephron begins in the Bowman's capsule. The filtrate created in the Bowman's capsule travels first into the proximal tubule, then the loop of Henle, the distal tubule, and either the cortical or medullary collecting ducts. The structural arrangement of the tubule allows the distal tubule to lie in close proximity to where the afferent and efferent arteriole respectively enter and leave the glomerulus. The distal tubular cells located in this area, known as the macula densa, function with the adjacent afferent arteriole and create what is known as the juxtaglomerular apparatus. This is the site of

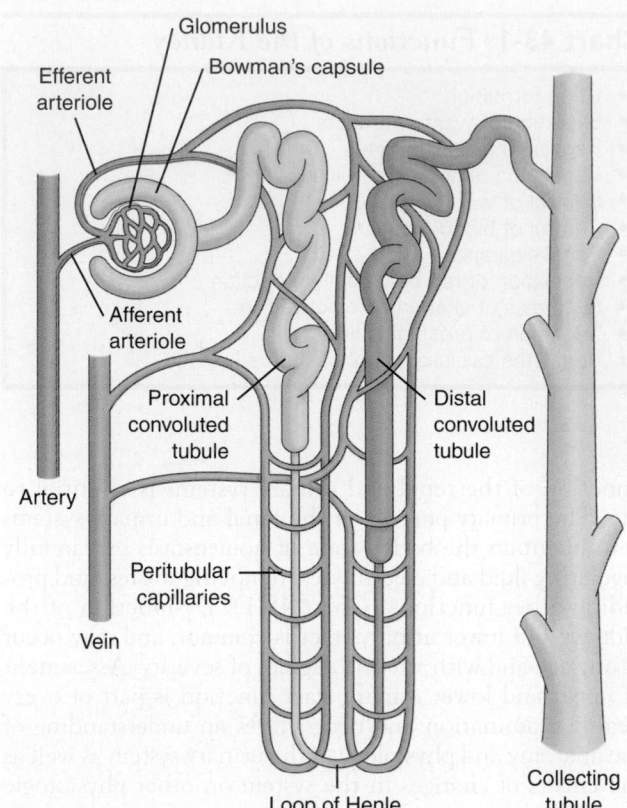

Figure 43-2 Representation of a nephron. Each kidney has about 1 million nephrons of two types: cortical and juxtamedullary. Cortical nephrons are located in the cortex of the kidney; juxtamedullary nephrons are adjacent to the medulla.

renin production. Renin is a hormone directly involved in the control of arterial blood pressure; it is essential for proper functioning of the glomerulus (see later discussion).

The tubular component consists of the Bowman's capsule, the proximal tubule, the descending and ascending limbs of the loop of Henle, and the cortical and medullary collecting ducts. This portion of the nephron is responsible for making adjustments in the filtrate based on the body's needs. Changes are continually made as the filtrate travels through the tubules until it enters the collecting system and is expelled from the body (see Fig. 43-2).

Ureters, Bladder, and Urethra

The urine formed in the nephrons flows into the renal pelvis and then into the ureters, which are long fibromuscular tubes that connect each kidney to the bladder. These narrow tubes, each 24 to 30 cm long, originate at the lower portion of the renal pelvis and terminate in the trigone of the bladder wall.

The left ureter is slightly shorter than the right ureter. The lining of the ureters is made up of transitional cell epithelium called urothelium. The urothelium prevents reabsorption of urine. The movement of urine from each renal pelvis through the ureter into the bladder is facilitated by peristaltic contraction of the smooth muscles in the ureter wall. There are three narrowed areas of each ureter: the ureteropelvic junction, the ureteral segment near the sacroiliac junction, and the ureterovesical junction. These three areas of the ureters have a propensity for obstruction by renal calculi (kidney stones) or stricture. Obstruction of the ureteropelvic junction is the most serious because of its close proximity to the kidney and the risk of associated kidney dysfunction.

The urinary bladder is a muscular, hollow sac located just behind the pubic bone. The capacity of the adult bladder is 400 to 500 mL (Bickley, 2007). The bladder is characterized by its central, hollow area, called the vesicle, which has two inlets (the ureters) and one outlet (the urethra). The area surrounding the bladder neck is called the urethrovesical junction. The angling of the ureterovesical junction is the primary means of providing antegrade, or downward, movement of urine, also referred to as efflux of urine. This angling prevents vesicoureteral reflux (retrograde, or backward, movement of urine) from the bladder, up the ureter, toward the kidney.

The wall of the bladder contains four layers. The outermost layer is the adventitia, which is made up of connective tissue. Immediately beneath the adventitia is a smooth muscle layer known as the detrusor. Beneath the detrusor is a submucosal layer of loose connective tissue that serves as an interface between the detrusor and the innermost layer, a mucosal lining. The inner layer contains specialized transitional cell epithelium, a membrane that is impermeable to water and prevents reabsorption of urine stored in the bladder. The bladder neck contains bundles of involuntary smooth muscle that form a portion of the urethral sphincter known as the internal sphincter. An important portion of the sphincteric mechanism that helps maintain continence is the external urinary sphincter at the anterior urethra, the segment most distal from the bladder (Porth & Matfin, 2009). During voiding **(micturition),** increased intravesical pressure keeps the ureterovesical junction closed and keeps urine within the ureters. As soon as micturition is completed, intravesical pressure returns to its normal low baseline value, allowing efflux of urine to resume. Therefore, the only time that the bladder is completely empty is in the last seconds of micturition, before efflux of urine resumes.

The urethra arises from the base of the bladder: In the male, it passes through the penis; in the female, it opens just anterior to the vagina. In the male, the prostate gland, which lies just below the bladder neck, surrounds the urethra posteriorly and laterally.

Function of the Renal and Urinary Tract Systems

Urine Formation

The healthy human body is composed of approximately 60% water. Water balance is regulated by the kidneys and results in the formation of urine. Urine is formed in the nephrons through a complex three-step process: **glomerular filtration, tubular reabsorption,** and **tubular secretion** (Fig. 43-3). The various substances normally filtered by the glomerulus, reabsorbed by the tubules, and excreted in the urine include sodium, chloride, bicarbonate, potassium, glucose, urea, creatinine, and uric acid. Within the tubule, some of these substances are selectively reabsorbed into the blood. Others are secreted from the blood into the filtrate as it travels down the tubule.

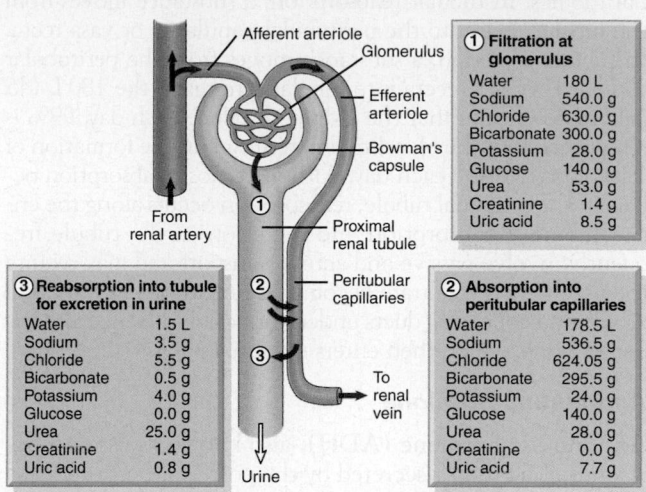

Physiology ■■■ Pathophysiology

Figure 43-3 Urine is formed in the nephrons in a three-step process: filtration, reabsorption, and excretion. Water, electrolytes, and other substances, such as glucose and creatinine, are filtered by the glomerulus; varying amounts of these substances are reabsorbed in the renal tubule or excreted in the urine. Approximate normal volumes of these substances during the steps of urine formation are shown at the top. Wide variations may occur in these values depending on diet.

Amino acids and glucose are usually filtered at the level of the glomerulus and reabsorbed so that neither is excreted in the urine. Normally, glucose does not appear in the urine. However, **renal glycosuria** (recurring or persistent excretion of glucose in the urine) occurs if the amount of glucose in the blood and glomerular filtrate exceeds the amount that the tubules are able to reabsorb. Renal glycosuria occurs in diabetes, the most common condition that causes the blood glucose level to exceed the kidney's reabsorption capacity. Renal glycosuria is also common in pregnancy.

Protein molecules also are not usually found in the urine; however, low-molecular-weight proteins (globulins and albumin) may periodically be excreted in small amounts. Protein in the urine is referred to as **proteinuria.**

Glomerular Filtration

The normal blood flow through the kidneys is about 1200 mL/min. As blood flows into the glomerulus from an afferent arteriole, filtration occurs. The filtered fluid, also known as filtrate or ultrafiltrate, then enters the renal tubules. Under normal conditions, about 20% of the blood passing through the glomeruli is filtered into the nephron, amounting to about 180 L/day of filtrate. The filtrate normally consists of water, electrolytes, and other small molecules, because water and small molecules are allowed to pass, whereas larger molecules stay in the bloodstream. Efficient filtration depends on adequate blood flow that maintains a consistent pressure through the glomerulus. Many factors can alter this blood flow and pressure, including hypotension, decreased oncotic pressure in the blood, and increased pressure in the renal tubules from an obstruction.

Tubular Reabsorption and Tubular Secretion

The second and third steps of urine formation occur in the renal tubules. In tubular reabsorption, a substance moves from the filtrate back into the peritubular capillaries or vasa recta. In tubular secretion, a substance moves from the peritubular capillaries or vasa recta into tubular filtrate. Of the 180 L (45 gallons) of filtrate that the kidneys produce each day, 99% is reabsorbed into the bloodstream, resulting in the formation of 1 L to 2 L of urine each day. Although most reabsorption occurs in the proximal tubule, reabsorption occurs along the entire tubule. Reabsorption and secretion in the tubule frequently involve passive and active transport and may require the use of energy. Filtrate becomes concentrated in the distal tubule and collecting ducts under hormonal influence and becomes urine, which then enters the renal pelvis.

Antidiuretic Hormone

Antidiuretic hormone (ADH), also known as vasopressin, is a hormone that is secreted by the posterior portion of the pituitary gland in response to changes in osmolality of the blood. With decreased water intake, blood osmolality tends to increase, stimulating ADH release. ADH then acts on the kidney, increasing reabsorption of water and thereby returning the osmolality of the blood to normal. With excess water intake, the secretion of ADH by the pituitary is suppressed; therefore, less water is reabsorbed by the kidney tubule. This latter situation leads to increased urine volume **(diuresis).**

A dilute urine with a fixed specific gravity (about 1.010) or fixed osmolality (about 300 mOsm/L) indicates an inability to concentrate and dilute the urine, a common early sign of kidney disease.

Osmolarity and Osmolality

Osmolarity refers to the ratio of solute to water. The regulation of salt and water is paramount for control of the extracellular volume and both serum and urine osmolarity. Controlling either the amount of water or the amount of solute can change osmolarity. Osmolarity and ionic composition are maintained by the body within very narrow limits. As little as a 1% to 2% change in the serum osmolarity can cause a conscious desire to drink and conservation of water by the kidneys (Goertz, 2006).

The degree of dilution or concentration of the urine is also measured in terms of osmolality, the number of osmoles (the standard unit of osmotic pressure) dissolved per kilogram of solution. The filtrate in the glomerular capillary normally has the same osmolality as the blood, 280 to 300 mOsm/kg. Serum and urine osmolality and osmolarity are discussed in more detail in Chapter 14.

Regulation of Water Excretion

Regulation of the amount of water excreted is an important function of the kidney. With high fluid intake, a large volume of dilute urine is excreted. Conversely, with a low fluid intake, a small volume of concentrated urine is excreted. A person normally ingests about 1300 mL of oral liquids and 1000 mL of water in food per day. Of the fluid ingested, approximately 900 mL is lost through the skin and lungs (called insensible loss), 50 mL through sweat, and 200 mL

through feces. It is important to consider all fluid gained and lost when evaluating total fluid status. Daily weight measurements are a reliable means of determining overall fluid status. One pound equals approximately 500 mL, so a weight change of as little as 1 lb could suggest an overall fluid gain or loss of 500 mL.

Regulation of Electrolyte Excretion

When the kidneys are functioning normally, the volume of electrolytes excreted per day is equal to the amount ingested. For example, the average American daily diet contains 6 to 8 g each of sodium chloride (salt) and potassium chloride, and approximately the same amounts are excreted in the urine.

The regulation of sodium volume excreted depends on **aldosterone,** a hormone synthesized and released from the adrenal cortex. With increased aldosterone in the blood, less sodium is excreted in the urine, because aldosterone fosters renal reabsorption of sodium. Release of aldosterone from the adrenal cortex is largely under the control of angiotensin II. Angiotensin II levels are in turn controlled by renin, an enzyme that is released from specialized cells in the kidneys (Fig. 43-4). This complex system is activated when pressure in the renal arterioles falls below normal levels, as occurs with shock, dehydration, or decreased sodium chloride delivery to the tubules. Activation of this system increases the retention of water and expansion of the intravascular fluid volume, thereby maintaining enough pressure within the glomerulus to ensure adequate filtration.

The regulation of serum sodium and potassium are discussed in detail in Chapter 14.

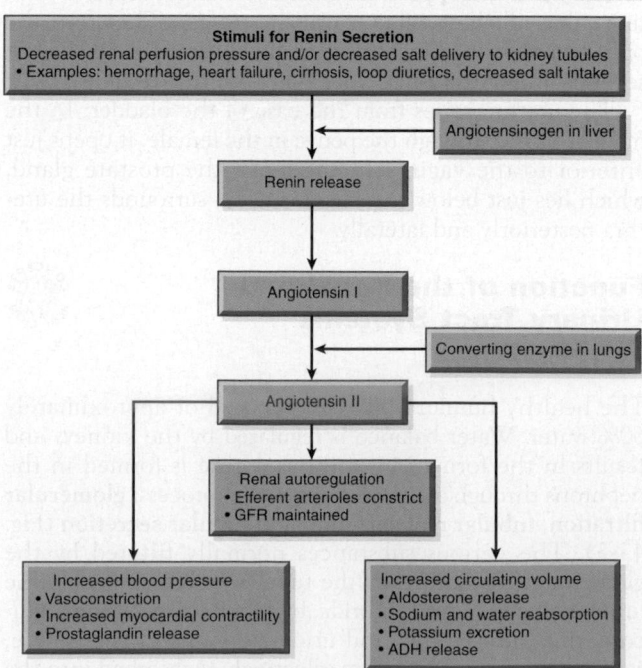

Figure 43-4 The renin–angiotensin system. ADH, antidiuretic hormone; GFR, glomerular filtration rate.

Regulation of Acid–Base Balance

The normal serum pH is about 7.35 to 7.45 and must be maintained within this narrow range for optimal physiologic function. The kidney performs two major functions to assist in this balance. The first is to reabsorb and return to the body's circulation any bicarbonate from the urinary filtrate; the second is to excrete acid in the urine. Because bicarbonate is a small ion, it is freely filtered at the glomerulus. The renal tubules actively reabsorb most of the bicarbonate in the urinary filtrate. To replace any lost bicarbonate, the renal tubular cells generate new bicarbonate through a variety of chemical reactions. This newly generated bicarbonate is then reabsorbed by the tubules and returned to the body.

The body's acid production is the result of catabolism, or breakdown, of proteins, which produces acid compounds, in particular phosphoric and sulfuric acids. The normal daily diet also includes a certain amount of acid materials. Unlike carbon dioxide (CO_2), phosphoric and sulfuric acids cannot be eliminated by the lungs. Because accumulation of these acids in the blood lowers pH (making the blood more acidic) and inhibits cell function, they must be excreted in the urine. A person with normal kidney function excretes about 70 mEq of acid each day. The kidney is able to excrete some of this acid directly into the urine until the urine pH reaches 4.5, which is 1000 times more acidic than blood.

However, more acid usually needs to be eliminated from the body than can be secreted directly as free acid in the urine. These excess acids are bound to chemical buffers so that they can be excreted in the urine. Two important chemical buffers are phosphate ions and ammonia (NH_3). When buffered with acid, ammonia becomes ammonium (NH_4). Phosphate is present in the glomerular filtrate, and ammonia is produced by the cells of the renal tubules and secreted into the tubular fluid. Through the buffering process, the kidney is able to excrete large quantities of acid in a bound form, without further lowering the pH of the urine.

Autoregulation of Blood Pressure

Regulation of blood pressure is an important function of the kidney. Specialized vessels of the kidney, called the vasa recta, constantly monitor blood pressure as blood begins its passage into the kidney. When the vasa recta detect a decrease in blood pressure, specialized juxtaglomerular cells called denta cells, near the afferent arteriole, distal tubule, and efferent arteriole secrete the hormone renin. Renin converts angiotensinogen to angiotensin I, which is then converted to angiotensin II, the most powerful vasoconstrictor known; angiotensin II causes the blood pressure to increase (Goshorn, 2005). The adrenal cortex secretes aldosterone in response to stimulation by the pituitary gland, which occurs in response to poor perfusion or increasing serum osmolality. The result is an increase in blood pressure. When the vasa recta recognize the increase in blood pressure, renin secretion stops. Failure of this feedback mechanism is one of the primary causes of hypertension (see Fig. 43-4).

Renal Clearance

Renal clearance refers to the ability of the kidneys to clear solutes from the plasma. A 24-hour collection of urine is the primary test of renal clearance used to evaluate how well the kidney performs this important excretory function. Renal clearance depends on several factors: how quickly the substance is filtered across the glomerulus, how much of the substance is reabsorbed along the tubules, and how much of the substance is secreted into the tubules. It is possible to measure the renal clearance of any substance, but the one measure that is particularly useful is the creatinine clearance.

Creatinine is an endogenous waste product of skeletal muscle that is filtered at the glomerulus, passed through the tubules with minimal change, and excreted in the urine. Hence, creatinine clearance is a good measure of the glomerular filtration rate (GFR). To calculate creatinine clearance, a 24-hour urine specimen is collected. Midway through the collection, the serum creatinine level is measured. The following formula is then used to calculate the creatinine clearance:

$$\frac{(\text{Volume of urine [mL/min]} \times \text{urine creatinine [mL/dL]})}{\text{Serum creatinine (mg/dL)}}$$

The adult GFR can vary from a normal of approximately 125 mL/min (1.67 to 2.0 mL/sec) to a high of 200 mL/min (Porth & Matfin, 2009). Creatinine clearance is an excellent measure of renal function; as renal function declines, creatinine clearance decreases.

Regulation of Red Blood Cell Production

When the kidneys detect a decrease in the oxygen tension in renal blood flow, they release erythropoietin. Erythropoietin is a glycoprotein from the kidney that stimulates the bone marrow to produce red blood cells (RBCs) that carry oxygen throughout the body.

Vitamin D Synthesis

The kidneys are also responsible for the final conversion of inactive vitamin D to its active form, 1,25-dihydroxycholecalciferol. Vitamin D is necessary for maintaining normal calcium balance in the body.

Secretion of Prostaglandins

The kidneys also produce prostaglandin E and prostacyclin, which have a vasodilatory effect and are important in maintaining renal blood flow.

Excretion of Waste Products

The kidneys eliminate the body's metabolic waste products. The major waste product of protein metabolism is urea, of which about 25 to 30 g are produced and excreted daily. All of this urea must be excreted in the urine; otherwise, it accumulates in body tissues. Other waste products of metabolism that must be excreted are creatinine, phosphates, and sulfates. Uric acid, formed as a waste product of purine metabolism, is also eliminated in the urine. The kidneys serve as the primary mechanism for excreting drug metabolites.

Urine Storage

The bladder is the reservoir for urine. Both filling and emptying of the bladder are mediated by coordinated sympathetic and parasympathetic nervous system control mechanisms involving the detrusor muscle and the bladder outlet.

Conscious awareness of bladder filling occurs as a result of sympathetic neuronal pathways that travel via the spinal cord to the level of T10 through T12, where peripheral, hypogastric nerve innervation allows for continued bladder filling. As bladder filling continues, stretch receptors in the bladder wall are activated, coupled with the desire to void. This information from the detrusor muscle is relayed back to the cerebral cortex via the parasympathetic pelvic nerves at the level of S1 through S4 (Porth & Matfin, 2009). Overall bladder pressure remains low due to the bladder's compliance (ability to expand or collapse) as urine volume changes.

Bladder compliance is due in part to the smooth muscle lining of the bladder and collagen deposits within the wall of the bladder, as well as to neuronal mechanisms that inhibit the detrusor muscle from contracting (specifically, adrenergic receptors that mediate relaxation). To maintain adequate kidney filtration rates, bladder pressure during filling must remain lower than 40 cm H_2O. This low pressure allows the urine to freely leave the renal pelvis and enter the ureters. The sensation of bladder fullness is transmitted to the central nervous system when the bladder has reached about 150 to 200 mL in adults, and an initial desire to void occurs. A marked sense of fullness and discomfort with a strong desire to void usually occurs when the bladder reaches its functional capacity 300 mL to 500 mL of urine (Bickley, 2007). Neurologic changes to the bladder at the level of the supraspinal nerves, the spinal nerves, or the bladder wall itself can cause abnormally high volumes (up to 2000 mL) of urine to be stored due to a decreased or absent urge to void.

Under normal circumstances with average fluid intake of approximately 1 to 2 L/day, the bladder should be able to store urine for periods of 2 to 4 hours at a time during the day. At night, the release of vasopressin in response to decreased fluid intake causes a decrease in the production of urine and makes it more concentrated. This phenomenon usually allows the bladder to continue filling for periods of 6 to 8 hours in adolescents and adults, making them able to sleep for longer periods before needing to void. In older people, decreasing bladder compliance and decreased vasopressin levels often cause **nocturia** (the need to wake up during the night to urinate).

Bladder Emptying

Micturition (voiding) normally occurs approximately eight times in a 24-hour period. It is activated via the micturition reflex arc within the sympathetic and parasympathetic nervous systems, which causes a coordinated sequence of events. Initiation of voiding occurs when the efferent pelvic nerve, which originates in the S1 to S4 area, stimulates the bladder to contract, resulting in complete relaxation of the striated urethral sphincter. This is followed by a decrease in urethral pressure, contraction of the detrusor muscle, opening of the vesicle neck and proximal urethra, and flow of urine. This coordinated effort by the parasympathetic system is mediated by muscarinic and, to a lesser extent, cholinergic receptors within the detrusor muscle. The pressure generated in the bladder during micturition is about 20 to 40 cm H_2O in females. It is somewhat higher and more variable in males 45 years of age and older due to the normal hyperplasia of the cells of the middle lobes of the

prostate gland, which surround the proximal urethra. Any obstruction of the bladder outlet, such as in advanced benign prostatic hyperplasia (BPH), results in a high voiding pressure. High voiding pressures make it more difficult to start urine flow and maintain it.

If the spinal pathways from the brain to the urinary system are destroyed (eg, after a spinal cord injury), reflex contraction of the bladder is maintained, but voluntary control over the process is lost. In both situations, the detrusor muscle can contract and expel urine, but the contractions are generally insufficient to empty the bladder completely, so residual urine (urine left in the bladder after voiding) remains. Normally, residual urine amounts to no more than 50 mL in the middle-aged adult and less than 50 to 100 mL in the older adult.

Gerontologic Considerations

Upper and lower urinary tract function changes with age (Stanley, Blair & Beare, 2005). The GFR decreases, starting between 35 and 40 years of age, and a yearly decline of about 1 mL/min continues thereafter. The elderly are more susceptible to acute and chronic renal failure due to the structural and functional changes in the kidney. Examples include sclerosis of the glomerulus and renal vasculature, decreased blood flow, decreased GFR, altered tubular function, and acid–base imbalance. Although renal function usually remains adequate, renal reserve is decreased and may reduce the kidneys' ability to respond effectively to drastic or sudden physiologic changes. This steady decrease in glomerular filtration, combined with the use of multiple medications in which metabolites are cleared by the kidneys, puts the older person at higher risk for adverse drug effects and drug–drug interactions (Stanley, et al., 2005).

The elderly are more prone to develop hypernatremia and fluid volume deficit, because increasing age is also associated with diminished osmotic stimulation of thirst (Stanley, et al., 2005). Thirst is defined as one's awareness of the desire to drink. The sense of thirst is so protective that hypernatremia almost never occurs in adults younger than 60 years of age.

Structural or functional abnormalities that occur with aging may also prevent complete emptying of the bladder. This may be due to decreased bladder wall contractility; secondary to myogenic or neurogenic factors; or related to bladder outlet obstruction, such as in BPH or after prostatectomy (Ostaszkiewicz, 2007). Vaginal and urethral tissues atrophy (become thinner) in aging women due to decreased estrogen levels. This causes decreased blood supply to the urogenital tissues, resulting in urethral and vaginal irritation and urinary incontinence.

Urinary incontinence is the most common reason for admission to skilled nursing facilities. Many older people and their families are unaware that urinary incontinence stems from many causes. The nurse needs to inform the patient and family that, with appropriate evaluation, urinary incontinence can often be managed at home, and in many cases it can be eliminated. Many treatments are available for urinary incontinence in the elderly, including noninvasive, behavioral interventions that the patient or caregiver can carry out (Palmer & Newman, 2007). Treatment modalities for urinary incontinence are described in further detail in Chapter 45.

Preparation of the elderly patient for diagnostic tests must be managed carefully to prevent dehydration, which might precipitate renal failure in a patient with marginal renal function. Limitations in mobility may affect an elderly patient's ability to void adequately or to consume an adequate volume of fluids. The patient may limit fluid intake to minimize the frequency of voiding or the risk of incontinence. Teaching the patient and family about the dangers of an inadequate fluid intake is an important role of the nurse caring for the elderly incontinent patient.

Assessment of the Renal and Urinary Tract Systems

Health History

Obtaining a urologic health history requires excellent communication skills, because many patients are embarrassed or uncomfortable discussing genitourinary function or symptoms (Bickley, 2007; Weber & Kelley, 2007). It is important to use language the patient can understand and to avoid medical jargon. It is also important to review risk factors, particularly for those patients who are at high risk. For example, the nurse needs to be aware that multiparous women delivering their children vaginally have a high risk for stress urinary incontinence, which, if severe enough, can also lead to urge incontinence. Elderly women and people with neurologic disorders such as diabetic neuropathy, multiple sclerosis (MS), or Parkinson's disease often have incomplete emptying of the bladder and urinary stasis, which may result in urinary tract infection or increasing bladder pressure, leading to overflow incontinence, hydronephrosis, pyelonephritis, or chronic kidney disease (Burrows-Hudson, 2005). Risk factors for specific disorders and kidney and lower urinary tract dysfunction are summarized in Table 43-1 and discussed in Chapters 44 and 45.

When obtaining the health history, the nurse should inquire about the following:

- The patient's chief concern or reason for seeking health care, the onset of the problem, and its effect on the patient's quality of life
- The location, character, and duration of pain, if present, and its relationship to voiding; factors that precipitate pain, and those that relieve it
- History of urinary tract infections, including past treatment or hospitalization for urinary tract infection
- Fever or chills
- Previous renal or urinary diagnostic tests or use of indwelling urinary catheters
- **Dysuria** and when during voiding (ie, at initiation or at termination of voiding) it occurs
- Hesitancy, straining, or pain during or after urination
- Urinary incontinence (stress incontinence, urge incontinence, overflow incontinence, or functional incontinence)
- Hematuria or change in color or volume of urine
- Nocturia and its date of onset
- Renal calculi (kidney stones), passage of stones or gravel in urine

Table 43-1 **RISK FACTORS FOR SELECTED RENAL OR UROLOGIC DISORDERS**

Risk Factor	Possible Renal or Urologic Disorder
Childhood diseases: "strep throat" impetigo, nephrotic syndrome	Chronic kidney disease
Advanced age	Incomplete emptying of bladder, leading to urinary tract infection
Instrumentation of urinary tract, cystoscopy, catheterization	Urinary tract infection, incontinence
Immobilization	Kidney stone formation
Occupational, recreational, or environmental exposure to chemicals (plastics, pitch, tar, rubber)	Acute renal failure
Diabetes mellitus	Chronic kidney disease, neurogenic bladder
Hypertension	Renal insufficiency, chronic renal failure
Multiple sclerosis	Incontinence, neurogenic bladder
Parkinson's disease	Incontinence
Systemic lupus erythematosus	Nephritis, chronic kidney disease
Gout, hyperparathyroidism, Crohn's disease, ileostomy	Kidney stone formation
Sickle cell anemia, multiple myeloma	Chronic kidney disease
Benign prostatic hyperplasia	Obstruction to urine flow, leading to frequency, oliguria, anuria
Radiation therapy to pelvis	Cystitis, fibrosis of ureter, or fistula in urinary tract
Recent pelvic surgery	Inadvertent trauma to ureters or bladder
Pregnancy	Proteinuria, frequent voiding
Obstetric injury, tumors	Incontinence
Spinal cord injury	Neurogenic bladder, urinary tract infection, incontinence

- Female patients: number and type (vaginal or cesarean) of deliveries; use of forceps; vaginal infection, discharge, or irritation; contraceptive practices
- History of **anuria** (decreased urine production) or other renal problem
- Presence or history of genital lesions or sexually transmitted diseases
- Use of tobacco, alcohol, or recreational drugs
- Any prescription and over-the-counter medications (including those prescribed for renal or urinary problems)

Common Symptoms

Dysfunction of the kidney can produce a complex array of symptoms throughout the body. Pain, changes in voiding, and gastrointestinal symptoms are particularly suggestive of urinary tract disease.

Pain

Genitourinary pain is usually caused by distention of some portion of the urinary tract as a result of obstructed urine flow or inflammation and swelling of tissues. Severity of pain is related to the sudden onset rather than the extent of distention.

Table 43-2 lists the various types of genitourinary pain, characteristics of the pain, associated signs and symptoms,

Table 43-2 IDENTIFYING CHARACTERISTICS OF GENITOURINARY PAIN

Type	Location	Character	Associated Signs and Symptoms	Possible Etiology
Kidney	Costovertebral angle, may extend to umbilicus	Dull constant ache; if sudden distention of capsule, pain is severe, sharp, stabbing, and colicky in nature	Nausea and vomiting, diaphoresis, pallor, signs of shock	Acute obstruction, kidney stone, blood clot, acute pyelonephritis, trauma
Bladder	Suprapubic area	Dull, continuous pain, may be intense with voiding, may be severe if bladder full	Urgency, pain at end of voiding, painful straining	Overdistended bladder, infection, interstitial cystitis; tumor
Ureteral	Costovertebral angle, flank, lower abdominal area, testis, or labium	Severe, sharp, stabbing pain, colicky in nature	Nausea and vomiting, paralytic ileus	Ureteral stone, edema or stricture, blood clot
Prostatic	Perineum and rectum	Vague discomfort, feeling of fullness in perineum, vague back pain	Suprapubic tenderness, obstruction to urine flow; frequency, urgency, dysuria, nocturia	Prostatic cancer, acute or chronic prostatitis
Urethral	Male: along penis to meatus; female: urethra to meatus	Pain variable, most severe during and immediately after voiding	Frequency, urgency, dysuria, nocturia, urethral discharge	Irritation of bladder neck, infection of urethra, trauma, foreign body in lower urinary tract

and possible causes. However, kidney disease does not always involve pain. It tends to be diagnosed because of other symptoms that cause a patient to seek health care, such as pedal edema, shortness of breath, and changes in urine elimination (Stanley, et al., 2005).

Changes in Voiding

Micturition is normally a painless function that occurs approximately eight times in a 24-hour period. The average person voids 1 to 2 L of urine in 24 hours, although this amount varies depending on fluid intake, sweating, environmental temperature, vomiting, or diarrhea. Common problems associated with voiding include **frequency,** urgency, dysuria, hesitancy, incontinence, enuresis, polyuria, **oliguria,** and hematuria. These problems and others are described in Table 43-3. Increased urinary urgency and frequency coupled with decreasing urine volumes strongly suggest urine retention. Depending on the acuity of the onset of these symptoms, immediate bladder emptying via catheterization and evaluation may be necessary to prevent kidney dysfunction.

Table 43-3 PROBLEMS ASSOCIATED WITH CHANGES IN VOIDING

Problem	Definition	Possible Etiology
Frequency	Frequent voiding—more than every 3 h	Infection, obstruction of lower urinary tract leading to residual urine and overflow, anxiety, diuretics, benign prostatic hyperplasia, urethral stricture, diabetic neuropathy
Urgency	Strong desire to void	Infection, chronic prostatitis, urethritis, obstruction of lower urinary tract leading to residual urine and overflow, anxiety, diuretics, benign prostatic hyperplasia, urethral stricture, diabetic neuropathy
Dysuria	Painful or difficult voiding	Lower urinary tract infection, inflammation of bladder or urethra, acute prostatitis, stones, foreign bodies, tumors in bladder
Hesitancy	Delay, difficulty in initiating voiding	Benign prostatic hyperplasia, compression of urethra, outlet obstruction, neurogenic bladder
Nocturia	Excessive urination at night	Decreased renal concentrating ability, heart failure, diabetes mellitus, incomplete bladder emptying, excessive fluid intake at bedtime, nephrotic syndrome, cirrhosis with ascites
Incontinence	Involuntary loss of urine	External urinary sphincter injury, obstetric injury, lesions of bladder neck, detrusor dysfunction, infection, neurogenic bladder, medications, neurologic abnormalities
Enuresis	Involuntary voiding during sleep	Delay in functional maturation of central nervous system (bladder control usually achieved by 5 y of age), obstructive disease of lower urinary tract, genetic factors, failure to concentrate urine, urinary tract infection, psychological stress
Polyuria	Increased volume of urine voided	Diabetes mellitus, diabetes insipidus, use of diuretics, excess fluid intake, lithium toxicity, some forms of kidney disease (hypercalcemic and hypokalemic nephropathy)
Oliguria	Urine output less than 500 mL/day	Acute or chronic renal failure (see Chapter 44), inadequate fluid intake
Anuria	Urine output less than 50 mL/day	Acute or chronic renal failure (see Chapter 44), complete obstruction
Hematuria	Red blood cells in the urine	Cancer of genitourinary tract, acute glomerulonephritis, renal stones, renal tuberculosis, blood dyscrasia, trauma, extreme exercise, rheumatic fever, hemophilia, leukemia, sickle cell trait or disease
Proteinuria	Abnormal amounts of protein in the urine	Acute and chronic renal disease, nephrotic syndrome, vigorous exercise, heat stroke, severe heart failure, diabetic nephropathy, multiple myeloma

Gastrointestinal Symptoms

Gastrointestinal signs and symptoms are often associated with urologic conditions because of shared autonomic and sensory innervation and renointestinal reflexes (see Table 43-3). The proximity of the right kidney to the colon, duodenum, head of the pancreas, common bile duct, liver, and gallbladder may cause gastrointestinal disturbances. The proximity of the left kidney to the colon (splenic flexure), stomach, pancreas, and spleen may also result in intestinal symptoms. The most common signs and symptoms are nausea, vomiting, diarrhea, abdominal discomfort, and abdominal distention. Urologic symptoms can mimic such disorders as appendicitis, peptic ulcer disease, and cholecystitis; this can make diagnosis difficult, especially in the elderly, who have decreased neurologic innervation to this area (Goshorn, 2005).

Unexplained Anemia

Gradual kidney dysfunction can be insidious in its presentation, although fatigue is a common symptom. Fatigue, shortness of breath, and exercise intolerance all result from the condition known as "anemia of chronic disease." Although historically hematocrit has been the blood test of choice when assessing a patient for anemia, use of the hemoglobin level rather than hematocrit is currently recommended, because that measurement is a better assessment of the oxygen transport ability of the blood.

Past Health, Family, and Social History

Data collection about previous health problems or diseases provides the health care team with useful information for evaluating the patient's current urinary status. People with diabetes who have consistent hypertension and those with primary hypertension are at risk for renal dysfunction. Older men are at risk for prostatic enlargement, which causes urethral obstruction and can result in urinary tract infections and renal failure. People with a family history of urinary tract problems are at increased risk for renal disorders. Genetics may also influence renal conditions (Chart 43-2).

It is also important to assess the patient's psychosocial status, level of anxiety, perceived threats to body image, available support systems, and sociocultural patterns.

Physical Assessment

Several body systems can affect upper and lower urinary tract dysfunction, and conversely that dysfunction can affect several end organs; therefore, a head-to-toe assessment is indicated. Areas of emphasis include the abdomen, suprapubic region, genitalia, lower back, and lower extremities.

The kidneys are not usually palpable. However, palpation of the kidneys may detect an enlargement that could prove to be very important (Bickley, 2007). The correct technique for palpation is illustrated in Figure 43-5. It

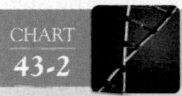

CHART 43-2

GENETICS IN NURSING PRACTICE
Renal and Urinary Tract Disorders

Various conditions that affect the renal system and urinary tract function are influenced by genetic factors. Some examples of these genetic disorders are:
- Alport syndrome
- Congenital absence of the vas deferens (caused by *CFTR* gene mutation for cystic fibrosis)
- Cystic, dysplastic kidneys
- Fabry disease
- Familial Wilms' tumor
- Focal and segmental glomerulosis
- Horseshoe kidney
- Polycystic kidney (autosomal dominant gene)
- Nephrosis of later onset
- Renal cystic disease in tuberous sclerosis complex

Nursing Assessments

Family History
- Inquire about other family members with renal and/or urinary tract malformations.
- Ask about family history of kidney disease with onset in third to fifth decade (polycystic kidney, autosomal dominant gene).
- Identify family history of male infertility and cystic fibrosis (congenital absence of vas deferens).
- Be alert for family members with history of early-onset renal (Wilms' tumor) or other cancers.

Physical Assessment
- Be alert for signs and symptoms of renal disease at an early age (hematuria, hypertension, abdominal mass).

- Assess for clinical findings suggesting that renal disease is a component of a genetic syndrome (eg, seizures, mental retardation, skin involvement).

Management Issues Specific to Genetics
- Inquire whether DNA mutation or other genetic testing has been performed on an affected family member.
- If indicated, refer for genetic counseling and evaluation so that the family can discuss concerns regarding inheritance, risks to other family members, availability of genetic testing, and gene-based interventions.
- Offer appropriate genetics information and resources (eg, Genetic Alliance Web site).
- Provide support to families newly diagnosed with gene-related renal and/or kidney disease.

Genetics Resources for Nurses and Their Patients on the Web

Genetic Alliance—a directory of support groups for patients and families with genetic conditions, www.geneticalliance.org
Gene Clinics—a listing of common genetic disorders with up-to-date clinical summaries and genetic counseling and testing information, www.geneclinics.org
National Organization of Rare Disorders—a directory of support groups and information for patients and families with rare genetic disorders, www.rarediseases.org
OMIM: Online Mendelian Inheritance in Man—a complete listing of inherited genetic conditions, www.ncbi.nlm.nih.gov/projects/omim

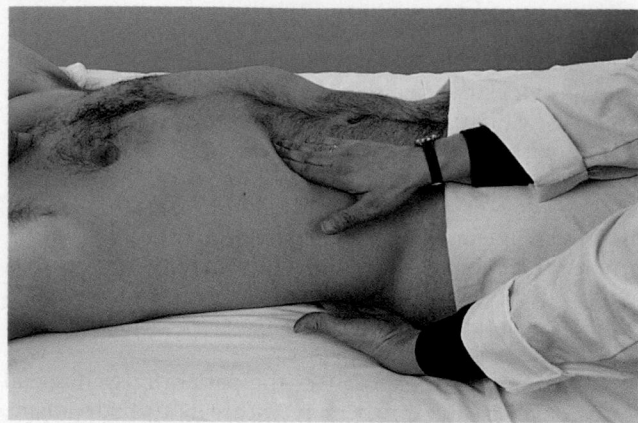

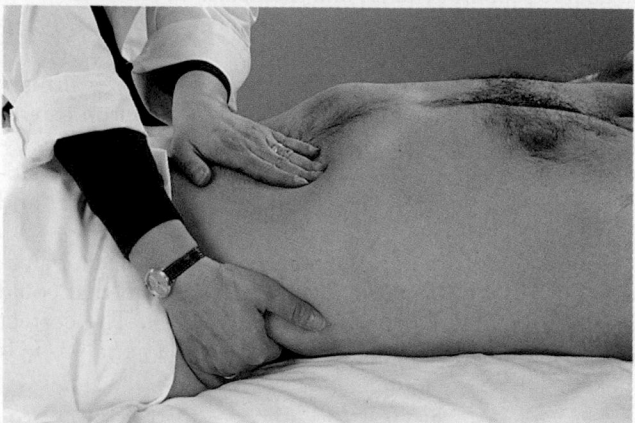

Figure 43-5 Technique for palpating the right kidney (*top*). Place one hand under the patient's back with the fingers under the lower rib. Place the palm of the other hand anterior to the kidney with fingers above the umbilicus. Push the hand on top forward as the patient inhales deeply. The left kidney (*bottom*) is palpated similarly by reaching over to the patient's left side and placing the right hand beneath the patient's lower left rib. From Weber, J. & Kelley, J. (2007). *Health assessment in nursing* (3rd ed.). Philadelphia: Lippincott Williams & Wilkins.

may be possible to palpate the smooth, rounded lower pole of the kidney between the hands. The right kidney is easier to detect, because it is somewhat lower than the left one. In obese patients, palpation of the kidneys is more difficult.

Renal dysfunction may produce tenderness over the costovertebral angle, which is the angle formed by the lower border of the 12th, or bottom, rib and the spine (Fig. 43-6). The abdomen (just slightly to the right and left of the midline in both upper quadrants) is auscultated to assess for bruits (low-pitched murmurs that indicate renal artery stenosis or an aortic aneurysm). The abdomen is also assessed for the presence of ascites (accumulation of fluid in the peritoneal cavity), which may occur with kidney as well as liver dysfunction.

To check for residual urine, the bladder should be percussed after the patient voids. Percussion of the bladder begins at the midline just above the umbilicus and proceeds downward. The sound changes from tympanic to dull when percussing over the bladder. The bladder, which can be palpated only if it is moderately distended, feels like a smooth,

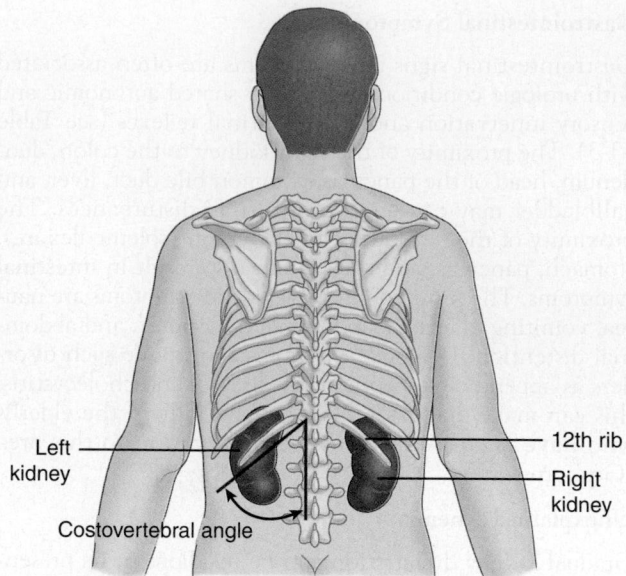

Figure 43-6 Location of the costovertebral angle.

firm, round mass rising out of the abdomen, usually at midline (Fig. 43-7). Dullness to percussion of the bladder after voiding indicates incomplete bladder emptying (Bickley, 2007; Weber & Kelley, 2007).

In older men, BPH or prostatitis can cause difficulty with urination (Stanley, et al., 2005). Because the signs and symptoms of prostate cancer can mimic those of

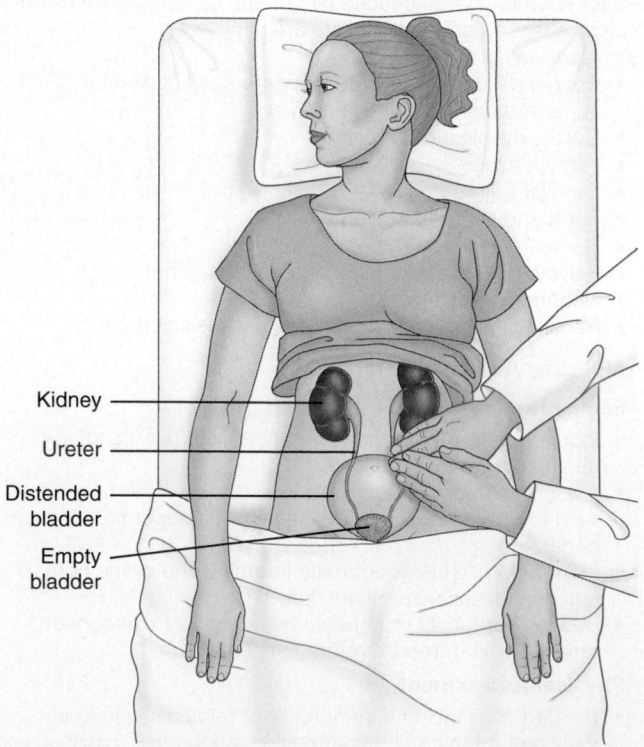

Figure 43-7 Palpation of the bladder.

BPH, the prostate gland is palpated by digital rectal examination (DRE) as part of the yearly physical examination in men 40 years of age and older (see Chapter 49). In addition, a blood specimen is obtained to test the prostate-specific antigen (PSA) level annually; the results of the DRE and PSA are then correlated. Blood is drawn for PSA before the DRE, because manipulation of the prostate can cause the PSA level to increase temporarily. The inguinal area is examined for enlarged nodes, an inguinal or femoral hernia, and varicocele (varicose veins of the spermatic cord).

In women, the vulva, urethral meatus, and vagina are examined (Bickley, 2007; Weber & Kelley, 2007). The urethra is palpated for diverticula, and the vagina is assessed for adequate estrogen effect and any of five types of herniation. Urethrocele is the bulging of the anterior vaginal wall into the urethra. Cystocele is the herniation of the bladder wall into the vaginal vault. Pelvic prolapse is bulging of the cervix into the vaginal vault. Enterocele is herniation of the bowel into the posterior vaginal wall. Rectocele is herniation of the rectum into the vaginal wall. These prolapses are graded depending on the degree of herniation (see Chapter 47 for more information).

The woman is asked to cough and perform a Valsalva maneuver to assess the urethra's system of muscular and ligament support. If urine leakage occurs, the index and middle fingers of the examiner's gloved hand are used to support either side of the urethra as the woman is asked to repeat the Valsalva maneuver; this is called the Marshall-Boney maneuver. If this produces urinary leakage, referral is suggested.

The patient is assessed for edema and changes in body weight. Edema may be observed, particularly in the face and dependent parts of the body, such as the ankles and sacral areas, and suggests fluid retention. An increase in body weight commonly accompanies edema. A 1-kg weight gain equals approximately 1000 mL of fluid (1 lb is approximately 500 mL).

The deep tendon reflexes of the knee are examined for quality and symmetry. This is an important part of testing for neurologic causes of bladder dysfunction, because the sacral area, which innervates the lower extremities, is the same peripheral nerve area responsible for urinary continence. The gait pattern of the person with bladder dysfunction is also noted, as well as the patient's ability to walk toe-to-heel. These tests evaluate possible supraspinal causes for urinary incontinence.

Diagnostic Evaluation

A comprehensive health history is used to determine the appropriate laboratory and diagnostic tests. The following sections review some of the tests that might be used.

Most patients undergoing urologic testing or imaging studies are apprehensive, even those who have had these tests in the past. Patients frequently feel discomfort and embarrassment about such a private and personal function as voiding. Voiding in the presence of others can frequently cause guarding, a natural reflex that inhibits voiding due to situational anxiety. Because the outcomes of these studies determine the plan of care, the nurse must help the patient relax by providing as much privacy and explanation about the procedure as possible (Chart 43-3). In addition, Chart 43-4 provides a plan of care for patients undergoing diagnostic testing.

Urinalysis and Urine Culture

The urinalysis provides important clinical information about kidney function and helps diagnose other diseases, such as diabetes. The urine culture determines whether bacteria are present in the urine, as well as their strains and concentration. Urine culture and sensitivity also identify the antimicrobial therapy that is best suited for the particular strains identified, taking into consideration the antibiotics that have the best rate of resolution in that particular geographic region. Appropriate evaluation of any abnormality can assist in detecting serious underlying diseases.

Components

Urine examination includes the following:
- Urine color (Table 43-4)
- Urine clarity and odor
- Urine pH and specific gravity
- Tests to detect protein, glucose, and ketone bodies in the urine (proteinuria, renal glycosuria, and ketonuria, respectively)
- Microscopic examination of the urine sediment after centrifugation to detect RBCs **(hematuria),** white blood cells **(pyuria),** casts (cylindruria), crystals (crystalluria), and bacteria **(bacteriuria)**

Researchers are working on additional noninvasive tests that can be performed on urine to detect conditions such as bladder cancer. For example, urine telomerase activity levels have been found to be sensitive and specific to detect bladder cancer in men (Sanchini, Gunelli, Nanni, et al., 2005). More research is needed before these tests are acceptable for routine use in patients.

Significance of Findings

Several abnormalities, such as hematuria and proteinuria, produce no symptoms but may be detected during a routine urinalysis using a dipstick. Normally, about 1 million RBCs pass into the urine daily, which is equivalent to one to three RBCs per high-power field. Hematuria (more than three RBCs per high-power field) can develop from an abnormality anywhere along the genitourinary tract and is more common in women than in men. Common causes include acute infection (cystitis, urethritis, or prostatitis), renal calculi, and neoplasm. Other causes include systemic disorders, such as bleeding disorders; malignant lesions; and medications, such as warfarin (Coumadin) and heparin (Heparin Sodium). Although hematuria may initially be detected using a dipstick test, further microscopic evaluation is necessary (Tierney & Henderson, 2005).

Proteinuria may be a benign finding, or it may signify serious disease (Burrows-Hudson, 2005). Occasional loss of

CHART
43-3

PATIENT EDUCATION
Before and After Urodynamic Testing

- A physician or nurse will conduct an in-depth interview. Questions related to your urologic symptoms and voiding habits will be asked.
- You will be asked to describe sensations felt during the procedure.
- During the procedure, you might be asked to change positions (eg, from supine to sitting or standing).
- You may be asked to cough or perform the Valsalva maneuver (bear down) during the procedure.
- You will probably need to have one or two urethral catheters inserted so that bladder pressure and bladder filling can be measured. Another catheter may be placed in the rectum or vagina to measure abdominal pressure.
- You may also have electrodes (surface, wire, or needle) placed in the perianal area for electromyography (EMG). This may be uncomfortable initially during insertion and later during position changes.
- Your bladder will be filled through the urethral catheter one or more times during the procedure.

- After the procedure, you may experience urinary frequency, urgency, or dysuria from the urethral catheters. Avoid caffeinated, carbonated, and alcoholic beverages after the procedure because these can further irritate the bladder. These symptoms usually decrease or subside by the day after the procedure.
- You might notice a slight hematuria (blood-tinged urine) right after the procedure (especially in men with benign prostatic hyperplasia). Drinking fluids will help to clear the hematuria.
- If the urinary meatus is irritated, a warm sitz bath may be helpful.
- Be alert for signs of a urinary tract infection after the procedure. Contact your physician if you experience fever, chills, lower back pain, or continued dysuria and hematuria.
- If you receive an antibiotic medication before the procedure, you should continue taking the complete course of medication after the procedure. This is a measure to prevent infection.

up to 150 mg/day of protein in the urine, primarily albumin and Tamm-Horsfall protein (also known as uromodulin), is considered normal and usually does not require further evaluation. A dipstick examination, which can detect from 30 to 1000 mg/dL of protein, should be used as a screening test only, because urine concentration, pH, hematuria, and radiocontrast materials all affect the results. Because dipstick analysis does not detect protein concentrations of less than 30 mg/dL, the test cannot be used for early detection of diabetic nephropathy. Microalbuminuria (excretion of 20 to 200 mg/dL of protein in the urine) is an early sign of diabetic nephropathy. Common benign causes of transient proteinuria are fever, strenuous exercise, and prolonged standing.

Causes of persistent proteinuria include glomerular diseases, malignancies, collagen diseases, diabetes mellitus, preeclampsia, hypothyroidism, heart failure, exposure to heavy metals, and use of medications, such as nonsteroidal anti-inflammatory drugs (NSAIDs) and angiotensin-converting enzyme (ACE) inhibitors (Karch, 2008).

Specific Gravity

Specific gravity measures the density of a solution compared to the density of water, which is 1.000. Specific gravity is altered by the presence of blood, protein, and casts in the urine. The normal range of urine specific gravity is 1.010 to 1.025.

Methods for determination of specific gravity include the following:

- Multiple-test dipstick (most common method), with a specific reagent area for specific gravity
- Urinometer (least accurate method), in which urine is placed in a small cylinder and the urinometer is floated in the urine; a specific gravity reading is obtained at the meniscus level of the urine

- Refractometer, an instrument used in a laboratory setting, which measures differences in the speed of light passing through air and the urine sample

Urine specific gravity depends largely on hydration status. When fluid intake decreases, specific gravity normally increases. With high fluid intake, specific gravity decreases. In patients with kidney disease, urine specific gravity does not vary with fluid intake, and the patient's urine is said to have a fixed specific gravity. Disorders or conditions that cause decreased urine specific gravity include diabetes insipidus, glomerulonephritis, and severe renal damage. Those that can cause increased specific gravity include diabetes mellitus, nephritis, and fluid deficit.

Osmolality

Osmolality is the most accurate measurement of the kidney's ability to dilute and concentrate urine. It measures the number of solute particles in a kilogram of water. Serum and urine osmolality are measured simultaneously to assess the body's fluid status. In healthy adults serum osmolality is 280 to 300 mOsm/kg, and normal urine osmolality is 200 to 800 mOsm/kg (Goertz, 2006). For a 24-hour urine sample, the normal value is 300 to 900 mOsm/kg.

Renal Function Tests

Renal function tests are used to evaluate the severity of kidney disease and to assess the status of the patient's kidney function. These tests also provide information about the effectiveness of the kidney in carrying out its excretory function. Renal function test results may be within normal limits until the GFR is reduced to less than 50% of normal. Renal function can be assessed most accurately if several tests are performed and their results are analyzed together. Common tests of renal function include renal concentration tests, creatinine clearance, and

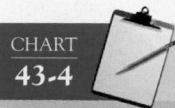

CHART 43-4

PLAN OF NURSING CARE
Care of the Patient Undergoing Diagnostic Testing of the Renal–Urologic System

NURSING DIAGNOSIS: Deficient knowledge about procedures and diagnostic tests
GOAL: Patient demonstrates increased understanding of the procedure and tests and expected behaviors

Nursing Interventions	Rationale	Expected Outcomes
1. Assess patient's level of understanding of planned diagnostic tests. 2. Provide a description of tests in language the patient can understand. 3. Assess patient's understanding of test results after their completion. 4. Reinforce information provided to patient about test results and implications for follow-up care.	1. Provides basis for teaching and gives indication of patient's perception of tests 2. Understanding what is expected enhances patient compliance and cooperation. 3. Apprehension may interfere with patient's ability to understand information and results provided by health care team. 4. Provides opportunity for patient to clarify information and anticipate follow-up care.	• States rationale for planned diagnostic tests and what tasks and behaviors are expected during the procedure • Complies with urine collection, fluid modifications, or other procedures required for diagnostic evaluation • Restates in own words results of diagnostic tests • Asks for clarification of terms and procedures • Explains rationale for follow-up care • Participates in follow-up care

NURSING DIAGNOSIS: Acute pain related to infection, edema, obstruction, or bleeding along urinary tract or related to invasive diagnostic tests
GOAL: Patient reports decrease in pain and absence of discomfort

Nursing Interventions	Rationale	Expected Outcomes
1. Assess level of pain: dysuria, burning on urination, abdominal or flank pain, bladder spasm. 2. Encourage fluid intake (unless contraindicated). 3. Encourage warm sitz baths. 4. Report increased pain to physician. 5. Administer analgesic and antispasmodic agents for pain and spasm as prescribed. 6. Assess voiding patterns and hygiene practices and provide instructions about recommended voiding patterns and hygienic practices.	1. Provides baseline for evaluation of pain relief strategies and progression of dysfunction 2. Promotes dilute urine and flushing of the lower urinary tract 3. Relieves local discomfort and promotes relaxation 4. May indicate progression or recurrence of dysfunction, or untoward signs (eg, bleeding, calculi) 5. Prescribed to relieve pain or spasm 6. Delayed emptying of the bladder and poor hygiene may contribute to pain secondary to renal or urinary tract dysfunction.	• Reports decreasing levels of pain • Reports absence of local symptoms • States ability to start and stop urinary stream without discomfort • Consumes increased fluid intake if indicated • Uses sitz bath as indicated • Identifies signs and symptoms to be reported to the health care provider • Takes medications as prescribed • Does not delay in emptying bladder • Uses appropriate hygienic measures, avoids use of bubble bath, uses appropriate hygiene after bowel movements

NURSING DIAGNOSIS: Fear related to potential alteration in renal function and embarrassment secondary to discussion of urinary function and invasion of genitalia
GOAL: Patient appears relaxed and reports decreased fear and anxiety

Nursing Interventions	Rationale	Expected Outcomes
1. Assess patient's level of fear and apprehension. 2. Explain all procedures and tests to patient. 3. Provide privacy and respect patient's modesty by closing doors and keeping patient covered. Keep urinal and bedpan covered and out of sight. 4. Use correct terminology in a factual manner when questioning patient about urinary tract dysfunction. 5. Assess patient's fears about perceived changes associated with tests and other procedures. 6. Instruct patient in relaxation techniques.	1. A high level of fear or apprehension can interfere with learning and cooperation. 2. Knowledge about what is expected helps reduce fear and apprehension. 3. Communicates that you are aware of and accept patient's need for privacy and modesty 4. Conveys that you are comfortable discussing patient's urinary dysfunction and symptoms with patient 5. May uncover fears and misconceptions of the patient that can be alleviated by correct understanding 6. Promotes relaxation and assists patient in coping with uncertainty about outcomes	• Appears relaxed with a low level of fear or apprehension • States rationale for tests and procedures in a calm, relaxed manner • Maintains usual privacy and modesty • Discusses own urinary tract dysfunction using correct terminology without overt indications of embarrassment or discomfort • Relates fears and concerns • Demonstrates correct understanding of procedures and possible outcomes • Appears relaxed with low level of fear and apprehension

Table 43-4   CHANGES IN URINE COLOR AND POSSIBLE CAUSES

Urine Color	Possible Cause
Colorless to pale yellow	Dilute urine due to diuretics, alcohol consumption, diabetes insipidus, glycosuria, excess fluid intake, renal disease
Yellow to milky white	Pyuria, infection, vaginal cream
Bright yellow	Multiple vitamin preparations
Pink to red	Hemoglobin breakdown, red blood cells, gross blood, menses, bladder or prostate surgery, beets, blackberries, medications (phenytoin, [Dilantin], rifampin [Rifadin], phenothiazine [Mellaril], cascara [Sagrada], senna products)
Blue, blue green	Dyes, methylene blue, Pseudomonas species organisms, medications (amitriptyline [Amitriptyline HCL], triamterine [Dyrenium])
Orange to amber	Concentrated urine due to dehydration, fever, bile, excess bilirubin or carotene, medications (pyridium [Phenazopyridium HCL], nitrofurantoin [Furadantin])
Brown to black	Old red blood cells, urobilinogen, bilirubin, melanin, porphyrin, extremely concentrated urine due to dehydration, medications (cascara, metronidazole [Flagyl], iron preparations, quinine [Quinine Sulfate], senna products, methyldopa [Aldomet], nitrofurantoin)

serum creatinine and blood **urea nitrogen** levels. Table 43-5 describes the purpose and gives the normal range for each test. Other tests for evaluating renal function that may be helpful include serum electrolyte levels (see Chapter 14).

Diagnostic Imaging

Kidney, Ureter, and Bladder Studies

An x-ray study of the abdomen or kidneys, ureters, and bladder (KUB) may be performed to delineate the size, shape, and position of the kidneys and to reveal urinary system abnormalities (Labus, 2008).

General Ultrasonography

Ultrasonography is a noninvasive procedure that uses sound waves passed into the body through a transducer to detect abnormalities of internal tissues and organs. Abnormalities such as fluid accumulation, masses, congenital malformations, changes in organ size, and obstructions can be identified. During the test, the lower abdomen and genitalia may need to be exposed. Ultrasonography requires a full bladder; therefore, fluid intake should be encouraged before the procedure. Because of its sensitivity, ultrasonography has replaced many other tests as the initial diagnostic procedure (Burrows-Hudson, 2005).

Bladder Ultrasonography

Bladder ultrasonography is a noninvasive method of measuring urine volume in the bladder. It may be indicated for urinary frequency, inability to void after removal of an indwelling urinary catheter, measurement of postvoiding residual urine volume, inability to void postoperatively, or assessment of the need for catheterization during the initial stages of an intermittent catheterization training program. Portable, battery-operated devices are available for bedside use. The scan head is placed on the patient's abdomen and

Table 43-5   RENAL FUNCTION TESTS

Test	Purpose	Normal Values		
Renal Concentration Tests				
Specific gravity	Evaluates ability of kidneys to concentrate solutes in urine.	1.010–1.025		
Urine osmolality	Concentrating ability is lost early in kidney disease; hence, these test findings may disclose early defects in renal function.	300–900 mOsm/kg/24 h, 50–1200 mOsm/kg random sample		
24-Hour Urine Test				
Creatinine clearance	Detects and evaluates progression of renal disease. Test measures volume of blood cleared of endogenous creatinine in 1 min, which provides an approximation of the glomerular filtration rate. Sensitive indicator of renal disease used to follow progression of renal disease.	Measured in mL/min/1.73 m²		
		Age	Male	Female
		Under 30	88–146	81–134
		30–40	82–140	75–128
		40–50	75–133	69–122
		50–60	68–126	64–116
		60–70	61–120	58–110
		70–80	55–113	52–105
Serum Tests				
Creatinine level	Measures effectiveness of renal function. Creatinine is end product of muscle energy metabolism. In normal function, level of creatinine, which is regulated and excreted by the kidneys, remains fairly constant in body.	0.6–1.2 mg/dL (50–110 mmol/L)		
Urea nitrogen (blood urea nitrogen [BUN])	Serves as index of renal function. Urea is nitrogenous end product of protein metabolism. Test values are affected by protein intake, tissue breakdown, and fluid volume changes.	7–18 mg/dL Patients >60 yrs: 8–20 mg/dL		
BUN-to-creatinine ratio	Evaluates hydration status. An elevated ratio is seen in hypovolemia; a normal ratio with an elevated BUN and creatinine is seen with intrinsic renal disease.	About 10:1		

directed toward the bladder. The device automatically calculates and displays urine volume.

Computed Tomography and Magnetic Resonance Imaging

Computed tomography (CT) scans and magnetic resonance imaging (MRI) are noninvasive techniques that provide excellent cross-sectional views of the anatomy of the kidney and urinary tract (Labus, 2008). They are used to evaluate genitourinary masses, nephrolithiasis, chronic renal infections, renal or urinary tract trauma, metastatic disease, and soft tissue abnormalities. Occasionally, an oral or intravenous (IV) radiopaque contrast agent is used in CT scanning to enhance visualization.

Preparation for Magnetic Resonance Imaging

Patient preparation should include teaching relaxation techniques and informing the patient that he or she will be able to communicate with the staff by means of a microphone located inside the scanner. Many MRI suites provide headphones so that patients can listen to the music of their choice during the procedure. Nursing care guidelines for patient preparation and test precautions for any imaging procedure that requires a contrast agent (contrast medium) are explained in Chart 43-5.

Before the patient enters the room where the MRI is to be performed, all metal objects and credit cards (the magnetic field can erase them) are removed. This includes

Chart 43-5 • *Patient Care During Urologic Testing With Contrast Agents*

For some patients, contrast agents are nephrotoxic and allergenic. The following guidelines can help the nurse and other health care providers respond quickly in the event of a problem.

Nursing Actions for Room Preparation

- Have emergency equipment and medications available in case the patient has an anaphylactic reaction to the contrast agent. Emergency supplies include epinephrine, corticosteroids, vasopressors, oxygen, and airway and suction equipment.

Nursing Actions for Patient Preparation

- Obtain the patient's allergy history with emphasis on allergy to iodine, shellfish, and other seafood, because many contrast agents contain iodine.
- Notify physician and radiologist if the patient is allergic or suspected to be allergic to iodine.
- Obtain health history. Contrast agents should be used with caution in older patients and patients who have diabetes mellitus, multiple myeloma, renal insufficiency, or volume depletion.
- Inform the patient that he or she may experience a temporary feeling of warmth, flushing of the face, and an unusual flavor (similar to that of seafood) in the mouth when the contrast agent is infused.
- Monitor patient closely for allergic reaction and monitor urine output.

medication patches (eg, nicotine and nitroglycerine) that have a metal backing, which can cause burns if they are not removed. No metal objects (eg, oxygen tanks, ventilators, stethoscopes) may be brought into the MRI room. The magnetic field is so strong that any metal-containing items will be pulled toward the magnet, causing severe injury and possible death. A patient history is obtained to determine the presence of any metal objects (eg, aneurysm clips, orthopedic hardware, pacemakers, artificial heart valves, intrauterine devices). These objects could malfunction, be dislodged, or heat up as they absorb energy. Cochlear implants are inactivated by MRI; therefore, other imaging procedures are considered. A sedative may be prescribed, because claustrophobia is a problem for some patients.

Prior to MRI of the urinary system the patient needs to be informed to avoid alcohol, caffeine-containing beverages, and smoking for at least 2 hours and food for at least 1 hour prior to the scan. Patients should continue taking their usual medication, except for iron supplements, which can interfere with the imaging (Labus, 2008).

Nuclear Scans

Nuclear scans require injection of a radioisotope (a technetium 99m–labeled compound or iodine 123 [^{123}I] hippurate) into the circulatory system; the isotope is then monitored as it moves through the blood vessels of the kidneys. A scintillation camera is placed behind the kidney with the patient in a supine, prone, or seated position. Hypersensitivity to the radioisotope is rare. The technetium scan provides information about kidney perfusion. The ^{123}I-hippurate renal scan provides information about kidney function, such as GFR.

Nuclear scans are used to evaluate acute and chronic renal failure, renal masses, and blood flow before and after kidney transplantation. The radioisotope is injected at a specified time to achieve the proper concentration in the kidneys. After the procedure is completed, the patient is encouraged to drink fluids to promote excretion of the radioisotope by the kidneys.

Intravenous Urography

IV urography includes various tests such as excretory urography, intravenous pyelography (IVP), and infusion drip pyelography. A radiopaque contrast agent is administered by IV. An IVP shows the kidneys, ureter, and bladder via x-ray imaging as the dye moves through the upper and then the lower urinary system. A nephrotomogram may be carried out as part of the study to visualize different layers of the kidney and the diffuse structures within each layer and to differentiate solid masses or lesions from cysts in the kidneys or urinary tract.

IV urography may be used as the initial assessment of many suspected urologic conditions, especially lesions in the kidneys and ureters. It also provides an approximate estimate of renal function. After the contrast agent (sodium diatrizoate or meglumine diatrizoate) is administered by IV, multiple x-rays are obtained to visualize drainage structures in the upper and lower urinary systems.

Infusion drip pyelography requires IV infusion of a large volume of a dilute contrast agent to opacify the renal parenchyma and fill the urinary tract. This examination method is useful when prolonged opacification of the drainage structures is desired so that tomograms (body-section radiography) can be made. Images are obtained at specified intervals after the start of the infusion. These images show the filled and distended collecting system. The patient preparation is the same as for excretory urography, except that fluids are not restricted.

Retrograde Pyelography

In retrograde pyelography, catheters are advanced through the ureters into the renal pelvis by means of cystoscopy. A contrast agent is then injected. Retrograde pyelography is usually performed if IV urography provides inadequate visualization of the collecting systems. It may also be used before extracorporeal shock wave lithotripsy and in patients with urologic cancer who need follow-up and have an allergy to IV contrast agents. Possible complications include infection, hematuria, and perforation of the ureter. Retrograde pyelography is used infrequently because of improved techniques in excretory urography.

Cystography

Cystography aids in evaluating vesicoureteral reflux (backflow of urine from the bladder into one or both ureters) and in assessing for bladder injury. A catheter is inserted into the bladder, and a contrast agent is instilled to outline the bladder wall. The contrast agent may leak through a small bladder perforation stemming from bladder injury, but such leakage is usually harmless. Cystography can also be performed with simultaneous pressure recordings inside the bladder.

Voiding Cystourethrography

Voiding cystourethrography uses fluoroscopy to visualize the lower urinary tract and assess urine storage in the bladder. It is commonly used as a diagnostic tool to identify vesicoureteral reflux. A urethral catheter is inserted, and a contrast agent is instilled into the bladder. When the bladder is full and the patient feels the urge to void, the catheter is removed, and the patient voids.

Renal Angiography

A renal angiogram, or renal arteriogram, provides an image of the renal arteries. The femoral (or axillary) artery is pierced with a needle, and a catheter is threaded up through the femoral and iliac arteries into the aorta or renal artery. A contrast agent is injected to opacify the renal arterial supply. Angiography is used to evaluate renal blood flow in suspected renal trauma, to differentiate renal cysts from tumors, and to evaluate hypertension. It is used preoperatively for renal transplantation. Before the procedure, a laxative may be prescribed to evacuate the colon so that unobstructed x-rays can be obtained. Injection sites (groin for femoral approach or axilla for axillary approach) may be shaved. The peripheral pulse sites (radial, femoral, and dorsalis pedis) are marked for easy access during postprocedural assessment. The patient is informed that there may be a brief sensation of warmth along the course of the vessel when the contrast agent is injected.

After the procedure, vital signs are monitored until stable. If the axillary artery was the injection site, blood pressure measurements are taken on the opposite arm. The injection site is examined for swelling and hematoma. Peripheral pulses are palpated, and the color and temperature of the involved extremity are noted and compared with those of the uninvolved extremity. Cold compresses may be applied to the injection site to decrease edema and pain. Possible complications include hematoma formation, arterial thrombosis or dissection, false aneurysm formation, and altered renal function.

Urologic Endoscopic Procedures

Endourology, or urologic endoscopic procedures, can be performed in one of two ways: using a cystoscope inserted into the urethra, or percutaneously, through a small incision.

The cystoscopic examination is used to directly visualize the urethra and bladder. The cystoscope, which is inserted through the urethra into the bladder, has an optical lens system that provides a magnified, illuminated view of the bladder (Fig. 43-8). The use of a high-intensity light and interchangeable lenses allows excellent visualization and permits still and motion pictures to be taken. The cystoscope is manipulated to allow complete visualization of the urethra and bladder as well as the ureteral orifices and prostatic urethra. Small ureteral catheters can be passed through the cystoscope for assessment of the ureters and the pelvis of each kidney.

The cystoscope also allows the urologist to obtain a urine specimen from each kidney to evaluate its function. Cup forceps can be inserted through the cystoscope for biopsy. Calculi may be removed from the urethra, bladder, and ureter using cystoscopy. If a lower tract cystoscopy is performed, the patient is usually conscious, and the procedure is usually no more uncomfortable than a catheterization. To

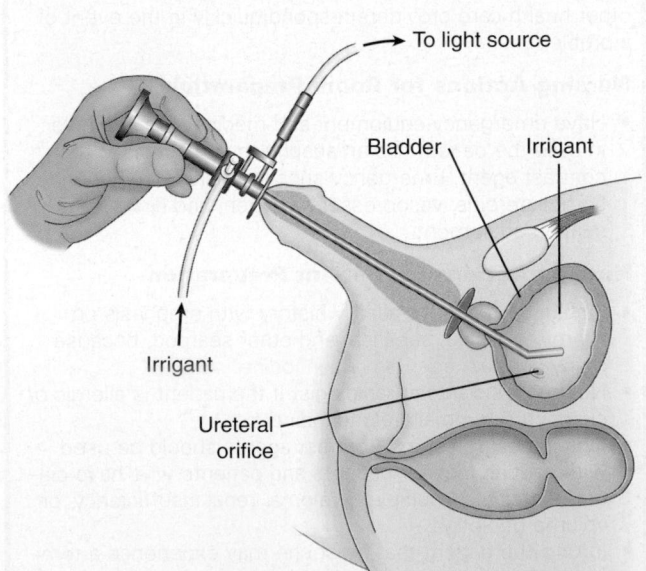

Figure 43-8 Cystoscopic examination. A rigid or semirigid cystoscope is introduced into the bladder. The upper cord is an electric line for the light at the distal end of the cystoscope. The lower tubing leads from a reservoir of sterile irrigant that is used to inflate the bladder.

minimize posttest urethral discomfort, viscous lidocaine is administered several minutes before the study. If the cystoscopy includes examination of the upper tracts, a sedative may be administered before the procedure. General anesthesia is usually administered to ensure that there are no involuntary muscle spasms when the scope is being passed through the ureters or kidney.

The nurse describes the procedure to the patient and family to prepare them and to allay their fears. If an upper cystoscopy is to be performed, the patient is usually restricted to nothing by mouth (NPO) for several hours beforehand.

Postprocedural management is directed at relieving any discomfort resulting from the examination. Some burning on voiding, blood-tinged urine, and urinary frequency from trauma to the mucous membranes can be expected. Moist heat to the lower abdomen and warm sitz baths are helpful in relieving pain and relaxing the muscles.

After a cystoscopic examination, the patient with obstructive pathology may experience urine retention if the instruments used during the examination caused edema. The nurse carefully monitors the patient with prostatic hyperplasia for urine retention. Warm sitz baths and antispasmodic medication, such as flavoxate (Urispas), may be prescribed to relieve temporary urine retention caused by poor relaxation of the urinary sphincter; however, intermittent catheterization may be necessary for a few hours after the examination. The nurse monitors the patient for signs and symptoms of urinary tract infection. Because edema of the urethra secondary to local trauma may obstruct urine flow, the patient is also monitored for signs and symptoms of obstruction.

Biopsy

Renal and Ureteral Brush Biopsy

Brush biopsy techniques provide specific information when abnormal x-ray findings of the ureter or renal pelvis raise questions about whether a defect is a tumor, a stone, a blood clot, or an artifact. First, a cystoscopic examination is conducted. Then, a ureteral catheter is introduced, followed by a biopsy brush that is passed through the catheter. The suspected lesion is brushed back and forth to obtain cells and surface tissue fragments for histologic analysis.

After the procedure, IV fluids may be administered to help clear the kidneys and prevent clot formation. Urine may contain blood (usually clearing in 24 to 48 hours) from oozing at the brushing site. Postoperative renal colic occasionally occurs and responds to analgesic agents.

Kidney Biopsy

Biopsy of the kidney is used to help diagnose and evaluate the extent of kidney disease. Indications for biopsy include unexplained acute renal failure, persistent proteinuria or hematuria, transplant rejection, and glomerulopathies. A small section of renal cortex is obtained either percutaneously (needle biopsy) or by open biopsy through a small flank incision. Before the biopsy is carried out, coagulation studies are conducted to identify any risk of postbiopsy bleeding. Contraindications to kidney biopsy include bleed-

ing tendencies, uncontrolled hypertension, a solitary kidney, and morbid obesity (Morton, Fontaine, Hudak, et al., 2005).

Procedure

The patient may be prescribed a fasting regimen 6 to 8 hours before the test. An IV line is established. A urine specimen is obtained and saved for comparison with the postbiopsy specimen.

If a needle biopsy is to be performed, the patient is instructed to breathe in and hold that breath (to prevent the kidney from moving) while the needle is being inserted. The sedated patient is placed in a prone position with a sandbag under the abdomen. The skin at the biopsy site is infiltrated with a local anesthetic agent. The biopsy needle is introduced just inside the renal capsule of the outer quadrant of the kidney. The location of the needle may be confirmed by fluoroscopy or by ultrasound, in which case a special probe is used.

With open biopsy, a small incision is made over the kidney, allowing direct visualization. Preparation for an open biopsy is similar to that for any major abdominal surgery.

CRITICAL THINKING EXERCISES

EBP **1** Two days after major surgery your patient complains of lower abdominal pain. Describe the assessment techniques appropriate to evaluate the pain. Review the possible causes, describe the actions you would take and the rationale for each action, and identify the evidence base that supports the actions. What criteria would you use to evaluate the strength of the evidence?

2 A 46-year-old patient with a history of smoking is admitted to the hospital for evaluation of urinary dysfunction and is scheduled for a urinary system MRI. Explain why the MRI is indicated for this patient and what, if any, precautions must be taken because the patient is trying to stop smoking. What nursing observations and assessments are indicated because of the history of smoking? What patient teaching is appropriate before the MRI?

EBP **3** You make a home visit to an elderly female patient who is incontinent. Identify assessments and possible interventions you would use to evaluate and manage the incontinence. Identify the evidence for the assessments and nursing interventions you chose and the strength of that evidence.

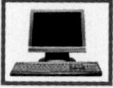

The Smeltzer suite offers these additional resources to enhance learning and facilitate understanding of this chapter:
- thePoint online resource, thepoint.lww.com/Smeltzer12E
- Student CD-ROM included with the book
- *Study Guide to Accompany Brunner & Suddarth's Textbook of Medical-Surgical Nursing*

REFERENCES AND SELECTED READINGS

*Asterisk indicates nursing research.

Books

Bickley, L. S. (2007). *Bates' guide to physical examination and history taking* (9th ed.). Philadelphia: Lippincott Williams & Wilkins.

Bulechek, G. M., Butcher, H. K. & Dochterman, J. M. (2008). *Nursing interventions classification (NIC)* (5th ed.). St. Louis: Mosby.

Goshorn, J. (2005). Acute renal failure. In M. L. Sole, D. G. Klein & M. J. Moseley (Eds.), *Introduction to critical care nursing*. St. Louis: Elsevier Saunders.

Karch, A. M. (2008). *Lippincott's nursing drug guide*. Philadelphia: Lippincott Williams & Wilkins.

Labus, D. M. (2008). *Portable diagnostic tests*. Philadelphia: Lippincott Williams & Wilkins.

Morton, P. G., Fontaine, D. K., Hudak, C. M., et al. (2005). *Critical care nursing: A holistic approach*. Philadelphia: Lippincott Williams & Wilkins.

Porth, C. M. & Matfin, G. (2009). *Pathophysiology: Concepts of altered health status* (8th ed.). Philadelphia: Lippincott Williams & Wilkins.

Stanley, M., Blair, K. A. & Beare, P. G. (2005). *Gerontological nursing: Promoting successful aging with older adults* (3rd ed.). Philadelphia: F. A. Davis.

Tanagho, E. & McAninch, J. (Eds.). (2007). *Smith's general urology* (17th ed.). New York: McGraw-Hill.

Tierney, L. M. & Henderson, M. C. (2005). *The patient history: Evidence-based approach*. New York: Lange Medical Books.

Weber, J. & Kelley, J. (2007). *Health assessment in nursing* (3rd ed.). Philadelphia: Lippincott Williams & Wilkins.

Journals and Electronic Documents

Burrows-Hudson, S. (2005). Chronic kidney disease: An overview: Early and aggressive treatment is vital. *American Journal of Nursing, 105*(2), 44–49.

Goertz, S. (2006). Gauging fluid balance with osmolality. *Nursing, 36*(10), 70–71.

Kohtz, C. & Thompson, M. (2007). Preventing contrast medium induced nephropathy. *American Journal of Nursing, 107*(9), 40–50.

Ostaszkiewicz, J. (2007). Incomplete bladder emptying in frail older adults: A clinical conundrum. *International Journal of Urologic Nursing, 1*(2), 87–91.

Palmer, M. H. & Newman, D. K. (2007) Urinary incontinence and estrogen: Is hormone replacement therapy an effective treatment? *American Journal of Nursing, 107*(3), 35–37.

Patraca, K. (2005). Measure bladder volume without catheterization. *Nursing, 35*(4), 46–47.

*Rassin, M., Dubches, L., Libshitz, A., et al. (2007). Levels of comfort and ease among patients suffering from urinary incontinence. *International Journal of Urologic Nursing, 1*(2), 64–70.

Sanchini, M. A., Gunelli, R., Nanni, O., et al. (2005). Relevance of urine telomerase in the diagnosis of bladder caner. *Journal of the American Medical Association, 294*(16), 2052–2056.

Stern, M. (2005). Aging with multiple sclerosis. *Physical Medicine and Rehabilitation Clinics of North America, 16*(1), 219–234.

Stevens, E. (2005). Bladder ultrasound: Avoiding unnecessary catheterizations. *MedSurg Nursing, 14*(4), 249–253.

RESOURCES

American Association of Kidney Patients, www.aakp.org

American Urological Association, www.auafoundation.org

National Kidney Foundation, www.kidney.org

National Institute of Diabetes and Digestive and Kidney Diseases, National Institutes of Health, www.niddk.nih.gov

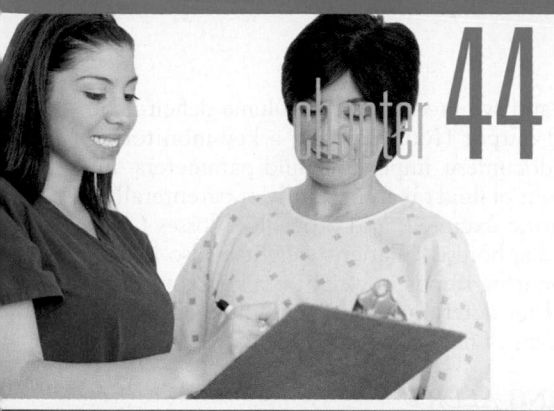

chapter 44

Management of Patients With Renal Disorders

LEARNING OBJECTIVES

On completion of this chapter, the learner will be able to:

1 Describe the key factors associated with the development of renal disorders.

2 Differentiate between the causes of chronic kidney disease and acute and chronic renal failure.

3 Compare and contrast the pathophysiology, clinical manifestations, medical management, and nursing management for patients with renal disorders.

4 Describe the nursing management of patients with acute and chronic renal failure.

5 Compare and contrast the renal replacement therapies including hemodialysis, peritoneal dialysis, and kidney transplantation.

6 Describe the nursing management of the hospitalized patient on dialysis.

7 Develop a postoperative plan of nursing care and teaching plan for the patient undergoing kidney surgery and transplantation.

GLOSSARY

acute nephritic syndrome: type of renal failure with glomerular inflammation

acute renal failure: sudden rapid deterioration of kidney function that is sometimes reversible

acute tubular necrosis: type of acute renal failure in which there is actual damage to the kidney tubules

anuria: total urine output less than 50 mL in 24 hours

arteriovenous fistula: type of vascular access for dialysis; created by surgically connecting an artery to a vein

arteriovenous graft: type of surgically created vascular access for dialysis by which a piece of biologic, semibiologic, or synthetic graft material connects the patient's artery to a vein

azotemia: abnormal concentration of nitrogenous wastes in the blood

chronic kidney disease: chronic progressive and irreversible diseases of the kidneys

continuous ambulatory peritoneal dialysis: method of peritoneal dialysis whereby a patient manually performs four or five complete exchanges or cycles throughout the day

GLOSSARY *(Continued)*

continuous cyclic peritoneal dialysis: method of peritoneal dialysis in which a peritoneal dialysis machine (cycler) automatically performs exchanges, usually while the patient sleeps

continuous renal replacement therapy: variety of methods used to replace normal kidney function by circulating the patient's blood through a filter and returning it to the patient

dialysate: solution that circulates through the dialyzer in hemodialysis and through the peritoneal membrane in peritoneal dialysis

dialyzer: "artificial kidney" or dialysis machine; contains a semipermeable membrane through which particles of a certain size can pass

diffusion: movement of solutes (waste products) from an area of higher concentration to an area of lower concentration

effluent: term used to describe the drained fluid from a peritoneal dialysis exchange

end-stage renal disease: final stage of renal failure that results in retention of uremic waste products and the need for renal replacement therapies

exchange (peritoneal dialysis): complete cycle of peritoneal dialysis includes fill, dwell, and drain phases

glomerulonephritis: inflammation of the glomerular capillaries

hemodialysis: procedure during which a patient's blood is circulated through a dialyzer to remove waste products and excess fluid

interstitial nephritis: inflammation within the renal tissue

nephrosclerosis: hardening of the renal arteries

nephrotic syndrome: type of renal failure with increased glomerular permeability and massive proteinuria

nephrotoxic: any substance, medication, or action that destroys kidney tissue

osmosis: movement of water through a semipermeable membrane from an area of lower solute concentration to an area of higher solute concentration

peritoneal dialysis: procedure that uses the lining of the patient's peritoneal cavity as the semipermeable membrane for exchange of fluid and solutes

peritonitis: inflammation of the peritoneal membrane (lining of the peritoneal cavity)

pyelonephritis: inflammation of the renal pelvis

ultrafiltration: process whereby water is removed from the blood by means of a pressure gradient between the patient's blood and the dialysate

uremia: an excess of urea and other nitrogenous wastes in the blood

urinary casts: proteins secreted by damaged kidney tubules

The renal system helps regulate the body's internal environment and is essential for the maintenance of life. Nurses working in any clinical setting may encounter patients with various renal disorders and thus need to be knowledgeable about these disorders. This chapter provides an overview of electrolyte imbalances that are common in patients with renal disorders. The main causes of kidney disease are discussed, together with management strategies to prevent damage and preserve renal function. Chronic kidney disease and acute and chronic renal failure are discussed, as is the care of patients with other renal conditions who require dialysis, transplantation, and kidney surgery.

FLUID AND ELECTROLYTE IMBALANCES IN RENAL DISORDERS

Patients with renal disorders commonly experience fluid and electrolyte imbalances and require careful assessment and close monitoring for signs of potential problems. The patient whose fluid intake exceeds the ability of the kidneys to excrete fluid is said to have fluid overload. If fluid intake is inadequate, the patient is said to be volume depleted and may show signs and symptoms of fluid volume deficit. The fluid intake and output (I&O) record, a key monitoring tool, is used to document important fluid parameters, including the amount of fluid taken in (orally or parenterally), the volume of urine excreted, and other fluid losses (diarrhea, vomiting, diaphoresis). Patient weight is also important, and documenting trends in weight is a key assessment strategy essential for determining the daily fluid allowance and indicating signs of fluid overload or deficit.

 NURSING ALERT

The most accurate indicator of fluid loss or gain in an acutely ill patient is weight. An accurate daily weight must be obtained and recorded. A 1-kg weight gain is equal to 1000 mL of retained fluid.

Clinical Manifestations

The signs and symptoms of common fluid and electrolyte disturbances that can occur in patients with renal disorders and their general management strategies are listed in Table 44-1. The nurse continually assesses, monitors, and informs appro-

Table 44-1	COMMON FLUID AND ELECTROLYTE DISTURBANCES IN RENAL DISORDERS	
Disturbance	**Manifestations**	**General Management Strategies**
Fluid volume deficit	Acute weight loss ≥5%, decreased skin turgor, dry mucous membranes, oliguria or anuria, increased hematocrit, blood urea nitrogen (BUN) level increased out of proportion to creatinine level, hypothermia	Fluid challenge, fluid replacement orally or parenterally
Fluid volume excess	Acute weight gain ≥5%, edema, crackles, shortness of breath, decreased BUN, decreased hematocrit, distended neck veins	Fluid and sodium restriction, diuretics, dialysis
Sodium deficit	Nausea, malaise, lethargy, headache, abdominal cramps, apprehension, seizures	Diet, normal saline or hypertonic saline solutions
Sodium excess	Dry, sticky mucous membranes, thirst, rough dry tongue, fever, restlessness, weakness, disorientation	Fluids, diuretics, dietary restriction
Potassium deficit	Anorexia, abdominal distention, paralytic ileus, muscle weakness, ECG changes, dysrhythmias	Diet, oral or parenteral potassium replacement therapy
Potassium excess	Diarrhea, colic, nausea, irritability, muscle weakness, ECG changes	Dietary restriction, diuretics, IV glucose, insulin and sodium bicarbonate, cation-exchange resin, calcium gluconate, dialysis
Calcium deficit	Abdominal and muscle cramps, stridor, carpopedal spasm, hyperactive reflexes, tetany, positive Chvostek's or Trousseau's sign, tingling of fingers and around mouth, ECG changes	Diet, oral or parenteral calcium salt replacement
Calcium excess	Deep bone pain, flank pain, muscle weakness, depressed deep tendon reflexes, constipation, nausea and vomiting, confusion, impaired memory, polyuria, polydipsia, ECG changes	Fluid replacement, etidronate, pamidronate, mithramycin, calcitonin, glucocorticoids, phosphate salts
Bicarbonate deficit	Headache, confusion, drowsiness, increased respiratory rate and depth, nausea and vomiting, warm flushed skin	Bicarbonate replacement, dialysis
Bicarbonate excess	Depressed respirations, muscle hypertonicity, dizziness, tingling of fingers and toes	Fluid replacement if volume depleted; ensure adequate chloride
Protein deficit	Chronic weight loss, emotional depression, pallor, fatigue, soft flabby muscles	Diet, dietary supplements, hyperalimentation, albumin
Magnesium deficit	Dysphagia, muscle cramps, hyperactive reflexes, tetany, positive Chvostek's or Trousseau's sign, tingling of fingers, dysrhythmias, vertigo	Diet, oral or parenteral magnesium replacement therapy
Magnesium excess	Facial flushing, nausea and vomiting, sensation of warmth, drowsiness, depressed deep tendon reflexes, muscle weakness, respiratory depression, cardiac arrest	Calcium gluconate, mechanical ventilation, dialysis
Phosphorus deficit	Deep bone pain, flank pain, muscle weakness and pain, paresthesia, apprehension, confusion, seizures	Diet, oral or parenteral phosphorus supplementation therapy
Phosphorus excess	Tetany, tingling of fingers and around mouth, muscle spasms, soft tissue calcification	Diet restriction, phosphate binders, normal saline solution, IV dextrose solution, and insulin

priate members of the health care team if the patient exhibits any of these signs. Management strategies for fluid and electrolyte disturbances in renal disease are discussed in greater depth later in this chapter (see also Chapter 14).

 Gerontologic Considerations

With aging, the kidney is less able to respond to acute fluid and electrolyte changes. Elderly patients may develop atypical and nonspecific signs and symptoms of disturbed renal function and fluid and electrolyte imbalances. A fluid balance deficit in the elderly can lead to constipation, falls, medication toxicity, urinary tract and respiratory tract infections, delirium, seizures, electrolyte imbalances, hyperthermia, and delayed wound healing (Mentes, 2006). Recognition of acute changes in fluid and electrolytes is further hampered by their association with preexisting disorders and the misconception that they are normal changes of aging.

RENAL DISORDERS

Chronic Kidney Disease

Chronic kidney disease (CKD) is an umbrella term that describes kidney damage or a decrease in the glomerular filtration rate (GFR) for 3 or more months (Thomas-Hawkins & Zazworsky, 2005). CKD is associated with decreased quality of life, increased health care expenditures, and premature death. Untreated CKD can result in **end-stage renal disease (ESRD)** and necessitate renal replacement therapy (dialysis or kidney transplantation). Risk factors include cardiovascular disease, diabetes, hypertension, and obesity. Recent research reported that 16.8% of the U.S. population aged 20 years and older have CKD (Centers for Disease Control and Prevention [CDC], 2007).

Diabetes is the primary cause of CKD. Between 25% and 40% of patients with type 1 diabetes and 5% to 40% of those with type 2 diabetes develop kidney damage (Thomas & Atkins, 2006). Diabetes is the leading cause of renal failure in patients starting renal replacement therapy. The second leading cause is hypertension, followed by glomerulonephritis and **pyelonephritis;** polycystic, hereditary, or congenital disorders; and renal cancers (U.S. Renal Data System [USRDS], 2007).

Pathophysiology

In the early stages of CKD there can be significant damage to the kidneys without signs or symptoms. The pathophysiology of CKD is not yet clearly understood, but the damage to the kidneys is thought to be caused by prolonged acute inflammation that is not organ specific and thus has subtle systemic manifestations.

Stages of Chronic Kidney Disease

CKD has been classified into five stages by the National Kidney Foundation (NKF) (Chart 44-1). Stage 5 results when the kidneys cannot remove the body's metabolic wastes or perform their regulatory functions and renal replacement therapies are required to sustain life. Screening

---

Chart 44-1• *Stages of Chronic Kidney Disease*

Stages are based on the glomerular filtration rate (GFR). The normal GFR is 125 mL/min/1.73 m^2.

Stage 1
GFR $\geq$ 90 mL/min/1.73 m^2
Kidney damage with normal or increased GFR

Stage 2
GFR = 60–89 mL/min/1.73 m^2
Mild decrease in GFR

Stage 3
GFR = 30–59 mL/min/1.73 m^2
Moderate decrease in GFR

Stage 4
GFR = 15–29 mL/min/1.73 m^2
Severe decrease in GFR

Stage 5
GFR < 15 mL/min/1.73 m^2
Kidney failure (end-stage renal disease [ESRD])

---

and early intervention are important, as not all patients progress to stage 5 CKD. Patients with CKD are at increased risk for cardiovascular disease, the leading cause of morbidity and mortality (Thomas & Atkins, 2006). Treatment of hypertension, anemia, and hyperglycemia and detection of proteinuria all help to slow disease progression and improve patient outcomes (Compton, 2007).

Clinical Manifestations

Elevated serum creatinine levels indicate underlying kidney disease; as the creatinine level increases, symptoms of chronic kidney disease begin. Anemia, due to decreased erythropoietin production by the kidney; metabolic acidosis; and abnormalities in calcium and phosphorus herald the development of CKD. Fluid retention, evidenced by both edema and congestive heart failure, develops. As the disease progresses, abnormalities in electrolytes occur, heart failure worsens, and hypertension becomes more difficult to control.

Assessment and Diagnostic Findings

The GFR is the amount of plasma filtered through the glomeruli per unit of time. Creatinine clearance is a measure of the amount of creatinine the kidneys are able to clear in a 24-hour period. Normal values differ in men and women. Calculation of GFR, an important assessment perimeter in CKD, is discussed in Chapter 43.

Medical Management

The management of patients with CKD includes treatment of the underlying causes. Regular clinical and laboratory assessment is important to keep the blood pressure (BP) below 130/80 mm Hg. Medical management also includes early referral for initiation of renal replacement therapies as indicated by the patient's renal status. Prevention of complications is accomplished by controlling cardiovascular risk factors; treating hyperglycemia; treating anemia; smoking cessation, weight loss, and exercise programs as needed; and reduction in salt and alcohol intake.

 Gerontologic Considerations

Changes in kidney function with normal aging increase the susceptibility of elderly patients to kidney dysfunction and renal failure (Miller, 2009). In addition, the incidence of systemic diseases, such as atherosclerosis, hypertension, heart failure, diabetes, and cancer, increases with advancing age, predisposing older adults to renal disease associated with these disorders. Therefore, acute problems need to be prevented if possible or recognized and treated quickly to avoid kidney damage. Thus, nurses in all settings need to be alert for signs and symptoms of renal dysfunction in elderly patients.

Elderly patients frequently take multiple prescription and over-the-counter medications. Because alterations in renal blood flow, glomerular filtration, and renal clearance increase the risk for medication-associated changes in renal function, precautions are indicated with all medications. When elderly patients undergo extensive diagnostic tests or when new medications (eg, diuretic agents) are added, precautions must be taken to prevent dehydration, which can compromise marginal renal function and lead to renal failure (Mentes, 2006).

Nephrosclerosis

Nephrosclerosis (hardening of the renal arteries) is most often due to prolonged hypertension and diabetes. Nephrosclerosis is a major cause of CKD and ESRD secondary to many disorders.

Pathophysiology

There are two forms of nephrosclerosis: malignant (accelerated) and benign. Malignant nephrosclerosis is often associated with significant hypertension (diastolic blood pressure higher than 130 mm Hg). It usually occurs in young adults and twice as often in men compared to women. Damage is caused by decreased blood flow to the kidney resulting in patchy necrosis of the renal parenchyma. Over time, fibrosis occurs and glomeruli are destroyed.

The disease process progresses rapidly. Without dialysis, more than half of patients die from **uremia** (an excess of urea and other nitrogenous wastes in the blood) in a few years. Benign nephrosclerosis can be found in older adults, associated with atherosclerosis and hypertension.

Assessment and Diagnostic Findings

Symptoms are rare early in the disease, even though the urine usually contains protein and occasional casts. Renal insufficiency and associated signs and symptoms occur late in the disease.

Medical Management

Treatment of nephrosclerosis is aggressive antihypertensive therapy. An angiotensin-converting enzyme (ACE) inhibitor, alone or in combination with other antihyperten-

sive medications, significantly reduces its incidence (Munar & Singh, 2007). See Chapter 32 for additional information on hypertension.

Primary Glomerular Diseases

Diseases that destroy the glomerulus of the kidney are the third most common cause of stage 5 CKD. In these disorders, the glomerular capillaries are primarily involved. Antigen–antibody complexes form in the blood and become trapped in the glomerular capillaries (the filtering portion of the kidney), inducing an inflammatory response. Immunoglobulin G (IgG), the major immunoglobulin (antibody) found in the blood, can be detected in the glomerular capillary walls. The major clinical manifestations of glomerular injury include proteinuria, hematuria, decreased GFR, decreased excretion of sodium, edema, and hypertension (Chart 44-2).

ACUTE NEPHRITIC SYNDROME

The **acute nephritic syndrome** is the clinical manifestation of glomerular inflammation (Porth & Matfin, 2009). **Glomerulonephritis** is an inflammation of the glomerular capillaries that can occur in acute and chronic forms.

Pathophysiology

Primary glomerular diseases include postinfectious glomerulonephritis, rapidly progressive glomerulonephritis, membrane proliferative glomerulonephritis, and membranous glomerulonephritis. Postinfectious causes are group A beta-hemolytic streptococcal infection of the throat that precedes the onset of glomerulonephritis by 2 to 3 weeks (Fig. 44-1). It may also follow impetigo (infection of the skin) and acute viral infections (upper respiratory tract infections, mumps, varicella zoster virus, Epstein-Barr virus, hepatitis B, and human immunodeficiency virus [HIV] infection). In some patients, antigens outside the body (eg, medications, foreign serum) initiate the process, resulting in antigen–antibody complexes being deposited in the glomeruli. In other patients, the kidney tissue itself serves as the inciting antigen.

Chart 44-2 • *Terms Typically Used When Describing Glomerular Disease*

Primary: Disease is mainly in glomeruli
Secondary: Glomerular diseases that are the consequence of systemic disease
Idiopathic: Cause is unknown
Acute: Occurs over days or weeks
Chronic: Occurs over months or years
Rapidly progressing: Constant loss of renal function with minimal chance of recovery
Diffuse: Involves all glomeruli
Focal: Involves some glomeruli
Segmental: Involves portions of individual glomeruli
Membranous: Evidence of thickened glomerular capillary walls
Proliferative: Number of glomerular cells involved is increasing

Physiology ■■■ Pathophysiology

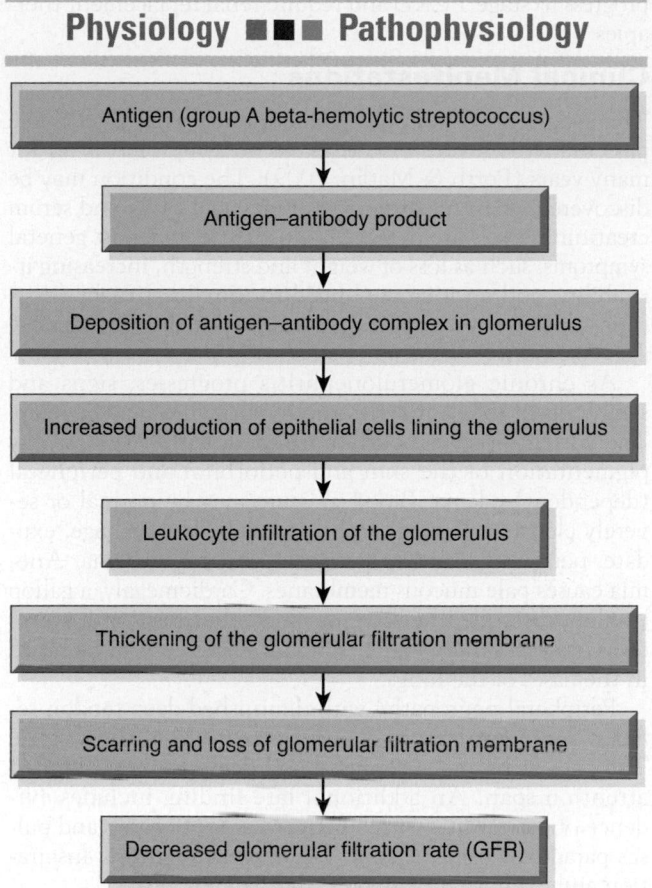

Antigen (group A beta-hemolytic streptococcus)

↓

Antigen–antibody product

↓

Deposition of antigen–antibody complex in glomerulus

↓

Increased production of epithelial cells lining the glomerulus

↓

Leukocyte infiltration of the glomerulus

↓

Thickening of the glomerular filtration membrane

↓

Scarring and loss of glomerular filtration membrane

↓

Decreased glomerular filtration rate (GFR)

Figure 44-1 Sequence of events in acute nephritic syndrome.

Clinical Manifestations

The primary presenting features of an acute glomerular inflammation are hematuria, edema, **azotemia**, an abnormal concentration of nitrogenous wastes in the blood, and proteinuria or excess protein in the urine (Porth & Matfin, 2009). The hematuria may be microscopic (identifiable only through microscopic examination) or macroscopic (visible to the eye). The urine may appear cola-colored because of red blood cells (RBCs) and protein plugs or casts; RBC casts indicate glomerular injury. Glomerulonephritis may be mild and the hematuria discovered incidentally through a routine urinalysis, or the disease may be severe, with acute renal failure (ARF) and oliguria.

Some degree of edema and hypertension is present in most patients. Marked proteinuria due to the increased permeability of the glomerular membrane may also occur, with associated pitting edema, hypoalbuminemia, hyperlipidemia, and fatty casts in the urine. Blood urea nitrogen (BUN) and serum creatinine levels may increase as urine output decreases. In addition, anemia may be present.

In the more severe form of the disease, patients also complain of headache, malaise, and flank pain. Elderly patients may experience circulatory overload with dyspnea, engorged neck veins, cardiomegaly, and pulmonary edema. Atypical symptoms include confusion, somnolence, and seizures, which are often confused with the symptoms of a primary neurologic disorder.

Assessment and Diagnostic Findings

In acute nephritic syndrome, the kidneys become large, edematous, and congested. All renal tissues including the glomeruli, tubules, and blood vessels are affected to varying degrees. Patients with an IgA nephropathy have an elevated serum IgA and low to normal complement levels. Electron microscopy and immunofluorescent analysis help identify the nature of the lesion; however, a kidney biopsy may be needed for definitive diagnosis. (See Chapter 43 for discussion of kidney biopsy.)

If the patient improves, the amount of urine increases and the urinary protein and sediment diminish. The percentage of adults who recover is unknown. Some patients develop severe uremia (an excess of urea and other nitrogenous wastes in the blood) within weeks and require dialysis for survival. Others, after a period of apparent recovery, insidiously develop chronic glomerulonephritis.

Complications

Complications of acute glomerulonephritis include hypertensive encephalopathy, heart failure, and pulmonary edema. Hypertensive encephalopathy is a medical emergency, and therapy is directed toward reducing the blood pressure without impairing renal function. This can occur in acute nephritic syndrome or preeclampsia with chronic hypertension of greater than 140/90 mm Hg. Rapidly progressive glomerulonephritis is characterized by a rapid decline in renal function. Without treatment, ESRD develops in a matter of weeks or months. Signs and symptoms are similar to those of acute glomerulonephritis (hematuria and proteinuria), but the course of the disease is more severe and rapid. Crescent-shaped cells accumulate in Bowman's space, disrupting the filtering surface. Plasma exchange (plasmapheresis) and treatment with high-dose corticosteroids and cytotoxic agents have been used to reduce the inflammatory response. Dialysis is initiated in acute glomerulonephritis if signs and symptoms of uremia are severe. The prognosis for patients with acute nephritic syndrome is excellent and rarely causes CKD (Porth & Matfin, 2009).

Medical Management

Management consists primarily of treating symptoms, attempting to preserve kidney function, and treating complications promptly. Treatment may include corticosteroids, managing hypertension, and controlling proteinuria (Glick, 2007). Pharmacologic therapy depends on the cause of acute glomerulonephritis. If residual streptococcal infection is suspected, penicillin is the agent of choice; however, other antibiotic agents may be prescribed. Dietary protein is restricted when renal insufficiency and nitrogen retention (elevated BUN) develop. Sodium is restricted when the patient has hypertension, edema, and heart failure.

Nursing Management

Although most patients with acute uncomplicated glomerulonephritis are cared for as outpatients, nursing care is important in every setting.

Providing Care in the Hospital

In a hospital setting, carbohydrates are given liberally to provide energy and reduce the catabolism of protein. I&O are carefully measured and recorded. Fluids are given based on the patient's fluid losses and daily body weight. Insensible fluid loss through the lungs (300 mL) and skin (600 mL) is considered when estimating fluid loss (see Chapter 14). If treatment is effective, diuresis will begin, resulting in decreased edema and blood pressure. Proteinuria and microscopic hematuria may persist for many months; in fact, 20% of patients have some degree of persistent proteinuria or decreased GFR 1 year after presentation (Porth & Matfin, 2009). Other nursing interventions focus on patient education about the disease process, explanations of laboratory and other diagnostic tests, and preparation for safe and effective self-care at home (Hughes, 2008).

Promoting Home and Community-Based Care

Teaching Patients Self-Care

Patient education is directed toward symptom management and monitoring for complications. Fluid and diet restrictions must be reviewed with the patient to avoid worsening of edema and hypertension. The patient is instructed verbally and in writing to notify the physician if symptoms of renal failure occur (eg, fatigue, nausea, vomiting, diminishing urine output) or at the first sign of any infection.

Continuing Care

The importance of follow-up evaluations of blood pressure, urinalysis for protein, and BUN and serum creatinine levels to determine if the disease has progressed is stressed to the patient. A referral for home care may be indicated; a visit from a home care nurse provides an opportunity for careful assessment of the patient's progress and detection of early signs and symptoms of renal insufficiency. If corticosteroids, immunosuppressant agents, or antibiotic medications are prescribed, the home care nurse or nurse in the outpatient setting uses the opportunity to review the dosage, desired actions, and adverse effects of medications and the precautions to be taken.

CHRONIC GLOMERULONEPHRITIS

Chronic glomerulonephritis may be due to repeated episodes of acute nephritic syndrome, hypertensive nephrosclerosis, hyperlipidemia, chronic tubulointerstitial injury, or hemodynamically mediated glomerular sclerosis. Secondary glomerular diseases that can have systemic effects include lupus erythematosus, Goodpasture's syndrome (caused by antibodies to the glomerular basement membrane), diabetic glomerulosclerosis, and amyloidosis.

Pathophysiology

The kidneys are reduced to as little as one-fifth their normal size (consisting largely of fibrous tissue). The cortex layer shrinks to 1 to 2 mm in thickness or less. Bands of scar tissue distort the remaining cortex, making the surface of the kidney rough and irregular. Numerous glomeruli and their tubules become scarred, and the branches of the renal artery are thickened. The resulting severe glomerular damage can

progress to stage 5 CKD and require renal replacement therapies.

Clinical Manifestations

The symptoms of chronic glomerulonephritis vary. Some patients with severe disease have no symptoms at all for many years (Porth & Matfin, 2009). The condition may be discovered when hypertension or elevated BUN and serum creatinine levels are detected. Most patients report general symptoms, such as loss of weight and strength, increasing irritability, and an increased need to urinate at night (nocturia). Headaches, dizziness, and digestive disturbances are also common.

As chronic glomerulonephritis progresses, signs and symptoms of CKD and chronic renal failure may develop. The patient appears poorly nourished, with a yellow-gray pigmentation of the skin and periorbital and peripheral (dependent) edema. Blood pressure may be normal or severely elevated. Retinal findings include hemorrhage, exudate, narrowed tortuous arterioles, and papilledema. Anemia causes pale mucous membranes. Cardiomegaly, a gallop rhythm, distended neck veins, and other signs and symptoms of heart failure may be present. Crackles can be heard in the bases of the lungs.

Peripheral neuropathy with diminished deep tendon reflexes and neurosensory changes occur late in the disease. The patient becomes confused and demonstrates a limited attention span. An additional late finding includes evidence of pericarditis with a pericardial friction rub and pulsus paradoxus (difference in blood pressure during inspiration and expiration of greater than 10 mm Hg).

Assessment and Diagnostic Findings

A number of laboratory abnormalities occur. Urinalysis reveals a fixed specific gravity of about 1.010, variable proteinuria, and **urinary casts** (proteins secreted by damaged kidney tubules). As renal failure progresses and the GFR falls below 50 mL/min, the following changes occur:

- Hyperkalemia due to decreased potassium excretion, acidosis, catabolism, and excessive potassium intake from food and medications
- Metabolic acidosis from decreased acid secretion by the kidney and inability to regenerate bicarbonate
- Anemia secondary to decreased erythropoiesis (production of RBCs)
- Hypoalbuminemia with edema secondary to protein loss through the damaged glomerular membrane
- Increased serum phosphorus level due to decreased renal excretion of phosphorus
- Decreased serum calcium level (calcium binds to phosphorus to compensate for elevated serum phosphorus levels)
- Mental status changes
- Impaired nerve conduction due to electrolyte abnormalities and uremia

Chest x-rays may show cardiac enlargement and pulmonary edema. The electrocardiogram (ECG) may be normal or may indicate left ventricular hypertrophy associated with hypertension and signs of electrolyte disturbances, such as tall, tented (or peaked) T waves associated with hyperkalemia. Computed tomography (CT) and magnetic resonance imaging (MRI) scans show a decrease in the size of the renal cortex.

Medical Management

Management of symptoms guides the treatment. If the patient has hypertension, efforts are made to reduce the blood pressure with sodium and water restriction, antihypertensive agents, or both. Weight is monitored daily, and diuretic medications are prescribed to treat fluid overload. Proteins of high biologic value (dairy products, eggs, meats) are provided to promote good nutritional status. Adequate calories are provided to spare protein for tissue growth and repair. Urinary tract infections (UTIs) must be treated promptly to prevent further renal damage.

Dialysis is initiated early in the course of the disease to keep the patient in optimal physical condition, prevent fluid and electrolyte imbalances, and minimize the risk of complications of renal failure. The course of dialysis is smoother if treatment begins before the patient develops complications.

Nursing Management

Whether the patient is hospitalized or cared for in the home, the nurse observes the patient for common fluid and electrolyte disturbances in renal disease (see Table 44-1). Changes in fluid and electrolyte status and in cardiac and neurologic status are reported promptly to the physician. Anxiety levels are often extremely high for both the patient and family. Throughout the course of the disease and treatment, the nurse gives emotional support by providing opportunities for the patient and family to verbalize their concerns, have their questions answered, and explore their options.

Promoting Home and Community-Based Care

Teaching Patients Self-Care

The nurse has a major role in teaching the patient and family about the prescribed treatment plan and the risks associated with noncompliance. Instructions to the patient include explanations and scheduling for follow-up evaluations: blood pressure, urinalysis for protein and casts, and laboratory studies of BUN and serum creatinine levels. If long-term dialysis is needed, the nurse teaches the patient and family about the procedure, how to care for the access site, dietary restrictions, and other necessary lifestyle modifications. These topics are discussed later in this chapter.

Periodic hospitalization, visits to the outpatient clinic or office, and home care referrals provide the nurse in each setting with the opportunity for careful assessment of the patient's progress and continued education about changes to report to the primary health care provider (worsening signs and symptoms of renal failure, such as nausea, vomiting, and diminished urine output). Specific teaching may include explanations about recommended diet and fluid modifications and medications (purpose, desired effects, adverse effects, dosage, and administration schedule).

Continuing Care

Periodic laboratory evaluations of creatinine clearance and BUN and serum creatinine levels are carried out to assess residual renal function and the need for dialysis or trans-

plantation. If dialysis is initiated, the patient and family require considerable assistance and support in dealing with therapy and its long-term implications. The patient and family are reminded of the importance of participation in health promotion activities, including health screening. The patient is instructed to inform all health care providers about the diagnosis of glomerulonephritis so that all medical management, including pharmacologic therapy, is based on altered renal function.

NEPHROTIC SYNDROME

Nephrotic syndrome is a type of renal failure characterized by increased glomerular permeability and is manifested by massive proteinuria (Porth & Matfin, 2009). Clinical findings include a marked increase in protein (particularly albumin) in the urine (proteinuria), a decrease in albumin in the blood (hypoalbuminemia), diffuse edema, high serum cholesterol, and low-density lipoproteins (hyperlipidemia).

The syndrome is apparent in any condition that seriously damages the glomerular capillary membrane and results in increased glomerular permeability to plasma proteins. Although the liver is capable of increasing the production of albumin, it cannot keep up with the daily loss of albumin through the kidneys. Thus, hypoalbuminemia results (Fig. 44-2).

Pathophysiology

Nephrotic syndrome occurs with many intrinsic renal diseases and systemic diseases that cause glomerular damage. It is not a specific glomerular disease but a constellation of clinical findings that result from the glomerular damage (Porth & Matfin, 2009).

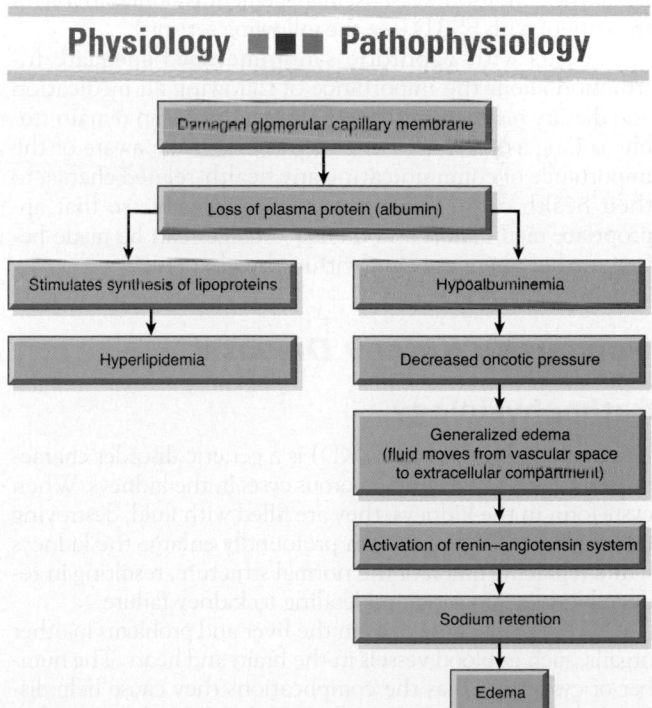

Figure 44-2 Sequence of events in nephrotic syndrome.

Clinical Manifestations

The major manifestation of nephrotic syndrome is edema. It is usually soft and pitting and commonly occurs around the eyes (periorbital), in dependent areas (sacrum, ankles, and hands), and in the abdomen (ascites). Patients may also exhibit irritability, headache, and malaise.

Assessment and Diagnostic Findings

Proteinuria (predominately albumin) exceeding 3.5 g/day is the hallmark of the diagnosis of nephrotic syndrome (Porth & Matfin, 2009). Protein electrophoresis and immunoelectrophoresis may be performed on the urine to categorize the type of proteinuria. The urine may also contain increased white blood cells (WBCs) as well as granular and epithelial casts. A needle biopsy of the kidney may be performed for histologic examination of renal tissue to confirm the diagnosis.

Complications

Complications of nephrotic syndrome include infection (due to a deficient immune response), thromboembolism (especially of the renal vein), pulmonary emboli, ARF (due to hypovolemia), and accelerated atherosclerosis (due to hyperlipidemia).

Medical Management

Treatment is focused on treating the underlying disease state causing proteinuria, slowing progression of CKD, and relieving symptoms. Typical treatment includes diuretics for edema, ACE inhibitors to reduce proteinuria, and lipid-lowering agents for hyperlipidemia.

Nursing Management

In the early stages of nephrotic syndrome, nursing management is similar to that of the patient with acute glomerulonephritis, but as the condition worsens, management is similar to that of the patient with ESRD (see the following section).

Patients with nephrotic syndrome need adequate instruction about the importance of following all medication and dietary regimens so that their condition can remain stable as long as possible. Patients must be made aware of the importance of communicating any health-related change to their health care providers as soon as possible so that appropriate medication and dietary changes can be made before further changes occur within the glomeruli.

Polycystic Kidney Disease

Pathophysiology

Polycystic kidney disease (PKD) is a genetic disorder characterized by the growth of numerous cysts in the kidneys. When cysts form in the kidneys, they are filled with fluid, destroying the nephrons. PKD cysts can profoundly enlarge the kidneys while replacing much of the normal structure, resulting in reduced kidney function and leading to kidney failure.

PKD can also cause cysts in the liver and problems in other organs, such as blood vessels in the brain and heart. The number of cysts as well as the complications they cause help distinguish PKD from the usually harmless "simple" cysts that can form in the kidneys in later years of life. In the United

States, PKD and cystic diseases are the fifth leading cause of kidney failure. Two major inherited forms of PKD exist:

*   *Autosomal dominant PKD* is the most common inherited form. Symptoms usually develop between the ages of 30 and 40, but they can begin earlier, even in childhood. About 90% of all PKD cases are autosomal dominant PKD.
*   *Autosomal recessive PKD* is a rare inherited form. Symptoms of autosomal recessive PKD begin in the earliest months of life or in utero.

When autosomal dominant PKD causes kidneys to fail, which usually happens after many years, the patient requires dialysis or kidney transplantation. About one half of people with the most common type of PKD progress to CKD stage 5, requiring renal replacement.

Clinical Manifestations

Signs and symptoms of PKD result from loss of renal function and the increasing size of the kidneys as the cysts grow. Renal damage can result in hematuria, polyuria (large amounts of urine), hypertension, development of renal calculi and associated urinary tract infections, and proteinuria. The growing cysts are noted with reports of abdominal fullness and flank pain (back and lower sides).

Assessment and Diagnostic Findings

Since PKD is a genetic disease, careful evaluation of family history is necessary. Palpation of the abdomen will often reveal enlarged cystic kidneys. Diagnosis is usually made with ultrasound imaging of the kidney (Porth & Matfin, 2009).

Medical Management

PKD has no cure and treatment is largely supportive including blood pressure control, pain control, and antibiotics to resolve infections. Once the kidneys fail, renal replacement therapy is indicated. Genetic testing and counseling may be indicated.

RENAL CANCER

Renal cancer accounts for about 3% of all cancers in adult men and 2% in adult woman in the United States (American Cancer Society, 2009). In the United States, the incidence of renal cancer at all stages has increased in the past two decades. The incidence of renal cell carcinoma is higher in both men and women with an increased body mass index. Tobacco use continues to be a significant risk factor for renal carcinoma (Chart 44-3).

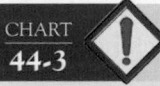

| CHART 44-3 | ⚠ | *Risk Factors for Renal Cancer* |

*   Gender: Affects men more than women
*   Tobacco use
*   Occupational exposure to industrial chemicals, such as petroleum products, heavy metals, and asbestos
*   Obesity
*   Unopposed estrogen therapy
*   Polycystic kidney disease

The most common type of renal carcinoma arises from the renal epithelium and accounts for more than 85% of all kidney tumors. These tumors may metastasize early to the lungs, bone, liver, brain, and contralateral kidney. One quarter of patients have metastatic disease at the time of diagnosis. Although enhanced imaging techniques account for improved detection of early-stage kidney cancer, it is unknown why the rate of late-stage kidney cancers is high (Cohen & McGovern, 2005).

Clinical Manifestations

Many renal tumors produce no symptoms and are discovered on a routine physical examination as a palpable abdominal mass. The classic signs and symptoms, which occur in only 10% of patients, include hematuria, pain, and a mass in the flank (Cohen & McGovern, 2005). The usual sign that first calls attention to the tumor is painless hematuria, which may be either intermittent and microscopic or continuous and gross. There may be a dull pain in the back from the pressure produced by compression of the ureter, extension of the tumor into the perirenal area, or hemorrhage into the kidney tissue. Colicky pains occur if a clot or mass of tumor cells passes down the ureter. Symptoms from metastasis may be the first manifestations of renal tumor and may include unexplained weight loss, increasing weakness, and anemia.

Assessment and Diagnostic Findings

The diagnosis of a renal tumor may require intravenous (IV) urography, cystoscopic examination, nephrotomograms, renal angiograms, ultrasonography, or a CT scan. These tests may be exhausting for patients already debilitated by the systemic effects of a tumor as well as for elderly patients and those who are anxious about the diagnosis and outcome. The nurse assists the patient to prepare physically and psychologically for these procedures and monitors carefully for signs and symptoms of dehydration and exhaustion.

Medical Management

The goal of management is to eradicate the tumor before metastasis occurs.

Surgical Management

Nephrectomy

A radical nephrectomy is the preferred treatment if the tumor can be removed. This includes removal of the kidney (and tumor), adrenal gland, surrounding perinephric fat and Gerota's fascia, and lymph nodes. Laparoscopic nephrectomy can be performed for removal of the kidney with a small tumor. This procedure incurs less morbidity and a shorter recovery time. Radiation therapy, hormonal therapy, or chemotherapy may be used along with surgery. Immunotherapy may also be helpful. For patients with bilateral tumors or cancer of a functional single kidney, nephron-sparing surgery (partial nephrectomy) may be considered. Favorable results have been achieved in patients with small local tumors and a normal contralateral kidney (Cohen & McGovern, 2005).

Nephron-sparing surgery is increasingly being used to treat patients with solid renal lesions. The technical success

rate of nephron-sparing surgery is excellent, and operative morbidity and mortality are low.

Patients with upper tract transitional cell carcinoma may benefit from laparoscopic nephroureterectomy. Although it is a lengthier surgical procedure, it has the same efficacy and is better tolerated by patients than open nephroureterectomy.

Renal Artery Embolization

In patients with metastatic renal carcinoma, the renal artery may be occluded to impede the blood supply to the tumor and thus kill the tumor cells. After angiographic studies are completed, a catheter is advanced into the renal artery, and embolizing materials (eg, Gelfoam, autologous blood clot, steel coils) are injected into the artery and carried with the arterial blood flow to occlude the tumor vessels mechanically. This decreases the local blood supply, making removal of the kidney (nephrectomy) easier. It also stimulates an immune response because infarction of the renal cell carcinoma releases tumor-associated antigens that enhance the patient's response to metastatic lesions. The procedure may also reduce the number of tumor cells entering the venous circulation during surgical manipulation.

After renal artery embolization and tumor infarction, a characteristic symptom complex called postinfarction syndrome occurs, lasting 2 to 3 days. The patient has pain localized to the flank and abdomen, elevated temperature, and gastrointestinal (GI) symptoms. Pain is treated with parenteral analgesic agents, and acetaminophen (Tylenol) is administered to control fever. Antiemetic medications, restriction of oral intake, and IV fluids are used to treat the GI symptoms.

Pharmacologic Therapy

Currently, no pharmacologic agents are in widespread use for treatment of renal cell carcinoma, which is refractory to most chemotherapeutic agents. However, depending on the stage of the tumor, percutaneous partial or radical nephrectomy may be followed by treatment with chemotherapeutic agents. Radiation therapy may be used for palliation in patients who are not candidates for surgery.

Treatment with biologic response modifiers such as interleukin-2 (IL-2) is effective. IL-2, a protein that regulates cell growth, is used alone or in combination with lymphokine-activated killer cells (WBCs that have been stimulated by IL-2 to increase their ability to kill cancer cells). Interferon, another biologic response modifier, appears to have a direct antiproliferative effect on renal tumors. Temsirolimus (Torisel) is administered by IV infusion on a weekly basis to treat advanced renal cell carcinoma (Aschenbrenner, 2007).

Another promising experimental approach to renal cell carcinoma is a vaccination to stimulate immune response, with autologous tumor cells with IL-2–, granulocyte-macrophage stimulating factor–, and dendritic cell–type vaccines. If patients with renal cancer do not respond to immunotherapy, allogeneic stem cell transplantation may be indicated (Cohen & McGovern, 2005).

Nursing Management

The patient with a renal tumor usually undergoes extensive diagnostic and therapeutic procedures. Treatment includes surgery, radiation therapy, and medications. After surgery, the patient usually has catheters and drains in place to maintain a patent urinary tract, to remove drainage, and to permit accurate measurement of urine output. Because of the location of the surgical incision, the patient's position during surgery, and the nature of the surgical procedure, pain and muscle soreness are common. Pharmacologic management often includes immunosuppressant agents; therefore, patients are monitored for infection (Aschenbrenner, 2007).

The patient requires frequent analgesia during the postoperative period and assistance with turning, coughing, use of incentive spirometry, and deep breathing to prevent atelectasis and other pulmonary complications. The patient and family require assistance and support to cope with the diagnosis and uncertain prognosis. (See this chapter for discussion of postoperative care of the patient undergoing kidney surgery and Chapter 16 for discussion of care of the patient with cancer.)

Promoting Home and Community-Based Care

Teaching Patients Self-Care

The nurse teaches the patient to inspect and care for the incision and perform other general postoperative care including activity and lifting restrictions, driving, and pain management. Instructions are provided about when to notify the physician about problems (eg, fever, breathing difficulty, wound drainage, blood in the urine, pain or swelling of the legs).

The nurse encourages the patient to eat a healthy diet and to drink adequate liquids to avoid constipation and to maintain an adequate urine volume. Education and emotional support are provided related to the diagnosis, treatment, and continuing care because many patients are concerned about the loss of the other kidney, the possible need for dialysis, or the recurrence of cancer.

Continuing Care

Follow-up care is essential to detect signs of metastases and to reassure the patient and family about the patient's status and well-being. The patient who has had surgery for renal carcinoma should have a yearly physical examination and chest x-ray, because late metastases are not uncommon. All subsequent symptoms should be evaluated with possible metastases in mind.

If follow-up chemotherapy is necessary, the patient and family are informed about the treatment plan or chemotherapy protocol, what to expect with each visit, and when to notify the physician. Evaluation of remaining renal function (creatinine clearance, BUN and serum creatinine levels) may also be carried out periodically. A home care nurse may monitor the patient's physical status and psychological well-being and coordinate other indicated services and resources.

RENAL FAILURE

Renal failure results when the kidneys cannot remove the body's metabolic wastes or perform their regulatory functions. The substances normally eliminated in the urine ac-

cumulate in the body fluids as a result of impaired renal excretion, affecting endocrine and metabolic functions as well as fluid, electrolyte, and acid–base disturbances. Renal failure is a systemic disease and is a final common pathway of many different kidney and urinary tract diseases. Each year, the number of deaths from irreversible renal failure increases (USRDS, 2007).

Acute Renal Failure

Acute renal failure (ARF) is a rapid loss of renal function due to damage to the kidneys. Depending on the duration and severity of ARF, a wide range of potentially life-threatening metabolic complications can occur, including metabolic acidosis as well as fluid and electrolyte imbalances. Treatment is aimed at replacing renal function temporarily to minimize potentially lethal complications and reduce potential causes of increased renal injury with the goal of minimizing long-term loss of renal function. ARF is a problem seen in hospitalized patients and those in outpatient settings. A widely accepted criterion for ARF is a 50% or greater increase in serum creatinine above baseline (normal creatinine is less than 1.0 mg/dL) (Best & Counselman, 2008). Urine volume may be normal, or changes may occur. Possible changes include oliguria (less than 500 mL/day), nonoliguria (greater than 800 mL/day), or **anuria** (less than 50 mL/day) (Counts, 2008).

Pathophysiology

Although the pathogenesis of ARF and oliguria is not always known, many times there is a specific underlying problem. Some of the factors may be reversible if identified and treated promptly, before kidney function is impaired. This is true of the following conditions that reduce blood flow to the kidney and impair kidney function: (1) hypovolemia; (2) hypotension; (3) reduced cardiac output and heart failure; (4) obstruction of the kidney or lower urinary tract by tumor, blood clot, or kidney stone; and (5) bilateral obstruction of the renal arteries or veins. If these conditions are treated and corrected before the kidneys are permanently damaged, the increased BUN and creatinine levels, oliguria, and other signs may be reversed.

Although renal stones are not a common cause of ARF, some types may increase the risk for ARF. Some hereditary stone diseases (see Chapter 45), primary struvite stones, and infection-related urolithiasis associated with anatomic and functional urinary tract anomalies and spinal cord injury may cause recurrent bouts of obstruction as well as crystal-specific damage to tubular epithelial cells and interstitial renal cells.

Categories of Acute Renal Failure

The major categories of ARF are prerenal (hypoperfusion of kidney), intrarenal (actual damage to kidney tissue), and postrenal (obstruction to urine flow). Prerenal ARF, which occurs in 60% to 70% of cases, is the result of impaired blood flow that leads to hypoperfusion of the kidney and a decrease in the GFR. Intrarenal ARF is the result of actual parenchymal damage to the glomeruli or kidney tubules. **Acute tubular necrosis (ATN)** is the most common type of intrinsic ARF. Characteristics of ATN are intratubular obstruction, tubular back leak (abnormal reabsorption of filtrate and decreased urine flow through the tubule), vasoconstriction, and changes in glomerular permeability. These processes result in a decrease of GFR, progressive azotemia, and fluid and electrolyte imbalances. CKD, diabetes, heart failure, hypertension, and cirrhosis can lead to ATN (Bednarski, Castner & Douglas, 2008). Postrenal ARF usually results from obstruction distal to the kidney. Pressure rises in the kidney tubules and eventually, the GFR decreases. Common causes of each type of ARF are summarized in Chart 44-4.

Chart 44-4 • *Causes of Acute Renal Failure*

Prerenal Failure

- Volume depletion resulting from:
  Hemorrhage
  Renal losses (diuretics, osmotic diuresis)
  Gastrointestinal losses (vomiting, diarrhea, nasogastric suction)
- Impaired cardiac efficiency resulting from:
  Myocardial infarction
  Heart failure
  Dysrhythmias
  Cardiogenic shock
- Vasodilation resulting from:
  Sepsis
  Anaphylaxis
  Antihypertensive medications or other medications that cause vasodilation

Intrarenal Failure

- Prolonged renal ischemia resulting from:
  Pigment nephropathy (associated with the breakdown of blood cells containing pigments that in turn occlude kidney structures)
  Myoglobinuria (trauma, crush injuries, burns)
  Hemoglobinuria (transfusion reaction, hemolytic anemia)
- Nephrotoxic agents such as:
  Aminoglycoside antibiotics (gentamicin, tobramycin)
  Radiopaque contrast agents
  Heavy metals (lead, mercury)
  Solvents and chemicals (ethylene glycol, carbon tetrachloride, arsenic)
  Nonsteroidal anti-inflammatory drugs (NSAIDs)
  Angiotensin-converting enzyme inhibitors (ACE inhibitors)
- Infectious processes such as:
  Acute pyelonephritis
  Acute glomerulonephritis

Postrenal Failure

- Urinary tract obstruction, including:
  Calculi (stones)
  Tumors
  Benign prostatic hyperplasia
  Strictures
  Blood clots

Phases of Acute Renal Failure

There are four phases of ARF: initiation, oliguria, diuresis, and recovery.

- The initiation period begins with the initial insult and ends when oliguria develops.
- The oliguria period is accompanied by an increase in the serum concentration of substances usually excreted by the kidneys (urea, creatinine, uric acid, organic acids, and the intracellular cations [potassium and magnesium]). The minimum amount of urine needed to rid the body of normal metabolic waste products is 400 mL. In this phase uremic symptoms first appear and life-threatening conditions such as hyperkalemia develop.

Some patients have decreased renal function with increasing nitrogen retention, yet actually excrete normal amounts of urine (2 L/day or more). This is the nonoliguric form of renal failure and occurs predominantly after exposure of the patient to nephrotoxic agents, burns, traumatic injury, and the use of halogenated anesthetic agents.

- The diuresis period is marked by a gradual increase in urine output, which signals that glomerular filtration has started to recover. Laboratory values stabilize and eventually decrease. Although the volume of urinary output may reach normal or elevated levels, renal function may still be markedly abnormal. Because uremic symptoms may still be present, the need for expert medical and nursing management continues. The patient must be observed closely for dehydration during this phase; if dehydration occurs, the uremic symptoms are likely to increase.
- The recovery period signals the improvement of renal function and may take 3 to 12 months. Laboratory values return to the patient's normal level. Although a permanent 1% to 3% reduction in the GFR is common, it is not clinically significant.

Clinical Manifestations

Almost every system of the body is affected with failure of the normal renal regulatory mechanisms. The patient may appear critically ill and lethargic. The skin and mucous membranes are dry from dehydration. Central nervous system signs and symptoms include drowsiness, headache, muscle twitching, and seizures. Table 44-2 summarizes common clinical characteristics in all three categories of ARF.

Assessment and Diagnostic Findings

Assessment of the patient with ARF includes evaluation for changes in the urine, diagnostic tests that evaluate the kidney contour, and a variety of laboratory values. See Chapter 43 for information about the normal characteristics of urine, diagnostic findings, and laboratory values in the renal system.

In ARF, urine output varies from scanty to a normal volume, hematuria may be present, and the urine has a low specific gravity (compared with a normal value of 1.010 to 1.025). One of the earliest manifestations of tubular damage is the inability to concentrate the urine (Porth & Matfin, 2009). Patients with prerenal azotemia have a decreased amount of sodium in the urine (less than 20 mEq/L) and

Table 44-2	COMPARING CLINICAL CHARACTERISTICS OF ACUTE RENAL FAILURE		
	Categories		
Characteristics	Prerenal	Intrarenal	Postrenal
Etiology	Hypoperfusion	Parenchymal damage	Obstruction
Blood urea nitrogen value	Increased (out of normal 20:1 proportion to creatinine)	Increased	Increased
Creatinine	Increased	Increased	Increased
Urine output	Decreased	Varies, often decreased	Varies, may be decreased, or sudden anuria
Urine sodium	Decreased to <20 mEq/L	Increased to >40 mEq/L	Varies, often decreased to 20 mEq/L or less
Urinary sediment	Normal, few hyaline casts	Abnormal casts and debris	Usually normal
Urine osmolality	Increased to 500 mOsm	About 350 mOsm similar to serum	Varies, increased or equal to serum
Urine specific gravity	Increased	Low normal	Varies

normal urinary sediment. Patients with intrarenal azotemia usually have urinary sodium levels greater than 40 mEq/L with urinary casts and other cellular debris.

Ultrasonography is a critical component of the evaluation of patients with renal failure. A renal sonogram or a CT or MRI scan may show evidence of anatomic changes.

The BUN level increases steadily at a rate dependent on the degree of catabolism (breakdown of protein), renal perfusion, and protein intake. Serum creatinine levels are useful in monitoring kidney function and disease progression and increase with glomerular damage.

With a decline in the GFR, oliguria, and anuria, patients are at high risk for hyperkalemia. Protein catabolism results in the release of cellular potassium into the body fluids, causing severe hyperkalemia (high serum potassium levels). Hyperkalemia may lead to dysrhythmias, such as ventricular tachycardia and cardiac arrest. Sources of potassium include normal tissue catabolism, dietary intake, blood in the GI tract, or blood transfusion and other sources (eg, IV infusions, potassium penicillin, and extracellular shift in response to metabolic acidosis).

Progressive metabolic acidosis occurs in renal failure because patients cannot eliminate the daily metabolic load of acid-type substances produced by the normal metabolic processes. In addition, normal renal buffering mechanisms fail. This is reflected by a decrease in the serum CO_2-combining power and blood pH.

There may be an increase in blood phosphate concentrations; calcium levels may be low due to decreased absorption of calcium from the intestine and as a compensatory mechanism for the elevated blood phosphate levels. Anemia is another common laboratory finding in ARF, as a result of reduced erythropoietin production, uremic GI lesions, reduced RBC lifespan, and blood loss from the GI tract.

Prevention

ARF has a high mortality rate that ranges from 25% to 90%. Factors that influence mortality include increased age, comorbid conditions, and preexisting renal and vascular diseases (Dirkes & Hodge, 2007). Therefore, prevention of ARF is essential (Chart 44-5).

A careful history is obtained to identify exposure to nephrotoxic agents or environmental toxins. The kidneys are susceptible to the adverse effects of medications because the kidneys are repeatedly exposed to substances in the blood. Patients taking nephrotoxic medications (eg, aminoglycosides, gentamicin, tobramycin, colistimethate, polymyxin B, amphotericin B, vancomycin, amikacin, cyclosporine) should be monitored closely for changes in renal function. BUN and serum creatinine levels should be obtained at baseline within 24 hours after initiation of these medications and at least twice a week while the patient is receiving them.

Chart 44-5 • *Preventing Acute Renal Failure*

1. Provide adequate hydration to patients at risk for dehydration including:
   Before, during, and after surgery
   Patients undergoing intensive diagnostic studies requiring fluid restriction and contrast agents (eg, barium enema, intravenous pyelograms), especially elderly patients who may have marginal renal reserve
   Patients with neoplastic disorders or disorders of metabolism (eg, gout) and those receiving chemotherapy
2. Prevent and treat shock promptly with blood and fluid replacement.
3. Monitor central venous and arterial pressures and hourly urine output of critically ill patients to detect the onset of renal failure as early as possible.
4. Treat hypotension promptly.
5. Continually assess renal function (urine output, laboratory values) when appropriate.
6. Take precautions to ensure that the appropriate blood is administered to the correct patient in order to avoid severe transfusion reactions, which can precipitate renal failure.
7. Prevent and treat infections promptly. Infections can produce progressive renal damage.
8. Pay special attention to wounds, burns, and other precursors of sepsis.
9. To prevent infections from ascending in the urinary tract, give meticulous care to patients with indwelling catheters. Remove catheters as soon as possible.
10. To prevent toxic drug effects, closely monitor dosage, duration of use, and blood levels of all medications metabolized or excreted by the kidneys.

Any agent that reduces renal blood flow (eg, long-term analgesic use) may cause renal insufficiency. Chronic use of analgesic agents, particularly nonsteroidal anti-inflammatory drugs (NSAIDs), may cause **interstitial nephritis** (inflammation within the renal tissue) and papillary necrosis. Patients with heart failure or cirrhosis with ascites are at particular risk for NSAID-induced renal failure. Increased age, preexisting renal disease, and the simultaneous administration of several nephrotoxic agents increase the risk for kidney damage.

Radiocontrast-induced nephropathy (CIN) is a major cause of hospital-acquired ARF. Patients undergo more than 1 million radiocontrast studies in the United States annually; of these approximately 150,000 will experience CIN, and at least 1% of these will require dialysis and experience a prolonged hospital stay (Barreto, 2007). This is a potentially preventable condition. Baseline levels of creatinine greater than 2 mg/dL identify patients at high risk. Limiting the patient's exposure to contrast agents and nephrotoxic medications will reduce the risk of CIN (Steward, 2007). Administration of N-acetylcysteine and sodium bicarbonate before and during procedures reduces risk, but prehydration with saline is considered the most effective method to prevent CIN (Barreto, 2007).

 Gerontologic Considerations

About half of all patients who develop ARF during hospitalization are older than 60 years. The etiology of ARF in older adults includes prerenal causes such as dehydration, intrarenal causes such as **nephrotoxic** agents (eg, medications, contrast agents), and complications of major surgery (Steward, 2007). Suppression of thirst, enforced bed rest, lack of access to drinking water, and confusion all contribute to the older patient's failure to consume adequate fluids and may lead to dehydration, further compromising already decreased renal function.

ARF in the elderly is also often seen in the community setting. Nurses in the ambulatory setting need to be aware of the risk. All medications need to be monitored for potential side effects that could result in damage to the kidney either through reduced circulation or nephrotoxicity. Outpatient procedures that require fasting or a bowel preparation may cause dehydration and therefore require careful monitoring.

Medical Management

The kidneys have a remarkable ability to recover from insult. The objectives of treatment of ARF are to restore normal chemical balance and prevent complications until repair of renal tissue and restoration of renal function can occur. Management includes eliminating the underlying cause; maintaining fluid balance; avoiding fluid excesses; and, when indicated, providing renal replacement therapy. Prerenal azotemia is treated by optimizing renal perfusion, whereas postrenal failure is treated by relieving the obstruction. Intrarenal azotemia is treated with supportive therapy, with removal of causative agents, aggressive management of prerenal and postrenal failure, and avoidance of associated risk factors. Shock and infection, if present, are treated promptly (see Chapter 15).

Maintenance of fluid balance is based on daily body weight, serial measurements of central venous pressure, serum and urine concentrations, fluid losses, blood pressure, and the clinical status of the patient. The parenteral and oral intake and the output of urine, gastric drainage, stools, wound drainage, and perspiration are calculated and are used as the basis for fluid replacement. The insensible fluid produced through the normal metabolic processes and lost through the skin and lungs is also considered in fluid management.

Fluid excesses can be detected by the clinical findings of dyspnea, tachycardia, and distended neck veins. The patient's lungs are auscultated for moist crackles. Because pulmonary edema may be caused by excessive administration of parenteral fluids, extreme caution must be used to prevent fluid overload. The development of generalized edema is assessed by examining the presacral and pretibial areas several times daily. Mannitol (Osmitrol), furosemide (Lasix), or ethacrynic acid (Edecrin) may be prescribed to initiate diuresis.

Adequate renal blood flow in patients with prerenal causes of ARF may be restored by IV fluids or transfusions of blood products. If ARF is caused by hypovolemia secondary to hypoproteinemia, an infusion of albumin may be prescribed. Dialysis may be initiated to prevent complications of ARF, such as hyperkalemia, metabolic acidosis, pericarditis, and pulmonary edema. Dialysis corrects many biochemical abnormalities; allows for liberalization of fluid, protein, and sodium intake; diminishes bleeding tendencies; and promotes wound healing. **Hemodialysis** (a procedure that circulates the patient's blood through a dialyzer to remove waste products and excess fluid), **peritoneal dialysis** (PD) (a procedure that uses the patient's peritoneal membrane [the lining of the peritoneal cavity] as the semipermeable membrane to exchange fluid and solutes), or a variety of **continuous renal replacement therapies** (CRRTs) (methods used to replace normal kidney function by circulating the patient's blood through a hemofilter) may be performed. These and other treatment modalities for patients with renal dysfunction are discussed later in this chapter.

Pharmacologic Therapy

Hyperkalemia is the most life-threatening of the fluid and electrolyte changes that occur in patients with renal disturbances. Therefore, the patient is monitored for hyperkalemia through serial serum electrolyte levels (potassium value greater than 5.0 mEq/L [5 mmol/L]), ECG changes (tall, tented, or peaked T waves), and changes in clinical status (see Chapter 14). Other symptoms of hyperkalemia include irritability, abdominal cramping, diarrhea, paresthesia, and generalized muscle weakness. Muscle weakness may present as slurred speech, difficulty breathing, paresthesia, and paralysis. As the potassium level increases, both cardiac and other muscular function declines, making this a true medical emergency (Counts, 2008).

The elevated potassium levels may be reduced by administering cation-exchange resins (sodium polystyrene sulfonate [Kayexalate]) orally or by retention enema. Kayexalate works by exchanging sodium ions for potassium ions in the intestinal tract. Sorbitol may be administered in combination with Kayexalate to induce a diarrhea-type effect (it induces water loss in the GI tract). If a Kayexalate retention enema is administered (the colon is the major site of potassium exchange), a rectal catheter with a balloon may be used to facilitate retention if necessary. The patient should retain the Kayexalate for 30 to 45 minutes to promote potassium removal. Afterward, a cleansing enema may be prescribed to remove remaining medication as a precaution against fecal impaction.

If the patient is hemodynamically unstable (low blood pressure, changes in mental status, dysrhythmia), IV dextrose 50%, insulin, and calcium replacement may be administered to shift potassium back into the cells. Albuterol sulfate (Ventolin HFA) by nebulizer can lower plasma potassium concentration by 0.5 to 1.5 mEq/L (Best & Counselman, 2008). The shift of potassium into the intracellular space is temporary, so arrangements for dialysis need to be made on an emergent basis.

Since many medications are eliminated through the kidneys, dosages must be reduced when a patient has ARF. Examples of commonly used agents that require adjustment are antibiotic medications (especially aminoglycosides), digoxin, ACE inhibitors, and magnesium-containing agents.

In addition, many medications have been used in patients with ARF in an attempt to improve patient outcomes. Diuretic agents are often used to control fluid volume, but they have not been shown to improve recovery from ARF (Dirkes & Hodge, 2007).

In patients with severe acidosis, the arterial blood gases and serum bicarbonate levels (CO_2-combining power) must be monitored because the patient may require sodium bicarbonate therapy or dialysis. If respiratory problems develop, appropriate ventilatory measures must be instituted. The elevated serum phosphate level may be controlled with phosphate-binding agents (eg, calcium or lanthanum carbonate) that help prevent a continuing rise in serum phosphate levels by decreasing the absorption of phosphate from the intestinal tract.

Nutritional Therapy

ARF causes severe nutritional imbalances (because nausea and vomiting contribute to inadequate dietary intake), impaired glucose use and protein synthesis, and increased tissue catabolism. The patient is weighed daily and loses 0.2 to 0.5 kg (0.5 to 1 lb) daily if the nitrogen balance is negative (ie, caloric intake falls below caloric requirements). If the patient gains or does not lose weight or develops hypertension, fluid retention should be suspected.

Nutritional support is based on the underlying cause of ARF, the catabolic response, the type and frequency of renal replacement therapy, comorbidities, and nutritional status. Replacement of dietary proteins is individualized to provide the maximum benefit and minimize uremic symptoms. Caloric requirements are met with high-carbohydrate meals, because carbohydrates have a protein-sparing effect (ie, in a high-carbohydrate diet, protein is not used for meeting energy requirements but is "spared" for growth and tissue healing). Foods and fluids containing potassium or phosphorus (eg, bananas, citrus fruits and juices, coffee) are restricted.

The oliguric phase of ARF may last 10 to 20 days and is followed by the diuretic phase, at which time urine output begins to increase, signaling that kidney function is returning. Results of blood chemistry tests are used to determine the amounts of sodium, potassium, and water needed for replacement, along with assessment for overhydration or underhydration. Following the diuretic phase, the patient is placed on a high-protein, high-calorie diet and is encouraged to resume activities gradually.

Nursing Management

The nurse has an important role in caring for the patient with ARF. The nurse monitors for complications, participates in emergency treatment of fluid and electrolyte imbalances, assesses the patient's progress and response to treatment, and provides physical and emotional support. Additionally, the nurse keeps family members informed about the patient's condition, helps them understand the treatments, and provides psychological support. Although the development of ARF may be the most serious problem, the nurse continues to provide nursing care indicated for the primary disorder (eg, burns, shock, trauma, obstruction of the urinary tract).

Monitoring Fluid and Electrolyte Balance

Because of the serious fluid and electrolyte imbalances that can occur with ARF, the nurse monitors the patient's serum electrolyte levels and physical indicators of these complications during all phases of the disorder. Hyperkalemia is the most immediate life-threatening imbalance seen in ARF. Parenteral fluids, all oral intake, and all medications are screened carefully to ensure that hidden sources of potassium are not inadvertently administered or consumed. IV solutions must be carefully selected based on the patient's fluid and electrolyte status. The patient's cardiac function and musculoskeletal status are monitored closely for signs of hyperkalemia.

The nurse monitors fluid status by paying careful attention to fluid intake (IV medications should be administered in the smallest volume possible), urine output, apparent edema, distention of the jugular veins, alterations in heart sounds and breath sounds, and increasing difficulty in breathing. Accurate daily weights, as well as I&O records, are essential. Indicators of deteriorating fluid and electrolyte status are reported immediately to the physician, and preparation is made for emergency treatment. Severe fluid and electrolyte disturbances may be treated with hemodialysis, PD, or CRRT.

Reducing Metabolic Rate

The nurse takes steps to reduce the patient's metabolic rate. Bed rest may be indicated to reduce exertion and the metabolic rate during the most acute stage of the disorder. Fever and infection, both of which increase the metabolic rate and catabolism, are prevented or treated promptly.

Promoting Pulmonary Function

Attention is given to pulmonary function, and the patient is assisted to turn, cough, and take deep breaths frequently to prevent atelectasis and respiratory tract infection. Drowsiness and lethargy may prevent the patient from moving and turning without encouragement and assistance.

Preventing Infection

Asepsis is essential with invasive lines and catheters to minimize the risk of infection and increased metabolism. An indwelling urinary catheter is avoided whenever possible due to the high risk of UTI associated with its use but may be required to provide ongoing data required to monitor fluid I&O.

Providing Skin Care

The skin may be dry or susceptible to breakdown as a result of edema; therefore, meticulous skin care is important. Additionally, excoriation and itching of the skin may result from the deposit of irritating toxins in the patient's tissues. Bathing the patient with cool water, frequent turning, and keeping the skin clean and well moisturized and the fingernails trimmed to avoid excoriation are often comforting and prevent skin breakdown.

Providing Psychosocial Support

The patient with ARF may require treatment with hemodialysis, PD, or CRRT. The length of time that these treatments are necessary varies with the cause and extent of damage to the kidneys. The patient and family need assistance, explanation, and support during this period. The purpose of the treatment is explained to the patient and family by the physician. However, high levels of anxiety and fear may necessitate repeated explanation and clarification by the nurse. The family members may initially be afraid to touch and talk to the patient during these procedures but should be encouraged and assisted to do so.

In an intensive care setting, many of the nurse's functions are devoted to the technical aspects of patient care; however, it is essential that the psychological needs and other concerns of the patient and family be addressed. Continued assessment of the patient for complications of ARF and precipitating causes is essential.

Chronic Renal Failure (End-Stage Renal Disease)

When a patient has sustained enough kidney damage to require renal replacement therapy on a permanent basis, the patient has moved into the fifth or final stage of CKD, also referred to as chronic renal failure (CRF) or ESRD.

Pathophysiology

As renal function declines, the end products of protein metabolism (normally excreted in urine) accumulate in the blood. Uremia develops and adversely affects every system in the body. The greater the buildup of waste products, the more pronounced the symptoms are.

The rate of decline in renal function and progression of ESRD is related to the underlying disorder, the urinary excretion of protein, and the presence of hypertension. The disease tends to progress more rapidly in patients who excrete significant amounts of protein or have elevated blood pressure than in those without these conditions.

Clinical Manifestations

Because virtually every body system is affected in ESRD, patients exhibit a number of signs and symptoms (Broscious & Castagnola, 2006). The severity of these signs and symptoms depends in part on the degree of renal impairment, other underlying conditions, and the patient's age. Cardiovascular disease is the predominant cause of death in patients with ESRD (Burrows & Muller, 2007). Peripheral neuropathy, a disorder of the peripheral nervous system, is present in some patients. Patients complain of severe pain and discomfort. Restless leg syndrome and burning feet can occur in the early stage of uremic peripheral neuropathy (Phillips & Ryr, 2005; Slack & Landis, 2006). The precise mechanisms for many of these systemic signs and symptoms have not been identified. However, it is generally thought that the accumulation of uremic waste products is the probable cause. Chart 44-6 summarizes the systemic signs and symptoms.

Assessment and Diagnostic Findings

Glomerular Filtration Rate

As the GFR decreases (due to nonfunctioning glomeruli), the creatinine clearance decreases, while the serum creatinine and BUN levels increase. Serum creatinine is a more sensitive indicator of renal function than BUN. The BUN is affected not only by renal disease but also by protein intake in the diet, catabolism (tissue and RBC breakdown), parenteral nutrition, and medications such as corticosteroids.

Sodium and Water Retention

The kidney cannot concentrate or dilute the urine normally in ESRD. Appropriate responses by the kidney to changes in the daily intake of water and electrolytes, therefore, do not occur. Some patients retain sodium and water, increasing the risk for edema, heart failure, and hypertension. Hypertension may also result from activation of the renin–angiotensin–aldosterone axis and the concomitant increased aldosterone secretion. Other patients have a tendency to lose sodium and run the risk of developing hypotension and hypovolemia. Vomiting and diarrhea may cause sodium and water depletion, which worsens the uremic state.

Acidosis

Metabolic acidosis occurs in ESRD because the kidneys are unable to excrete increased loads of acid. Decreased acid secretion results from the inability of the kidney tubules to excrete ammonia (NH_3^-) and to reabsorb sodium bicarbonate (HCO_3^-). There is also decreased excretion of phosphates and other organic acids.

Anemia

Anemia develops as a result of inadequate erythropoietin production, the shortened lifespan of RBCs, nutritional deficiencies, and the patient's tendency to bleed, particularly from the GI tract. Erythropoietin, a substance normally produced by the kidneys, stimulates bone marrow to produce RBCs (Brattich, 2007). In ESRD, erythropoietin production decreases and profound anemia results, producing fatigue, angina, and shortness of breath.

Chart 44-6•*Assessing for End-stage Renal Disease*

Be alert for the following signs and symptoms:

Neurologic

- Weakness and fatigue
- Confusion
- Inability to concentrate
- Disorientation
- Tremors
- Seizures
- Asterixis
- Restlessness of legs
- Burning of soles of feet
- Behavior changes

Integumentary

- Gray-bronze skin color
- Dry, flaky skin
- Pruritus
- Ecchymosis
- Purpura
- Thin, brittle nails
- Coarse, thinning hair

Cardiovascular

- Hypertension
- Pitting edema (feet, hands, sacrum)
- Periorbital edema
- Pericardial friction rub
- Engorged neck veins
- Pericarditis
- Pericardial effusion
- Pericardial tamponade
- Hyperkalemia
- Hyperlipidemia

Pulmonary

- Crackles
- Thick, tenacious sputum
- Depressed cough reflex
- Pleuritic pain
- Shortness of breath
- Tachypnea
- Kussmaul-type respirations
- Uremic pneumonitis

Gastrointestinal

- Ammonia odor to breath ("uremic fetor")
- Metallic taste
- Mouth ulcerations and bleeding
- Anorexia, nausea, and vomiting
- Hiccups
- Constipation or diarrhea
- Bleeding from gastrointestinal tract

Hematologic

- Anemia
- Thrombocytopenia

Reproductive

- Amenorrhea
- Testicular atrophy
- Infertility
- Decreased libido

Musculoskeletal

- Muscle cramps
- Loss of muscle strength
- Renal osteodystrophy
- Bone pain
- Bone fractures
- Foot drop

Calcium and Phosphorus Imbalance

Another abnormality seen in ESRD is a disorder in calcium and phosphorus metabolism (McCarley & Arjomand, 2008). Serum calcium and phosphate levels have a reciprocal relationship in the body: As one increases, the other decreases. With a decrease in filtration through the glomerulus of the kidney, there is an increase in the serum phosphate level and a reciprocal or corresponding decrease in the serum calcium level. The decreased serum calcium level causes increased secretion of parathormone from the parathyroid glands. However, in renal failure, the body does not respond normally to the increased secretion of parathormone; as a result, calcium leaves the bone, often producing bone changes and bone disease as well as calcification of major blood vessels in the body. In addition, the active metabolite of vitamin D (1,25-dihydroxycholecalciferol) normally manufactured by the kidney decreases as renal failure progresses (Gesek & Desmond, 2008). Uremic bone disease, often called renal osteodystrophy, develops from the complex changes in calcium, phosphate, and parathormone balance. There is also evidence of calcification of blood vessels.

Complications

Potential complications of chronic renal failure that concern the nurse and necessitate a collaborative approach to care include the following:

- Hyperkalemia due to decreased excretion, metabolic acidosis, catabolism, and excessive intake (diet, medications, fluids)
- Pericarditis, pericardial effusion, and pericardial tamponade due to retention of uremic waste products and inadequate dialysis
- Hypertension due to sodium and water retention and malfunction of the renin–angiotensin–aldosterone system
- Anemia due to decreased erythropoietin production, decreased RBC lifespan, bleeding in the GI tract from irritating toxins and ulcer formation, and blood loss during hemodialysis
- Bone disease and metastatic and vascular calcifications due to retention of phosphorus, low serum calcium levels, abnormal vitamin D metabolism, and elevated aluminum levels

Medical Management

The goal of management is to maintain kidney function and homeostasis for as long as possible. All factors that contribute to ESRD and all factors that are reversible (eg, obstruction) are identified and treated. Management is accomplished primarily with medications and diet therapy, although dialysis may also be needed to decrease the level of uremic waste products in the blood and to control electrolyte balance.

Pharmacologic Therapy

Complications can be prevented or delayed by administering prescribed phosphate-binding agents, calcium supplements, antihypertensive and cardiac medications, antiseizure medications, and erythropoietin (Epogen).

Calcium and Phosphorus Binders

Hyperphosphatemia and hypocalcemia are treated with medications that bind dietary phosphorus in the GI tract. Binders such as calcium carbonate (Os-Cal) or calcium acetate (PhosLo) are prescribed, but there is a risk of hypercalcemia. If calcium is high or the calcium–phosphorus product exceeds 55 mg/dL, a polymeric phosphate binder such as sevelamer hydrochloride (Renagel) may be prescribed (Zonderman & Doyle, 2006). These medications bind dietary phosphorus in the intestinal tract. All binding agents must be administered with food to be effective. Magnesium-based antacids are avoided to prevent magnesium toxicity.

Antihypertensive and Cardiovascular Agents

Hypertension is managed by intravascular volume control and a variety of antihypertensive agents. Heart failure and pulmonary edema may also require treatment with fluid restriction, low-sodium diets, diuretic agents, inotropic agents such as digoxin (Lanoxin) or dobutamine (Dobutrex), and dialysis. The metabolic acidosis of ESRD usually produces no symptoms and requires no treatment; however, sodium bicarbonate supplements or dialysis may be needed to correct the acidosis if it causes symptoms (Molzahn & Butera, 2006).

Antiseizure Agents

Neurologic abnormalities may occur, so the patient must be observed for early evidence of slight twitching, headache, delirium, or seizure activity. If seizures occur, the onset of the seizure is recorded along with the type, duration, and general effect on the patient. The physician is notified immediately. IV diazepam (Valium) or phenytoin (Dilantin) is usually administered to control seizures. The side rails of the bed should be raised and padded to protect the patient. The nursing management of the patient with seizures is discussed in Chapter 61.

Erythropoietin

Anemia associated with ESRD is treated with recombinant human erythropoietin (Epogen). Patients with anemia (hematocrit less than 30%) present with nonspecific symptoms, such as malaise, general fatigability, and decreased activity tolerance. Erythropoietin therapy is initiated to achieve a hematocrit of 33% to 38% and a target hemoglo-bin of 12 g/dL, which generally alleviates the symptoms of anemia (Brattich, 2007).

Erythropoietin is administered intravenously or subcutaneously three times a week in ESRD. It may take 2 to 6 weeks for the hematocrit to increase; therefore, the medication is not indicated for patients who need immediate correction of severe anemia. Adverse effects seen with erythropoietin therapy include hypertension (especially during early stages of treatment), increased clotting of vascular access sites, seizures, and depletion of body iron stores (Zonderman & Doyle, 2006).

Management involves adjustment of heparin to prevent clotting of the lines during hemodialysis treatments, frequent monitoring of hemoglobin and hematocrit, and periodic assessment of serum iron and transferrin levels. Because adequate stores of iron are necessary for an adequate response to erythropoietin, supplementary iron may be prescribed. Common iron supplements include iron sucrose (Venofer) and ferric gluconate (Ferrlecit). In addition, the patient's blood pressure and serum potassium level are monitored to detect hypertension and increasing serum potassium levels, which may occur with therapy and the increasing RBC mass. The occurrence of hypertension requires initiation or adjustment of the patient's antihypertensive therapy. Hypertension that cannot be controlled is a contraindication to recombinant erythropoietin therapy.

Patients who have received erythropoietin therapy have reported decreased levels of fatigue, increased feelings of well-being, better tolerance of dialysis, higher energy levels, and improved exercise tolerance. Additionally, this therapy has decreased the need for transfusion and its associated risks, including bloodborne infectious disease, antibody formation, and iron overload.

Nutritional Therapy

Dietary intervention is necessary with deterioration of renal function and includes careful regulation of protein intake, fluid intake to balance fluid losses, sodium intake to balance sodium losses, and some restriction of potassium. At the same time, adequate caloric intake and vitamin supplementation must be ensured. Protein is restricted because urea, uric acid, and organic acids—the breakdown products of dietary and tissue proteins—accumulate rapidly in the blood when there is impaired renal clearance. The allowed protein must be of high biologic value (dairy products, eggs, meats). High-biologic-value proteins are those that are complete proteins and supply the essential amino acids necessary for growth and cell repair.

Usually, the fluid allowance per day is 500 mL to 600 mL more than the previous day's 24-hour urine output. Calories are supplied by carbohydrates and fat to prevent wasting. Vitamin supplementation is necessary because a protein-restricted diet does not provide the necessary complement of vitamins. Additionally, the patient on dialysis may lose water-soluble vitamins during the dialysis treatment.

Hyperkalemia is usually prevented by ensuring adequate dialysis treatments with potassium removal and careful monitoring of diet, medications, and fluids for their potassium content. Sodium polystyrene sulfonate (Kayexalate), a cation-exchange resin, may be needed for acute hyperkalemia.

Dialysis

The patient with increasing symptoms of renal failure is referred to a dialysis and transplantation center early in the course of progressive renal disease. Dialysis is usually initiated when the patient cannot maintain a reasonable lifestyle with conservative treatment.

Nursing Management

The patient with ESRD requires astute nursing care to avoid the complications of reduced renal function and the stresses and anxieties of dealing with a life-threatening illness.

Nursing care is directed toward assessing fluid status and identifying potential sources of imbalance, implementing a dietary program to ensure proper nutritional intake within the limits of the treatment regimen, and promoting positive feelings by encouraging increased self-care and greater independence. It is extremely important to provide explanations and information to the patient and family concerning ESRD, treatment options, and potential complications. A great deal of emotional support is needed by the patient and family because of the numerous changes experienced. Specific interventions, along with rationale and evaluation criteria, are presented in more detail in the plan of nursing care for the patient with chronic renal failure (Chart 44-7).

Promoting Home and Community-Based Care

Teaching Patients Self-Care

The nurse plays an important role in teaching the patient with ESRD. Because of the extensive teaching needed, the home care nurse, dialysis nurse, and nurses in the hospital and outpatient settings all provide ongoing education and reinforcement while monitoring the patient's progress and compliance with the treatment regimen.

A referral to a nutritionist is made because of the dietary changes required. The patient is taught how to check the vascular access device for patency and appropriate precautions, such as avoiding venipuncture and blood pressure measurements on the arm with the access device.

Additionally, the patient and family need to know what problems to report to the health care provider. These include the following:

- Worsening signs and symptoms of renal failure (nausea, vomiting, change in usual urine output [if any], ammonia odor on breath)
- Signs and symptoms of hyperkalemia (muscle weakness, diarrhea, abdominal cramps)
- Signs and symptoms of access problems (clotted fistula or graft, infection)

These signs and symptoms of decreasing renal function, in addition to increasing BUN and serum creatinine levels, may indicate a need to alter the dialysis prescription. The dialysis nurses also provide ongoing education and support at each treatment visit.

Continuing Care

The importance of follow-up examinations and treatment is stressed to the patient and family because of changing physical status, renal function, and dialysis requirements. Referral for home care provides the home care nurse with the opportunity to assess the patient's environment and emotional status and the coping strategies used by the patient and family to deal with the changes in family roles often associated with chronic illness.

The home care nurse also assesses the patient for further deterioration of renal function and signs and symptoms of complications resulting from the primary renal disorder, the resulting renal failure, and effects of treatment strategies (eg, dialysis, medications, dietary restrictions). Patients need education and reinforcement of the dietary restrictions required, including fluid, sodium, potassium, and protein restriction. Reminders about the need for health promotion activities and health screening are an important part of nursing care for the patient with renal failure.

Gerontologic Considerations

Diabetes, hypertension, chronic glomerulonephritis, interstitial nephritis, and urinary tract obstruction are the causes of ESRD in the elderly. The signs and symptoms of renal disease in the elderly are often nonspecific. The occurrence of symptoms of other disorders (heart failure, dementia) can mask the symptoms of renal disease and delay or prevent diagnosis and treatment. Patients often develop signs and symptoms of nephrotic syndrome, such as edema and proteinuria.

Hemodialysis and PD are used effectively in treating elderly patients. The number of elderly patients initiating dialysis has dramatically increased in the past decade (Kurella, Covinsky, Collins, et al., 2007). Although there is no specific age limitation for renal transplantation, concomitant disorders (eg, coronary artery disease, peripheral vascular disease) have made it a less common treatment for the elderly. However, the outcome is comparable to that of younger patients. Some elderly patients elect not to undergo dialysis or transplantation. Conservative management, including nutritional therapy, fluid control, and medications such as phosphate binders, may be considered in patients who are not suitable for or elect not to have dialysis or transplantation.

RENAL REPLACEMENT THERAPIES

The use of renal replacement therapies becomes necessary when the kidneys can no longer remove wastes, maintain electrolytes, and regulate fluid balance. This can occur rapidly or over a long period of time and the need for replacement therapy can be acute (short term) or chronic (long term). The main renal replacement therapies include the various types of dialysis and kidney transplantation.

Dialysis

Types of dialysis include hemodialysis, CRRT, and PD. Acute dialysis is indicated when there is a high and increasing level of serum potassium, fluid overload, or impending pulmonary edema, increasing acidosis, pericarditis, and severe confusion. It may also be used to remove medications or toxins (poisoning or medication overdose) from

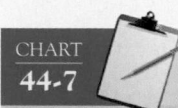

CHART
44-7

PLAN OF NURSING CARE
The Patient With Chronic Renal Failure

NURSING DIAGNOSIS: Excess fluid volume related to decreased urine output, dietary excesses, and retention of sodium and water
GOAL: Maintenance of ideal body weight without excess fluid

Nursing Interventions	Rationale	Expected Outcomes

1. Assess fluid status:
   a. Daily weight
   b. Intake and output balance
   c. Skin turgor and presence of edema
   d. Distention of neck veins
   e. Blood pressure, pulse rate, and rhythm
   f. Respiratory rate and effort
2. Limit fluid intake to prescribed volume.
 	
3. Identify potential sources of fluid:
   a. Medications and fluids used to take or administer medications: oral and intravenous
   b. Foods
4. Explain to patient and family rationale for fluid restriction.
 	
5. Assist patient to cope with the discomforts resulting from fluid restriction.
6. Provide or encourage frequent oral hygiene.
	1. Assessment provides baseline and ongoing database for monitoring changes and evaluating interventions.
	
	2. Fluid restriction will be determined on basis of weight, urine output, and response to therapy.
	3. Unrecognized sources of excess fluids may be identified.
	
	4. Understanding promotes patient and family cooperation with fluid restriction.
	5. Increasing patient comfort promotes compliance with dietary restrictions.
	6. Oral hygiene minimizes dryness of oral mucous membranes.
		• Demonstrates no rapid weight changes
		• Maintains dietary and fluid restrictions
		• Exhibits normal skin turgor without edema
		• Exhibits normal vital signs
		• Exhibits no neck vein distention
		• Reports no difficulty breathing or shortness of breath
		• Performs oral hygiene frequently
		• Reports decreased thirst
		• Reports decreased dryness of oral mucous membranes

NURSING DIAGNOSIS: Imbalanced nutrition: less than body requirements related to anorexia, nausea, vomiting, dietary restrictions, and altered oral mucous membranes
GOAL: Maintenance of adequate nutritional intake

Nursing Interventions	Rationale	Expected Outcomes

1. Assess nutritional status:
   a. Weight changes
   b. Laboratory values (serum electrolyte, BUN, creatinine, protein, transferrin, and iron levels)
2. Assess patient's nutritional dietary patterns:
   a. Diet history
   b. Food preferences
   c. Calorie counts
3. Assess for factors contributing to altered nutritional intake:
   a. Anorexia, nausea, or vomiting
   b. Diet unpalatable to patient
   c. Depression
   d. Lack of understanding of dietary restrictions
   e. Stomatitis
4. Provide patient's food preferences within dietary restrictions.
5. Promote intake of high-biologic-value protein foods: eggs, dairy products, meats.
	1. Baseline data allow for monitoring of changes and evaluating effectiveness of interventions.
	
	2. Past and present dietary patterns are considered in planning meals.
	
	3. Information about other factors that may be altered or eliminated to promote adequate dietary intake is provided.
	
	4. Increased dietary intake is encouraged.
	5. Complete proteins are provided for positive nitrogen balance needed for growth and healing.
		• Consumes protein of high biologic value
		• Chooses foods within dietary restrictions that are appealing
		• Consumes high-calorie foods within dietary restrictions
		• Explains in own words rationale for dietary restrictions and relationship to urea and creatinine levels
		• Takes medications on schedule that does not produce anorexia or feeling of fullness
		• Consults written lists of acceptable foods
		• Reports increased appetite at meals
		• Exhibits no rapid increases or decreases in weight
		• Demonstrates normal skin turgor without edema; wound healing and acceptable plasma albumin levels

Continued on following page

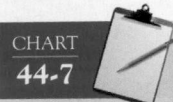

CHART
44-7

PLAN OF NURSING CARE
The Patient With Chronic Renal Failure (Continued)

Nursing Interventions	Rationale	Expected Outcomes
6. Encourage high-calorie, low-protein, low-sodium, and low-potassium snacks between meals.	6. Reduces source of restricted foods and proteins and provides calories for energy, sparing protein for tissue growth and healing.	
7. Alter schedule of medications so that they are not given immediately before meals.	7. Ingestion of medications just before meals may produce anorexia and feeling of fullness.	
8. Explain rationale for dietary restrictions and relationship to kidney disease and increased urea and creatinine levels.	8. Promotes patient understanding of relationships between diet and urea and creatinine levels to renal disease	
9. Provide written lists of foods allowed and suggestions for improving their taste without use of sodium or potassium.	9. Lists provide a positive approach to dietary restrictions and a reference for patient and family to use when at home.	
10. Provide pleasant surroundings at meal-times.	10. Unpleasant factors that contribute to patient's anorexia are eliminated.	
11. Weigh patient daily.	11. Allows monitoring of fluid and nutritional status	
12. Assess for evidence of inadequate protein intake: a. Edema formation b. Delayed wound healing c. Decreased serum albumin levels	12. Inadequate protein intake can lead to decreased albumin and other proteins, edema formation, and delay in wound healing.	

NURSING DIAGNOSIS: Deficient knowledge regarding condition and treatment
GOAL: Increased knowledge about condition and related treatment

Nursing Interventions	Rationale	Expected Outcomes
1. Assess understanding of cause of renal failure, consequences of renal failure, and its treatment: a. Cause of patient's renal failure b. Meaning of renal failure c. Understanding of renal function d. Relationship of fluid and dietary restrictions to renal failure e. Rationale for treatment (hemodialysis, peritoneal dialysis, transplantation)	1. Provides baseline for further explanations and teaching	• Verbalizes relationship of cause of renal failure to consequences • Explains fluid and dietary restrictions as they relate to failure of kidney's regulatory functions • States in own words relationship of renal failure and need for treatment • Asks questions about treatment options, indicating readiness to learn • Verbalizes plans to continue as normal a life as possible • Uses written information and instructions to clarify questions and seek additional information
2. Provide explanation of renal function and consequences of renal failure at patient's level of understanding and guided by patient's readiness to learn.	2. Patient can learn about renal failure and treatment as he or she becomes ready to understand and accept the diagnosis and consequences.	
3. Assist patient to identify ways to incorporate changes related to illness and its treatment into lifestyle.	3. Patient can see that his or her life does not have to revolve around the disease.	
4. Provide oral and written information as appropriate about: a. Renal function and failure b. Fluid and dietary restrictions c. Medications d. Reportable problems, signs, and symptoms e. Follow-up schedule f. Community resources g. Treatment options	4. Provides patient with information that can be used for further clarification at home	

Continued

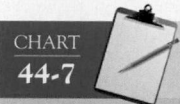

CHART 44-7

PLAN OF NURSING CARE
The Patient With Chronic Renal Failure (Continued)

NURSING DIAGNOSIS: Activity intolerance related to fatigue, anemia, retention of waste products, and dialysis procedure
GOAL: Participation in activity within tolerance

Nursing Interventions	Rationale	Expected Outcomes

1. Assess factors contributing to activity intolerance:
  a. Fatigue
  b. Anemia
  c. Fluid and electrolyte imbalances
  d. Retention of waste products
  e. Depression
2. Promote independence in self-care activities as tolerated; assist if fatigued.
3. Encourage alternating activity with rest.
4. Encourage patient to rest after dialysis treatments.
	1. Indicates factors contributing to severity of fatigue
	
	2. Promotes improved self-esteem
	
	3. Promotes activity and exercise within limits and adequate rest
	4. Adequate rest is encouraged after dialysis treatments, which are exhausting to many patients.
		• Participates in increasing levels of activity and exercise
		• Reports increased sense of well-being
		• Alternates rest and activity
		• Participates in selected self-care activities

NURSING DIAGNOSIS: Risk for situational low self-esteem related to dependency, role changes, change in body image, and change in sexual function
GOAL: Improved self-esteem

Nursing Interventions	Rationale	Expected Outcomes

1. Assess patient's and family's responses and reactions to illness and treatment.
2. Assess relationship of patient and significant family members.
3. Assess usual coping patterns of patient and family members.
 	
4. Encourage open discussion of concerns about changes produced by disease and treatment:
  a. Role changes
  b. Changes in lifestyle
  c. Changes in occupation
  d. Sexual changes
  e. Dependence on health care team
5. Explore alternate ways of sexual expression other than sexual intercourse.
6. Discuss role of giving and receiving love, warmth, and affection.
	1. Provides data about problems encountered by patient and family in coping with changes in life
	2. Identifies strengths and supports of patient and family
	3. Coping patterns that may have been effective in past may be harmful in view of restrictions imposed by disease and treatment.
	4. Encourages patient to identify concerns and steps necessary to deal with them
	
	5. Alternative forms of sexual expression may be acceptable.
	
	6. Sexuality means different things to different people, depending on stage of maturity.
		• Identifies previously used coping styles that have been effective and those no longer possible due to disease and treatment (alcohol or drug use; extreme physical exertion)
		• Patient and family identify and verbalize feelings and reactions to disease and necessary changes in their lives
		• Seeks professional counseling, if necessary, to cope with changes resulting from renal failure
		• Reports satisfaction with method of sexual expression

COLLABORATIVE PROBLEMS: Hyperkalemia; pericarditis, pericardial effusion, and pericardial tamponade; hypertension; anemia; bone disease and metastatic calcifications
GOAL: Absence of complications

Nursing Interventions	Rationale	Expected Outcomes
Hyperkalemia 1. Monitor serum potassium levels. Notify physician if level greater than 5.5 mEq/L, and prepare to treat hyperkalemia. 2. Assess patient for muscle weakness, diarrhea, ECG changes (tall-tented T waves and widened QRS).	1. Hyperkalemia causes potentially life-threatening changes in the body. 2. Cardiovascular signs and symptoms are characteristic of hyperkalemia.	• Patient has normal potassium level • Experiences no muscle weakness or diarrhea • Exhibits normal ECG pattern • Vital signs are within normal limits

Continued on following page

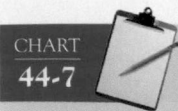

CHART
44-7

PLAN OF NURSING CARE
The Patient With Chronic Renal Failure (*Continued*)

Nursing Interventions	Rationale	Expected Outcomes
Pericarditis, Pericardial Effusion, and Pericardial Tamponade		
1. Assess patient for fever, chest pain, and a pericardial friction rub (signs of pericarditis) and, if present, notify physician.	1. About 30%–50% of patients with chronic renal failure develop pericarditis due to uremia; fever, chest pain, and a pericardial friction rub are classic signs.	• Has strong and equal peripheral pulses • Absence of a paradoxical pulse • Absence of pericardial effusion or tamponade on cardiac ultrasound • Patient has normal heart sounds

2. If patient has pericarditis, assess for the following every 4 hours:
    a. Paradoxical pulse >10 mm Hg
    b. Extreme hypotension
    c. Weak or absent peripheral pulses
    d. Altered level of consciousness
    e. Bulging neck veins
	2. Pericardial effusion is a common fatal sequela of pericarditis. Signs of an effusion include a paradoxical pulse (>10 mm Hg drop in blood pressure during inspiration) and signs of shock due to compression of the heart by a large effusion. Cardiac tamponade exists when the patient is severely compromised hemodynamically.	

3. Prepare patient for cardiac ultrasound to aid in diagnosis of pericardial effusion and cardiac tamponade.	3. Cardiac ultrasound is useful in visualizing pericardial effusions and cardiac tamponade.	
4. If cardiac tamponade develops, prepare patient for emergency pericardiocentesis.	4. Cardiac tamponade is a life-threatening condition, with a high mortality rate. Immediate aspiration of fluid from the pericardial space is essential.	
Hypertension		
1. Monitor and record blood pressure as indicated.	1. Provides objective data for monitoring. Elevated levels may indicate nonadherence to the treatment regimen.	• Blood pressure within normal limits • Reports no headaches, visual problems, or seizures • Edema is absent • Demonstrates compliance with dietary and fluid restrictions
2. Administer antihypertensive medications as prescribed.	2. Antihypertensive medications play a key role in treatment of hypertension associated with chronic renal failure.	
3. Encourage compliance with dietary and fluid restriction therapy.	3. Adherence to diet and fluid restrictions and dialysis schedule prevents excess fluid and sodium accumulation.	
4. Teach patient to report signs of fluid overload, vision changes, headaches, edema, or seizures.	4. These are indications of inadequate control of hypertension and the need to alter therapy.	
Anemia		
1. Monitor RBC count, hemoglobin, and hematocrit levels as indicated.	1. Provides assessment of degree of anemia	• Patient has a normal skin color without pallor • Exhibits hematology values within acceptable limits • Experiences no bleeding from any site
2. Administer medications as prescribed, including iron and folic acid supplements, Epogen, and multivitamins.	2. RBCs need iron, folic acid, and vitamins to be produced. Epogen stimulates the bone marrow to produce RBC.	
3. Avoid drawing unnecessary blood specimens.	3. Anemia is worsened by drawing numerous specimens.	
4. Teach patient to prevent bleeding: avoid vigorous nose blowing and contact sports, and use a soft toothbrush.	4. Bleeding from anywhere in the body worsens anemia.	
5. Administer blood component therapy as indicated.	5. Blood component therapy may be needed if the patient has symptoms.	

Continued

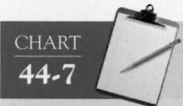

CHART 44-7

PLAN OF NURSING CARE
The Patient With Chronic Renal Failure (Continued)

Nursing Interventions	Rationale	Expected Outcomes
Bone Disease and Metastatic Calcifications 1. Administer the following medications as prescribed: phosphate binders, calcium supplements, vitamin D supplements. 2. Monitor serum lab values as indicated (calcium, phosphorus, aluminum levels) and report abnormal findings to physician. 3. Assist patient with an exercise program.	1. Chronic renal failure causes numerous physiologic changes affecting calcium, phosphorus, and vitamin D metabolism. 2. Hyperphosphatemia, hypocalcemia, and excess aluminum accumulation are common in chronic renal failure. 3. Bone demineralization increases with immobility.	• Exhibits serum calcium, phosphorus, and aluminum levels within acceptable ranges • Exhibits no symptoms of hypocalcemia • Has no bone demineralization on bone scan • Discusses importance of maintaining activity level and exercise program

the blood or for edema that does not respond to other treatment, hepatic coma, hyperkalemia, hypercalcemia, hypertension, and uremia (Mosenkis, Kirk & Berns, 2006).

Chronic or maintenance dialysis is indicated in advanced CKD and ESRD in the following instances: the presence of uremic signs and symptoms affecting all body systems (nausea and vomiting, severe anorexia, increasing lethargy, mental confusion), hyperkalemia, fluid overload not responsive to diuretics and fluid restriction, and a general lack of well-being. An urgent indication for dialysis in patients with renal failure is pericardial friction rub.

The decision to initiate dialysis should be reached only after thoughtful discussion among the patient, family, physician, and others as appropriate. Many potentially life-threatening issues are associated with the need for dialysis. The nurse can assist the patient and family by answering their questions, clarifying the information provided, and supporting their decision.

Successful kidney transplantation eliminates the need for dialysis. Not only is the quality of life much improved in patients with ESRD who undergo transplantation, but physiologic function is improved as well. Patients who undergo renal transplantation from living donors before dialysis is initiated generally have longer survival of the transplanted kidney than patients who receive transplantation after dialysis treatment is initiated.

HEMODIALYSIS

Hemodialysis is used for patients who are acutely ill and require short-term dialysis (days to weeks) and for patients with advanced CKD and ESRD who require long-term or permanent renal replacement therapy. Hemodialysis prevents death but does not cure renal disease and does not compensate for the loss of endocrine or metabolic activities of the kidneys. More than 90% of patients requiring long-term renal replacement therapy are on chronic hemodialysis (USRDS, 2007). Most patients receive intermittent hemodialysis that involves treatments three times a week with the average treatment duration of 3 to 4 hours in an outpatient setting. Hemodialysis can also be performed at home by the patient and a caregiver. With home dialysis, treatment time and frequency can be adjusted to meet optimal patient needs.

The objectives of hemodialysis are to extract toxic nitrogenous substances from the blood and to remove excess water. A **dialyzer** (also referred to as an artificial kidney) serves as a synthetic semipermeable membrane, replacing the renal glomeruli and tubules as the filter for the impaired kidneys. In hemodialysis, the blood, laden with toxins and nitrogenous wastes, is diverted from the patient to a machine, a dialyzer, where toxins are filtered out and removed and the blood is returned to the patient.

Diffusion, osmosis, and ultrafiltration are the principles on which hemodialysis is based (see Chapter 14). The toxins and wastes in the blood are removed by **diffusion**—that is, they move from an area of higher concentration in the blood to an area of lower concentration in the **dialysate.** The dialysate is a solution made up of all the important electrolytes in their ideal extracellular concentrations. The electrolyte level in the patient's blood can be brought under control by properly adjusting the dialysate bath. The semipermeable membrane impedes the diffusion of large molecules, such as RBCs and proteins.

Excess water is removed from the blood by **osmosis,** in which water moves from an area of low concentration potential (the blood) to an area of high concentration potential (the dialysate bath). In **ultrafiltration,** water moves under high pressure to an area of lower pressure. This process is much more efficient than osmosis at water removal and is accomplished by applying negative pressure or a suctioning force to the dialysis membrane. Because patients with renal disease usually cannot excrete water, this force is necessary to remove fluid to achieve fluid balance.

The body's buffer system is maintained using a dialysate bath made up of bicarbonate (most common) or acetate, which is metabolized to form bicarbonate. The anticoagulant heparin is administered to keep blood from clotting in the dialysis circuit. Cleansed blood is returned to the body. By the end of the dialysis treatment, many waste products have been removed, the electrolyte balance has been restored to normal, and the buffer system has been replenished.

Dialyzers

Dialyzers are hollow-fiber devices containing thousands of tiny strawlike tubes that carry the blood through the dialyzer. The tubes are porous and act as a semipermeable membrane

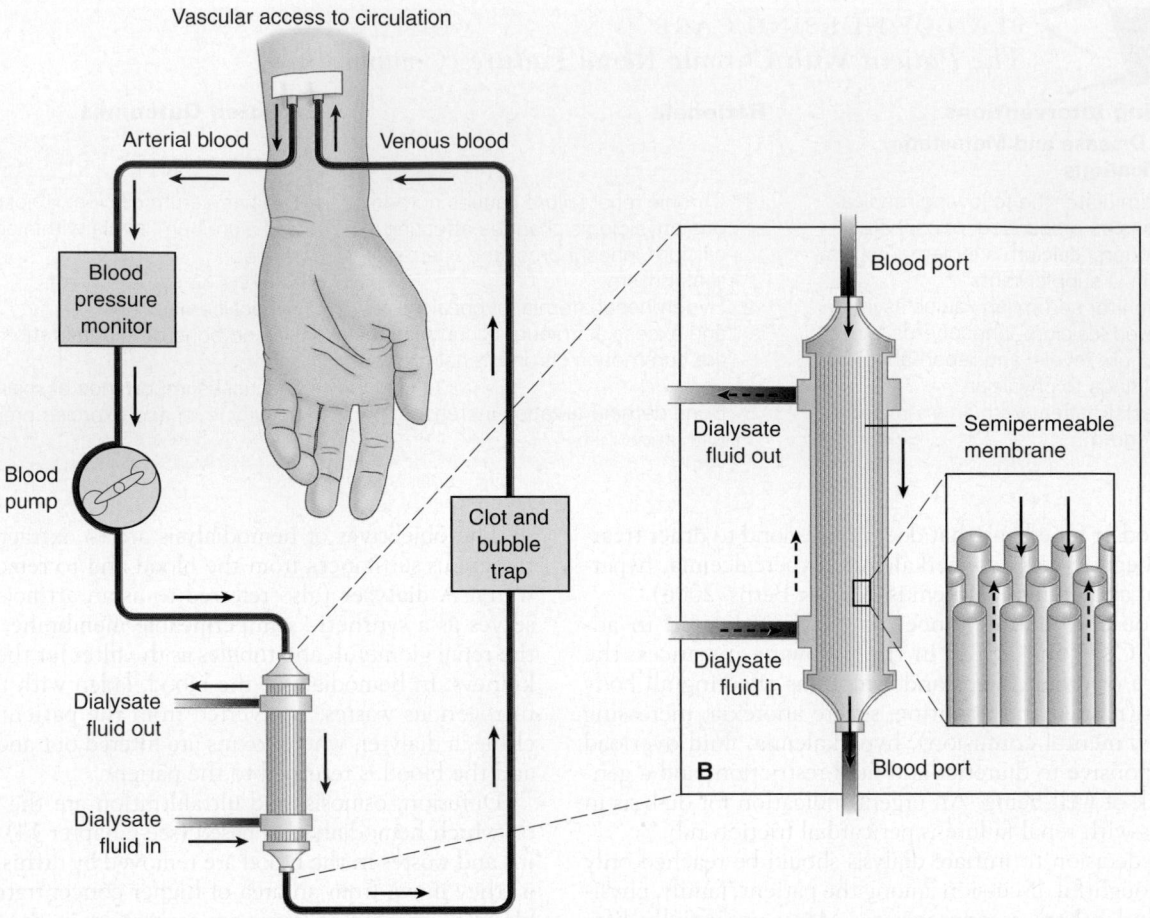

Figure 44-3 Hemodialysis system. **A,** Blood from an artery is pumped into **(B)** a dialyzer where it flows through the cellophane tubes, which act as the semipermeable membrane (*inset*). The dialysate, which has the same chemical composition as the blood except for urea and waste products, flows in around the tubules. The waste products in the blood diffuse through the semipermeable membrane into the dialysate.

allowing toxins, fluid, and electrolytes to pass through. The constant flow of the solution maintains the concentration gradient to facilitate the exchange of wastes from the blood through the semipermeable membrane into the dialysate solution, where they are removed and discarded (Fig. 44-3).

Dialyzers have undergone many technologic changes in performance and biocompatibility. High-flux dialysis uses highly permeable membranes to increase the clearance of low- and mid-molecular-weight molecules. These special membranes are used with higher than traditional rates of flow for the blood entering and exiting the dialyzer (500 to 550 mL/min). High-flux dialysis increases the efficiency of treatments while shortening their duration and reducing the need for heparin.

Vascular Access

Access to the patient's vascular system must be established to allow blood to be removed, cleansed, and returned to the patient's vascular system at rates between 300 and 800 mL/min. Several types of access are available.

Vascular Access Devices

Immediate access to the patient's circulation for acute hemodialysis is achieved by inserting a double-lumen, noncuffed, large-bore catheter into the subclavian, internal jugular, or femoral vein by the physician (Fig. 44-4). This method of vascular access involves some risk (eg, hematoma, pneumothorax, infection, thrombosis of the subclavian vein, inadequate flow). The catheter is removed when no longer needed (eg, because the patient's condition has improved or another type of access has been established). Double-lumen, cuffed catheters may also be inserted, usually by either a surgeon or interventional radiologist, into the internal jugular vein of the patient. Since these catheters have cuffs under the skin, the insertion site heals, sealing the wound and reducing the risk for ascending infection. This feature makes these catheters safe for longer-term use. Infection rates, however, remain high and septicemia continues to be a common cause for hospital admission.

Arteriovenous Fistula

The preferred method of permanent access is an **arteriovenous fistula (AVF)** that is created surgically (usually in the forearm) by joining (anastomosing) an artery to a vein, either side to side or end to side (Fig. 44-5A). Needles are inserted into the vessel to obtain blood flow adequate to pass through the dialyzer. The arterial segment of the fistula is used for arterial flow to the dialyzer and the venous segment for reinfusion of the dialyzed blood. This

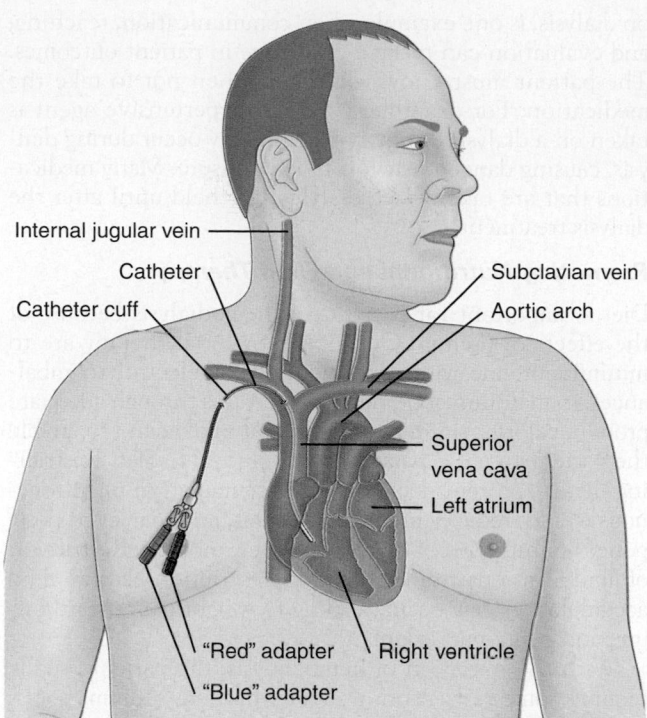

Figure 44-4 Double-lumen, cuffed hemodialysis catheter used in acute hemodialysis. The red adapter is attached to a blood line through which blood is pumped from the patient to the dialyzer. After the blood passes through the dialyzer (artificial kidney), it returns to the patient through the blue adaptor.

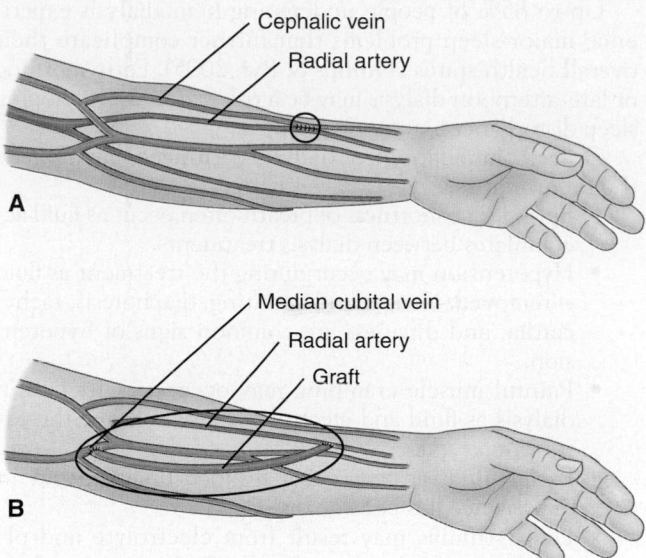

Figure 44-5 A, Arteriovenous fistulas are created by anastomosing a patient's vein to an artery. This illustrates a side-to-side anastomosis. **B,** Arteriovenous grafts are established by placing synthetic tubing between the artery and vein.

> ⚑ **NURSING ALERT**
>
> Failure of the permanent dialysis access (fistula or graft) accounts for most hospital admissions of patients undergoing chronic hemodialysis. Thus, protection of the access is of high priority.

access will need time, (2 to 3 months) to "mature" before it can be used. As the AVF matures, the venous segment dilates due to the increased blood flow coming directly from the artery. Once sufficiently dilated it will then accommodate two large-bore (14-, 15-, or 16-gauge) needles that are inserted for each dialysis treatment. The patient is encouraged to perform hand exercises to increase the size of these vessels (ie, squeezing a rubber ball for forearm fistulas) to accommodate the large-bore needles. Once established, this access has the longest useful life and thus is the best option for vascular access for the chronic hemodialysis patient.

Arteriovenous Graft

An **arteriovenous graft** can be created by subcutaneously interposing a biologic, semibiologic, or synthetic graft material between an artery and vein (Fig. 44-5B). Usually a graft is created when the patient's vessels are not suitable for creation of an AV fistula. Patients with compromised vascular systems (eg, from diabetes) will require a graft because their native vessels are not suitable for creation of an AV Fistula. Grafts are usually placed in the arm but may be placed in the thigh or chest area. Stenosis, infection, and thrombosis are the most common complications that result in loss of this access. It is not at all uncommon to see a dialysis patient with numerous "old" or "nonfunctioning" accesses present on their arms. The patient is asked to identify which is the current access in use and it is checked carefully for the presence of a bruit and thrill.

Complications

While hemodialysis can prolong life indefinitely, it does not alter the natural course of the underlying CKD, nor does it completely replace kidney function. The CKD complications previously discussed will continue to worsen and require more aggressive treatment. With the initiation of dialysis, disturbances of lipid metabolism (hypertriglyceridemia) are accentuated and contribute to cardiovascular complications. Heart failure, coronary heart disease, angina, stroke, and peripheral vascular insufficiency may occur and can incapacitate the patient. Cardiovascular disease remains the leading cause of death in patients receiving dialysis (Burrows & Muller, 2007).

Anemia is compounded by blood lost during hemodialysis. Gastric ulcers may result from the physiologic stress of chronic illness, medication, and preexisting medical conditions (eg, diabetes). Patients with uremia report a metallic taste and nausea when they require dialysis. Vomiting may occur during the hemodialysis treatment when rapid fluid shifts and hypotension occur. These contribute to the malnutrition seen in patients on dialysis. Worsening calcium metabolism and renal osteodystrophy can result in bone pain and fractures, interfering with mobility. As time on dialysis continues, calcification of major blood vessels has been reported and linked to hypertension and other vascular complications. Phosphorus deposits in the skin can occur and cause itching.

Up to 85% of people undergoing hemodialysis experience major sleep problems that further complicate their overall health status (Phillips & Ryr, 2005). Early-morning or late-afternoon dialysis may be a risk factor for developing sleep disturbances.

Other complications of dialysis treatment may include the following:

- Episodes of shortness of breath often occur as fluid accumulates between dialysis treatments.
- Hypotension may occur during the treatment as fluid is removed. Nausea and vomiting, diaphoresis, tachycardia, and dizziness are common signs of hypotension.
- Painful muscle cramping may occur, usually late in dialysis as fluid and electrolytes rapidly leave the extracellular space.
- Exsanguination may occur if blood lines separate or dialysis needles become dislodged.
- Dysrhythmias may result from electrolyte and pH changes or from removal of antiarrhythmic medications during dialysis.
- Air embolism is rare but can occur if air enters the vascular system.
- Chest pain may occur in patients with anemia or arteriosclerotic heart disease.
- Dialysis disequilibrium results from cerebral fluid shifts. Signs and symptoms include headache, nausea and vomiting, restlessness, decreased level of consciousness, and seizures. It is more likely to occur in acute renal failure or when blood urea nitrogen levels are very high (exceeding 150 mg/dL).

Nursing Management

The nurse in the dialysis unit has an important role in monitoring, supporting, assessing, and educating the patient. During dialysis, the patient, the dialyzer, and the dialysate bath require constant monitoring because numerous complications are possible, including clotting of the circuit, air embolism, inadequate or excessive ultrafiltration hypotension, cramping, vomiting, blood leaks, contamination, and access complications. Nursing care of the patient and maintenance of the vascular access device are especially important and are discussed later in this chapter in the section titled Special Considerations: Nursing Management of the Hospitalized Patient on Dialysis.

Promoting Pharmacologic Therapy

Many medications are removed from the blood during hemodialysis; therefore, dosage or timing of the medication administration may require adjustment. Medications that are water soluble are readily removed during hemodialysis treatment and those that are fat soluble or adhere to other substances (like albumin) are not dialyzed out very well. This is the reason some drug overdoses are treated with emergency hemodialysis and others are not.

Patients undergoing hemodialysis who require medications (eg, cardiac glycosides, antibiotic agents, antiarrhythmic medications, antihypertensive agents) are monitored closely to ensure that blood and tissue levels of these medications are maintained without toxic accumulation. Antihypertensive therapy, often part of the regimen of patients

on dialysis, is one example when communication, teaching, and evaluation can make a difference in patient outcomes. The patient must know when and when not to take the medication. For example, if an antihypertensive agent is taken on a dialysis day, hypotension may occur during dialysis, causing dangerously low blood pressure. Many medications that are taken once daily can be held until after the dialysis treatment.

Promoting Nutritional and Fluid Therapy

Diet is important for patients on hemodialysis because of the effects of uremia. Goals of nutritional therapy are to minimize uremic symptoms and fluid and electrolyte imbalances; to maintain good nutritional status through adequate protein, calorie, vitamin, and mineral intake; and to enable the patient to eat a palatable and enjoyable diet. Restricting dietary protein decreases the accumulation of nitrogenous wastes, reduces uremic symptoms, and may even postpone the initiation of dialysis for a few months. Restriction of fluid is also part of the dietary prescription because fluid accumulation may occur, leading to weight gain, heart failure, and pulmonary edema.

With the initiation of hemodialysis, the patient usually requires some restriction of dietary protein, sodium, potassium, and fluid intake. Protein intake is restricted to about 1.2 to 1.3 g/kg ideal body weight per day; therefore, protein must be of high biologic quality. Sodium is usually restricted to 2 to 3 g/day; fluids are restricted to an amount equal to the daily urine output plus 500 mL/day. The goal for patients on hemodialysis is to keep their interdialytic (between dialysis treatments) weight gain under 1.5 kg (Welch & Perkins, 2006). Potassium restriction depends on the amount of residual renal function and the frequency of dialysis. Dietary restriction is an unwelcome change in lifestyle for many patients with chronic renal failure. Patients can feel stigmatized in social situations because there may be few food choices available for their diet. If the restrictions are ignored, life-threatening complications, such as hyperkalemia and pulmonary edema, may result. Thus, the patient may feel punished for responding to basic human drives to eat and drink. The nurse who cares for a patient with symptoms or complications resulting from dietary indiscretion must avoid harsh, judgmental, or punitive tones when communicating with him or her. Regular education with reinforcement is needed to achieve this difficult change in life style (Welch & Perkins, 2006) (Chart 44-8).

Meeting Psychosocial Needs

Patients requiring long-term hemodialysis are often concerned about the unpredictability of the illness and the disruption of their lives. They often have financial problems, difficulty holding a job, waning sexual desire and impotence, depression from being chronically ill, and fear of dying. Younger patients worry about marriage, having children, and the burden that they bring to their families. The regimented lifestyle that frequent dialysis treatments and restrictions in food and fluid intake impose is often demoralizing to the patient and family.

Dialysis alters the lifestyle of the patient and family. The amount of time required for dialysis and physician visits and being chronically ill can create conflict, frustration, guilt,

CHART
44-8
NURSING RESEARCH PROFILE
Hemodialysis and Nonadherence

Belguzar, K., Kayser, C. & Kilic, S. (2007). Nonadherence with diet and fluid restrictions and perceived social support in patients receiving hemodialysis. *Journal of Nursing Scholarship, 39*(3), 243–248.

Purpose

Nonadherence to diet and fluid restrictions has adverse consequences for patients receiving hemodialysis. The purpose of this study was to describe nonadherence with diet and fluid restrictions and the level of perceived social support in hemodialysis patients. Nonadherence often occurs when a person's behavior conflicts with medical advice regarding taking medications, following diets, or other lifestyle changes.

Design

This descriptive study surveyed 160 patients on hemodialysis in three centers in Turkey. Participants were asked about personal characteristics, and data were collected using the Dialysis Diet and Fluid Nonadherence Questionnaire (DDFQ) and Multidimensional Scale of Perceived Social Support (MSP). Data were collected during the patient's regularly scheduled dialysis session. The DDFQ is a four-item self-report questionnaire that assesses the frequency of nonadherence to diet and fluid restrictions for the previous 14 days. The MSP is a 12-item scale used to assess emotional support and the degree of satisfaction with perceived social support from family, friends, and significant others.

Findings

Adherence to fluid restriction is a difficult and stressful aspect of hemodialysis treatment, and most patients in this study showed some degree of nonadherence to fluid restrictions (68%) and diet (58%). Participants perceived total social support as low. Nonadherence was most common with younger patients, those who were married, and those with lower levels of perceived social support.

Nursing Implications

Nurses working in hemodialysis centers need to consider social support and how it affects adherence in patients receiving hemodialysis. The results of this study suggest that younger, married patients may require assistance to develop the levels of social support needed to adhere to fluid and diet restrictions between hemodialysis sessions.

---

and depression. It may be difficult for the patient, spouse, and family to express anger and negative feelings.

The nurse needs to give the patient and family the opportunity to express feelings of anger and concern about the limitations that the disease and treatment impose, possible financial problems, and job insecurity. If anger is not expressed, it may be directed inward and lead to depression, despair, and attempts at suicide (suicide is more prevalent in patients on dialysis); however, if anger is projected outward to other people, it may destroy already threatened family relationships.

Although these feelings are normal in this situation, they are often profound and overwhelming. Counseling and psychotherapy may be necessary. Depression may require treatment with antidepressant agents. Referring the patient and family to a mental health provider with expertise in the care of patients receiving dialysis may also be helpful. Clinical nurse specialists, psychologists, and social workers may be helpful in assisting the patient and family to cope with the changes brought about by renal failure and its treatment.

The "sense of loss" that the patient experiences cannot be underestimated because every aspect of a "normal life" is disrupted. Some patients use denial to deal with the overwhelming array of medical problems (eg, infections, hypertension, anemia, neuropathy). Staff who are tempted to label the patient as noncompliant must consider the impact of renal failure and its treatment on the patient and family and the coping strategies that they may use.

Palliative care principles that focus on symptom control are becoming increasingly important as greater attention is focused on quality-of-life issues (Cohen, Moss, Weisord, et al., 2006). Patients and their families should be encouraged to discuss end-of-life options and have developed advanced directives or living wills.

Promoting Home and Community-Based Care

Teaching Patients Self-Care

Preparing a patient for hemodialysis is challenging. Often the patient does not fully comprehend the impact of dialysis, and learning needs may go unrecognized. Good communication between dialysis staff and home care nurses is essential.

Assessment helps identify the learning needs of the patient and family members. In many cases, the patient is discharged home before learning needs and readiness to learn can be thoroughly evaluated; therefore, hospital-based nurses, dialysis staff, and home care nurses must work together to provide appropriate teaching that meets the patient's and family's changing needs and readiness to learn.

The diagnosis of chronic renal failure and the need for dialysis often overwhelm the patient and family. In addition, many patients with ESRD have depressed mentation, a shortened attention span, a decreased level of concentration, and altered perception. Therefore, teaching must occur in brief, 10- to 15-minute sessions, with time added for clarification, repetition, reinforcement, and questions from the patient and family. The nurse needs to convey a nonjudgmental attitude to enable the patient and family to discuss options and their feelings about those options. Team conferences are helpful for sharing information and providing every team member the opportunity to discuss the needs of the patient and family.

Home Hemodialysis

Most patients who undergo hemodialysis do so in an outpatient setting, but home hemodialysis is an option for some. Home hemodialysis requires a highly motivated patient who is willing to take responsibility for the procedure and is able to adjust each treatment to meet the body's changing needs. It also requires the commitment and cooperation of a caregiver to assist the patient. However, many patients are not comfortable imposing on others this way and do not wish to subject family members to the feeling that their home is being turned into a clinic. The health care team never forces a patient to use home hemodialysis because this treatment requires significant changes in the home and family. Home hemodialysis must be the patient's and family's decision (American Nephrology Nurses Association, 2007a).

The patient undergoing home hemodialysis and the caregiver assisting that patient must be trained to prepare, operate, and disassemble the dialysis machine; maintain and clean the equipment; administer medications (eg, heparin) into the machine lines; and handle emergency problems (hemodialysis dialyzer rupture, electrical or mechanical problems, hypotension, shock, and seizures). Because home hemodialysis places primary responsibility for the treatment on the patient and the family member, they must understand and be capable of performing all aspects of the hemodialysis procedure (Chart 44-9).

Before home hemodialysis is initiated, the home environment, household and community resources, and ability and willingness of the patient and family to carry out this treatment are assessed. The home is surveyed to see if electrical outlets, plumbing facilities, and storage space are adequate. Modifications may be needed to enable the patient and assistant to perform dialysis safely and to deal with emergencies.

Once home hemodialysis is initiated, the home care nurse must visit periodically to evaluate compliance with the recommended techniques, to assess the patient for complications, to reinforce previous teaching, and to provide reassurance.

Continuing Care

The health care team's goal in treating patients with chronic renal failure is to maximize their vocational potential, functional status, and quality of life. To facilitate renal rehabilitation, appropriate follow-up and monitoring by members of the health care team (physicians, dialysis nurses, social worker, psychologist, home care nurses, and others as appropriate) are essential to identify and resolve problems early on. Many patients with chronic renal failure can resume relatively normal lives, doing the things that are important to them: traveling, exercising, working, or actively participating in family activities. If appropriate interventions are available early in the course of dialysis, the potential for better health improves, and the patient can remain active in family and community life. Outcome goals for renal rehabilitation include employment for those able to work, improved physical functioning of all patients, improved understanding about adaptation and options for living well, increased control over the effects of kidney disease and dialysis, and resumption of activities enjoyed before dialysis.

CONTINUOUS RENAL REPLACEMENT THERAPIES

Continuous renal replacement therapies (CRRTs) may be indicated for patients with acute or chronic renal failure who are too clinically unstable for traditional hemodialysis,

---

CHART 44-9 🏠 **HOME CARE CHECKLIST**
Hemodialysis

At the completion of the home care instruction, the patient or caregiver will be able to:	PATIENT	CAREGIVER
• Discuss renal failure and its effects on the body.	✔	✔
• Describe the cause of renal failure and why hemodialysis is necessary.	✔	✔
• Describe the basic principles of hemodialysis.	✔	✔
• Discuss common problems that may occur during hemodialysis and their prevention and management.	✔	✔
• Demonstrate knowledge about prescribed medications and the reason for their use, potential side effects, guidelines on when to notify physician, and the schedule of medications on dialysis and nondialysis days.	✔	✔
• Acknowledge dietary and fluid restrictions, rationale, and consequences of noncompliance.	✔	✔
• Describe commonly measured laboratory values, results, and implications.	✔	✔
• List guidelines for prevention and detection of fluid overload, meaning of "dry" weight, and how to weigh self.	✔	✔
• Demonstrate vascular access care, how to check patency, signs and symptoms of infection, and prevention of complications.	✔	✔
• Discuss strategies for detection, management, and relief of pruritus, neuropathy, and other complications of renal failure.	✔	✔
• Develop strategies to manage or reduce anxiety and maintain independence.	✔	✔
• Coordinate financial arrangements for dialysis and strategies to identify and obtain resources.	✔	✔

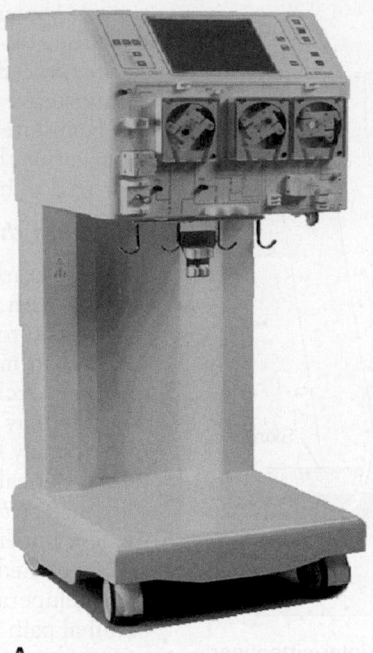
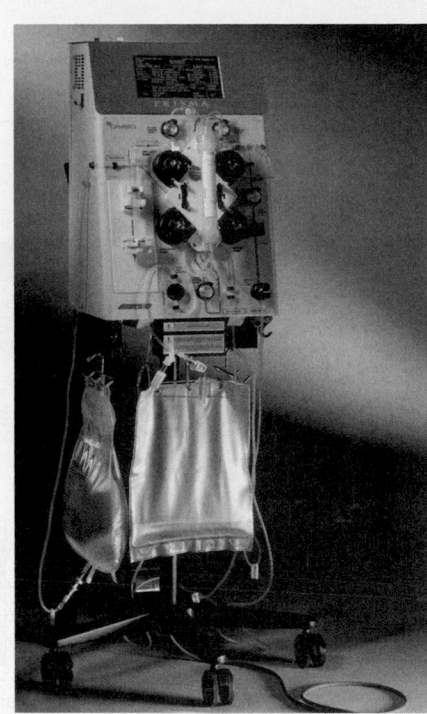

Figure 44-6 Devices for administering continuous renal replacement therapy (CRRT) offer an integrated fluid warmer for the heating of infusion and dialysate fluids, a weighing system to reduce the possibility of error in assessing fluid balance, and a battery backup that allows treatments to continue when the patient is moved. **A,** Diapact CRRT System, B-Braun Medical, Inc., Bethlehem, PA. **B,** PRISMA, Gambro Corporation, Lakewood, CO.

A

B

for patients with fluid overload secondary to oliguric (low urine output) renal failure, and for patients whose kidneys cannot handle their acutely high metabolic or nutritional needs. CRRT does not produce rapid fluid shifts, does not require dialysis machines or dialysis personnel to carry out the procedures, and can be initiated quickly. Several types of CRRT are available and widely used in critical care units (Fig. 44-6). The methods are similar as they require access to the circulation and blood to pass through an artificial filter. A hemofilter (an extremely porous blood filter containing a semipermeable membrane) is used in all types.

Continuous Venovenous Hemofiltration

Continuous venovenous hemofiltration (CVVH) is used to manage acute renal failure. Blood from a double-lumen venous catheter is pumped (using a small blood pump) through a hemofilter and then returned to the patient through the same catheter. CVVH provides continuous slow fluid removal (ultrafiltration); therefore, hemodynamic effects are mild and better tolerated by patients with unstable conditions. CVVH does not require arterial access, and critical care nurses can set up, initiate, maintain, and terminate the system.

Continuous Venovenous Hemodialysis

Continuous venovenous hemodialysis (CVVHD) is similar to CVVH. Blood is pumped from a double-lumen venous catheter through a hemofilter and returned to the patient through the same catheter. In addition to the benefits of ultrafiltration, CVVHD uses a concentration gradient to facilitate the removal of uremic toxins and fluid. No arterial access is required, hemodynamic effects are usually mild,

and critical care nurses can set up, initiate, maintain, and terminate the system (Martin & Jurschak, 2007).

Examples of less frequently used CRRT include slow continuous ultrafiltration (SCUF), continuous arteriovenous hemofiltration (CAVH), and continuous arteriovenous hemodialysis (CAVHD) (Martin & Jurschak, 2007).

PERITONEAL DIALYSIS

The goals of PD are to remove toxic substances and metabolic wastes and to reestablish normal fluid and electrolyte balance. PD may be the treatment of choice for patients with renal failure who are unable or unwilling to undergo hemodialysis or renal transplantation. Patients who are susceptible to the rapid fluid, electrolyte, and metabolic changes that occur during hemodialysis experience fewer of these problems with the slower rate of PD. Therefore, patients with diabetes or cardiovascular disease, many older patients, and those who may be at risk for adverse effects of systemic heparin are likely candidates for PD. Additionally, severe hypertension, heart failure, and pulmonary edema not responsive to usual treatment regimens have been successfully treated with PD. Less than 8% of patients with ESRD receive PD as their treatment modality (USRDS, 2007).

In PD, the peritoneal membrane that covers the abdominal organs and lines the abdominal wall serves as the semipermeable membrane. Sterile dialysate fluid is introduced into the peritoneal cavity through an abdominal catheter at intervals (Fig. 44-7). Once the sterile solution is in the peritoneal cavity, uremic toxins such as urea and creatinine begin to be cleared from the blood. Diffusion and osmosis occur as waste products move from an area of higher concentration (the blood stream) to an area of lesser

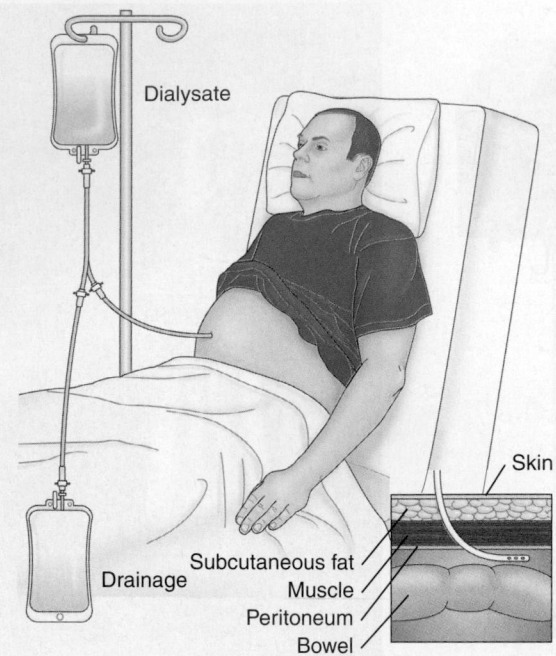

Dialysate

Skin

Drainage

Subcutaneous fat

Muscle

Peritoneum

Bowel

Figure 44-7 In peritoneal dialysis and in acute intermittent peritoneal dialysis, dialysate is infused into the peritoneal cavity by gravity, after which the clamp on the infusion line is closed. After a dwell time (when the dialysate is in the peritoneal cavity), the drainage tube is unclamped and the fluid drains from the peritoneal cavity, again by gravity. A new container of dialysate is infused as soon as drainage is complete. The duration of the dwell time depends on the type of peritoneal dialysis.

concentration (the dialysate fluid) through a semipermeable membrane (the peritoneum). This movement of solute from the blood into the dialysate fluid is called clearance. Since substances cross the peritoneal membrane at different rates, adjustments in dwell time and amount of fluid used are made to facilitate the process. Ultrafiltration (water removal) occurs in PD through an osmotic gradient created by using a dialysate fluid with a higher glucose concentration. PD usually takes 36 to 48 hours to achieve what hemodialysis accomplishes in 6 to 8 hours.

Procedure

As with other forms of treatment, the decision to begin PD is made by the patient and family in consultation with the physician. The patient may be acutely ill, thus requiring short-term treatment to correct severe disturbances in fluid and electrolyte status, or may have ESRD and need to receive ongoing treatments.

Preparing the Patient

The nurse's preparation of the patient and family for PD depends on the patient's physical and psychological status, level of alertness, previous experience with dialysis, and understanding of and familiarity with the procedure.

The nurse explains the procedure to the patient and assists in obtaining signed consent. Baseline vital signs, weight, and serum electrolyte levels are recorded. Evaluation of the abdomen for placement of the catheter is done to facilitate self-care. Typically the catheter is placed on the nondominant side to allow the patient easier access to the

catheter connection site when exchanges are done. The patient is encouraged to empty the bladder and bowel to reduce the risk of puncture of internal organs during the insertion procedure. Broad-spectrum antibiotic agents may be administered to prevent infection. The peritoneal catheter can be inserted in interventional radiology, in the operating room, or at the bedside. Depending on the situation, this will need to be explained to the patient and family.

Preparing the Equipment

In addition to assembling the equipment for PD, the nurse consults with the physician to determine the concentration of dialysate to be used and the medications to be added to it. Heparin may be added to prevent fibrin formation and resultant occlusion of the peritoneal catheter. Potassium chloride may be prescribed to prevent hypokalemia. Antibiotics may be added to treat **peritonitis** (inflammation of the peritoneal membrane) caused by infection. Regular insulin may be added for patients with diabetes. Aseptic technique is imperative whenever medications are added.

Before medications are added, the dialysate is warmed to body temperature to prevent patient discomfort and abdominal pain and to dilate the vessels of the peritoneum to increase urea clearance. Solutions that are too cold cause pain, cramping, and vasoconstriction and reduce clearance. Dry heating (heating cabinet, incubator, or heating pad) is recommended. Methods not recommended include soaking the bags of solution in warm water (can introduce bacteria to the exterior of the bags of solution and increase the chance of peritonitis) and use of a microwave to heat the fluid (increases the danger of burning the peritoneum).

Immediately before initiating dialysis, using aseptic technique, the nurse assembles the administration set and tubing. The tubing is filled with the prepared dialysate to reduce the amount of air entering the catheter and peritoneal cavity, which could increase abdominal discomfort and interfere with instillation and drainage of the fluid.

Inserting the Catheter

Ideally, the peritoneal catheter is inserted in the operating room or radiology suite to maintain surgical asepsis and minimize the risk of contamination. However, in some circumstances, the physician may insert the rigid stylet catheter at the bedside using strict asepsis. Whenever a rigid catheter is used, careful securing and close observation for bowel perforation is essential to minimize complications.

Catheters for long-term use (eg, Tenckhoff, Swan, or Cruz) are usually soft and flexible and made of silicone with a radiopaque strip to permit visualization on x-ray. These catheters have three sections: (1) an intraperitoneal section, with numerous openings and an open tip to let dialysate flow freely; (2) a subcutaneous section that passes from the peritoneal membrane and tunnels through muscle and subcutaneous fat to the skin; and (3) an external section for connection to the dialysate system. Most of these catheters have two cuffs, which are made of Dacron polyester. The cuffs stabilize the catheter, limit movement, prevent leaks, and provide a barrier against microorganisms. One cuff is placed just distal to the peritoneum, and the other cuff is placed subcutaneously. The subcutaneous tunnel (5 to 10 cm long) further protects against bacterial infection (Fig. 44-8).

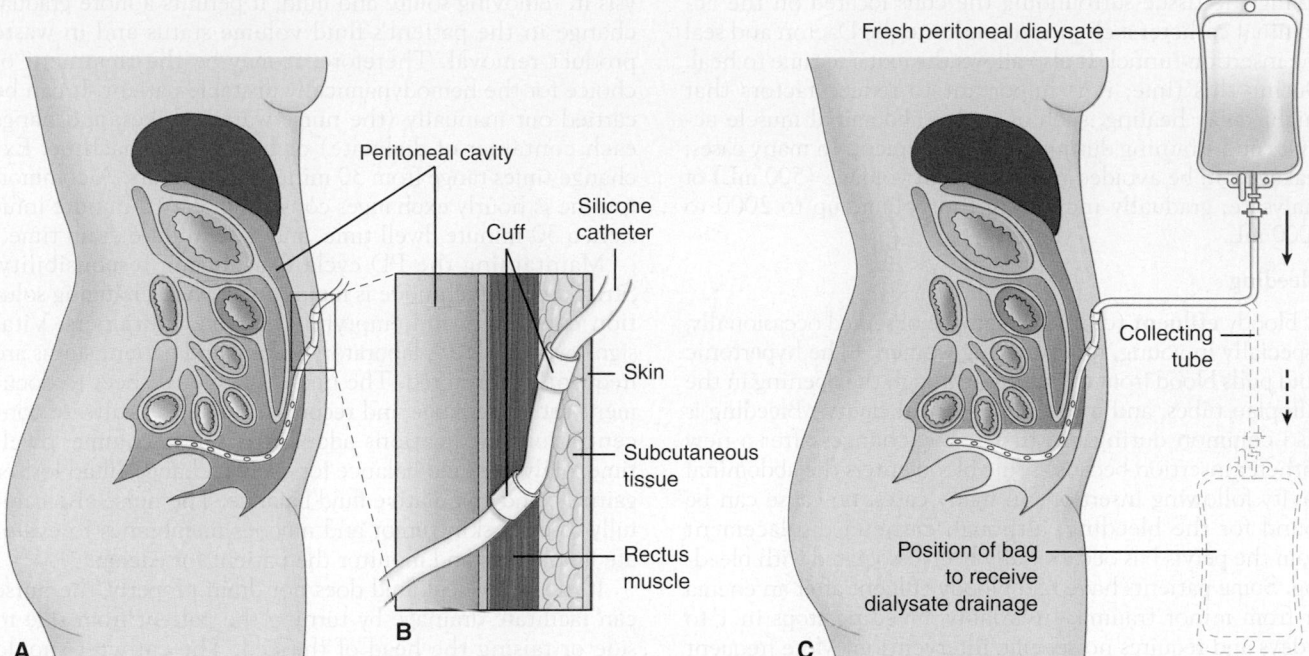

Figure 44-8 Continuous ambulatory peritoneal dialysis. **A,** The peritoneal catheter is implanted through the abdominal wall. **B,** Dacron cuffs and a subcutaneous tunnel provide protection against bacterial infection. **C,** Dialysate flows by gravity through the peritoneal catheter into the peritoneal cavity. After a prescribed period of time, the fluid is drained by gravity and discarded. New solution is then infused into the peritoneal cavity until the next drainage period. Dialysis thus continues on a 24-hour-a-day basis, during which the patient is free to move around and engage in his or her usual activities.

Performing the Exchange

PD involves a series of exchanges or cycles. An **exchange** is defined as the infusion (fill), dwell, and drainage of the dialysate. This cycle is repeated throughout the course of the dialysis. The dialysate is infused by gravity into the peritoneal cavity. A period of about 5 to 10 minutes is usually required to infuse 2 to 3 L of fluid. The prescribed dwell, or equilibration, time allows diffusion and osmosis to occur. At the end of the dwell time, the drainage portion of the exchange begins. The tube is unclamped and the solution drains from the peritoneal cavity by gravity through a closed system. Drainage is usually completed in 10 to 20 minutes. The drainage fluid is normally colorless or straw-colored and should not be cloudy. Bloody drainage may be seen in the first few exchanges after insertion of a new catheter but should not occur after that time. The number of cycles or exchanges and their frequency are prescribed based on monthly laboratory values and presence of uremic symptoms.

The removal of excess water during PD occurs because dialysate has a high dextrose concentration, making it hypertonic. An osmotic gradient is created between the blood and the dialysate solution. Dextrose solutions of 1.5%, 2.5%, and 4.25% are available in several volumes, from 1000 mL to 3000 mL. The higher the dextrose concentration, the greater the osmotic gradient and the more water will be removed. Selection of the appropriate solution is based on the patient's fluid status.

Complications

Most complications of PD are minor, but several, if unattended, can have serious consequences.

Acute Complications

Peritonitis

Peritonitis is the most common and serious complication of PD. The first sign of peritonitis is cloudy dialysate drainage fluid. Diffuse abdominal pain and rebound tenderness occur much later. Hypotension and other signs of shock may also occur with advancing infection. The patient with peritonitis may be treated as an inpatient or outpatient (most common), depending on the severity of the infection and the patient's clinical status. Drainage fluid is examined for cell count; Gram stain and culture are used to identify the organism and guide treatment. Antibiotic agents (aminoglycosides or cephalosporins) are usually added to subsequent exchanges until Gram stain or culture results are available for appropriate antibiotic determination. Intraperitoneal administration of antibiotics is as effective as IV administration and therefore most often used. Antibiotic therapy continues for 10 to 14 days. Careful selection and calculation of the antibiotic dosage are needed to prevent nephrotoxicity and further compromise of residual renal function.

Regardless of which organism causes peritonitis, the patient with peritonitis loses large amounts of protein through the peritoneum. Acute malnutrition and delayed healing may result. Therefore, attention must be given to detecting and promptly treating peritonitis.

Leakage

Leakage of dialysate through the catheter site may occur immediately after the catheter is inserted. Usually, the leak stops spontaneously if dialysis is withheld for several days, giving the tissue surrounding the cuffs located on the abdominal catheter a chance to infiltrate the Dacron and seal the insertion tunnel. It also allows the exit site time to heal. During this time, it is important to reduce factors that might delay healing, such as undue abdominal muscle activity and straining during bowel movement. In many cases, leakage can be avoided by using small volumes (500 mL) of dialysate, gradually increasing the volume up to 2000 to 3000 mL.

Bleeding

A bloody **effluent** (drainage) may be observed occasionally, especially in young, menstruating women. (The hypertonic fluid pulls blood from the uterus, through the opening in the fallopian tubes, and into the peritoneal cavity.) Bleeding is also common during the first few exchanges after a new catheter insertion because some blood enters the abdominal cavity following insertion. In many cases, no cause can be found for the bleeding, although catheter displacement from the pelvis has occasionally been associated with bleeding. Some patients have had bloody effluent after an enema or from minor trauma. Invariably, bleeding stops in 1 to 2 days and requires no specific intervention. More frequent exchanges and the addition of heparin to the dialysate during this time may be necessary to prevent blood clots from obstructing the catheter.

Long-Term Complications

Hypertriglyceridemia is common in patients undergoing long-term PD, suggesting that the therapy may accelerate atherogenesis. Despite this, the use of cardioprotective medications is relatively uncommon, and many patients have suboptimal blood pressure control. Given the high burden of disease in these patients, beta-blockers and ACE inhibitors should be used to control hypertension or protect the heart, and the use of aspirin and statins should be considered.

Other complications that may occur with long-term PD include abdominal hernias (incisional, inguinal, diaphragmatic, and umbilical), probably resulting from continuously increased intra-abdominal pressure. The persistently elevated intra-abdominal pressure also aggravates symptoms of hiatal hernia and hemorrhoids. Low back pain and anorexia from fluid in the abdomen and a constant sweet taste related to glucose absorption may also occur.

Mechanical problems occasionally occur and may interfere with instillation or drainage of the dialysate. Formation of clots in the peritoneal catheter and constipation are factors that may contribute to these problems.

Approaches

PD can be performed using several different approaches: acute intermittent peritoneal dialysis, **continuous ambulatory peritoneal dialysis (CAPD),** and **continuous cyclic peritoneal dialysis (CCPD).**

Acute Intermittent Peritoneal Dialysis

Indications for acute intermittent PD, a variation of PD, include uremic signs and symptoms (nausea, vomiting, fatigue, altered mental status), fluid overload, acidosis, and hyperkalemia. Although PD is not as efficient as hemodial-

ysis in removing solute and fluid, it permits a more gradual change in the patient's fluid volume status and in waste product removal. Therefore, it may be the treatment of choice for the hemodynamically unstable patient. It can be carried out manually (the nurse warms, spikes, and hangs each container of dialysate) or by a cycler machine. Exchange times range from 30 minutes to 2 hours. A common routine is hourly exchanges consisting of a 10-minute infusion, a 30-minute dwell time, and a 20-minute drain time.

Maintaining the PD cycle is a nursing responsibility. Strict aseptic technique is maintained when changing solution containers and emptying drainage containers. Vital signs, weight, I&O, laboratory values, and patient status are frequently monitored. The nurse uses a flow sheet to document each exchange and records vital signs, dialysate concentration, medications added, exchange volume, dwell time, dialysate fluid balance for each exchange (fluid lost or gained), and cumulative fluid balance. The nurse also carefully assesses skin turgor and mucous membranes to evaluate fluid status and monitor the patient for edema.

If the peritoneal fluid does not drain properly, the nurse can facilitate drainage by turning the patient from side to side or raising the head of the bed. The catheter should never be pushed further into the peritoneal cavity. Other measures to promote drainage include checking the patency of the catheter by inspecting for kinks, closed clamps, or an air lock. The nurse monitors for complications, including peritonitis, bleeding, respiratory difficulty, and leakage of peritoneal fluid. Abdominal girth may be measured periodically to determine if the patient is retaining large amounts of dialysis solution. Additionally, the nurse must ensure that the PD catheter remains secure and that the dressing remains dry. Physical comfort measures, frequent turning, and skin care are provided. The patient and family are educated about the procedure and are kept informed about progress (fluid loss, weight loss, laboratory values). Emotional support and encouragement are given to the patient and family during this stressful and uncertain time.

Continuous Ambulatory Peritoneal Dialysis

CAPD is the second most common form of dialysis for patients with ESRD to be started on (USRDS, 2007). CAPD is performed at home by the patient or a trained caregiver who is usually a family member. The procedure allows the patient reasonable freedom and control of daily activities but requires a serious commitment to be successful. Chart 44-10 discusses suitability for CAPD.

CAPD works on the same principles as other forms of PD: diffusion and osmosis. Less extreme fluctuations in the patient's laboratory values occur with CAPD than with intermittent PD or hemodialysis because the dialysis is constantly in progress. The serum electrolyte levels usually remain in the normal range.

Procedure

The patient performs exchanges four or five times a day, 24 hours a day, 7 days a week, at intervals scheduled throughout the day. Different manufacturers supply different equipment. Most commonly used is a Y-shaped system, in which a bag containing dialysate solution comes connected to one branch of the "Y" and a sterile empty

Chart 44-10 • *Considerations in CAPD*

Although CAPD is not suitable for all patients with end-stage renal disease (ESRD), it is a viable therapy for those who can perform self-care and exchanges and who can fit therapy into their own routines. Often, patients report having more energy and feeling healthier once they begin CAPD. Nurses can be instrumental in helping patients with ESRD find the dialysis therapy that best suits their lifestyle. Those considering CAPD need to understand the advantages and disadvantages along with the indications and contraindications for this form of therapy.

Advantages

- Freedom from a dialysis machine
- Control over daily activities
- Opportunities to avoid dietary restrictions, increase fluid intake, raise serum hematocrit values, improve blood pressure control, avoid venipuncture, and gain a sense of well-being

Disadvantages

- Continuous dialysis 24 hours a day, 7 days a week

Indications

- Patient's willingness, motivation, and ability to perform dialysis at home
- Strong family or community support system (essential for success), particularly if the patient is an older adult

- Special problems with long-term hemodialysis, such as dysfunctional or failing vascular access devices, excessive thirst, severe hypertension, postdialysis headaches, and severe anemia requiring frequent transfusion
- Interim therapy while awaiting kidney transplantation
- ESRD secondary to diabetes because hypertension, uremia, and hyperglycemia are easier to manage with CAPD than with hemodialysis

Contraindications

- Adhesions from previous surgery (adhesions reduce clearance of solutes) or systemic inflammatory disease
- Chronic backache and preexisting disk disease, which could be aggravated by the continuous pressure of dialysis fluid in the abdomen
- Risk of complications, for example, in patients receiving immunosuppressive medications, which impede healing of the catheter site, and in patients with a colostomy, ileostomy, nephrostomy, or ileal conduit because of the risk of peritonitis. The risk for complications is not an absolute contraindication for CAPD therapy.
- Diverticulitis because CAPD has been associated with rupture of the diverticulum
- Severe arthritis or poor hand strength necessitating assistance in performing the exchange. However, blind or partially blind patients and those with other physical limitations can learn to perform CAPD.

---

bag is connected to the second branch. This leaves the third part of the "Y" open and available for connection to the transfer set on the PD catheter. To perform an exchange, the patient (or person doing the exchange) washes his or her hands, dons a mask, and then removes the cap from the transfer set while maintaining sterility. The open end of the "Y" set is connected to the end of the transfer set and the dialysate infused where it will dwell. After the dialysate is infused, the patient clamps off the transfer set and the tubing set, disconnects the tubing set, and applies a new cap to the transfer set, making it a closed system. The patient drains the fluid (effluent) from the peritoneal cavity through the catheter (over about 20 to 30 minutes) into an empty bag. Once the effluent has been fully drained, fresh fluid is instilled into the peritoneal cavity.

The longer the dwell time, the better the clearance of uremic toxins is. If dwell time is excessive, the patient will absorb some of the effluent back into the body simply because the osmotic gradient is lost. Once equilibrium is reached, the movement of fluid and toxins stops.

Complications

To reduce the risk of peritonitis, the patient (and all caregivers) must use meticulous care to avoid contaminating the catheter, fluid, or tubing and to avoid accidentally disconnecting the catheter from the tubing. Whenever a connection/disconnection is made, hands must be washed and a mask worn by anyone within 6 feet of the area to avoid contamination with airborne bacteria. Excess manipulation

should be avoided and meticulous care of the catheter entry site is provided using a standardized protocol.

Continuous Cyclic Peritoneal Dialysis

CCPD uses a machine called a cycler to provide the exchanges. It is programmed as to how much fluid to use and how long and how many exchanges need to be done. Since it is programmed, it also keeps track of the total amounts removed and will sound an alarm if limits are not met. It requires that a person set up and break down the system for use, which typically takes about 15 minutes.

CCPD combines overnight intermittent PD with a prolonged dwell time during the day. The peritoneal catheter is connected to a cycler machine every evening, usually just before the patient goes to sleep for the night. Because the machine is very quiet, the patient can sleep, and the extra-long tubing allows the patient to move and turn normally during sleep.

In the morning, the patient disconnects from the cycler. Sometimes dialysate is left in the abdominal cavity for a longer day dwell cycle. This day exchange is drained during the day either by using a "Y" set or reattaching to the cycler. This process is done every day to achieve the effects of dialysis required.

CCPD has a lower infection rate than other forms of PD because there are fewer opportunities for contamination with bag changes and tubing disconnections. It also allows the patient to be free from exchanges throughout the day, making it possible to engage in work and activities of daily living more freely.

Nursing Management

Meeting Psychosocial Needs

In addition to the complications of PD previously described, patients who elect to do PD may experience altered body image because of the presence of the abdominal catheter, bag, tubing, and cycler. Waist size increases from 1 to 2 inches (or more) with fluid in the abdomen. This affects clothing selection and may make the patient feel "fat." Body image may be so altered that patients do not want to look at or care for the catheter for days or weeks. The nurse may arrange for the patient to talk with other patients who have adapted well to PD. Although some patients have no psychological problems with the catheter—they think of it as their lifeline and as a life-sustaining device—other patients feel they are doing exchanges all day long and have no free time, particularly in the beginning. They may experience depression because they feel overwhelmed with the responsibility of self-care.

Patients undergoing PD may also experience altered sexuality patterns and sexual dysfunction. The patient and partner may be reluctant to engage in sexual activities, partly because of the catheter being psychologically "in the way" of sexual performance. The peritoneal catheter, drainage bag, and about 2 L of dialysate may interfere with the patient's sexual function and body image as well. In patients on CCPD, the presence of the dialysis cycler in the bedroom and the continual connection during the sleeping hours can also cause interference with intimacy. Although these problems may resolve with time, some problems may warrant special counseling. Questions by the nurse about concerns related to sexuality and sexual function often provide the patient with a welcome opportunity to discuss these issues and a first step toward their resolution.

Promoting Home and Community-Based Care

Teaching Patients Self-Care

Patients are taught as inpatients or outpatients to perform PD once their condition is medically stable. Training usually takes 5 days to 2 weeks. Patients are taught according to their own learning ability and knowledge level and only as much at one time as they can handle without feeling uncomfortable or becoming overwhelmed. Education topics for the patient and family who will be performing PD at home are described in Chart 44-11. The use of an adult learning theory–based curriculum may decrease peritonitis and exit site infection rates.

CHART 44-11	HOME CARE CHECKLIST *Peritoneal Dialysis (CAPD or CCPD)*		
At the completion of the home care instruction, the patient or caregiver will be able to:		**PATIENT**	**CAREGIVER**
• Discuss basic information about normal kidney function.		✔	✔
• Discuss basic information about the disease process.		✔	✔
• Discuss the basic principles of peritoneal dialysis.		✔	✔
• Demonstrate catheter and exit site care.		✔	✔
• Demonstrate measurement of vital signs and weight measurement.		✔	✔
• Discuss monitoring and management of fluid balance.		✔	✔
• Discuss basic principles of aseptic technique.		✔	✔
• Demonstrate the CAPD exchange procedure using aseptic technique (CCPD patients should also demonstrate exchange procedure in case of failure or unavailability of cycling machine).		✔	✔
• Demonstrate cycler set-up procedure and maintenance if on CCPD.		✔	✔
• Discuss complications of peritoneal dialysis; prevention, recognition, and management of complications.		✔	✔
• Demonstrate procedure for adding medications to the dialysis solution.		✔	✔
• Demonstrate procedure for obtaining sterile dialysis fluid samples.		✔	✔
• Discuss routine laboratory tests needed and implications of results.		✔	✔
• Discuss dietary restrictions.			
• Discuss medications: name of medications, their actions, potential side effects, and when to contact physician.		✔	✔
• Discuss ordering, storage, and inventory of dialysis supplies.		✔	✔
• Describe plan for follow-up care.		✔	✔
• Demonstrate maintenance of home dialysis records.		✔	✔
• Describe actions in case of emergency.		✔	✔

Because of protein loss with continuous PD, the patient is instructed to eat a high-protein, well-balanced diet. The patient is also encouraged to increase his or her daily fiber intake to help prevent constipation, which can impede the flow of dialysate into or out of the peritoneal cavity. Many patients gain 3 to 5 lb within a month of initiating PD, so they may be asked to limit their carbohydrate intake to avoid excessive weight gain. Potassium, sodium, and fluid restrictions are not usually needed. Patients commonly lose about 2 to 3 L of fluid over and above the volume of dialysate infused into the abdomen during a 24-hour period, permitting a normal fluid intake even in an anephric patient (a patient without kidneys).

Continuing Care

Follow-up care through phone calls, visits to the outpatient department, and continuing home care assists patients in the transition to home and promotes their active participation in their own health care. Patients often depend on checking with the nurse to see if they are making the correct choices about dialysate or control of blood pressure, or simply to discuss a problem.

Patients may be seen by the PD team as outpatients once a month or more often if needed. The exchange procedure is evaluated at that time to see that strict aseptic technique is being used. Blood chemistry values are followed closely to make certain the therapy is adequate for the patient.

If a referral is made for home care, the home care nurse assesses the home environment and suggests modifications to accommodate the equipment and facilities needed to carry out PD. In addition, the nurse assesses the patient's and family's understanding of PD and evaluates their technique in performing PD. Assessments include checking for changes related to renal disease, complications such as peritonitis, and treatment-related problems such as heart failure, inadequate drainage, and weight gain or loss. The nurse continues to reinforce and clarify teaching about PD and renal disease and assesses the patient's and family's progress in coping with the procedure. This is also an opportunity to remind patients about the need to participate in appropriate health promotion activities and health screening (eg, gynecologic examinations, colonoscopy).

Because of the projected high numbers of elderly patients who will develop ESRD, the nursing home or extended care facility is likely to become an increasingly important site for both rehabilitation and long-term management of patients with renal failure.

SPECIAL CONSIDERATIONS: NURSING MANAGEMENT OF THE HOSPITALIZED PATIENT ON DIALYSIS

Whether undergoing hemodialysis or PD, the patient may be hospitalized for treatment of complications related to the dialysis treatment, the underlying renal disorder, or health problems not related to renal dysfunction or its treatment.

Protecting Vascular Access

When the patient undergoing hemodialysis is hospitalized for any reason, care must be taken to protect the vascular access. The nurse assesses the vascular access for patency and takes precautions to ensure that the extremity with the vascular access is not used for measuring blood pressure or for obtaining blood specimens; tight dressings, restraints, or jewelry over the vascular access must be avoided as well.

The bruit, or "thrill," over the venous access site must be evaluated at least every 8 hours. Absence of a palpable thrill or audible bruit may indicate blockage or clotting in the vascular access. Clotting can occur if the patient has an infection anywhere in the body (serum viscosity increases) or if the blood pressure has dropped. When blood flow is reduced through the access for any reason (hypotension, application of blood pressure cuff or tourniquet), the access can clot. If a patient has a hemodialysis catheter or implanted hemodialysis access device, the nurse must observe for signs and symptoms of infection such as redness, swelling, drainage from the exit site, fever, and chills. The nurse must assess the integrity of the dressing and change it as needed. Patients with renal disease are more prone to infection; therefore, infection control measures must be used for all procedures.

Taking Precautions During Intravenous Therapy

When the patient needs IV therapy, the rate of administration must be as slow as possible and should be strictly controlled by a volumetric infusion pump. Because patients on dialysis cannot excrete water, rapid or excessive administration of IV fluid can result in pulmonary edema. Accurate intake and output records are essential.

Monitoring Symptoms of Uremia

As metabolic end products accumulate, symptoms of uremia worsen. Patients whose metabolic rate accelerates (those receiving corticosteroid medications or parenteral nutrition, those with infections or bleeding disorders, those undergoing surgery) accumulate waste products more quickly and may require daily dialysis. These same patients are more likely than other patients receiving dialysis to experience complications.

Detecting Cardiac and Respiratory Complications

Cardiac and respiratory assessment must be conducted frequently. As fluid builds up, fluid overload, heart failure, and pulmonary edema develop. Crackles in the bases of the lungs may indicate pulmonary edema.

Pericarditis may result from the accumulation of uremic toxins. If not detected and treated promptly, this serious complication may progress to pericardial effusion and cardiac tamponade. Pericarditis is detected by the patient's report of substernal chest pain (if the patient can communicate), low-grade fever (often overlooked), and pericardial friction rub. A pulsus paradoxus (a decrease in blood pressure of more than 10 mm Hg during inspiration) is often present. When pericarditis progresses to effusion, the friction rub disappears, heart sounds become distant and muffled, ECG waves show very low voltage, and the pulsus paradoxus worsens.

The effusion may progress to life-threatening cardiac tamponade, noted by narrowing of the pulse pressure in addition to muffled or inaudible heart sounds, crushing chest pain, dyspnea, and hypotension. Although pericarditis, pericardial effusion, and cardiac tamponade can be detected by chest x-ray, they should also be detected through astute nursing assessment. Because of their clinical significance, assessment of the patient for these complications is a priority.

Controlling Electrolyte Levels and Diet

Electrolyte alterations are common, and potassium changes can be life-threatening. All IV solutions and medications to be administered are evaluated for their electrolyte content. Serum laboratory values are assessed daily. If blood transfusions are required, they may be administered during hemodialysis, if possible, so that excess potassium can be removed. Dietary intake must also be monitored. The patient's frustrations related to dietary restrictions typically increase if the hospital food is unappetizing. The nurse needs to recognize that this may lead to dietary indiscretion and hyperkalemia.

Hypoalbuminemia is an indicator of malnutrition in patients undergoing long-term or maintenance dialysis. Although some patients can be treated with adequate nutrition alone, some patients remain hypoalbuminemic for reasons that are poorly understood.

Managing Discomfort and Pain

Complications such as pruritus and pain secondary to neuropathy must be managed. Antihistamine agents, such as diphenhydramine hydrochloride (Benadryl), are commonly used, and analgesic medications may be prescribed. However, because elimination of the metabolites of medications occurs through dialysis rather than through renal excretion, medication dosages may need to be adjusted. Keeping the skin clean and well moisturized using bath oils, superfatted soap, and creams or lotions helps promote comfort and reduce itching. Teaching the patient to keep the nails trimmed to avoid scratching and excoriation also promotes comfort.

Monitoring Blood Pressure

Hypertension in renal failure is common. It is usually the result of fluid overload and, in part, oversecretion of renin. Many patients undergoing dialysis receive some form of antihypertensive therapy and require ongoing teaching about its purpose and adverse effects. The trial-and-error approach that may be necessary to identify the most effective antihypertensive agent and dosage may confuse the patient if no explanation is provided. Antihypertensive agents must be withheld before dialysis to avoid hypotension due to the combined effect of the dialysis and the medication.

Typically these patients require single or multiple antihypertensive agents to achieve normal blood pressure, thus adding to the total number of medications needed on an ongoing basis.

Preventing Infection

Patients with ESRD commonly have low WBC counts (and decreased phagocytic ability), low RBC counts (anemia), and impaired platelet function. Together, these pose a high risk for infection and potential for bleeding after even minor trauma. Preventing and controlling infection are essential because the incidence of infection is high. Infection of the vascular access site and pneumonia are common.

Caring for the Catheter Site

Patients receiving CAPD usually know how to care for the catheter site; however, the hospital stay is an opportunity to assess catheter care technique and correct misperceptions or deviations from recommended technique. Recommended daily or three-or-four-times-weekly routine catheter site care is typically performed during showering or bathing. The exit site should not be submerged in bath water. The most common cleaning method is soap and water; liquid soap is recommended. During care, the nurse and patient need to make sure that the catheter remains secure to avoid tension and trauma. The patient may wear a gauze or semi-transparent dressing over the exit site.

Administering Medications

All medications and the dosage prescribed for any patient on dialysis must be closely monitored to avoid those that are toxic to the kidneys and may threaten remaining renal function. Medications are also scrutinized for potassium and magnesium content, because medications containing potassium or magnesium must be avoided. Care must be taken to evaluate all problems and symptoms that the patient reports without automatically attributing them to renal failure or to dialysis therapy.

Providing Psychological Support

Patients undergoing dialysis for a while may begin to reevaluate their status, the treatment modality, their satisfaction with life, and the impact of these factors on their families and support systems. Nurses must provide opportunities for these patients to express their feelings and reactions and to explore options. The decision to begin dialysis does not require that dialysis be continued indefinitely, and it is not uncommon for patients to consider discontinuing treatment. These feelings and reactions must be taken seriously, and the patient should have the opportunity to discuss them with the dialysis team as well as with a psychologist, psychiatrist, psychiatric nurse, trusted friend, or spiritual advisor. The patient's informed decision about discontinuing treatment, after thoughtful deliberation, should be respected.

KIDNEY SURGERY

A patient may undergo surgery to remove obstructions that affect the kidney (tumors or calculi), to insert a tube for draining the kidney (nephrostomy, ureterostomy), or to remove the kidney involved in unilateral kidney disease, renal carcinoma, or kidney transplantation.

Management of Patients Undergoing Kidney Surgery

Preoperative Considerations

Surgery is performed only after a thorough evaluation of renal function. Patient preparation to ensure that optimal renal function is maintained is essential. Fluids are encouraged to promote increased excretion of waste products before surgery unless contraindicated because of preexisting renal or cardiac dysfunction. If kidney infection is present preoperatively, broad-spectrum antimicrobial agents may be prescribed to prevent bacteremia. Antibiotic agents must be given with extreme care because many are toxic to the kidneys. Coagulation studies (prothrombin time, partial thromboplastin time, platelet count) may be indicated if the patient has a history of bruising and bleeding. The preoperative preparation is similar to that described in Chapter 18.

Because many patients facing kidney surgery are apprehensive, the nurse encourages the patient to recognize and verbalize concerns. Confidence is reinforced by establishing a relationship of trust and by providing expert care. Patients faced with the prospect of losing a kidney may think that they will be dependent on dialysis for the rest of their lives. It is important to teach the patient and family that normal function may be maintained by a single healthy kidney.

Perioperative Concerns

Renal surgery requires various patient positions to expose the surgical site adequately. Three surgical approaches are common: flank, lumbar, and thoracoabdominal (Fig. 44-9). During surgery, plans are carried out for managing altered urinary drainage. These may include inserting a nephrostomy or other drainage tube.

Postoperative Management

Because the kidney is a highly vascular organ, hemorrhage and shock are the chief complications of renal surgery. Fluid and blood component replacement is frequently necessary in the immediate postoperative period to treat intraoperative blood loss.

Abdominal distention and paralytic ileus are fairly common after renal and ureteral surgery and are thought to be due to a reflex paralysis of intestinal peristalsis and manipulation of the colon or duodenum during surgery. Abdominal distention is relieved by decompression through a nasogastric tube (see Chapter 38 for treatment of paralytic ileus). Oral fluids are permitted when the passage of flatus is noted.

If infection occurs, antibiotics are prescribed after a culture reveals the causative organism. The toxic effects that antibiotic agents have on the kidneys (nephrotoxicity) must be kept in mind when assessing the patient. Low-dose heparin therapy may be initiated postoperatively to prevent thromboembolism in patients who had any type of urologic surgery.

Nursing Management

In addition to those interventions listed in this section, Chart 44-12 provides a plan of nursing care for the patient undergoing kidney surgery.

Providing Immediate Postoperative Care

Immediate postoperative care of the patient who has undergone surgery of the kidney includes assessment of all body systems. Respiratory and circulatory status, pain level, fluid and electrolyte status, and patency and adequacy of urinary drainage systems are assessed.

Respiratory Status

As with any surgery, the use of anesthesia increases the risk for respiratory complications. Noting the location of the surgical incision assists the nurse in anticipating respiratory problems and pain. Respiratory status is assessed by monitoring the rate, depth, and pattern of respirations. The location of the incision frequently causes pain on inspiration and coughing; therefore, the patient tends to splint the chest wall and take shallow respirations. Auscultation is performed to assess normal and adventitious breath sounds.

Circulatory Status and Blood Loss

The patient's vital signs and arterial or central venous pressure are monitored. Skin color and temperature and urine output provide information about circulatory status. The surgical incision and drainage tubes are observed frequently to help detect unexpected blood loss and hemorrhage.

Pain

Postoperative pain is a major problem for the patient because of the location of the surgical incision and patient's

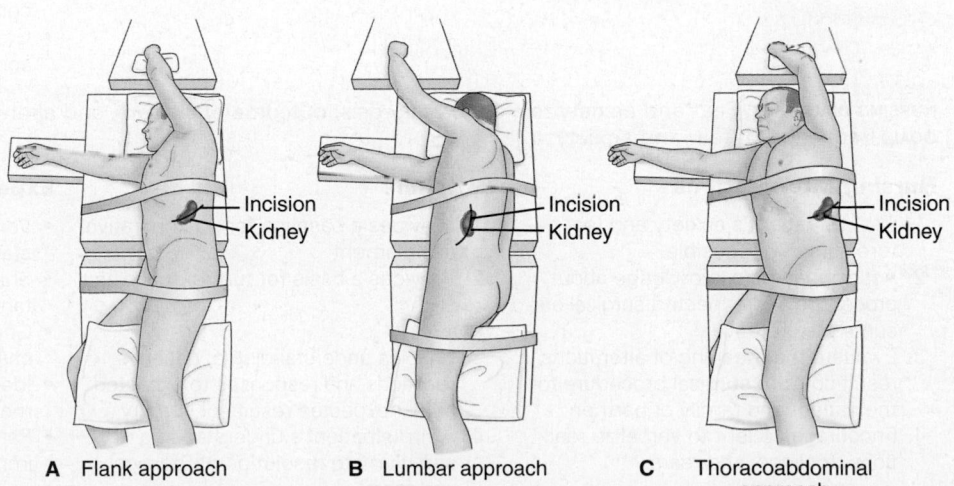

Figure 44-9 Patient positioning and incisional approaches (**A**, flank; **B**, lumbar; **C**, thoracoabdominal) for kidney surgery are associated with significant postoperative discomfort.

A Flank approach   **B** Lumbar approach   **C** Thoracoabdominal approach

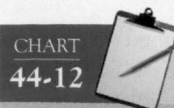

CHART 44-12

PLAN OF NURSING CARE
Care of Patient Undergoing Kidney Surgery

NURSING DIAGNOSIS: Ineffective airway clearance related to pain of high abdominal or flank incision, abdominal discomfort, and immobility; risk for ineffective breathing pattern related to high abdominal incision
GOAL: Improved airway clearance

Nursing Interventions	Rationale	Expected Outcomes
1. Administer analgesic agent as prescribed.	1. Enables patient to take deep breaths and cough	• Takes deep breaths and coughs adequately when encouraged and assisted
2. Splint incision with hands or pillow to assist patient in coughing.	2. Splints incision and promotes adequate cough and prevention of atelectasis	• Exhibits respiratory rate of 12–18 breaths/min
3. Assist patient to change positions frequently.	3. Promotes drainage and inflation of all lobes of the lungs	• Exhibits normal breath sounds without adventitious sounds
4. Encourage use of incentive spirometer if indicated or prescribed.	4. Encourages adequate deep breaths	• Exhibits full thoracic excursion without shallow respirations
5. Assist with and encourage early ambulation.	5. Mobilizes pulmonary secretions	• Uses incentive spirometer with encouragement
		• Splints incision while taking deep breaths and coughing
		• Reports progressively less pain and discomfort with coughing and deep breaths
		• Exhibits normal blood gas levels and chest x-ray
		• Exhibits normal body temperature with no signs of atelectasis or pneumonia on assessment

NURSING DIAGNOSIS: Acute pain and discomfort related to surgical incision, positioning, and stretching of muscles during kidney surgery
GOAL: Relief of pain and discomfort

Nursing Interventions	Rationale	Expected Outcomes
1. Assess level of pain.	1. Provides baseline for later evaluation of pain relief strategies	• Reports relief of severe pain and discomfort
2. Administer analgesic agents as prescribed.	2. Promotes pain relief	• Takes analgesia as prescribed
3. Splint incision with hands or pillow during movement or deep breathing and coughing exercises.	3. Minimizes sensation of pulling or tension on incision and provides sense of support to the patient	• Exercises aching muscles within recommendations
		• Uses distraction, relaxation exercises, and imagery to relieve pain
4. Assist and encourage early ambulation.	4. Promotes resumption of muscle activity exercise	• Exhibits no behavioral manifestations of pain and discomfort (eg, restlessness, perspiration, verbal expressions of pain)
		• Participates in deep-breathing and coughing exercises
		• Gradually increases physical activity and exercise

NURSING DIAGNOSIS: Fear and anxiety related to diagnosis, outcome of surgery, and alteration in urinary function
GOAL: Reduction of fear and anxiety

Nursing Interventions	Rationale	Expected Outcomes
1. Assess patient's anxiety and fear before surgery if possible.	1. Provides a baseline for postoperative assessment	• Verbalizes reactions and feelings to staff
2. Assess patient's knowledge about procedure and expected surgical outcome preoperatively.	2. Provides a basis for further teaching	• Shares reactions and feelings with family or partner
3. Evaluate the meaning of alterations resulting from surgical procedure for the patient and family or partner.	3. Enables understanding of patient's reactions and responses to expected and unexpected results of surgery	• Grieves appropriately for self and for changes in role and function
		• Identifies information needed to promote own adaptation and coping
4. Encourage patient to verbalize reactions, feelings, and fears.	4. Affirms patient's understanding of and ultimate resolution of feelings and fears	• Participates in activities and events in immediate environment

Continued

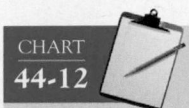

CHART
44-12

PLAN OF NURSING CARE
Care of Patient Undergoing Kidney Surgery (Continued)

Nursing Interventions	Rationale	Expected Outcomes
5. Encourage patient to share feelings with spouse or partner. 6. Offer and arrange for visit from member of support group (eg, ostomy group, if indicated).	5. Enables patient and partner to receive mutual support and reduces sense of isolation from each other 6. Provides support from another person who has encountered the same or a similar surgical procedure and an example of how others have coped with the alteration	• Accepts visit from ostomy group if indicated • Identifies support person or support group

NURSING DIAGNOSIS: Impaired urinary elimination related to urinary drainage; risk for infection related to altered urinary drainage
GOAL: Maintenance of urinary elimination; infection-free urinary tract

Nursing Interventions	Rationale	Expected Outcomes
1. Assess urinary drainage system immediately.	1. Provides basis for further assessment and action	• Exhibits adequate urinary output and patent drainage system
2. Assess adequacy of urinary output and patency of drainage system.	2. Provides baseline	• Exhibits urinary output consistent with fluid intake
3. Use asepsis and hand hygiene when providing care and manipulating drainage system.	3. Prevents or reduces risk of contamination of urinary drainage system	• Demonstrates normal laboratory values: BUN, serum creatinine levels, urine specific gravity, and osmolality
4. Maintain closed urinary drainage system.	4. Reduces risk of bacterial contamination and infection	• Exhibits sterile urine on urine culture
5. If irrigation of the drainage system is necessary, use sterile gloves and sterile irrigating solution and a closed drainage and irrigation system.	5. Permits irrigation when necessary while maintaining closed drainage system, minimizing risk of infection	• Exhibits clear, dilute urine without debris or encrustation in the drainage system
6. If irrigation is necessary and prescribed, perform it gently with sterile saline and the prescribed amount of irrigating fluid.	6. Maintains patency of the catheter or drainage system and prevents sudden increases in pressure in the urinary tract that may cause trauma, pressure on sutures or urinary tract structures, and pain	• States rationale for avoiding manipulation of catheter, drainage, or irrigation system • Exhibits normal placement of urinary stent or ureteral catheters until removed by physician
7. Assist patient in turning and moving in bed and when ambulating to prevent displacement or inadvertent removal of urinary stent or ureteral catheters if in place.	7. Prevents trauma from accidental displacement of urinary stent or ureteral catheter necessitating repeated instrumentation of the urinary tract (eg, cystoscopy) to replace them	• Maintains closed urinary drainage system • Exhibits normal body temperature without signs or symptoms of urinary tract infection
8. Observe urine color, volume, odor, and components.	8. Provides information about adequacy of urine output, condition and patency of drainage system, and debris in urine	• Cleans catheter with soap and water • Consumes adequate fluid intake (6 to 8 glasses of water or more per day, unless contraindicated)
9. Minimize trauma and manipulation of catheter, drainage system, and urethra.	9. Reduces risk of contamination of drainage system and eliminates site of bacterial invasion	• Urinary drainage system remains in place until physician removes or discontinues it
10. Clean catheter gently with soap during bath, avoiding any to-and-fro movement of catheter.	10. Removes debris and encrustations without causing trauma to or contamination of urethra	• Maintains urinary drainage system without infection or obstruction
11. Anchor drainage tube.	11. Prevents movement or slipping of drainage tube, minimizing trauma to and contamination of urethra or catheter	• Maintains urinary diversion as instructed
12. Maintain adequate fluid intake.	12. Promotes adequate urine output and prevents urinary stasis	• Maintains self-care so that environment is odor-free
13. Assist with and encourage early ambulation while ensuring placement of urinary drainage system.	13. Minimizes cardiovascular and pulmonary complications while preventing loss, dislodging, or disruption of drainage system	• States rationale for close follow-up and maintains recommended schedule of appointments with health care providers
14. If patient is to be discharged with urinary drainage system (catheter) in place or a urinary diversion, instruct patient and family member in care.	14. Knowledge and understanding of the drainage system or urinary diversion are essential to prevent infection and other complications.	

Continued on following page

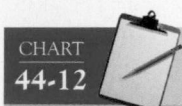

PLAN OF NURSING CARE

CHART 44-12   *Care of Patient Undergoing Kidney Surgery (Continued)*

NURSING DIAGNOSIS: Risk for imbalanced fluid volume related to surgical fluid loss, altered urinary output, parenteral fluid administration

GOAL: Normal fluid balance will be maintained

Nursing Interventions	Rationale	Expected Outcomes
1. Weigh patient daily.	1. Daily weight is the most sensitive indicator of fluid loss or gain.	• Patient's weight will be within 2–3 lb of patient's baseline.
2. Take accurate intake and output measurements.	2. Detects fluid retention due to poor cardiac or renal output	• Intake that exceeds output will be detected early.
3. Place all parenteral therapy on an infusion pump.	3. Ensures that the patient does not receive excess or insufficient intravenous fluids	• The exact amount of solution is infused with no adverse effects resulting from overinfusion or underinfusion.
4. Monitor amount and characteristics of urine.	4. Assists in early detection of possible complications of surgery or tube insertion	• Urine is clear and absent of blood, pus, or any foreign substances.
5. Monitor vital signs: temperature, pulse, respirations, and blood pressure.	5. When fluid volume or cardiac output is altered, vital signs are affected.	• Temperature, pulse, respiration, and blood pressure are normal.
6. Auscultate heart and lungs every shift.	6. When fluid volume is increased because of poor cardiac or renal output, fluid accumulates in the lungs. Also, heart sounds change as heart failure develops; frequent auscultation ensures early detection.	• Normal heart and lung sounds are present.

position on the operating table to permit access to the kidney. The location and severity of pain are assessed before and after analgesic medications are administered. Abdominal distention, which increases discomfort, is also noted.

Urinary Drainage

Urine output and drainage from tubes inserted during surgery are monitored for amount, color, and type or characteristics. Decreased or absent drainage is promptly reported to the physician because it may indicate obstruction that could cause pain, infection, and disruption of the suture lines.

Monitoring and Managing Potential Complications

Bleeding is a major complication of kidney surgery. If undetected and untreated it can result in hypovolemia and hemorrhagic shock. The nurse's role is to observe for these complications, to report their signs and symptoms, and to administer prescribed parenteral fluids and blood and blood components. Monitoring of vital signs, skin condition, the urinary drainage system, the surgical incision, and the level of consciousness is necessary to detect evidence of bleeding, decreased circulating blood, and fluid volume and cardiac output. Frequent monitoring of vital signs (initially monitored at least at hourly intervals) and urinary output is necessary for early detection of these complications.

If bleeding goes undetected or is not detected promptly, the patient may lose significant amounts of blood and may experience hypoxemia. In addition to hypovolemic shock due to hemorrhage, this type of blood loss may precipitate a myocardial infarction or transient ischemic attack. Bleeding may be suspected when the patient experiences fatigue and when urine output is less than 30 mL/h. As bleeding

persists, late signs of hypovolemia occur, such as cool skin, flat neck veins, and change in level of consciousness or responsiveness. Transfusions of blood components are indicated, along with surgical repair of the bleeding vessel.

Pneumonia may be prevented through use of an incentive spirometer, adequate pain control, and early ambulation. Early signs of pneumonia include fever, increased heart and respiratory rates, and adventitious breath sounds.

Preventing infection is the rationale for using asepsis when changing dressings and handling and preparing catheters, other drainage tubes, central venous catheters, and IV catheters for administration of fluids. Insertion sites are monitored closely for signs and symptoms of inflammation: redness, drainage, heat, and pain. Special care must be taken to prevent urinary tract infection, which is associated with the use of indwelling urinary catheters. Catheters and other invasive tubes are removed as soon as they are no longer needed.

Antibiotics are commonly administered postoperatively to prevent infection. If antibiotic agents are prescribed, serum creatinine and BUN values must be monitored closely because many antibiotic agents are toxic to the kidney or can accumulate to toxic levels if renal function is decreased.

Preventing fluid imbalance is critical when caring for a patient undergoing kidney surgery, because both fluid loss and fluid excess are possible adverse effects of the surgery. Fluid loss may occur during surgery as a result of excessive urinary drainage when the obstruction is removed, or it may occur if diuretic agents are used. Such loss may also occur with GI losses, with diarrhea resulting from antibiotic use, or with nasogastric drainage. When postoperative IV therapy is inadequate to match the output or fluids lost, a fluid deficit results. Fluid excess, or overload, may result from cardiac effects of anesthesia, administration of excessive amounts of fluids, or the patient's inability to excrete fluid because of changes in renal function. Decreased urine output may be an indication of fluid excess.

Astute assessment skills are needed to detect early signs of fluid excess (such as weight gain, pedal edema, urine output below 30 mL/h, and slightly elevated pulmonary wedge pressure, if available) before they become severe (appearance of adventitious breath sounds, shortness of breath).

Fluid excess may be treated with fluid restriction and administration of furosemide (Lasix) or other diuretic agents. If renal insufficiency is present, these medications may prove ineffective; therefore, dialysis may be necessary to prevent heart failure and pulmonary edema.

Deep venous thrombosis (DVT) may occur postoperatively because of surgical manipulation of the iliac vessels during surgery or prolonged immobility. Anti-embolism stockings are applied, and the patient is monitored closely for signs and symptoms of thrombosis and encouraged to exercise the legs. Heparin may be administered postoperatively to reduce the risk of thrombosis.

Promoting Home and Community-Based Care

Teaching Patients Self-Care

If the patient has a drainage system in place, measures are taken to ensure that both the patient and family understand the importance of maintaining the system correctly at home and preventing infection. Verbal and written instructions and guidelines are provided to the patient and family at the time of hospital discharge. The patient may be asked to demonstrate management of the drainage system to ensure understanding. The importance of strategies to prevent postoperative complications (urinary tract infection and obstruction, DVT, atelectasis, and pneumonia) is stressed to the patient and family. Those signs, symptoms, problems, and questions that should be referred to the physician or other primary health care provider are reviewed by the nurse with the patient and family.

Continuing Care

The need for postoperative assessment and care after renal surgery continues regardless of the setting: the home, subacute care unit, outpatient clinic or office, or rehabilitation facility. Referral for home care is indicated for the patient going home with a urinary drainage system in place. During the home visit, the home care nurse reviews the instructions and guidelines given to the patient at hospital discharge. The nurse assesses the patient's ability to carry out the instructions in the home and answers questions that the patient or family has about management of the drainage system and the surgical incision.

Additionally, the home care nurse obtains vital signs and assesses the patient for signs and symptoms of urinary tract infection and obstruction. The nurse also ensures that pain is adequately controlled and that the patient is complying with recommendations. The home care nurse encourages adequate fluid intake and increased levels of activity. Together the nurse, patient, and family review the signs, symptoms, problems, and questions that should be referred to the physician or other primary health care provider. If the patient has a drainage tube in place, the nurse assesses the site and the patency of the system and monitors the patient for complications, such as DVT, bleeding, or pneumonia.

Because it is easy for the patient, family, and health care team to focus on the patient's immediate disorder to the exclusion of other health issues, the nurse reminds the patient and family about the importance of participating in health promotion activities, including health screening.

Kidney Transplantation

Kidney transplantation has become the treatment of choice for most patients with ESRD. During the past 40 years, more than 400,000 kidney transplantations have been performed worldwide, and approximately 9000 are performed in the United States each year. In the United States, there are many more patients on the waiting list for kidney transplantation than there are organ donors (Danovitch, 2005). Patients choose kidney transplantation for various reasons, such as the desire to avoid dialysis or to improve their sense of well-being and the wish to lead a more normal life. Additionally, the cost of maintaining a successful transplantation is one-third the cost of dialysis treatment. Kidney transplantation is an elective procedure, not an emergency life-saving procedure. Therefore, patients should be in the best possible condition prior to transplantation.

Kidney transplantation involves transplanting a kidney from a living donor or deceased donor to a recipient who no longer has renal function (Chart 44-13). A living donor is a person who is alive at the time of donation and may or may not be related to the recipient. A deceased or cadaveric transplant comes from someone who has died and donated his or her organs. Transplantation from well-matched living donors who are related to the patient (those with compatible ABO and human leukocyte antigens) is slightly more successful than from cadaver donors. The success rate further increases if kidney transplantation from a living donor is performed before dialysis is initiated (Danovitch, 2005).

Prior to either receiving or donating an organ, an extensive medical evaluation is performed. Not everyone is suitable

---

Chart 44-13 • *Kidney Donation*

An inadequate number of available kidneys remains the greatest limitation to treating patients with end-stage renal disease successfully. For those interested in donating a kidney, the National Kidney Foundation provides written information describing the organ donation program and a card specifying the organs to be donated in the event of death.

The organ donation card is signed by the donor and two witnesses and should be carried by the donor at all times. Procurement of an adequate number of kidneys for potential recipients is still a major problem, despite national legislation that requires relatives of deceased patients or patients declared brain-dead to be asked if they would consider organ donation.

In some states in the United States, drivers can indicate their desire to be organ donors on their driver's license application or renewal.

for a kidney transplant. Contraindications include recent malignancy, active or chronic infection, severe irreversible extrarenal disease (eg, inoperable cardiac disease, chronic lung disease, severe peripheral vascular disease), active autoimmune disease (eg, HIV, hepatitis B and C), morbid obesity (body mass index greater than 35), current substance abuse, inability to give informed consent, and history of nonadherence to treatment regimens (Counts, 2008). Donors may be rejected for the same reasons or any condition that is determined to have an impact on the remaining kidney. Examples include hypertension and diabetes mellitus since both are known causes of renal disease. It is imperative when donors are evaluated that serious consideration be given to the overall long-term health of the donor. Every precaution must be taken to ensure that the remaining kidney in the donor will remain healthy. If these conditions are met, the donor should remain healthy after donation and have a normal lifespan. Since one kidney can easily handle the body's needs, no long-term adjustments will need to be made.

The patient's native kidneys are not usually removed. The transplanted kidney is placed in the patient's iliac fossa anterior to the iliac crest because it allows for easier access to the blood supply needed to perfuse the kidney. The ureter of the newly transplanted kidney is transplanted into the bladder or anastomosed to the ureter of the recipient (Fig. 44-10). Once the blood supply has been reestablished to the transplanted kidney in the operating room, urine should begin to flow. The production of urine at this stage is an important indicator of the overall success of the procedure and ultimate long-term outcome.

Preoperative Management

Preoperative management goals include bringing the patient's metabolic state to a level as close to normal as possible, making sure that the patient is free of infection, and preparing the patient for surgery and the postoperative course.

Medical Management

A complete physical examination is performed to detect and treat any conditions that could cause complications after transplantation. Tissue typing, blood typing, and antibody screening are performed to determine compatibility of the tissues and cells of the donor and recipient. Other diagnostic tests must be completed to identify conditions requiring treatment before transplantation. The lower urinary tract is studied to assess bladder neck function and to detect ureteral reflux.

The patient must be free of infection at the time of renal transplantation, because after surgery medications to prevent transplant rejection will be prescribed. These medications suppress the immune response, leaving the patient immunosuppressed and at risk for infection. Therefore, the patient is evaluated and treated for any infections, including gingival (gum) disease and dental caries.

A psychosocial evaluation is conducted to assess the patient's ability to adjust to the transplant, coping styles, social history, social support available, and financial resources. A history of psychiatric illness is important to obtain because psychiatric conditions are often aggravated by the corticosteroids needed for immunosuppression after transplantation. If a dialysis routine has been established, hemodialysis is often performed the day before the scheduled transplantation procedure to optimize the patient's physical status.

Nursing Management

The nursing aspects of preoperative care for the patient undergoing renal transplant are similar to those for patients undergoing other types of kidney or elective abdominal surgery. Preoperative teaching can be conducted in a variety of settings, including the outpatient preadmission area, the hospital, or the transplantation clinic during the preliminary workup phase. Patient teaching addresses postoperative pulmonary hygiene, pain management options, dietary

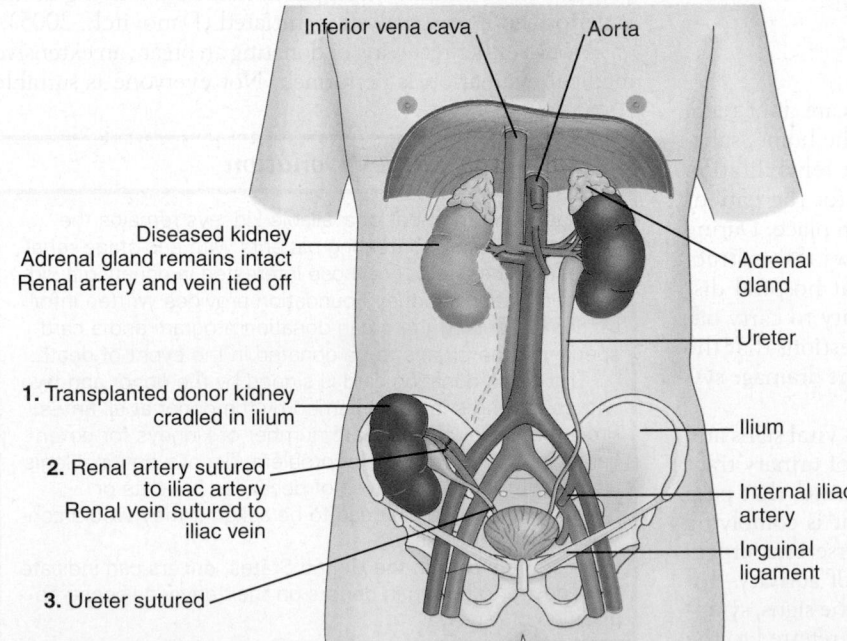

Diseased kidney
Adrenal gland remains intact
Renal artery and vein tied off

Inferior vena cava

Aorta

Adrenal gland

Ureter

1. Transplanted donor kidney cradled in ilium

2. Renal artery sutured to iliac artery
Renal vein sutured to iliac vein

Ilium

Internal iliac artery

Inguinal ligament

3. Ureter sutured

Figure 44-10 Renal transplantation: **1,** The transplanted kidney is placed in the iliac fossa. **2,** The renal artery of the donated kidney is sutured to the ileac artery, and the renal vein is sutured to the iliac vein. **3,** The ureter of the donated kidney is sutured to the bladder or to the patient's ureter.

restrictions, IV and arterial lines, tubes (indwelling catheter and possibly a nasogastric tube), and early ambulation. The patient who receives a kidney from a living related donor may be concerned about the donor and how the donor will tolerate the surgical procedure.

Most patients have been on dialysis for months or years before transplantation. Many have waited months to years for a kidney transplant and are anxious about the surgery, possible rejection, and the need to return to dialysis. Helping the patient to deal with these concerns is part of the nurse's role in preoperative management, as is teaching the patient about what to expect after surgery.

Postoperative Management

The goal of care is to maintain homeostasis until the transplanted kidney is functioning well. The patient whose kidney functions immediately has a more favorable prognosis than the patient whose kidney does not.

Medical Management

After a kidney transplant, rejection and failure can occur within 24 hours (hyperacute), within 3 to 14 days (acute), or after many years. The long-term survival of a transplanted kidney depends on how well it matches the recipient and how well the body's immune response is controlled. Since the body's immune system views the transplanted kidney as "foreign," it continually works to reject it. To overcome or minimize the body's defense mechanisms, immunosuppressive agents are administered. Optimally, medications modify the immune system enough to prevent rejection, but not enough to allow infections or malignancies to occur.

Combinations of glucocorticoids and medications specifically developed to affect the action of lymphocytes are used to minimize the body's reaction to the transplanted organ. Treatment with combinations of new agents has dramatically improved survival rates, and now 90% to 95% of transplanted kidneys still function after 1 year (American Nephrology Nurses Association, 2007b). Doses of immunosuppressive agents are often adjusted depending on the patient's immunologic response to the transplant. However, the patient will be required to take some form of immunosuppressive therapy for the entire time that he or she has the transplanted kidney.

The risks associated with taking these medications include nephrotoxicity, hypertension, hyperlipidemia, hirsutism, tremors, blood dyscrasias, cataracts, gingival hyperplasia, and several types of cancer (American Nephrology Nurses Association, 2006).

Nursing Management

Assessing the Patient for Transplant Rejection

After kidney transplantation, the nurse assesses the patient for signs and symptoms of transplant rejection: oliguria, edema, fever, increasing blood pressure, weight gain, and swelling or tenderness over the transplanted kidney or graft. Patients receiving cyclosporine may not exhibit the usual signs and symptoms of acute rejection. In these patients, the only sign may be an asymptomatic rise in the serum creatinine level (more than a 20% rise is considered acute rejection).

Preventing Infection

The results of blood chemistry tests and leukocyte and platelet counts are monitored closely because immunosuppression depresses the formation of leukocytes and platelets. The patient is closely monitored for infection because of susceptibility to impaired healing and infection related to immunosuppressive therapy and complications of renal failure. Clinical manifestations of infection include shaking chills, fever, rapid heartbeat (tachycardia), and respirations (tachypnea), as well as either an increase or a decrease in WBCs (leukocytosis or leukopenia).

Infection may be introduced through the urinary tract, the respiratory tract, the surgical site, or other sources. Urine cultures are performed frequently because of the high incidence of bacteriuria during early and late stages of transplantation. Any type of wound drainage should be viewed as a potential source of infection because drainage is an excellent culture medium for bacteria. Catheter and drain tips may be cultured when removed by cutting off the tip of the catheter or drain (using aseptic technique) and placing the tip in a sterile container to be taken to the laboratory for culture (Chart 44-14).

The nurse ensures that the patient is protected from exposure to infection by hospital staff, visitors, and other

Chart 44-14 • *Renal Transplant Rejection and Infection*

Renal graft rejection and failure may occur within 24 hours (hyperacute), within 3 to 14 days (acute), or after many years (chronic). It is not uncommon for rejection to occur during the first year after transplantation.

Detecting Rejection

Ultrasonography may be used to detect enlargement of the kidney; percutaneous renal biopsy (most reliable) and x-ray techniques are used to evaluate transplant rejection. If the body rejects the transplanted kidney, the patient needs to return to dialysis. The rejected kidney may or may not be removed, depending on when the rejection occurs (acute versus chronic) and the risk for infection if the kidney is left in place.

Potential Infection

About 75% of kidney transplant recipients have at least one episode of infection in the first year after transplantation because of immunosuppressant therapy. Immunosuppressants of the past made the transplant recipient more vulnerable to opportunistic infections (candidiasis, cytomegalovirus, *Pneumocystis* pneumonia) and infection with other relatively nonpathogenic viruses, fungi, and protozoa, which can be a major hazard. Cyclosporine therapy has reduced the incidence of opportunistic infections because it selectively exerts its effect, sparing T cells that protect the patient from life-threatening infections. In addition, combination immunosuppressant therapy and improved clinical care have produced 1-year patient survival rates approaching 100% and graft survival exceeding 90%. Infections, however, remain a major cause of death at all points in time for kidney transplant recipients (Danovitch, 2005).

patients with active infections. Attention to hand hygiene by all who come in contact with the patient is imperative.

Monitoring Urinary Function

A kidney from a living donor related to the patient usually begins to function immediately after surgery and may produce large quantities of dilute urine. A kidney from a cadaver donor may undergo acute tubular necrosis and therefore may not function for 2 or 3 weeks, during which time anuria, oliguria, or polyuria may be present. During this stage, the patient may experience significant changes in fluid and electrolyte status. Therefore, careful monitoring is indicated. The output from the urinary catheter (connected to a closed drainage system) is measured every hour. IV fluids are administered on the basis of urine volume and serum electrolyte levels and as prescribed by the physician. Hemodialysis may be necessary postoperatively to maintain homeostasis until the transplanted kidney is functioning well. It also may be required if fluid overload and hyperkalemia occur. After successful renal transplantation, the vascular access device may clot, possibly from improved coagulation with the return of renal function. The vascular access for hemodialysis is monitored to ensure patency and to evaluate for evidence of infection.

Addressing Psychological Concerns

The rejection of a transplanted kidney is of great concern to the patient, the family, and the health care team for many months. The fear of kidney rejection and the complications of immunosuppressive therapy (Cushing's syndrome, diabetes, capillary fragility, osteoporosis, glaucoma, cataracts, acne, nephrotoxicity) place tremendous psychological stress on the patient. Anxiety and uncertainty about the future and difficult posttransplantation adjustment are often sources of stress for the patient and family.

An important nursing function is the assessment of the patient's stress and coping. The nurse uses each visit with the patient to determine if the patient and family are coping effectively and the patient is adhering to the prescribed medication regimen. If indicated or requested, the nurse refers the patient for counseling.

Monitoring and Managing Potential Complications

The patient undergoing kidney transplantation is at risk for the postoperative complications that are associated with any surgical procedure. In addition, the patient's physical condition may be compromised because of the effects of long-standing renal failure and its treatment. Therefore, careful assessment for the complications related to renal failure and those associated with a major surgery are important aspects of nursing care. Breathing exercises, early ambulation, and care of the surgical incision are important aspects of postoperative care.

GI ulceration and corticosteroid-induced bleeding may occur. Fungal colonization of the GI tract (especially the mouth) and urinary bladder may occur secondary to corticosteroid and antibiotic therapy. Closely monitoring the patient and notifying the physician about the occurrence of these complications are important nursing interventions. In addition, the patient is monitored closely for signs and symptoms of adrenal insufficiency if the treatment has included use of corticosteroids.

Promoting Home and Community-Based Care

Teaching Patients Self-Care. The nurse works closely with the patient and family to be sure that they understand the need for continuing immunosuppressive therapy as prescribed. Additionally, the patient and family are instructed to assess for and report signs and symptoms of transplant rejection, infection, or significant adverse effects of the immunosuppressive regimen. These include decreased urine output; weight gain; malaise; fever; respiratory distress; tenderness over the transplanted kidney; anxiety; depression; changes in eating, drinking, or other habits; and changes in blood pressure. The patient is instructed to inform other health care providers (eg, dentist) about the kidney transplant and the use of immunosuppressive agents.

Continuing Care. The patient needs to know that follow-up care after transplantation is a lifelong necessity. Individual verbal and written instructions are provided concerning diet, medication, fluids, daily weight, daily measurement of urine, management of I&O, prevention of infection, resumption of activity, and avoidance of contact sports in which the transplanted kidney may be injured. Because of the risk for other potential complications, the patient is followed closely.

Cardiovascular disease is the major cause of morbidity and mortality after transplantation, due in part to the increasing age of patients with transplants. An additional problem is possible malignancy; patients receiving long-term immunosuppressive therapy are at higher risk for cancers than the general population. So the patient is reminded of the importance of health promotion and health screening.

The American Association of Kidney Patients (listed at the end of this chapter) is a nonprofit organization that serves the needs of those with kidney disease. It can provide many helpful suggestions for patients and family members learning to cope with dialysis and transplantation.

RENAL TRAUMA

The kidneys are protected by the rib cage and musculature of the back posteriorly and by a cushion of abdominal wall and viscera anteriorly. They are highly mobile and are fixed only at the renal pedicle (stem of renal blood vessels and the ureter). With traumatic injury, the kidneys can be thrust against the lower ribs, resulting in contusion and rupture. Rib fractures or fractures of the transverse process of the upper lumbar vertebrae may be associated with renal contusion or laceration. Failure to wear seat belts contributes to the incidence of renal trauma in motor vehicle crashes. Up to 80% of patients with renal trauma have associated injuries of other internal organs.

Injuries may be blunt (automobile and motorcycle crashes, falls, athletic injuries, assaults) or penetrating (gunshot wounds, stabbings). Blunt renal trauma accounts for 80% to 90% of all renal injuries; penetrating renal trauma accounts for the remaining 10% to 20%.

Blunt renal trauma is classified into one of four groups, as follows:

- Contusion: bruises or hemorrhages under the renal capsule; capsule and collecting system intact

- Minor laceration: superficial disruption of the cortex; renal medulla and collecting system are not involved
- Major laceration: parenchymal disruption extending into cortex and medulla, possibly involving the collecting system
- Vascular injury: tears of renal artery or vein

The most common renal injuries are contusions, lacerations, ruptures, and renal pedicle injuries or small internal lacerations of the kidney (Fig. 44-11). The kidneys receive half of the blood flow from the abdominal aorta; therefore, even a fairly small renal laceration can produce massive bleeding. About 70% of patients are in shock when admitted to the hospital. In some cases, there is an isolated renal artery thrombosis.

Clinical manifestations include pain, renal colic (due to blood clots or fragments obstructing the collecting system), hematuria, mass or swelling in the flank, ecchymoses, and lacerations or wounds of the lateral abdomen and flank. Hematuria is the most common manifestation of renal trauma; its presence after trauma suggests renal injury. There is no relationship between the degree of hematuria and the degree of injury. Hematuria may not occur, or it may be detectable only on microscopic examination. Signs and symptoms of hypovolemia and shock are likely with significant hemorrhage.

Medical Management

The goals of management in patients with renal trauma are to control hemorrhage, pain, and infection as well as to preserve and restore renal function. All urine is saved and sent to the laboratory for analysis to detect RBCs and to evaluate the course of bleeding. Hematocrit and hemoglobin levels are monitored closely; decreasing values indicate hemorrhage.

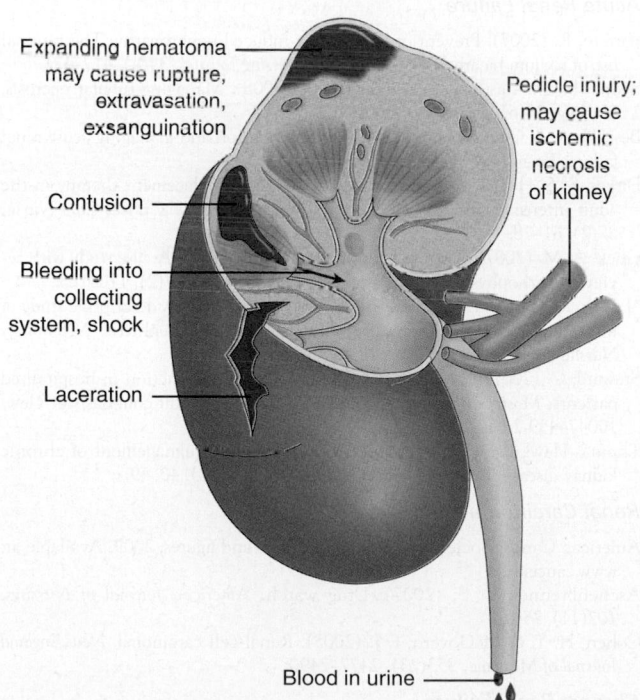

Expanding hematoma may cause rupture, extravasation, exsanguination

Contusion

Bleeding into collecting system, shock

Laceration

Pedicle injury; may cause ischemic necrosis of kidney

Blood in urine

Figure 44-11 Types and pathophysiologic effects of renal injuries: contusions, lacerations, rupture, and pedicle injury.

The patient is monitored for oliguria and signs of hemorrhagic shock, because a pedicle injury or shattered kidney can lead to rapid exsanguination (lethal blood loss). An expanding hematoma may cause rupture of the kidney capsule. To detect hematoma, the area around the lower ribs, upper lumbar vertebrae, flank, and abdomen is palpated for tenderness. A palpable flank or abdominal mass with local tenderness, swelling, and ecchymosis suggests renal hemorrhage. The area of the original mass can be outlined with a marking pen so that the examiner can evaluate the area for change.

Renal trauma is often associated with other injuries to the abdominal organs (liver, colon, small intestines); therefore, the patient is assessed for skin abrasions, lacerations, and entry and exit wounds of the upper abdomen and lower thorax because these may be associated with renal injury.

With a contusion of the kidney, healing may take place with conservative measures. If the patient has microscopic hematuria and a normal IV urogram, outpatient management is possible. If gross hematuria or a minor laceration is present, the patient is hospitalized and kept on bed rest until the hematuria clears. Antimicrobial medications may be prescribed to prevent infection from perirenal hematoma or urinoma (a cyst containing urine). Patients with retroperitoneal hematomas may develop low-grade fever as absorption of the clot takes place.

Surgical Management

In renal trauma, any sudden change in the patient's condition suggests hemorrhage and requires rapid surgical intervention. Depending on the patient's condition and the nature of the injury, major lacerations may be treated through surgical intervention or conservatively (bed rest, no surgery). Vascular injuries require immediate exploratory surgery because of the high incidence of involvement of other organ systems and the serious complications that may result if these injuries are untreated. The patient is often in shock and requires aggressive fluid resuscitation. The damaged kidney may have to be removed (nephrectomy).

Early postoperative complications (within 6 months) include rebleeding, perinephritic abscess formation, sepsis, urine extravasation, and fistula formation. Other complications include stone formation, infection, cysts, vascular aneurysms, and loss of renal function. Hypertension can be a complication of any renal surgery but usually is a late complication of renal injury.

Nursing Management

The patient with renal trauma must be assessed frequently during the first few days after injury to detect flank and abdominal pain, muscle spasm, and swelling over the flank. During this time, the patient who has undergone surgery is instructed about care of the incision and the importance of an adequate fluid intake. In addition, instructions about changes that should be reported to the physician, such as fever, hematuria, flank pain, or any signs and symptoms of decreasing kidney function, are provided. Guidelines for gradually increasing activity, lifting, and driving are also provided in accordance with the physician's prescription.

Follow-up nursing care includes monitoring the blood pressure to detect hypertension and advising the patient to restrict activities for about 1 month after trauma to minimize the incidence of delayed or secondary bleeding. The patient should be advised to schedule periodic follow-up assessments of renal function (creatinine clearance, BUN and serum creatinine analyses). If a nephrectomy was necessary, the patient is advised to wear medical identification.

CRITICAL THINKING EXERCISES

1 You are a staff nurse in an outpatient dialysis facility. A 50-year-old woman with ESRD is scheduled to be seen in the clinic; it is anticipated that she will need dialysis in the near future. The patient lives alone and will require teaching about the dialysis options. Develop a teaching plan to explain the different types of dialysis, goals, and level of involvement on the part of the patient.

EBP 2 A 45-year-old married man visits the nephrology department to discuss options for dealing with his ESRD. His brother has begun the workup to donate one of his kidneys and the preliminary reports show that a match is possible. The patient states that he does not want his brother to go through the process of kidney donation if dialysis is possible. Identify the evidence for and the criteria used to evaluate the strength of the evidence for dialysis compared to kidney transplantation.

3 You are caring for a 35-year-old woman who has been recently diagnosed with renal cancer. Identify possible treatment options. What nursing assessment and interventions should you make at this time? What explanations would you give the patient about renal cancer?

4 A 55-year-old man who is blind has just had a catheter placed for PD. His wife, his primary caretaker, is deaf. Develop a teaching plan to explain peritoneal dialysis, goals, and level of involvement to the patient and family.

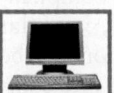

The Smeltzer suite offers these additional resources to enhance learning and facilitate understanding of this chapter:
- thePoint online resource, thepoint.lww.com/Smeltzer12E
- Student CD-ROM included with the book
- *Study Guide to Accompany Brunner & Suddarth's Textbook of Medical-Surgical Nursing*
- *Handbook for Brunner & Suddarth's Textbook of Medical-Surgical Nursing*

REFERENCES AND SELECTED READINGS

*Asterisk indicates nursing research.

Books

Bickley, L. S. (2007). *Bates' guide to physical examination and history taking* (9th ed.). Philadelphia: Lippincott Williams & Wilkins.

Counts, C. S. (2008). *ANNA core curriculum for nephrology nursing* (5th ed.). Pitman, NJ: American Nephrology Nurses Association.

Danovitch, G. M. (Ed.). (2005). *Handbook of kidney transplantation.* Philadelphia: Lippincott Williams & Wilkins.

Miller, C. A. (2009). *Nursing for wellness in older adults* (5th ed.). Philadelphia: Lippincott Williams & Wilkins.

Molzahn, A. & Butera, E. (2006). *Contemporary nephrology nursing: Principles and practice* (2nd ed.). Pitman, NJ: American Nephrology Nurses' Association.

Porth, C. M. & Matfin, G. (2009). *Pathophysiology: Concepts of altered health states* (8th ed.). Philadelphia: Lippincott Williams & Wilkins.

Zonderman, J. & Doyle, R. (2006). *Springhouse nurse's drug guide 2006.* Philadelphia: Lippincott Williams & Wilkins.

Journals and Electronic Documents

General

Hughes, R. G. (2008). *Patient safety and quality: An evidence-based handbook for nurses.* AHRQ Publication No. 08-0043. Rockville, MD: Agency for Healthcare Research and Quality. www.ahrq.gov/qual/nurseshdbk/

Phillips, B. & Ryr, D. B. (2005). Diagnosis and management of restless leg syndrome. *Clinical Reviews, 15*(11), 92–106.

Slack, C. B. & Landis, C. A. (2006). Improving outcomes for restless leg syndrome. *The Nurse Practitioner, 31*(5), 26–35.

Chronic Kidney Disease

Broscious, S. K. & Castagnola, J. (2006). Chronic kidney disease: Acute manifestations and role of critical care nurses. *Critical Care Nurse, 26*(4), 17–28.

Burrows, L. & Muller, R. (2007). Chronic kidney disease and cardiovascular disease: Pathophysiological links. *Nephrology Nursing Journal, 34*(1), 55–65.

Centers for Disease Control and Prevention (CDC). (2007). Prevalence of chronic kidney disease and associated risk factors. *MMWR: Morbidity and Mortality Weekly Report, 56*(8), 161–165.

Coresh, J., Selvin, E., Stevens, L., et al. (2007). Prevalence of chronic kidney disease in the United States. *Journal of the American Medical Association, 298*(17), 2038–2047.

Legg, V. (2005). Complications of chronic kidney disease. *American Journal of Nursing, 102*(6), 40–50.

McCarley, P. B. & Burrows-Hudson, S. (2006). Chronic kidney disease and cardiovascular disease using the ANNA standards and practice guidelines to improve care. *Nephrology Nursing Journal, 33*(6), 666–675.

McCarley, P. B. & Salai, P. B. (2007). Chronic kidney disease and cardiovascular disease: A case presentation. *Nephrology Nursing Journal, 34*(2), 187–200.

Mosenkis, A., Kirk, D. & Berns, J. S. (2006). When chronic kidney disease becomes advanced. *Postgraduate Medicine, 119*(1), 83–91.

Munar, M. & Singh, H. (2007). Drug dosing adjustments in patients with chronic kidney disease. *American Family Physician, 75*(10), 1487–1496.

Acute Renal Failure

Barreto, R. (2007). Prevention of contrast-induced nephropathy: The rational use of sodium bicarbonate. *Nephrology Nursing Journal, 34*(4), 417–421.

Bednarski, D., Castner, D. & Douglas, C. (2008). Managing tubular necrosis. *Nursing, 38*(6), 56hn1–56hn6.

Best, H. A. & Counselman, F. L. (2008). Evaluation and managing acute renal failure. *Emergency Medicine, 40*(5), 16–20.

Dirkes, S. & Hodge, K. (2007). Continuous renal replacement therapy in the adult intensive care unit. History and current trends. *Critical Care Nurse, 27*(2), 61–78.

Glick, A. M. (2007). Focal segmental glomerulosclerosis: A case study with review of pathophysiology. *Nephrology Nursing Journal, 34*(2), 176–183.

*Lu, D., McCarthy, A. M., Lanning, L. D., et al. (2007). A descriptive study of individuals with membranoproliferative glomerulonephritis. *Nephrology Nursing Journal, 34*(3), 295–302.

Steward, C. (2007). Preventing the decline of kidney function in hospitalized patients. *Mosby's Nursing Consult.* www.nursingconsult.com/das/stat/view/100474459-2/cup

Thomas-Hawkins, C. & Zazworsky, D. (2005). Self-management of chronic kidney disease. *American Journal of Nursing, 105*(10), 40–49.

Renal Carcinoma

American Cancer Society (2009). Cancer facts and figures: 2009. Available at: www.cancer.org

Aschenbrenner, D. S. (2007). Drug watch. *American Journal of Nursing, 107*(11), 25–26.

Cohen, H. T. & McGovern, F. J. (2005). Renal-cell carcinoma. *New England Journal of Medicine, 353*(23), 2477–2490.

Chronic Renal Failure

Brattich, M. (2007). Comorbid diseases in patients on dialysis: The impact on anemia. *Nephrology Nursing Journal, 34*(1), 72–75, 98.

Carver, M., Cardner, J., Hartwell, L., et al. (2008). Management of mineral and bone disorders in patients: A team approach to improving outcomes. *Nephrology Nursing Journal, 35*(3), 265–270.

Cohen, L. M., Moss, A. H., Weisord, S. D., et al. (2006). Renal palliative care. *Journal of Palliative Medicine, 9*(4), 977–992.

Compton, A. (2007). Chronic kidney disease. *Clinical Reviews, 17*(5), 38–44.

Gesek, F. & Desmond, J. S. (2008). Improved patient outcomes in chronic kidney disease: Optimizing vitamin D therapy. *Nephrology Nursing Journal, 35*(2S), 5S–23S.

Thomas, M. C. & Atkins, R. C. (2006). Blood pressure lowering for the prevention and treatment of diabetic kidney disease. *Drugs, 66*(17), 2213–2234.

Renal Replacement Therapies

American Nephrology Nurses' Association. (2007a). Home hemodialysis fact sheet. Pitman, NJ: Author. www.annanurse.org

*Belguzar, K., Kayser, C. & Kilic, S. (2007). Nonadherence with diet and fluid restrictions and perceived social support in patients receiving hemodialysis. *Journal of Nursing Scholarship, 39*(3), 243–248.

Kurella, M., Covinsky, K. E., Collins, A. J., et al. (2007). Octogenarians and nonagenarians starting dialysis in the United States. *Annals of Internal Medicine, 146*(3), 177–183.

Martin, R. K. & Jurschak, J. (2007). Nursing management of continuous renal replacement therapy. *Seminars in Dialysis, 9*(2), 192–199.

McCarley, P. B. & Arjomand, M. (2008). Mineral and bone disorders in patients on dialysis: Physiology and clinical consequences. *Nephrology Nursing Journal, 35*(1), 59–64.

Mentes, J. (2006). Oral hydration in older adults. *American Journal of Nursing, 106*(6), 40–48.

Munoz, C. & Hilgenberg, C. (2005). Ethnopharmacology: Understanding how ethnicity can affect drug response is essential to providing culturally competent care. *American Journal of Nursing, 105*(8), 40–49.

United States Renal Data System (USRDS). (2007). *2007 Annual report.* www.usrds.org/2007/ref/A_incidence_07.pdf

Welch, J. L. & Perkins, S. M. (2006). Patterns of interdialytic weight gain during the first year of hemodialysis. *Nephrology Nursing Journal, 33*(5), 493–498.

Kidney Transplantation

American Nephrology Nurses' Association. (2006). *Chronic kidney disease fact sheet.* Pitman NJ: Author. www.annanurse.org

American Nephrology Nurses' Association. (2007b). *Chronic kidney disease. What every nurse should know. Module 6: The post transplant patient.* Pitman, NJ: Author.

*Zarifian, A. (2006). Symptom occurrence, symptom distress, and quality of life in renal transplant recipients. *Nephrology Nursing Journal, 33*(6), 609–618.

RESOURCES

American Association of Kidney Patients, www.aakp.org

American Nephrology Nurses' Association, www.annanurse.org

American Foundation for Urologic Disease, www.afud.org

American Kidney Fund, www.arbon.com/kidney

AV Fistula First, www.fistulafirst.org

National Institute of Diabetes and Digestive and Kidney Diseases, www.niddk.nih.gov

National Kidney and Urologic Diseases Information Clearinghouse, www.niddk.nih.gov

National Kidney Foundation, www.kidney.org

United Network for Organ Sharing, www.unos.org

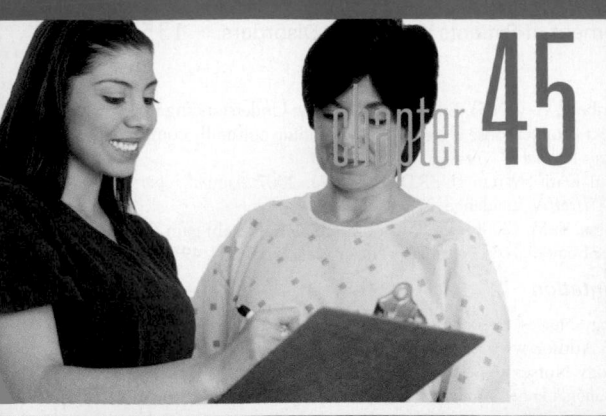

chapter 45

Management of Patients With Urinary Disorders

LEARNING OBJECTIVES

On completion of this chapter, the learner will be able to:

1 Identify factors contributing to upper and lower urinary tract infections (UTIs).

2 Use the nursing process as a framework for care of the patient with a UTI.

3 Differentiate between the various adult dysfunctional voiding patterns.

4 Develop a patient education plan for a patient who has mixed (stress and urge) urinary incontinence.

5 Identify potential causes of an obstruction of the urinary tract and management of the patient with this condition.

6 Develop a teaching plan for the patient undergoing treatment for renal calculi (kidney stones).

7 Formulate preoperative and postoperative nursing diagnoses for the patient undergoing surgery for urinary diversion.

GLOSSARY

bacteriuria: more than 10^5 colonies of bacteria per milliliter of urine

cystectomy: removal of the urinary bladder

cystitis: inflammation of the urinary bladder

frequency: voiding more often than every 3 hours

ileal conduit: transplantation of the ureters to an isolated section of the terminal ileum, with one end of the ureters brought to the abdominal wall

interstitial cystitis: inflammation of the bladder wall that eventually causes disintegration of the lining and loss of bladder elasticity

micturition: voiding or urination

neurogenic bladder: bladder dysfunction that results from a disorder or dysfunction of the nervous system; may result in either urinary retention or bladder overactivity, resulting in urinary urgency and urge incontinence

nocturia: awakening at night to urinate

overflow incontinence: involuntary urine loss associated with overdistention of the bladder due to mechanical or anatomic bladder outlet obstruction

prostatitis: inflammation of the prostate gland

pyelonephritis: inflammation of the renal pelvis

pyuria: white blood cells in the urine

residual urine: urine that remains in the bladder after voiding

suprapubic catheter: a urinary catheter that is inserted through a suprapubic incision into the bladder

ureterosigmoidostomy: transplantation of the ureters into the sigmoid colon, allowing urine to flow through the colon and out the rectum

ureterovesical or **vesicoureteral reflux:** backward flow of urine from the bladder into one or both ureters

urethritis: inflammation of the urethra

urethrovesical reflux: backward flow of urine from the urethra into the bladder

urinary incontinence: involuntary or uncontrolled loss of urine from the bladder sufficient to cause a social or hygienic problem

urosepsis: sepsis resulting from infected urine, most often a UTI

The urinary system is responsible for providing the route for drainage of urine formed by the kidneys. Care of the patient with disorders of the urinary tract requires an understanding of the anatomy, physiology, diagnostic testing, nursing care, and rehabilitation of patients with the multiple processes that affect the urinary system. Nurses care for patients with urologic disorders in all settings. This chapter focuses on the nursing management of patients with common urinary dysfunctions, including infections, dysfunctional voiding patterns, urolithiasis, genitourinary trauma, cancer of the urinary tract, and urinary diversions.

INFECTIONS OF THE URINARY TRACT

Urinary tract infections (UTIs) are caused by pathogenic microorganisms in the urinary tract (the normal urinary tract is sterile above the urethra). UTIs are generally classified as infections involving the upper or lower urinary tract and further classified as uncomplicated or complicated, depending on other patient-related conditions (Chart 45-1).

Lower UTIs include bacterial **cystitis** (inflammation of the urinary bladder), bacterial **prostatitis** (inflammation of the prostate gland), and bacterial **urethritis** (inflammation of the urethra). There can be acute or chronic nonbacterial causes of inflammation in any of these areas that can be misdiagnosed as bacterial infections. Upper UTIs are much less common and include acute or chronic **pyelonephritis** (inflammation of the renal pelvis), interstitial nephritis (inflammation of the kidney), and renal abscesses. Upper and lower UTIs are further classified as uncomplicated or complicated, depending on whether the UTI is recurrent and the duration of the infection. Most uncomplicated UTIs are community acquired. Complicated UTIs usually occur in people with urologic abnormalities or recent catheterization and are often acquired during hospitalization.

A UTI is the second most common infection in the body. Most cases occur in women; one out of every five women in the United States will develop a UTI during her lifetime. The urinary tract is the most common site of nosocomial infection, accounting for greater than 40% of the total number reported by hospitals and affecting about 600,000 patients each year. In most of these hospital-acquired UTIs, instrumentation of the urinary tract or catheterization is the precipitating cause. More than 250,000 cases of acute pyelonephritis occur in the United States each year, with 100,000 patients requiring hospitalization. Approximately 11.3 million women are diagnosed with UTIs in the United States annually, representing an expenditure of about $1.6 billion in direct heath care costs. This amount does not include the indirect costs associated with time lost from work and the negative impact on the person's lifestyle (National Kidney and Urologic Diseases Information Clearinghouse, 2005).

Lower Urinary Tract Infections

Several mechanisms maintain the sterility of the bladder: the physical barrier of the urethra, urine flow, ureterovesical junction competence, various antibacterial enzymes and antibodies, and antiadherent effects mediated by the mucosal cells of the bladder. Abnormalities or dysfunctions of these mechanisms are contributing risk factors for lower UTIs (Chart 45-2).

Pathophysiology

For infection to occur, bacteria must gain access to the bladder, attach to and colonize the epithelium of the urinary tract to avoid being washed out with voiding, evade host

---

Chart 45-1• *Classifying Urinary Tract Infections*

Urinary tract infections (UTIs) are classified by location: the lower urinary tract (which includes the bladder and structures below the bladder) or the upper urinary tract (which includes the kidneys and ureters). They can also be classified as uncomplicated or complicated UTIs.

Lower UTIs

Cystitis, prostatitis, urethritis

Upper UTIs

Acute pyelonephritis, chronic pyelonephritis, renal abscess, interstitial nephritis, perirenal abscess

Uncomplicated Lower or Upper UTIs

Community-acquired infection; common in young women and not usually recurrent

Complicated Lower or Upper UTIs

Often nosocomial (acquired in the hospital) and related to catheterization; occur in patients with urologic abnormalities, pregnancy, immunosuppression, diabetes mellitus, and obstructions and are often recurrent

---

 **CHART 45-2** *Risk Factors for Urinary Tract Infection*

- Inability or failure to empty the bladder completely
- Obstructed urinary flow caused by:
   Congenital abnormalities
   Urethral strictures
   Contracture of the bladder neck
   Bladder tumors
   Calculi (stones) in the ureters or kidneys
   Compression of the ureters
- Decreased natural host defenses or immunosuppression
- Instrumentation of the urinary tract (eg, catheterization, cystoscopic procedures)
- Inflammation or abrasion of the urethral mucosa
- Contributing conditions such as:
   Diabetes mellitus (increased urinary glucose levels create an infection-prone environment in the urinary tract)
   Pregnancy
   Neurologic disorders
   Gout
   Altered states caused by incomplete emptying of the bladder and urinary stasis

defense mechanisms, and initiate inflammation. Many UTIs result from fecal organisms ascending from the perineum to the urethra and the bladder and then adhering to the mucosal surfaces.

Bacterial Invasion of the Urinary Tract

By increasing the normal slow shedding of bladder epithelial cells (resulting in bacteria removal), the bladder can clear large numbers of bacteria. Glycosaminoglycan (GAG), a hydrophilic protein, normally exerts a nonadherent protective effect against various bacteria. The GAG molecule attracts water molecules, forming a water barrier that serves as a defensive layer between the bladder and the urine. GAG may be impaired by certain agents (cyclamate, saccharin, aspartame, and tryptophan metabolites). The normal bacterial flora of the vagina and urethral area also interfere with adherence of *Escherichia coli*. Urinary immunoglobulin A (IgA) in the urethra may also provide a barrier to bacteria.

Reflux

An obstruction to free-flowing urine is a condition known as **urethrovesical reflux,** which is the reflux (backward flow) of urine from the urethra into the bladder (Fig. 45-1). With coughing, sneezing, or straining, the bladder pressure increases, which may force urine from the bladder into the urethra. When the pressure returns to normal, the urine

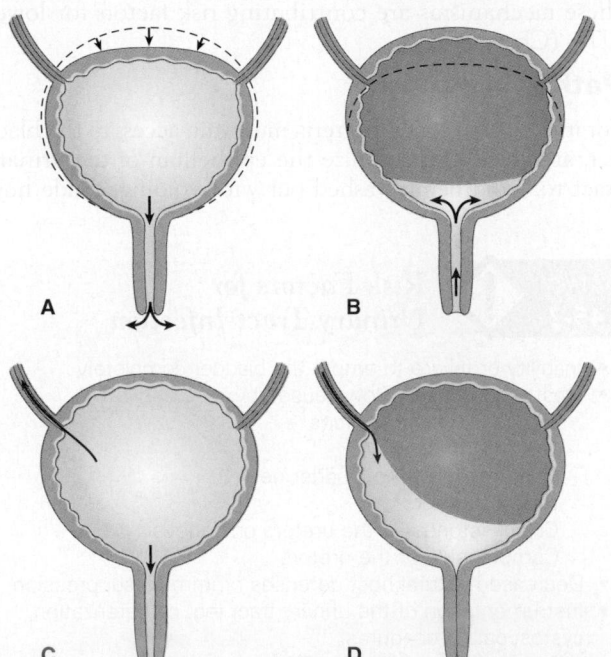

Figure 45-1 Mechanisms of urethrovesical and ureterovesical reflux may cause urinary tract infection. **Urethrovesical reflux:** With coughing and straining, bladder pressure rises, which may force urine from the bladder into the urethra. **A,** When bladder pressure returns to normal, the urine flows back to the bladder **(B),** which introduces bacteria from the urethra to the bladder. **Ureterovesical reflux:** With failure of the ureterovesical valve, urine moves up the ureters during voiding **(C)** and flows into the bladder when voiding stops **(D).** This prevents complete emptying of the bladder. It also leads to urinary stasis and contamination of the ureters with bacteria-laden urine.

flows back into the bladder, bringing into the bladder bacteria from the anterior portions of the urethra. Urethrovesical reflux is also caused by dysfunction of the bladder neck or urethra. The urethrovesical angle and urethral closure pressure may be altered with menopause, increasing the incidence of infection in postmenopausal women. Reflux is most often noted in young children, and treatment is based on its severity.

Ureterovesical or **vesicoureteral reflux** refers to the backward flow of urine from the bladder into one or both ureters (see Fig. 45-1). Normally, the ureterovesical junction prevents urine from traveling back into the ureter. The ureters tunnel into the bladder wall so that the bladder musculature compresses a small portion of the ureter during normal voiding. When the ureterovesical valve is impaired by congenital causes or ureteral abnormalities, the bacteria may reach the kidneys and eventually destroy them.

Uropathogenic Bacteria

Bacteriuria is generally defined as more than 10^5 colonies of bacteria per milliliter of urine. Because urine samples (especially in women) are commonly contaminated by the bacteria normally present in the urethral area, a bacterial count exceeding 10^5 colonies/mL of clean-catch midstream urine is the measure that distinguishes true bacteriuria from contamination. In men, contamination of the collected urine sample occurs less frequently; hence, bacteriuria is defined as 10^4 colonies/mL urine. Community-acquired UTIs are among the most common bacterial infections in women (Porth & Matfin, 2009).

The organisms most frequently responsible for UTIs are those normally found in the lower gastrointestinal (GI) tract, usually *E. coli.* However, isolation of *E. coli* is decreasing compared with previous observations, especially in males and in patients with indwelling bladder catheters, who instead have higher rates of *Pseudomonas* and *Enterococcus* organisms than females and noncatheterized patients (Porth & Matfin, 2009).

Routes of Infection

Bacteria enter the urinary tract in three ways: by the transurethral route (ascending infection), through the bloodstream (hematogenous spread), or by means of a fistula from the intestine (direct extension).

The most common route of infection is transurethral, in which bacteria (often from fecal contamination) colonize the periurethral area and subsequently enter the bladder by means of the urethra. In women, the short urethra offers little resistance to the movement of uropathogenic bacteria. Sexual intercourse forces the bacteria from the urethra into the bladder. This accounts for the increased incidence of UTIs in sexually active women. Bacteria may also enter the urinary tract by means of the blood from a distant site of infection or through direct extension by way of a fistula from the intestinal tract.

Clinical Manifestations

A variety of signs and symptoms are associated with UTI. About half of all patients with bacteriuria have no symptoms. Signs and symptoms of an uncomplicated lower UTI (cystitis) include burning on urination, **frequency** (voiding more than every 3 hours), urgency, **nocturia** (awakening at night to urinate), incontinence, and suprapubic or pelvic pain. Hematuria and back pain may also be present. In older people, these symptoms are less common (see Gerontologic Considerations).

In patients with complicated UTIs, manifestations can range from asymptomatic bacteriuria to gram-negative sepsis with shock. Complicated UTIs often are caused by a broader spectrum of organisms, have a lower response rate to treatment, and tend to recur. Many patients with catheter-associated UTIs are asymptomatic; however, any patient with a catheter who suddenly develops signs and symptoms of septic shock should be evaluated for **urosepsis** (sepsis resulting from infected urine).

 ### Gerontologic Considerations

The incidence of bacteriuria in the elderly differs from that in younger adults. Bacteriuria increases with age and disability, and women are affected more frequently than men. UTI is the most common cause of acute bacterial sepsis in patients older than 65 years of age, in whom gram-negative sepsis carries a mortality rate exceeding 50%. Urologists see many asymptomatic patients with bacteriuria and 20% are women older than 65 years. In older patients who reside in nursing homes, 25% to 50% of females and 15% to 40% of males have chronic bacteriuria (Juthani-Mehta, 2007; Miller, 2009).

In the elderly population at large, structural abnormalities secondary to decreased bladder tone and neurogenic bladder (dysfunctional bladder) secondary to stroke or autonomic neuropathy of diabetes may prevent complete emptying of the bladder and increase the risk for UTI (Morton, Fontaine, Hudak, et al., 2005). When indwelling catheters are used, the risk of UTI increases dramatically. Elderly women often have incomplete emptying of the bladder and urinary stasis. In the absence of estrogen, postmenopausal women are susceptible to colonization and increased adherence of bacteria to the vagina and urethra. Oral or topical estrogen has been used to restore the glycogen content of vaginal epithelial cells and an acidic pH for some postmenopausal women with recurrent cystitis.

The antibacterial activity of prostatic secretions that protect men from bacterial colonization of the urethra and bladder decreases with aging. Although UTIs are rare in men, the prevalence of infection in men older than 50 years of age approaches that of women in the same age group. The increase of UTIs in men as they age is largely a result of prostatic hyperplasia or carcinoma, strictures of the urethra, and neuropathic bladder. The use of catheterization or cystoscopy in evaluation or treatment may also contribute to the higher incidence of UTIs in this group. The incidence of bacteriuria increases in men with confusion, dementia, or bowel or bladder incontinence. The most common cause of recurrent UTIs in elderly males is chronic bacterial prostatitis. Resection of the prostate gland may help reduce its incidence (see Chapter 49).

In institutionalized elderly patients, such as those in long-term care facilities, infecting pathogens are often resistant to many antibiotics. Chart 45-3 lists other factors that may contribute to UTI in elderly patients in these en-

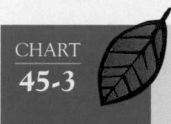

vironments. Diligent hand hygiene, careful perineal care, and frequent toileting may decrease the incidence of UTIs.

The organisms responsible for UTIs in the institutionalized elderly may differ from those found in patients residing in the community; this is thought to result in part from the frequent use of antibiotic agents by patients in long-term care facilities. *E. coli* is the most common organism seen in elderly patients in the community or hospital. However, patients with indwelling catheters are more likely to be infected with *Proteus, Klebsiella, Pseudomonas,* or *Staphylococcus* species. Patients who have been previously treated with antibiotics may be infected with *Enterococcus* species. Frequent reinfections are common in older adults.

The most common subjective presenting symptom of UTI in older adults is generalized fatigue. The most common objective finding is a change in cognitive functioning, especially in those with dementia, because these patients usually exhibit even more profound cognitive changes with the onset of a UTI.

Controversy continues about the need for treatment of asymptomatic bacteriuria in institutionalized elderly patients, because resulting antibiotic-resistant organisms and sepsis may be greater threats to patients. Most experts now recommend withholding antibiotics unless symptoms develop. However, treatment regimens are generally the same as those for younger adults, although age-related changes in the intestinal absorption of medications and decreased renal function and hepatic flow may necessitate alterations in the antimicrobial regimen. Renal function must be monitored, and medication dosages should be altered accordingly.

 NURSING ALERT

Elderly patients often lack the typical symptoms of UTI and sepsis. Although frequency and urgency may occur, nonspecific symptoms, such as altered sensorium, lethargy, anorexia, new incontinence, hyperventilation, and low-grade fever, may be the only clues.

Assessment and Diagnostic Findings

Results of various tests, such as bacterial colony counts, cellular studies, and urine cultures, help confirm the diagnosis of UTI. In an uncomplicated UTI, the strain of bacteria determines the antibiotic of choice.

Urine Cultures

Urine cultures are useful for documenting a UTI and identifying the specific organism present. UTI is diagnosed by bacteria in the urine culture. A colony count of at least 10^5

colony-forming units (CFU) per milliliter of urine on a clean-catch midstream or catheterized specimen is a major criterion for infection (Smythe, Moore & Goldsmith, 2006). However, UTI and subsequent sepsis have occurred with lower bacterial colony counts. About one third of women with symptoms of acute infections have negative midstream urine culture results and may go untreated if 10^5 CFU/mL is used as the criterion for infection. The presence of any bacteria in specimens obtained by suprapubic needle aspiration of the urinary bladder or catheterization (insertion of a tube into the urinary bladder) is considered indicative of infection.

The following groups of patients should have urine cultures obtained when bacteriuria is present:

- All men (because of the likelihood of structural or functional abnormalities)
- All children
- Women with a history of compromised immune function or renal problems
- Patients with diabetes mellitus
- Patients who have undergone recent instrumentation (including catheterization) of the urinary tract
- Patients who have been recently hospitalized or who live in long-term care facilities
- Patients with prolonged or persistent symptoms
- Patients with three or more UTIs in the previous year
- Pregnant women
- Postmenopausal women
- Women who are sexually active
- Women who have new sexual partners

Cellular Studies

Microscopic hematuria is present in about half of patients with an acute UTI (see Chapter 43). **Pyuria** (greater than 4 white blood cells [WBCs] per high-power field) occurs in all patients with UTI; however, it is not specific for bacterial infection. Pyuria can also be seen with kidney stones, interstitial nephritis, and renal tuberculosis.

Other Studies

A multiple-test dipstick often includes testing for WBCs, known as the leukocyte esterase test, and nitrite testing. Urine hydroxyproline, an amino acid found mainly in collagen, may be tested for in disorders characterized by bone resorption (Karpoff & Labus, 2008).

Tests for sexually transmitted diseases (STDs), also referred to as sexually transmitted infections (STIs), may be performed because acute urethritis caused by sexually transmitted organisms (ie, *Chlamydia trachomatis, Neisseria gonorrhoeae*, herpes simplex) or acute vaginitis infections (caused by *Trichomonas* or *Candida* species) may be responsible for symptoms similar to those of UTIs.

Diagnostic studies such as computed tomography (CT) and ultrasonography are useful diagnostic tools. A CT scan may detect pyelonephritis or abscesses, and ultrasonography is extremely sensitive for detecting obstruction, abscesses, tumors, and cysts. Transrectal ultrasonography (to assess the prostate and bladder) is the procedure of choice for men with recurrent or complicated UTIs. A cystourethroscopy may be indicated to visualize the ureters or to detect strictures, calculi, or tumors (Karpoff & Labus, 2008).

Medical Management

Management of UTIs typically involves pharmacologic therapy and patient education. The nurse teaches the patient about prescribed medication regimens and infection prevention measures.

Acute Pharmacologic Therapy

The ideal medication for treatment of UTI is an antibacterial agent that eradicates bacteria from the urinary tract with minimal effects on fecal and vaginal flora, thereby minimizing the incidence of vaginal yeast infections. (Yeast vaginitis occurs in as many as 25% of patients treated with antimicrobial agents that affect vaginal flora. Yeast vaginitis can cause more symptoms and be more difficult and costly to treat than the original UTI.) Additionally, the antibacterial agent should be affordable and should have few adverse effects and low resistance. Because the organism in initial, uncomplicated UTIs in women is most likely *E. coli* or other fecal flora, the agent should be effective against these organisms (Mehnert-Kay, 2005). Various treatment regimens have been successful in treating uncomplicated lower UTIs in women: single-dose administration, short-course (3 to 4 days) regimens, or 7- to 10-day regimens. The trend is toward a shortened course of antibiotic therapy for uncomplicated UTIs, because most cases are cured after 3 days of treatment. Patients in institutional settings may require 7 to 10 days of medication for the treatment to be effective. Some of the medications commonly used to treat UTIs are listed in Table 45-1. Regardless of the regimen prescribed, the patient is instructed to take all the doses prescribed, even if relief of symptoms occurs promptly. Longer medication courses are indicated for men, pregnant women, and women with pyelonephritis and other types of complicated UTIs. Hospitalization and intravenous (IV) antibiotics are occasionally necessary (Karch, 2008).

Long-Term Pharmacologic Therapy

Although brief pharmacologic treatment of UTIs for 3 days is usually adequate in women, infection recurs in about 20% of women treated for uncomplicated UTIs. Infections that recur within 2 weeks of therapy do so because organisms of the original offending strain remain. Relapses suggest that the source of bacteriuria may be the upper urinary tract or that initial treatment was inadequate or administered for too short a time. Recurrent infections in men are usually caused by persistence of the same organism; further evaluation and treatment are indicated.

Reinfection with new bacteria is the reason for more than 90% of recurrent UTIs in women. If the diagnostic evaluation reveals no structural abnormalities in the urinary tract, the woman with recurrent UTIs may be instructed to begin treatment on her own whenever symptoms occur and to contact her health care provider only when symptoms persist, fever occurs, or the number of treatment episodes exceeds four in a 6-month period. The patient may be taught to use dip-slide culture devices to detect bacteria.

If infection recurs after completing antimicrobial therapy, another short course (3 to 4 days) of full-dose antimicrobial therapy followed by a regular bedtime dose of an antimicrobial agent may be prescribed. If there is no recurrence, medication is taken every other night for 6 to

Table 45-1	EXAMPLES OF MEDICATIONS USED TO TREAT UTIs AND PYELONEPHRITIS	
Drug Classes	**Generic (Brand) Name**	**Major Indications**
Antibiotic Cephalosporin (first generation)	Cephalexin (Keflex)	Genitourinary infections
Antibiotic	Ampicillin (Principen)	UTI—not commonly used alone due to *Escherichia coli* resistance Pyelonephritis
Antibiotic	Amoxicillin (Amoxil)	UTI—not commonly used alone due to *E. coli* resistance
Trimethoprim-sulfamethoxazole combination	Cotrimoxazole (TMP-SMZ, Bactrim Septra)	UTI Pyelonephritis
Antibiotic Urinary tract anti-infective	Nitrofurantoin (Macrodantin, Furadantin)	UTI
Fluoroquinolone Antibiotic	Ciprofloxacin (Cipro)	UTI Pyelonephritis
Fluoroquinolone	Levofloxacin (Levaquin)	Uncomplicated UTI
Urinary analgesic agent	Phenazopyridine (Pyridium)	For relief of burning, burning, pain and other symptoms associated with UTI

UTI, urinary tract infection.

Compiled using information from Karch, A. (2008). 2008 *Lippincott's nursing drug guide*. Philadelphia: Lippincott Williams & Wilkins; and Mehnert-Kay, S. A. (2005). Diagnosis and management of uncomplicated urinary tract infections. *American Family Physician, 72*(3), 451–456.

7 months. Long-term use of antimicrobial agents decreases the risk of reinfection and may be indicated in patients with recurrent infections.

If recurrence is caused by persistent bacteria from preceding infections, the cause (ie, kidney stone, abscess), if known, must be treated. After treatment and sterilization of the urine, low-dose preventive therapy (trimethoprim with or without sulfamethoxazole) each night at bedtime is often prescribed.

Current evidence about the effectiveness of daily intake of cranberry juice to prevent UTIs is inconclusive (Mc-Murdo, Bissett, Price, et al., 2005). Patients who like cranberry juice can be encouraged to include it in their increased fluid intake to help flush bacteria (Dudek, 2006).

NURSING PROCESS

THE PATIENT WITH A LOWER URINARY TRACT INFECTION

Nursing care of the patient with a lower UTI focuses on treating the underlying infection and preventing its recurrence.

Assessment

A history of signs and symptoms related to UTI is obtained from the patient with a suspected UTI. The presence of pain, frequency, urgency, hesitancy, and changes in urine are assessed, documented, and reported. The patient's usual pattern of voiding is assessed to detect factors that may predispose him or her to UTI. Infrequent emptying of the bladder, the association of symptoms of UTI with sexual intercourse, contraceptive practices, and personal hygiene are assessed. The patient's knowledge about prescribed antimicrobial medications and preventive health care measures is also assessed. Additionally, the urine is assessed for volume, color, concentration, cloudiness, and odor, all of which are altered by bacteria in the urinary tract.

Diagnosis

Nursing Diagnoses

Based on the assessment data, the nursing diagnoses may include the following:

- Acute pain related to infection within the urinary tract
- Deficient knowledge about factors predisposing the patient to infection and recurrence, detection and prevention of recurrence, and pharmacologic therapy

Collaborative Problems/Potential Complications

Based on assessment data, the following complications may develop:

- Sepsis (urosepsis)
- Renal failure, which may occur as the long-term result of either an extensive infective or inflammatory process

Planning and Goals

Major goals for the patient may include relief of pain and discomfort, increased knowledge of preventive measures and treatment modalities, and absence of complications.

Nursing Interventions

Relieving Pain

The pain associated with UTI is quickly relieved once effective antimicrobial therapy is initiated. Antispasmodic agents may also be useful in relieving bladder irritability and pain. Analgesic agents and the application of heat to the perineum help relieve pain and spasm. The patient is encouraged to drink liberal amounts of fluids (water is the best choice) to promote renal blood flow and to flush the bacteria from the urinary tract. Urinary tract irritants (eg, coffee, tea, citrus, spices, colas, alcohol) are avoided. Frequent voiding (every 2 to 3 hours) is encouraged to empty the bladder completely because this can significantly lower urine bacterial counts, reduce urinary stasis, and prevent reinfection.

Monitoring and Managing Potential Complications

Early recognition of UTI and prompt treatment are essential to prevent recurrent infection and the possibility of complications, such as renal failure, sepsis (urosepsis), strictures, and obstructions. The goal of treatment is to prevent infection from progressing and causing permanent renal damage and renal failure. Thus, the patient must be taught to recognize early signs and symptoms, to test for bacteriuria, and to initiate treatment as prescribed. Appropriate antimicrobial therapy, liberal fluid intake, frequent voiding, and hygienic measures are commonly prescribed for managing UTIs. The patient is instructed to notify the primary health care provider if fatigue, nausea, vomiting, or pruritus occurs. Periodic monitoring of renal function and evaluation for strictures, obstructions, or stones may be indicated for patients with recurrent UTIs.

Patients with UTIs are at increased risk for gram-negative sepsis. Indwelling catheters should be avoided if possible and removed at the earliest opportunity. However, if an indwelling catheter is necessary, the following specific nursing interventions are initiated to prevent infection and urosepsis:

- Using strict aseptic technique during insertion of the smallest catheter possible
- Securing the catheter with tape to prevent movement
- Frequently inspecting urine color, odor, and consistency
- Performing meticulous daily perineal care with soap and water
- Maintaining a closed system
- Following the manufacturer's instructions when using the catheter port to obtain urine specimens

Careful assessment of vital signs and level of consciousness may alert the nurse to kidney involvement or impending sepsis. Positive blood cultures and elevated WBC counts must be reported immediately. At the same time, appropriate antibiotic therapy and increased fluid intake are prescribed (IV antibiotic therapy and fluids may be required). Aggressive early treatment is the key to reducing the mortality rate associated with gram-negative sepsis, especially in elderly patients.

Promoting Home and Community-Based Care

TEACHING PATIENTS SELF-CARE. In helping patients learn about and prevent or manage a recurrent UTI, the nurse implements teaching that meets the patient's needs. Health-related behaviors that help prevent recurrent UTIs include practicing careful personal hygiene, increasing fluid intake to promote voiding and dilution of urine, urinating regularly and more frequently, and adhering to the therapeutic regimen. For a detailed discussion of patient teaching, see Chart 45-4.

Evaluation

Expected Patient Outcomes

Expected patient outcomes may include:

1. Experiences relief of pain
   a. Reports absence of pain, urgency, frequency, nocturia, or hesitancy on voiding
   b. Takes analgesic, antispasmodic, and antibiotic agents as prescribed
2. Explains UTIs and their treatment
   a. Demonstrates knowledge of preventive measures and prescribed treatments
   b. Drinks 8 to 10 glasses of fluids daily
   c. Voids every 2 to 3 hours
   d. Produces urine that is clear and odorless
3. Experiences no complications
   a. Reports no symptoms of infection (fever, frequency)
   b. Has normal renal function, negative urine and blood cultures
   c. Exhibits normal vital signs and temperature; no signs or symptoms of sepsis (urosepsis)
   d. Maintains adequate urine output more than 30 mL/h

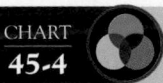

CHART
45-4

PATIENT EDUCATION
Preventing Recurrent Urinary Tract Infections

Hygiene

- Shower rather than bathe in tub because bacteria in the bath water may enter the urethra.
- After each bowel movement, clean the perineum and urethral meatus from front to back. This will help reduce concentrations of pathogens at the urethral opening and, in women, the vaginal opening.

Fluid Intake

- Drink liberal amounts of fluids daily to flush out bacteria.
- Avoid coffee, tea, colas, alcohol, and other fluids that are urinary tract irritants.

Voiding Habits

- Void every 2 to 3 hours during the day and completely empty the bladder. This prevents overdistention of the bladder and compromised blood supply to the bladder wall. Both predispose the patient to UTI. Precautions expressly for women include voiding immediately after sexual intercourse.

Therapy

- Take medication *exactly* as prescribed. Special timing of administration may be required.
- If bacteria continue to appear in the urine, long-term antimicrobial therapy may be required to prevent colonization of the periurethral area and recurrence of infection.
- For recurrent infection, consider acidification of the urine through ascorbic acid (vitamin C), 1000 mg daily, or cranberry juice.
- If prescribed, test urine for presence of bacteria following manufacturer's and health care provider's instructions.
- Notify the primary health care provider if fever occurs or if signs and symptoms persist.
- Consult the primary health care provider regularly for follow-up.

Upper Urinary Tract Infections

Pyelonephritis is a bacterial infection of the renal pelvis, tubules, and interstitial tissue of one or both kidneys. Causes involve either the upward spread of bacteria from the bladder or spread from systemic sources reaching the kidney via the bloodstream. Pathogenic bacteria from a bladder infection can ascend into the kidney, resulting in pyelonephritis. An incompetent ureterovesical valve or obstruction occurring in the urinary tract increases the susceptibility of the kidneys to infection (see Fig. 45-1), because static urine provides a good medium for bacterial growth. Bladder tumors, strictures, benign prostatic hyperplasia, and urinary stones are some potential causes of obstruction that can lead to infections. Systemic infections (such as tuberculosis) can spread to the kidneys and result in abscesses.

Pyelonephritis may be acute or chronic. Acute pyelonephritis is usually manifested by enlarged kidneys with interstitial infiltrations of inflammatory cells. Abscesses may be noted on or within the renal capsule and at the corticomedullary junction. Eventually, atrophy and destruction of tubules and the glomeruli may result. When pyelonephritis becomes chronic, the kidneys become scarred, contracted, and nonfunctioning. Chronic pyelonephritis is a cause of chronic kidney disease that can result in the need for renal replacement therapies such as transplantation or dialysis (Burrows-Hudson, 2005).

ACUTE PYELONEPHRITIS

Clinical Manifestations

The patient with acute pyelonephritis is acutely ill with chills, fever, leukocytosis, bacteriuria, and pyuria. Low back pain, flank pain, nausea and vomiting, headache, malaise, and painful urination are common findings. Physical examination reveals pain and tenderness in the area of the costovertebral angle (see Chapter 43, Fig. 43-6). In addition, symptoms of lower urinary tract involvement, such as urgency and frequency, are common.

Assessment and Diagnostic Findings

An ultrasound study or a CT scan may be performed to locate any obstruction in the urinary tract. Relief of obstruction is essential to prevent the complications and eventual kidney damage. An IV pyelogram may be indicated with pyelonephritis if functional and structural renal abnormalities are suspected (Karpoff & Labus, 2008). Radionuclide imaging with gallium citrate and indium-111 (^{111}In)–labeled WBCs may be useful to identify sites of infection that may not be visualized on CT scan or ultrasound. Urine culture and sensitivity tests are performed to determine the causative organism so that appropriate antimicrobial agents can be prescribed.

Medical Management

Patients with acute uncomplicated pyelonephritis are most often treated on an outpatient basis if they are not exhibiting dehydration, nausea or vomiting, or symptoms of sepsis. In addition, they must be responsible and reliable to ensure that all medications will be taken as prescribed. For outpatients, a 2-week course of antibiotics is recommended because renal parenchymal disease is more difficult to eradicate than mucosal bladder infections. Commonly prescribed agents include some of the same medications prescribed for the treatment of UTIs (see Table 45-1).

Pregnant women may be hospitalized for 2 or 3 days of parenteral antibiotic therapy. Oral antibiotic agents may be prescribed once the patient is afebrile and showing clinical improvement.

A possible issue in acute pyelonephritis treatment is a chronic or recurring symptomless infection persisting for months or years. After the initial antibiotic regimen, the patient may need antibiotic therapy for up to 6 weeks if a relapse occurs. A follow-up urine culture is obtained 2 weeks after completion of antibiotic therapy to document clearing of the infection.

Hydration with oral or parenteral fluids is essential in all patients with UTIs when there is adequate kidney function. Hydration helps facilitate "flushing" of the urinary tract and reduces pain and discomfort.

CHRONIC PYELONEPHRITIS

Repeated bouts of acute pyelonephritis may lead to chronic pyelonephritis.

Clinical Manifestations

The patient with chronic pyelonephritis usually has no symptoms of infection unless an acute exacerbation occurs. Noticeable signs and symptoms may include fatigue, headache, poor appetite, polyuria, excessive thirst, and weight loss. Persistent and recurring infection may produce progressive scarring of the kidney, resulting in renal failure (see Chapter 44).

Assessment and Diagnostic Findings

The extent of the disease is assessed by an IV urogram and measurements of creatinine clearance, blood urea nitrogen, and creatinine levels. Bacteria, if detected in the urine, are eradicated if possible.

Complications

Complications of chronic pyelonephritis include end-stage renal disease (from progressive loss of nephrons secondary to chronic inflammation and scarring), hypertension, and formation of kidney stones (from chronic infection with urea-splitting organisms).

Medical Management

Long-term use of prophylactic antimicrobial therapy may help limit recurrence of infections and renal scarring. Impaired renal function alters the excretion of antimicrobial agents and necessitates careful monitoring of renal function, especially if the medications are potentially toxic to the kidneys.

Nursing Management

The patient may require hospitalization or may be treated as an outpatient. When the patient requires hospitalization, fluid intake and output are carefully measured and recorded. Unless contraindicated, 3 to 4 L of fluids per day is encouraged to dilute the urine, decrease burning on urination, and prevent dehydration. The nurse assesses the patient's temperature every 4 hours and administers antipyretic and antibiotic agents as prescribed. Symptomatic patients are often more comfortable on bed rest.

Patient teaching focuses on prevention of further infection by consuming adequate fluids, emptying the bladder regularly, and performing recommended perineal hygiene. The importance of taking antimicrobial medications exactly as prescribed is stressed, as is the need for keeping follow-up appointments.

ADULT VOIDING DYSFUNCTION

Both neurogenic and non-neurogenic disorders can cause adult voiding dysfunction (Table 45-2). The **micturition** (voiding or urination) process involves several highly coordinated neurologic responses that mediate bladder function. A functional urinary system allows for appropriate bladder filling and complete bladder emptying (see Chapter 43). If voiding dysfunction goes undetected and untreated, the upper urinary system may be compromised. Chronic incomplete bladder emptying from poor detrusor pressure results in recurrent bladder infection. Incomplete bladder emptying due to bladder outlet obstruction (such as benign prostatic hyperplasia), causing high-pressure detrusor contractions, can result in hydronephrosis from the high detrusor pressure that radiates up the ureters to the renal pelvis.

Urinary Incontinence

More than 17 million adults in the United States are estimated to have **urinary incontinence** (involuntary loss of urine from the bladder), with most of them experiencing overactive bladder syndrome, making this disorder more prevalent than diabetes or ulcer disease (Vinsnes, Harkless & Nyronning, 2007). Despite widespread media coverage, urinary incontinence remains underdiagnosed and under-reported. Patients may be too embarrassed to seek help, causing them to ignore or conceal symptoms. Many patients resort to using absorbent pads or other devices without having their condition properly diagnosed and treated. Health care providers must be alert to subtle cues of urinary incontinence and stay informed about current management strategies.

The cost of urologic care in the United States is more than 11 billion dollars (Carson, 2007). The costs of care for patients with urinary incontinence include the expenses of absorbent products, medications, and surgical or nonsurgical treatment modalities, as well as psychosocial costs (ie, embarrassment, loss of self-esteem, and social isolation).

Although urinary incontinence is commonly regarded as a condition that occurs in older multiparous women, it can occur in young nulliparous women, especially during vigorous high-impact activity. Age, gender, and number of vaginal deliveries are established risk factors that explain, in part, the increased incidence in women (Chart 45-5). Urinary incontinence is a symptom of many possible disorders.

Types of Urinary Incontinence

This section provides some of the more common terms used to describe the many types of urinary incontinence (Miller, 2009; Muller, 2005).

Stress incontinence is the involuntary loss of urine through an intact urethra as a result of sneezing, coughing, or changing position (Miller, 2009). It predominantly affects women who have had vaginal deliveries and is thought to be the result of decreasing ligament and pelvic floor support of the urethra and decreasing or absent estrogen levels

Table 45-2	CONDITIONS CAUSING ADULT VOIDING DYSFUNCTION	
Condition	**Voiding Dysfunction**	**Treatment**
Neurogenic Disorders		
Cerebellar ataxia	Incontinence or dyssynergia	Timed voiding; anticholinergic agents
Cerebrovascular accident	Retention or incontinence	Anticholinergic agents; bladder retraining
Dementia	Incontinence	Prompted voiding; anticholinergic agents
Diabetes mellitus	Incontinence and/or incomplete bladder emptying	Timed voiding; EMG/biofeedback; pelvic floor nerve stimulation; anticholinergic/antispasmodic agents; well-controlled blood glucose levels
Multiple sclerosis	Incontinence or incomplete bladder emptying	Timed voiding; EMG/biofeedback to learn pelvic muscle exercises and urge inhibition; pelvic floor nerve stimulation; antispasmodic agents
Parkinson's disease	Incontinence	Anticholinergic/antispasmodic agents
Spinal Cord Dysfunction		
Acute injury	Urinary retention	Indwelling catheter
Degenerative disease	Incontinence and/or incomplete bladder emptying	EMG/biofeedback; pelvic floor nerve stimulation; anticholinergic agents
Non-Neurogenic Disorders		
"Bashful bladder"	Inability to initiate voiding in public bathrooms	Relaxation therapy; EMG/biofeedback
Overactive bladder	Urgency, frequency, and/or urge incontinence	EMG/biofeedback; pelvic floor nerve stimulation; bladder drill (see Chart 45-8); anticholinergic agents
Post-general surgery	Acute urine retention	Catheterization
Postprostatectomy	Incontinence	*Mild:* biofeedback; bladder drill (see Chart 45-8); pelvic floor nerve stimulation *Moderate/severe:* surgery—artificial sphincter
Stress incontinence	Incontinence with cough, laugh, sneeze, position change	*Mild:* biofeedback: bladder drill (see Chart 45-8); periurethral bulking with collagen *Moderate/severe:* surgery

CHART 45-5 — Risk Factors for Urinary Incontinence

- Pregnancy: vaginal delivery, episiotomy
- Menopause
- Genitourinary surgery
- Pelvic muscle weakness
- Incompetent urethra due to trauma or sphincter relaxation
- Immobility
- High-impact exercise
- Diabetes mellitus
- Stroke
- Age-related changes in the urinary tract
- Morbid obesity
- Cognitive disturbances: dementia, Parkinson's disease
- Medications: diuretics, sedatives, hypnotics, opioids
- Caregiver or toilet unavailable

within the urethral walls and bladder base. In men, stress incontinence is often experienced after a radical prostatectomy for prostate cancer because of the loss of urethral compression that the prostate had supplied before the surgery, and possibly bladder wall irritability.

Urge incontinence is the involuntary loss of urine associated with a strong urge to void that cannot be suppressed. The patient is aware of the need to void but is unable to reach a toilet in time (Miller, 2009). An uninhibited detrusor contraction is the precipitating factor. This can occur in a patient with neurologic dysfunction that impairs inhibition of bladder contraction or in a patient without overt neurologic dysfunction.

Functional incontinence refers to those instances in which lower urinary tract function is intact but other factors, such as severe cognitive impairment (eg, Alzheimer's dementia), make it difficult for the patient to identify the need to void

or physical impairments make it difficult or impossible for the patient to reach the toilet in time for voiding.

Iatrogenic incontinence refers to the involuntary loss of urine due to extrinsic medical factors, predominantly medications. One such example is the use of alpha-adrenergic agents to decrease blood pressure. In some people with an intact urinary system, these agents adversely affect the alpha receptors responsible for bladder neck closing pressure; the bladder neck relaxes to the point of incontinence with a minimal increase in intra-abdominal pressure, thus mimicking stress incontinence. As soon as the medication is discontinued, the apparent incontinence resolves.

Mixed urinary incontinence, which encompasses several types of urinary incontinence, is involuntary leakage associated with urgency and also with exertion, effort, sneezing, or coughing (Miller, 2009).

Only with appropriate recognition of the problem, assessment, and referral for diagnostic evaluation and treatment can the outcome of incontinence be determined. All people with incontinence should be considered for evaluation and treatment.

Gerontologic Considerations

Although urinary incontinence is not a normal consequence of aging, age-related changes in the urinary tract do predispose the older person to incontinence. However, if nurses and other health care providers accept incontinence as an inevitable part of illness or aging or consider it irreversible and untreatable, it cannot be treated successfully. Collaborative, interdisciplinary efforts are essential in assessing and effectively treating urinary incontinence (Specht, 2005). Chart 45-6 presents research about improving urinary incontinence in frail elderly patients. Urinary incontinence can decrease an elderly person's ability to maintain an independent lifestyle, which increases dependence on caregivers and may lead to institutionalization. Between 25% and 50% of all nursing home residents have urinary incontinence.

CHART 45-6 — NURSING RESEARCH PROFILE
Improving Urinary Incontinence in Frail Elderly Patients

Vinsnes, A. G., Harkless, G. E. & Nyronning, S. (2007). Unit-based intervention to improve urinary incontinence in frail elderly. *Journal of Nursing Research & Clinical Studies, 27*(3), 53–56.

Purpose

Of the many health challenges that frail elderly people face, urinary incontinence is one of the most common. The purpose of this study was to determine the effect of a unit-based educational program in a nursing home on urinary incontinence in frail elderly people.

Design

This quantitative study used a quasi-experimental design and involved 18 patients (16 women, 2 men) with a mean age of 83 years who were all experiencing urinary incontinence before the study began. The intervention was a systemic educational program for staff delivered over 14 weeks, which included regular coaching about caring for elders with urinary incontinence. Outcome measures were postvoid residual

urine volumes, urinary pad weights, oral fluid intake patterns, and urinary tract infections.

Findings

The education sessions were successful. Both the average and maximum incontinence pads weighed less following the intervention. Average postvoiding residual urine did not change, but the average minimum amount per resident decreased in volume. Daily fluid volume intake remained the same; however, more patients received drinks at night after the intervention with no subsequent increase in overall amount of incontinence.

Nursing Implications

This small study demonstrates the potential of using a unit-based educational program to improve care and change outcomes for patients. Future work is needed to expand the research to a larger, more diverse patient population; develop better tools and strategies for investigation; and enhance treatment and evaluation methods in the frail elderly population.

Many older people experience transient episodes of incontinence that tend to be abrupt in onset. When this occurs, the nurse should question the patient, as well as the family if possible, about the onset of symptoms and any signs or symptoms of a change in other organ systems. Acute UTI, infection elsewhere in the body, constipation, decreased fluid intake, and a change in a chronic disease pattern, such as elevated blood glucose levels in patients with diabetes or decreased estrogen levels in menopausal women, can provoke the onset of urinary incontinence. If the cause is identified and modified or eliminated early at the onset of incontinence, the incontinence itself may be eliminated. Although the bladder of the older person is more vulnerable to altered detrusor activity, age alone is not a risk factor for urinary incontinence (Vinsnes, et al., 2007).

Decreased bladder muscle tone is a normal age-related change found in the elderly. This leads to decreased bladder capacity, increased residual urine, and an increase in urgency (Miller, 2009).

Many medications affect urinary continence in addition to causing other unwanted or unexpected effects. All medications need to be assessed for potential interactions.

Assessment and Diagnostic Findings

Once incontinence is recognized, a thorough history is necessary. This includes a detailed description of the problem and a history of medication use. The patient's voiding history, a diary of fluid intake and output, and bedside tests (eg, residual urine, stress maneuvers) may be used to help determine the type of urinary incontinence involved. Extensive urodynamic tests may be performed (see Chapter 43). Urinalysis and urine culture are performed to identify infection.

Urinary incontinence may be transient or reversible if the underlying cause is successfully treated and the voiding pattern reverts to normal. Chart 45-7 provides causes of transient incontinence.

Medical Management

Management depends on the type of urinary incontinence and its causes. Management of urinary incontinence may be behavioral, pharmacologic, or surgical.

Behavioral Therapy

Behavioral therapies are the first choice to decrease or eliminate urinary incontinence (Chart 45-8). In using these

---

Chart 45-7 • *Causes of Transient Incontinence: DIAPPERS*

Delirium
Infection of urinary tract
Atrophic vaginitis, urethritis
Pharmacologic agents (anticholinergic agents, sedatives, alcohol, analgesic agents, diuretics, muscle relaxants, adrenergic agents)
Psychological factors (depression, regression)
Excessive urine production (increased intake, diabetes insipidus, diabetic ketoacidosis)
Restricted activity
Stool impaction

---

techniques, health care professionals help patients avoid potential adverse effects of pharmacologic or surgical interventions. Pelvic floor muscle exercises (sometimes called Kegel exercises) represent the cornerstone of behavioral intervention for addressing symptoms of stress, urge, and mixed incontinence. Other behavioral treatments include use of a voiding diary, biofeedback, verbal instruction (prompted voiding), and physical therapy (Miller, 2009).

Pharmacologic Therapy

Pharmacologic therapy works best when used as an adjunct to behavioral interventions. Anticholinergic agents inhibit bladder contraction and are considered first-line medications for urge incontinence. Several tricyclic antidepressant medications (eg, amitriptyline [Endep], amoxapine [Asendin]) can also decrease bladder contractions as well as increase bladder neck resistance (Karch, 2008). Pseudoephedrine sulfate (Sudafed), which acts on alpha-adrenergic receptors, causing urinary retention, may be used to treat stress incontinence; it needs to be used with caution in men with prostatic hyperplasia. Hormone therapy (eg, estrogen) taken orally, transdermally, or topically was once the treatment of choice for urinary incontinence in postmenopausal women because it restores the mucosal, vascular, and muscular integrity of the urethra. However, the results of the Women's Health Initiative showed that after 1 year of therapy, incontinence had increased, especially in women taking estrogen alone compared to placebo (Mennick, 2005). More research is needed in this area.

Surgical Management

Surgical correction may be indicated in patients who have not achieved continence using behavioral and pharmacologic therapy. Surgical options vary according to the underlying anatomy and the physiologic problem. Most procedures involve lifting and stabilizing the bladder or urethra to restore the normal urethrovesical angle or to lengthen the urethra.

Women with stress incontinence may undergo an anterior vaginal repair, retropubic suspension, or needle suspension to reposition the urethra. Procedures to compress the urethra and increase resistance to urine flow include sling procedures and placement of periurethral bulking agents such as artificial collagen.

Periurethral bulking is a semipermanent procedure in which small amounts of artificial collagen are placed within the walls of the urethra to enhance the closing pressure of the urethra. This procedure takes only 10 to 20 minutes and may be performed under local anesthesia or moderate sedation. A cystoscope is inserted into the urethra. An instrument is inserted through the cystoscope to deliver a small amount of collagen into the urethral wall at locations selected by the urologist. The patient is usually discharged home after voiding. There are no restrictions following the procedure, although occasionally more than one collagen bulking session may be necessary if the initial procedure did not halt stress incontinence. Collagen placement anywhere in the body is considered semipermanent because its durability averages between 12 and 24 months, until the body absorbs the material. Periurethral bulking with collagen offers an alternative to surgery, as in a frail, elderly person.

Chart 45-8 • *Behavioral Interventions for Urinary Incontinence*

Behavioral strategies are largely carried out, coordinated, and monitored by the nurse. These interventions may or may not be augmented by the use of medications.

Fluid Management

An adequate daily fluid intake of approximately 50 to 60 ounces (1500 to 1600 mL), taken as small increments between breakfast and the evening meal, helps to reduce urinary urgency related to concentrated urine production, decreases the risk of urinary tract infection, and maintains bowel functioning. (Constipation, resulting from inadequate daily fluid intake, can increase urinary urgency and urine retention.) The best fluid is water. Fluids containing caffeine, carbonation, alcohol, or artificial sweetener should be avoided because they irritate the bladder wall, thus resulting in urinary urgency. Some patients who have heart failure or end-stage renal disease need to discuss their daily fluid limit with their primary health care provider.

Standardized Voiding Frequency

After establishing a patient's natural voiding and urinary incontinence tendencies, voiding on a schedule can be very effective in those with and without cognitive impairment, although patients with cognitive impairment may require assistance with this technique from nursing personnel or family members. The object is to purposely empty the bladder before the bladder reaches the critical volume that would cause an urge or stress incontinence episode. This approach involves the following:

- **Timed voiding** involves establishing a set voiding frequency (such as every 2 hours if incontinent episodes tend to occur 2 or more hours after voiding). The individual chooses to "void by the clock" at the given interval while awake, rather than wait until a voiding urge occurs.
- **Prompted voiding** is timed voiding that is carried out by staff or family members when the individual has cognitive difficulties that make it difficult to remember to void at set intervals. The caregiver checks the patient to assess if he or she has remained dry and, if so, assists the patient to use the bathroom while providing positive reinforcement for remaining dry.
- **Habit retraining** is timed voiding at an interval that is more frequent than the individual would usually choose. This technique helps to restore the sensation of the need to void in individuals who are experiencing diminished sensation of bladder filling due to various medical conditions such as a mild cerebrovascular accident (CVA).
- **Bladder retraining,** also known as "bladder drill," incorporates a timed voiding schedule and urinary urge inhibition exercises to inhibit voiding, or leaking urine, in an attempt to remain dry for a set time. When the first timing interval is easily reached on a consistent basis without urinary urgency or incontinence, a new voiding interval, usually 10 to 15 minutes beyond the last, is established. Again, the individual practices urge inhibition exercises to delay voiding or avoid incontinence until the next preset interval arrives. When an acceptable voiding interval is reached, the patient continues that timed voiding sequence throughout the day.

Pelvic Muscle Exercise (PME)

Also known as Kegel exercises, PME aims to strengthen the voluntary muscles that assist in bladder and bowel continence in both men and women. Research shows that written or verbal instruction alone is usually inadequate to teach an individual how to identify and strengthen the pelvic floor for sufficient bladder and bowel control. Biofeedback-assisted PME uses either electromyography or manometry to help the individual identify the pelvic muscles as he or she attempts to learn which muscle group is involved when performing PME. The biofeedback method also allows assessment of the strength of this muscle area.

PME involves gently tightening the same muscles used to stop flatus or the stream of urine for 5- to 10-second increments, followed by 10-second resting phases. To be effective, these exercises need to be performed two or three times a day for at least 6 weeks. Depending on the strength of the pelvic musculature when initially evaluated, anywhere from 10 to 30 repetitions of PME are prescribed at each session. Elderly patients may need to exercise for an even longer time to strengthen the pelvic floor muscles. Pelvic muscle exercises are helpful for women with stress, urge, or mixed incontinence and for men who have undergone prostate surgery.

Vaginal Cone Retention Exercises

Vaginal cone retention exercises are an adjunct to the Kegel exercises. Vaginal cones of varying weight are inserted intravaginally twice a day. The patient tries to retain the cone for 15 minutes by contracting the pelvic muscles.

Transvaginal or Transrectal Electrical Stimulation

Commonly used to treat urinary incontinence, electrical stimulation is known to elicit a passive contraction of the pelvic floor musculature, thus re-educating these muscles to provide enhanced levels of continence. This modality is often used with biofeedback-assisted pelvic muscle exercise training and voiding schedules. At high frequencies, it is effective for stress incontinence. At low frequencies, electrical stimulation can also relieve symptoms of urinary urgency, frequency, and urge incontinence. Intermediate ranges are used for mixed incontinence.

Neuromodulation

Neuromodulation via transvaginal or transrectal nerve stimulation of the pelvic floor inhibits detrusor overactivity and hypersensory bladder signals and strengthens weak sphincter muscles.

It is also an option for people who are seeking help with stress incontinence who prefer to avoid surgery and who do not have access to behavioral therapies.

An artificial urinary sphincter can be used to close the urethra and promote continence. Two types of artificial sphincters are a periurethral cuff and a cuff inflation pump.

Men with overflow and stress incontinence may undergo a transurethral resection to relieve symptoms of prostatic enlargement. An artificial sphincter can be used after prostatic surgery for sphincter incompetence (Fig. 45-2). After surgery, periurethral bulking agents can be injected into the periurethral area to increase compression of the urethra.

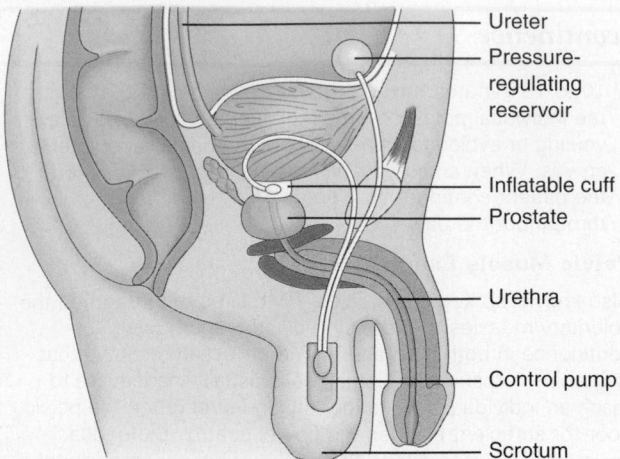

Ureter
Pressure-regulating reservoir
Inflatable cuff
Prostate
Urethra
Control pump
Scrotum

Figure 45-2 Male artificial urinary sphincter. An inflatable cuff is inserted surgically around the urethra or neck of the bladder. To empty the bladder, the cuff is deflated by squeezing the control pump located in the scrotum.

Nursing Management

Nursing management is based on the premise that incontinence is not inevitable with illness or aging and that it is often reversible and treatable. The nursing interventions are determined in part by the type of treatment that is undertaken. For behavioral therapy to be effective, the nurse must provide support and encouragement, because it is easy for the patient to become discouraged if therapy does not quickly improve the level of continence. Patient teaching is important and should be provided verbally and in writing (Chart 45-9). The patient should be taught to develop and use a log or diary to record timing of pelvic floor muscle exercises, frequency of voiding, any changes in bladder function, and any episodes of incontinence (Miller, 2009).

If pharmacologic treatment is used, its purpose is explained to the patient and family. It is important to tell patients with mixed incontinence that anticholinergic and antispasmodic agents can help decrease urinary urgency and frequency and urge incontinence but do not decrease the urinary incontinence related to stress incontinence. If surgical correction is undertaken, the procedure and its desired outcomes are described to the patient and family. Follow-up

contact with the patient enables the nurse to answer the patient's questions and to provide reinforcement and encouragement.

Urinary Retention

Urinary retention is the inability to empty the bladder completely during attempts to void. Chronic urine retention often leads to **overflow incontinence** (from the pressure of the retained urine in the bladder). **Residual urine** is urine that remains in the bladder after voiding. In a healthy adult younger than 60 years of age, complete bladder emptying should occur with each voiding. In adults older than 60 years of age, 50 to 100 mL of residual urine may remain after each voiding because of the decreased contractility of the detrusor muscle.

Urinary retention can occur postoperatively in any patient, particularly if the surgery affected the perineal or anal regions and resulted in reflex spasm of the sphincters. General anesthesia reduces bladder muscle innervation and suppresses the urge to void, impeding bladder emptying.

Pathophysiology

Urinary retention may result from diabetes, prostatic enlargement, urethral pathology (infection, tumor, calculus), trauma (pelvic injuries), pregnancy, or neurologic disorders such as stroke, spinal cord injury, multiple sclerosis, or Parkinson's disease. Some medications cause urinary retention, either by inhibiting bladder contractility or by increasing bladder outlet resistance (Karch, 2008).

Assessment and Diagnostic Findings

The assessment of a patient for urinary retention is multifaceted because the signs and symptoms are challenging to detect. The following questions serve as a guide in assessment:

- What was the time of the last voiding, and how much urine was voided?
- Is the patient voiding small amounts of urine frequently?
- Is the patient dribbling urine?
- Does the patient complain of pain or discomfort in the lower abdomen? (Discomfort may be relatively mild if the bladder distends slowly.)
- Is the pelvic area rounded and swollen (could indicate urine retention and a distended bladder)?

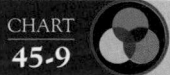

CHART 45-9   **PATIENT EDUCATION**
Strategies for Promoting Urinary Continence

- Increase your awareness of the amount and timing of all fluid intake.
- Avoid taking diuretics after 4 PM.
- Avoid bladder irritants, such as caffeine, alcohol, and aspartame (NutraSweet).
- Take steps to avoid constipation: Drink adequate fluids, eat a well-balanced diet high in fiber, exercise regularly, and take stool softeners if recommended.
- Void regularly, five to eight times a day (about every 2 to 3 hours):

    First thing in the morning
    Before each meal
    Before retiring to bed
    Once during the night if necessary
- Perform all pelvic floor muscle exercises as prescribed, every day.
- Stop smoking (smokers usually cough frequently, which increases incontinence).

- Does percussion of the suprapubic region elicit dullness (possibly indicating urine retention and a distended bladder)?
- Are other indicators of urinary retention present, such as restlessness and agitation?
- Does a postvoid bladder ultrasound test reveal residual urine?

The patient may verbalize an awareness of bladder fullness and a sensation of incomplete bladder emptying. Signs and symptoms of UTI (hematuria, urgency, frequency, and nocturia) may be present. A series of urodynamic studies, described in Chapter 43, may be performed to identify the type of bladder dysfunction and to aid in determining appropriate treatment. A voiding diary can be used to provide a written record of the amount of urine voided and the frequency of voiding. Postvoid residual urine may be assessed either using straight catheterization or an ultrasound bladder scanner and is considered diagnostic of urinary retention if there is more than 100 mL of residual urine.

Complications

Urine retention can lead to chronic infections that if unresolved predispose the patient to renal calculi (urolithiasis or nephrolithiasis), pyelonephritis, sepsis, or hydronephrosis. In addition, urine leakage can lead to perineal skin breakdown, especially if regular hygiene measures are neglected.

Nursing Management

Strategies are instituted to prevent overdistention of the bladder and to treat infection or correct obstruction. However, many complications can be prevented with careful assessment and appropriate nursing interventions. The nurse explains to the patient why normal voiding is not occurring and monitors urine output closely. The nurse also provides reassurance about the temporary nature of retention and successful management strategies.

Promoting Urinary Elimination

Nursing measures to encourage normal voiding patterns include providing privacy, ensuring an environment and body position conducive to voiding, and assisting the patient with the use of the bathroom or bedside commode, rather than a bedpan, to provide a more natural setting for voiding. If his condition allows, the male patient may stand beside the bed to use the urinal; most men find this position more comfortable and natural.

Additional measures include applying warmth to relax the sphincters (ie, sitz baths, warm compresses to the perineum, showers), giving the patient hot tea, and offering encouragement and reassurance. Simple trigger techniques, such as turning on the water faucet while the patient is trying to void, may also be used. Other examples of trigger techniques are stroking the abdomen or inner thighs, tapping above the pubic area, and dipping the patient's hands in warm water. After surgery or childbirth, prescribed analgesic agents should be administered because pain in the perineal area can make voiding difficult. A combination of techniques may be necessary to initiate voiding.

When the patient cannot void, catheterization is used to prevent overdistention of the bladder (see later discussion of neurogenic bladder and catheterization). In the case of prostatic obstruction, attempts at catheterization (by the urologist) may not be successful, requiring insertion of a **suprapubic catheter** (catheter inserted through a small abdominal incision into the bladder). After urinary drainage is restored, bladder retraining is initiated for the patient who cannot void spontaneously.

Promoting Home and Community-Based Care

In addition to the strategies listed for promoting urinary continence found in Chart 45-9, modifications to the home environment can provide simple and effective ways to assist in treating urinary incontinence and retention. For example, the patient may need to remove obstacles, such as throw rugs or other objects, to provide easy, safe access to the bathroom. Other modifications that the nurse may recommend include installing support bars in the bathroom; placing a bedside commode, bedpan, or urinal within easy reach; leaving lights on in the bedroom and bathroom; and wearing clothing that is easy to remove quickly.

Neurogenic Bladder

Neurogenic bladder is a dysfunction that results from a lesion of the nervous system and leads to urinary incontinence. It may be caused by spinal cord injury, spinal tumor, herniated vertebral disk, multiple sclerosis, congenital disorders (spina bifida or myelomeningocele), infection, or complications of diabetes mellitus (see Chapters 41, 63, and 64).

Pathophysiology

The two types of neurogenic bladder are spastic (or reflex) bladder and flaccid bladder. Spastic bladder is the more common type and is caused by any spinal cord lesion above the voiding reflex arc (upper motor neuron lesion). The result is a loss of conscious sensation and cerebral motor control. A spastic bladder empties on reflex, with minimal or no controlling influence to regulate its activity.

Flaccid bladder is caused by a lower motor neuron lesion, commonly resulting from trauma. This form of neurogenic bladder is also increasingly being recognized in patients with diabetes mellitus. The bladder continues to fill and becomes greatly distended, and overflow incontinence occurs. The bladder muscle does not contract forcefully at any time. Because sensory loss may accompany a flaccid bladder, the patient feels no discomfort.

Assessment and Diagnostic Findings

Evaluation for neurogenic bladder involves measurement of fluid intake, urine output, and residual urine volume; urinalysis; and assessment of sensory awareness of bladder fullness and degree of motor control. Comprehensive urodynamic studies are also performed.

Complications

The most common complication of neurogenic bladder is infection resulting from urinary stasis and catheterization. Long-term complications include urolithiasis (stones in the urinary tract), vesicoureteral reflux, and hydronephrosis, all of which can lead to destruction of the kidney.

Medical Management

The problems resulting from neurogenic bladder disorders vary considerably from patient to patient and are a major challenge to the health care team. Several long-term objectives appropriate for all types of neurogenic bladders include preventing overdistention of the bladder, emptying the bladder regularly and completely, maintaining urine sterility with no stone formation, and maintaining adequate bladder capacity with no reflux.

Specific interventions include continuous, intermittent, or self-catheterization (discussed later in this chapter); use of an external condom-type catheter; a diet low in calcium (to prevent calculi); and encouragement of mobility and ambulation. A liberal fluid intake is encouraged to reduce the urinary bacterial count, reduce stasis, decrease the concentration of calcium in the urine, and minimize the precipitation of urinary crystals and subsequent stone formation.

A bladder retraining program may be effective in treating a spastic bladder or urine retention. Use of a timed, or habit, voiding schedule may be established. To further enhance emptying of a flaccid bladder, the patient may be taught to "double void." After each voiding, the patient is instructed to remain on the toilet, relax for 1 to 2 minutes, and then attempt to void again in an effort to further empty the bladder.

Pharmacologic Therapy

Parasympathomimetic medications, such as bethanechol (Urecholine), may help to increase the contraction of the detrusor muscle.

Surgical Management

In some cases, surgery may be carried out to correct bladder neck contractures or vesicoureteral reflux or to perform some type of urinary diversion procedure.

Catheterization

In patients with a urologic disorder or with marginal kidney function, care must be taken to ensure that urinary drainage is adequate and that kidney function is preserved. When urine cannot be eliminated naturally and must be drained artificially, catheters may be inserted directly into the bladder, the ureter, or the renal pelvis (Senese, Hendricks, Morrison, et al., 2006). Catheters vary in size, shape, length, material, and configuration. The type of catheter used depends on its purpose.

Catheterization is performed to achieve the following:
- Relieve urinary tract obstruction
- Assist with postoperative drainage in urologic and other surgeries
- Provide a means to monitor accurate urine output in critically ill patients
- Promote urinary drainage in patients with neurogenic bladder dysfunction or urine retention
- Prevent urinary leakage in patients with stage III to IV pressure ulcers (see Chapter 11)

A patient should be catheterized only if necessary, because catheterization commonly leads to UTI. Catheters

impede most of the natural defenses of the lower urinary tract by obstructing the periurethral ducts, irritating the bladder mucosa, and providing an artificial route for organisms to enter the bladder. Organisms may be introduced from the urethra into the bladder during catheterization, or they may migrate along the epithelial surface of the urethra or external surface of the catheter. In addition, urinary catheters have been associated with other complications, such as bladder spasms, urethral strictures, and pressure necrosis.

Indwelling Catheters

When an indwelling catheter cannot be avoided, a closed drainage system is essential. This drainage system is designed to prevent any disconnections, thereby reducing the risk of contamination. Triple-lumen catheters are commonly used after transurethral prostate surgery (see Chapter 49). This system has a triple-lumen indwelling urethral catheter attached to a closed sterile drainage system. With the triple-lumen catheter, urinary drainage occurs through one channel. The retention balloon of the catheter is inflated with water or air through the second channel, and the bladder is continuously irrigated with sterile irrigating solution through the third channel.

The spout (or drainage port) of any urinary drainage bag can become contaminated when opened to drain the bag. Bacteria enter the urinary drainage bag, multiply rapidly, and then migrate to the drainage tubing, catheter, and bladder. By keeping the drainage bag lower than the patient's bladder and not allowing urine to flow back into the bladder, this risk is reduced.

Suprapubic Catheters

Suprapubic catheterization allows bladder drainage by inserting a catheter or tube into the bladder through a suprapubic (above the pubis) incision or puncture (Fig. 45-3). The catheter or suprapubic drainage tube is then threaded into the bladder and secured with sutures or tape, and the area around the catheter is covered with a sterile dressing. The catheter is connected to a sterile closed drainage system, and the tubing is secured to prevent tension on the catheter. This may be a temporary measure to divert the flow of urine from the urethra when the urethral route is impassable (because of injuries, strictures, prostatic obstruction), after gynecologic or other abdominal surgery when bladder dysfunction is likely to occur, and occasionally after pelvic fractures.

Suprapubic bladder drainage may be maintained continuously for several weeks. When the patient's ability to void is to be tested, the catheter is clamped for 4 hours, during which time the patient attempts to void. After the patient voids, the catheter is unclamped, and the residual urine is measured. If the amount of residual urine is less than 100 mL on two separate occasions (morning and evening), the catheter is usually removed. However, if the patient complains of pain or discomfort, the suprapubic catheter is usually left in place until the patient can void successfully.

Suprapubic drainage offers certain advantages. Patients can usually void sooner after surgery than those with urethral catheters, and they may be more comfortable. The catheter allows greater mobility, permits measurement of

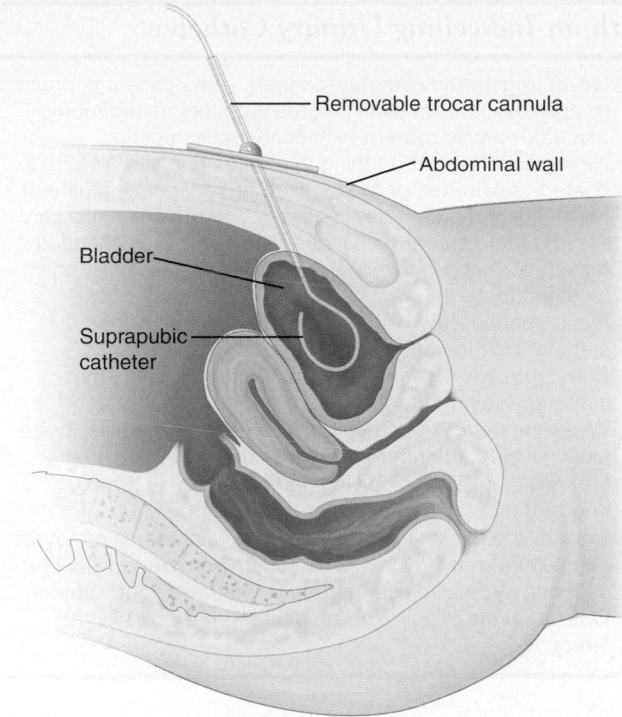

Figure 45-3 Suprapubic bladder drainage. A trocar cannula is used to puncture the abdominal and bladder walls. The catheter is threaded through the trocar cannula, which is then removed, leaving the catheter in place. The catheter is secured by tape or sutures to prevent unintentional removal.

residual urine without urethral instrumentation, and presents less risk of bladder infection. The suprapubic catheter is removed when it is no longer required, and a sterile dressing is placed over the site.

The patient requires liberal amounts of fluid to prevent encrustation around the catheter. Other potential problems include the formation of bladder stones, acute and chronic infections, and problems collecting urine. A wound care specialist/enterostomal therapist, also referred to as a wound-ostomy-continence nurse (WOCN), may be consulted to assist the patient and family in selecting the most suitable urine collection system and to teach them about its use and care.

Nursing Management

Assessing the Patient and the System

For patients with indwelling catheters, the nurse assesses the drainage system to ensure that it provides adequate urinary drainage. The color, odor, and volume of urine are also monitored. An accurate record of fluid intake and urine output provides essential information about the adequacy of renal function and urinary drainage.

Patients at high risk for UTI from catheterization need to be identified and monitored carefully. These include women; older adults; and patients who are debilitated, malnourished, chronically ill, immunosuppressed, or have diabetes. They are observed for signs and symptoms of UTI: cloudy malodorous urine, hematuria, fever, chills, anorexia, and malaise. Any drainage and excoriation in the area

Physiology ■■■ Pathophysiology

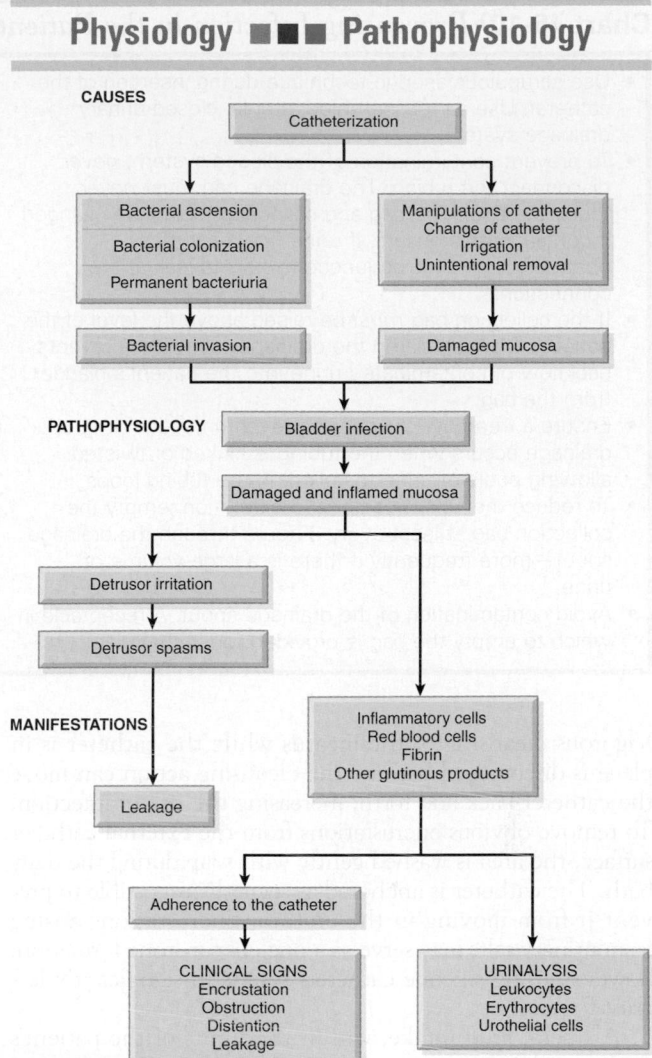

Figure 45-4 Pathophysiology and manifestations of bladder infection with long-term catheterization in elderly patients.

around the urethral orifice is noted. Urine cultures provide the most accurate means of assessing a patient for infection.

 Gerontologic Considerations

The elderly patient with an indwelling catheter may not exhibit the typical signs and symptoms of infection. Therefore, any subtle change in physical condition or mental status must be considered a possible indication of infection and promptly investigated because sepsis may occur before the infection is diagnosed. Figure 45-4 summarizes the sequence of events leading to infection and leakage of urine that often follow long-term use of an indwelling catheter in an elderly patient.

Preventing Infection

Certain principles of care are essential to prevent infection in patients with a closed urinary drainage system (Chart 45-10). The catheter is a foreign body in the urethra and produces a reaction in the urethral mucosa with some urethral discharge.

Chart 45-10 • *Preventing Infection in the Patient With an Indwelling Urinary Catheter*

- Use scrupulous aseptic technique during insertion of the catheter. Use a preassembled, sterile, closed urinary drainage system.
- To prevent contamination of the closed system, *never* disconnect the tubing. The drainage bag must *never* touch the floor. The bag and collecting tubing are changed if contamination occurs, if urine flow becomes obstructed, or if tubing junctions start to leak at the connections.
- If the collection bag *must* be raised above the level of the patient's bladder, clamp the drainage tube. This prevents backflow of contaminated urine into the patient's bladder from the bag.
- Ensure a free flow of urine to prevent infection. Improper drainage occurs when the tubing is kinked or twisted, allowing pools of urine to collect in the tubing loops.
- To reduce the risk of bacterial proliferation, empty the collection bag at least every 8 hours through the drainage spout—more frequently if there is a large volume of urine.
- Avoid contamination of the drainage spout. A receptacle in which to empty the bag is provided for each patient.

- Never irrigate the catheter routinely. If the patient is prone to obstruction from clots or large amounts of sediment, use a three-way system with continuous irrigation.
- Never disconnect the tubing to obtain urine samples, to irrigate the catheter, or to ambulate or transport the patient.
- Never leave the catheter in place longer than is necessary.
- Avoid routine catheter changes. The catheter is changed only to correct problems such as leakage, blockage, or encrustations.
- Avoid unnecessary handling or manipulation of the catheter by the patient or staff.
- Carry out hand hygiene before and after handling the catheter, tubing, or drainage bag.
- Wash the perineal area with soap and water at least twice a day; avoid a to-and-fro motion of the catheter. Dry the area well, but avoid applying powder because it may irritate the perineum.
- Monitor the patient's voiding when the catheter is removed. The patient must void within 8 hours; if unable to void, the patient may require catheterization with a straight catheter.
- Obtain a urine specimen for culture at the first sign of infection.

Vigorous cleansing of the meatus while the catheter is in place is discouraged because the cleansing action can move the catheter back and forth, increasing the risk of infection. To remove obvious encrustations from the external catheter surface, the area is washed gently with soap during the daily bath. The catheter is anchored as securely as possible to prevent it from moving in the urethra. Encrustations arising from urinary salts may serve as a nucleus for stone formation; however, using silicone catheters results in significantly less crust formation.

A liberal fluid intake, within the limits of the patient's cardiac and renal reserve, and an increased urine output must be ensured to flush the catheter and to dilute urinary substances that might form encrustations (Senese, et al., 2006).

Urine cultures are obtained as prescribed or indicated when monitoring the patient for infection; many catheters have an aspiration (puncture) port from which a specimen can be obtained.

Bacteriuria is considered inevitable in patients with indwelling catheters; therefore, controversy remains about the usefulness of taking cultures and treating asymptomatic bacteriuria, because overtreatment may lead to resistant strains of bacteria. Continual observation for fever, chills, and other signs and symptoms of systemic infection is necessary. Infections are treated aggressively.

Minimizing Trauma

Trauma to the urethra can be minimized by:
- Using an appropriate-sized catheter
- Lubricating the catheter adequately with a water-soluble lubricant during insertion
- Inserting the catheter far enough into the bladder to prevent trauma to the urethral tissues when the retention balloon of the catheter is inflated

Manipulation of the catheter is the most common cause of trauma to the bladder mucosa in the catheterized patient. Infection can occur when urine invades the damaged mucosa.

The catheter is secured properly to prevent it from moving, causing traction on the urethra, or being unintentionally removed, and care is taken to ensure that the catheter position permits leg movement. In male patients, the drainage tube (not the catheter) is taped laterally to the thigh to prevent pressure on the urethra at the penoscrotal junction, which can eventually lead to formation of an urethrocutaneous fistula. In female patients, the drainage tubing attached to the catheter is taped to the thigh to prevent tension and traction on the bladder.

Special care should be taken to ensure that any patient who is confused does not remove the catheter with the retention balloon still inflated, because this could cause bleeding and considerable injury to the urethra.

Retraining the Bladder

When an indwelling urinary catheter is in place, the detrusor muscle does not actively contract the bladder wall to stimulate emptying because urine is continuously draining from the bladder. As a result, the detrusor may not immediately respond to bladder filling when the catheter is removed, resulting in either urine retention or urinary incontinence. This condition, known as postcatheterization detrusor instability, can be managed with bladder retraining (Chart 45-11).

Immediately after the indwelling catheter is removed, the patient is placed on a timed voiding schedule, usually every 2 to 3 hours. At the given time interval, the patient is instructed to void. The bladder is then scanned using a portable ultrasonic bladder scanner, and if the bladder has not emptied completely, straight catheterization may be performed (Altschuler & Diaz, 2006). After a few days, as the nerve endings in the bladder wall become resensitized to the bladder filling and emptying, bladder function usually

Chart 45-11 • *Bladder Retraining After Indwelling Catheterization*

- Instruct the patient to drink a measured amount of fluid from 8 AM to 10 PM to avoid bladder overdistention. Offer no fluids (except sips) after 10 PM.
- At specific times, ask the patient to void by applying pressure over the bladder, tapping the abdomen, or running water to trigger the bladder.
- Immediately after the voiding attempt, catheterize the patient to determine the amount of residual urine.
- Measure the volumes of urine voided and obtained by catheterization.
- Palpate the bladder at repeated intervals to assess for distention.
- Instruct the patient who has no voiding sensation to be alert for any signs that indicate a full bladder, such as perspiration, cold hands or feet, or feelings of anxiety.
- Lengthen the intervals between catheterizations as the volume of residual urine decreases. Catheterization is usually discontinued when the volume of residual urine is less than 100 mL.

returns to normal. If the person has had an indwelling catheter in place for an extended period, bladder retraining will take longer; in some cases, function may never return to normal and long-term intermittent catheterization may become necessary.

Assisting With Intermittent Self-Catheterization

Intermittent self-catheterization provides periodic drainage of urine from the bladder. By promoting drainage and eliminating excessive residual urine, intermittent catheterization protects the kidneys, reduces the incidence of UTIs, and improves continence. It is the treatment of choice in some patients with spinal cord injury and other neurologic disorders, such as multiple sclerosis, when the ability to empty the bladder is impaired. Self-catheterization promotes independence, results in few complications, and enhances self-esteem and quality of life.

When teaching the patient how to perform self-catheterization, the nurse must use aseptic technique to minimize the risk of cross-contamination. However, the patient may use a "clean" (nonsterile) technique at home, where the risk of cross-contamination is reduced. Either antibacterial liquid soap or povidone-iodine (Betadine) solution is recommended for cleaning urinary catheters at home. The catheter is thoroughly rinsed with tap water after soaking in the cleaning solution. It must dry before reuse. It should be kept in its own container, such as a plastic food-storage bag.

In teaching the patient, the nurse emphasizes the importance of frequent catheterization and emptying the bladder at the prescribed time. The average daytime clean intermittent catheterization schedule is every 4 to 6 hours and just before bedtime. If the patient is awakened at night with an urge to void, catheterization may be performed after an attempt is made to void normally.

The female patient assumes a Fowler's position and uses a mirror to help locate the urinary meatus. She lubricates the catheter and inserts it 7.5 cm (3 inches) into the urethra, in a downward and backward direction. The male patient assumes a Fowler's or sitting position, lubricates the catheter, and retracts the foreskin of the penis with one hand while grasping the penis and holding it at a right angle to the body. (This maneuver straightens the urethra and makes it easier to insert the catheter.) He inserts the catheter 15 to 25 cm (6 to 10 inches) until urine begins to flow. After removal, the catheter is cleaned, rinsed, dried, and placed in a plastic bag or case. Patients who follow an intermittent catheterization routine should consult a primary health care provider at regular intervals to assess urinary function and to detect complications. If the patient cannot perform intermittent self-catheterization, a family member or caregiver may be taught to carry out the procedure at regular intervals during the day.

An alternative to self-catheterization is creation of the Mitrofanoff umbilical appendicovesicostomy, which provides easy access to the bladder, but requires an extensive surgical procedure. In this procedure, the bladder neck is closed and the appendix is used to create access to the bladder from the skin surface through a submucosal tunnel created with the appendix. One end of the appendix is brought to the skin surface and used as a stoma and the other end is tunneled into the bladder. The appendix serves as an artificial urinary sphincter when an alternative is necessary to empty the bladder. A surgically prepared continent urine reservoir with a sphincter mechanism is required in cases of bladder cancer and severe **interstitial cystitis** (inflammation of the bladder wall). Various types of urologic stomas may be used when a radical **cystectomy** (surgical removal of the bladder) is necessary.

UROLITHIASIS AND NEPHROLITHIASIS

Urolithiasis and nephrolithiasis refer to stones (calculi) in the urinary tract and kidney, respectively. Urinary stones account for more than 320,000 hospital admissions each year. The occurrence of urinary stones occurs predominantly in the third to fifth decades of life and affects men more than women. About half of patients with a single renal stone have another episode within 5 years (Colella, Kochis, Galli, et al., 2005).

Pathophysiology

Stones are formed in the urinary tract when urinary concentrations of substances such as calcium oxalate, calcium phosphate, and uric acid increase. Referred to as supersaturation, this is dependent on the amount of the substance, ionic strength, and pH of the urine. Stones may be found anywhere from the kidney to the bladder and may vary in size from minute granular deposits, called sand or gravel, to bladder stones as large as an orange. The different sites of calculi formation in the urinary tract are shown in Figure 45-5.

Stone formation is not clearly understood, and there are a number of theories about their causes. One theory is that there is a deficiency of substances that normally prevent crystallization in the urine, such as citrate, magnesium, nephrocalcin, and uropontin (Porth & Matfin, 2009). Another theory relates to fluid volume status of the patient

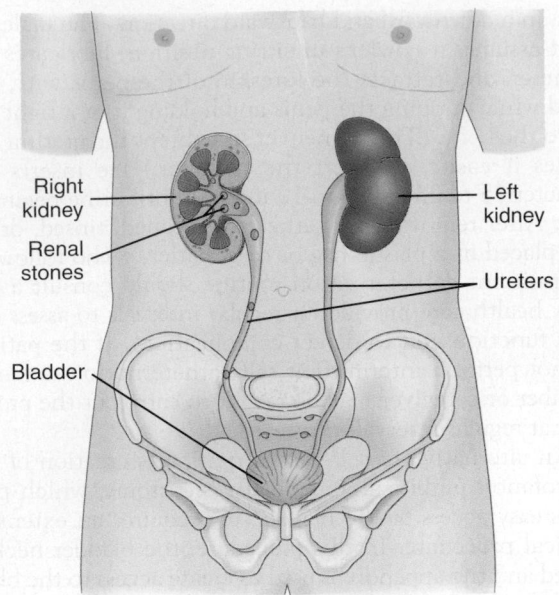

Figure 45-5 Examples of potential sites of calculi formation (urolithiasis) in the urinary tract.

Labels: Right kidney, Renal stones, Bladder, Left kidney, Ureters

(stones tend to occur more often in dehydrated patients). Certain factors favor the formation of stones, including infection, urinary stasis, and periods of immobility, all of which slow renal drainage and alter calcium metabolism. In addition, increased calcium concentrations in the blood and urine promote precipitation of calcium and formation of stones (about 75% of all renal stones are calcium based). Causes of hypercalcemia (high serum calcium) and hypercalciuria (high urine calcium) may include the following:

- Hyperparathyroidism
- Renal tubular acidosis
- Cancers
- Granulomatous diseases (eg, sarcoidosis, tuberculosis), which may cause increased vitamin D production by the granulomatous tissue
- Excessive intake of vitamin D
- Excessive intake of milk and alkali
- Myeloproliferative diseases (leukemia, polycythemia vera, multiple myeloma), which produce an unusual proliferation of blood cells from the bone marrow

For patients with stones containing uric acid, struvite, or cystine, a thorough physical examination and metabolic workup are indicated because of associated disturbances contributing to the stone formation. Uric acid stones (5% to 10% of all stones) may be seen in patients with gout or myeloproliferative disorders. Struvite stones account for 15% of urinary calculi and form in persistently alkaline, ammonia-rich urine caused by the presence of urease-splitting bacteria such as *Proteus, Pseudomonas, Klebsiella, Staphylococcus,* or *Mycoplasma* species. Predisposing factors for struvite stones include neurogenic bladder, foreign bodies, and recurrent UTIs. Cystine stones (1% to 2% of all stones) occur exclusively in patients with a rare inherited defect in renal absorption of cystine (an amino acid) (Porth & Matfin, 2009).

Several conditions as well as certain metabolic risk factors predispose patients to stone formation. These include anatomic derangements such as polycystic kidney disease, horseshoe kidneys, chronic strictures, and medullary sponge disease. Urinary stone formation can occur in patients with inflammatory bowel disease and in those with an ileostomy or bowel resection because these patients absorb more oxalate. Medications known to cause stones in some patients include antacids, acetazolamide (Diamox), vitamin D, laxatives, and high doses of aspirin (Karch, 2008). However, in many patients, no cause may be found.

Clinical Manifestations

Signs and symptoms of stones in the urinary system depend on the presence of obstruction, infection, and edema. When stones block the flow of urine, obstruction develops, producing an increase in hydrostatic pressure and distending the renal pelvis and proximal ureter. Infection (pyelonephritis and UTI with chills, fever, and frequency) can be a contributing factor with struvite stones (Porth & Matfin, 2009). Some stones cause few, if any, symptoms while slowly destroying the functional units (nephrons) of the kidney; others cause excruciating pain and discomfort.

Stones in the renal pelvis may be associated with an intense, deep ache in the costovertebral region. Hematuria is often present; pyuria may also be noted. Pain originating in the renal area radiates anteriorly and downward toward the bladder in the female and toward the testis in the male. If the pain suddenly becomes acute, with tenderness over the costovertebral area, and nausea and vomiting appear, the patient is having an episode of renal colic. Diarrhea and abdominal discomfort may occur. These GI symptoms are due to renointestinal reflexes and the anatomic proximity of the kidneys to the stomach, pancreas, and large intestine.

Stones lodged in the ureter (ureteral obstruction) cause acute, excruciating, colicky, wavelike pain, radiating down the thigh and to the genitalia. Often, the patient has a desire to void, but little urine is passed, and it usually contains blood because of the abrasive action of the stone. This group of symptoms is called ureteral colic. Colic is mediated by prostaglandin E, a substance that increases ureteral contractility and renal blood flow and that leads to increased intraureteral pressure and pain. In general, the patient spontaneously passes stones 0.5 to 1 cm in diameter. Stones larger than 1 cm in diameter usually must be removed or fragmented (broken up by lithotripsy) so that they can be removed or passed spontaneously.

Stones lodged in the bladder usually produce symptoms of irritation and may be associated with UTI and hematuria. If the stone obstructs the bladder neck, urinary retention occurs. If infection is associated with a stone, the condition is far more serious, with urosepsis threatening the patient's life.

Assessment and Diagnostic Findings

The diagnosis is confirmed by x-rays of the kidneys, ureters, and bladder (KUB) or by ultrasonography, IV urography, or retrograde pyelography. Blood chemistries and a 24-hour urine test for measurement of calcium, uric acid, creatinine, sodium, pH, and total volume are part of the diagnostic workup. Dietary and medication histories and family history of renal stones are obtained to identify factors predisposing the patient to the formation of stones.

When stones are recovered (stones may be freely passed by the patient or removed through special procedures), chemical analysis is carried out to determine their composition. Stone analysis can provide a clear indication of the underlying disorder. For example, calcium oxalate or calcium phosphate stones usually indicate disorders of oxalate or calcium metabolism, whereas urate stones suggest a disturbance in uric acid metabolism (Porth & Matfin, 2009).

Medical Management

The goals of management are to eradicate the stone, determine the stone type, prevent nephron destruction, control infection, and relieve any obstruction that may be present. The immediate objective of treatment of renal or ureteral colic is to relieve the pain until its cause can be eliminated. Opioid analgesic agents are administered to prevent shock and syncope that may result from the excruciating pain. Nonsteroidal anti-inflammatory drugs (NSAIDs) are effective in treating renal stone pain because they provide specific pain relief. They also inhibit the synthesis of prostaglandin E, reducing swelling and facilitating passage of the stone. Generally once the stone has passed, the pain is relieved. Hot baths or moist heat to the flank areas may also be helpful. Unless the patient is vomiting or has heart failure or any other condition requiring fluid restriction, fluids are encouraged. This increases the hydrostatic pressure behind the stone, assisting it in its downward passage. A high, around-the-clock fluid intake reduces the concentration of urinary crystalloids, dilutes the urine, and ensures a high urine output.

Nutritional Therapy

Nutritional therapy plays an important role in preventing renal stones (Dudek, 2006) (Chart 45-12). Fluid intake is the mainstay of most medical therapy for renal stones.

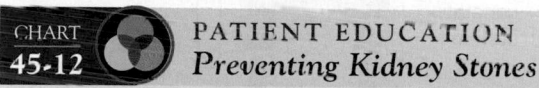

CHART 45-12   PATIENT EDUCATION
Preventing Kidney Stones

- Avoid protein intake; usually protein is restricted to 60 g/day to decrease urinary excretion of calcium and uric acid.
- A sodium intake of 3 to 4 g/day is recommended. Table salt and high-sodium foods should be reduced, because sodium competes with calcium for reabsorption in the kidneys.
- Low-calcium diets are not generally recommended, except for true absorptive hypercalciuria. Evidence shows that limiting calcium, especially in women, can lead to osteoporosis and does not prevent renal stones.
- Avoid intake of oxalate-containing foods (eg, spinach, strawberries, rhubarb, tea, peanuts, wheat bran).
- During the day, drink fluids (ideally water) every 1 to 2 hours.
- Drink two glasses of water at bedtime and an additional glass at each nighttime awakening to prevent urine from becoming too concentrated during the night.
- Avoid activities leading to sudden increases in environmental temperatures that may cause excessive sweating and dehydration.
- Contact your primary health care provider at the first sign of a urinary tract infection.

Unless fluids are contraindicated, patients with renal stones should drink eight to ten 8-ounce glasses of water daily or have IV fluids prescribed to keep the urine dilute. A urine output exceeding 2 L/day is advisable.

Calcium Stones

Historically, patients with calcium-based renal stones were advised to restrict calcium in their diet. However, recent evidence has questioned the advisability of this practice, except for patients with type II absorptive hypercalciuria (half of all patients with calcium stones), in whom stones are clearly the result of excess dietary calcium. Liberal fluid intake is encouraged along with dietary restriction of protein and sodium; however, dietary changes cannot be recommended with confidence because of insufficient evidence. It was once thought that a high-protein diet was associated with increased urinary excretion of calcium and uric acid, thereby causing a supersaturation of these substances in the urine. Similarly, a high sodium intake was thought to increase the amount of calcium in the urine. These beliefs have not been supported by research (Flagg, 2007). Medications such as ammonium chloride may be used, and if increased parathormone production (resulting in increased serum calcium levels in blood and urine) is a factor in the formation of stones, therapy with thiazide diuretics may be beneficial in reducing the calcium loss in the urine and lowering the elevated parathormone levels (Porth & Matfin, 2009).

Uric Acid Stones

For uric acid stones, the patient is placed on a low-purine diet to reduce the excretion of uric acid in the urine. Foods high in purine (shellfish, anchovies, asparagus, mushrooms, and organ meats) are avoided, and other proteins may be limited. Allopurinol (Zyloprim) may be prescribed to reduce serum uric acid levels and urinary uric acid excretion.

Cystine Stones

A low-protein diet is prescribed, the urine is alkalinized, and fluid intake is increased.

Oxalate Stones

A dilute urine is maintained and the intake of oxalate is limited. Many foods contain oxalate; however, only certain foods increase the urinary excretion of oxalate. These include spinach, strawberries, rhubarb, chocolate, tea, peanuts, and wheat bran.

Interventional Procedures

If the stone does not pass spontaneously or if complications occur, common interventions include endoscopic or other procedures. For example, ureteroscopy, extracorporeal shock wave lithotripsy (ESWL), or endourologic (percutaneous) stone removal may be necessary.

Ureteroscopy (Fig. 45-6A) involves first visualizing the stone and then destroying it. Access to the stone is accomplished by inserting a ureteroscope into the ureter and then inserting a laser, electrohydraulic lithotriptor, or ultrasound device through the ureteroscope to fragment and remove the stones. A stent may be inserted and left in place for 48 hours or more after the procedure to keep the ureter

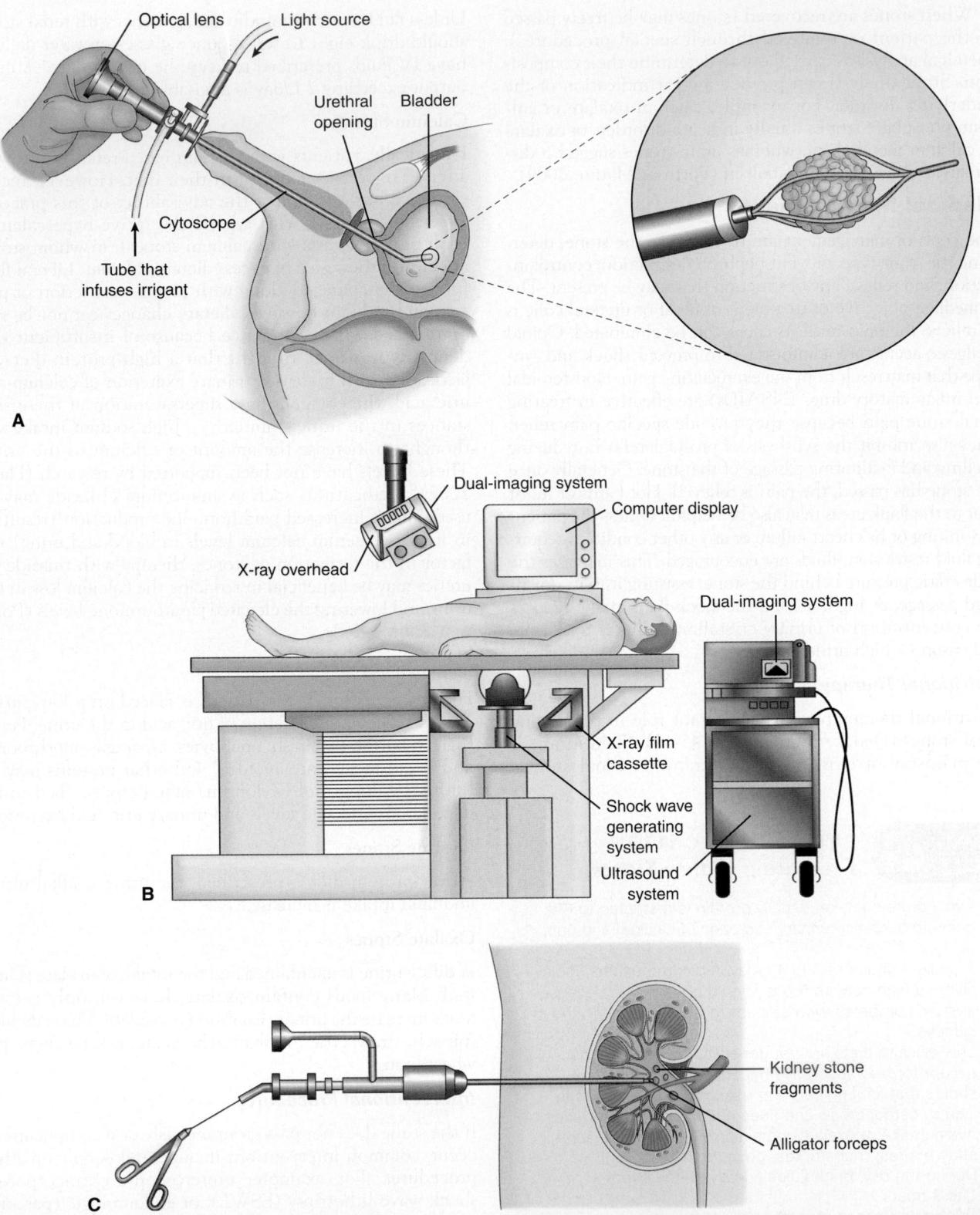

Figure 45-6 Methods of treating renal stones. **A,** During a cystoscopy, which is used for removing small stones located in the ureter close to the bladder, a ureteroscope is inserted into the ureter to visualize the stone. The stone is then fragmented or captured and removed. **B,** Extracorporeal shock water lithotripsy (ESWL) is used for most symptomatic, nonpassable upper urinary stones. Electromagnetically generated shock waves are focused over the area of the renal stone. The high-energy dry shock waves pass through the skin and fragment the stone. **C,** Percutaneous nephrolithotomy is used to treat larger stones. A percutaneous tract is formed and a nephroscope is inserted through it. Then the stone is extracted or pulverized.

patent. Hospital stays are generally brief, and some patients can be treated as outpatients.

ESWL is a noninvasive procedure used to break up stones in the calyx of the kidney (Fig. 45-6B). After the stones are fragmented to the size of grains of sand, the remnants of the stones are spontaneously voided. In ESWL, a high-energy amplitude of pressure, or shock wave, is generated by the abrupt release of energy and transmitted through water and soft tissues. When the shock wave encounters a substance of different intensity (a renal stone), a compression wave causes the surface of the stone to fragment. Repeated shock waves focused on the stone eventually reduce it to many small pieces that are excreted in the urine.

Discomfort from the multiple shocks may occur, although the shock waves usually do not cause damage to other tissue. The patient is observed for obstruction and infection resulting from blockage of the urinary tract by stone fragments. All urine is strained after the procedure; voided gravel or sand is sent to the laboratory for chemical analysis. Several treatments may be necessary to ensure disintegration of stones. Although lithotripsy is a costly treatment, its cost is offset by a decrease in the length of hospital stay and avoidance of a surgical procedure.

Endourologic methods of stone removal (Fig. 45-6C) may be used to extract renal calculi that cannot be removed by other procedures. A percutaneous nephrostomy or a percutaneous nephrolithotomy (which are similar procedures) may be performed. A nephroscope is introduced through a percutaneous route into the renal parenchyma. Depending on its size, the stone may be extracted with forceps or by a stone retrieval basket. If the stone is too large to initially be removed, an ultrasound probe inserted through a nephrostomy tube is used to pulverize the stone. Small stone fragments and stone dust are then removed.

Electrohydraulic lithotripsy is a similar method in which an electrical discharge is used to create a hydraulic shock wave to break up the stone. A probe is passed through the cystoscope, and the tip of the lithotriptor is placed near the stone. The strength of the discharge and pulse frequency can be varied. This procedure is performed under topical anesthesia. After the stone is extracted, the percutaneous nephrostomy tube is left in place for a time to ensure that the ureter is not obstructed by edema or blood clots. The most common complications are hemorrhage, infection, and urinary extravasation. After the tube is removed, the nephrostomy tract usually closes spontaneously.

Chemolysis, stone dissolution using infusions of chemical solutions (eg, alkylating agents, acidifying agents) for the purpose of dissolving the stone, is an alternative treatment sometimes used in patients who are at risk for complications with other types of therapy, who refuse to undergo other methods, or who have stones (struvite) that dissolve easily. A percutaneous nephrostomy is performed, and the warm chemical solution is allowed to flow continuously onto the stone. The solution exits the renal collecting system by means of the ureter or the nephrostomy tube. The pressure inside the renal pelvis is monitored during the procedure.

Several of these treatment modalities may be used in combination to ensure removal of the stones.

Surgical Management

Surgical removal was the major mode of therapy before the advent of lithotripsy. However, today, surgery is performed in only 1% to 2% of patients. Surgical intervention is indicated if the stone does not respond to other forms of treatment. It may also be performed to correct anatomic abnormalities within the kidney to improve urinary drainage. If the stone is in the kidney, the surgery performed may be a nephrolithotomy (incision into the kidney with removal of the stone) or a nephrectomy, if the kidney is nonfunctional secondary to infection or hydronephrosis. Stones in the kidney pelvis are removed by a pyelolithotomy, those in the ureter by ureterolithotomy, and those in the bladder by cystotomy. If the stone is in the bladder, an instrument may be inserted through the urethra into the bladder, and the stone crushed. Such a procedure is called a cystolitholapaxy. Nursing management following kidney surgery is discussed in Chapter 44.

NURSING PROCESS

THE PATIENT WITH KIDNEY STONES

Assessment

The patient with suspected renal stones is assessed for pain and discomfort as well as associated symptoms, such as nausea, vomiting, diarrhea, and abdominal distention. The severity and location of pain are determined, along with any radiation of the pain. Nursing assessment also includes observing for signs and symptoms of UTI (chills, fever, frequency, and hesitancy) and obstruction (frequent urination of small amounts, oliguria, or anuria). The urine is inspected for blood and is strained for stones or gravel.

The history focuses on factors that predispose the patient to urinary tract stones or that may have precipitated the current episode of renal or ureteral colic. The patient's knowledge about renal stones and measures to prevent their occurrence or recurrence is also assessed.

Diagnosis

Nursing Diagnoses

Based on the assessment data, the nursing diagnoses in the patient with renal stones may include the following:

- Acute pain related to inflammation, obstruction, and abrasion of the urinary tract
- Deficient knowledge regarding prevention of recurrence of renal stones

Collaborative Problems/Potential Complications

Based on assessment data, potential complications that may develop include the following:

- Infection and urosepsis (from UTI and pyelonephritis)
- Obstruction of the urinary tract by a stone or edema with subsequent acute renal failure

Planning and Goals

The major goals for the patient may include relief of pain and discomfort, prevention of recurrence of renal stones, and absence of complications.

Nursing Interventions

Relieving Pain

Severe acute pain is often the presenting symptom of a patient with renal and urinary calculi and requires immediate attention. Opioid analgesic agents (IV or intramuscular) may be prescribed and administered to provide rapid relief along with an IV NSAID. The patient is encouraged and assisted to assume a position of comfort. If activity brings pain relief, the patient is assisted to ambulate. The pain level is monitored closely, and an increase in severity is reported promptly to the physician so that relief can be provided and additional treatment initiated.

Monitoring and Managing Potential Complications

Increased fluid intake is encouraged to prevent dehydration and increase hydrostatic pressure within the urinary tract to promote passage of the stone. If the patient cannot take adequate fluids orally, IV fluids are prescribed. The total urine output and patterns of voiding are monitored. Ambulation is encouraged as a means of moving the stone through the urinary tract.

All urine is strained through gauze because uric acid stones may crumble. Any blood clots passed in the urine should be crushed and the sides of the urinal and bedpan inspected for clinging stones. Because renal stones increase the risk of infection, sepsis, and obstruction of the urinary tract, the patient is instructed to report decreased urine volume, bloody or cloudy urine, fever, and pain.

Patients with calculi require frequent nursing observation to detect the spontaneous passage of a stone. The patient is instructed to immediately report any sudden increases in pain intensity because of the possibility of a stone fragment obstructing a ureter. Vital signs, including temperature, are monitored closely to detect early signs of infection. UTIs may be associated with renal stones due to an obstruction from the stone or from the stone itself. All infections should be treated with the appropriate antibiotic agent before efforts are made to dissolve the stone.

Promoting Home and Community-Based Care

TEACHING PATIENTS SELF-CARE. Because the risk of recurring renal stones is high, the nurse provides education about the causes of kidney stones and recommendations to prevent their recurrence (see Chart 45-12). The patient is encouraged to follow a regimen to avoid further stone formation, including maintaining a high fluid intake because stones form more readily in concentrated urine. A patient who has shown a tendency to form stones should drink enough fluid to excrete greater than 2000 mL (preferably 3000 to 4000 mL) of urine every 24 hours.

Urine cultures may be performed every 1 to 2 months the first year and periodically thereafter. Recurrent UTI is treated vigorously. Because prolonged immobilization slows renal drainage and alters calcium metabolism, increased mobility is encouraged whenever possible. In addition, excessive ingestion of vitamins (especially vitamin D) and minerals is discouraged.

If lithotripsy, percutaneous stone removal, ureteroscopy, or other surgical procedures for stone removal have been performed, the nurse instructs the patient about the signs and symptoms of complications that need to be reported to the physician. The importance of follow-up to assess kidney function and to ensure the eradication or removal of all kidney stones is emphasized to the patient and family.

If ESWL has been performed, the nurse must provide instructions for home care and necessary follow-up. The patient is encouraged to increase fluid intake to assist in the passage of stone fragments, which may occur for 6 weeks to several months after the procedure. The patient and family are instructed about signs and symptoms of complications. It is also important to inform the patient to expect hematuria (it is anticipated in all patients), but it should disappear within 4 to 5 days. If the patient has a stent in the ureter, hematuria may be expected until the stent is removed. The patient is instructed to check his or her temperature daily and notify the physician if the temperature is greater than 38°C (about 101°F) or the pain is unrelieved by the prescribed medication. The patient is also informed that a bruise may be observed on the treated side of the back.

CONTINUING CARE. Close monitoring of the patient in follow-up care ensures that treatment has been effective and that no complications have developed. The nurse has the opportunity to assess the patient's understanding of ESWL and possible complications. Additionally, the nurse has the opportunity to assess the patient's understanding of factors that increase the risk of recurrence of renal calculi and strategies to reduce those risks.

It is necessary to assess the patient's ability to monitor urinary pH and interpret the results during follow-up visits. Because of the high risk of recurrence, the patient with renal stones needs to understand the signs and symptoms of stone formation, obstruction, and infection and the importance of reporting these signs promptly. If medications are prescribed for the prevention of stone formation, the nurse explains their actions, importance, and side effects to the patient.

Evaluation

Expected Patient Outcomes

Expected patient outcomes may include:

1. Reports relief of pain
2. States increased knowledge of health-seeking behaviors to prevent recurrence
   a. Consumes increased fluid intake (at least eight 8-ounce glasses of fluid per day)
   b. Participates in appropriate activity
   c. Consumes diet prescribed to reduce dietary factors predisposing to stone formation
   d. Recognizes symptoms (fever, chills, flank pain, hematuria) to be reported to health care provider
   e. Monitors urinary pH as directed
   f. Takes prescribed medication as directed to reduce stone formation
3. Experiences no complications
   a. Reports no signs or symptoms of infection or urosepsis
   b. Voids 200 to 400 mL per voiding of clear urine without evidence of bleeding
   c. Experiences absence of urgency, frequency, and hesitancy
   d. Maintains normal body temperature

GENITOURINARY TRAUMA

Various types of injuries of the flank, back, or upper abdomen may result in trauma to the ureters, bladder, or urethra. Approximately 10% of all injuries seen in the emergency department involve the genitourinary system (Tanagho & McAninch, 2007). (Renal trauma is discussed in Chapter 44.)

Specific Injuries

Ureteral Trauma

Penetrating trauma and unintentional injury during surgery are the major causes of trauma to the ureters. Gunshot wounds account for 95% of ureteral injuries, which may range from contusions to complete transection. Unintentional injury to the ureter may occur during gynecologic or urologic surgery. There are no specific signs or symptoms of ureteral injury; many traumatic injuries are discovered during exploratory surgery. If the ureteral trauma is not detected and urine leakage continues, fistulas can develop.

IV urography detects 90% of ureteral injuries and can be performed on the operating table in patients undergoing emergency surgery. Surgical repair with placement of stents (to divert urine away from an anastomosis) is usually necessary.

Bladder Trauma

Injury to the bladder may occur with pelvic fractures and multiple trauma or from a blow to the lower abdomen when the bladder is full. Blunt trauma may result in contusion evident as an ecchymosis—a large bruise resulting from escape of blood into the tissues and involving a segment of the bladder wall—or in rupture of the bladder extraperitoneally, intraperitoneally, or both. Complications from these injuries include hemorrhage, shock, sepsis, and extravasation of blood into the tissues, which must be treated promptly.

Urethral Trauma

Urethral injuries usually occur with blunt trauma to the lower abdomen or pelvic region. Many patients also have associated pelvic fractures. The classic triad of symptoms comprises blood at the urinary meatus, inability to void, and a distended bladder.

Medical Management

The goals of management in patients with genitourinary trauma are to control hemorrhage, pain, and infection and to maintain urinary drainage. Genitourinary trauma is frequently associated with renal trauma (see Chapter 44). Hematocrit and hemoglobin levels are monitored closely; decreasing values can indicate hemorrhage within the genitourinary system. The patient is also monitored for oliguria, signs of hemorrhagic shock, and signs and symptoms of acute peritonitis.

Surgical Management

In urethral trauma, unstable patients who need monitoring of urine output may need a suprapubic catheter inserted. The patient is catheterized after urethrography has been performed to minimize the risk of urethral disruption and extensive, long-term complications, such as stricture, incontinence, and impotence. Surgical repair may be performed immediately or at a later time. Delayed surgical repair tends to be the favored procedure because it is associated with fewer long-term complications, such as impotence, strictures, and incontinence. After surgery, an indwelling urinary catheter may remain in place for up to 1 month.

Nursing Management

The patient with genitourinary trauma should be assessed frequently during the first few days after injury to detect flank and abdominal pain, muscle spasm, and swelling over the flank.

During this time, patients can be instructed about care of the incision and the importance of an adequate fluid intake. In addition, instructions about changes that should be reported to the physician, such as fever, hematuria, flank pain, or any signs and symptoms of decreasing kidney function, are provided. The patient with a ruptured bladder may have gross bleeding for several days after repair. Guidelines for increasing activity gradually, lifting, and driving are also provided in accordance with the physician's prescription.

Follow-up nursing care includes monitoring the blood pressure to detect hypertension and advising the patient to restrict activities for about 1 month after trauma to minimize the incidence of delayed or secondary bleeding.

URINARY TRACT CANCERS

In 2009, the American Cancer Society (ACS) estimated that there were more than 131,000 new cases in the urinary system. Urinary tract cancers include those of the urinary bladder; kidney and renal pelvis; ureters; and other urinary structures, such as the prostate. (Renal cancer is discussed in Chapter 44, and prostate cancer is discussed in Chapter 49.) Malignant tumors include transitional cell carcinomas (90%), squamous cell carcinomas (5% to 8%), adenocarcinomas (1% to 2%), sarcomas (less than 1%), and other types of cancers.

Cancer of the Bladder

Cancer of the urinary bladder is more common in people older than 55 years of age. It affects more men than women (4:1) and is more common in Caucasians than in African Americans. Bladder cancer is the fourth leading cause of cancer in American men, accounting for more than 14,000 deaths in the United States annually, and has a high incidence worldwide (ACS, 2009).

Bladder cancer, combined with prostatic cancer, is the most common urologic malignancy, accounting for 90% of all tumors seen. Cancers arising from the prostate, colon, and rectum in males and from the lower gynecologic tract in females may metastasize to the bladder.

Tobacco use continues to be a leading risk factor for all urinary tract cancers. People who smoke develop bladder cancer twice as often as those who do not smoke (Chart 45-13) (ACS, 2009).

Risk Factors for Bladder Cancer

- Cigarette smoking: risk proportional to pack-years of smoking
- Exposure to environmental carcinogens: dyes, rubber, leather, ink, or paint
- Recurrent or chronic bacterial infection of the urinary tract
- Bladder stones
- High urinary pH
- High cholesterol intake
- Pelvic radiation therapy
- Cancers arising from the prostate, colon, and rectum in males

Clinical Manifestations

Bladder tumors usually arise at the base of the bladder and involve the ureteral orifices and bladder neck. Visible, painless hematuria is the most common symptom of bladder cancer. Infection of the urinary tract is a common complication, producing frequency and urgency. However, any alteration in voiding or change in the urine may indicate cancer of the bladder. Pelvic or back pain may occur with metastasis.

Assessment and Diagnostic Findings

The diagnostic evaluation includes cystoscopy (the mainstay of diagnosis), excretory urography, CT, ultrasonography, and bimanual examination with the patient anesthetized. Biopsies of the tumor and adjacent mucosa are the definitive diagnostic procedures. Transitional cell carcinomas and carcinomas in situ shed recognizable cancer cells. Cytologic examination of fresh urine and saline bladder washings provide information about the prognosis and staging, especially for patients at high risk for recurrence of primary bladder tumors.

Although the mainstay diagnostic tools such as cytology and CT have a high detection rate, they are costly. Newer diagnostic tools such as bladder tumor antigens, nuclear matrix proteins, adhesion molecules, cytoskeletal proteins, and growth factors are being studied to support the early detection and diagnosis of bladder cancer (ACS, 2009).

Medical Management

Treatment of bladder cancer depends on the grade of the tumor (the degree of cellular differentiation), the stage of tumor growth (the degree of local invasion and the presence or absence of metastasis), and the multicentricity (having many centers) of the tumor. The patient's age and physical, mental, and emotional status are considered when determining treatment modalities.

Surgical Management

Transurethral resection or fulguration (cauterization) may be performed for simple papillomas (benign epithelial tumors). These procedures, described in more detail in Chapter 49, eradicate the tumors through surgical incision or electrical current with the use of instruments inserted through the urethra. After this bladder-sparing surgery, intravesical adminis-

tration of bacille Calmette-Guérin (BCG) is the treatment of choice. BCG is an attenuated live strain of *Mycobacterium bovis*, the causative agent in tuberculosis. The exact action of BCG is unknown, but it is thought to produce a local inflammatory as well as a systemic immunologic response (Sharma, Old & Allison, 2007).

Management of superficial bladder cancers presents a challenge because there are usually widespread abnormalities in the bladder mucosa. The entire lining of the urinary tract, or urothelium, is at risk because carcinomatous changes can occur in the mucosa of the bladder, renal pelvis, ureter, and urethra. About 25% to 40% of superficial tumors recur after transurethral resection or fulguration. Patients with benign papillomas should undergo cytology and cystoscopy periodically for the rest of their lives because aggressive malignancies may develop from these tumors.

A simple cystectomy or a radical cystectomy is performed for invasive or multifocal bladder cancer. Radical cystectomy in men involves removal of the bladder, prostate, and seminal vesicles and immediate adjacent perivesical tissues. In women, radical cystectomy involves removal of the bladder, lower ureter, uterus, fallopian tubes, ovaries, anterior vagina, and urethra. It may include removal of pelvic lymph nodes. Removal of the bladder requires a urinary diversion procedure, which is described later in this chapter.

Although radical cystectomy remains the standard of care for invasive bladder cancer in the United States, researchers are exploring trimodality therapy—transurethral resection of the bladder tumor, radiation, and chemotherapy—in an effort to spare patients the need for cystectomy. This approach to transitional cell bladder cancer mandates lifelong surveillance with periodic cystoscopy. Although most patients respond completely and their bladders remain free from invasive relapse, one fourth develop a relapse of noninvasive disease. This may be managed with transurethral resection of the bladder tumor and intravesical therapies but carries an additional risk that a late cystectomy may be required.

Pharmacologic Therapy

Chemotherapy with a combination of methotrexate (Rheumatrex), 5-fluorouracil (5-FU), vinblastine (Velban), doxorubicin (Adriamycin), and cisplatin (Platinol) has been effective in producing partial remission of transitional cell carcinoma of the bladder in some patients. IV chemotherapy may be accompanied by radiation therapy. Topical chemotherapy (intravesical chemotherapy or instillation of antineoplastic agents into the bladder, resulting in contact of the agent with the bladder wall) is considered when there is a high risk of recurrence, when cancer in situ is present, or when tumor resection has been incomplete. Topical chemotherapy delivers a high concentration of medication (thiotepa [Thioplex], doxorubicin, mitomycin [Mutamycin], and BCG [TheraCys]) to the tumor to promote tumor destruction. Bladder cancer may also be treated by direct infusion of the cytotoxic agent through the bladder's arterial blood supply to achieve a higher concentration of the chemotherapeutic agent with fewer systemic toxic effects.

BCG is now considered the most effective intravesical agent for recurrent bladder cancer, especially superficial transitional cell carcinoma, because it is an immunotherapeutic agent that enhances the body's immune response to cancer. BCG has a 43% advantage in preventing tumor recurrence, a significantly better rate than the 16% to 21% advantage of intravesical chemotherapy. In addition, BCG is particularly effective in the treatment of carcinoma in situ, eradicating it in more than 80% of cases. In contrast to intravesical chemotherapy, BCG has also been shown to decrease the risk of tumor progression (Sharma, et al., 2007).

The optimal course of BCG appears to be a 6-week course of weekly instillations, followed by a 3-week course at 3 months for tumors that do not respond. In high-risk cancers, maintenance BCG administered in a 3-week course at 6, 12, 18, and 24 months may limit recurrence and prevent progression (Sharma, et al., 2007). However, the adverse effects associated with this prolonged therapy may limit its widespread applicability.

The patient is allowed to eat and drink before the instillation procedure. Once the bladder is full, the patient must retain the intravesical solution for 2 hours before voiding. At the end of the procedure, the patient is encouraged to void and to drink liberal amounts of fluid to flush the medication from the bladder.

Radiation Therapy

Radiation of the tumor may be performed preoperatively to reduce microextension of the neoplasm and viability of tumor cells, thus reducing the chances that the cancer may recur in the immediate area or spread through the circulatory or lymphatic systems. Radiation therapy is also used in combination with surgery or to control the disease in patients with inoperable tumors.

For more advanced bladder cancer or for patients with intractable hematuria (especially after radiation therapy), a large, water-filled balloon placed in the bladder produces tumor necrosis by reducing the blood supply of the bladder wall (hydrostatic therapy). The instillation of formalin, phenol, or silver nitrate relieves hematuria and strangury (slow and painful discharge of urine) in some patients.

Investigational Therapy

The use of photodynamic techniques in treating superficial bladder cancer is under investigation. This procedure involves systemic injection of a photosensitizing material (hematoporphyrin), which the cancer cell picks up. A laser-generated light then changes the hematoporphyrin in the cancer cell into a toxic agent. This process has received renewed interest with regulatory approval of several photosensitizing medications and light applicators as potential palliative and curative treatments (Huang, 2005).

URINARY DIVERSIONS

Urinary diversion procedures are performed to divert urine from the bladder to a new exit site, usually through a surgically created opening (stoma) in the skin. These procedures are primarily performed when a bladder tumor necessitates cystectomy. Urinary diversion has also been used in managing pelvic malignancy, birth defects, strictures, trauma to the ureters and urethra, neurogenic bladder, chronic infection causing severe ureteral and renal damage, and

intractable interstitial cystitis. It may also be used as a last resort in managing incontinence.

Controversy exists about the best method of establishing permanent diversion of the urinary tract. New techniques are frequently introduced in an effort to improve patient outcomes and quality of life. The age of the patient, condition of the bladder, body build, degree of obesity, degree of ureteral dilation, status of renal function, and the patient's learning ability and willingness to participate in postoperative care are all taken into consideration when determining the appropriate surgical procedure.

The extent to which the patient accepts urinary diversion depends to a large degree on the location or position of the stoma, whether the drainage device (pouch or bag) establishes a watertight seal to the skin, and the patient's ability to manage the pouch and drainage apparatus.

There are two types of urinary diversion. In a cutaneous urinary diversion, urine drains through an opening created in the abdominal wall and skin (Fig. 45-7). In a **continent urinary diversion,** a portion of the intestine is used to create a new reservoir for urine (Fig. 45-8).

Cutaneous Urinary Diversions

ILEAL CONDUIT

The **ileal conduit** (ileal loop) is the oldest and most common of the urinary diversion procedures in use because of the low number of complications and surgeons' familiarity with the procedure. In an ileal conduit, the urine is diverted by implanting the ureter into a 12-cm loop of ileum that is led out through the abdominal wall. This loop of ileum is a simple conduit (passageway) for urine from the ureters to the surface. A loop of the sigmoid colon may also be used. An ileostomy bag is used to collect the urine. The resected (cut) ends of the remaining intestine are anastomosed (connected) to provide an intact bowel (Diepenbrock, 2007).

Stents, usually made of thin, pliable tubing, are placed in the ureters to prevent occlusion secondary to postsurgical edema. The bilateral ureteral stents allow urine to drain from the kidney to the stoma and provide a method for accurate measurement of urine output. They may be left in place 10 to 21 days postoperatively. Jackson-Pratt tubes or other types of drains are inserted to prevent the accumulation of fluid in the space created by removal of the bladder.

After surgery, a skin barrier and a transparent, disposable urinary drainage bag are applied around the conduit and connected to drainage. A custom-cut appliance is used until the edema subsides and the stoma shrinks to normal size. The clear bag allows the stoma to be inspected and the patency of the stent and the urine output to be monitored. The ileal bag drains urine (not feces) continuously. The appliance (bag) usually remains in place as long as it is watertight; it is changed when necessary to prevent leakage of urine.

Complications

Complications that may follow placement of an ileal conduit include wound infection or wound dehiscence, urinary leakage, ureteral obstruction, hyperchloremic acidosis, small bowel obstruction, ileus, and gangrene of the stoma. Delayed

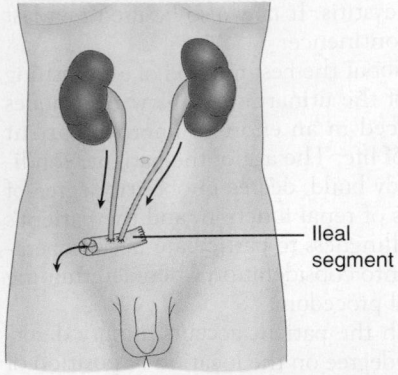

A Conventional ileal conduit.
The surgeon transplants the ureters to an isolated section of the terminal ileum (ileal conduit), bringing one end to the abdominal wall. The ureter may also be transplanted into the transverse sigmoid colon (colon conduit) or proximal jejunum (jejunal conduit).

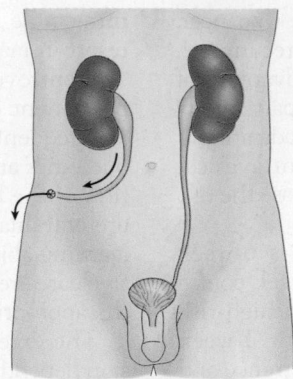

B Cutaneous ureterostomy.
The surgeon brings the detached ureter through the abdominal wall and attaches it to an opening in the skin.

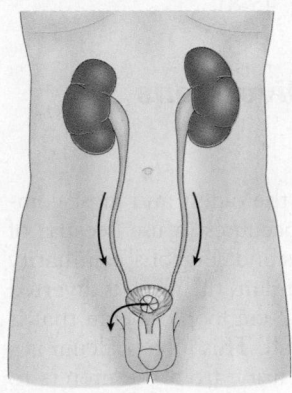

C Vesicostomy.
The surgeon sutures the bladder to the abdominal wall and creates an opening (stoma) through the abdominal and bladder walls for urinary drainage.

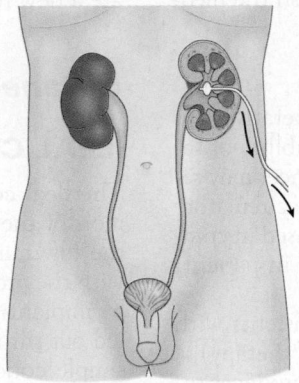

D Nephrostomy.
The surgeon inserts a catheter into the renal pelvis via an incision in the flank or by percutaneous catheter placement into the kidney.

Figure 45-7 Types of cutaneous diversions include **(A)** the conventional ileal conduit, **(B)** cutaneous ureterostomy, **(C)** vesicostomy, and **(D)** nephrostomy.

complications include ureteral obstruction, contraction or narrowing of the stoma (stenosis), renal deterioration due to chronic reflux, pyelonephritis, and renal calculi.

Nursing Management

In the immediate postoperative period, urine volumes are monitored hourly. Throughout the patient's hospitalization, the nurse monitors closely for complications, reports signs and symptoms of them promptly, and intervenes quickly to prevent their progression.

A urine output below 30 mL/h may indicate dehydration or an obstruction in the ileal conduit, with possible backflow or leakage from the ureteroileal anastomosis. After the physician's order is obtained, a catheter may be inserted through the urinary conduit to monitor the patient for possible stasis or residual urine from a constricted stoma. Urine may drain through the bilateral ureteral stents as well as around the stents. If the ureteral stents are not draining, the nurse may be instructed to carefully irrigate with 5 to 10 mL

sterile normal saline solution, being careful not to exert tension that could dislodge the stent. Hematuria may be noted in the first 48 hours after surgery but usually resolves spontaneously.

Providing Stoma and Skin Care

Because the patient requires specialized care, a consultation is initiated with a WOCN. The stoma is inspected frequently for color and viability. A healthy stoma is pink or red. A change from this normal color to purple, brown, or black suggests that the vascular supply may be compromised. If cyanosis and a compromised blood supply persist, surgical intervention may be necessary. The stoma is not sensitive to touch, but the skin around the stoma becomes sensitive if urine or the appliance irritates it. The skin is inspected for (1) signs of irritation and bleeding of the stoma mucosa, (2) encrustation and skin irritation around the stoma (from alkaline urine coming in contact with exposed skin), and (3) wound infections.

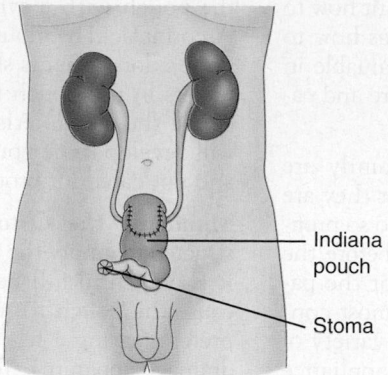

A Indiana pouch.
The surgeon introduces the ureters into
a segment of ileum and cecum. Urine
is drained periodically by inserting a
catheter into the stoma.

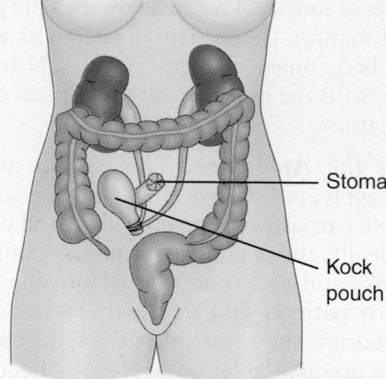

B Continent ileal urinary diversions (Kock pouch).
The surgeon transplants the ureters to an isolated
segment of small bowel, ascending colon, or
ileocolonic segment and develops an effective
continence mechanism or valve. Urine is drained
by inserting a catheter into the stoma.

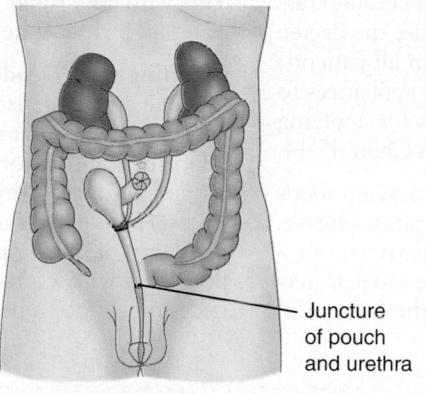

C
In male patients, the Kock pouch can be
modified by attaching one end of the
pouch to the urethra, allowing more
normal voiding. The female urethra is
too short for this modification.

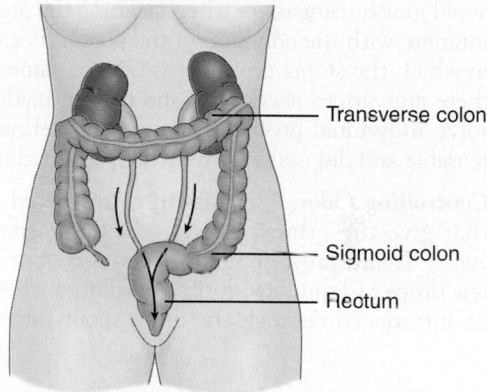

D Ureterosigmoidostomy.
The surgeon introduces the ureters into the
sigmoid colon, thereby allowing urine to flow
through the colon and out of the rectum.

Figure 45-8 Types of continent urinary diversions include **(A)** the Indiana pouch; **(B, C)** the Kock pouch,
also called a continent ileal diversion;
and **(D)** ureterosigmoidostomy.

Testing Urine and Caring for the Ostomy

Moisture in bed linens or clothing or the odor of urine
around the patient should alert the nurse to the possibility
of leakage from the appliance, potential infection, or a
problem in hygienic management. Because severe alkaline
encrustation can accumulate rapidly around the stoma, the
urine pH is kept below 6.5 by administration of ascorbic
acid by mouth. Urine pH is determined by testing the urine
draining from the stoma, not from the collecting appliance.
A properly fitted appliance is essential to prevent exposure
of the skin around the stoma to urine. If the urine is foul-
smelling, the stoma is catheterized, if prescribed, to obtain a
urine specimen for culture and sensitivity testing.

Encouraging Fluids and Relieving Anxiety

Because mucous membrane is used in forming the conduit,
the patient may excrete a large amount of mucus mixed
with urine. This causes anxiety in many patients. To help
relieve this anxiety, the nurse reassures the patient that this

is a normal occurrence after an ileal conduit procedure. The
nurse encourages adequate fluid intake to flush the ileal
conduit and decrease the accumulation of mucus.

Selecting the Ostomy Appliance

Various urine collection appliances are available, and the
nurse is instrumental (often with consultation with a
WOCN) in selecting an appropriate one. The urinary appliance may consist of one or two pieces and may be disposable (usually used once and discarded) or reusable. The
choice of appliance is determined by the location of the
stoma and by the patient's normal activity, manual dexterity, visual function, body build, economic resources, and
preference.

Promoting Home and Community-Based Care

Teaching Patients Self-Care

Patient education begins in the hospital but continues into
the home setting because patients are usually discharged

within days of surgery. The nurse teaches the patient how to assess and manage the urinary diversion as well as how to deal with body image changes. A WOCN is invaluable in consulting with the nurse on various aspects of care and patient education.

Changing the Appliance. The patient and family are taught to apply and change the appliance so that they are comfortable carrying out the procedure and can do so proficiently. Ideally, the appliance system is changed before the system leaks and at a time that is convenient for the patient. Many patients find that early morning is most convenient because the urine output is reduced. A variety of appliances are available; an average collecting appliance lasts 3 to 7 days before leakage occurs.

Regardless of the type of appliance used, a skin barrier is essential to protect the skin from irritation and excoriation. To maintain skin integrity, a skin barrier or leaking pouch is never patched with tape to prevent accumulation of urine under the skin barrier or faceplate. The patient is instructed to avoid moisturizing soaps when cleaning the area because they interfere with the adhesion of the pouch. Because the degree to which the stoma protrudes is not the same in all patients, there are various accessories and custom-made appliances to solve individual problems. Patient guidelines for applying reusable and disposable systems are presented in Chart 45-14.

Controlling Odor. The patient is instructed to avoid foods that give the urine a strong odor (eg, asparagus, cheese, eggs). Today, most appliances contain odor barriers, but a few drops of liquid deodorizer or diluted white vinegar may be introduced through the drain spout into the bottom of the pouch with a syringe or eyedropper to reduce odors. Ascorbic acid by mouth helps acidify the urine and suppress urine odor. Patients should be cautioned not to put aspirin tablets in the pouch to control odor because they may ulcerate the stoma. Also, the patient is reminded that odor will develop if the pouch is worn longer than recommended and not cared for properly.

Managing the Ostomy Appliance. The patient is instructed to empty the pouch by means of a drain valve when it is one-third full because the weight of more urine will cause the pouch to separate from the skin. Some patients prefer wearing a leg bag attached with an adapter to the drainage apparatus. To promote uninterrupted sleep, a collecting bottle and tubing (one unit) are snapped onto an adapter that connects to the ileal appliance. A small amount of urine is left in the bag when the adapter is attached to prevent the bag from collapsing against itself. The tubing may be threaded down the pajama or pants leg to prevent kinking. The collecting bottle and tubing are rinsed daily with cool water and once a week with a 3:1 solution of water and white vinegar.

Cleaning and Deodorizing the Appliance. Usually, the reusable appliance is rinsed in warm water and soaked in a 3:1 solution of water and white vinegar or a commercial deodorizing solution for 30 minutes. It is rinsed with tepid water and air-dried away from direct sunlight. (Hot water and exposure to direct sunlight dry the pouch and increase the incidence of cracking.) After drying, the appliance may be powdered with cornstarch and stored. Two appliances are necessary—one to be worn while the other is air-drying.

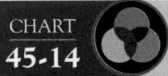

CHART 45-14   **PATIENT EDUCATION**
Using Urinary Diversion Collection Appliances

Applying a Reusable Pouch System

1 Gather all necessary supplies.
2. Prepare new appliance according to the manufacturer's directions.
   • Apply double-faced adhesive disk that has been properly sized to fit the reusable pouch face-plate. Remove paper backing and set pouch aside, or apply thin layer of contact cement to one side of the reusable pouch faceplate. Set pouch aside.
3. Remove soiled pouch gently. Lay aside to clean later.
4. Clean peristomal skin (skin around stoma) with small amount of soap and water. Rinse thoroughly and dry. If a film of soap remains on the skin and the site does not dry, the appliance will not adhere adequately.
5. Use a wick (rolled gauze pad or tampon) over the stoma to absorb urine and keep the skin dry throughout the appliance change.
6. Inspect peristomal skin for irritation.
7. A skin protector wipe or barrier ring may be applied before centering the faceplate opening directly over the stoma.
8. Position appliance over stoma and press gently into place.
9. If desired, use a pouch cover or apply cornstarch under the pouch to prevent perspiration and skin irritation.
10. Clean soiled pouch and prepare for reuse.

Applying a Disposable Pouch System

1. Gather all necessary supplies.
2. Measure stoma and prepare an opening in the skin barrier about an $\frac{1}{8}$-inch larger than the stoma and the same shape as the stoma.
3. Remove paper backing from skin barrier and set aside.
4. Gently remove old appliance and set aside.
5. Clean peristomal skin with warm water and dry thoroughly.
6. Inspect peristomal skin (skin around stoma) for irritation.
7. Use a wick (rolled gauze pad or tampon) over the stoma to absorb urine and keep the skin dry during the appliance change.
8. Center opening of skin barrier over stoma and apply with firm, gentle pressure to attain a water-tight seal.
9. If using a two-piece system, snap pouch onto the flanged wafer that adheres to skin.
10. Close drainage tap or spout at bottom of pouch.
11. A pouch cover can be used or cornstarch applied under pouch to prevent perspiration and skin irritation.
12. Apply hypoallergenic tape around the skin barrier in a picture-frame manner.
13. Dispose of soiled appliance.

Continuing Care

Follow-up care is essential to determine how the patient has adapted to the altered body image changes and lifestyle changes. Referral for home care is indicated to determine how well the patient and family are coping with the changes necessitated by altered urinary drainage. The home care nurse assesses the patient's physical status and emotional response to urinary diversion. Additionally, the nurse assesses the ability of the patient and family to manage the urinary diversion and appliance, reinforces previous teaching, and provides additional information (eg, community resources, sources of ostomy supplies, insurance coverage for supplies).

As the postoperative edema subsides, the home care nurse assists in determining the appropriate changes needed in the ostomy appliance. The size of the stoma is measured every 3 to 6 weeks for the first few months postoperatively. The correct appliance size is determined by measuring the widest part of the stoma with a ruler. The permanent appliance should be no more than 1.6 mm (1/8 inch) larger than the diameter of the stoma and the same shape as the stoma to prevent contact of the skin with drainage.

The nurse teaches the patient and family about resources (see the list of resources at end of this chapter). Local chapters of the ACS can provide medical equipment and supplies and other resources for the patient who has undergone ostomy surgery for cancer.

The home care nurse assesses the patient for potential long-term complications such as ureteral obstruction, stenosis, hernias, or deterioration of renal function. The nurse also reinforces previous teaching about these complications.

CUTANEOUS URETEROSTOMY

A cutaneous ureterostomy (see Fig. 45-7), in which the ureters are directed through the abdominal wall and attached to an opening in the skin, is used for selected patients with ureteral obstruction (ie, advanced pelvic cancer) because it requires less extensive surgery than other urinary diversion procedures. It is also an appropriate procedure for patients who have had previous abdominal irradiation.

A urinary appliance is fitted immediately after surgery. The management of the patient with a cutaneous ureterostomy is similar to the care of the patient with an ileal conduit, although the stomas are usually flush with the skin or retracted.

Continent Urinary Diversions

CONTINENT ILEAL URINARY RESERVOIR (INDIANA POUCH)

The most common continent urinary diversion is the Indiana pouch, created for the patient whose bladder is removed or no longer functions. The Indiana pouch uses a segment of the ileum and cecum to form the reservoir for urine (see Fig. 45-8A). The ureters are tunneled through the muscular bands of the intestinal pouch and anastomosed. The reservoir is made continent by narrowing the efferent portion of the ileum and sewing the terminal ileum to the subcutaneous tissue, forming a continent stoma flush with the skin. The pouch is sewn to the anterior abdominal wall around a cecostomy tube. Urine collects in the pouch until a catheter is inserted and the urine is drained (Diepenbrock, 2007).

The pouch must be drained at regular intervals by a catheter to prevent absorption of metabolic waste products from the urine, reflux of urine to the ureters, and UTI. Postoperative nursing care of the patient with a continent ileal urinary pouch is similar to nursing care of the patient with an ileal conduit. However, these patients usually have additional drainage tubes (cecostomy catheter from the pouch, stoma catheter exiting from the stoma, ureteral stents, and Penrose drain, as well as a urethral catheter). All drainage tubes must be carefully monitored for patency and amount and type of drainage. In the immediate postoperative period, the cecostomy tube is irrigated two or three times daily to remove mucus and prevent blockage.

Other variations of continent urinary reservoirs include the **Kock pouch** (U-shaped pouch constructed of ileum, with a nipplelike one-way valve; see Fig. 45-8B, C) and the **Charleston pouch** (uses the ileum and ascending colon as the pouch, with the appendix and colon junction serving as the one-way valve mechanism). With both of these methods, the pouch must be drained at regular intervals by a catheter.

URETEROSIGMOIDOSTOMY

Ureterosigmoidostomy, another form of continent urinary diversion, is an implantation of the ureters into the sigmoid colon (see Fig. 45-8D). It is usually performed in patients who have had extensive pelvic irradiation, previous small bowel resection, or coexisting small bowel disease.

After surgery, voiding occurs from the rectum (for life), and an adjustment in lifestyle will be necessary because of urinary frequency. Drainage has a consistency equivalent to watery diarrhea, and the patient has some degree of nocturia. Patients usually need to plan activities around the frequent need to urinate, which in turn may affect the patient's social life. However, patients have the advantage of urinary control without having to wear an external appliance.

Nursing Management

In addition to the usual preoperative regimen, the patient may be placed on a liquid diet for several days preoperatively to reduce residue in the colon. Antibiotic agents (neomycin, kanamycin) are administered to disinfect the bowel. Ureterosigmoidostomy requires a competent anal sphincter, adequate renal function, and active renal peristalsis. The degree of anal sphincter control may be determined by assessing the patient's ability to retain enemas.

The postoperative regimen initially includes placing a catheter in the rectum to drain the urine and prevent reflux of urine into the ureters and kidneys. The tube is taped to the buttocks, and special skin care is given around the anus to prevent excoriation. Irrigations of the rectal tube may be prescribed, but force is never used because of the danger of introducing bacteria into the newly implanted ureters.

Monitoring Fluid and Electrolytes

In ureterosigmoidostomy, larger areas of the bowel mucosa are exposed to urine and electrolyte reabsorption. As a result, electrolyte imbalance and acidosis may occur. Potassium and magnesium in the urine may cause diarrhea. Fluid and electrolyte balance is maintained in the immediate postoperative period by closely monitoring the serum electrolyte levels and administering appropriate IV fluids. Acidosis may be prevented by placing the patient on a low-chloride diet supplemented with sodium potassium citrate.

The patient should be instructed never to wait longer than 2 to 3 hours before emptying urine from the intestine. This keeps rectal pressure low and minimizes the absorption of urinary constituents from the colon. It is essential to teach the patient about the symptoms of UTI: fever, flank pain, urgency, and frequency.

Retraining the Anal Sphincter

After the rectal catheter is removed, the patient learns to control the anal sphincter through special sphincter exercises. At first, urination is frequent. With reassurance and encouragement and the passage of time, the patient gains greater control and learns to differentiate between the need to void and the need to defecate.

Promoting Dietary Measures

Specific dietary instructions include avoidance of gas-forming foods (flatus can cause stress incontinence and offensive odors). Other ways to avoid gas are to avoid chewing gum, smoking, and any other activity that involves swallowing air. Salt intake may be restricted to prevent hyperchloremic acidosis. Potassium intake is increased through foods and medication because potassium may be lost in acidosis.

Monitoring and Managing Potential Complications

Pyelonephritis (upper UTI) due to reflux of bacteria from the colon is fairly common. Long-term antibiotic therapy may be prescribed to prevent infection. A late complication is adenocarcinoma of the sigmoid colon, possibly from cellular changes due to exposure of the colonic mucosa to urine. Urinary carcinogens promote late malignant transformation of the colon after a ureterosigmoidostomy, warranting lifelong medical follow-up.

Other Urinary Diversion Procedures

Variations in urinary diversion surgical procedures are devised frequently in an effort to identify and perfect procedures that will improve patient outcomes and reduce the incidence of postoperative problems. These include cecal, patched cecal, and Mainz reservoirs. These techniques involve isolating a part of the large intestine to form a reservoir for urine and creating an abdominal stoma. Another surgical procedure, the Camey procedure, uses a portion of the ileum as a bladder substitute. In this procedure, the isolated ileum serves as the reservoir for urine; it is anastomosed directly to the portion of the remaining urethra after cystectomy. This procedure permits emptying of the bladder through the urethra. However, the Camey procedure applies only to men because the entire urethra is removed when a cystectomy is performed in women.

NURSING PROCESS

THE PATIENT UNDERGOING URINARY DIVERSION SURGERY

Preoperative Assessment

The following are key preoperative nursing assessment concerns:

- Cardiopulmonary function assessments are performed because patients undergoing cystectomy are often older people who may be at greater risk for cardiac and respiratory complications.
- A nutritional status assessment is important because of possible poor nutritional intake related to underlying health problems.
- Learning needs are assessed in consultation with a WOCN to evaluate the patient's and the family's understanding of the procedure as well as the changes in physical structure and function that result from the surgery. The patient's self-concept and self-esteem are assessed, in addition to methods for coping with stress and loss. The patient's mental status, manual dexterity and coordination, and preferred method of learning are noted because they affect postoperative self-care.

Preoperative Nursing Diagnoses

Based on the assessment data, the preoperative nursing diagnoses for the patient undergoing urinary diversion surgery may include the following:

- Anxiety related to anticipated losses associated with the surgical procedure
- Imbalanced nutrition, less than body requirements related to inadequate nutritional intake
- Deficient knowledge about the surgical procedure and postoperative care

Preoperative Planning and Goals

The major goals for the patient may include relief of anxiety, improved preoperative nutritional status, and increased knowledge about the surgical procedure, expected outcomes, and postoperative care.

Preoperative Nursing Interventions

Relieving Anxiety

The threat of cancer and removal of the bladder create anxiety related to changes in body image. Patients may face problems adapting to an external appliance, a stoma, a surgical incision, and altered toileting habits. Men must also adapt to sexual impotency; a penile implant is considered if the patient is a candidate for the procedure. Women also have anxiety related to altered appearance, body image, and self-esteem. A supportive approach, both physical and psychosocial, is needed and includes assessing the patient's self-concept and manner of coping with stress and loss; helping the patient to identify ways to maintain his or her lifestyle and independence with as few changes as possible; and encouraging the patient to express fears and anxieties about the ramifications of the upcoming surgery. A visitor from the Ostomy Visitation Program of the ACS can provide emotional support and make adaptation easier both before and after surgery.

Ensuring Adequate Nutrition

In addition to cleansing the bowel to minimize fecal stasis, decompress the bowel, and minimize postoperative ileus, a low-residue diet is prescribed. In addition, antibiotic medications are administered to reduce pathogenic flora in the bowel and to reduce the risk of infection. Because the patient undergoing a urinary diversion procedure for cancer may be severely malnourished due to the tumor, radiation enteritis, and anorexia, enteral or parenteral nutrition may be prescribed to promote healing. Adequate preoperative hydration is imperative to ensure urine flow during surgery and to prevent hypovolemia during the prolonged surgical procedure.

Explaining Surgery and Its Effects

Participation of a WOCN is invaluable for informed preoperative teaching and postoperative care planning. Explanations of the surgical procedure, the appearance of the stoma, the rationale for preoperative bowel preparation, the reasons for wearing a collection device, and the anticipated effects of the surgery on sexual functioning are part of patient teaching. The placement of the stoma site is planned preoperatively with the patient standing, sitting, and lying down to locate the stoma away from bony prominences, skin creases, and folds. The stoma should also be placed away from old scars, the umbilicus, and the belt line.

For ease of self-care, the patient must be able to see and reach the site comfortably. The site is marked with indelible ink so that it can be located easily during surgery. The patient is assessed for allergies or sensitivity to tape or adhesives. Patch testing of certain appliances may be necessary before the ostomy equipment is selected. This is particularly important if the patient is or may be allergic to latex (see Chapter 18).

Preoperative Evaluation

To measure the effectiveness of care, the nurse evaluates the patient's preoperative anxiety level and nutritional status as well as preexisting knowledge and expectations of surgery.

Expected Patient Outcomes

Expected patient outcomes may include:

1. Exhibits reduced anxiety about surgery and expected losses
   a. Verbalizes fears with health care team and family
   b. Expresses positive attitude about outcome of surgery
2. Exhibits adequate nutritional status
   a. Maintains adequate intake before surgery
   b. Maintains body weight
   c. States rationale for enteral or parenteral nutrition if needed
   d. Exhibits normal skin turgor, moist mucous membranes, adequate urine output, and absence of excessive thirst

3. Demonstrates knowledge about the surgical procedure and postoperative course
   a. Identifies limitations expected after surgery
   b. Discusses expected immediate postoperative environment (tubes, equipment, nursing surveillance)
   c. Practices deep-breathing, coughing, and foot exercises

Postoperative Assessment

The role of the nurse in the immediate postoperative period is to prevent complications and to assess the patient carefully for any signs and symptoms of complications. The catheters and any drainage devices are monitored closely. Urine volume, patency of the drainage system, and color of the drainage are assessed. A sudden decrease in urine volume or increase in drainage is reported promptly to the physician because these may indicate obstruction of the urinary tract, inadequate blood volume, or bleeding. In addition, the patient's need for pain control is assessed regularly as with all postoperative patients.

Postoperative Diagnosis

Nursing Diagnoses

Based on the assessment data, the major postoperative nursing diagnoses for the patient following urinary diversion surgery may include the following:

- Risk for impaired skin integrity related to problems in managing the urine collection appliance
- Acute pain related to surgical incision
- Disturbed body image related to urinary diversion
- Potential for sexual dysfunction related to structural and physiologic alterations
- Deficient knowledge about management of urinary function

Collaborative Problems/Potential Complications

Potential complications may include the following:

- Peritonitis due to disruption of anastomosis
- Stoma ischemia and necrosis due to compromised blood supply to stoma
- Stoma retraction and separation of mucocutaneous border due to tension or trauma

Postoperative Planning and Goals

The major goals for the patient may include maintaining skin integrity, relieving pain, increasing self-esteem, developing appropriate coping mechanisms to accept and deal with altered urinary function and sexuality, increasing knowledge about management of urinary function, and preventing potential complications.

Postoperative Nursing Interventions

Postoperative management focuses on monitoring urinary function, preventing postoperative complications (infection and sepsis, respiratory complications, fluid and electrolyte imbalances, fistula formation, and urine leakage), and promoting patient comfort. Catheters or drainage systems are monitored, and urine output is monitored carefully. A nasogastric tube is inserted during surgery to decompress the GI tract and to relieve pressure on the intestinal anastomosis. It is usually kept in place for several days after surgery. As soon as bowel function resumes, as indicated by bowel sounds, the passage of flatus, and a soft abdomen, oral fluids are permitted. Until that time, IV fluids and electrolytes are administered. The patient is assisted to ambulate as soon as possible to prevent complications of immobility.

Maintaining Skin Integrity

Strategies to promote skin integrity begin with reducing and controlling those factors that increase the patient's risk of poor nutrition and poor healing. As indicated previously, meticulous skin care and management of the drainage system are provided by the nurse until the patient can manage them and is comfortable doing so. Care is taken to keep the drainage system intact to protect the skin from exposure to drainage. Supplies must be readily available to manage the drainage in the immediate postoperative period. Consistency in implementing the skin care program throughout the postoperative period results in maintenance of skin integrity and patient comfort. Additionally, maintenance of skin integrity around the stoma enables the patient and family to adjust more easily to the alterations in urinary function and helps them learn skin care techniques.

Relieving Pain

Analgesic medications are administered liberally postoperatively to relieve pain and promote comfort, thereby allowing the patient to turn, cough, and perform deep-breathing exercises. Patient-controlled analgesia and regular administration of analgesic agents around the clock are two options that may be used to ensure adequate pain relief. A pain intensity scale is used to evaluate the adequacy of the medication and the approach to pain management.

Improving Body Image

The patient's ability to cope with the changes associated with the surgery depends to some degree on his or her body image and self-esteem before the surgery and the support and reaction of others. Allowing the patient to express concerns and anxious feelings can help, especially in adjusting to the changes in toileting habits. The nurse can also help improve the patient's self-concept by teaching the skills needed to be independent in managing the urinary drainage devices. Education about ostomy care is conducted in a private setting to encourage the patient to ask questions without fear of embarrassment. Explaining why the nurse must wear gloves when performing ostomy care can prevent the patient from misinterpreting the use of gloves as a sign of aversion to the stoma.

Exploring Sexuality Issues

Patients who experience altered sexual function as a result of the surgical procedure may mourn this loss. Encouraging the patient and partner to share their feelings about this loss with each other and acknowledging the importance of sexual function and expression may encourage the patient and partner to seek sexual counseling and to explore alternative ways of expressing sexuality. A visit from another "ostomate" who is functioning fully in society and family life may also assist the patient and family in recognizing that full recovery is possible.

Monitoring and Managing Potential Complications

Complications are not unusual because of the complexity of the surgery, the underlying reason (cancer, trauma) for the urinary diversion procedure, and the patient's frequently less-than-optimal nutritional status. Complications may include respiratory disorders (eg, atelectasis, pneumonia), fluid and electrolyte imbalances, breakdown of any anastomosis, sepsis, fistula formation, fecal or urine leakage, and skin irritation. If these occur, the patient will remain hospitalized for an extended length of time and will probably require parenteral nutrition, GI decompression by means of nasogastric suction, and further surgery. The goals of management are to establish drainage, provide adequate nutrition for healing to occur, and prevent sepsis.

PERITONITIS. Peritonitis can occur postoperatively if urine leaks at the anastomosis. Signs and symptoms include abdominal pain and distention, muscle rigidity with guarding, nausea and vomiting, paralytic ileus (absence of bowel sounds), fever, and leukocytosis.

Urine output must be monitored closely, because a sudden decrease in output with a corresponding increase in drainage from the incision or drains may indicate urine leakage. In addition, the urine drainage device is observed for leakage. The pouch is changed if a leak is observed. Small leaks in the anastomosis may seal themselves, but surgery may be needed for larger leaks.

Vital signs (blood pressure, pulse and respiratory rates, temperature) are monitored. Changes in vital signs, as well as increasing pain, nausea and vomiting, and abdominal distention, are reported to the physician and may indicate peritonitis.

STOMA ISCHEMIA AND NECROSIS. The stoma is monitored because ischemia and necrosis of the stoma can result from tension on the mesentery blood vessels, twisting of the bowel segment (conduit) during surgery, or arterial insufficiency. The new stoma must be inspected at least every 4 hours to assess the adequacy of its blood supply. The stoma should be red or pink. If the blood supply to the stoma is compromised, the color changes to purple, brown, or black. These changes are reported immediately to the physician. The physician or WOCN may insert a small, lubricated tube into the stoma and shine a flashlight into the lumen of the tube to assess for superficial ischemia or necrosis. A necrotic stoma requires surgical intervention. If the ischemia is superficial, the dusky stoma is observed and may slough its outer layer in several days.

STOMA RETRACTION AND SEPARATION. Stoma retraction and separation of the mucocutaneous border can occur as a result of trauma or tension on the internal bowel segment used for creation of the stoma. In addition, mucocutaneous separation can occur if the stoma does not heal as a result of accumulation of urine on the stoma and mucocutaneous border. Using a collection drainage pouch with an antireflux valve is helpful because the valve prevents urine from pooling on the stoma and mucocutaneous border. Meticulous skin care to keep the area around the stoma clean and dry promotes healing. If a separation of the mucocutaneous border occurs, surgery is not usually needed. The separated area is protected by applying karaya powder, stoma adhesive paste, and a properly fitted skin barrier and pouch. By protecting the separation, healing is promoted. If the stoma retracts into the peritoneum, surgical intervention is mandatory.

If surgery is needed to manage these complications, the nurse provides explanations to the patient and family. The need for additional surgery is usually perceived as a setback by the patient and family. Emotional support of the patient and family is provided along with physical preparation of the patient for surgery.

Promoting Home and Community-Based Care

TEACHING PATIENTS SELF-CARE. A major postoperative objective is to assist the patient to achieve the highest level of independence and self-care possible. The nurse and WOCN work closely with the patient and family to instruct and assist them in all phases of managing the ostomy. Adequate supplies and complete instruction are necessary to enable the patient and a family member to develop competence and confidence in their skills. Written and verbal instructions are provided, and the patient is encouraged to contact the nurse or physician with follow-up questions. Follow-up telephone calls from the nurse to the patient and family after discharge may provide added support and provide another opportunity to answer their questions. Follow-up visits and reinforcement of correct skin care and appliance management techniques also promote skin integrity. Specific techniques for managing the appliance are described in Chart 45-14.

The patient is encouraged to participate in decisions regarding the type of collecting appliance and the time of day to change the appliance. The patient is assisted and encouraged to look at and touch the stoma early to overcome any fears. The patient and family need to know the characteristics of a normal stoma:

- Pink and moist, like the inside of the mouth
- Insensitive to pain because it has no nerve endings
- Vascular, which means it may bleed when cleaned

Additionally, if a segment of the GI tract was used to create the urinary diversion, mucus may be visible in the urine. By learning what is normal, the patient and family become familiar with what signs and symptoms they should report to the physician or nurse and what problems they can handle themselves.

Information provided to the patient and the extent of involvement in self-care are determined by the patient's physical recovery and ability to accept and acquire the knowledge and skill needed for independence. Verbal and written instructions are provided, and the patient is given the opportunity to practice and demonstrate the knowledge and skills needed to manage urinary drainage.

CONTINUING CARE. Follow-up care is essential to determine how the patient has adapted to the body image changes and lifestyle adjustments. Visits from a home care nurse are important to assess the patient's adaptation to the home setting and management of the ostomy. Teaching and reinforcement may assist the patient and family to cope with altered urinary function. It is also necessary to assess for long-term complications that may occur, such as pouch leakage or rupture, stone formation, stenosis of the stoma, deterioration in renal function, or incontinence.

Long-term monitoring for anemia is performed to identify vitamin B deficiency, which may occur when a significant portion of the terminal ileum is removed. This may take several years to develop and can be treated with vitamin B injections. The patient and family are informed about the United Ostomy Association and any local ostomy support groups to provide ongoing support, assistance, and education.

Postoperative Evaluation

Expected Patient Outcomes

Expected patient outcomes may include:

1. Maintains skin integrity
   a. Maintains intact skin and demonstrates skill in managing drainage system and appliance
   b. States actions to take if skin excoriation occurs
2. Reports relief of pain
3. Exhibits improved body image as evidenced by the following:
   a. Voices acceptance of urinary diversion, stoma, and appliance
   b. Demonstrates increasingly independent self-care, including hygiene and grooming
   c. States acceptance of support and assistance from family members, health care providers, and other ostomates
4. Copes with sexuality issues
   a. Verbalizes concern about possible alterations in sexuality and sexual function
   b. Reports discussion of sexual concerns with partner and appropriate counselor
5. Demonstrates knowledge needed for self-care
   a. Performs self-care and proficient management of urinary diversion and appliance
   b. Asks questions relevant to self-management and prevention of complications
   c. Identifies signs and symptoms needing care from physician, nurse, or other health care providers
6. Absence of complications as evidenced by the following:
   a. Reports absence of pain or tenderness in abdomen
   b. Has temperature within normal range
   c. Reports no urine leakage from incision or drains
   d. Has urine output within desired volume limits
   e. Maintains stoma that is red or pink, moist, and appropriate in size without edema
   f. Has intact and healed border of the stoma

CRITICAL THINKING EXERCISES

EBP **1** As the head nurse in a long-term care facility, you are approached by the daughter of one of the residents. She requests that her mother, who can ambulate with assistance, have an indwelling urinary catheter inserted "for convenience sake." What is the evidence base that determines your response? Identify the criteria used to evaluate the strength of the evidence.

EBP **2** As one of the nurses in a busy urology practice, you often care for elderly women with incontinence. Describe the major types of incontinence and compare and contrast them. What are the evidence-based management techniques used in treating the different types of incontinence?

3 A 35-year-old man is admitted to a medical-surgical nursing unit with a suspected renal stone. Describe the pathophysiology of renal stone formation. What diagnostic tests should be performed to confirm the diagnosis? What is the most common priority nursing diagnosis in the patient admitted with a renal stone? What history and physical findings are common in the patient who is trying to pass the stone? If the patient does not pass the stone or develops complications, what are the interventional procedures available for stone removal?

4 You are caring for a 78-year-old patient after the creation of an ileal conduit. What is the best description of the ileal conduit? Describe the complications that may follow the placement of an ileal conduit. What assessments do you commonly perform in the immediate postoperative period? What is the role of a WOCN in the care of this patient?

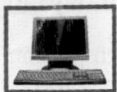

The Smeltzer suite offers these additional resources to enhance learning and facilitate understanding of this chapter:
- thePoint online resource, thepoint.lww.com/Smeltzer12E
- Student CD-ROM included with the book
- *Study Guide to Accompany Brunner & Suddarth's Textbook of Medical-Surgical Nursing*
- *Handbook for Brunner & Suddarth's Textbook of Medical-Surgical Nursing*

REFERENCES AND SELECTED READINGS

Asterisk indicates nursing research.

Books

Bickley, L. S. (2007). *Bates' guide to physical examination and history taking* (9th ed.). Philadelphia: Lippincott Williams & Wilkins.

Diepenbrock, N. H. (2007). *Quick reference to critical care* (3rd ed.). Philadelphia: Lippincott Williams & Wilkins.

Dudek, S. G. (2006). *Nutrition essentials for nursing practice* (5th ed.). Philadelphia: Lippincott Williams & Wilkins.

Karch, A. (2008). *2008 Lippincott's nursing drug guide*. Philadelphia: Lippincott Williams & Wilkins.

Karpoff, S. & Labus, D. (Eds.). (2008). *Portable diagnostic tests*. Philadelphia: Lippincott Williams & Wilkins.

McFarlane, M. T. (2006). *Urology*. Philadelphia: Lippincott Williams & Wilkins.

Miller, C. A. (2009). *Nursing for wellness in older adults*. Philadelphia: Lippincott Williams & Wilkins.

Morton, P. G., Fontaine, D. K., Hudak, C. M., et al. (2005). *Critical care nursing: A holistic approach* (8th ed.). Philadelphia: Lippincott Williams & Wilkins.

Porth, C. M. & Matfin, G. (2009). *Pathophysiology: Concepts of altered health status* (8th ed.). Philadelphia: Lippincott Williams & Wilkins.

Schnell, Z., Leeuwen, A. & Kranpitz, T. (2006). *Davis's comprehensive handbook of laboratory and diagnostic tests with nursing implications* (2nd ed.). Philadelphia: F. A. Davis.

Stanley, M., Blair, K. A. & Beare, P. G. (2005). *Gerontological nursing: Promoting successful aging with older adults* (3rd ed.). Philadelphia: F. A. Davis.

Tanagho, E. & McAninch, J. (Eds.). (2007). *Smith's general urology* (17th ed.). New York: McGraw-Hill.

Journals and Electronic Documents

General

Altschuler, V. & Diaz, L. (2006). Bladder ultrasound. *MedSurg Nursing, 15*(5), 317–318.

Burrows-Hudson, S. (2005). Chronic kidney disease: An overview: Early and aggressive treatment is vital. *American Journal of Nursing, 105*(2), 40–49.

Carson, C. C. (2007). The cost of urologic care in America: 11 billion and growing. *Contemporary Urology, 19*(11), 6.

Toughill, E. (2005). Indwelling catheters: Common mechanical and pathogenic problems. *American Journal of Nursing, 105*(5), 35–37.

Infections of the Urinary Tract

Blakely, M. (2008). Reducing the percentage of Foley catheters in patients 65 and older. *Clinical Nurse Specialist, 22*(2), 101–102.

Jackson, M. A. (2007). Evidence-based practice for evaluation and management of female urinary tract infections. *Urologic Nursing, 27*(2), 133–136.

Juthani-Mehta, M. (2007). Asymptomatic bacteriuria and urinary tract infection in older adults. *Clinics in Geriatric Medicine, 23*(3), 585–594.

Juthani-Mehta, M., Tinetti, M., Perrelli, E., et al. (2007). Diagnostic accuracy of criteria for urinary tract infection in a cohort of nursing home residents. *Journal of the American Geriatrics Society, 55*(7), 1072–1077.

McMurdo, M. E., Bissett, L. Y., Price, R. J., et al. (2005). Does ingestion of cranberry juice reduce symptomatic urinary tract infections in older people in hospital? *Age and Ageing, 34*(3), 256–261.

Mehnert-Kay, S. A. (2005). Diagnosis and management of uncomplicated urinary tract infections. *American Family Physician, 72*(3), 451–456.

National Kidney and Urologic Diseases Information Clearinghouse. (2005). *Urinary tract infection in adults*. National Institute of Diabetes and Digestive and Kidney Diseases, National Institutes of Health (NIH) Publication No. 07–2097. Available at: http://kidney.niddk.nih.gov/Kudiseases/pubs/pdf/KU-03.pdf

Senese, V., Hendricks, M. B., Morrison, M., et al. (2006). Clinical practice guidelines: Care of the patient with an indwelling catheter. *Urologic Nursing, 26*(1), 80–81.

Smythe, M., Moore, J. E. & Goldsmith, C. E. (2006). Urinary tract infections: Role of the clinical microbiology laboratory. *Urologic Nursing, 26*(3), 198–203.

Adult Voiding Dysfunction

*Cheater, F. M. Baker, R., Gillies, C., et al. (2008). The nature and impact of urinary incontinence experienced by patients receiving community nursing services: A cross-sectional study. *International Journal of Nursing Studies, 45*(3), 339.

*Klay, M. & Marfyak, K. (2005). Use of a continence nurse specialist in an extended care facility. *Urologic Nursing, 25*(2), 101–108.

Mennick, F. (2005). Urinary incontinence worsens with menopausal hormone therapy. *American Journal of Nursing, 105*(7), 22.

*Muller, N. (2005). What Americans understand and how they are affected by bladder control problems: Highlights of recent nationwide consumer research. *Urologic Nursing, 25*(2), 109–115.

Specht, J. (2005). Nine myths of incontinence in older adults. *American Journal of Nursing, 105*(6), 58–70.

*Vinsnes, A. G., Harkless, G. E. & Nyronning, S. (2007). Unit-based intervention to improve urinary incontinence in frail elderly. *Journal of Nursing Research & Clinical Studies, 27*(3), 53–56.

Urolithiasis and Nephrolithiasis

Colella, J., Kochis, E., Galli, B., et al. (2005). Urolithiasis/Nephrolithiasis: What's it all about? *Urologic Nursing, 25*(6), 427–448, 475.

Flagg, L. R. (2007). Dietary and holistic treatment of recurrent calcium oxalate kidney stones. *Urologic Nursing, 27*(2), 113–123.

Straub, D. A. (2007). Calcium supplementation in clinical practice: A review of forms, doses and indications. *Nutrition in Clinical Practice, 22*(3), 286–296.

Taylor, E. N. & Curhan, G. C. (2008). Fructose consumption and the risk of kidney stones. *Kidney International, 73*(2), 207–212.

Urinary Tract Cancers

American Cancer Society. (2009) *Cancer facts and figures 2009*. www.cancer.org

Hoffman, P., Roumeguere, T., Schulman, C., et al. (2006). Use of statins and outcome of BCG treatment for bladder cancer. *New England Journal of Medicine, 355*(25), 2705–2507.

Huang, Z. (2005). A review of progress in clinical photodynamic therapy. *Technology in Cancer Research and Treatment, 4*(3), 283–293.

Sharma, P., Old, L. J. & Allison, J. P. (2007). Immunotherapeutic strategies for high-risk bladder cancer. *Seminars in Oncology, 34*(2), 165–172.

Torpy, J. M., Lynm, C. & Glass, R. M. (2005). Bladder cancer. *Journal of the American Medical Association, 293*(7), 890.

Genitourinary Trauma

Alders, L. L., Sedler, K. D., Bedrick, E. J., et al. (2007). Factors related to genital tract trauma in normal spontaneous vaginal births. *Birth, 33*(2), 94–100.

Wald, H. L., Radcliff, T. A. & Kramer, A. M. (2008). Extended use of urinary catheters in older surgical patients: A patient safety problem? *Infection Control & Hospital Epidemiology, 29*(2), 116–124.

Ziran, B., Chamberlin, E., Shuler, F. D., et al. (2005). Delays and difficulty in the diagnosis of lower urologic injuries in the context of pelvic fractures. *Journal of Trauma-Injury and Critical Care, 58*(3), 533–537.

Urinary Diversions

Fulham, J. (2008). Providing dietary advice for the individual with a stoma. *British Journal of Nursing, 17*(2), S22–S27.

Marchese, K. (2006). Using Peplau's theory of interpersonal relations to guide the education of patient undergoing urinary diversion. *Urologic Nursing, 26*(5), 363–370.

Pullen, R. L. (2007). Replacing a urostomy drainage pouch. *Nursing, 37*(6), 14.

RESOURCES

American Cancer Society, www.cancer.org
American Urological Association, www.auanet.org
National Association for Continence, www.nafc.org
National Institute of Diabetes and Digestive and Kidney Diseases (NIDDK), National Institutes of Health, www.niddk.nih.gov
National Kidney Foundation, www.kidney.org

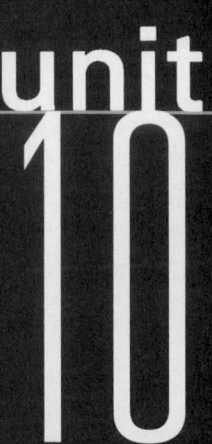

Reproductive Function

Case Study • Applying Concepts From NANDA, NIC, and NOC

A Patient With a Difficult Health Care Choice Involving Losses

Mrs. Cole is a 49-year-old woman who has been undergoing cancer staging after positive breast biopsy results. The surgeon has informed her that she has stage IIB infiltrating ductal carcinoma. The surgeon has discussed with her two different surgical approaches—breast conserving or modified radical mastectomy (MRM). If she chooses MRM, Mrs. Cole must decide whether she will undergo breast reconstruction or use a breast prosthesis. The nurse notes that Mrs. Cole is trembling and near tears. Mrs. Cole tells the nurse that she is uncertain about how her husband will respond if she chooses MRM. She is also concerned that she will not feel feminine after MRM but states she is very frightened about anything less since a friend died of metastatic breast cancer.

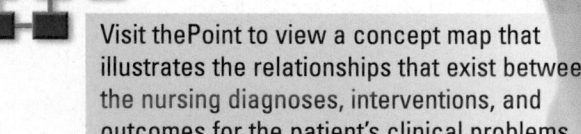

Visit thePoint to view a concept map that illustrates the relationships that exist between the nursing diagnoses, interventions, and outcomes for the patient's clinical problems.

Nursing Classifications and Languages

NANDA NURSING DIAGNOSES	NIC NURSING INTERVENTIONS	NOC NURSING OUTCOMES
		Return to functional baseline status, stabilization of, or improvement in:
DECISIONAL CONFLICT—Uncertainty about course of action to be taken when choice among competing actions involves risk, loss, or challenge to personal life values	**ACTIVE LISTENING**—Attending closely to and attaching significance to a patient's verbal and nonverbal messages	**DECISION MAKING**—Ability to make judgments and choose between two or more alternatives
ANTICIPATORY GRIEVING—Intellectual and emotional responses and behaviors by which individuals, families, and communities work through the process of modifying self-concept based on the perception of potential loss	**DECISION-MAKING SUPPORT**—Providing information and support for a patient who is making a decision regarding health care	**GRIEF RESOLUTION**—Adjustment to actual or impending loss
	ANTICIPATORY GUIDANCE—Preparation of a patient for an anticipated developmental and/or situational crisis **GRIEF WORK FACILITATION**—Assistance with the resolution of a significant loss **EMOTIONAL SUPPORT**—Provision of reassurance, acceptance and encouragement during times of stress	**PSYCHOSOCIAL ADJUSTMENT: LIFE CHANGE**—Adaptive psychosocial response of an individual to a significant life change

Bulechek, G. M., Butcher, H. K., & Dochterman, J. M. (2008). *Nursing interventions classification (NIC)* (5th ed.). St. Louis: Mosby.
Johnson, M., Bulechek, G., Butcher, H. K., et al. (2006). *NANDA, NOC, and NIC linkages* (2nd ed.). St. Louis: Mosby.
Moorhead, S., Johnson, M., Mass, M. L., et al. (2008). *Nursing outcomes classification (NOC)* (4th ed.). St. Louis: Mosby.
NANDA International. (2007). *Nursing diagnoses: Definitions & classification 2007–2008*. Philadelphia: North American Nursing Diagnosis Association.

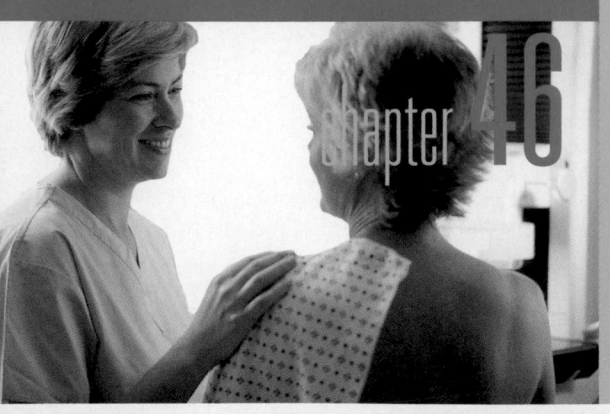

chapter 46

Assessment and Management of Female Physiologic Processes

On completion of this chapter, the learner will be able to:

1 Describe female reproductive function.

2 Describe approaches to effective sexual assessment.

3 Describe indicators of domestic violence and abuse of women and methods of identifying and treating women who are survivors of abuse.

4 Identify the diagnostic examinations and tests used to determine alteration in female reproductive function and describe the nurse's role before, during, and after these examinations and procedures.

5 Identify types of menstrual disorders and related nursing implications.

6 Describe nursing care for patients with premenstrual syndrome.

7 Develop a teaching plan for women who are approaching or have completed menopause.

8 Describe methods of contraception and implications for health care and education.

9 Describe the nursing management of the patient having an abortion.

10 Describe the causes and management of infertility.

11 Use the nursing process to plan for the care of the patient with an ectopic pregnancy.

12 Discuss the healthy older woman and health teaching related to aging.

GLOSSARY

adnexa: the fallopian tubes and ovaries

amenorrhea: absence of menstrual flow

androgens: hormones produced by the ovaries and adrenals that affect many aspects of female health, including follicle development, libido, oiliness of hair and skin, and hair growth

cervix: bottom (inferior) part of the uterus that is located in the vagina

chandelier sign: pain on gentle movement of the cervix; associated with pelvic infection

corpus luteum: site of a follicle that changes after ovulation to produce progesterone

cystocele: weakness of the anterior vaginal wall that allows the bladder to protrude into the vagina

GLOSSARY *(Continued)*

dysmenorrhea: painful menstruation

dyspareunia: difficult or painful sexual intercourse

endometrial ablation: procedure performed through a hysteroscope in which the lining of the uterus is burned away or ablated to treat abnormal uterine bleeding

endometriosis: condition in which endometrial tissue implants in other areas of the pelvis; may produce dysmenorrhea or infertility

endometrium: lining of the uterus

estrogen: hormone that develops and maintains the female reproductive system

follicle-stimulating hormone (FSH): hormone released by the pituitary gland to stimulate estrogen production and ovulation

fornix: upper part of the vagina

fundus: body of the uterus

graafian follicle: cystic structure that develops on the ovary as ovulation begins

hymen: tissue that covers the vaginal opening partially or completely before vaginal penetration

hysteroscopy: a procedure performed using a long telescope-like instrument inserted through the cervix to diagnose uterine problems

introitus: perineal opening to the vagina

luteal phase: stage in the menstrual cycle in which the endometrium becomes thicker and more vascular

luteinizing hormone (LH): hormone released by the pituitary gland that stimulates progesterone production

menarche: beginning of menstrual function

menopause: permanent cessation of menstruation resulting from the loss of ovarian follicular activity

menstruation: sloughing and discharge of the lining of the uterus if conception does not take place

ovaries: almond-shaped reproductive organs that produce eggs at ovulation and play a major role in hormone production

ovulation: discharge of a mature ovum from the ovary

perimenopause: the period immediately prior to menopause and the first year after menopause

polyp (cervical or endometrial): growth of tissue on the cervix or endometrial lining; usually benign

progesterone: hormone produced by the corpus luteum

proliferative phase: stage in the menstrual cycle before ovulation when the endometrium proliferates

rectocele: weakness of the posterior vaginal wall that allows the rectal cavity to protrude into the submucosa of the vagina

secretory phase: stage of the menstrual cycle in which the endometrium becomes thickened, more vascular, and edematous

uterine prolapse: relaxation of pelvic tone that allows the cervix and uterus to descend into the lower vagina

Women are becoming more knowledgeable about their health. Nurses who work with them need to understand normal female anatomy and physiology and the physical, developmental, psychological, and sociocultural influences on women's health, health practices, and use of health care resources. Health assessment, maintenance, and promotion across the lifespan must consider women's growth and development, sexuality, contraception, preconception care, conception, prenatal care, effects of pregnancy on health, perimenopause, menopause, and aging. It is also necessary to consider how medications and diseases affect women. In addition, women's sexuality is complex and often affected by many factors, and related issues need careful evaluation and treatment. Because women use the health care system more often than men and make up the majority of health care workers, addressing women's health needs and concerns improves quality and access for women and their families.

ROLE OF NURSES IN WOMEN'S HEALTH

As their presence in the labor market continues to increase, women face challenges in their roles, lifestyles, and family patterns. Furthermore, they encounter environmental hazards and stress, prompting greater attention on health and health-promoting practices. As a result, many women are taking a greater interest in and responsibility for their own health and health care, although not all women have the time, finances, or other resources to do so.

In recent years, many women have delayed pregnancy and childbearing until well after they have established careers, in part because of the wide variety of contraceptive methods that are available. Advances in the treatment of infertility have enabled many women previously unable to have children to become pregnant and have allowed couples well into their 40s to have children. Women who have many roles and multiple responsibilities (eg, workers, wives, mothers, parental caretakers) often "multitask"; they have little time for themselves and often put the needs of others before their own health needs. Nurses must be sensitive to these needs and knowledgeable about preventive health care for women. Nurses are in an ideal position to encourage women to determine their own health goals and behaviors, teach about health promotion and illness prevention, offer intervention strategies, and provide support, counseling, and ongoing monitoring. Areas of special interest in health promotion include the following:

- Normal physical changes and optimal personal hygiene
- Strategies for detecting and preventing disease, especially sexually transmitted diseases (STDs), also referred to as sexually transmitted infections (STIs), including human immunodeficiency virus (HIV) infection and acquired immunodeficiency syndrome (AIDS)
- Issues related to sexuality and sexual function, such as contraception; preconception, prenatal, and postnatal care; sexual satisfaction; and menopause

- Diet, exercise, and health-promoting practices that maintain and enhance health, including having a normal weight for height
- Appropriate stress management to reduce the detrimental effects of stress on health and well-being
- Treatment for substance abuse and smoking

Nurses need to model a healthy lifestyle for their patients. It is important that nurses promote positive practices and behaviors related to the reproductive and sexual health of all patients. Necessary strategies include the following:

- Recommending regular examinations to promote health, detect health problems at an early stage, assess problems related to gynecologic and reproductive function, and discuss questions or concerns related to sexual function and sexuality
- Providing an open, nonjudgmental environment (crucial in providing nursing and health care, especially when patients are discussing personal issues). Nurses must convey understanding and sensitivity and be alert to cues about unspoken patient concerns.
- Recognizing signs and symptoms of abuse and screening all patients in a private and safe environment
- Recognizing cultural differences and beliefs and respecting sexual orientation

ASSESSMENT OF THE FEMALE REPRODUCTIVE SYSTEM

Anatomic and Physiologic Overview

Anatomy of the Female Reproductive System

The female reproductive system consists of external and internal pelvic structures. Other anatomic structures that affect the female reproductive system include the hypothalamus and pituitary gland of the endocrine system.

External Genitalia

The external genitalia (the vulva) include two thick folds of tissue called the labia majora and two smaller lips of delicate tissue called the labia minora, which lie within the labia majora. The upper portions of the labia minora unite, forming a partial covering for the clitoris, a highly sensitive organ composed of erectile tissue. Between the labia minora, below and posterior to the clitoris, is the urinary meatus, the external opening of the female urethra, which is about 3 cm (less than 1.5 in) long. Below this orifice is a larger opening, the vaginal orifice or **introitus** (Fig. 46-1). On each side of the vaginal orifice is a vestibular (Bartholin's) gland, a bean-sized structure that empties its mucous secretion through a small duct. The opening of the duct lies within the labia minora, external to the hymen. The area between the vagina and rectum is called the perineum.

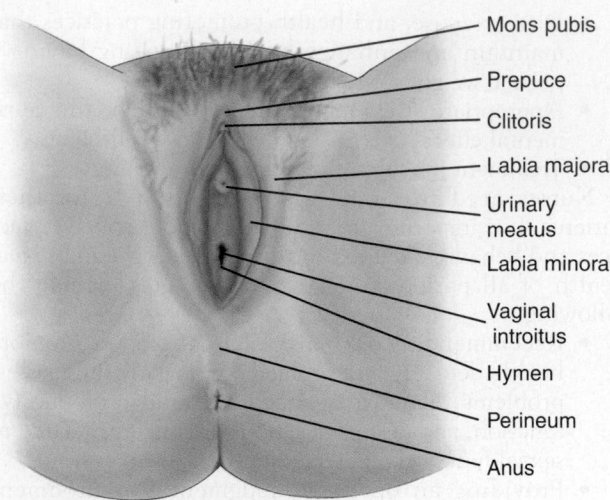

Figure 46-1 External female genitalia.

Mons pubis
Prepuce
Clitoris
Labia majora
Urinary meatus
Labia minora
Vaginal introitus
Hymen
Perineum
Anus

Internal Reproductive Structures

The internal structures consist of the vagina, uterus, ovaries, and fallopian or uterine tubes (Fig. 46-2).

Vagina

The vagina, a canal lined with mucous membrane, is 7.5 to 10 cm (3 to 4 in) long and extends upward and backward from the vulva to the cervix. Anterior to it are the bladder and the urethra, and posterior to it lies the rectum. The anterior and posterior walls of the vagina normally touch each other. The upper part of the vagina, the **fornix,** surrounds the **cervix** (the inferior part of the uterus).

Uterus

The uterus, a pear-shaped, muscular organ, is about 7.5 cm (3 in) long and 5 cm (2 in) wide at its upper part. Its walls are about 1.25 cm (0.5 in) thick. The size of the uterus varies, depending on parity (number of viable births) and uterine abnormalities (eg, fibroids, which are a type of tumor that may distort the uterus). A nulliparous woman

(one who has not completed a pregnancy to the stage of fetal viability) usually has a smaller uterus than a multiparous woman (one who has completed two or more pregnancies to the stage of fetal viability). The uterus lies posterior to the bladder and is held in position by several ligaments. The round ligaments extend anteriorly and laterally to the internal inguinal ring and down the inguinal canal, where they blend with the tissues of the labia majora. The broad ligaments are folds of peritoneum extending from the lateral pelvic walls and enveloping the fallopian tubes. The uterosacral ligaments extend posteriorly to the sacrum. The uterus has two parts: the cervix, which projects into the vagina, and a larger upper part, the **fundus** or body, which is covered posteriorly and partly anteriorly by peritoneum. The triangular inner portion of the fundus narrows to a small canal in the cervix that has constrictions at each end, referred to as the external os and internal os. The upper lateral parts of the uterus are called the cornua. From here, the oviducts or fallopian (or uterine) tubes extend outward, and their lumina are internally continuous with the uterine cavity (Porth & Matfin, 2009).

Ovaries

The **ovaries** lie behind the broad ligaments and behind and below the fallopian tubes. They are oval bodies about 3 cm (1.2 in) long. At birth, they contain thousands of tiny egg cells, or ova. The ovaries and the fallopian tubes together are referred to as the **adnexa.**

Function of the Female Reproductive System

Ovulation

At puberty (usually between 12 and 14 years of age, but earlier for some; 10 or 11 years of age is not uncommon), the ova begin to mature and menstrual cycles begin. In the follicular phase, an ovum enlarges as a type of cyst called a **graafian follicle** until it reaches the surface of the ovary, where transport occurs. The ovum (or oocyte) is discharged into the peritoneal cavity. This periodic discharge of matured ovum is referred to as **ovulation.** The ovum usually finds its way into the fallopian tube, where it is carried to the uterus. If it is penetrated by a spermatozoon, the male reproductive cell, a union occurs and conception takes place. After the discharge of the ovum, the cells of the graafian follicle undergo a rapid change. Gradually, they become yellow **(corpus luteum)** and produce **progesterone,** a hormone that prepares the uterus for receiving the fertilized ovum. Ovulation usually occurs 2 weeks prior to the next menstrual period.

Menstrual Cycle

The menstrual cycle is a complex process involving the reproductive and endocrine systems. The ovaries produce steroid hormones, predominantly estrogens and progesterone. Several different **estrogens** are produced by the ovarian follicle, which consists of the developing ovum and its surrounding cells. The most potent of the ovarian

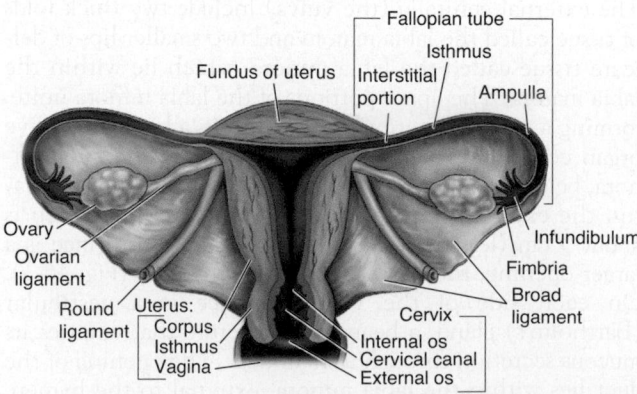

Figure 46-2 Internal female reproductive structures.

Fundus of uterus
Fallopian tube
Isthmus
Interstitial portion
Ampulla
Ovary
Ovarian ligament
Round ligament
Uterus:
Corpus
Isthmus
Vagina
Cervix
Internal os
Cervical canal
External os
Infundibulum
Fimbria
Broad ligament

estrogens is estradiol. Estrogens are responsible for developing and maintaining the female reproductive organs and the secondary sex characteristics associated with the adult female. Estrogens play an important role in breast development and in monthly cyclic changes in the uterus (Porth & Matfin, 2009).

Progesterone is also important in regulating the changes that occur in the uterus during the menstrual cycle. It is secreted by the corpus luteum, which is the ovarian follicle after the ovum has been released. Progesterone is the most important hormone for conditioning the **endometrium** (the mucous membrane lining the uterus) in preparation for implantation of a fertilized ovum. If pregnancy occurs, the progesterone secretion becomes largely a function of the placenta and is essential for maintaining a normal pregnancy. In addition, progesterone, working with estrogen, prepares the breast for producing and secreting milk. **Androgens** are also produced by the ovaries and adrenal glands, but only in small amounts. These hormones are involved in the early development of the follicle and also affect the female libido (Porth & Matfin, 2009).

Two gonadotropic hormones are released by the pituitary gland: **follicle-stimulating hormone (FSH)** and **luteinizing hormone (LH).** FSH is primarily responsible for stimulating the ovaries to secrete estrogen. LH is primarily responsible for stimulating progesterone production. Feedback mechanisms, in part, regulate FSH and LH secretion. For example, elevated estrogen levels in the blood inhibit FSH secretion but promote LH secretion, whereas elevated progesterone levels inhibit LH secretion. In addition, gonadotropin-releasing hormone (GnRH) from the hypothalamus affects the rate of FSH and LH release.

The secretion of ovarian hormones follows a cyclic pattern that results in changes in the uterine endometrium and in **menstruation** (Fig. 46-3, Table 46-1). This cycle is typically 28 days in length, but there are many normal variations (from 21 to 42 days). In the **proliferative phase** at the beginning of the cycle (just after menstruation), FSH output increases, stimulating estrogen secretion. This causes the endometrium to thicken and become more vascular. In the **secretory phase** near the middle portion of the cycle (day 14 in a 28-day cycle), LH output increases, stimulating ovulation. Under the combined stimulus of estrogen and progesterone, the endometrium reaches the peak of its thickening and vascularization. In the **luteal phase,** which begins after ovulation, progesterone is secreted by the corpus luteum.

If the ovum is fertilized, estrogen and progesterone levels remain high, and the complex hormonal changes of pregnancy follow. If the ovum has not been fertilized, FSH and LH output diminishes, estrogen and progesterone secretion falls, the ovum disintegrates, and the endometrium, which has become thick and congested, becomes hemorrhagic. The product, menstrual flow, consisting of old blood, mucus, and endometrial tissue, is discharged through the cervix and into the vagina. After the menstrual flow stops, the cycle begins again; the endometrium proliferates and thickens from estrogenic

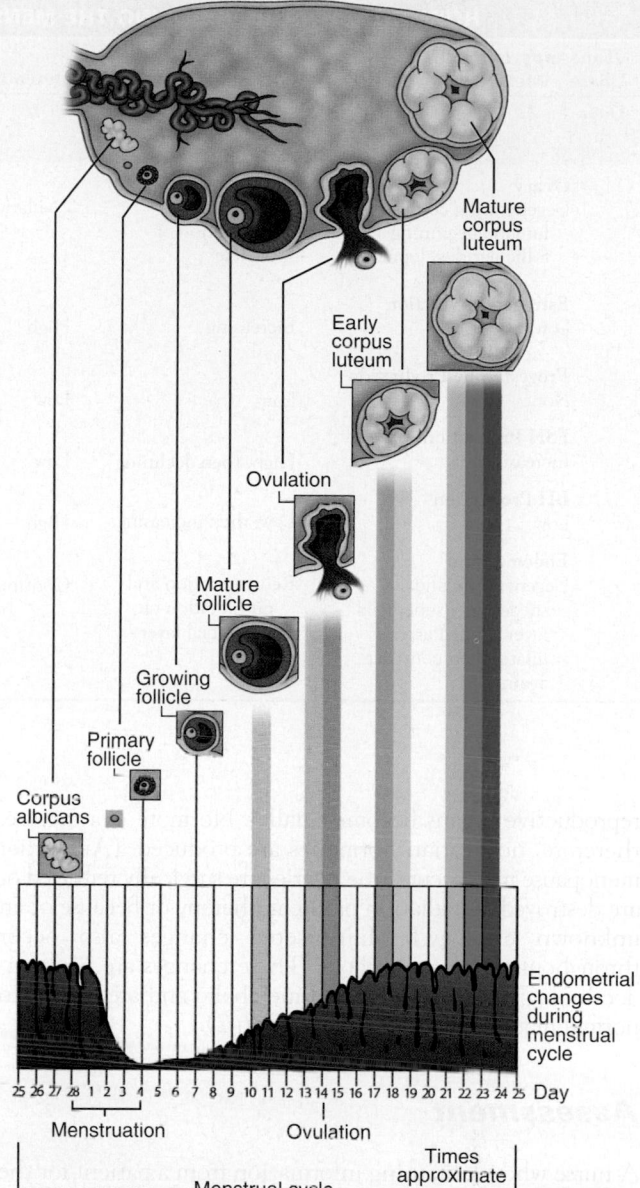

Figure 46-3 One menstrual cycle and the corresponding changes in the endometrium.

stimulation, and ovulation recurs (Porth & Matfin, 2009).

Menopausal Period

The menopausal period marks the end of a woman's reproductive capacity. It usually occurs between 45 and 52 years of age but may occur as early as 42 or as late as 55; the median age is 51 years. Perimenopause precedes this and can begin as early as 35 years of age. Physical, emotional, and menstrual changes may occur, and this transition offers another opportunity for health promotion and disease prevention teaching and counseling. **Menopause** is not a pathologic phenomenon but a normal part of aging and maturation. Menstruation ceases, and because the ovaries are no longer active, the

Table 46-1 **HORMONAL CHANGES DURING THE MENSTRUAL CYCLE**

(Times approximate) Phase	Menstrual	Follicular	Ovulation	Luteal	Premenstrual
Days	1 2 3 4 5 6 7 8	9 10 11 12 13	14 15 16 17 18	19 20 21 22 23	24 25 26 27 28 1 2
Ovary	Degenerating corpus luteum; beginning follicular development	Growth and maturation of follicle	Ovulation	Active corpus luteum	Degenerating corpus luteum
Estrogen Production	Low	Increasing	High	Declining, then a secondary rise	Decreasing
Progesterone Production	None	Low	Low	Increasing	Decreasing
FSH Production	Increasing	High, then declining	Low	Low	Increasing
LH Production	Low	Low, then increasing	High	High	Decreasing
Endometrium	Degeneration and shedding of superficial layer. Coiled arteries dilate, then constrict again.	Reorganization and proliferation of superficial layer	Continued growth	Active secretion and glandular dilation; highly vascular; edematous	Vasoconstriction of coiled arteries; beginning degeneration

reproductive organs become smaller. No more ova mature; therefore, no ovarian hormones are produced. (An earlier menopause may occur if the ovaries are surgically removed or are destroyed by radiation or chemotherapy or because of an unknown etiology.) Multifaceted changes also occur throughout the woman's body. These changes are neuroendocrinologic, biochemical, and metabolic and are related to normal maturation or aging (Table 46-2).

Assessment

A nurse who is obtaining information from a patient for the health history and performing physical assessment is in an ideal position to discuss the woman's general health issues, health promotion, and health-related concerns. Relevant topics include fitness, nutrition, cardiovascular risks, health screening, sexuality, menopause, abuse, health risk behaviors, emotional well-being, and immunizations. Recommendations for health screening are summarized in Chart 46-1.

Health History

In addition to the general health history, the nurse asks about past illnesses and experiences specific to a woman's health. Data should be collected about the following:

- Menstrual history (including **menarche,** length of cycles, duration and amount of flow, presence of cramps or pain, bleeding between periods or after intercourse, bleeding after menopause)
- Pregnancies (number of pregnancies, outcomes of pregnancies)

Table 46-2 **AGE-RELATED CHANGES IN THE FEMALE REPRODUCTIVE SYSTEM**

	Physiologic Changes	Signs and Symptoms
Cessation of ovarian function and decreased estrogen production	Decreased ovulation	Decreased/loss of ability to conceive; increased infertility
	Onset of menopause	Irregular menses with eventual cessation of menses
	Vasomotor instability and hormonal fluctuations	Hot flashes or flushing; night sweats, sleep disturbances; mood swings; fatigue
	Decreased bone formation	Bone loss and increased risk for osteoporosis and osteoporotic fractures; loss of height
	Decreased vaginal lubrication	Dyspareunia, resulting in lack of interest in sex
	Thinning of urinary and genital tracts	Increased risk for urinary tract infection
	Increased pH of vagina	Increased incidence of inflammation (atrophic vaginitis) with discharge, itching, and vulvar burning
	Thinning of pubic hair and shrinking of labia	
Relaxation of pelvic musculature	Prolapse of uterus, cystocele, rectocele	Dyspareunia, incontinence, feelings of perineal pressure

Chart 46-1 • *Summary of Health Screening and Counseling Issues for Women*

Ages 19–39

Sexuality and Reproductive Issues

Annual pelvic examination
Annual clinical breast examination
Contraceptive options
High-risk sexual behaviors

Health and Risk Behaviors

Hygiene
Injury prevention
Nutrition
Exercise patterns
Risk for domestic abuse
Use of tobacco, drugs, and alcohol
Life stresses
Immunizations

Diagnostic Testing*

Pap smear every 3 years after onset of sexual intercourse
STD/STI screening as indicated

Ages 40–64

Sexuality and Reproductive Issues

Annual pelvic examination
Annual clinical breast examination
Contraceptive options
High-risk sexual behaviors
Menopausal concerns

Health and Risk Behaviors

Hygiene
Bone loss and injury prevention
Nutrition
Exercise patterns
Risk for domestic abuse
Use of tobacco, drugs, and alcohol
Life stresses
Immunizations

Diagnostic Testing*

Pap smear every 2 to 3 years after three consecutive
    negative tests if no history of cervical abnormalities,
    HIV infection, or DES exposure
Mammography
Cholesterol and lipid profile
Colorectal cancer screening
Bone mineral density testing
Thyroid-stimulating hormone testing
Hearing and eye examinations

Ages 65 and Over

Sexuality and Reproductive Issues

Annual pelvic examination
Annual clinical breast examination
High-risk sexual behaviors

Health and Risk Behaviors

Hygiene
Injury prevention
Nutrition
Exercise patterns
Risk for domestic abuse
Use of tobacco, drugs, and alcohol
Life stresses
Immunizations

Diagnostic Testing*

Pap smear every 2 to 3 years after three consecutive
    negative tests if no history of cervical abnormalities,
    HIV infection, or DES exposure
Mammography
Cholesterol and lipid profile
Colorectal cancer screening
Bone mineral density testing
Thyroid-stimulating hormone testing
Hearing and eye examinations

*Each individual's risks (family history, personal history) influence the need for specific assessments and their frequency.

- Exposure to medications (diethylstilbestrol [DES], immunosuppressive agents, others)
- Pain with menses (**dysmenorrhea**), pain with intercourse (**dyspareunia**), pelvic pain
- Symptoms of vaginitis (ie, odor or itching)
- Problems with urinary function, including frequency, urgency, and incontinence
- Bowel problems
- Sexual history
- STDs and methods of treatment
- Current or previous sexual abuse or physical abuse
- Past surgery or other procedures on reproductive tract structures (including female genital mutilation or female circumcision)
- Chronic illness or disability that may affect health status, reproductive health, need for health screening, or access to health care
- Presence of or family history of a genetic disorder. Chart 46-2 presents information about genetic reproductive disorders.

In collecting data related to reproductive health, the nurse can teach the patient about normal physiologic processes, such as menstruation and menopause, and assess possible abnormalities. Many problems experienced by young or middle-age women can be corrected easily. However, if they are not treated, they may result in anxiety and health problems. Issues related to sexuality and sexual function are typically more often brought to the attention of the gynecologic or women's health care provider than other health care providers; however, nurses caring for all women should consider these issues part of routine health assessment.

Sexual History

A sexual assessment includes both subjective and objective data. Health and sexual histories, physical examination findings, and laboratory results are all part of the database. The purpose of a sexual history is to obtain information that provides a picture of a woman's sexuality and sexual practices and to promote sexual health. The sexual history may enable a patient to discuss sexual matters openly and

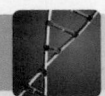

GENETICS IN NURSING PRACTICE
CHART 46-2
Reproductive Disorders

Various reproductive disorders are influenced by genetic factors. Some examples are:

- Hereditary breast or ovarian cancer syndromes
- Hereditary nonpolyposis colon cancer syndrome (risk for uterine cancer)
- Müllerian aplasia
- 21-Hydroxylase deficiency (female masculinization)
- Turner syndrome (45,XO)
- Klinefelter syndrome (47,XXY)

Nursing Assessments

Family History Assessment

- Assess family history for other family members with similar reproductive problems/abnormalities.
- Inquire about ethnic background (eg, Ashkenazi Jewish populations and hereditary breast/ovarian cancer mutations).
- Inquire about relatives with other cancers, including early-onset ovarian, uterine, renal, prostate cancers.

Patient Assessment

- In females with delayed puberty or primary amenorrhea, assess for clinical features of Turner syndrome (short stature, webbing of the neck, widely spaced nipples).
- In males with delayed puberty or infertility, assess for clinical features of Klinefelter syndrome (tall stature, gynecomastia, learning disabilities).
- Assess for other congenital anomalies in females with Müllerian defect, including renal and vertebral anomalies.

Management Issues Specific to Genetics

- Inquire whether genetics testing (DNA chromosomal, metabolic) has been carried out on affected family member(s).
- If indicated, refer for further genetics counseling and evaluation so that family members can discuss inheritance,

risk to other family members, availability of genetics testing, and gene-based interventions.

- Offer appropriate genetics information and resources.
- Assess patient's understanding of genetics information.
- Provide support to families with newly diagnosed gene-related reproductive disorders.
- Participate in management and coordination of care of patients with genetic conditions, individuals predisposed to develop or pass on a genetic condition.

Genetics Resources for Nurses and their Patients on the Web

Genetic Alliance—a directory of support groups for patients and families with genetic conditions, www.geneticalliance.org

American Cancer Society—offers general information about cancer and support resources for families, www.cancer.org

Gene Clinics—a listing of common genetic disorders with up-to-date clinical summaries, genetic counseling and testing information, www.geneclinics.org

National Organization of Rare Disorders—a directory of support groups and information for patients and families with rare genetic disorders, www.rarediseases.org

National Cancer Institute—current information about cancer research, treatment, resources for health care providers, individuals and families, www.nci.nih.gov

OMIM: Online Mendelian Inheritance in Man—a complete listing of inherited genetic conditions, www.ncbi.nlm.nih.gov/omim/stats/html

---

to discuss sexual concerns with an informed health professional. This information can be obtained after the gynecologic–obstetric or genitourinary history is completed. By incorporating the sexual history into the general health history, the nurse can move from areas of lesser sensitivity to areas of greater sensitivity after establishing initial rapport.

Taking the sexual history becomes a dynamic process reflecting an exchange of information between the patient and the nurse and provides the opportunity to clarify myths and explore areas of concern that the patient may not have felt comfortable discussing in the past. In obtaining a sexual history, the nurse must not assume the patient's sexual preference until clarified. When asking about sexual health, the nurse also cannot assume that the patient is married or unmarried. Asking a patient to label herself as single, married, widowed, or divorced may be considered by some women as inappropriate. Asking about a partner or about current meaningful relationships may be a less offensive way to initiate a sexual history.

The PLISSIT (permission, limited information, specific suggestions, intensive therapy) model of sexual assess-

ment and intervention may be used to provide a framework for nursing interventions (Annon, 1976). The assessment begins by introducing the topic and asking the woman for permission to discuss issues related to sexuality with her.

The nurse can begin by explaining the purpose of obtaining a sexual history (eg, "I ask all my patients about their sexual health. May I ask you some questions about this?"). History taking continues by inquiring about present sexual activity and sexual orientation (eg, "Are you currently having sex? With a man, a woman, or both?"). Inquiries about possible sexual dysfunction may include, "Are you having any problems related to your current sexual activity?" Such problems may be related to medication, life changes, disability, or the onset of physical or emotional illness. A patient can be asked about her thoughts on what is causing the current problem.

Information about sexual function can be introduced during the health history. As the discussion progresses, the nurse may offer specific suggestions for interventions. A professional who specializes in sex therapy may provide more intensive therapy if necessary. By initiating an assessment about sexual concerns, the nurse communicates to the patient that issues about changes or problems in sexual functioning are valid health issues, which provides a safe environment for discussing these sensitive topics. Young women may be apprehensive about having irregular periods, may be concerned about STDs, or may need contraception. They may want information about using tampons, emergency contraception, or issues related to pregnancy. Perimenopausal women may have concerns about irregular menses. Menopausal women may be concerned about vaginal dryness and discomfort with intercourse. Women of any age may have concerns about relationships, sexual satisfaction, orgasm, or masturbation.

Risk of STDs can be assessed by asking about the number of sexual partners in the past year or in the patient's lifetime. An open-ended question related to the patient's need for further information should be included (eg, "Do you have any questions or concerns about your sexual health?"). Women can be advised that intercourse should never be painful; pain should be investigated by a care provider. They should also be encouraged to talk openly about their sexual feelings with their partner; in an intimate relationship, feelings are facts (Sarrel, 2005).

Female Genital Mutilation or Cutting

Female genital mutilation (FGM), or cutting, refers to the partial or total removal of the external female genitalia or other injury to female organs. Over 140 million girls and women have been subjected to this practice. Some cultures accept FGM as a rite of passage to womanhood and believe that this practice promotes hygiene, protects virginity and family honor, prevents promiscuity, improves female attractiveness and male sexual pleasure, and enhances fertility. FGM is considered an acceptable practice in many cultures, mostly in Africa and the Middle East. However, FGM is illegal in the United States and many organizations (eg, World Health Organization, Amnesty International) consider it a health and human rights issue and are working to end it. An increasing number of women entering the United States health care system underwent FGM before coming to the United States (Turner, 2007), and others have undergone FGM since their arrival in this country. Some of these women think that the practice is acceptable and do not consider themselves mutilated, whereas others believe it to be harmful and feel that they have been traumatized.

FGM is usually performed when a girl is between 4 and 10 years of age, but it may be performed on a newborn, adolescent, at the time of marriage, or during the first pregnancy. Short-term complications of FGM include hemorrhage, cellulitis, lacerations, urinary dysfunction, and infection. Long-term complications include urinary dysfunction, chronic vaginitis and pelvic infections, inability to undergo pelvic examination, painful intercourse, impaired sexual response, anemia, increased risk of HIV infection due to tearing of scar tissue, and psychological and psychosexual sequelae. Because FGM can affect sexual function, menstrual hygiene, and bladder function, the possibility of FGM must be considered in the sexual history, particularly in women from cultures and countries where the practice is common.

Nurses who care for patients who have undergone FGM need to be sensitive, empathetic, knowledgeable, culturally competent, and nonjudgmental (Turner, 2007). Respect for others' health beliefs, practices, and behaviors, and recognition of the complexity of issues involved is crucial. The nurse should use the woman's terminology. "Cutting" is a more acceptable term than mutilation. Speculums are not used in some developing countries; the function of this instrument should be explained and an appropriate-sized speculum used to examine women who have experienced FGM.

Domestic Violence

Domestic violence is a broad term that includes child abuse, elder abuse, and abuse of women and men. Abuse can be emotional, physical, sexual, or economic. Abuse involves fear of one partner by another and control by threats, intimidation, and physical abuse. Abuse is related to the need to maintain control of a partner and is rooted in sex role inequality.

More than 6 million women experience domestic violence each year, and battered women are encountered daily in nursing practice. Battering involves repeated physical or sexual assault in a context of coercive control and, more broadly, emotional degradation, threats, and intimidation. Violence is rarely a one-time occurrence in a relationship; it usually continues and escalates in severity. This is an important point to emphasize when a woman states that her partner has hurt her but has promised to change. Batterers can change their behavior but not without extensive counseling and motivation. If a woman states that she is being hurt, sensitive care is required (Chart 46-3).

By knowing about this major public health problem, being alert to abuse-related problems, and learning how to elicit information from women about abuse in their lives, nurses can offer intervention for a problem that might otherwise go undetected and can save lives by making women safer through education and support. Asking each woman about violence in her life in a safe environment (ie, a private room with the door closed) is part of a comprehensive assessment and universal screening. Asking about abuse directly is effective in identifying the presence of abuse and should be included in the health history of all women (Chart 46-4). The third and fourth questions of the screening questionnaire are specifically directed at abuse in women with disabilities.

No specific signs or symptoms are diagnostic of battering; however, nurses may see an injury that does not fit the account of how it happened (eg, a bruise on the side of the upper arm after "I walked into a door"). Manifestations of abuse may involve suicide attempts, drug and alcohol abuse, frequent emergency department visits, vague pelvic pain, somatic complaints, and depression. However, there may be no obvious signs or symptoms. Women in abusive situations often report that they do not feel well, possibly because of the stress of fear and anticipation of impending abuse.

The assessment for abuse by health professionals has lagged behind community awareness and response (Alpert, 2007). In addition to asking about domestic abuse, nurses need to provide resources and referral, as well as to follow written protocols of their institution or agency to ensure

Chart 46-3 • *Managing Reported Domestic Abuse*

1. Reassure the woman that she is not alone. *Rationale: Women often believe that they are alone in experiencing abuse at the hands of their partners.*
2. Express your belief that no one should be hurt, that abuse is the fault of the batterer and is against the law. *Rationale: Doing so lets the woman know that no one deserves to be abused and that she has not caused the abuse.*
3. Assure the woman that her information is confidential, although it does become part of her medical record. *If children are suspected of being abused or are being abused, the law requires that this be reported to the authorities.* Some states require reporting of spousal or partner abuse. Domestic violence agencies and medical and nursing groups disagree with this policy and are trying to have it changed. Serious opposition is based on the fact that reporting does not and cannot currently guarantee a woman's safety and may place her in more danger. It may also interfere with a patient's willingness to discuss her personal life and concerns with care providers. This places a serious barrier in the way of comprehensive nursing care. If nurses are in doubt about laws on reporting abuse, they need to check with their local or state domestic violence agency. *Rationale: Women are often afraid that their information will be reported to the police or protective services and their children may be taken away.*

4. Document the woman's statement of abuse and take photographs of any visible injuries if written formal consent has been obtained. (Emergency departments usually have a camera available if one is not on the nursing unit.) *Rationale: Doing so provides documentation of injuries that may be needed for later legal or criminal proceedings.*
5. Provide teaching. *Rationale: The following options may be life-saving for the woman and her children:*
   - Inform the woman that shelters are available to ensure safety for her and her children. (Lengths of stay in shelters vary by state but are often up to 2 months. Staff often assist with housing, jobs, and the emotional distress that accompanies the break-up of the family.) Provide list of shelters.
   - Inform the woman that violence gets worse, not better.
   - If the woman chooses to go to a shelter, let her make the call.
   - If the woman chooses to return to the abuser, remain nonjudgmental and provide information that will make her safer than she was before disclosing her situation.
   - Make sure that the woman has a 24-hour hotline telephone number that provides information and support (Spanish translation and a device for the deaf are also available), police number, and 911.
   - Assist her to set up a safety plan in case she decides to return home. (A safety plan is an organized plan for departure with packed bags and important papers hidden in a safe spot.)

---

comprehensive care (Furniss, McCaffrey, Parnell, et al., 2007).

Incest and Childhood Sexual Abuse

More than one in five women has experienced incest or childhood sexual abuse, and nurses frequently encounter women who have been sexually traumatized. It has been reported that female survivors of sexual abuse have more health problems and undergo more surgery than women

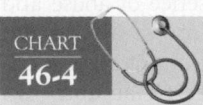

CHART 46-4

Screening for Abuse

Abuse Assessment Screen-Disability (AAS-D)

- Within the last year, have you been hit, slapped, kicked, pushed, shoved, or otherwise physically hurt by someone?
- Within the last year, has anyone forced you to have sexual activities?
- Within the last year, has anyone prevented you from using a wheelchair, cane, respiratory, or other assistive devices?
- Within the last year, has anyone you depend on refused to help you with an important personal need, such as taking your medicine, getting to the bathroom, getting out of bed, bathing, getting dressed, or getting food or drink?

Center for Research on Women with Disabilities. Abuse Assessment Screen-Disability. www.bcm.edu/crowd/?PMID=1325m

who were not victims of abuse. Victims of childhood sexual abuse are reported to experience more chronic depression, posttraumatic stress disorder, morbid obesity, marital instability, gastrointestinal problems, and headaches, as well as use health care services more frequently than people who were not victims. In women, chronic pelvic pain is often associated with physical violence, emotional neglect, and sexual abuse in childhood (McFarlane, Malecha, Watson, et al., 2005). Women who have experienced rape or sexual abuse may be very anxious about pelvic examinations, labor, pelvic or breast irradiation, or any treatment or examination that involves hands-on treatment or requires removal of clothing. Nurses should be prepared to offer support and referral to psychologists, community resources, and self-help groups.

Rape and Sexual Assault

Sexual assault occurs about every 2 minutes in the United States (U.S. Department of Justice, 2007). Men, women, and children may be victims. Many rapes occur on dates. Sexual assault nurse examiners, emergency department staff, and gynecologists perform the painstaking collection of forensic evidence that is needed for criminal prosecution. Oral, anal, and genital tissue is examined for evidence of trauma, semen, or infection. Saliva, hair, and fingernail evidence is also collected. Cultures are obtained for STDs, and prophylactic antibiotics are prescribed. The postexposure prophylaxis recommended by the Centers for Disease Control and Prevention (CDC) consists of ceftriaxone (Rocephin), metronidazole (Flagyl), and azithromycin (Zithromax) (CDC, 2006, 2007). The first injection of hepatitis B vaccine may also be given if the patient is not already immune, with subsequent doses given at 1 to 2 months and 4 to 6 months (CDC, 2006). HIV testing is offered and is repeated in 3 to 6 months. HIV prophylaxis is not universally recommended but is considered when mucosal exposure to contamination has occurred. Prophylaxis against chlamydia and gonorrhea is provided. Emergency contraception is explained and provided if requested and appropriate. Emotional counseling is provided, and follow-up treatment visits are arranged. Rape trauma syndrome is the emotional reaction to a sexual assault and may consist of shock, sleep disturbances, nightmares, flashbacks, anxiety, anger, mood swings, and depression. It is important and helpful for survivors to discuss the experience and to obtain professional counseling.

Screening for abuse, rape, and violence should be part of routine assessment because women often do not report or seek treatment for assault. Often, the assailant is a partner, husband, or date. Nurses may encounter women with infections or pregnancies related to sexual assault who require support, understanding, and comprehensive care.

Health Issues in Women With Disabilities

Approximately 20% of women have disabilities and encounter physical, architectural, and attitudinal barriers that may limit their full participation in society. Women with disabilities may experience stereotyping and increased risk of abuse. They have reported that others, including health care providers, often equate them with their disability. Studies have shown that women with disabilities receive less primary health care and preventive health screening than other women, often because of access problems and health care providers who focus on the causes of disability rather than on health issues that are of concern to all women (Smeltzer, 2006, 2007). To address these issues, the health history must include questions about barriers to health care encountered by women with disabilities and the effect of their disability on their health status and health care. Other issues to be addressed are identified in Chart 46-5. If a patient has hearing loss, vision loss, or another disability that affects communication, it may be necessary to obtain the assistance of an interpreter or to establish another method of communication. Nurses assessing women with disabilities may require additional time and the assistance of others to be certain that accurate information is obtained in a sensitive and unhurried manner (Smeltzer, 2007; Smeltzer & Sharts-Hopko, 2005). Women with disabilities may have had previous negative experiences with health care providers (Smeltzer, Sharts-Hopko, Ott, et al., 2007), and it is important that nurses provide them with knowledgeable and sensitive care. See Chapter 10 for further discussion of health care of patients with disabilities.

 Gerontologic Considerations

Care of older women with gynecologic concerns requires knowledge and understanding. Many older women are functioning at various levels across the health spectrum; some function at a high level in their jobs or families, whereas others may be very ill. Nurses need to be prepared to care for older women who may be bright, energetic, and ambitious or who are coping with multiple family crises,

---

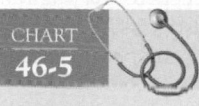

CHART 46-5 *Assessing a Woman With a Disability*

Health History

Address questions directly to the woman herself rather than to people accompanying her. Ask about:

- Self-care limitations resulting from her disability (ability to feed and dress self, use of assistive devices, transportation requirements, other assistance needed)
- Sensory limitations (lack of sensation, low vision, deaf or hard of hearing)
- Accessibility issues (ability to get to health care provider, transfer to examination table, accessibility of office/clinic of health care provider, previous experiences with health care providers, health screening practices; her understanding of physical examination)
- Cognitive or developmental changes that affect understanding
- Limitations secondary to disability that affect general health issues and reproductive health and health care
- Sexual function and concerns (those of all women and those that may be affected by the presence of a disabling condition)
- Menstrual history and menstrual hygiene practices
- Physical, sexual, or psychological abuse (including abuse by care providers; abuse by neglect, withholding or withdrawing assistive devices or personal or health care)

- Presence of secondary disabilities (ie, those resulting from the patient's primary disability: pressure ulcers, spasticity, osteoporosis, etc.)
- Health concerns related to aging with a disability

Physical Assessment

Provide instructions directly to the woman herself rather than to people accompanying her; provide written or audiotaped instructions.

Ask the woman what assistance she needs for the physical examination and provide assistance if needed:
  —Undressing and dressing
  —Providing a urine specimen
  —Standing on scale to be weighed (provide alternative means of obtaining weight if she is unable to stand on scale)
  —Moving on and off the examination table
  —Assuming, changing, and maintaining positions

Consider the fatigue experienced by the woman during a lengthy examination and allow rest.

Provide assistive devices and other aids/methods needed to allow adequate communication with the patient (interpreters, signers, large-print written materials).

Complete examination that would be indicated for any other woman; having a disability is *never* justification for omitting parts of the physical examination, including the pelvic examination.

including their own health issues as well as for those who are experiencing a life-altering or life-threatening health problem. Older women are at risk for several conditions, including diabetes, dyslipidemia, hypertension, and thyroid disease, all of which have symptoms that may be dismissed as typical aging. Nurses can help prevent morbidity and mortality from these conditions by encouraging women to obtain regular health screenings (Thakur & Supiano, 2007). In addition, knowledge related to heart disease prevention, pharmacology, diet, signs of dementia or cognitive decline, fall prevention, osteoporosis prevention, gynecologic and breast cancers, and sexuality are important for providing high-level nursing care. Health disparities, cultural competency, and end-of-life issues also need to be considered.

Physical Assessment

Periodic examinations and routine cancer screening are important for all women. Annual breast and pelvic examinations are important for all women 18 years of age or older and for those who are sexually active, regardless of age. Patients deserve understanding and support because of the emotional and physical considerations associated with gynecologic examinations. Women may be embarrassed by the usual questions asked by a gynecologist or women's health care provider. Because gynecologic conditions are of a personal and private nature to most women, such information is shared only with those directly involved in patient care (as is true with all patient information).

Throughout the examination, the nurse explains the procedures to be performed. This not only encourages the woman to relax but also provides an opportunity for her to ask questions and minimizes the negative feelings that many women associate with gynecologic examinations.

The first pelvic examination is often anxiety producing; the nurse can alleviate many of these feelings with explanations and teaching (Chart 46-6). It may be helpful to emphasize that a pelvic examination should not usually be un-

---

CHART 46-6

PATIENT EDUCATION
The Pelvic Examination

A pelvic examination includes assessment of the appearance of the vulva, vagina, and cervix and the size and shape of the uterus and ovaries to ensure reproductive health and absence of illness. The following should make the examination proceed more smoothly:

- You may have a feeling of fullness or pressure during the examination, but you should not feel pain. It is important to relax, because if you are very tense, you may feel discomfort.
- It is normal to feel uncomfortable and apprehensive.
- A narrow, warmed speculum will be inserted to visualize the cervix.
- A Papanicolaou (Pap) smear will be obtained and should not be uncomfortable.
- You may watch the examination with a mirror if you choose.
- The examination usually takes no longer than 5 minutes.
- Draping will be used to minimize exposure and reduce embarrassment.

---

comfortable. Before the examination begins, the patient is asked to empty her bladder and to provide a urine specimen if urine tests are part of the total assessment. Voiding ensures patient comfort and eases the examination because a full bladder can make palpation of pelvic organs uncomfortable for the patient and difficult for the examiner.

Positioning

Although several positions may be used for the pelvic examination, the supine lithotomy position is used most commonly, although the upright lithotomy position (in which the woman assumes a semisitting posture) may also be used. This position offers several advantages:

- It is more comfortable for some women.
- It allows better eye contact between patient and examiner.
- It may provide an easier means for the examiner to carry out the bimanual examination.
- It enables the woman to use a mirror to see her anatomy (if she chooses) to visualize any conditions that require treatment or to learn about using certain types of contraceptive methods.

In the supine lithotomy position, the patient lies on the table with her feet on foot rests or stirrups. She is encouraged to relax so that her buttocks are positioned at the edge of the examination table, and she is asked to relax and spread her thighs as widely apart as possible. If the patient is unable to lie safely on the examination table or unable to maintain the supine lithotomy position because of acute illness or disability, the Sims' position (or alternate positions) may be used. In Sims' position, the patient lies on her left side with her right leg bent at a 90-degree angle. The right labia may be retracted to gain adequate access to the vagina. The presence of a disability does not justify skipping any parts of the physical assessment, including the pelvic examination.

The following equipment is obtained and readily available: a good light source; a vaginal speculum; clean examination gloves; lubricant, spatula, cytobrush, glass slides, fixative solution or spray; and diagnostic testing supplies for screening for occult rectal blood if the woman is older than 40 years of age. Latex-free gloves should be available if the patient or clinician is allergic to latex. This allergy is becoming more prevalent in nurses and other health care providers and patients and is potentially life-threatening. Patients should be questioned about previous reactions to latex. (See Chapter 18 for a latex screening form and Chapter 53 for more information on latex allergy.)

Inspection

After the patient is prepared, the examiner inspects the labia majora and minora, noting the epidermal tissue of the labia majora; the skin fades to the pink mucous membrane of the vaginal introitus. Lesions of any type (eg, venereal warts, pigmented lesions [melanoma]) are evaluated. In the nulliparous woman, the labia minora come together at the opening of the vagina. In a woman who has delivered children vaginally, the labia minora may gape and vaginal tissue may protrude.

Trauma to the anterior vaginal wall during childbirth may have resulted in incompetency of the musculature, and a bulge caused by the bladder protruding into the submucosa of the anterior vaginal wall **(cystocele)** may be seen. Childbirth trauma may also have affected the posterior vaginal wall, producing a bulge caused by rectal cavity protrusion **(rectocele).** The cervix may descend under pressure through the vaginal canal and be seen at the introitus **(uterine prolapse).** See Chapter 47 for a discussion of these structural changes. To identify such protrusions, the examiner asks the patient to "bear down."

The introitus should be free of superficial mucosal lesions. The labia minora may be separated by the fingers of the gloved hand and the lower part of the vagina palpated. In women who have not had vaginal intercourse, a **hymen** of variable thickness may be felt circumferentially within the vaginal opening. The hymenal ring usually permits the insertion of one finger. Rarely, the hymen totally occludes the vaginal entrance **(imperforate hymen).**

In women who have had intercourse, a rim of scar tissue representing the remnants of the hymenal ring may be palpated circumferentially around the vagina near its opening. The greater vestibular glands (Bartholin's glands) lie between the labia minora and the remnants of the hymenal ring. An abscess of the Bartholin's gland can cause discomfort and requires incision and drainage.

Speculum Examination

The bivalved speculum, either metal or plastic, is available in many sizes. Metal specula are soaked, scrubbed, and sterilized between patients. Some clinicians and some patients prefer plastic specula, which permit one-time use. The speculum can be warmed with a heating pad or warm water to make insertion more comfortable for the patient. The speculum is not usually lubricated because commercial lubricants may interfere with cervical cytology (Papanicolaou [Pap] smear) findings.

The speculum is gently inserted into the posterior portion of the introitus and slowly advanced to the top of the vagina; this should not be painful or uncomfortable for the woman. The speculum is then slowly opened and the setscrew of the thumb rest is tightened to hold the speculum open (Fig. 46-4).

Inspecting the Cervix

The cervix is inspected. In nulliparous women, the cervix usually is 2 to 3 cm wide and smooth. In women who have borne children, the cervix may have a laceration, usually transverse, giving the cervical os a "fishmouth" appearance. Epithelium from the endocervical canal may have grown onto the surface of the cervix, appearing as beefy-red surface

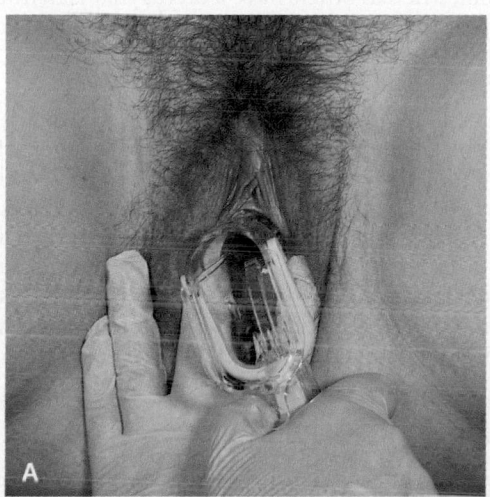

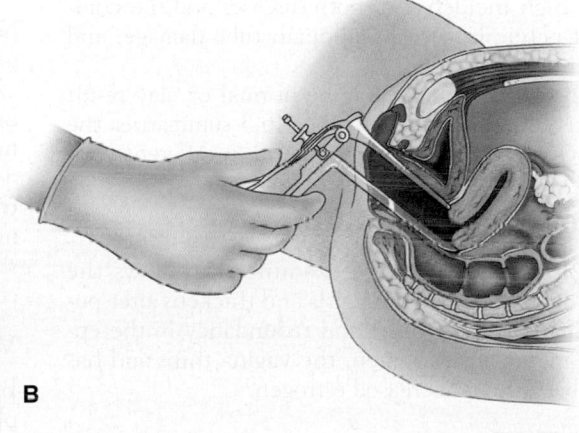

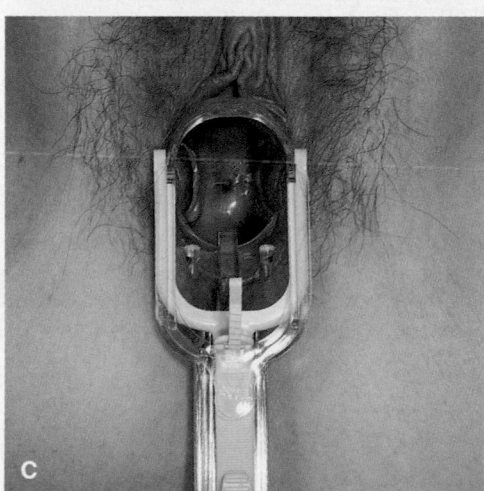

Figure 46-4 Technique for speculum examination of the vagina and cervix. **A,** The labia are spread apart with a gloved left hand, while the speculum is grasped in the right hand and turned counterclockwise before being inserted into the vagina. Once the speculum is inserted, the blades are then spread apart (**B**) to reveal the cervical os (**C**).

epithelium circumferentially around the os. Occasionally, the cervix of a woman whose mother took DES during pregnancy has a hooded appearance (a peaked aspect superiorly or a ridge of tissue surrounding it); this is evaluated by colposcopy when identified.

Malignant changes may not be obviously differentiated from the rest of the cervical mucosa. Small, benign cysts may appear on the cervical surface. These are usually bluish or white and are called nabothian cysts. A **polyp** of endocervical mucosa may protrude through the os and usually is dark red. Polyps can cause irregular bleeding; they are rarely malignant and usually are removed easily in an office or clinic setting. A carcinoma may appear as a cauliflower-like growth that bleeds easily when touched. Bluish coloration of the cervix is a sign of early pregnancy (Chadwick's sign).

Obtaining Pap Smears and Other Samples

A Pap smear is obtained by rotating a small spatula at the os, followed by a cervical brush rotated in the os. The material obtained is spread on a glass slide and sprayed/fixed immediately, or inserted into liquid (thin "prep"). A small broomlike device can also be used to obtain specimens for the Pap smear.

A specimen of any purulent material appearing at the cervical os is obtained for culture. A sterile applicator is used to obtain the specimen, which is immediately placed in an appropriate medium for transfer to a laboratory. In a patient who has a high risk of infection, routine cultures for gonococcal and chlamydial organisms are recommended because of the high incidence of both diseases and the complications of pelvic infection, fallopian tube damage, and subsequent infertility.

Vaginal discharge, which may be normal or may result from vaginitis, may be present. Table 46-3 summarizes the characteristics of vaginal discharge found in different conditions.

Inspecting the Vagina

The vagina is inspected as the examiner withdraws the speculum. It is smooth in young girls and thickens after puberty, with many rugae (folds) and redundancy in the epithelium. In menopausal women, the vagina thins and has fewer rugae because of decreased estrogen.

Bimanual Palpation

To complete the pelvic examination, the examiner performs a bimanual examination, usually from a standing position. The fingers are advanced vertically along the vaginal canal, and the vaginal wall is palpated. Any firm part of the vaginal wall may represent old scar tissue from childbirth trauma but may also require further evaluation.

Cervical Palpation

The cervix is palpated and assessed for its consistency, mobility, size, and position. The normal cervix is uniformly firm but not hard. Softening of the cervix is a finding in early pregnancy. Hardness and immobility of the cervix may reflect invasion by a neoplasm. Pain on gentle movement of the cervix is called a positive **chandelier sign** or positive cervical motion tenderness (recorded as +CMT) and usually indicates a pelvic infection.

Uterine Palpation

To palpate the uterus, the examiner places the opposite hand on the abdominal wall halfway between the umbilicus and the pubis and presses firmly toward the vagina. Movement of the abdominal wall causes the body of the uterus to descend, and the organ becomes freely movable between the hand used to examine the abdomen and the fingers of the hand used to examine the pelvis. Uterine size, mobility, and contour can be estimated through palpation. Fixation of the uterus in the pelvis may be a sign of **endometriosis** or malignancy.

The body of the uterus is normally twice the diameter and twice the length of the cervix, curving anteriorly toward the abdominal wall. Some women have a retroverted or retroflexed uterus, which tips posteriorly toward the sacrum, whereas others have a uterus that is neither anterior nor posterior and is described as midline.

Adnexal Palpation

Next, the right and left adnexal areas are palpated to evaluate the fallopian tubes and ovaries. The fingers of the hand examining the pelvis are moved first to one side, then to the other, while the hand palpating the abdominal area is moved correspondingly to either side of the abdomen and downward. The adnexa (ovaries and fallopian tubes) are trapped between the two hands and palpated for an obvious mass, tenderness, and mobility. Commonly, the ovaries are slightly tender, and the patient is informed that slight discomfort on palpation is normal.

Vaginal and Rectal Palpation

Bimanual palpation of the vagina and cul-de-sac is accomplished by placing the index finger in the vagina and the middle finger in the rectum. To prevent cross-contamination between the vaginal and rectal orifices, the examiner puts on new gloves. A gentle movement of these fingers toward each other compresses the posterior vaginal wall and the anterior rectal wall and assists the examiner in identifying the integrity of these structures. During this procedure, the patient may sense an urge to defecate. The nurse assures the

Table 46-3	CHARACTERISTICS OF VAGINAL DISCHARGE		
Cause of Discharge	**Symptoms**	**Odor**	**Consistency/Color**
Physiologic	None	None	Mucus/white
Candida species infection	Itching, irritation	Yeast odor or none	Thin to thick, curdlike/white
Bacterial vaginosis	Odor	Fishy, often noticed after intercourse	Thin/grayish or yellow
Trichomonas species infection	Irritation, odor	Malodorous	Copious, often frothy/yellow-green
Atrophic	Vulvar or vaginal dryness	Occasional mild malodor	Usually scant and mucoid/may be blood-tinged

patient that this is unlikely to occur. Ongoing explanations are provided to reassure and educate the patient about the procedure.

 Gerontologic Considerations

Yearly examinations are important; they identify problems of the reproductive tract in aging women early. Some older women do not have regular gynecologic examinations. For example, a woman who delivered her children at home may never have had a pelvic examination. Some women regard it as an embarrassing and unpleasant procedure. Nurses play an important role; they can encourage all women to have an annual gynecologic examination. Nurses can make the examination a time for education and reassurance rather than a time of embarrassment.

Perineal pruritus is abnormal in elderly women and should be evaluated because it may indicate a disease process (diabetes or malignancy). Vulvar dystrophy, a thickened or whitish discoloration of tissue, may be visible, and biopsy is needed to rule out abnormal cells. Topical cortisone and hormone creams may be prescribed for symptomatic relief.

With relaxing pelvic musculature, uterine prolapse and relaxation of the vaginal walls can occur. Appropriate evaluation and surgical repair can provide relief if the patient is a candidate for surgery. After surgery, the patient should know that tissue repair and healing may require more time with aging. Pessaries (latex devices that provide support) are often used if surgery is contraindicated or before surgery to see if surgery can be avoided. They are fitted by a health care provider and may reduce discomfort and pressure. Use of a pessary requires the patient to have routine gynecologic examinations to monitor for irritation or infection. The patient must be assessed for allergy prior to insertion of a latex pessary (see Chapter 47 for details about pessaries).

Diagnostic Evaluation

Cytologic Test for Cancer (Pap Smear)

The Pap smear is used to detect cervical cancer. Cervical secretions are gently removed from the cervical os and may be transferred to a glass slide and fixed immediately by spraying with a fixative or immersed in solution (Fig. 46-5). If the Pap smear reveals atypical cells, the liquid method allows for human papillomavirus (HPV) testing (see Chapter 47 for further discussion of HPV, a commonly transmitted STD that can cause venereal warts or cervical cancer). HPV DNA testing is helpful in that it can detect high-risk types that may require careful monitoring. HPV infection is often temporary, especially in healthy young women.

The proper technique for obtaining a cervical specimen for cytologic study is described in Chart 46-7. A Pap smear should be performed when a patient is not menstruating, because blood usually interferes with interpretation. To avoid washing away cellular material, the patient should be instructed not to douche before having a Pap smear taken.

Terminology used to describe findings includes the following categories:

- Normal
- Atypical squamous cells of undetermined significance (ASCUS), either HPV + or –
- Low-grade squamous intraepithelial lesion (LSIL), which is equivalent to cervical intraepithelial neoplasia (CIN; grade 1) and to mild changes related to exposure to HPV
- High-grade squamous intraepithelial lesion (HGSIL), which equates to moderate and severe dysplasia, carcinoma in situ (CIS), as well as CIN grade 2 and CIN grade 3

The terms in the last category are precursors to invasive carcinoma of the cervix that indicate the need for evaluation and treatment.

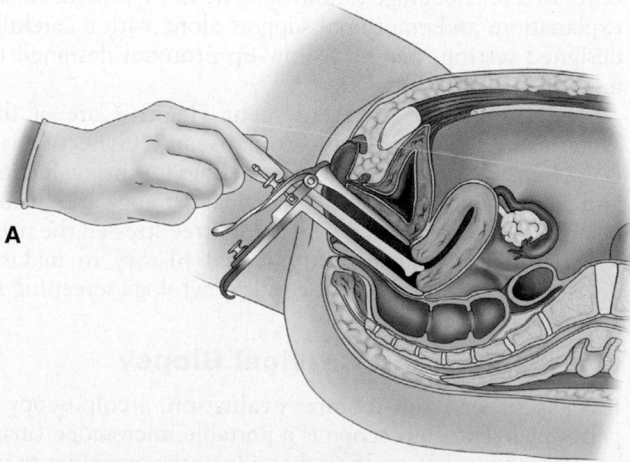
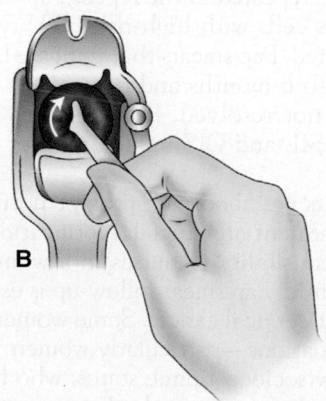
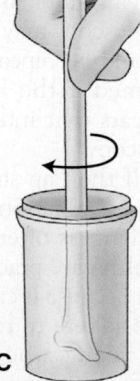

Figure 46-5 Method of using an Ayre spatula to obtain cervical secretions for cytology. **A,** Speculum in place and the Ayre spatula in position at the cervical os. **B,** The tip of the spatula is placed in the cervical os and the spatula rotated 360 degrees, firmly but non-traumatically. **C,** Instead of the cells being smeared on a slide, the sampling device is rinsed or twirled in the small vial containing the transport medium and sent to the laboratory.

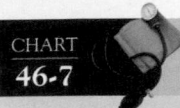

CHART 46-7 Guidelines for Obtaining an Optimal Pap Smear

Equipment Needed

- Speculum
- Gloves
- Slide, spatula, and cytobrush or thin prep kit

Implementation

Nursing Action	Rationale
1. Do not obtain a Pap smear if the woman is menstruating or has other frank bleeding (exception: high suspicion of neoplasia).	1. Blood obscures a proper reading of cells.
2. If performing more than one test (eg, Pap and GC), obtain the Pap smear first.	2. By performing the Pap smear first, the chance of a bloody smear is avoided.
3. Label the frosted end of the slide with the patient's name in pencil or label Thin-prep Pap bottle.	3. Ink may rub off or blur. Labeling with a pencil prevents improper identification.
4. Put on gloves before gently inserting the unlubricated speculum. (Speculum may be moistened with warm water.)	4. Gloves provide protection and warm water prevents discomfort. Lubricants may obscure cells on Pap smear.
5. Place the longer end of the Ayre spatula in the cervical canal and rotate it in a full circle to obtain a sample from the exocervix. Spread the material obtained onto the Pap smear slide.	5. This technique obtains a sampling of the exocervix and squamocolumnar junction.
6. Insert a cytobrush 2 cm into the cervical canal and rotate 180 degrees. Roll the brush onto the Pap smear slide. (With Thin-prep Pap smears, the brushings are not spread onto a slide. The spatula and brush are placed in a bottle of fixative and swirled.)	6. This technique obtains a sampling of the endocervical cells and may sample cells from the squamocolumnar junction if it is high in the canal.
7. In women who have had a hysterectomy for a gynecological cancer, use a cotton applicator moistened with saline solution to obtain a sampling of cells from the vaginal cuff or posterior vagina. Women who have had a hysterectomy for benign conditions do not require frequent Pap smears.	7. Saline solution prevents drying, which makes interpretation difficult for the cytologist and prevents absorption of cells into the cotton, increasing the yield on the slide.
8. Immediately spray the slide or, if a Thin-prep, swirl the brush and spatula in the solution.	8. Exposure to light or air causes distortion of cells.

The patient may incorrectly assume that an abnormal Pap smear signifies cancer. If the Pap smear (liquid immersion method) shows atypical cells and no high-risk HPV types, the next Pap smear is performed in 1 year. If a specific infection is causing inflammation, it is treated appropriately, and the Pap smear is repeated. If the repeat Pap smear reveals atypical squamous cells with high-risk HPV types, colposcopy may be indicated. Pap smears that indicate LSIL should be repeated in 4 to 6 months and colposcopy performed if the LSIL has not resolved. Patients with Pap smears that indicate HGSIL and CIS require prompt colposcopy.

If the Pap smear results are abnormal, prompt notification, evaluation, and treatment are crucial. Notification of patients is often the responsibility of nurses in a women's health care practice or clinic. Pap smear follow-up is essential because it can prevent cervical cancer. Some women do not adhere to recommendations—particularly women who are young, who are of low socioeconomic status, who have difficulty coping with the diagnosis, or who have no social support. Fear, lack of understanding, and child care responsibilities have all been identified by women as reasons for poor follow-up. Women with a history of abuse, obese women, and women who have had a negative gynecologic experience may also find returning for follow-up difficult. Interventions are tailored to meet the needs of the particular patient. Intensive telephone counseling, tracking systems, brochures, videos, and financial incentives have all been used to encourage follow-up. The nurse provides clear explanations and emotional support along with a carefully designed setting-specific follow-up protocol designed to meet the needs of the patient.

The Committee on Adolescent Health Care of the American College of Obstetricians and Gynecologists (ACOG, 2006b) issued a set of guidelines for the evaluation and management of abnormal cervical cytology and histology in adolescent females. The committee stressed the need for a complete and accurate sexual history in making decisions about initiation of cervical cytology screening in adolescents.

Colposcopy and Cervical Biopsy

If a Pap smear result requires evaluation, a colposcopy is performed. The colposcope is a portable microscope (magnification from 10X to 25X) that allows the examiner to visualize the cervix and obtain a sample of abnormal tissue for analysis. Nurse practitioners and gynecologists require special training in this diagnostic technique.

After inserting a speculum and visualizing the cervix and vaginal walls, the examiner applies acetic acid to the cervix. Subsequent abnormal findings that indicate the need for biopsy include leukoplakia (white plaque visible before applying acetic acid), acetowhite tissue (white epithelium after applying acetic acid), punctation (dilated capillaries occurring in a dotted or stippled pattern), mosaicism (a tilelike pattern), and atypical vascular patterns. If biopsy specimens show premalignant cells or CIN, the patient usually requires cryotherapy, laser therapy, or a cone biopsy (excision of an inverted tissue cone from the cervix).

Cryotherapy and Laser Therapy

Cryotherapy (freezing cervical tissue with nitrous oxide) and laser treatment are used in the outpatient setting. Cryotherapy may result in cramping and occasional feelings of faintness (vasovagal response). A watery discharge is normal for a few weeks after the procedure as the cervix heals.

Cone Biopsy and Loop Electrosurgical Excision Procedure

If endocervical curettage findings indicate abnormal changes or if the lesion extends into the canal, the patient may undergo a cone biopsy. This can be performed surgically or with a procedure called loop electrosurgical excision procedure (LEEP), which uses a laser beam.

Usually performed in the outpatient setting, LEEP is associated with a high success rate in removal of abnormal cervical tissue. The gynecologist excises a small amount of cervical tissue, and the pathologist examines the borders of the specimen to determine if disease is present. A patient who has received anesthesia for a surgical cone biopsy is advised to rest for 24 hours after the procedure and to leave any vaginal packing in place until it is removed (usually the next day). The patient is instructed to report any excessive bleeding.

The nurse or physician provides guidelines regarding postoperative sexual activity, bathing, and other activities. Because open tissue may be potentially exposed to HIV and other pathogens, the patient is cautioned to avoid intercourse until healing is complete and verified at follow-up. LEEP has a low incidence of complications, but there is a slight increase in the risk of later cervical stenosis or premature deliveries.

Endometrial (Aspiration) Biopsy

Endometrial biopsy, a method of obtaining endometrial tissue, is performed as an outpatient procedure. This procedure is usually indicated in cases of midlife irregular bleeding, postmenopausal bleeding, and irregular bleeding while taking hormone therapy or tamoxifen. A tissue sample obtained through biopsy permits diagnosis of cellular changes in the endometrium.

Women who undergo endometrial biopsy may experience slight discomfort. The examiner may apply a tenaculum (a clamplike instrument that stabilizes the uterus) after the pelvic examination and then inserts a thin, hollow, flexible suction tube (Pipelle or sampler) through the cervix into the uterus.

Findings on aspiration may include normal endometrial tissue, hyperplasia, or endometrial cancer. Simple hyperplasia is an overgrowth of the uterine lining and is usually treated with progesterone. Complex hyperplasia, which refers to overgrowth of cells with abnormal features, is a risk factor for uterine cancer and is treated with progesterone and careful follow-up. Women who are overweight, who are older than 45 years of age, who have a history of nulliparity and infertility, or who have a family history of colon cancer seem to be at higher risk for hyperplasia. Endometrial cancer is discussed in Chapter 47.

Dilation and Curettage

Dilation and curettage (D & C) may be diagnostic (identifies the cause of irregular bleeding) or therapeutic (often temporarily stops irregular bleeding). The cervical canal is widened with a dilator, and the uterine endometrium is scraped with a curette. The purpose of the procedure is to secure endometrial or endocervical tissue for cytologic examination, to control abnormal uterine bleeding, and as a therapeutic measure for incomplete abortion.

Because D & C is usually carried out under anesthesia and requires surgical asepsis, it is usually performed in the operating room. However, it may take place in the outpatient setting with the patient receiving a local anesthetic supplemented with diazepam (Valium) or midazolam (Versed).

The nurse explains the procedure, preparation, and expectations regarding postoperative discomfort and bleeding. The patient is instructed to void before the procedure. The patient is placed in the lithotomy position, the cervix is dilated with a dilating instrument, and endometrial scrapings are obtained by a curette. A perineal pad is placed over the perineum after the procedure, and excessive bleeding is reported. No restrictions are placed on dietary intake. If pelvic discomfort or low back pain occurs, mild analgesics usually provide relief. The physician indicates when sexual intercourse may be safely resumed. To reduce the risk of infection and bleeding, most physicians advise no vaginal penetration or use of tampons for 2 weeks.

Endoscopic Examinations

Laparoscopy (Pelvic Peritoneoscopy)

A laparoscopy involves inserting a laparoscope (a tube about 10 mm wide and similar to a small periscope) into the peritoneal cavity through a 2-cm (0.75-in) incision below the umbilicus to allow visualization of the pelvic structures (Fig. 46-6). Laparoscopy may be used for diagnostic purposes (eg, in cases of pelvic pain when no cause can be found) or treatment. Laparoscopy facilitates many surgical procedures, such as tubal ligation, ovarian biopsy, myomectomy, hysterectomy, and lysis of adhesions (scar tissue that can cause pelvic discomfort). A surgical instrument (intrauterine sound or cannula) may be positioned inside the uterus to permit manipulation or movement during laparoscopy, affording better visualization. The pelvic organs can be visualized after the injection of carbon dioxide intraperitoneally into the cavity. Called insufflation, this technique separates the intestines from the pelvic organs. If a patient is undergoing sterilization, the fallopian or uterine tubes may be electrocoagulated, sutured, or ligated and a segment removed for histologic verification (clips are an alternative device for occluding the tubes).

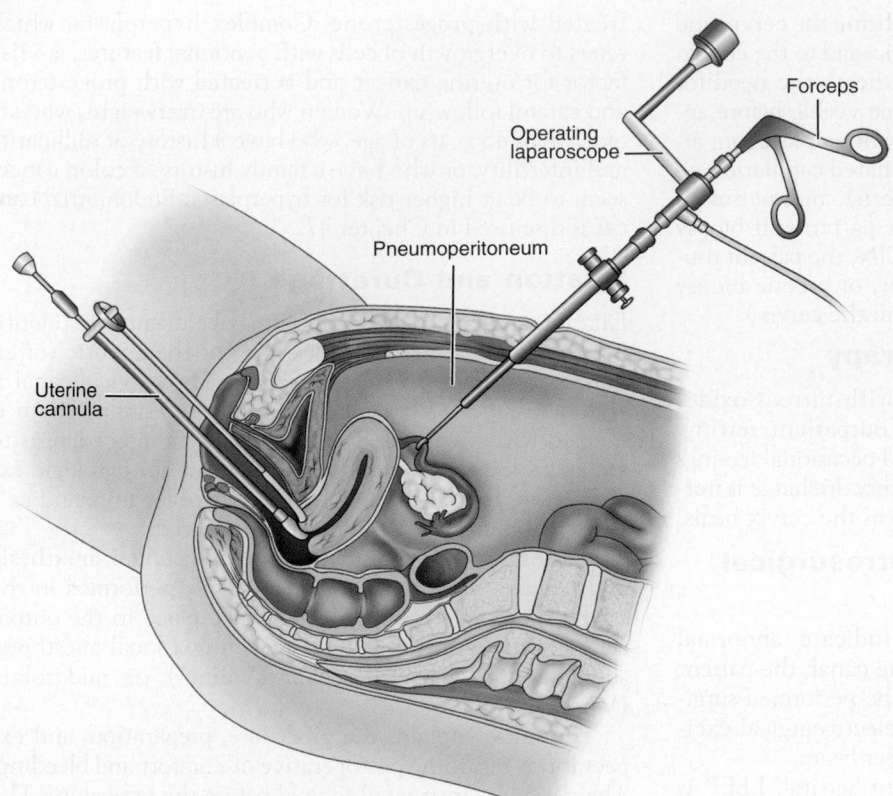

Operating
laparoscope

Forceps

Pneumoperitoneum

Uterine
cannula

Figure 46-6 Laparoscopy. The laparoscope (*right*) is inserted through a small incision in the abdomen. A forceps is inserted through the scope to grasp the fallopian tube. To improve the view, a uterine cannula (*left*) is inserted into the vagina to push the uterus upward. Insufflation of gas creates an air pocket (pneumoperitoneum), and the pelvis is elevated (note the angle), which forces the intestines higher in the abdomen.

After the laparoscopy is completed, the laparoscope is withdrawn, carbon dioxide is allowed to escape through the outer cannula, the small skin incision is closed with sutures or a clip, and the incision is covered with an adhesive bandage. The patient is carefully monitored for several hours to detect any untoward signs indicating bleeding (most commonly from vascular injury to the hypogastric vessels), bowel or bladder injury, or burns from the coagulator. These complications are rare, making laparoscopy a cost-effective and safe short-stay procedure. The patient may experience abdominal or shoulder pain related to the use of carbon dioxide gas.

Hysteroscopy

Hysteroscopy (transcervical intrauterine endoscopy) allows direct visualization of all parts of the uterine cavity by means of a lighted optical instrument. The procedure is best performed about 5 days after menstruation ceases, in the estrogenic phase of the menstrual cycle. The vagina and vulva are cleansed, and a paracervical anesthetic block is performed or lidocaine spray is used. The instrument used for the procedure, a hysteroscope, is passed into the cervical canal and advanced 1 or 2 cm under direct vision. Uterine-distending fluid (normal saline solution or 5% dextrose in water) is infused through the instrument to dilate the uterine cavity and enhance visibility. Hysteroscopy, which has few complications, is useful for evaluating endometrial pathology.

Hysteroscopy may be indicated as an adjunct to a D & C and laparoscopy in cases of infertility, unexplained bleeding, retained intrauterine device (IUD), and recurrent early pregnancy loss. Treatment for some conditions (eg, fibroid

tumors) can be accomplished during this procedure, and sterilization may also be performed. Hysteroscopy is contraindicated in patients with cervical or endometrial carcinoma or acute pelvic inflammation.

Endometrial ablation (destruction of the uterine lining) is performed with a hysteroscope and resector (cutting loop), roller ball (a barrel-shaped electrode), or laser beam in cases of severe bleeding not responsive to other therapies. Performed in an outpatient setting under general, regional, or local anesthesia, this rapid procedure is an alternative to hysterectomy for some patients. Following uterine distension with fluid infusion, the lining of the uterus is destroyed. Hemorrhage, perforation, and burns can occur.

Other Diagnostic Procedures

Many diagnostic procedures are helpful in evaluating pelvic conditions. These may include x-rays, barium enemas, gastrointestinal x-ray series, intravenous urography, and cystography studies. In addition, because the uterus, ovaries, and fallopian tubes are near the structures of the urinary tract, urologic diagnostic studies, such as x-ray study of the kidney, ureters, and bladder (KUB) and pyelography are used, as are angiography and radioisotope scanning, if needed. Other diagnostic procedures include hysterosalpingography and computed tomography (CT) scanning.

Hysterosalpingography or Uterotubography

Hysterosalpingography (HSG) is an x-ray study of the uterus and the fallopian tubes after injection of a contrast agent. The diagnostic procedure is performed to evaluate infertility or tubal patency and to detect any abnormal condition in the uterine cavity. Sometimes the procedure is therapeutic because the flowing contrast agent flushes debris or loosens adhesions.

Prior to hysterosalpingography, laxatives and an enema may be administered to evacuate the intestinal tract so that gas shadows do not distort the x-ray findings. A mild sedative or an analgesic agent, such as ibuprofen (Advil, Motrin) may be prescribed. The patient is placed in the lithotomy position and the cervix is exposed with a bivalved speculum. A cannula is inserted into the cervix and the contrast agent is injected into the uterine cavity and the fallopian tubes. X-rays are taken to show the path and the distribution of the contrast agent.

Some patients experience nausea, vomiting, cramps, and faintness. After the test, the patient is advised to wear a perineal pad for several hours, because the radiopaque contrast agent may stain clothing.

Computed Tomography

CT has several advantages over ultrasonography (described below), even though it involves radiation exposure and is more costly. It is more effective than ultrasonography for obese patients or for patients with a distended bowel. CT can also demonstrate a tumor and any extension into the retroperitoneal lymph nodes and skeletal tissue, although it has limited value in diagnosing other gynecologic abnormalities.

Ultrasonography

Ultrasonography (or ultrasound) is a useful adjunct to the physical examination, particularly in obstetric patients or in patients with abnormal pelvic examination findings. It is a simple procedure based on sound wave transmission that uses pulsed ultrasonic waves at frequencies exceeding 20,000 Hz (formerly cycles per second) by way of a transducer placed in contact with the abdomen (abdominal scan) or a vaginal probe (vaginal ultrasound). Mechanical energy is converted into electrical impulses, which in turn are amplified and recorded on an oscilloscope screen while a photograph or video recording of the patterns is taken. The entire procedure takes usually less than 10 minutes and involves no ionizing radiation and no discomfort other than a full bladder, which is necessary for good visualization during an abdominal scan. (A vaginal ultrasound or sonogram does not require a full bladder; however, the vaginal probe can cause mild discomfort in some women.) Saline may be instilled into the uterus (saline infusion sonogram) to help delineate endometrial polyps or fibroids.

Magnetic Resonance Imaging

Magnetic resonance imaging (MRI) produces patterns that are finer and more definitive than other imaging procedures, and it does not expose patients to radiation. However, MRI is more costly.

> ◥ **NURSING ALERT**
>
> All metal devices, including medication skin patches with foil backing, must be removed before MRI is performed to avoid burns.

MANAGEMENT OF FEMALE PHYSIOLOGIC PROCESSES

Many health concerns of women are related to normal changes or abnormalities of the menstrual cycle and may result from women's lack of understanding of the menstrual cycle, developmental changes, and factors that may affect the pattern of the menstrual cycle. Educating women about the menstrual cycle and changes over time is an important aspect of the nurse's role in providing quality care to women. Teaching should begin early, so that menstruation and the lifelong changes in the menstrual cycle can be anticipated and accepted as a normal part of life.

Menstruation

Menstruation, a cyclic vaginal flow of tissue that lines the uterus, occurs about every 28 days during the reproductive years, although normal cycles can vary from 21 to 42 days. The flow usually lasts 4 to 5 days, during which time 50 to 60 mL (4 to 12 tsp) of blood are lost.

A perineal pad or tampon is generally used to absorb menstrual discharge. Tampons are used extensively. There is no significant evidence of untoward effects from their use, provided that there is no difficulty in inserting them. However, tampons should not be used for more than 4 to 6 hours, and superabsorbent tampons should not be used because of their association with toxic shock syndrome. If a tampon is difficult to remove or shreds when removed, less absorbent tampons should be used. If the string breaks or retracts, the woman should squat in a comfortable position, insert one finger into the vagina, try to locate the tampon, and remove it. If she feels uncomfortable attempting this maneuver or cannot remove the tampon, she should consult a gynecologic health care provider promptly.

Psychosocial Considerations

Girls who are approaching menarche (the onset of menstruation) should be instructed about the normal process of the menstrual cycle before it occurs. Psychologically, it is much healthier and appropriate to refer to this event as a "period" rather than as "being sick." With adequate nutrition, rest, and exercise, most women feel little discomfort, although some report breast tenderness and a feeling of fullness 1 or 2 days before menstruation begins. Others report fatigue and some discomfort in the lower back, legs, and pelvis on the first day and temperament or mood changes. Slight deviations from a usual pattern of daily living are considered normal, but excessive deviation may require evaluation. Regular exercise and a healthy diet have been found to decrease discomfort for some women. Heating pads or nonsteroidal anti-inflammatory drugs (NSAIDs) may be very effective for cramps. For women with excessive cramping or dysmenorrhea, referral to a women's health care provider is appropriate; following evaluation, practitioners may prescribe oral contraceptives.

Cultural Considerations

Culture refers to knowledge, beliefs, customs, and values acquired as members of a racial, ethnic, religious, or social group. The United States is becoming more culturally diverse. Various aspects of culture affect many health care encounters, and these encounters can be positive if nurses understand the various cultures of their patients.

Cultural views and beliefs about menstruation differ. Some women believe that it is detrimental to change a pad or tampon too frequently; they think that allowing the discharge to accumulate increases the flow, which is considered desirable. Some women believe they are vulnerable to illness during menstruation. Others believe it is harmful to swim, shower, have their hair permed, have their teeth filled, or eat certain foods during menstruation. They may also avoid using contraception during menstruation.

In such situations, nurses are in a position to provide women with facts in an accepting and culturally sensitive manner. The objective is to be mindful of these unexpressed, deep-rooted beliefs and to provide the facts with care. Aspects of gynecologic problems cannot always be expressed easily. The nurse needs to convey confidence and openness and to offer facts to facilitate communication. Suggestions to improve care include overcoming language barriers, providing appropriate materials in the patient's language, asking about traditional beliefs and dietary practices, and asking about fears regarding care. Patience, sensitivity, and a desire to learn about other cultures and groups will enhance the nursing care of all women (Chart 46-8).

Perimenopause

Perimenopause is the period extending from the first signs of menopause—usually hot flashes, vaginal dryness, or irregular menses—to beyond the complete cessation of menses. It has also been defined as the period around menopause, lasting to 1 year after the last menstrual period. Women often have varied beliefs about aging, and these must be considered when caring for or educating perimenopausal patients.

Nursing Management

Perimenopausal women often benefit from information about the subtle physiologic changes they are experiencing.

Perimenopause has been described as an opportune time for teaching women about health promotion and disease prevention strategies. When discussing health-related concerns with midlife women, nurses should consider the following issues:

- Sexuality, fertility, contraception, and STDs
- Unintended pregnancy (if contraception is not used correctly and consistently)
- Oral contraceptive use. Oral contraceptives provide perimenopausal women with protection against uterine cancer, ovarian cancer, anemia, pregnancy, and fibrocystic breast changes as well as relief from perimenopausal symptoms. This option should be discussed with perimenopausal women. (Women who smoke and are 35 years of age or older should not take oral contraceptives because of an increased risk of cardiovascular disease.) Contraception is discussed in detail later in this chapter.
- Breast health. About 16% of cases of breast cancer occur in perimenopausal women, so breast self-examination, routine physical examinations, and mammograms are essential.

Women in their 40s are often less concerned with menopause and more interested in their health, well-being, and appearance. They view taking care of themselves as one way to look and feel younger (Beyene, Gilliss & Lee, 2007).

Menopause

Menopause is the permanent physiologic cessation of menses associated with declining ovarian function; during this time, reproductive function diminishes and ends. Postmenopause is the period beginning from about 1 year after menses cease. Menopause may be associated with some atrophy of breast tissue and genital organs, loss in bone density, and vascular changes.

Menopause starts gradually and is usually signaled by changes in menstruation. The monthly flow may increase or

---

Chart 46-8 • *Health Care for Women Who Are Lesbians*

Lesbians can generally be defined as women who have sex with or primary emotional partnerships with women, but there is no universally accepted definition; variability exists in relationships and sexual preferences. Lesbians are found in every ethnic group and socioeconomic class. They can be single, celibate, divorced, and are seen in all age groups, including teens and seniors. Most experts believe that sexual orientation is not a conscious choice.

Lesbians have often encountered insensitivity in health care encounters. When they are asked if they are sexually active and respond affirmatively, contraception is immediately urged as health care providers may assume incorrectly that they practice heterosexual intercourse. Similar to many other marginalized groups of women, they often feel invisible and underuse health care. Whether heterosexual or homosexual, nurses need to consider lesbianism within the continuum of human sexual behavior and need to use gender-neutral questions and terms that are nonjudgmental

and accepting. Lesbian teens are at risk for suicide and STDs. Many lesbians do participate in heterosexual activity and often consider themselves at low risk for STDs. Because HPV, herpes infections, and other organisms implicated in STDs are transmitted by secretions and contact, they may need information on STDs and contraception. If sex toys are used and not cleaned, pelvic infections can occur.

Lesbians have lower health screening rates than other women. They are at high risk for cancer, heart disease, depression, and alcohol abuse. They may have a higher body mass index, may bear fewer or no children, and often have fewer health preventive screenings than heterosexual women. These factors may increase the risk of colon, endometrial, ovarian, and breast cancer, as well as cardiovascular disease and diabetes. Adolescent lesbians are at risk for smoking and suicide/depression. Nurses need to understand the unique needs of this population and provide appropriate and sensitive care (Roberts, 2006).

decrease, become irregular, and finally cease. Often, the interval between periods is longer; a lapse of several months between periods is not uncommon. Changes signaling menopause begin to occur as early as the late 30s, when ovulation occurs less frequently, estrogen levels fluctuate, and FSH levels increase in an attempt to stimulate estrogen production.

Clinical Manifestations

Because of these hormonal changes, some women notice irregular menses, breast tenderness, and mood changes long before menopause occurs. The hot or warm flashes and night sweats reported by some women are thought to be caused by hormonal changes and denote vasomotor instability. They may vary in intensity from a barely perceptible warm feeling to a sensation of extreme warmth accompanied by profuse sweating, causing discomfort, sleep disturbances, and subsequent fatigue. Other physical changes may include increased bone loss (discussed later in this chapter).

The entire genitourinary system is affected by the reduced estrogen level. Changes in the vulvovaginal area may include a gradual thinning of pubic hair and a gradual shrinkage of the labia. Vaginal secretions decrease, and women may report dyspareunia (discomfort during intercourse). The vaginal pH increases during menopause, predisposing women to bacterial infections and atrophic vaginitis. Discharge, itching, and vulvar burning may result.

Some women report fatigue, forgetfulness, weight gain, irritability, trouble sleeping, feeling "blue," and feelings of panic. Menopausal complaints need to be evaluated carefully because they may indicate other disorders. Most women have few problems and are relieved to be free from menstrual periods.

Psychological Considerations

Women's reactions and feelings related to loss of reproductive capacity may vary. Some women may experience role confusion, whereas others experience a sense of sexual and personal freedom. Women may be relieved that the childbearing phase of their lives is over. Each woman's personal views about menopause and circumstances affect her response and must be considered on an individual basis. Nurses need to be sensitive to all possibilities and take their cues from the patient. Chart 46-9 describes how women with disabilities may view menopause.

Medical Management

Women approaching menopause often have many concerns about their health. Some have concerns based on a family history of heart disease, osteoporosis, or cancer. Each woman needs to be as knowledgeable as possible about her health options and should be encouraged to discuss her

---

CHART 46-9 NURSING RESEARCH PROFILE
Perceptions of Women With Disabilities About Menopause

Harrison, T. & Becker, H. (2007). A qualitative study of menopause among women with disabilities. *Advances in Nursing Science, 30*(2), 123–138.

Purpose

Because of preexisting impairments and treatments associated with disabling conditions, women with disabilities may experience menopause in ways that differ from women without disabilities. Little information about menopause in women with disabilities or their experiences related to menopause is available. The purpose of this study was to examine the perceptions of women with mobility impairments about menopause—how they understand and react to menopause.

Design

A total of 19 women between 42 and 64 years of age were included in this qualitative, decisional support menopause intervention study. The women were interviewed by telephone using a semistructured questionnaire that addressed their experience with menopause, the effect of menopause on their daily lives, their responses to menopause, their prior knowledge about menopause, and their sources of information about menopause. Interviews were audiotaped and then transcribed verbatim. Data were analyzed using qualitative methods to identify and categorize both themes and patterns of the women's experiences.

Results

The women reported concerns about medical issues related to menopause. They viewed menopause as having possible negative effects on their health and well-being because of disorders (eg, osteoporosis) that occur in women with mobility limitations well before the onset of menopause. In most cases, they indicated a desire to make decisions about medical management of menopause and its symptoms. Nevertheless, they considered menopause to be a minor issue compared to the other physical issues they face related to their disability. They indicated that information was their best defense; in addition, they found that knowledge of their own body could be helpful. They reported that they try to avoid health care providers.

Nursing Implications

The concerns related to menopause expressed by women with disabilities should be further explored by nurses. Because women desire a major role in medical decision making related to menopause, they need to be provided with accurate, up-to-date information about results of studies related to all methods of symptom management. Furthermore, the women's view that they know their own bodies better than anyone else needs to be recognized and taken into consideration when providing care. Lastly, some women with disabilities reported that avoidance of health care providers might be beneficial. This suggests that nurses should take every opportunity to discuss health-related issues and concerns of women with disabilities.

concerns with her primary health care provider so that she can make an informed decision about managing menopausal symptoms and maintaining her health.

Hormone Therapy

Until recently, hormone therapy (HT) was prescribed to prevent hot flashes, reduce the risk of osteoporotic fractures, and decrease the risk of cardiovascular disease. Contrary to long-held beliefs, HT or menopausal hormonal therapy (North American Menopause Society, 2007) (previously referred to as hormone replacement therapy [HRT]) has been found to increase some health disorders and to be less effective in preventing others than previously believed. Although HT decreases hot flashes and reduces the risk of osteoporotic fractures as well as colorectal cancer, studies have shown that it increases the risk of breast cancer, heart attack, stroke, and blood clots (Heiss, Wallace, Anderson, et al., 2008; Writing Group for Women's Health Initiative Investigators, 2002). Thus, the benefits of HT are inadequate given the increased risk of these other disorders. Because of these findings, many women have discontinued HT or are reluctant to begin HT. Although some women have elected to use HT in low doses on the advice of their health care providers, the effect of these low doses has not been studied. The current recommendation for treatment of hot flashes with HT is to use the lowest dose possible for the shortest time possible.

Nurses need to be knowledgeable about HT-related issues to be able to respond to women's questions about HT use.

Methods of Administration

Both estrogen and progestin are prescribed for women who have not had a hysterectomy; progestin prevents proliferation of the uterine lining and hyperplasia. Women who no longer have a uterus because of hysterectomy can take estrogen without progestin (ie, unopposed estrogen) because there is no longer a risk of estrogen-induced hyperplasia of the uterine lining. Although there is a slight increase of risk of stroke in women taking estrogen alone following hysterectomy, the risk of breast cancer is unchanged (Heiss, et al., 2008).

Some women take both estrogen and progestin daily; others take estrogen for 25 consecutive days each month, with progestin taken in cycles (eg, 10 to 14 days of the month). Women who take HT for 25 days often experience bleeding after completing the progestin. Other women take estrogen and progestin every day and usually experience no bleeding. They occasionally have irregular spotting, which should be evaluated by their health care provider. Progestin administration may be oral, transdermal, vaginal, or intrauterine.

Estrogen patches, which are replaced once or twice weekly, are another option but require a progestin along with them if the woman still has a uterus. Another type of patch provides estrogen and progestin treatment. Skin should be dry at the area of application, and cleansing the site with alcohol may improve adhesiveness. Vaginal treatment with an estrogen cream, suppository, or an estradiol ring (Estring) may be used for vaginal dryness or atrophic vaginitis. The estradiol ring is a small, flexible vaginal ring

that slowly releases estrogen in small doses over 3 months. Vaginal estrogen preparations may improve vulvovaginal sensation; however, women who use them should be monitored for endometrial hyperplasia (Speroff & Fritz, 2005).

Risks and Benefits

HT is contraindicated in women with a history of breast cancer, vascular thrombosis, impaired liver function, uterine cancer, and undiagnosed abnormal vaginal bleeding. Because the risk of thromboembolic phenomena is increased with HT, women who elect to take it should be taught the signs and symptoms of deep vein thrombosis and pulmonary embolism and instructed to report these signs and symptoms immediately. Women who take HT should be assessed for leg redness, tenderness, chest pain, and shortness of breath. Furthermore, they need to be informed about the importance of regular follow-up care, including a yearly physical examination and mammogram. An endometrial biopsy is indicated for any irregular bleeding. Because the risk of complications increases the longer HT is used, HT should be used for the shortest time possible (American Heart Association, 2007). Estrogen alone or in combination with a progestin does not reduce risk of dementia or cognitive impairment.

Alternative Therapy for Hot Flashes

Because women often seek information about alternatives to HT use, nurses must be knowledgeable about other approaches women can use to promote their health in the perimenopausal and postmenopausal period. Problematic hot flashes have been treated with venlafaxine (Effexor), paroxetine (Paxil), gabapentin (Neurontin), and clonidine (Catapres). Similarly, vitamin B_6 and vitamin E may be effective. Some women have expressed interest in other alternative treatments (eg, natural estrogens and progestins, black cohosh, ginseng, dong quai, soy products, and several other herbal preparations); however, few data exist about their safety or effectiveness. Therefore, assessment of menopausal women should address their use of complementary and alternative therapies and supplements. The North American Menopause Society provides additional suggestions. Glucose levels also affect hot flashes; thus, nurses can encourage patients to maintain stable glucose levels (Dormire & Becker, 2007).

Maintaining Bone Health

Acceleration of bone loss resulting in osteoporosis and microarchitectural deterioration of bone tissue occurs at menopause and leads to increased bone fragility and risk of fracture. Other factors that increase a woman's risk of osteoporosis include a thin body frame, race (Caucasian or Asian), family history of osteoporosis, nulliparity, early menopause, moderate to heavy alcohol ingestion, smoking, caffeine use, sedentary lifestyle, and a diet low in calcium. About 80% of people with osteoporosis are women, and about half of these women will experience a fracture related to osteoporosis during her lifetime (National Osteoporosis Foundation, 2008). Thus, women are advised to remain active and to begin or continue a regular exercise program of weight-bearing activity, such as walking, which helps maintain bone mass; to take a calcium supplement; to decrease or stop smoking; and to discuss with their health care provider the use of pharmacologic agents to reduce bone loss if indicated. Osteoporosis and its treatment are described in detail in Chapter 68.

Maintaining Cardiovascular Health

The American Heart Association (2007) recommends a variety of strategies to lower the risk of heart disease in women. These include lifestyle changes and behavioral strategies. Diet, exercise, stress reduction, and a healthy lifestyle all contribute to older women's cardiac health and are an essential part of health promotion. Regular physical exercise increases the heart rate and high-density lipoprotein levels. Weight-bearing exercise (eg, walking, jogging) at least four times a week is recommended. Pharmacologic therapy (eg, aspirin, beta-blockers, "statins," angiostatin-converting enzyme inhibitors) may be indicated in women who have cardiovascular disease or are at high risk for it. Prevention and treatment of cardiovascular disease are discussed in detail in Chapter 26.

Behavioral Strategies

As previously stated, regular physical exercise is beneficial. It may also reduce stress, enhance well-being, and improve self-image. In addition, weight-bearing exercise may prevent loss of muscle tissue and bone tissue.

Women are also encouraged to participate in other health-promoting activities. These include regular health screening recommended for women at the time of menopause: gynecologic examinations, mammograms, colonoscopy, fecal occult blood testing, and bone mineral density testing if at risk for osteoporosis.

Nutritional Therapy

Women are encouraged to decrease their fat and caloric intake and increase their intake of whole grains, fiber, fruit, and vegetables. Women of all ages tend to ingest less than the recommended amount of calcium; therefore, they should be encouraged to increase their intake of foods high in calcium (eg, nonfat yogurt, green leafy vegetables, seafood, and calcium-fortified foods). Calcium and vitamin D supplementation may be helpful in reducing bone loss and preventing the morbidity associated with osteoporotic fractures (National Osteoporosis Foundation, 2008).

Nursing Management

Nurses can encourage women to view menopause as a natural change resulting in freedom from symptoms related to menses. No relationship exists between menopause and mental health problems; however, social circumstances (eg, adolescent children, ill partners, and dependent or ill parents) that may coincide with menopause can be stressful.

Measures should be taken to promote general health. The nurse explains to the patient that cessation of menses is a normal occurrence that is rarely accompanied by nervous symptoms or illness. The current expected lifespan after menopause for the average woman is 30 to 35 years, which may encompass as many years as the childbearing phase of her life. Normal sexual urges continue, and women retain their usual response to sex long after menopause. Many women enjoy better health after menopause than before, especially those who have experienced dysmenorrhea. The individual woman's evaluation of herself and her worth, now and in the future, is likely to affect her emotional reaction to menopause. Patient teaching and counseling regarding healthy lifestyles, health promotion, and health screening are of paramount importance (Chart 46-10).

Menstrual Disorders

Menstrual disorders may include premenstrual syndrome (PMS); dysmenorrhea; amenorrhea; and excessive bleeding, irregular bleeding, or bleeding between cycles or unrelated to cycles. These disorders need to be discussed with a health care provider and managed individually. Menstrual-related disorders have been reported in as many as 19% of women who report feeling more anxious, sad, nervous, restless, hopeless, and worthless than those without complaints. Affected women are more likely to smoke cigarettes, drink alcohol to excess, and be overweight (Strine, Chapman & Ahluwalia, 2005). Dysmenorrhea may result from endometriosis or anatomic abnormalities or it can be a normal variation. Amenorrhea may be related to pregnancy, thyroid disorders, anatomic abnormalities, and eating disorders. Excessive bleeding may be caused by fibroids, clotting disorders, thyroid disorders, and miscarriage. Irregular bleeding may be secondary to hormonal changes in adolescence or perimenopause or may result from pregnancy, threatened abortion, or a variety of other factors.

PREMENSTRUAL SYNDROME

Premenstrual symptoms are common in ovulating women and can influence quality of life. Symptoms occur in the luteal phase and disappear with the onset of menses. PMS is a combination of bothersome symptoms, and premenstrual dysphoric disorder is a severe type of premenstrual disorder that significantly impairs normal activity (Chart 46-11). The cause of these conditions is unknown; they are diagnosed if symptoms occur during the 5 days prior to the onset of menses, disappear within 4 days of the onset of menses, and occur through several cycles. PMS tends to become less symptomatic with menopause.

Clinical Manifestations

Major symptoms of PMS include physical symptoms such as headache, fatigue, low back pain, painful breasts, and a feeling of abdominal fullness. Behavioral and emotional symptoms may include general irritability, mood swings, fear of losing control, binge eating, and crying spells. Symptoms vary widely from one woman to another and from one cycle to the next in the same woman. Great variability is found in the degree of symptoms. Many women are affected to some degree, but some are severely affected.

A generally stressful life and problematic relationships may be related to the intensity of physical symptoms. Some women report moderate to severe life disruption secondary to PMS that negatively affects their interpersonal relationships. PMS may also be a factor in reduced productivity, work-related injuries, and absenteeism.

CHART 46-10 — HOME CARE CHECKLIST
The Woman Approaching Menopause

At the completion of the home care instruction, the patient or caregiver will be able to:	PATIENT	CAREGIVER
• Describe menopause as a normal period in a woman's life.	✔	✔
• State that fatigue and stress may worsen hot flashes.	✔	✔
• State that a nutritious diet and weight control will enhance physical and emotional well-being.	✔	✔
• State the importance of exercising for at least 30 minutes three or four times a week to maintain good health.	✔	✔
• Describe involvement in outside activities as beneficial in reducing anxiety and tension.	✔	✔
• Identify the following as changes that often occur in midlife: departure of children, aging, dependence of parents, possible loss of loved ones.	✔	✔
• Describe this phase of life as having the potential for intellectual growth, personal accomplishment, and initiation of new activities.	✔	✔
• State the following points about sexual activity: Frequent sexual activity helps to maintain the elasticity of the vagina. Contraception is advised until 1 year passes without menses. Safer sex is important at any age. Sexual functioning may be enhanced at midlife.	✔	
• Identify the importance of an annual physical examination to screen for problems and to promote general health.	✔	
• Identify strategies and methods to prevent or manage the following problems: Itching or burning of vulvar areas: see primary health care provider to rule out dermatologic abnormalities and, if appropriate, to obtain a prescription for a lubricating or hormonal cream.	✔	
Dyspareunia (painful intercourse) due to vaginal dryness; use a water-soluble lubricant, such as K-Y Jelly, Astro-Glide, Replens, hormone cream, or contraceptive foam.	✔	
Decreased perineal muscle tone and bladder control: practice Kegel exercises daily (contract the perineal muscles as though stopping urination; hold for 5–10 seconds and release; repeat frequently during the day).	✔	
Dry skin: use mild emollient skin cream and lotions to prevent dry skin.	✔	
Weight control: join a weight-reduction support group such as Weight Watchers or a similar group if appropriate, or consult a registered dietitian for guidance about the tendency to gain weight, particularly around the hips, thighs, and abdomen.	✔	
Osteoporosis: observe recommended calcium and vitamin D intake, including calcium supplements, if indicated, to slow the process of osteoporosis; avoid smoking, alcohol, and excessive caffeine, all of which increase bone loss. Perform weight-bearing exercises. Undergo bone density testing when appropriate.	✔	
Risk for urinary tract infection (UTI): drink 6 to 8 glasses of water daily and take vitamin C (500 mg) as a possible way to reduce the incidence of UTI related to atrophic changes of the urethra.	✔	
Vaginal bleeding: report any bleeding after 1 year of no menses to a primary health care provider *immediately, no matter how minimal.*	✔	

Medical Management

Because there is no single treatment or known cure for PMS, women should chart their symptoms so they can anticipate and therefore cope with them. Regular exercise may be helpful. Although women have been advised to avoid caffeine, high-fat foods, and refined sugars, little research demonstrates the efficacy of dietary changes. Alternative therapies that have been used include vitamins B and E, magnesium, and oil of evening primrose cap-

sules. No studies have evaluated the effectiveness of these therapies.

Pharmacologic remedies include selective serotonin reuptake inhibitors (eg, fluoxetine [Prozac, Sarafem]), GnRH agonists, prostaglandin inhibitors (eg, ibuprofen and naproxen [Anaprox, Aleve]), diuretics, antianxiety agents, and calcium supplements. Oral contraceptives containing drospirenone (a synthetic progestin) and extended regimens also may be effective (Coffee, Kuehl, Willis, et al., 2006; Lopez, Kaptein & Helmerhorst, 2008).

Chart 46-11 • *Causes, Manifestations, and Treatment of Premenstrual Syndrome*

Cause

- Unknown; may be related to hormonal changes combined with other factors (diet, stress, and lack of exercise)
- Many women have some symptoms related to menses, but PMS affects 2% to 5% of women and is a complex of symptoms that result in dysfunction.

Physical Symptoms

- Fluid retention (eg, bloating, breast tenderness)
- Headache

Affective Symptoms

- Depression
- Anger
- Irritability
- Anxiety
- Confusion

- Withdrawal
- Symptoms begin in the 5 days preceding menses and relief occurs within 4 days of onset of menses. Dysfunction usually occurs in relationships, parenting, work, or school.

Treatment

- Use of social support and family resources
- Nutritious diet consisting of whole grains, fruits, and vegetables; increased water intake may help
- Serotonin reuptake inhibitors
- Alprazolam (Xanax) has been effective but risk of physical and psychological dependence is high.
- Spironolactone, a diuretic, may be effective in treating fluid retention.
- Initiation/maintenance of exercise program
- Stress reduction techniques

Nursing Management

The nurse obtains a health history, noting the time when symptoms began and their nature and intensity. The nurse then determines whether symptoms occur before or shortly after the menstrual flow begins. In addition, the nurse can show the patient how to record the timing and intensity of symptoms. A nutritional history is also elicited to determine if the diet is high in salt, caffeine, or alcohol or low in essential nutrients.

The patient's goals may include reduction of anxiety, mood swings, crying, binge eating, fear of losing control, improved coping with day-to-day stressors, improved relationships with family and coworkers, and increased knowledge about PMS. Positive coping measures are promoted. This may involve encouraging the woman's partner to offer support and assistance with child care. The patient can try to plan her working time to accommodate the days she is less productive because of PMS. The nurse encourages the patient to use exercise, meditation, imagery, and creative activities to reduce stress. The nurse also encourages the patient to take medications as prescribed and provides instructions about the desired effects of the medications. Enrolling in a PMS group may help the patient learn to recognize and cope with this condition.

If the patient has severe symptoms of PMS or premenstrual dysphoric disorder, the nurse assesses her for suicidal, uncontrollable, and violent behavior. An immediate psychiatric evaluation is necessary for women with any suggestions of suicidal tendencies. In rare cases, uncontrollable behavior may lead to violence toward family members. If abuse of children or other members of a patient's family is suspected, it is important to implement and follow reporting protocols. Referral for immediate psychiatric or psychological care and counseling is required.

DYSMENORRHEA

Primary dysmenorrhea is painful menstruation, with no identifiable pelvic pathology. It occurs at the time of menarche or shortly thereafter. It is characterized by crampy pain that begins before or shortly after the onset of menstrual flow and continues for 48 to 72 hours. Pelvic examination findings are normal. Dysmenorrhea is thought to result from excessive production of prostaglandins, which causes painful contraction of the uterus and arteriolar vasospasm. Psychological factors, such as anxiety and tension, may also contribute to dysmenorrhea. As women become older, dysmenorrhea often decreases and frequently completely resolves after childbirth.

In secondary dysmenorrhea, pelvic pathology such as endometriosis, tumor, or pelvic inflammatory disease (PID) contributes to symptoms. Patients frequently have pain that occurs several days before menses, with ovulation, and occasionally with intercourse.

Assessment and Diagnostic Findings

A pelvic examination is performed to rule out possible disorders, such as endometriosis, PID, adenomyosis, and uterine fibroids. A laparoscopy may be required to identify organic causes.

Management

In primary dysmenorrhea, the reason for the discomfort is explained, and the patient is assured that menstruation is a normal function of the reproductive system. If the patient is young and accompanied by her mother, the mother may also need reassurance. Many young women expect to have painful periods if their mothers did. The discomfort of cramps can be treated once anxiety and concern about its cause are dispelled by adequate explanation. Symptoms usually subside with appropriate medication. Aspirin, a mild prostaglandin inhibitor, may be taken at recommended doses every 4 hours. Other useful prostaglandin antagonists include NSAIDs such as ibuprofen, naproxen, and mefenamic acid (Ponstel). If one medication does not provide relief, another may be recommended. Usually these medications are well tolerated, but some women experience gastrointestinal side effects. Contraindications include allergy, peptic ulcer history, sensitivity to aspirinlike medications, asthma, and pregnancy. Low-dose oral contraceptives provide relief in more than 90% of patients and may be prescribed for women with dysmenorrhea who are sexually active but do not desire pregnancy.

Continuous low-level local heat may also be effective in relieving primary dysmenorrhea. Heat therapy and medication have been found to work well in combination. The patient is encouraged to continue her usual activities and to increase physical exercise if possible because this relieves discomfort for some women. Taking analgesic agents before cramps start, in anticipation of discomfort, is advised.

Management of secondary dysmenorrhea is directed at diagnosis and treatment of the underlying cause (eg, endometriosis or PID).

AMENORRHEA

Amenorrhea (absence of menstrual flow) is a symptom of a variety of disorders and dysfunctions. Primary amenorrhea (delayed menarche) refers to the situation in which young women older than 16 years of age have not begun to menstruate but otherwise show evidence of sexual maturation, or in which young women have not begun to menstruate and have not begun to show development of secondary sex characteristics by 14 years of age. Amenorrhea may be of considerable concern but often occurs as a result of minor variations in body build, heredity, environment, and physical, mental, and emotional development.

The nurse encourages the patient to express her concerns and anxiety about this problem because the patient may feel that she is different from her peers. A complete physical examination, careful health history, and simple laboratory tests help rule out possible causes, such as metabolic or endocrine disorders and systemic diseases. Treatment is directed toward correcting any abnormalities.

Secondary amenorrhea (an absence of menses for three cycles or 6 months after a normal menarche) may be caused by pregnancy, emotional upset, eating disorder, or excessive exercise. In adolescents, secondary amenorrhea can be caused by minor emotional upset related to being away from home, attending college, tension due to schoolwork, or interpersonal problems. However, the second most common cause is pregnancy, so a pregnancy test is almost always indicated.

Secondary nutritional disturbances may also be factors. Obesity can result in anovulation and subsequent amenorrhea. Eating disorders, such as anorexia and bulimia, often result in lack of menses because the decrease in body fat and caloric intake affects hormonal function. Intense exercise can induce menstrual disturbances. Competitive female athletes often experience amenorrhea. If they do, they may be placed on HT to prevent bone loss related to low estrogen levels. On occasion, a pituitary or thyroid dysfunction may cause amenorrhea. These dysfunctions can be treated successfully by treatment of the underlying endocrine disorder. Infrequent periods (oligomenorrhea) may be related to thyroid disorders, polycystic ovarian syndrome, or premature ovarian failure. Women who are HIV positive are apt to miss menstrual periods and need to be evaluated for pregnancy, thyroid disorders, hyperprolactinemia, and menopause (if appropriate) (Cejtin, Kalinowski, Bacchetti, et al., 2006).

ABNORMAL UTERINE BLEEDING

Dysfunctional uterine bleeding is abnormal bleeding that has no known organic cause. The bleeding is defined as irregular, painless bleeding of endometrial origin that may be excessive, prolonged, or without pattern. Dysfunctional uterine bleeding can occur at any age but is most common at opposite ends of the reproductive lifespan. It is usually secondary to anovulation (lack of ovulation) and is common in adolescents and women approaching menopause.

Adolescents account for many cases of abnormal uterine bleeding; they often do not ovulate regularly as the pituitary–ovarian axis matures. Perimenopausal women also experience this condition because of irregular ovulation secondary to decreasing ovarian hormone production. Other causes may include fibroids, obesity, and hypothalamic dysfunction.

Abnormal or unusual vaginal bleeding that is atypical in time or amount must be evaluated because it could possibly be a manifestation of a major disorder. A physical examination is performed, and the patient is evaluated for conditions such as pregnancy, neoplasm, infection, anatomic abnormalities, endocrine disorders, trauma, blood dyscrasias, platelet dysfunction, and hypothalamic disorders.

Menorrhagia

Menorrhagia is prolonged or excessive bleeding at the time of the regular menstrual flow. In young women the cause is usually related to endocrine disturbance, whereas in later life it usually results from inflammatory disturbances, tumors of the uterus, or hormonal imbalance.

Women with menorrhagia are urged to see a primary health care provider and to describe the amount of bleeding by pad count and saturation (ie, absorbency of perineal pad or tampon and number saturated hourly). Persistent heavy bleeding can result in anemia. It can also be a sign of a bleeding disorder or a result of anticoagulant therapy. Hysterectomy can be challenging in these women; endometrial ablation has been found to be less risky (El-Nashar, Hopkins, Feitoza, et al., 2007).

Metrorrhagia

Metrorrhagia (vaginal bleeding between regular menstrual periods) is probably the most significant form of menstrual dysfunction because it may signal cancer, benign tumors of the uterus, or other gynecologic problems. This condition warrants prompt evaluation and treatment. Although bleeding between menstrual periods by women taking oral contraceptives is usually not serious, irregular bleeding by women taking HT should be evaluated.

Menometrorrhagia is heavy vaginal bleeding between and during periods. It, too, requires evaluation.

Postmenopausal Bleeding

Bleeding 1 year after menses cease at menopause must be investigated, and a malignant condition must be considered until proven otherwise. A vaginal ultrasound can be used to measure the thickness of the endometrial lining. The uterine lining in postmenopausal women should be thin because of low estrogen levels. A lining thicker than 5 mm usually warrants evaluation by endometrial biopsy or a D & C.

Dyspareunia

Dyspareunia (difficult or painful intercourse) can be superficial, deep, primary, or secondary and may occur at the beginning of, during, or after intercourse. Dyspareunia may be related to many factors, including injury during childbirth; lack of vaginal lubrication; a history of incest, sexual abuse, or assault; endometriosis; pelvic infection; vaginal atrophy with menopause; gastrointestinal disorders; fibroids; urinary tract infection; STDs; or vulvodynia (vulvar pain that affects women of all ages without any discernible physical cause). Depending on the cause of dyspareunia, counseling, extra lubrication, or antidepressants may be prescribed. Women's health issues related to sexuality may be affected by many factors. Thus, these issues need to be taken seriously, carefully assessed, and treated.

Contraception

Each year, more than half of the pregnancies in the United States are unintended; this is the highest rate among industrialized nations. Although unintended pregnancies occur in women of all ages, incomes, and racial and ethnic groups, the highest rates occur among adolescents and perimenopausal women. Adolescents are more likely to experience pregnancy complications and are more prone to have low-birthweight babies. In addition, adolescent mothers are less likely to obtain a high school diploma and are more likely subsequently to live in poverty. One of two unplanned pregnancies end in abortion (Paru, Boatwright, Tozer, et al., 2006).

Women may fail to use effective methods of contraception consistently or at all. Of the women who undergo abortions, many were not using contraception when they became pregnant, and others have never used any method of contraception. Decreasing unwanted pregnancies may reduce the number of abortions, abused children, stressed families, and infant mortality and morbidity.

Nurses can assist with information and support. Women can be asked directly when they plan to have their next pregnancy and about their need for contraception. Many women who are sexually active or who are considering becoming sexually active can benefit from learning about contraception. Nurses who are involved in helping patients make contraceptive choices need to listen, take time to answer questions, and teach and assist patients in choosing the method they prefer. It is important for women to receive unbiased and nonjudgmental information, understand the benefits and risks of each method, learn about alternatives and how to use them, and receive positive reinforcement and acceptance of their choice. Some women have received misinformation (ie, contraception causes cancer or weight gain). Adolescents who worry that they may be unable to become pregnant may not be willing to use contraception. Factors related to this fear include a history of an STD, an older partner, a partner who desires a pregnancy, and the adolescent's desire for pregnancy (White, Rosengard, Weitzen, et al., 2006).

ABSTINENCE

Abstinence, or celibacy, is the only completely effective means of preventing pregnancy. Abstinence may not be a desired or available option for many women because of cultural expectations and their own and their partner's values and sexual needs.

STERILIZATION

After abstinence, sterilization by bilateral tubal occlusion or vasectomy is the most effective means of contraception. Both procedures must be considered permanent because neither is easily reversible. Women and men who choose these methods should be certain that they no longer wish to have children, no matter how the circumstances in their life may change. Often, decisions made hastily may be regretted later. Some gynecologists suggest a waiting period to ensure that patients are certain about a potentially irreversible decision.

Tubal Ligation

Sterilization by tubal ligation is one of the most common surgical procedures performed on women. Tubal ligation is usually performed as a same-day surgical procedure and is carried out by laparoscopy or hysteroscopy, with the patient receiving a general or local anesthetic. After the laparoscope is inserted, the fallopian tubes are visualized and may be coagulated, sutured (Pomeroy procedure), or ligated with silicone bands or a spring clip, thereby disrupting their patency. The use of spring clips is associated with the highest rate of pregnancy following sterilization. In another procedure, transcervical tubal occlusion procedure, a 0.6-inch metal coil or spring is inserted into the fallopian tubes through the cervix, thus avoiding the need for laparoscopy or a surgical incision. This method, referred to as the Essure procedure, is performed via hysteroscopy and obstructs the tubes by inducing scar tissue. Women who have had this procedure should abstain from unprotected intercourse for 3 months to avoid pregnancy until the scar tissue develops and the effectiveness of the procedure is verified by HSG.

Despite a very high rate of effectiveness, all women who have undergone tubal ligation but miss a period should be tested for pregnancy because ectopic and intrauterine pregnancies, although rare, may occur. Ovulation and menstruation are not affected by sterilization, although some women report heavier menstrual bleeding and more cramping after tubal ligation.

Before undergoing tubal ligation, the patient should be informed that an IUD, if present, will be removed. If the patient is taking oral contraceptives, she usually continues them up to the time of the procedure. If a laparoscopic procedure is performed, the patient may experience postoperative abdominal or shoulder discomfort for a few days, related to the carbon dioxide gas and the manipulation of organs. The patient is instructed to report heavy bleeding, fever, or pain that persists or increases. She should avoid intercourse, strenuous exercise, and lifting for 2 weeks. Risks associated with tubal ligation are minimal and are more often related to anesthesia than to the surgery itself. Risk is increased in women with diabetes, previous abdominal or pelvic surgery, or obesity.

Vasectomy

Vasectomy (male sterilization) and hysteroscopic/laparoscopic tubal ligation are compared in Table 46-4. See Chapter 49 for a discussion of vasectomy.

Table 46-4	COMPARISON OF STERILIZATION METHODS	
Sterilization Method	Advantages	Disadvantages
Vasectomy	• Highly effective • Relieves female of contraceptive burden • Inexpensive in long run • Permanent • Highly acceptable procedure to most patients • Very safe • Quickly performed	• Expensive in short term • Serious long-term effects suggested (although currently unproved) • Permanent (although reversal is possible, it is expensive and requires highly technical and major surgery, and results cannot be guaranteed) • Regret in 5%–10% of patients • No protection against STDs, including HIV • Not effective until sperm remaining in reproductive system are ejaculated
Hysteroscopic and laparoscopic tubal sterilization	• Low incidence of complications • Short recovery • Leaves small or no scar • Quickly performed	• Permanent • Reversal difficult and expensive • Sterilization procedures technically difficult • Requires surgeon, operating room (aseptic conditions), trained assistants, medications, surgical equipment (Essure [insertion of coil or spring in fallopian tubes] requires hysteroscopy rather than surgery) • Expensive at the time performed • If failure, high probability of ectopic pregnancy • No protection against STDs, including HIV

HORMONAL CONTRACEPTION

Oral contraceptives block ovarian stimulation by preventing the release of FSH from the anterior pituitary gland. In the absence of FSH, a follicle does not ripen, and ovulation does not occur. Progestins (synthetic forms of progesterone) suppress the LH surge, prevent ovulation, and also render the cervical mucus impenetrable to sperm. Hormonal contraceptive agents may be oral, transdermal, vaginal, or injectable. Combined oral contraceptives that contain both estrogens and progestins are currently used by many women to prevent pregnancy.

Benefits and Risks

Benefits of combined hormonal contraceptive use include a reduction in the incidence of benign breast disease; improvement in acne; and reduced risk of uterine and ovarian cancers, anemia, and pelvic infection. In general, prolonged hormonal contraceptive use has resulted in no definite long-term undesirable effects, although there is an increased risk of gallbladder problems (eg, cholestasis). Resumption of normal menses is delayed 2 to 3 months or longer in about 20% of hormonal contraceptive users. Risks include venous thromboembolism, although its incidence has decreased because the estrogen concentrations used today are less than that used in early preparations. Venous thromboembolism is less than half as likely with hormonal contraceptives than with pregnancy. Fetal anomalies do not appear to be an issue, and normal reproductive tract function and fertility resume after hormonal contraceptive use is discontinued. However, most health care providers recommend that women who wish to become pregnant use a barrier contraceptive method for 1 to 2 months after stopping hormonal contraceptives before attempting to become pregnant to permit a normal period for accurate dating of the pregnancy.

A few patients experience adverse reactions when using hormonal contraceptives. These include nausea, depression, headache, leg cramps, and breast soreness. Usually, these symptoms subside after 3 or 4 months. Because such symptoms are sometimes related to sodium and water retention caused by estrogen, a smaller dose of the hormone or a different hormonal combination may alleviate the problem. Many patients experience spotting in the first month of use of hormonal contraceptive or if they use it irregularly, so they need to be reassured and advised to use it as prescribed. Chart 46-12 compares different oral contraceptive regimens, and Chart 46-13 describes the benefits and risks of oral contraceptive use.

Contraindications

Absolute contraindications to hormonal contraceptives include current or past thromboembolic disorder, cerebrovascular disease, or artery disease; migraine headaches with visual auras; known or suspected breast cancer; known or suspected current or past estrogen-dependent neoplasia; pregnancy; current or past benign or malignant liver tumors; liver dysfunction; clotting disorders; congenital hyperlipidemia; and abnormal vaginal bleeding (ACOG, 2006c).

Relative contraindications include hypertension, bile-induced jaundice, acute phase of mononucleosis, and sickle cell disease. Controlled hypertension in otherwise healthy young nonsmokers is generally not a contraindication to use of combination agents but does require a low dose and careful blood pressure monitoring. Women older than 35 years of age who smoke are at risk for cardiac problems and should not use hormonal contraceptives. Occasionally, neuro-ocular complications arise, but a cause-and-effect relationship has not been established. If visual disturbances occur, hormonal contraceptives should be discontinued.

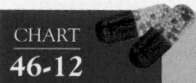

CHART 46-12

PHARMACOLOGY
Comparison of Hormonal Contraceptive Regimens

There are two kinds of hormonal contraceptives: combined (consisting of an estrogen and a progestin) and progestin only.

Combined Preparations (pills, transdermal patches, vaginal rings)

- Monophasic preparations supply the same dose of estrogen and progestin for 21 days.
- Biphasic preparations and triphasic pills vary the amount of hormonal components during the cycle.
- Usually leads to a lighter-than-normal menstrual flow, which results from withdrawal.

Progestin-Only "Mini" Preparations

- Preparations provide less protection against conception than combined preparations.
- About 40% of women taking progestin-only preparations have ovulatory cycles.
- Progestin-only preparations are useful for women who have had estrogen-related side effects (eg, headaches, hypertension, leg pain, chloasma or skin discoloration, weight gain, or nausea) on combination pills.
- Progestin-only preparations are useful for lactating women who need a hormonal contraceptive method.
- Depo-Provera, a progestin-only injection, lasts for 3 months.
- Implanon, a subdermal implant lasts for 3 years.

Chart 46-14 summarizes patient education guidelines that are important for women using combination hormonal contraceptives.

Coexisting medical disorders may make contraception a complex issue. These disorders include chronic hypertension, lipid disorders, diabetes, migraines, fibroids, obesity, lupus, depression, seizures, and HIV infection or AIDS. Contraception needs to be addressed individually in women with these conditions, and clinicians may prescribe injectable hormonal contraceptives (eg, Depo-Provera) or IUDs (ACOG, 2006c).

Methods of Hormonal Contraception

Various hormonal methods of birth control are approved by the U.S. Food and Drug Administration (FDA). Combination methods include the combination of oral contraceptive pills, vaginal ring (NuvaRing), and transdermal patch (Ortho Evra). Progestin-only methods include the progestin-only pills or minipills, progestin-only emergency contraception (Plan B), once-every-3-month injection (Depo-Provera), levonorgestrel-releasing intrauterine system (Mirena), and single-rod subdermal implant (Implanon).

 NURSING ALERT

Patients need to be aware that hormonal contraceptives protect them from pregnancy but not from STDs or HIV infection. In addition, sex with multiple partners or sex without a condom may also result in chlamydial and other infections, including HIV infection.

Oral Contraceptives

Many women currently use oral contraceptive preparations of synthetic estrogens and progestins. A variety of formulations are available. Extended regimens of oral hormonal contraceptive agents are an option for women who have heavy or uncomfortable menstrual bleeding or who wish to have fewer periods. With the use of these regimens, women may have an increased occurrence of breakthrough bleeding; the blood may be dark brown rather than red. It may be more difficult to tell if a pregnancy occurs with this method, although pregnancy is unlikely if pills are taken as prescribed. Studies are ongoing to assess the risks of exposure to increased estrogen resulting from this method.

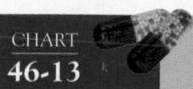

CHART 46-13

PHARMACOLOGY
Benefits and Risks of Combination Hormonal Contraceptives

Benefits

- Decreased cramps and bleeding
- Regular bleeding cycle
- Decreased incidence of anemia
- Decrease in acne with some formulations
- Protection from uterine and ovarian cancer
- Decreased incidence of ectopic pregnancy
- Protection from benign breast disease
- Decreased incidence of pelvic infection

Risks

- Rare in healthy women
- Bothersome side effects (eg, breakthrough bleeding, breast tenderness)
- Nausea, weight gain, mood changes
- Small increased risk of developing blood clots, stroke, or heart attack, related more to smoking than to oral contraceptive use alone
- Possible increased incidence of benign liver tumors and gallbladder disorders
- No protection from STDs/STIs (possible increased risk with unsafe sex)

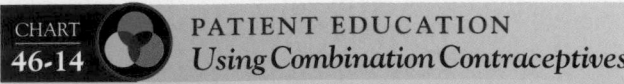

Transdermal Contraceptives

Ortho Evra is a thin, beige, matchbook-size skin patch that releases an estrogen and a progestin continuously. It is changed every week for 3 weeks, and no patch is used during the fourth week, resulting in withdrawal bleeding. The effectiveness of Ortho Evra is comparable to that of oral contraceptives. Its risks are similar to those of oral contraceptives and include an increased risk of blood clots. The patch may be applied to the torso, chest, arms, or thighs; it should not be applied to the breasts. The patch is convenient and more easily remembered than a daily pill but is not as effective for women who weigh more than 198 lb (90 kg). In addition, it may also irritate skin conditions (eg, psoriasis) in some women and results in higher blood estrogen levels than oral contraceptives.

Vaginal Contraceptives

NuvaRing (etonogestrel/ethinyl estradiol vaginal ring) is a combination hormonal contraceptive that releases estrogen and progestin. It is inserted in the vagina for 3 weeks and then removed, resulting in withdrawal bleeding. It is as effective as oral contraceptives and results in lower hormone blood levels than oral contraceptives. NuvaRing is flexible, does not require sizing or fitting, and is effective when placed anywhere in the vagina. Patients are occasionally reluctant to consider vaginal methods of contraception unless discussed openly and as a convenient alternative to other routes of administration. Some women are uncomfortable with this method and may fear that the ring may migrate or be uncomfortable or be noticed by a partner. The nurse can be helpful in dispelling misconceptions. The patient can be informed that while some women notice a slight increase in vaginal discharge, this effective method of contraception has been found to increase the vaginal health-promoting lactobacillus (ACOG, 2006d; Roumen, 2008). NuvaRing is usually more expensive than oral contraceptives.

Injectable Contraceptives

An intramuscular injection of Depo-Provera (a long-acting progestin) every 3 months inhibits ovulation and provides a reliable, private, and convenient contraceptive method. A subcutaneous formulation is also available. It can be used by lactating women and those with hypertension, liver disease, migraine headaches, heart disease, and hemoglobinopathies.

With continued use, women must be prepared for irregular bleeding episodes and spotting decrease, or amenorrhea.

Advantages of Depo-Provera include reduction of menorrhagia, dysmenorrhea, and anemia due to heavy menstrual bleeding. It may reduce the risk of pelvic infection, has been associated with improvement in hematologic status in women with sickle cell disease, and does not interfere with the efficacy of antiseizure agents. It decreases the risk of endometrial cancer, PID, endometriosis, and uterine fibroids.

Possible side effects of Depo-Provera include irregular menstrual bleeding, bloating, headaches, hair loss, decreased sex drive, bone loss, and weight loss or weight gain. The contraceptive does not protect against STDs. Fertility may be delayed when women discontinue this method; therefore, other methods of contraception may be more appropriate for the woman who wishes to conceive within a year of discontinuing contraception. While Depo-Provera is used, bone density is decreased, and this may be a risk factor for future osteoporosis. Severe allergic response is rare but possible following injection (Haider & Darney, 2007).

Depo-Provera is contraindicated in women who are pregnant and those who have abnormal vaginal bleeding of unknown cause, breast or pelvic cancer, or sensitivity to synthetic progestin. The long-term effects on infants of nursing mothers who use Depo-Provera are unknown but are thought to be negligible.

Implants

Implanon is a single-rod subdermal implant that is usually placed inside the upper arm via a small incision. It is effective for 3 years. Implanon may cause irregular bleeding but may improve dysmenorrhea, and it does not affect bone density. This contraceptive can be used by lactating women.

INTRAUTERINE DEVICE

An IUD is a small plastic device, usually T-shaped, that is inserted into the uterine cavity to prevent pregnancy. A string attached to the IUD is visible and palpable at the cervical os. An IUD prevents conception by causing a local inflammatory reaction that is toxic to spermatozoa and blastocysts, thus preventing fertilization. The IUD does not work by causing abortion.

Advantages include effectiveness over a long period of time, few if any systemic effects, and reduction of patient error. This reversible method of birth control is as effective as sterilization and more effective than barrier methods.

Disadvantages include possible excessive bleeding, cramps, and backaches; a slight risk of tubal pregnancy; slight risk of pelvic infection on insertion; displacement of the device; and, rarely, perforation of the cervix and uterus. If a pregnancy occurs with an IUD in place, the device is removed immediately to avoid infection. Spontaneous abortion (miscarriage) may occur on removal. An IUD is not usually used in women who have not had children because a small nulliparous uterus may not tolerate it. Women with multiple partners, women with heavy or crampy periods, or those with a history of ectopic pregnancy or pelvic infection should be encouraged to use other methods of contraception.

Some clinicians test for chlamydia and gonorrhea prior to insertion to prevent PID.

The ParaGard T 380A, an IUD that has been available for 15 years, is effective for at least 10 years. It prevents fertilization by impairing sperm function as copper has an antispermatic effect. The Levonorgestrel Intrauterine System (LNG-IUS; Mirena), another IUD, releases levonorgestrel, a synthetic progestin used in oral contraceptives, and is effective for at least 5 years. It works by impairing sperm function, thickening cervical mucus, and suppressing the endometrium. It has also been used therapeutically to reduce heavy bleeding; it may prevent the need for hysterectomy in some women with heavy vaginal bleeding. LNG-IUS is also helpful in women with menorrhagia, dysmenorrhea, endometriosis, and fibroids (ACOG, 2006d).

MECHANICAL BARRIERS

Diaphragm

The diaphragm is an effective contraceptive device that consists of a round, flexible spring (50 to 90 mm wide) covered with a domelike latex rubber cup. A spermicidal (contraceptive) jelly or cream is used to coat the concave side of the diaphragm before it is inserted deep into the vagina, covering the cervix completely. The spermicide inhibits spermatozoa from entering the cervical canal. The diaphragm is not felt by the user or her partner when properly fitted and inserted. Because women vary in size, the diaphragm must be sized and fitted by an experienced clinician. The woman is instructed in using and caring for the device. A return demonstration ensures that the woman can insert the diaphragm correctly and that it covers the cervix.

Each time the woman uses the diaphragm, she should examine it carefully. By holding it up to a bright light, she should ensure that it has no pinpoint holes, cracks, or tears. She then applies spermicidal jelly or cream and inserts the diaphragm. The diaphragm should remain in place at least 6 hours after coitus (no more than 12 hours). Additional spermicide is necessary if more than 6 hours have passed before intercourse occurs and before each act of repeated intercourse. On removal, the diaphragm should be cleansed thoroughly with mild soap and water, rinsed, and dried before being stored in its original container.

Disadvantages include allergic reactions in those who are sensitive to latex and an increased incidence of urinary tract infections. Toxic shock syndrome has been reported in some diaphragm users but is rare.

> ◢ **NURSING ALERT**
>
> The nurse must assess the woman for possible latex allergy because use of latex barrier methods (eg, diaphragm, cervical cap, male condoms) may cause severe allergic reactions, including anaphylaxis, in patients with latex allergy.

Cervical Cap

The cervical cap is much smaller (22 to 35 mm) than the diaphragm and covers only the cervix. If a woman can feel her cervix, she can usually learn to use a cervical cap. The

chief advantage is that the cap may be left in place for 2 days after coitus. Although convenient to use, the cervical cap may cause cervical irritation; therefore, before fitting a cap, most clinicians obtain a Pap smear and repeat the smear after 3 months. The cap is used with a spermicide and does not require additional spermicide for repeated intercourse.

Contraceptive Sponge

The sponge, another barrier method of contraception, is made of soft, disposable polyurethane foam that is moistened with water and inserted into the vagina before intercourse. It contains and releases a spermicide (eg, nonoxynol-9) that is continuously released into the vagina in small amounts through a 24-hour wear time. The sponge is left in place in the vagina for at least 6 hours after intercourse and can be kept in place for up to 24 additional hours without the need to replace it with repeated acts of intercourse during that period of time. The sponge is sold over the counter and does not require a prescription or special fitting by a health care provider. The sponge should not be used by women with allergy to polyurethane. It should not be used during menstruation. Women who have a history of toxic shock syndrome should not use the contraceptive sponge.

Female Condom

The female condom was developed to give control of barrier protection to women—to provide them with protection from STDs and HIV as well as pregnancy. The female condom (Reality) consists of a cylinder of polyurethane enclosed at one end by a closed ring that covers the cervix and at the other end by an open ring that covers the perineum (Fig. 46-7). (New, improved models are currently pending approval by the FDA.) Advantages include some degree of protection from STDs (HPV, herpes simplex virus, and HIV). Disadvantages include the inability to use the female condom with some positions (ie, standing). Women have found that it can be noisy and slippery.

Spermicides

Spermicides are made from nonoxynol-9 or octoxynol and are available over the counter as foams, gels, films, and suppositories and also on condoms. Spermicides do not protect women from HIV or other STDs (Alan Guttmacher Institute, 2008). In fact, nonoxynol-9 has been found to be associated with minute tears in vaginal tissue with frequent use (eg, daily), possibly increasing the possibility of contracting HIV from an infected partner.

Male Condom

The male condom is an impermeable, snug-fitting cover applied to the erect penis before it enters the vaginal canal. The tip of the condom is pinched while being applied to leave space for ejaculate. If no space is left, ejaculation may cause a tear or hole in the condom and reduce its effectiveness. The penis, with the condom held in place, is removed from the vagina while still erect to prevent the ejaculate from leaking. Condoms are now available in large and small sizes.

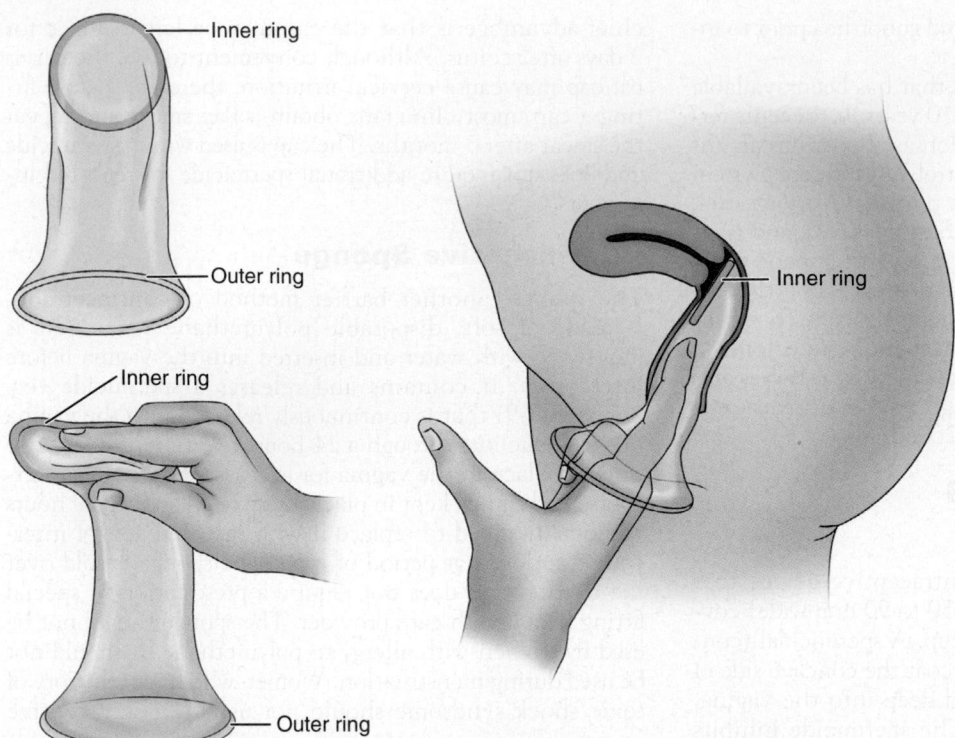

Figure 46-7 Female condom. To insert the female condom, hold the inner ring between the thumb and middle finger. Put the index finger on the pouch between the thumb and other fingers and squeeze the ring. Slide the condom into the vagina as far as it will go. The inner ring keeps the condom in place.

The latex condom also creates a barrier against transmission of STDs (gonorrhea, chlamydial infection, and HIV) by body fluids and may reduce the risk of herpes virus transmission. However, natural condoms (those made from animal tissue) do not protect against HIV infection. Nurses need to reassure women that they have a right to insist that their male partners use condoms and a right to refuse sex without condoms, although women in abusive relationships may increase their risk of abuse by doing so. Some women carry condoms with them to be certain that one is available. Nurses should be familiar and comfortable with instructions about using condoms because many women need to know about this way of protecting themselves from HIV and other STDs. Condoms do not provide complete protection from STDs because HPV may be transmitted by skin-to-skin contact. Other STDs may be transmitted if any abraded skin is exposed to body fluids. This information should be included in patient teaching.

The nurse needs to consider the possibility of latex allergy. Swelling and itching can also occur. Possible warning signs of latex allergy include oral itching after blowing up a balloon or eating kiwis, bananas, pineapples, passion fruit, avocados, or chestnuts. Because many contraceptives are made of latex, patients who experience burning or itching while using latex contraceptives are instructed to see their primary health care provider. Alternatives to latex condoms may include the female condom (Reality) and the male condom (Avanti), made of polyurethane.

COITUS INTERRUPTUS OR WITHDRAWAL

Coitus interruptus (removing the penis from the vagina before ejaculation) requires careful control by the male partner. Although it is a frequently used method of preventing pregnancy and better than no method, it is considered an unreliable method of contraception.

RHYTHM AND NATURAL METHODS

Natural family planning is any method of conception regulation that is based on awareness of signs and symptoms of fertility during a menstrual cycle. The advantages of natural contraceptive methods include: (1) they are not hazardous to health, (2) they are inexpensive, and (3) they are approved by some religions that do not approve of other methods of contraception. The disadvantage is that they require discipline by the couple, who must monitor the menstrual cycle and abstain from sex during the fertile phase.

Current methods include the calendar method, the basal body temperature method, the ovulation method, and the symptothermal method. The calendar and basal body temperature methods are older than the ovulation method and the symptothermal method. Combinations of these methods are often used (Fehring, Schneider, Raviele, et al., 2007). The fertile phase (in which sexual abstinence is required) is estimated to occur about 14 days before menstruation, although it may occur between the 10th and 17th days. Spermatozoa can fertilize an ovum up to 72 hours after intercourse, and the ovum can be fertilized for 24 hours after leaving the ovary. The pregnancy rate with the rhythm (ie, calendar) method is about 40% yearly.

Women who carefully determine their "safe period," based on a precise recording of menstrual dates for at least 1 year, and who follow a carefully worked-out formula may achieve very effective protection. A long abstinence period during each cycle is required. These prerequisites require more time and control than many couples have. Changes in cervical mucus and basal body temperature due to hormonal changes related to ovulation form the scientific basis for the sympothermal method of ovulatory timing. Courses in natural family planning are offered at many Catholic hospitals and some family planning clinics.

Ovulation detection methods (eg, Clearblue Easy Fertility Monitor) are available in most pharmacies. The presence of the enzyme guaiacol peroxidase in cervical mucus signals ovulation 6 days beforehand and also affects mucosal viscosity. Over-the-counter test kits are easy to use and reliable but can be expensive. Ovulation prediction kits are more effective for planning conception than for avoiding it. But if they are used in combination with cervical mucus changes and the calendar method, they may be effective; further research is needed (Fehring, et al., 2007).

Douching is not a contraceptive method and may enhance rather than decrease the chances of conception.

EMERGENCY CONTRACEPTION

The need for emergency contraception may arise after an episode of unprotected sexual intercourse. Therefore, nurses need to be aware of emergency contraception as an option for women and the indications for its use. It is clearly not suitable for long-term avoidance of pregnancy because it is not as effective as oral contraceptives or other reliable methods used regularly. However, it is valuable following intercourse when a pregnancy is not intended and in emergency situations such as rape, a defective or torn condom or diaphragm, or other situations that may result in unwanted conception. Women need to be made aware of emergency contraception and how to obtain it.

Methods of Emergency Contraception

Hormonal Methods

A properly timed, adequate dose of estrogen and a progestin or progestin-only medication after intercourse without effective contraception, or when a method has failed, can prevent pregnancy by inhibiting or delaying ovulation. This method does not interrupt an established pregnancy and does not cause an abortion.

Generally, emergency contraception is currently available only with prescription and is not available over the counter. Emergency contraceptives may be dispensed by pharmacists without a prescription in some states. The sooner emergency contraception is taken, the more effective it is. It is considered safe and effective by the FDA and can be prescribed or purchased as Plan B (progestin only) packages of emergency contraception with patient literature. It can also be prescribed as a specific number of contraceptive pills, depending on the medication and dose used.

This method must be used not more than 5 days following intercourse. Nausea, a common side effect, can be minimized by taking the medication with meals and with an antiemetic agent. Other side effects, such as breast soreness and irregular bleeding, may occur but are transient. Patients who use this method should be advised of the potential failure rate and also counseled about other contraceptive methods. There are no known contraindications to the use of this method, except an established pregnancy (Allen & Goldberg, 2007).

The nurse reviews with the patient instructions for emergency contraception based on the medication regimen prescribed. If the woman is breastfeeding, a progestin-only formulation is prescribed. To avoid exposing infants to synthetic hormones through breast milk, the patient can manually express milk and bottle feed for 24 hours after treatment. The patient should be informed that her next menstrual period may begin a few days earlier or a few days later than expected. She is instructed to return for a pregnancy test if she has not had a menstrual period in 3 weeks and should be offered another visit to provide a regular method of contraception if she does not have one currently.

Postcoital Intrauterine Device Insertion

Postcoital IUD insertion, another form of emergency contraception, involves insertion of a copper-bearing IUD within 5 days of coitus in women who want this method of contraception; however, it may be inappropriate for some women or if contraindications exist. The mechanism of action is unknown, but it is thought that the IUD interferes with fertilization (Allen & Goldberg, 2007). The patient may experience discomfort on insertion and may have heavier menstrual periods and increased cramping. Contraindications include a confirmed or suspected pregnancy or any contraindication to regular copper IUD use. The patient must be informed that there is a risk that insertion of an IUD may disrupt a pregnancy that is already present.

Nursing Management

Patients who use emergency contraception may be anxious, embarrassed, and lacking information about birth control. The nurse must be supportive and nonjudgmental and provide facts and appropriate patient teaching. If the patient repeatedly uses this method of birth control, she should be informed that the failure rate with this method is higher than with a regularly used method. A toll-free telephone information service (1-888-NOT-2-LATE) operates 24 hours a day in English and Spanish and provides information and referrals to health care providers. Nurses can educate and inform women about emergency contraception options to reduce unwanted pregnancies and abortions. See the list of resources at the end of this chapter for more information.

Abortion

Interruption of pregnancy or expulsion of the product of conception before the fetus is viable is called abortion. The fetus is generally considered to be viable any time after the 5th to 6th month of gestation.

SPONTANEOUS ABORTION

It is estimated that 1 of every 5 to 10 conceptions ends in spontaneous abortion. Most of these occur because an abnormality in the fetus makes survival impossible. Other causes may include systemic diseases, hormonal imbalance, or anatomic abnormalities. If a pregnant woman experiences bleeding and cramping, a threatened abortion is diagnosed because an actual abortion is usually imminent.

Spontaneous abortion occurs most commonly in the 2nd or 3rd month of gestation.

There are various types of spontaneous abortion, depending on the nature of the process (threatened, inevitable, incomplete, or complete). In a threatened abortion, the cervix does not dilate. With bed rest and conservative treatment, the abortion may be prevented. If not, an abortion is imminent. If only some of the tissue is passed, the abortion is referred to as incomplete. An emptying or evacuation procedure (D & C, or dilation and evacuation [D & E]) or administration of oral misoprostol (Cytotec) is usually required to remove the remaining tissue. If the fetus and all related tissue are spontaneously evacuated, the abortion is termed complete, and no further treatment is required.

Habitual Abortion

Habitual or recurrent abortion is defined as successive, repeated, spontaneous abortions of unknown cause. As many as 60% of abortions may result from chromosomal anomalies. After two consecutive abortions, the patient is referred for genetic counseling and testing and other possible causes are explored.

If bleeding occurs in a pregnant woman with a past history of habitual abortion, conservative measures, such as bed rest and administration of progesterone to support the endometrium, are attempted to save the pregnancy. Supportive counseling is crucial in this stressful condition. Bed rest, sexual abstinence, a light diet, and no straining on defecation may be recommended in an effort to prevent spontaneous abortion. If infection is suspected, antibiotics may be prescribed.

In the condition known as incompetent or dysfunctional cervix, the cervix dilates painlessly in the second trimester of pregnancy, often resulting in a spontaneous abortion. In such cases, a surgical procedure called cervical cerclage may be used to prevent the cervix from dilating prematurely, although its effectiveness is unclear. It involves placing a purse-string suture around the cervix at the level of the internal os. Bed rest is usually advised to keep the weight of the uterus off the cervix. About 2 to 3 weeks before term or at the onset of labor, the suture is cut. Delivery is usually by cesarean section.

Medical Management

After a spontaneous abortion, all tissue passed vaginally is saved for examination if possible. The patient and all personnel who care for her are alerted to save any discharged material. In the rare case of heavy bleeding, the patient may require blood component transfusions and fluid replacement. An estimate of the bleeding volume can be determined by recording the number of perineal pads and the degree of saturation over 24 hours. When an incomplete abortion occurs, oxytocin may be prescribed to cause uterine contractions before D & E or uterine suctioning.

Nursing Management

Because patients experience loss and anxiety, emotional support and understanding are important aspects of nursing care. Women may be grieving or relieved, depending on their feelings about the pregnancy. Providing opportunities for the patient to talk and express her emotions is helpful and also provides clues for the nurse in planning more specific care.

ELECTIVE ABORTION

A voluntary induced termination of pregnancy is called an elective abortion and is usually performed by skilled health care providers. In 1973, the U.S. Supreme Court in *Roe v. Wade* ruled that decisions about abortion reside with a woman and her physician in the first trimester. During the second trimester, the state may regulate practice in the interest of a woman's health, and during the final weeks of pregnancy may choose to protect the life of the fetus, except when necessary to preserve the life or health of the woman.

The U.S. rate of abortion is among the highest in the industrialized Western world. These numbers indicate the need for effective contraceptive education, information about emergency contraception, and counseling.

Medical Management

Before the abortion procedure is performed (Chart 46-15), a nurse or counselor trained in pregnancy counseling should talk with the patient and explore her fears, feelings, and options. The nurse then identifies the patient's choice (ie, continuing pregnancy and parenthood; continuing pregnancy followed by adoption; or terminating pregnancy by abortion). If abortion is chosen, the patient has a pelvic examination to determine uterine size. A pelvic ultrasound may also be performed. Laboratory studies before an abortion must include a pregnancy test to confirm the pregnancy, hematocrit to rule out anemia, and Rh determination. Patients with anemia may need an iron supplement, and patients who are Rh-negative may require RhoGAM to prevent isoimmunization. Before the procedure, all patients should be screened for STDs to prevent introducing pathogens upward through the cervix during the procedure.

> ▶ **NURSING ALERT**
>
> Women who have resorted to unskilled attempts to end a pregnancy are often critically ill because of infection, hemorrhage, or uterine rupture. If a woman has undergone such efforts to end a pregnancy, prompt medical attention, broad-spectrum antibiotics, and replacement of fluids and blood components may be required before careful attempts are made to evacuate the uterus.

Surgical terminations include D & C or vacuum aspiration of uterine contents. Medications can also be used. Mifepristone (RU-486, Mifeprex) is used only in early pregnancy (up to 49 days from the last menstrual period). It works by blocking progesterone. Cramping and bleeding similar to a heavy menstrual period occur. After counseling and consent and often a sonogram to confirm the pregnancy, mifepristone is administered. This is followed by a dose of misoprostol orally or vaginally. If the pregnancy persists, a suction aspiration is performed. Contraindications include ectopic pregnancy, adrenal failure, allergy to the medications, bleeding disorder, irritable bowel syndrome, or uncontrolled seizure disorders. Several deaths from sepsis have occurred following medical abortion; researchers and the FDA

Chart 46-15 • *Types of Elective Abortions*

Vacuum Aspiration

- The cervix is dilated manually with instrumentation or by laminaria (small suppositories made of seaweed that swells as it absorbs water).
- A uterine aspirator is introduced.
- Suction is applied, and tissue is removed from the uterus.

This is the most common type of termination procedure and is used early in pregnancy, up to 14 weeks. Laminaria may be used to soften and dilate the cervix prior to the procedure.

Dilation and Evacuation

Cervical dilation with laminaria followed by vacuum aspiration

Labor Induction

These procedures account for less than 1% of all terminations and generally take place in an inpatient setting.
1. Installation of saline or urea results in uterine contractions.
   - Although rare, serious complications can occur, including cardiovascular collapse, cerebral edema, pulmonary edema, renal failure, and disseminated intravascular coagulopathy (DIC).
2. Prostaglandins
   - Prostaglandins are introduced into the amniotic fluid or by vaginal suppository or intramuscular injection in later pregnancy.
   - Strong uterine contractions begin within 4 hours and usually result in abortion.
   - Gastrointestinal side effects (eg, nausea, vomiting, diarrhea, and abdominal cramping) and fever can occur.
3. Intravenous oxytocin
   Used for later abortions for genetic indications. Requires patient to go through labor.

Medical Abortion

Mifepristone

- Mifepristone (formerly known as RU-486) is a progesterone antagonist that prevents implantation of the ovum.
- Administered orally within 10 days of an expected menstrual period, mifepristone produces a medical abortion in most patients.
- Combined with a prostaglandin suppository, mifepristone causes abortion in up to 95% of patients.
- Prolonged bleeding may occur. Other side effects may include abdominal pain, nausea, vomiting, and diarrhea. This method may not be used in women with adrenal failure, asthma, long-term corticosteroid therapy, an IUD in place, porphyria, or a history of allergy to mifepristone or other prostaglandins. It is less effective when used in pregnancies more than 49 days from the beginning of the last menstrual period.

Methotrexate

- Methotrexate has also been used to terminate pregnancy because it is a teratogen that is lethal to the fetus. It has been found to have minimal risk and few side effects in the woman. Its low cost may provide an alternative for some women.

Misoprostol

- Misoprostol is a synthetic prostaglandin analog that produces cervical effacement and uterine contractions.
- Inserted vaginally, misoprostol is effective in terminating a pregnancy in about 75% of cases.
- When combined with methotrexate or mifepristone, misoprostol's effectiveness rate is high.

---

are closely monitoring the morbidity and mortality associated with medical abortion. Currently, there is no evidence that a previous medical or surgical abortion increases the risk of adverse future pregnancy outcomes (Virk, Zhang & Olsen, 2007).

Nursing Management

Patient teaching is an important aspect of care for women who elect to terminate a pregnancy. A patient undergoing elective abortion is informed about what the procedure entails and the expected course after the procedure. The patient is scheduled for a follow-up appointment 2 weeks after the procedure and is instructed about signs and symptoms (ie, fever, heavy bleeding, or pain) that should be reported.

Available contraceptive methods are reviewed with the patient at this time. Effectiveness depends on the method used and the extent to which the woman and her partner follow the instructions for use. A woman who has used any method of birth control should be assessed for her understanding of the method and its potential side effects as well as her satisfaction with the method. If the woman has not been using contraception, the nurse explains all methods and their benefits and risks and helps the patient make a contraceptive choice for use after abortion. Related teaching issues, such as the need to use barrier contraceptive devices (ie, condoms) for protection against transmission of STDs and HIV infection and the availability of emergency contraception, are becoming increasingly important.

Psychological support is another important aspect of nursing care. The nurse needs to be aware that women terminate pregnancies for many reasons. Some women terminate pregnancies because of severe genetic defects. Women who have been raped or impregnated in incestuous relationships or by an abusive partner may elect to terminate their pregnancies. The care of a woman undergoing termination of pregnancy is stressful, and assistance needs to be provided in a safe and nonjudgmental way. Nurses have the right to refuse to participate in a procedure that is against their religious beliefs but are professionally obligated not to impose their beliefs or judgments on their patients.

Infertility

Infertility is defined as a couple's inability to achieve pregnancy after 1 year of unprotected intercourse. Primary infertility refers to a couple who has never had a child. Secondary infertility means that at least one conception has occurred, but currently the couple cannot achieve a pregnancy. In the United States, infertility affects 6 million couples. It is often a complex physical problem, and its causes are usually related to azoospermia, anovulation, or tubal obstruction.

Pathophysiology

Ovarian and Ovulation Factors

Diagnostic studies performed to determine if ovulation is regular and whether the progestational endometrium is adequate for implantation may include a serum progesterone level and an ovulation index. The ovulation index involves a urine-stick test to determine whether the surge in LH that precedes follicular rupture has occurred. Ovulatory dysfunction is complex, but many women with ovulation disorders have polycystic ovary syndrome, described in Chapter 47, and may be treated with clomiphene (Clomid) to induce ovulation or insulin sensitizing agents. Once insulin levels are normalized, ovulation often occurs. Some women have high prolactin levels, which inhibit ovulation, and they are treated with dopaminergic drugs after a pituitary adenoma is ruled out by MRI. If a woman has premature ovarian failure, oocyte donation may be considered.

Tubal and Uterine Factors

HSG is used to rule out uterine or tubal abnormalities. A contrast agent injected into the uterus through the cervix produces an outline of the shape of the uterine cavity and the patency of the tubes. This process sometimes removes mucus or tissue that is lodged in the tubes. Laparoscopy permits direct visualization of the tubes and other pelvic structures and can assist in identifying conditions that may interfere with fertility (eg, endometriosis).

Fibroids, polyps, and congenital malformations are possible causative factors affecting the uterus. Their presence may be determined by pelvic examination, hysteroscopy, saline sonogram (a variation of a sonogram), and HSG. Endometriosis, even if mild, is associated with reduced fertility.

Male Factors

An analysis of semen provides information about the number of sperm (density), percentage of moving forms, quality of forward movement (forward progression), and morphology (shape and form). From 2 to 6 mL of watery alkaline semen is normal. A normal count has 60 to 100 million sperm/mL. However, the incidence of impregnation is lessened only when the count decreases to less than 20 million sperm/mL.

Men may also be affected by varicoceles, varicose veins around the testicle, which decrease semen quality by increasing testicular temperature. Retrograde ejaculation or ejaculation into the bladder is assessed by urinalysis after ejaculation. Blood tests for male partners may include measuring testosterone; FSH and LH (both of which are involved in maintaining testicular function); and prolactin levels.

Medical Management

The treatment of infertility is complex and often requires advanced technology. The specific type of treatment depends on the cause of the problem, if it can be identified. Many infertile couples have normal test results for ovulation, sperm production, and fallopian tube patency.

Pharmacologic Therapy

Pharmacologically induced ovulation is undertaken when women do not ovulate on their own or ovulate irregularly. Women older than 37 years are less likely to be fertile. These couples are often treated with clomiphene to stimulate ovulation. Gonadotropin treatment may also be used if conception does not occur. Various other medications are used, depending on the primary cause of infertility (Chart 46-16).

CHART 46-16

PHARMACOLOGY
Medications That Induce Ovulation

- Clomiphene citrate (Clomid, Serophene) is an estrogen antagonist that increases gonadotropin release, resulting in follicular rupture or ovulation. Clomiphene is used when the hypothalamus is not stimulating the pituitary gland to release follicle-stimulating hormone (FSH) and luteinizing hormone (LH). This medication stimulates follicles in the ovary. It is usually taken for 5 days beginning on the 5th day of the menstrual cycle. Ovulation should occur 4 to 8 days after the last dose. Patients receive instructions about timing intercourse to facilitate fertilization.
- Menotropins (Repronex, Pergonal), a combination of FSH and LH, may be used to stimulate the ovaries to produce eggs. These agents are used for women with deficiencies in FSH and LH. When followed by administration of human chorionic gonadotropin, menotropins stimulates the ovaries, so monitoring by ultrasound and hormone levels is essential because overstimulation may occur.
- Follitropin-alpha (Gonal-F), follitropin-beta (Follistim), and urofollitropin (Bravelle) may be used to treat ovulation disorders or to stimulate a follicle and egg production for

intrauterine insemination or in vitro fertilization or other assisted reproductive technologies.
- Gonadotropin-releasing hormone agonists (leuprolide [Lupron, Synarel]) suppress FSH, prevent premature egg release, and shrink fibroids.
- Bromocriptine (Parlodel) may be used in treatment of infertility due to elevated prolactin levels.
- Progesterone (Prometrium Crinone, progesterone in oil) vaginal suppositories help improve the uterine lining after ovulation.
- Urofollitropin (Metrodin, Bravelle), which contains FSH with a small amount of LH, is used in some disorders (eg, polycystic ovarian syndrome) to stimulate follicle growth. Clomiphene is then used to stimulate ovulation.
- Chorionic gonadotropin (Ovidrel, Novarel, Pregnyl), which mimics LH, releases an egg after hyperstimulation and supports the corpus luteum.
- Metformin (Glucophage, Fortamet) may be used in polycystic ovarian syndrome to induce regular ovulation.
- Aspirin and heparin may be used to prevent recurrent pregnancy loss in patients with elevated antiphospholipid antibodies.

Blood tests and ultrasounds are used to monitor ovulation. Multiple pregnancies (ie, twins, triplets or more) may occur with use of these medications. Ovarian hyperstimulation syndrome (OHSS) may also occur. This condition is characterized by enlarged multicystic ovaries and is complicated by a shift of fluid from the intravascular space into the abdominal cavity. The fluid shift can result in ascites, pleural effusion, and edema; hypovolemia may also occur. Risk factors include younger age, history of polycystic ovarian syndrome, high serum estradiol levels, a larger number of follicles, and pregnancy.

Artificial Insemination

Artificial insemination is the deposit of semen into the female genital tract by artificial means. If the sperm cannot penetrate the cervical canal normally, artificial insemination using a partner's or husband's semen or that of a donor may be considered. When the sperm of the woman's partner is defective or absent (azoospermia) or when there is a risk of transmitting a genetic disease, donor sperm may be used. Safeguards are put in place to address legal, ethical, emotional, and religious issues. Written consent is obtained to protect all parties involved, including the woman, the donor, and the resulting child. The donor's semen is frozen, and the donor is evaluated to ensure that he is free of genetic disorders and STDs, including HIV infection.

Certain conditions must be met before semen is transferred to the vagina or uterus. The woman must have no abnormalities of the genital system, the fallopian tubes must be patent, and ova must be available. In the male, sperm need to be normal in shape, amount, motility, and endurance. The time of ovulation should be determined as accurately as possible so that the 2 or 3 days during which fertilization is possible each month can be targeted for treatment.

Ultrasonography and blood studies of varying hormone levels are used to pinpoint the best time for insemination and to monitor for OHSS. Fertilization seldom occurs from a single insemination. Usually, insemination is attempted between days 10 and 17 of the cycle; three different attempts may be made during one cycle. The woman may have received clomiphene or other medications to stimulate ovulation before insemination. The recipient is placed in the lithotomy position on the examination table, a speculum is inserted, and the vagina and cervix are swabbed with a cotton-tipped applicator to remove any excess secretions. The sperm are washed before insertion to remove biochemicals and to select the most active sperm. Semen is drawn into a sterile syringe, and a cannula is attached. The semen is then directed to the external os. In IUI, semen is placed into the uterine cavity.

In Vitro Fertilization

In vitro fertilization (IVF) involves ovarian stimulation, egg retrieval, fertilization, and embryo transfer. This procedure is accomplished by first stimulating the ovary to produce multiple eggs or ova, usually with medications, because success rates are greater with more than one embryo. Many different protocols exist for inducing ovulation with one or more agents. Patients are carefully selected and evaluated, and cycles are carefully monitored using ultrasound and monitoring hormone levels. At the appropriate time, the ova are recovered by transvaginal ultrasound retrieval. Sperm and eggs are coincubated for up to 36 hours, and the embryos are transferred about 48 hours after retrieval. Implantation should occur in 3 to 5 days.

Gamete intrafallopian transfer (GIFT), a variation of IVF, is the treatment of choice for patients with ovarian failure. GIFT is considered in unexplained infertility and when there is religion-based discomfort with IVF. The most common indications for IVF and GIFT are irreparable tubal damage, endometriosis, unexplained infertility, inadequate sperm, and exposure to DES. Success rates for GIFT vary from 20% to 30%.

Other Assisted Reproductive Technologies

In intracytoplasmic sperm injection (ICSI), an ovum is retrieved as described previously, and a single sperm is injected through the zona pellucida, through the egg membrane, and into the cytoplasm of the oocyte. The fertilized egg is then transferred back to the donor. ICSI is the treatment of choice in severe male factor infertility.

Women who cannot produce their own eggs (ie, premature ovarian failure) have the option of using the eggs of a donor after stimulation of the donor's ovaries. The recipient also receives hormones in preparation for these procedures. Couples may also choose this modality if the female partner has a genetic disorder that may be passed on to children.

Nursing Management

Nursing interventions that are appropriate when working with couples during infertility evaluations include assisting in reducing stress in the relationship, encouraging cooperation, protecting privacy, fostering understanding, and referring the couple to appropriate resources when necessary. Because infertility evaluations and treatments are expensive, time-consuming, invasive, stressful, and not always successful, couples need support in working together to deal with this process.

Resolve, Inc., a nonprofit self-help group that provides information and support for infertile patients, was founded by a nurse who experienced difficulty conceiving. The literature on infertility that is produced by this group is an important resource for patients and professionals. Most areas of the country have local support groups. More information can be obtained by visiting the Resolve Web site or contacting Resolve, Inc.

Smoking is strongly discouraged because it has an adverse effect on the success of assisted reproduction. Diet, exercise, stress reduction techniques, folic acid supplementation, health maintenance, and disease prevention are emphasized in many infertility programs. Couples may also consider adoption, child-free living, and gestational carriers (use of surrogate to carry the fetus for the infertile couple). Nurses can be helpful listeners and information resources in these deliberations.

Preconception/Periconception Health Care

Nurses can be instrumental in encouraging all women of childbearing age, including those with chronic illness or disabilities, to consider issues that may affect health during pregnancy (Smeltzer, 2007; Smeltzer & Wetzel-Effinger,

2009). Women who plan their pregnancies and are healthy and well informed tend to have better outcomes. This is an important issue because half of all pregnancies in the United States are unplanned.

Nurses can make a difference through education and counseling; preconception counseling can decrease the incidence of birth defects. Women who smoke should be encouraged to stop smoking, and it may help to offer smoking cessation classes. Women should take folic acid supplements to prevent neural tube defects. Women with diabetes should have good glycemic control prior to conception. It is necessary to assess rubella immunity and other immunizations as well as a family history of genetic defects; genetic counseling may be appropriate. Women taking teratogenic medications and women concerned about genetic disorders should be encouraged to discuss effective contraception and childbearing plans with their health care provider (see Chart 46-2).

Ectopic Pregnancy

The incidence of ectopic pregnancy and the risk of death due to ectopic pregnancy are decreasing. However, ectopic pregnancy remains the leading cause of pregnancy-related death in the first trimester. Ectopic pregnancy occurs when a fertilized ovum (a blastocyst) becomes implanted on any tissue other than the uterine lining (eg, the fallopian tube, ovary, abdomen, cervix or scar tissue from previous caesarean section). The most common site of ectopic implantation is the fallopian tube (Fig. 46-8).

Possible causes of ectopic pregnancy include salpingitis, peritubal adhesions (after pelvic infection, endometriosis, appendicitis), structural abnormalities of the fallopian tube (rare and usually related to DES exposure), previous ectopic pregnancy, previous tubal surgery, multiple previous induced abortions (particularly if followed by infection), tumors that distort the tube, and IUD and progestin-only contraceptives. PID appears to be the major risk factor. Improved antibiotic therapy for PID usually prevents total tubal closure but may leave a stricture or narrowing, predisposing to ectopic implantation. The odds of recurrent ectopic pregnancy are three times higher if an infectious pathology caused the first ectopic pregnancy. After a second ectopic pregnancy occurs, assisted reproduction is considered.

Risk factors are important, but all women need to be educated about early treatment and have a high index of suspicion in the case of a period that does not seem normal, the presence of pain, or pain with a suspected pregnancy. Women may have fatal hemorrhage with ruptured ectopic pregnancies if they delay seeking attention or if their health care providers are not alert to the possibility of this diagnosis.

Clinical Manifestations

Signs and symptoms vary depending on whether tubal rupture has occurred. Delay in menstruation from 1 to 2 weeks followed by slight bleeding (spotting) or a report of a slightly abnormal period suggests the possibility of an ectopic pregnancy. Symptoms may begin late, with vague soreness on the affected side (probably due to uterine contractions and distention of the tube), and may proceed to sharp, colicky pain. Most patients experience some pelvic or abdominal pain and some spotting or bleeding. Gastrointestinal symptoms, dizziness, or lightheadedness may occur. Patients may think the abnormal bleeding is a menstrual period, especially if a recent period occurred and was normal.

If implantation occurs in the fallopian tube, the tube becomes more and more distended and can rupture if the ectopic pregnancy remains undetected for 4 to 6 weeks or longer after conception. When the tube ruptures, the ovum is discharged into the abdominal cavity, and the woman experiences agonizing pain, dizziness, faintness, and nausea and vomiting due to the peritoneal reaction to blood escaping from the tube. Air hunger and symptoms of shock may occur, and the signs of hemorrhage—rapid and thready pulse, decreased blood pressure, subnormal temperature, restlessness, pallor, and sweating—are evident. Later, the pain becomes generalized in the abdomen and radiates to the shoulder and neck because of accumulating intraperitoneal blood that irritates the diaphragm.

Assessment and Diagnostic Findings

Ectopic pregnancies must be diagnosed promptly to prevent life-threatening hemorrhage, the major complication of rupture. During vaginal examination, a large mass of clotted blood that has collected in the pelvis behind the uterus or a tender adnexal mass may be palpable, although there are often no abnormal findings. If an ectopic pregnancy is suspected, the patient is evaluated by sonography and human chorionic gonadotropin (hCG) levels. If the ultrasound results are inconclusive, the hCG test is repeated. The levels of hCG (the diagnostic hormone of pregnancy) double in early normal pregnancies every 3 days but are reduced in abnormal or ectopic pregnancies. A less-than-normal increase is cause for suspicion. Serum progesterone levels are also measured. Levels less than 5 ng/mL are considered abnormal; levels greater than 25 ng/mL are associated with a normally developing pregnancy.

Ultrasound, the usual method of diagnosis, can detect a pregnancy between 5 and 6 weeks from the time of the last menstrual period. Detectable fetal heart movement outside

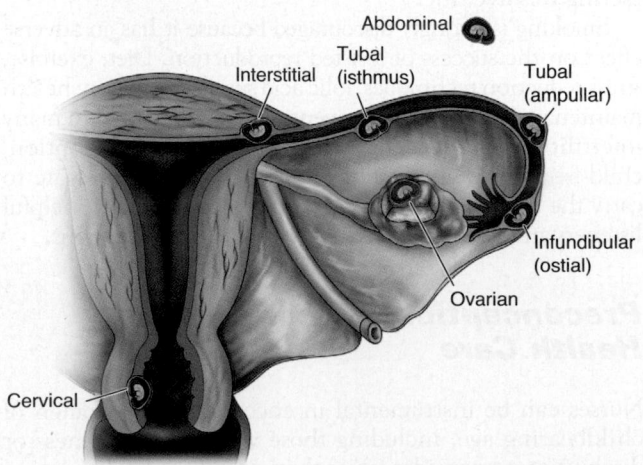

Abdominal

Tubal
(isthmus)

Interstitial

Tubal
(ampullar)

Infundibular
(ostial)

Ovarian

Cervical

Figure 46-8 Sites of ectopic pregnancy.

the uterus on ultrasound is firm evidence of an ectopic pregnancy. On occasion, an ultrasound study is not definitive and the diagnosis must be made with combined diagnostic aids (beta-hCG and progesterone levels, ultrasound, pelvic examination, and clinical judgment).

Occasionally, the clinical picture makes the diagnosis relatively easy. However, when the clinical signs and symptoms are inconclusive, which is often the case, other procedures may be needed. Laparoscopy can be used because the physician can visually detect an unruptured tubal pregnancy and thereby circumvent the risk of its rupture.

Medical Management

Surgical Management

When surgery is performed early, almost all patients recover rapidly; if tubal rupture occurs, mortality increases. The type of surgery is determined by the size and extent of local tubal damage. Conservative surgery includes "milking" an ectopic pregnancy from the tube. Resection of the involved fallopian tube with end-to-end anastomosis may be effective. Some surgeons attempt to salvage the tube with a salpingotomy, which involves opening and evacuating the tube and controlling bleeding. More extensive surgery includes removing the tube alone (salpingectomy) or with the ovary (salpingo-oophorectomy). Depending on the amount of blood lost, blood component therapy and treatment of hemorrhagic shock may be necessary before and during surgery. Surgery may also be indicated in women unlikely to comply with close monitoring or those who live too far away from a health care facility to obtain the monitoring needed with nonsurgical management.

Methotrexate (Trexall), a chemotherapeutic agent and folic acid antagonist, may be used after surgery to treat any remaining embryonic or early pregnancy tissue, as indicated by a persistent or increasing beta-hCG level. The beta-hCG test is repeated 2 weeks after surgery to ensure that the level is decreasing.

Pharmacologic Therapy

Another option is the use of methotrexate without surgery. Because methotrexate stops the pregnancy from progressing by interfering with DNA synthesis and the multiplication of cells, it interrupts early, small, unruptured ectopic pregnancies. The patient must be hemodynamically stable, have no active renal or hepatic disease, have no evidence of thrombocytopenia or leukopenia, and have a very small, unruptured ectopic pregnancy on ultrasound. Other indications may include no fetal cardiac activity, no active bleeding, and a beta-hCG level of less than 2000 mIU/mL. The medication is administered intramuscularly or orally. Some patients may be treated with intratubal injection of methotrexate. Complete blood count and tests of liver and renal function are conducted to monitor the patient; blood typing is performed in anticipation of the need for transfusions.

Until the pregnancy is resolved, the patient is advised to refrain from alcohol, intercourse, and vitamins containing folic acid, because these may exacerbate the adverse effects of methotrexate. Abdominal pain may occur within 5 to 10 days and may indicate termination of the pregnancy. This requires careful assessment by the health care provider. Serum levels of beta-hCG are monitored carefully, and these levels should gradually decrease. Ultrasound may also be used for monitoring. Side effects of methotrexate include abdominal cramping, mucositis, and renal and hepatic damage. Allergic reactions have occurred in patients receiving high doses.

NURSING PROCESS

THE PATIENT WITH AN ECTOPIC PREGNANCY

Assessment

The health history includes the menstrual pattern and any (even slight) bleeding since the last menstrual period. The nurse elicits the patient's description of pain and its location. The nurse asks the patient whether any sharp, colicky pains have occurred. Then the nurse notes whether pain radiates to the shoulder and neck (possibly caused by rupture and pressure on the diaphragm).

In addition, the nurse monitors vital signs, level of consciousness, and the nature and amount of vaginal bleeding. If possible, the nurse assesses how the patient is coping with the abnormal pregnancy and likely loss.

Diagnosis

Nursing Diagnoses

Based on the assessment data, major nursing diagnoses may include the following:

- Acute pain related to the progression of the tubal pregnancy
- Anticipatory grieving related to the loss of pregnancy and effect on future pregnancies
- Deficient knowledge related to the treatment and effect on future pregnancies

Collaborative Problems/Potential Complications

Based on the assessment data, major complications may include the following:

- Hemorrhage
- Hemorrhagic shock

Planning and Goals

The major goals may include relief of pain; acceptance and resolution of grief and pregnancy loss; increased knowledge about ectopic pregnancy, its treatment, and its outcome; and absence of complications.

Nursing Interventions

Relieving Pain

The abdominal pain associated with ectopic pregnancy may be described as cramping or severe continuous pain. If the patient is to have surgery, preanesthetic medications may provide pain relief. Postoperatively, analgesic agents are administered liberally; this promotes early ambulation and enables the patient to cough and take deep breaths.

Supporting the Grieving Process

Patients' distress levels vary. If the pregnancy was desired, loss may or may not be expressed verbally by the patient and her partner. The impact may not be fully realized until much later. The nurse should be available to listen and provide support. The patient's partner, if appropriate, should participate in this process. Even if the pregnancy was unplanned, a loss has been experienced, and a grief reaction may occur.

Monitoring and Managing Potential Complications

Potential complications of ectopic pregnancy are hemorrhage and shock. Careful assessment is essential to detect the development of these complications. Continuous monitoring of vital signs, level of consciousness, amount of bleeding, and intake and output provides information about the possibility of hemorrhage and the need to prepare for intravenous (IV) therapy. Bed rest is indicated. Hematocrit, hemoglobin, and blood gases are monitored to assess hematologic status and adequacy of tissue perfusion. Significant deviations in these laboratory values are reported immediately, and the patient is prepared for possible surgery. Blood component therapy may be required if blood loss has been rapid and extensive. If hypovolemic shock occurs, the treatment is directed toward reestablishing tissue perfusion and adequate blood volume. See Chapter 15 for a discussion of the IV fluids and medications used in treating shock.

The nurse has an important role in prevention by being alert to patients with abnormal bleeding who may be at risk for an ectopic pregnancy and referring them immediately for care. It is necessary to keep a high index of suspicion in daily practice when a woman of childbearing age, particularly one who is not using an effective method of contraception consistently, reports abdominal discomfort or abnormal bleeding.

Promoting Home and Community-Based Care

TEACHING PATIENTS SELF-CARE. If the patient has experienced life-threatening hemorrhage and shock, these complications are addressed and treated before any in-depth teaching can begin. At this time, the patient's and the nurse's attention is focused on the crisis, not on learning. At a later time, the patient begins to ask questions about what happened and why certain procedures were performed. Procedures are explained in terms that the distressed and apprehensive patient can understand. The patient's partner is included in teaching and explanations when possible. After the patient recovers from postoperative discomfort, it may be more appropriate to address any questions and concerns that she and her partner have, including the effect of this pregnancy or its treatment on future pregnancies. The patient should be advised that ectopic pregnancies may recur. The patient is informed about possible complications and instructed to report early signs and symptoms. It is important to review signs and symptoms with the patient and instruct her to report an abnormal menstrual period promptly.

CONTINUING CARE. Because of the risk of subsequent ectopic pregnancies, the patient is advised to seek preconception counseling before considering future pregnancies and to seek early prenatal care. Follow-up contact allows the nurse to answer questions and clarify information for the patient and her partner.

Evaluation

Expected Patient Outcomes

Expected patient outcomes may include:

1. Experiences relief of pain
   a. Reports a decrease in pain and discomfort
   b. Ambulates as prescribed; performs coughing and deep breathing
2. Begins to accept loss of pregnancy and expresses grief by verbalizing feelings and reactions to loss
3. Verbalizes an understanding of the causes of ectopic pregnancy
4. Experiences no complications
   a. Exhibits no signs of bleeding, hemorrhage, or shock
   b. Has decreased amounts of discharge (on perineal pad)
   c. Has normal skin color and turgor
   d. Exhibits stable vital signs and adequate urine output
   e. Levels of beta-hCG return to normal

CRITICAL THINKING EXERCISES

EBP **1** A 50-year-old woman has been experiencing severe hot flashes and resultant insomnia. She is considering beginning hormone therapy (HT) but is concerned about its risks. What information would you give to her? What is the evidence base for that information? What criteria would you use to assess the strength of the evidence? What resources would you recommend to her?

2 A 19-year-old female college student comes to the student health clinic for a gynecologic examination because she anticipates having sex with her new girlfriend. She asks you for advice about avoiding sexually transmitted diseases. What advice would you give her? How would you modify your teaching if she informed you that her new partner has other partners? What other teaching would you provide?

EBP **3** You are working in a women's health practice and are responsible for educating women about menopause and health promotion. Your 48-year-old patient has mild diabetes, and she is obese and has hypertension. She takes oral antidiabetic and antihypertensive medications. She reports that she has a strong family history of heart disease. She is concerned about menopause because her mother and sisters experienced "difficult" menopause. She indicates that she has little time for exercise and eats mostly fast food because of her high-pressure job. What health promotion strategies would you suggest to assist the patient in improving her health status as she approaches menopause? What is the evidence base for those strategies? How would you use that evidence to develop a teaching plan for her?

4 At a health clinic, you meet a 45-year-old woman with postpolio syndrome who uses a battery-powered scooter most of the time because of increasing muscle weakness. She is approaching menopause and is concerned about how her physical limitations secondary to postpolio syndrome might affect her health related to menopause. Describe what health promotion issues would be relevant and the actions, including patient teaching, that are warranted.

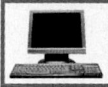 The Smeltzer suite offers these additional resources to enhance learning and facilitate understanding of this chapter:

- thePoint online resource, thepoint.lww.com/Smeltzer12E
- Student CD-ROM included with the book
- *Study Guide to Accompany Brunner & Suddarth's Textbook of Medical-Surgical Nursing*

REFERENCES AND SELECTED READINGS

Asterisk indicates nursing research.
**Double asterisk indicates classic reference.*

Books

American Cancer Society. (2009). *Cancer facts and figures 2009.* Atlanta: Author.

Andrews, M. & Boyle, J. (Eds.). (2007). *Transcultural concepts in nursing care* (5th ed.). Philadelphia: Lippincott William & Wilkins.

**Annon, J. S. (1974). *The behavioral treatment of sexual problems* (1st ed.). Honolulu, HI: Enabling Systems.

Gibbs, R. S., Karlan, B. Y., Haney, A. F., et al. (2008). *Danforth's obstetrics and gynecology* (10th ed.). Philadelphia: Lippincott Williams & Wilkins.

Hawkins, J., Roberto-Nichols, D. & Stanley-Haney, J. (2007). *Protocols for nurse practitioners in gynecologic settings* (9th ed.). New York: Tiresias Press.

Katz, V. L., Lentz, G., Lobo, R. A., et al. (2007). *Comprehensive gynecology: Text with online access.* St. Louis: Mosby Elsevier.

National Osteoporosis Foundation. (2008). *Clinician's guide to prevention and treatment of osteoporosis.* Washington, DC: Author.

North American Menopause Society (2007) *Menopause practice: A clinician's guide.* Cleveland, OH: Author.

Orshan, S. (2006). *Maternal newborn and women's health nursing: Comprehensive care across the life span.* Philadelphia: Lippincott Williams & Wilkins.

Porth, C. M. & Matfin, G. (2009). *Pathophysiology: Concepts of altered health states* (8th ed.). Philadelphia: Lippincott Williams & Wilkins.

Smeltzer, S. C. & Sharts-Hopko, N. C. (2005). *A providers' guide for the care of women with physical disabilities and chronic health conditions.* Chapel Hill, NC: North Carolina Office on Disability & Health.

Speroff, L. & Darney, P. A. (2005). *Clinical guide for contraception* (4th ed.). Philadelphia: Lippincott Williams & Wilkins.

Speroff, L. & Fritz, M. (2005). *Clinical gynecologic endocrinology and infertility* (7th ed.). Philadelphia: Lippincott Williams & Wilkins.

U.S. Department of Health and Human Services. (2005). *The surgeon general's call to action to improve the health and wellness of persons with disabilities.* Rockville, MD: Author.

World Health Organization Department of Reproductive Health and Research (WHO/RHR) and Johns Hopkins Bloomberg School of Public Health/Center for Communication Programs (CCP), INFO Project. (2007). *Family planning: A global handbook for providers.* Baltimore and Geneva: Author.

Journals and Electronic Documents

General

American College of Obstetricians and Gynecologists (ACOG). (2006a). ACOG Committee on Gynecologic Practice. Routine cancer screening. ACOG Committee Opinion No. 356. *Obstetrics & Gynecology, 108*(6), 1611–1622.

Beyene, Y., Gilliss, C. & Lee, K. (2007). "I take the good with the bad, and I moisturize": Defying middle age in the new millennium. *Menopause: Journal of the North American Menopause Society, 14*(4), 734–741.

Centers for Disease Control and Prevention (CDC). (2006). Sexually transmitted diseases treatment guidelines, 2006. *MMWR Morbidity and Mortality Weekly Report, 55*(RR-11), 1–94.

Centers for Disease Control and Prevention (CDC). (2007). Update to CDC's *Sexually transmitted diseases treatment guidelines, 2006.* Fluoroquinolones no longer recommended for treatment of gonococcal infections. *MMWR Morbidity and Mortality Weekly Report, 56*(14), 332–336.

Dormire, S. & Becker, H. (2007). Menopause health decision support for women with physical disabilities. *Journal of Obstetric, Gynecologic & Neonatal Nursing, 36*(1), 97–104.

Katz, A. (2007). When sex hurts: Menopause-related dyspareunia. Vaginal dryness and atrophy can be treated. *American Journal of Nursing, 107*(7), 34–36, 39.

*Lee, K. A. (2009). Sleep in midlife women. *Journal of Obstetric, Gynecologic, & Neonatal Nursing, 38*(3), 331–332.

*Minarik, P. A. (2009). Sleep disturbance in midlife women. *Journal of Obstetric, Gynecologic, & Neonatal Nursing, 38*(3), 333–343.

North American Menopause Society. (2007). *Menopause core curriculum study guide.* Cleveland: Author. Available at: www.menopause.org

Oriet, P., Cudney, S. & Weinert, C. L. (2007). *NursePractitioner, 32*(6), 37–40.

Sarrel, P. M. (2005). Sexual dysfunction: Treat or refer. *Obstetrics & Gynecology, 106*(4), 834–839.

Smeltzer, S. C. (2006). Preventive health screening for breast and cervical cancer and osteoporosis in women with physical disabilities. *Family and Community Health, 29*(1 Suppl), 35S–43S.

Smeltzer, S. C. (2007). Pregnancy in women with physical disabilities. *Journal of Obstetrical, Gynecologic, and Neonatal Nursing, 36*(1), 88–96.

Smeltzer, S. C. & Wetzel-Effinger, L. (2009). Pregnancy in women with spinal cord injury. *Topics in Spinal Cord Injury Rehabilitation. 15*(1), 29–42.

Smeltzer, S. C., Sharts-Hopko, N. C., Ott, B., et al. (2007). Perspectives of women with disabilities on reaching those who are hard to reach. *Journal of Neuroscience Nursing, 39*(3), 163–171.

Abortion

Fischer, M., Bhatnagar, J., Guarner, J., et al. (2005). Fatal toxic shock syndrome associated with *Clostridium sordellii* after medical abortion. *New England Journal of Medicine, 353*(22), 2352–2360.

Kulier, R., Fekih, A., Hofmeyr, G., et al. (2007). Surgical methods for first trimester termination of pregnancy. *Cochrane Database of Systematic Reviews, 4,* CD002900.

Lohr, P. A., Hayes, J. L. & Gemzell-Danielsson, K. (2008). Surgical versus medical methods for second trimester induced abortion. *Cochrane Database of Systematic Reviews, 1,* CD0067.

Say, L., Kulier, R., Gulmezoglu, M., et al. (2007). Medical versus surgical methods for first trimester termination of pregnancy. *Cochrane Database of Systematic Reviews, 4,* CD003037.

Virk, J., Zhang, J. & Olsen J. (2007). Medical abortion and the risk of subsequent adverse pregnancy outcomes. *New England Journal of Medicine, 357*(7), 648–653.

Conception Control

American College of Obstetricians and Gynecologists (ACOG). (2006c). Use of hormonal contraception in women with coexisting medical conditions. ACOG practice bulletin 73. *Obstetrics & Gynecology, 107*(6), 1453–1472.

American College of Obstetricians and Gynecologists (ACOG) Committee on Gynecologic Practice. (2006d). ACOG Committee Opinion 337. Noncontraceptive uses of the levonorgestrel intrauterine system. *Obstetrics & Gynecology, 107*(6), 1479–1482.

Alan Guttmacher Institute. (2008). Facts on contraceptive use. Available at: www.guttmacher.org

Allen, R. & Goldberg, A. (2007). Emergency contraception: A clinical review. *Clinical Obstetrics and Gynecology, 50*(4), 927–936.

Fantasia, H. C. (2008). Options for intrauterine contraception. *Journal of Obstetrical, Gynecologic, and Neonatal Nursing, 37*(3), 375–383.

*Fehring, R., Schneider, M., Raviele, K., et al. (2007). Efficacy of cervical mucus observations plus electronic hormonal fertility monitoring as a method of natural family planning. *Journal of Obstetrical, Gynecologic, and Neonatal Nursing, 36*(2), 152–160.

Haider, S. & Darney, P. (2007). Injectable contraception. *Clinical Obstetrics and Gynecology, 50*(4), 898–906.

Hoffman, H. & Creinin, M. (2007). The contraceptive implant. *Clinical Obstetrics and Gynecology, 50*(4), 907–917.

Kiley, J. & Hammond, C. (2007). Combined oral contraceptives: A comprehensive review. *Clinical Obstetrics and Gynecology, 50*(4), 868–877.

Lopez, L. M., Kaptein, A. & Helmerhorst, F. M. (2008). Oral contraceptives containing drospirenone for premenstrual syndrome. *Cochrane Database of Systematic Reviews, 1*, CD006586.

Noone, J. (2007). Strategies for contraceptive success. *Nurse Practitioner, 32*(6), 29–35.

Paru, S., Boatwright, E., Tozer, B., et al. (2006). Hormonal contraception update. *Mayo Clinic Proceedings, 81*(7), 949–955.

Roumen, F. J. M. E. (2008). Review of the combined contraceptive vaginal ring, NuvaRing. *Therapeutics and Clinical Risk Management, 4*(2), 441–451.

Tangm, O. S. & Ho, P. C. (2006). Clinical applications of mifepristone. *Gynecology and Endocrinology, 22*(12), 655–659.

White, E., Rosengard, C., Weitzen, S., et al. (2006). Fear of inability to conceive in pregnant adolescents. *Obstetrics & Gynecology, 108*(6), 1411–1416.

Zurawin, R. & Ayensu-Coker, L. (2007). Innovations in contraception: A review. *Clinical Obstetrics, 50*(2), 425–439.

Cultural Differences in Health Care of Women

Cooper, M., Grywalski, M., Lamp, J., et al. (2007). Enhancing cultural competence. *Nursing for Women's Health, 11*(2), 148–159.

Roberts, S. (2006). Health care recommendations for lesbian women. *Journal of Obstetrical, Gynecologic, and Neonatal Nursing, 35*(5), 583–591.

Stevens, W., Betancourt, J., Wynia, J., et al. (2007). Recommendations for teaching about racial and ethnic disparities in health and health care. *Annals of Internal Medicine, 147*(9), 654–665.

Menstruation, Irregular Bleeding, Perimenopause, PMS, and Menopause

Alexander, I. (2007). Overview of current HT recommendations using evidence-based decision making. *American Journal of Nurse Practitioners, 11*(10), 29–41.

American Heart Association. (2007). Evidence-based guidelines for cardiovascular disease prevention in women. 2007 Update. *Circulation, 115*(11), 1481–1501.

Cejtin, H., Kalinowski, A., Bacchetti, P., et al. (2006). Effects of human immunodeficiency virus on protracted amenorrhea and ovarian dysfunction. *Obstetrics & Gynecology, 108*(6), 1423–1430.

Coffee, A., Kuehl, T., Willis, S., et al. (2006). Oral contraceptives and premenstrual symptoms: Comparison of a 21/7 and extended regimen. *American Journal of Obstetrics and Gynecology, 195*(5), 1311–1319.

*Dormire, S. & Howharn, C. (2007). The effect of dietary intake on hot flashes in menopausal women. *Journal of Obstetrical, Gynecologic, and Neonatal Nursing, 36*(3), 255–262.

El-Nashar, S., Hopkins, M., Feitoza, S., et al. (2007). Global endometrial ablation for menorrhagia in women with bleeding disorders. *Obstetrics & Gynecology, 109*(6), 1381–1386.

Finkler. K. (2007). An application of the theory of life's lesions to the study of the menopausal transition. *Menopause, 14*(4), 769–776.

*Harrison, T. & Becker, H. (2007). A qualitative study of menopause among women with disabilities. *Advances in Nursing Science, 30*(2), 123–138.

Heiss, G., Wallace, R., Anderson, G. L., et al. (2008). Health risks and benefits 3 years after stopping randomized treatment with estrogen and progestin. *Journal of American Medical Association, 299*(9), 1036–1045.

Lopez, L. M., Kaptein, A. & Helmerhorst, F. M. (2008). Oral contraceptives containing drospirenone for premenstrual syndrome. *Cochrane Database of Systematic Reviews, 1*, CD006586.

Strine, T., Chapman, D. & Ahluwalia, I. B. (2005). Menstrual-related problems and psychological distress among women in the United States. *Journal of Women's Health, 14*(4), 316–323.

Thakur, S. & Supiano, M. (2007). Screening for common clinical conditions in older women. *Clinical Obstetrics & Gynecology, 50*(3), 767–775.

*Twiss, J., Wegner, J., Hunter, M., et al. (2007). Perimenopausal symptoms, quality of life, and health behaviors in users and non users of hormone therapy. *Journal of the American Academy of Nurse Practitioners, 19*(11), 602–613.

**Writing Group for Women's Health Initiative Investigators. (2002). Risks and benefits of estrogen plus progestin in healthy postmenopausal women: Principal results from the Women's Health Initiative randomized controlled trial. *Journal of the American Medical Association, 288*(3), 321–333.

Mutilation, Domestic Violence, Physical and Sexual Assault

Alpert, E. (2007). Addressing domestic violence: The long road ahead. *Annals of Internal Medicine, 147*(9), 666–667.

Catania, L., Abdulcadir, O., Puppo,V., et al. (2007). Pleasure and orgasm in women with female genital mutilation. *Journal of Sexual Medicine, 4*(6), 1666–1678.

Feerick, M. & Snow, K. (2005). The relationships between childhood sexual abuse, social anxiety and symptoms of posttraumatic stress disorder in women. *Journal of Family Violence, 20*(6), 409–419.

Furniss, K., McCaffrey, M., Parnell, V., et al. (2007). Nurses and barriers to screening for intimate partner violence. *American Journal of Maternal Child Nursing, 32*(4), 238–243.

*McFarlane, J., Malecha, A., Watson, K., et al. (2005). Intimate partner sexual assault against women: Frequency, health consequences, and treatment outcomes. *Obstetrics & Gynecology, 105*(1), 99–108.

Turner, D. (2007). Female genital cutting. *Nursing for Women's Health, 11*(4), 366–372.

U.S. Department of Justice. (2007). 2007 national crime victimization survey. Available at: www.ojp.usdoj.gov/bjs/pub/pdf/cv07.pdf

Pap Smears and Follow-Up Treatment

American College of Obstetricians and Gynecologists (ACOG) Committee on Adolescent Health Care. (2006b). Evaluation and management of abnormal cervical cytology and histology in the adolescent. ACOG Committee Opinion 330. *Obstetrics & Gynecology, 107*(4), 963–968.

Moore, D. H. (2006). Cervical cancer. *Obstetrics & Gynecology, 107*(5), 1152–1161.

Wright, T., Massad, L., Dunton, C., et al. (2007). 2006 consensus guidelines for the management of women with abnormal cervical cancer screening results. *American Journal of Obstetrics & Gynecology, 197*(4), 346–355.

RESOURCES

American College of Obstetricians and Gynecologists (ACOG), www.acog.org

American Society for Reproductive Medicine (ASRM), www.asrm.org

Amnesty International (resource for activists to end female genital mutilation), www.amnesty.org

Association of Reproductive Health Professionals, www.arhp.org

Association of Women's Health, Obstetrical and Neonatal Nurses (AWHONN), www.awhonn.org

DES Action USA, www.desaction.org

Emergency Contraception, opr.princeton.edu/ec

Family Violence Prevention Fund, www.endabuse.org

Female Genital Mutilation Education and Networking Project (provides fact sheets, state policies, periodicals), www.fgmnetwork.org

Guttmacher Institute, www.guttmacher.org

Health Promotion for Women with Disabilities Project, Villanova University College of Nursing, www.nurseweb.villanova.edu/womenwithdisabilities

National Association of Nurse Practitioners in Women's Health (NPWH), www.npwh.org

National Coalition Against Domestic Violence, www.ncadv.org

North American Menopause Society, www.menopause.org

Planned Parenthood Federation of America, www.plannedparenthood.org

Resolve National Headquarters, www.resolve.org

Sexuality Information and Education Council of the United States, www.siecus.org

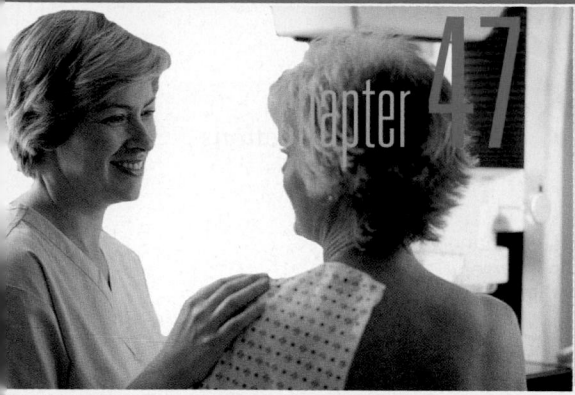

Chapter 47

Management of Patients With Female Reproductive Disorders

LEARNING OBJECTIVES

On completion of this chapter, the learner will be able to:

1 Compare the various types of vaginal infections and the signs, symptoms, and treatments of each.

2 Develop a teaching plan for the patient with a vaginal infection.

3 Use the nursing process as a framework for care of the patient with a vulvovaginal infection.

4 Use the nursing process as a framework for care of the patient with genital herpes.

5 Discuss the signs and symptoms, management, and nursing care implications of malignant disorders of the female reproductive tract.

6 Use the nursing process as a framework for care of the patient undergoing a hysterectomy.

7 Describe indications for a wide excision of the vulva, or vulvectomy, and the preoperative and postoperative nursing interventions.

8 Compare nursing interventions indicated for the patient undergoing radiation therapy and chemotherapy for cancer of the female reproductive tract.

GLOSSARY

abscess: a collection of purulent material

acquired immunodeficiency syndrome (AIDS): a disease transmitted by body fluids that results in impaired immune response

Bartholin's cyst: a cyst in a paired vestibular gland in the vulva

brachytherapy: radiation delivered by an internal device placed close to the tumor

candidiasis: infection caused by *Candida* species or yeast; also referred to as monilial vaginitis or yeast infection

colporrhaphy: repair of the vagina

condylomata: warty growths indicative of the human papillomavirus (HPV)

conization: procedure in which a cone-shaped piece of cervical tissue is removed as a result of detection of abnormal cells; also called cone biopsy

cryotherapy: destruction of tissue by freezing (eg, with liquid nitrogen)

cystocele: bulging of the bladder downward into the vagina

douche: rinsing the vaginal canal with fluid

dysplasia: term related to abnormal cell changes found on Pap smear and cervical biopsy reports

endocervicitis: inflammation of the mucosa and the glands of the cervix

GLOSSARY *(Continued)*

endometriosis: endometrial tissue in abnormal locations; causes pain with menstruation, scarring, and possible infertility

enterocele: is a protrusion of the intestinal wall into the vagina

fibroid tumor: usually benign tumor of the uterus that may cause irregular bleeding; also called myoma or leiomyoma

fistula: abnormal opening between two organs or sites (eg, vesicovaginal, between bladder and vagina; rectovaginal, between rectum and vagina)

hyphae: microscopic findings that indicate monilia

hysterectomy: surgical removal of the uterus

lactobacilli: vaginal bacteria that limit the growth of other bacteria by producing hydrogen peroxide

laparoscope: surgical device inserted through a periumbilical incision to facilitate visualization and surgical procedures

lichen sclerosus: benign disorder of the vulva that usually occurs when estrogen levels are low; characterized by itching

liposomal therapy: chemotherapy delivered in a liposome, a nontoxic drug carrier

loop electrocautery excision procedure (LEEP): procedure in which laser energy is used to remove a portion of cervical tissue after abnormal biopsy findings

mucopurulent cervicitis: inflammation of the cervix with exudate; almost always related to a chlamydial infection

myomectomy: removal of uterine fibroids though an abdominal incision

oophorectomy: surgical removal of an ovary

pelvic exenteration: major surgical procedure in which the pelvic organs are removed

pelvic inflammatory disease (PID): infection of uterus and fallopian tubes, usually from a sexually transmitted disease

perineorrhaphy: surgical repair of perineal lacerations

polycystic ovary syndrome (PCOS): disorder in the hypothalamic-pituitary and ovarian network, resulting in chronic anovulation, androgen excess, and polycystic ovaries

rectocele: bulging of the rectum into the vagina

salpingitis: inflammation of the fallopian tube

salpingo-oophorectomy: removal of the ovary and its fallopian tube (removal of the fallopian tube alone is a salpingectomy)

vaginal vault: term used to describe the vagina following a hysterectomy, which involves removal of the uterus including the cervix

vaginitis: inflammation of the vagina, usually secondary to infection

vestibulitis: inflammation of the vulvar vestibule, or tissue around the opening of the vagina, that often causes pain with intercourse (dyspareunia)

vestibulodynia: most common type of vulvodynia, characterized by sharp pain in response to pressure applied to the vestibular area of the vulva.

vulvar dystrophy: thickening or lesions of the vulva; usually causes itching and may require biopsy to exclude malignancy

vulvectomy: removal of the tissue of the vulva

vulvitis: inflammation of the vulva, usually secondary to infection or irritation

vulvodynia: painful condition that affects the vulva

Disorders of the female reproductive system can be minor or serious but are usually anxiety producing and often distressing. Some disorders are self-limited and cause only minor inconvenience to the woman; others are life-threatening and require immediate attention and long-term therapy. Many disorders are managed by the patient at home, whereas others require hospitalization and surgical intervention. All disorders require that nurses have knowledge, understanding, and skill in patient teaching. Nurses must also be sensitive to the woman's concerns and possible discomfort in discussing and dealing with these disorders.

VULVOVAGINAL INFECTIONS

Vulvovaginal infections are common, and nurses have an important role in providing information that may prevent their occurrence. To help prevent these infections, women need to understand their own anatomy and vulvovaginal health.

The vagina is protected against infection by its normally low pH (3.5 to 4.5), which is maintained in part by the actions of *Lactobacillus acidophilus,* the dominant bacteria in a healthy vaginal ecosystem. These bacteria suppress the growth of anaerobes and produce lactic acid, which maintains normal pH. They also produce hydrogen peroxide, which is toxic to anaerobes. The risk of infection increases if a woman's resistance is reduced by stress or illness, if the pH is altered, or if a pathogen is introduced. Continued research into causes and treatments is needed, along with better ways to encourage growth of **lactobacilli.**

The epithelium of the vagina is highly responsive to estrogen, which induces glycogen formation. The subsequent breakdown of glycogen into lactic acid assists in producing a low vaginal pH. When estrogen decreases during lactation and menopause, glycogen also decreases. With reduced glycogen formation, infections may occur. In addition, as estrogen production ceases during the perimenopausal and postmenopausal periods, the vagina and labia may atrophy (thin), making the vaginal area more susceptible to infection. When patients are treated with antibiotics, the normal vaginal flora are reduced. This results in altered pH and growth of fungal organisms. Other factors that may initiate or predispose to infections include contact with an infected partner and wearing tight, nonabsorbent, and heat-retaining and moisture-retaining clothing (Chart 47-1).

Vaginitis (inflammation of the vagina) is a group of conditions that cause vulvovaginal symptoms such as itching, irritation, burning, and abnormal discharge. Bacterial vaginosis is the most common cause (22% to 50% of symptomatic women), followed by vulvovaginal candidiasis (17% to 39%) and trichomoniasis (4% to 35%) (American College of Obstetricians and Gynecologists [ACOG], 2006a). (Table 47-1). Other types include desquamative vaginitis, atrophic vaginitis, various vulvar dermatologic conditions, and vulvodynia. The normal vaginal discharge, which may occur in slight amounts during ovulation or just before the onset of menstruation, becomes more profuse when vaginitis occurs. Urethritis may accompany vaginitis because of the proximity of the urethra to the vagina. Discharge that occurs with vaginitis may produce itching, odor, redness,

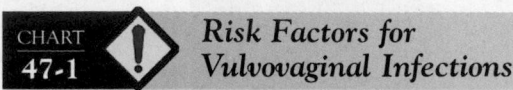

CHART 47-1 **Risk Factors for Vulvovaginal Infections**

- Premenarche
- Pregnancy
- Perimenopause/Menopause
- Poor personal hygiene
- Tight undergarments
- Synthetic clothing
- Frequent douching
- Allergies
- Use of oral contraceptives
- Use of broad-spectrum antibiotics
- Diabetes mellitus
- Low estrogen levels
- Intercourse with infected partner
- Oral–genital contact (yeast can inhabit the mouth and intestinal tract)
- HIV infection

burning, or edema, which may be aggravated by voiding and defecation. After the causative organism has been identified, appropriate treatment (discussed later) is prescribed. This may include an oral medication or a local medication that is inserted into the vagina using an applicator.

Candidiasis

Vulvovaginal **candidiasis** is a fungal or yeast infection caused by strains of Candida (see Table 47-1). *Candida albicans* accounts for most cases, but other strains, such as *Candida glabrata,* may also be implicated. Many women with a healthy vaginal ecosystem harbor Candida but are asymptomatic. Certain conditions favor the change from an asymptomatic state to colonization with symptoms. For example, use of antibiotics decreases bacteria, thereby altering the natural protective organisms usually present in the vagina. Although infections can occur at any time, they occur more commonly in pregnancy or with a systemic condition such as diabetes mellitus or human immunodeficiency virus (HIV) infection, or when patients are taking medications such as corticosteroids or oral contraceptives.

Clinical Manifestations

Clinical manifestations include a vaginal discharge that causes pruritus (itching) and subsequent irritation. The discharge may be watery or thick but has a white, cottage cheese–like appearance. Symptoms are usually more severe just before menstruation and may be less responsive to treatment during pregnancy. Diagnosis is made by microscopic identification of spores and **hyphae** on a glass slide prepared from a discharge specimen mixed with potassium hydroxide. With candidiasis, the pH is 4.5 or less.

Medical Management

The goal of management is to eliminate symptoms. Treatments include antifungal agents such as miconazole (Monistat), nystatin (Mycostatin), clotrimazole (Gyne-Lotrimin), and terconazole (Terazol) cream. These agents are inserted into the vagina with an applicator at bedtime. There are

Table 47-1 VAGINAL INFECTIONS AND VAGINITIS

Infection	Cause	Clinical Manifestations	Management Strategies
Candidiasis	*Candida albicans, glabrata,* or *tropicalis*	Inflammation of vaginal epithelium, producing itching, reddish irritation White, cheeselike discharge clinging to epithelium	Eradicate the fungus by administering an antifungal agent. Frequently used brand names of vaginal creams and suppositories are Monistat, Femstat, Terazol, and Gyne-Lotrimin. Review other causative factors (eg, antibiotic therapy, nylon underwear, tight clothing, pregnancy, oral contraceptives). Assess for diabetes and HIV infection in patients with recurrent monilia.
Gardnerella-associated bacterial vaginosis	*Gardnerella vaginalis* and vaginal anaerobes	Usually no edema or erythema of vulva or vagina Gray-white to yellow-white discharge clinging to external vulva and vaginal walls	Administer metronidazole (Flagyl), with instructions about avoiding alcohol while taking this medication. If infection is recurrent may treat partner.
Trichomonas vaginalis vaginitis (STD)	*Trichomonas vaginalis*	Inflammation of vaginal epithelium, producing burning and itching Frothy yellow-white or yellow-green vaginal discharge	Relieve inflammation, restore acidity, and reestablish normal bacterial flora; provide oral metronidazole for patient and partner.
Bartholinitis (infection of greater vestibular gland)	*Escherichia coli* *Trichomonas vaginalis* Staphylococcus Streptococcus Gonococcus	Erythema around vestibular gland Swelling and edema Abscessed vestibular gland	Drain the abscess; provide antibiotic therapy; excise gland of patients with chronic bartholinitis.
Cervicitis: acute and chronic	Chlamydia Gonococcus Streptococcus Many pathogenic bacteria	Profuse purulent discharge Backache Urinary frequency and urgency	Determine the cause: perform cytologic examination of cervical smear and appropriate cultures. Eradicate the gonococcal organism, if present: penicillin (as directed) or spectinomycin or tetracycline, if patient is allergic to penicillin. Tetracycline, doxycycline (Vibramycin) to eradicate chlamydia. Eradicate other causes.
Atrophic vaginitis	Lack of estrogen; glycogen deficiency	Discharge and irritation from alkaline pH of vaginal secretions	Provide topical vaginal estrogen therapy; improve nutrition if necessary; relieve dryness through use of moisturizing medications.

1-night, 3-night, and 7-night treatment courses available. Oral medication (fluconazole [Diflucan]) is also available in a one-pill dose. Relief should be noted within 3 days.

Some vaginal creams are available without a prescription; however, patients are cautioned to use these creams only if they are certain that they have a yeast or monilial infection. Patients often use these remedies for problems other than yeast infections. If a woman is uncertain about the cause of her symptoms or if relief has not been obtained after using these creams, she should be instructed to seek health care promptly. Yeast infections can become recurrent or complicated. Women may have more than four infections in a year and severe symptoms due to preexisting conditions such as diabetes or immunosuppression. Cell-mediated immunity may be a factor. Women with recurrent yeast infections benefit from a comprehensive gynecologic assessment.

Bacterial Vaginosis

Bacterial vaginosis is caused by an overgrowth of anaerobic bacteria and *Gardnerella vaginalis* normally found in the vagina and an absence of lactobacilli (see Table 47-1). Risk factors include douching after menses, smoking, multiple sex partners, and other sexually transmitted diseases (STDs) (also referred to as sexually transmitted infections [STIs]).

Clinical Manifestations

Bacterial vaginosis can occur throughout the menstrual cycle and does not produce local discomfort or pain. More than half of patients with bacterial vaginosis do not notice any symptoms. Discharge, if noticed, is heavier than normal and gray to yellowish white in color. It is characterized by a fishlike odor that is particularly noticeable after sexual intercourse or during menstruation as a result of an increase in vaginal pH. The pH of the discharge is usually greater than 4.7 because of the amines that result from enzymes from anaerobes. The fishlike odor can be detected readily by adding a drop of potassium hydroxide to a glass slide with a sample of vaginal discharge, which releases amines; this is referred to as a positive "whiff" test. Under the microscope, vaginal cells are coated with bacteria and are described as "clue cells." Lactobacilli, which serve as a natural host defense, are usually absent. Bacterial vaginosis is not usually considered a serious condition, although it can be associated with premature labor, premature rupture of membranes, endometritis, and recurrent urinary tract infection.

Medical Management

Metronidazole (Flagyl), administered orally twice a day for 1 week, is effective; a vaginal gel is also available. Clindamycin (Cleocin) vaginal cream or ovules (oval suppositories) are also effective. Treatment of patients' partners does not seem to be effective, but use of condoms may be helpful.

Trichomoniasis

Trichomonas vaginalis is a flagellated protozoan that causes a common, usually sexually transmitted vaginitis that is often called "trich"; about 7.4 million cases occur each year (ACOG, 2006a). Trichomoniasis may be transmitted by an asymptomatic carrier who harbors the organism in the urogenital tract (see Table 47-1). It may increase the risk of contracting HIV from an infected partner and may play a role in development of cervical neoplasia, postoperative infections, adverse pregnancy outcomes, pelvic inflammatory disease (PID), and infertility.

Clinical Manifestations

Clinical manifestations include a vaginal discharge that is thin (sometimes frothy), yellow to yellow-green, malodorous, and very irritating. An accompanying vulvitis may result, with vulvovaginal burning and itching. Diagnosis is made most often by microscopic detection of the motile causative organisms or less frequently by culture. Inspection with a speculum often reveals vaginal and cervical erythema (redness) with multiple small petechiae ("strawberry spots"). Testing of a trichomonal discharge demonstrates a pH greater than 4.5.

Medical Management

The most effective treatment for trichomoniasis is metronidazole or tinidazole (Tindamax). Both partners receive a one-time loading dose or a smaller dose three times a day for 1 week. The one-time dose is more convenient; consequently, compliance tends to be greater. The week-long treatment has occasionally been noted to be more effective. Some patients complain of an unpleasant but transient metallic taste when taking metronidazole. Nausea and vomiting, as well as a hot, flushed feeling (disulfiram-like reaction), occur when this medication is taken with an alcoholic beverage. In view of these side effects, patients taking metronidazole are strongly advised to abstain from alcohol.

Metronidazole is not prescribed without examination. It is contraindicated in patients with some blood dyscrasias or central nervous system diseases, in the first trimester of pregnancy, and in women who are breastfeeding. Tinidazole is not considered safe in pregnancy.

 ## Gerontologic Considerations

After menopause, the vaginal mucosa becomes thinner and may atrophy. This condition can be complicated by infection from pyogenic bacteria, resulting in atrophic vaginitis (see Table 47-1). Leukorrhea (vaginal discharge) may cause itching and burning. Management is similar to that for bacterial vaginosis if bacteria are present. Estrogenic hormones, either taken orally or inserted into the vagina in a cream form, can also be effective in restoring the epithelium.

NURSING PROCESS

The Patient With a Vulvovaginal Infection

Assessment

The woman with vulvovaginal symptoms should be examined as soon as possible after the onset of symptoms. She should be instructed not to **douche** because doing so removes the vaginal discharge needed to make the diagnosis. The area is observed for erythema, edema, excoriation, and discharge. Each of the infection-producing organisms produces its own characteristic discharge and effect (see Table 47-1). The patient is asked to describe any discharge and other symptoms, such as odor, itching, or burning. Dysuria often occurs as a result of local irritation of the urinary meatus. A urinary tract infection may need to be ruled out by obtaining a urine specimen for culture and sensitivity testing.

The patient is asked about the occurrence of factors that may contribute to vulvovaginal infection:
- Physical and chemical factors, such as constant moisture from tight or synthetic clothing, perfumes and powders, soaps, bubble bath, poor hygiene, and use of feminine hygiene products
- Psychogenic factors (eg, stress, fear of STDs, abuse)
- Medical conditions or endocrine factors, such as a predisposition to *Monilia* in a patient who has diabetes
- Use of medications such as antibiotics, which may alter the vaginal flora and allow an overgrowth of monilial organisms
- New sex partner, multiple sex partners, previous vaginal infection

The patient is also asked about factors that could contribute to infection, including hygiene practices (douching), and use or nonuse of condoms and other barrier methods of birth control.

The nurse may prepare a vaginal smear (wet mount) to assist in diagnosing the infection. A common method for preparing the smear is to collect vaginal secretions with an applicator and place the secretions on two separate glass slides. A drop of saline solution is added to one slide and a drop of 10% potassium hydroxide is added to another slide for examination under a microscope. If bacterial vaginosis is present, the slide with normal saline solution added shows epithelial cells dotted with bacteria (clue cells). If *Trichomonas* species is present, small motile cells are seen. In the presence of yeast, the potassium hydroxide slide reveals typical characteristics. Discharge associated with bacterial vaginosis produces a strong odor when mixed with potassium hydroxide. Testing the pH of the discharge with Nitrazine paper assists in proper diagnosis.

Diagnosis

Nursing Diagnoses

Based on the nursing assessment and other data, major nursing diagnoses may include the following:

- Discomfort related to burning, odor, or itching from the infectious process
- Anxiety related to stressful symptoms
- Risk for infection or spread of infection
- Deficient knowledge about proper hygiene and preventive measures

Planning and Goals

Major goals may include relief of discomfort, reduction of anxiety related to symptoms, prevention of reinfection or infection of sexual partner, and acquisition of knowledge about methods for preventing vulvovaginal infections and managing self-care.

Nursing Interventions

Relieving Discomfort

Treatment with the appropriate medication usually relieves discomfort. Sitz baths may be occasionally recommended and may provide temporary relief of symptoms.

Reducing Anxiety

Vulvovaginal infections are upsetting and require treatment. The patient who experiences such an infection may be very anxious about the significance of the symptoms and possible causes. Explaining the cause of symptoms may reduce anxiety related to fear of a more serious illness. Discussing ways to help prevent vulvovaginal infections may help patients adopt specific strategies to decrease infection and the related symptoms.

Preventing Reinfection or Spread of Infection

The patient needs to be informed about the importance of adequate treatment of herself and her partner, if indicated. Other strategies to prevent persistence or spread of infection include abstaining from sexual intercourse when infected, treatment of sexual partners, and minimizing irritation of the affected area. When medications such as antibiotic agents are prescribed for any infection, the nurse instructs the patient about the usual precautions related to using these agents. If vaginal itching occurs several days after use, the patient can be reassured that this is usually not an allergic reaction but may be a yeast or monilial infection resulting from altered vaginal bacteria. Treatment for monilial infection is prescribed.

Another goal of treatment is to reduce tissue irritation caused by scratching or wearing tight clothing. The area needs to be kept clean by daily bathing and adequate hygiene after voiding and defecation. The use of a hairdryer on a cool setting will dry the area and application of topical corticosteroids may decrease irritation.

When teaching the patient about medications such as suppositories and devices such as applicators to dispense cream or ointment, the nurse may demonstrate the procedure by using a plastic model of the pelvis and vagina. The nurse should also stress the importance of hand washing before and after each administration of medication. To prevent the medication from escaping from the vagina, the patient

should recline for 30 minutes after it is inserted, if possible. The patient is informed that seepage of medication may occur, and the use of a perineal pad may be helpful.

Promoting Home and Community-Based Care

TEACHING PATIENTS SELF-CARE. Vulvovaginal conditions are treated on an outpatient basis unless a patient has other medical problems. Patient teaching, tact, and reassurance are important aspects of nursing care. Women may express embarrassment, guilt, or anger and may be concerned that the infection could be serious or that it may have been acquired from a sex partner. (In some instances, treatment plans include the partner.)

In addition to reviewing ways of relieving discomfort and preventing reinfection, the nurse assesses each patient's learning needs relative to the immediate problem. The patient needs to know the characteristics of normal as opposed to abnormal discharge. Questions often arise about douching. Normally, douching and use of feminine hygiene sprays are unnecessary because daily baths or showers and proper hygiene after voiding and defecating keep the perineal area clean. Douching tends to eliminate normal flora, reducing the body's ability to ward off infection. In addition, repeated douching may result in vaginal epithelial breakdown and chemical irritation and has been associated with other pelvic disorders. No studies show any benefit from douching (ACOG, 2006a). In the case of recurrent yeast infections, the perineum should be kept as dry as possible. Loose-fitting cotton instead of tight-fitting synthetic, nonabsorbent, heat-retaining underwear is recommended. Use of talcum powder should be discouraged.

Vulvar self-examination is a good health practice for all women. Becoming familiar with one's own anatomy and reporting anything that seems new or different may result in early detection and treatment of any new disorders. Nurses can also play a role in teaching women about the risks of unprotected intercourse, particularly with partners who have had sex with others.

Evaluation

Expected Patient Outcomes

Expected patient outcomes may include:

1. Experiences reduced discomfort
   a. Cleans the perineum as instructed
   b. Reports that itching is relieved
   c. Maintains urine output within normal limits and without dysuria
2. Experiences relief of anxiety
3. Remains free from infection
   a. Has no signs of inflammation, pruritus, odor, or dysuria
   b. Notes that vaginal discharge appears normal (thin, clear, not frothy)
4. Participates in self-care
   a. Takes medication as prescribed
   b. Wears absorbent underwear
   c. Avoids unprotected sexual intercourse
   d. Douches only as prescribed
   e. Performs vulvar self-examination regularly and reports any new findings to care provider

Human Papillomavirus

Human papillomavirus (HPV) infection is sexually transmitted and is the most common STD in young, sexually active people. An estimated 6.2 million patients acquire these infections every year (Centers for Disease Control and Prevention [CDC], 2006a, 2007). Most infections are self-limiting and without symptoms, and others can cause cervical and anogenital cancers. Infections can be latent (asymptomatic and detected only by DNA hybridization tests for HPV), subclinical (visualized only after application of acetic acid followed by inspection under magnification), or clinical (visible condylomata acuminata).

Pathophysiology

More than 100 types of HPV exist. The most common strains of HPV, 6 and 11, usually cause **condylomata** (warty growths) on the vulva. These are often visible or may be palpable by patients. Condylomata are rarely premalignant but are an outward manifestation of the virus. Strains 6 and 11 are associated with a low risk for cervical cancer. Some HPV strains (16, 18, 31, 33, and 45) may not cause condylomata but do affect the cervix, resulting in abnormal Papanicolaou (Pap) smears. The effects of these strains are usually invisible on examination but may be seen on colposcopy. They may cause cervical changes that may appear as koilocytosis on Pap smear. Seventy percent of all cervical cancers are caused by strains 16 and 18 (Wright, Massad, Dunton, et al., 2007). However, most women with HPV infection do not develop cervical cancer.

The incidence of HPV in young, sexually active women is high. The infection often disappears as the result of an effective immune system response. It is thought that two proteins produced by high-risk types of HPV interfere with tumor suppression by normal cells. Risk factors include being young, being sexually active, having multiple sex partners, and having sex with a partner who has or has had multiple partners.

In 2006, the Advisory Committee on Immunization Practices (ACIP) of the CDC recommended that a newly licensed vaccine (Gardasil) against the four strains of HPV that cause the majority of cases of cervical cancer be routinely administered to girls 11 to 12 years of age—that is, before they become sexually active. Although this vaccine is considered an important medical breakthrough, it does not replace other strategies important in prevention of HPV or the need for cervical cancer screening. It is administered in three intramuscular doses, with the initial dose followed by second dose in 2 months and a third dose 6 months after the first dose. This vaccine, along with regular Pap smears, has the potential to decrease the impact of HPV-related disease (ACOG, 2006b; CDC, 2006a, 2007; Markowitz, Dunne, Saraiya, et al., 2007).

Medical Management

Treatment of external genital warts includes topical application of trichloroacetic acid, podophyllin (Podofin, Podocon), and chemotherapeutic agents, as well as injections of interferon administered by a health care provider.

Topical agents that can be applied by patients to external lesions include podofilox (Condylox) and imiquimod (Aldara). Because the safety of podophyllin, imiquimod, and podofilox during pregnancy has not been determined, these agents should not be used during pregnancy. Electrocautery and laser therapy are alternative therapies that may be indicated for patients with a large number or area of genital warts (CDC, 2007).

Treatment usually eradicates perineal warts or condylomata. However, they may resolve spontaneously without treatment and may also recur even with treatment.

If the treatment includes application of a topical agent by the patient, she needs to be carefully instructed in the use of the agent prescribed and must be able to identify the warts and be able to apply the medication to them. The patient is instructed to anticipate mild pain or local irritation with the use of these agents.

Women with HPV should have annual Pap smears because of the potential of HPV to cause **dysplasia** (changes in cervical cells). Much remains unknown about subclinical and latent HPV disease. Women are often exposed to HPV by partners who are unknowing carriers. Use of condoms can reduce the likelihood of transmission, but transmission can also occur during skin-to-skin contact in areas not covered by condoms.

In many cases, patients are angry about having warts or HPV and do not know who infected them because the incubation period can be long and partners may have no symptoms. Acknowledging the emotional distress that occurs when an STD is diagnosed and providing support and facts are important nursing actions.

Herpesvirus Type 2 Infection (Herpes Genitalis, Herpes Simplex Virus)

Herpes genitalis is a recurrent, life-long viral infection that causes herpetic lesions (blisters) on the external genitalia and occasionally the vagina and cervix. It is an STD but may also be transmitted asexually from wet surfaces or by self-transmission (ie, touching a cold sore and then touching the genital area). The initial infection is usually very painful and lasts about 1 week, but it can also be asymptomatic. Recurrences are less painful and usually produce minor itching and burning. Some patients have few or no recurrences, whereas others have frequent bouts. Recurrences are often associated with stress, sunburn, dental work, or inadequate rest or nutrition—all situations that may tax the immune system.

Since the late 1970s, the incidence of herpes infection has increased fivefold among Caucasian adolescents and young adults. At least 50 million people in the United States have genital herpes infection and most have not been diagnosed (CDC, 2006a). The prevalence of other STDs has decreased slightly, possibly because of increased condom use, but herpes can be transmitted by contact with skin not covered by a condom. Transmission is possible even when a carrier does not have symptoms (subclinical shedding). Lesions increase vulnerability to HIV infection and other STDs. Vaccines for herpes genitalis are in clinical trials.

Pathophysiology

Of the known herpesviruses, six affect humans: (1) herpes simplex type 1 (HSV-1), which usually causes cold sores of the lips; (2) herpes simplex type 2 (HSV-2), or genital herpes; (3) varicella zoster, or shingles; (4) Epstein-Barr virus; (5) cytomegalovirus (CMV); and (6) human B-lymphotrophic virus. HSV-2 appears to be the cause of about 80% of genital and perineal lesions; HSV-1 may cause about 20%.

There is considerable overlap between HSV-1 and HSV-2, which are clinically indistinguishable. Close human contact by the mouth, oropharynx, mucosal surface, vagina, or cervix appears necessary to acquire the infection. Other susceptible sites are skin lacerations and conjunctivae. Usually, the virus is killed at room temperature by drying. When viral replication diminishes, the virus ascends the peripheral sensory nerves and remains inactive in the nerve ganglia. Another outbreak may occur when the host is subjected to stress. In pregnant women with active herpes, infants delivered vaginally may become infected with the virus. There is a risk of fetal morbidity and mortality if this occurs; therefore, a cesarean delivery may be performed if the virus recurs near the time of delivery.

Clinical Manifestations

Itching and pain occur as the infected area becomes red and edematous. Primary infection may begin with macules and papules and progress to vesicles and ulcers. The vesicular state often appears as a blister, which later coalesces, ulcerates, and encrusts. In women, the labia are the usual primary site, although the cervix, vagina, and perianal skin may be affected. In men, the glans penis, foreskin, or penile shaft is typically affected. Influenza-like symptoms may occur 3 or 4 days after the lesions appear. Inguinal lymphadenopathy (enlarged lymph nodes in the groin), minor temperature elevation, malaise, headache, myalgia (aching muscles), and dysuria (pain on urination) are often noted. Pain is evident during the first week and then decreases. The lesions subside in about 1 to 2 weeks unless secondary infection occurs.

Rarely, complications may arise from extragenital spread, such as to the buttocks, upper thighs, or even the eyes as a result of touching lesions and then touching other areas. Patients should be advised to wash their hands after contact with lesions. Other potential problems are aseptic meningitis, neonatal transmission, and severe emotional stress related to the diagnosis.

Medical Management

There is currently no cure for HSV-2 infection, but treatment is aimed at relieving the symptoms. Management goals include preventing the spread of infection, making patients comfortable, decreasing potential health risks, and initiating a counseling and education program. The antiviral agents acyclovir (Zovirax), valacyclovir (Valtrex), and famciclovir (Famvir) can suppress symptoms and shorten the course of the infection. These are effective at reducing the duration of lesions and preventing recurrences. Resistance and long-term side effects do not appear to be major problems. Recurrent episodes are often milder than the initial episode.

NURSING PROCESS

THE PATIENT WITH A GENITAL HERPESVIRUS INFECTION

Assessment

The health history and a physical and pelvic examination are important in establishing the nature of the infectious condition. In addition, patients are assessed for risk of STDs. The perineum is inspected for painful lesions. Inguinal nodes are assessed and are often enlarged and tender during an occurrence of HSV.

Diagnosis

Nursing Diagnoses

Based on the assessment data, major nursing diagnoses may include the following:
- Acute pain related to the genital lesions
- Risk for infection or spread of infection
- Anxiety related to the diagnosis
- Deficient knowledge about the disease and its management

Planning and Goals

Major goals may include relief of pain and discomfort, control of infection and its spread, relief of anxiety, knowledge of and adherence to the treatment regimen and self-care, and knowledge about implications for the future.

Nursing Interventions

Relieving Pain

The lesions should be kept clean, and proper hygiene practices are advocated. Sitz baths ease discomfort. Clothing should be clean, loose, soft, and absorbent. Aspirin and other analgesics are usually effective in controlling pain. Occlusive ointments and powders are avoided because they prevent the lesions from drying.

If there is considerable pain and malaise, bed rest may be required. The patient is encouraged to increase fluid intake, to be alert for possible bladder distention, and to contact her primary health care provider immediately if she cannot void because of discomfort. Painful voiding may occur if urine comes in contact with the herpes lesions. Discomfort with urination can be reduced by pouring warm water over the vulva during voiding or by sitz baths. When oral acyclovir or other antiviral agents are prescribed, the patient is instructed about when to take the medication and what side effects to note, such as rash and headache. Rest, fluids, and a nutritious diet are recommended to promote recovery.

Preventing Infection and Its Spread

The risk of reinfection and spread of infection to others or to other structures of the body can be reduced by hand washing, use of barrier methods with sexual contact, and adherence to prescribed medication regimens. Avoidance of contact when obvious lesions are present does not eliminate the risk because the virus can be shed in the absence of symptoms, and lesions may not be visible to women.

Relieving Anxiety

Concern about the presence of herpes infection, future occurrences of lesions, and the impact of the infection on future relationships and childbearing may cause considerable patient anxiety. Nurses can be an important support, listening to patients' concerns and providing information and instruction. The patient may be angry with her partner if the partner is the probable source of the infection. The patient may need assistance and support in discussing the infection and its implications with her current sexual partners and in future sexual relationships. The nurse can refer the patient to a support group to assist in coping with the diagnosis (see Resources at the end of the chapter).

Increasing Knowledge About the Disease and Its Treatment

Patient teaching is an essential part of nursing care of the patient with a genital herpes infection. This includes an adequate explanation about the infection and how it is transmitted, management and treatment strategies, strategies to minimize spread of infection, the importance of adherence to the treatment regimen, and self-care strategies. Because of the increased risk of HIV and other STDs in the presence of skin lesions, an important part of patient education involves instructing the patient to protect herself from exposure to HIV and other STDs (Chart 47-2).

Promoting Home and Community-Based Care

TEACHING PATIENTS SELF-CARE. Self-care measures for people with genital herpes appear in Chart 47-2.

Evaluation

Expected Patient Outcomes

Expected patient outcomes may include:

1. Experiences a reduction in pain and discomfort
2. Keeps infection under control
   a. Demonstrates proper hygiene techniques
   b. Takes medication as prescribed
   c. Consumes adequate fluids
   d. Assesses own current lifestyle (diet, adequate fluid intake, safer sex practices, stress management)
3. Uses strategies to reduce anxiety
   a. Verbalizes issues and concerns related to genital herpes infection
   b. Discusses strategies to deal with issues and concerns with current and future sexual partners
   c. Initiates contact with support group if indicated

CHART 47-2	HOME CARE CHECKLIST *The Patient With Genital Herpes*		
At the completion of the home care instruction, the patient or caregiver will be able to:		**PATIENT**	**CAREGIVER**
• State that herpes is transmitted mainly by direct contact.		✔	✔
• State that abstinence from sex is required for a brief period (intercourse is avoided during treatment, but other options such as hand holding and kissing are acceptable).		✔	✔
• State that intercourse during a herpes outbreak not only increases the risk of transmission but also increases the likelihood of contracting HIV and other STDs.		✔	✔
• State that transmission is possible even in the absence of active lesions.		✔	✔
• State that condoms may provide some protection against viral transmission.		✔	✔
• Explain that obstetric care provider should be informed about the history of herpes. In cases of recurrence at time of delivery, cesarean section may be considered.		✔	✔
• Describe appropriate hygiene practices (hand washing, perineal cleanliness, gentle washing of lesions with mild soap and running water and lightly drying lesions) and importance of avoiding occlusive ointments, strong perfumed soaps, or bubble bath.		✔	✔
• State that control of the condition may require changes in sexual behavior and use of medications.		✔	✔
• Describe strategies to avoid self-infection (eg, avoid touching lesions during an outbreak).		✔	✔
• Explain rationale for avoiding self-infection (ie, lesions can become infected from germs on the hand, and the virus from the lesion can be transmitted from the hand to another area of the body or another person).		✔	✔
• Describe health promotion strategies: wear loose, comfortable clothing; eat a balanced diet; get adequate rest and relaxation.		✔	✔
• State rationale for avoiding exposure to the sun as it can cause recurrences (and skin cancer).		✔	✔
• Identify importance of taking medications as prescribed, keeping follow-up appointments with health care provider, and reporting repeated recurrences (may not be as severe as the initial episode).		✔	✔
• Describe possible benefits of joining a group to share solutions and experiences and hear about newer treatments, such as HELP (Herpetics Engaged in Living Productively).		✔	✔

4. Demonstrates knowledge about genital herpes and strategies to control and minimize recurrences
   a. Identifies methods of transmission of herpes infection and strategies to prevent transmission to others
   b. Discusses strategies to reduce recurrence of lesions
   c. Takes medications as prescribed
   d. Reports no recurrence of lesions

Endocervicitis and Cervicitis

Endocervicitis is an inflammation of the mucosa and the glands of the cervix that may occur when organisms gain access to the cervical glands after intercourse and, less often, after procedures such as abortion, intrauterine manipulation, or vaginal delivery. If untreated, the infection may extend into the uterus, fallopian tubes, and pelvic cavity. Inflammation can irritate the cervical tissue, resulting in spotting or bleeding and **mucopurulent cervicitis.**

Chlamydia and Gonorrhea

Chlamydia and gonorrhea are the most common causes of endocervicitis, although *Mycoplasma* may also be involved. Chlamydia causes about 3 million infections every year in the United States; it is most commonly found in young, sexually active people with more than one partner and is transmitted through sexual intercourse. It can result in serious complications, including pelvic infection, an increased risk for ectopic pregnancy, and infertility. As many as 40% of untreated women develop PID. One in 20 women of reproductive age in the United States is infected (CDC, 2006a). Chlamydial infections of the cervix often produce no symptoms, but cervical discharge, dyspareunia, dysuria, and bleeding may occur. Other complications include conjunctivitis and perihepatitis. If pregnant women are infected, stillbirth, neonatal death, and premature labor may occur. Infants born to infected mothers may experience prematurity, conjunctivitis, and pneumonia.

Chlamydial infection and gonorrhea often coexist. As many as 25% of females who have chlamydial infections also have gonorrhea (CDC, 2006a). The inflamed cervix that results from this infection may leave a woman more vulnerable to HIV transmission from an infected partner. Gonorrhea is also a major cause of PID, tubal infertility, ectopic pregnancy, and chronic pelvic pain. Fifty percent of women with gonorrhea have no symptoms, but without treatment, 40% may develop PID. In males, urethritis and epididymitis may occur. Diagnosis can be confirmed by culture, smear, or other methods, using a swab to obtain a sample of cervical discharge or penile discharge from the patient's partner.

Medical Management

The CDC recommends treating chlamydia with doxycycline (Vibramycin) for 1 week or with a single dose of azithromycin (Zithromax). Because of the high incidence of coinfection with chlamydia and gonorrhea, treatment for gonorrhea should include treatment for chlamydia as well (CDC, 2006a). Partners must also be treated. Pregnant women are cautioned not to take tetracycline because of potential adverse effects on the fetus. In these cases, erythromycin may be prescribed. Results are usually good if treatment begins early. Possible complications from delayed treatment are tubal disease, ectopic pregnancy, PID, and infertility.

The CDC no longer recommends fluoroquinolones (eg, ciprofloxacin [Cipro], ofloxacin [Floxin], or levofloxacin [Levaquin]) for the treatment of gonorrhea and associated conditions (eg, PID). Instead, the CDC (2007) recommends cephalosporins for the treatment of gonorrhea.

Cultures for chlamydia and other STDs should be obtained from all patients who have been sexually assaulted when they first seek medical attention; patients are treated prophylactically. Cultures should then be repeated in 2 weeks. Annual screening for chlamydia is recommended for all sexually active young women and older women with new sex partners or multiple partners (CDC, 2006a).

Nursing Management

All sexually active women may be at risk for chlamydia, gonorrhea, and other STDs, including HIV. Nurses can assist patients in assessing their own risk. Recognition of risk is a first step before changes in behavior occur. Patients should be discouraged from assuming that a partner is "safe" without open, honest discussion. Nonjudgmental attitudes, educational counseling, and role playing may be helpful.

Because chlamydia, gonorrhea, and other STDs may have a serious effect on future health and fertility and because many of these disorders can be prevented by the use of condoms and spermicides and careful choice of partners, nurses can play a major role in counseling patients about safer sex practices. Exploring options with patients, addressing knowledge deficits, and correcting misinformation may reduce morbidity and mortality.

Promoting Home and Community-Based Care

Teaching Patients Self-Care

Nurses can educate women and help them develop communication skills and initiate discussions about sex with their partners. Communicating with partners about sex, risk, postponing intercourse, and using safer sex behaviors, including use of condoms, may be lifesaving. Some young women report having sex but not being comfortable enough to discuss sexual risk issues. Nurses can help women to advocate for their own health by discussing safety with partners prior to sexual activity.

Reinforcing the need for annual screening for chlamydia and other STDs is an important part of patient teaching. Instructions also include the need for the patient to abstain from sexual intercourse until all of her sex partners are treated (CDC, 2006a). The CDC recommends rescreening of all women with chlamydial infections 3 to 4 months after treatment is completed to reduce the risks of infertility.

Pelvic Infection (Pelvic Inflammatory Disease)

Pelvic inflammatory disease (PID) is an inflammatory condition of the pelvic cavity that may begin with cervicitis and may involve the uterus (endometritis), fallopian tubes (**salpingitis**), ovaries (oophoritis), pelvic peritoneum, or pelvic vascular system. Infection, which may be acute, subacute, recurrent, or chronic and localized or widespread, is usually caused by bacteria but may be attributed to a virus, fungus, or parasite. Gonorrheal and chlamydial organisms are the most likely causes. CMV has also been implicated. This condition can result in the fallopian tubes becoming narrowed and scarred, which increases the risk of ectopic pregnancy (fertilized eggs become trapped in the tube), infertility, recurrent pelvic pain, tubo-ovarian **abscess,** and recurrent disease. Rupture of a tubo-ovarian abscess has a 5% to 10% mortality rate and usually necessitates a complete hysterectomy. PID is a common gynecologic cause of hospital admissions in the United States. The true incidence of PID is unknown because some cases are asymptomatic.

Pathophysiology

The exact pathogenesis of PID has not been determined, but it is presumed that organisms usually enter the body through the vagina, pass through the cervical canal, colonize the endocervix, and move upward into the uterus. Under various conditions, the organisms may proceed to one or both fallopian tubes and ovaries and into the pelvis. In bacterial infections that occur after childbirth or abortion, pathogens are disseminated directly through the tissues that support the uterus by way of the lymphatics and blood vessels (Fig. 47-1). In pregnancy, the increased blood supply required by the placenta provides more pathways for infection. These postpartum and postabortion infections tend to be unilateral. Infections can cause perihepatic inflammation when the organism invades the peritoneum.

In gonorrheal infections, the gonococci pass through the cervical canal and into the uterus, where the environment, especially during menstruation, allows them to multiply rapidly and spread to the fallopian tubes and into the pelvis (see Fig. 47-1). The infection is usually bilateral.

In rare instances, organisms (eg, tuberculosis) gain access to the reproductive organs by way of the bloodstream from the lungs (see Fig. 47-1). One of the most common causes of salpingitis (inflammation of the fallopian tube) is chlamydia, possibly accompanied by gonorrhea.

Pelvic infection is most commonly caused by sexual transmission but can also occur with invasive procedures such as endometrial biopsy, surgical abortion, hysteroscopy, or insertion of an intrauterine device. Bacterial vaginosis, a vaginal infection, may predispose women to pelvic infection. Risk factors include early age at first intercourse, multiple sexual partners, frequent intercourse, intercourse without condoms, sex with a partner with an STD, and a history of STDs or previous pelvic infection.

Clinical Manifestations

Symptoms of pelvic infection usually begin with vaginal discharge, dyspareunia, lower abdominal pelvic pain, and tenderness that occurs after menses. Pain may increase with voiding or with defecation. Other symptoms include fever, general malaise, anorexia, nausea, headache, and possibly vomiting. On pelvic examination, intense tenderness may be noted on palpation of the uterus or movement of the cervix (cervical motion tenderness). Symptoms may be acute and severe or low grade and subtle.

Complications

Pelvic or generalized peritonitis, abscesses, strictures, and fallopian tube obstruction may develop. Obstruction may cause an ectopic pregnancy in the future if a fertilized egg cannot pass a tubal stricture, or scar tissue may occlude the tubes, resulting in sterility. Adhesions are common and often result in chronic pelvic pain; they eventually may require removal of the uterus, fallopian tubes, and ovaries. Other complications include bacteremia with septic shock and thrombophlebitis with possible embolization.

Medical Management

Broad-spectrum antibiotic therapy is prescribed, usually a combination of ceftriaxone (Ceftin), azithromycin, or doxycycline. Women with mild infections may be treated as outpatients, but hospitalization may be necessary. Intensive therapy includes bed rest, intravenous (IV) fluids, and IV

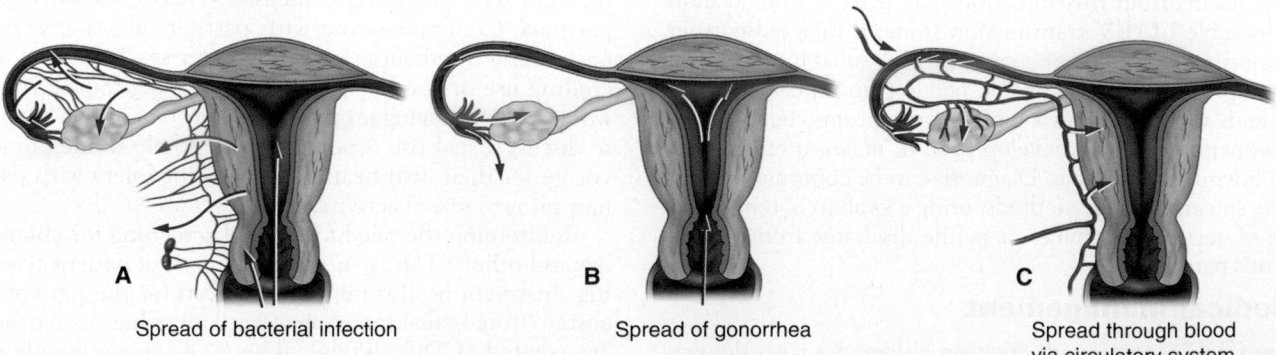

Spread of bacterial infection   Spread of gonorrhea   Spread through blood via circulatory system

Figure 47-1 Pathway by which micro-organisms spread in pelvic infections. **A,** Bacterial infection spreads up the vagina into the uterus and through the lymphatics. **B,** Gonorrhea spreads up the vagina into the uterus and then to the tubes and ovaries. **C,** Bacterial infection can reach the reproductive organs through the bloodstream (hematogenous spread).

antibiotic therapy. If the patient has abdominal distention or ileus, nasogastric intubation and suction are initiated. Careful monitoring of vital signs and symptoms assists in evaluating the status of the infection. Treatment of sexual partners is necessary to prevent reinfection.

Nursing Management

Infection takes a toll, both physically and emotionally. The patient may feel well one day and experience vague symptoms and discomfort the next. She may also suffer from constipation and menstrual difficulties.

A hospitalized patient is maintained on bed rest and is usually placed in the semi-Fowler's position to facilitate dependent drainage. Accurate recording of vital signs and the characteristics and amount of vaginal discharge is necessary as a guide to therapy.

The nurse administers analgesic agents as prescribed for pain relief. Heat applied safely to the abdomen may also provide some pain relief and comfort. In addition, the nurse minimizes the transmission of infection to others by carefully handling perineal pads with gloves, discarding the soiled pad according to hospital guidelines for disposal of biohazardous material, and performing meticulous hand hygiene.

Promoting Home and Community-Based Care

Teaching Patients Self-Care

The patient must be informed of the need for precautions and must be encouraged to take part in procedures to prevent infecting others and protect herself from reinfection. If a partner is not well known or has had other sexual partners recently, use of condoms is essential to prevent infection and sequelae. If reinfection occurs or if the infection spreads, symptoms may include abdominal pain, nausea and vomiting, fever, malaise, malodorous purulent vaginal discharge, and leukocytosis. Patient teaching consists of explaining how pelvic infections occur, how they can be controlled and avoided, and their signs and symptoms. Guidelines and instructions provided to the patient are summarized in Chart 47-3.

All patients who have had PID need to be informed of the signs and symptoms of ectopic pregnancy (pain, abnormal bleeding, delayed menses, faintness, dizziness, and shoulder pain) because they are prone to this complication. (See Chapter 46 for a discussion of ectopic pregnancy.)

Human Immunodeficiency Virus Infection and Acquired Immunodeficiency Syndrome

Any discussion of vulvovaginal infections and STDs must include the topic of HIV and **acquired immunodeficiency syndrome (AIDS),** which is described in Chapter 52. Because HIV infection may be detected through prenatal testing and screening for STDs, nurses and other women's health care clinicians are often the first professionals to provide care for a woman with HIV infection (ACOG, 2007a). Thus, they need to be knowledgeable about this disorder and sensitive to women's issues and concerns.

The incidence of HIV infection and AIDS in women is increasing. If rates of new cases of HIV infection continue to increase, infections in women will outnumber men with HIV (CDC, 2006b). Most women with HIV infection are in the reproductive age group. Heterosexual transmission is the leading cause of new HIV infection in women, surpassing IV/injection drug use as the most common mode of transmission. Younger women are disproportionately at higher risk; 25% to 50% of all women who acquire HIV heterosexually do so in adolescence or in their early 20s. Women are nine times more likely to contract HIV from men than men are from women. The presence of genital ulcers (eg, a herpetic or syphilitic lesion) or a friable cervix increases risk. Intercourse during menses may also increase risk. Syphilis appears to accelerate in HIV-positive patients and proceeds directly from primary to tertiary disease in some patients. Chlamydia is associated with a high risk of HIV (which may be related to inflammatory changes of the cervix, providing

---

CHART 47-3	HOME CARE CHECKLIST *The Patient With Pelvic Inflammatory Disease*		
At the completion of the home care instruction, the patient or caregiver will be able to:		**PATIENT**	**CAREGIVER**
• State that any pelvic pain or abnormal discharge, particularly after sexual exposure, childbirth, or pelvic surgery, should be evaluated as soon as possible.		✔	✔
• State that antibiotics may be prescribed after insertion of intrauterine devices (IUDs).		✔	✔
• Describe proper perineal care procedures (wiping from front to back after defecation or urination).		✔	✔
• State that douching reduces the natural flora that combat infecting organisms and may introduce bacteria upward.		✔	✔
• Identify the importance of consulting a health care provider if unusual vaginal discharge or odor is noted.		✔	✔
• Discuss the importance of following health practices (ie, proper nutrition, exercise, and weight control), and safer sex practices (ie, using condoms, avoiding multiple sexual partners).		✔	✔
• Explain the importance of consistent use of condoms before intercourse or any penile–vaginal contact if there is any chance of transmitting infection.		✔	✔
• State that a gynecologic examination should be performed at least once a year.		✔	✔

entry sites). HIV-positive women have a higher rate of HPV. Infections with HPV and HIV together increase the risk of malignant transformation and cervical cancer. Thus, women with HIV infection should have frequent Pap smears. HIV-positive women also have larger and more painful herpes lesions with more recurrences, probably related to immunosuppression from their disease. Many HIV-infected women have gynecologic disorders, including candidiasis, PID, anogenital warts, and cervical dysplasia (CDC, 2006a).

Women with HIV and women with partners who have HIV must be counseled about safer sex and informed about the dangers of unprotected sex. Inconsistent use of condoms results in a higher seroconversion rate. Because there is a risk of perinatal transmission, decisions to conceive or to use contraception must be based on teaching, accurate information, and care. Pregnant women are advised to have an HIV test. The use of antiretroviral agents by pregnant women significantly decreases perinatal transmission of HIV infection. Therefore, the use of these agents during pregnancy is critical and must also be discussed. For women who choose to avoid conception, use of condoms alone and with oral contraceptives are possible choices.

After informed consent is obtained, women who are at risk for HIV are offered testing by a nurse or counselor. Because patients may be reluctant to discuss risk-taking behavior, routine screening should be offered to all women. Early detection permits early treatment to delay progression of the disease.

Use of antiretroviral therapy has been improving, but barriers to use of health services by disadvantaged women include lack of insurance, current drug use, and difficulty keeping appointments. Depression and abuse are issues that affect women's use of health care services. Prevention of cervical neoplasia and PID need to be part of the teaching for women at risk. The nurse also needs to remember that many women do not see themselves as at risk for acquiring HIV infection. See Chapter 52 for further discussion of HIV infection and AIDS.

STRUCTURAL DISORDERS

Fistulas of the Vagina

A **fistula** is an abnormal, tortuous opening between two internal hollow organs or between an internal hollow organ and the exterior of the body. The name of the fistula indicates the two areas that are connected abnormally: a vesicovaginal fistula is an opening between the bladder and the vagina, and a rectovaginal fistula is an opening between the rectum and the vagina (Fig. 47-2). Fistulas may be congenital in origin. However, in adults, breakdown usually occurs because of tissue damage resulting from injury sustained during surgery, vaginal delivery, irritable bowel disease, radiation therapy, or disease processes such as carcinoma (Rivadeneira, Ruffo, Amrani, et al., 2007).

Clinical Manifestations

Symptoms depend on the specific defect. For example, in a patient with a vesicovaginal fistula, urine escapes continuously into the vagina. With a rectovaginal fistula, there is fecal incontinence, and flatus is discharged through the

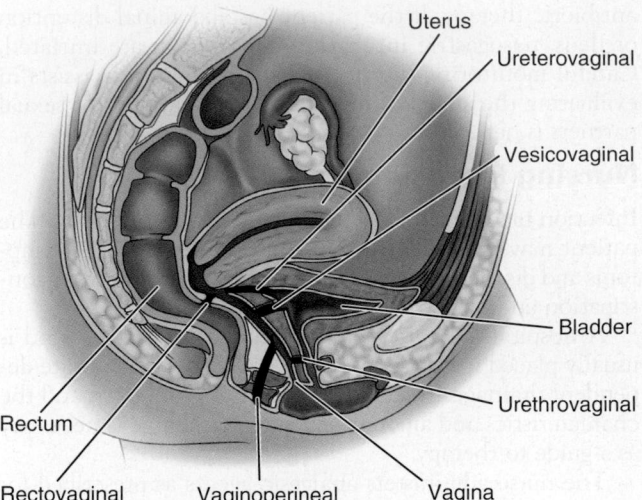

Figure 47-2 Common sites for vaginal fistulas: *Vesicovaginal*—bladder and vagina. *Urethrovaginal*—urethra and vagina. *Vaginoperineal*—vagina and perineal area. *Ureterovaginal*—ureter and vagina. *Rectovaginal*—rectum and vagina.

vagina. The combination of fecal discharge with leukorrhea results in malodor that is difficult to control.

Assessment and Diagnostic Findings

A history of the symptoms experienced by the patient is important to identify the structural alterations and to assess the impact of the symptoms on the patient's quality of life. In addition, the use of methylene blue dye helps delineate the course of the fistula. In vesicovaginal fistula, the dye is instilled into the bladder and appears in the vagina. After a negative methylene blue test result, indigo carmine is injected intravenously; the appearance of the dye in the vagina indicates a ureterovaginal fistula. Cystoscopy or IV pyelography may then be used to determine the exact location.

Medical Management

The goal is to eliminate the fistula and to treat infection and excoriation. A fistula may heal without surgical intervention, but surgery is often required. If the primary care provider determines that a fistula will heal without surgical intervention, care is planned to relieve discomfort, prevent infection, and improve the patient's self-concept and self-care abilities. Measures to promote healing include proper nutrition, cleansing douches and enemas, rest, and administration of prescribed intestinal antibiotics. A rectovaginal fistula heals faster when the patient eats a low-residue diet and when the affected tissue drains properly. Warm perineal irrigations promote healing.

Sometimes a fistula does not heal on its own and cannot be surgically repaired. In this situation, care must be planned and implemented on an individual basis. Cleanliness, frequent sitz baths, and deodorizing douches are required, as are perineal pads and protective undergarments. Meticulous skin care is necessary to prevent excoriation. Applying bland creams or lightly dusting with cornstarch may be soothing. In addition, attending to the patient's social and psychological needs is an essential aspect of care.

If the patient is to have a fistula repaired surgically, preoperative treatment of any existing vaginitis is important to ensure success. Usually, the vaginal approach is used to repair vesicovaginal and urethrovaginal fistulas; the abdominal approach is used to repair fistulas that are large or complex. Fistulas that are difficult to repair or that are very large may require surgical repair with a urinary or fecal diversion. Tissue transfer techniques (skin or tissue grafting) may be used (Rivadeneira, et al., 2007).

Because fistulas usually are typically related to obstetric, surgical, or radiation trauma, occurrence in a patient without previous vaginal delivery or a history of surgery must be evaluated carefully. Crohn's disease or lymphogranuloma venereum may be the cause.

Despite the best surgical intervention, fistulas may recur. After surgery, medical follow-up continues for at least 2 years to monitor for a possible recurrence.

Pelvic Organ Prolapse: Cystocele, Rectocele, Enterocele

Age and parity can put strain on the ligaments and structures that make up the female pelvis and pelvic floor. Childbirth can result in tears of the levator sling musculature, resulting in structural weakness. Hormone deficiency also may play a role. Some degree of prolapse (weakening of the vaginal walls allowing the pelvic organs to descend and protrude into the vaginal canal) may be found in many older women. Risk factors include age, parity, and vaginal delivery, and there may also be a familial predisposition (Buschbaum, Duecy, Kerr, et al., 2006).

Cystocele is a downward displacement of the bladder toward the vaginal orifice (Fig. 47-3), resulting from damage to the anterior vaginal support structures. It usually results from injury and strain during childbirth. The condition usually appears some years later when genital atrophy associated with aging occurs, but younger, multiparous, premenopausal women may also be affected.

Rectocele is an upward pouching of the rectum that pushes the posterior wall of the vagina forward. Both rectoceles and perineal lacerations, which occur because of muscle tears below the vagina, may affect the muscles and tissues of the pelvic floor and may occur during childbirth. Sometimes the lacerations may completely sever the fibers of the anal sphincter (complete tear). An **enterocele** is a protrusion of the intestinal wall into the vagina. Prolapse results from a weakening of the support structures of the uterus itself; the cervix drops and may protrude from the vagina. (If complete prolapse occurs, it may also be referred to as procidentia.)

Clinical Manifestations

Because a cystocele causes the anterior vaginal wall to bulge downward, the patient may report a sense of pelvic pressure, fatigue, and urinary problems such as incontinence, frequency, and urgency. Back pain and pelvic pain may occur as well. The symptoms of rectocele resemble those of cystocele, with one exception: instead of urinary symptoms, patients may experience rectal pressure. Constipation, uncontrollable gas, and fecal incontinence may occur in patients with complete tears. Prolapse can result in feelings of pressure and ulcerations and bleeding. Dyspareunia may occur with these disorders.

Medical Management

Kegel exercises, which involve contracting or tightening the vaginal muscles, are prescribed to help strengthen these weakened muscles. The exercises are more effective in the early stages of a cystocele. Kegel exercises are easy to perform and are recommended for all women, including those with strong pelvic floor muscles (Chart 47-4).

A pessary can be used to avoid surgery. This device is inserted into the vagina and positioned to keep an organ, such as the bladder, uterus, or intestine, properly aligned when a cystocele, rectocele, or prolapse has occurred. Pessaries are usually ring shaped or doughnut shaped and are made of various materials, such as rubber or plastic (Fig. 47-4). Rubber pessaries must be avoided in women with latex allergy. The size and type of pessary are selected and fitted by a gynecologic health care provider. The patient should have the pessary removed, examined, and cleaned by her health care provider at prescribed intervals. At these checkups, vaginal walls should be examined for pressure points or

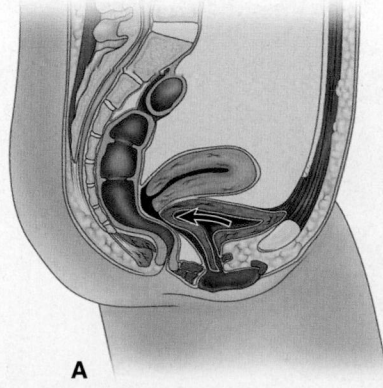 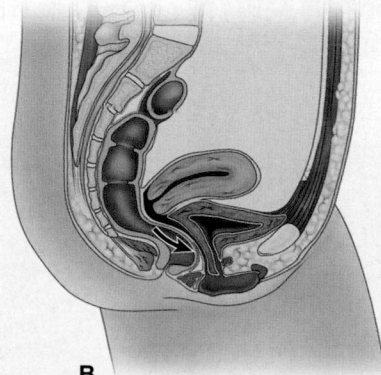 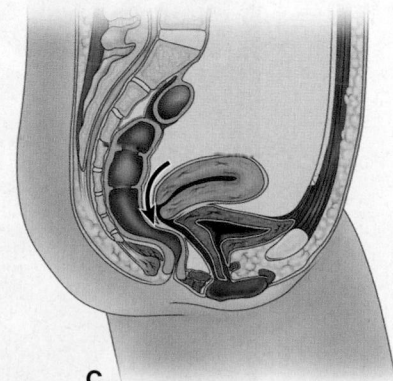

A **B** **C**

Figure 47-3 Diagrammatic representation of the three most common types of pelvic floor relaxation: **A,** cystocele, **B,** rectocele, and **C,** enterocele. *Arrows* depict sites of maximum protrusion.

CHART 47-4

PATIENT EDUCATION
Performing Kegel (Pelvic Muscle) Exercises

Purposes: To strengthen and maintain the tone of the pubo-coccygeal muscle, which supports the pelvic organs; reduce or prevent stress incontinence and uterine prolapse; enhance sensation during sexual intercourse; and hasten postpartum healing

1. Become aware of pelvic muscle function by "drawing in" the perivaginal muscles and anal sphincter as if to control urine or defecation, but not contracting the abdominal, buttock, or inner thigh muscles.
2. Sustain contraction of the muscles for up to 10 seconds, followed by at least 10 seconds of relaxation.
3. Perform these exercises 30–80 times a day.

---

signs of irritation. Normally, the patient experiences no pain, discomfort, or discharge with a pessary, but if chronic irritation occurs, alternative measures may be needed.

A Colpexin sphere is another nonsurgical device used to treat pelvic organ prolapse. This intravaginal device is similar to a pessary, but it supports the pelvic floor muscles and facilitates exercise of these muscles. It is removed daily for cleaning.

Surgical Management

In many cases, surgery helps correct structural abnormalities. The procedure to repair the anterior vaginal wall is called anterior **colporrhaphy,** repair of a rectocele is called a posterior colporrhaphy, and repair of perineal lacerations is called a **perineorrhaphy.** These repairs are frequently performed laparoscopically, resulting in short hospital stays and good outcomes. A **laparoscope** is inserted through a small abdominal incision, the pelvis is visualized, and surgical repairs are performed.

Uterine Prolapse

Usually the uterus and the cervix lie at right angles to the long axis of the vagina with the body of the uterus inclined slightly forward. The uterus is normally freely movable on examination. Individual variations may result in an anterior, middle, or posterior uterine position. A backward positioning of the uterus, known as retroversion and retroflexion, is not uncommon (Fig. 47-5).

If the structures that support the uterus weaken (typically from childbirth), the uterus may work its way down the vaginal canal (prolapse) and even appear outside the vaginal orifice (procidentia) (Fig. 47-6). As the uterus descends, it may pull the vaginal walls and even the bladder and rectum with it. Symptoms include pressure and urinary problems (incontinence or retention) from displacement of the bladder. The symptoms are aggravated when a woman coughs, lifts a heavy object, or stands for a long time. Normal activities, even walking up stairs, may aggravate the symptoms.

Medical Management

Surgery and pessaries are two options for treatment. With surgery, the uterus is sutured back into place and repaired to strengthen and tighten the muscle bands. In postmenopausal women, the uterus may be removed **(hysterectomy)** or repaired by colpopexy. Colpocleisis, or vaginal closure, may be an option for women who do not wish to have sexual intercourse or to bear children and want to avoid hysterectomy (ACOG, 2007b). Pessaries may be the treatment of choice in elderly women or those who are too ill to tolerate surgery.

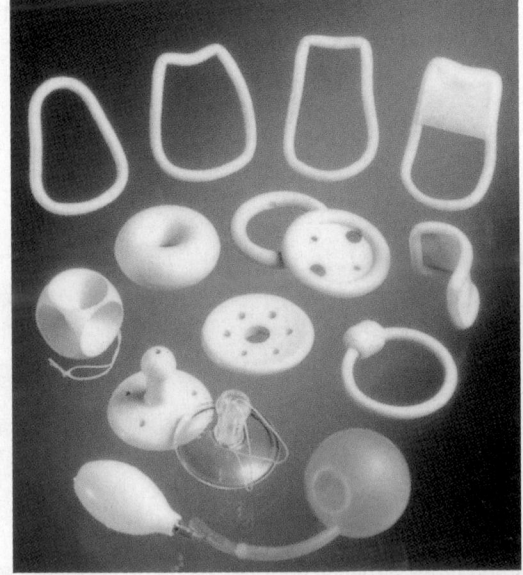

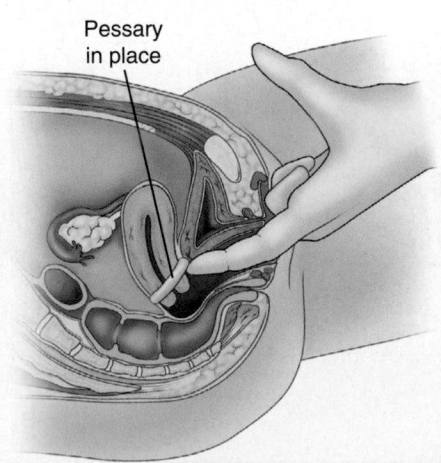

Pessary in place

Figure 47-4 Examples of pessaries. **A,** Various shapes and sizes of pessaries available. **B,** Insertion of one type of pessary.

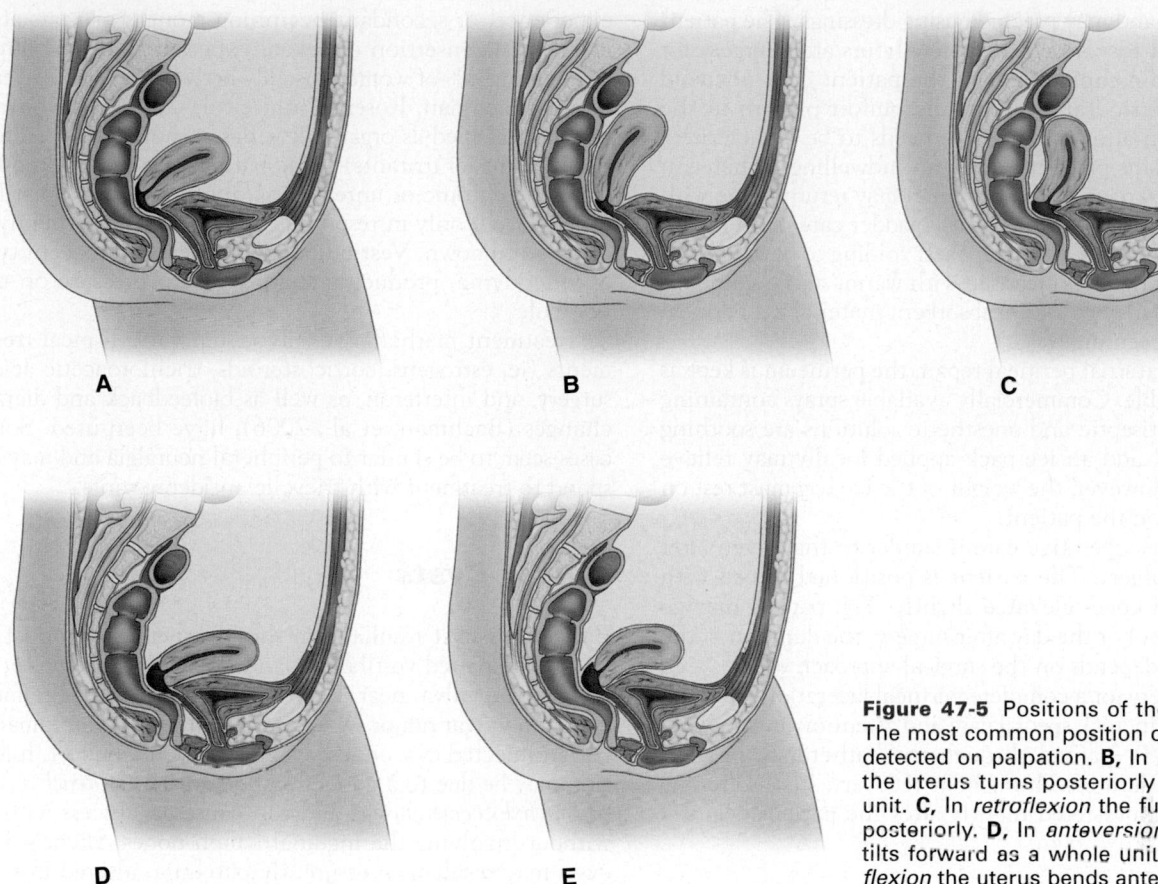

Figure 47-5 Positions of the uterus. **A,** The most common position of the uterus detected on palpation. **B,** In *retroversion* the uterus turns posteriorly as a whole unit. **C,** In *retroflexion* the fundus bends posteriorly. **D,** In *anteversion* the uterus tilts forward as a whole unit. **E,** In *anteflexion* the uterus bends anteriorly.

Nursing Management

Implementing Preventive Measures

Some disorders related to "relaxed" pelvic muscles (cystocele, rectocele, and uterine prolapse) may be prevented.

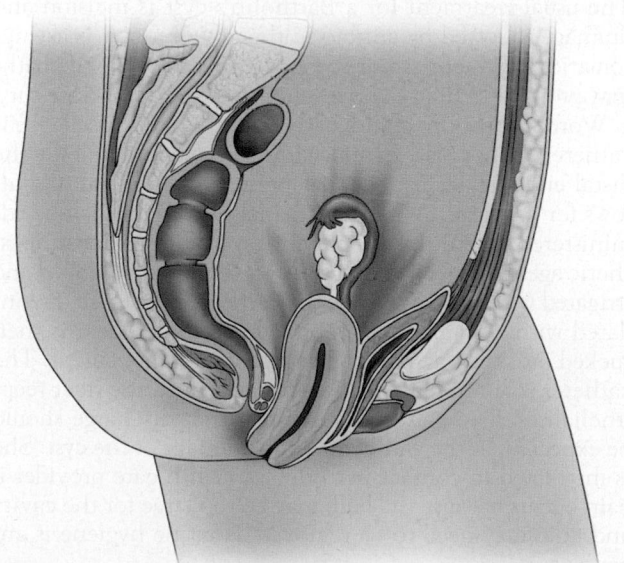

Figure 47-6 Complete prolapse of the uterus through the introitus.

During pregnancy, early visits to the health care provider permit early detection of problems. During the postpartum period, the woman can be taught to perform Kegel exercises to strengthen the muscles that support the uterus and then to continue them as a preventive action.

Delays in obtaining evaluation and treatment may result in complications such as infection, cervical ulceration, cystitis, and hemorrhoids. The nurse encourages the patient to obtain prompt treatment for these structural disorders.

Implementing Preoperative Nursing Care

Before surgery, the patient needs to know the extent of the proposed surgery, the expectations for the postoperative period, and the effect of surgery on future sexual function. In addition, the patient having a rectocele repair needs to know that before surgery, a laxative and a cleansing enema may be prescribed. She may be asked to administer these at home the day before surgery. A perineal shave may be prescribed as well. The patient is usually placed in a lithotomy position for surgery, with special attention given to moving both legs in and out of the stirrups simultaneously to prevent muscle strain and excess pressure on the legs and thighs. Other preoperative interventions are similar to those described in Chapter 18.

Initiating Postoperative Nursing Care

Immediate postoperative goals include preventing infection and pressure on any existing suture line. This may require perineal care and may preclude using dressings. The patient is encouraged to void within a few hours after surgery for cystocele and complete tear. If the patient does not void within this period and reports discomfort or pain in the bladder region after 6 hours, she needs to be catheterized. Some physicians prefer to leave an indwelling catheter in place for 2 to 4 days, so some women may return home with a catheter in place. Various other bladder care methods are described in Chapter 45. After each voiding or bowel movement, the perineum is cleansed with warm, sterile saline solution and dried with sterile absorbent material if a perineal incision has been made.

After an external perineal repair, the perineum is kept as clean as possible. Commercially available sprays containing combined antiseptic and anesthetic solutions are soothing and effective, and an ice pack applied locally may relieve discomfort. However, the weight of the ice bag must rest on the bed, not on the patient.

Routine postoperative care is similar to that given after abdominal surgery. The patient is positioned in bed with her head and knees elevated slightly. The patient may go home the day of or the day after surgery; the duration of the hospital stay depends on the surgical approach used.

After surgery for a complete perineal laceration (through the rectal sphincter), special care and attention are required. The bladder is drained through the catheter to prevent strain on the sutures. Throughout recovery, stool-softening agents are administered nightly after the patient begins a soft diet.

Promoting Home and Community-Based Care

Teaching Patients Self-Care

Predischarge instructions include information pertaining to the gynecologist's postoperative instructions related to cleanliness, prevention of constipation, recommended exercises, and avoiding lifting heavy objects or standing for prolonged periods. The patient is instructed to report any pelvic pain, unusual discharge, inability to carry out personal hygiene, and vaginal bleeding.

Continuing Care

The patient is advised to continue with perineal exercises, which are recommended to improve muscle strength and tone. She is reminded to return to the gynecologist for a follow-up visit and to consult with the physician about when it is safe to resume sexual intercourse.

BENIGN DISORDERS

Vulvitis and Vulvodynia

Vulvitis, an inflammation of the vulva, may occur with other disorders, such as diabetes, dermatologic problems, or poor hygiene, or it may be secondary to irritation from a vaginal discharge related to a specific vaginitis.

Vulvodynia is a chronic vulvar pain syndrome (ACOG, 2006c). Symptoms may include burning, stinging, irritation, or stabbing pain. The syndrome has been described as primary, with onset at first tampon insertion or sexual

experience, or secondary, beginning months or years after first tampon insertion or sexual experience. It may affect more than 18% of women, usually between 18 and 25 years of age (Bachman, Rosen, Pinn, et al., 2006). Vulvodynia may be classified as organic if it has a known cause (infection, trauma, or irritants) or idiopathic if no cause is known. It can be chronic or unremitting, intermittent or episodic, or may occur only in response to contact. The pathophysiology is unknown. **Vestibulodynia** is the most frequent type of vulvodynia, producing sharp pain on pressure on the vestibule.

Treatment methods for vulvodynia vary. Topical treatments (ie, estrogens, corticosteroids, trichloroacetic acid), surgery, and interferon, as well as biofeedback and dietary changes (Bachman, et al., 2006), have been used. Some cases seem to be similar to peripheral neuralgia and may respond to treatment with tricyclic antidepressants.

Vulvar Cysts

Bartholin's cyst results from the obstruction of a duct in one of the paired vestibular glands located in the posterior third of the vulva, near the vestibule. This cyst is the most common vulvar tumor. A simple cyst may be asymptomatic, but an infected cyst or abscess may cause discomfort. Infection may be due to a gonococcal organism, *Escherichia coli*, or *Staphylococcus aureus* and can cause an abscess with or without involving the inguinal lymph nodes. Skene's duct cysts may result in pressure, dyspareunia, altered urinary stream, and pain, especially if infection is present. Vestibular cysts, located inferior to the hymen, may also occur. Cysts can be treated by resection or with laser, ablation with silver nitrate, and puncture. Asymptomatic cysts do not require treatment. Malignancy can occur, usually in women older than 50 years of age, so drainage and biopsy may be considered.

Medical Management

The usual treatment for a Bartholin's cyst is incision and drainage followed by antibiotic therapy. If a cyst is asymptomatic, treatment is unnecessary. Moist heat or sitz baths may promote drainage and resolution. If surgery is necessary, a Word Bartholin gland catheter is usually used. This catheter, a short latex stem with an inflatable bulb at the distal end, creates a tract that preserves the gland and allows for drainage. A nonopioid analgesic agent may be administered before this outpatient procedure. A local anesthetic agent is injected, and the cyst is incised or lanced and irrigated with normal saline; the catheter is inserted and inflated with 2 to 3 mL of water. The catheter stem is then tucked into the vagina to allow freedom of movement. The catheter is left in place for 4 to 6 weeks until the tract reepithelializes. The patient is informed that discharge should be expected, as the catheter allows drainage of the cyst. She is instructed to contact her primary health care provider if pain occurs because the bulb may be too large for the cavity and fluid may need to be removed. Routine hygiene is encouraged.

Skene's duct cysts can be excised or drained with a Word catheter. Vestibular cysts are excised if symptomatic.

Vulvar Dystrophy

Vulvar dystrophy is a condition found in older women that causes dry, thickened skin on the vulva or slightly raised, whitish papules, fissures, or macules. Symptoms usually consist of varying degrees of itching, but some patients have no symptoms. A few patients with vulvar cancer have associated dystrophy (vulvar cancer is discussed later in this chapter). Biopsy with careful follow-up is the standard intervention. Benign dystrophies include lichen planus, simplex chronicus, **lichen sclerosus,** squamous cell hyperplasia, vulvar **vestibulitis,** and other dermatoses.

Medical Management

Topical corticosteroids (ie, hydrocortisone creams) are the usual treatment. Petrolatum jelly may relieve pruritus. Use is decreased as symptoms resolve. Topical corticosteroids are effective in treating squamous cell hyperplasia. Treatment is often complete in 2 to 3 weeks; this condition is not likely to recur after treatment is completed.

If malignant cells are detected on biopsy, local excision, laser therapy, local chemotherapy, and immunologic treatment are used. Vulvectomy is avoided, if possible, to spare the patient from the stress of disfigurement and possible sexual dysfunction.

Nursing Management

Key nursing responsibilities for patients with vulvar dystrophies focus on teaching. Important topics include hygiene and self-monitoring for signs and symptoms of complications.

Promoting Home and Community-Based Care

Teaching Patients Self-Care

Instructions for patients with benign vulvar dystrophies include the importance of maintaining good personal hygiene and keeping the vulva dry. Lanolin or hydrogenated vegetable oil is recommended for relief of dryness. Sitz baths may help but should not be overused because dryness may result or increase. The patient is instructed to notify her primary health care provider about any change or ulceration because biopsy may be necessary to rule out squamous cell carcinoma.

By encouraging all patients to perform genital self-examinations regularly and have any itching, lesions, or unusual symptoms assessed by a health care provider, nurses can help prevent complications and progression of vulvar lesions.

Ovarian Cysts

The ovary is a common site for cysts, which may be simple enlargements of normal ovarian constituents, the graafian follicle, or the corpus luteum, or they may arise from abnormal growth of the ovarian epithelium. The risk of malignancy is much greater in postmenopausal women than in premenopausal patients. Almost all pelvic masses in premenopausal women are benign (ACOG, 2007c).

Ovarian cysts are often detected on routine pelvic examination. Although these cysts are typically benign, they nevertheless should be evaluated to exclude ovarian cancer, particularly in postmenopausal women (ACOG, 2007c).

The patient may or may not report acute or chronic abdominal pain. Symptoms of a ruptured cyst mimic various acute abdominal emergencies, such as appendicitis or ectopic pregnancy. Larger cysts may produce abdominal swelling and exert pressure on adjacent abdominal organs.

Postoperative nursing care after surgery to remove an ovarian cyst is similar to that after abdominal surgery, with one exception. The marked decrease in intra-abdominal pressure resulting from removal of a very large cyst usually leads to considerable abdominal distention. This may be prevented to some extent by applying a snug-fitting abdominal binder.

Some surgeons discuss the option of a hysterectomy when a woman is undergoing bilateral ovary removal because of a suspicious mass; it may increase life expectancy and avoid a later second surgery. Patient preference is a priority in determining its appropriateness.

Polycystic ovary syndrome (PCOS) is another type of cystic disorder that affects the ovaries. This complex endocrine condition involves a disorder in the hypothalamic–pituitary and ovarian network or axis, resulting in chronic anovulation and clinical androgen excess, along with multiple small ovarian cysts called polycystic ovaries. Onset of PCOS may be at menarche or later; it occurs in approximately 5% to 10% of women of childbearing age (Stankiewicz & Norman, 2006). Features include obesity, insulin resistance, impaired glucose tolerance, dyslipidemia, sleep apnea, and infertility. Symptoms are related to androgen excess. Irregular menstrual periods, resulting from lack of regular ovulation, infertility, obesity, and hirsutism, may be a presenting complaint. Cysts form in the ovaries because the hormonal milieu cannot cause ovulation on a regular basis. Women with PCOS may develop insulin resistance and metabolic syndrome, and they may be at higher risk for diabetes and cardiac disorders in later life. Metformin (Glucophage) is also used to decrease the hyperinsulinemia that occurs with PCOS.

Medical Management

The treatment of large ovarian cysts is usually surgical removal. However, oral contraceptives may be used in young, healthy patients to suppress ovarian activity and resolve small cysts that appear to be fluid filled or physiologic.

Oral contraceptives are also usually prescribed to treat PCOS. When pregnancy is desired, medications to stimulate ovulation (clomiphene [Clomid]) are often effective. Lifestyle modification is critical, and weight management is part of the treatment plan.

Benign Tumors of the Uterus: Fibroids (Leiomyomas, Myomas)

Myomatous or **fibroid tumors** of the uterus are estimated to occur in 20% to 40% of women during their reproductive years. It is thought that women are genetically predisposed to develop this condition, which is almost always benign. Fibroids arise from the muscle tissue of the uterus and can be solitary or multiple, in the lining (intracavitary), muscle wall (intramural), and outside surface (serosal) of the uterus. They usually develop slowly in women between 25

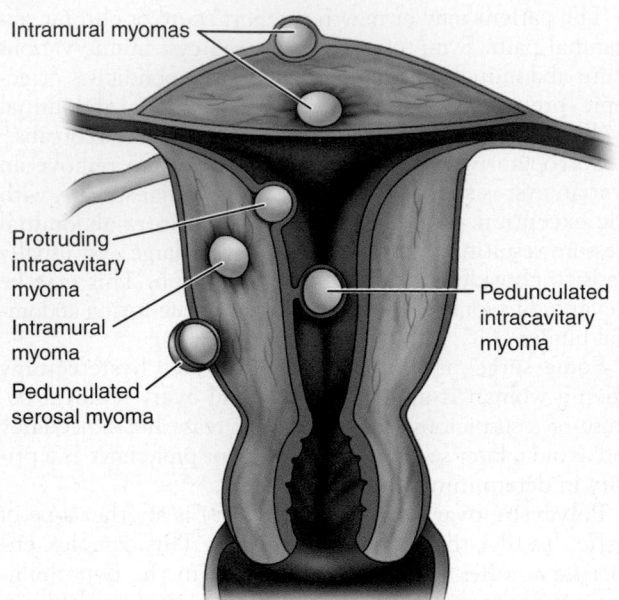

Intramural myomas

Protruding intracavitary myoma

Intramural myoma

Pedunculated serosal myoma

Pedunculated intracavitary myoma

Figure 47-7 Myomas (fibroids). Those that impinge on the uterine cavity are called intracavitary myomas.

and 40 years of age and may become quite large. A growth spurt with enlargement of the fibroid tumor may occur in the decade before menopause, possibly related to anovulatory cycles and high levels of unopposed estrogen. Fibroids are a common reason for hysterectomy because they often result in menorrhagia, which can be difficult to control.

Clinical Manifestations

Fibroids may cause no symptoms, or they may produce abnormal vaginal bleeding. Other symptoms result from pressure on the surrounding organs and include pain, backache, pressure, bloating, constipation, and urinary problems. Menorrhagia (excessive bleeding) and metrorrhagia (irregular bleeding) may occur because fibroids may distort the uterine lining (Fig. 47-7). Fibroids may interfere with fertility.

Medical Management

Treatment of uterine fibroids may include medical or surgical intervention and depends to a large extent on the size, symptoms, and location, as well as the woman's age and her reproductive plans. Fibroids usually shrink and disappear during menopause, when estrogen is no longer produced. Simple observation and follow-up may be all the management that is necessary. The patient with minor symptoms is closely monitored. If she plans to have children, treatment is as conservative as possible. As a rule, large tumors that produce pressure symptoms should be removed **(myomectomy)**. A hysterectomy may be performed if symptoms are bothersome and childbearing is completed (see later discussion of nursing care for a patient having a hysterectomy).

Several other alternatives to hysterectomy have been developed for the treatment of excessive bleeding due to fibroids (ACOG, 2007d). These include the following:

- Hysteroscopic resection of myomas: a laser is used through a hysteroscope passed through the cervix; no incision or overnight stay is needed

- Laparoscopic myomectomy: removal of a fibroid through a laparoscope inserted through a small abdominal incision
- Laparoscopic myolysis: a laser or electrical needles are used to cauterize and shrink the fibroid
- Laparoscopic cryomyolysis: electric current is used to coagulate the fibroid
- Uterine artery embolization (UAE): polyvinyl alcohol or gelatin particles are injected into the blood vessels that supply the fibroid via the femoral artery, resulting in infarction and resultant shrinkage. This percutaneous image–guided therapy offers an alternative to hormone therapy or surgery. UAE may result in infrequent but serious complications such as pain, infection, amenorrhea, necrosis, and bleeding. Although rare, deaths and ovarian failure may occur. Women need to weigh the risks and benefits carefully, especially if they have not completed childbearing. This procedure has been found to cause fewer complications than hysterectomy, but women may need further treatment in the future (Dutton, Hirst, McPherson, et al., 2008).
- Magnetic resonance–guided focused ultrasound surgery (MRgFUS): ultrasonic energy is passed through the abdominal wall to target and destroy the fibroid. Although not yet widely used, this noninvasive procedure is approved by the U.S. Food and Drug Administration for premenopausal women with bothersome symptoms due to fibroids and who do not want more children. It is an outpatient treatment (Stewart, Gostout, Rabinovici, et al., 2007).

Medications (eg, leuprolide [Lupron]) or other gonadotropin-releasing hormone (GnRH) analogues, which induce a temporary menopause-like environment, may be prescribed to shrink the fibroids. This treatment consists of monthly injections, which may cause hot flashes and vaginal dryness. Treatment is usually short term (ie, before surgery) to shrink the fibroids, allowing easier surgery, and to alleviate anemia, which may occur as a result of heavy menstrual flow. This treatment is used on a temporary basis because it leads to vasomotor symptoms and loss of bone density.

Antifibrotic agents are under investigation for long-term treatment of fibroids. Mifepristone (RU-486, Mifeprex), a progesterone antagonist, has also been prescribed; it appears to be effective (Fiscella, Eisinger, Meldrum, et al., 2006).

Endometriosis

Endometriosis is a chronic disease that affects between 5% to 15% of women of reproductive age. A benign lesion or lesions with cells similar to those lining the uterus grow aberrantly anywhere in the pelvic cavity outside the uterus. Often, extensive endometriosis causes few symptoms, whereas an isolated lesion may produce severe symptoms. It is a major cause of chronic pelvic pain and infertility.

Endometriosis has been diagnosed more frequently as a result of the increased use of laparoscopy, but diagnosis can often be delayed, and women with this problem often feel as if their complaints are being dismissed. Before laparoscopy became widely available, major surgery was necessary before a diagnosis could be made. There is a high incidence among patients who bear children late and among those who have fewer children. In countries where tradition favors early marriage and early childbearing, endometriosis is rare. There also appears to be a familial predisposition to endometriosis; it is more common in women whose close female relatives are affected. Other factors that may suggest increased risk include a shorter menstrual cycle (less than every 27 days), flow longer than 7 days, outflow obstruction, and younger age at menarche. Characteristically, endometriosis is found in young, nulliparous women between 25 and 35 years of age and in adolescents, particularly those with dysmenorrhea that does not respond to nonsteroidal anti-inflammatory drugs (NSAIDs) or oral contraceptives.

Pathophysiology

Misplaced endometrial tissue responds to and depends on ovarian hormonal stimulation. During menstruation, this ectopic tissue bleeds, mostly into areas having no outlet, which causes pain and adhesions. The lesions are typically small and puckered, with a blue/brown/gray powder-burn appearance and brown or blue-black appearance, indicating concealed bleeding.

Endometrial tissue contained within an ovarian cyst has no outlet for the bleeding; this formation is referred to as a pseudocyst or chocolate cyst. Adhesions, cysts, and scar tissue may result, causing pain and infertility. Endometriosis may increase the risk of ovarian, renal, thyroid, and breast cancer (Melin, Sparén & Bergqvist, 2008).

Currently the best-accepted theory regarding the origin of endometrial lesions is the transplantation theory, which suggests that a backflow of menses (retrograde menstruation) transports endometrial tissue to ectopic sites through the fallopian tubes. Why some women with retrograde menstruation develop endometriosis and others do not is unknown. Endometrial tissue can also be spread by lymphatic or venous channels.

Clinical Manifestations

Symptoms vary but include dysmenorrhea, dyspareunia, and pelvic discomfort or pain. Dyschezia (pain with bowel movements) and radiation of pain to the back or leg may occur. Depression, loss of work due to pain, and relationship difficulties may result. Infertility may occur because of fibrosis and adhesions or because of a variety of substances (prostaglandins, cytokines, other factors) produced by the implants.

Assessment and Diagnostic Findings

A health history, including an account of the menstrual pattern, is necessary to elicit specific symptoms. On bimanual pelvic examination, fixed tender nodules are sometimes palpated, and uterine mobility may be limited, indicating adhesions. Laparoscopic examination confirms the diagnosis and helps stage the disease. In stage 1, patients have superficial or minimal lesions; stage 2, mild involvement; stage 3, moderate involvement; and stage 4, extensive involvement and dense adhesions, with obliteration of the cul-de-sac.

Medical Management

Treatment depends on the symptoms, the patient's desire for pregnancy, and the extent of the disease. If the woman does not have symptoms, routine examination may be all that is required. Other therapy for varying degrees of symptoms may be NSAIDs, oral contraceptives, GnRH agonists, or surgery. Pregnancy often alleviates symptoms because neither ovulation nor menstruation occurs.

Pharmacologic Therapy

Palliative measures include use of medications, such as analgesic agents and prostaglandin inhibitors, for pain. Hormonal therapy is effective in suppressing endometriosis and relieving dysmenorrhea (menstrual pain). Oral contraceptives are often used. Infrequently, side effects may occur with oral contraceptives, such as fluid retention, weight gain, and nausea. These can usually be managed by changing brands or formulations. Depo-Provera, an injectable contraceptive agent, may also be used.

Several types of hormonal therapy are also available in addition to oral contraceptives. A synthetic androgen, danazol (Danocrine), causes atrophy of the endometrium and subsequent amenorrhea. The medication inhibits the release of gonadotropin with minimal overt sex hormone stimulation. The drawbacks of this medication are that it is expensive and may cause troublesome side effects such as fatigue, depression, weight gain, oily skin, decreased breast size, mild acne, hot flashes, and vaginal atrophy. GnRH agonists decrease estrogen production and cause subsequent amenorrhea. Side effects are related to low estrogen levels (eg, hot flashes and vaginal dryness). Loss of bone density is often offset by concurrent use of estrogen. Leuprolide, an GnRH agonist, is injected monthly to suppress hormones and induce an artificial menopause, thus avoiding menstrual effects and relieving endometriosis. Some clinicians prescribe a combination of therapies. Most women continue treatment despite side effects, and symptoms diminish for 80% to 90% of women with mild to moderate endometriosis. Hormonal medications are not used in patients with a history of abnormal vaginal bleeding or liver, heart, or kidney disease. Bone density is followed carefully because of the risk of bone loss; hormone therapy is usually short term.

Surgical Management

If conservative measures are not helpful, surgery may be necessary to relieve pain and enhance the possibility of pregnancy. Surgery may be combined with use of medical therapy. The procedure selected depends on the patient. Laparoscopy may be used to fulgurate (cut with high-frequency current) endometrial implants and to release adhesions. Laser surgery is another option made possible by laparoscopy. Laser therapy vaporizes or coagulates the endometrial implants, thereby destroying this tissue. Other surgical options include endocoagulation and electrocoagulation, laparotomy, abdominal hysterectomy, **oophorectomy,** bilateral **salpingo-oophorectomy,** and appendectomy. For women older than 35 years of age or those willing to sacrifice reproductive capability, total hysterectomy is an option. Endometriosis recurs in many women.

Nursing Management

The health history and physical examination focus on specific symptoms (eg, pain) and when and how long they have been bothersome, the effect of prescribed medications, and the woman's reproductive plans. This information helps in determining the treatment plan. Explaining the various diagnostic procedures may help to alleviate the patient's anxiety. Patient goals include relief of pain, dysmenorrhea, dyspareunia, and avoidance of infertility.

As the treatment progresses, the woman with endometriosis and her partner may find that pregnancy is not easily possible, and the psychosocial impact of this realization must be recognized and addressed. Alternatives, such as in vitro fertilization or adoption, may be discussed at an appropriate time and referrals offered.

The nurse's role in patient education is to dispel myths and encourage the patient to seek care if dysmenorrhea or dyspareunia occurs. The Endometriosis Association (see Resources at the end of this chapter) is a helpful resource for patients seeking further information and support for this condition, which can cause disabling pain and severe emotional distress.

Chronic Pelvic Pain

Chronic pelvic pain is a common disorder of women that may be related to several of the previously discussed gynecologic disorders. Fifteen percent to 20% of women have chronic pelvic pain—that is, pelvic pain that persists for more than 6 months. It may be cyclic or intermittent and noncyclic. Causes may be reproductive, genitourinary, or gastrointestinal. A history of abuse, PID, endometriosis, interstitial cystitis, musculoskeletal disorders, irritable bowel syndrome, and previous surgery resulting in abdominal adhesions may be associated with chronic pelvic pain. Dysmenorrhea, dyspareunia, and lower abdominal pain may also be associated with sexual and physical abuse (Pikarinen, Saisto, Schei, et al., 2007).

Chronic pelvic pain is often difficult to treat. Treatment depends on physical and diagnostic test results and may include antidepressants, analgesics, oral contraceptives, GnRH agonists, exercise, and surgery.

Adenomyosis

In adenomyosis, the tissue that lines the endometrium invades the uterine wall. The incidence is highest in women 40 to 50 years of age. Symptoms include hypermenorrhea (excessive and prolonged bleeding), acquired dysmenorrhea, polymenorrhea (abnormally frequent bleeding), and premenstrual staining. Physical examination findings on palpation include an enlarged, firm, and tender uterus. Treatment depends on the severity of bleeding and pain. Hysterectomy may offer greater relief than more conservative therapies.

Endometrial Hyperplasia

This condition, a build-up of endometrial tissue, can be a precursor to endometrial cancer and often results from unopposed estrogen from any source. Estrogen therapy alone without progesterone in a woman with a uterus can cause this condition. Women with anovulatory cycles, PCOS, or obesity may all have high circulating levels of estrogen. Tamoxifen (Nolvadex) may also be a causative factor (ACOG, 2006d). Diagnosis is by biopsy or ultrasound findings of thickness of the endometrium. Hyperplasia with atypia on a pathology or biopsy report indicates risk of progression. Progestin treatment may be effective, but hysterectomy may be advised if pathology from an endometrial biopsy shows atypia. Abnormal bleeding is the most common symptom.

MALIGNANT CONDITIONS

The projected incidence and estimated mortality for female reproductive cancers in the United States are (American Cancer Society [ACS], 2009):
- Cervical cancer: about 11,300 new cases and 4,100 deaths
- Uterine cancer: about 42,100 new cases and 7,800 deaths
- Ovarian cancer: about 21,600 new cases and 14,600 deaths
- Vaginal cancer: about 2,160 new cases and 770 deaths
- Vulvar cancer: about 3,600 new cases and 900 deaths

Cervical cancer is the second most prevalent cancer in women worldwide and the fifth leading cause of cancer deaths. Worldwide, the incidence is declining. Pap smears in developed countries have resulted in increased detection of preinvasive lesions and decreased cancer death rates. Eighty percent of all cases of cervical cancer are found in developing countries, where early detection methods are often not available (U.S. Cancer Statistics Working Group, 2007).

Although death rates from all cancers are decreasing in the United States and other developed countries, cancer in developing countries is increasing. Many of these cases affect women. Although infectious diseases and HIV are often high priorities in these countries, the toll of increasing malignancies needs to be considered.

Although some cancers are difficult to detect or prevent, annual pelvic examination with a Pap smear is a painless and relatively inexpensive method of early detection. Health care providers can encourage women to follow this health practice by providing nonstressful examinations that are educational and supportive and offer women an opportunity to ask questions and clarify misinformation. If more women understood that gynecologic examinations and Pap smears do not have to be uncomfortable or embarrassing, early detection rates would likely improve and lives would be saved.

Many women diagnosed with gynecologic malignancies experience depression and anxiety. The occurrence of physical symptoms may cause psychological distress. Intervention directed toward physical and psychological symptoms requires a multidisciplinary approach.

Nurses should be aware of ongoing clinical trials that are being conducted to identify effective treatments for many conditions. They are often in a position to answer questions about clinical trials and to encourage patients to consider participation if appropriate. Women's participation in cancer research may occur in part because women are unaware of ongoing relevant research.

Cancer of the Cervix

Carcinoma of the cervix is predominantly squamous cell cancer. Cervical cancer is less common than it once was because of early detection of cell changes by Pap smear. However, it is still the third most common female reproductive cancer and is estimated to affect more than 11,300 women in the United States every year (ACS, 2009). Risk factors are presented in Chart 47-5.

Preventive measures include regular pelvic examinations and Pap tests for all women, especially older women past childbearing age. This decreases the chance of dying from cervical cancer from 1 in 250 to 1 in 2,000. Preventive counseling should encourage delaying first intercourse, avoiding HPV infection, participating in safer sex only, smoking cessation, and receiving HPV immunization (see earlier discussion).

There are several different types of cervical cancer. Most of these cancers are squamous cell carcinomas and the remainder are adenocarcinomas or mixed adenosquamous carcinomas. Adenocarcinomas begin in mucus-producing glands and are often due to HPV infection. Most cervical cancers, if not detected and treated, spread to regional pelvic lymph nodes, and local recurrence is not uncommon.

Clinical Manifestations

Early cervical cancer rarely produces symptoms. If symptoms are present, they may go unnoticed as a thin watery vaginal discharge often noticed after intercourse or douching. When symptoms such as discharge, irregular bleeding, or pain or bleeding after sexual intercourse occur, the disease may be advanced. Advanced disease should not occur if all women have access to gynecologic care and avail themselves of it. The nurse's role in access to care and its utilization is crucial.

In advanced cervical cancer, the vaginal discharge gradually increases and becomes watery and, finally, dark and foul-smelling from necrosis and infection of the tumor. The bleeding, which occurs at irregular intervals between periods (metrorrhagia) or after menopause, may be slight (just enough to spot the undergarments) and occurs usually after mild trauma or pressure (eg, intercourse, douching, or bearing down during defecation). As the disease continues, the bleeding may persist and increase. Leg pain, dysuria, rectal bleeding, and edema of the extremities signal advanced disease.

As the cancer advances, it may invade the tissues outside the cervix, including the lymph glands anterior to the sacrum. In one third of patients with invasive cervical cancer, the disease involves the fundus. The nerves in this region may be affected, producing excruciating pain in the back and the legs that is relieved only by large doses of opioid analgesics. If the disease progresses, it often produces extreme emaciation and anemia, usually accompanied by fever due to secondary infection and abscesses in the ulcerating mass, and by fistula formation. Because the survival rate for in situ cancer is 100% and the rate for women with more advanced stages of cervical cancer decreases dramatically, early detection is essential.

Assessment and Diagnostic Findings

Diagnosis may be made on the basis of abnormal Pap smear results, followed by biopsy results identifying severe dysplasia (cervical intraepithelial neoplasia type III [CIN III], high-grade squamous intraepithelial lesions [HGSIL; also referred to as HSIL], or carcinoma in situ; see below). HPV infections are usually implicated in these conditions. Carcinoma in situ is technically classified as severe dysplasia and is defined as cancer that has extended through the full thickness of the epithelium of the cervix, but not beyond. This is often referred to as preinvasive cancer.

In its very early stages, invasive cervical cancer is found microscopically by Pap smear. In later stages, pelvic examination may reveal a large, reddish growth or a deep, ulcerating lesion. The patient may report spotting or bloody discharge.

When the patient has been diagnosed with invasive cervical cancer, clinical staging estimates the extent of the disease so that treatment can be planned more specifically and prognosis reasonably predicted. The tumor, nodes, and metastases (TNM) system is the most widely used staging system. The TNM classification is also used in describing cancer stages. In this system, T refers to the extent of the primary tumor, N to lymph node involvement, and M to metastasis, or spread of the disease.

Signs and symptoms are evaluated, and x-rays, laboratory tests, and special examinations, such as punch biopsy and colposcopy, are performed. Depending on the stage of the cancer, other tests and procedures may be performed to determine the extent of disease and appropriate treatment. These tests may include dilation and curettage (D & C),

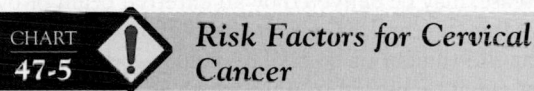

| CHART 47-5 | ⚠ | *Risk Factors for Cervical Cancer* |

- Sexual activity:
  Multiple sex partners
  Early age (younger than 20) at first coitus (exposes the vulnerable young cervix to potential viruses from a partner)
- Sex with uncircumcised males
- Sexual contact with males whose partners have had cervical cancer
- Early childbearing
- Exposure to human papillomavirus, types 16 and 18
- HIV infection and other causes of immunodeficiency
- Smoking and exposure to secondhand smoke
- Exposure to diethylstilbestrol (DES) in utero
- Family history of cervical cancer
- Low socioeconomic status (may be related to early marriage and early childbearing)
- Nutritional deficiencies (folate, beta-carotene, and vitamin C levels are lower in women with cervical cancer than in women without it)
- Chronic cervical infection
- Overweight status

computed tomography (CT), magnetic resonance imaging (MRI), IV urography, cystography, positron emission tomography, and barium x-ray studies.

Medical Management

Precursor or Preinvasive Lesions

When precursor lesions, such as low-grade squamous intraepithelial lesion (LGSIL; also referred to as LSIL) (CIN I and II or mild to moderate dysplasia), are found by colposcopy and biopsy, careful monitoring by frequent Pap smears or conservative treatment is possible. Conservative treatment may consist of monitoring, **cryotherapy** (freezing with nitrous oxide), or laser therapy. A **loop electrocautery excision procedure (LEEP)** may also be used to remove abnormal cells. In this procedure, a thin wire loop with laser is used to cut away a thin layer of cervical tissue. LEEP is an outpatient procedure usually performed in a gynecologist's office; it takes only a few minutes. Analgesia is given before the procedure, and a local anesthetic agent is injected into the area. This procedure allows the pathologist to examine the removed tissue sample to determine if the borders of the tissue are disease free. Another procedure called a cone biopsy or **conization** (removing a cone-shaped portion of the cervix) is performed when biopsy findings demonstrate CIN III or HGSIL (equivalent to severe dysplasia) and carcinoma in situ.

If preinvasive cervical cancer (carcinoma in situ) occurs when a woman has completed childbearing, a simple hysterectomy (removal of the uterus only) is usually recommended. If a woman has not completed childbearing and invasion is less than 1 mm, conization may be sufficient. Frequent follow-up examinations are necessary to monitor for recurrence.

Patients who have precursor or premalignant lesions need reassurance that they do not have invasive cancer. However, the importance of close follow-up is emphasized because the condition, if untreated for a long time, may progress to cancer. Patients with cervical cancer in situ also need to know that this is usually a slow-growing and nonaggressive type of cancer that is not expected to recur after appropriate treatment.

Invasive Cancer

Treatment of invasive cervical cancer depends on the stage of the lesion, the patient's age and general health, and the judgment and experience of the physician. Surgery and radiation treatment (intracavitary and external) are most often used. Surgical procedures that may be used to treat cervical cancer are summarized in Chart 47-6. When tumor invasion is less than 3 mm, a hysterectomy is often sufficient. Invasion exceeding 3 mm usually requires a radical hysterectomy with pelvic node dissection and aortic node assessment. Stage 1B1 tumors are treated with radical hysterectomy and radiation. Stage 1B2 tumors are treated individually, because no single correct course of treatment has been identified and many variable options may be considered.

A procedure called a radical trachelectomy is an alternative to hysterectomy in women with invasive cervical cancer who are young and want to have children. In this procedure, the cervix is gripped with retractors and pulled

---

Chart 47-6 • *Surgical Procedures for Cervical Cancer*

- Total hysterectomy—removal of the uterus, cervix, and ovaries
- Radical hysterectomy—removal of the uterus, ovaries, fallopian tubes, proximal vagina, and bilateral lymph nodes through an abdominal incision (*Note:* "radical" indicates that an extensive area of the paravaginal, paracervical, parametrial, and uterosacral tissues is removed with the uterus.)
- Radical vaginal hysterectomy—vaginal removal of the uterus, ovaries, fallopian tubes, and proximal vagina
- Bilateral pelvic lymphadenectomy—removal of the common iliac, external iliac, hypogastric, and obturator lymphatic vessels and nodes
- Pelvic exenteration—removal of the pelvic organs, including the bladder or rectum and pelvic lymph nodes, and construction of diversional conduit, colostomy, and vagina
- Radical trachelectomy—removal of the cervix and selected nodes to preserve childbearing capacity in a woman of reproductive age with cervical cancer

---

down into the vagina until it is visible. The affected tissue is excised while the rest of the cervix and uterus remain intact. A drawstring suture is used to close the cervix.

Frequent follow-up after surgery by a gynecologic oncologist is imperative because the risk of recurrence is 35% after treatment for invasive cervical cancer. Recurrence usually occurs within the first 2 years. Recurrences are often in the upper quarter of the vagina, and ureteral obstruction may be a sign. Weight loss, leg edema, and pelvic pain may be signs of lymphatic obstruction and metastasis. Micrometastases have been found in patients with negative lymph nodes.

Radiation, which is often part of treatment to reduce recurrent disease, may be delivered by an external beam or by **brachytherapy** (method by which the radiation source is placed near the tumor) or both. The field to be irradiated and dose of radiation are determined by stage, volume of tumor, and lymph node involvement. Treatment can be administered daily for 4 to 6 weeks followed by one or two treatments of intracavitary radiation. Interstitial therapy may be used when vaginal placement has become impossible because of tumor or stricture.

Platinum-based agents are being used to treat advanced cervical cancer. They are often used in combination with radiation therapy, surgery, or both. Studies are ongoing to find the best approach to treat advanced cervical cancer. Vaginal stenosis is a frequent side effect of radiation. Sexual activity, with lubrication, is preventive, as is use of a vaginal dilator to avoid severe permanent vaginal stenosis.

Some patients with recurrences of cervical cancer are considered for **pelvic exenteration,** in which a large portion of the pelvic contents is removed. This is a complex, extensive surgical procedure that is reserved for women with a high likelihood of cure. Unilateral leg edema, sciatica, and ureteral obstruction indicate likely disease progression. Patients with these symptoms have advanced disease and are not considered candidates for this major surgical procedure.

Surgery is often complex because it is performed close to the bowel, bladder, ureters, and great vessels. Complications can be considerable and include pulmonary emboli, pulmonary edema, myocardial infarction, cerebrovascular accident, hemorrhage, sepsis, small bowel obstruction, fistula formation, obstruction of the ileal conduit, bladder dysfunction, and pyelonephritis, most often in the first 18 months. Vein constriction must be avoided postoperatively. Patients with varicose veins or a history of thromboembolic disease may be treated prophylactically with heparin. Antiembolism stockings are prescribed to reduce the risk of deep vein thrombosis (DVT). Nursing care of these patients is complex and requires coordination and care by experienced health care professionals. Pelvic exenteration is discussed in further detail later in this chapter.

Cancer of the Uterus (Endometrium)

Although the incidence of cancer of the uterine endometrium (fundus or corpus) has stabilized, the death rate from this cancer has increased, possibly because of increased lifespan and coexisting comorbidities. This cancer is the most frequently occurring gynecological cancer in the United States. After breast, colorectal, and lung cancer, endometrial cancer is the fourth most common cancer in women. More than 42,100 new cases of uterine cancer occur each year, with more than 7,800 deaths (ACS, 2009). Most women are diagnosed between 55 and 64 years of age. Seventy percent of women with endometrial cancer are obese; obesity increases the risk of morbidity and mortality from this disease. This disease occurs twice as often in Caucasian women as in African American women, who have a less favorable prognosis, and research is needed to explain this disparity (Sorosky, 2008). Cumulative exposure to estrogen is considered the major risk factor (Chart 47-7). This exposure occurs with the use of estrogen therapy without the use of progestin, early menarche, late menopause, nulliparity, and anovulation. Other risk factors include obesity, infertility, and diabetes, as well as use of tamoxifen. This medication, taken for treatment or prevention of breast cancer, may cause proliferation of the uterine lining (ACOG, 2006d). Women who take it should be monitored by their oncologists and gynecologic health care providers.

| CHART 47-7 | **Risk Factors for Uterine Cancer** |

- Age: at least 55 years; median age, 61 years
- Obesity that results in increased estrone levels (related to excess weight) resulting from conversion of androstenedione to estrone in body fat, which exposes the uterus to unopposed estrogen
- Unopposed estrogen therapy (estrogen used without progesterone, which offsets the risk of unopposed estrogen)
- Other: nulliparity, truncal obesity, late menopause (after 52 years of age) and use of tamoxifen

Pathophysiology

Most uterine cancers are endometrioid (ie, originating in the lining of the uterus). There are three types. Type 1, which accounts for the majority of cases, is estrogen related and occurs in younger, obese, and perimenopausal women. It is usually low grade and endometrioid. Type 2, which occurs in about 10% of cases, is high grade and usually serous cell or clear cell. It affects older women and African American women. Type 3, which also occurs in about 10% of cases, is the hereditary and genetic types, some of which are related to Lynch II syndrome. (This syndrome is associated with the occurrence of breast, ovarian, colon, endometrial, and other cancers throughout a family.)

Assessment and Diagnostic Findings

All women should be encouraged to have annual checkups, including a gynecologic examination. Any woman who is experiencing irregular bleeding should be evaluated promptly. If a menopausal woman experiences bleeding, an endometrial aspiration or biopsy is performed to rule out hyperplasia, a possible precursor of endometrial cancer. The procedure is quick and usually painless. Ultrasonography can also be used to measure the thickness of the endometrium. (Postmenopausal women should have a very thin endometrium due to low levels of estrogen; a thicker lining warrants further investigation.) A biopsy or aspiration for tissue pathology is diagnostic.

Medical Management

Treatment of endometrial cancer consists of total or radical hysterectomy (discussed later in this chapter) and bilateral salpingo-oophorectomy and node sampling. It is necessary to monitor cancer antigen 125 (CA-125) levels, because elevated levels are a significant predictor of extrauterine disease or metastasis. Depending on the stage, the therapeutic approach is individualized and is based on stage, type, differentiation, degree of invasion, and node involvement. Adjuvant radiation may be used in a patient who is considered high risk. Vaginal brachytherapy is being studied as adjuvant therapy. Whole pelvis radiotherapy may be used if there is any spread beyond the uterus. Recurrent cancer usually occurs inside the **vaginal vault** or in the upper vagina, and metastasis usually occurs in lymph nodes or the ovary. Recurrent lesions in the vagina are treated with surgery and radiation. Recurrent lesions beyond the vagina are treated with hormonal therapy or chemotherapy. Progestin therapy is used frequently. Patients should be prepared for such side effects as nausea, depression, rash, or mild fluid retention with progestin therapy.

Cancer of the Vulva

Primary cancer of the vulva represents 4% of all gynecologic malignancies and is seen mostly in postmenopausal women, although its incidence in younger women is increasing. The median age for cancer limited to the vulva is 50 years, whereas the median age for invasive vulvar cancer is 70 years. Possible risk factors include smoking, HPV infection, HIV infection, and immunosuppression. Squamous cell carcinoma accounts for most primary vulvar tumors. Less common are Bartholin's gland cancer, vulvar sarcoma, and malignant melanoma. Little is known about what causes this disease; however, increased risk may be related to chronic vulvar irritation. In younger women, HPV infection may be implicated, especially types 16, 18, and 31. Prevention includes delaying onset of sexual activity to avoid early exposure to HPV and avoidance of smoking. Regular pelvic examinations, Pap smears, and vulvar self-examination are helpful in early detection. Women with persistent irritation or itching should be encouraged to seek evaluation.

Clinical Manifestations

Long-standing pruritus and soreness are the most common symptoms of vulvar cancer. Itching occurs in half of all patients with vulvar malignancy. Bleeding, foul-smelling discharge, and pain may also be present and are usually signs of advanced disease. Cancerous lesions of the vulva are visible and accessible and grow relatively slowly. Early lesions appear as a chronic dermatitis; later, patients may note a lump that continues to grow and becomes a hard, ulcerated, cauliflower-like growth. Biopsy should be performed on any vulvar lesion that persists, ulcerates, or fails to heal quickly with proper therapy. Vulvar malignancies may appear as a lump or mass, redness, or a lesion that fails to heal.

Nurses are in an ideal position to encourage women to perform vulvar self-examinations regularly. Using a mirror, patients can see what constitutes normal female anatomy and learn about changes that should be reported (eg, lesions, ulcers, masses, and persistent itching). Nurses must urge women to seek health care if they notice anything abnormal, because vulvar cancer is one of the most curable of all malignant conditions.

Medical Management

Vulvar intraepithelial lesions are preinvasive and are also called vulvar carcinoma in situ. They may be treated by local excision, laser ablation, application of chemotherapeutic creams, or cryosurgery.

When invasive vulvar carcinoma exists, primary treatment may include wide excision or removal of the vulva **(vulvectomy)**. An effort is made to individualize treatment, depending on the extent of the disease. A wide excision is performed only if lymph nodes are normal. More pervasive lesions require vulvectomy with deep pelvic node dissection. Vulvectomy is very effective at prolonging life but is frequently followed by complications (ie, scarring, wound breakdown, leg swelling, vaginal stenosis, or rectocele). To reduce complications, only necessary tissue is removed. External beam radiation may be used, resulting in sunburn-like irritation that usually resolves in 6 to 12 months. Laser therapy and chemotherapy are other possible treatment options.

If a widespread area is involved or the disease is advanced, a radical vulvectomy with bilateral groin dissection may be performed. Antibiotic and heparin prophylaxis may be prescribed preoperatively and continued postoperatively to prevent infection, DVT, and pulmonary emboli. Antiembolism stockings are applied to reduce the risk of DVT.

Although the role of systemic chemotherapy in the treatment of vulvar cancer remains to be determined, chemotherapy may be useful when used in combination with radiation therapy for the treatment of advanced disease. The combination of radiation and chemotherapy may reduce the size of the cancer, resulting in less extensive subsequent surgery (ACS, 2009).

Clinical trials to determine the most effective treatment are difficult to conduct because there are few patients with this condition. Morbidity with recurrence of the disease is high, and patterns of recurrence vary. Reconstruction after vulvectomy is performed by plastic surgeons when appropriate and desired.

Nursing Management

Assessment

The health history is a valuable tool for establishing rapport with the patient. The reason the patient is seeking health care is apparent. What the nurse can tactfully elicit is the reason why a delay, if any, occurred, in seeking health care—for example, because of modesty, economics, denial, neglect, or fear (abusive partners sometimes prevent women from seeking health care). Factors involved in any delay in seeking health care and treatment may also affect recovery. The patient's health habits and lifestyle are assessed, and her receptivity to teaching is evaluated. Psychosocial factors are also assessed. Preoperative preparation and psychological support begin at this time.

Preoperative Nursing Interventions

Relieving Anxiety

Prior to surgery, the patient must be allowed time to talk and ask questions. Fear often decreases when a woman who is to undergo wide excision of the vulva or vulvectomy learns that the possibility for subsequent sexual relations is good and that pregnancy is possible after a wide excision. The nurse reinforces the information the physician has given to the patient and addresses the patient's questions and concerns.

Preparing Skin for Surgery

Skin preparation may include cleansing the lower abdomen, inguinal areas, upper thighs, and vulva with a detergent germicide for several days before the surgical procedure. The patient may be instructed to do this at home.

Postoperative Nursing Interventions

Relieving Pain

Because of the wide excision, the patient may experience severe pain and discomfort even with minimal movement. Therefore, analgesic agents are administered preventively (ie, around the clock at designated times) to relieve pain, increase the patient's comfort level, and allow mobility. Patient-controlled analgesia (see Chapter 13) may be used to relieve pain and promote patient comfort. Careful positioning using pillows usually increases comfort, as do soothing back rubs. A low Fowler's position or, occasionally, a pillow placed under the knees reduces pain by relieving tension on the incision; however, efforts must be made to avoid pressure behind the knees, which increases the risk of DVT. Positioning the patient on her side, with pillows between her legs and against the lumbar region, provides comfort and reduces tension on the surgical wound.

Improving Skin Integrity

A pressure-reducing mattress may be used to prevent pressure ulcers. Moving from one position to another requires time and effort; use of an overbed trapeze bar may help the patient move herself more easily. Ambulation may be attempted on the second day.

The extent of the surgical incision and the type of dressing are considered when choosing strategies to promote skin integrity. Intact skin needs to be protected from drainage and moisture. Dressings are changed as needed to ensure patient comfort, to perform wound care and irrigation (if prescribed), and to permit observation of the surgical site.

The wound is usually cleansed daily with warm, normal saline irrigations or other antiseptic solutions as prescribed, or a transparent dressing may be in place over the wound to minimize exposure to the air and subsequent pain. The appearance of the surgical site and the characteristics of drainage are assessed and documented. After the dressings are removed, a bed cradle may be used to keep the bed linens away from the surgical site. The patient is always protected from exposure when visitors arrive or someone else enters the room.

Supporting Positive Sexuality and Sexual Function

The patient who undergoes vulvar surgery usually experiences concerns about body image, sexual attractiveness, and functioning. Establishing a trusting nurse–patient relationship is important for the patient to feel comfortable expressing her concerns and fears. The patient is encouraged to discuss her concerns with her sexual partner.

Because alterations in sexual sensation and functioning depend on the extent of surgery, the nurse needs to know about any structural and functional changes resulting from the surgery. Referral of the patient and her partner to a sex counselor may help them address these changes and resume satisfying sexual activity.

Monitoring and Managing Potential Complications

Location, extent, and exposure of the surgical site and incision put the patient at risk for contamination of the site and infection and sepsis. The patient is monitored closely for local and systemic signs and symptoms of infection: purulent drainage, redness, increased pain, fever, and increased white blood cell count. The nurse assists in obtaining specimens for culture if infection is suspected and administers antibiotic agents as prescribed. Hand hygiene, always a crucial infection-preventing measure, is of particular importance along with wearing masks whenever there is an extensive area of exposed tissue. Catheters, drains, and dressings are handled carefully with gloves on to avoid cross-contamination. A low-residue diet prevents straining on defecation and wound contamination.

The patient is at risk for DVT because of the positioning required during surgery, postoperative edema, and the usually prolonged immobility needed to promote healing. Antiembolism stockings are applied, and the patient is encouraged and reminded to perform ankle exercises to minimize venous pooling, which leads to DVT. The patient is encouraged and assisted in changing positions by using the overhead trapeze bar. Pressure behind the knees is avoided when positioning the patient because this may increase venous pooling. The patient is assessed for signs and symptoms of DVT (leg pain, redness, warmth, edema) and pulmonary embolism (chest pain, tachycardia, dyspnea). Fluid intake is encouraged to prevent dehydration, which also increases the risk of DVT.

The extent of the surgical incision and possibly wide excision of tissue increase the risk of postoperative bleeding and hemorrhage. Although the pressure dressings that are applied after surgery minimize the risk, the patient must be monitored closely for signs of hemorrhage and resulting hypovolemic shock. These signs may include decreased blood pressure; increased pulse rate; decreased urine output; decreased mental status; and cold, clammy skin.

If hemorrhage and shock occur, interventions include fluid replacement, blood component therapy, and vasopressor medications. Laboratory results (eg, hematocrit and hemoglobin levels) and hemodynamic monitoring are used to assess the patient's response to treatment. Depending on the specific cause of hemorrhage, the patient may be returned to the operating room. See Chapter 15 for a detailed discussion of shock.

Promoting Home and Community-Based Care

Teaching Patients Self-Care

Preparing the patient for hospital discharge begins before hospital admission. The patient and family are informed about what to expect during the immediate postoperative and recovery periods. Depending on the changes resulting from the surgery, the patient and her family may need instruction about wound care, urinary catheterization, and possible complications. The patient is encouraged to share her concerns and to assume increasing responsibility for her own care. She is encouraged and assisted in learning to care for the surgical site. A referral for home care is made as indicated.

Continuing Care

Shortened hospital stays may result in the patient's discharge during the early postoperative recovery stage to home or a subacute facility. During this phase, the patient's physical status and psychological responses to the surgery are assessed. In addition, the patient is assessed for complications and healing of the surgical site. During home visits, the nurse assesses the home to determine if modifications are needed to facilitate care. The home visit is used to reinforce previous teaching and to assess the patient's and the family's understanding of and adherence to the prescribed treatment strategies. Follow-up phone calls by the nurse to the patient between home visits are usually reassuring to the patient and family, who may be responsible for performing complex care procedures. Attention to the patient's psychological responses is important because the patient may become discouraged and depressed because of alterations in body image and a slow recovery. Communication between the nurse involved in the patient's immediate postoperative care and the home care nurse is essential to ensure continuity of care.

Cancer of the Vagina

Cancer of the vagina is rare and usually takes years to develop. Primary cancer of the vagina is usually squamous in origin. Malignant melanoma and sarcomas can occur. Risk factors include previous cervical cancer, in utero exposure to diethylstilbestrol (DES), previous vaginal or vulvar cancer, previous radiation therapy, history of HPV, or pessary use. Any patient with previous cervical cancer should be examined regularly for vaginal lesions.

Before 1970, vaginal cancer occurred primarily in postmenopausal women. In the 1970s, it was shown that maternal ingestion of DES, prescribed from 1938 to 1971 to enhance pregnancy outcomes, affected female offspring who were exposed in utero. DES was prescribed under many brand names, and it is unclear how many pregnant women received it. All patients should be asked about DES exposure if they were born or were pregnant between 1938 and 1971. Benign genital tract abnormalities, such as vaginal adenosis (abnormal tissue growth), cervical irregularities (collars, hoods, septae, cockscombs), and uterine abnormalities, have occurred in approximately one third of exposed women. Clear cell carcinoma of the vagina or cervix may also occur as a result of DES exposure; the risk is 0.14 to 1.4 in 1000 women. However, most female offspring of mothers who took DES are now between 40 and 75 years of age, and diagnosis of this condition has been decreasing. Vigilance is still necessary because it is unknown how long women remain at risk (ACS, 2009). Colposcopy is indicated for all women exposed to DES in utero. If colposcopic examination discloses adenosis or a significant cervical or vaginal lesion, follow-up is essential. In addition, health care providers should be aware that men who were exposed to DES in utero may have an increased risk of developing epididymal cysts.

Vaginal pessaries, used to support prolapsed tissues, can be a source of chronic irritation. As such, they have been associated with vaginal cancer, but only when the devices were not cared for properly (ie, the device was not cleaned regularly or the patient did not return to the health care provider regularly for vaginal examinations).

Patients often do not have symptoms but may report slight bleeding after intercourse, spontaneous bleeding, vaginal discharge, pain, and urinary or rectal symptoms (or both). Diagnosis is often by Pap smear of the vagina. Encouraging close follow-up by health care providers is the primary focus of nursing interventions with women who were exposed to DES in utero. Emotional support for mothers who received DES before its risks were discovered and their daughters who were exposed to DES in utero is essential.

Medical Management

Treatment of early lesions may include local excision, topical chemotherapy, or laser. Laser therapy is a common treatment option in early vaginal and vulvar cancer. Surgery for more advanced lesions depends on the size and the stage of the cancer. If radical vaginectomy is required, a vagina can be reconstructed with tissue from the intestine, muscle, or skin grafts. After vaginal reconstructive surgery and radiation, regular intercourse may be helpful in preventing vaginal stenosis. Water-soluble lubricants are helpful in reducing pain with intercourse (dyspareunia).

Following surgery, radiation therapy may be administered by a variety of methods, including external beam radiation, which is usually an outpatient procedure, or brachytherapy, which is internal radiation therapy. Internal radiation may be given with intracavitary radioactive material contained in a seed, wire, needle, or tube, which is placed into a cavity such as the uterus or vagina. Interstitial radiation is another type of internal radiation treatment in which the radioactive material is placed in or near the cancer but not into a body cavity and is used in cervical and ovarian malignancies. These treatments may be high dose for a short period or low dose, which may take longer. Treatment during hospitalization or during outpatient therapy depends on several factors, including the status of the patient and the mode of delivery.

Cancer of the Fallopian Tubes

Malignancies of the fallopian tube are the least common type of genital cancer. Although this type of cancer can occur at any age, the average age at diagnosis is 55 years. Symptoms include abdominal pain, abnormal bleeding, and vaginal discharge. An enlarged fallopian tube may be found on sonogram if dilated and fluid filled or it may appear or be palpated as a mass. Surgery followed by radiation therapy is the usual treatment.

Cancer of the Ovary

Ovarian cancer is the leading cause of gynecological cancer deaths in the United States (Jemal, Siegel, Ward, et al., 2007). Despite careful physical examination, ovarian tumors are often difficult to detect because they are usually deep in the pelvis. No early screening mechanism exists at present, although tumor markers are being explored. Transvaginal ultrasound and CA-125 antigen testing may be reassuring for women who have a high risk for this condition, and clinical trials are under way to evaluate the effect of these screening modalities on mortality from ovarian cancer. Tumor-associated antigens are helpful in determining follow-up care after diagnosis and treatment but not in early general screening.

Epidemiology

One woman in 70 will develop ovarian cancer in her lifetime. The incidence of this type of cancer increases after 40 years of age and peaks in the early 80s; the median age of affected women is 63 years. The frequency of ovarian cancer is highest in industrialized countries, except for Japan, where it is low. The incidence seems to be remaining constant, and 5-year survival has improved (Bhoola & Hoskins, 2006). Pregnancy and use of oral contraceptives decrease risk. Mutations of BRCA1 and BRCA2 increase risk; the lifetime risk for women with these mutations is 28% to 40% (the higher percentage is in Ashkenazi Jews).

A woman with ovarian cancer has a threefold to fourfold increased risk of breast cancer, and a woman with breast cancer has an increased risk of ovarian cancer. A family history, older age, low parity, and obesity may increase risk of ovarian cancer. However, most women who develop ovarian cancer have no known risk factors, and no definitive causative factors have been determined.

Genetic testing is indicated when three or more cases of closely related family members have premenopausal breast cancer or ovarian cancer. One member with cancer is tested, and if the results are positive, other members without cancer may undergo testing. This testing is available at centers with genetics counselors or nurses with expertise in genetics counseling. Many health care providers advocate pelvic examinations every 6 months for women who have one or two relatives with ovarian cancer. It is recommended that women with a family history of breast or ovarian cancer undergo periodic screening.

Much more needs to be learned about the risks associated with some mutations, the reliability of testing, and the efficacy of follow-up. Confidentiality and insurance risks are ethical issues that need clarification. Because there are no primary methods of preventing breast or ovarian cancer, emotional distress is also an issue. Patients with concerns about their family history should be referred to a cancer genetics center to obtain information and testing, if indicated. Women with inherited types of ovarian cancer tend to be younger when the diagnosis is made than the average age at the time of diagnosis. Prophylactic oophorectomy in women with genetic mutations has been found to be associated with decreased risk of ovarian and other gynecologic cancers as well as breast cancer and is an option for women who have completed childbearing (ACOG, 2008a). Hereditary nonpolyposis colon cancer increases the risk of uterine cancer and slightly increases the risk of ovarian cancer.

Pathophysiology

Types of tumors include germ cell tumors, which arise from the cells that produce eggs; stromal cell tumors, which arise in connective tissue cells that produce hormones; and epithelial tumors, which originate from the outer surface of the ovary. Most ovarian cancers are epithelial in origin. Of the many different cell types in ovarian cancer, epithelial tumors constitute 90%. Germ cell tumors and stromal tumors make up the other 10%.

Primary peritoneal carcinoma is closely related to ovarian cancer. Extraovarian primary peritoneal carcinoma (EOPPC) resembles ovarian cancer histologically and can occur in women with and without ovaries. Symptoms and treatment are similar. Because of the possibility of EOPPC, oophorectomy does not guarantee that the patient will not develop carcinoma following hysterectomy.

Clinical Manifestations

Symptoms of ovarian cancer are nonspecific and may include increased abdominal girth, pelvic pressure, bloating, back pain, constipation, abdominal pain, urinary urgency, indigestion, flatulence, increased waist size, leg pain, and pelvic pain. Symptoms are often vague, so many women tend to ignore them. Ovarian cancer is often silent, but enlargement of the abdomen from an accumulation of fluid is the most common sign. All women with gastrointestinal symptoms and without a known diagnosis must be evaluated

for potential ovarian cancer. Vague, undiagnosed, persistent gastrointestinal symptoms should alert the nurse to the possibility of an early ovarian malignancy. A palpable ovary in a woman who has gone through menopause is investigated immediately because ovaries normally become smaller and less palpable after menopause.

Assessment and Diagnostic Findings

Any enlarged ovary must be investigated. Pelvic examination often does not detect early ovarian cancer, and pelvic imaging techniques are not always definitive. Ovarian tumors are classified as benign if there is no proliferation or invasion, borderline if there is proliferation but no invasion, and malignant if there is invasion. Fifteen percent of all new cases of ovarian tumors are classified as borderline and have low malignancy potential. However, by the time of diagnosis, most ovarian cancers are advanced (Ryerson, Eheman, Burton, et al., 2007).

Surgical Management

Surgical staging, exploration, and reduction of tumor mass are the basics of treatment. Surgical removal is the treatment of choice; the preoperative workup may include a barium enema or colonoscopy, upper gastrointestinal series, MRI, ultrasound, chest x-rays, and IV urography. CT may be used preoperatively to rule out intra-abdominal metastasis. Staging the tumor by the TNM system is performed to guide treatment (Chart 47-8). Likely treatment involves a total abdominal hysterectomy with removal of the fallopian tubes and ovaries and possibly the omentum (bilateral salpingo-oophorectomy and omentectomy); tumor debulking; para-aortic and pelvic lymph node sampling; diaphragmatic biopsies; random peritoneal biopsies; and cytologic washings. Postoperative management may include taxanes or platinum-based chemotherapy (discussed in next section).

Borderline tumors resemble ovarian cancer but have much more favorable outcomes. Women diagnosed with this type of cancer tend to be younger (early 40s). A conservative surgical approach is now used. The affected ovary is removed, but the uterus and the contralateral ovary may remain in place. Adjuvant therapy may not be warranted.

Chart 47-8 • *Stages of Ovarian Cancer*

I Cancer is contained within the ovary (or ovaries).

II Cancer is in one or both ovaries and has involved other organs (ie, uterus, fallopian tubes, bladder, the sigmoid colon, or the rectum) within the pelvis.

III Cancer involves one or both ovaries, and one or both of the following are present: (1) cancer has spread beyond the pelvis to the lining of the abdomen; (2) cancer has spread to lymph nodes.

IV The most advanced stage of ovarian cancer. Cancer is in one or both ovaries. There is distant metastasis to the liver, lungs, or other organs outside the peritoneal cavity; ovarian cancer cells in the pleural cavity are evidence of stage IV disease.

Pharmacologic Therapy

Chemotherapy is usually administered IV on an outpatient basis using a combination of platinum and taxane agents. Paclitaxel (Taxol) plus carboplatin (Paraplatin) are most often used because of their excellent clinical benefits and manageable toxicity. Leukopenia, neurotoxicity, and fever may occur.

Because paclitaxel often causes leukopenia, patients may need to take granulocyte colony-stimulating factor as well. Paclitaxel is contraindicated in patients with hypersensitivity to medications formulated in polyoxyethylated castor oil and in patients with baseline neutropenia. Because of possible adverse cardiac effects, paclitaxel is not used in patients with cardiac disorders. Hypotension, dyspnea, angioedema, and urticaria indicate severe reactions that usually occur soon after the first and second doses are administered. The nurse must be prepared to assist in treating anaphylaxis. Patients should be prepared for inevitable hair loss.

Carboplatin may be used in the initial treatment and in patients with recurrence. It should be used with caution in patients with renal impairment. Usually, six cycles are given. A positive clinical response is normalization of the tumor marker CA-125, negative CT results, and a normal physical and gynecologic examination.

Liposomal therapy, delivery of chemotherapy in a liposome, allows the highest possible dose of chemotherapy to the tumor target with a reduction in adverse effects. Liposomes are used as drug carriers because they are nontoxic, biodegradable, easily available, and relatively inexpensive. This encapsulated chemotherapy allows increased duration of action and better targeting. The encapsulation of doxorubicin (Doxil) lessens the incidence of nausea, vomiting, and alopecia. Patients must be monitored for bone marrow suppression and gastrointestinal and cardiac effects.

Combination IV and intraperitoneal chemotherapy is an option for some patients. However, this treatment may result in pain; fatigue; and hematologic, gastrointestinal, metabolic, and neurologic toxicities, thus decreasing the quality of life (ACOG, 2008b). Because of these effects, the decision to use intraperitoneal chemotherapy is individualized.

Genetic engineering and identification of cancer genes may make gene therapy a future possibility; gene therapy is under investigation. Emerging proteomic technologies (tissue-based protein analysis) look promising; they may allow earlier diagnosis and treatment decision making. New biomarkers need further validation, but protein signature patterns are now being tested. These technologies may result in individualized treatment strategies for epithelial ovarian cancer.

Recurrence of ovarian cancer is common, and many patients may require treatment with multiple agents. Therefore, ovarian cancer may be considered a chronic disease, with treatment directed toward control of the cancer, maintenance of quality of life, and palliation. Liposomal preparations, intraperitoneal drug administration, anti-cancer vaccines, monoclonal antibodies directed against cancer antigens, gene therapy, and antiangiogenic treatments (to prevent formation of new blood vessels in an effort to halt growth of ovarian cancer) may be used in the treatment of recurrence. Gemcitabine (Gemzar), topotecan (Hycamtin), paclitaxel, carboplatin, and doxorubicin are all being studied in clinical trials in advanced ovarian cancer (Bhoola & Hoskins, 2006).

Nursing Management

Nursing measures include those related to the patient's treatment plan, which may include surgery, chemotherapy, palliative care, or a combination of these. Emotional support, comfort measures, and information, plus attentiveness and caring, are important components of nursing care for the patient and her family (Bohnenkamp, LeBaron & Yoder, 2007a).

Nursing interventions after pelvic surgery to remove the tumor are similar to those after other abdominal surgeries. If ovarian cancer occurs in a young woman and the tumor is unilateral, it is removed. Childbearing, if desired, is encouraged in the near future. After childbirth, surgical reexploration may be performed, and the remaining ovary may be removed. If both ovaries are involved, bilateral oophorectomy is performed and chemotherapy follows. Chart 47-9 describes symptom clusters in women who are survivors of ovarian cancer.

Patients with advanced ovarian cancer may develop ascites and pleural effusion. Nursing care may include administering IV fluids prescribed to alleviate fluid and electrolyte imbalances, administering parenteral nutrition to provide adequate nutrition, providing postoperative care after intestinal bypass to alleviate any obstruction, controlling pain, and managing drainage tubes. Comfort measures for women with ascites may include providing small frequent meals, decreasing fluid intake, administering diuretic agents, and providing rest. Patients with pleural effusion may experience shortness of breath, hypoxia, pleuritic chest pain, and cough. Thoracentesis is usually performed to relieve these symptoms. The patient with ovarian cancer often has complex needs and benefits from the assistance and support of an oncology nurse specialist (Bohnenkamp, LeBaron & Yoder, 2007b).

Hysterectomy

Hysterectomy is the surgical removal of the uterus to treat cancer, dysfunctional uterine bleeding, endometriosis, nonmalignant growths, persistent pain, pelvic relaxation and prolapse, and previous injury to the uterus. In the United States, approximately 5.5 of every 1000 women undergo hysterectomy each year (Wu, Wechter, Geller, et al., 2007). The number is thought to be leveling off because the number of other therapeutic options (ie, laser therapy, endometrial ablation, UAE, and medications to shrink fibroid tumors) has increased.

A total hysterectomy involves removal of the uterus and the cervix. Hysterectomy can be supracervical or subtotal, in which the uterus is removed but the cervix is spared. Radical hysterectomy involves removal of the uterus as well as the surrounding tissue, including the upper third of the vagina and pelvic lymph nodes. The procedure can be performed through the vagina, through an abdominal incision,

CHART 47-9

NURSING RESEARCH PROFILE
Quality of Life in Survivors of Ovarian Cancer

Fox, S. W. & Lyon, D. (2007). Symptom clusters and quality of life in survivors of ovarian cancer. *Cancer Nursing, 30*(5), 270–282.

Purpose

The purpose of this study was to identify relationships among depression, fatigue, and pain in survivors of ovarian cancer to determine if a possible cluster of symptoms exists in patients with ovarian cancer. Further, the researchers examined the relationship of a cluster of symptoms to quality of life (QOL) in women with ovarian cancer. Few studies have addressed symptoms in women with ovarian cancer, even though it is the fourth leading cause of cancer-related deaths in the United States.

Design

This correlational study involved secondary data analysis from 76 women with ovarian cancer. The study from which the data were obtained addressed the psychometric properties of a new health-related QOL instrument. The subjects were recruited from an online information and support group. The Short Form-36 Health Status Survey (SF-36) was used to address symptoms of depression, fatigue, and bodily pain. The Fox Simple Quality of Life Scale (FSQOLS) was used to measure QOL. The reliability and validity of both the SF-36 and the FSQOLS have been established. Statistical analysis, including multiple regression, was used to identify possible symptom clusters and the relationship of clusters with QOL.

Findings

Scores of women were compared to those of other groups. The scores on pain and depression of the ovarian cancer survivors were similar to those of a group of similar age of a well population; however, they had significantly greater fatigue than the well population. Depression was significantly correlated with fatigue ($r = .49$), and fatigue was significantly correlated with pain ($r = .35$). Although the sample of 76 women with ovarian cancer had a mean QOL score of 99 (on a scale of 25 to 125, with higher scores representing better QOL), depression ($r = .58$) and fatigue ($r = .51$) were significantly correlated with QOL. There was not a significant correlation of pain with QOL. Together, depression and fatigue explained 41% of the variance in QOL, with the depression accounting for most of the variance in QOL scores.

Nursing Implications

Because fatigue and depression are common in patients with ovarian cancer and significantly affect QOL, nurses need to address these issues in their care of patients who are ovarian cancer survivors. The results of this study may help nurses and other health care providers target the symptoms that have the greatest effect on QOL. Most women in this study were not actively engaged in treatment; thus, other symptom clusters might be more relevant in patients who are in different phases of treatment.

---

or laparoscopically (in which the uterus is removed in sections through small incisions using a laparoscope). Malignant conditions usually require a total abdominal hysterectomy and bilateral salpingo-oophorectomy (removal of fallopian tubes and ovaries).

A laparoscopically assisted approach can also be used for vaginal hysterectomy, with excellent results and rapid recovery. This procedure is performed as a short-stay procedure or ambulatory surgery in carefully selected patients.

Preoperative Management

Patients are advised to discontinue anticoagulant medications, NSAIDs such as aspirin, and vitamin E prior to surgery to reduce the risk of bleeding. Pregnancy is ruled out on the day of surgery. Prophylactic antibiotics may be administered prior to surgery and discontinued the next day. Prevention of thromboembolic events is critical, and methods may include heparin and use of anti-embolism stockings or an intermittent pneumatic compression device.

Postoperative Management

The principles of general postoperative care for abdominal surgery apply. Major risks are infection and hemorrhage. In addition, because the surgical site is close to the bladder, voiding problems may occur, particularly after a vaginal hysterectomy. Also, edema or nerve trauma may cause temporary loss of bladder tone (bladder atony), and an indwelling catheter may be inserted.

NURSING PROCESS

THE PATIENT UNDERGOING A HYSTERECTOMY

Assessment

The health history and the physical and pelvic examination are completed, and laboratory tests are performed. Additional assessment data include the patient's psychosocial responses, because the need for a hysterectomy may elicit strong emotional reactions. If the hysterectomy is performed to remove a malignant tumor, anxiety related to fear of cancer and its consequences adds to the stress of the patient and her family. Women who have had a hysterectomy may be at risk for psychological and physical symptoms. Alternatively, women may note improved physical and mental health after hysterectomy as troublesome symptoms may be alleviated.

Diagnosis

Nursing Diagnoses

Based on all the assessment data, the major nursing diagnoses may include the following:

- Anxiety related to the diagnosis of cancer, fear of pain, possible perception of loss of femininity or childbearing potential
- Disturbed body image related to altered fertility and fears about sexuality and relationships with partner and family

- Acute pain related to surgery and other adjuvant therapy
- Deficient knowledge of the perioperative aspects of hysterectomy and postoperative self-care

Collaborative Problems/Potential Complications

Based on assessment data, potential complications may include the following:

- Hemorrhage
- DVT
- Bladder dysfunction
- Infection

Planning and Goals

The major goals may include relief of anxiety, acceptance of loss of the uterus, absence of pain or discomfort, increased knowledge of self-care requirements, and absence of complications.

Nursing Interventions

Relieving Anxiety

Anxiety stems from several factors: unfamiliar environment, the effects of surgery on body image and reproductive ability, fear of pain and other discomfort, and, possibly, feelings of embarrassment about exposure of the genital area in the perioperative period. The nurse determines what the experience means to the patient and encourages her to verbalize her concerns. Throughout the preoperative, postoperative, and recovery periods, explanations are given about physical preparations and procedures that are performed.

Patient education addresses the outcomes of surgery, possible feelings of loss, and options for management of symptoms of menopause. Women vary in their preferences; many want a choice of treatment options, a part in decision making, accurate and useful information at the appropriate time, support from their health care providers, and access to professional and lay support systems (Bohnenkamp, et al., 2007a).

Improving Body Image

The patient may have strong emotional reactions to having a hysterectomy and strong personal feelings related to the diagnosis, views of significant others who may be involved (family, partner), religious beliefs, and fears about prognosis. Concerns such as the inability to have children and the effect on femininity may surface, as may questions about the effects of surgery on sexual relationships, function, and satisfaction. The patient needs reassurance that she will still have a vagina and that she can experience sexual intercourse after temporary postoperative abstinence while tissues heal. Information that sexual satisfaction and orgasm arise from clitoral stimulation rather than from the uterus reassures many women. Most women note some change in sexual feelings after hysterectomy, but they vary in intensity. In some cases, the vagina is shortened by surgery, and this may affect sensitivity or comfort.

When hormonal balance is upset, as often occurs with reproductive system disorders, the patient may experience depression and heightened emotional sensitivity to people and situations. The nurse needs to approach and evaluate each patient individually in light of these factors. A nurse who exhibits interest, concern, and willingness to listen to the patient's fears will help the patient progress through the surgical experience.

Relieving Pain

Postoperative pain and discomfort are common. Therefore, the nurse assesses the intensity of the patient's pain and assists the patient with analgesia as prescribed. Excision of a large tumor could cause edema because of the sudden release of pressure. In the postoperative period, fluids and food may be restricted for 1 or 2 days. If the patient has abdominal distention or flatus, a rectal tube and application of heat to the abdomen may be prescribed. When abdominal auscultation reveals return of bowel sounds and peristalsis, additional fluids and a soft diet are permitted. Early ambulation facilitates the return of normal peristalsis (Bohnenkamp, et al., 2007b).

Monitoring and Managing Potential Complications

HEMORRHAGE. Vaginal bleeding and hemorrhage may occur after hysterectomy. To detect these complications early, the nurse counts the perineal pads used, assesses the extent of saturation with blood, and monitors vital signs. Abdominal dressings are monitored for drainage if an abdominal surgical approach was used. In preparation for hospital discharge, the nurse gives prescribed guidelines for activity restrictions to promote healing and to prevent postoperative bleeding. Because many women may go home the day of surgery or within a day or two, they are instructed to contact the nurse or surgeon if bleeding is excessive.

DEEP VEIN THROMBOSIS. Because of positioning during surgery, postoperative edema, and decreased activity postoperatively, the patient is at risk for DVT and pulmonary embolism (PE). To minimize the risk, anti-embolism stockings are applied. In addition, the patient is encouraged and assisted to change positions frequently, although pressure under the knees is avoided, and to exercise her legs and feet while in bed. The nurse helps the patient ambulate early in the postoperative period. In addition, the nurse assesses for DVT or phlebitis (leg pain, redness, warmth, edema) and PE (chest pain, tachycardia, dyspnea). If the patient is being discharged home soon after surgery, she is instructed to avoid prolonged sitting in a chair with pressure at the knees, sitting with crossed legs, and inactivity. Furthermore, she is instructed to contact her health care provider if symptoms of DVT or PE occur.

BLADDER DYSFUNCTION. Because of possible difficulty in voiding postoperatively, occasionally an indwelling catheter may be inserted before or during surgery and is left in place in the immediate postoperative period. If a catheter is in place, it is usually removed shortly after the patient begins to ambulate. After the catheter is removed, urinary output is monitored; additionally, the abdomen is assessed for distention. If the patient does not void within a prescribed time, measures are initiated to encourage voiding (eg, assisting the patient to the bathroom, pouring warm water over the perineum). If the patient cannot void, catheterization may be necessary. On rare occasions, the patient may be discharged home with the catheter in place and is instructed in its management.

Promoting Home and Community-Based Care

TEACHING PATIENTS SELF-CARE. The information provided to the patient is tailored to her needs. She must know what limitations or restrictions, if any, to expect. She is instructed to check the surgical incision daily and to contact her primary health care provider if redness or purulent drainage or discharge occurs. She is informed that her periods are now over but that she may have a slightly bloody discharge for a few days; if bleeding recurs after this time, it should be reported immediately. The patient is instructed about the importance of an adequate oral intake and of maintaining bowel and urinary tract function. The patient is informed that she is likely to recover quickly, but that postoperative fatigue is not unusual.

The patient should resume activities gradually. This does not mean sitting for long periods, because doing so may cause blood to pool in the pelvis, increasing the risk of thromboembolism. The nurse explains that showers are preferable to tub baths to reduce the possibility of infection and to avoid the dangers of injury that may occur when getting in and out of the bathtub. The patient is instructed to avoid straining, lifting, having sexual intercourse, or driving until her surgeon permits these activities (Bohnenkamp, et al., 2007b). Vaginal discharge, foul odor, excessive bleeding, any leg redness or pain, or an elevated temperature should be reported to the primary health care provider promptly. The nurse reinforces information given to patients by their surgeons regarding activities and restrictions.

CONTINUING CARE. Follow-up telephone contact provides the nurse with the opportunity to determine whether the patient is recovering without problems and to answer any questions that may have arisen. The patient is reminded about postoperative follow-up appointments. If the patient's ovaries were removed and she finds vasomotor symptoms troublesome, hormone therapy (HT, previously referred to as hormone replacement therapy [HRT]) may be considered. Providing information about the findings of the Women's Health Initiative (2002) study about the benefits and risks of HT promotes informed decision making about its use. Estrogen alone does not seem to increase the risk of breast cancer and may decrease coronary plaques but may increase the risk of Alzheimer's dementia and thromboses (Heiss, Wallace, Anderson, et al., 2008). The patient is reminded to discuss risks and benefits of HT and alternative therapies with her primary care provider. Decisions about use of HT need to be made individually in consultation with this provider.

Evaluation

Expected Patient Outcomes

Expected patient outcomes may include:

1. Experiences decreased anxiety
2. Has improved body image
   a. Discusses changes resulting from surgery with her partner
   b. Verbalizes understanding of her disorder and the treatment plan
   c. Displays minimal depression or anxiety
3. Experiences minimal pain and discomfort

   a. Reports relief of abdominal pain and discomfort
   b. Ambulates without pain
4. Verbalizes knowledge and understanding of self-care
   a. Practices deep-breathing, turning, and leg exercises as instructed
   b. Increases activity and ambulation daily
   c. Reports adequate fluid intake and adequate urinary output
   d. Identifies reportable symptoms
   e. Schedules and keeps follow-up appointments
5. Absence of complications
   a. Has minimal vaginal bleeding and exhibits normal vital signs
   b. Ambulates early
   c. Notes no chest or calf pain and no redness, tenderness, or swelling in the extremities
   d. Reports no urinary problems or abdominal distention

Radiation Therapy

Radiation may be used in the treatment of cervical, uterine, and ovarian cancers either alone or in combination with surgery and chemotherapy. Several approaches are used to deliver radiation to the female reproductive system: external radiation, intraoperative radiation therapy (IORT), and internal (intracavitary) irradiation or brachytherapy. The cervix and uterus can serve as a receptacle for radioactive sources for internal radiation therapy.

Methods of Radiation Therapy

External Radiation Therapy

This method of delivering radiation destroys cancerous cells at the skin surface or deeper in the body. Other methods of delivering radiation therapy are more commonly used to treat cancer of the female reproductive system than this method.

Intraoperative Radiation Therapy

IORT allows radiation to be applied directly to the affected area during surgery. An electron beam is directed at the disease site. This direct-view irradiation may be used when para-aortic nodes are involved or for unresectable (inoperable) or partially resectable neoplasms. Benefits include accurate beam direction (which precisely limits the radiation to the tumor) and the ability during treatment to block sensitive organs from radiation. IORT is usually combined with external beam irradiation preoperatively or postoperatively.

Internal (Intracavitary) Irradiation

After the patient receives an anesthetic agent and an examination, specially prepared applicators are inserted into the endometrial cavity and vagina. These devices are not loaded with radioactive material until the patient returns to her room. X-rays are obtained to verify the precise relationship of the applicator to the normal pelvic anatomy and to the tumor. When this step is completed, the radiation oncologist loads the applicators with predetermined amounts of radioactive material. This procedure, called afterloading,

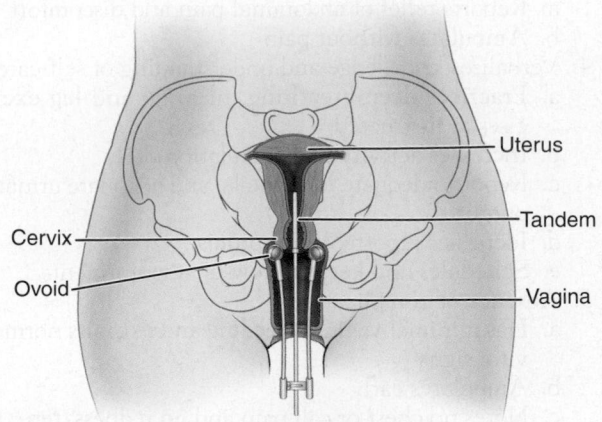

Figure 47-8 Placement of tandem and ovoids for internal radiation therapy.

allows for precise control of the radiation exposure received by the patient, with minimal exposure of physicians, nurses, and other health care personnel. A patient undergoing internal radiation treatment remains isolated in a private room until the application is completed. Adjacent rooms may need to be evacuated and a lead shield placed at the doorway to the patient's room.

Of the various applicators developed for intracavitary treatment, some are inserted into the endometrial cavity and endocervical canal as multiple small irradiators (eg, Heyman capsules). Others consist of a central tube (a tandem or intrauterine "stem") placed through the dilated endocervical canal into the uterine cavity, which remains in a fixed relationship with the irradiators placed in the upper vagina on each side of the cervix (vaginal ovoids) (Fig. 47-8).

When the applicator is inserted, an indwelling urinary catheter is also inserted. Vaginal packing is inserted to keep the applicator in place and to keep other organs, such as the bladder and rectum, as far from the radioactive source as possible. The objective of the internal treatment is to maintain the distribution of internal radiation at a fixed dosage throughout the application, which may last 24 to 72 hours, depending on dose calculations made by the radiation physicist.

Automated high-dose rate (HDR) intracavitary brachytherapy systems have been developed that allow outpatient radiation therapy. Treatment time is shorter, thereby decreasing patient discomfort. Staff exposure to radiation is also avoided. Isotopes of radium and cesium are used for intracavitary irradiation.

Nursing Considerations for Radiation Safety

Special precautions for the safety of the patient and the nurse are important considerations when the patient is receiving radiation therapy. The Radiation Safety Department will identify specific safety precautions to those people who will be in contact with the patient, including health care providers and family. Of the many nursing concerns, primary concerns include providing the patient with emotional support and physical comfort. Further details about nursing management are provided in Chapter 16.

CRITICAL THINKING EXERCISES

EBP **1** A 55-year-old patient has been diagnosed with ovarian cancer. She reports that she has a strong family history of cancer; two sisters have breast cancer. Her mother died of cancer when the patient was a child, and she is not certain of the type of cancer. Because of her strong family history, she is concerned about the health status of her twin daughters who are in their early 30s. She has asked you to discuss the risks for cancer with them. Explain what counseling and education you will provide to the patient and her daughters. Identify the evidence base for the counseling and education and the strength of that evidence. How will you approach your counseling and education?

2 A 65-year-old woman with rheumatoid arthritis who has had surgery for breast cancer is scheduled to undergo radical vulvectomy to treat vulvar cancer. She reports that she is very anxious because of her previous surgery. Describe the preoperative teaching for her and the postoperative care that can be anticipated. How will her history of breast cancer and rheumatoid arthritis affect her care? What modifications in care, postoperative teaching, and discharge planning may be necessary because of these health issues? How will your discharge planning be modified if the patient tells you that she provides care at home for her husband who has signs of early Alzheimer's disease?

3 A 38-year-old woman with a diagnosis of fibroids has been admitted to the outpatient surgery center for uterine artery embolization. When you are completing the preoperative admission procedures, she asks you about the effect of the procedure on future sexual relationships and on her ability to become pregnant in the future. What teaching is indicated for this woman based on her concerns and on her risk for future fertility? What nursing care is important to minimize the risk of complications?

EBP **4** A 17-year-old patient is seeking contraception. She explains that she has not had a sexual relationship but wants to be prepared for future sexual relationships. She also asks you for your recommendation about receiving the new HPV vaccine. What recommendations would you give her about contraception and the HPV vaccine? What is the evidence base for your recommendations? How would you approach the topic of safer sex, contraception, and HPV vaccine with her in responding to her request for information?

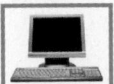

The Smeltzer suite offers these additional resources to enhance learning and facilitate understanding of this chapter:
- thePoint online resource, thepoint.lww.com/Smeltzer12E
- Student CD-ROM included with the book
- *Study Guide to Accompany Brunner & Suddarth's Textbook of Medical-Surgical Nursing*
- *Handbook for Brunner & Suddarth's Textbook of Medical-Surgical Nursing*

REFERENCES AND SELECTED READINGS

Asterisk indicates nursing research.
**Double asterisk indicates classic reference.*

Books

American Cancer Society (ACS). (2009). *Cancer facts and figures.* Atlanta, GA: Author.

American College of Obstetricians and Gynecologists (ACOG). (2008). *Compendium of selected publications.* Washington, DC: Author.

Emans, J., Laufer, M. & Goldstein, D. (2008). *Pediatric and adolescent gynecology* (4th ed.). Philadelphia: Lippincott Williams & Wilkins.

Gibbs, R. S., Karlan, B. Y., Haney, A. F., et al. (2008). *Danforth's Obstetrics and Gynecology* (10th ed.). Philadelphia: Lippincott Williams & Wilkins.

Katz, V. L., Lentz, G., Lobo, R. A., et al. (2007). *Comprehensive gynecology.* St. Louis: Mosby Elsevier.

Orshan, S. (2008). *Maternal, newborn and women's health nursing: Comprehensive care across the life span.* Philadelphia: Lippincott Williams & Wilkins.

Speroff, L. & Darney, P. D. (2005). *A clinical guide for contraception* (4th ed.). Philadelphia: Lippincott Williams & Wilkins.

World Health Organization Department of Reproductive Health and Research (WHO/RHR) and Johns Hopkins Bloomberg School of Public Health/Center for Communication Programs (CCP), INFO Project. (2007). *Family planning: A global handbook for providers.* Baltimore and Geneva: CCP and WHO.

Journals and Electronic Documents

General

Buschbaum, G., Duecy, E., Kerr, L., et al. (2006). Pelvic organ prolapse in nulliparous women and their parous sisters. *Obstetrics & Gynecology, 108*(6), 1388–1393.

Fernando, R., Thankar, R., Sultan, A., et al. (2006). Effect of vaginal pessaries on symptoms associated with pelvic organ prolapse. *Obstetrics & Gynecology, 108*(1), 93–99.

Heiss, G., Wallace, R., Anderson, G., et al. (2008). Health risks and benefits 3 years after stopping randomized treatment with estrogen and progestin. *Journal of the American Medical Association, 299*(9), 1036–1045.

Pikarinen, U., Saisto, T., Schei, B., et al. (2007). Experiences of physical and sexual abuse and their implications for current health. *Obstetrics & Gynecology, 109*(5), 1116–1122.

Rivadeneira, D. E., Ruffo, B., Amrani, S., et al. (2007). Rectovaginal fistulas: Current surgical management. *Clinics in Colon and Rectal Surgery, 20*(2), 96–101.

**Women's Health Initiative. (2002). Risks and benefits of estrogen plus progestin in healthy postmenopausal women: Principal results from the Women's Health Initiative randomized controlled trial. *Journal of the American Medical Association, 288*(3), 321–333.

Benign Vulvar Disorders

American College of Obstetricians and Gynecologists (ACOG). (2006c). ACOG committee opinion 345. Vulvodynia. *Obstetrics & Gynecology, 108*(4), 1049–1052.

Bachman, G., Rosen, R., Pinn, V., et al. (2006). Vulvodynia: A state of the art consensus on definitions, diagnosis and management. *Journal of Reproductive Medicine, 51*(6), 447–456.

Bergeron, S., Khalife, S., Glazer, H., et al. (2008). Surgical and behavioral treatments for vestibulodynia. *Obstetrics & Gynecology, 111*(1), 159–166.

Benign Ovarian Disorders

American College of Obstetricians and Gynecologists (ACOG). (2007c). Practice bulletin 83. Management of adnexal masses. *Obstetrics & Gynecology, 110*(1), 201–214.

Stankiewicz, M. & Norman, R. (2006). Diagnosis and management of polycystic ovary syndrome: A practical guide. *Drugs, 66*(7), 903–912.

Benign Uterine Disorders, Endometriosis, Prolapse, Fibroids

American College of Obstetricians and Gynecologists (ACOG). (2007d). ACOG practice bulletin 81. Endometrial ablation. *Obstetrics & Gynecology, 109*(5), 1233–1248.

American College of Obstetricians and Gynecologists (ACOG). (2007b). ACOG practice bulletin 79. Pelvic organ prolapse. *Obstetrics & Gynecology, 109*(2 Pt. 1), 461–473.

Fiscella, K., Eisinger, S. H., Meldrum, S., et al. (2006). Effect of mifepristone for symptomatic leiomyomata on quality of life and uterine size: A randomized controlled trial. *Obstetrics & Gynecology, 108*(6), 1381–1387.

Goodwin, S., Spies, J., Worthington-Kirsch, R., et al. for the Fibroid Registry for Outcomes Data (FIBROID) Registry Steering Committee and Core Site Investigators. (2008). Uterine artery embolization for the treatment of leiomyomata: Long term-outcomes from the FIBROID registry. *Obstetrics & Gynecology, 111*(1), 22–33.

McDaniel, C. (2007). Uterine fibroid embolization: The less invasive alternative. *Nursing, 37*(5), 26–27.

Melin, A., Sparén, P. & Bergqvist, A. (2008). The risk of cancer and the role of parity among women with endometriosis. *Obstetrical and Gynecological Survey, 63*(3), 156–157.

Rotveit, G., Brown, J., Thom, D., et al. (2007). Symptomatic pelvic organ prolapse. *Obstetrics & Gynecology, 109*(6), 1396–1403.

Stewart, E. A., Gostout, B., Rabinovici, J., et al. (2007). Sustained relief of leiomyoma symptoms by using focused ultrasound surgery. *Obstetrics & Gynecology, 110*(2 Pt. 1), 279–287.

Human Papillomavirus

American College of Obstetricians and Gynecologists (ACOG). (2006b). ACOG committee opinion 344. Human papillomavirus vaccination. *Obstetrics & Gynecology, 108*(3 Pt. 1), 699–704.

Centers for Disease Control and Prevention (CDC). (2007). Human papillomavirus: HPV information for clinicians. Atlanta: Author. www.cdc.gov/std/hpv/common-clinicians/ClinicianBro.txt

Markowitz, L. E, Dunne, E. F., Saraiya, M., et al. (2007). Quadrivalent human papillomavirus vaccine: Recommendations of the Advisory Committee on Immunization Practices (ACIP). *MMWR Morbidity and Mortality Weekly Report, 56*(RR-02), 1–24.

U.S. Cancer Statistics Working Group. (2007). *United States Cancer Statistics: 2004 Incidence and Mortality.* Atlanta: Department of Health and Human Services, Centers for Disease Control and Prevention, and National Cancer Institute.

World Health Organization. (n.d.). Women, girls, HIV and AIDS. HIV unit. www.searo.who.int/LinkFiles/World_AIDS_Day_women-hiv.pdf

UNAIDS. (2006). Report on the global AIDS epidemic. Executive summary. http://data.unaids.org/pub/GlobalReport/2006/2006_GR-Executive Summary_en.pdf

Wright, T. C., Massad, L. S., Dunton, C. J., et al. (2007). 2006 consensus guidelines for the management of women with abnormal cervical cancer screening tests. *American Journal of Obstetrics and Gynecology, 197*(4), 346–355.

Hysterectomy

Dutton, S., Hirst, A., McPherson, K., et al. (2008). A UK multicenter retrospective cohort study comparing hysterectomy and uterine artery embolization for the treatment of symptomatic uterine fibroids (HOPEFUL study): Main results on medium-term safety and efficacy. *Obstetrical and Gynecological Survey, 63*(2), 87–88.

Kim, K. H. & Lee, K. A. (2009). Sleep and fatigue symptoms in women before and 6 weeks after hysterectomy. *Journal of Obstetrics, Gynecologic, & Neonatal Nursing, 38*(3), 344–352.

Wu, J. M., Wechter, M. E., Geller, E. J., et al. (2007). Hysterectomy rates in the United States, 2003. *Obstetrics and Gynecology, 110*(5), 1091–1095.

Reproductive Malignancy

American College of Obstetricians and Gynecologists (ACOG). (2006d). ACOG committee opinion 336. Tamoxifen and uterine cancer. *Obstetrics & Gynecology, 107*(6), 1475–1478.

American College of Obstetricians and Gynecologists (ACOG). (2007a). Practice bulletin 84. Prevention of deep vein thrombosis and pulmonary embolism. *Obstetrics & Gynecology, 110*(2 Pt 1), 429–440.

American College of Obstetricians and Gynecologists (ACOG). (2008a). Practice bulletin 89. Elective and risk reducing salpingo-oophorectomy. *Obstetrics & Gynecology, 111*(1), 231–240.

American College of Obstetricians and Gynecologists (ACOG). (2008b). Committee Opinion #396. Intraperitoneal therapy for ovarian cancer. *Obstetrics & Gynecology, 111*(1), 249–250.

Bhoola, S. & Hoskins, W. J. (2006). Diagnosis and management of epithelial ovarian cancer. *Obstetrics & Gynecology, 107*(6), 1399–1410.

Bohnenkamp, S., LeBaron, V. & Yoder, L. H. (2007a). The medical-surgical nurse's guide to ovarian cancer: Part I. *MedSurg Nursing, 16*(4), 259–266.

Bohnenkamp, S., LeBaron, V. & Yoder, L. H. (2007b). The medical-surgical nurse's guide to ovarian cancer: Part II. *MedSurg Nursing, 16*(5), 323–331.

Hordern, A. (2008). Intimacy and sexuality after cancer. A critical review of the literature. *Cancer Nursing, 31*(2), E9–E17.

Jemal, A., Siegel, R., Ward, E., et al. (2007). Cancer statistics 2007. *CA: A Cancer Journal for Clinicians, 57*(1), 43–66.

Ryerson, A., Eheman, C., Burton, J., et al. (2007). Symptoms, diagnoses and time to key diagnostic procedures among older U.S. women with ovarian cancer. *Obstetrics & Gynecology, 109*(5), 1053–1061.

Sorosky, J. (2008). Endometrial cancer. *Obstetrics & Gynecology, 112*(2 Pt. 1), 436–447.

STDs, Vaginitis, and Vulvovaginal Infections and Pelvic Infections

American College of Obstetricians and Gynecologists (ACOG). (2006a). Practice bulletin 72. Vaginitis. *Obstetrics & Gynecology, 107*(5), 1195–1206.

American College of Obstetricians and Gynecologists (ACOG). (2007a). ACOG committee opinion 389. Human immunodeficiency virus. *Obstetrics & Gynecology, 110*(6), 1473–1478.

Centers for Disease Control and Prevention (CDC). (2006a). Sexually transmitted diseases treatment guideline, 2006. *MMWR Morbidity and Mortality Weekly Report, 55*(RR-11), 1–94.

Centers for Disease Control and Prevention (CDC). (2006b). Epidemiology of HIV/AIDS—United States, 1981–2005. *MMWR Morbidity Mortality Weekly Report, 55*(21), 589–592.

Centers for Disease Control and Prevention (CDC). (2007). Update to CDC's *Sexually Transmitted Diseases Treatment Guidelines, 2006:* Fluoroquinolones no longer recommended for treatment of gonococcal infections. *MMWR Morbidity and Mortality Weekly Report, 56*(24), 332–336.

Gibbs, R. (2007). Asymptomatic bacterial vaginosis: Is it time to treat? *American Journal of Obstetrics & Gynecology, 196*(6), 495–496.

Goodman, P., Herman, J., Murdaugh, C., et al. (2007). Role of decision making in women's self diagnosis and management of vaginitis. *Women's Health Care, 6*(2), 57–63.

Livengood, C. H., Ferris, D. G., Wiesenfeld, H. C., et al. (2007). Effectiveness of two tinidazole regimens in treatment of bacterial vaginosis. *Obstetrics & Gynecology, 110*(2), 302–309.

RESOURCES

American Cancer Society, www.cancer.org

American Social Health Association, www.ashastd.org/hpv_overview.cfm

Association of Reproductive Health Professionals, www.arhp.org

Association of Women's Health, Obstetrical and Neonatal Nurses (AWHONN), www.awhonn.org

Centers for Disease Control and Prevention, Office of Women's Health, www.cdc.gov/women/

Endometriosis Association, www.endometriosisassn.org

Gay and Lesbian Medical Association, www.glma.org

Herpes Hotline: (919) 361-8488.

National Ovarian Cancer Coalition, www.ovarian.org

National STD Hotline: (800) 227-8922 or (800) 342-2437

Ovarian Cancer National Alliance, www.ovariancancer.org

Planned Parenthood Federation of America, www.plannedparenthood.org/sti

Resolve: The National Infertility Association, www.resolve.org

Women's Cancer Network, Gynecologic Cancer Foundation, www.wcn.org

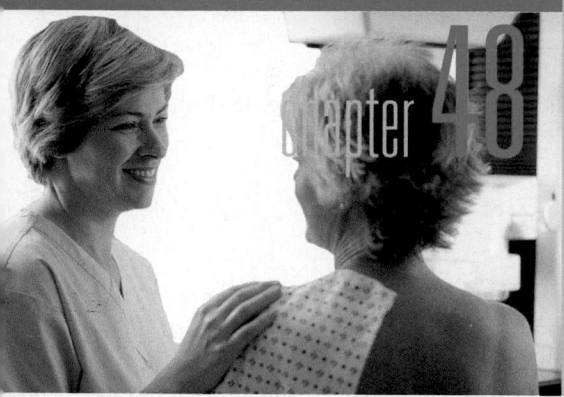

Chapter 48

Assessment and Management of Patients With Breast Disorders

LEARNING OBJECTIVES

On completion of this chapter, the learner will be able to:

1 Summarize the guidelines for the early detection of breast cancer.

2 Develop a teaching plan for breast self-examination for patients and consumer groups.

3 Identify and describe the different types of breast disorders, both benign and malignant.

4 Identify the examinations and biopsy procedures used to diagnose breast disorders.

5 Describe the different modalities used to treat breast cancer.

6 Use the nursing process as a framework for care of the patient undergoing surgery for the treatment of breast cancer.

7 Describe the physical, psychosocial, and rehabilitative needs of the patient who has had breast surgery for the treatment of breast cancer.

GLOSSARY

adjuvant chemotherapy: use of anticancer medications in addition to other treatments to delay or prevent a recurrence of the disease

adjuvant hormonal therapy: use of synthetic hormones or other medications given after primary treatment to increase the chances of a cure by stopping or slowing the growth of certain cancers that are affected by hormone stimulation (sometimes called endocrine or antiestrogen therapy)

aromatase inhibitors: medications that block the production of estrogens by the adrenal glands

atypical hyperplasia: abnormal increase in the number of cells in a specific area within the ductal or lobular areas of the breast; this abnormal proliferation increases the risk for cancer

benign proliferative breast disease: various types of atypical, yet noncancerous, breast tissue that increase the risk for breast cancer

brachytherapy: form of partial breast radiation in which a radioactive source is placed within the lumpectomy site

BRCA1 and ***BRCA2*:** genes on chromosome 17 that, when damaged or mutated, increase a woman's risk for breast and/or ovarian cancer compared with women without the mutation

breast conservation treatment: surgery to remove a breast tumor and a margin of tissue around the tumor without removing any other part of the breast; may or may not include lymph node removal and radiation therapy

dose-dense chemotherapy: administration of chemotherapeutic agents at standard doses with shorter time intervals between each cycle of treatment

ductal carcinoma in situ (DCIS): cancer cells starting in the ductal system of the breast not penetrating surrounding tissue

GLOSSARY *(Continued)*

estrogen and progesterone receptor assay: test to determine whether the breast tumor is nourished by hormones; this information helps to determine prognosis and treatment

fibrocystic breast changes: term used to describe certain benign changes in the breast, typically associated with palpable nodularity, lumpiness, swelling, or pain

fine-needle aspiration (FNA): removal of fluid for diagnostic analysis from a cyst or cells from a mass using a needle and syringe

galactography: use of mammography after an injection of radiopaque dye to diagnose problems in the ductal system of the breast

gynecomastia: overdeveloped breast tissue typically seen in adolescent boys

lobular carcinoma in situ (LCIS): atypical change and proliferation of the lobular cells of the breast; previously considered a premalignant condition but now considered a marker of increased risk for invasive breast cancer

lymphedema: chronic swelling of an extremity due to interrupted lymphatic circulation, typically from an axillary lymph node dissection

mammoplasty: surgery to reconstruct or change the size or shape of the breast; can be performed for reduction or augmentation

mastalgia: breast pain, usually related to hormonal fluctuations or irritation of a nerve

mastitis: inflammation or infection of the breast

modified radical mastectomy: removal of the breast tissue, nipple–areola complex, and a portion of the axillary lymph nodes

Paget's disease: form of breast cancer that begins in the ductal system and involves the nipple, areola, and surrounding skin

prophylactic mastectomy: removal of the breast to reduce the risk of breast cancer in women considered to be at high risk

sentinel lymph node: first lymph node(s) in the lymphatic basin that receives drainage from the primary tumor in the breast; identified by a radioisotope and/or blue dye

stereotactic core biopsy: computer-guided method of core needle biopsy that is useful when masses in the breast cannot be felt but can be visualized using mammography

surgical biopsy: Surgical removal of all or a portion of a mass for microscopic examination by a pathologist

tissue expander followed by permanent implant: series of breast-reconstructive surgeries after a mastectomy; involves stretching the skin and muscle before inserting the permanent implant

total mastectomy: removal of the breast tissue and nipple–areola complex

transverse rectus abdominis myocutaneous (TRAM) flap: method of breast reconstruction in which a flap of skin, fat, and muscle from the lower abdomen, with its attached blood supply, is rotated to the mastectomy site

ultrasonography: imaging method using high-frequency sound waves to diagnose whether masses are solid or fluid filled

In many cultures, the breast plays a significant role in a woman's sexuality and self-identity. A breast disorder, whether benign or malignant, can cause great anxiety and fear of potential disfigurement, loss of sexual attractiveness, and even death. Nurses, therefore, must have expertise in the assessment and management of not only the physical symptoms but also the psychosocial symptoms associated with breast disorders.

BREAST ASSESSMENT

Anatomic and Physiologic Overview

Male and female breasts mature comparably until puberty, when in females estrogen and other hormones initiate breast development. This development usually occurs from 10 to 16 years of age, although the range can vary from 9 to 18 years. Stages of breast development are described as Tanner stages 1 through 5.

- Stage 1 describes a prepubertal breast.
- Stage 2 is breast budding, the first sign of puberty in a female.
- Stage 3 involves further enlargement of breast tissue and the areola (a darker tissue ring around the nipple).
- Stage 4 occurs when the nipple and areola form a secondary mound on top of the breast tissue.
- Stage 5 is the continued development of a larger breast with a single contour.

The breasts are located between the second and sixth ribs over the pectoralis muscle from the sternum to the midaxillary line. An area of breast tissue, called the tail of Spence, extends into the axilla. Fascial bands, called Cooper's ligaments, support the breast on the chest wall. The inframammary fold (or crease) is a ridge of fat at the bottom of the breast.

Each breast contains 12 to 20 cone-shaped lobes, which are made up of glandular elements (lobules and ducts) and separated by fat and fibrous tissue that binds the lobes together. Milk is produced in the lobules and then carried through the ducts to the nipple. Figure 48-1 shows the anatomy of the fully developed breast.

Assessment

Health History

When a patient presents with a breast problem, the nurse conducts a general health assessment, including history of medical disorders and previous surgery; family history of diseases, particularly cancer; gynecologic and obstetric history; present medications (including prescriptions, vitamins, and herbal); past and present use of hormonal contraceptives, hormone therapy (HT) (formerly referred to as hormone replacement therapy [HRT]), or fertility treatments; and social habits (eg, smoking, drinking alcohol). Psychosocial information, such as the patient's marital status, occupation, and availability of resources and support people, is obtained. Any recent x-rays or other diagnostic tests are noted. Focused questions pertaining to the breast disorder are asked concerning the onset of the disorder and the length of time it has been present. In addition, the patient is asked if any masses are palpable and if there is any associated pain, swelling, redness, nipple discharge, or skin changes. Knowledge and comfort in practicing breast self-examination (BSE) should also be ascertained from the patient.

Physical Assessment: Female Breast

A female breast examination can be conducted during any general physical or gynecologic examination or whenever the patient reports an abnormality. The American Cancer Society (ACS) recommends that women at average risk for breast cancer undergo a clinical breast examination at least every 3 years while in their 20s and 30s and then annually thereafter (Smith, Cokkinides & Brawley, 2008). A thorough breast examination, including instruction in BSE, takes at least 10 minutes.

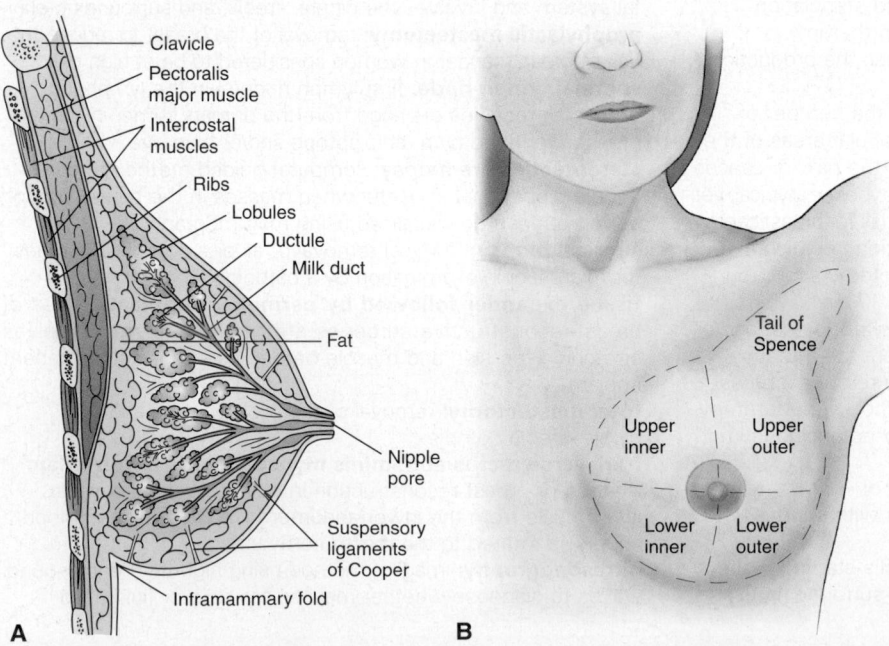

A

B

Figure 48-1 A, Anatomy of the breast. **B,** Areas of breast, including the tail of Spence.

Inspection

Examination begins with inspection. The patient is asked to disrobe to the waist and sit in a comfortable position facing the examiner. The breasts are inspected for size and symmetry. A slight variation in the size of each breast is common and generally normal. The skin is inspected for color, venous pattern, thickening, or edema. Erythema (redness) may indicate benign local inflammation or superficial lymphatic invasion by a neoplasm. A prominent venous pattern can signal increased blood supply required by a tumor. Edema and pitting of the skin may result from a neoplasm blocking lymphatic drainage, giving the skin an orange-peel appearance (peau d'orange), a classic sign of advanced breast cancer. Nipple inversion of one or both breasts is not uncommon and is significant only when of recent origin. Ulceration, rashes, or spontaneous nipple discharge requires evaluation. Examples of abnormal breast findings on inspection can be found in Chart 48-1.

To elicit skin dimpling or retraction that may otherwise go undetected, the examiner instructs the patient to raise both arms overhead. This maneuver normally elevates both breasts equally. The patient is then instructed to place her hands on her waist and push in. These movements, which cause contraction of the pectoral muscles, do not normally alter the breast contour or nipple direction. Any dimpling or retraction during these position changes suggests an underlying mass. The clavicular and axillary regions are inspected for swelling, discoloration, lesions, or enlarged lymph nodes.

Palpation

The breasts are palpated with the patient sitting up (upright) and lying down (supine). In the supine position the patient's shoulder is first elevated with a small pillow to help balance the breast on the chest wall. Failure to do this allows the breast tissue to slip laterally, and a breast mass may be missed. The entire surface of the breast and the axillary tail is systematically palpated using the flat part (pads) of the second, third, and fourth fingertips, held together, making dime-size circles. The examiner may choose to proceed in a clockwise direction, following imaginary concentric circles from the outer limits of the breast toward the nipple. Other acceptable methods are to palpate from each number on the face of the clock toward the nipple in a clockwise fashion or along imaginary vertical lines on the breast (Fig. 48-2).

Palpation of the axillary and clavicular areas is easily performed with the patient seated (Fig. 48-3). To examine the axillary lymph nodes, the examiner gently abducts the patient's arm from the thorax. With the left hand, the patient's left forearm is grasped and supported. The right hand is then free to palpate the axillae. Any lymph nodes that may be lying against the thoracic wall are noted. Normally, these lymph nodes are not palpable, but if they are enlarged, their location, size, mobility, and consistency are noted. During palpation, the examiner notes any patient-reported tenderness or masses. If a mass is detected, it is described by its location (eg, left breast, 2 cm from the nipple at 2 o'clock position). Size, shape, consistency, border delineation, and mobility are included in the description.

The breast tissue of the adolescent is usually firm and lobular, whereas that of the postmenopausal woman is more likely to feel thinner and fattier. During pregnancy and lactation, the breasts are firmer and larger with lobules that are more distinct. Hormonal changes cause the areola to darken. Cysts are commonly found in menstruating women and are usually well defined and freely movable. Premenstrually, cysts may be larger and more tender. Malignant tumors, on the other hand, tend to be hard, poorly defined, and nontender. A physician should further evaluate any abnormalities detected during inspection and palpation.

Physical Assessment: Male Breast

Breast cancer can occur in men. Examination of the male breast and axillae should be included in a physical examination. The nipple and areola are inspected for masses and nipple discharge. The same procedure for palpating the female axillae is used when assessing the male axillae.

Gynecomastia is the firm enlargement of glandular tissue beneath and immediately surrounding the areola of the male. This is different from the enlargement of soft, fatty tissue, which is caused by obesity.

Diagnostic Evaluation

Breast Self-Examination

The nurse plays an important role in BSE education, a modality used for the early detection of breast cancer. BSE can be taught in a variety of settings—either on a one-to-one basis or in a group. It can also be initiated by a health care practitioner during a patient's routine physical examination.

Variations in breast tissue occur during the menstrual cycle, pregnancy, and the onset of menopause. Women on HT can also experience fluctuations. Normal changes must be distinguished from those that may signal disease. Most women notice increased tenderness and lumpiness before their menstrual periods; therefore, BSE is best performed after menses (day 5 to day 7, counting the first day of menses as day 1). Also, many women have grainy-textured breast tissue, but these areas are usually less nodular after menses. Younger women may find BSE particularly difficult because of the density of their breast tissue. As women age, their breasts become fattier and may be easier to examine.

It is estimated that only 25% to 30% of women perform BSE proficiently and regularly each month. Some find BSE to be anxiety producing; others find it too difficult to differentiate between normal changes and worrisome findings. Even women who perform BSE and detect a change may delay seeking medical attention because of fear, economic factors, lack of education, and modesty. Despite these factors, many women discover their own breast cancers. For this reason, BSE should be taught and encouraged but not overemphasized. The ACS recommends that women, beginning in their early 20s, be told about the benefits and limitations of BSE. It is then up to the individual woman whether to perform BSE regularly, irregularly, or not at all (Smith, et al., 2008).

Instructions about BSE should also be provided to men if they have a family history of breast cancer, because they may have an increased risk of male breast cancer.

Chart 48-1 • *Abnormal Findings During Inspection of the Breasts*

Retraction Signs

- Signs include skin dimpling, creasing, or changes in the contour of the breast or nipple
- May be secondary to contraction of fibrotic tissue that can occur with underlying malignancy
- May be secondary to scar tissue formation after breast surgery
- Retraction signs may appear only with position changes

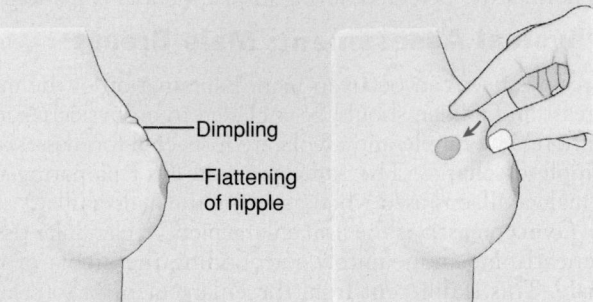

Retraction signs   Retraction with compression

Increased Venous Prominence

- Unilateral localized increase in venous pattern associated with malignant tumors
- Normal with bilateral and symmetrical breast enlargement associated with pregnancy and lactation

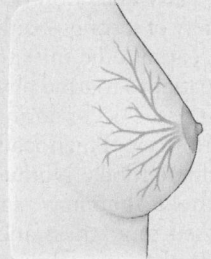

Increased venous prominence

Peau d'Orange (Edema)

- Associated with inflammatory breast cancer
- Caused by interference with lymphatic drainage
- Breast skin has orange peel appearance
- Skin pores enlarge
- May be noted on the areola
- Skin becomes thick, hard, and immobile

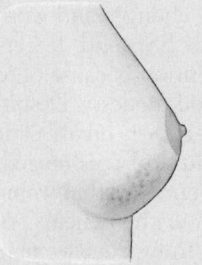

Peau d'orange

Nipple Inversion

- Considered normal if long-standing
- Associated with fibrosis and malignancy if recent development

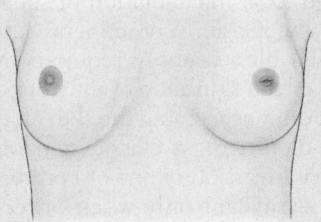

Nipple inversion

Acute Mastitis (Inflammation of the Breasts)

- Associated with lactation but may occur at any age
- Nipple cracks or abrasions noted
- Breast skin reddened and warm to touch
- Tenderness
- Systemic signs include fever and increased pulse

Paget's Disease (Malignancy of Mammary Ducts)

- Early signs: erythema of nipple and areola
- Late signs: thickening, scaling, and erosion of the nipple and areola

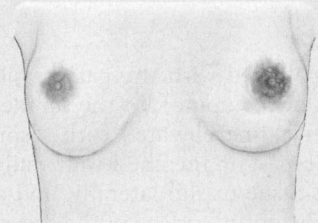

Paget's disease

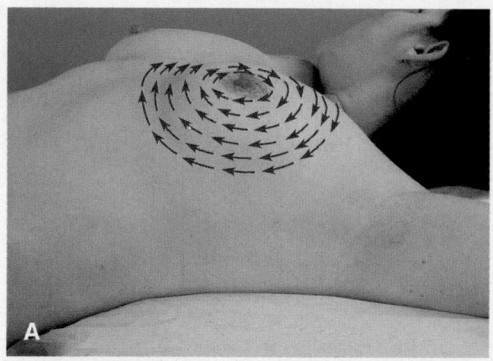
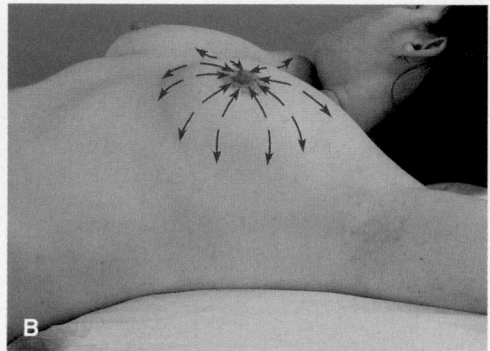
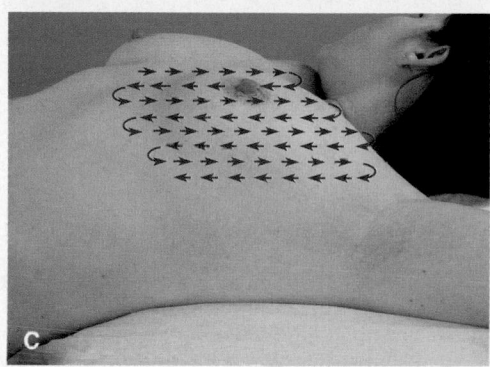

Figure 48-2 Breast examination with the woman in a supine position. The entire surface of the breast is palpated from the outer edge of the breast to the nipple; palpation patterns are **(A)** circular or clockwise, **(B)** wedge, and **(C)** vertical strip.

Patients who elect to perform BSE should receive proper instruction on technique (Chart 48-2). They should be informed that routine BSE will help them become familiar with their "normal abnormalities." If a change is detected, they should seek medical attention.

Patients should be instructed about optimal timing for BSE (5 to 7 days after menses begin for premenopausal women and once monthly for postmenopausal women). When demonstrating examination techniques, the feel of normal breast tissue should be reviewed and ways to identify breast changes discussed. Patients should then perform a BSE demonstration on themselves or on a breast model. Patients who have had breast cancer surgery should be instructed to examine their breast or chest wall for any new changes or nodules that may indicate a recurrence of the disease.

BSE videos, shower cards, and pamphlets can be obtained from local chapters of the ACS.

Mammography

Mammography is a breast-imaging technique that has been shown to reduce breast cancer mortality rates. It can detect nonpalpable lesions and assist in diagnosing palpable masses. The procedure takes about 15 minutes and can be performed in a hospital radiology department or independent imaging center. Two views are taken of each breast. The breast is mechanically compressed from top to bottom (craniocaudal view) and side to side (mediolateral oblique view) (Fig. 48-4). Women may experience some fleeting discomfort because maximum compression is necessary for proper visualization. The new mammogram is compared with previous mammograms, and any changes may indicate a need for further investigation. Mammography may detect a breast tumor before it is clinically palpable (ie, smaller than 1 cm); however, it has limitations. The false-negative rate ranges between 5% and 10%. Younger women, or those taking HT, may have dense breast tissue, making it more difficult to detect lesions with mammography.

Patients scheduled for a mammogram may voice concern about exposure to radiation. The radiation exposure is equivalent to about 1 hour of exposure to sunlight, so patients would have to have many mammograms in a year to increase their cancer risk. The benefits of this test outweigh the risks. To ensure that a mammogram is reliable, it is important that a woman find a reputable facility. A facility that is certified by the Mammography Quality Standards Act must meet stringent quality standards, be accredited by the U.S. Food and Drug Administration (FDA) and be inspected annually.

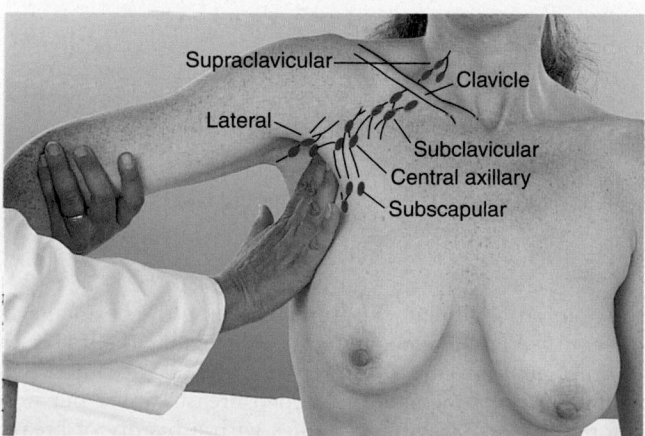

Supraclavicular
Clavicle
Lateral
Subclavicular
Central axillary
Subscapular

Figure 48-3 Palpating axillary nodes in breast examination.

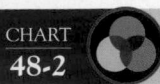

CHART 48-2

PATIENT EDUCATION
Breast Self-Examination (BSE)

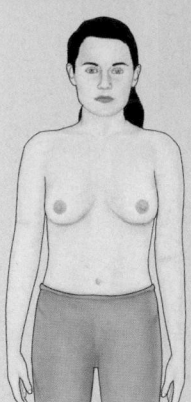

Step 1

1. Stand in front of a mirror.
2. Check both breasts for anything unusual.
3. Look for discharge from the nipple, puckering, dimpling, or scaling of the skin.

The next two steps are done to check for any changes in the contour of your breasts. As you do them, you should be able to feel your muscles tighten.

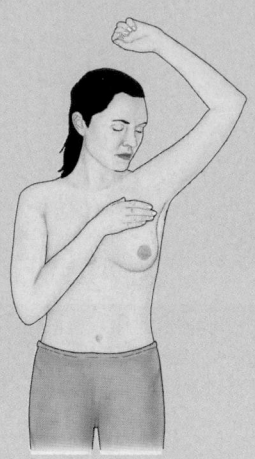

Step 2

1. Watch closely in the mirror as you clasp your hands behind your head and press your hands forward.
2. Note any change in the contour of your breasts.

Step 4

1. Raise your left arm.
2. Use three or four fingers of your right hand to feel your left breast firmly, carefully, and thoroughly.
3. Beginning at the outer edge, press the flat part of your fingers in small circles, moving the circles slowly around the breast.
4. Gradually work toward the nipple.
5. Be sure to cover the whole breast.
6. Pay special attention to the area between the breast and the underarm, including the underarm itself.
7. Feel for any unusual lumps or masses under the skin.
8. If you have any spontaneous discharge during the month—whether or not it is during your BSE—see your doctor.
9. Repeat the examination on your right breast.

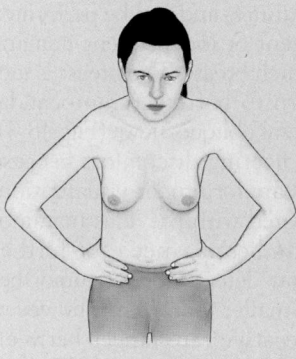

Step 3

1. Next, press your hands firmly on your hips and bow slightly toward the mirror as you pull your shoulders and elbows forward.
2. Note any change in the contour of your breasts.

Some women do the next part of the examination in the shower. Your fingers will glide easily over soapy skin, so you can concentrate on feeling for changes inside the breast.

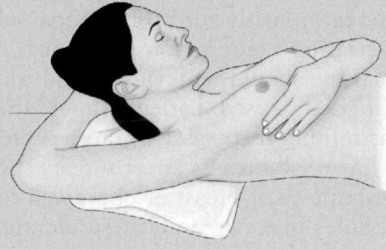

Step 5

1. Step 4 should be repeated lying down.
2. Lie flat on your back with your left arm over your head and a pillow or folded towel under your left shoulder. (This position flattens your breast and makes it easier to check.)
3. Use the same circular motion described above.
4. Repeat on your right breast.

Adapted from U.S. Department of Health and Human Services, Public Health Service, *What you need to know about breast cancer.* Bethesda, MD: National Institutes of Health.

Current mammographic screening guidelines of the ACS recommend a mammogram every year beginning at 40 years of age. There is no upper age limit at which mammography should be discontinued as long as the woman is in good health (Smith, et al., 2008). Women who are at increased risk because of a strong family history should seek the opinion of a breast specialist regarding the optimal age to begin screening mammography. A general guideline is to begin screening 10 years earlier than the age at which the youngest family member developed breast cancer but not before 25 years of age. In families with a history of breast cancer, a downward shift in age of diagnosis of about

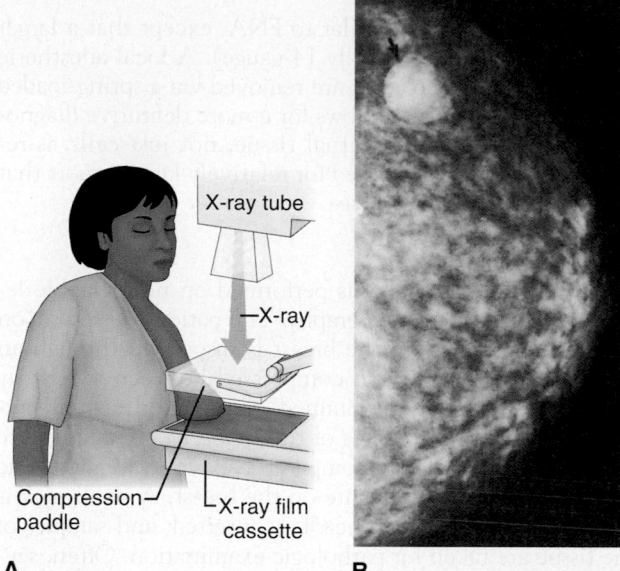

A   **B**

Figure 48-4 The mammography procedure (**A**) relies on x-ray imaging to produce the mammogram (**B**), which in this case reveals a breast lump.

10 years is seen (eg, grandmother diagnosed with breast cancer at 48 years of age, mother diagnosed with breast cancer at 38 years of age, then daughter should begin screening at age 28 years of age).

Despite the decreased mortality rates associated with mammographic screening, many women are not undergoing this simple procedure. Only 52.9% of non-Hispanic white women older than 40 years of age reported having mammography within the past year. Recent data also suggest a decline in the use of mammography. The screening rate in 2000 was 70% and decreased to 66% in 2005 (Breen, Cronin, Meissner, et al., 2007). The percentage was even lower for women in racial and ethnic minority groups, particularly in those who immigrated to the United States in the past 10 years. Low rates of screening were also seen in women with less education and no health insurance. The implementation of screening programs such as the National Breast and Cervical Cancer Early Detection Program of the Centers for Disease Control and Prevention (CDC) helps low-income, uninsured, and underserved women gain access not only to mammograms but to clinical breast examinations, Papanicolaou (Pap) tests, diagnostic testing for abnormal screening tests, and surgical consultation (CDC, 2007). The program was established in 1991 and has provided more than 7 million screening examinations and diagnosed more than 30,000 patients with breast cancer. Nurses are in key positions to educate women about the current ACS screening guidelines and the benefits of mammography. They can also help identify and provide information to women who may benefit from such screening programs as the one operated by the CDC.

Newer techniques for breast screening include digital mammography and computer-assisted detection (CAD) programs. Digital mammography records x-ray images on a computer instead of on film, thus allowing radiologists to adjust the contrast and focus on an image without having to take additional x-rays. Compared with conventional film mammography, digital mammography has been shown to be significantly better at detecting breast cancer in women younger than 50 years of age, women with dense breast tissue, and premenopausal and perimenopausal women. CAD is designed to assist radiologists in the identification of suspicious areas on a mammogram. Trials of CAD programs have generally, but not always, shown improvements in detection rates (Helvie, 2007). The effectiveness of both digital mammography and CAD continues to be evaluated.

Galactography

Galactography is a diagnostic procedure that involves injection of less than 1 mL of radiopaque material through a cannula inserted into a ductal opening on the areola, which is followed by a mammogram. It is performed to evaluate an abnormality within the duct when the patient has bloody nipple discharge on expression, spontaneous nipple discharge, or a solitary dilated duct noted on mammography.

Ultrasonography

Ultrasonography (ultrasound) is used as a diagnostic adjunct to mammography to help distinguish fluid-filled cysts from other lesions. A thin coating of lubricating jelly is spread over the area to be imaged. A transducer is then placed on the breast. The transducer transmits high-frequency sound waves through the skin toward the area of concern. The sound waves that are reflected back form a two-dimensional image, which is then displayed on a computer screen. No radiation is emitted during the procedure.

Ultrasonography has advantages and disadvantages. Although it can diagnose cysts with great accuracy, it cannot definitively rule out malignant lesions. Microcalcifications, which are detectable on mammography, cannot be identified on ultrasonography. Finally, examination techniques and interpretation criteria are not standardized.

Magnetic Resonance Imaging

Magnetic resonance imaging (MRI) of the breast is rapidly gaining in popularity. This highly sensitive test has become a useful diagnostic adjunct to mammography. A magnet is linked to a computer that creates detailed images of the breast without exposure to radiation. An intravenous (IV) injection of gadolinium, a contrast dye, is given to improve visibility. The patient lies face down and the breast is placed through a depression in the table. A coil is placed around the breast, and the patient is placed inside the MRI machine. The entire procedure takes about 30 to 40 minutes.

MRI is most useful in patients with proven breast cancer when assessing for multifocal (more than one tumor in the same quadrant of the breast) or multicentric (more than one tumor in different quadrants of the breast) disease, chest wall involvement, tumor recurrence, or response to chemotherapy. The procedure can also identify occult (undetectable) breast cancer and determine the integrity of saline or silicone breast implants. Recent studies have shown that MRI is a highly sensitive screening tool that can be used to identify breast cancer in women at high risk for the disease (Orel, 2008). The ACS now recommends an annual MRI scan in addition to mammography in women at high risk for breast cancer (ie, those with greater than 20% lifetime risk). Candidates include women who have a *BRCA1* or *BRCA2* mutation, a first-degree relative with either of these mutations, certain rare genetic syndromes, or radiation to the chest between 10 and 30 years of age (Saslow, Boetes, Burke, et al., 2007). MRI should be used in addition to mammography, not instead of it.

Some disadvantages of MRI include high cost, variations in technique and interpretation, and the potential for patient claustrophobia. The procedure cannot always accurately distinguish between malignant and benign breast conditions. MRI is contraindicated in patients with implantable metal devices (eg, aneurysm clips, pacemakers, ports of tissue expanders) because of the metallic force. Foil-backed medication patches (eg, nicotine, nitroglycerine, fentanyl) must be removed prior to MRI to avoid burns to the skin.

Procedures for Tissue Analysis

Percutaneous Biopsy

Percutaneous biopsy is performed on an outpatient basis to sample palpable and nonpalpable lesions. Less invasive than a surgical biopsy, percutaneous biopsy is a needle or core biopsy that obtains tissue by making a small puncture in the skin. Table 48-1 outlines the different types of biopsies that can be performed to obtain a tissue diagnosis.

Fine-Needle Aspiration

Fine-needle aspiration (FNA) is a noninvasive biopsy technique that is generally well tolerated by most women. A local anesthetic may or may not be used. A small gauge needle (25- or 22-gauge) attached to a syringe is inserted into the mass or area of nodularity. Suction is applied to the syringe, and multiple passes are made through the mass. A simple cyst often disappears on aspiration, and the fluid is usually discarded. If no fluid is obtained, any cellular material obtained in the hub of the needle is spread on a glass slide or placed in a preservative and sent to the laboratory for analysis. For nonpalpable masses, the same procedure can be performed by a radiologist using ultrasound guidance (ultrasound-guided FNA).

FNA is less expensive than other diagnostic methods and results are usually available quickly. However, false-negative or false-positive results are possible, and appropriate follow-up depends on the clinical judgment of the treating physician.

Core Needle Biopsy

Core needle biopsy is similar to FNA, except that a larger gauge needle is used (usually 14-gauge). A local anesthetic is applied, and tissue cores are removed via a spring-loaded device. This procedure allows for a more definitive diagnosis than FNA, because actual tissue, not just cells, is removed. It is often performed for relatively large tumors that are close to the skin surface.

Stereotactic Core Biopsy

Stereotactic core biopsy is performed on nonpalpable lesions detected by mammography. The patient lies prone on the stereotactic table. The breast is suspended through an opening in the table and compressed between two x-ray plates. Images are then obtained using digital mammography. The exact coordinates of the lesion to be sampled are located with the aid of a computer. Next, a local anesthetic is injected into the entry site on the breast. A small nick is made in the skin, a core needle is inserted, and samples of the tissue are taken for pathologic examination. Often, several passes are taken to ensure that the lesion is well sampled. Postbiopsy films are then taken to check that sampling has been adequate. A small titanium clip is often placed at the biopsy site so that the site can easily be located if further treatment is indicated.

Stereotactic biopsy is quite accurate and often allows the patient to avoid a surgical biopsy. However, there is a small false-negative rate. Appropriate follow-up depends on the final pathologic diagnosis and the clinical judgment of the treating physician. Use of a titanium clip does not preclude subsequent MRIs.

Ultrasound-Guided Core Biopsy

The principles for ultrasound-guided core biopsy are similar to those of stereotactic core biopsy, but by using ultrasound guidance, computer coordination and mammographic compression are not necessary. Ultrasound-guided core biopsy does not use radiation and is also faster and less expensive than stereotactic core biopsy.

Magnetic Resonance Imaging–Guided Core Biopsy

Recently, the technology has become available to perform core biopsies under MRI guidance. The number of facilities that are equipped to perform this procedure is increasing.

Table 48-1	TYPES OF BREAST BIOPSIES		
Procedure	Palpable Mass	Health Professional Who Performs Procedure	Nature of Breast Tissue Removed
Fine-needle aspiration	Yes	Surgeon	Cellular material
Core needle biopsy	Yes	Surgeon	Tissue core
Stereotactic core biopsy	No	Radiologist	Tissue core
Ultrasound-guided core biopsy	No	Radiologist	Tissue core
MRI-guided core biopsy	No	Radiologist	Tissue core
Excisional biopsy	Yes	Surgeon	Entire mass
Incisional biopsy	Yes	Surgeon	Tissue core
Wire needle localization biopsy; may be guided by mammogram, ultrasound, or MRI	No	Radiologist inserts wire, surgeon performs biopsy	Entire mass

Surgical Biopsy

Surgical biopsy is usually performed using local anesthesia and IV sedation. After an incision is made, the lesion is excised and sent to a laboratory for pathologic examination.

Types of Surgical Breast Biopsy

Excisional Biopsy. Excisional biopsy is the standard procedure for complete pathological assessment of a palpable breast mass. The entire mass, plus a margin of surrounding tissue, is removed. This type of biopsy may also be referred to as a lumpectomy. Depending on the clinical situation, a frozen section analysis of the specimen may be performed at the time of the biopsy by the pathologist, who does an immediate reading intraoperatively and provides a provisional diagnosis. This can help confirm a diagnosis in a patient who had no previous tissue analysis performed.

Incisional Biopsy. Incisional biopsy surgically removes a portion of a mass. This is performed to confirm a diagnosis and to conduct special studies (eg, ER/PR, HER-2/neu [also referred to as ERBB2]; see later discussion for explanation of these terms) that will aid in determining treatment, which are discussed later in this chapter. Complete excision of the area may not be possible or immediately beneficial to the patient, depending on the clinical situation. This procedure is often performed on women with locally advanced breast cancer or on women with suspected cancer recurrence, whose treatment may depend on the results of these special studies. However, pathological information may be easily obtained from core needle biopsy, and incisional biopsy is becoming less common.

Wire Needle Localization. Wire needle localization is a technique used to locate nonpalpable masses or suspicious calcium deposits detected on a mammogram, ultrasound, or MRI that require an excisional biopsy. The radiologist inserts a long, thin wire through a needle, which is then inserted into the area of abnormality using x-ray or ultrasound guidance (whichever imaging technique originally identified the abnormality). The wire remains in place after the needle is withdrawn to ensure the precise location. The patient is then taken to the operating room, where the surgeon follows the wire to the tip and excises the area.

Nursing Management

During the preoperative visit, the nurse assesses the patient for any specific educational, physical, or psychosocial needs that she may have. This can be accomplished by reviewing her medical and psychosocial history and encouraging her to verbalize her fears, concerns, and questions. Patients are often worried not only about the procedure but also about the potential implications of the pathology results. Providing a thorough explanation about what to expect in a supportive manner can help alleviate anxiety. Patients often have difficulty absorbing all the information given to them; therefore, written materials should be provided to reinforce teaching.

The nurse instructs the patient to discontinue any agents that can increase the risk of bleeding, including products containing aspirin, nonsteroidal anti-inflammatory drugs (NSAIDs), vitamin E supplements, herbal substances (such as ginkgo biloba and garlic supplements), and warfarin (Coumadin). The patient may be instructed not to eat or drink for several hours or after midnight the night before the procedure, depending on the type of biopsy planned. Most breast biopsy procedures today are performed with the use of moderate sedation and local anesthesia.

Immediate postoperative assessment includes monitoring the effects of the anesthesia and inspecting the surgical dressing for any signs of bleeding. Once the sedation has worn off, the nurse reviews the care of the biopsy site, pain management, and activity restrictions with the patient. Prior to discharge from the ambulatory surgical center or the office, the patient must be able to tolerate fluids, ambulate, and void. The patient must have somebody to accompany her home. The dressing covering the incision is usually removed after 48 hours, but the Steri-Strips, which are applied directly over the incision, should remain in place for approximately 7 to 10 days. The use of a supportive bra following surgery is encouraged to limit movement of the breast and reduce discomfort. A follow-up telephone call from the nurse 24 to 48 hours after the procedure can provide the patient with the opportunity to ask any questions and can be a source of great comfort and reassurance.

Most women return to their usual activities the day after the procedure but are encouraged to avoid jarring or high-impact activities for 1 week to promote healing of the biopsy site. Discomfort is usually minimal, and most women find acetaminophen (Tylenol) sufficient for pain relief, although a mild opioid may be prescribed if needed.

Follow-up after the biopsy includes a return visit to the surgeon for discussion of the final pathology report and assessment of the healing of the biopsy site. Depending on the results of the biopsy, the nurse's role varies. If the pathology report is benign, the nurse reviews incision care and explains what the patient should expect as the biopsy site heals (ie, changes in sensation may occur weeks or months after the biopsy due to nerve injury within the breast tissue). If a diagnosis of cancer is made, the nurse's role changes dramatically. This is discussed in depth later in this chapter.

CONDITIONS AFFECTING THE NIPPLE

Nipple Discharge

Nipple discharge in a woman who is not lactating may be related to many causes, such as carcinoma, papilloma, pituitary adenoma, cystic breasts, and various medications. Oral contraceptives, pregnancy, HT, chlorpromazine (Thorazine)-type medications, and frequent breast stimulation may be contributing factors. In some athletic women, nipple discharge may occur during running or aerobic exercises. Nipple discharge should be evaluated by a health care provider, but it is not often a cause for alarm. One in three women has clear discharge on expression, which is usually normal. A green discharge could indicate an infection. Any discharge that is spontaneous, persistent, or unilateral is of more concern. Although bloody discharge can indicate a malignancy, it is often caused by a benign wartlike growth on the lining of the duct called an intraductal papilloma.

Nipple discharge should be evaluated for the presence of occult (hidden) blood by performing a guaiac test. A galactogram can also be performed to detect abnormalities within the duct that may be causing the discharge. If there is a high level of suspicion, a surgical biopsy called a duct excision may be indicated.

Fissure

A fissure is a longitudinal ulcer that may develop in breastfeeding women. If the nipple becomes irritated, a painful, raw area may form and become a site of infection. Daily washing with water, massage with breast milk or lanolin, and exposure to air are helpful. Breastfeeding can be continued with the use of a nipple shield if necessary. If the fissure is severe or extremely painful, the woman is advised to stop breastfeeding. A breast pump can be used until breastfeeding can be resumed. Persistent ulceration requires further diagnosis and therapy. Guidance from a nurse or lactation consultant may be helpful because nipple irritation can result from improper positioning (ie, the infant has not grasped the areola fully) during breastfeeding.

BREAST INFECTIONS

Mastitis

Mastitis, an inflammation or infection of breast tissue, occurs most commonly in breastfeeding women, although it may also occur in nonlactating women. The infection may result from a transfer of micro-organisms to the breast by the patient's hands or from a breastfed infant with an oral, eye, or skin infection. Mastitis may also be caused by blood-borne organisms. As inflammation progresses, the breast texture becomes tough or doughy, and the patient complains of dull to severe pain in the infected region. A nipple that is discharging purulent material, serum, or blood should be investigated.

Treatment consists of antibiotics and local application of cold compresses to relieve discomfort. A broad-spectrum antibiotic agent may be prescribed for 7 to 10 days. The patient should wear a snug bra and perform personal hygiene carefully. Adequate rest and hydration are important aspects of management.

Lactational Abscess

A breast abscess may develop as a consequence of acute mastitis. The area affected becomes tender and red. Purulent matter can usually be aspirated with a needle, but incision and drainage may be required. Specimens of the aspirated material are obtained for culture so that an organism-specific antibiotic can be prescribed.

BENIGN CONDITIONS OF THE BREAST

Breast Pain

Breast pain **(mastalgia)** may be cyclical or noncyclical. Cyclical pain is usually related to hormonal fluctuations and accounts for nearly 75% of all complaints. Noncyclical pain is far less common and does not vary with the menstrual cycle. Women who experience injury or trauma to the breast or those who had a breast biopsy may experience noncyclical pain. Patients should be reassured that breast pain is rarely indicative of cancer. However, if the pain persists after menses begins, the patient should see her primary health care provider.

Nursing Management

The nurse may recommend that the patient wear a supportive bra both day and night for a week, decrease her salt and caffeine intake, and take ibuprofen (Advil) as needed for its anti-inflammatory actions. Vitamin E supplements or oil of evening primrose (an over-the-counter herbal preparation) may also be helpful.

Cysts

Cysts are fluid-filled sacs that develop as breast ducts dilate. Cysts occur most commonly in women 30 to 55 years of age and may be exacerbated during perimenopause. Although their cause is unknown, cysts usually disappear after menopause, suggesting that estrogen is a factor. Cystic areas often fluctuate in size and are usually larger premenstrually. They may be painless or may become very tender premenstrually. Occasionally, a patient may report an intermittent shooting sensation or a dull ache. Various breast masses are compared in Table 48-2. Cysts that are confirmed on an ultrasound and are not bothersome can often be left alone. To confirm a diagnosis or to relieve pain, FNA can be performed. Cysts do not increase the risk of breast cancer.

Fibrocystic breast changes, which is often called fibrocystic breast disease, is a nonspecific term used to describe an array of benign findings. The changes do not necessarily indicate a cystic process.

Fibroadenomas

Fibroadenomas are firm, round, movable, benign tumors. They can occur from puberty to menopause with a peak incidence at 30 years of age. These masses are nontender and are sometimes removed for definitive diagnosis.

Benign Proliferative Breast Disease

The two most common diagnoses of **benign proliferative breast disease** found on biopsy are atypical hyperplasia and lobular carcinoma in situ. These diagnoses increase a woman's risk of breast cancer.

Table 48-2 COMPARISON OF VARIOUS BREAST MASSES

The most common breast masses are due to cysts, fibroadenomas, or malignancy. Biopsy is usually needed for confirmation, but the following characteristics are diagnostic clues:

Characteristics	Cysts	Fibroadenomas	Malignancy
Age	30–55 years, regress after menopause except with use of estrogen therapy	Puberty to menopause	30–90 years; most common, 40–80 years
Number	Single or multiple	Usually single	Usually single
Shape	Round	Round, disk, or lobular	Irregular or stellate
Consistency	Soft to firm, usually elastic	Usually firm	Firm or hard
Mobility	Mobile	Mobile	May be fixed to skin or underlying tissues
Tenderness	Usually tender	Usually nontender	Usually nontender
Retraction signs	Absent	Absent	May be present

Atypical Hyperplasia

Atypical hyperplasia is an abnormal increase in the ductal (atypical ductal hyperplasia) or lobular (atypical lobular hyperplasia) cells in the breast and is usually found incidentally in mammographic abnormalities. Atypical hyperplasia increases a woman's risk of breast cancer about four to five times compared with that of the general population (Hanby & Hughes, 2008).

Lobular Carcinoma in Situ

Lobular carcinoma in situ (LCIS) is characterized by a proliferation of cells within the breast lobules. LCIS is usually found incidentally on pathologic diagnosis because it cannot be seen on mammography and does not form a palpable lump. The term LCIS is misleading because it is not a carcinoma. Historically, LCIS was considered a premalignant condition but is now considered a marker for increased risk of invasive carcinoma. A patient with LCIS may later develop an invasive carcinoma in either breast that is either ductal or lobular in origin. LCIS increases a woman's risk of breast cancer about 8 to 10 times compared with that of the general population (Hanby & Hughes, 2008).

Other Benign Conditions

Cystosarcoma phyllodes is a rare fibroepithelial lesion that tends to grow rapidly. It is rarely malignant and is treated with surgical excision. If it is malignant, mastectomy may follow. Lymph node removal is usually not performed because metastasis is rare.

Fat necrosis is a condition of the breast that is often associated with a history of trauma. Surgical procedures such as a breast biopsy can cause fat necrosis. It may be indistinguishable from carcinoma, and the entire mass is usually excised.

Intraductal papilloma is a wartlike growth that often involves the large milk ducts near the nipple, causing bloody nipple discharge. Surgery usually involves removal of the papilloma and a segment of the duct where the papilloma is found.

Superficial thrombophlebitis of the breast (Mondor disease) is an uncommon condition that is usually associated with pregnancy, trauma, or breast surgery. Pain and redness occur as a result of a superficial thrombophlebitis in the vein that drains the outer part of the breast. The mass is usually linear, tender, and erythematous. Treatment consists of analgesics and heat.

MALIGNANT CONDITIONS OF THE BREAST

Breast cancer is a major health problem in the United States. At present, there is no cure. It is estimated that more than 190,000 women and 1900 men develop the disease and more than 40,000 die of it annually (ACS, 2009). Incidence rates, however, have decreased by 3.5% per year from 2001 to 2004 after increasing since 1980. Between 1990 and 2002, the mortality rate for breast cancer decreased by 2.2%, suggesting that the combination of early detection and improved treatment modalities had an effect on overall survival.

Current statistics indicate that over an entire lifetime (birth to death), a woman's risk of developing breast cancer is one in eight. When broken down by age, the risk by 39 years of age is 1 in 210, and it increases to 1 in 26 by 59 years of age. Approximately 80% of breast cancers are diagnosed in women older than 50 years of age (Jemal, et al., 2008).

Types of Breast Cancer

Ductal Carcinoma in Situ

The increased use of mammography as a screening tool has contributed to the dramatic increase in the diagnosis of **ductal carcinoma in situ (DCIS)**. An estimated 67,000 new cases are diagnosed annually (Jemal, et al., 2008). DCIS is characterized by the proliferation of malignant cells inside the milk ducts without invasion into the surrounding tissue. Therefore, it is a noninvasive form of cancer (also called intraductal carcinoma). DCIS is frequently manifested on a mammogram with the appearance of calcifications, and it is considered breast cancer stage 0.

If DCIS is left untreated, there is an increased likelihood that it will progress to invasive cancer. Deciding on the best surgical treatment option can be very complex. DCIS can be categorized in terms of its aggressiveness depending on a variety of factors, including histological subtype (comedo is more aggressive than noncomedo), size of tumor, and whether it is multicentric (present in different quadrants of the breast). These factors, together with patient preference, are important determinants in making treatment decisions. The most traditional treatment is total or simple mastectomy (removal of the breast only), with a cure rate of 98% to 99% (Boughey, Gonzalez, Bonner, et al., 2007). The trend today is toward less aggressive surgery; **breast conservation treatment** (limited surgery followed by radiation) is being performed with increasing frequency. In rare cases, lumpectomy alone is an option. The National Surgical Adjuvant Breast and Bowel Project B-24 study demonstrated that the addition of tamoxifen (Nolvadex) significantly reduced local recurrence rates after surgery and radiation (Daly, 2006). The medication is usually prescribed for 5 years.

Invasive Cancer

The National Comprehensive Cancer Network (NCCN), a nonprofit group of the world's 21 leading cancer centers, disseminates estimates for various types of cancer.

Infiltrating Ductal Carcinoma

Infiltrating ductal carcinoma, the most common histologic type of breast cancer, accounts for 80% of all cases. The tumors arise from the duct system and invade the surrounding tissues. They often form a solid irregular mass in the breast.

Infiltrating Lobular Carcinoma

Infiltrating lobular carcinoma accounts for 10% to 15% of breast cancers. The tumors arise from the lobular epithelium and typically occur as an area of ill-defined thickening in the breast. They are often multicentric and can be bilateral.

Medullary Carcinoma

Medullary carcinoma accounts for about 5% of breast cancers, and it tends to be diagnosed more often in women younger than 50 years of age. The tumors grow in a capsule inside a duct. They can become large and may be mistaken for a fibroadenoma. The prognosis is often favorable.

Mucinous Carcinoma

Mucinous carcinoma accounts for about 3% of breast cancers and often presents in postmenopausal women 75 years of age and older. A mucin producer, the tumor is also slow growing and thus the prognosis is more favorable than in many other types.

Tubular Ductal Carcinoma

Tubular ductal carcinoma accounts for about 2% of breast cancers. Because axillary metastases are uncommon with this histology, prognosis is usually excellent.

Inflammatory Carcinoma

Inflammatory carcinoma is a rare (1% to 3%) and aggressive type of breast cancer that has unique symptoms. The cancer is characterized by diffuse edema and brawny erythema of the skin, often referred to as peau d'orange (resembling an orange peel). This is caused by malignant cells blocking the lymph channels in the skin. An associated mass may or may not be present; if there is a mass, it is often a large area of indiscrete thickening. Inflammatory carcinoma can be confused with an infection because of its presentation. The disease can spread to other parts of the body rapidly. Chemotherapy often plays an initial role in controlling disease progression, but radiation and surgery may also be useful.

Paget's Disease

Paget's disease of the breast accounts for 1% of diagnosed cases of breast cancer. Symptoms typically include a scaly, erythematous, pruritic lesion of the nipple. Paget's disease often represents ductal carcinoma in situ of the nipple but may have an invasive component. If no lump can be felt in the breast tissue and the biopsy shows DCIS without invasion, the prognosis is very favorable.

Risk Factors

There is no single, specific cause of breast cancer. A combination of genetic, hormonal, and possibly environmental factors may increase the risk of its development (Table 48-3). More than 80% of all cases of breast cancer are sporadic, meaning that patients have no known family history of the disease. The remaining cases are either familial (there is a family history of breast cancer but it is not passed on genetically) or genetically acquired. There is no evidence that smoking, silicone breast implants, use of antiperspirants, underwire bras, or abortion (induced or spontaneous) increases the risk of the disease.

As stated previously, breast cancer can be genetically inherited, resulting in significant risk. Approximately 5% to 10% of breast cancer cases develop as a result of genetic mutations. Factors that may indicate a genetic link include multiple first-degree relatives with early-onset breast

Table 48-3 RISK FACTORS FOR BREAST CANCER

Risk Factor	Comments
Female gender	99% of cases occur in women.
Increasing age	Increasing age is associated with an increased risk.
Personal history of breast cancer	Once treated for breast cancer, the risk of developing breast cancer in same or opposite breast is significantly increased.
Family history of breast cancer	Having first-degree relative with breast cancer (mother, sister, daughter) increases the risk twofold; having two first-degree relatives increases the risk fivefold. The risk is higher if the relative was premenopausal at the time of diagnosis.
	The risk is increased if a father or brother had breast cancer (exact risk is unknown).
Genetic mutation	*BRCA1* and *BRCA2* mutations account for the majority of inherited cases of breast cancer (see additional information in text).
Hormonal Factors	
• Early menarche	Before 12 years of age
• Late menopause	After 55 years of age
• Nulliparity	No full-term pregnancies
• Late age at first full-term pregnancy	After 30 years of age
• Hormone therapy (formerly referred to as hormone replacement therapy)	Current or recent use of combined postmenopausal hormone therapy (estrogen and progesterone) Long-term use (several years or more)
Exposure to ionizing radiation during adolescence and early adulthood	The risk is highest if breast tissue was exposed while still developing (during adolescence) such as women who received mantle radiation (to the chest area) for treatment of Hodgkin lymphoma in their younger years.
History of benign proliferative breast disease	Having had atypical ductal or lobular hyperplasia or lobular carcinoma in situ increases the risk.
Obesity	Obesity and weight gain during adulthood increases the risk of postmenopausal breast cancer. During menopause, estrogen is primarily produced in fat tissue. More fat tissue can increase estrogen levels, thereby increasing breast cancer risk.
High-fat diet (controversial)	More research is needed.
Alcohol intake (beer, wine, or liquor)	Two to five drinks daily increases the risk about one and a half times.

cancer, breast and ovarian cancer in the same family, male breast cancer, and Ashkenazi Jewish background. **BRCA1** and **BRCA2** are tumor suppressor genes that normally function to identify damaged DNA and thereby restrain abnormal cell growth. Mutations in these genes are responsible for the majority of hereditary breast cancer in the United States. *BRCA1* mutations have been associated with a 65% to 87% estimated lifetime risk, and *BRCA2* mutations have been associated with a 45% to 84% risk. Carriers also have a significantly increased risk for ovarian cancer, approaching 30% (Turnbull & Rahman, 2008). Men with *BRCA* mutations, particularly the *BRCA2* mutation, also have an increased risk of breast cancer. A recent study reported that there is a broad variation in breast cancer risk among carriers of *BRCA1* and *BRCA2* when different variables are considered. A gene carrier was found to be at significantly higher risk if a relative was diagnosed with breast cancer at an early age (Begg, Haile & Borg, 2008).

Protective Factors

Certain factors may be protective in relation to the development of breast cancer. A systematic review of 48 studies showed that physical activity reduced the risk of breast cancer in postmenopausal women by 20% to 80%; the evidence was much weaker for premenopausal women with the disease (Monninkhof, Elias, Vlems, et al., 2007). Studies to determine the most effective exercises and how often to perform them are ongoing.

Breastfeeding is also thought to decrease risk because it prevents the return of menstruation, thereby decreasing exposure to endogenous estrogen. Having completed a full-term pregnancy before 30 years of age is also thought to be protective.

Breast Cancer Prevention Strategies in the High-Risk Patient

Patients often overestimate or underestimate their risk of developing breast cancer. A consultation with a breast specialist is of paramount importance prior to embarking on any of the prevention strategies that follow. Once patients have an accurate assessment of their risk, along with the knowledge of the pros and cons of each prevention strategy, they can make a decision that is most appropriate for their situation.

Long-Term Surveillance

Long-term surveillance is a form of secondary prevention that focuses on early detection of the disease. As recommended by the ACS, women with a 20% or greater lifetime risk benefit from additional screening with MRI (Saslow, et al., 2007). Clinical breast examinations may be performed twice a year starting as early as 25 years of age. Mammograms may also be performed as early as 25 years of age. Data concerning the effectiveness of BSE are limited. In addition to yearly mammography and MRI, other screening tests, including ultrasonography, may be useful.

Chemoprevention

Chemoprevention is a primary prevention modality that aims to prevent the disease. In April 1998, the results of the Breast Cancer Prevention Trial were released to the general public. This national, randomized, double-blind clinical trial evaluated tamoxifen (20 mg daily for 5 years) versus a placebo in more than 13,000 women considered to be at high risk for breast cancer. The women who received tamoxifen had a 49% reduction in the incidence of breast cancer (Fisher, Constantino, Wickerham, et al., 1998), suggesting that tamoxifen was an effective chemopreventive agent. Subsequently, the FDA approved its use in high-risk women. Nurses can help women who are considering this option by providing them with information about the benefits, risks, and possible side effects of tamoxifen.

Raloxifene (Evista) is a medication that is used for the prevention and treatment of osteoporosis. The results of the Multiple Outcomes of Raloxifene Evaluation trial in postmenopausal women with osteoporosis showed that women who received raloxifene instead of placebo had a 76% reduction in invasive breast cancer (Cummings, Eckert, Krueger, et al., 1999).

A national, randomized clinical trial, the Study of Tamoxifen and Raloxifene (STAR), compared these two agents for the prevention of breast cancer in postmenopausal women (Vogel, Costantino, Wickerham, et al., 2006). Results showed that raloxifene is as effective as tamoxifen in reducing breast cancer risk and has fewer side effects, including fewer uterine cancers, blood clots, and cataracts. In September 2007 the FDA approved the use of raloxifene as a chemopreventive agent in postmenopausal women.

Prophylactic Mastectomy

Prophylactic mastectomy is another primary prevention modality. This procedure can reduce the risk of breast cancer by 90% (Alschuler, Nekhlyudov, Rolnick, et al., 2008) and is sometimes referred to as a "risk-reducing" mastectomy. The procedure consists of a total mastectomy (removal of breast tissue only) and is usually accompanied by immediate breast reconstruction. Possible candidates include women with a strong family history of breast cancer, a diagnosis of LCIS or atypical hyperplasia, a mutation in a BRCA gene, an extreme fear of cancer ("cancer phobia"), or previous cancer in one breast.

A patient who is considering prophylactic mastectomy is often faced with a very controversial and emotional decision. A multidisciplinary approach should be used to help the patient arrive at a decision that is best for her. Consultation with a genetics counselor, plastic surgeon, medical oncologist, and psychiatrist can be invaluable. The patient needs to understand that this surgery is elective and not emergent. The nurse can play a valuable role in providing the patient with information, clarification, and support during the decision-making process.

Clinical Manifestations

Breast cancers can occur anywhere in the breast but are usually found in the upper outer quadrant, where the most breast tissue is located. Generally, the lesions are nontender, fixed rather than mobile, and hard with irregular borders. Complaints of diffuse breast pain and tenderness with menstruation are usually associated with benign breast disease.

With the increased use of mammography, more women are seeking treatment at earlier stages of the disease. These women often have no signs or symptoms other than a mammographic abnormality. Unfortunately, some women with advanced disease seek initial treatment after ignoring symptoms. Advanced signs may include skin dimpling, nipple retraction, or skin ulceration.

Assessment and Diagnostic Findings

Techniques to determine the diagnosis of breast cancer include various types of biopsy, which have been described previously. Tumor staging and analysis of additional prognostic factors are used to determine the prognosis and optimal treatment regimen (see below).

Staging

Staging involves classifying the cancer by the extent of disease. Clinical staging involves the physician's estimate of the size of the breast tumor and the extent of axillary lymph node involvement. Such staging is determined by physical examination and imaging studies. Pathological staging is done when the pathologist examines the surgically excised breast tissue under the microscope and determines the exact size of the breast tumor and the exact number of lymph nodes involved.

The staging of breast cancer has become complex. Classification of tumors that are stage 0 (DCIS, LCIS, or Paget's disease of the nipple with no invasion), stage I (tumors that are 2 cm or less with no involvement of axillary lymph nodes), and stage IV (tumors of any size, with distant metastases) is fairly straightforward. However, classification of tumors that are stage II and stage III, which represent a wide spectrum of breast cancers, is more difficult. Factors that play a role in determining stages II and III include the number and characteristics of axillary lymph nodes, the status of other regional lymph nodes such as internal mammary nodes or supraclavicular nodes, and the presence or absence of involvement of the skin or underlying muscle. Based on these factors, stage II and stage III breast cancers are further subdivided into stage IIA, IIB, IIIA, IIIB, and IIIC. For a detailed explanation of the staging system, the reader is referred to the *American Joint Committee on Cancer Staging Manual* (Greene, Page, Fleming, et al., 2002) or to the ACS Web site (see Resources below).

Other diagnostic tests may be performed before or after the surgery to help in the staging of the disease. The extent of testing often depends on the clinical presentation of the disease and may include chest x-rays, computed tomography (CT), MRI, positron emission tomography (PET) scan, bone scans, and blood work (complete blood count, comprehensive metabolic panel, tumor markers [ie, carcinoembryonic antigen, cancer antigen 15-3]).

Prognosis

Several different factors must be taken into consideration when determining the prognosis of a patient with breast cancer. The two most important factors are tumor size and whether the tumor has spread to the lymph nodes under the arm (axilla).

Generally, the smaller the tumor, the better the prognosis. Carcinoma of the breast is not a pathologic entity that develops overnight. It starts with a genetic alteration in a single cell and takes time to divide and double in size. A carcinoma may double in size 30 times to become 1 cm or larger, at which point it becomes clinically apparent. Doubling time varies, but breast tumors are often present for several years before they become palpable. Nurses can reassure patients that once breast cancer is diagnosed, they have a safe period of several weeks to make decisions regarding treatment.

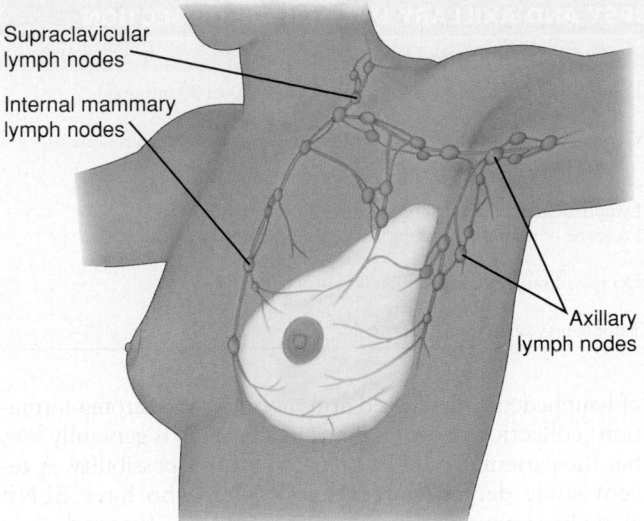

Supraclavicular
lymph nodes

Internal mammary
lymph nodes

Axillary
lymph nodes

Figure 48-5 Lymphatic drainage of the breast.

Prognosis also depends on the extent of spread of the breast cancer. The 5-year survival rate can be as high as 98.1% for a stage I breast cancer and as low as 27.1% for a stage IV breast cancer (National Cancer Institute, 2008). The most common route of regional spread is to the axillary lymph nodes. Other sites of lymphatic spread include the internal mammary and supraclavicular nodes (Fig. 48-5). Distant metastasis can affect any organ, but the most common sites are bone, lung, liver, pleura, adrenals, skin, and brain.

In addition to the type of breast cancer and the stage, other factors may help determine prognosis (Chart 48-3). Excessive number of copies of certain genes (amplification) or excessive amounts of their protein product (overexpression) may represent a poorer prognosis. The HER-2/neu (also known as ERBB2) oncogene is the classic example; approximately 25% to 30% of invasive breast cancers, which typically involve the more aggressive tumors, have amplification or overexpression of the HER-2/neu gene (Dawood, Broglio, Esteva, et al., 2008). Research concerning the prognostic usefulness of the proliferative rate (S-phase fraction) and DNA content (ploidy) of a tumor is ongoing.

Surgical Management

The main goal of surgery is to gain local control of the disease. With breast cancer being diagnosed today at earlier stages, options for less invasive surgical procedures are avail-

Chart 48-3 • *Pathologic Factors Associated With Favorable Prognosis for Breast Cancer*

- Noninvasive tumors or invasive tumors less than 1 cm
- Negative axillary lymph nodes
- Estrogen receptor (ER) and progesterone receptor (PR) proteins
- Well-differentiated tumors
- Low expression of HER-2/neu oncogene (also known as ERBB2)
- No vascular or lymphatic invasion
- Diploid tumors with low S-phase fraction

Table 48-4 SURGICAL TREATMENT OPTIONS FOR NONINVASIVE AND INVASIVE BREAST CANCER	
Noninvasive Breast Cancer	**Invasive Breast Cancer**
Breast conservation* alone	Breast conservation* with one of the following: Sentinel lymph node biopsy Axillary lymph node dissection
Total mastectomy alone	Total mastectomy with sentinel lymph node biopsy or Modified radical mastectomy

*Breast conservation treatment includes lumpectomy, wide excision, partial or segmental mastectomy, and quadrantectomy. These are relatively synonymous terms that describe removal of varying amounts of breast tissue.

able. Surgical treatment options for noninvasive and invasive breast cancer are summarized in Table 48-4.

Modified Radical Mastectomy

Modified radical mastectomy is performed to treat invasive breast cancer. The procedure involves removal of the entire breast tissue, including the nipple–areola complex. In addition, a portion of the axillary lymph nodes are also removed in axillary lymph node dissection (ALND). If immediate breast reconstruction is desired, the patient is referred to a plastic surgeon prior to the mastectomy so that she has the opportunity to explore all available options. In modified radical mastectomy, the pectoralis major and pectoralis minor muscles are left intact, unlike in radical mastectomy, in which the muscles are removed. Radical mastectomy is rarely performed today.

Total Mastectomy

Like modified radical mastectomy, **total mastectomy** (ie, simple mastectomy) also involves removal of the breast and nipple–areola complex but does not include ALND. Total mastectomy may be performed in patients with noninvasive breast cancer (eg, DCIS), which does not have a tendency to spread to the lymph nodes. It may also be performed prophylactically in patients who are at high risk for breast cancer (eg, LCIS, BRCA mutation). A total mastectomy may also be performed in conjunction with sentinel lymph node biopsy (SLNB) for patients with invasive breast cancer.

Breast Conservation Treatment

The goal of breast conservation treatment (ie, lumpectomy, wide excision, partial or segmental mastectomy, quadrantectomy) is to excise the tumor in the breast completely and obtain clear margins while achieving an acceptable cosmetic result. If the procedure is being performed to treat a noninvasive breast cancer, lymph node removal is not necessary. For an invasive breast cancer, lymph node removal (SLNB or ALND) is indicated. The lymph nodes are removed through a separate semicircular incision in the axilla. In 1990, the National Institutes of Health (NIH) issued a consensus statement that breast conservation along with radiation therapy in stage I and stage II breast cancer resulted in a survival rate equal to that of modified radical mastectomy.

Table 48-5 COMPARISON OF SENTINEL LYMPH NODE BIOPSY AND AXILLARY LYMPH NODE DISSECTION	
Sentinel Lymph Node Biopsy (SLNB)	**Axillary Lymph Node Dissection (ALND)**
Shorter operating room time (approximately 15 to 30 minutes)	Longer operating room time (approximately 60 to 90 minutes)
No surgical drain	Surgical drain
Local anesthesia with IV moderate sedation as outpatient surgery (unless being performed in conjunction with total mastectomy)	General anesthesia; usually overnight admission (sometimes done as outpatient surgery)
Lymphedema incidence approximately 0% to 8%	Lymphedema incidence approximately 10% to 30%
Presence of neuropathic sensations postoperatively (prevalence lower than after axillary lymph node dissection)	Presence of neuropathic sensations postoperatively
Decreased range of motion in affected arm unlikely postoperatively but may occur	Decreased range of motion likely postoperatively
Seroma (collection of serous fluid in the axilla) may occur postoperatively	Seroma may occur postoperatively

Sentinel Lymph Node Biopsy

As previously discussed, the status of the lymph nodes is the most important prognostic factor in breast cancer. Approximately two thirds of women with early-stage breast cancer who have an ALND have negative nodes. In the mid-1990s, SLNB emerged as a less invasive alternative to ALND and is now considered a standard of care for the treatment of early-stage breast cancer. ALND is associated with potential morbidity, including lymphedema, cellulitis, decreased arm mobility, and sensory changes. Studies have shown that SLNB is highly accurate and is associated with a local recurrence rate similar to that of ALND (Bergkvist, deBoniface, Jonsson, et al., 2008; Krag, Anderson, Julian, et al., 2007). Table 48-5 compares sentinel lymph node biopsy and axillary lymph node dissection.

The **sentinel lymph node,** which is the first node (or nodes) in the lymphatic basin that receives drainage from the primary tumor in the breast, is identified by injecting a radioisotope and/or blue dye into the breast; the radioisotope or dye then travels via the lymphatic pathways to the node. In SLNB, the surgeon uses a hand-held probe to locate the sentinel lymph node, excises it, and sends it for pathologic analysis, which is often performed immediately during the surgery using frozen section analysis. If the sentinel lymph node is positive, the surgeon can proceed with an immediate ALND, thus sparing the patient a return trip to the operating room and additional anesthesia. (The patient could also opt to return for additional surgery at a later time.) If the sentinel lymph node is negative, a standard ALND is not needed, thus sparing the patient the sequelae of the procedure. After the operation is complete, all the specimens are sent to pathology for more thorough analysis.

Nursing Management

Patients who undergo SLNB in conjunction with breast conservation are generally discharged the same day. Patients who undergo SLNB with total mastectomy usually stay in the hospital overnight, possibly longer if breast reconstruction is being performed. The patient must be informed that although frozen section analysis is highly accurate, false-negative results can occur. A negative sentinel lymph node on frozen section analysis may show metastatic disease on subsequent analysis, indicating that ALND is still necessary. The patient should also be reassured that the radioisotope and blue dye are generally safe. The patient may notice a blue-green discoloration in the urine or stool for the first 24 hours as the blue dye is excreted. The incidence of lymphedema, decreased arm mobility, and seroma formation (collection of serous fluid) in the axilla is generally low, but the patient should be prepared for this possibility. A recent study demonstrated that women who have SLNB alone have neuropathic sensations similar to those who undergo ALND, although the prevalence and severity of these sensations and the resulting distress are lower with SLNB (Baron, Fey, Borgen, et al., 2007).

The nurse must not overlook the psychosocial needs of the patient who has undergone SLNB. Although SLNB is a less invasive procedure than ALND and results in a shorter recovery period, a patient who has undergone SLNB also has many difficult issues surrounding her breast cancer diagnosis and treatment. The nurse must listen, provide emotional support, and refer the patient to appropriate specialists when indicated.

NURSING PROCESS

THE PATIENT UNDERGOING SURGERY FOR BREAST CANCER

Assessment

The health history is a valuable tool to assess the patient's reaction to the diagnosis and her ability to cope with it. Pertinent questions include the following:
- How is the patient responding to the diagnosis?
- What coping mechanisms does she find most helpful?
- What psychological or emotional supports does she have and use?
- Is there a partner, family member, or friend available to assist her in making treatment choices?
- What are her educational needs?
- Is she experiencing any discomfort?

Diagnosis

Preoperative Nursing Diagnoses

Based on the health history and other assessment data, major preoperative nursing diagnoses may include the following:
- Deficient knowledge about the planned surgical treatments
- Anxiety related to the diagnosis of cancer
- Fear related to specific treatments and body image changes

- Risk for ineffective coping (individual or family) related to the diagnosis of breast cancer and related treatment options
- Decisional conflict related to treatment options

Postoperative Nursing Diagnoses

Based on the health history and other assessment data, major postoperative nursing diagnoses may include the following:

- Pain and discomfort related to surgical procedure
- Disturbed sensory perception related to nerve irritation in affected arm, breast, or chest wall
- Disturbed body image related to loss or alteration of the breast
- Risk for impaired adjustment related to the diagnosis of cancer and surgical treatment
- Self-care deficit related to partial immobility of upper extremity on operative side
- Risk for sexual dysfunction related to loss of body part, change in self-image, and fear of partner's responses
- Deficient knowledge: drain management after breast surgery
- Deficient knowledge: arm exercises to regain mobility of affected extremity
- Deficient knowledge: hand and arm care after ALND

Collaborative Problems/Potential Complications

Based on the assessment data, potential complications may include the following:

- Lymphedema
- Hematoma/seroma formation
- Infection

Planning and Goals

The major goals may include increased knowledge about the disease and its treatment; reduction of preoperative and postoperative fear, anxiety, and emotional stress; improvement of decision-making ability; pain management; improvement in coping abilities; improvement in sexual function; and the absence of complications.

Preoperative Nursing Interventions

Providing Education and Preparation about Surgical Treatments

Patients with newly diagnosed breast cancer are expected to absorb an abundance of new information during a very emotionally difficult time. The nurse plays a key role in reviewing treatment options by reinforcing information provided to the patient and answering any questions. The nurse fully prepares the patient for what to expect before, during, and after surgery. Patients undergoing breast conservation with ALND, or a total or modified radical mastectomy, generally remain in the hospital overnight (or longer if they have immediate reconstruction). Surgical drains will be inserted in the mastectomy incision and in the axilla if the patient undergoes an ALND. A surgical drain is generally not needed after a SLNB. The patient should be informed that she will go home with the drain(s) and that complete instructions about drain care will be provided prior to discharge. In addition, the patient should be informed that she will often have decreased arm and shoulder mobility after an ALND and that she will be shown range-of-motion exercises prior to discharge. The patient should also be reassured that appropriate analgesia and comfort measures will be provided to alleviate any postoperative discomfort.

Reducing Fear and Anxiety and Improving Coping Ability

The nurse must help the patient cope with the physical as well as the emotional effects of surgery. Many fears may emerge during the preoperative phase. These can include fear of pain, mutilation (after mastectomy), and loss of sexual attractiveness; concern about inability to care for oneself and one's family; concern about taking time off from work; and coping with an uncertain future. Providing the patient with realistic expectations about the healing process and expected recovery can help alleviate fears. Maintaining open communication and assuring the patient that she can contact the nurse at any time with questions or concerns can be a source of comfort. The patient should also be made aware of available resources at the treatment facility as well as in the breast cancer community such as social workers, psychiatrists, and support groups. Some women find it helpful and reassuring to talk to a breast cancer survivor who has undergone similar treatments.

Promoting Decision-Making Ability

The patient may be eligible for more than one therapeutic approach; she may be presented with treatment options and then asked to make a choice. This can be very frightening for some patients, and they may prefer to have someone else make the decision for them (eg, surgeon, family member). The nurse can be instrumental in ensuring that the patient and family members truly understand their options. The nurse can then help the patient weigh the risks and benefits of each option. The patient may be presented with the option of having breast conservation treatment followed by radiation or a mastectomy. The nurse can explore the issues with the individual patient by asking questions such as the following:

- How would you feel about losing your breast?
- Are you considering breast reconstruction?
- If you choose to retain your breast, would you consider undergoing radiation treatments 5 days a week for 5 to 6 weeks?

Questions such as these can help the patient focus. Once the patient's decision is made, it is very important to support it.

Postoperative Nursing Interventions

Relieving Pain and Discomfort

Many patients tolerate the breast surgery quite well and have minimal pain during the postoperative period. This is particularly true of the less invasive procedures such as breast conservation treatment with SLNB. However, all patients must be carefully assessed, because individual patients can have varying degrees of pain. Patients who have had more invasive procedures such as a modified radical mastectomy with immediate reconstruction may have considerably more pain. All patients are discharged home with analgesic medication (eg, oxycodone and acetaminophen [Percocet] or propoxyphene and acetaminophen [Darvocet]) and are encouraged to take it if needed. An over-the-counter analgesic such as acetaminophen may provide sufficient relief. Sometimes patients complain of a slight increase in pain after the first few days of surgery; this may occur as patients regain sensation around the surgical site and become more active. However, patients who report excruciating pain must be evaluated to rule out any potential complications such as infection or a hematoma. Alternative methods of pain management such as taking warm showers and using distraction methods (eg, guided imagery) may also be helpful.

Managing Postoperative Sensations

Because nerves in the skin and axilla are often cut or injured during breast surgery, patients experience a variety of sensations. Common sensations include tenderness, soreness, numbness, tightness, pulling, and twinges. These sensations may occur along the chest wall, in the axilla, and along the inside aspect of the upper arm. After mastectomy, some patients experience phantom sensations and report a feeling that the breast or nipple is still present. Overall, patients do not find these sensations severe or distressing (Baron, et al., 2007). Chart 48-4 presents specific information from this study. Sensations usually persist for several months and then begin to diminish, although some may persist for as long as 5 years and possibly longer. Patients should be reassured that this is a normal part of healing and that these sensations are not indicative of a problem.

Promoting Positive Body Image

Patients who have undergone mastectomy often find it very difficult to view the surgical site for the first time. No matter how prepared the patient may think she is, the appearance of an absent breast can be very emotionally distressing. Ideally, the patient sees the incision for the first time when she is with the nurse or another health care provider who is available for support.

The nurse first assesses the patient's readiness and provides gentle encouragement. It is important to maintain the patient's privacy while assisting her as she views the incision; this allows her to express feelings safely to the nurse. Asking the patient what she perceives, acknowledging her feelings, and allowing her to express her emotions are important nursing actions. Reassuring the patient that her feelings are a normal response to breast cancer surgery may be comforting. If the patient has not had immediate reconstruction, providing her with a temporary breast form to place in her bra on discharge can help alleviate feelings of embarrassment or self-consciousness.

Promoting Positive Adjustment and Coping

Providing ongoing assessment of how the patient is coping with her diagnosis of breast cancer and her surgical treatment is important in determining her overall adjustment. Assisting the patient in identifying and mobilizing her support systems can be beneficial to her well-being. The patient's spouse or partner may also need guidance, support, and education. The patient and partner may benefit from a wide network of available community resources, including

---

NURSING RESEARCH PROFILE
48-4   *Sensory Morbidity After Breast Cancer Surgery*

Baron, R. H., Fey, J. V., Borgen, P. I., et al. (2007). Eighteen sensations after breast cancer surgery: A 5-year comparison of sentinel lymph node biopsy and axillary lymph node dissection. *Annals of Surgical Oncology, 14*(5), 1653–1661.

Purpose

Women with breast cancer often report a variety of sensations following surgery and question whether these sensations are normal. The purpose of this study was to compare the prevalence, severity, and level of distress associated with sensations after sentinel lymph node biopsy (SLNB) with axillary lymph node dissection (ALND) at 3 to 15 days (baseline) and 5 years after breast cancer surgery. Long-term differences in sensations after SLNB and ALND have rarely been addressed by researchers, making it difficult for clinicians to provide effective guidance and symptom management.

Design

This descriptive study prospectively evaluated sensations in 133 women who had SLNB and in 54 women who had more extensive ALND. Researchers used the Breast Sensation Assessment Scale, a Likert-type scale to assess the presence and severity of 18 sensations and posed an additional question about the prevalence, severity, and resulting distress of phantom sensations. Study participants completed the scale six times over a 5-year period, beginning 3 to 15 days after surgery during their initial postoperative visit and by mail at

3, 6, 12, 24, and 60 months after surgery. Although the investigators had conducted previous studies of women using a larger sample, only women described in the present study provided data at all six data collection points. These women represent 47% of the original sample; loss to follow-up from the previous studies was similar in the SLNB and ALND groups.

Findings

The prevalence and severity of sensations and the resulting level of distress were lower in women who had SLNB compared with those who had ALND. Tenderness and twinges were prevalent at baseline after SLNB and remained so over 5 years. Numbness and tightness were prevalent after ALND and continued over 5 years; however, these sensations decreased in prevalence over time. In general, the majority of sensations were reportedly neither severe nor distressing. In women who underwent mastectomy, the severity and resulting distress caused by phantom sensations were low.

Nursing Implications

Nurses can use the results of this study to provide women undergoing SLNB and ALND with accurate information about postoperative sensations. It is important to provide this information to help women anticipate these sensations and understand that they are a normal part of the healing process.

the Reach to Recovery program of the ACS, advocacy groups, or a spiritual advisor. Encouraging the patient to discuss issues and concerns with other patients who have had breast cancer may help her to understand that her feelings are normal and that other women who have had breast cancer can provide invaluable support and understanding.

The patient may also have considerable anxiety about the treatments that will follow surgery (ie, chemotherapy and radiation) and their implications. Providing her with information about the plan of care and referring her to the appropriate members of the health care team also promote coping during recovery. Some women require additional support to adjust to their diagnosis and the changes that it brings. If a woman displays ineffective coping, consultation with a mental health practitioner may be indicated.

Improving Sexual Function

Once discharged from the hospital, most patients are physically allowed to engage in sexual activity. However, any change in the patient's body image, self-esteem, or the response of her partner may increase her anxiety level and affect sexual function. Some partners may have difficulty looking at the incision, whereas others may be completely unaffected. Encouraging the patient to openly discuss how she feels about herself and about possible reasons for a decrease in libido (eg, fatigue, anxiety, self-consciousness) may help clarify issues for her. Helpful suggestions for the patient may include varying the time of day for sexual activity (when the patient is less tired), assuming positions that are more comfortable, and expressing affection using alternative measures (eg, hugging, kissing, manual stimulation).

Most patients and their partners adjust with minimal difficulty if they openly discuss their concerns. However, if issues cannot be resolved, a referral for counseling (eg, psychologist, psychiatrist, psychiatric clinical nurse specialist, social worker, sex therapist) may be helpful. The ambulatory care nurse in the outpatient clinic or hospital should inquire whether the patient is having difficulty with sexuality issues because many patients are reluctant or embarrassed to bring it up themselves.

Monitoring and Managing Potential Complications

LYMPHEDEMA. Lymphedema occurs in about 10% to 30% of patients who undergo ALND and in about 0% to 8% of patients who have SLNB (Langer, Guller, Berclaz, et al., 2007; Lucci, McCall, Beitsch, et al., 2007). Risk factors for lymphedema include increasing age, obesity, presence of

extensive axillary disease, radiation treatment, and injury or infection to the extremity (Warren, Brorson, Borud, et al., 2007). Lymphedema results if functioning lymphatic channels are inadequate to ensure a return flow of lymph fluid to the general circulation. After axillary lymph nodes are removed, collateral circulation must assume this function. Transient edema in the postoperative period occurs until collateral circulation has completely taken over this function, which generally occurs within a month. Performing prescribed exercises, elevating the arm above the heart several times a day, and gentle muscle pumping (making a fist and releasing) can help reduce the transient edema. The patient needs reassurance that this transient swelling is not lymphedema.

Once lymphedema develops, it tends to be chronic, so preventive strategies are vital. After ALND, the patient is taught hand and arm care to prevent injury or trauma to the affected extremity, thus decreasing the likelihood for lymphedema development (Chart 48-5). The patient is instructed to follow these guidelines for the rest of her life. She is also instructed to contact the physician or a nurse immediately if she suspects that she has lymphedema, because early intervention provides the best chance for control. If allowed to progress without treatment, the swelling can become more difficult to manage. Treatment may consist of a course of antibiotics if an infection is present. A referral to a rehabilitation specialist (eg, occupational or physical therapist) may be necessary for a compression sleeve or glove, exercises, manual lymph drainage, and a discussion of ways to modify daily activities to avoid worsening lymphedema.

HEMATOMA OR SEROMA FORMATION. Hematoma formation (collection of blood inside a cavity) may occur after either mastectomy or breast conservation and usually develops within the first 12 hours after surgery. The nurse assesses for signs and symptoms of a hematoma at the surgical site, which may include swelling, tightness, pain, and bruising of the skin. The surgeon should be notified immediately if there is gross swelling or increased bloody output from the drain. Depending on the surgeon's assessment, a compression wrap may be applied to the incision for approximately 12 hours, or the patient may be returned to the operating room so that the incision may be reopened to identify the source of bleeding. Some hematomas are small, and the body absorbs the blood naturally. The patient may take warm showers or apply warm compresses to

---

CHART 48-5

PATIENT EDUCATION
Hand and Arm Care After Axillary Lymph Node Dissection

- Avoid blood pressures, injections, and blood draws in affected extremity.
- Use sunscreen (higher than 15 SPF) for extended exposure to sun.
- Apply insect repellent to avoid insect bites.
- Wear gloves for gardening.
- Use cooking mitt for removing objects from oven.
- Avoid cutting cuticles; push them back during manicures.

- Use electric razor for shaving armpit.
- Avoid lifting objects greater than 5–10 pounds.
- If a trauma or break in the skin occurs, wash the area with soap and water, and apply an over-the-counter antibacterial ointment (Bacitracin or Neosporin).
- Observe the area and extremity for 24 hours; if redness, swelling, or a fever occurs, call the surgeon or nurse.

help increase the absorption. A hematoma usually resolves in 4 to 5 weeks.

A seroma, a collection of serous fluid, may accumulate under the breast incision after mastectomy or breast conservation or in the axilla. Signs and symptoms may include swelling, heaviness, discomfort, and a sloshing of fluid. Seromas may develop temporarily after the drain is removed or if the drain is in place and becomes obstructed. Seromas rarely pose a threat and may be treated by unclogging the drain or manually aspirating the fluid with a needle and syringe. Large, long-standing seromas that have not been aspirated could lead to infection. Small seromas that are not bothersome to the patient usually resolve on their own.

INFECTION. Although infection is rare, it is a risk after any surgical procedure. This risk may be higher in patients with conditions such as diabetes, immune disorders, and advanced age, as well as in those with poor hygiene. Patients are taught to monitor for signs and symptoms of infection (redness, warmth around incision, tenderness, foul-smelling drainage, temperature greater than 40°C [100.4°F], chills) and to contact the surgeon or nurse for evaluation. Treatment consists of oral or IV antibiotics (for more severe infections) for 1 or 2 weeks. Cultures are taken of any foul-smelling discharge.

Promoting Home and Community-Based Care

TEACHING PATIENTS SELF-CARE. Patients who undergo breast cancer surgery receive a tremendous amount of information preoperatively and postoperatively. It is often difficult for the patient to absorb all of the information, partly because of the emotional distress that often accompanies the diagnosis and treatment. Prior to discharge, the nurse must assess the patient's readiness to assume self-care responsibilities and identify any gaps in knowledge. A review of teaching, with reinforcement, may be required to ensure that the patient and family are prepared to manage the necessary care at home. The nurse reiterates symptoms the patient should report, such as infection, seroma, hematoma, or arm swelling. All teaching should be reinforced during office visits and by telephone.

Most patients are discharged 1 or 2 days after ALND or mastectomy (possibly later if they have had immediate reconstruction) with surgical drains in place. Initially, the drainage fluid appears bloody, but it gradually changes to a serosanguineous and then a serous fluid over the next several days. The patient is given instructions about drainage management at home (Chart 48-6). If the patient lives alone and drainage management is difficult, a referral for a home care nurse should be made. The drains are usually removed when the output is less than 30 mL in a 24-hour period (approximately 7 to 10 days). The home care nurse also reviews pain management and incision care.

Generally, the patient may shower on the second postoperative day and wash the incision and drain site with soap and water to prevent infection. If immediate reconstruction has been performed, showering may be contraindicated until the drain is removed. A dry dressing may be applied to the incision each day for 7 days. The patient should realize that sensation may be decreased in the operative area because the nerves were disrupted during surgery and should be informed that gentle care is needed to avoid injury. After the incision has completely healed (usually after 4 to 6 weeks), lotions or creams may be applied to the area to increase skin elasticity. The patient can begin to use deodorant on the affected side, although many women note that they no longer perspire as much as before the surgery.

After ALND, patients are taught arm exercises on the affected side to restore range of motion (Chart 48-7). After SLNB, patients may also benefit from these exercises, although they are less likely to have decreased range of motion than those who have undergone ALND. Range-of-motion exercises are initiated on the second postoperative day, although instruction often occurs on the first postoperative day. The goals of the exercise regimen are to increase circulation and muscle strength, prevent joint stiffness and contractures, and restore full range of motion. The patient is instructed to perform range-of-motion exercises at home three times a day for 20 minutes at a time until full range of motion is restored (generally 4 to 6 weeks). Most patients find that after the drain is removed, range of motion returns quickly if they have adhered to their exercise program.

If the patient is having any discomfort, taking an analgesic 30 minutes before beginning the exercises can be helpful. Taking a warm shower before exercising can also loosen stiff muscles and provide comfort. When exercising, the patient is encouraged to use the muscles in both arms and to maintain proper posture. Specific exercises may need to be prescribed and introduced gradually if the patient has had skin grafts; has a tense, tight surgical incision; or has

---

CHART 48-6	HOME CARE CHECKLIST *Surgical Breast Cancer Patient With a Drainage Device*		
At the completion of the home care instruction, the patient or caregiver will be able to:		**PATIENT**	**CAREGIVER**
• Demonstrate how to empty and measure fluid from the drainage device.		✔	✔
• Demonstrate how to milk clots through the tubing of the drainage device.		✔	✔
• State observations that require contacting the physician or nurse (eg, sudden change in color of drainage, sudden cessation of drainage, signs or symptoms of an infection).		✔	✔
• Care for the drain site as per surgeon's recommendation.		✔	✔
• Identify when the drain is ready for removal (usually when draining less than 30 mL for a 24-hour period).		✔	✔

CHART
48-7

PATIENT EDUCATION
Exercise After Breast Surgery

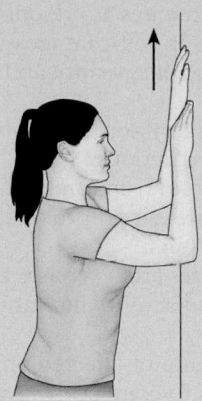

1. *Wall handclimbing.* Stand facing the wall with feet apart and toes as close to the wall as possible. With elbows slightly bent, place the palms of the hand on the wall at shoulder level. By flexing the fingers, work the hands up the wall until arms are fully extended. Then reverse the process, working the hands down to the starting point.

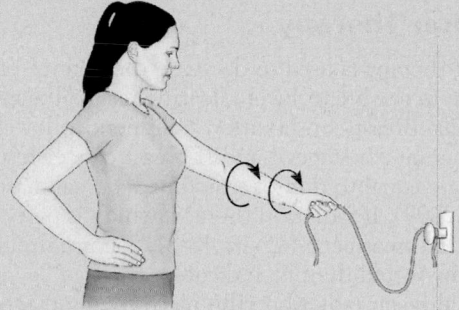

2. *Rope turning.* Tie a light rope to a doorknob. Stand facing the door. Take the free end of the rope in the hand on the side of surgery. Place the other hand on the hip. With the rope-holding arm extended and held away from the body (nearly parallel with the floor), turn the rope, making as wide swings as possible. Begin slowly at first; speed up later.

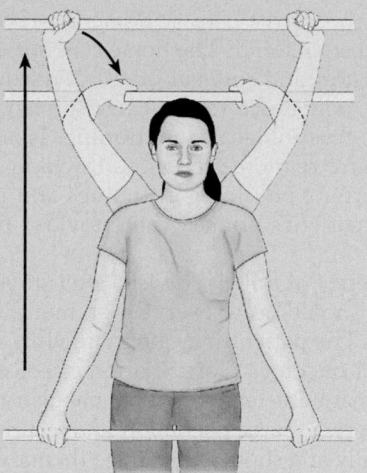

3. *Rod or broomstick lifting.* Grasp a rod with both hands, held about 2 feet apart. Keeping the arms straight, raise the rod over the head. Bend elbows to lower the rod behind the head. Reverse maneuver, raising the rod above the head, then return to the starting position.

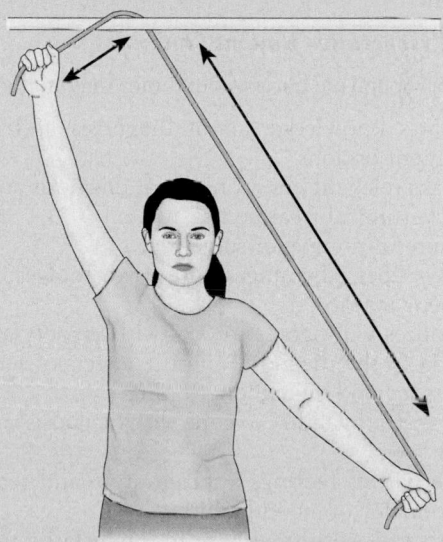

4. *Pulley tugging.* Toss a light rope over a shower curtain rod or doorway curtain rod. Stand as nearly under the rope as possible. Grasp an end in each hand. Extend the arms straight and away from the body. Pull the left arm up by tugging down with the right arm, then the right arm up and the left down in a see-sawing motion.

had immediate reconstruction. Self-care activities, such as brushing the teeth, washing the face, and brushing the hair, are physically and emotionally therapeutic because they aid in restoring arm function and provide a sense of normalcy for the patient.

The patient is instructed about postoperative activity limitation. Generally, heavy lifting (more than 5 to 10 lb) is avoided for about 4 to 6 weeks, although normal house-hold and work-related activities are promoted to maintain muscle tone. Brisk walking, use of stationary bikes and stepping machines, and stretching exercises may begin as soon as the patient feels comfortable. Once the drain is removed, the patient may begin to drive if she has full arm range of motion and is no longer taking opioid analgesics. General guidelines for activity focus on the gradual introduction of previous activities (eg, bowling, weight training) once fully healed, although checking with the physician or nurse beforehand is recommended.

CONTINUING CARE. Patients who have difficulty managing their postoperative care at home may benefit from a home health care referral. The home care nurse assesses the patient's incision and surgical drain(s), adequacy of pain management, adherence to the exercise plan, and overall physical and psychological functioning. In addition, the home care nurse reinforces previous teaching and communicates important physiologic findings and psychosocial issues to the patient's primary care provider, nurse, or surgeon.

The frequency of follow-up visits after surgery may vary but generally should occur every 3 to 6 months for the first several years. The patient may alternate visits with the surgeon, medical oncologist, or radiation oncologist, depending on the treatment regimen. The ambulatory care nurse can also be a great source of comfort and security for the patient and family and should encourage them to telephone if they have any questions or concerns. It is common for people to ignore routine health care when a major health issue arises, so women who have been treated for breast cancer should be reminded of the importance of participating in routine health screening.

Evaluation

Expected Preoperative Patient Outcomes

Expected preoperative patient outcomes may include:

1. Exhibits knowledge about diagnosis and surgical treatment options
   a. Asks relevant questions about diagnosis and available surgical treatments
   b. States rationale for surgery
   c. Describes advantages and disadvantages of treatment options
2. Verbalizes willingness to deal with anxiety and fears related to the diagnosis and the effects of surgery on self-image and sexual functioning
3. Demonstrates ability to cope with diagnosis and treatment
   a. Verbalizes feelings appropriately and recognizes normalcy of mood lability
   b. Proceeds with treatment in timely fashion
   c. Discusses impact of diagnosis and treatment on family and work
4. Makes decisions regarding treatment options in timely fashion

Expected Postoperative Patient Outcomes

Expected postoperative patient outcomes may include:

1. Reports that pain has decreased and states pain and discomfort management strategies are effective
2. Identifies postoperative sensations and recognizes that they are a normal part of healing
3. Exhibits clean, dry, and intact surgical incisions without signs of inflammation or infection
4. Lists the signs and symptoms of infection to be reported to the nurse or surgeon
5. Verbalizes feelings regarding change in body image

6. Discusses meaning of the diagnosis, surgical treatment, and fears appropriately
7. Participates actively in self-care measures
   a. Performs exercises as prescribed
   b. Participates in self-care measures as prescribed
8. Discusses issues of sexuality and resumption of sexual relations
9. Demonstrates knowledge of postdischarge recommendations and restrictions
   a. Describes follow-up care and activities
   b. Demonstrates appropriate care of incisions and drainage system
   c. Demonstrates arm exercises and describes exercise regimen and activity limitations during postoperative period
   d. Describes care of affected arm and hand and lists indications to contact the surgeon or nurse
10. Experiences no complications
    a. Identifies signs and symptoms of reportable complications (eg, redness, heat, pain, edema)
    b. Explains how to contact appropriate health care providers in case of complications

Radiation Therapy

Radiation therapy is used to decrease the chance of a local recurrence in the breast by eradicating residual microscopic cancer cells. Breast conservation treatment followed by radiation therapy for stages I and II breast cancer results in a survival rate equal to that of a modified radical mastectomy (NCCN, 2009). If radiation therapy, which is part of breast conservation treatment (Chart 48-8), is contraindicated, a mastectomy would then be indicated.

External-beam radiation (the most common type) typically begins about 6 weeks after breast conservation to allow the surgical site to heal. If systemic chemotherapy is indicated, radiation therapy usually begins after its completion. Before radiation begins, the patient undergoes a planning session called a simulation in which the anatomic areas to be treated are mapped out and then identified with small permanent ink markings. External-beam radiation, which delivers high-energy photons from a linear accelerator, is administered to the entire breast region (whole breast radiation). Each treatment lasts only a few minutes and is

---

Chart 48-8 • *Contraindications to Breast-Conservation Treatment*

Note: Breast-conservation treatment includes both surgery and radiation.

Absolute Contraindications

- First or second trimester of pregnancy
- Presence of multicentric disease in the breast
- Prior radiation to the breast or chest region

Relative Contraindications

- History of collagen vascular disease
- Large tumor-to-breast ratio
- Tumor beneath nipple

generally given 5 days a week for 5 to 6 weeks. After completion of radiation to the entire breast, many patients receive a "boost," a dose of radiation to the lumpectomy site where the cancer cells were located. The boost consists of the same dose of radiation but is less penetrating and directed to a smaller area. The treatments are not painful.

Because most breast cancer recurrences appear at or near the lumpectomy site, the need for whole breast radiation is now being questioned. Partial breast radiation (radiation to the lumpectomy site alone) is now being evaluated at some institutions in carefully selected patients. One approach is **brachytherapy,** which delivers partial breast radiation by placing a radioactive source within the lumpectomy site. This technique can lead to an improved quality of life because the treatments are administered over 4 to 5 days instead of 5 to 6 weeks. Another approach is intraoperative radiation therapy (IORT), in which a single intense dose of radiation is delivered to the surgical site in the operating room immediately following the lumpectomy. Short-term results of both of these approaches are promising with regard to rates of local recurrence and overall survival (Sauer, Sautter-Bihl, Budach, et al., 2007). Many questions remain unanswered, and longer follow-up with larger studies is needed to document the long-term effectiveness and potential side effects of these techniques. In the meantime, whole breast radiation remains the standard treatment of choice.

Although not widely used today after mastectomy, postoperative radiation is indicated for women at high risk for cancer recurrence (ie, chest wall involvement, four or more positive lymph nodes, tumors larger than 5 cm, positive surgical margins).

Side Effects

Generally, radiation therapy is well tolerated. Acute side effects consist of mild to moderate erythema, breast edema, and fatigue. Occasionally, skin breakdown may occur in the inframammary fold or near the axilla toward the end of treatment. Fatigue can be depressing, as can the frequent trips to the radiation oncology unit for treatment. The patient needs to be reassured that the fatigue is normal and not a sign of recurrence. Side effects usually resolve within a few weeks to a few months after treatment is completed. Rare long-term effects of radiation therapy include pneumonitis, rib fracture, and breast fibrosis.

Nursing Management

Self-care instructions for patients receiving radiation are provided to assist in the maintenance of skin integrity during the treatments and for several weeks after completion. They pertain only to the area being treated and not to the rest of the body.

- Use mild soap with minimal rubbing.
- Avoid perfumed soaps or deodorants.
- Use hydrophilic lotions (Lubriderm, Eucerin, Aquaphor) for dryness.
- Use a nondrying, antipruritic soap (Aveeno) if pruritus occurs.
- Avoid tight clothes, underwire bras, excessive temperatures, and ultraviolet light.

Follow-up care includes teaching the patient to minimize sun exposure to the treated area (ie, using sunblock

with sun protection factor [SPF] 15 or above) and reassuring the patient that minor twinges and shooting pain in the breast are normal after radiation treatment.

Systemic Treatments

Chemotherapy

Adjuvant chemotherapy involves the use of anticancer agents in addition to other treatments (ie, surgery, radiation) to delay or prevent a recurrence of breast cancer. It is recommended for patients who have positive lymph nodes or who have invasive tumors greater than 1 cm in size, regardless of nodal status. It is considered in patients with tumors that are 0.6 cm to 1 cm, are moderately to poorly differentiated, or have unfavorable features (NCCN, 2009). Table 48-6 outlines general indications for adjuvant chemotherapy. A survival benefit has been shown in premenopausal and postmenopausal women who received chemotherapy, although data are limited in women older than 70 years of age. Chemotherapy is most commonly initiated after breast surgery and before radiation.

Chemotherapy regimens for breast cancer combine several agents (polychemotherapy), generally administered over a period of 3 to 6 months. Decisions regarding the optimal regimen are based on a variety of factors, including tumor characteristics (ie, tumor size, lymph node status, hormone receptor status, HER-2/neu status) and the patient's age, physical status, and existing comorbid conditions. A regimen that includes cyclophosphamide (Cytoxan), methotrexate (Trexall), and fluorouracil (Fluoroplex) (CMF) has been the most widely used adjuvant therapy. It is usually well tolerated and may be considered for patients with a low risk of recurrence. CMF also may be considered for use in patients who have a high risk for cardiac toxicity (a potential side effect of anthracycline-based regimens) or who have other limiting comorbidities. Anthracycline-based regimens (eg, doxorubicin [Adriamycin],

Table 48-6	GENERAL INDICATIONS FOR ADJUVANT CHEMOTHERAPY FOR BREAST CANCER	
Nodal Status, Tumor Size	**Adjuvant Chemotherapy**
Node negative, 0.5 cm or less	None
Node negative 0.6–1 cm (well differentiated)	None
Node negative, 0.6–1 cm (moderately or poorly differentiated and/or unfavorable features)	Consider chemotherapy
Node negative, greater than 1 cm	Chemotherapy
Node positive, any tumor size	Chemotherapy

- In addition to chemotherapy, patients with HER-2/neu positive tumors will receive trastuzumab if they have node positive disease; or node negative disease with a tumor greater than 1 cm. Trastuzumab is a monoclonal antibody that targets and inactivates the HER-2/neu protein. HER-2/neu is overproduced in 25% to 30% of tumors and is associated with rapid growth and poor prognosis.
- Following chemotherapy, patients with hormone receptor positive (ER+/PR+) tumors will receive hormonal therapy (tamoxifen or aromatase inhibitor) if they have either node positive disease; node negative disease with a tumor >1cm; or node negative with a tumor 0.6cm–1cm and moderately or poorly differentiated and/or unfavorable features.

Note: These are only general guidelines. Recommendations may vary depending on factors such as prognostic variables, patient age, and comorbid conditions.

epirubicin [Ellence]) were associated with a decrease in the annual breast cancer death rate by 38% in women younger than 50 years and 20% in women ages 50 to 69 (McArthur & Hudis, 2007a). Cyclophosphamide, doxorubicin, and fluorouracil (CAF) and doxorubicin and cyclophosphamide (AC) are examples of combination regimens often administered to higher risk patients.

The taxanes (paclitaxel [Taxol], docetaxel [Taxotere]) are generally incorporated into treatment regimens for patients with larger, node-negative cancers and for those with positive axillary lymph nodes. The addition of four cycles of paclitaxel after a standard course of AC (regimen known as ACT) has been found to increase the disease-free period and improve overall survival in patients with operable breast cancer and positive lymph nodes (DeLaurentis, Cancello, D'Agostino, et al., 2008).

Much attention has been focused on **dose-dense chemotherapy,** the administration of chemotherapeutic agents at standard doses with shorter time intervals between each cycle of treatment. Patients who received ACT every 2 weeks, compared with those who received it on the conventional schedule of every 3 weeks, had an improved disease-free and overall survival (McArthur & Hurdis, 2007b). Long-term follow-up of this study and other clinical trials are ongoing to determine optimal treatment regimens, doses, and timing.

Side Effects

Today, many of the side effects of adjuvant chemotherapy can be managed well, allowing patients to maintain their daily routines and work schedules. In large part, this has been a result of the meticulous educational and psychological preparation provided to patients and their families by oncology nurses, oncologists, social workers, and other members of the health care team. In addition, strides have been made in the effectiveness of antiemetic agents used to alleviate nausea and vomiting and the use of hematopoietic growth factors to treat neutropenia and anemia.

Common physical side effects of chemotherapy for breast cancer may include nausea, vomiting, bone marrow suppression, taste changes, alopecia (hair loss), mucositis, neuropathy, skin changes, and fatigue. A weight gain of more than 10 lb occurs in about half of all patients; the cause is unknown. Premenopausal women may also experience temporary or permanent amenorrhea.

Specific side effects vary with the type of chemotherapeutic agent used. In general, CMF and the taxanes are better tolerated than the anthracyclines. However, the taxanes can cause peripheral neuropathy, arthralgias, and myalgias, particularly at high doses. During taxane administration, hypersensitivity reactions may occur; therefore, the patient must be premedicated. Alopecia is also common. The side effects of the anthracyclines may be severe and include cardiotoxicity in addition to nausea and vomiting, bone marrow suppression, and alopecia. Their vesicant properties can lead to tissue necrosis if infiltration of the medication infusion occurs.

Nursing Management

Nurses play an important role in helping patients manage the physical and psychosocial sequelae of chemotherapy.

(Chapter 16 provides an in-depth discussion of side-effect management.) Instructing the patient about the use of antiemetics and reviewing the optimal dosage schedule can help minimize nausea and vomiting. The different classes of antiemetic agents include serotonin (5-HT-3) receptor antagonists (palonosetron [Aloxi], granisetron [Kytril], ondansetron [Zofran]); neurokinin-1 receptor antagonists (aprepitant [Emend]); dopamine receptor antagonists (prochlorperazine [Compazine], metoclopramide [Reglan]); benzodiazepines (lorazepam [Ativan]); and corticosteroids (dexamethasone [Decadron]). Measures to ease the symptoms of mucositis may include rinsing with normal saline or sodium bicarbonate solution, avoiding hot and spicy foods, and using a soft toothbrush.

Some patients may require hematopoietic growth factors to minimize the effects of chemotherapy-induced neutropenia and anemia. Granulocyte colony-stimulating factors (G-CSFs) boost the white blood cell count, helping reduce the incidence of neutropenic fever and infection. The short-acting form, filgrastim (Neupogen), is injected subcutaneously for 7 to 10 days after chemotherapy administration. The long-acting form, pegfilgrastim (Neulasta), is injected once, 24 hours after chemotherapy. Erythropoietin growth factor increases the production of red blood cells, thus decreasing the symptoms of anemia. The short-acting form, epoetin alfa (Epogen) is usually administered weekly. The long-acting form, darbepoetin alfa (Aranesp), can be administered every 2 to 3 weeks. The nurse instructs the patient and family on proper injection technique of hematopoietic growth factors and about symptoms that require follow-up with a physician (Chart 48-9).

To prevent some of the emotional trauma associated with alopecia, it often helps to have a patient obtain a wig before hair loss begins to occur. The nurse may provide a list of wig suppliers in the patient's geographic region. Familiarity with creative ways to use scarves and turbans may also help minimize the patient's distress. The patient needs reassurance that new hair will grow back when treatment is completed, although the color and texture may be different. The ACS offers a program called Look Good, Feel Better that provides useful tips for applying cosmetics during the period a patient is receiving chemotherapy.

Chemotherapy may negatively affect the patient's self-esteem, sexuality, and sense of well-being. This, combined with the stress of a potentially life-threatening disease, can be overwhelming. Providing support and promoting open communication are important aspects of nursing care. Referring the patient to the dietitian, social worker, psychiatrist, or spiritual advisor can provide additional support. Numerous community support and advocacy groups are available for patients and their families. Complementary therapies, such as guided imagery, meditation, and relaxation exercises, can also be used in conjunction with conventional treatments.

Hormonal Therapy

The use of **adjuvant hormonal therapy,** with or without the addition of chemotherapy, is considered in women who have hormone receptor–positive tumors. Its use can be determined by the results of an **estrogen and progesterone receptor assay.** About two thirds of breast cancers are dependent

CHART 48-9	HOME CARE CHECKLIST *Self-Administration of Hematopoietic Growth Factors*		
At the completion of the home care instruction, the patient or caregiver will be able to:		**PATIENT**	**CAREGIVER**
• State the purpose for the injections.		✔	✔
• Identify the equipment necessary for self-injection.		✔	✔
• Identify appropriate body sites for self-injection.		✔	✔
• Demonstrate how to draw up the solution in a syringe if indicated (note: darbepoetin and pegfilgrastim come in prefilled syringes).		✔	✔
• Demonstrate how to give an injection properly.		✔	✔
• State possible side effects of medication.		✔	✔
• Demonstrate correct disposal of sharps.		✔	✔
• Describe proper storage of supplies.		✔	✔
• State reasons for contacting the physician or nurse (eg, excessive pain, fever).		✔	✔

on estrogen for growth and express a nuclear receptor that binds to the estrogen; thus, they are estrogen receptor–positive (ER+). Similarly, tumors that express the progesterone receptor are progesterone receptor–positive (PR+). Hormonal therapy involves the use of medications that compete with estrogen by binding to the receptor sites (selective estrogen receptor modulators [SERMs]), or by blocking estrogen production (**aromatase inhibitors**). Generally, tumors that are ER+/PR+ have the greatest likelihood of responding to hormonal therapy and have a more favorable prognosis than those that are ER−/PR−. Premenopausal and perimenopausal women are more likely to have non–hormone-dependent lesions, whereas postmenopausal women are more likely to have hormone-dependent lesions.

Traditionally, the SERM tamoxifen has been the primary hormonal agent used in treatment of premenopausal and postmenopausal breast cancer and remains the mainstay in premenopausal women. As a SERM, tamoxifen has estrogen antagonistic (estrogen-blocking) and agonistic (estrogen-like) effects on certain tissues. Its antagonistic effects in the breast prevent estrogen from binding to the receptor sites, thus preventing tumor growth. Tamoxifen has positive agonistic effects on blood lipid profiles and bone mineral density in postmenopausal women. It also has agonistic effects on endometrial tissue and blood coagulation processes, leading to an increased incidence of endometrial

cancer and thromboembolic events (eg, deep vein thrombosis, superficial phlebitis, pulmonary embolism). Nevertheless, the benefits of tamoxifen in most women with breast cancer outweigh the risks.

The aromatase inhibitors anastrazole (Arimidex), letrozole (Femara), and exemestane (Aromasin) are important components in the hormonal management of postmenopausal women. Most of the circulating estrogens in postmenopausal women are derived from the conversion of the adrenal androgen androstenedione to estrone and the conversion of testosterone to estradiol. Aromatase inhibitors work by blocking the enzyme aromatase from performing the conversion, thereby decreasing the level of circulating estrogen in peripheral tissues. Clinical trials have demonstrated that the aromatase inhibitors are superior to tamoxifen in terms of disease-free survival. Benefits were seen in patients who received an aromatase inhibitor as their initial adjuvant therapy, as therapy given after 2 to 3 years of tamoxifen, or when given for 5 years after receiving tamoxifen for 5 years (Carpenter, 2008). These data ensure that aromatase inhibitors will play an increasingly central role in the long-term management and follow-up of early-stage breast cancer. Trials are ongoing to determine the optimal treatment regimen and the timing of the treatment. Table 48-7 outlines the adverse effects of adjuvant hormonal therapy. Chart 48-10 outlines appropriate patient education to manage the adverse effects.

Table 48-7	ADVERSE REACTIONS ASSOCIATED WITH ADJUVANT HORMONAL THERAPY USED TO TREAT BREAST CANCER
Therapeutic Agent	**Adverse Reactions/Side Effects**
Selective Estrogen Receptor Modulator	
Tamoxifen (Nolvadex)	Hot flashes, vaginal dryness/discharge/bleeding, irregular menses, nausea, mood disturbances; increased risk for endometrial cancer; increased risk for thromboembolic events (deep vein thrombosis, pulmonary embolism, superficial phlebitis)
Aromatase Inhibitors	
Anastrozole (Arimidex) Letrozole (Femara) Exemestane (Aromasin)	Musculoskeletal symptoms (arthritis, arthralgia, myalgia), increased risk of osteoporosis/fractures, nausea/vomiting, hot flashes, fatigue, mood disturbances

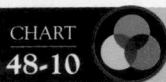

PATIENT EDUCATION
Managing Side Effects of Adjuvant Hormonal Therapy in Breast Cancer

CHART 48-10

Hot Flashes

- Wear breathable, layered clothing.
- Avoid caffeine and spicy foods.
- Perform breathing exercises (paced respirations).
- Consider medications (vitamin E, antidepressants) or acupuncture.

Vaginal Dryness

- Use vaginal moisturizers for everyday dryness (eg, Replens, Vitamin E suppository).
- Apply vaginal lubrication during intercourse (eg, Astroglide, K-Y jelly).

Nausea and Vomiting

- Consume a bland diet.
- Try to take medication in the evening.

Musculoskeletal Symptoms

- Take nonsteroidal analgesics as recommended.
- Take warm baths.

Risk of Endometrial Cancer

- Report any irregular bleeding to a gynecologist for evaluation.

Risk for Thromboembolic Events

- Report any redness, swelling, or tenderness in the lower extremities, or any unexplained shortness of breath.

Risk for Osteoporosis or Fractures

- Undergo a baseline bone density scan.
- Perform regular weight-bearing exercises.
- Take calcium supplements with vitamin D.
- Take bisphosphonates (eg, alendronate) or calcitonin as prescribed.

Targeted Therapy

One of the most exciting areas of research in the systemic treatment of breast cancer involves the use of targeted therapies. Trastuzumab (Herceptin) is a monoclonal antibody that binds specifically to the HER-2/neu protein. This protein, which regulates cell growth, is present in small amounts on the surface of normal breast cells and in most breast cancers. Approximately 25% to 30% of tumors overexpress (overproduce) the HER-2/neu protein and are associated with rapid growth and poor prognosis. Trastuzumab targets and inactivates the HER-2/neu protein, thus slowing tumor growth.

Unlike chemotherapy, trastuzumab spares the normal cells and has limited adverse reactions, which may include fever, chills, nausea, vomiting, diarrhea, and headache. However, when trastuzumab is administered to patients who have previously been treated with an anthracycline, the risk of cardiac toxicity is increased. The medication has been shown to improve survival rates in women with HER-2/neu–positive metastatic breast cancer and is now regarded as standard therapy. It may be administered as a single agent or in combination with chemotherapy. More recently, trastuzumab has been shown to be effective in treating early-stage breast cancer that is HER-2/neu positive. Adding trastuzumab to standard chemotherapy reduces the risk of recurrence by 52% and death by 33% (Romond, Perez, Bryant, et al., 2005). Patients with node-positive disease or node-negative disease with a tumor greater than 1 cm in size should receive trastuzumab for 1 year (Piccart-Gebhart, Procter, Leyland-Jones, et al., 2005). Another monoclonal antibody, bevacizumab (Avastin), is used in combination with paclitaxel to treat metastatic breast cancer (NCCN, 2007). It interferes with the vascular endothelial growth factor (VEGF), thus preventing the growth of new blood vessels that supply tumor cells with blood, oxygen, and nutrients that they need to grow. It is generally well tolerated but can cause hypertension and proteinuria.

Treatment of Recurrent and Metastatic Breast Cancer

Despite the advances made in the treatment of breast cancer, it may recur locally (on the chest wall or in the conserved breast), regionally (in the remaining lymph nodes), or systemically (in distant organs). In metastatic disease, the bone, usually the hips, spine, ribs, skull, or pelvis, is the most common site of spread. Other sites of metastasis include the lungs, liver, pleura, and brain.

The overall prognosis and optimal treatment are determined by a variety of factors such as the site and extent of recurrence, the time to recurrence from the original diagnosis, history of prior treatments, the patient's performance status, and any existing comorbid conditions. Patients with bone metastases generally have a longer overall survival compared with metastases in visceral organs.

Local recurrence in the absence of systemic disease is treated aggressively with surgery, radiation, and hormonal therapy. Chemotherapy may also be used for tumors that are not hormonally sensitive. Local recurrence may be an indicator that systemic disease will develop in the future, particularly if it occurs within 2 years of the original diagnosis.

Metastatic breast cancer involves control of the disease rather than cure. Treatment includes hormonal therapy, chemotherapy, and targeted therapy. Surgery or radiation may be indicated in select situations. Premenopausal women who have hormonally dependent tumors may eliminate the production of estrogen by the ovaries through oophorectomy (removal of the ovaries) or suppression of estrogen production by medications such as leuprolide (Lupron) or goserelin (Zoladex).

Patients with advanced breast cancer are monitored closely for signs of disease progression. Baseline studies are obtained at the time of recurrence. These may include complete blood count; comprehensive metabolic panel; tumor markers (ie, carcinoembryonic antigen, cancer antigen 15-3); bone scan; CT of the chest, abdomen, and pelvis;

and MRI of symptomatic areas. Additional x-rays may be performed to evaluate areas of pain or abnormal areas seen on bone scan (eg, long bones, pelvis). These studies are repeated at regular intervals to assess for effectiveness of treatment and to monitor progression of disease.

Nursing Management

Nurses play an important role in not only educating patients and managing their symptoms but also in providing emotional support. Many patients find that recurrence of the disease is more distressing than the initial cancer diagnosis. They not only have to contend with another round of treatments but are faced with a greater uncertainty about their future and long-term survival. The nurse can help the patient identify coping strategies and set priorities to optimize quality of life. Family members and significant others should be included in the treatment plan and follow-up care. Referrals to support groups, psychiatry or psychiatric clinical nurse specialist, social work, and complementary medicine programs (eg, guided imagery, meditation, yoga) should be made as indicated.

Nurses also play important roles in providing palliative care, if indicated. The highest priorities should include alleviating pain and providing comfort measures. A frank discussion with the patient and family regarding their preferences for end-of-life care should occur before the need arises to ensure a smooth transition without disruption of care. Referrals to hospice and home health care should be initiated as necessary. Chapter 16 provides more information on the general care of the patient with advanced cancer. Chapter 17 discusses end-of-life care.

Reconstructive Procedures After Mastectomy

Breast reconstruction can provide a significant psychological benefit for women who are already struggling with the emotional distress of losing a breast. A consultation with a plastic surgeon can help the patient understand procedures for which she is a candidate and the pros and cons of each. Factors to consider include body size and shape, comorbid conditions (eg, hypertension, diabetes mellitus, obesity), personal habits such as smoking, and patient preference. The patient must be informed that although breast reconstruction can provide a good cosmetic result, it will never precisely duplicate the natural breast. Realistic preparation can help the patient avoid unrealistic expectations. Once reconstruction

is complete, the opposite breast may require augmentation, reduction, or mastopexy to achieve symmetry on both sides. The patient must also be informed that breast reconstruction neither will interfere with breast cancer treatments nor affect the risk of cancer recurrence. Reconstruction is considered an integral component in the surgical treatment of breast cancer and is usually covered by insurance companies.

Many women elect immediate reconstruction at the time of the mastectomy operation. This can be beneficial in that it saves the woman from undergoing general anesthesia a second time and it saves the cost and stress of future hospitalizations. However, it does increase the length of the surgical procedure. Delayed reconstruction is preferable in women who are having a difficult time deciding on the type of reconstruction they desire. It may also be preferable in patients with advanced disease such as inflammatory breast cancer, where the breast cancer treatments should begin without delay. Any delays in healing after immediate reconstruction may interfere with the initiation of treatment.

Tissue Expander Followed by Permanent Implant

Breast reconstruction using a **tissue expander followed by a permanent implant** is the simplest and most common method used today (Fig. 48-6). To accommodate an implant, the skin remaining after a mastectomy and the underlying muscle must gradually be stretched by a process called tissue expansion. The surgeon places a balloonlike device called a tissue expander through the mastectomy incision underneath the pectoralis muscle. A small amount of saline is injected through a metal port intraoperatively to partially inflate the expander. Then, for about 6 to 8 weeks, at weekly intervals, the patient receives additional saline injections through the port until the expander is fully inflated. It remains fully expanded for about 6 weeks to allow the skin to loosen. The expander is then exchanged for a permanent implant. This is usually performed as an outpatient surgical procedure.

Advantages of this expansion procedure are a shorter operating time and a shorter recuperation period than for autologous reconstruction (see Tissue Transfer Procedures below). A disadvantage is a tendency for the implant to feel firm and round, with little natural ptosis (sag). Women with a small to medium opposite breast with little ptosis are good candidates for this procedure. Women who have had radiation or who have connective tissue disease are not good candidates because of the decreased elasticity of the skin.

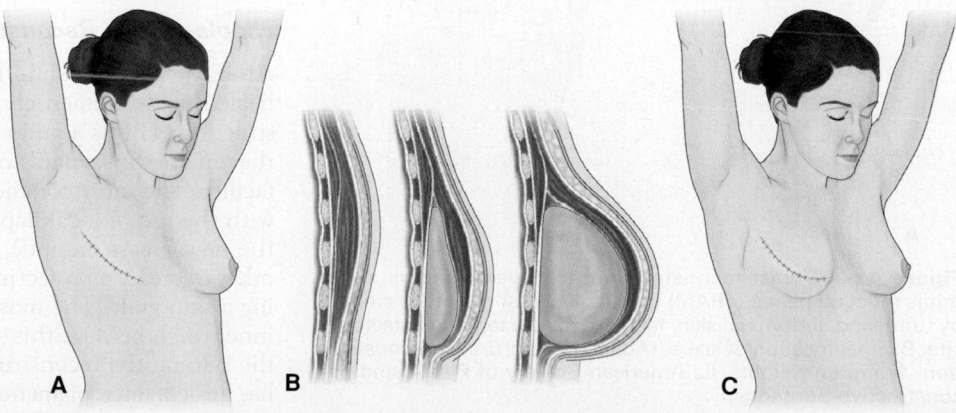

Figure 48-6 Breast reconstruction with tissue expander. **A,** Mastectomy incision line prior to tissue expansion. **B,** The expander is placed under the pectoralis muscle and is gradually filled with saline solution through a port to stretch the skin enough to accept a permanent implant. **C,** The breast mound is restored. Although permanent, scars will fade with time. The nipple and areola are reconstructed later. (Adapted from *Breast reconstruction.* Arlington Heights, IL: American Society of Plastic and Reconstructive Surgeons.)

A   B   C

⚑ **NURSING ALERT**

The patient must be cautioned not to have an MRI while the tissue expander is in place because the port contains metal. This is not an issue once the permanent implant is in place because it does not contain any metal.

The patient should be informed that for the rest of her life she should not engage in any exercises that will develop the pectoralis muscle because this can result in distortion of the reconstructed breast.

Tissue Transfer Procedures

Autologous reconstruction is the use of the patient's own tissue to create a breast mound. A flap of skin, fat, and muscle with its attached blood supply is rotated to the mastectomy site to create a mound that simulates the breast. Donor sites may include the **transverse rectus abdominis myocutaneous (TRAM) flap** (abdominal muscle) (Fig. 48-7), gluteal flap (buttock muscle), or the latissimus dorsi flap (back muscle) (Fig. 48-8). The results more closely resemble a real breast because the skin and fat from the donor sites are similar in consistency to a natural breast. These procedures avoid the use of synthetic material. However, they are far more complex and involve longer operative time (ranging from about 5 to 10 hours total time for the mastectomy and reconstruction) and longer recuperation than a tissue expander procedure. The risk of potential complications (eg, infection, bleeding, flap necrosis) is also greater. Therefore, patients must be in relatively good health, and those with medical conditions (eg, atherosclerosis, pulmonary disease, heart failure) that affect circulation or compromise oxygen delivery are not good candidates. Other poor candidates include those with uncontrolled type 1 diabetes mellitus or morbid obesity and heavy smokers.

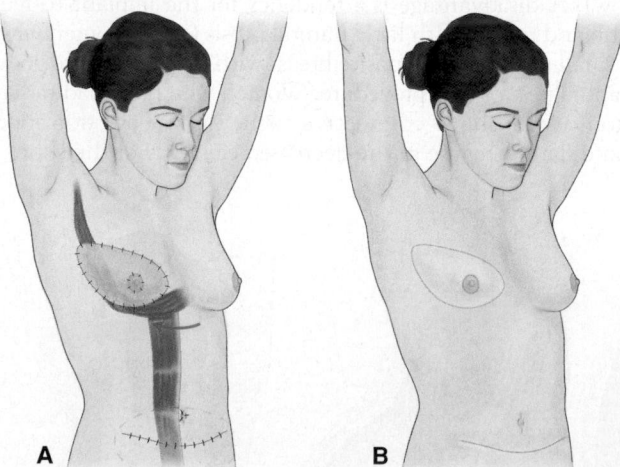

Figure 48-7 Breast reconstruction: transverse rectus abdominis myocutaneous (TRAM) flap. **A,** A breast mound is created by tunneling abdominal skin, fat, and muscle to the mastectomy site. **B,** Final location of scars. (Adapted from *Breast reconstruction.* Arlington Heights, IL: American Society of Plastic and Reconstructive Surgeons.)

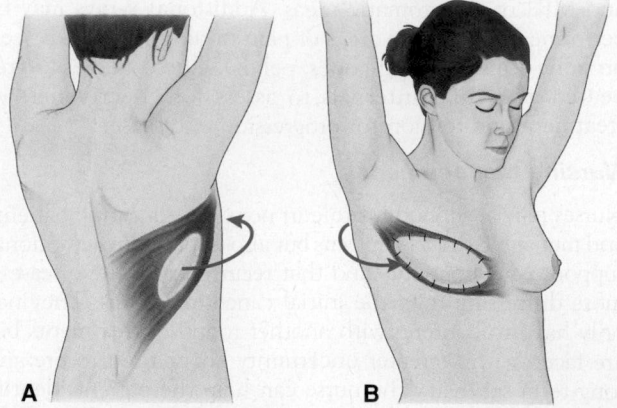

Figure 48-8 Breast reconstruction: latissimus dorsi flap. **A,** The latissimus muscle with an ellipse of skin is rotated from the back to the mastectomy site. **B,** Because the flap is usually not bulky enough to provide an adequate breast mound, an implant is often also required. (Adapted from *Breast reconstruction.* Arlington Heights, IL: American Society of Plastic and Reconstructive Surgeons.)

The TRAM flap is the most commonly performed tissue transfer procedure. A free TRAM procedure may also be performed; in this case, the skin, fat, muscle, and blood supply are completely detached from the body and then transplanted to the mastectomy site using microvascular surgery (use of a microscope to reconnect the vessels). Postoperatively, patients who have undergone TRAM procedures often face a lengthy recovery (often 6 to 8 weeks) and have incisions both at the mastectomy site and at the donor site in the abdomen. The nurse must assess the newly constructed breast site for changes in color, circulation, and temperature because flap loss is a potential complication. Mottling or an obvious decrease in skin temperature is reported to the surgeon immediately. Breathing and leg exercises are essential because the patient is more limited in her activity and is at greater risk for respiratory complications and deep vein thrombosis. Measures to help the patient reduce tension on the abdominal incision during the first postoperative week include elevating the head of the bed 45 degrees and flexing the patient's knees.

Once the patient is able to ambulate, she can protect the surgical incision by splinting it and will gradually achieve a more upright position. The patient is instructed to avoid high-impact activities and lifting (more than 5 to 10 lb for 6 to 8 weeks after surgery) to prevent stress on the incision.

Nipple–Areola Reconstruction

After the breast mound has been created and the site has healed, some women choose to have nipple–areola reconstruction. This is a minor surgical procedure carried out either in the physician's office or at an outpatient surgical facility. The most common method of creating a nipple is with the use of local flaps (skin and fat from the center of the new breast mound), which are wrapped around each other to create a projecting nipple. The areola is created using a skin graft. The most common donor site is the upper inner thigh because this skin has darker pigmentation than the skin on the reconstructed breast. After the nipple graft has healed, micropigmentation (tattooing) can be performed to achieve a more natural color. The surgeon can usually match the reconstructed nipple–areola complex with that of the contralateral breast for an acceptable cosmetic result.

Prosthetics

Not all patients desire or are candidates for reconstructive surgery. A breast prosthesis, an external form that simulates the breast, is another option. Prostheses are available in different shapes, sizes, colors, and materials, although they are most often made of silicone. They can be placed inside a pocket in a bra or can adhere directly to the chest wall. The nurse can provide the patient with the names of shops where she can be fitted for a prosthesis, or the patient can call the Reach to Recovery program of the ACS for appropriate referrals. The patient should be encouraged to find a shop with a comfortable, supportive atmosphere that employs a certified prosthetics consultant. Generally, medical supply shops are not recommended because often they do not have the appropriate resources to ensure the proper fitting of a prosthesis.

Prior to discharge from the hospital, the nurse usually provides the patient with a temporary, lightweight, cotton-filled form that can be worn until the surgical incision is well healed (4 to 6 weeks). After that, the patient can be fitted for a prosthesis. Insurance companies generally cover the cost of the prosthesis and the special bras that hold it in place. A breast prosthesis can provide a psychological benefit and assist the woman in resuming proper posture because it helps balance the weight of the remaining breast.

Special Issues in Breast Cancer Management

Implications of Genetic Testing

The rapid advancement in genetics has brought new knowledge about genetically inherited breast cancer, but it has also raised potential ethical and psychosocial issues. Although the actual testing for the *BRCA1* and *BRCA2* genes involves a simple blood test, it is these issues that must be addressed. Before undergoing genetic testing, a person should meet either with a clinician who has expertise in this area or with a certified genetics counselor to discuss risk factors as well as the benefits, sequelae, and limitations of testing.

How people react when they receive their actual test results is not always easy to predict. A negative test in a person who comes from a family with a known mutation may lead to enormous relief. However, a negative test in a family with no known mutation may be a source of undue reassurance; the possibility of existing genes that cannot yet be detected remains. A negative test may also lead to feelings of guilt in a person whose family members did not receive favorable test results; this is known as survivor's guilt. A positive test could act as a motivator in a person to pursue appropriate screening or treatment, or it could cause tremendous anxiety, depression, and worry.

In addition, test results may be ambiguous, leading to feelings of confusion and uncertainty. People must be informed that not all gene carriers develop breast cancer (incomplete penetrance) and that not all noncarriers are protected.

Other issues include those of cost: Who should pay for genetics testing and the services that relate to it? Difficult ethical questions arise concerning whether the person who is tested should disclose the test results. Is it ethical to withhold results from family members who may be at risk? If they are told, what effect will it have on them? People considering testing must be informed that there is no guarantee that test results will remain confidential. Once confidentiality is breached, it could unleash potential discrimination in employment and insurability. There are laws now, however, in many states to protect the individual if this should happen. People must be well informed of all of the issues and potential implications prior to undergoing genetics testing. Nurses play a role in educating and counseling patients and their family members about the implications of genetic testing. Nurses provide support and clarification and make referrals to appropriate specialists when indicated.

Pregnancy and Breast Cancer

Breast cancer during pregnancy is defined as breast cancer diagnosed during gestation or within 1 year of childbirth and occurs in 1 in 3000 women (NCCN, 2007). Because of increased levels of hormones produced during pregnancy and subsequent lactation, the breast tissue becomes tender and swollen, making it more difficult to detect a mass. If a mass is found during pregnancy, ultrasound is the preferred diagnostic method because it involves no exposure to radiation. If indicated, mammography with appropriate shielding, FNA, and biopsy can be performed. Modified radical mastectomy remains the most common form of surgical treatment. SLNB is typically not performed because of the unknown effects of the radioisotope and the blue dye on the fetus. Breast conservation treatment may be considered if the breast cancer is diagnosed during the third trimester. Radiation can then be delayed until after delivery because it is contraindicated during pregnancy. Chemotherapy should be avoided during the first trimester; the fetal organs are still developing, and it poses a great risk for fetal malformations. However, chemotherapy has been administered during the second and third trimesters with few reported abnormalities. Long-term effects on the fetus are still being studied. If a woman is close to term, a cesarean section may be performed as soon as maturation of the fetus allows, and then treatment is initiated. If aggressive disease is detected early in pregnancy and chemotherapy is advised, termination of the pregnancy may be considered. If a mass is found while a woman is breastfeeding, she is urged to stop to allow the breast to involute (return to its baseline state) before any type of surgery is performed.

Fertility issues and the future desire for children are major concerns of young breast cancer survivors. Certain chemotherapeutic agents, particularly cyclophosphamide, can lead to amenorrhea. Even if the woman is still fertile, many physicians recommend postponing pregnancy for 2 to 3 years after primary treatment because recurrence rates are the highest during this time. Women taking tamoxifen for 5 years are cautioned to avoid pregnancy because of potential effects on the fetus. This waiting period may make it more difficult for the woman to later become pregnant as she advances in age. These issues should be discussed with the patient prior to initiating treatment. There are options today that may help preserve a woman's fertility, and prior to the onset of chemotherapy she should seek the opinion of a reproductive specialist (Partridge & Ruddy, 2007). Fertile Hope, a national nonprofit organization, can also provide updated information on reproduction (see Resources at the end of the chapter).

Quality of Life and Survivorship

With increased early detection and improved treatment modalities, women with breast cancer have become the largest group of cancer survivors. However, the treatment or simply the diagnosis of breast cancer may have long-term effects that negatively affect the patient and her family. The patient should be prepared early on for the potential long-term effects of the disease so she has realistic expectations and can make informed decisions.

Breast cancer survivors may experience a variety of issues as a result of their diagnosis and treatment. Estrogen withdrawal from chemotherapy-induced menopause and hormonal treatments can lead to a variety of symptoms, including hot flashes, vaginal dryness, urinary tract infections, weight gain, decreased sex drive, and increased risk of osteoporosis. HT to alleviate symptoms is contraindicated in women with breast cancer. Certain chemotherapeutic agents can cause long-term cardiac effects and neuropathy. In addition, patients may experience impaired cognitive functioning such as difficulty concentrating (often referred to as chemobrain). Rare long-term effects of radiation can include pneumonitis and rib fractures. Long-term sequelae after breast surgery may include lymphedema (mainly after ALND), pain, and sensory disturbances. Once lymphedema develops, it tends to be a chronic problem, so prevention strategies (discussed earlier) are vital. Patients have also reported sensations such as tenderness and soreness 5 years after their surgical procedure (Baron, et al., 2007).

Some of these symptoms can also lead to fatigue and sleep disturbances. Long-term psychosocial sequelae may include anxiety, depression, uncertainty about the future, and fear of recurrence. In the workplace, the patient may suffer from fear of discrimination, concern over coworkers' reactions, fear of losing insurance benefits, and lack of physical stamina. Studies have found, however, that many of these issues are not recognized or addressed (Khatcheressian & Swainey, 2008).

 Gerontologic Considerations

When deciding on the optimal treatment modality for an elderly patient, age alone should not be the single determining factor. Many older women, regardless of their advancing chronological age, remain in excellent health. Therefore, the woman's treatment preferences should play a strong role in the decision-making process. It should not be assumed that elderly women are less concerned about their appearance than their younger counterparts. One study surveyed 75 women who were 60 years of age or older about their thoughts on breast reconstruction (Bowman, Lennox, Clugston, et al., 2006). More than 90% of the women believed that age should not be taken into consideration before being offered the option of breast reconstruction. Of the women who were not told about immediate reconstruction at the time of their diagnosis, 100% believed that it should have been discussed. Research studies on women older than 70 years of age are lacking. Nurses can play an important role in conducting research on this older population, thus adding to the knowledge base.

A thorough assessment must be performed before any treatment is initiated, and careful monitoring must occur throughout the course of treatment to avoid complications. The physical and psychosocial assessment of the older woman should include general health, currently existing comorbidities, performance status, cognitive status, current medications, available resources, and support systems.

Breast Health of Women With Disabilities

Women with a variety of disabilities may be unable to detect changes in their own breasts. Those with decreased sensation in their fingers may be unable to palpate even large breast masses, and those with vision loss may be unable to detect changes in the appearance of their breasts. Women with disabilities tend to undergo mammography less often than recommended (Poulos, Balandin, Llewellyn, et al., 2006). They may lack transportation to the imaging facility, and they may be unable to undress without assistance, stand, or maintain positioning for a mammogram. Many imaging facilities do not have accessible mammography equipment, and staff members may be unfamiliar with modifications in positioning needed to obtain acceptable scans (Smeltzer & Sharts-Hopko, 2005). Furthermore, health care providers often neglect to recommend health screening for women with disabilities, despite the fact that they have the same risks for breast cancer as other women and generally have a normal or near-normal life expectancy (U.S. Department of Human Services, 2005). The more severe the disability, the less likely that a woman will undergo mammography. For those women who cannot be adequately positioned for a mammogram, ultrasound may be used as an alternative; however, these women may need more frequent clinical breast examinations.

Women with disabilities who are diagnosed with breast cancer tend to be offered breast conservation surgery less often than other women. However, they have the same concerns about body image as other women.

An essential role of the nurse is to assist women with disabilities to identify accessible health screening and to advocate for greater accessibility of imaging centers and other health care facilities. Reminding women of the need for recommended clinical breast examinations and mammograms is an important part of nursing care.

RECONSTRUCTIVE BREAST SURGERY

Breast reconstruction is elective surgery that can enhance a woman's self-image and sense of well-being. Women desire reconstruction for a variety of physical and psychological reasons. Therefore, it is important that the health care team conduct a thorough assessment prior to reconstructive surgery to evaluate the woman's underlying desire, motivation, and expectations. Preparing a woman realistically could help her to avoid potential disappointment. A variety of reconstructive options are available today for women who desire a correction in the size or the shape of the breast, including reduction **mammoplasty** (breast reduction), augmentation mammoplasty (breast enlargement), and mastopexy (breast lift). Several options are also available to reconstruct the breast after a mastectomy.

Reduction Mammoplasty

Reduction mammoplasty is usually performed on women who have breast hypertrophy (excessively large breasts). The weight of the enlarged breasts can cause discomfort, fatigue, embarrassment, and poor posture.

Reduction mammoplasty is an outpatient procedure that is performed under general anesthesia. Most commonly, an anchor-shaped incision that circles the areola is made, extending downward and following the natural curve of the crease beneath the breast (inframammary fold). Depending on the size of the breast, the nipple may be moved up to a higher position while still attached to the breast tissue or it may be separated and transplanted to a new location. Drains are placed in the incision and remain for 2 to 5 days.

During the preoperative consultation, the patient should be informed that there is a possibility that sensory changes of the nipple (such as numbness) may occur. These sensations are normal and usually resolve after several months but can sometimes persist. The procedure may also make breastfeeding impossible, although some women have breastfed successfully. The patient must also be aware that if she gains weight (usually more than 10 lb), her breasts may also enlarge.

After reduction mammoplasty, many women verbalize feelings of extreme satisfaction, possibly because of the relief they experience. The patient is instructed to wear a supportive bra 24 hours a day for 2 weeks to prevent tension on the swollen breast and incision line. Vigorous exercise (eg, jumping, jogging) should be avoided for about 6 weeks after surgery.

Augmentation Mammoplasty

Augmentation mammoplasty is requested by women who desire larger or fuller breasts. The procedure is performed by placing a breast implant either under the pectoralis muscle (subpectoral) or under the breast tissue (subglandular). The subpectoral approach is preferred because it interferes less with clinical breast examinations and mammograms. The incision line can be placed in the inframammary fold, in the axilla, or around the areola. The procedure is performed as an outpatient procedure under general anesthesia. A drain is not necessary. Postoperative instructions are the same as for reduction mammoplasty.

Saline implants are typically used for augmentation mammoplasty. Because of concerns that silicone implants could cause autoimmune diseases, they were removed from the market in 1992. In November 2006 the FDA approved the use of silicone implants as long as they were manufactured by two specific companies. This approval covered women of all ages for breast reconstruction and women 22 years of age and older for breast augmentation (U.S. FDA, 2007). Women with breast implants should be aware that mammograms may be more difficult to read, and they should seek experienced breast radiologists.

Mastopexy

Mastopexy is performed when the patient is happy with the size of her breasts but wishes to have the shape improved and a lift performed. This is also an outpatient surgical procedure, and postoperative instructions are the same as for reduction mammoplasty.

DISEASES OF THE MALE BREAST

Gynecomastia

Gynecomastia, or overdeveloped breast tissue, is the most common breast condition in the male. Adolescent boys can be affected by this condition because of hormones secreted by the testes. This type of gynecomastia is virtually always benign and resolves spontaneously in 1 to 2 years. Gynecomastia can also occur in older men and usually presents as a firm, tender mass underneath the areola. In these patients, gynecomastia may be diffuse and related to use of certain medications (eg, digitalis, ranitidine [Zantac]). It may also be associated with certain conditions, including feminizing testicular tumors, infection in the testes, and liver disease resulting from factors such as alcohol abuse or a parasitic infection.

Patients in their late teens to late 40s presenting with idiopathic (unknown cause) gynecomastia should have a testicular examination and possibly a testicular ultrasound. Treatment of the enlarged breast tissue is based on patient preference and is usually reserved for those men who cannot tolerate the cosmetic appearance of the breast or who have severe pain associated with the condition. Observation is acceptable in most cases because gynecomastia may resolve on its own. Surgical removal of the tissue through a small incision around the areola is the best treatment option. Liposuction performed by a plastic surgeon is another possibility, although this does not allow for pathologic examination of the tissue.

Male Breast Cancer

Cancer of the male breast accounts for less than 1% of all cases of breast cancer. The average age at the time of diagnosis is 67 years, but the disease may occur in younger men, especially if there is a genetic link (Nahleh & Girnius, 2006). There is a well-documented link to mutations in the BRCA2 gene in men with breast cancer; men 70 years of age with a BRCA2 mutation have an estimated cumulative risk of breast cancer of 6.8% (Tai, Domchek, Parmigiani, et al., 2007). In sporadic cases of male breast cancer (no known family history), risk factors may include a history of mumps orchitis, radiation exposure, and Klinefelter's syndrome (a chromosomal condition reflecting decreased testosterone levels). Liver disease due to factors such as alcohol abuse or a parasitic infection, which compromises estrogen metabolism, may also lead to an increase in rates of male breast cancer. Symptoms include a painless lump beneath the areola, nipple retraction, bloody nipple discharge, or skin ulceration. Diagnostic tests and treatment modalities are similar to those used for women.

Early detection is uncommon in male breast cancer because of the rare nature of the disease. Neither patient nor physician suspects male breast cancer early in its development. Treatment generally consists of a total mastectomy with either SLNB or ALND. As in women with breast cancer, prognosis depends on the stage of disease at presentation. Involvement of the axillary lymph nodes is the most important prognostic indicator. Male breast cancers are very likely to be ER+, and tamoxifen, although it has several side effects, is a mainstay of treatment.

Because breast cancer is primarily a disease of women, men may feel that a certain stigma is attached to their diagnosis. Health care professionals must be sensitive to their needs and provide information and support.

CRITICAL THINKING EXERCISES

EBP **1** You are reviewing early detection guidelines with a 65-year-old woman who has a *BRCA1* mutation. She had an MRI 1 week ago that was normal. Because of this, she asks you if she can skip having her mammogram. What would you advise? What screening modalities would you recommend to her on a yearly basis? What is the evidence base for your recommendations? How would you determine the strength of that evidence?

EBP **2** A 45-year-old woman tells you that nobody in her family has breast cancer. She is relieved, she says, because now she does not have to worry about getting it either. How would you respond to this woman? What is the evidence related to the risk of breast cancer with and without a family history? What is the strength of that evidence?

3 A 50-year-old woman had a right lumpectomy and an axillary lymph node dissection for breast cancer 12 years ago. She calls you in a panic because she accidentally burned her right hand while cooking. What advice would you give her?

4 A 28-year-old woman was just diagnosed with breast cancer. She will need surgery and most likely chemotherapy. She desperately wants to have children. How would you address this issue? What resources would be appropriate to provide to the patient?

EBP **5** A 54-year-old woman with breast cancer has completed surgery, chemotherapy, and radiation treatment. She tolerated the treatments very well both physically and emotionally. She is now taking tamoxifen, which she started 6 months ago, and she feels very depressed and anxious. What would you recommend for this woman? What is the evidence base for the recommendations you would provide? How would you determine the strength of that evidence?

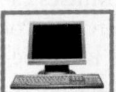 The Smeltzer suite offers these additional resources to enhance learning and facilitate understanding of this chapter:
- thePoint online resource, thepoint.lww.com/Smeltzer12E
- Student CD-ROM included with the book

- *Study Guide to Accompany Brunner & Suddarth's Textbook of Medical-Surgical Nursing*
- *Handbook for Brunner & Suddarth's Textbook of Medical-Surgical Nursing*

REFERENCES AND SELECTED READINGS

Asterisk indicates nursing research.
**Double asterisk indicates classic reference.*

Books

American Cancer Society (ACS). (2009). *Breast cancer facts and figures, 2009.* Atlanta: Author.

*Berger, A. M., Treat Marunda, H. A. & Agrawal, S. (2009). Influence of menopausal status on sleep and hot flashes throughout breast cancer adjuvant chemotherapy. *Journal of Obstetric, Gynecologic, & Neonatal Nursing,* 38(3), 353–366.

Bickley, L. S. (2007). *Bates' guide to physical examination and history taking* (9th ed.). Philadelphia: Lippincott Williams & Wilkins.

Dow, K. H. (2005). *Pocket guide to breast cancer* (3rd ed.). Boston: Jones & Bartlett.

Greene, F. L., Page, D. L., Fleming, I. D., et al. (2002). *AJCC cancer staging manual* (6th ed.). New York: Springer-Verlag.

Love, S. M. & Lindsey, K. (2005). *Dr. Susan Love's breast book* (4th ed.). Cambridge, MA: Da Capo Press.

National Comprehensive Cancer Network (NCCN). (2007). *Breast cancer treatment guidelines for patients.* Version IX. Atlanta: American Cancer Society.

National Comprehensive Cancer Network (NCCN). (2009). *NCCN practice guidelines in oncology. Breast cancer.* Version 1. Atlanta: American Cancer Society.

Smeltzer, S. C. & Sharts-Hopko, N. C. (2005). *A provider's guide for the care of women with physical disabilities and chronic health conditions.* Chapel Hill, NC: North Carolina Office on Disability & Health.

U.S. Department of Health and Human Services. (2005). *The surgeon general's call to action to improve the health and wellness of persons with disabilities.* Washington, DC: U.S. Department of Health and Human Services, Office of the Surgeon General.

Weber, J. & Kelley, J. (2006). *Health assessment in nursing* (3rd ed.). Philadelphia: Lippincott Williams & Wilkins.

Yarbro, C. H., Frogge, M. H. & Goodman, M. (Eds.) (2005). *Cancer nursing: Principles and practices* (6th ed.). Sudbury, MA: Jones & Bartlett.

Journals and Electronic Documents

*Allard, N. C. (2007). Day surgery for breast cancer: Effects of a psychoeducational telephone intervention on functional status and emotional distress. *Oncology Nursing Forum,* 34(1), 133–141.

Alschuler, A., Nekhlyudov, L., Rolnick, S. J., et al. (2008). Positive, negative, and disparate—Women's differing long-term psychosocial experiences of bilateral or contralateral prophylactic mastectomy. *The Breast Journal,* 14(1), 25–32.

*Baron, R. H., Fey, J. V., Borgen, P. I., et al. (2007). Eighteen sensations after breast cancer surgery: A five-year comparison of sentinel lymph node biopsy and axillary lymph node dissection. *Annals of Surgical Oncology,* 14(5), 1653–1661.

Begg, C. B., Haile, R. W. & Borg, A. (2008). Variation of breast cancer risk among BRCA1/2 carriers. *Journal of the American Medical Association,* 299(2), 194–201.

Bergkvist, L., deBoniface, J., Jonsson, P. E., et al. (2008). Axillary recurrence rate after sentinel node biopsy in breast cancer: Three-year follow-up of the Swedish Multicenter Cohort Study. *Annals of Surgery,* 247(1), 150–156.

Boughey, J. C., Gonzalez, R. J., Bonner, E., et al. (2007). Current treatment and clinical trial developments for ductal carcinoma in situ of the breast. *The Oncologist,* 12(11), 1276–1287.

Bowman, C. C., Lennox, P. A., Clugston, P. A., et al. (2006). Breast reconstruction in older women: Should age be an exclusion criterion? *Plastic and Reconstructive Surgery,* 118(1), 16–22.

Breen, N., Cronin, K. A., Meissner, H. I., et al. (2007). Reported drop in mammography: Is this cause for concern? *Cancer,* 109(12), 2405–2409.

Carpenter, R. (2008). Choosing early adjuvant therapy for postmenopausal women with hormone sensitive breast cancer: Aromatase inhibitors versus tamoxifen. *European Journal of Surgical Oncology,* 34(7), 746–755.

Centers for Disease Control and Prevention (CDC). (2007). The National Breast and Cervical Cancer early detection program. Available at: www.cdc.gov/cancer/nbccedp/about.htm

**Cummings, S. R., Eckert, S., Krueger, K. A., et al. (1999). The effect of raloxifene on risk of breast cancer in postmenopausal women: Results from the MORE randomized trial. *Journal of the American Medical Association*, 281(23), 2189–2197.

Daly, M. B. (2006). Tamoxifen in ductal carcinoma in situ. *Seminars in Oncology*, 33(6), 647–649.

Dawood, S., Broglio, K., Esteva, F. J., et al. (2008). Defining prognosis for women with breast cancer and CNS metastases by HER2 status. *Annals of Oncology*, 19(7), 1242–1248.

DeLaurentis, M., Cancello, G., D'Agostino, D., et al. (2008). Taxane-based combinations as adjuvant chemotherapy of early breast cancer: A meta-analysis of randomized trials. *Journal of Clinical Oncology*, 26(1), 44–53.

Diedrich, J. Depke, J. & Engle, J. (2007). What every nurse needs to know about breast cancer: An overview and update of breast cancer screening, diagnosis, and treatment. *American Nurse Today*, 2(10), 32–37.

**Fisher, B., Costantino, J. P., Wickerham, D. L., et al. (1998). Tamoxifen for prevention of breast cancer. Report of the National Surgical Adjuvant Breast and Bowel Project P-1 study. *Journal of the National Cancer Institute*, 90(18), 1371–1388.

Hanby, A. M. & Hughes, T. A. (2008). In situ and invasive neoplasia of the breast. *Histiopathology*, 52(1), 58–66.

Hayes, D. F. (2007). Follow-up of patients with early breast cancer. *New England Journal of Medicine*, 356(24), 2505–2513.

Helvie, M. (2007). Improving mammographic interpretation: Double reading and computer-aided diagnosis. *Radiologic Clinics of North America*, 45(5), 801–811.

Horning, K. M. & Guhde, J. (2007). Lymphedema: An undertreated problem. *MedSurg Nursing*, 16(4), 221–227.

Iezzoni, L., Ngo, L., Li, D., et al. (2008). Early stage breast cancer treatments for younger Medicare beneficiaries with different disabilities. *Health Services Research*, 43(5), 1752–1767.

Jemal, A., Siegel, R., Ward, E., et al. (2008). Cancer statistics, 2008. *CA: A Cancer Journal for Clinicians*, 58(2), 71–96.

Khatcheressian, J. & Swainey, C. (2008). Breast cancer follow-up in the adjuvant setting. *Current Oncology Reports*, 10(1), 38–46.

*Koren, M. E. & Hertz, J. E. (2007). Older women's breast screening behaviors: What nurses need to know. *MedSurg Nursing*, 16(2), 80–85.

Krag, D. N., Anderson, S. J., Julian, T. B., et al. (2007). Technical outcomes of sentinel-lymph-node resection and conventional axillary-lymph-node dissection in patients with clinically node-negative breast cancer: results from the NSABP B-32 randomized phase III trial. *The Lancet Oncology*, 8(10), 881–888.

Lacovara, J. E. & Yoder, L. H. (2006). Secondary lymphedema in the cancer patient. *MedSurg Nursing*, 15(5), 302–306.

Langer, I., Guller, U., Berclaz, G., et al. (2007). Morbidity of sentinel lymph node biopsy (SLN) alone versus SLN and completion axillary lymph node dissection after breast cancer surgery. *Annals of Surgery*, 245(3), 452–461.

Lucci, A., McCall, M. M., Beitsch, P. D., et al. (2007). Surgical complications associated with sentinel lymph node dissection (SLND) plus axillary lymph node dissection compared with SLND alone in the American College of Surgeons Oncology Group trial Z0011. *Journal of Clinical Oncology*, 25(24), 3657–3663.

McArthur, H. L. & Hudis, C. A. (2007a). Breast cancer chemotherapy. *The Cancer Journal*, 13(3), 141–147.

McArthur, H. L. & Hudis, C. A. (2007b). Dose-dense therapy in the treatment of early-stage breast cancer: An overview of the data. *Clinical Breast Cancer*, 8(Suppl 1), S6–S10.

Monninkhof, E. M., Elias, S. G., Vlems, F. A., et al. (2007). Physical activity and breast cancer: A systematic review. *Epidemiology*, 18(1), 137–157.

Nahleh, Z. & Girnius. (2006). Male breast cancer: A gender issue. *Nature Clinical Practice Oncology*, 3(8), 428–437.

National Cancer Institute (NCI). (2008). Surveillance, epidemiology and end results: SEER stat fact sheet. Available at: http://seer.cancer.gov/statfacts/html/breast.html

Orel, S. (2008). Who should have breast magnetic resonance imaging evaluation? *Journal of Clinical Oncology*, 26(5), 703–711.

Partridge, A. H. & Ruddy, K. J. (2007). Fertility and adjuvant treatment in young women with breast cancer. *The Breast*, 16(Suppl 2), S175–S181.

Piccart-Gebhart, M. J., Procter, M., Leyland-Jones, B., et al. (2005). Trastuzumab after adjuvant chemotherapy in HER2-positive breast cancer. *New England Journal of Medicine*, 353(16), 1659–1672.

Poulos, A. E., Balandin, S., Llewellyn, G., et al. (2006). Women with cerebral palsy and breast cancer screening by mammography. *Archives of Physical Medicine and Rehabilitation*, 87(2), 304–307.

Punglia, R. S., Morrow, M., Winer, E. P., et al. (2007). Local therapy and survival in breast cancer. *New England Journal of Medicine*, 356(23), 2399–2405.

Ravdin, P. M., Cronin, K. A., Howlader, N., et al. (2007). The decrease in breast-cancer incidence in 2003 in the United States. *New England Journal of Medicine*, 356(16), 1670–1674.

Romond, E. H., Perez, E. A., Bryant, J., et al. (2005). Trastuzumab plus adjuvant chemotherapy for operable HER2-positive breast cancer. *New England Journal of Medicine*, 353(16), 1673–1684.

Saslow, D., Boetes, C., Burke, W., et al. (2007). American Cancer Society guidelines for breast screening with MRI as an adjunct to mammography. *CA: A Cancer Journal for Clinicians*, 57(2), 75–89.

Sauer, R., Sautter-Bihl, M. L., Budach, W., et al. (2007). Accelerated partial breast irradiation: Consensus statement of 3 German oncology societies. *Cancer*, 110(6), 1187–1194.

Smith, R. A., Cokkinides, V. & Brawley, O. W. (2008). Cancer screening in the United States, 2008: A review of current American Cancer Society guidelines and cancer screening issues. *CA: A Cancer Journal for Clinicians*, 58(3), 161–179.

Tai, Y. C., Domchek, S., Parmigiani, G., et al. (2007). Breast cancer risk among male BRCA1 and BRCA2 mutation carriers. *Journal of the National Cancer Institute*, 99(23), 1811–1814.

Turnbull, C. & Rahman, N. (2008). Genetic predisposition to breast cancer: Past, present, and future. *Annual review of Genomics and Human Genetics*, 9, 321–345.

U.S. Food and Drug Administration (FDA). (2007). Silicone gel-filled implants approved. *FDA Consumer Magazine*, 41(1), 8–9.

Vogel, V. G., Costantino, J. P., Wickerham, D. L., et al. (2006). Effects of tamoxifen vs raloxifene on the risk of developing invasive breast cancer and other disease outcomes. The NSABP study of tamoxifen and raloxifene (STAR) P-2 trial. *Journal of the American Medical Association*, 295(23), 2727–2741.

Warren, A. G., Brorson, H., Borud, L. J., et al. (2007). Lymphedema: A comprehensive review. *Annals of Plastic Surgery*, 59(4), 464–472.

RESOURCES

American Cancer Society, www.cancer.org

American Society of Plastic and Reconstructive Surgeons, www.plasticsurgery.org

Cancer Care, Inc. (provides free professional support services to anyone affected by cancer), www.cancercare.org

Fertile Hope, www.fertilehope.org

National Breast Cancer Coalition (This activist group has raised funds and consciousness levels regarding breast cancer and was instrumental in obtaining funds for research on prevention), www.natlbcc.org

National Cancer Institute, www.cancer.gov/cancertopics/types/breast

National Lymphedema Network, www.lymphnet.org

Oncology Nursing Society, www.ons.org

Reach to Recovery Program—I Can Cope Program. (Information available through local American Cancer Society chapters).

Susan G. Komen for the Cure, ww5.komen.org

Y-ME Breast Cancer Organization, www.y-me.org

Young Survival Coalition, www.youngsurvival.org

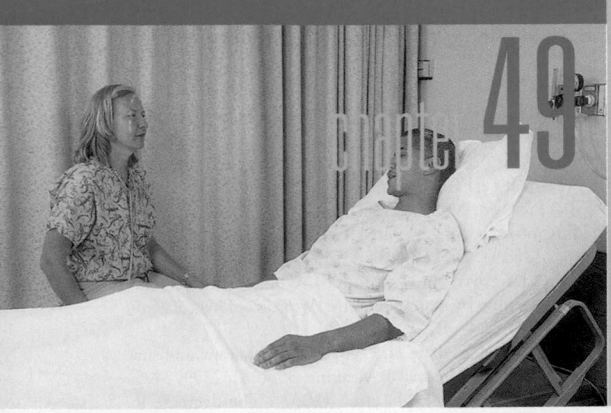

Assessment and Management of Problems Related to Male Reproductive Processes

Chapter 49

LEARNING OBJECTIVES

On completion of this chapter, the learner will be able to:

1 Describe structures and function of the male reproductive system.

2 Discuss nursing assessment of the male reproductive system and identify diagnostic tests that complement assessment.

3 Discuss the causes and management of male sexual dysfunction.

4 Compare the types of prostatectomy with regard to advantages and disadvantages.

5 Use the nursing process as a framework for care of the patient undergoing prostatectomy.

6 Describe the nursing management of patients with testicular cancer.

7 Describe the various conditions affecting the penis, including pathophysiology, clinical manifestations, and management.

GLOSSARY

androgen deprivation therapy (ADT): surgical (orchiectomy) or medical castration (eg, with luteinizing hormone–releasing hormone agonists)

benign prostatic hyperplasia (BPH): noncancerous enlargement or hypertrophy of the prostate; the most common pathologic condition in older men

brachytherapy: delivery of radiation therapy through internal implants called seeds to a localized area of tissue

circumcision: excision of the foreskin, or prepuce, of the glans penis

cryosurgery of the prostate: localized treatment of the prostate by application of freezing temperatures

cystostomy: surgical creation of an opening into the urinary bladder

cryptorchidism: most common congenital defect in males; characterized by failure of one or both of the testes to descend into the scrotum

epididymitis: infection of the epididymis that usually descends from an infected prostate or urinary tract; also may develop as a complication of gonorrhea

erectile dysfunction: also called impotence; the inability to either achieve or maintain an erection sufficient to accomplish sexual intercourse

hydrocele: a collection of fluid, generally in the tunica vaginalis of the testis, although it also may collect within the spermatic cord

GLOSSARY *(Continued)*

minimally invasive therapy: treatments such as laparoscopic and robotic prostatectomy, cryotherapy, and high-intensity focused ultrasound (HIFU); are less invasive than other procedures with less morbidity, lower blood loss, and more rapid recovery

orchiectomy: surgical removal of one or both of the testes

orchitis: inflammation of the testes (testicular congestion) caused by pyogenic, viral, spirochetal, parasitic, traumatic, chemical, or unknown factors

penile cancer: malignancy that can involve the glans, the body of the penis, the urethra, and regional or distant lymph nodes

Peyronie's disease: buildup of fibrous plaques in the sheath of the corpus cavernosum, causing curvature of the penis when it is erect

phimosis: condition in which the foreskin is constricted so that it cannot be retracted over the glans; can occur congenitally or from inflammation and edema

priapism: an uncontrolled, persistent erection of the penis from either neural or vascular causes, including medications, sickle cell thrombosis, leukemic cell infiltration, spinal cord tumors, and tumor invasion of the penis or its vessels

prostate cancer: A common type of cancer in men; involves the prostate gland

prostatectomy: open or laparoscopic surgical removal of the entire prostate, the prostate urethra, the attached seminal vesicles plus the ampulla of the vas deferens

prostate-specific antigen (PSA): substance that is produced by the prostate gland; is used in combination with digital rectal examination to screen for prostate cancer

prostatism: obstructive and irritative symptom complex that includes increased frequency and hesitancy in starting urination, a decrease in the volume and force of the urinary stream, acute urinary retention, and recurrent urinary tract infections

prostatitis: inflammation of the prostate gland caused by infectious agents (bacteria, fungi, mycoplasma) or various other problems (eg, urethral stricture, prostatic hyperplasia)

spermatogenesis: production of sperm in the testes

testicular cancer: cancer of one or both testes

testosterone: male sex hormone secreted by the testes; induces and preserves the male sex characteristics

transurethral resection of the prostate (TURP): resection of the prostate through endoscopy; the surgical and optical instrument is introduced directly through the urethra to the prostate, and the gland is then removed in small chips with an electrical cutting loop

varicocele: an abnormal dilation of the veins of the pampiniform venous plexus in the scrotum (the network of veins from the testis and the epididymis, which constitute part of the spermatic cord)

vasectomy: also called male sterilization; ligation and transection of part of the vas deferens, with or without removal of a segment of the vas, to prevent the passage of the sperm from the testes

Disorders of the male reproductive system include a wide variety of conditions that usually affect both urinary and reproductive systems. Because these disorders involve the genitalia and often affect sexuality, the patient may experience anxiety and embarrassment. The nurse must be aware of the patient's need for privacy as well as his need for education and support. This requires an openness to discuss critical and sensitive issues with the patient, including his partner when appropriate, as well as effective assessment, management, and communication. Nurses must be comfortable when examining male genitalia and must recognize their own attitudes and perceptions about male reproductive problems. Education of the patient and partner about treatment and self-care strategies is essential (Zang, Chung & Wong, 2008).

ASSESSMENT OF THE MALE REPRODUCTIVE SYSTEM

Anatomic and Physiologic Overview

In the male, several organs serve as parts of both the urinary tract and the reproductive system. Disorders in the male reproductive organs may interfere with the functions of one or both of these systems. As a result, diseases of the male reproductive system are usually treated by a urologist. The structures in the male reproductive system include the (1) external male genitalia, consisting of the testes, epididymides, scrotum, and penis, and the (2) internal male genitalia, consisting of the vas deferens (ductus deferens), ejaculatory duct, and prostatic and membranous sections of the urethra, seminal vesicles, and certain accessory glands, such as the prostate gland and Cowper glands (bulbourethral glands) (Fig. 49-1).

The testes have a dual function: **spermatogenesis** (production of sperm) and secretion of the male sex hormone **testosterone,** which induces and preserves the male sex characteristics. The testes are formed in the embryo, within the abdominal cavity, near the kidney. During the last month of fetal life, they descend posterior to the peritoneum and pierce the abdominal wall in the groin. Later, they progress along the inguinal canal into the scrotal sac. In this descent, they are accompanied by blood vessels, lymphatics, nerves, and ducts, which support the tissue and make up the spermatic cord. This cord extends from the internal inguinal ring through the abdominal wall and the inguinal canal to the scrotum. As the testes descend into the scrotum, a tubular extension of peritoneum accompanies them. Normally, this tissue is obliterated during fetal development; only the tunica vaginalis, which covers the testes, remains. If the peritoneal process remains open into the abdominal cavity, a potential sac remains into which abdominal contents may enter to form an indirect inguinal hernia.

The testes, or ovoid sex glands, are encased in the scrotum, which keeps them at a slightly lower temperature than the rest of the body to facilitate spermatogenesis. The testes consist of numerous seminiferous tubules in which the spermatozoa form. Collecting tubules transmit the spermatozoa into the epididymis, a hoodlike structure lying on the testes and containing winding ducts that lead into the vas deferens. This firm, tubular structure passes upward through the inguinal canal to enter the abdominal cavity behind the peritoneum. It then extends downward toward the base of the bladder. An outpouching from this structure is the seminal vesicle, which acts as a reservoir for testicular secretions. The tract is continued as the ejaculatory duct, which passes through the prostate gland to enter the urethra. Testicular secretions take this pathway when they exit the penis during ejaculation.

The penis is the organ for both copulation and urination. It consists of the glans penis, the body, and the root. The glans penis is the soft, rounded portion at the distal end of the penis. The urethra, the tube that carries urine, opens at the tip of the glans. The glans is naturally covered by elongated penile skin—the foreskin—which may be retracted to expose the glans. However, many men as newborns have had the foreskin removed (**circumcision**). The body of the

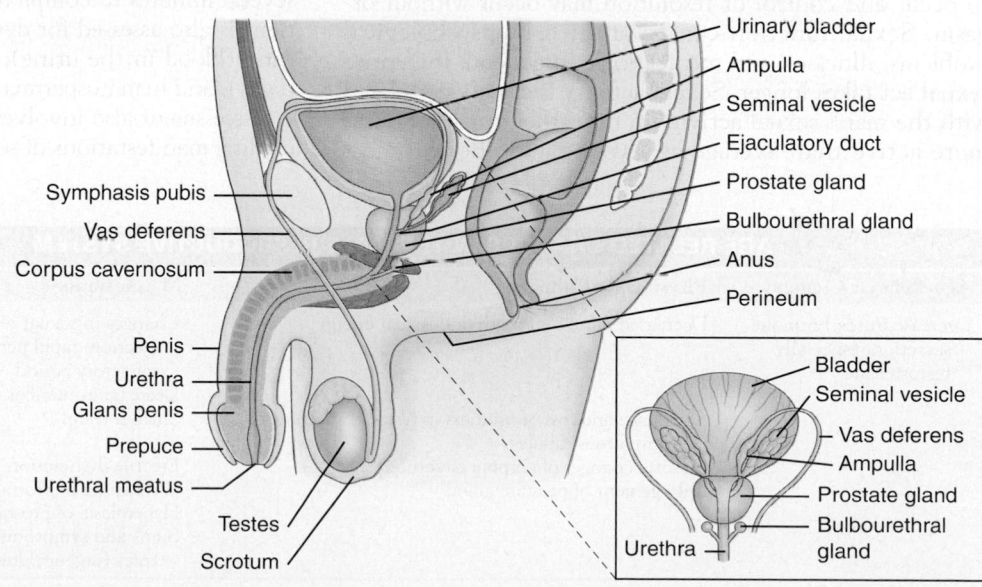

Figure 49-1 Structures of the male reproductive system.

Labels (main figure): Symphasis pubis, Vas deferens, Corpus cavernosum, Penis, Urethra, Glans penis, Prepuce, Urethral meatus, Testes, Scrotum, Urinary bladder, Ampulla, Seminal vesicle, Ejaculatory duct, Prostate gland, Bulbourethral gland, Anus, Perineum

Labels (inset): Bladder, Seminal vesicle, Vas deferens, Ampulla, Prostate gland, Bulbourethral gland, Urethra

penis is composed of erectile tissues containing numerous blood vessels that become dilated, leading to an erection during sexual excitement. The urethra, which passes through the penis, extends from the bladder through the prostate to the distal end of the penis.

The prostate gland, lying just below the neck of the bladder, is composed of four zones and four lobes. It surrounds the urethra and is traversed by the ejaculatory duct, a continuation of the vas deferens. This gland produces a secretion that is chemically and physiologically suitable to the needs of the spermatozoa in their passage from the testes. Cowper glands lie below the prostate, within the posterior aspect of the urethra. This gland empties its secretions into the urethra during ejaculation, providing lubrication.

 ### Gerontologic Considerations

As men age, the prostate gland enlarges, prostate secretion decreases; the scrotum hangs lower; the testes decrease in weight, atrophy, and become softer; and pubic hair becomes sparser and stiffer. Changes in gonadal function include a decline in plasma testosterone levels and reduced production of progesterone (Table 49-1). Other changes include decreasing sexual function, decreased libido (sexual desire), slower sexual response, longer time before sexual arousal can occur again, increased incidence of genitourinary tract cancer, and urinary incontinence. Libido and potency often decrease in as many as two thirds of men older than 70 years of age (Tabloski, 2006). Vascular problems cause about half of the cases of impotence in men older than 50 years of age.

However, male reproductive capability is maintained with advancing age. Although degenerative changes occur in the seminiferous tubules and sperm production decreases, spermatogenesis continues, allowing men to produce viable sperm throughout their lives (McCance & Huether, 2005).

Male hypogonadism (decreased function of the testes) starts gradually at approximately 50 years of age, resulting in decreased testosterone production. The older man notices that the sexual response slows, erection takes longer, full erections may not be attained, and ejaculation takes longer to occur and control or resolution may occur without orgasm. Sexual function can be affected by psychological problems, illnesses, and medications. In general, the entire sexual act takes longer. Sexual activity is closely correlated with the man's sexual activity in his earlier years; if he was more active than average as a young man, he will most

likely continue to be more active than average in his later years.

Men older than 50 years of age are at risk for cancer of the kidney, bladder, prostate, and penis. The digital rectal examination (DRE), prostate-specific antigen (PSA) test, and urinalysis, which screens for hematuria, may uncover a higher percentage of malignancies at earlier stages and lead to lower treatment-associated morbidity as well as a lower mortality.

Urinary incontinence occurs in one fifth of community-dwelling older men and rises to nearly 50% in men in long-term care settings (Tabloski, 2006). Therefore, older adults admitted to acute care settings should be screened for this problem. Urinary incontinence may have many causes, including medications, neurologic disease, or benign prostatic hyperplasia (BPH). Diagnostic tests are performed to exclude reversible causes. New-onset urinary incontinence is a nursing priority that requires evaluation.

Assessment

Health History

Male sexuality is a complex phenomenon that is strongly influenced by personal, cultural, religious, and social factors. Sexuality and male reproductive function become concerns in the presence of illness and disability (Bruner & Calvano, 2007). Throughout the assessment process, the nurse must recognize the importance of sexuality to the patient. Assessment of male reproductive function begins with an evaluation of urinary function and symptoms. The patient is asked about his usual state of health and any recent change in general physical and sexual activity. Any symptoms or changes in function are explored fully and described in detail. Symptoms related to bladder function and urination, collectively referred to as **prostatism,** are explored further. They may occur with an obstruction caused by an enlarged prostate gland: increased urinary frequency, decreased force of urine stream, and "double" or "triple" voiding (the patient needs to urinate two or three times over a period of several minutes to completely empty his bladder). The patient is also assessed for dysuria (painful urination), hematuria (blood in the urine), nocturia (urination during the night), and hematospermia (blood in the ejaculate).

Assessment also involves addressing sexual function, including manifestations of sexual dysfunction. The extent of

Table 49-1	AGE-RELATED CHANGES IN THE MALE REPRODUCTIVE SYSTEM	
Age-Related Changes	**Physiologic Changes**	**Manifestations**
Decrease in sex hormone secretion, especially testosterone	Decreased muscle strength and sexual energy	Changes in sexual response: prolonged time to reach full erection, rapid penile detumescence and prolonged refractory period
		Decrease in number of viable sperm
	Shrinkage and loss of firmness of testes; thickening of seminiferous tubules	Smaller testes
	Fibrotic changes of corpora cavernosa	Erectile dysfunction
	Enlargement of prostate gland	Weakening of prostatic contractions
		Hyperplasia of prostate gland
		Signs and symptoms of obstruction of lower urinary tract (urgency, frequency, nocturia)

the history depends on the patient's presenting symptoms and the presence of factors that may affect sexual function such as chronic illnesses or disability (eg, diabetes, multiple sclerosis, stroke, cardiac disease), use of medications that affect sexual function (eg, antihypertensive and anticholesterolemic medications, psychotropic agents), stress, use of alcohol, and patient's willingness to discuss sexual issues.

By initiating an assessment about sexual concerns, the nurse conveys the message that changes in sexual functioning are valid topics and provides a safe environment for discussing these sensitive topics. A number of models are available to assist in assessing patient's problems and concerns. The PLISSIT (permission, limited information, specific suggestions, intensive therapy) model of sexual assessment and intervention may be used to provide a framework for nursing interventions (Annon, 1976). It provides a graded counseling approach that allows health care professionals to deal with sexual issues with a level of comfort and expertise. The model begins by asking the patient's permission (P) to discuss sexual functioning. Limited information (LI) about sexual function may then be provided to the patient. As the discussion progresses, the nurse may offer specific suggestions (SS) for interventions. A professional who specializes in sex therapy may provide more intensive therapy (IT) as needed. The BETTER (bringing up the topic, explaining, telling, timing, educate about treatment-related sexual side effects, recording) model was developed more recently to assist health care professionals to include sexuality in the assessment of patients with cancer (Katz, 2005, 2007).

Patients may find it difficult to express their feelings and concerns regarding their sexuality, especially after a body image change. Discussing sexuality with patients who have an illness or disability can be uncomfortable for nurses and other health care providers; this, in turn, makes discussion of these issues more difficult and uncomfortable for patients. Health care professionals may unconsciously have stereotypes about the sexuality of people who are ill or have a disability (eg, the belief that people with disabilities are asexual or should be sexually inactive). In addition, patients are often embarrassed to initiate a discussion about sexual issues with their health care providers (Zang, et al., 2008).

Physical Assessment

In addition to the usual aspects of the physical examination, two essential components address disorders of the male genital or reproductive system: the DRE and the testicular examination.

Digital Rectal Examination

The DRE is used to screen for prostate cancer and is recommended annually for every man older than 50 years of age (45 years of age for men at high risk [African American men and men with a strong family history of prostate cancer]) annually (American Cancer Society [ACS], 2009). The DRE enables the skilled examiner, using a lubricated, gloved finger placed in the rectum, to assess the size, symmetry, shape, and consistency of the posterior surface of the prostate gland (Fig. 49-2). The clinician assesses for tenderness of the prostate gland on palpation and for the presence and consistency of any nodules. The DRE may be performed with the patient leaning over an examination table or positioning the man in a

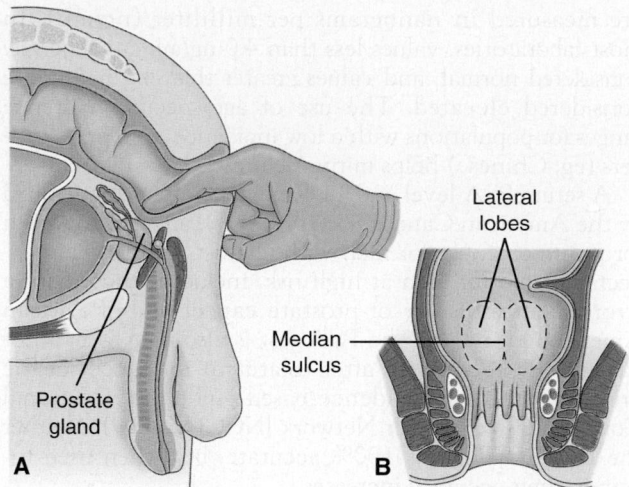

Figure 49-2 A, Palpation of the prostate gland during digital rectal examination (DRE) enables the examiner to assess the size, shape, and texture of the gland. **B,** The prostate is round, with a palpable median sulcus or groove separating the lateral lobes. It should feel rubbery and free of nodules and masses.

side-lying position with legs flexed toward the abdomen or supine with legs resting in stirrups. To minimize discomfort and relax the anal sphincter during the rectal examination, the patient is instructed to take a deep breath and exhale slowly as the practitioner inserts a finger. If possible, he should turn his feet inward so his toes are touching. Although this examination may be uncomfortable and embarrassing for the patient, it is an important screening tool.

Testicular Examination

The male genitalia are inspected for abnormalities and palpated for masses. The scrotum is palpated carefully for nodules, masses, or inflammation. Examination of the scrotum can reveal such disorders as hydrocele, inguinal hernia, testicular torsion, orchitis, epididymitis, or a tumor of the testis. The penis is inspected and palpated for ulcerations, nodules, inflammation, discharge, and curvature. If the patient is uncircumcised, the foreskin should be retracted for visualization of the glans penis. The testicular examination provides an excellent opportunity to instruct the patient on how to perform a testicular self-examination (TSE) and its importance in early detection of testicular cancer. TSE should begin during adolescence.

Diagnostic Evaluation

Prostate-Specific Antigen Test

The cells within the prostate gland produce a protein that can be measured in the blood called the **prostate-specific antigen (PSA).** It is a sensitive but not specific test for prostate cancer. In the absence of prostate cancer, serum PSA levels vary with age, race, and prostate volume. Increased levels may indicate prostate cancer. However, a number of other conditions such as BPH, acute urinary retention, and acute prostatitis may cause high PSA levels. Values of PSA may also increase after ejaculation. PSA levels are measured in nanograms per milliliter (ng/mL). In most laboratories, values less than 4.0 ng/mL are generally considered normal, and values greater than 4.0 ng/mL are considered elevated. The use of age-specific reference ranges for populations with a low incidence of prostate cancers (eg, Chinese) helps minimize unnecessary biopsies.

A serum PSA level and a DRE, which are recommended by the American Cancer Society (2009), are used to screen for prostate cancer for men with at least a 10-year life expectancy and for men at high risk, including those with a strong family history of prostate cancer and of African American ethnicity. The PSA test is also used to monitor patients for recurrence after treatment for cancer of the prostate, based on evidence-based guidelines (National Comprehensive Cancer Network [NCCN], 2009). Neither the DRE nor PSA is 100% accurate, but when used together, their accuracy increases.

Ultrasonography

Transrectal ultrasound (TRUS) may be performed in patients with abnormalities detected by DRE and in those with elevated PSA levels. After DRE has been completed, a lubricated, condom-covered, rectal probe transducer is inserted into the rectum, along the anterior wall. Water may be introduced into the condom to help transmit sound waves to the prostate. TRUS may be used in detecting nonpalpable prostate cancers and in staging localized prostate cancer. Needle biopsies of the prostate are commonly guided by TRUS.

Prostate Fluid or Tissue Analysis

Specimens of prostate fluid or tissue may be obtained for culture if disease or inflammation of the prostate gland is suspected. A biopsy of the prostate gland may be necessary to obtain tissue for histologic examination. This may be performed at the time of prostatectomy or by means of a perineal or transrectal needle biopsy. Six to 12 biopsies from all four prostate zones may be obtained during a TRUS-guided biopsy.

Tests of Male Sexual Function

If the patient cannot engage in sexual intercourse to his satisfaction, a detailed history is obtained. Nocturnal erections occur in healthy males of all ages. Nocturnal penile tumescence tests may be conducted in a sleep laboratory to monitor changes in penile circumference during sleep using various methods to determine number, duration, rigidity, and circumference of penile erections; the results help identify whether the erectile dysfunction is caused by physiologic or psychologic factors. Additional tests, including psychological evaluations, are also part of the diagnostic workup and are usually conducted by a specialized team of health care providers.

DISORDERS OF MALE SEXUAL FUNCTION

Erectile Dysfunction

Erectile dysfunction, also called impotence, is the inability to achieve or maintain an erect penis (Seftel, Miner, Kloner, et al., 2007). The man may report decreased frequency of erections, inability to achieve a firm erection, or rapid detumescence (subsiding of erection). In the United States, 30 million men experience erectile dysfunction; more than half of men 40 to 70 years of age are unable to attain or maintain an erection sufficient for satisfactory sexual performance (Tanagho & McAninch, 2008). The physiology of erection and ejaculation is complex and involves parasympathetic and sympathetic components. Erection involves the release of nitric oxide into the corpus cavernosum during sexual stimulation. Its release activates cyclic guanosine monophosphate (cGMP), causing smooth muscle relaxation. This allows flow of blood into the corpus cavernosum, resulting in erection (Beckman, Abu-Lebdeh & Mynderse, 2006; Porth & Matfin, 2009).

Erectile dysfunction has both psychogenic and organic causes. Psychogenic causes include anxiety, fatigue, depression, pressure to perform sexually, negative body image, absence of desire, privacy, and trust and relationship issues. Organic causes include cardiovascular disease, endocrine disease (diabetes, pituitary tumors, testosterone deficiency, hyperthyroidism, and hypothyroidism), cirrhosis, chronic renal failure, genitourinary conditions (radical pelvic surgery), hematologic conditions (Hodgkin lymphoma, leukemia), neurologic disorders (neuropathies, parkinsonism, spinal cord injury, multiple sclerosis), trauma to the pelvic or genital area, alcohol, smoking, medications (Chart 49-1), and drug abuse.

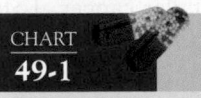

CHART 49-1

PHARMACOLOGY
Classes of Medications Associated With Erectile Dysfunction

- Antiadrenergics and antihypertensives: guanethidine (Ismelin), clonidine (Catapres), hydralazine (Apresoline), metoprolol (Lopressor)
- Anticholinergics and phenothiazines: prochlorperazine (Compazine), trihexyphenidyl (Artane)
- Antiseizure agents: carbamazepine (Tegretol)
- Antifungals: ketoconazole (Nizoral)
- Antihormone (prostate cancer treatment): flutamide (Eulexin), leuprolide (Lupron)
- Antipsychotics: haloperidol (Haldol), chlorpromazine (Thorazine)
- Antispasmodics: oxybutynin (Ditropan)
- Anxiolytics, sedative–hypnotics, tranquilizers: lorazepam (Ativan), triazolam (Halcion)

- Beta-blockers: nadolol (Corgard)
- Calcium channel blockers: nifedipine (Adalat, Procardia)
- Carbonic anhydrase inhibitors: acetazolamide (Diamox)
- H₂ antagonists: nizatidine (Axid)
- Nonsteroidal anti-inflammatory drugs: naproxen (Naprosyn)
- Diuretics: hydrochlorothiazide (HydroDIURIL), furosemide (Lasix), spironolactone (Aldactone)
- Antidepressants: tricyclic antidepressants: amitriptyline (Elavil), desipramine (Norpramin); selective serotonin reuptake inhibitors: fluoxetine (Prozac), sertraline (Zoloft)
- Parkinson's disease medications: levodopa (Sinemet)
- Antihistamines: diphenhydramine (Benadryl)

Assessment and Diagnostic Findings

The diagnosis of erectile dysfunction requires a sexual and medical history; an analysis of presenting symptoms; a physical examination, including a neurologic examination; a detailed assessment of all medications, alcohol, and drugs used; and various laboratory studies. Nocturnal penile tumescence tests are conducted to monitor changes in penile circumference. This test can help to determine if erectile impotence has an organic or a psychological cause. In healthy men, nocturnal penile erections closely parallel rapid eye movement (REM) sleep in occurrence and duration. Organically impotent men show inadequate sleep-related erections that correspond to their waking performance. Arterial blood flow to the penis is measured using a Doppler probe. In addition, nerve conduction tests and extensive psychological evaluations may be carried out. Figure 49-3 describes the evaluation and treatment of erectile dysfunction.

Medical Management

Treatment can be medical, surgical, or both, depending on the cause. The American Urological Association (AUA) guidelines on treatment of erectile dysfunction suggest that therapy for associated disorders (eg, alcoholism, diabetes) or adjustment of medications may be necessary (AUA, 2005). Endocrine therapy instituted to treat erectile dysfunction secondary to hypothalamic-pituitary-gonadal dysfunction may reverse the condition. Insufficient penile blood flow may be treated with vascular surgery. Patients with erectile dysfunction from psychogenic causes are referred to a health care provider or therapist who specializes in sexual dysfunction. Patients with erectile dysfunction secondary to organic causes may be candidates for penile implants.

Currently available therapies for the treatment of erectile dysfunction include pharmacologic therapy (including urethral suppositories), penile implants, and vacuum constriction devices (Table 49-2). These options should be considered in a stepwise fashion, with increasing invasiveness and risk balanced against the likelihood of efficacy. The patient and, if possible, his partner, should be informed of the relevant treatment options and their associated risks and benefits. The choice of treatment is made jointly by the physician, patient, and partner, taking into consideration patient preferences and expectations.

Pharmacologic Therapy

Phosphodiesterase-5 (PDE-5) inhibitors, oral medications that are used to treat erectile dysfunction, are first-line therapy (AUA, 2005). Currently available PDE-5 inhibitors include sildenafil (Viagra), vardenafil (Levitra), and tadalafil (Cialis). Each of these agents has a similar mechanism of action but a different pharmacologic action and clinical use. Erection involves the release of nitrous oxide in the vasculature of the corpus cavernosum as a result of sexual stimulation. This subsequently leads to smooth muscle relaxation in blood vessels supplying the corpus cavernosum, resulting in increased blood flow and an erection. During sexual stimulation, PDE-5 inhibitors increase blood flow to the penis (Carson, 2007; Porth & Matfin, 2009).

When PDE-5 inhibitors are taken about 1 hour before sexual activity, they are effective in producing an erection with

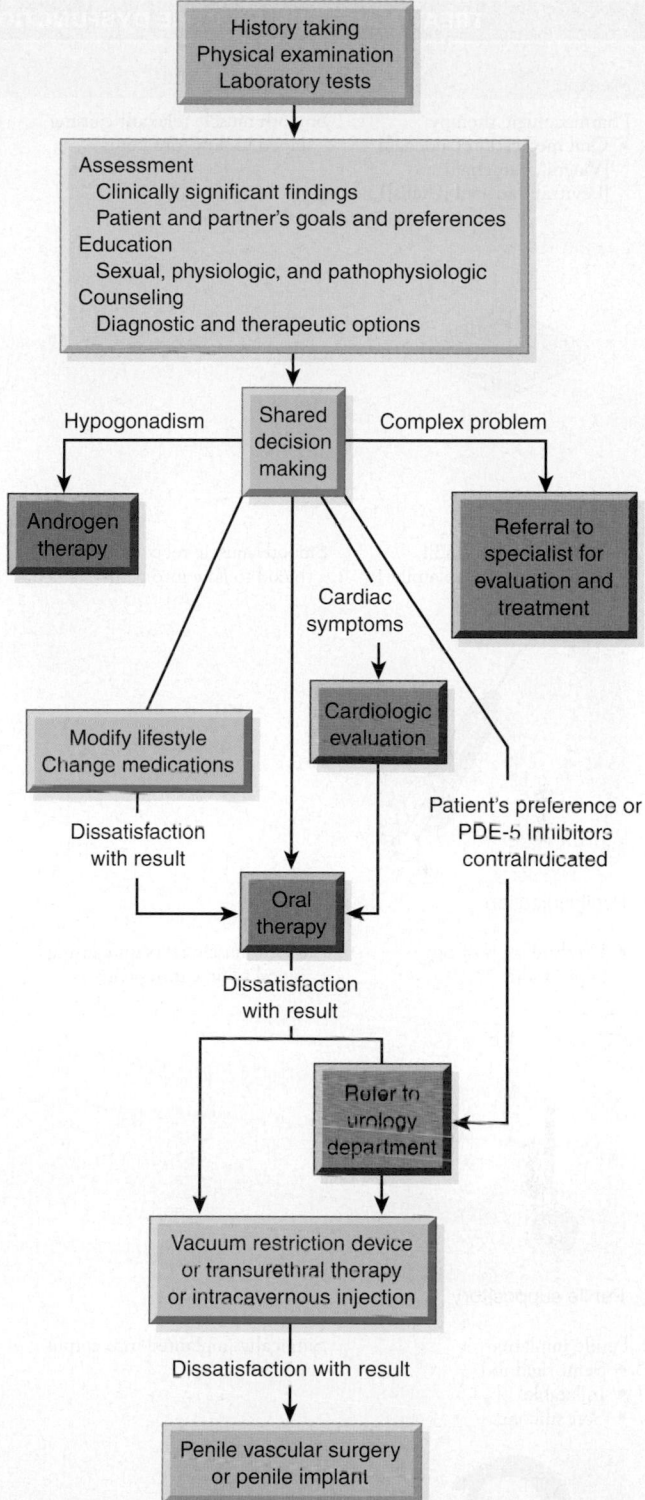

Figure 49-3 Evaluation and treatment of men with erectile dysfunction. (Redrawn from Lue, T. F. (2000). Erectile dysfunction. *New England Journal of Medicine, 342*(24), 1807. © 2000 Massachusetts Medical Society. All rights reserved. Used with permission.)

sexual stimulation; the erection can last about 1 to 2 hours. The most common side effects of these medications include headache, flushing, dyspepsia, diarrhea, nasal congestion, and lightheadedness. These agents are contraindicated in men

Table 49-2   TREATMENTS FOR ERECTILE DYSFUNCTION

Method	Description	Advantages and Disadvantages	Duration
Pharmacologic therapy • Oral medication (sildenafil [Viagra]; vardenafil [Levitra]; tadalafil [Cialis])	Smooth muscle relaxant causing blood to flow into penis	Can cause headache and diarrhea Contraindicated for men taking nitrate medications Used with caution in patients with retinopathy, especially diabetic retinopathy	Taken orally 1 hour before intercourse Stimulation is required to achieve erection Erection can last 1 hour

Oral medication

Method	Description	Advantages and Disadvantages	Duration
• Injection (alprostadil, papaverine, phentolamine)	Smooth muscle relaxant causing blood to flow into penis	Firm erections are achievable in more than 50% of cases Pain at injection site; plaque formation, risk of priapism	Injection 20 minutes before intercourse Erection can last up to 1 hour

Penile injection

Method	Description	Advantages and Disadvantages	Duration
• Urethral suppository (alprostadil)	Smooth muscle relaxant causing blood to flow into penis	May be used twice a day Urethral and genital pain; risk of hypertension and syncope Not recommended with pregnant partners	Inserted 10 minutes before intercourse Erection can last up to 1 hour

Penile suppository

Method	Description	Advantages and Disadvantages	Duration
Penile implants • Semi-rigid rod • Inflatable • Soft silicone	Surgically implanted into corpus cavernosum	Reliable Requires surgery Healing takes up to 3 weeks Subsequent cystoscopic surgery is difficult Semirigid rod results in permanent semierection	Indefinite Inflatable prosthesis: saline returns from penile receptacle to reservoir

Penile implant

Table 49-2	TREATMENTS FOR ERECTILE DYSFUNCTION (Continued)		
Method	Description	Advantages and Disadvantages	Duration
Negative-pressure (vacuum) devices	Induction of erection with vacuum; maintained with constriction band around base of penis	Few side effects Cumbersome to use before intercourse Vasocongestion of penis can cause pain or numbness	To prevent penile injury, constriction band must not be left in place for longer than 1 hour

Penile vacuum pump

who take organic nitrates (eg, isosorbide [Isordil, Nitro-Dur], nitroglycerin), because taken together, these medications can cause side effects such as severe hypotension (Beckman, et al., 2006; Carson, 2007; Porth & Matfin, 2009). In addition, PDE-5 inhibitors must be used with caution in patients with retinopathy, especially in those with diabetic retinopathy. Patient teaching about the use of these medications and their side effects is summarized in Table 49-3.

For patients in whom PDE-5 inhibitors are contraindicated or ineffective, other pharmacologic measures to induce erections include injecting vasoactive agents, such as alprostadil, papaverine, and phentolamine, directly into the penis. Complications include **priapism** (a persistent abnormal erection) and development of fibrotic plaques at the injection sites. Alprostadil is also formulated in a gel pellet that can be inserted into the tip of the urethra using an applicator to create an erection.

Penile Implants

Two general types of penile implants are available: the malleable, noninflatable, nonhydraulic prosthesis (also called the semirigid rod); and the inflatable, hydraulic prostheses (AUA, 2006; Henry & Wilson, 2007). The semirigid rod (eg, the Small-Carrion prosthesis) results in a permanent semierection but can be bent into an unnoticeable position when appropriate. The inflatable prosthesis simulates natural erections and natural flaccidity. Complications after implantation include infection, erosion of the prosthesis through the skin (more common with the semirigid rod than with the inflatable prosthesis), and persistent pain, which may require removal of the implant. Subsequent cystoscopic surgery, such as transurethral resection of the prostate (TURP), is more difficult with a semirigid rod than with the inflatable prosthesis.

Factors to consider in choosing a penile prosthesis are the patient's activities of daily living, social activities, and the expectations of the patient and his partner. Ongoing counseling for the patient and his partner is usually necessary to help them adapt to the prosthesis.

Negative-Pressure Devices

Negative-pressure (vacuum) devices may also be used to induce an erection. A plastic cylinder is placed over the flaccid penis, and negative pressure is applied. When an erection is attained, a constriction band is placed around the base of the penis to maintain the erection. The patient is instructed not to leave the constricting band in place for longer than 1 hour to avoid penile injury. Only devices with a vacuum limiter are recommended for use (AUA, 2005). Although many men find this method satisfactory, others experience premature loss of penile rigidity or pain when applying suction or during intercourse.

Nursing Management

Personal satisfaction and the ability to sexually satisfy a partner are common concerns of patients. Men with illnesses and disabilities may need the assistance of a sex therapist to identify, implement, and integrate their sexual beliefs and behaviors into a healthy and satisfying lifestyle. The nurse can inform patients about support groups for men with erectile dysfunction and their partners. Information about Impotence Anonymous for patients and I-Anon for their partners can be found at the end of this chapter.

Disorders of Ejaculation

Premature ejaculation (PE) is defined as the occurrence of ejaculation sooner than desired, either before or shortly after penetration, causing distress to either one or both partners (AUA, 2004). It is one of the most common complaints of men or couples, affecting 20% to 30% of men (Schuster, 2006; Waldinger, 2007). The spectrum of responses ranges from occasional ejaculation with intercourse or self-stimulation to complete inability to ejaculate under any circumstances. A variety of forms of PE have been identified: (1) lifelong PE caused by neurobiological or genetic conditions, (2) acquired PE (medical or psychological), (3) natural variable PE (normal variation), and (4) premature-like ejaculatory dysfunction (psychological). Other ejaculatory problems may include inhibited (delayed or retarded) ejaculation, which is the involuntary inhibition of the ejaculatory reflex. Retrograde ejaculation occurs when semen travels toward the bladder instead of exiting through the penis, resulting in infertility. This form of PE may occur after prior prostate or urethral surgery or with diabetes and use of medications such as antihypertensives.

Table 49-3   **PHARMACOLOGIC TREATMENT OF ERECTILE DYSFUNCTION**

	Sildenafil (Viagra)	Vardenafil (Levitra)	Tadalafil (Cialis)
Recommended dose	Initial dose is 25 mg Usual dose is 50 mg Maximal dose is 100 mg/24 hours	Usual dose is 10 mg Maximum dose is 20 mg/24 hours If you are 65 years of age or older, the starting dose is 5 mg	Dosage range is 5–20 mg, based on individual response Maximum dose is 20 mg/24 hours Maximum dose is 10 mg every 48 hours if you have decreased liver or kidney function
When to take	Take the medication 30 minutes to 4 hours before intercourse. *There must be sexual stimulation to produce an erection.*	Follow the same directions as with sildenafil; take the medication 1 hour before intercourse. The peak action occurs in 30 to 120 minutes. *There must be sexual stimulation to produce an erection.*	Take the medication before sexual activity. Effect peaks at 30 minutes to 6 hours; effect may last up to 36 hours. *There must be sexual stimulation to produce an erection.*
Frequency of use	If you take this medication more than once a day, it will not have an increased effect. You may take it 7 days per week if you wish, but only once in 24 hours. It does not build up in your bloodstream. Remember to take it only when you want to have intercourse.	The recommended frequency for this medication is 10 mg in 24 hours.	The effects of this medication may last up to 36 hours. This allows for increased spontaneity in the sexual experience.
Side effects	Side effects include headache, flushing, indigestion, nasal congestion, abnormal vision, diarrhea, dizziness, and rash. You may also have low blood sugar and abnormal liver function tests; your physician can determine this.	Side effects include headache, flushing, runny nose, indigestion, sinusitis, flulike syndrome, dizziness, nausea, back pain, and joint pain. Tell your physician if you experience any of these effects. You may also have abnormally elevated liver enzymes; your physician can determine this.	Side effects are similar to those of sildenafil and vardenafil. Tadalafil may also cause back pain and muscle aches. Tell your physician if you experience any of these side effects.
Contraindications	Do not take if you are taking nitrate medications such as nitroglycerine (eg, Nitro-Bid) or isosorbide mononitrate (eg, Imdur). Do not take if you have high uncontrolled blood pressure, coronary artery disease, or have had a heart attack within the past 6 months. Do not take if you have been diagnosed with a cardiac dysrhythmia or kidney or liver dysfunction.		
Drug interactions	This medication can react with other medications that you may be taking. Provide your physician and pharmacist with a complete list of all prescribed as well as over-the-counter medications that you are using.		
Use of PDE-5 inhibitors with penile injections or urethral suppositories	The use of PDE-5 inhibitors with other forms of therapy for erectile dysfunction has not been tested and should be avoided.		

Evaluation of PE involves a thorough sexual history focusing on the duration of symptoms, time to ejaculation, degree of voluntary control over ejaculation, frequency of occurrence, and course of the problem since the first sexual encounter (Schuster, 2006; Waldinger, 2007). Treatment, which depends on the nature and severity of PE and perceived distress it causes, includes behavioral and psychological approaches, as well as pharmacologic therapy that attempts to alter the sensory input or retard the ejaculatory response. Behavioral therapy (eg, counseling, sex therapy, psychoeducation, and couples therapy) often involves both the man and his sexual partner. The couple is encouraged to identify their sexual needs and to communicate those needs to each other. Pharmacologic management involves selective serotonin reuptake inhibitors, alpha$_1$ adrenoceptor antagonists, the tricyclic antidepressant clomipramine (Anafranil), and topical anesthetics. In some cases, a combination of pharmacologic and behavioral therapy may be effective.

Inhibited ejaculation is most often caused by psychological factors, neurologic disorders (eg, spinal cord injury [SCI], multiple sclerosis, neuropathy secondary to diabetes), surgery (prostatectomy), and medications. Chemical, vibratory, and electrical methods of stimulation have been used with some success. Treatment usually addresses the physical and psychological factors involved in inhibited ejaculation (Schuster, 2006). Although outpatient therapy may involve numerous sessions (12 to 18), it often results in a success rate of 70% to 80%. The outcome depends on a previous satisfying sexual experience history, a short duration of the ejaculatory problem, feelings of sexual desire, feelings of attraction to one's sexual partner, motivation for treatment, and absence of serious psychological problems.

For men with retrograde ejaculation, the urine may be collected shortly after ejaculation, revealing a large amount of sperm in the urine. This urine may also be collected to obtain adequate viable sperm for use in artificial insemination. In men with SCI, techniques that may be used to obtain sperm for artificial insemination include self-stimulation, vibratory stimulation, or electroejaculation. Electroejaculation involves the use of a specially designed probe that is inserted into the rectum next to the prostate. The probe delivers a current that stimulates the nerves and produces contraction of the pelvic muscles and ejaculation. However, spontaneous or stimulated ejaculation may cause autonomic dysreflexia (AD) (overstimulation of the autonomic nervous system) in patients with SCI at T6 or above, creating a life-threatening situation. If this disorder is not treated promptly, it may lead to seizures, stroke, and even death.

INFECTIONS OF THE MALE GENITOURINARY TRACT

Acute uncomplicated cystitis in adult men is uncommon but occasionally occurs in men whose sexual partners have vaginal infections with *Escherichia coli*. Asymptomatic bacteriuria may also result from genitourinary manipulation, catheterization, or instrumentation. Urinary tract infections (UTIs) are discussed in Chapter 45.

According to the Centers for Disease Control and Prevention (CDC, 2008), more than 19 million people develop sexually transmitted diseases (STDs) or sexually transmitted infections (STIs) annually in the United States; almost half of all STDs occur in people 18 to 24 years of age. The incidence of STDs has declined over the past several years, except in specific populations, including men who have sex with men. STDs affect people from all walks of life—from all social, educational, economic, and racial backgrounds. The single greatest risk factor for contracting an STD is the number of sexual partners. As the number of partners increases, so does the risk of exposure to a person infected with an STD. For men who have sex with men, the CDC recommends annual testing for human immunodeficiency virus (HIV), syphilis, *Chlamydia*, and gonorrhea (CDC, 2006).

Several diseases are classified as STDs: urethritis (gonococcal and nongonococcal), genital ulcers (genital herpes infections, primary syphilis, chancroid, granuloma inguinale, and lymphogranuloma venereum), genital warts (human papillomavirus [HPV]), scabies, pediculosis pubis, molluscum contagiosum, hepatitis and enteric infections, proctitis, and acquired immunodeficiency syndrome (AIDS). Trichomoniasis and STDs characterized by genital ulcers are thought to increase susceptibility to HIV infection. Trichomoniasis is associated with nonchlamydial, nongonococcal urethritis.

Current treatment guidelines for STDs are available from the CDC (2006, 2007). Treatment must target the patient as well as his sexual partners and sometimes an unborn child. A thorough history, including a sexual history, is crucial to identify patients at risk and to direct care and teaching. Partners of men with STDs must also be examined, treated, and counseled to prevent reinfection and complications in both partners and to limit the spread of the disease. Sexual abstinence during treatment and recovery is advised to prevent the transmission of STDs. Use of synthetic condoms for at least 6 months after completion of treatment is recommended to decrease transmission of HPV infection as well as other STDs. It is important to assess and test for other STDs because patients who have one STD may also have another. Use of spermicides with nonoxynol 9 (known as N-9) is discouraged; these agents do not protect against HIV infection and may increase the risk of transmission of the virus. See Chapters 52 and 70 for more detailed discussions of HIV infection and AIDS and other STDs.

CONDITIONS OF THE PROSTATE

Prostatitis

Prostatitis is an inflammation of the prostate gland that is often associated with lower urinary tract symptoms and symptoms of sexual discomfort and dysfunction. The condition affects 5% to 10% of men. It is the most common urologic diagnosis in men younger than 50 years of age and the third most common such diagnosis in men older than 50 years (Potts & Payne, 2007; Wein, Kavoussi, Novick, et al., 2007). Prostatitis may be caused by infectious agents (bacteria, fungi, mycoplasma) or other conditions (eg, urethral stricture, benign prostatic hyperplasia). *E. coli* is the most commonly isolated organism, although *Klebsiella* and *Proteus* species are also found (Potts & Payne, 2007). The micro-organisms colonize the urinary tract and ascend to the prostate, ultimately causing infection. The causal pathogen is usually the same in recurrent infections.

There are four types of prostatitis: acute bacterial prostatitis (type I); chronic bacterial prostatitis (type II); chronic prostatitis/chronic pelvic pain syndrome (CP/CPPS) (type III), and asymptomatic inflammatory prostatitis (type IV). Type III, which occurs in more than 90% of cases, is further classified as type IIIA or type IIIB, depending on the presence (type IIIA) or absence (type IIIB) of white blood cells in semen after prostate massage.

Clinical Manifestations

Acute prostatitis is characterized by the sudden onset of fever, dysuria, perineal prostatic pain and severe lower urinary tract symptoms: dysuria, frequency, urgency, hesitancy, and nocturia. Approximately 5% of cases of type I prostatitis (acute prostatitis) progress to type II prostatitis (chronic bacterial prostatitis) (Wein, et al., 2007). Patients with type II disease are typically asymptomatic between episodes. Patients with type III prostatitis often have no bacteria in the urine in the presence of genitourinary pain. Patients with type IV prostatitis are usually diagnosed incidentally during a workup for infertility, an elevated PSA test, or other disorders.

Medical Management

The goal of treatment is to eradicate the causal organisms. Hospital admission may be necessary for patients with unstable vital signs, sepsis, or intractable pelvic pain; those who are frail or immunosuppressed; or those who have diabetes or renal insufficiency. Specific treatment is based on the type of prostatitis and on the results of culture and sensitivity testing of the urine (Potts & Payne, 2007). If bacteria are cultured from the urine, antibiotics, including trimethoprim-sulfamethoxazole (TMP-SMZ) or a fluoroquinolone (eg, ciprofloxacin [Cipro]), may be prescribed, and continuous therapy with low-dose antibiotics may be used to suppress the infection. If the patient is afebrile and has a normal urinalysis, anti-inflammatory agents may be used. Alpha-adrenergic blocker therapy (eg, tamsulosin [Flomax]), may be prescribed to promote bladder and prostate relaxation.

Factors contributing to prostatitis, including stress, neuromuscular factors, and myofascial pain, are also addressed. Supportive, nonpharmacologic therapies may be prescribed. These include biofeedback, pelvic floor training, physical therapy, reduction of prostatic fluid retention by ejaculation through sexual intercourse or masturbation, sitz baths, stool softeners, and evaluation of sexual partners to reduce the possibility of cross-infection.

Nursing Management

If the patient experiences symptoms of acute prostatitis (fever, severe pain and discomfort, inability to urinate, malaise), he may be hospitalized for intravenous (IV) antibiotic therapy. Nursing management includes administration of prescribed antibiotics and provision of comfort measures, including prescribed analgesic agents and sitz baths.

The patient with chronic prostatitis is usually treated on an outpatient basis and needs to be instructed about the importance of continuing antibiotic therapy and recognizing recurrent signs and symptoms of prostatitis.

Promoting Home and Community-Based Care

Teaching Patients Self-Care

The nurse instructs the patient to complete the prescribed course of antibiotics. If IV antibiotics are to be administered at home, the nurse instructs the patient and family about correct and safe administration. Arrangements for a home care nurse to oversee administration may be needed. Hot sitz baths (10 to 20 minutes) may be taken several times daily. Fluids are encouraged to satisfy thirst but are not "forced," because an effective medication level must be maintained in the urine. Foods and liquids with diuretic action or that increase prostatic secretions, such as alcohol, coffee, tea, chocolate, cola, and spices, should be avoided. A suprapubic catheter may be necessary for severe urinary retention. During periods of acute inflammation, sexual arousal and intercourse should be avoided. To minimize discomfort, the patient should avoid sitting for long periods. Medical follow-up is necessary for at least 6 months to 1 year because prostatitis caused by the same or different organisms can recur. The patient is advised that the UTI may recur and is taught to recognize its symptoms.

Benign Prostatic Hyperplasia (Enlarged Prostate)

Benign prostatic hyperplasia (BPH) is one of the most common diseases in aging men. It can cause bothersome lower urinary tract symptoms that affect quality of life by in-

terfering with normal daily activities and sleep patterns (AUA, 2006; Kaplan, 2006). BPH typically occurs in men older than 40 years of age. By the time they reach 60 years of age, 50% of men have BPH. It affects as many as 90% of men by 85 years of age. BPH is the second most common cause of surgical intervention in men older than 60 years of age.

Pathophysiology

The cause of BPH is not well understood, but testicular androgens have been implicated. Dihydrotestosterone (DHT), a metabolite of testosterone, is a critical mediator of prostatic growth. Estrogens may also play a role in the cause of BPH; BPH generally occurs when men have elevated estrogen levels and when prostate tissue becomes more sensitive to estrogens and less responsive to DHT. Smoking, heavy alcohol consumption, obesity, reduced activity level, hypertension, heart disease, diabetes, and a Western diet (high in animal fat and protein and refined carbohydrates, low in fiber) are risk factors for BPH (Parsons, 2007).

BPH develops over a prolonged period; changes in the urinary tract are slow and insidious. BPH is a result of complex interactions involving resistance in the prostatic urethra to mechanical and spastic effects, bladder pressure during voiding, detrusor muscle strength, neurologic functioning, and general physical health (McCance & Huether, 2005). The hypertrophied lobes of the prostate may obstruct the bladder neck or urethra, causing incomplete emptying of the bladder and urinary retention. As a result, a gradual dilation of the ureters (hydroureter) and kidneys (hydronephrosis) can occur. Urinary retention may result in UTIs because urine that remains in the urinary tract serves as a medium for infective organisms.

Clinical Manifestations

BPH may or may not lead to lower urinary tract symptoms; if symptoms occur, they may range from mild to severe. Severity of symptoms increases with age, and half of men with BPH report having moderate to severe symptoms. Obstructive and irritative symptoms may include urinary frequency, urgency, nocturia, hesitancy in starting urination, decreased and intermittent force of stream and the sensation of incomplete bladder emptying, abdominal straining with urination, a decrease in the volume and force of the urinary stream, dribbling (urine dribbles out after urination), and complications of acute urinary retention (more than 60 mL of urine remaining in the bladder after urination), and recurrent UTIs. Ultimately, chronic urinary retention and large residual volumes can lead to azotemia (accumulation of nitrogenous waste products) and renal failure.

Generalized symptoms may also be noted, including fatigue, anorexia, nausea, vomiting, and pelvic discomfort. Other disorders that produce similar symptoms include urethral stricture, prostate cancer, neurogenic bladder, and urinary bladder stones.

Assessment and Diagnostic Findings

The health history focuses on the urinary tract, previous surgical procedures, general health issues, family history of prostate disease, and fitness for possible surgery (AUA, 2006).

A patient voiding diary is used to record voiding frequency and urine volume. A DRE often reveals a large, rubbery, and nontender prostate gland. A urinalysis to screen for hematuria and UTI is recommended. A PSA level is obtained if the patient has at least a 10-year life expectancy and for whom knowledge of the presence of prostate cancer would change management. The AUA Symptom Index or International Prostate Symptom Score (IPSS) can be used to assess the severity of symptoms (AUA, 2006).

Other diagnostic tests may include urinary flow-rate recording and the measurement of postvoid residual (PVR) urine. If invasive therapy is considered, urodynamic studies, urethrocystoscopy, and ultrasound may be performed. Complete blood studies are performed. Cardiac status and respiratory function are assessed because a high percentage of patients with BPH have cardiac or respiratory disorders because of their age.

Medical Management

The goals of medical management of BPH are to improve quality of life, improve urine flow, relieve obstruction, prevent disease progression, and minimize complications. Treatment depends on the severity of symptoms, the cause of disease, the severity of the obstruction, and the patient's condition.

If a patient is admitted on an emergency basis because he is unable to void, he is immediately catheterized. The ordinary catheter may be too soft and pliable to advance through the urethra into the bladder. In such cases, a thin wire (stylet) is introduced (by a urologist) into the catheter to prevent the catheter from collapsing when it encounters resistance. A metal catheter with a pronounced prostatic curve may be used if obstruction is severe. An incision into the bladder (a suprapubic **cystostomy**) may be needed to provide urinary drainage.

Discussion of all treatment options by the physician enables the patient to make an informed decision based on symptom severity, the effect of BPH on his quality of life, and preference. Patients with mild symptoms and patients with moderate or severe symptoms who are not bothered by them and have not developed complications may be managed with watchful waiting. With this approach, the patient is monitored and reexamined annually but receives no active intervention (Kaplan, 2006). Other therapeutic choices include pharmacologic treatment, minimally invasive procedures, and surgery.

Pharmacologic Therapy

Pharmacologic treatment for BPH includes use of alpha-adrenergic blockers and 5-alpha-reductase inhibitors (AUA, 2006). Alpha-adrenergic blockers, which include alfuzosin (Uroxatral), terazosin (Hytrin), doxazosin (Cardura), and tamsulosin, relax the smooth muscle of the bladder neck and prostate. This improves urine flow and relieves symptoms of BPH. Side effects include dizziness, headache, asthenia/fatigue, postural hypotension, rhinitis, and sexual dysfunction (Kaplan, 2006; Lepor, 2007).

Another method of treatment involves hormonal manipulation with antiandrogen agents. The 5-alpha-reductase inhibitors, finasteride (Proscar) and dutasteride (Avodart), are used to prevent the conversion of testosterone to DHT and decrease prostate size. Side effects include decreased libido, ejaculatory dysfunction, erectile dysfunction, gynecomastia (breast enlargement), and flushing. Combination therapy (doxazosin and finasteride) has decreased symptoms and reduced clinical progression of BPH (AUA, 2006; Kaplan, 2006).

Use of phytotherapeutic agents and other dietary supplements (*Serenoa repens* [saw palmetto berry] and *Pygeum africanum* [African plum]) are not recommended, although they are commonly used. They may function by interfering with the conversion of testosterone to DHT. In addition, *S. repens* may directly block the ability of DHT to stimulate prostate cell growth. These agents should not be used with finasteride, dutasteride, or estrogen-containing medications.

Surgical Treatment

Other treatment options include minimally invasive procedures and resection of the prostate gland.

Minimally Invasive Therapy

Several forms of **minimally invasive therapy** may be used to treat BPH. Transurethral microwave heat treatment (TUMT) involves the application of heat to prostatic tissue. High-energy TUMT devices (CoreTherm, Prostatron, Targis) and low-energy devices (TherMatrx) are available (AUA, 2006). A transurethral probe is inserted into the urethra, and microwaves are directed to the prostate tissue. The targeted tissue becomes necrotic and sloughs. To minimize damage to the urethra and decrease the discomfort from the procedure, some systems have a water-cooling apparatus.

Other minimally invasive treatment options include (transurethral needle ablation [TUNA]) by radiofrequency energy and the UroLume stent. TUNA uses low-level radiofrequencies delivered by thin needles placed in the prostate gland to produce localized heat that destroys prostate tissue while sparing other tissues. The body then resorbs the dead tissue. Prostatic stents are associated with significant complications (eg, eucrustation, infection, chronic pain); therefore, they are used only for patients with urinary retention and in patients who are poor surgical risks (AUA, 2006).

Surgical Resection

Surgical resection of the prostate gland is another option for patients with moderate to severe lower urinary tract symptoms of BPH and for those with acute urinary retention or other complications. The specific surgical approach (open or endoscopic) and the energy source (electrocautery versus laser) are based on the surgeon's experience, the size of the prostate gland, the presence of other medical disorders, and the patient's preference. If surgery is to be performed, all clotting defects must be corrected and medications for anticoagulation withheld because bleeding is a complication of prostate surgery.

Transurethral resection of the prostate (TURP) remains the benchmark for surgical treatment of BPH. It involves the surgical removal of the inner portion of the prostate through an endoscope inserted through the urethra; no external skin incision is made. It can be performed with ultrasound guidance. The treated tissue either vaporizes or becomes necrotic and sloughs. The procedure is performed in the outpatient setting and usually results in less postoperative bleeding than a traditional surgical prostatectomy.

Other surgical options for BPH include transurethral incision of the prostate (TUIP), transurethral electrovaporization, laser therapy, and open prostatectomy (AUA, 2006; Kaplan, 2006). TUIP is an outpatient procedure used to treat smaller prostates. One or two cuts are made in the prostate and prostate capsule to reduce constriction of the urethra and decrease resistance to flow of urine out of the bladder, and no tissue is removed. Open prostatectomy involves the surgical removal of the inner portion of the prostate via a suprapubic, retropubic, or perineal (rare) approach for large prostate glands. Prostatectomy may also be performed laparoscopically or by a robot-assisted laparoscopy.

Nursing management of patients undergoing these procedures is described later in this chapter.

Cancer of the Prostate

Prostate cancer is the most common cancer in men other than nonmelanoma skin cancer. It is the second most common cause of cancer death in American men, exceeded only by lung cancer, and is responsible for 10% of cancer-related deaths in men. Among men diagnosed with prostate cancer, 98% survive at least 5 years, 84% survive at least 10 years, and 56% survive 15 years (ACS, 2009).

Prostate cancer is common in the United States and northwestern Europe but is rare in Africa, Central America, South America, China, and other parts of Asia. African American men have a high risk of prostate cancer; furthermore, they are twice as likely to die of prostate cancer than men of any other racial or ethnic group. The findings of the African-American Hereditary Prostate Cancer Study suggest that a strong genetic link increases the risk of early-onset disease (Jones, Underwood & Rivers, 2007). Other risk factors in African American men include their lower level of engagement in the health care system, disparities in health care, and cultural and structural barriers. These findings support the need for education about prostate cancer and screening in African American men (Weinrich, Vijayakumar, Powell, et al., 2007). Culturally sensitive promotional campaigns, teaching and counseling about prostate cancer, screening, and treatment are important in increasing awareness of the high incidence of prostate cancer and mortality rates in African American men (Chart 49-2).

Other risk factors for prostate cancer include increasing age; the incidence of prostate cancer increases rapidly after the age of 50 years. More than 70% of cases occur in men older than 65 years of age. A familial predisposition may occur in men who have a father or brother previously diagnosed with prostate cancer, especially if their relatives were

NURSING RESEARCH PROFILE
CHART 49-2 *Knowledge About Hereditary Prostate Cancer in African American Men*

Weinrich, S., Vijayakumar, S., Powell, I. J., et al. (2007). Knowledge of hereditary prostate cancer among high-risk African American men. *Oncology Nursing Forum, 34*(4), 854–860.

Purpose

Because African American men develop prostate cancer 50% to 60% more often than Caucasians and die from it at twice the rate of any other ethnic group, it is critical for this group to be aware of their increased risk and the need for screening for early detection of prostate cancer. The purpose of this study was to measure the level of knowledge about hereditary prostate cancer in a group of high-risk African American men.

Design

For this cross-sectional, correlational pilot study, investigators recruited a sample of 79 high-risk African American men (defined as those with four or more men in their families with prostate cancer) from four geographic areas. These men, who were also participants in the African American Hereditary Prostate Cancer Study, came from all educational levels, and their average age was 54 years. Almost half (n = 38, 48%) of them had received a diagnosis of prostate cancer. Researchers conducted telephone interviews using a scripted telephone protocol and a true-false, nine-item questionnaire, called the "Knowledge of Hereditary Prostate Cancer Scale," developed by the first author. Each man's individual answers were scored as correct or incorrect, with a range of possible total scores ranging from 0 to 9. To reach each participant, an average of 2.5 calls was needed; each call lasted an average of 15 minutes.

Findings

Data analysis revealed a range of scores from 3.5 to 9, with a mean score of 6.34 (standard deviation = 1.11). The authors interpreted this as a low level of knowledge about hereditary prostate cancer; answering six of nine questions correctly would produce a score of 67%.

Nursing Implications

The authors interpreted the high percentage of incorrect responses to questions about genetic testing, prevention, and risk based on a positive family history as indicating a need for education. They proposed that cancer fatalism (eg, the belief that death is inevitable when cancer is present) may account for a high percentage of incorrect or unanswered responses to a question measuring risk probability based on a positive prostate cancer test. In the current genomic health care system, a critical need exists for nurses to have a sound understanding of genetics and to educate high-risk African American men and their families about hereditary prostate cancer. The lack of knowledge exhibited by the participants in this study suggests a decreased likelihood of prostate cancer screening. The American Cancer Society recommends prostate cancer screening at 45 years of age for African American men and men with a positive family history (5 years earlier than the recommended age for men in the general population). Nurses can encourage early prostate screening. They have a valuable role in promoting healthy behaviors among high-risk African American men through education and other innovative strategies.

diagnosed at a young age. Genes that may be associated with increased risk of prostate cancer include hereditary prostate cancer 1 (*HPC1*) and *BRCA1* and *BRCA2* mutations (Jones, et al., 2007; Lessick & Katz, 2006). The risk of prostate cancer is also greater in men whose diet contains excessive amounts of red meat or dairy products that are high in fat (ACS, 2009). Endogenous hormones, such as androgens and estrogens, also may be associated with the development of prostate cancer.

Several large-scale studies have examined the ability of 5-alpha reductase inhibitors (finasteride and dutasteride) to delay or prevent prostate cancer (Tindall & Rittmaster, 2008).

Clinical Manifestations

Cancer of the prostate in its early stages rarely produces symptoms. Usually symptoms that develop from urinary obstruction occur in advanced disease. Prostate cancer tends to vary in its course. If the cancer is large enough to encroach on the bladder neck, signs and symptoms of urinary obstruction occur (difficulty and frequency of urination, urinary retention, and decreased size and force of the urinary stream). Other symptoms may include blood in the urine or semen and painful ejaculation. Hematuria may occur if the cancer invades the urethra or bladder. Sexual dysfunction is common before the diagnosis is made.

Prostate cancer can spread to lymph nodes and bone. Symptoms of metastases include backache, hip pain, perineal and rectal discomfort, anemia, weight loss, weakness, nausea, oliguria (decreased urine output), and spontaneous pathologic fractures. These symptoms may be the first indications of prostate cancer.

Assessment and Diagnostic Findings

If prostate cancer is detected early, the likelihood of cure is high. It can be diagnosed through an abnormal finding with the DRE, serum PSA, and ultrasound-guided TRUS with biopsy. Detection is more likely with use of combined diagnostic procedures. Routine repeated DRE (preferably by the same examiner) is important because early cancer may be detected as a nodule within the gland or as an extensive hardening in the posterior lobe. The more advanced lesion is "stony hard" and fixed. DRE also provides useful clinical information about the rectum, anal sphincter, and quality of stool.

The diagnosis of prostate cancer is confirmed by a histologic examination of tissue removed surgically by TURP, open prostatectomy, or ultrasound-guided transrectal needle biopsy. Fine-needle aspiration is a quick, painless method of obtaining prostate cells for cytologic examination and determining the stage of disease.

Most prostate cancers are detected when a man seeks medical attention for symptoms of urinary obstruction or are found by routine DRE and PSA testing. Cancer detected incidentally when TURP is performed for clinically benign disease and lower urinary tract symptoms occurs in about 1 of 10 cases. Abnormal DRE and elevated levels of PSA may raise suspicion of prostate cancer, but detection requires confirmation with a prostate biopsy.

TRUS helps detect nonpalpable prostate cancers and assists with staging of localized prostate cancer. Needle biopsies of the prostate are commonly guided by TRUS. The biopsies are examined by a pathologist to both determine if cancer is present and to grade the tumor. The most commonly used tumor grading system is the Gleason score. This system assigns a grade of 1 to 5 for the most predominant architectural pattern of the glands of the prostate and a secondary grade of 1 to 5 to the second most predominant pattern. The Gleason score is then reported as, for example, 2 + 4; the combined value can range from 2 to 10. With each increase in Gleason score, there is an increase in tumor aggressiveness. Lower Gleason scores indicate well-differentiated and less aggressive tumor cells; higher Gleason scores indicate undifferentiated cells and more aggressive cancer. A total score of 8 to 10 indicates a high-grade cancer (AUA, 2007).

Categorization of low-risk, intermediate-risk, and high-risk prostate cancer is determined by the extent of cancer in the prostate gland, whether or not the cancer is localized to the prostate, the aggressiveness of the cells, and the spread to the lymph nodes and beyond. Level of risk, in turn, is used to determine treatment options.

Bone scans, skeletal x-rays, and magnetic resonance imaging (MRI) may be used to identify metastatic bone disease. Pelvic computed tomography (CT) may be performed to determine if the cancer has spread to the lymph nodes. The radiolabeled monoclonal antibody capromab pendetide with indium 111 (ProstaScint) is an antibody that can be used to detect either recurrent prostate cancer at low PSA levels or metastatic disease (NCCN, 2008).

Medical Management

Treatment is based on the patient's life expectancy, symptoms, risk of recurrence after definitive treatment, size of the tumor, Gleason score, PSA level, likelihood of complications, and patient preference. Therapy is often guided by the use of a nomogram or risk stratification scheme suggested by the NCCN (2008) and AUA (2007) clinical practice guidelines. A multidisciplinary team approach is essential for the development of appropriate treatment. Management may be nonsurgical and involve watchful waiting or be surgical and entail **prostatectomy.** Nursing care of the patient with cancer of the prostate is summarized in the plan of nursing care in Chart 49-3.

Patients with prostate cancer may also choose nonsurgical watchful waiting. This approach involves actively monitoring the course of disease and intervening only if the cancer progresses or if symptoms warrant other intervention. It is an option for patients with life expectancy of less than 5 years and low-risk cancers. Advantages include absence of side effects of more aggressive treatment, improved quality of life, avoidance of unnecessary treatment, and decreased initial costs. Disadvantages include missed chance at cure, risk of metastasis, subsequent need for more aggressive treatment, anxiety about living with untreated cancer, and need for frequent monitoring (Bailey, Wallace & Mishel, 2007; NCCN, 2008).

Surgical Management

Radical prostatectomy is considered the standard first-line treatment for prostate cancer and is used with patients whose tumor is confined to the prostate. It is the complete surgical removal of the prostate, seminal vesicles, tips of the vas deferens, and often the surrounding fat, nerves, and

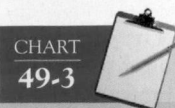

CHART
49-3

PLAN OF NURSING CARE
The Patient With Prostate Cancer

NURSING DIAGNOSIS: Anxiety related to concern and lack of knowledge about the diagnosis, treatment plan, and prognosis
GOAL: Reduced stress and improved ability to cope

Nursing Interventions	Rationale	Expected Outcomes
1. Obtain health history to determine the following: a. Patient's concerns b. His level of understanding of his health problem c. His past experience with cancer d. Whether he knows his diagnosis of malignancy and its prognosis e. His support systems and coping methods	1. Nurse clarifies information and facilitates patient's understanding and coping.	• Appears relaxed • States that anxiety has been reduced or relieved • Demonstrates understanding of illness, diagnostic tests, and treatment when questioned • Engages in open communication with others
2. Provide education about diagnosis and treatment plan: a. Explain in simple terms what diagnostic tests to expect, how long they will take, and what will be experienced during each test. b. Review treatment plan and allow patient to ask questions.	2. Helping the patient to understand the diagnostic tests and treatment plan will help decrease his anxiety and promote cooperation.	
3. Assess his psychological reaction to his diagnosis/prognosis and how he has coped with past stresses.	3. This information provides clues in determining appropriate measures to facilitate coping.	
4. Provide information about institutional and community resources for coping with prostate cancer: social services, support groups, community agencies.	4. Institutional and community resources can help the patient and family cope with the illness and treatment on an ongoing basis.	

NURSING DIAGNOSIS: Urinary retention related to urethral obstruction secondary to prostatic enlargement or tumor and loss of bladder tone due to prolonged distention/retention
GOAL: Improved pattern of urinary elimination

Nursing Interventions	Rationale	Expected Outcomes
1. Determine patient's usual pattern of urinary function. 2. Assess for signs and symptoms of urinary retention: amount and frequency of urination, suprapubic distention, complaints of urgency and discomfort. 3. Catheterize patient to determine amount of residual urine. 4. Initiate measures to treat retention: a. Encourage assuming normal position for voiding. b. Recommend using Valsalva maneuver preoperatively, if not contraindicated. c. Administer prescribed cholinergic agent. d. Monitor effects of medication. 5. Consult with physician regarding intermittent or indwelling catheterization; assist with procedure as required. 6. Monitor catheter function; maintain sterility of closed system; irrigate as required. 7. Prepare patient for surgery if indicated.	1. Provides a baseline for comparison and goal to work toward 2. Voiding 20 to 30 mL frequently and output less than intake suggest retention. 3. Determines amount of urine remaining in bladder after voiding. 4. Promotes voiding: a. Usual position provides relaxed conditions conducive to voiding. b. Valsalva maneuver exerts pressure to force urine out of bladder. c. Stimulates bladder contraction. d. If unsuccessful, another measure may be required. 5. Catheterization will relieve urinary retention until the specific cause is determined; it may be an obstruction that can be corrected only surgically. 6. Adequate functioning of catheter is to be ensured to empty bladder and to prevent infection. 7. Surgical removal of obstruction may be necessary.	• Voids at normal intervals • Reports absence of frequency, urgency, or bladder fullness • Displays no palpable suprapubic distention after voiding • Maintains balanced intake and output

Continued

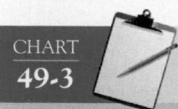

CHART 49-3	PLAN OF NURSING CARE
	The Patient With Prostate Cancer (Continued)

NURSING DIAGNOSIS: Deficient knowledge related to the diagnosis of: cancer, urinary difficulties, and treatment modalities
GOAL: Understanding of the diagnosis and ability to care for self

Nursing Interventions	Rationale	Expected Outcomes
1. Encourage communication with the patient.	1. This is designed to establish rapport and trust.	• Discusses his concerns and problems freely
2. Review the anatomy of the involved area.	2. Orientation to one's anatomy is basic to understanding its function.	• Asks questions and shows interest in his disorder
3. Be specific in selecting information that is relevant to the patient's particular treatment plan.	3. This is based on the treatment plan; as it varies with each patient, individualization is desirable.	• Describes activities that help or hinder recovery
4. Identify ways to reduce pressure on the operative area after prostatectomy:	4. This is to prevent bleeding; such precautions are in order for 6 to 8 weeks postoperatively.	• Identifies ways of attaining/maintaining bladder control
a. Avoid prolonged sitting (in a chair, long automobile rides), standing, walking.		• Demonstrates satisfactory technique and understanding of catheter care
b. Avoid straining, such as during exercises, bowel movement, lifting, and sexual intercourse.		• Lists signs and symptoms that must be reported should they occur
5. Familiarize patient with ways of attaining/maintaining bladder control.	5. These measures will help control frequency and dribbling and aid in preventing retention.	
a. Encourage urination every 2 to 3 hours; discourage voiding when supine.	a. By sitting or standing, patient is more likely to empty his bladder.	
b. Avoid drinking cola and caffeine beverages; urge a cutoff time in the evening for drinking fluids to minimize frequent voiding during the night.	b. Spacing the kind and amount of liquid intake will help to prevent frequency.	
c. Describe perineal exercises to be performed every hour.	c. Exercises will assist him in starting and stopping the urinary stream.	
d. Develop a schedule with patient that will fit into his routine.	d. A schedule will assist in developing a workable pattern of normal activities.	
6. Demonstrate catheter care; encourage his questions; stress the importance of position of urinary receptacle.	6. By requiring a return demonstration of care, collection, and emptying of the device, he will become more independent and also can prevent backflow of urine, which can lead to infection.	

NURSING DIAGNOSIS: Imbalanced nutrition: less than body requirements related to decreased oral intake because of anorexia, nausea, and vomiting caused by cancer or its treatment
GOAL: Maintain optimal nutritional status

Nursing Interventions	Rationale	Expected Outcomes
1. Assess the amount of food eaten.	1. This assessment will help determine nutrient intake.	• Responds positively to his favorite foods
2. Routinely weigh patient.	2. Weighing the patient on the same scale under similar conditions can help monitor changes in weight.	• Assumes responsibility for his oral hygiene
3. Elicit patient's explanation of why he is unable to eat more.	3. His explanation may present easily corrected practices.	• Reports absence of nausea and vomiting
4. Cater to his individual food preferences (eg, avoiding foods that are too spicy or too cold).	4. He will be more likely to consume larger servings if food is palatable and appealing.	• Notes increase in weight after improved appetite
5. Recognize effect of medication or radiation therapy on appetite.	5. Many chemotherapeutic agents and radiation therapy promote anorexia.	

Continued on following page

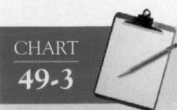

PLAN OF NURSING CARE
The Patient With Prostate Cancer (*Continued*)

CHART
49-3

Nursing Interventions	Rationale	Expected Outcomes
6. Inform patient that alterations in taste can occur.	6. Aging and the disease process can reduce taste sensitivity. In addition, smell and taste can be altered as a result of the body's absorption of byproducts of cellular destruction (brought on by malignancy and its treatment).	

7. Use measures to control nausea and vomiting:
  a. Administer prescribed anti-emetics, around the clock if necessary.
  b. Provide oral hygiene after vomiting episodes.
  c. Provide rest periods after meals.
	7. Prevention of nausea and vomiting can stimulate appetite.	

8. Provide frequent small meals and a comfortable and pleasant environment.	8. Smaller portions of food are less overwhelming to the patient.	
9. Assess patient's ability to obtain and prepare foods.	9. Disability or lack of social support can hinder the patient's ability to obtain and prepare foods.	

NURSING DIAGNOSIS: Sexual dysfunction related to effects of therapy: chemotherapy, hormonal therapy, radiation therapy, surgery

GOAL: Ability to resume/enjoy modified sexual functioning

Nursing Interventions	Rationale	Expected Outcomes
1. Determine from nursing history what effect patient's medical condition is having on his sexual functioning.	1. Usually decreased libido and, later, impotence may be experienced.	• Describes the reasons for changes in sexual functioning • Discusses with appropriate health care personnel alternative approaches and methods of sexual expression • Includes partner in discussions related to changes in sexual function
2. Inform patient of the effects of prostate surgery, orchiectomy (when applicable), chemotherapy, irradiation, and hormonal therapy on sexual function.	2. Treatment modalities may alter sexual function, but each is evaluated separately with regard to its effect on a particular patient.	
3. Include his partner in developing understanding and in discovering alternative, satisfying close relations with each other.	3. The bonds between a couple may be strengthened with new appreciation and support that had not been evident before the current illness.	

NURSING DIAGNOSIS: Pain related to progression of disease and treatment modalities

GOAL: Relief of pain

Nursing Interventions	Rationale	Expected Outcomes
1. Evaluate nature of patient's pain, its location and intensity using pain rating scale.	1. Determining nature and causes of pain and its intensity helps to select proper pain-relief modality and provide baseline for later comparison.	• Reports relief of pain • Expects exacerbations, reports their quality and intensity, and obtains relief • Uses pain relief strategies appropriately and effectively • Identifies strategies to avoid complications of analgesic use (eg, constipation)
2. Avoid activities that aggravate or worsen pain.	2. Bumping the bed is an example of an action that can intensify the patient's pain.	
3. Because pain is usually related to bone metastasis, ensure that patient's bed has a bed board on a firm mattress. Also, protect the patient from falls/injuries.	3. This will provide added support and is more comfortable. Protecting the patient from injury protects him from additional pain.	
4. Provide support for affected extremities.	4. More support, coupled with reduced movement of the part, helps in pain control.	
5. Prepare patient for radiation therapy if prescribed.	5. Radiation therapy may be effective in controlling pain.	

Continued

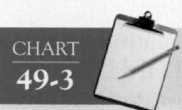

CHART 49-3

PLAN OF NURSING CARE

The Patient With Prostate Cancer (Continued)

Nursing Interventions	Rationale	Expected Outcomes
6. Administer analgesics or opioids at regularly scheduled intervals as prescribed.	6. Analgesics alter perception of pain and provide comfort. Regularly scheduled analgesics around the clock rather than PRN provide more consistent pain relief.	
7. Initiate bowel program to prevent constipation.	7. Opioid analgesics and inactivity contribute to constipation.	

NURSING DIAGNOSIS: Impaired physical mobility and activity intolerance related to tissue hypoxia, malnutrition, and exhaustion and to spinal cord or nerve compression from metastases
GOAL: Improved physical mobility

Nursing Interventions	Rationale	Expected Outcomes
1. Assess for factors causing limited mobility (eg, pain, hypercalcemia, limited exercise tolerance).	1. This information offers clues to the cause; if possible, cause is treated.	• Achieves improved physical mobility • Relates that short-term goals are encouraging him because they are attainable
2. Provide pain relief by administering prescribed medications.	2. Analgesics/opioids allow the patient to increase his activity more comfortably.	
3. Encourage use of assistive devices: cane, walker.	3. Support may offer the security needed to become mobile.	
4. Involve significant others in helping patient with range-of-motion exercises, positioning, and walking	4. Assistance from partner or others encourages patient to repeat activities and achieve goals.	
5. Provide positive reinforcement for achievement of small gains.	5. Encouragement stimulates improvement of performance.	
6. Assess nutritional status.	6. See Nursing Diagnosis: Imbalanced nutrition: less than body requirements.	

COLLABORATIVE PROBLEMS: Hemorrhage, infection, bladder neck obstruction
GOAL: Absence of complications

Nursing Interventions	Rationale	Expected Outcomes
1. Alert the patient to changes that may occur (after discharge) and that need to be reported: a. Continued bloody urine; passing blood clots. b. Pain; burning around the catheter. c. Frequency of urination. d. Diminished urinary output. e. Increasing loss of bladder control.	1. Certain changes signal beginning complications, which call for nursing and medical interventions. a. Hematuria with or without blood clot formation may occur postoperatively. b. Indwelling urinary catheters may be a source of infections. c. Urinary frequency may be caused by urinary tract infections or by bladder neck obstruction, resulting in incomplete voiding. d. Bladder neck obstruction decreases the amount of urine that is voided. e. Urinary incontinence may be a result of urinary retention.	• Experiences no bleeding or passage of blood clots • Reports no pain around the catheter • Experiences normal frequency or urination • Reports normal urinary output • Maintains bladder control

blood vessels. Laparoscopic radical prostatectomy and robotic-assisted laparoscopic radical prostatectomy have become the standard surgical approaches for localized cancer of the prostate. Although sexual impotence is a common side effect, these laparoscopic radical prostatectomy approaches result in low morbidity and more favorable postoperative outcomes, including improved quality of life and less sexual dysfunction if the nerves are spared. (Surgical approaches are discussed in detail later in this chapter.)

Radiation Therapy

Two major forms of radiation therapy are used to treat cancer of the prostate: teletherapy (external) and brachytherapy (internal). Teletherapy (external beam radiation therapy [EBRT]) may be given for 5 days per week for 7 to 8 weeks. It is a treatment option for patients with low-risk prostate cancer; progression-free survival is similar to that of low-risk patients treated with radical prostatectomy.

Patients with intermediate-risk and high-risk cancers receive higher doses of EBRT and may be candidates for both pelvic lymph node irradiation and androgen deprivation therapy (NCCN, 2008). Intensity modulated radiation therapy (IMRT) is one method of delivery of EBRT. IMRT sets a dose for the target volume and restricts the dose to surrounding tissue. A new approach to delivery of radiation uses a computer-controlled robotic arm to deliver a course of radiotherapy (ie, stereotactic radiosurgery) to localized prostate cancer. This method, referred to as the CyberKnife, is being evaluated in clinical trials and compared with other methods of delivering radiation to treat prostate cancer.

Brachytherapy (internal implants) involves the implantation of interstitial radioactive seeds under anesthesia. It has become a commonly used monotherapy treatment option for early, clinically organ-confined prostate cancer. The surgeon uses ultrasound guidance to place 80 to 100 seeds (depending on the prostate volume), and the patient returns home after the procedure. Exposure of others to radiation is minimal, but the patient should avoid close contact with pregnant women and infants for up to 2 months. Radiation safety guidelines include straining urine for seeds and using a condom during sexual intercourse for 2 weeks after implantation to catch any seeds that pass through the urethra. This approach can be completed in one day, with little lost time from normal activities. Brachytherapy may be combined with EBRT with or without neoadjuvant androgen deprivation therapy for patients considered at intermediate risk. High-risk patients are considered poor candidates for permanent brachytherapy (NCCN, 2008).

Although cure rates with radiation are comparable to those of radical prostatectomy, radiation therapy possesses its own unique set of side effects, which differ depending on the method of radiation administration. Patients receiving EBRT or brachytherapy may experience inflammation of the rectum, bowel, and bladder (proctitis, enteritis, and cystitis) because of the proximity of these structures to the prostate and the radiation doses. Inflammation and mucosal loss at the bladder neck, prostate, and urethra can cause acute urinary dysfunction. Both irritative and obstructive urinary symptoms can cause pain with urination and ejaculation until the irritation subsides. Rectal urgency, diarrhea, and tenesmus may occur as a result of radiation of the anterior rectal wall. Late side effects include rectal proctitis, bleeding, and rectal fistula, painless hematuria, chronic interstitial cystitis, urethral stricture erectile dysfunction, and, rarely, secondary cancers of the rectum and bladder (Michaelson, Cotter, Gargollo, et al., 2008).

Hormonal Strategies

The number of survivors of prostate cancer in the United States is estimated at 2 million; approximately one third of these men currently receive **androgen deprivation therapy (ADT)** (Michaelson, et al., 2008). ADT is commonly used to suppress androgenic stimuli to the prostate by decreasing the level of circulating plasma testosterone or interrupting the conversion to or binding of DHT. As a result, the prostatic epithelium atrophies (decreases in size). This effect is accomplished either by surgical castration (bilateral **orchiectomy,** removal of the testes), which has traditionally been the mainstay of hormonal treatment, or by medical

castration with the administration of medications, such as luteinizing hormone–releasing hormone (LHRH) agonists. Bilateral orchiectomy decreases plasma testosterone levels significantly because approximately 93% of circulating testosterone is of testicular origin (7% is from the adrenal glands). Thus, the testicular stimulus required for continued prostatic growth is removed, resulting in prostatic atrophy.

However, orchiectomy often results in significant morbidity. Although the procedure does not cause the side effects associated with other hormonal therapies (described later), it is associated with considerable emotional impact. Because patients who have prostate cancer are living longer with the disease, health care providers have now begun to focus their attention on effective therapeutic modalities that promote an acceptable quality of life. Patients may be given the option for testicular prostheses to be placed during surgery.

LHRH agonists include leuprolide (Lupron) and goserelin (Zoladex). Additional hormonal manipulation with antiandrogens may be prescribed for patients who do not show adequate serum testosterone suppression (less than 50 ng/mL) with medical or surgical castration. Antiandrogen receptor antagonists include flutamide (Eulexin), bicalutamide (Casodex), and nilutamide (Nilandron). LHRH agonists suppress testicular androgen, whereas antiandrogen receptor antagonists cause adrenal androgen suppression. When LHRH agonists are initiated, a testosterone flare may occur, causing pain in bony metastatic disease. Antiandrogens given for the first 7 days may reduce this uncomfortable symptom. The most common uses of LHRH agonists are the following: (1) in the adjuvant and neoadjuvant setting in combination with radiation therapy; (2) after radical prostatectomy; and (3) in the treatment of recurrence indicated by an elevation in the PSA but without clinical or x-ray evidence. Medical and surgical castration causes hot flushing because these treatment modalities increase hypothalamic activity, which stimulates the thermoregulatory centers of the body.

The management of hormone-refractory prostate cancer remains somewhat controversial. Another category of medication used as a second-line hormonal intervention is called adrenal ablating drugs. Ketoconazole (Nizoral) is used to inhibit cytochrome P450 enzymes, which are required for the synthesis of androgens and other steroids. High-dose ketoconazole lowers testosterone by decreasing both testicular and endocrine production of androgen. Administration of this medication requires steroid supplementation to prevent adrenal insufficiency.

Hypogonadism is responsible for the adverse effects of ADT, which include vasomotor flushing, loss of libido, decreased bone density (resulting in osteoporosis and fractures), anemia, fatigue, increased fat mass, lipid alterations, decreased muscle mass, gynecomastia (increased breast tissue), and mastodynia (breast/nipple tenderness). Hypogonadism is associated with an increased risk of diabetes, resulting from insulin resistance, metabolic syndrome, and cardiovascular disease (Michaelson, et al., 2008).

Chemotherapy

Recent studies have shown clear benefits in terms of survival with chemotherapy treatment that includes a docetaxel-based regimen for non–androgen-dependent prostate cancer (NCCN, 2008; Pienta & Smith, 2005). Other studies are under way to determine the importance of the vascular endothelial growth factor system. Tumor angiogenesis is essential for tumor growth, including growth of prostate carcinomas and other high-grade cancers. Therefore, antiangiogenic treatment in combination with conventional therapies may play a future role in treatment. Gene-based therapy in prostate cancer is an emerging and promising adjuvant to conventional treatment strategies.

Complications related to chemotherapy are specific to the type of chemotherapy administered. These are discussed in detail in Chapter 16.

Other Therapies

Cryosurgery of the prostate is used to ablate prostate cancer in patients who cannot tolerate surgery and in those with recurrent prostate cancer. Transperineal probes are inserted into the prostate under ultrasound guidance to freeze the tissue directly.

Keeping the urethral passage patent may require repeated TURPs. If this is impractical, catheter drainage is instituted by way of the suprapubic or transurethral route. For men with advanced prostate cancer, palliative measures are indicated. Although cure is unlikely with advanced prostate cancer, many men survive for long periods, free of debilitating symptoms.

Bone lesions that result from metastasis of prostate cancer can be very painful and result in pathologic fractures. Opioid and nonopioid medications are used to control bone pain. EBRT can be delivered to skeletal lesions to relieve pain. Radiopharmaceuticals, such as strontium or samarium, can be injected intravenously to treat multiple sites of bone metastasis. Antiandrogen therapies are used in an effort to reduce the circulating androgens. If antiandrogen therapies are not effective, medications such as prednisone have been effective in reducing pain and improving quality of life. Bisphosphonate therapy with pamidronate (Aredia) can be administered to reduce the risk of pathologic fracture. In advanced prostate cancer, blood transfusions are administered to maintain adequate hemoglobin levels when bone marrow is replaced by tumor.

More than one third of men with a diagnosis of prostate cancer elect to use some form of complementary and alternative medicine (CAM). Because of lack of research on many forms of CAM, patients often rely on anecdotal information to make decisions about its use. Nurses play a vital role in assisting patients to locate and evaluate available information about CAM to ensure that harmful forms are avoided. The National Center for Complementary and Alternative Medicine's Web site (see Resources at the end of the chapter) can assist nurses in providing patients with evidence-based information.

The Patient Undergoing Prostate Surgery

Prostate surgery may be indicated for the patient with BPH or prostate cancer. The objectives before prostate surgery are to assess the patient's general health status and to establish optimal renal function. Prostate surgery should be performed before acute urinary retention develops and damages the upper urinary tract and collecting system or, in the case of prostate cancer, before cancer progresses.

Surgical Procedures

Several approaches can be used to remove the hypertrophied portion of the prostate gland: TURP, suprapubic prostatectomy, perineal prostatectomy, retropubic prostatectomy, TUIP, and laparoscopic radical prostatectomy and robotic-assisted laparoscopic radical prostatectomy (Table 49-4). With these approaches, the surgeon removes all cancerous or hyperplastic tissue, leaving behind only the capsule of the prostate. The transurethral approaches (TURP, TUIP) are closed procedures; the other three are open procedures (ie, a surgical incision is required) and the two laparoscopic approaches are minimally invasive. The procedure chosen depends on the underlying disorder, the patient's age and physical status, patient preference, and the skill of the surgeon.

Transurethral Resection of the Prostate

TURP, the most common procedure used, can be carried out through endoscopy. The surgical and optical instrument is introduced directly through the urethra to the prostate, which can then be viewed directly. The gland is removed in small chips with an electrical cutting loop (Fig. 49-4A). This procedure eliminates the risk of transurethral resection syndrome (hyponatremia, hypovolemia). Transurethral resection syndrome is a potential but rare complication of TURP that occurs in approximately 2% of men who undergo the procedure (Chart 49-4).

TURP usually requires an overnight hospital stay. Urethral strictures are more frequent than with non-transurethral procedures, and repeated procedures may be necessary because the residual prostatic tissue grows back. TURP rarely causes erectile dysfunction but may trigger retrograde ejaculation, because removal of prostatic tissue at the bladder neck can cause the seminal fluid to flow backward into the bladder rather than forward through the urethra during ejaculation.

Suprapubic Prostatectomy

In suprapubic prostatectomy, an incision is made into the bladder, and the prostate gland is removed from above (Fig. 49-4B). Such an approach can be used for a gland of any size, and few complications occur, although blood loss may be greater than with the other methods. Another disadvantage is the need for an abdominal incision, which has the risks associated with any major abdominal surgical procedure.

Perineal Prostatectomy

In perineal prostatectomy, the prostate gland is removed through an incision in the perineum (Fig. 49-4C). This procedure is practical when other approaches are not possible and is useful for an open biopsy. However, incontinence, sexual dysfunction, and rectal injury are more likely with this approach.

Retropubic Prostatectomy

Retropubic prostatectomy is used more commonly than the suprapubic approach. The surgeon makes a low abdominal incision and approaches the prostate gland between the

Table 49-4   COMPARING SURGICAL APPROACHES FOR TREATMENT OF PROSTATE DISORDERS

The surgical approach of choice depends on (1) the size of the gland, (2) the severity of the obstruction, (3) the age of the patient, (4) the condition of the patient, and (5) the presence of associated diseases.

Surgical Approach	Advantages	Disadvantages	Nursing Implications
Transurethral resection (TURP) (Removal of prostatic tissue by instrument introduced through urethra; used for glands of varying size. Ideal for patients who are poor surgical risks.)	Avoids abdominal incision Safer for surgical-risk patient Shorter hospitalization and recovery periods Lower morbidity rate Causes less pain Can be used as a palliative approach with history of radiation therapy	Requires highly skilled surgeon Recurrent obstruction, urethral trauma, and stricture may develop Delayed bleeding may occur	Monitor for hemorrhage Observe for symptoms of urethral stricture (dysuria, straining, weak urinary stream)
Open surgical removal Suprapubic approach (Removal of prostatic tissue through abdominal incision; can be used for gland of any size.)	Technically simple Offers wide area of exploration Permits exploration for cancerous lymph nodes Allows more complete removal of obstructing gland Permits treatment of associated bladder lesions	Requires surgical approach through the bladder Control of hemorrhage difficult Urine may leak around the suprapubic tube. Recovery may be prolonged and uncomfortable.	Monitor for indications of hemorrhage and shock. Provide meticulous aseptic care to the area around suprapubic tube.
Perineal approach (Removal of gland through an incision in the perineum; preferred approach for obese patients.)	Offers direct anatomic approach Permits gravity drainage Particularly effective for radical cancer therapy Allows hemostasis under direct vision Low mortality rate Low incidence of shock Ideal for very old, frail, and poor surgical-risk patients with large prostate	Higher postoperative incidence of impotence and urinary incontinence Possible damage to rectum and external sphincter Restricted operative field Greater potential for contamination and infection of incision	Avoid using rectal tubes or thermometers and enemas after perineal surgery Use drainage pads to absorb excess urinary drainage Provide foam rubber ring for patient comfort in sitting Anticipate urinary leakage around the wound for several days after the catheter is removed
Retropubic approach (Low abdominal incision; bladder is not entered.)	Avoids incision into the bladder Permits surgeon to see and control bleeding Shorter recovery period Less bladder sphincter damage Suitable for removal of large glands	Cannot treat associated bladder disease Increased incidence of hemorrhage from prostatic venous plexus; pubic osteitis	Monitor for hemorrhage Anticipate posturinary leakage for several days after removing the catheter
Transurethral incision (TUIP) (Urethral approach; 1–2 cuts are made in the prostate and prostate capsule to reduce pressure on the urethra and to reduce urethral constriction.)	Results comparable to TURP Low incidence of erectile dysfunction and retrograde ejaculation No bladder neck contracture	Requires highly skilled surgeon Recurrent obstruction and urethral trauma Delayed bleeding	Monitor for hemorrhage
Laparoscopic radical prostatectomy	Minimally invasive technique Improved patient satisfaction and quality of life Shorter hospital stay Short convalescence More rapid return to normal activity Short indwelling catheter duration Decreased blood loss to 400 mL Reduced infection risk Less scarring Better visualization of surgical field than other approaches	Lack of tactile sensation available with open prostatectomy Inability to palpably assess for induration and palpable nodules Inability to delineate the proximity of involvement of the neurovascular bundles due to lack of palpation Technically demanding Long surgical time (4–5 hours)	Observe for symptoms of urethral stricture (dysuria), straining, weak urinary stream Monitor for hemorrhage and shock Provide meticulous aseptic care to the area around suprapubic tube Monitor for changes in bowel function Avoid using rectal tubes or thermometers and enemas after perineal surgery Use drainage pads to absorb excess urinary drainage Provide foam rubber ring for patient comfort in sitting Anticipate urinary leakage around the wound for several days after the catheter is removed

Table 49-4	COMPARING SURGICAL APPROACHES FOR TREATMENT OF PROSTATE DISORDERS (Continued)		
Surgical Approach	**Advantages**	**Disadvantages**	**Nursing Implications**
Robotic-assisted laparoscopic radical prostatectomy (Involves using computer console and da Vinci robotic system. Six small incisions are made in the abdomen; laparoscopic instruments inserted through the incisions are used to dissect the prostate.)	Minimally invasive technique Improved patient satisfaction and quality of life Shorter hospital stay Short convalescence More rapid return to normal activity Short indwelling catheter duration Decreased blood loss to 150 mL Improved magnification of operative field, using a 3-dimensional view (includes, magnification, high resolution and depth perception) Less postoperative pain Reduced infection risk Less scarring Laparoscopic instruments have six degrees of movement with joints, allowing extensive range of motion and precision Nerve-sparing with less incontinence and sexual dysfunction	Lack of tactile sensation available with open prostatectomy Inability to palpably assess for induration and palpable nodules Inability to delineate the proximity of involvement of the neurovascular bundles due to lack of palpation Technically demanding	Observe for symptoms of urethral stricture (dysuria), straining, weak urinary stream Monitor for hemorrhage and shock Provide meticulous aseptic care to the area around suprapubic tube Monitor for changes in bowel function Avoid using rectal tubes or thermometers and enemas after perineal surgery Use drainage pads to absorb excess urinary drainage Provide foam rubber ring for patient comfort in sitting Anticipate urinary leakage around the wound for several days after the catheter is removed

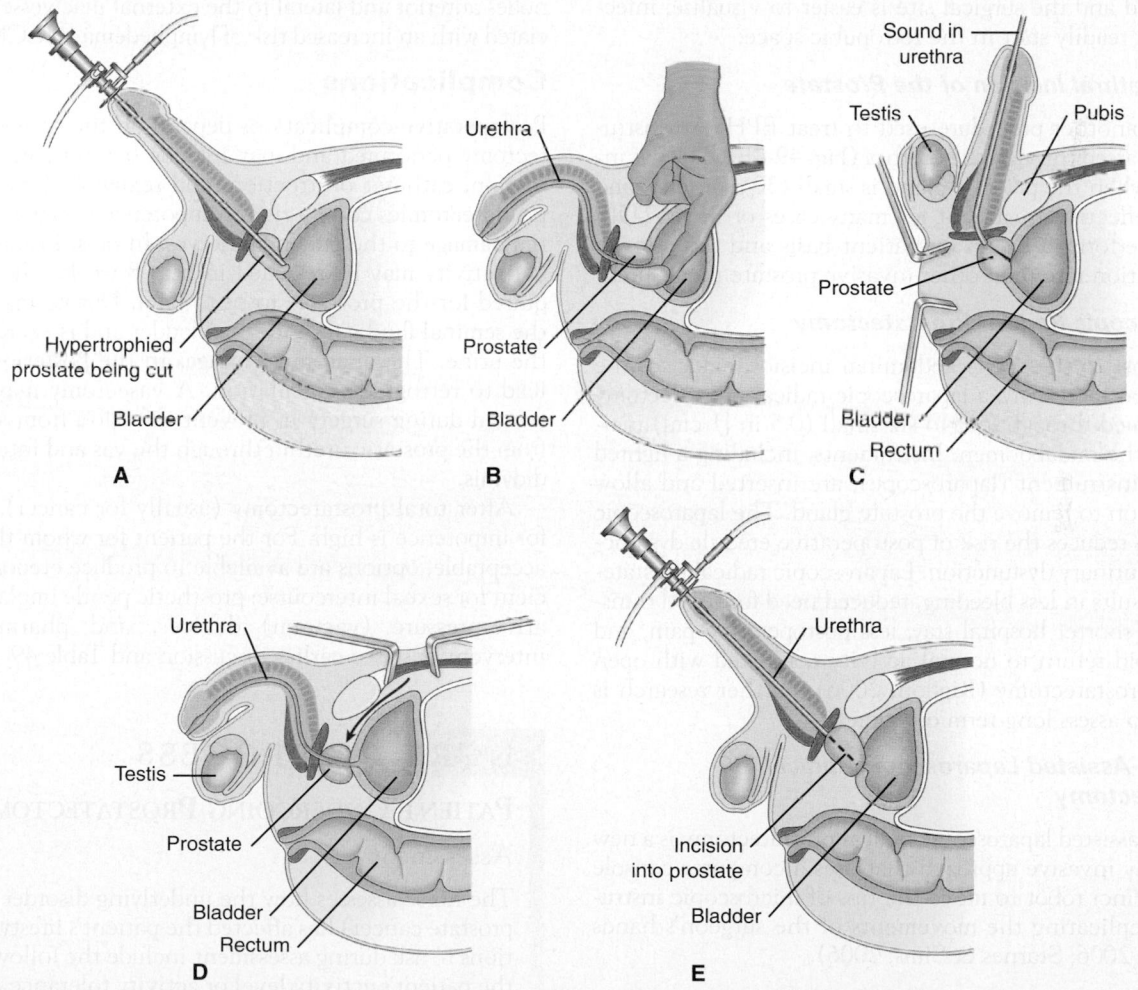

Figure 49-4 Prostate surgery procedures. **A,** Transurethral resection (TUR). A loop of wire connected with a cutting current is rotated in the cystoscope to remove shavings of prostate at the bladder orifice. **B,** Suprapubic prostatectomy. With an abdominal approach, the prostate is shelled out of its bed. **C,** Perineal prostatectomy. Two retractors on the left spread the perineal incision to provide a view of the prostate. **D,** Retropubic prostatectomy is performed through a low abdominal incision. Note two abdominal retractors and arrow pointing to the prostate gland. **E,** Transurethral incision of prostate (TUIP) involves one or two incisions into the prostate to reduce pressure on the urethra.

Chart 49-4 • *Transurethral Resection Syndrome*

Transurethral resection syndrome is a rare but potentially serious complication of transurethral prostatectomy (TURP). Signs and symptoms are caused by neurologic, cardiovascular, and electrolyte imbalances associated with absorption of the solution used to irrigate the surgical site during the surgical procedure. Hyponatremia, hypovolemia, and occasionally hyperammonemia may occur (Eaton, 2003).

Signs and Symptoms

- Lethargy and confusion
- Hypotension
- Tachycardia
- Nausea and vomiting
- Collapse
- Headache
- Muscle spasms
- Seizures

Interventions

- Discontinue irrigation
- Administer diuretics as prescribed
- Replace bladder irrigation with normal saline
- Monitor intake and output
- Monitor the patient's vital signs and level of consciousness
- Differentiate lethargy and confusion of TUR syndrome from postoperative disorientation and hyponatremia
- Maintain patient safety during times of confusion
- Assess lung and heart sounds for indications of pulmonary edema, heart failure, or both as fluid moves back into the intravascular space

pubic arch and the bladder without entering the bladder (Fig. 49-4D). This procedure is suitable for large glands located high in the pelvis. Although blood loss can be better controlled and the surgical site is easier to visualize, infections can readily start in the retropubic space.

Transurethral Incision of the Prostate

TUIP is another procedure used to treat BPH. An instrument is passed through the urethra (Fig. 49-4E). TUIP is indicated when the prostate gland is small (30 g or less), and it is an effective treatment for many cases of BPH. TUIP can be performed on an outpatient basis and has a lower complication rate than other invasive prostate procedures.

Laparoscopic Radical Prostatectomy

In contrast to the single abdominal incision made for the radical prostatectomy, a laparoscopic radical prostatectomy is performed through four to six small (0.5 in [1 cm]) incisions in the midabdomen. Instruments, including a lighted viewing instrument (laparoscope), are inserted and allow the surgeon to remove the prostate gland. The laparoscopic approach reduces the risk of postoperative erectile dysfunction and urinary dysfunction. Laparoscopic radical prostatectomy results in less bleeding, reduced need for blood transfusion, a shorter hospital stay, less postoperative pain, and more rapid return to normal activity compared with open radical prostatectomy (Rigdon, 2006). Further research is needed to assess long-term outcomes.

Robotic-Assisted Laparoscopic Radical Prostatectomy

Robotic-assisted laparoscopic radical prostatectomy is a new minimally invasive approach that uses a computer console and da Vinci robot to move the tips of microscopic instruments, replicating the movements of the surgeon's hands (Rigdon, 2006; Starnes & Sims, 2006).

Pelvic Lymph Node Dissection

Pelvic lymph node dissection (PLND) is not always performed. It may be used in some patients to provide information for staging the tumor and to remove an area of microscopic metastasis. The planned treatment may influence the surgeon's decision to perform PLND and the extent (limited versus extended) of the dissection. Dissection of nodes anterior and lateral to the external iliac vessels is associated with an increased risk of lymphedema (NCCN, 2009).

Complications

Postoperative complications depend on the type of prostatectomy performed and may include hemorrhage, clot formation, catheter obstruction, and sexual dysfunction. All prostatectomies carry a risk of impotence because of potential damage to the pudendal nerves. In most instances, sexual activity may be resumed in 6 to 8 weeks, the time required for the prostatic fossa to heal. During ejaculation, the seminal fluid goes into the bladder and is excreted with the urine. The anatomic changes in the posterior urethra lead to retrograde ejaculation. A vasectomy may be performed during surgery to prevent infection from spreading from the prostatic urethra through the vas and into the epididymis.

After total prostatectomy (usually for cancer), the risk for impotence is high. For the patient for whom this is unacceptable, options are available to produce erections sufficient for sexual intercourse: prosthetic penile implants, negative-pressure (vacuum) devices, and pharmacologic interventions (see earlier discussion and Table 49-2).

NURSING PROCESS

PATIENT UNDERGOING PROSTATECTOMY

Assessment

The nurse assesses how the underlying disorder (BPH or prostate cancer) has affected the patient's lifestyle. Questions to ask during assessment include the following: Has the patient's activity level or activity tolerance changed? What is his presenting urinary problem (described in the patient's own words)? Has he experienced decreased force of urinary flow, decreased ability to initiate voiding, urgency, frequency, nocturia, dysuria, urinary retention, or hematuria? Does the patient report back pain, flank pain, and lower abdominal or suprapubic discomfort? Possible causes of such discomfort include infection, retention, and renal colic. Has the patient experienced erectile dysfunction or changes in frequency or enjoyment of sexual activity?

The nurse obtains further information about the patient's family history of cancer and heart or kidney disease, including hypertension. Has he lost weight? Does he appear pale? Can he raise himself out of bed and return to bed without assistance? Can he perform usual activities of daily living? This information helps determine how soon the patient will be able to return to normal activities after prostatectomy.

Diagnosis

Preoperative Nursing Diagnoses

Based on the assessment data, the patient's major nursing diagnoses may include the following.
- Anxiety about surgery and its outcome
- Acute pain related to bladder distention
- Deficient knowledge about factors related to the disorder and the treatment protocol

Postoperative Nursing Diagnoses

- Acute pain related to the surgical incision, catheter placement, and bladder spasms
- Deficient knowledge about postoperative care

Collaborative Problems/Potential Complications

Based on the assessment data, the potential complications may include the following:
- Hemorrhage and shock
- Infection
- Deep vein thrombosis
- Catheter obstruction
- Sexual dysfunction

Planning and Goals

The major preoperative goals for the patient may include reduced anxiety and learning about his prostate disorder and the perioperative experience. The major postoperative goals may include maintenance of fluid volume balance, relief of pain and discomfort, ability to perform self-care activities, and absence of complications.

Preoperative Nursing Interventions

Reducing Anxiety

The patient is frequently admitted to the hospital or surgical center on the morning of surgery. Because contact with the patient may be limited before surgery, the nurse must establish communication with the patient to assess his understanding of the diagnosis and of the planned surgical procedure. The nurse clarifies the nature of the surgery and expected postoperative outcomes. In addition, the nurse familiarizes the patient with the preoperative and postoperative routines and initiates measures to reduce anxiety. Because the patient may be sensitive and embarrassed discussing problems related to the genitalia and sexuality, the nurse provides privacy and establishes a trusting and professional relationship. Guilt feelings often surface if the patient falsely assumes a cause-and-effect relationship between sexual practices and his current problems. He is encouraged to verbalize his feelings and concerns.

Relieving Discomfort

If the patient experiences discomfort before surgery, bed rest is prescribed, analgesic agents are administered, and measures are initiated to relieve anxiety. If he is hospitalized, the nurse monitors his voiding patterns, watches for bladder distention, and assists with catheterization if indicated. An indwelling catheter is inserted if the patient has continuing urinary retention or if close monitoring is needed because of laboratory test results that indicate azotemia (accumulation of nitrogenous waste products in the blood). The catheter can help decompress the bladder gradually over several days, especially if the patient is elderly and hypertensive and has diminished renal function or urinary retention that has existed for many weeks. For a few days after the bladder begins draining, the blood pressure may fluctuate and renal function may decline. If the patient cannot tolerate a urinary catheter, he is prepared for a cystostomy (and insertion of a suprapubic catheter).

Providing Instruction

Before surgery, the nurse reviews with the patient the anatomy of the affected structures and their function in relation to the urinary and reproductive systems, using diagrams and other teaching aids if indicated. This instruction often takes place during the preadmission testing visit or in the urologist's office. The nurse explains what will take place while the patient is prepared for diagnostic tests and then for surgery (depending on the type of prostatectomy planned). The nurse also reinforces information given by the surgeon about the type of incision, which varies with the surgical approach (directly over the bladder, low on the abdomen, or in the perineal area; four to six small incisions with laparoscopic and robotic-assisted approaches; and no incision with a transurethral procedure), and describes the likely type of urinary drainage system (urethral or suprapubic) and the recovery room procedure. The amount of information given is based on the patient's needs and questions. The nurse explains procedures expected to occur during the immediate perioperative period, answers questions the patient or family may have, and provides emotional support. In addition, the nurse provides the patient with information about postoperative pain management.

Preparing the Patient

If the patient is scheduled for a prostatectomy, the preoperative preparation described in Chapter 18 is provided. Antiembolism stockings are applied before surgery and are particularly important to prevent deep vein thrombosis (DVT) if the patient is placed in a lithotomy position during surgery. An enema is usually administered at home on the evening before surgery or on the morning of surgery to prevent postoperative straining, which can induce bleeding.

Postoperative Nursing Interventions

Maintaining Fluid Balance

During the postoperative period, the patient is at risk for imbalanced fluid volume because of the irrigation of the surgical site during and after surgery. With irrigation of the urinary catheter to prevent its obstruction by blood clots, fluid may be absorbed through the open surgical site and retained, increasing the risk of excessive fluid retention, fluid imbalance, and water intoxication. The urine output and the amount of fluid used for irrigation must be closely monitored to determine whether irrigation fluid is being retained and to ensure an adequate urine output. An intake and output record, including the amount of fluid used for irrigation, must be maintained. The patient is also monitored for electrolyte imbalances (eg, hyponatremia), increasing blood pressure, confusion, and respiratory distress. These signs and symptoms are documented and reported to the surgeon. The risk of fluid and electrolyte imbalance is greater in elderly patients with preexisting cardiovascular or respiratory disease.

Relieving Pain

After a prostatectomy, the patient is assisted to sit and dangle his legs over the side of the bed on the day of surgery. The next morning, he is assisted to ambulate. If pain is present, the cause and location are determined and the severity of pain and discomfort is assessed. The pain may be related to the incision or may be the result of excoriation of the skin at the catheter site. It may be in the flank area, indicating a kidney problem, or it may be caused by bladder spasms. Bladder irritability can initiate bleeding and result in clot formation, leading to urinary retention.

Patients experiencing bladder spasms may report an urgency to void, a feeling of pressure or fullness in the bladder, and bleeding from the urethra around the catheter. Medications that relax the smooth muscles can help ease the spasms, which can be intermittent and severe; these medications include flavoxate (Urispas) and oxybutynin (Ditropan). Warm compresses to the pubis or sitz baths may also relieve the spasms.

The nurse monitors the drainage tubing and irrigates the system as prescribed to relieve any obstruction that may cause discomfort. Usually, the catheter is irrigated with 50 mL of irrigating fluid at a time. It is important to make sure that the same amount is recovered in the drainage receptacle. Securing the catheter drainage tubing to the leg or abdomen can help decrease tension on the catheter and prevent bladder irritation. Discomfort may be caused by dressings that are too snug, saturated with drainage, or improperly placed. Analgesic agents are administered as prescribed. The nurse notifies the physician if the analgesic medications do not relieve the patient's pain and obtains a prescription for new doses or different medications.

After the patient is ambulatory, he is encouraged to walk but not to sit for prolonged periods, because this increases intra-abdominal pressure and the possibility of discomfort and bleeding. Prune juice and stool softeners are provided to ease bowel movements and to prevent excessive straining. An enema, if prescribed, is administered with caution to avoid rectal perforation.

Monitoring and Managing Potential Complications

After prostatectomy, the patient is monitored for major complications such as hemorrhage, infection, DVT, catheter obstruction, and sexual dysfunction.

HEMORRHAGE. Although patients have discontinued all aspirin, nonsteroidal anti-inflammatory drugs, and platelet inhibitors 10 to 14 days before the surgery to prevent excessive bleeding, bleeding and hemorrhagic shock remain the greatest risks. The risk is increased with BPH because a hyperplastic prostate gland is very vascular. Bleeding may occur from the prostatic bed. Bleeding may also result in the formation of clots, which then obstruct urine flow. The drainage normally begins as reddish-pink and then clears to a light pink within 24 hours after surgery. Bright red bleeding with increased viscosity and numerous clots usually indicates arterial bleeding. Venous blood appears darker and less viscous. Arterial hemorrhage usually requires surgical intervention (eg, suturing or transurethral coagulation of bleeding vessels), whereas venous bleeding may be controlled by applying prescribed traction to the catheter so that the balloon holding the catheter in place applies pressure to the prostatic fossa. The surgeon applies traction by securely taping the catheter to the patient's thigh if hemorrhage occurs. Less blood loss (150 mL) is expected with robotic-assisted laparoscopic radical prostatectomy, compared with 500 to 900 mL, which may occur with open prostatectomy.

Nursing management includes assistance in implementing strategies to stop the bleeding and to prevent or reverse hemorrhagic shock. If blood loss is extensive, fluids and blood component therapy may be administered. If hemorrhagic shock occurs, treatments described in Chapter 15 are initiated.

Nursing interventions include closely monitoring vital signs; administering medications, IV fluids, and blood component therapy as prescribed; maintaining an accurate record of intake and output; and carefully monitoring drainage to ensure adequate urine flow and patency of the drainage system. The patient who experiences hemorrhage and his family are often anxious and benefit from explanations and reassurance about the event and the procedures that are performed.

INFECTION. After perineal prostatectomy, the surgeon usually changes the dressing on the first postoperative day. Further dressing changes may become the responsibility of the nurse or home care nurse. Careful aseptic technique is used because the potential for infection is great. Dressings can be held in place by a double-tailed, T-binder bandage or a padded athletic supporter. The tails cross over the incision to give double thickness, and then each tail is drawn up on either side of the scrotum to the waistline and fastened.

Rectal thermometers, rectal tubes, and enemas are avoided because of the risk of injury and bleeding in the prostatic fossa. After the perineal sutures are removed, the perineum is cleansed as indicated. A heat lamp may be directed to the perineal area to promote healing. The scrotum is protected with a towel while the heat lamp is in use. Sitz baths are also used to promote healing.

UTIs and epididymitis are possible complications after prostatectomy. The patient is assessed for their occurrence; if they occur, the nurse administers antibiotics as prescribed. Because the risk of infection continues after discharge from the hospital, the patient and family need to be instructed to monitor for signs and symptoms of infection (fever, chills, sweating, myalgia, dysuria, urinary frequency, and urgency). The patient and family are instructed to contact the urologist if these symptoms occur.

DEEP VEIN THROMBOSIS. Patients undergoing prostatectomy are at risk for DVT and pulmonary embolism; therefore, the nurse assesses the patient frequently after surgery for manifestations of DVT. Further, anti-embolism stockings are used to reduce the risk of DVT and pulmonary embolism. Early postoperative ambulation is essential to reduce the risk of DVT. Nursing and medical management of DVT and pulmonary embolism are described in Chapters 31 and 23, respectively. In addition, if the patient is at high risk for clot formation, IV heparin or subcutaneous enoxaparin (Lovenox) may be administered.

OBSTRUCTED CATHETER. After a TURP, the catheter must drain well; an obstructed catheter produces distention of the prostatic capsule and resultant hemorrhage. Furosemide (Lasix) may be prescribed to promote urination and initiate postoperative diuresis, thereby helping to keep the catheter patent.

The nurse observes the lower abdomen to ensure that the catheter has not become blocked. A distinct, rounded swelling above the pubis is a manifestation of an overdistended bladder.

The drainage bag, dressings, and surgical incision are examined for bleeding. The color of the urine is noted and documented; a change in color from pink to amber indicates reduced bleeding. Blood pressure, pulse, and respirations are monitored and compared with baseline preoperative vital signs to detect hypotension. The nurse also observes the patient for restlessness, diaphoresis, pallor, any drop in blood pressure, and an increasing pulse rate.

Drainage of the bladder may be accomplished by gravity through a closed sterile drainage system. A three-way drainage system is useful in irrigating the bladder and preventing clot formation (Fig. 49-5). Continuous irrigation may be used with TURP. Some urologists leave an indwelling catheter attached to a dependent drainage system. Gentle irrigation of the catheter may be prescribed to remove any obstructing clots.

If the patient complains of pain, the tubing is examined. The drainage system is irrigated with irrigating fluid (usually 50 mL), if indicated and prescribed, to clear any obstruction. The amount of fluid recovered in the drainage bag must equal the amount of fluid instilled. Overdistention of the bladder is avoided because it can induce secondary hemorrhage by stretching the coagulated blood vessels in the prostatic capsule.

To prevent traction on the bladder, the drainage tube (not the catheter) is taped to the shaved inner thigh. If a cystostomy catheter is in place, it is taped to the abdomen. The nurse explains the purpose of the catheter to the patient and assures him that the urge to void results from the presence of the catheter and from bladder spasms. He is cautioned not to pull on the catheter because this causes bleeding and subsequent catheter blockage, which leads to urinary retention.

COMPLICATIONS WITH CATHETER REMOVAL. After the catheter is removed (usually when the urine appears clear), urine may leak around the wound for several days in the patient who has undergone perineal, suprapubic, or retropubic surgery. The cystostomy tube may be removed before or after the urethral catheter is removed. Some urinary incontinence may occur after catheter removal, and the patient is informed that this is likely to subside over time (see below).

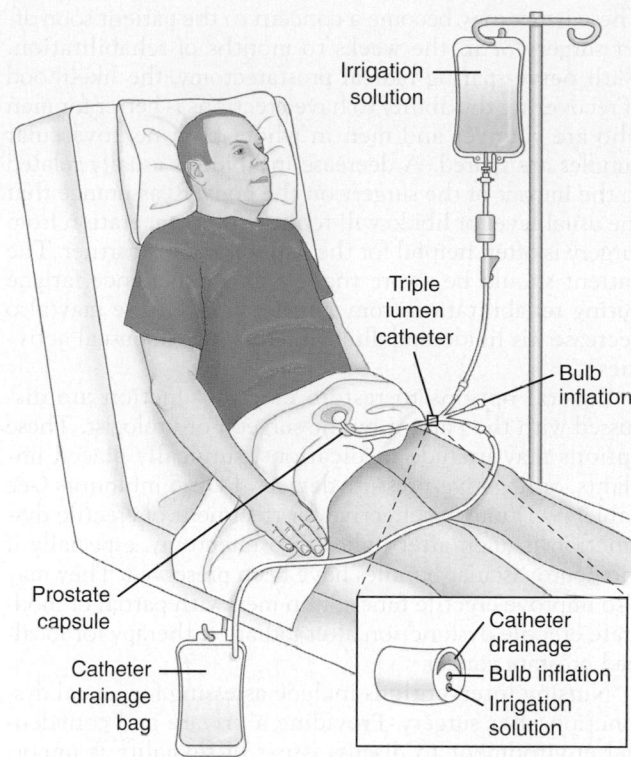

Figure 49-5 A three-way system for bladder irrigation.

URINARY INCONTINENCE. Postoperative urinary incontinence, a devastating complication of prostatectomy, occurs in 80% to 95% of patients. Urinary incontinence often decreases over time—although it may last as long as 1 to 2 years following surgery. Factors associated with postoperative continence are younger age, preservation of both neurovascular bundles, absence of an anastomotic stricture, eversion of the bladder neck, and a smaller prostate volume. The nurse can encourage the patient who experiences incontinence to take steps to prevent incontinence, improve continence, anticipate leakage, and cope with lack of complete control (Yu Ko & Sawatzky, 2008). Preventing incontinence involves increasing voiding frequency, avoiding positions that encourage the urge to void, and decreasing fluid intake prior to activities. Promoting continence involves pelvic floor exercises (see Teaching Patients Self-Care below), biofeedback, and electrical stimulation. Anticipating leakage may entail lifestyle modifications such as using absorbent pads and carrying extra clothes to prevent urinary accidents; this can improve confidence when bathroom access is limited. It also helps to know the location of public bathrooms. Coping long term with complete lack of control may involve collagen injections, artificial sphincter implants, medications, and leg bags (Michaelson, et al., 2008; Yu Ko & Sawatzky, 2008).

SEXUAL DYSFUNCTION. Depending on the type of surgery, the patient may experience sexual dysfunction related to erectile dysfunction, decreased libido, and fatigue.

These issues may become a concern to the patient soon after surgery or in the weeks to months of rehabilitation. With nerve-sparing radical prostatectomy, the likelihood of recovering the ability to have erections is better for men who are younger and men in whom both neurovascular bundles are spared. A decrease in libido is usually related to the impact of the surgery on the body. Reassurance that the usual level of libido will return after recuperation from surgery is often helpful for the patient and his partner. The patient should be aware that he may experience fatigue during rehabilitation from surgery. This fatigue may also decrease his libido and alter his enjoyment of usual activities.

Several options to restore erectile function are discussed with the patient by the surgeon or urologist. These options may include medications, surgically placed implants, or negative-pressure devices. PDE-5 inhibitors (see Table 49-3) may be effective for treatment of erectile dysfunction in men after radical prostatectomy, especially if the neurovascular bundles have been preserved. They may also improve erectile function in men with partial or moderate erectile dysfunction after radiation therapy for localized prostate cancer.

Nursing interventions include assessing for sexual dysfunction after surgery. Providing a private and confidential environment to discuss issues of sexuality is important. The emotional challenges of prostate surgery and its consequences need to be carefully explored with the patient and his partner. Providing the opportunity to discuss these issues can be very beneficial to the patient. For patients who have significant difficulty adjusting to sexual dysfunction, a referral to a sex therapist may be indicated.

Promoting Home and Community-Based Care

TEACHING PATIENTS SELF-CARE. The patient undergoing prostatectomy may be discharged within several days. The length of the hospital stay depends on the surgical approach used and may range from 1 to 2 days for robotic-assisted laparoscopic prostatectomy to 3 to 5 days for open prostatectomy. The patient and family require instructions about how to manage the drainage system, how to assess for complications, and how to promote recovery. The nurse provides verbal and written instructions about the need to maintain the drainage system and to monitor urinary output, about wound care, and about strategies to prevent complications, such as infection, bleeding, and thrombosis. In addition, the patient and family need to know about signs and symptoms that should be reported to the physician (eg, blood in urine, decreased urine output, fever, change in wound drainage, calf tenderness).

As the patient recovers and drainage tubes are removed, he may become discouraged and depressed because he cannot regain bladder control immediately. Furthermore, urinary frequency and burning may occur after the catheter is removed. Teaching the patient the following exercises may help him regain urinary control:

- Tense the perineal muscles by pressing the buttocks together, hold this position, and then relax. This exercise can be performed 10 to 20 times each hour while sitting or standing.
- Try to interrupt the urinary stream after starting to void; wait a few seconds and then continue to void.

Perineal exercises should continue until the patient gains full urinary control. The patient is instructed to urinate as soon as he feels the first urge to do so. It is important that the patient know that regaining urinary control is a gradual process; he may continue to "dribble" after being discharged from the hospital, but this should gradually diminish (usually within 1 year). The urine may be cloudy for several weeks after surgery but should clear as the prostate area heals.

While the prostatic fossa heals (6 to 8 weeks), the patient should avoid activities that produce Valsalva effects (straining, heavy lifting) because this may increase venous pressure and produce hematuria. He should avoid long motor trips and strenuous exercise, which increase the tendency to bleed. He should also know that spicy foods, alcohol, and coffee may cause bladder discomfort. The patient should be cautioned to drink enough fluids to avoid dehydration, which increases the tendency for a blood clot to form and obstruct the flow of urine. Signs of complications, such as bleeding, passage of blood clots, a decrease in the urinary stream, urinary retention, or symptoms of UTIs, should be reported to the physician (Chart 49-5). Patients who have undergone robotic-assisted prostatectomy are often able to return to their usual activities in approximately 7 to 10 days (Rigdon, 2006).

CHART 49-5 HOME CARE CHECKLIST
Postprostatectomy Care

At the completion of the home care instruction, the patient or caregiver will be able to:	PATIENT	CAREGIVER
• Demonstrate appropriate measures to relieve postoperative pain and discomfort.	✔	✔
• Demonstrate appropriate care of urinary catheter and collection receptacle.	✔	✔
• Demonstrate appropriate wound care.	✔	✔
• Demonstrate performance of perineal muscle exercises to facilitate bladder control.	✔	
• Demonstrate increased activity and ambulation.	✔	
• Identify activities to avoid, such as lifting heavy objects.	✔	✔
• Identify signs and symptoms of complications that should be reported to surgeon.	✔	✔

CONTINUING CARE. Referral for home care may be indicated if the patient is elderly or has other health problems, if the patient and family cannot provide care in the home, or if the patient lives alone without available supports. The home care nurse assesses the patient's physical status (cardiovascular and respiratory status, fluid and nutritional status, patency of the urinary drainage system, wound and nutritional status) and provides catheter and wound care, if indicated. The nurse reinforces previous teaching and assesses the ability of the patient and family to manage required care. The home care nurse encourages the patient to ambulate and to carry out perineal exercises as prescribed. The patient may need to be reminded that return of bladder control may take time.

The patient is reminded about the importance of routine health screening and other health promotion activities. If the prostatectomy was performed to treat prostate cancer, the patient and family are also instructed about the importance of follow-up and monitoring with the physician.

Evaluation

Expected Preoperative Patient Outcomes

Expected preoperative patient outcomes may include the following:

1. Demonstrates reduced anxiety
2. States that pain and discomfort are decreased
3. Relates understanding of the surgical procedure and postoperative course and practices perineal muscle exercises and other techniques useful in facilitating bladder control

Expected Postoperative Patient Outcomes

Expected postoperative patient outcomes may include the following:

1. Reports relief of discomfort
2. Exhibits fluid and electrolyte balance
   a. Irrigation fluid and urinary output are within parameters determined by surgeon
   b. Experiences no signs or symptoms of fluid retention
3. Participates in self-care measures
   a. Increases activity and ambulation daily
   b. Produces urine output within normal ranges and consistent with intake
   c. Performs perineal exercises and interrupts urinary stream to promote bladder control
   d. Avoids straining and lifting heavy objects
4. Is free of complications
   a. Maintains vital signs within normal limits
   b. Exhibits wound healing, without signs of inflammation or hemorrhage
   c. Maintains acceptable level of urinary elimination
   d. Maintains optimal drainage of catheter and other drainage tubes
   e. Reports understanding of changes in sexual function

CONDITIONS AFFECTING THE TESTES AND ADJACENT STRUCTURES

Orchitis

Orchitis is a rare, acute inflammatory response of one or both testes as a complication of systemic infection or as an extension of an associated epididymitis caused by bacterial, viral, spirochetal, or parasitic organisms. Micro-organisms may reach the testes through the blood, lymphatic system, or, more commonly, by traveling through the urethra, vas deferens, and epididymis; bacteria usually spread from an associated epididymitis in sexually active men. Causative organisms include *Neisseria gonorrhoeae*, *Chlamydia trachomatis*, *E. coli*, *Klebsiella*, *Pseudomonas aeruginosa*, *Staphylococcus* species, and *Streptococcus* species. A more common cause of isolated orchitis is mumps. Orchitis develops in approximately 30% of postpubertal men with mumps 4 to 6 days after parotitis starts, and one third of men have some testicular atrophy.

Signs and symptoms of orchitis include fever; pain, which may range from mild to severe; tenderness in one or both testicles; bilateral or unilateral testicular swelling; penile discharge; blood in the semen; and leukocytosis.

Treatment of orchitis is based on whether the causative organism is bacterial or viral. Bacterial orchitis is treated with antibiotics and supportive comfort measures. If the cause of the orchitis is an STD, the partner should be treated as well. Viral orchitis is treated using supportive treatments of rest, elevation of the scrotum, ice packs to reduce scrotal edema, analgesic agents, and anti-inflammatory medications. Bilateral orchitis can cause sterility in some men. Mumps vaccination is recommended for postpubertal men who have not had mumps or received inadequate immunization in childhood.

Epididymitis

Epididymitis is an infection of the epididymis, which usually spreads from an infected urethra, bladder, or prostate. The incidence is less than 1 in 1000 males per year. Prevalence is greatest in men 19 to 35 years of age. Acute epididymitis occurs bilaterally in 5% to 10% of affected patients. Risk factors for epididymitis include recent surgery or a procedure involving the urinary tract, participation in high-risk sexual practices, personal history of an STD, past prostate infections or UTIs, lack of circumcision, history of an enlarged prostate, and the presence of a chronic indwelling urinary catheter.

Pathophysiology

A causative organism can be identified in 80% of patients. In prepubertal males, older men, and homosexual men, the predominate causal organism is *E. coli*, although in older men, the condition may also be a result of urinary obstruction. In sexually active men ages 35 years of age and younger, the pathogens usually are related to bacteria associated with STDs (eg, *C. trachomatis*, *N. gonorrhoeae*). The infection moves in an upward direction, through the urethra and the ejaculatory duct, and then along the vas deferens to the epididymis.

Clinical Manifestations

Epididymitis often slowly develops over 1 to 2 days, beginning with a low-grade fever, chills, and heaviness in the affected testicle. The testicle becomes increasingly tender to pressure and traction. The patient may report unilateral pain, soreness in the inguinal canal along the course of the vas deferens, and pain and swelling in the scrotum and the groin. The epididymis becomes increasingly swollen, with extreme pain in the lower abdomen and pelvis. Occasionally, there may be discharge from the urethra, blood in the semen, pus (pyuria) and bacteria (bacteriuria) in the urine, and pain during intercourse and ejaculation. The patient may report urinary frequency, urgency, or dysuria, and testicular pain aggravated by bowel movement.

Assessment and Diagnostic Findings

Laboratory assessment includes urinalysis, complete blood cell count, Gram stain of urethral drainage, urethral culture or DNA probe, and referral for syphilis and HIV testing in sexually active patients. Acute testicular pain should never be ignored, and it should be distinguished from testicular torsion, which is a surgical emergency.

Medical Management

The selection of an antibiotic depends on the causative organism; if epididymitis is associated with an STD, the patient's partner should also receive antimicrobial therapy. The spermatic cord may be infiltrated with a local anesthetic agent to relieve pain if the patient is seen within the first 24 hours after onset of pain. Supportive interventions also include reduction in physical activity, scrotal support and elevation, ice packs, anti-inflammatory agents, analgesics, including nerve blocks, and sitz baths. Urethral instrumentation (eg, catheter insertion) is avoided. The patient is observed for scrotal abscess formation as well.

In chronic epididymitis, a 4- to 6-week course of antibiotics for bacterial pathogens is prescribed. An epididymectomy (excision of the epididymis from the testis) may be performed for patients who have recurrent, refractory, incapacitating episodes of this infection. With long-term epididymitis, the passage of sperm may be obstructed. If the obstruction is bilateral, infertility may result.

Nursing Management

Bed rest is prescribed, and the scrotum is elevated with a scrotal bridge or folded towel to prevent traction on the spermatic cord, to promote venous drainage, and to relieve pain. Antimicrobial agents are administered as prescribed until the acute inflammation subsides. Intermittent cold compresses to the scrotum may help ease the pain. Later, local heat or sitz baths may help resolve the inflammation. Analgesic medications are administered for pain relief as prescribed.

The nurse instructs the patient to avoid straining, lifting, and sexual stimulation until the infection is under control. He should continue taking analgesic agents and antibiotics as prescribed and using ice packs if necessary to relieve

discomfort. He needs to know that it may take 4 weeks or longer for the inflammation to resolve.

Testicular Torsion

Testicular torsion is a surgical emergency requiring immediate diagnosis to avoid loss of the testicle. Torsion of the testis is rotation of the testis, which twists the blood vessels in the spermatic cord, and, therefore, impedes the arterial and venous supply to the testicle and surrounding structures in the scrotum. The patient presents with sudden pain in the testicle, developing over 1 to 2 hours, with or without a predisposing event. Nausea, lightheadedness, and swelling of the scrotum may develop. On physical examination, testicular tenderness, an elevated testis, a thickened spermatic cord, and a swollen, painful scrotum may be present. If the torsion cannot be reduced manually, surgery to untwist the spermatic cord and anchor both testes in their correct position to prevent recurrence should occur within 6 hours of the onset of symptoms in order to save the testis. After 6 hours of impaired blood supply, the risk for loss of the testicle increases.

Testicular Cancer

Although only accounting for about 1% of all cancers in men, **testicular cancer** is the most common cancer diagnosed in men between 15 and 35 years of age; approximately 8400 new cases and 380 deaths occur in the United States annually (ACS, 2009). It is the second most common malignancy in those 35 to 39 years of age. For unknown reasons, worldwide incidence of testicular tumors has more than doubled in the past 40 years. Because of advances in cancer therapy, testicular cancer is a highly treatable and usually curable form of cancer. The 5-year relative survival rate for all testicular cancers is more than 95% and approaches 99% if the cancer has not spread outside of the testes (ACS, 2009). After treatment, most patients with testicular cancer have a near-normal life expectancy.

Classification of Testicular Tumors

The testicles contain several types of cells, each of which may develop into one or more types of cancer. The type of cancer cell determines the appropriate treatment and affects the prognosis. Testicular cancer is classified as germinal or nongerminal (stromal). Secondary testicular cancers may also occur.

Germinal Tumors

Germinal tumors make up approximately 90% of all cancers of the testis; germinal tumors are further classified as seminomas or nonseminomas. These cancers grow from the germ cells that produce sperm, thus the name germinal tumors. Seminomas are slow-growing forms of testicular cancer that are usually found in men in their 30s and 40s. Although seminomas can spread to the lymph nodes, the cancer is usually localized in the testes. Nonseminomas are more common and tend to grow more quickly than seminomas. Nonseminomas are often made up of different cell types and are identified according to the cells in which they start to grow. Nonseminoma testicular cancers include choriocarcinomas (rare), embryonal carcinomas, teratomas, and yolk sac tumors. It is crucial to distinguish between seminomas and nonseminomas because the differences affect prognosis and treatment.

Nongerminal Tumors

Nongerminal tumors account for less than 10% of testicular cancers. These cancers may develop in the supportive and hormone-producing tissues, or stroma, of the testicles. The two main types of stromal tumors are Leydig cell tumors and Sertoli cell tumors. Although these tumors infrequently spread beyond the testicle, a small number metastasize and tend to be resistant to chemotherapy and radiation therapy.

Secondary Testicular Tumors

Secondary testicular tumors are those that have metastasized to the testicle from other organs. Lymphoma is the most common cause of secondary testicular cancer. Cancers may also spread to the testicles from the prostate gland, lung, skin (melanoma), kidney, and other organs. The prognosis with these cancers is usually poor because they typically also spread to other organs. Treatment depends on the specific type of cancer (ACS, 2009).

Risk Factors

Risk factors for testicular cancer include undescended testicles (**cryptorchidism**), family history of testicular cancer, and personal history of testicular cancer (ACS, 2009; Gilligan, 2007). Other risk factors include race and ethnicity: Caucasian American men have a five times greater risk than African American men and more than two to three times greater risk than Asian, Native American, and Hispanic American men. The risk of developing testicular cancer is higher in HIV-positive men (ACS, 2009). Occupational hazards, including exposure to chemicals encountered in mining, oil and gas production, and leather processing, have been suggested as possible risk factors. No evidence has linked testicular cancer to prenatal exposure to diethylstilbestrol or to vasectomy (ACS, 2009).

Clinical Manifestations

The symptoms appear gradually, with a mass or lump on the testicle and usually painless enlargement of the testis. The patient may report heaviness in the scrotum, inguinal area, or lower abdomen. Backache (from retroperitoneal node extension), abdominal pain, weight loss, and general weakness may result from metastasis. Enlargement of the testis without pain is a significant diagnostic finding. Some testicular tumors tend to metastasize early, spreading from the testis to the lymph nodes in the retroperitoneum and to the lungs.

Assessment and Diagnostic Findings

At this time, screening for testicular cancer is not recommended; however, educating young men about testicular cancer and the need for urgent evaluation of any mass or enlargement or unexplained testicular pain is key to early detection (Gilligan, 2007). Teaching TSE, starting in adolescence, alerts men to the importance of seeking medical attention if a testicle becomes indurated, enlarged, atrophied, nodular, or painful (Chart 49-6). TSE should be performed monthly. Testicular cancers generally grow rapidly and are easily detected against a typically smooth and homogeneous texture. Annual testicular examination by a clinician can reveal signs and lead to early diagnosis and treatment of testicular cancer. Promoting awareness of this disease is an important health promotion intervention; men should seek medical evaluation for signs or symptoms of testicular cancer without delay (Gilligan, 2007). Any suspicious testicular mass warrants prompt evaluation with a thorough history and physical examination, focusing on palpation of the affected testicle.

The tumor markers alpha-fetoprotein (AFP) and beta-human chorionic gonadotropin (beta-hCG) may be elevated in patients with testicular cancer. Tumor marker levels in the blood are used for diagnosis, staging, and monitoring the response to treatment. Blood chemistry, including lactate dehydrogenase, is also necessary.

A chest x-ray to assess for metastasis in the lungs and a transscrotal testicular ultrasound will be performed. Microscopic analysis of tissue is the only definitive way to determine if cancer is present, but it is usually performed at the time of surgery rather than as a part of the diagnostic workup to reduce the risk of promoting spread of the cancer (ACS, 2009). Inguinal orchiectomy is the standard way to establish the diagnosis of testicular cancer. Other staging tests to determine the extent of the disease in the retroperitoneum, pelvis, and chest include an abdominal/pelvic CT and chest CT (if the abdominal CT or chest x-ray is abnormal). A brain MRI and bone scan may be obtained if indicated (NCCN, 2008). Discussion of the option to bank sperm should take place prior to orchiectomy and treatment.

Medical Management

Testicular cancer, one of the most curable solid tumors, is highly responsive to treatment. Early-stage disease is curable more than 95% of the time; thus, prompt diagnosis and treatment are essential. The NCCN practice consensus guidelines for testicular cancer are used to guide diagnostic workup, primary treatment, follow-up, and salvage therapy (treatment given when the cancer does not respond to standard treatment) for both seminomas and nonseminomas (NCCN, 2008). The goals of management are to eradicate the disease and achieve a cure. Therapy is based on the cell type, the stage of the disease, and risk classification tables (determined as good, intermediate, and poor risk). Primary treatment includes removal of the affected testis by orchiectomy through an inguinal incision with a high ligation of the spermatic cord. The patient is offered the option of implantation of a testicular prosthesis during the orchiectomy. Although most patients experience no impairment of endocrine function after unilateral orchiectomy for testicular cancer, some patients have decreased hormonal levels, suggesting that the unaffected testis is not functioning normally. Retroperitoneal lymph node dissection (RPLND) may be performed after orchiectomy to diagnose and prevent lymphatic spread of the cancer. Alternatives to the more invasive open RPLND for

---

**CHART
49-6**

PATIENT EDUCATION
Testicular Self-Examination

Testicular self-examination (TSE) is to be performed once a month. The test is neither difficult nor time-consuming. A convenient time is usually after a warm bath or shower when the scrotum is more relaxed.

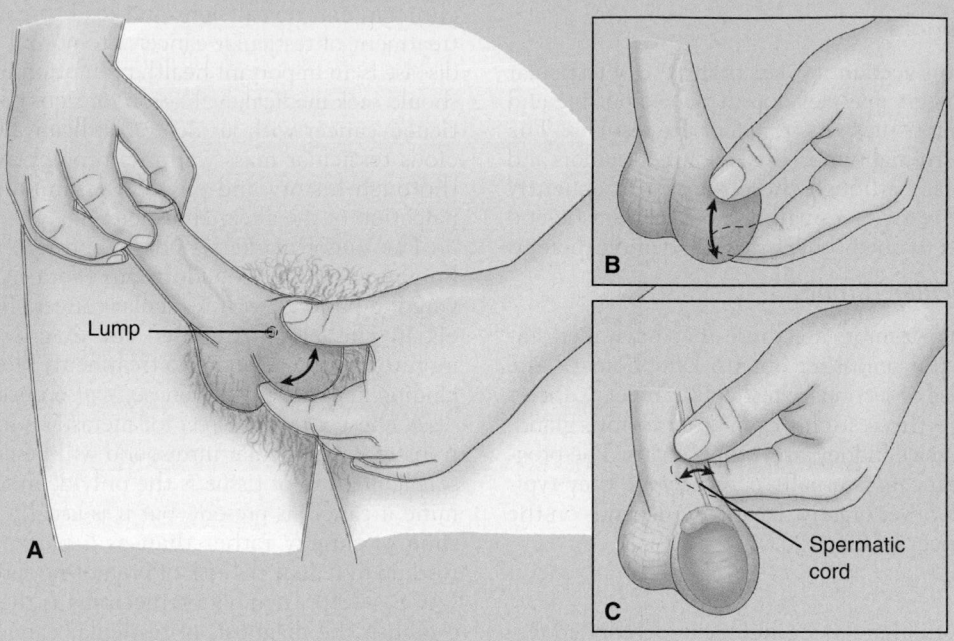

1. Use both hands to palpate the testis. The normal testicle is smooth and uniform in consistency.
2. With the index and middle fingers under the testis and the thumb on top, roll the testis gently in a horizontal plane between the thumb and fingers **(A)**.
3. Feel for any evidence of a small lump or abnormality.
4. Follow the same procedure and palpate upward along the testis **(B)**.
5. Locate and palpate the epididymis **(C)**, a cordlike structure on the top and back of the testicle that stores and transports sperm. Also locate and palpate the spermatic cord.
6. Repeat the examination for the other testis, epididymis, and spermatic cord. It is normal to find that one testis is larger than the other.
7. If you find any evidence of a small, pealike lump or if the testis is swollen (possibly from an infection or tumor), consult your physician.

---

early-stage germ cell testicular cancer include nerve-sparing and laparoscopic RPLND, which improve sexual function and promote rapid recovery (Tanagho & McAninch, 2008). Although libido and orgasm are usually unimpaired after RPLND, ejaculatory dysfunction with resultant infertility may develop. Two thirds of men who are newly diagnosed with testicular cancer may be considering future fatherhood, and sperm quality is reduced in men with testicular cancer; therefore, sperm banking before treatment may be considered (Fossa & Dahl, 2008; Girasole, Cookson, Smith, et al., 2006). Half of patients will not recover fertility as a result of radiation therapy, cytotoxic therapy, unilateral excision of a testis, and RPLND. Counseling about fertility issues may help the patient make the appropriate choices (Brydøy, Fosså, Klepp, et al., 2005; Gospodarowicz, 2008).

Radiation therapy is more effective with seminomas than with nonseminomas. Postoperatively, radiation may be used in early-stage seminomas. It is delivered only to the affected side; the other testis is shielded from radiation to preserve fertility. Radiation is also used in patients whose disease does not respond to chemotherapy and in those for whom lymph node surgery is not recommended.

Chemotherapy may be used for seminomas, nonseminomas, and advanced metastatic disease. Cisplatin (Platinol-AQ) can be used in combination with other chemotherapeutic agents, such as etoposide (Toposar), bleomycin (Blenoxane), paclitaxel (Taxol), ifosfamide (Ifex), and vinblastine (Velban), and results in a high percentage of complete remissions. With nonseminomas, aggressive surgical resection of all residual masses following chemotherapy is standard therapy. Good results may also be obtained by combining different types of treatment, including surgery, radiation therapy, and chemotherapy. Even with metastatic testicular cancer, the prognosis is favorable because of advances in treatment. However, for patients who do not respond to high-dose salvage chemotherapy, the cancer is nearly always incurable.

A patient with a history of one testicular tumor has a greater chance of developing subsequent tumors. Late relapse of testicular cancer is currently defined as tumor recurrence more than 2 years after complete remission following primary treatment that included chemotherapy. The most common site of recurrence is the retroperitoneum. Follow-up studies include chest x-rays, excretory urography, radioimmunoassay of beta-hCG and AFP levels, and examination of lymph nodes.

Long-term side effects associated with treatment for testicular cancer include renal insufficiency from kidney damage, hearing problems, gonadal damage, peripheral neuropathy, and, rarely, secondary cancers. Management of a patient with testicular carcinoma is therapy aimed at cure followed by close monitoring to detect and promptly treat any recurrences (NCCN, 2008). Investigations of new medications, combinations of chemotherapeutic agents, and stem cell transplantation are ongoing.

Nursing Management

Nursing management includes assessment of the patient's physical and psychological status and monitoring of the patient for response to and possible effects of surgery, chemotherapy, and radiation therapy (see Chapter 16). Preoperative and postoperative care is described in Chapters 18 and 20, respectively. In addition, because the patient may have difficulty coping with his condition, issues related to body image and sexuality should be addressed.

Patients may be required to endure a long course of therapy and will need encouragement to maintain a positive attitude. Once patients complete treatment, they enter a follow-up surveillance period. Nurses educate these cancer survivors about the importance of adhering to follow-up appointments for early detection of cancer recurrence (most often occurring within 2 years posttreatment), evaluation of late effects of treatment, including secondary cancers, infertility, cardiotoxicity, neurotoxicity, nephrotoxicity, pulmonary toxicity, metabolic syndrome, and alterations in quality of life (Gospodarowicz, 2008; Zoltick, Jacobs & Vaughn, 2005). The nurse reminds the patient about the importance of performing TSE in the treated or remaining testis. The patient is encouraged to participate in healthy behaviors, including smoking cessation, healthy diet, minimization of alcohol intake, and cancer screening activities (Shinn, Basen-Engquist, Thornton, et al., 2007). Most experts agree that couples should use birth control for 18 to 24 months after the last cycle of chemotherapy (Paduch, 2006).

Hydrocele

A **hydrocele** is a collection of fluid most commonly located between the visceral and parietal layers of the tunica vaginalis of the testis, although it may also collect within the spermatic cord. This condition is the most common cause of scrotal swelling. At birth, 1 in 10 infants has a hydrocele, which usually resolves without treatment within the first year of life. Acute hydroceles primarily develop in adults older than 40 years of age; they may occur in association with inflammation (eg, radiation therapy), infection, epididymitis, local injury, or systemic infectious disease (eg,

mumps). Chronic hydroceles may occur related to the imbalance between fluid secretion and reabsorption in the tunica vaginals. On physical examination, an easily transilluminated, painless, extratesticular mass is found. Hydrocele can be differentiated from a hernia by transillumination; a hydrocele transmits light, whereas a hernia does not. Ultrasonography is recommended for large hydroceles to differentiate them from testicular tumors.

Treatment is usually not required unless the hydrocele is large, bulky, tense, or uncomfortable; compromises testicular circulation; or causes an undesirable appearance. Treatment may involve surgical excision or needle aspiration. Surgical excision (hydrocelectomy) may be performed in an outpatient setting under general or spinal anesthesia with the goal of prevention of recurrence by excising the tunica vaginalis or sclerosing the visceral and parietal layers. Surgical excision involves resection or suturing together the two layers. A drainage tube may be required, and the patient is advised to wear a bulky dressing over the incisional site for a few days after the procedure. To reduce swelling, ice packs are applied to the scrotal area during the first 24 hours. A scrotal athletic supporter may be worn for a period of time postoperatively for comfort and support. Surgical risks include hematoma in the loose scrotal tissues, infection, or injury to the scrotum.

Needle aspiration is another option used to remove the fluid in the scrotum. Because it is common for fluid to reaccumulate, this treatment may be followed by the injection of a sclerosing agent to prevent this recurrence. This option may be used for men who are poor surgical risks. Potential risks include infection and scrotal pain.

Varicocele

A **varicocele** is an abnormal dilation of the pampiniform venous plexus and the internal spermatic vein in the scrotum (the network of veins from the testis and the epididymis that constitute part of the spermatic cord). Varicoceles occur in approximately 15% to 20% of healthy adult men and 40% of infertile men, the large majority (95%) in the left testicle. Although men may report scrotal pain, tenderness, heaviness in the inguinal area, and infertility, varicoceles are often asymptomatic.

If the varicocele is mild and fertility is not an issue, no treatment is required, and a scrotal support is usually sufficient to relieve symptoms of heaviness. If the condition results in ongoing, distressing symptoms or fertility is an issue, the varicocele can be corrected surgically. Postprocedural education and care include an ice pack applied to the scrotum for the first few hours after surgery to relieve edema, dressing removal after 48 hours, nonstrenuous exercise for the first 2 days, scrotal support, pain control, and reporting complications such as infection and hematoma.

Vasectomy

Vasectomy, or male sterilization, involves the surgical interruption of both vas deferens, which are the tubes that carry the sperm from the testicles and epididymis to the

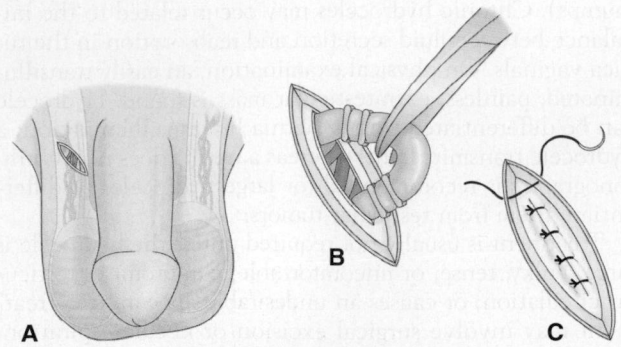

Figure 49-6 A vasectomy is a resection of the vas deferens to prevent passage of sperm from the testes to the urethra during ejaculation. **A,** An incision or small puncture is made to expose the vas deferens. **B,** The vas deferens is isolated and severed. **C,** The severed ends are occluded with ligatures or clips, or the lumen of each vas is sealed by electrocautery and the incision is sutured closed. (Suturing may not be required if a puncture approach has been used.)

seminal vesicles, to prevent fertilization of an egg after ejaculation. During the outpatient procedure, the surgeon exposes the vas deferens through a small surgical opening or puncture in the scrotum using a sharp, curved hemostat (Fig. 49-6). The vas is then ligated (cut) or cauterized (burned), with the severed ends occluded by ties or clips to seal the lumens and then placed back into the scrotum. A section of the vas deferens may or may not be removed. The spermatozoa, which are manufactured in the testes, cannot travel up the vas deferens after this surgery.

Because seminal fluid is manufactured predominantly in the seminal vesicles and prostate gland, which are unaffected by vasectomy, no noticeable decrease in the amount of ejaculate occurs (volume decreases approximately 3%), even though it contains no spermatozoa. Because the sperm cells have no exit, they are resorbed into the body. A vasectomy usually has no effect on sexual potency, erection, ejaculation, or production of male hormones and provides no protection against STDs.

Couples who were once worried about pregnancy resulting from contraceptive failure often report a decrease in concern and an increase in spontaneous sexual arousal after vasectomy. Concise and factual preoperative explanations may minimize or relieve the patient's concerns related to pain and reduced masculinity. The patient is advised that he will be sterile but that potency will not be altered after a bilateral vasectomy. On rare occasions, a spontaneous reanastomosis of the vas deferens occurs, making it possible to impregnate a partner.

Complications of vasectomy include scrotal ecchymoses and swelling, superficial wound infection, vasitis (inflammation of the vas deferens), epididymitis or epididymoorchitis, hematomas, chronic pain, and spermatic granuloma. A spermatic granuloma is an inflammatory response to the collection of sperm leaking from the severed end of the proximal vas deferens into the scrotal tissue. A painless small lump is formed, which usually does not require surgical intervention.

Nursing Management

Nursing education focuses on self-management of swelling and discomfort postvasectomy. Applying ice bags intermittently to the scrotum for several hours after surgery can reduce swelling and relieve discomfort. The nurse advises the patient to wear snug, cotton underwear or a scrotal support for added comfort and support. Explanation of expected discoloration of the scrotal skin and superficial swelling may alleviate anxiety and concerns. These conditions may be relieved by sitz baths.

Sexual intercourse may be resumed as desired, usually after 1 week. Fertility remains for a varying time after vasectomy until the spermatozoa stored distally in the seminal vesicles have been evacuated. Sterility is often achieved after 10 to 20 ejaculations after the vasectomy procedure but may take longer. A reliable method of contraception should be used until infertility is confirmed by examination of an ejaculate specimen in the urologist's office at a follow-up appointment, usually 4 to 8 weeks after the vasectomy.

Vasovasostomy (Sterilization Reversal)

Although men choosing to undergo vasectomy should not consider the surgical procedure as reversible, microsurgical techniques can be used to reverse a vasectomy (vasovasostomy) and restore patency to the vas deferens. Many men have sperm in their ejaculate after a reversal, and 50% to 70% can impregnate a partner. The success of the procedure depends on the vasectomy method performed and the amount of time since the vasectomy. The procedure can be very costly, is not covered by insurance, is not permanent with occlusion of the vas recurring 2 or more years after vasovasotomy, and results in sperm counts at lower than prevasectomy levels.

Semen Cryopreservation (Sperm Banking)

Storing fertile semen in a sperm bank before a vasectomy is an option for men who experience a major life change and may want to father a child at a later time. In addition, if a man is about to undergo a procedure or treatment (eg, radiation therapy to the pelvis, chemotherapy, orchiectomy) that may affect his fertility, sperm banking may be considered. This procedure usually requires several visits to the facility where the sperm is stored under hypothermic conditions. The semen is obtained by masturbation and collected in a sterile container for storage. Insurance carriers rarely cover the cost of semen collection and banking. The costs of semen cryopreservation vary according to facility, method of sperm retrieval, number of specimens, and length of time in storage, making the process cost-prohibitive for some men.

CONDITIONS AFFECTING THE PENIS

Phimosis

Phimosis is a condition in which the foreskin (prepuce) cannot be retracted over the glans in uncircumcised males. With the trend away from routine circumcision of newborns, early instruction should be given to parents about cleansing the foreskin and the need for retraction to cleanse the glans. If the glans is not cleaned, secretions accumulate, causing inflammation of the glans penis (balanitis), which can later lead to adhesions and fibrosis. Phimosis often develops in adults as a result of inflammation, edema, and constriction because of poor hygiene or underlying medical conditions such as diabetes mellitus. The thickened secretions (smegma) can become encrusted with urinary salts and calcify, forming calculi in the prepuce and increasing the risk of penile carcinoma. Treatment for phimosis secondary to inflammation is the application of steroidal cream to the foreskin to soften and correct the narrowness, resulting in decreased constriction. Although phimosis is the most common indication for adult circumcision, it is rarely necessary to surgically correct the condition by loosening or removing the foreskin.

Paraphimosis is a condition in which the foreskin, once retracted over the glans, cannot be returned to its usual position. Chronic inflammation under the foreskin leads to formation of a tight ring of skin when the foreskin is retracted behind the glans, causing venous congestion, edema, and enlargement of the glans, which makes the condition worse. As the condition progresses, arterial occlusion and necrosis of the glans may occur. Paraphimosis usually can be treated by firmly compressing the glans for 5 minutes to reduce the tissue edema and size and then pushing the glans back while simultaneously moving the foreskin forward (manual reduction). The constricting skin ring may require incision under local anesthesia. Circumcision is usually indicated after the inflammation and edema subside (Tanagho & McAninch, 2008).

Cancer of the Penis

Penile cancer is rare, occurring in less than 1% of cancers among men in the United States. It accounts for an estimated 1290 new cancer cases and 300 expected deaths each year (ACS, 2009). The 5-year survival rates for cancer localized to the penis approaches 80%, but this statistic drops to 52% if the lymph nodes are involved and to 18% if the cancer has spread beyond the inguinal lymph nodes (Tanagho & McAninch, 2008). Penile cancer is much more common in some parts of Africa and South America, where it accounts for up to 10% of cancers in men. Because the penis contains different cell types, penile cancer can arise in each type of cell, which determines the prognosis. Types of penile cancer include squamous cell carcinoma (most common; 95% of cases), epidermoid penile cancer, verrucous carcinoma, adenocarcinoma, in situ carcinomas (erythroplasia of Queyrat and Bowen's disease), basal cell penile cancer, melanoma, and sarcomas (Blanco-Yarosh, 2007). Several risk factors for penile cancer have been identified, including lack of circumcision, poor genital hygiene, phimosis, HPV, smoking, ultraviolet light treatment of psoriasis on the penis, increasing age (two thirds of cases occur in men older than 65 years of age), lichen sclerosus, and balanitis xerotica obliterans. However, the exact cause remains unclear.

Because of the rarity of penile cancer, there has been little improvement in diagnostic and staging tests, understanding of risk factors, and development of treatment modalities.

Clinical Manifestations

The penile lesion usually alerts the patient to the presence of penile cancer; however, a man may delay seeking treatment for more than a year because of embarrassment, fear, or lack of understanding. Common clinical presentations are a painless lump, ulcer, or wartlike growth on the skin of the penis; a change in skin color such as a red rash, bluish growths, or whitish patches; and malodorous and persistent discharge in late stages.

Assessment and Diagnostic Findings

Penile cancer involves the glans most frequently (48%), followed by lesions of the foreskin (21%), the coronal sulcus (6%), the penile shaft (less than 2%), the urethra, and regional or distant lymph nodes (Wein, et al., 2007). A thorough physical examination is necessary, including assessment and palpation of the penis and the inguinal lymph nodes. The size, location, borders, consistency, fixation, and character and time of onset of the penile lesions should be noted. Incisional or excisional biopsy is performed to determine the cell types of the penile cancer. Further staging tests using ultrasonography, MRI, or CT may be obtained to determine the extent of local lesions, if metastatic disease is present, and treatment options.

Prevention

The best way to reduce the risk of penile cancer is to avoid known risk factors whenever possible (ACS, 2009). Avoidance of sexual practices that are likely to result in HPV infection may reduce the risk of penile cancer. Gardasil, a vaccine that protects against infection with HPV, the cause of 90% of genital warts, is being evaluated for possible use in males. Although uncircumcised men have a greater incidence of penile cancer than circumcised men, the more important factor in preventing penile cancer is good genital hygiene. Circumcision is not recommended as a prevention strategy (ACS, 2009).

Medical Management

Treatment varies depending on the type and stage of penile cancer, location of the lesion, overall physical health, and personal preferences about treatments and side effects. During the past 25 years, therapeutic options have largely remained unchanged (Busby & Pettaway, 2005). The goal of treatment in invasive penile cancer is complete excision with adequate margins. Surgery is the most common treatment method used in all forms of the disease. Depending on the stage and invasiveness of the cancer, therapeutic options may include simple excision, electrodesiccation and curettage, cryosurgery, Mohs' surgery (microscopically controlled surgery), yttrium aluminum garnet (YAG) laser surgery, wide local excision, circumcision, and surgical removal of part of the penis or the entire penis (penectomy). Organ-sparing surgical approaches are preferable. Partial penectomy is preferred to total penectomy because patients can then participate in sexual intercourse, stand for urination, and maintain cosmesis. Modern reconstructive surgical techniques are providing more options for patients. The shaft of the penis can still respond to sexual arousal with an erection and has the sensory capacity for orgasm and ejaculation. Total penectomy is indicated if the tumor is not amenable to conservative treatment. After a total penectomy, the patient may still experience orgasm with stimulation of the perineum and scrotal area.

Topical chemotherapy with 5-fluorouracil cream or biologic therapy may also be effective. Radiation therapy is used to treat small squamous cell carcinomas of the penis and for palliation in advanced tumors or cases of lymph node metastasis.

Penile cancer spreads primarily to the inguinal lymph nodes; thus, appropriate lymph node management plays a significant role in survival. Because enlarged inguinal lymph nodes are caused by inflammation in 50% of cases, patients who present with enlarged lymph nodes should undergo treatment of the primary lesion followed by a 4- to 6-week course of oral broad-spectrum antibiotics. Persistent enlarged lymph nodes after antibiotic therapy should be considered to be metastatic disease and treated with either a sentinel lymph node biopsy (to determine presence of cancer) or with bilateral inguinal and PLND. If extensive pelvic lymph node involvement is present, the patient should receive adjuvant or neoadjuvant chemotherapy and postoperative radiation therapy (Micali, Nasca, Innocenzi, et al., 2006).

Priapism

Priapism, a relatively uncommon disorder, is defined as a persistent penile erection that may or may not be related to sexual stimulation. The penis becomes large, hard, and painful. Priapism results from either neural or vascular causes, including sickle cell disease, leukemic cell infiltration, polycythemia, spinal cord tumors or injury, and tumor invasion of the penis or its vessels. It may also occur with use of vasoactive agents that affect the central nervous system, antihypertensive agents, antipsychotic and antidepressant medications, substances injected into the penis to treat erectile dysfunction, alcohol, and cocaine. There are three forms of priapism: ischemic (veno-occlusive; low flow), nonischemic (high flow), and stuttering (intermittent).

The ischemic form, which is described as nonsexual, persistent erection with little or no cavernous blood flow, must be treated promptly to prevent permanent damage to the penis. The goal of therapy is to improve venous drainage of the corpora cavernosa to prevent ischemia, fibrosis, and impotence. The initial treatment is directed at relieving the erection, preventing penile damage and simultaneously treating the underlying disease. Recommended treatment is aspiration of the corpora cavernosa (with or without irrigation) or intracavernous injection of sympathomimetics (eg, phenylephrine). Repeated injections may be needed to resolve priapism. Surgical shunts are used to reestablish penile

circulation if repeated injections of the sympathomimetic are ineffective (Burnett & Bivalacqua, 2007).

Nonischemic priapism and stuttering are generally not considered emergencies and often resolve without treatment. Conservative treatment (eg, application of ice and site-specific compression to the injury) may be used. If repeated episodes occur, surgical shunting is considered. Patients with the intermittent form of priapism may be instructed in intracavernosal self-injection of phenylephrine.

Peyronie's Disease

Peyronie's disease is an acquired, benign condition that involves the buildup of fibrous plaques in the sheath of the corpus cavernosum. These plaques are not visible when the penis is relaxed. However, when the penis is erect, curvature occurs that can be painful and can make sexual intercourse difficult or impossible. Peyronie's disease typically begins between 45 and 65 years of age. Medical management in the first year of active disease includes systemic, topical, intralesional, or extracorporeal techniques, with 50% of men experiencing spontaneous resolution. Surgical removal of mature plaques is used to treat severe disease. Patients should be fully informed of available treatment options and their likely outcomes (Taylor & Levine, 2007).

Urethral Stricture

Urethral stricture is a condition in which a section of the urethra is narrowed. It can occur congenitally or from a scar along the urethra. Traumatic injury to the urethra (eg, from instrumentation or infections) can result in strictures that restrict urine flow and decrease the urinary stream, leading to spraying or double stream, postvoiding dribbling, and dilation of the proximal urethra and prostatic ducts. Prostatitis is a common complication. Treatment involves dilation of the urethra or, in severe cases, urethrotomy (surgical removal of the stricture). Antimicrobial agents are necessary for resolution of UTIs, followed by long-term prophylactic therapy until the stricture is corrected. Treatment should not be considered successful until at least 1 year has passed, because strictures may recur anytime during that period (Tanagho & McAninch, 2008).

Circumcision

Circumcision is the surgical excision of the foreskin (prepuce) of the glans penis. One of the oldest surgical procedures, it is the fifth most common procedure preformed in the United States. In adults, circumcision may be indicated as part of treatment for phimosis, paraphimosis, and recurrent infections of the glans and foreskin. It also may be performed at the patient's request.

The primary method of circumcision in adults is surgical excision. Postoperatively, a petrolatum (Vaseline) gauze dressing is applied and changed as indicated. The patient is observed for bleeding. Because considerable pain may occur after circumcision, analgesic agents are administered as needed.

CRITICAL THINKING EXERCISES

1 One of your patients, a 59-year-old man who has diabetes and a history of cardiac disease, asks about various treatments of erectile dysfunction. How would you respond, and what information would you give him about medications and nonpharmacologic methods to treat erective dysfunction? How would your approach differ if your patient was a 32-year-old man with sexual dysfunction caused by multiple sclerosis and who has limited hand dexterity?

EBP **2** During a community health fair, you are approached by a 44-year-old African American man who asks you about his risk of prostate cancer and the risk to his 20-year-old son. His father has been recently diagnosed with prostate cancer and is scheduled for surgery the following week. How would you address this issue with him at the health fair? Provide a rationale for your plan. How would your responses differ if you saw the patient during an office visit to follow-up an elevated prostate-specific antigen (PSA) test result? What health counseling is indicated for the man and his son? What is the evidence base for the health advice you develop?

EBP **3** A 63-year-old biology professor has been diagnosed with prostate cancer. His Gleason score is 6 and he is currently undergoing tests to determine if there is any metastasis of the cancer beyond the prostate gland. He is struggling to make a decision about treatment and has asked for further information about strategies that he has discussed with his physician: radical prostatectomy, suprapubic prostatectomy, and robotic-assisted radical prostatectomy. Compare the advantages and disadvantages of these three treatment strategies with watchful waiting. Identify the evidence for each of these strategies and how you would explain them to the patient.

4 A 26-year-old patient is scheduled for surgery to treat testicular cancer. He is depressed and apprehensive about the outcomes of surgery related to sexual function and fertility. Describe your approach to caring for this patient preoperatively and postoperatively. What recommendations for follow-up health care and preventive screening are relevant for this patient?

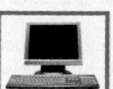

The Smeltzer suite offers these additional resources to enhance learning and facilitate understanding of this chapter:
- thePoint online resource, thepoint.lww.com/Smeltzer12E
- Student CD-ROM included with the book
- *Study Guide to Accompany Brunner & Suddarth's Textbook of Medical-Surgical Nursing*
- *Handbook for Brunner & Suddarth's Textbook of Medical-Surgical Nursing*

REFERENCES AND SELECTED READINGS

*Asterisk indicates nursing research.
**Double asterisk indicates classic reference.

Books

American Cancer Society (ACS). (2009). *Cancer facts and figures 2008*. Atlanta: Author.
**Annon, J. S. (1976). *Behavioral treatment of sexual problems: Brief therapy*. Hagerstown, MD: Harper & Row.
Katz, A. (2007). *Breaking the silence on cancer and sexuality*. Pittsburgh: Oncology Nursing Society.
Langhorne, M., Fulton, J. & Otto, S. E. (Eds.). (2007). *Oncology nursing* (5th ed.). St. Louis: Mosby.
McCance, K. L. & Huether, S. E. (Eds.). (2005). *Pathophysiology: The biologic basis for disease in adults and children* (5th ed.). St. Louis: Mosby.
Porth, C. M. & Matfin, G. (2009). *Pathophysiology: Concepts of altered health states* (8th ed.). Philadelphia: Lippincott Williams & Wilkins.
Tabloski, P. A. (2006). *Gerontological nursing*. Upper Saddle River, NJ: Pearson Education.
Tanagho. E. A. & McAninch, J. W. (2008). *Smith's general urology* (17th ed.). New York: McGraw Hill.
Wein, A. J., Kavoussi, L. R., Novick, A. C., et al. (Eds.). (2007). *Campbell-Walsh urology* (9th ed.). Philadelphia: Saunders Elsevier.

Journals and Electronic Documents

General

Eaton, J. (2003). Detection of hyponatremia in the PACU. *Journal of Perianethesia Nursing*, 18(6), 392–397.
Gates, T. J., Beelen, M. J. & Hershey, C. L. (2008). Cancer screening in men. *Nursing Clinics of North America*, 43(4), 283–306.
Lin, K., Lipsitz, R., Miller, T., et al. (2008). Benefits and harms of prostate-specific antigen screening for prostate cancer: An evidence update for the U.S. preventive services task force. *Annals of Internal Medicine*, 149(3), 192–199.
Smith, J. F., Walsh, T. J. & Lue, T. F. (2008). Peyronie's disease: A critical appraisal of current diagnosis and treatment. *International Journal of Impotence Research*, 20(5), 445–449.
Zang, Y., Chung, L. Y. & Wong, T. K. (2008). A review of the psychosocial issues for nurses in male genitalia-related care. *Journal of Clinical Nursing*, 17(8), 983–998.

Benign Prostatic Hyperplasia

American Urological Association (AUA). (2006). Guideline on the management of benign prostatic hyperplasia (BPH). http://www.auanet.org/content/guidelines-and-quality-care/clinical-guidelines.cfm?sub=bph
Kaplan, S. A. (2006). Update on the American Urological Association guidelines for the treatment of benign prostatic hyperplasia. *Reviews in Urology*, 8(Suppl 4), S10–S17.
Lepor, H. (2007). Alpha blockers for the treatment of benign prostatic hyperplasia. *Review in Urology*, 9(4), 181–190.
Parsons, J. K. (2007). Modifiable risk factors for benign prostatic hyperplasia and lower urinary tract symptoms: New approaches to old problems. *Journal of Urology*, 178(2), 395–401.

Sexual Dysfunction

American Urological Association (AUA). (2005). *The management of erectile dysfunction: An update*. www.auanet.org/content/guidelines-and-quality-care/clinical-guidelines.cfm?sub=bph
Bruner, D. W. & Calvano, T. (2007). The sexual impact of cancer and cancer treatments in men. *Nursing Clinics of North America*, 42(4), 555–580.
Burnett, A. L. & Bivalacqua, T. J. (2007). Priapism: Current principles and practice. *Urologic Clinics of North America*, 34(4), 631–642.
Fossa, S. D. & Dahl, A. A. (2008). Fertility and sexuality in young cancer survivors who have adult-onset malignancies. *Hematology/Oncology Clinics of North America*, 22(2), 291–303.
Henry, G. D. & Wilson, S. K. (2007). Updates in inflatable penile prostheses. *Urologic Clinics of North America*, 34(4), 535–547.
Katz, A. (2005). The sounds of silence: Sexuality information for cancer patients. *Journal of Clinical Oncology*, 23(1), 238–241.
Schuster, T. G. (2006). Premature ejaculation. *Urologic Nursing*, 26(4), 245–249.
Shell, J. A. (2007). Including sexuality in your nursing practice. *Nursing Clinics of North America*, 42(4), 685–696.

Taylor, F. L. & Levine, L. A. (2007). Peyronie's disease. *Urologic Clinics of North America, 34*(4), 517–534.

Waldinger, M. D. (2007). Premature ejaculation: State of the art. *Urologic Clinics of North America 34*(4), 591–599.

Sexually Transmitted Diseases

Centers for Disease Control and Prevention (CDC). (2006). Sexually transmitted diseases treatment guidelines, 2006. *MMWR Morbidity and Mortality Weekly Report, 55*(RR-11), 1–94.

Centers for Disease Control and Prevention (CDC). (2007). Update to CDC's sexually transmitted diseases treatment guidelines, 2006. Fluoroquinolones no longer recommended for treatment of gonococcal infections. *MMWR Morbidity and Mortality Weekly Report, 56*(14), 332–336.

Centers for Disease Control and Prevention (CDC). (2008). National Center for HIV/AIDS, Viral Hepatitis, STD, and TB Prevention. 2006 disease profile. www.cdc.gov/NCHHSTP/Publications/docs/2006_Disease_Profile_508_ FINAL.pdf

Workowshi, K. A. & Berman, S. M. (2006). Sexually transmitted diseases treatment guidelines, 2006. *MMWR Morbidity and Mortality Weekly Report, 55*(RR11), 1–94.

Erectile Dysfunction

American Urological Association (AUA). (2004). Premature ejaculation: Guideline on the pharmacologic management of premature ejaculation. www.auanet.org/content/guidelines-and-quality-care/clinical-guidelines/main-reports/pme/pme_2004.pdf

American Urological Association (AUA). (2007). Erectile Dysfunction. The management of erectile dysfunction: An update. www.auanet.org/content/guidelines-and-quality-care/clinical-guidelines.cfm?sub=ed

Beckman, T. J., Abu-Lebdeh, H. S. & Mynderse, L. A. (2006). Evaluation and medical management of erectile dysfunction. *Mayo Clinical Proceedings, 81*(3), 385–390.

Carson, C. (2007). Phosphodiesterase type 5 inhibitors: State of the therapeutic class. *Urologic Clinics of North America, 34*(4), 507–515.

Seftel, A. D., Miner, M. M., Kloner, R. A., et al. (2007). Office evaluation of male sexual dysfunction. *Urologic Clinics of North America, 34*(4), 463–482.

Cancer of the Penis

Blanco-Yarosh, M. (2007). Penile cancer: An overview. *Urologic Nursing, 27*(4), 286–290.

Busby, J. E. & Pettaway, C. A. (2005). What's new in the management of penile cancer? *Current Opinion in Urology, 15*(5), 350–357.

Micali, G., Nasca, M. R., Innocenzi, D., et al. (2006). Penile cancer. *Journal of American Academy of Dermatology, 54*(3), 369–390.

Prostate Cancer

American Urological Association (AUA). (2007). Guideline for the management of clinically localized prostate cancer: 2007 update. www. auanet.org/content/guidelines-and-quality-care/clinical-guidelines/main-reports/proscan07/content.pdf

*Bailey, D. E., Wallace, M. & Mishel, M. H. (2007). Watching, waiting and uncertainty in prostate cancer. *Clinical Journal of Nursing, 16*(4), 734–741.

*Eller, L. S., Lev, E. L., Gejerman, G., et al. (2006). Prospective study of quality of life of patients receiving treatment for prostate cancer. *Nursing Research, 55*(2S), S23–S36.

*Hawes, S. M., Malcarne, V. L., Ko, C. M., et al. (2006). Identifying problems faced by spouses and partners of patients with prostate cancer. *Oncology Nursing Forum, 33*(4), 807–814.

Jones, R. A., Underwood, S. M. & Rivers, B. M. (2007). Reducing prostate cancer morbidity and mortality in African American men: Issues and challenges. *Clinical Journal of Oncology Nursing, 11*(6), 865–872.

Lessick, M. & Katz, A. (2006). A genetics perspective on prostate cancer. *Urologic Nursing, 26*(6), 454–460.

Michaelson, M. D., Cotter, S. E., Gargollo, P. C., et al. (2008). Management of complications of prostate cancer treatment. *CA A Cancer Journal for Clinicians, 58*(4), 196–213.

National Comprehensive Cancer Network (NCCN). (2008). Clinical practice guidelines in oncology: Prostate cancer, version 2.2009. http://www.nccn.org/professionals/physician_gls/PDF/prostate.pdf

Pienta, K. J. & Smith, D. C. (2005). Advances in prostate cancer chemotherapy: A new era begins. *CA A Cancer Journal for Clinicians, 55*(5), 300–318.

Sanders, S., Pedro, L. W., Bantum, E. O., et al. (2006). Couples surviving prostate cancer: Long-term intimacy needs and concerns following treatment. *Clinical Journal of Oncology Nursing, 10*(4), 503–508.

Tindall, D. J. & Rittmaster, R. S. (2008). The rationale for inhibiting 5alpha-reductase isoenzymes in the prevention and treatment of prostate cancer. *The Journal of Urology, 179*(4), 1235–1242.

*Weinrich, S., Vijayakumar, S., Powell, I. J., et al. (2007). Knowledge of hereditary prostate cancer among high-risk African-American men. *Oncology Nursing Forum, 34*(4), 854–860.

Prostate Surgery

Barqawi, A. B. & Crawford, D. (2007). The current use and future trends of focal surgical therapy in the management of localized prostate cancer. *The Cancer Journal, 13*(5), 313–317.

Darst, E. H. (2007). Sexuality and prostatectomy: Nursing assessment and intervention. *Urologic Nursing, 27*(6), 534–541.

Joseph, A. C. (2006). Noninvasive therapies for treating post-prostatectomy urinary incontinence. *Urologic Nursing, 26*(4), 271–269.

Rigdon, J. L. (2006). Robotic-assisted laparoscopic radial prostatectomy. *AORN Journal, 84*(5), 760–770.

Schober, P., Meuleman, E. J. H. & Boer, C. (2008). Transurethral resection syndrome detected and managed using transesophageal Doppler. *Anesthesia & Analgesia, 107*(3), 921–925.

Starnes, D. N. & Sims, T. W. (2006). Care of the patient undergoing robotic-assisted prostatectomy. *Urologic Nursing, 26*(2), 129–136.

*Ward-Smith, P. & Mehl, J. (2007). Quality of life before and after prostatectomy as treatment for localized cancer. *Urologic Nursing, 27*(6), 542–547.

Yu Ko, W. F. & Sawatzky, J. V. (2008). Understanding urinary incontinence after radical prostatectomy: a nursing framework. *Clinical Journal of Oncology Nursing, 12*(4), 647-654.

Prostatitis

Giubilei, G., Mondaini, N., Minervini, A., et al. (2007). Physical activity of men with chronic prostatitis/chronic pelvic pain syndrome not satisfied with conventional treatments—Could it represent a valid option? The physical activity and male pelvic pain trial: a double-blind, randomized study. *Journal of Urology, 177*(1), 159–165.

Müller, A. & Mulhall, J. P. (2005). Sexual dysfunction in the patient with prostatitis. *Current Opinion in Urology, 15*(6), 404–409.

Potts, J. & Payne, R. E. (2007). Prostatitis: Infection, neuromuscular disorder, or pain syndrome? Proper patient classification is key. *Cleveland Clinic Journal of Medicine, 74*(Suppl 3), S63–S71.

Testicular Cancer

American Urologic Association (AUA). (2007). Erectile dysfunction guideline. The management of erectile dysfunction: An update. http://www.auanet.org/content/guidelines-and-quality-care/clinical-guidelines/mainreports/edmgmt/content.pdf

Brydøy, M., Fosså, S. D., Klepp, O., et al. (2005). Paternity following treatment for testicular cancer. *Journal of National Cancer Institute, 97*(21), 1580–1588.

Feldman, D. R., Bosl, G. J., Sheinfeld, J., et al. (2008). Medical treatment of advanced testicular cancer. *Journal of the American Medical Association, 299*(6), 672–684.

Gilligan, T. (2007). Testis cancer: Rare, but curable with prompt referral. *Cleveland Clinic Journal of Medicine, 74*(11), 817–824.

Girasole, C. R., Cookson, M. S., Smith, J. A., et al. (2006). Sperm banking: Use and outcomes in patients treated for testicular cancer. *BJU International, 99*(1), 33–36.

*Gleason, A. M. (2006). Racial disparities in testicular cancer: Impact on health promotion. *Journal of Transcultural Nursing, 17*(1), 58–64.

Gospodarowicz, M. (2008). Testicular cancer patients: Considerations in long-term follow-up. *Hematology/Oncology Clinics of North America, 22*(2), 247–255.

National Comprehensive Cancer Network (NCCN). (2009). Clinical practice guidelines in oncology: Testicular cancer, version 2.2009. http://www.nccn.org/professionals/physician_gls/PDF/testicular.pdf

Paduch, D. A. (2006). Testicular cancer and male infertility. *Current Opinion in Urology, 16*(6), 419–427.

Shinn, E. H., Basen-Engquist, B. & Thornton, B., et al. (2007). Health behavior and depressive symptoms in testicular cancer survivors. *Urology, 69*(4), 748–753.

Zoltick, B. H., Jacobs, L. A. & Vaughn, D. J. (2005). Cardiovascular risk in testicular cancer survivors treated with chemotherapy: Incidence, significance and practice implications. *Oncology Nursing Forum, 32*(5), 1005–1009.

RESOURCES

American Cancer Society, www.cancer.org
American Urological Association Foundation, www.auafoundation.org, www.urologyhealth.org
CancerCare, www.cancercare.org
Centers for Disease Control and Prevention, www.cdc.gov/cancer

Hartford Institute for Geriatric Nursing, www.hartfordign.org
Hartford Institute for Geriatric Nursing www.consultgerirn.org/topics/urinary_incontinence/want_to_know_more
Impotence Institute of America, www.bodyandfitness.com/Information/Menhealth/impotence1.htm
National Center for Complementary and Alternative Therapy, http://nccam.nih.gov
National Cancer Institute, www.nci.nih.gov
National Comprehensive Cancer Network, www.nccn.org
National Prostate Cancer Coalition, www.fightprostatecancer.org
Us TOO International Prostate Cancer Education and Support Network, www.ustoo.org

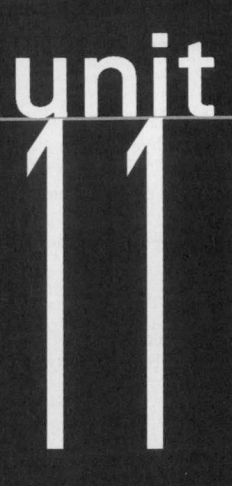

unit 11

Immunologic Function

Case Study • Applying Concepts From NANDA, NIC, and NOC

An Immunosuppressed Patient With a History of Oral Infections

Mrs. Baker is a 52-year-old mother of three with severe rheumatoid arthritis. She has been taking prednisone, 10 mg daily for 6 months, as part of a treatment plan that will also include nonsteroidal anti-inflammatory drugs (NSAIDs) and disease-modifying antirheumatic drugs (DMARDs). Although her physician has tried to taper the prednisone, each time the dose is reduced Mrs. Baker experiences a painful flare-up of her rheumatoid arthritis and symptoms of steroid withdrawal. Mrs. Baker states that when her symptoms flare, she takes an extra dose of prednisone. She has had oral candidal disease twice in the preceding 3 months and has had frequent upper respiratory tract infections.

Visit thePoint to view a concept map that illustrates the relationships that exist between the nursing diagnoses, interventions, and outcomes for the patient's clinical problems.

Nursing Classifications and Languages

NANDA NURSING DIAGNOSES	NIC NURSING INTERVENTIONS	NOC NURSING OUTCOMES
		Return to functional baseline status, stabilization of, or improvement in:
RISK FOR INFECTION—At risk for being invaded by pathogenic organisms	**INFECTION PROTECTION**—Prevention and early detection of infection in a patient at risk	**INFECTION SEVERITY**—Severity of infection and associated symptoms
IMPAIRED ORAL MUCOUS MEMBRANE—Disruption of the lips and soft tissues of the oral cavity	**INFECTION CONTROL**—Minimizing the acquisition and transmission of infectious agents	**TISSUE INTEGRITY: SKIN AND MUCOUS MEMBRANES**—Structural intactness and normal physiologic function of skin and mucous membranes
RISK FOR INEFFECTIVE THERAPEUTIC REGIMEN MANAGEMENT—Having the potential for developing a pattern of regulating and integrating into daily living a program for treatment of illness and the sequelae of illness that is unsatisfactory for meeting specific health goals	**ORAL HEALTH MAINTENANCE**—Maintenance and promotion of oral hygiene and dental health for the patient at risk for developing oral or dental lesions	**KNOWLEDGE: TREATMENT REGIMEN**—Extent of understanding conveyed about the safe use of medication
	TEACHING: PRESCRIBED MEDICATION—Preparing a patient to safely take prescribed medications and monitor their effects	

Bulechek, G. M., Butcher, H. K., & Dochterman, J. M. (2008). *Nursing interventions classification (NIC)* (5th ed.). St. Louis: Mosby.
Johnson, M., Bulechek, G., Butcher, H. K., et al. (2006). *NANDA, NOC, and NIC linkages* (2nd ed.). St. Louis: Mosby.
Moorhead, S., Johnson, M., Mass, M. L., et al. (2008). *Nursing outcomes classification (NOC)* (4th ed.). St. Louis: Mosby.
NANDA International. (2007). *Nursing diagnoses: Definitions & classification 2007–2008*. Philadelphia: North American Nursing Diagnosis Association.

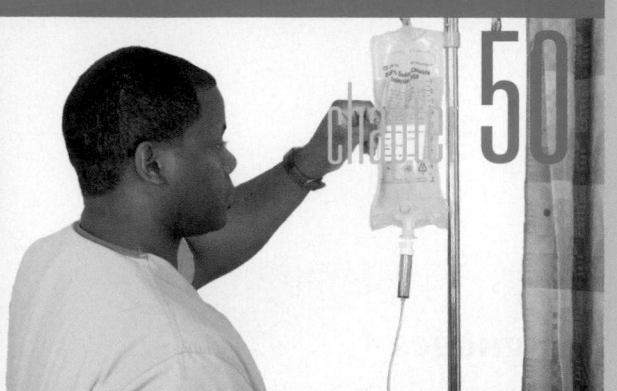

50

Assessment of Immune Function

On completion of this chapter, the learner will be able to:

1 Describe the body's general immune responses.

2 Discuss the stages of the immune response.

3 Differentiate between cellular and humoral immune responses.

4 Describe the effects of selected variables on function of the immune system.

5 Use assessment parameters for determining the status of patients' immune function.

GLOSSARY

agglutination: clumping effect occurring when an antibody acts as a cross-link between two antigens

antibody: a protein substance developed by the body in response to and interacting with a specific antigen

antigen: substance that induces the production of antibodies

antigenic determinant: the specific area of an antigen that binds with an antibody combining site and determines the specificity of the antigen–antibody reaction

apoptosis: programmed cell death that results from the digestion of deoxyribonucleic acid by endonucleases

B cells: cells that are important for producing a humoral immune response

cellular immune response: the immune system's third line of defense, involving the attack of pathogens by T cells

complement: series of enzymatic proteins in the serum that, when activated, destroy bacteria and other cells

cytokines: generic term for nonantibody proteins that act as intercellular mediators, as in the generation of immune response

cytotoxic T cells: lymphocytes that lyse cells infected with virus; also play a role in graft rejection

epitope: any component of an antigen molecule that functions as an antigenetic determinant by permitting the attachment of certain antibodies

GLOSSARY (Continued)

genetic engineering: emerging technology designed to enable replacement of missing or defective genes

helper T cells: lymphocytes that attack foreign invaders (antigens) directly

humoral immune response: the immune system's second line of defense; often termed the antibody response

immune response: the coordinated response of the components of the immune system to a foreign agent or organism

immune system: the collection of organs, cells, tissues, and molecules that mediate the immune response

immunity: the body's specific protective response to a foreign agent or organism; resistance to disease, specifically infectious diseases

immunopathology: study of diseases resulting in dysfunctions within the immune system

immunoregulation: complex system of checks and balances that regulates or controls immune responses

interferons: proteins formed when cells are exposed to viral or foreign agents; capable of activating other components of the immune system

lymphokines: substances released by sensitized lymphocytes when they come in contact with specific antigens

memory cells: cells that are responsible for recognizing antigens from previous exposure and mounting an immune response

natural killer (NK) cells: lymphocytes that defend against microorganisms and malignant cells

null lymphocytes: lymphocytes that destroy antigens already coated with the antibody

opsonization: the coating of antigen–antibody molecules with a sticky substance to facilitate phagocytosis

phagocytic cells: cells that engulf, ingest, and destroy foreign bodies or toxins

phagocytic immune response: the immune system's first line of defense, involving white blood cells that have the ability to ingest foreign particles

stem cells: precursors of all blood cells; reside primarily in bone marrow

suppressor T cells: lymphocytes that decrease B-cell activity to a level at which the immune system is compatible with life

T cells: cells that are important for producing a cellular immune response

The term **immunity** refers to the body's specific protective response to a foreign agent or organism. The **immune system** functions as the body's defense mechanism against invasion and allows a rapid response to foreign substances in a specific manner. Genetic and cellular responses result. Any qualitative or quantitative change in the components of the immune system can produce profound effects on the integrity of the human organism. Immune function is affected by a variety of factors, such as central nervous system integrity, general physical and emotional status, medications, dietary patterns, and the stress of illness, trauma, or surgery. Dysfunctions involving the immune system occur across the lifespan. Many are genetically based; others are acquired. Immune memory is a property of the immune system that provides protection against harmful microbial agents despite the timing of re-exposure to the agent. Tolerance is the mechanism by which the immune system is programmed to eliminate foreign substances such as microbes, toxins, and cellular mutations but maintains the ability to accept self-antigens. Some credence is given to the concept of surveillance, in which the immune system is in a perpetual state of vigilance, screening and rejecting any invader that is recognized as foreign to the host. The term **immunopathology** refers to the study of diseases that result from dysfunctions within the immune system. Disorders of the immune system may stem from excesses or deficiencies of immunocompetent cells, alterations in the function of these cells, immunologic attack on self-antigens, or inappropriate or exaggerated responses to specific antigens (Table 50-1).

A growing number of patients with immunologic disorders live to adulthood. Thus, nurses in many practice settings need to understand how the immune system functions as well as immunopathologic processes. In addition, knowledge about assessment and care of people with immunologic disorders enables nurses to make appropriate management decisions.

Anatomic and Physiologic Overview

Anatomy of the Immune System

The immune system is composed of an integrated collection of various cell types, each with a designated function in defending against infection and invasion by other organisms.

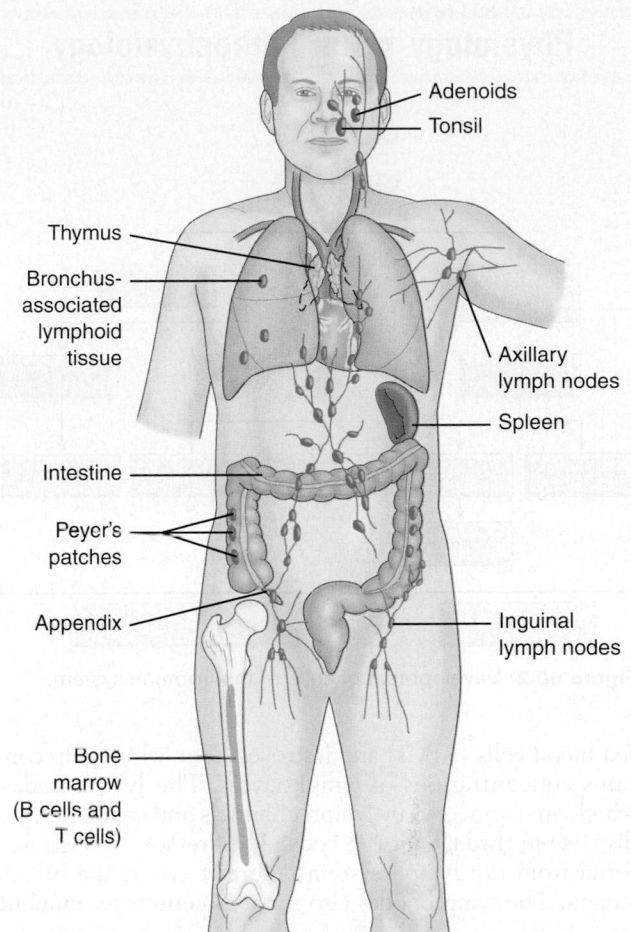

Figure 50-1 Central and peripheral lymphoid organs, tissues, and cells. Adapted from Porth, C. M. & Matfin, G. (2009). *Pathophysiology: Concepts of altered health states* (8th ed., p. 371). Philadelphia: Lippincott Williams & Wilkins.

Supporting this system are molecules that are responsible for the interactions, modulations, and regulation of the system. These molecules and cells participate in specific interactions with immunogenic **epitopes** (antigenic determinants) present on foreign materials, initiating a series of actions in a host, including the inflammatory response, the lysis of microbial agents, and the disposal of foreign toxins. The major components of the immune system include central and peripheral organs, tissues, and cells (Fig. 50-1).

Bone Marrow

The white blood cells (WBCs) involved in immunity are produced in the bone marrow (Fig. 50-2). Like other blood cells, lymphocytes are generated from **stem cells**, which are undifferentiated cells. There are two types of lymphocytes—B lymphocytes (**B cells**) and T lymphocytes (**T cells**) (Fig. 50-3). B lymphocytes mature in the bone marrow and then enter the circulation. T lymphocytes move from the bone marrow to the thymus, where they mature into several kinds of cells with different functions.

Lymphoid Tissues

The spleen, composed of red and white pulp, acts somewhat like a filter. The red pulp is the site where old and injured

Table 50-1	IMMUNE SYSTEM DISORDERS
Disorder	**Description**
Autoimmunity	Normal protective immune response paradoxically turns against or attacks the body, leading to tissue damage
Hypersensitivity	Body produces inappropriate or exaggerated responses to specific antigens
Gammopathies	Immunoglobulins are overproduced
Immune deficiencies	
Primary	Deficiency results from improper development of immune cells or tissues; usually congenital or inherited
Secondary	Deficiency results from some interference with an already developed immune system; usually acquired later in life

Physiology ■■■ Pathophysiology

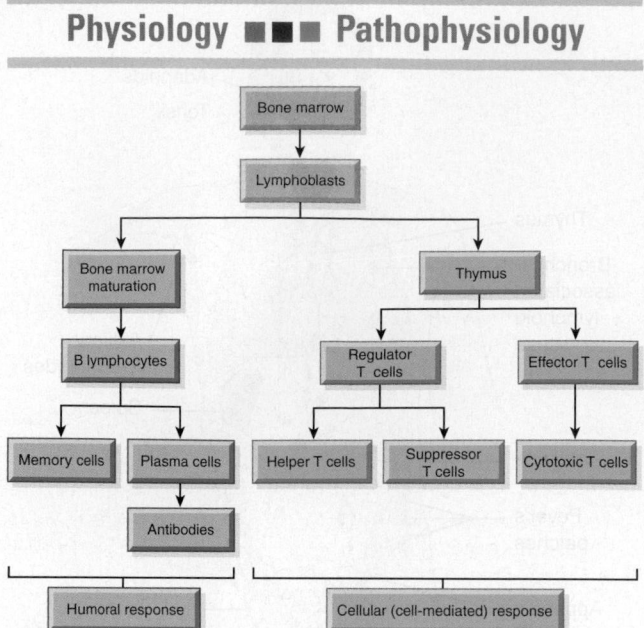

Figure 50-2 Development of cells of the immune system.

red blood cells (RBCs) are destroyed. The white pulp contains concentrations of lymphocytes. The lymph nodes, which are connected by lymph channels and capillaries, are distributed throughout the body. They remove foreign material from the lymph system before it enters the bloodstream. The lymph nodes also serve as centers for immune

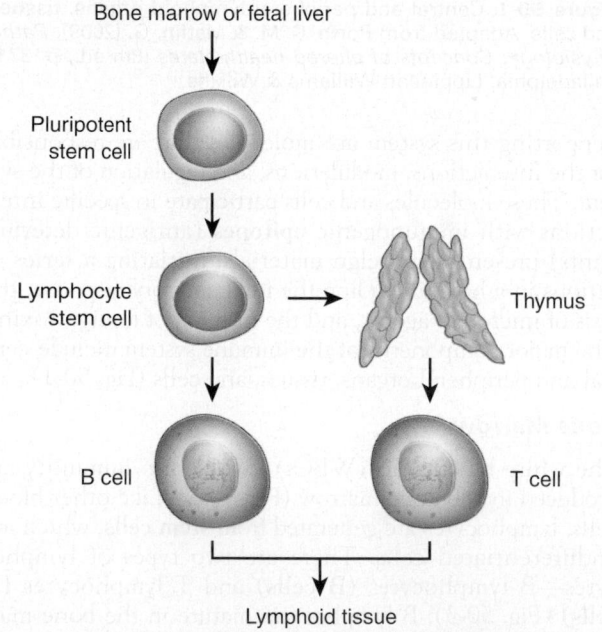

Figure 50-3 Lymphocytes originate from stem cells in the bone marrow. B lymphocytes mature in the bone marrow before entering the bloodstream, whereas T lymphocytes mature in the thymus, where they also differentiate into cells with various functions. Redrawn from Porth, C. M. & Matfin, G. (2009). *Pathophysiology: Concepts of altered health states* (8th ed., p. 362). Philadelphia: Lippincott Williams & Wilkins.

cell proliferation. The remaining lymphoid tissues contain immune cells that defend the body's mucosal surfaces against microorganisms (Levinson, 2008).

Function of the Immune System

The basic function of the immune system is to remove foreign antigens such as viruses and bacteria to maintain homeostasis. There are two general types of immunity, natural (innate) and acquired (adaptive). Natural immunity or nonspecific immunity is present at birth. Acquired or specific immunity develops after birth. Each type of immunity has a distinct role in defending the body against harmful invaders, but the various components are usually interdependent (Levinson, 2008).

Natural Immunity

Natural immunity, which is nonspecific, provides a broad spectrum of defense against and resistance to infection. It is considered the first line of host defense following antigen exposure, because it protects the host without "remembering" prior contact with an infectious agent (Kin & Sanders, 2006). Responses to a foreign invader are very similar from one encounter to the next, regardless of the number of times the invader is encountered. Natural (innate) immunity co-coordinates the initial response to pathogens through the production of cytokines and other effector molecules, which either activate cells for control of the pathogen (by elimination) or promote the development of the acquired **immune response.** The cells involved in this response are monocytes, macrophages, dendritic cells, **natural killer (NK) cells,** basophils, eosinophils, and granulocytes. The early events in this process are critical in determining the nature of the adaptive immune response. Natural immune mechanisms can be divided into two stages: immediate (generally occurring within 4 hours) and delayed (occurring between 4 and 96 hours after exposure) (Madoff & Kasper, 2008).

White Blood Cell Action

Cellular response is key to the effective initiation of the immune response. WBCs, or leukocytes, participate in both the natural and the acquired immune responses. Granular leukocytes, or granulocytes (so called because of granules in their cytoplasm), fight invasion by foreign bodies or toxins by releasing cell mediators, such as histamine, bradykinin, and prostaglandins, and engulfing the foreign bodies or toxins. Granulocytes include neutrophils, eosinophils, and basophils.

Neutrophils (polymorphonuclear leukocytes [PMNs]) are the first cells to arrive at the site where inflammation occurs. Eosinophils and basophils, other types of granulocytes, increase in number during allergic reactions and stress responses. Nongranular leukocytes include monocytes or macrophages (referred to as histiocytes when they enter tissue spaces) and lymphocytes. Monocytes also function as **phagocytic cells,** engulfing, ingesting, and destroying greater numbers and quantities of foreign bodies or toxins than granulocytes do. Lymphocytes, consisting of B cells and T cells, play major roles in humoral and cell-mediated immune responses. About 60% to 70% of lymphocytes in the blood are T cells, and about 10% to 20% are B cells (Abbas, Lichtman & Baker, 2008).

Inflammatory Response

The inflammatory response is a major function of the natural immune system that is elicited in response to tissue injury or invading organisms. Chemical mediators assist this response by minimizing blood loss, walling off the invading organism, activating phagocytes, and promoting formation of fibrous scar tissue and regeneration of injured tissue. The inflammatory response (discussed further in Chapter 6) is facilitated by physical and chemical barriers that are part of the human organism.

Physical and Chemical Barriers

Activation of the natural immunity response is enhanced by processes inherent in physical and chemical barriers. Physical surface barriers include intact skin, mucous membranes, and cilia of the respiratory tract, which prevent pathogens from gaining access to the body. The cilia of the respiratory tract, along with coughing and sneezing responses, filter and clear pathogens from the upper respiratory tract before they can invade the body further. Chemical barriers, such as mucus, acidic gastric secretions, enzymes in tears and saliva, and substances in sebaceous and sweat secretions, act in a nonspecific way to destroy invading bacteria and fungi. Viruses are countered by other means, such as interferon (see discussion later in chapter).

Immune Regulation

Regulation of the immune response involves balance and counterbalance. Dysfunction of the natural immune system can occur when the immune components are inactivated or when they remain active long after their effects are beneficial. A successful immune response eliminates the responsible antigen. If an immune response fails to develop and clear an antigen sufficiently, the host is considered to be immunocompromised or immunodeficient. If it is overtly robust or misdirected, allergies, asthma, or autoimmune disease results. The immune system's recognition of one's own tissues as "foreign" rather than as self is the basis of many autoimmune disorders. Despite the fact that the immune response is critical to the prevention of disease, it must be well controlled to curtail immunopathology. Most microbial infections induce an inflammatory response mediated by T cells and cytokines, which, in excess, can cause tissue damage. Therefore, regulatory mechanisms must be in place to suppress or halt the immune response. This is mainly achieved by the production of cytokines and transformation of growth factor that inhibits macrophage activation. In some cases, T-cell activation is so overwhelming that these mechanisms fail, and pathology develops. Ongoing research on **immunoregulation** holds the promise of preventing graft rejection and aiding the body in eliminating cancerous or infected cells (Kin & Sanders, 2006). Although natural immunity can effectively combat infections, many pathogenic microbes have evolved that resist natural immunity. Acquired immunity is necessary to defend against these resistant agents.

Acquired Immunity

Acquired (adaptive) immunity usually develops as a result of prior exposure to an antigen through immunization (vaccination) or by contracting a disease, both of which generate a protective immune response. Weeks or months after exposure to the disease or vaccine, the body produces an immune response that is sufficient to defend against the disease on re-exposure. In contrast to the rapid but nonspecific natural immune response, this form of immunity relies on the recognition of specific foreign antigens. The acquired immune response is broadly divided into two mechanisms: (1) the cell-mediated response, involving T-cell activation, and (2) effector mechanisms, involving B-cell maturation and production of antibodies.

The two types of acquired immunity are known as active and passive and are strongly interrelated. Active acquired immunity refers to immunologic defenses developed by the person's own body. This immunity typically lasts many years or even a lifetime. Passive acquired immunity is temporary immunity transmitted from a source outside the body that has developed immunity through previous disease or immunization. Examples are immune globulin or immunity resulting from the transfer of antibodies from the mother to an infant in utero or through breast-feeding. Active and passive acquired immunity involve humoral and cellular (cell-mediated) immunologic responses (described later).

Response to Invasion

When the body is invaded or attacked by bacteria, viruses, or other pathogens, it has three means of defense:
- The phagocytic immune response
- The humoral or antibody immune response
- The cellular immune response

The first line of defense, the **phagocytic immune response,** primarily involves the WBCs (granulocytes and macrophages), which have the ability to ingest foreign particles and destroy the invading agent; eosinophils are only weakly phagocytic. Phagocytes also remove the body's own dying or dead cells. Cells in necrotic tissue that are dying release substances that trigger an inflammatory response. **Apoptosis,** or programmed cell death, is the body's way of destroying worn-out cells such as blood or skin cells or cells that need to be renewed.

A second protective response, the **humoral immune response** (sometimes called the **antibody** response), begins with the B lymphocytes, which can transform themselves into plasma cells that manufacture antibodies. These antibodies are highly specific proteins that are transported in the bloodstream and attempt to disable invaders. The third mechanism of defense, the **cellular immune response,** also involves the T lymphocytes, which can turn into special cytotoxic (or killer) T cells that can attack the pathogens.

The structural part of the invading or attacking organism that is responsible for stimulating antibody production is called an **antigen** (or an immunogen). For example, an antigen can be a small patch of proteins on the outer surface of a microorganism. Not all antigens are naturally immunogenic; some must be coupled to other molecules to stimulate the immune response. A single bacterium or large molecule, such as a diphtheria or tetanus toxin, may have several

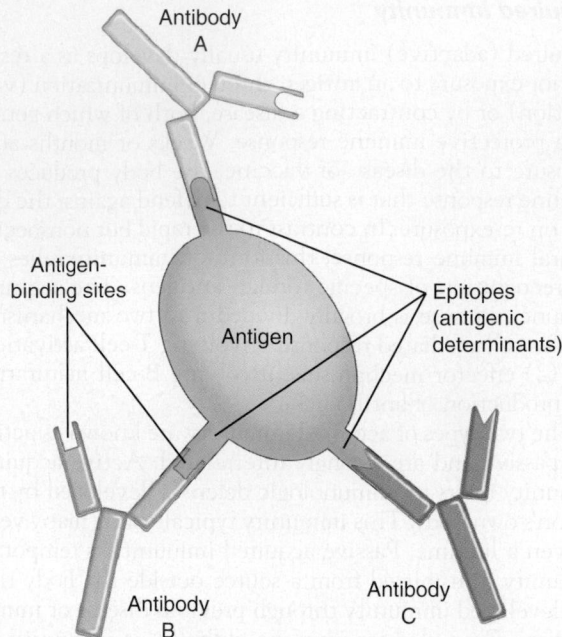

Figure 50-4 Complement-mediated immune responses. Redrawn from Porth, C. M. & Matfin, G. (2009). *Pathophysiology: Concepts of altered health states* (8th ed.). Philadelphia: Lippincott Williams & Wilkins.

antigens, or markers, on its surface, thus inducing the body to produce a number of different antibodies. Once produced, an antibody is released into the bloodstream and carried to the attacking organism. There, it combines with the antigen, binding with it like an interlocking piece of a jigsaw puzzle (Fig. 50-4). There are four well-defined stages in an immune response: recognition, proliferation, response, and effector (Fig. 50-5).

Recognition Stage

Recognition of antigens as foreign, or non-self, by the immune system is the initiating event in any immune response. Recognition involves the use of lymph nodes and lymphocytes for surveillance. Lymph nodes are widely distributed internally throughout the body and in the circulating blood, as well as externally near the body's surfaces. They continuously discharge small lymphocytes into the bloodstream. These lymphocytes patrol the tissues and vessels that drain the areas served by that node. Lymphocytes recirculate from the blood to lymph nodes and from the lymph nodes back into the bloodstream, in a continuous circuit. The exact way in which they recognize antigens on foreign surfaces is not known; however, recognition is thought to depend on specific receptor sites on the surface of the lymphocytes. Macrophages play an important role in helping the circulating lymphocytes process the antigens. Both macrophages and neutrophils have receptors for antibodies and complement; as a result, they coat microorganisms with antibodies, complement, or both, thereby enhancing phagocytosis.

In a streptococcal throat infection, for example, the streptococcal organism gains access to the mucous membranes of the throat. A circulating lymphocyte moving through the tissues of the throat comes in contact with the organism. The lymphocyte recognizes the antigens on the microbe as different (non-self) and the streptococcal organism as antigenic (foreign). This triggers the second stage of the immune response—proliferation.

Proliferation Stage

The circulating lymphocytes containing the antigenic message return to the nearest lymph node. Once in the node, these sensitized lymphocytes stimulate some of the resident T and B lymphocytes to enlarge, divide, and proliferate. T lymphocytes differentiate into cytotoxic (or killer) T cells, whereas B lymphocytes produce and release antibodies. Enlargement of the lymph nodes in the neck in conjunction with a sore throat is one example of the immune response.

Response Stage

In the response stage, the differentiated lymphocytes function in either a humoral or a cellular capacity. This stage begins with the production of antibodies by the B lymphocytes in response to a specific antigen. The cellular response stimulates the resident lymphocytes to become cells that attack microbes directly rather than through the action of antibodies. These transformed lymphocytes are known as cytotoxic (killer) T cells.

Viral rather than bacterial antigens induce a cellular response. This response is manifested by the increasing number of T lymphocytes (lymphocytosis) seen in the blood tests of people with viral illnesses such as infectious mononucleosis. (Cellular immunity is discussed in further detail later in this chapter.) Most immune responses to antigens involve both humoral and cellular responses, although one usually predominates. For example, during transplant rejection, the cellular response predominates, whereas in the bacterial pneumonias and sepsis, the humoral response plays the dominant protective role (Chart 50-1).

Effector Stage

In the effector stage, either the antibody of the humoral response or the cytotoxic (killer) T cell of the cellular response reaches and connects with the antigen on the surface of the foreign invader. This initiates activities involving interplay of antibodies (humoral immunity), complement, and action by the cytotoxic T cells (cellular immunity).

Humoral Immune Response

The humoral response is characterized by the production of antibodies by B lymphocytes in response to a specific antigen. While B lymphocytes are responsible for the production of antibodies, both the macrophages of natural immunity and the special T lymphocytes of cellular immunity are involved in recognition.

Antigen Recognition

Several theories explain the mechanisms by which B lymphocytes recognize the invading antigen and respond by producing antibodies. It is known that B lymphocytes recognize and respond to invading antigens in more than one way.

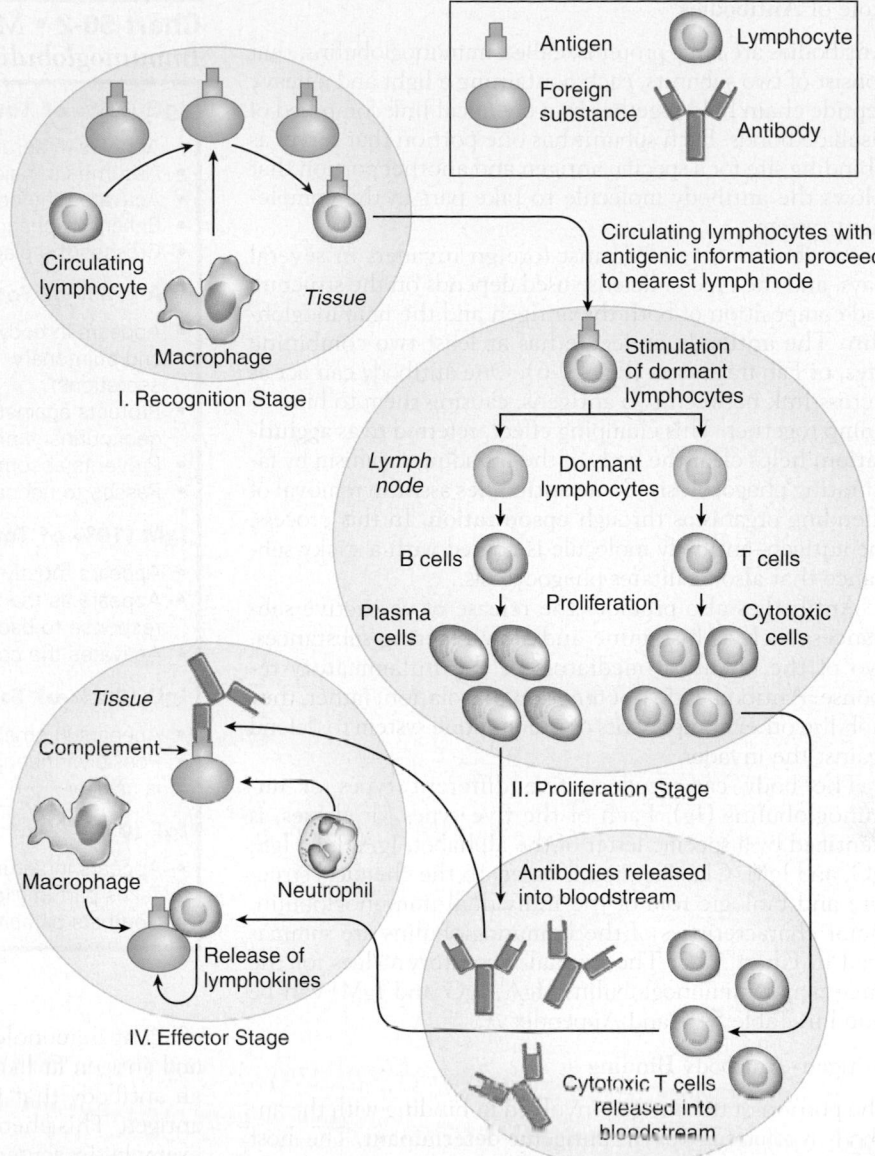

Figure 50-5 Stages of the immune response. **I,** In the *recognition stage,* antigens are recognized by circulating lymphocytes and macrophages. **II,** In the *proliferation stage,* the dormant lymphocytes proliferate and differentiate into cytotoxic (killer) T cells or B cells responsible for formation and release of antibodies. **III,** In the *response stage,* the cytotoxic T cells and the B cells perform cellular and humoral functions, respectively. **IV,** In the *effector stage,* antigens are destroyed or neutralized through the action of antibodies, complement, macrophages, and cytotoxic T cells.

Chart 50-1 • *Comparison of Cellular and Humoral Immune Responses*

Humoral Responses (B Cells)

- Bacterial phagocytosis and lysis
- Anaphylaxis
- Allergic hay fever and asthma
- Immune complex disease
- Bacterial and some viral infections

Cellular Responses (T Cells)

- Transplant rejection
- Delayed hypersensitivity (tuberculin reaction)
- Graft-versus-host disease
- Tumor surveillance or destruction
- Intracellular infections
- Viral, fungal, and parasitic infections

The B lymphocytes respond to some antigens by directly triggering antibody formation; however, in response to other antigens, they need the assistance of T cells to trigger antibody formation. With the help of macrophages, the T lymphocytes are believed to recognize the antigen of a foreign invader. The T lymphocyte picks up the antigenic message, or "blueprint," of the antigen and returns to the nearest lymph node with that message. B lymphocytes stored in the lymph nodes are subdivided into thousands of clones, which are stimulated to enlarge, divide, proliferate, and differentiate into plasma cells capable of producing specific antibodies to the antigen. Other B lymphocytes differentiate into B-lymphocyte clones with a memory for the antigen. These memory cells are responsible for the more exaggerated and rapid immune response in a person who is repeatedly exposed to the same antigen.

Role of Antibodies

Antibodies are large proteins, called immunoglobulins, that consist of two subunits, each containing a light and a heavy peptide chain held together by a chemical link composed of disulfide bonds. Each subunit has one portion that serves as a binding site for a specific antigen and another portion that allows the antibody molecule to take part in the complement system.

Antibodies defend against foreign invaders in several ways, and the type of defense used depends on the structure and composition of both the antigen and the immunoglobulin. The antibody molecule has at least two combining sites, or Fab fragments (Fig. 50-6). One antibody can act as a cross-link between two antigens, causing them to bind or clump together. This clumping effect, referred to as **agglutination,** helps clear the body of the invading organism by facilitating phagocytosis. Some antibodies assist in removal of offending organisms through **opsonization.** In this process, the antigen–antibody molecule is coated with a sticky substance that also facilitates phagocytosis.

Antibodies also promote the release of vasoactive substances, such as histamine and slow-reacting substances, two of the chemical mediators of the inflammatory response. Antibodies do not function in isolation; rather, they mobilize other components of the immune system to defend against the invader.

The body can produce five different types of immunoglobulins (Ig). Each of the five types, or classes, is identified by a specific letter of the alphabet, IgA, IgD, IgE, IgG, and IgM. Classification is based on the chemical structure and biologic role of the individual immunoglobulin. Major characteristics of the immunoglobulins are summarized in Chart 50-2. The normal laboratory values for the three major immunoglobulins (IgA, IgG and IgM) can be found in Table 54-1 and Appendix A.

Antigen–Antibody Binding

The portion of the antigen involved in binding with the antibody is referred to as the **antigenic determinant.** The most

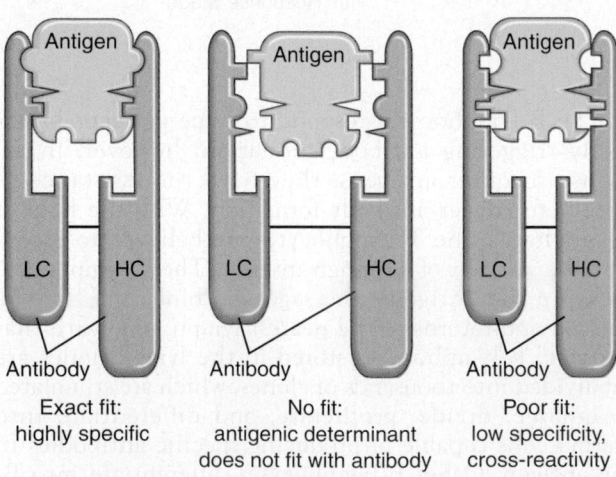

Figure 50-6 Antigen–antibody binding. (*Left*) A highly specific antigen–antibody complex. (*Center*) No match and, therefore, no immune response. (*Right*) Poor fit or match with low specificity; antibody reacts to antigen with similar characteristics, producing cross-reactivity. HC = heavy chain; LC = light chain.

Exact fit: highly specific

No fit: antigenic determinant does not fit with antibody binding site

Poor fit: low specificity, cross-reactivity

Chart 50-2 • *Major Characteristics of the Immunoglobulins*

IgG (75% of Total Immunoglobulin)

- Appears in serum and tissues (interstitial fluid)
- Assumes a major role in bloodborne and tissue infections
- Activates the complement system
- Enhances phagocytosis
- Crosses the placenta

IgA (15% of Total Immunoglobulin)

- Appears in body fluids (blood, saliva, tears, breast milk, and pulmonary, gastrointestinal, prostatic, and vaginal secretions)
- Protects against respiratory, gastrointestinal, and genitourinary infections
- Prevents absorption of antigens from food
- Passes to neonate in breast milk for protection

IgM (10% of Total Immunoglobulin)

- Appears mostly in intravascular serum
- Appears as the first immunoglobulin produced in response to bacterial and viral infections
- Activates the complement system

IgD (0.2% of Total Immunoglobulin)

- Appears in small amounts in serum
- Possibly influences B-lymphocyte differentiation, but role is unclear

IgE (0.004% of Total Immunoglobulin)

- Appears in serum
- Takes part in allergic and some hypersensitivity reactions
- Combats parasitic infections

---

efficient immunologic responses occur when the antibody and antigen fit like a lock and key. Poor fit can occur with an antibody that was produced in response to a different antigen. This phenomenon is known as cross-reactivity. For example, in acute rheumatic fever, the antibody produced against *Streptococcus pyogenes* in the upper respiratory tract may cross-react with the patient's heart tissue, leading to heart valve damage.

Cellular Immune Response

The T lymphocytes are primarily responsible for cellular immunity. Stem cells continuously migrate from the bone marrow to the thymus gland, where they develop into T cells. Despite the partial degeneration of the thymus gland that occurs at puberty, T cells continue to develop here. Several types of T cells exist, each with designated roles in the defense against bacteria, viruses, fungi, parasites, and malignant cells. T cells attack foreign invaders directly rather than by producing antibodies.

Cellular reactions are initiated, with or without the assistance of macrophages, by the binding of an antigen to an antigen receptor located on the surface of a T cell. The T cells then carry the antigenic message, or blueprint, to the lymph nodes, where the production of other T cells is stimulated. Some T cells remain in the lymph nodes and retain a memory for the antigen. Other T cells migrate from the lymph nodes into the general circulatory system and ultimately to the tissues, where they remain until they either come in contact with their respective antigens or die (Sompayrac, 2008).

Types of T Lymphocytes

T cells include effector T cells, suppressor T cells, and memory T cells. The two major categories of effector T cells—helper T cells and cytotoxic T cells—participate in the destruction of foreign organisms. T cells interact closely with B cells, indicating that humoral and cellular immune responses are not separate, unrelated processes, but rather branches of the immune response that interact.

Helper T cells are activated on recognition of antigens and stimulate the rest of the immune system. When activated, helper T cells secrete **cytokines,** which attract and activate B cells, cytotoxic T cells, NK cells, macrophages, and other cells of the immune system. Separate subpopulations of helper T cells produce different types of cytokines and determine whether the immune response will be the production of antibodies or a cell-mediated immune response. Helper T cells also produce **lymphokines,** one category of cytokines (Table 50-2).

Cytotoxic T cells (killer T cells) attack the antigen directly by altering the cell membrane and causing cell lysis (disintegration) and by releasing cytolytic enzymes and cytokines. Lymphokines can recruit, activate, and regulate other lymphocytes and WBCs. These cells then assist in destroying the invading organism. Delayed-type hypersensitivity is an example of an immune reaction that protects the body from antigens through the production and release of lymphokines (see later discussion).

Suppressor T cells have the ability to decrease B-cell production, thereby keeping the immune response at a level that is compatible with health (eg, sufficient to fight infection adequately without attacking the body's healthy tissues). **Memory cells** are responsible for recognizing antigens from previous exposure and mounting an immune response (Table 50-3).

Null Lymphocytes and Natural Killer Cells

Null lymphocytes and NK cells are other lymphocytes that assist in combating organisms. These cells are distinct from B cells and T cells and lack the usual characteristics of those cells. **Null lymphocytes,** a subpopulation of lymphocytes, destroy antigens already coated with antibody. These cells have special receptor sites on their surface that allow them to connect with the end of antibodies; this is known as antibody-dependent, cell-mediated cytotoxicity.

NK cells are a class of lymphocytes that recognize infected and stressed cells and respond by killing these cells and by secreting macrophage-activating cytokine. The helper T cells contribute to the differentiation of null and NK cells.

Complement System

Circulating plasma proteins, known as **complement,** are made in the liver and activated when an antibody connects with its antigen. Complement plays an important role in

Table 50-2	CYTOKINES AND THEIR BIOLOGIC ACTIVITY
Cytokine*	**Biologic Activity**
Interleukin-1 (α and β)	Promotes differentiation of T and B lymphocytes, natural killer (NK) cells, and null cells
Interleukin-2	Stimulates growth of T lymphocytes and special activated killer lymphocytes (known as lymphocyte-activated killer cells [LAK cells])
Interleukin-3	Stimulates growth of mast cells and other blood cells
Interleukin-4	Stimulates growth of T and B lymphocytes, mast cells, and macrophages
Interleukin-5	Stimulates antibody responses
Interleukin-6	Stimulates growth and function of B lymphocytes and antibodies
Interleukin-7	Stimulates growth of pre-B, CD4+ and CD8+ T lymphocytes and activates mature T lymphocytes
Interleukin-8	Promotes chemotaxis and activation of neutrophils
Interleukin-9	Stimulates growth and proliferation of T lymphocytes
Interleukin-10	Inhibits interferon-gamma and mononuclear cell inflammation
Interleukin-11	Promotes induction of acute phase proteins
Interleukin-12	Introduces helper T lymphocytes
Interleukin-13	Inhibits mononuclear phagocyte inflammation and promotes differentiation of B cells
Interleukin-16	Promotes chemotaxis CD4+ T lymphocytes and eosinophils
Permeability factor	Increases vascular permeability, allowing white cells into area
Interferon-γ	Activates macrophages; increases expression of class I and II MHC antigen processing and presentation
Interferon (type 1α and type β)	Exerts antiviral activity in body cells; induces class I antigen expression; activates NK cells
Migration inhibitory factor	Suppresses movement of macrophages, keeping macrophages in area of foreign cells
Skin reactive factor	Induces inflammatory response
Cytotoxic factor (lymphotoxin)	Kills certain antigenic cells
Macrophage chemotactic factor	Attracts macrophages into the area
Lymphocyte blastogenic factor	Stimulates more lymphocytes, recruiting additional lymphocytes into the area
Macrophage aggregation factor	Causes clumping of macrophages and lymphocytes
Macrophage activation factor	Allows macrophages to adhere to surfaces more readily
Proliferation inhibitor factor	Inhibits growth of certain antigenic cells
Cytophilic antibody	Binds to an Fc receptor on macrophages, thereby permitting macrophages to bind to antigens
Tumor necrosis factor-alpha	Stimulates inflammation, wound healing, and tissue remodeling
Tumor necrosis factor-beta	Mediates inflammation and graft rejection

*Cytokines are biologically active substances that are released by cells to regulate growth and function of other cells within the immune system.

Lymphocytes produce lymphokines, and monocytes and macrophages produce monokines. This table lists some of the cytokines that play a role in immune system functioning. MHC = major histocompatibility complex.

Table 50-3 LYMPHOCYTES INVOLVED IN IMMUNE RESPONSES

Type of Immune Response	Cell Type	Function
Humoral	B lymphocyte	Produces antibodies or immunoglobulins (IgA, IgD, IgE, IgG, IgM)
Cellular	T lymphocyte	
	Helper T	Attacks foreign invaders (antigens) directly
		Initiates and augments inflammatory response
	Helper T_1	Increases activated cytotoxic T cells
	Helper T_2	Increases B cell antibody production
	Suppressor T	Suppresses the immune response
	Memory T	Remembers contact with an antigen and on subsequent exposures mounts an immune response
	Cytotoxic T (killer T)	Lyses cells infected with virus; plays a role in graft rejection
Nonspecific	Non-T or non-B lymphocyte	
	Null cell	Destroys antigens already coated with antibody
	Natural killer (NK) cell (granular lymphocyte)	Defends against microorganisms and some types of malignant cells; produces cytokines

the defense against microbes. Destruction of an invading or attacking organism or toxin is not achieved merely by the binding of the antibody and antigens; it also requires activation of complement, the arrival of killer T cells, or the attraction of macrophages. Complement has three major physiologic functions: defending the body against bacterial infection, bridging natural and acquired immunity, and disposing of immune complexes and the byproducts associated with inflammation (Porth & Matfin, 2009).

The proteins that comprise complement interact sequentially with one another in a cascading effect. The complement cascade is important to modifying the effector arm of the immune system. Activation of complement allows important events, such as removal of infectious agents and initiation of the inflammatory response, to take place. These events involve active parts of the pathway that enhance chemotaxis of macrophages and granulocytes, alter blood vessel permeability, change blood vessel diameters, cause cells to lyse, alter blood clotting, and cause other points of modification. These macrophages and granulocytes continue the body's defense by devouring the antibody-coated microbes and by releasing bacterial products.

The complement cascade may be activated by any of three pathways: classic, lectin, and alternative. The classic pathway is triggered after antibodies bind to microbes or other antigens and is part of the humoral type of adaptive immunity. The lectin pathway is activated when a plasma protein (mannose-binding lectin) binds to terminal mannose residue on the surface glycoproteins of microbes. The alternative pathway is triggered when complement proteins are activated on microbial surfaces. This pathway is part of natural immunity.

Complement components, prostaglandins, leukotrienes, and other inflammatory mediators all contribute to the recruitment of inflammatory cells, as do chemokines, a group of cytokines. The activated neutrophils pass through the vessel walls to accumulate at the site of infection, where they phagocytose complement-coated microbes (Abbas, et al., 2008). This response is usually therapeutic and can be lifesaving if the cell attacked by the complement system is a true foreign invader. However, if that cell is part of the human organism, the result can be devastating disease and even death. Many autoimmune diseases and disorders characterized by chronic infection are thought to be caused in part by continued or chronic activation of complement, which in turn results in chronic inflammation. The RBCs and platelets have complement receptors and, as a result, play an important role in the clearance of immune complexes that consist of antigen, antibody, and components of the complement system (Abbas, et al., 2008).

Immunomodulators

While antimicrobial agents and vaccines have yielded considerable therapeutic success and the immune system usually works effectively, many infectious diseases remain difficult clinical challenges. Treatment success may be compromised by defects of the immune system; in this case, enhancement of the host immune response may be therapeutically beneficial. An immunomodulator (also known as a biologic response modifier) affects the host via direct or indirect effects on one or more components of the immunoregulatory network. Interferons and colony-stimulating factors are two of the more commonly used immunomodulators (Liles, 2005).

Interferons

Interferon, one type of biologic response modifier, is a nonspecific viricidal protein that is naturally produced by the body and is capable of activating other components of the immune system. These substances continue to be investigated to determine their roles in the immune system and their potential therapeutic effects in disorders characterized by disturbed immune responses. Interferons have antiviral and antitumor properties. In addition to responding to viral infection, interferons are produced by T lymphocytes, B lymphocytes, and macrophages in response to antigens. They are thought to modify the immune response by suppressing antibody production and cellular immunity. They also facilitate the cytolytic role of macrophages and NK cells. Interferons are used to treat immune-related disorders (eg, multiple sclerosis) and chronic inflammatory conditions (eg, chronic hepatitis). Research continues to evaluate the effectiveness of interferons in treating tumors and acquired immunodeficiency syndrome (AIDS).

Colony-Stimulating Factors

Colony-stimulating factors are a group of naturally occurring glycoprotein cytokines that regulate production, differentiation, survival, and activation of hematopoietic cells. Erythropoietin stimulates RBC production. Thrombopoietin plays a key regulatory role in the growth and differentiation of bone marrow cells. Interleukin-5 (IL-5) stimulates the growth and survival of eosinophils and basophils.

Stem cell factor and IL-3 serve as stimuli for multiple hematopoietic cell lines. Granulocyte colony-stimulating factor, granulocyte-macrophage colony-stimulating factor, and macrophage colony-stimulating factor all serve as growth factors for specific cell lines. These cytokines have attracted considerable interest for their potential role in immunomodulation (McInnes, 2005; Nelson, 2007).

Advances in Immunology

Genetic Engineering

One of the more remarkable evolving technologies is **genetic engineering,** which uses recombinant deoxyribonucleic acid (DNA) technology. Two facets of this technology exist. The first permits scientists to combine genes from one type of organism with genes of a second organism. This type of technology allows cells and microorganisms to manufacture proteins, monokines, and lymphokines, which can alter and enhance immune system function. The second facet of recombinant DNA technology involves gene therapy. If a particular gene is abnormal or missing, experimental recombinant DNA technology may be capable of restoring normal gene function. For example, a recombinant gene is inserted onto a virus particle. When the virus particle splices its genes, the virus automatically inserts the missing gene and theoretically corrects the genetic anomaly. Extensive research into recombinant DNA technology and gene therapy is ongoing (Abbas, et al., 2008).

Stem Cells

Stem cells are capable of self-renewal and differentiation; they continually replenish the body's entire supply of both RBCs and WBCs. Some stem cells, described as totipotent cells, have tremendous capacity to self-renew and differentiate. Embryonic stem cells, described as pluripotent, give rise to numerous cell types that are able to form tissues. Research has shown that stem cells can restore an immune system that has been destroyed. Stem cell transplantation has been carried out in humans with certain types of immune dysfunction, such as severe combined immunodeficiency (SCID); clinical trials using stem cells are under way in patients with a variety of disorders having an autoimmune component, including systemic lupus erythematosus, rheumatoid arthritis, scleroderma, and multiple sclerosis. Research with embryonic stem cells has enabled investigators to make substantial gains in developmental biology, gene therapy, therapeutic tissue engineering, and the treatment of a variety of diseases. However, along with these remarkable opportunities, many ethical challenges arise, which are largely based on concerns about safety, efficacy, resource allocation, and human cloning (Goldman, 2007).

Assessment of the Immune System

An assessment of immune function begins during the health history and physical examination. Areas to be assessed include nutritional status; infections and immunizations; allergies; disorders and disease states, such as autoimmune disorders, cancer, and chronic illnesses; surgeries; medications; and blood transfusions. In addition to inspection of general characteristics, palpation of the lymph nodes and examinations of the skin, mucous membranes, and respiratory, gastrointestinal, musculoskeletal, genitourinary, cardiovascular, and neurosensory systems are performed (Moorhead, Johnson, Mass, et al., 2008) (Chart 50-3).

Health History

The history should note the patient's age along with information about past and present conditions and events that may provide clues to the status of the patient's immune system.

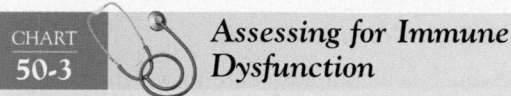

CHART 50-3 *Assessing for Immune Dysfunction*

Be alert for the following signs and symptoms:

Respiratory System

- Changes in respiratory rate
- Cough (dry or productive)
- Abnormal lung sounds (wheezing, crackles, rhonchi)
- Rhinitis
- Hyperventilation
- Bronchospasm

Cardiovascular System

- Hypotension
- Tachycardia
- Dysrhythmia
- Vasculitis
- Anemia

Gastrointestinal System

- Hepatosplenomegaly
- Colitis
- Vomiting
- Diarrhea

Genitourinary System

- Frequency and burning on urination
- Hematuria
- Discharge

Musculoskeletal System

- Joint mobility, edema, and pain

Skin

- Rashes
- Lesions
- Dermatitis
- Hematomas or purpura
- Edema or urticaria
- Inflammation
- Discharge

Neurosensory System

- Cognitive dysfunction
- Hearing loss
- Visual changes
- Headaches and migraines
- Ataxia
- Tetany

Gender

There are differences in the immune system functions of men and women. For example, many autoimmune diseases have a higher incidence in females than in males, a phenomenon believed to be correlated with sex hormones. Sex hormones have long been recognized for their role in reproductive function, and in the past two decades research has revealed that these hormones are integral signaling modulators of the immune system. Sex hormones play definitive roles in lymphocyte maturation, activation, and synthesis of antibodies and cytokines. In autoimmune disease, expression of sex hormones is altered, and this change contributes to immune dysregulation (Ackerman, 2006).

Gerontologic Considerations

Immunosenescence is a complex route in which the aging process stimulates changes in the immune system. The immune system undergoes age-associated alterations that lead to a progressive deterioration in the ability to respond to infections. The capacity for self-renewal of hematopoietic stem cells diminishes. There is a notable decline in the total number of phagocytes, coupled with an intrinsic reduction in their activity. The cytotoxicity of NK cells decreases, contributing to a decline in humoral immunity (Kovalou & Gribeck-Loebenstein, 2006). Acquired immunity may be negatively affected; the efficacy of vaccines is frequently decreased in older adults. Natural immunity, however, continues to function reasonably well, perhaps as an adaptive response to the deterioration of cell-mediated immunity in old age (Aw, Silva & Palmer, 2007).

The incidence of autoimmune diseases also increases with age, possibly from a decreased ability of antibodies to differentiate between self and non-self. Failure of the surveillance system to recognize mutant or abnormal cells also

may be responsible, in part, for the high incidence of cancer associated with increasing age.

Age-related changes in many body systems also contribute to impaired immunity (Table 50-4). Decreased gastric secretions and motility allow normal intestinal flora to proliferate and produce infection, causing gastroenteritis and diarrhea. Decreased renal circulation, filtration, absorption, and excretion contribute to the risk for urinary tract infections. Moreover, prostatic enlargement or a neurogenic bladder can impede urine passage and impair bacterial clearance through the urinary system. Urinary stasis permits the growth of microorganisms (Bengmark, 2006). Prolonged exposure to tobacco and environmental toxins impairs pulmonary function and decreases the elasticity of lung tissue, the effectiveness of cilia, and the ability to cough effectively. These impairments hinder the removal of infectious organisms and toxins, increasing the older person's susceptibility to pulmonary infections and cancers. The skin becomes thinner and less elastic. Impaired skin integrity predisposes older people to infection from organisms that are part of normal skin flora. Secondary changes, including malnutrition and poor circulation, as well as the breakdown of natural mechanical barriers such as the skin, place the aging immune system at even greater disadvantage against infection. In addition, the increased incidence of peripheral neuropathy and the accompanying decreased sensation and circulation may lead to stasis ulcers, pressure ulcers, abrasions, and burns.

The effects of the aging process and psychological stress interact, with the potential to negatively influence immune integrity (Graham, Christian & Kiecolt-Glaser, 2006; Sandman-Goddard, Peeva & Shoenfeld, 2007). Consequently, continual assessment of the physical and emotional status of the elderly is imperative, because early recognition and management of factors influencing immune response

Table 50-4	AGE-RELATED CHANGES IN IMMUNOLOGIC FUNCTION	
Body System	**Changes**	**Consequences**
Immune	Impaired function of B and T lymphocytes	Suppressed responses to pathogenic organisms with increased risk for infection
	Failure of lymphocytes to recognize mutant or abnormal cells	Increased incidence of cancers
	Decreased antibody production	Anergy (lack of response to antigens applied to the skin [allergens])
	Failure of immune system to differentiate "self" from "non-self"	Increased incidence of autoimmune diseases
	Suppressed phagocytic immune response	Absence of typical signs and symptoms of infection and inflammation
		Dissemination of organisms usually destroyed or suppressed by phagocytes (eg, reactivation or spread of tuberculosis)
Gastrointestinal	Decreased gastric secretions and motility	Proliferation of intestinal organisms resulting in gastroenteritis and diarrhea
	Decreased phagocytosis by the liver's Kupffer cells	Increased incidence and severity of hepatitis B; increased incidence of liver abscesses
	Altered nutritional intake with inadequate protein intake	Suppressed immune response
Urinary	Decreased kidney function and changes in lower urinary tract function (enlargement of prostate gland, neurogenic bladder). Altered genitourinary tract flora	Urinary stasis and increased incidence of urinary tract infections
Pulmonary	Impaired ciliary action due to exposure to smoke and environmental toxins	Impaired clearance of pulmonary secretions; increased incidence of respiratory infections
Integumentary	Thinning of skin with less elasticity; loss of adipose tissue	Increased risk of skin injury, breakdown, and infection
Circulatory	Impaired microcirculation	Stasis and pressure ulcers
Neurologic function	Decreased sensation and slowing of reflexes	Increased risk of injury, skin ulcers, abrasions, and burns

may prevent or mitigate the high morbidity and mortality seen with illness in the elderly population (Pawelec, 2006; Woodland & Blackman, 2006).

Nutrition

The relationship of infection to nutritional status is a key determinant of human health. Traditionally, this relationship focused on the effect of nutrients on host defenses and the effect of infection on nutritional needs. This has expanded in scope to encompass the role of specific nutrients in acquired immune function—the modulation of inflammatory processes and the virulence of the infectious agent itself. Iron may have beneficial or deleterious effects on the immune system, and further research is needed (Munoz, Rios, Olivos, et al., 2007). The list of nutrients affecting infection, immunity, inflammation, and cell injury has expanded from traditional proteins to several vitamins, multiple minerals, and more recently specific lipid components of the diet (Puertollano, Puertollano, Alvarez de Cienfuegos, et al., 2007). Vitamin D deficiency has been associated with increased risk of common cancers, autoimmune diseases, and infectious diseases (Maggini, Wintergerst, Beveridge, et al., 2007). More recently, the role of micronutrients and fatty acids on the response of cells and tissues to hypoxic and toxic damage has been recognized, suggesting that there is another dimension to the relationship. Micronutrients such as zinc, copper, manganese, and selenium may have widespread negative effects on the immune response, which can be reversed by supplementation (Overbeck, Rink & Hasse, 2008).

The effects exerted by polyunsaturated fatty acids on immune system functions are under investigation. Studies show that these elements play a role in diminishing the incidence and severity of inflammatory disorders. Recent studies show that diets high in olive oil are not as immunosuppressive as diets rich in fish oil. The contribution of immune modulation by lipids to the high risk of infectious complications associated with the use of parenteral nutrition is unclear (Hise, Compher, Harlan, et al., 2006).

Depletion of protein reserves results in atrophy of lymphoid tissues, depression of antibody response, reduction in the number of circulating T cells, and impaired phagocytic function. As a result, susceptibility to infection is greatly increased. During periods of infection or serious illness, nutritional requirements may be further altered, potentially contributing to depletion of protein, fatty acid, vitamin, and trace elements and causing even greater risk of impaired immune response and sepsis. Nutritional intake that supports a competent immune response plays an important role in reducing the incidence of infections; patients whose nutritional status is compromised have a delayed postoperative recovery and often experience more severe infections and delayed wound healing. The nurse must assess the patient's nutritional status, caloric intake, and quality of foods ingested. There is evidence that nutrition plays a role in the development of cancer and that diet and lifestyle can alter the risk of cancer development as well as other chronic diseases (Valdes-Ramos, Benitez & Alejandra, 2007). The nurse is responsible for assuming a proactive role in ensuring the best possible nutritional intake for all patients as a vital step in preventing disease and poor outcomes (Morse & High, 2005).

Infection and Immunization

The patient is asked about childhood and adult immunizations, including vaccinations, to provide protection against influenza, pneumococcal disease (Pneumovax), pertussis, herpes simplex, and the usual childhood diseases (eg, measles, mumps). Herpes simplex virus (HSV) infections have a significant impact on health, causing a wide range of diseases (eg, oral and genital herpes). Teaching about the importance of adhering to the recommended schedule for these vaccines should be initiated. Known past or present exposure to tuberculosis is assessed, and the dates and results of any tuberculin tests (purified protein derivative [PPD] or tine test) and chest x-rays are documented. Recent exposure to any infections and the exposure dates are elicited. It is important for the nurse to assess whether the patient has been exposed to any sexually transmitted diseases (STDs) or bloodborne pathogens such as hepatitis A, B, C, D, and E viruses and human immunodeficiency virus (HIV). A history of STDs such as gonorrhea, syphilis, human papillomavirus (HPV) infection, and chlamydia can alert the nurse that the patient may have been exposed to HIV or hepatitis. A history of past and present infections and the dates and types of treatments, along with a history of any multiple persistent infections, fevers of unknown origin, lesions or sores, or any type of drainage, as well as the response to treatment are obtained.

Allergy

The patient is asked about any allergies, including types of allergens (eg, pollens, dust, plants, cosmetics, food, medications, vaccines, latex), the symptoms experienced, and seasonal variations in occurrence or severity in the symptoms. A history of testing and treatments, including prescribed and over-the-counter medications that the patient has taken or is currently taking for these allergies and the effectiveness of the treatments, is obtained. All medication and food allergies are listed on an allergy alert sticker and placed on the front of the patient's health record or chart to alert others. Continued assessment for potential allergic reactions in the patient is vital.

Disorders and Diseases

Autoimmune Disorders

Autoimmune disorders affect people of both genders of all ages, ethnicities, and social classes. Specific autoimmune disorders affect approximately 5% of the U.S. population. As mentioned previously, they tend to be more common in women because estrogen tends to enhance immunity. Androgen, on the other hand, tends to be immunosuppressive. Autoimmune diseases are the fifth leading cause of death by disease in females of reproductive age.

The patient is asked about any autoimmune disorders, such as lupus erythematosus, rheumatoid arthritis, multiple sclerosis, or psoriasis. The onset, severity, remissions and exacerbations, functional limitations, treatments that the patient has received or is currently receiving, and effectiveness of the treatments are described. The occurrence of different autoimmune diseases within a family strongly suggests a genetic predisposition to more than one autoimmune disease (Hawker, 2008; Yurasov & Nussenzweig, 2007).

Neoplastic Disease

If there is a history of cancer in the family, the type of cancer, age at onset, and relationship (maternal or paternal) of the patient to the affected family members is noted. Dates and results of any cancer screening tests for the patient are documented. A history of cancer in the patient is also obtained, along with the type of cancer, date of diagnosis, and treatment modalities used. Immunosuppression contributes to the development of cancers; however, cancer itself is immunosuppressive, as is the treatment for cancer. Large tumors can release antigens into the blood, and these antigens combine with circulating antibodies and prevent them from attacking the tumor cells. Furthermore, tumor cells may possess special blocking factors that coat tumor cells and prevent their destruction by killer T lymphocytes. During the early development of tumors, the body may fail to recognize the tumor antigens as foreign and subsequently fail to initiate destruction of the malignant cells. Hematologic cancers, such as leukemia and lymphoma, are associated with altered production and function of WBCs and lymphocytes.

All treatments that the patient has received or is currently receiving, such as radiation or chemotherapy, are recorded in the health history. In addition, the nurse should elicit information related to complementary or alternative modalities that have been used and the response to these efforts. Radiation destroys lymphocytes and decreases the ability to mount an effective immune response. The size and extent of the irradiated area determine the extent of immunosuppression. Whole-body irradiation may leave the patient totally immunosuppressed. Chemotherapy also affects bone marrow function, destroying cells that contribute to an effective immune response and resulting in immunosuppression (Sompayrac, 2008).

Chronic Illness and Surgery

The health assessment includes a history of chronic illness, such as diabetes mellitus, renal disease, chronic obstructive pulmonary disease (COPD), or fibromyalgia. The onset and severity of illnesses, as well as treatment that the patient is receiving for the illness, are obtained. Chronic illness may contribute to immune system impairments in various ways. Renal failure is associated with a deficiency in circulating lymphocytes. In addition, immune defenses may be altered by acidosis and uremic toxins. In diabetes, an increased incidence of infection has been associated with vascular insufficiency, neuropathy, and poor control of serum glucose levels. Recurrent respiratory tract infections are associated with COPD as a result of altered inspiratory and expiratory function and ineffective airway clearance. Additionally, a history of organ transplantation or surgical removal of the spleen, lymph nodes, or thymus is noted, because these conditions may place the patient at risk for impaired immune function (Doering, Martinez-Maza, Vredevoe, et al., 2008).

Special Problems

Conditions such as burns and other forms of injury and infection may contribute to altered immune system function. Major burns cause impaired skin integrity and compromise the body's first line of defense. Loss of large amounts of serum occurs with burn injuries and depletes the body of essential proteins, including immunoglobulins. The physiologic and psychological stressors associated with surgery or injury stimulate cortisol release from the adrenal cortex; increased serum cortisol also contributes to suppression of normal immune responses (Shankar, Melstrom & Gamelli, 2007).

Medications and Blood Transfusions

A list of past and present medications is obtained. In large doses, antibiotics, corticosteroids, cytotoxic agents, salicylates, nonsteroidal anti-inflammatory drugs (NSAIDs), and anesthetic agents can cause immune suppression (Table 50-5).

A history of blood transfusions is obtained, because previous exposure to foreign antigens through transfusion may be associated with abnormal immune function. Additionally, although the risk of HIV transmission through blood transfusion is extremely low in patients who received a transfusion after 1985 (when testing of blood for HIV was initiated in the United States), a small risk remains.

The patient is also asked about use of herbal agents and over-the-counter medications. Because many of these products have not been subjected to rigorous testing, their effects have not been fully identified. It is important, therefore, to ask patients about their use of these substances, to document their use, and to educate patients about untoward effects that may alter immune responsiveness.

Lifestyle Factors

Like any other body system, the functions of the immune system depend on other body systems. Poor nutritional status, smoking, excessive consumption of alcohol, illicit drug use, STDs, and occupational or residential exposure to environmental radiation and pollutants have been associated with impaired immune function and are assessed in a detailed patient history. Although factors that are not consistent with a healthy lifestyle are predominately responsible for ineffective immune function, positive lifestyle factors can also negatively affect immune function and require assessment. For example, rigorous exercise or competitive exercise—usually considered a positive lifestyle factor—can be a physiologic stressor and cause negative effects on immune response (Friedrich, 2008). This outcome is compounded if the person also faces stressful environmental conditions while undergoing exercise. Given the cumulative impact of various environmental stressors on the immune system, every effort should be made to minimize the person's exposure to stressors other than the exercise performed (Raso, Benard, Da Silva Duarte, et al., 2007).

Psychoneuroimmunologic Factors

Patient assessment must also address psychoneuroimmunologic factors. The bidirectional pathway between the brain and immune system is referred to as psychoneuroimmunology, a field that has been the focus of research and discussion over the last several decades (Starkweather, Witek-Janusek, Peterson, et al., 2006; Steel, Geller, Gamblin, et al., 2007). It is thought that the immune response is regulated and modulated in part by neuroendocrine influences. Lymphocytes and macrophages have receptors that are capable of responding to neurotransmitters and endocrine hormones.

Table 50-5 — SELECTED MEDICATIONS AND EFFECTS ON THE IMMUNE SYSTEM

Drug Classification (and Examples)	Effects on the Immune System
Antibiotics (in large doses)	**Bone Marrow Suppression**
ceftriaxone (Rocefin)	Eosinophilia, hemolytic anemia, hypoprothrombinemia, neutropenia, thrombocytopenia
cefuroxime sodium (Ceftin)	Eosinophilia, hemolytic anemia, hypoprothrombinemia, neutropenia, thrombocytopenia
chloramphenicol (Chloromycetin)	Leukopenia, aplastic anemia
dactinomycin (Cosmogen)	Agranulocytosis, neutropenia
fluoroquinolones (Cipro, Levaquin, Tequin)	Hemolytic anemia, methemoglobinemia, eosinophilia, leukopenia, pancytopenia
gentamicin sulfate (Garamycin)	Agranulocytosis, granulocytosis
macrolides (erythromycin, Zithromax, Biaxin)	Neutropenia, leukopenia
penicillins	Agranulocytosis
streptomycin	Leukopenia, neutropenia, pancytopenia
vancomycin (Vancocin, Vancoled)	Transient leukopenia
Antithyroid Drugs	
propylthiouracil (PTU)	Agranulocytosis, leukopenia
Nonsteroidal Anti-inflammatory Drugs (NSAIDs) (in large doses)	**Inhibit Prostaglandin Synthesis or Release**
aspirin	Agranulocytosis
COX-2 inhibitors	Anemia, allergy, no major other adverse affects to the immune system
ibuprofen (Advil, Motrin)	Leukopenia, neutropenia
indomethacin (Indocid, Indocin)	Agranulocytosis, leukopenia
phenylbutazone	Pancytopenia, agranulocytosis, aplastic anemia
Adrenal Corticosteroids	**Immunosuppression**
prednisone	
Antineoplastic Agents (cytotoxic agents)	**Immunosuppression**
alkylating agents	Leukopenia, bone marrow suppression
cyclophosphamide (Cytoxan)	Leukopenia, neutropenia
mechlorethamine HCl (Mustargen)	Agranulocytosis, neutropenia
cyclosporine	Leukopenia, inhibits T-lymphocyte function
Antimetabolites	**Immunosuppression**
fluorouracil (pyrimidine antagonist)	Leukopenia, eosinophilia
methotrexate (folic acid antagonist)	Leukopenia, aplastic bone marrow
mercaptopurine (6-MP) (purine antagonist)	Leukopenia, pancytopenia

Lymphocytes can produce and secrete adrenocorticotropic hormone and endorphinlike compounds. Cells in the brain, especially in the hypothalamus, can recognize prostaglandins, interferons, and interleukins as well as histamine and serotonin, which are released during the inflammatory process. Like all other biologic systems functioning to maintain homeostasis, the immune system is integrated with other psychophysiologic processes and is subject to regulation and modulation by the brain. These relationships may have immunologic consequences (Chart 50-4).

Conversely, the immune processes can affect neural and endocrine function, including behavior. Growing evidence indicates that a measurable immune system response can be positively influenced by biobehavioral strategies such as relaxation and imagery techniques, biofeedback, humor, hypnosis, and conditioning (Stephenson, Swanson, Dalton, et al., 2007). Therefore, the assessment should address the patient's general psychological status and the patient's use of and response to these strategies.

Physical Assessment

On physical examination (see Chart 50-3), the skin and mucous membranes are assessed for lesions, dermatitis, purpura (subcutaneous bleeding), urticaria, inflammation, or any discharge. Any signs of infection are noted. The patient's temperature is recorded, and the patient is observed for chills and sweating. The anterior and posterior cervical, axillary, and inguinal lymph nodes are palpated for enlargement; if palpable nodes are detected, their location, size, consistency, and reports of tenderness on palpation are noted. Joints are assessed for tenderness, swelling, increased warmth, and limited range of motion. The patient's respiratory, cardiovascular, genitourinary, gastrointestinal, and neurosensory systems are evaluated for signs and symptoms indicative of immune dysfunction. Any functional limitations or disabilities the patient may have are also assessed.

Diagnostic Evaluation

A series of blood tests and skin tests and a bone marrow biopsy may be performed to evaluate the patient's immune competence. Specific laboratory and diagnostic tests are discussed in greater detail along with individual disease processes in subsequent chapters in this unit. Selected laboratory and diagnostic tests used to evaluate immune competence are summarized in Chart 50-5.

CHART 50-4 NURSING RESEARCH PROFILE
Factors Affecting Immune Responses in Breast Cancer

Von Ah, D., Hang, D. & Carpenter, J. (2007). Stress, optimism and social support: Impact on immune responses in breast cancer. *Research in Nursing and Health, 30*(1), 72–83.

Purpose

The stress of a breast cancer diagnosis and initial surgical treatment can produce a variety of negative sequelae and impaired immune responses. The purpose of this study was to examine the roles of stress, optimism, and satisfaction with social support and their interactions in relation to immune responses in women who had been diagnosed with breast cancer and who had undergone surgical treatment.

Design

Researchers used a correlational, cross-sectional design to study the hypothesized relationships. They recruited, from one outpatient breast health center, a convenience sample of 54 women, 19 years of age and older, newly diagnosed with stage 0 or ductal carcinoma in situ, who were postsurgery (at least 7 days) and who had not received any other treatment. To collect demographic and medical data, investigators relied on self-report questionnaires and verified the results using medical record review. They used various measures of psychological factors: the Impact of Event Scale for perceived stress, the Life Orientation Test for optimism, and the Social Support Questionnaire for satisfaction with social support. Immunologic assessments measured natural killer cells and cytokine levels that are known to promote cell-mediated immunity and enhance natural killer cell activity.

Findings

The mean age of the participants was 55 years. They represented the racial diversity of the local population, and the majority of women were married and well educated, with a middle-income level. Women had stage I or II breast cancer and were surgically treated with either lumpectomy or modified mastectomy. Although they reported moderately significant levels of stress, the women were generally optimistic and had exceptionally high levels of satisfaction with their social support. Women with higher levels of perceived stress had lower natural killer cell activity and cytokine levels than women with lower levels of stress. Optimism and satisfaction with social support did not have direct main effects on any of the immune responses examined.

The most robust finding was the significant negative relationship between stress and natural killer cell activity and cytokine level that underscores the negative sequelae of cancer-specific stress on immune responses in women following breast cancer surgery. In addition, the study partially supported the hypothesis that optimism and social support moderated the relationship of stress on natural killer cell activity and cytokine level. Stress significantly interacted with optimism to predict natural killer cell activity. In the significant interaction between stress and optimism, natural killer cell activity was lowest when the participant reported greater stress and lower optimism. Satisfaction with social support did not have a stress-buffering effect on any of the immune indices examined in the study.

Nursing Implications

This study illustrates the need to identify supportive interventions that will have a positive effect on the issues faced by women who are undergoing surgical treatment for breast cancer. Interventions directed to the reduction of stress and enhancing optimism in women with breast cancer are warranted to achieve quality outcomes in these patients.

Nursing Management

The nurse needs to be aware that patients undergoing evaluation for possible immune system disorders experience not only physical pain and discomfort with certain types of diagnostic procedures, but also many psychological reactions. It is the nurse's role to counsel, educate, and support patients throughout the diagnostic process. Many patients may be extremely anxious about the results of diagnostic tests and the possible implications of those results for their employment, insurance, and personal relationships. This is an ideal time for the nurse to provide counseling and education, should these interventions be warranted.

Chart 50-5 • *Selected Tests for Evaluating Immunologic Status*

Various laboratory tests may be performed to assess immune system activity or dysfunction. The studies assess leukocytes and lymphocytes, humoral immunity, cellular immunity, phagocytic cell function, complement activity, hypersensitivity reactions, specific antigen–antibodies, or human immunodeficiency virus (HIV) infection.

Humoral (Antibody-mediated) Immunity Tests

- B-cell quantification with monoclonal antibody
- In vivo immunoglobulin synthesis with T-cell subsets
- Specific antibody response
- Total serum globulins and individual immunoglobulins (electrophoresis, immunoelectrophoresis, single radial immun-

odiffusion, nephelometry, and isohemagglutinin techniques)

Cellular (Cell-mediated) Immunity Tests

- Total lymphocyte count
- T-cell and T-cell-subset quantification with monoclonal antibody
- Delayed hypersensitivity skin test
- Cytokine production
- Lymphocyte response to mitogens, antigens, and allogenic cells
- Helper and suppressor T-cell functions

CRITICAL THINKING EXERCISES

1 A 70-year-old woman is referred to the allergy and immunology clinic for evaluation of her immune status. In addition to the eight medications she routinely takes, she has received several courses of antibiotics in the previous months for recurrent infections. What diagnostic tests would you expect to be ordered? What is the rationale for these? What further assessment data would you want to obtain from this patient?

EBP **2** A 38-year-old woman is hospitalized for a heart transplant, and immunosuppressant medications are prescribed. Describe how her altered immune function would affect the care that you provide. Develop an evidence-based teaching plan for the patient and her family before hospital discharge. Discuss the criteria used to assess the strength of the evidence for your teaching plan.

3 A 24-year-old woman is diagnosed with systemic lupus erythematosus (SLE), and corticosteroids are prescribed. What nursing observations and assessments are indicated? Identify patient teaching that is appropriate for the new diagnosis and prescription of steroids.

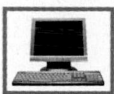 The Smeltzer suite offers these additional resources to enhance learning and facilitate understanding of this chapter:
• thePoint online resource, thepoint.lww.com/Smeltzer12E
• Student CD-ROM included with the book
• *Study Guide to Accompany Brunner & Suddarth's Textbook of Medical-Surgical Nursing*

REFERENCES AND SELECTED READINGS

Asterisk indicates nursing research.

Books

Abbas, A., Lichtman, A. & Baker, D. (2008). *Basic immunology, functions and disorders of the immune system* (3rd ed.). Philadelphia: W. B. Saunders.

Bulechek, G. M., Butcher, H. K. & Dochterman, J. M. (2008). *Nursing interventions classification (NIC)* (5th ed.). St. Louis: Mosby.

Goldman, C. (2007). *Medicine* (23rd ed.). Philadelphia: W. B. Saunders.

Harvey, R., Champe, P., Finkel, R., et al. (2008). *Lippincott's illustrated reviews, pharmacology.* Philadelphia: Lippincott Williams & Wilkins.

Huether, S. & McCance, K. (2008). *Understanding pathophysiology* (4th ed.). St. Louis: Mosby/Elsevier.

Levinson, W. (2008). *Review of medical microbiology and immunology* (10th ed.). Hollywood, CA: Lange Publishers.

Liles, W. C. (2005). Immunomodulators. In Mandell, G. L., Bennett, J. E. & Dolin, R. (Eds.). *Principles and practices of infectious diseases* (6th ed.). Philadelphia: Elsevier/Churchill Livingstone.

Madoff, L. & Kasper, D. (2008). The immune response. In Fauci, A., Braunwald, E., Kasper, D., et al. (Eds.). *Harrison's principles of internal medicine* (17th ed.). New York: McGraw-Hill Medical.

McInnes, I. B. (2005). Cytokines. In *Harris, Kelley's textbook of rheumatology* (7th ed.). Philadelphia: Saunders/Elsevier.

Moorhead, S., Johnson, M., Mass, M. L., et al. (2008). *Nursing outcomes classification (NOC)* (4th ed.). St. Louis: Mosby.

Morse, C. G. & High, K. P. (2005). Nutrition immunity and infection. In Mandell, G. L., Bennett, J. E. & Dolin, R. (Eds.). *Principles and practices of infectious diseases* (6th ed.). Philadelphia: Elsevier/Churchill Livingstone.

Porth, C. M. & Matfin, G. (2009). *Pathophysiology: Concepts of altered health states* (8th ed.). Philadelphia: Lippincott Williams & Wilkins.

Sompayrac, L. (2008). *How the immune system works* (3rd ed.). Malden, MA: Blackwell Publishers.

Stein, C. M. (2005). Immunoregulatory drugs. In *Harris, Kelley's textbook of rheumatology* (7th ed.). Philadelphia: W. B. Saunders.

Journals and Electronic Documents

Ackerman, L. (2006). Sex hormones and the genesis of autoimmunity. *Archives of Dermatology, 142*(3), 371–376.

Aw, D., Silva, A. & Palmer, D. (2007). Immunosenescence emerging challenges for an ageing population. *Immunology, 120*(4), 435–46.

Bartlett, J. (2006). Update in infectious diseases. *Annals of Internal Medicine, 144*(1), 49–56.

Bengmark, S. (2006). Impact of nutrition on ageing and disease. *Current Opinion in Clinical Nutrition and Metabolic Care, 9*(1), 2–7.

*Doering, L., Martinez-Maza, O., Vredevoe, D., et al. (2008). Relation of depression, natural killer cell function and infections after coronary artery bypass in women. *European Journal of Cardiovascular Nursing, 7*(1), 52–58.

Donaldson, T. (2007). Immune responses to infection. *Critical Care Nursing Clinics of North America, 19*(1), 1–8.

Friedrich, M. (2008). Exercise may boost aging immune system. *Journal of the American Medical Association, 299*(2), 160–161.

Graham, J., Christian, L. & Kiecolt-Glaser, J. (2006). Stress, age and immune function. Toward a lifespan approach. *Journal of Behavioral Medicine, 29*(4), 389–400.

Hawker, K. (2008). B-cell targeted treatment for multiple sclerosis. Mechanism of action and clinical data. *Current Opinion in Neurology, 21*(suppl 1), S19–S25.

Hise, M., Compher, C., Harlan, L., et al. (2006). Inflammatory mediators and immune function are altered in home parenteral nutrition patients. *Nutrition, 22*(2), 97–103.

*Hughes, D., Lada, E., Rooney C., et al. (2008). Massage therapy as a supportive care intervention for children with cancer. *Oncology Nursing Forum, 35*(3), 431–442.

Hughes, S. & Kelly, P. (2006). Interactions of malnutrition and immune impairment with specific reference to immunity against parasites. *Parasite Immunology, 28*(11), 577–588.

Kin, N. & Sanders, V. (2006). It takes nerve to tell T and B cells what to do. *Journal of Leukocyte Biology, 79*(6), 1093–1104.

Kovalou, R. & Gribeck-Loebenstein, B. (2006). Age-associated changes within CD4 T cells. *Immunology Letters, 107*(1), 8–14.

Linag, S. & Mackowiak, P. (2007). Infections in the elderly. *Clinics in Geriatric Medicine, 23*(2), 441–456.

*Lusk, B. & Lash, A. (2005). The stress response, psychoneuroimmunology and stress among ICU patients. *Dimensions in Critical Care Nursing, 24*(1), 25–31.

Maggini, S., Wintergerst, E., Beveridge, S., et al. (2007). Selected vitamins and trace elements support immune function by strengthening epithelial barriers and cellular and humoral immune responses. *British Journal of Nutrition, 98*(Suppl 1), S29–S35.

Munoz, C., Rios, E., Olivos, J., et al. (2007). Iron, copper and immunocompetence. *British Journal of Nutrition, 98*(suppl 1), S24–S28.

Nelson, L. (2007). Use of granulocyte-macrophage colony stimulating factor to reverse anergy in otherwise immunologically healthy children. *Annals of Allergy, Asthma and Immunology, 98*(4), 373–382.

Overbeck, S., Rink, L. & Hasse, H. (2008). Modulating the immune response by oral zinc supplementation: A single approach for multiple diseases (2008). *Archivum Immunologiae et Therapiae Experimentalis, 56*(1), 15–30.

Pawelec, G. (2006). Immunity and ageing in man. *Experimental Gerontology, 41*(12), 1239–1242.

Puertollano, M., Puertollano, E., Alvarez de Cienfuegos, G., et al. (2007). Significance of olive oil in the host immune resistance to infection. *British Journal of Nutrition, 98*(suppl 1), S54–S58.

Raso, V., Benard, G., Da Silva Duarte, A., et al. (2007). Effect of resistance training on immunological parameters of healthy elderly women. *Medicine and Science in Sports and Exercise, 39*(12), 2152–2159.

Sandman-Goddard, G., Peeva, E. & Shoenfeld, Y. (2007). Gender and autoimmunity. *Autoimmunity Reviews, 6*(6), 366–372.

Shankar, R., Melstrom, K. & Gamelli, R. (2007). Inflammation and sepsis. Past, present and future. *Journal of Burn Care and Research, 28*(4), 566–571.

*Starkweather, A., Witek-Janusek, L., Peterson, J., et al. (2006). Impact of psychological and immune factors on sciatic pain. A randomized, controlled trial among herniated disc patients. *SIC Nursing, 23*(3), 1–11.

Steel, J., Geller, D., Gamblin, T., et al. (2007). Depression, immunity and survival in patients with hepatobiliary carcinoma. *Journal of Clinical Oncology, 125*(27), 2397–2405.

*Stephenson, N., Swanson, M., Dalton, J., et al. (2007). Partner-delivered reflexology. Effects on cancer pain and anxiety. *Oncology Nursing Forum, 34*(1), 127–132.

Valdes-Ramos, R., Benitez, A. & Alejandra, D. (2007). Nutrition and immunity in cancer. *British Journal of Nutrition, 98*(suppl 1), S127–S132.

Vasto, S., Candore, G., Blaisteri, C., et al. (2007). Inflammatory networks in ageing, age-related diseases and longevity. *Mechanisms of Ageing and Development, 128*(1), 83–91.

Versleijen, M., Oyen, W., van Emst-deVries, S., et al. (2008). Immune function and leukocyte sequestration under the influence of parenteral lipid emulsions in healthy humans: A placebo-controlled crossover study. *American Journal of Clinical Nutrition, 87*(3), 539–547.

*Von Ah, D., Kang, D. & Carpenter, J. (2007). Stress, optimism and social support: Impact on immune responses in breast cancer. *Research in Nursing and Health, 30*(1), 72–83.

Woodland, D. & Blackman, M. (2006). Immunity and age: Living in the past? *Trends in Immunology, 27*(7), 303–307.

Yurasov, S. & Nussenzweig, M. (2007). Regulation of autoreactive antibodies. *Current Opinion in Rheumatology, 19*(5), 421–426.

Zandman-Goddard, G., Peeva, E. & Shoenfeld, Y. (2007). Gender and autoimmunity. *Autoimmunity Reviews, 6*(6), 366–372.

RESOURCES

Centers for Disease Control and Prevention, www.cdc.gov
National Institute of Allergy and Infectious Disease, www3.niaid.nih.gov/
National Institutes of Health, www.nih.gov/health/infoline.htm
U.S. Department of Health and Human Services, www.hhs.gov

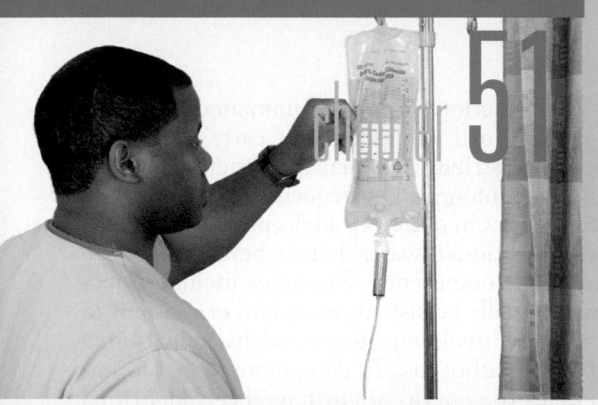

Management of Patients With Immunodeficiency

LEARNING OBJECTIVES

On completion of this chapter, the learner will be able to:

1 Compare the different types of primary immunodeficiency disorders and their causes, clinical manifestations, potential complications, and treatment modalities.

2 Describe the nursing management of the patient with an immunodeficiency.

3 Identify the essential teaching needs for a patient with an immunodeficiency.

GLOSSARY

agammaglobulinemia: disorder marked by an almost complete lack of immunoglobulins or antibodies

angioneurotic edema: condition marked by development of urticaria and an edematous area of skin, mucous membranes, or viscera

ataxia: loss of muscle coordination

ataxia-telangiectasia: autosomal recessive disorder affecting T- and B-cell immunity primarily seen in children and resulting in a degenerative brain disease

hypogammaglobulinemia: lack of one or more of the five immunoglobulins; caused by B-cell deficiency

immunocompromised host: person with a secondary immunodeficiency and associated immunosuppression

panhypoglobulinemia: general lack of immunoglobulins in the blood

severe combined immunodeficiency disease: disorder involving a complete absence of humoral and cellular immunity resulting from an X-linked or autosomal genetic abnormality

telangiectasia: vascular lesions caused by dilated blood vessels

thymic hypoplasia: T-cell deficiency that occurs when the thymus gland fails to develop normally during embryogenesis; also known as DiGeorge syndrome

Wiskott-Aldrich syndrome: immunodeficiency characterized by thrombocytopenia and the absence of T and B cells

Immunodeficiency disorders may be caused by a defect in or a deficiency of phagocytic cells, B lymphocytes, T lymphocytes, or the complement system. The specific symptoms and their severity, age at onset, and prognosis depend on the immune system components affected and their degree of functional impairment. Regardless of the underlying cause, the cardinal symptoms of immunodeficiency include chronic or recurrent and severe infections, infections caused by unusual organisms or by organisms that are normal body flora, poor response to standard treatment for infections, and chronic diarrhea. In addition, the patient is susceptible to a variety of secondary disorders, including autoimmune disease and lymphoreticular malignancies (Cooper & Schroeder, 2008).

Immunodeficiencies may be acquired spontaneously or as a consequence of medical treatment. These disorders can be classified as either primary or secondary and by the affected components of the immune system. Primary immunodeficiency diseases are genetic in origin and result from intrinsic defects in the cells of the immune system. In contrast, secondary immunodeficiencies result from external factors such as infection. Effective nursing care reflects knowledge of the immune system, potential secondary disorders, relevant assessment parameters, and strategies for symptom management, as well as sensitivity and responsiveness to the learning needs of the patient and caregiver.

PRIMARY IMMUNODEFICIENCIES

Primary immunodeficiencies represent inborn errors of immune function that predispose people to frequent, severe infections; autoimmunity; and cancer. Advances in medical treatment have meant that patients with primary immunodeficiencies live longer, thus increasing their overall risk of developing cancer (Salavoura, Koloalexi, Tsangaris, et al., 2008). The type of malignancy depends on the immunodeficiency, the age of the patient, and possible viral infection, which suggests that different pathogenic mechanisms are implicated in each case. Non-Hodgkin lymphomas account for the majority of cancers. The primary immunodeficiencies known to be associated with increased incidence of malignancy are common variable immunodeficiency, immunoglobulin A (IgA) deficiency, and deoxyribonucleic acid (DNA) repair disorders. More recently, investigators have shown that **severe combined immunodeficiency disease (SCID)** and **Wiskott-Aldrich syndrome** (thrombocytopenia and the absence of T and B cells) may also lead to cancer (Salavoura, et al., 2008). People with various primary immunodeficiencies, who are predisposed to cancer, exhibit immune deficits that also increase their susceptibility to fungal infections. A number of yeasts, molds, and fungi may cause infections in patients with chronic granulomatous disease, SCID, chronic mucocutaneous candidiasis, and common variable immunodeficiency (CVID); these infections may occasionally be the presenting clinical manifestation of a primary immunodeficiency. If the immune condition is misdiagnosed or mistreated, it can lead to significant morbidity and mortality (Antachopoulos, Walsh & Rollides, 2007).

The majority of primary immunodeficiencies are diagnosed in infancy, with a male-to-female ratio of 5 to 1.

However, a large fraction of primary immunodeficiencies are not diagnosed until adolescence or early adulthood, when the gender distribution equalizes. Diagnosis at this stage frequently is confounded by frequent use of antibiotics that mask symptoms. On occasion, adults present with clinical episodes of infectious diseases that are beyond the scope of normal immunocompetence. Examples include infections that are unusually persistent, recurrent, or resistant to treatment and those involving unexpected dissemination of disease or atypical pathogens. To date, more than 120 immunodeficiencies of genetic origin have been identified (Verbsky & Grossman, 2006).

Common primary immunodeficiencies include disorders of humoral immunity (affecting B-cell differentiation or antibody production), T-cell defects, combined B- and T-cell defects, phagocytic disorders, and complement deficiencies. These disorders may involve one or more components of the immune system. Symptoms of immune deficiency disorders are related to the deficient component (Table 51-1). Major signs and symptoms include multiple infections despite aggressive treatment, infections with unusual or opportunistic organisms, failure to thrive or poor growth, and a positive family history (Cooper & Schroeder, 2008).

Phagocytic Dysfunction

Pathophysiology

A variety of primary defects of phagocytes may occur; almost all of them are genetic in origin and affect the natural (innate) immune system. In some types of phagocytic disorders, the neutrophils are impaired so that they cannot exit the circulation and travel to sites of infection. As a result, the person cannot initiate a normal inflammatory response against pathogenic organisms. In some disorders, the neutrophil count may be very low; in others, it may be very high because the neutrophils remain in the vascular system. Phagocytic cell disorders are characterized by disease-specific infections, such as chronic granulomatous disease (Abbas, Lichtman & Baker, 2008).

Clinical Manifestations

In phagocytic cell disorders there is an increased incidence of bacterial and fungal infections caused by organisms that are normally nonpathogenic. People with these disorders may also develop fungal infections from *Candida* organisms and viral infections from herpes simplex or herpes zoster. These patients experience recurrent cutaneous abscesses, chronic eczema, bronchitis, pneumonia, chronic otitis media, and sinusitis. In one rare type of phagocytic disorder, hyperimmunoglobulinemia E syndrome (formerly known as Job syndrome), white blood cells cannot initiate an inflammatory response to infectious organisms. This results in recurrent bacterial infections of the skin and lung; abnormalities of connective tissue, skeleton, and dentition; and extremely elevated levels of IgE (Freeman & Holland, 2008).

Although patients with phagocytic cell disorders may be asymptomatic, severe neutropenia may present and may be accompanied by deep and painful mouth ulcers, gingivitis, stomatitis, and cellulitis. Death from overwhelming infection

Table 51-1 SELECTED PRIMARY IMMUNODEFICIENCY DISORDERS

Immune Component	Disorder	Major Symptoms	Treatment
Phagocytic cells	Hyperimmunoglobulinemia E (HIE) syndrome	Bacterial, fungal, and viral infections; deep-seated cold abscesses	Antibiotic therapy and treatment for viral and fungal infections Granulocyte-macrophage colony-stimulating factor (GM-CSF); granulocyte colony-stimulating factor (G-CSF)
B lymphocytes	Sex-linked agammaglobulinemia (Bruton's disease)	Severe pyogenic infections soon after birth	Passive pooled plasma or gamma-globulin
	Common variable immunodeficiency (CVID)	Bacterial infections, infection with *Giardia lamblia*	Intravenous immunoglobulin (IVIG) Metronidazole (Flagyl) Quinacrine HCl (Atabrine)
		Pernicious anemia	Vitamin B$_{12}$
		Chronic respiratory infections	Antimicrobial therapy
	Immunoglobulin A (IgA) deficiency	Predisposition to recurrent infections, adverse reactions to blood transfusions or immunoglobulin, autoimmune diseases, hypothyroidism	None
	IgC$_2$ deficiency	Heightened incidence of infectious diseases	Pooled immunoglobulin
T lymphocytes	Thymic hypoplasia (DiGeorge syndrome)	Recurrent infections; hypoparathyroidism, hypocalcemia, tetany, convulsions, congenital heart disease, possible renal abnormalities; abnormal facies	Thymus graft

	Chronic mucocutaneous candidiasis	*Candida albicans* infections of mucous membrane, skin, and nails; endocrine abnormalities (hypoparathyroidism, Addison's disease)	Antifungal agents:
			  Topical: miconazole
			  Oral: clotrimazole, ketoconazole
			  IV: amphotericin B

B and T lymphocytes	Ataxia-telangiectasia	Ataxia with progressive neurologic deterioration, telangiectasia (vascular lesions), recurrent infections; malignancies	Antimicrobial therapy; management of presenting symptoms; fetal thymus transplant, IVIG
	Nezelof's syndrome	Severe infections, malignancies	Antimicrobial therapy; IVIG, bone marrow transplantation; thymus transplantation; thymus factors
	Wiskott-Aldrich syndrome	Thrombocytopenia, resulting in bleeding, infections; malignancies	Antimicrobial therapy; splenectomy with continuous antibiotic prophylaxis; IVIG and bone marrow transplantation
	Severe combined immunodeficiency disease (SCID)	Overwhelming severe fatal infections soon after birth (also includes opportunistic infections)	Antimicrobial therapy; IVIG and bone marrow transplantation
Complement system	Angioneurotic edema	Episodes of edema in various parts of the body, including respiratory tract and bowels	Pooled plasma, androgen therapy
	Paroxysmal nocturnal hemoglobinuria (PNH)	Lysis of erythrocytes due to lack of decay-accelerating factor (DAF) on erythrocytes	None

occurs in about 10% of patients with severe neutropenia. Chronic granulomatous disease, another type of primary phagocytic disorder, produces recurrent or persistent infections of the soft tissues, lungs, and other organs; these are resistant to aggressive treatment with antibiotics (Tierney, McPhee & Papadakis, 2008).

Assessment and Diagnostic Findings

Diagnosis is based on the history, signs and symptoms (see Chart 50-3), and laboratory analysis by the nitroblue tetrazolium reductase test, which indicates the cytocidal (causing death of cells) activity of the phagocytic cells. A history of recurrent infection and fever, including the treatment given, in a child, and occasionally in an adult, is an impor-

tant key to diagnosis; timely intervention can prevent morbidity and mortality (DeSilva, Gunawardena, Wickremesinghe, et al., 2007). Failure of an infection to resolve with the usual treatment is an important indicator. Warning signs of primary immunodeficiency disorders are summarized in Figure 51-1.

Medical Management

Patients with neutropenia continue to be at increased risk for development of severe infections despite substantial advances in supportive care. Epidemiologic shifts occur periodically and need to be detected early because they influence prophylactic, empiric, and specific strategies for medical management. Attention to infection control practices is

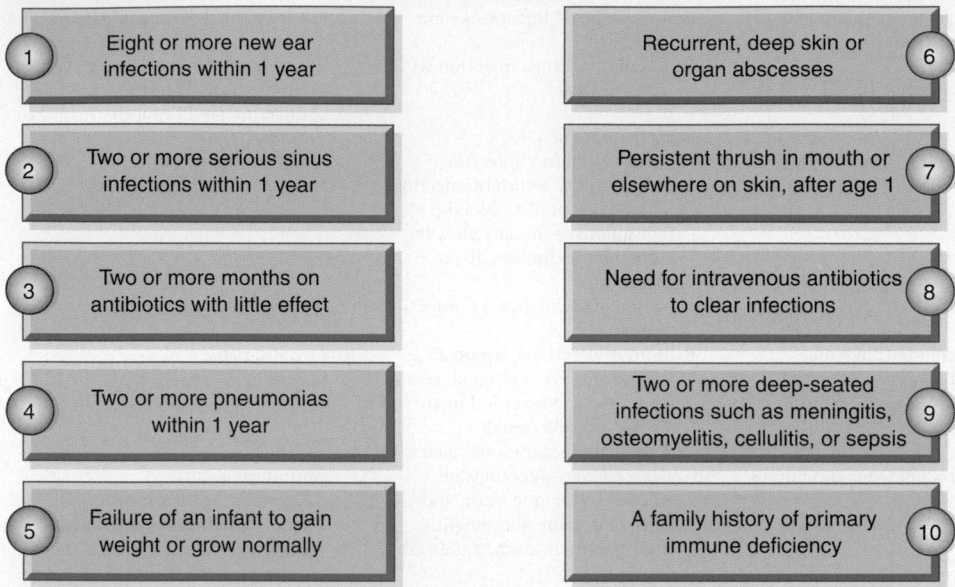

Primary immune deficiency causes children and adults to have infections that come back frequently or are unusually hard to cure. In America alone, up to half a million people suffer from one or more of the 70 known primary immune deficiency diseases.

If you or your child is affected by more than one of the following conditions, speak to your doctor about the possible presence of primary immune deficiency.

1. Eight or more new ear infections within 1 year
2. Two or more serious sinus infections within 1 year
3. Two or more months on antibiotics with little effect
4. Two or more pneumonias within 1 year
5. Failure of an infant to gain weight or grow normally
6. Recurrent, deep skin or organ abscesses
7. Persistent thrush in mouth or elsewhere on skin, after age 1
8. Need for intravenous antibiotics to clear infections
9. Two or more deep-seated infections such as meningitis, osteomyelitis, cellulitis, or sepsis
10. A family history of primary immune deficiency

Though the primary immune deficiency diseases can be serious, they are rarely fatal and can generally be controlled. Primary immune deficiency should not be confused with AIDS. Primary immune deficiency can be diagnosed through blood tests and should be detected as soon as possible to prevent avoidable permanent damage. As with all disease, only direct examination by a physician should be used to determine the presence of primary immune deficiency.

Figure 51-1 The 10 warning signs of primary immune deficiency. Education materials developed by the Jeffrey Modell Foundation Medical Advisory Board, New York. Used with permission.

important, especially with the emergence of multidrug-resistant organisms. Although it is effective in preventing some bacterial and some fungal infections, prophylactic drug treatment must be used with caution, because it has been implicated in the emergence of resistant organisms. The choices for empiric therapy include combination regimens and monotherapy. Specific choices depend on local factors (epidemiology, susceptibility/resistance patterns, availability, cost). Home and inpatient settings are also available and the selection of setting depends on the patient's risk category. Early diagnosis and appropriate treatment of many fungal and viral infections remains suboptimal in many cases (Saria & Gosselin-Acomb, 2007).

While granulocyte transfusions are used as a medical treatment, they are seldom successful because of the short half-life of these cells. Treatment with granulocyte-macrophage colony-stimulating factor (GM-CSF) or granulocyte colony-stimulating factor (G-CSF) may prove successful, because these proteins draw nonlymphoid stem cells from the bone marrow and hasten their maturation. Cell therapy, which refers to the provision of living cells to patients for the prevention of human disease, may be effective. (The infusion of blood and blood products is the best established and most widely practiced form of cell therapy.)

Hematopoietic stem cell transplantation (HSCT), another form of cell therapy, has proven to be a successful curative modality. The stem cells may be from embryos or adults. However, toxicity and reduced efficacy are frequent limitations of HSCT (Antachopoulos, et al., 2007; DeSilva, et al., 2007). Another emerging therapy involves the use of cells as vehicles for the delivery of genes or gene products. However, gene therapy has many side effects and needs further improvement (Santilli, Thompson, Kinnon, et al., 2008).

B-Cell Deficiencies

Pathophysiology

Two types of inherited B-cell deficiencies exist. The first type results from lack of differentiation of B-cell precursors into mature B cells. As a result, plasma cells are absent, and the germinal centers from all lymphatic tissues disappear, leading to a complete absence of antibody production against invading bacteria, viruses, and other pathogens. This syndrome is called X-linked **agammaglobulinemia** (Bruton's disease), because all antibodies disappear from the patient's plasma. B cells in the peripheral blood and IgG,

IgM, IgA, IgD, and IgE are low or absent. Infants born with this disorder suffer from severe infections starting soon after birth. Males are at a high risk for having X-linked agammaglobulinemia if they have an affected male relative. More than 10% of patients with X-linked agammaglobulinemia are hospitalized for infection when they are younger than 6 months of age; prognosis depends on prompt recognition and treatment (Levinson, 2008).

Autosomal agammaglobulinemia refers to a rare instance in which normal hypogammaglobulinemia of infancy is prolonged. It can result from mutations in a variety of genes whose products are required for differentiation of B cells. However, IgG levels do rise eventually. Periodic immunologic assessment is needed to differentiate transient hypogammaglobulinemia from other forms of antibody deficiency.

The second type of B-cell deficiency results from a lack of differentiation of B cells into plasma cells. Only diminished antibody production occurs with this disorder. Although plasma cells are the most vigorous producers of antibodies, affected patients have normal lymph follicles and many B lymphocytes that produce some antibodies. This syndrome, called **hypogammaglobulinemia,** is a frequently occurring immunodeficiency. It is also called CVID; this disorder encompasses a variety of defects ranging from IgA deficiency, in which only the plasma cells that produce IgA are absent, to the other extreme, in which there is severe **panhypoglobulinemia** (general lack of immunoglobulins in the blood) (Stewart, Tian, Notorangelo, et al., 2008).

CVID is the most common primary immunodeficiency seen in adults; it can occur in people of either gender. Although it usually presents within the first two decades of life, most patients are diagnosed as adults, because CVID often goes unrecognized. Several T- and B-cell defects have been described, but the underlying cause is still unknown; the etiology is believed to be multifactorial. Patients usually have normal B-cell lymphocyte counts, but the cells are clinically diverse and immature. Although they can recognize antigens and mount a response, their ability to become memory B cells and mature plasma cells is impaired.

Clinical Manifestations

Infants with X-linked agammaglobulinemia usually become symptomatic after the natural loss of maternally transmitted immunoglobulins, which occurs at about 5 to 6 months of age. Symptoms of recurrent pyogenic infections usually occur by that time.

Besides recurrent infection, patients with CVID are at increased risk for autoimmune disease, granulomatous disease, and malignancy, indicating that CVID is a disease of abnormal immune regulation as well as of immunodeficiency. Approximately 20% to 22% of patients develop autoimmune diseases, notably autoimmune thrombocytopenic purpura and autoimmune hemolytic anemia (Seve, Bourdillon, Sarrot-Reynauld, et al., 2008). Other autoimmune diseases, such as arthritis and hypothyroidism, frequently occur. Associated fever, weight loss, anemia, thrombocytopenia, splenomegaly, lymphadenopathy, and lymphocytosis may suggest underlying lymphoid malignancy.

More than 50% of patients with CVID develop pernicious anemia. Lymphoid hyperplasia of the small intestine and spleen as well as gastric atrophy, which is detected by biopsy of the stomach, are common findings. Gastrointestinal malabsorption may occur. Young adults who develop the disease also have an increased incidence of chronic lung disease, hepatitis, gastric cancer, and malabsorption that results in chronic diarrhea. CVID must be distinguished from secondary immunodeficiency diseases caused by protein-losing enteropathy, nephrotic syndrome, or burns.

Patients with CVID are susceptible to infections with encapsulated bacteria, such as *Haemophilus influenzae*, *Streptococcus pneumoniae*, and *Staphylococcus aureus*. Frequent respiratory tract infections typically lead to chronic progressive bronchiectasis and pulmonary failure. Commonly, infection with *Giardia lamblia* occurs. Opportunistic infections with *Pneumocystis jiroveci* pneumonia (PCP), however, are seen only in patients who have a concomitant deficiency in T-cell immunity.

Assessment and Diagnostic Findings

X-linked agammaglobulinemia may be diagnosed by the marked deficiency or complete absence of all serum immunoglobulins. The diagnosis of CVID is based on the history of repeated bacterial infections, quantification of B-cell activity, and reported signs and symptoms. The number of B lymphocytes as well as the total and specific immunoglobulin levels are measured. Measuring only the total serum globulin level is inadequate, because a compensatory overproduction of one globulin may mask the loss of another globulin or the deficiency of a globulin that is present in very low amounts. Antibody titers to confirm successful childhood vaccination are determined by specific serologic tests. Previous successful childhood immunization indicates that B cells were functioning adequately earlier in life. If the patient exhibits signs and symptoms suggestive of pernicious anemia, hemoglobin and hematocrit levels are also obtained. Biopsies of the small intestine, spleen, and stomach may also be obtained to assess for lymphoid hyperplasia.

Medical Management

Patients with primary phagocytic disorders may be treated with intravenous immunoglobulin (IVIG) (Chart 51-1). Its administration is an essential part of the prevention and treatment of complications of CVID (Kishiyama, 2005). Antibody replacement therapy is recommended for severe, recurrent infections. Other interventions aimed at overcoming the immunologic defects in CVID, such as interleukin-2 therapy, are being studied (Garcia, Espanol, Gurbindo, et al., 2007).

T-Cell Deficiencies

Pathophysiology

Defects in T cells lead to opportunistic infections. Most primary T-cell immunodeficiencies are genetic in origin. Partial T-cell immunodeficiencies constitute a heterogeneous cluster of disorders characterized by an incomplete reduction in T-cell number or activity. Unlike severe T-cell immunodeficiencies, however, partial immunodeficiencies are commonly associated with hyperimmune dysregulation,

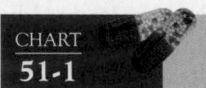

CHART
51-1

PHARMACOLOGY
Managing an Intravenous Immunoglobulin (IVIG) Infusion

IVIG has become an important treatment for a variety of disease states that are characterized by deficient production of antibodies. It may have other indications but is commonly used for the treatment of DiGeorge syndrome, common variable immunodeficiency disease (CVID), severe combined immunodeficiency disease (SCID), Wiskott-Aldrich syndrome, and idiopathic thrombocytopenic purpura. Previously available only for intramuscular injection, immunoglobulin can now be administered for replacement therapy as an IV infusion in greater, more effective doses without painful side effects, and it can safely be given in outpatient as well as inpatient settings. Variables affecting the risk and intensity of adverse events associated with the administration of IVIG include patient age, underlying condition, history of migraine, and cardiovascular and/or renal disease; dose, concentration, and rate of infusion; and specific data related to the precise lot of the product. The nurse must assess all of these variables before starting the IVIG infusion and during the infusion process. He or she must anticipate adverse effects if any of these variables are present (Shelton, et al., 2006).

How Supplied

Immunoglobulin is supplied in a 5% solution or a lyophilized powder with a reconstituting diluent prepared from Cohn fraction II obtained from pools of 1000 to 10,000 donors. Currently, a number of different IV preparations are approved for use and have been shown to be effective and safe by the U.S. Food and Drug Administration.

Dosage

The optimal dose is determined by the patient's response. In most instances, an IV dose of 100 to 400 mg/kg of body weight is administered monthly or more frequently to ensure adequate serum levels of immunoglobulin G.

Adverse Effects

*   Complaints of flank and back pain, shaking chills, dyspnea, and tightness in the chest; headache, fever, and local reaction at the infusion site
*   Serious conditions, including aseptic meningitis, renal failure, thromboembolic events, and anaphylaxis. Anaphylactic reactions typically occur 30 to 60 minutes after the start of the infusion. The potential increases as the dose of IVIG increases.
*   Hypotension (possible with severe reactions)

Guidelines for Nursing Management

*   Pretreatment assessments should be performed before each infusion.
*   Obtain height and weight before treatment to verify accurate dosing.
*   Assess baseline vital signs before, during, and after treatment. An elevated temperature at the beginning of treatment may be an indication to delay the infusion to avoid misinterpretation as a reaction to the infusion.
*   Premedicate with acetaminophen and diphenhydramine as prescribed 30 minutes before the start of the infusion.
*   Understand that long-term tolerance of an older IVIG product does not necessarily imply tolerance to a newer product, even if it is technically superior. Caution should be exercised when changing IVIG products because they are not biologically equivalent.
*   Be aware that corticosteroids may be used to prevent possible severe reactions in patients who are perceived to be at risk.
*   Administer the IV infusion at a slow rate, not to exceed 3 mL/min.
*   Continually assess the patient for adverse reactions; be especially aware of complaints of a tickle or lump in the throat as the precursor to laryngospasm that precedes bronchoconstriction.
*   Stop the infusions at the first sign of reaction and initiate the institutional protocol to be followed in this emergent situation.
*   Be aware that patients with low gammaglobulin levels have more severe reactions than those with normal levels (eg, patients who receive gammaglobulin for thrombocytopenia or Kawasaki disease).
*   Keep in mind that patients who have an immunoglobulin A (IgA) deficiency have IgE antibodies to IgA, which requires administration of plasma or immunoglobulin replacement from IgA-deficient patients. Because all IV immunoglobulin preparations contain some IgA, they may cause an anaphylactic reaction in patients with IgE anti-IgA antibodies.
*   Recognize that the pharmacokinetics of IgG differ when smaller doses are given more frequently, as is commonly done with subcutaneous regimens. Differences include lower peaks and higher troughs, which may be preferable for some patients.
*   Remember that the risk of transmission of hepatitis, HIV, or other known viruses is extremely low.

including autoimmune disorders, inflammatory diseases, and elevated IgG production (Liston, Enders & Siggs, 2008). Although an increased susceptibility to infection is common, symptoms can vary considerably, depending on the type of T-cell defect. Because the T cells play a regulatory role in immune system function, the loss of T-cell function is usually accompanied by some loss of B-cell activity.

DiGeorge syndrome, or **thymic hypoplasia,** is an example of a primary T-cell immunodeficiency. This rare, complex, multisystem genetic abnormality, which affects multiple organ systems, has been mapped to chromosomes 10 or 22. The symptom variation is a result of differences in the amount of genetic material affected. T-cell deficiency occurs when the thymus gland fails to develop normally during embryogenesis. The syndrome often manifests in the neonatal period as a cardiac anomaly, although hypocalcemic tetany and facial abnormalities may also occur. It is one of the few immunodeficiency disorders with symptoms that manifest almost immediately after birth (McLean-Tooke, Barge, Spickett, et al., 2008; Sullivan, 2008).

Chronic mucocutaneous candidiasis is a rare T-cell disorder, which is thought to be an autosomal recessive disorder that affects both males and females. It is considered an autoimmune disorder involving the thymus and other endocrine glands. The disease causes extensive morbidity resulting from endocrine dysfunction.

Clinical Manifestations

Infants born with DiGeorge syndrome have hypoparathyroidism with resultant hypocalcemia resistant to standard therapy, congenital heart disease, cleft palate and lip, dysmorphic facial features, and possibly renal abnormalities. These infants are susceptible to yeast, fungal, protozoan, and viral infections and are particularly susceptible to childhood diseases (chickenpox, measles, rubella), which are usually severe and may be fatal. Infection with *Candida albicans* is almost universal in patients with severe deficiencies in T cell–mediated immunity. Many affected infants are also born with congenital heart defects, which can result in heart failure. The most frequent presenting sign in patients with DiGeorge syndrome is hypocalcemia that is resistant to standard therapy. It usually occurs within the first 24 hours of life (McLean-Tooke, et al., 2008; Sullivan, 2008).

The initial presentation of chronic mucocutaneous candidiasis may be a result of either chronic candidal infection or idiopathic endocrinopathy. The disease is characterized by persistent or recurrent candidal infections of the skin, nails, and mucous membranes or by a variable combination of endocrine failure as well as immunodeficiency (Liu & Hua, 2007). Patients may survive to the second or third decade of life. Problems may include hypocalcemia and tetany secondary to hypofunction of the parathyroid glands (see Chapter 14). Hypofunction of the adrenal cortex (Addison's disease) is the major cause of death in these patients; it may develop suddenly and without any history of previous symptoms.

Assessment and Diagnostic Findings

Prompt diagnosis is necessary for appropriate management. A comprehensive immunologic laboratory analysis is necessary. Findings in children with DiGeorge syndrome include cardiac, nutritional, and developmental abnormalities (Sullivan, 2008).

Medical Management

Patients with T-cell deficiency should receive prophylaxis for PCP. General care includes management of hypocalcemia and correction of cardiac abnormalities. Hypocalcemia is controlled by oral calcium supplementation in conjunction with administration of vitamin D or parathyroid hormone. Congenital heart disease frequently results in heart failure, and these patients may require immediate surgical intervention in a tertiary care center. Transplantation of fetal thymus, postnatal thymus, or human leukocyte antigen (HLA)-matched bone marrow has been used for permanent reconstitution of T-cell immunity (Mazzolari, Forino, Guerci, et al, 2007). In children with DiGeorge syndrome, attention must be given to cardiac, nutritional, and developmental needs (Sullivan, 2008). IVIG may be used if an antibody deficiency exists. This therapy may also be used to control recurrent infections. T-cell function improves with age and often is normal by 5 years of age. Prolonged survival has been reported after spontaneous remission of immunodeficiency, which occurs in some patients (Markert, 2008).

Combined B-Cell and T-Cell Deficiencies

Pathophysiology

T-cell and B-cell immune deficiencies comprise a heterogeneous group of disorders, all characterized by profound impairment in the development or function of the cellular, the humoral, or both parts of the immune system. A variety of inherited (autosomal recessive and X-linked) conditions fit this description. These conditions are typified by disruption of the normal communication system of B cells and T cells and impairment of the immune response, and they appear early in life (Cooper & Schroeder, 2008).

Ataxia-telangiectasia is an autosomal recessive neurodegenerative disorder characterized by cerebellar **ataxia** (loss of muscle coordination), **telangiectasia** (vascular lesions caused by dilated blood vessels), and immune deficiency. The immunologic defects reflect abnormalities of the thymus. The disorder is characterized by some degree of T-cell deficiency, which becomes more severe with advancing age. In 40% of patients, a selective IgA deficiency exists. In addition, IgG and IgE deficiencies have been identified. Immunodeficiency is manifested by recurrent and chronic sinus and pulmonary infections, leading to bronchiectasis. Frequent causes of death are chronic pulmonary disease and malignancy. While lymphomas are most common, other carcinomas occur. The disease is also associated with neurologic, vascular, endocrine, hepatic, and cutaneous abnormalities (Levinson, 2008).

Severe combined immunodeficiency disease is a disorder in which both B cells and T cells are missing. Consequently, both cell-mediated and humoral functions are affected. In addition, SCID is marked by susceptibility to serious fungal, bacterial, and viral infections. It refers to a wide variety of congenital and hereditary immunologic defects characterized by early onset of infections, defects in both B-cell and T-cell systems, lymphoid aplasia, and thymic dysplasia. It is one of the most common causes of primary immunodeficiencies. Inheritance of this disorder can be X linked, autosomal recessive, or sporadic. The exact incidence of SCID is unknown; it is recognized as a rare disease in most population groups, with an incidence of about 1 case in 1,000,000. This illness occurs in all racial groups and both genders.

Wiskott-Aldrich syndrome (WAS), a variation of SCID, is an inherited immunodeficiency caused by a variety of mutations in the gene encoding the WAS protein. It is characterized by frequent infections, thrombocytopenia with small platelets, eczema, and increased risk of autoimmune disorders and malignancies. Vasculitides and autoimmune hemolytic anemia are the two most common autoimmune manifestations and often cause considerable morbidity and mortality. The prognosis is poor, because most affected people develop overwhelming fatal infections.

Clinical Manifestations

The onset of ataxia and telangiectasia occurs in the first 4 years of life. Many patients, however, remain symptom-free for 10 years or longer. As the patient approaches the second decade of life, chronic lung disease, cognitive impairment, neurologic symptoms, and physical disability become severe. Long-term survivors develop progressive deterioration of immunologic and neurologic functions. Some affected patients have lived until the fifth decade of life. The primary causes of death in these patients are overwhelming infection and lymphoreticular or epithelial cancer.

The onset of symptoms occurs within the first 3 months of life in most patients with SCID. Symptoms include respiratory infections and pneumonia (often secondary to PCP infection), thrush, diarrhea, and failure to thrive. Many of these infections are resistant to treatment. Shedding of viruses such as respiratory syncytial virus or cytomegalovirus from the respiratory and gastrointestinal tracts is persistent. Maculopapular and erythematous skin rashes may occur. Vomiting, fever, and a persistent rash are also common manifestations (Geha & Rosen, 2007).

Medical Management

Treatment of ataxia-telangiectasia includes early management of infections with antimicrobial therapy, management of chronic lung disease with postural drainage and physical therapy, and management of other presenting symptoms. Other treatments include transplantation of fetal thymus tissue and IVIG administration (see Chart 51-1).

Treatment options for SCID include stem cell and bone marrow transplantation. HSCT is the definitive therapy for SCID; the best outcome is achieved if the disease is recognized and treated early in life. Improvements continue in the use of HSCT to treat patients with SCID, as well as other primary immunodeficiencies. The ideal donor is an HLA-identical sibling. Evidence demonstrates that transplantation of allogeneic hematopoietic stem cells can cause an enhanced improvement over time. Other treatment

options include administration of IVIG or thymus-derived factors and thymus gland transplantation. Gene therapy has been used, but the results have been disappointing (Dvorak & Cowan, 2008). For the most common forms of combined immune deficiency, gene therapy can lead to immune reconstitution in most patients, but a minority derive minimal clinical benefit and some have suffered severe adverse effects, including death (Santilli, et al., 2008; Sokolic, Kesserwan & Candotti, 2008). As treatment improves, an increasing number of patients who previously would have died in infancy are living to adulthood. Newborn screening is proposed as a means to make a prompt diagnosis and initiate treatment in all affected infants (Puck, 2007).

Nursing Management

Many patients require immunosuppression to ensure engraftment of depleted bone marrow during transplantation procedures. For this reason, nursing care must be meticulous. Appropriate infection control precautions and thorough hand hygiene are essential (Chart 51-2). Institutional policies and procedures related to protective care must be followed scrupulously until definitive evidence demonstrates that precautions are unnecessary. Continual monitoring of the patient's condition is critical, so early signs of impending infection may be detected and treated before they seriously compromise the patient's status. It also is imperative that attention be given to appropriate application of standard precautions (previously known as universal precautions), which have become one of the first-line tools for decreasing transmission of disease, whether from nurse to patient, patient to patient, or patient to nurse. Standard precautions are based on the principle that all blood and body fluids, secretions, and excretions may contain transmissible infectious agents. Some of the key elements of

---

CHART 51-2	**NURSING RESEARCH PROFILE**

Implementation of New Hygiene Practices and the Resultant Impact on Infection Rates

Larson, E., Quiros, D. & Lin, S. (2007). Dissemination of the CDC's hand hygiene guideline and impact on infection rates. *American Journal of Infection Control, 35*(10), 666–675.

Purpose

Most hospitalized patients are at high risk for infection. This study was undertaken to measure the impact of national evidence-based guidelines on practice. The objectives were to (1) evaluate implementation and compliance with clinical practices recommended in the hand hygiene guidelines of the Centers for Disease Control and Prevention (CDC), (2) compare rates of health care–associated infections (HAIs) before and after implementation of the guidelines, and (3) examine the patterns and correlates of changes in the rates of HAIs.

Design

The investigators used pre- and postguideline implementation site visits and surveys in 40 U.S. hospitals that were members of the national nosocomial infections surveillance system. They measured HAI rates 1 year before and after publication of the CDC guidelines. In addition, they used hand hygiene compliance and guideline implementation scores as outcome measures.

Findings

The 40 hospitals had changed their policies and procedures and provided products in compliance with the recommended guidelines. Of 1359 staff members surveyed anonymously, 89.8% reported that they were familiar with the guidelines. However, in 44.2% of the hospitals, there was no evidence of a multidisciplinary program to improve compliance. Hand hygiene rates remained low (56.6%), similar to the rates reported for the past few decades. Rates of central line–associated bloodstream infections were significantly lower in hospitals with higher rates of hand hygiene compliance ($p < .001$). No impact of guideline implementation or hand hygiene compliance on other HAI rates was identified.

Nursing Implications

This study confirms the observation that institutional adoption of a guideline does not guarantee practice changes. The incidence of health care–associated infections has grown significantly and has resulted in increased patient morbidity and mortality. This increase has contributed to escalating costs of hospital care. It is the professional responsibility of every practitioner to deliver care consistent with standards of safety and quality.

standard precautions include performing hand hygiene, as previously mentioned; using appropriate personal protective equipment, depending on the expected type of exposure; and using safe injection practices (Tarrac, 2008).

Deficiencies of the Complement System

The complement system is an integral part of the immune system, and deficiencies in normal levels of C2 and C3 complement result in increased susceptibility to infectious diseases and immune-mediated disorders. Improved techniques to identify the individual components of the complement system have led to a steady increase in the number of deficiencies identified.

Hereditary **angioneurotic edema** results from the deficiency of C1-esterase inhibitor, which opposes the release of inflammatory mediators. The clinical picture of this autosomal dominant disorder includes recurrent attacks of edema formation in the subcutaneous tissue, gastrointestinal tract, and upper airway (Farkas, Varga, Szeplaki, et al., 2007). Although the disease is mild in childhood and becomes more severe after puberty, first episodes have been reported later in life. Food allergy has often been linked to this disorder, although recent evidence has implicated a C1-esterase inhibitor deficiency. The fluctuations in hormone levels at the beginning of adolescence, in the perimenopausal period, during pregnancy, and during the use of oral contraceptives can precipitate edematous attacks that usually disappear after the onset of menopause. Fresh-frozen plasma has been used as a treatment option, with variable results (Prematta, Gibbs, Pratt, et al., 2007).

Paroxysmal nocturnal hemoglobinuria is an acquired clonal stem cell disorder resulting from a somatic mutation in the hematopoietic stem cell. An absent glycosylphosphatidylinositol (GPI)-anchored receptor prevents several proteins from binding to the erythrocyte membrane. These include the complement-regulatory proteins, CD55 and CD59, the absence of which results in enhanced complement-mediated lysis. Clinical manifestations may be indolent or life-threatening. The disorder is characterized by hemoglobinuria that increases during sleep, as well as intravascular hemolysis, cytopenia, infections, bone marrow hyperplasia, and a high incidence of life-threatening venous thrombosis, which occurs most commonly in the abdominal and cerebral veins. Severe fatigue, abdominal pain, and esophageal spasm may also be present. Leukopenia, thrombocytopenia, and episodic crises are common. Severe infection can occur as a result of aplastic bone marrow and splenic thrombosis. Laboratory diagnosis can include specialized tests, such as the sucrose hemolysis test, Ham acid hemolysis test, and fluorescent-activated cell analysis. A coagulation profile is also indicated.

SECONDARY IMMUNODEFICIENCIES

Secondary immunodeficiencies are more common than primary immunodeficiencies and frequently occur as a result of underlying disease processes or the treatment of these disorders. The immune system can be affected by a variety of intrinsic factors, including immunosuppressive agents, harsh environmental conditions, hereditary disorders other than primary immunodeficiencies, and acquired metabolic disorders that cause secondary immunodeficiencies. Common causes of secondary immunodeficiencies include chronic stress, burns, uremia, diabetes mellitus, certain autoimmune disorders, certain viruses, exposure to immunotoxic medications and chemicals, and self-administration of recreational drugs and alcohol. Perhaps the best-known secondary immunodeficiency results from human immunodeficiency virus (HIV) infection, which causes acquired immunodeficiency syndrome (AIDS); however, the most prevalent cause of immunodeficiency worldwide is severe malnutrition. AIDS, the most common secondary disorder, is discussed in detail in Chapter 52.

In secondary immunodeficiencies, abnormalities of the immune system affect both natural and acquired immunity, may be subtle, and are usually heterogeneous in their clinical manifestations. Patients with secondary immunodeficiencies are known as **immunocompromised hosts.**

Medical Management

Medical management of secondary immunodeficiencies includes diagnosis and treatment of the underlying disease process. Treatment of the primary condition often results in the improvement of the affected immune components (Chinen & Shearer, 2008). Factors that contribute to immunosuppression are identified and infection is treated. Additional treatment includes HSCT, monoclonal antibody therapy, and anticoagulation therapy as indicated. HSCT may be curative (Brodsky, 2008; Woolhead, Deepak, Patel, et al., 2008).

NURSING MANAGEMENT FOR PATIENTS WITH IMMUNODEFICIENCIES

Nursing management includes assessment, patient teaching, selected interventions, and supportive care. Assessment of the patient for infection and timely initiation of treatment are essential. Nursing care of patients with primary and secondary immunodeficiencies depends on the underlying cause of the immunodeficiency, the type of immunodeficiency, and its severity. Because immunodeficiencies result in a compromised immune system and pose a high risk for infection, careful assessment of the patient's immune status is essential. The assessment focuses on the history of past infections, particularly the type and frequency of infection; methods of and response to past treatments; signs and symptoms of any current skin, respiratory, oral, gastrointestinal, or genitourinary infection; and measures taken by the patient to prevent infection. The nurse assesses and monitors the patient for signs and symptoms of infection (Chart 51-3).

Many patients develop oral manifestations and need education about promoting good dental hygiene to diminish the oral discomfort and complications that frequently result in inadequate nutritional intake. Involving patients in their daily oral assessment and care helps them become proactive in preventing complications. To implement individualized care strategies, it is essential to provide patients with the skills to promote health and limit the incidence of disease.

Because the inflammatory response may be blunted, the patient is observed for subtle and unusual signs and changes in physical status. Vital signs and the development of pain,

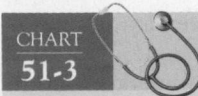

CHART 51-3

Assessing for Infection

Be alert for the following signs and symptoms:
- Fever with or without chills
- Cough with or without sputum
- Shortness of breath
- Difficulty breathing
- Difficulty swallowing
- White patches in the oral cavity
- Swollen lymph nodes
- Nausea with or without vomiting
- Persistent diarrhea
- Frequency, urgency, or pain on urination
- Change in the character of the urine
- Lesions on the face, lips, or perianal area
- Redness, swelling, or drainage from skin lesions
- Persistent vaginal discharge with or without perianal itching
- Persistent abdominal pain

neurologic signs, cough, and skin and oral lesions are monitored and reported immediately. Pulse rate and respiratory rate should be counted for a full minute, because subtle changes can signal deterioration in the patient's clinical status. Auscultation of the breath sounds is important to detect changes in respiratory status that signal an existing or impending infection. Any unusual response to treatment or a significant change in the patient's clinical condition must be promptly reported to the physician (Jarvis, 2008).

The nurse continuously monitors laboratory values for changes indicative of infection. Culture and sensitivity reports from wound drainage, lesions, sputum, stool, urine, and blood are monitored to identify pathogenic organisms and appropriate antimicrobial therapy. Changes in laboratory results and subtle changes in clinical status must be reported to the physician, because the immunocompromised patient may fail to develop typical signs and symptoms of infection.

Assessment also focuses on nutritional status; stress level and coping skills; use of alcohol, drugs, or tobacco; and general hygiene practices, all of which may affect immune function. Strategies the patient has used to reduce the risk of infection are identified and evaluated for their appropriateness and effectiveness (Dudek, 2006). Other aspects of nursing care are directed toward reducing the patient's risk for infection, assisting with medical measures aimed at improving immune status and treating infection, achieving optimal nutritional status, and maintaining respiratory, bowel, and bladder function. The patient's ability to demonstrate good hand hygiene must be assessed, and the patient is encouraged to cough and perform deep-breathing exercises at regular intervals. Teaching good dental hygiene measures reduces the potential for oral lesions, as do instructions on measures to protect the integrity of the skin. Attention to strict aseptic technique when performing invasive procedures, such as dressing changes, venipunctures, and bladder catheterizations, is essential. Other aspects of nursing care include assisting the patient to manage stress, to incorporate lifelong patterns of physiologic safety, and to adopt behaviors that strengthen immune system function.

Gene defects that cause many of the currently recognized immunodeficiency disorders are being identified, and genetic testing is becoming available for many of these disorders. Although this testing is rarely indicated in the initial workup for immunodeficiency (Lehman, Hernandez-Trujillo & Ballow, 2008), nurses should be aware of it and

CHART 51-4

HOME CARE CHECKLIST
Infection Prevention for the Patient With Immunodeficiency

At the completion of the home care instruction, the patient or caregiver will be able to:	PATIENT	CAREGIVER
• Identify signs and symptoms of infection to report to the health care provider, such as fever; chills; wet or dry cough; breathing problems; white patches in the mouth; swollen glands; nausea; vomiting; persistent abdominal pain; persistent diarrhea; problems with urination or changes in the character of the urine; red, swollen, or draining wounds; sores or lesions on the body; persistent vaginal discharge with or without itching; and severe fatigue.	✔	✔
• Demonstrate correct handwashing procedure.	✔	✔
• State rationale for thorough handwashing before eating, after using the bathroom, and before and after performing health care procedures.	✔	✔
• State rationale for use of cream and emollients to prevent or manage dry, chafed, or cracked skin.	✔	✔
• Demonstrate recommended personal hygiene in bathing and foot care to prevent bacterial and fungal diseases.	✔	✔
• State rationale for avoiding contact with people who have known illness or who have recently been vaccinated.	✔	✔
• Verbalize understanding of ways to maintain a well-balanced diet and adequate calories.	✔	✔
• State the reason for avoiding the eating of raw fruits and vegetables, cooking all foods thoroughly, and immediately refrigerating all leftover food.	✔	✔
• Identify the rationale for frequent cleaning of kitchen and bathroom surfaces with disinfectant.	✔	✔
• Identify rationale and benefits of avoiding alcohol, tobacco, and unprescribed medications.	✔	✔
• State rationale for taking prescribed medications as directed.	✔	✔
• Verbalize ways to cope with stress successfully, plans for regular exercise, and rationale for obtaining adequate rest.	✔	✔

CHART 51-5	HOME CARE CHECKLIST *Home Infusion of Intravenous Immunoglobulin (IVIG)*		
At the completion of the home care instruction, the patient or caregiver will be able to:		**PATIENT**	**CAREGIVER**
• Identify the benefits and expected outcome of IVIG.		✔	✔
• Demonstrate how to check for patency of the IV access device.		✔	✔
• Demonstrate how to prepare IVIG.		✔	✔
• Demonstrate how to infuse IVIG.		✔	✔
• Demonstrate how to clean and maintain IV equipment.		✔	✔
• Identify side effects and adverse effects of IVIG.		✔	✔
• State rationale for prophylactic use of acetaminophen (Tylenol) and diphenhydramine (Benadryl) before treatment begins.		✔	✔
• Verbalize understanding of emergency measures for anaphylactic shock.		✔	✔

knowledgeable about it. Some deficiencies can be diagnosed by phenotype and functional assays. Genetic testing can establish or confirm a suspected diagnosis of some primary immune deficiencies. In addition, it also may predict future disease risk prior to the onset of clinical signs and symptoms and guide clinicians in selecting the most appropriate therapeutic options (Morra, Geigenmuller, Curran, et al., 2008). Genetic testing is not typically required in CVID because known genetic defects cause only a small number of cases of CVID, and results would not alter treatment. To perform genetic testing, informed consent from the patient or legal guardian is necessary. It can be accomplished using whole blood samples and mouth swab samples.

If the patient is a candidate for any of the newer or experimental therapies (gene therapy, bone marrow transplantation, immunomodulators such as interferon-γ), the patient and family must be informed about the potential risks and benefits of the treatment regimen. A major role of the nurse is to develop and maintain a knowledge base in these evolving treatment modalities, to help the patient and family understand the treatment options and cope with the uncertainties of treatment outcomes.

Promoting Home and Community-Based Care

Teaching Patients Self-Care

The patient and caregivers require instruction about the signs and symptoms that indicate infection and about the potential for occurrence of atypical symptoms secondary to underlying immunosuppression. They must be informed of the need for continuous monitoring for subtle changes in the patient's physical health status and of the importance of seeking immediate health care if changes are detected. Patients should be advised that they know themselves best; therefore, whenever they experience a symptom that is not typical for them, they should contact their health care provider, who will determine and initiate appropriate therapy. Instruction needs to be provided about prophylactic medication regimens, including dosage, indications, times, actions, potential interactions, and side effects. Patients and their families are also instructed about the importance of continuing treatment regimens without interruption and

incorporating these routines into their daily living patterns. The patient is instructed about the importance of avoiding others with infections and avoiding crowds, and about other ways to prevent infection (Chart 51-4).

The patient who is to receive IVIG at home will need information about the expected benefits and outcomes of the treatment as well as expected adverse reactions and their management (Chart 51-5). Patients who can perform self-infusion at home must be instructed in sterile technique, medication dosages, administration rate, and detection and management of adverse reactions (Shelton, Griffin & Goldman, 2006).

Continuing Care

Encouraging the patient and family to be active partners in the management of the immunodeficiency is the key to successful outcomes and a favorable prognosis. The patient must be made aware that all health-related instructions are lifelong, that follow-up with all scheduled appointments is essential, and that it is the patient's responsibility to notify the primary care provider of any early signs or symptoms of infection, however subtle they may be. If the patient's treatment includes IVIG and the patient or family cannot administer treatment, a referral for home care or an infusion service is warranted.

CRITICAL THINKING EXERCISES

EBP 1 You are the charge nurse on a medical critical care unit. A new nurse approaches you for advice on the best infection control practices to use with a patient with cancer who has just been admitted and is immunosuppressed. Identify the infection control measures that are indicated. Describe the evidence base for the infection control measures you identified and the criteria used to evaluate the strength of that evidence.

2 The mother of your 7-year-old neighbor contacts you to discuss his frequent illnesses. She asks whether there may be something serious underlying the nine ear infections he has had in the previous year. Identify the 10 warning signs of primary immune deficiency that you would consider when responding to this mother's dilemma.

3 You are caring for a 20-year-old man who has an immunodeficiency and has been hospitalized multiple times. Describe the assessment parameters and the nursing plan of care for this patient. Identify the laboratory values that are important to monitor and report. Describe the plan for continuing care for this patient.

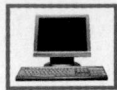

The Smeltzer suite offers these additional resources to enhance learning and facilitate understanding of this chapter:

• thePoint online resource, thepoint.lww.com/Smeltzer12E
• Student CD-ROM included with the book
• *Study Guide to Accompany Brunner & Suddarth's Textbook of Medical-Surgical Nursing*

REFERENCES AND SELECTED READINGS

Asterisk indicates nursing research.

Books

Abbas, A., Lichtman, A. & Baker, D. (2008). *Basic immunology: Functions and disorders of the immune system* (3rd ed.). Philadelphia, W. B. Saunders.

Cooper, M. & Schroeder, H. (2008). *Primary immune deficiency disease*. In Fauci, A., Braunwald, E., Kasper, D., et al. (Eds.). *Harrison's principles of internal medicine* (17th ed.). New York: McGraw-Hill Medical.

Dudek, S. G. (2006). *Nutrition essentials for nursing practice* (5th ed.). Philadelphia: Lippincott Williams & Wilkins.

Geha, R. & Rosen, F. (2007). *Case studies in immunology* (5th ed.). New York: Garland Publishing Company.

Jarvis, C. (2008). *Physical examination and health assessment*. Philadelphia: W. B. Saunders.

Kishiyama, J. (2005). Disorders of the immune system. In *Lange's pathophysiology of disease*. New York: McGraw-Hill.

Levinson, W. (2008). Congenital Immunodeficiencies. In *Lange's microbiology and immunology review*. New York: McGraw-Hill Medical.

Tierney, L. M., McPhee, S. J. & Papadakis, M. A. (2008). *Current medical diagnosis and treatment* (47th ed.). Stamford, CT: Appleton & Lange.

Journals and Electronic Documents

Antachopoulos, C., Walsh, T. & Rollides, E. (2007). Fungal infections in primary immunodeficiencies. *European Journal of Pediatrics*, 166(11), 1099–1117.

Barrett, J. (2006). Update in infectious diseases. *Annals of Internal Medicine*, 111(1), 49–56.

Brodsky, R. (2008). Narrative review: Paroxysmal nocturnal hemoglobinuria, the physiology of complement-related hemolytic anemia. *Annals of Internal Medicine*, 148(8), 587–595.

Centers for Disease Control and Prevention. (2007). *Guideline for isolation precautions: Preventing transmission of infectious agents in healthcare settings 2007*. Available at: www.cdc.gov/ncidod/dhqp/gl_isolation.html

Chinen, J. & Shearer, W. (2008). Secondary immunodeficiencies. *Journal of Allergy and Clinical Immunology*, 121(2 Suppl), S388–S392.

DeSilva, R., Gunawardena, S., Wickremesinghe, G., et al. (2007). Primary immune deficiency among patients with recurrent infections. *Ceylon Medical Journal*, 52(3), 83–86.

Dvorak, C. & Cowan, M. (2008). Hematopoietic stem cell transplantation for primary immunodeficiency disease. *Bone Marrow Transplantation*, 41(2), 119–126.

Farkas, H., Varga, L., Szeplaki, G., et al. (2007). Management of hereditary angioedema in pediatric patients. *Pediatrics*, 120(3), e713–e722.

Freeman, A. & Holland, S. (2008). The hyper – IgE syndromes. *Immunology and Allergy Clinics of North America*, 28(2), 277–291.

Garcia, J., Espanol, T., Gurbindo, M., et al. (2007). Update on the treatment of primary immunodeficiencies. *Allergologia et Immunopathologia*, 35(5), 184–192.

*Larson, E., Quiros, D. & Lin, S. (2007). Dissemination of the CDC's hand hygiene guideline and impact on infection rates. *American Journal of Infection Control*, 35(10), 666–675.

Lehman, H., Hernandez-Trujillo, V. & Ballow, M. (2008). The use of commercially available genetic tests in immunodeficiency disorders. *Annals of Allergy, Asthma & Immunology*, 101(2), 212–218.

Liston, A., Enders, A. & Siggs, O. (2008). Unraveling the association of partial T cell immunodeficiency and immune dysregulation. *Nature Reviews*, 8(7), 545–558.

Liu, X. & Hua, H. (2007). Oral manifestations of chronic mucocutaneous candidiasis: Seven case reports. *Journal of Oral Pathology and Medicine*, 36(9), 528–532.

Markert, M. (2008). Treatment of infants with complete DiGeorge anomaly. *Journal of Allergy and Clinical Immunology*, 121(4), 1063.

Mazzolari, E., Forino, C., Guerci, S., et al. (2007). Long-term immune reconstitution and clinical outcome after stem cell transplantation for severe T cell immunodeficiency. *Journal of Clinical Allergy and Immunology*, 120(4), 892–899.

McLean-Tooke, A., Barge, D., Spickett, G., et al. (2008). Immunologic defects in 22q11.2 deletion syndrome. *Journal of Allergy and Clinical Immunology*, 122(2), 362–367.

Morra, M., Geigenmuller, U., Curran, J., et al. (2008). Genetic diagnosis of primary immune deficiencies. *Immunology and Allergy Clinics of North America*, 28(2), 387–412.

Notarengelo, L., Miao, C. & Ochs, H. (2008). Wiskott-Aldrich syndrome. *Current Opinion in Hematology*, 15(1), 30–36.

Prematta, M., Gibbs, J., Pratt, E., et al. (2007). Fresh frozen plasma for the treatment of hereditary angioedema. *Annals of Allergy, Asthma and Immunology*, 98(4), 383–388.

Puck, J. (2007). Neonatal screening for severe combined immune deficiency. *Current Opinion in Allergy and Clinical Immunology*, 7(6), 522–527.

*Quiros, D., Lin, S. & Larson, E. (2007). Attitudes toward practice guidelines among intensive care unit personnel: A cross sectional anonymous survey. *Heart and Lung*, 36(4), 287–297.

Salavoura, K., Koloalexi, A., Tsangaris, G., et al. (2008). Development of cancer in patients with primary immunodeficiencies. *Anticancer Research*, 28(2B), 1263–1269.

Sandlin, D. (2007). Did you wash your hands? *Journal of PeriAnesthesia Nursing*, 22(2), 139–141.

Santilli, G., Thompson, S., Kinnon, C., et al. (2008). Gene therapy of inherited immunodeficiencies. *Expert Opinion on Biological Therapy*, 8(4), 397–407.

Saria, M. & Gosselin-Acomb, T. K. (2007). Hematopoietic stem cell transplantation: Implications for critical care nurses. *Clinical Journal of Oncology Nursing*, 11(1), 53–63.

Seve, P., Bourdillon, L., Sarrot-Reynauld, F., et al. (2008). Autoimmune hemolytic anemia and common variable immunodeficiency: A case control study of 18. *Medicine*, 87(3), 177–184.

Shelton, B., Griffin, J. & Goldman, F. (2006). Immune globulin IV therapy: Optimizing care of patients in the oncology setting. *Oncology Nursing Forum*, 33(5), 911–921.

Sokolic, R., Kesserwan, C. & Candotti, F. (2008). Recent advances in gene therapy for severe congenital immunodeficiency diseases. *Current Opinion in Hematology*, 15(4), 375–380.

Stewart, D., Tian, L., Notorangelo, L., et al. (2008). X-linked hypogammaglobulinemia and isolated growth hormone deficiency, an update. *Immunology Research*, 40(3), 262–270.

Sullivan, K. (2008). Chromosome 22q11.2 deletion syndrome, DiGeorge syndrome/velocardiofacial syndrome. *Immunology and Allergy Clinics of North America*, 28(2), 353–366.

Tarrac, S. (2008). Application of the updated CDC isolation guidelines for health care facilities. *AORN*, 87(3), 534–546.

Torgerson, T. (2008). Immune dysregulation in primary immunodeficiency disorders. *Immunology and Allergy Clinics of North America*, 28(2), 315–327.

Verbsky, J. & Grossman, W. (2006). Cellular and genetic basis of primary immune deficiencies. *Pediatric Clinics of North America*, 53(4), 649–684.

Woolhead, A., Deepak, H., Patel, M., et al. (2008). Paroxysmal haemgloginuria and its various manifestations. *Internet Journal of Anesthesiology*, 16(1), 8–16.

RESOURCES

Centers for Disease Control and Prevention, www.cdc.gov
Immune Deficiency Foundation (IDF), www.primaryimmune.org
National Institute of Allergy and Infectious Disease (NIAID), www.niaid.nih.gov
National Institutes of Health, www.nih.gov
National Library of Medicine, www.nlm.nih.gov
National Primary Immunodeficiency Resource Center/Jeffrey Modell Foundation, www.info4pi.org
U.S. Department of Health and Human Services, www.hhs.gov

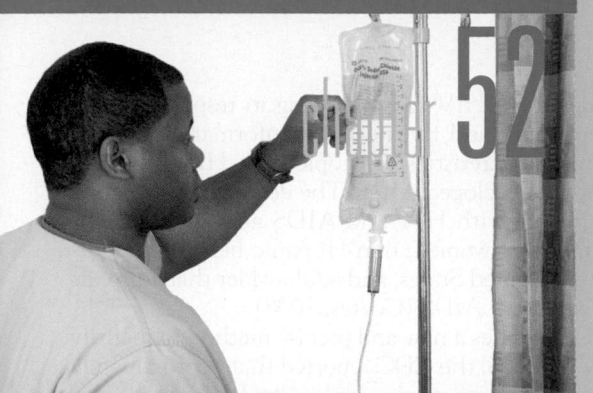

Management of Patients With HIV Infection and AIDS

chapter 52

LEARNING OBJECTIVES

On completion of this chapter, the learner will be able to:

1 Describe the modes of transmission of HIV infection and prevention strategies.

2 Describe the host/HIV interaction during primary infection.

3 Explain the pathophysiology associated with the clinical manifestations of HIV/AIDS.

4 Describe the clinical management of patients with HIV/AIDS.

5 Discuss the nursing interventions appropriate for patients with HIV/AIDS.

6 Use the nursing process as a framework for care of the patient with HIV/AIDS.

GLOSSARY

alpha-interferon: protein substance that the body produces in response to infection

B-cell lymphoma: common malignancy in patients with HIV/AIDS

candidiasis: yeast infection of skin or mucous membrane

CCR5: along with the CD4+ receptor, this cell surface molecule is used by HIV to fuse with the host's cell membranes

cytomegalovirus: a species-specific herpes virus that may cause retinitis in people with AIDS

EIA (enzyme immunoassay): a blood test that can determine the presence of antibodies to HIV in the blood or saliva; also referred to as **enzyme-linked immunosorbent assay (ELISA)**. Positive results must be validated, usually with Western blot test.

HIV-1: retrovirus isolated and recognized as the etiologic agent of AIDS

HIV-2: retrovirus identified in 1986 in AIDS patients in West Africa

HIV encephalopathy: degenerative neurologic condition characterized by a group of clinical presentations including loss of coordination, mood swings, loss of inhibitions, and widespread cognitive dysfunctions; formerly referred to as AIDS dementia complex (ADC)

human papillomavirus (HPV): viruses that cause various warts, including plantar and genital warts; some strains of HPV can also cause cervical cancer

immune reconstitution inflammatory syndrome: a syndrome that results from rapid restoration of pathogen-specific immune responses to opportunistic infections; most often occurs after starting antiretroviral therapy

Kaposi's sarcoma: malignancy that involves the epithelial layer of blood and lymphatic vessels

latent reservoir: the integrated HIV provirus within the CD4+ T cell during the resting memory state; does not express viral proteins and is invisible to the immune system and antiviral medications

GLOSSARY (Continued)

macrophage: large immune cell that devours invading pathogens and other intruders; can harbor large quantities of HIV without being killed, acting as a reservoir of the virus

monocyte: large white blood cell that ingests microbes or other cells and foreign particles. When a monocyte enters tissues, it develops into a macrophage.

***Mycobacterium avium* complex:** opportunistic infection caused by mycobacterial organisms that commonly causes a respiratory illness but can also infect other body systems

opportunistic infection: illness caused by various organisms, some of which usually do not cause disease in people with normal immune systems

p24 antigen: blood test that measures viral core protein; accuracy of test is limited because the p24 antibody binds with the antigen and makes it undetectable

peripheral neuropathy: disorder characterized by sensory loss, pain, muscle weakness, and wasting of muscles in the hands or legs and feet

***Pneumocystis* pneumonia or *Pneumocystis jiroveci* pneumonia (PCP):** common opportunistic lung infection caused by an organism, believed to be a fungus based on its structure

polymerase chain reaction: a sensitive laboratory technique that can detect and quantify HIV in a person's blood or lymph nodes

primary infection: 4- to 7-week period of rapid viral replication immediately following infection; also known as acute HIV infection

progressive multifocal leukoencephalopathy: opportunistic infection that infects brain tissue and causes damage to the brain and spinal cord

protease inhibitor: medication that inhibits the function of protease, an enzyme needed for HIV replication

provirus: viral genetic material in the form of DNA that has been integrated into the host genome. When it is dormant in human cells, HIV is in a proviral form.

retrovirus: a virus that carries genetic material in RNA instead of DNA and contains reverse transcriptase

reverse transcriptase: enzyme that transforms single-stranded RNA into a double-stranded DNA

viral load test: measures the quantity of HIV RNA in the blood

viral set point: amount of virus present in the blood after the initial burst of viremia and the immune response that follows

wasting syndrome: involuntary weight loss of 10% of baseline body weight with chronic diarrhea or chronic weakness and documented fever

Western blot assay: a blood test that identifies antibodies to HIV and is used to confirm the results of an EIA (ELISA) test

window period: time from infection with HIV until seroconversion detected on HIV antibody test

Although advances have been made in treating human immunodeficiency virus (HIV) infection and acquired immunodeficiency syndrome (AIDS), the epidemic remains a critical public health issue in all communities across the country and around the world. Prevention, early detection, and ongoing treatment remain important aspects of care for people with HIV infection and AIDS. Nurses in all settings encounter people who are positive for HIV infection; therefore, nurses need an understanding of the pathophysiology, knowledge of the physical and psychological consequences associated with the diagnosis, and expert assessment and clinical management skills to provide optimal care for people with HIV infection and AIDS.

In 1987, just 6 years after the first cases of AIDS were reported, the U.S. Food and Drug Administration (FDA) approved the first antiretroviral agent. In 1988, the first randomized controlled trial of primary prophylaxis of *Pneumocystis jiroveci* pneumonia (PCP; formerly *Pneumocystis carinii* pneumonia) appeared in the literature. Currently, more than 25 antiviral agents are approved for use in the United States (Eron, 2008); these agents interfere with the life cycle of HIV in variety of ways. HIV/AIDS is a chronic condition that requires daily medication. Although damage to the immune system is significant, survival rates have increased dramatically.

HIV INFECTION AND AIDS

Since AIDS was first identified almost 30 years ago, remarkable progress has been made in improving the quality and duration of life for people living with HIV disease. During the first decade, this progress was associated with the recognition and treatment of opportunistic diseases and introduction of prophylaxis against common **opportunistic infections.** The second decade witnessed progress in the development of highly active antiretroviral therapies (HAARTs) as well as continuing progress in the treatment of opportunistic infections. The third decade has focused on issues of adherence to antiretroviral therapy, development of second-generation medications that affect different stages of the viral life cycle, and continued need for an effective vaccine. The HIV antibody test, an enzyme immunoassay (EIA; formerly enzyme-linked immunosorbent assay [ELISA]), became available in 1984, allowing early diagnosis of the infection before onset of symptoms. Since then, HIV infection has been best managed as a chronic disease, most appropriately in an outpatient care setting, whereas AIDS may involve acute conditions that require hospital treatment.

Epidemiology

In the fall of 1982, after the first 100 cases were reported, the Centers for Disease Control and Prevention (CDC) issued a case definition of AIDS. Since then, the CDC has revised the case definition a number of times (1985, 1987, and 1993). All 50 states, the District of Columbia, U.S. dependencies and possessions, and independent nations in free association with the United States report AIDS cases to the CDC using a uniform surveillance case definition and case report form (CDC, 2005). Starting in the late 1990s, many more states began to implement HIV case reporting in response to the changing epidemic and the need for information on the numbers and characteristics of people with HIV infection who had not yet developed AIDS. The demographic characteristics of people with HIV and AIDS are changing; increasing numbers of women, non-Hispanic blacks, residents of the southern United States, and adults older than 45 years of age are dying from AIDS (Coates, 2008).

The CDC now uses a new and precise method to identify cases of HIV. In 2008, the CDC reported that approximately 56,300 new HIV infections occurred in the United States in 2006. This figure was roughly 40% higher than their former estimate of 40,000 HIV infections per year, which was based on limited data and less precise methods (CDC, 2008).

Almost 7000 people around the world still contract HIV infection every day (McConnell, 2008). Although the global percentage of people living with HIV has stabilized since 2000, the level remains unacceptably high. An estimated 33 million people are living with HIV/AIDS; however, the number of new infections declined from 3 million in 2001 to 2.7 million in 2007. Globally, the percentage of women among people with HIV/AIDS remains stable at 50% but is increasing in several countries (Joint United Nations Programme on HIV/AIDS [UNAIDS], 2008). Although there has been considerable progress worldwide in providing treatment to people with HIV/AIDS, there are still significant gaps. Sub-Saharan Africa continues to be most heavily affected by HIV/AIDS, with 67% of all people living with the disease. In 2007, 72% of the deaths from HIV/AIDS occurred in this region (UNAIDS, 2008).

HIV Transmission

HIV-1 is transmitted in body fluids that contain free virions and infected CD4+ T cells. These fluids include blood, seminal fluid, vaginal secretions, amniotic fluid, and breast milk. Inflammation and breaks in the skin or mucosa result in the increased probability that an exposure to HIV will lead to infection. The amount of HIV and infected cells in the body fluid is associated with the probability that the exposure will result in infection. Mother-to-child transmission of HIV-1 may occur in utero, at the time of delivery, or through breast-feeding, but most perinatal infections are thought to occur after exposure during delivery. HIV is not transmitted through casual contact (Chart 52-1).

Blood and blood products can transmit HIV to recipients. However, the risk associated with transfusions has been virtually eliminated as a result of voluntary self-deferral, completion of a detailed health history, extensive testing, heat treatment of clotting factor concentrates, and more

CHART 52-1   *Risk Behaviors Associated With HIV Infection and AIDS*

- Sharing infected injection drug use equipment
- Having sexual relations with infected individuals (both male and female)

Also at risk are people who received HIV-infected blood or blood products (especially before blood screening was instituted in 1985) and infants born to mothers with HIV infection.

effective virus inactivation methods. Donated blood is tested for antibodies to HIV-1, **HIV-2,** and **p24 antigen;** in addition, since 1999, nucleic acid amplification testing (NAT) has been performed.

Gerontologic Considerations

The number of people between the ages of 55 and 64 years living with AIDS more than doubled between the years 1998 and 2003 (from 19,258 to 38,997) (CDC, 2005). HIV infection in middle-aged and older populations may be underreported and underdiagnosed because health care professionals erroneously believe that older adults are not at risk for HIV infection. Also, HIV-related dementia in the older adult may mimic Alzheimer's disease and may be misdiagnosed. The characteristics of older people living with HIV infection reflect those of others in their country of origin who have HIV infection (Nokes, Rivero-Mendez, Valencia, et al., 2006).

Several factors put older adults at risk for HIV infection:
- Many older adults are sexually active but do not use condoms, viewing them only as a means of unneeded birth control.
- Many older adults do not consider themselves at risk for HIV infection.
- Older gay men, who grew up and lived in an era when disclosure of their sexual orientation was not acceptable and who have lost long-time partners, may begin new relationships with younger men.
- Older adults may be intravenous (IV)/injection drug users.
- Older adults may have received HIV-infected blood through transfusions before 1985.
- Normal age-related changes include a reduction in immune system function, which puts the older adult at greater risk for infections, cancers, and autoimmune disorders. Many older adults also experience the loss of loved ones, resulting in depression and bereavement, factors that are associated with depressed immune function.

Prevention of HIV Infection

Until an effective vaccine is developed, nurses need to prevent HIV infection by teaching patients how to eliminate or reduce risky behaviors. Although HIV prevention strategies have focused on individual behaviors, political, economic, and social determinants of risk also need to be considered (Horton & Das, 2008). A combination of evidence-based prevention strategies that include behavioral, structural, and biomedical approaches tempered by the wisdom and ownership of communities offers the best hope for prevention (Merson, O'Malley, Serwadda, et al., 2008).

Preventive Education

Evidence-based programs have been used to educate the public regarding safer sexual practices to decrease the risk of transmitting HIV infection to sexual partners (Chart 52-2). The CDC, through the HIV/AIDS Prevention Research Synthesis Project, has identified evidence-based behavioral interventions that can be applied in a number of settings. Other than abstinence, consistent and correct use of condoms (Chart 52-3) is the only effective method to decrease the risk of sexual transmission of HIV infection. When male condoms are used consistently during vaginal or anal intercourse, their effectiveness can be as high as 95% (Padian, Buve, Balkus, et al., 2008). Nonlatex condoms made of natural materials such as lambskin are available for people with latex allergy but will not protect against HIV infection. A male condom should be used for oral contact with the penis, and a dental dam (a flat piece of latex used by dentists to isolate a tooth for treatment) should be used for oral contact with the vagina or rectum. The polyurethane female condom, which is an effective contraceptive, provides a physical barrier that also prevents exposure to genital secretions containing HIV such as semen and vaginal fluid (Padian, et al., 2008). The female condom is the only barrier method that can be controlled by the woman (see Chapter 46).

Microbicides are chemical products such as gels, creams, films, or suppositories that are inserted into the vagina or

---

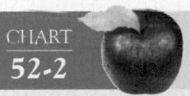

CHART 52-2

HEALTH PROMOTION
Safer Sexual Behaviors

- Advise patients to abstain from sharing sexual fluids.
- Advise patients to reduce the number of sexual partners to one.
- Advise patients to always use latex condoms. If the patient is allergic to latex, nonlatex condoms should be used.
- Advise patients to avoid reusing condoms.
- Advise patients to avoid using cervical caps or diaphragms without using a condom as well.
- Advise patients to always use dental dams for oral–genital or anal stimulation.
- Advise patients to avoid anal intercourse because this practice may injure tissues.
- Advise patients to avoid manual–anal intercourse ("fisting").
- Advise patients not to ingest urine or semen.

- Educate patients about nonpenetrative sexual activities, such as body massage, social kissing (dry), mutual masturbation, fantasy, and sex films.
- Advise patients to avoid sharing needles, razors, toothbrushes, sex toys, or blood-contaminated articles.
- Advise HIV-seropositive patients to inform previous, present, and prospective sexual and drug-using partners of their HIV-positive status. If the patient is concerned for his or her safety, advise the patient that many states have established mechanisms through the public health department in which professionals are available to notify exposed people.
- Advise HIV-seropositive patients to avoid having unprotected sex with another HIV-seropositive person. Cross-infection with that person's HIV can increase the severity of infection.
- Advise HIV-seropositive patients to avoid donating blood, plasma, body organs, or sperm.

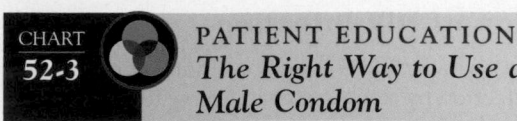

PATIENT EDUCATION
The Right Way to Use a Male Condom

1. Put on a new condom before any kind of sex.
2. Hold the condom by the tip to squeeze out the air.

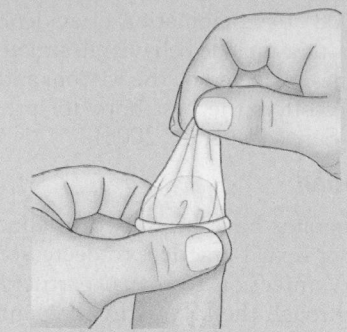

3. Unroll the condom all the way over the erect penis

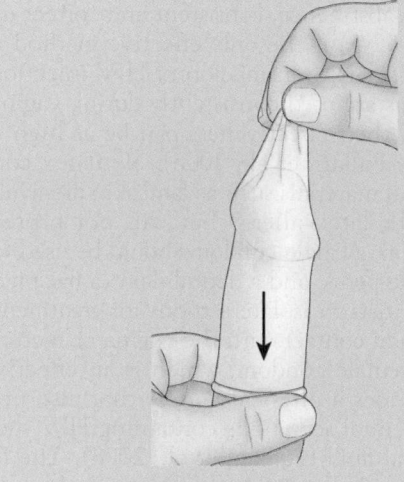

4. Have sex.
5. Hold the condom so it cannot come off the penis.
6. Pull out.
7. Use a new condom if you want to have sex again or if you want to have sex in a different place (eg, in the anus and then in the vagina).

   Keep condoms cool and dry. Never use skin lotions, baby oil, petroleum jelly, or cold cream with condoms. The oil in these products will cause the condom to break. Products made with water (such as K-Y jelly or glycerin) are safer to use.

rectum before sexual intercourse to prevent HIV transmission (Padian, et al., 2008). Nonoxynol-9 (N-9) was widely advocated to reduce the risk of HIV infection until a clinical trial conducted in almost 1000 female commercial sex workers in African countries revealed that those who used N-9 intravaginally along with condoms were 50% more likely to be infected with HIV than those who did not use the N-9 gel. Microbicide research is moving in three directions: (1) new microbicides that contain antiretroviral agents such as tenofovir gel or dapivirine gel and ring (International Partnership for Microbicides, 2009); (2) long-acting dispersal methods such as vaginal rings that remain

in place or do not require frequent applications; and (3) combination products with different mechanisms of action (Padian, et al., 2008).

In March 2007, based on the results of three clinical trials, the World Health Organization (WHO) and UNAIDS recommended that circumcision be recognized as an effective strategy to reduce the risk of HIV acquisition in men because the presence of the foreskin, which harbors HIV target cells, might facilitate survival and entry of the virus (Padian, et al., 2008). Other topics important in preventive education include the importance of avoiding sexual practices that might cut or tear the lining of the rectum, penis, or vagina and avoiding sexual contact with multiple partners or people who are known to be HIV positive or IV/injection drug users. In addition, people who are HIV positive or who use injection drugs should be instructed not to donate blood or share drug equipment with others.

The Harm Reduction Model recognizes that total abstinence from addictive drugs might not be a realistic short-term goal. This model recommends working with drug users to assist them to increase their healthy behaviors. Needle exchange programs are available in some locations so that IV/injection drug users can obtain sterile drug equipment at no cost. Extensive research has demonstrated that needle exchange programs do not promote increased drug use; on the contrary, they have been found to decrease the incidence of bloodborne infections in people who use IV/injection drugs. Nurses should refer clients to needle exchange programs in their neighborhood whenever available. In the absence of needle exchange programs, IV/injection drug users should be instructed on methods to clean their syringes and advised to avoid sharing cotton and other drug use equipment. Drug users interested in treatment programs should be referred to those programs.

Related Reproductive Education

Because HIV infection in women often occurs during the childbearing years, family planning issues need to be addressed. Attempts to achieve pregnancy by couples in which only one partner has HIV expose the unaffected partner to the virus. Efforts at artificial insemination using processed semen from an HIV-infected partner continue. Studies are needed, because HIV has been found in the spermatozoa of patients with AIDS, and it is possible that HIV can replicate in the male germ cell. Women considering pregnancy need to have accurate information about the risks of transmitting HIV infection to themselves, their partner, and their future children, and about the benefits of taking antiretroviral agents to reduce perinatal HIV transmission. Women who are HIV positive should be instructed not to breast-feed their infants, because HIV is transmitted through breast milk.

Certain contraceptive methods may pose additional health risks for women. Estrogen in oral contraceptives may increase a woman's risk of HIV infection. In addition, HIV-infected women who use estrogen-containing oral contraceptives have shown increased shedding of HIV in vaginal and cervical secretions. The intrauterine contraceptive device (IUD) may also increase the risk of HIV transmission because the string of the IUD may serve as a means to transmit the virus.

Transmission to Health Care Providers

Standard Precautions

To reduce the risk of exposure of health care workers to HIV, the CDC developed standard precautions (Chart 52-4). Specifically, standard precautions are designed to reduce the risk of transmission of bloodborne pathogens and of pathogens from moist body substances. Standard precautions are used when working with all patients in all health care settings, regardless of their diagnosis or presumed infectious status (Siegel, Rhinehart, Jackson, et al., 2007).

Postexposure Prophylaxis for Health Care Providers

Postexposure prophylaxis in response to the exposure of health care personnel to blood or other body fluids reduces the risk of HIV infection. The CDC recommends that all health care providers who have sustained a significant exposure to HIV be counseled and offered anti-HIV postexposure prophylaxis, if appropriate (Chart 52-5). Some clinicians are considering the use of postexposure prophylaxis for patients exposed to HIV as a result of high-risk sexual behavior or IV/injection drug use. This use of postexposure prophylaxis is controversial because of concern that it may be substituted for safer sex practices and safer IV/injection drug use. However, it may be advocated in high-risk situations, especially when the uninfected person has few options because of economic constraints and cultural norms.

Guidelines for treatment of health care workers with possible occupational exposure to HIV are available from the CDC. Treatment should be started as quickly as possible after exposure. Those who choose postexposure prophylaxis must be prepared for the side effects of the medications, as well as the unknown long-term risks, because HIV often becomes resistant to the medications used to treat it. The cost may be of concern; the cost of a medication regimen ranges from $500 to more than $1000, in addition to the costs of testing and counseling. However, the health care institution where the provider is employed usually covers these costs.

Vaccination

Despite enormous international efforts to develop an effective vaccine, the complexity of the science and challenges of HIV are proving formidable obstacles. Hopes were dashed when a vaccine efficacy trial was halted in September 2007, after interim results showed that the vaccine being tested did not protect against HIV and did not reduce viral load after infection (Senior, 2008). Cooperation among all nations continues to grow, and resources are being allocated to develop a vaccine and to create and support the infrastructure needed to facilitate vaccine testing.

Pathophysiology

Because HIV infection is an infectious disease, it is important to understand how HIV-1 integrates itself into a person's immune system and how immunity plays a role in the course of HIV disease. This knowledge is also essential for understanding medication therapy and vaccine development.

Viruses are intracellular parasites. HIV belongs to a group of viruses known as **retroviruses,** which carry their genetic material in the form of ribonucleic acid (RNA) rather than deoxyribonucleic acid (DNA). As shown in Figure 52-1A, HIV consists of a viral core containing the viral RNA, surrounded by an envelope consisting of protruding glycoproteins.

Chart 52-4 • Recommendations for Standard Precautions

1. **Hand hygiene:** Use after touching blood, body fluids, secretions, excretions, or contaminated items; immediately after removing gloves; and between patient contacts.
2. **Personal protective equipment (PPE)**
   - Gloves: Use for touching blood, body fluids, secretions, excretions, and contaminated items, and for touching mucous membranes and nonintact skin.
   - Gown: Use during procedures and patient care activities when contact of clothing/exposed skin with blood or body fluids, secretions, and excretions is anticipated.
   - Mask, eye protection (goggles), face shield*: Use during procedures and patient care activities likely to generate splashes or sprays of blood, body fluids, and secretions, especially suctioning or endotracheal intubation.
3. **Soiled patient care equipment:** Handle in a manner that prevents transfer of microorganisms to others and to the environment; wear gloves if visibly contaminated; and perform hand hygiene.
4. **Environmental control:** Develop procedures for routine care, cleaning, and disinfection of environmental surfaces, especially frequently touched surfaces in patient care areas.
5. **Textiles and laundry:** Handle in a manner that prevents transfer of microorganisms to others and to the environment.

Needles and other sharps: Do not recap, bend, break, or hand-manipulate used needles; if recapping is required, use a one-handed scoop technique only; use safety features when available; and place used sharps in a puncture-resistant container.
6. **Patient resuscitation:** Use mouthpiece, resuscitation bag, and other ventilation devices to prevent contact with mouth and oral secretions.
7. **Patient placement:** Prioritize for single-patient room if patient is at increased risk of transmission, is likely to contaminate the environment, does not maintain appropriate hygiene, or is at increased risk of acquiring infection or developing adverse outcome following infection.
8. **Respiratory hygiene/cough etiquette** (source containment of infectious respiratory secretions in symptomatic patients, beginning at initial point of encounter, such as triage and reception areas in emergency departments and physician offices): Instruct symptomatic people to cover mouth and nose when sneezing or coughing; use tissues and dispose in no-touch receptacle; observe hand hygiene after soiling of hands with respiratory secretions; and wear surgical mask if tolerated.

*During aerosol-generating procedures on patients with suspected or proven infections transmitted by respiratory aerosols (eg, severe acute respiratory syndrome [SARS]), wear a fit-tested N95 or higher respirator in addition to gloves, gown, and face/eye protection.
From the Centers for Disease Control and Prevention. www.cdc.gov/ncidod/dhqp/pdf/guidelines/Isolation2007.pdf

Chart 52-5 • *Postexposure Prophylaxis for Health Care Providers*

According to the Centers for Disease Control and Prevention (CDC; 2005), the average risk for HIV transmission to health care providers after a percutaneous exposure to HIV-infected blood is estimated to be approximately 0.3% and after a mucous membrane exposure, approximately 0.09%. If you sustain an occupational exposure to HIV, take the following actions immediately:

- Alert your supervisor/nursing faculty and initiate the injury-reporting system used in the setting.
- Identify the source patient, who may need to be tested for HIV, hepatitis B, and hepatitis C. State laws will determine whether written informed consent must be obtained from the source patient before his or her testing. OraQuick rapid testing should be used if possible if the HIV status of the source patient is unknown, because results can be available within 20 minutes.
- Report as quickly as possible to the employee health services, the emergency department, or other designated treatment facility. This visit should be documented in the health care worker's confidential medical record.
- Give consent for baseline testing for HIV, hepatitis B, and hepatitis C. Confidential HIV testing can be performed up to 72 hours after the exposure but should be performed as soon as the health care worker can give informed consent for baseline testing.
- Get postexposure prophylaxis for HIV in accordance with CDC guidelines. Start the prophylaxis medications within 2 hours after exposure. Make sure that you are being monitored for symptoms of toxicity. Practice safer sex until follow-up testing is complete. Continue the HIV medications for the full 4 weeks after exposure. The majority of HIV exposures will warrant a combination of antiretroviral agents. Combinations that may be prescribed for postexposure prophylaxis include zidovudine (ZDV) and lamivudine (3TC) or emtricitabine (FTC); stavudine (d4T) and 3TC or FTC; and tenofovir (TDF) and 3TC or FTC.
- Follow up with postexposure testing at 1 month, 3 months, and 6 months, and perhaps 1 year.
- Document the exposure in detail for your own records as well as for the employer.

Centers for Disease Control and Prevention. (2005). Updated U.S. Public Health Service guidelines for the management of occupational exposures to HIV and recommendations for postexposure prophylaxis. *MMWR–Morbidity and Mortality Weekly Report, 54*(RR-9), 1–17.

Physiology ■■■ Pathophysiology

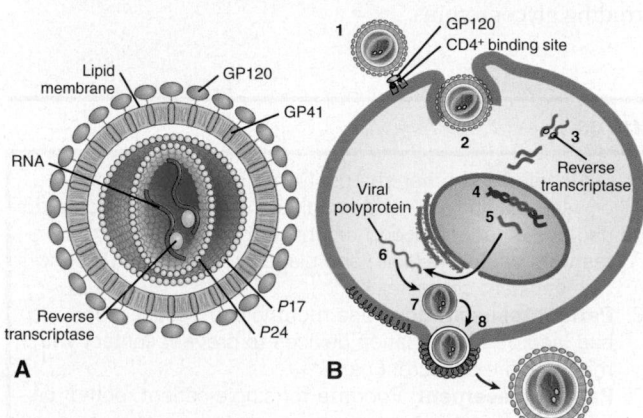

Figure 52-1 A, Structure of HIV-1. A glycoprotein envelope surrounds the virus, which carries its genetic material in RNA. Knobs, consisting of proteins GP120 and GP41, protrude from the envelope. These proteins are essential for binding the virus to the CD4+ T lymphocyte. **B,** Life cycle of HIV-1: (1) Attachment of the HIV virus to a CD4+ receptor; (2) internalization and uncoating of the virus with viral RNA and reverse transcriptase; (3) reverse transcription, which produces a mirror image of the viral RNA and double-stranded DNA molecule; (4) integration of viral DNA into host DNA using the integrase enzyme; (5) transcription of the inserted viral DNA to produce viral messenger RNA; (6) translation of viral messenger RNA to create viral polyprotein; (7) cleavage of viral polyprotein into individual viral proteins that make up the new virus; and (8) assembly and release of the new virus from the host cell. Redrawn from Porth, C. & Matfin, G. (2009). *Pathophysiology: Concepts of altered health states* (7th ed.). Philadelphia: Lippincott Williams & Wilkins.

All viruses target specific cells. HIV targets cells with CD4 receptors, which are expressed on the surface of T lymphocytes, **monocytes,** dendritic cells, and brain microglia. Mature T cells (T lymphocytes) are composed of two major subpopulations that are defined by cell surface receptors of CD4 or CD8. Approximately two thirds of peripheral blood T cells are CD4+, and approximately one third are CD8+. Most people have about 700 to 1000 CD4+ cells/mm^3, but a level as low as 500 cells/mm^3 can be considered within normal limits. During acute/recent infection, most varieties of HIV-1 use the chemokine receptor **CCR5** (R5 virus) for entry to T cells in addition to the CD4+ receptor, which suggests that the R5 variant is preferred to a different variant (CXCR4). Over the course of infection, viruses in the majority of untreated patients eventually exhibit a shift in coreceptor from CCR5 to either CXCR4 or both CCR5 and CXCR4 (dual- or mixed-tropic) receptors (1st International Reference Panel for HIV-1 RNA Genotypes Panel, 2004). The glycoproteins of HIV (GP120 and GP41) must attach to both the CD4+ and the CCR5 binding sites in order to bind to the CD4+ cell membrane, which results in fusion of HIV with the T cell.

Once HIV has attached to the host cell, the virus can replicate. The HIV life cycle is complex (see Fig. 52-1B) and consists of the following steps (Porth & Matfin, 2009):

1. Attachment. In this first step, the GP120 and GP41 glycoproteins of HIV bind with the host's uninfected CD4+ receptor and chemokine coreceptors, usually CCR5, which results in fusion of HIV with the CD4+ T-cell membrane.
2. Uncoating. The contents of HIV's viral core (two single strands of viral RNA and three viral enzymes: **reverse transcriptase,** integrase, and protease) are emptied into the CD4+ T cell.

3. DNA synthesis. HIV changes its genetic material from RNA to DNA through action of reverse transcriptase, resulting in double-stranded DNA that carries instruction for viral replication.

4. Integration. New viral DNA enters the nucleus of the CD4+ T cell and through action of integrase is blended with the DNA of the CD4+ T cell, resulting in permanent, lifelong infection. Prior to this step, the uninfected person has been only exposed to, not infected with, HIV. With this step, HIV infection is permanent.

5. Transcription. When the CD4+ T cell is activated, the double-stranded DNA forms single-stranded messenger RNA (mRNA), which builds new viruses.

6. Translation. The mRNA creates chains of new proteins and enzymes (polyproteins) that contain the components needed in the construction of new viruses.

7. Cleavage. The HIV enzyme protease cuts the polyprotein chain into the individual proteins that make up the new virus.

8. Budding. New proteins and viral RNA migrate to the membrane of the infected CD4+ T cell, exit from the cell, and start the process all over.

In resting (nondividing) CD4+ cells, HIV can survive in a latent state as an integrated **provirus** that produces few or no viral particles. These resting CD4+ T cells can be stimulated to produce new particles if something activates them. When a T cell that harbors this integrated DNA (also known as provirus) becomes activated against HIV or other microbes, the cell begins to produce new copies of both RNA and viral proteins. Activation of the infected cell may be achieved by antigens, mitogens, certain cytokines (tumor necrosis factor-alpha [TNF-α] or interleukin-1 [IL-1]), or virus gene products of such viruses as **cytomegalovirus (CMV)**, Epstein-Barr virus, herpes simplex virus, and hepatitis viruses. Consequently, whenever the infected CD4+ cell is activated, HIV replication and budding occur, which can destroy the host cell. Newly formed HIV released into the blood can infect other CD4+ cells (see Fig. 52-1B).

HIV-1 mutates quickly, at a relatively constant rate, with about 1% of the virus's genetic material changing annually. HIV-1 exhibits substantial genetic diversity and several different genotypes of HIV-1 exist. There is a major group (group M), which consists of subtypes A through L, and a more diverse collection of outliers, which has been referred to as groups N and O. Many of the early nucleic acid–based tests had a fairly narrow band of specificity targeted mainly at subtype B viruses, because these predominated in the western world (1st International Reference Panel for HIV-1 RNA Genotypes, 2004).

A mutation of CCR5 that is common in Caucasians, but not other ethnic groups, has been identified. About 1% of Caucasians lack functional CCR5 and are highly protected against HIV infection even if exposed (although protection is not absolute); about 18% are not markedly protected against infection but, if infected, demonstrate significantly slower rates of disease progression.

Stages of HIV Disease

The stage of HIV disease is based on clinical history, physical examination, laboratory evidence of immune dysfunction, signs and symptoms, and infections and malignancies. The CDC standard case definition of AIDS categorizes HIV infection and AIDS in adults and adolescents on the basis of clinical conditions associated with HIV infection and CD4+ T-cell counts. The classification system (Table 52-1) groups clinical conditions into one of three categories, denoted A, B, and C.

Primary Infection (Acute/Recent HIV Infection, Acute HIV Syndrome)

The period from infection with HIV to the development of HIV-specific antibodies is known as **primary infection.** Initially, there is a **window period** during which an HIV-positive person tests negative on the HIV antibody blood test, although he or she is infected and highly infectious, because his or her viral load is very high. After 2 to 3 weeks, antibodies to the glycoproteins of the HIV envelope can be detected in the sera of HIV-infected people, but most of these antibodies lack the ability to totally control the virus. By the time neutralizing antibodies can be detected, HIV-1 is firmly established in the host.

Primary infection is characterized by high levels of viral replication, widespread dissemination of HIV throughout the body, and destruction of CD4+ T cells. This leads to dramatic drops in CD4+ T-cell counts, which are normally 500 to 1500 cells/mm^3 of blood. The host is responding to the HIV infection through a CD4+ T-cell response that causes other immune cells, such as CD8+ lymphocytes, to increase their killing of infected, virus-producing cells. The body produces antibody molecules in an effort to contain the free HIV particles (outside cells) and assist in their removal. The remaining amount of virus in the body after this initial immune response is referred to as the **viral set point,** which results in a steady state of infection that lasts for years. The final level of the viral set point is inversely correlated with disease prognosis; that is, the higher the viral set point, the poorer the prognosis.

The primary infection stage is part of CDC category A and includes the acute symptomatic and early infection phases. During this stage, the virus is widely disseminated in lymphoid tissue, and a **latent reservoir** within resting memory CD4+ T cells is created (Zack & Park, 2008). An estimated 40% to 90% of patients who are acutely infected with HIV experience symptoms of acute retroviral syndrome characterized by fever, lymphadenopathy, pharyngitis, skin rash, myalgias/arthralgias, and other conditions (Panel on Antiretroviral Guidelines for Adults and Adolescents (Guidelines) (2008)).

HIV Asymptomatic (CDC Category A: More Than 500 CD4+ T Lymphocytes/mm^3)

After the viral set point is reached, HIV-positive people enter into a chronic stage in which the immune system cannot eliminate the virus despite its best efforts. This set point varies greatly from patient to patient and dictates the subsequent rate of disease progression; on average, 8 to 10 years pass before a major HIV-related complication develops. In

Table 52-1 CLASSIFICATION SYSTEM FOR HIV INFECTION AND EXPANDED AIDS SURVEILLANCE CASE DEFINITION FOR ADOLESCENTS AND ADULTS

Diagnostic Categories CD4+ T-Cell Category	Clinical Categories		
	A Asymptomatic, Acute (Primary) HIV or PGL	B Symptomatic, Not (A) or (C) Conditions	C AIDS-Indicator Conditions
(1) ≥500/μL	A1	B1	C1
(2) 200–499/μL	A2	B2	C2
(3) <200/μL AIDS-indicator T-cell count	A3	B3	C3

People with AIDS-indicator conditions (clinical category C) and those in categories A3 or B3 are considered to have AIDS.

Clinical Category A

Includes one or more of the following in an adult or adolescent with confirmed HIV infection and without conditions in clinical categories B and C:
- Asymptomatic HIV infection
- Persistent generalized lymphadenopathy (PGL)
- Acute (primary) HIV infection with accompanying illness or history of acute HIV infection

Clinical Category B

Examples of conditions in clinical category B include, but are not limited to, the following:
- Bacillary angiomatosis
- Candidiasis, oropharyngeal (thrush) or vulvovaginal (persistent, frequent, or poorly responsive to therapy)
- Cervical dysplasia (moderate or severe)/cervical carcinoma in situ
- Constitutional symptoms, such as fever (38.5°C) or diarrhea exceeding 1 mo in duration
- Hairy leukoplakia, oral
- Herpes zoster (shingles), involving at least two distinct episodes or more than one dermatome
- Idiopathic thrombocytopenic purpura
- Listeriosis
- Pelvic inflammatory disease, particularly if complicated by tubo-ovarian abscess
- Peripheral neuropathy

Clinical Category C

Examples of conditions in adults and adolescents include the following:
- Candidiasis of bronchi, trachea, or lungs; esophagus
- Cervical cancer, invasive
- Coccidioidomycosis, disseminated or extrapulmonary
- Cryptococcosis, extrapulmonary
- Cryptosporidiosis, chronic intestinal (exceeding 1 mo's duration)
- Cytomegalovirus disease (other than liver, spleen, or lymph nodes)
- Cytomegalovirus retinitis (with loss of vision)
- Encephalopathy, HIV related
- Herpes simplex: chronic ulcer(s) (exceeding 1 mo's duration); or bronchitis, pneumonitis, or esophagitis
- Histoplasmosis, disseminated or extrapulmonary
- Isosporiasis, chronic intestinal (exceeding 1 mo's duration)
- Kaposi's sarcoma
- Lymphoma, Burkitt's (or equivalent term); immunoblastic (or equivalent term); primary, of brain
- *Mycobacterium avium* complex or M. *kansasii*, disseminated or extrapulmonary
- *Mycobacterium tuberculosis*, any site (pulmonary or extrapulmonary)
- *Mycobacterium*, other species or unidentified species, disseminated or extrapulmonary
- *Pneumocystis jiroveci* pneumonia
- Pneumonia, recurrent
- Progressive multifocal leukoencephalopathy
- *Salmonella* septicemia, recurrent
- Toxoplasmosis of brain
- Wasting syndrome due to HIV

Adapted from Centers for Disease Control, U.S. Department of Health and Human Services. (1992). 1993 revised classification system for HIV infection and expanded surveillance case definition for AIDS among adolescents and adults. *MMWR Morbidity and Mortality Weekly Report, 41*(RR-17), 1–19.

this prolonged, chronic stage, patients feel well and have few, if any, symptoms. Apparent good health continues because CD4+ T-cell levels remain high enough to preserve immune defensive responses.

HIV Symptomatic (CDC Category B: 200 to 499 CD4 + T Lymphocytes/mm³)

Over time, the number of CD4+ T cells gradually falls. Category B consists of symptomatic conditions in HIV-infected patients that are not included in the conditions listed in category C. These conditions must also meet one of the following criteria: (1) the condition is caused by HIV infection or a defect in cellular immunity, or (2) the condition is considered to have a clinical course or to require management that is complicated by HIV infection. If a person was once treated for a category B condition and has not developed a category C disease but is now symptom-free, that person's stage of HIV disease is considered category B.

AIDS (CDC Category C: Fewer Than 200 CD4+ T Lymphocytes/mm³)

When the CD4+ T-cell level drops below 200 cells/mm³ of blood, the person is said to have AIDS. As levels decrease to fewer than 100 cells/mm³, the immune system is significantly impaired. Once a patient has had a category C condition, he or she remains in category C even if CD4+ T cells rebound with treatment. This classification has implications for entitlements (ie, disability benefits, housing, and food stamps), because these programs are often linked to an AIDS diagnosis. Although the 1993 classification emphasizes CD4+ T-cell counts, it allows for CD4+ percentages (percentage of CD4+ T cells compared with total lymphocytes). The CD4+ percentage is less subject to variation on repeated measurements than is the absolute CD4+ T-cell count. A CD4+ percentage of less than 14% of the total lymphocytes is consistent with a diagnosis of AIDS. The percentage, as compared with the absolute number of CD4+ T cells, becomes particularly important when the patient has a heightened immune response to infections in addition to HIV.

Assessment and Diagnostic Findings in HIV Infection

During the first stage of HIV infection, the patient may be asymptomatic or may exhibit various signs and symptoms. The patient's health history should alert the health care

Table 52-2 SELECTED LABORATORY TESTS FOR DIAGNOSING AND TRACKING HIV AND ASSESSING IMMUNE STATUS

Test	Findings in HIV Infection
EIA (enzyme immunoassay)	Antibodies are detected, resulting in positive results and marking the end of the window period
Western blot	Also detects antibodies to HIV; used to confirm EIA
Viral load	Measures HIV RNA in the plasma
CD4/CD8	These are markers found on lymphocytes. HIV kills CD4+ cells, which results in a significantly impaired immune system.

Chart 52-6• *HIV Test Results: Implications for Patients*

Interpretation of Positive Test Results

- Antibodies to HIV are present in the blood (the patient has been infected with the virus, and the body has produced antibodies).
- HIV is active in the body, and the patient can transmit the virus to others.
- Despite HIV infection, the patient does not necessarily have AIDS.
- The patient is not immune to HIV (the antibodies do not indicate immunity).

Interpretation of Negative Test Results

- Antibodies to HIV are not present in the blood at this time, which can mean that the patient has not been infected with HIV or, if infected, the body has not yet produced antibodies (window period—usually 3 weeks to 6 months).
- The patient should continue taking precautions. The test result does not mean that the patient is immune to the virus, nor does it mean the patient is not infected; it just means that the body may not have produced antibodies yet.

provider about the need for HIV screening based on the patient's sexual practices, IV/injection drug use, and receipt of blood transfusions. Additionally, exposure to body fluids containing infected blood while providing care to others with HIV infection (eg, through needlesticks) should alert health care providers to possible HIV infection. Patients who are in later stages of HIV infection may have a variety of symptoms related to their immunosuppressed state. Several screening tests are used to diagnose HIV infection. Others are used to assess the stage and severity of the infection. Table 52-2 identifies common blood tests.

HIV Antibody Tests

In 2006, the CDC issued recommendations for HIV testing in public and private health care settings (CDC, 2006), including hospital emergency departments, inpatient facilities, urgent care clinics, primary care settings, public health clinics, community clinics, substance abuse treatment clinics, and correctional health care facilities. The objectives of those recommendations were to increase HIV screening of patients, including pregnant women, in health care settings; foster earlier detection of HIV infection; identify and counsel people with unrecognized HIV infection and refer them to clinical and preventive services; and further reduce perinatal transmission of HIV. The major changes from previously published guidelines are:

1. HIV screening is recommended for patients (18 to 64 years of age) in all health care settings after the patient is notified that testing will be performed unless he or she declines (opt-out screening).
2. People at high risk for HIV infection should be screened for the disease at least annually.
3. Separate written consent for HIV testing should not be required; general consent for medical care should be considered sufficient to encompass consent for HIV testing.
4. Prevention counseling should not be required with HIV diagnostic testing or as part of HIV screening programs in health care settings.

Although these guidelines are already in effect in some states, they have not been implemented in others because they violate the states' existing HIV confidentiality laws.

Before an HIV antibody test is performed, the meaning of the test and possible test results are explained, and informed consent for the test is obtained from the patient. When the result of the HIV antibody test is received, it is carefully explained to the patient in private (Chart 52-6). All test results are kept confidential. Education and counseling about the test result and about preventing transmission are essential. The patient's psychological response to a positive test result may include feelings of panic, depression, and hopelessness. The social and interpersonal consequences of a positive test result can be devastating. The patient may lose his or her sexual partner, housing, and health insurance because of disclosure. He or she may experience discrimination in employment and housing, as well as social ostracism. For these reasons and others, patients who test positive may need ongoing counseling as well as referrals for social, financial, medical, and psychological support services. Patients whose test results are seronegative may develop a false sense of security, possibly resulting in continued high-risk behaviors or feelings that they are immune to the virus. These patients may need ongoing counseling to help modify high-risk behaviors and to encourage returns for repeated testing. Other patients may experience anxiety regarding the uncertainty of their status.

When a person is infected with HIV, the immune system responds by producing antibodies against the virus, usually within 3 to 12 weeks after infection. In 1985, the FDA licensed an HIV-1 antibody assay that uses approximately 5 to 7 mL of blood. Samples are tested using two different laboratory techniques to determine the presence of antibodies to HIV. The **EIA (enzyme immunoassay)** test, formerly referred to as the **ELISA (enzyme-linked immunosorbent assay)** test, identifies antibodies directed specifically against HIV. The **Western blot assay** is used to confirm seropositivity when the EIA result is positive. Adults whose blood contains antibodies for HIV are seropositive.

In addition to this HIV-1 antibody assay, two additional techniques are now available. The OraSure test uses saliva to perform an EIA antibody test. Using less than a drop of blood, the OraQuick Rapid HIV-1 Antibody Test quickly (approximately 20 minutes) and reliably (99.6% accuracy) detects antibodies to HIV-1. The OraQuick test is becoming the standard method of testing in settings where a delay would seriously affect treatment, such as in labor and delivery rooms or in emergency departments when the HIV status of a sexual abuser is unknown.

Home-based testing for HIV antibodies using a small amount of blood was first proposed in 1985 and approved by the FDA in 1995. However, use of home testing kits raises concerns because of the lack of counseling and possible inaccurate results, including both false-positive and false-negative results.

Viral Load Tests

Target amplification methods quantify HIV RNA or DNA levels in the plasma and have replaced p24 antigen capture assays. Target amplification methods include reverse transcriptase–**polymerase chain reaction** (RT-PCR) and nucleic acid sequence–based amplification. A widely used **viral load test** measures plasma HIV RNA levels. Currently, these tests are used to track viral load and response to treatment of HIV infection. RT-PCR is also used to detect HIV in high-risk seronegative people before antibodies are measurable, to confirm a positive EIA result, and to screen neonates. HIV culture or quantitative plasma culture and plasma viremia are additional tests that measure viral burden, but they are used infrequently. Viral load is a better predictor of the risk of HIV disease progression than the CD4+ count. The lower the viral load, the longer the time to AIDS diagnosis and the longer the survival time.

Treatment of HIV Infection

Protocols on how and when to start treatment for HIV disease change relatively often. The U.S. Department of Health and Human Services Panel on Antiretroviral Guidelines for Adults and Adolescents (Guidelines, 2008) is composed of HIV specialists from across the country who meet periodically to review the latest scientific evidence. The CD4+ T-cell count is usually the most important consideration in deciding whether antiretroviral medications should be started. In general, antiretroviral medications should be offered to people with a T-cell count of less than 350 cells/mm^3 or plasma HIV RNA levels exceeding 100,000 copies/mL (Guidelines, 2008). Some clinicians and patients, however, are choosing not to start medications until the CD4+ cell count decreases to approximately 200 cells/mm^3. Monitoring the National Institutes of Health (NIH) Web site (see Resources at the end of the chapter) for frequent updates of the recommendations is essential before caring for patients with HIV/AIDS (Guidelines, 2008).

Clinicians, in partnership with patients, make treatment decisions based on a number of factors, including CD4+ T-cell count, viral load, severity of HIV/AIDS-related symptoms, and willingness of the patient to adhere to the lifelong treatment regimen. The increasing number of antiretroviral agents (Table 52-3) and the rapid evolution of new information have introduced extraordinary complexity into the treatment of HIV infection. More than 25 agents have been approved in the United States. Drugs from established classes (nucleoside/nucleotide reverse transcriptase inhibitors [NRTIs], non-nucleoside reverse transcriptase inhibitors [NNRTIs], and **protease inhibitors [PIs]**) continue to serve as the mainstays of antiretroviral therapy (Kuritzkes, 2008). In 2008, the integrate inhibitor (raltegravir [Isentress]) and the CCR5 antagonist (maraviroc [Selzentry]), a novel entry inhibitor, were approved and joined the other fusion inhibitors such as enfuvirtide (T-20), which inhibits entry of HIV into the CD4+ T cell (Moyle, Gatell, Perno, et al., 2008). In patients with resistant HIV disease, these new classes of antiretroviral agents offer considerable potential benefit because of the absence of cross-resistance (Cooper, Steigbiegel, Gatell, et al., 2008).

To achieve sustained viral suppression, patients must take more than one antiretroviral medication. Although HAART was defined originally as a regimen that included at least one PI, it has evolved to include any regimen with at least two to three different medications. Some pharmaceutical companies have combined two to three agents into one tablet or capsule, such as Kaletra (lopinavir and ritonavir) and Atripla (efavirenz, emtricitabine, and tenofovir) in a single tablet for once-a-day use. Simplifying treatment regimens and decreasing the number of medications that must be taken each day may increase patients' adherence to therapy.

Adherence to long-term treatment is required to manage HIV infection and many other chronic illnesses; however, overall adherence rates remain low (30% to 50%). Although antiretroviral regimens have become less complex, side effects create barriers to adherence, and this can lead to viral resistance. The goals of treatment include maximal and sustained suppression of viral load to a nondetectable level, restoration or preservation of immunologic function, improved quality of life, and reduction of HIV-related morbidity and mortality. Viral load testing is recommended at the time of diagnosis of HIV disease and every 3 to 4 months thereafter in the untreated person; T-cell counts should be measured at diagnosis and usually every 3 to 6 months thereafter (Guidelines, 2008). In the majority of patients, HAART leads to sustained reductions in HIV replication, a rise in CD4+ T-cell counts with reconstitution of immune function, and significant reductions in morbidity and mortality.

It is difficult to predict patients' adherence to medication regimens, but a positive relationship between the patient and health care provider is associated with better adherence. Individualized plans of care that take into consideration housing and social support issues, in addition to health indicators, are essential. Adherence to the antiretroviral treatment plan involves very complex behavior that can change over the duration of the medication regimen. Self-reported adherence measures can distinguish clinically meaningful patterns of medication-taking behaviors; therefore, nurses should ask patients if they are taking their medications as prescribed. Factors associated with nonadherence include active substance abuse, depression, and lack of social support. Gender, race, pregnancy, and history of past substance use have not been associated with nonadherence (Guidelines, 2008). Chart 52-7 summarizes various strategies that health care providers can encourage to promote

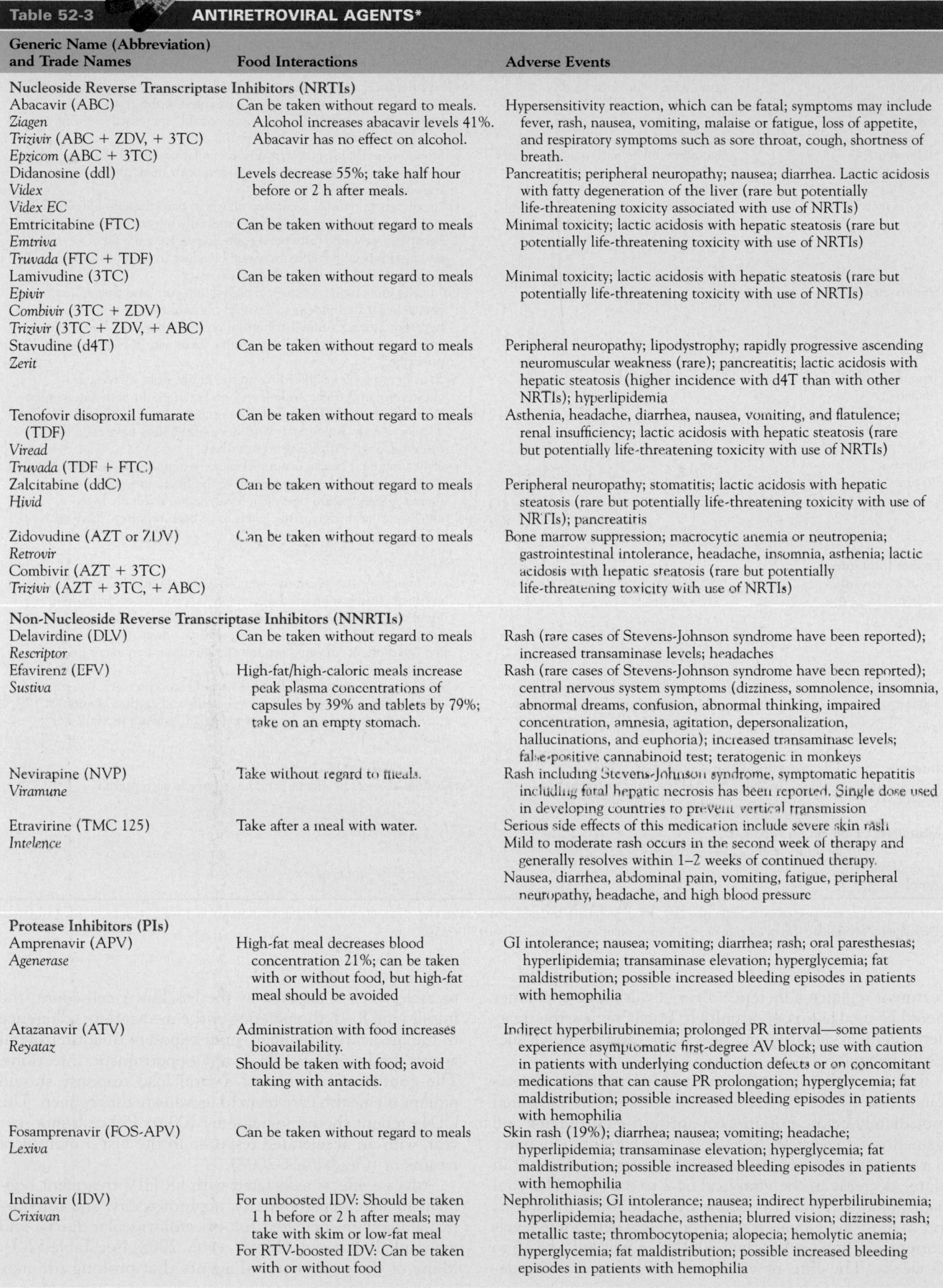

Table 52-3 | **ANTIRETROVIRAL AGENTS***

Generic Name (Abbreviation) and Trade Names	Food Interactions	Adverse Events
Nucleoside Reverse Transcriptase Inhibitors (NRTIs)		
Abacavir (ABC) *Ziagen* *Trizivir* (ABC + ZDV, + 3TC) *Epzicom* (ABC + 3TC)	Can be taken without regard to meals. Alcohol increases abacavir levels 41%. Abacavir has no effect on alcohol.	Hypersensitivity reaction, which can be fatal; symptoms may include fever, rash, nausea, vomiting, malaise or fatigue, loss of appetite, and respiratory symptoms such as sore throat, cough, shortness of breath.
Didanosine (ddl) *Videx* *Videx EC*	Levels decrease 55%; take half hour before or 2 h after meals.	Pancreatitis; peripheral neuropathy; nausea; diarrhea. Lactic acidosis with fatty degeneration of the liver (rare but potentially life-threatening toxicity associated with use of NRTIs)
Emtricitabine (FTC) *Emtriva* *Truvada* (FTC + TDF)	Can be taken without regard to meals	Minimal toxicity; lactic acidosis with hepatic steatosis (rare but potentially life-threatening toxicity with use of NRTIs)
Lamivudine (3TC) *Epivir* *Combivir* (3TC + ZDV) *Trizivir* (3TC + ZDV, + ABC)	Can be taken without regard to meals	Minimal toxicity; lactic acidosis with hepatic steatosis (rare but potentially life-threatening toxicity with use of NRTIs)
Stavudine (d4T) *Zerit*	Can be taken without regard to meals	Peripheral neuropathy; lipodystrophy; rapidly progressive ascending neuromuscular weakness (rare); pancreatitis; lactic acidosis with hepatic steatosis (higher incidence with d4T than with other NRTIs); hyperlipidemia
Tenofovir disoproxil fumarate (TDF) *Viread* *Truvada* (TDF + FTC)	Can be taken without regard to meals	Asthenia, headache, diarrhea, nausea, vomiting, and flatulence; renal insufficiency; lactic acidosis with hepatic steatosis (rare but potentially life-threatening toxicity with use of NRTIs)
Zalcitabine (ddC) *Hivid*	Can be taken without regard to meals	Peripheral neuropathy; stomatitis; lactic acidosis with hepatic steatosis (rare but potentially life-threatening toxicity with use of NRTIs); pancreatitis
Zidovudine (AZT or ZDV) *Retrovir* *Combivir* (AZT + 3TC) *Trizivir* (AZT + 3TC, + ABC)	Can be taken without regard to meals	Bone marrow suppression; macrocytic anemia or neutropenia; gastrointestinal intolerance, headache, insomnia, asthenia; lactic acidosis with hepatic steatosis (rare but potentially life-threatening toxicity with use of NRTIs)
Non-Nucleoside Reverse Transcriptase Inhibitors (NNRTIs)		
Delavirdine (DLV) *Rescriptor*	Can be taken without regard to meals	Rash (rare cases of Stevens-Johnson syndrome have been reported); increased transaminase levels; headaches
Efavirenz (EFV) *Sustiva*	High-fat/high-caloric meals increase peak plasma concentrations of capsules by 39% and tablets by 79%; take on an empty stomach.	Rash (rare cases of Stevens-Johnson syndrome have been reported); central nervous system symptoms (dizziness, somnolence, insomnia, abnormal dreams, confusion, abnormal thinking, impaired concentration, amnesia, agitation, depersonalization, hallucinations, and euphoria); increased transaminase levels; false-positive cannabinoid test; teratogenic in monkeys
Nevirapine (NVP) *Viramune*	Take without regard to meals.	Rash including Stevens-Johnson syndrome, symptomatic hepatitis including fatal hepatic necrosis has been reported. Single dose used in developing countries to prevent vertical transmission
Etravirine (TMC 125) *Intelence*	Take after a meal with water.	Serious side effects of this medication include severe skin rash Mild to moderate rash occurs in the second week of therapy and generally resolves within 1–2 weeks of continued therapy. Nausea, diarrhea, abdominal pain, vomiting, fatigue, peripheral neuropathy, headache, and high blood pressure
Protease Inhibitors (PIs)		
Amprenavir (APV) *Agenerase*	High-fat meal decreases blood concentration 21%; can be taken with or without food, but high-fat meal should be avoided	GI intolerance; nausea; vomiting; diarrhea; rash; oral paresthesias; hyperlipidemia; transaminase elevation; hyperglycemia; fat maldistribution; possible increased bleeding episodes in patients with hemophilia
Atazanavir (ATV) *Reyataz*	Administration with food increases bioavailability. Should be taken with food; avoid taking with antacids.	Indirect hyperbilirubinemia; prolonged PR interval—some patients experience asymptomatic first-degree AV block; use with caution in patients with underlying conduction defects or on concomitant medications that can cause PR prolongation; hyperglycemia; fat maldistribution; possible increased bleeding episodes in patients with hemophilia
Fosamprenavir (FOS-APV) *Lexiva*	Can be taken without regard to meals	Skin rash (19%); diarrhea; nausea; vomiting; headache; hyperlipidemia; transaminase elevation; hyperglycemia; fat maldistribution; possible increased bleeding episodes in patients with hemophilia
Indinavir (IDV) *Crixivan*	For unboosted IDV: Should be taken 1 h before or 2 h after meals; may take with skim or low-fat meal For RTV-boosted IDV: Can be taken with or without food	Nephrolithiasis; GI intolerance; nausea; indirect hyperbilirubinemia; hyperlipidemia; headache, asthenia; blurred vision; dizziness; rash; metallic taste; thrombocytopenia; alopecia; hemolytic anemia; hyperglycemia; fat maldistribution; possible increased bleeding episodes in patients with hemophilia

Continued on following page

Table 52-3	ANTIRETROVIRAL AGENTS* (Continued)	
Generic Name (Abbreviation) and Trade Names	**Food Interactions**	**Adverse Events**
Lopinavir + ritonavir (LPV/RTV) *Kaletra*	Should be taken with food	GI intolerance; nausea; vomiting; diarrhea; asthenia; hyperlipidemia (especially hypertriglyceridemia); elevated serum transaminase; hyperglycemia; fat maldistribution; possible increased bleeding episodes in patients with hemophilia
Nelfinavir (NFV) *Viracept*	Should be taken with a meal or snack	Diarrhea; hyperlipidemia; hyperglycemia; fat maldistribution; possible increased bleeding episodes in patients with hemophilia; serum transaminase elevation
Ritonavir (RTV) *Norvir*	Should be taken with food if possible; may improve tolerability	GI intolerance; nausea; vomiting; diarrhea; paresthesias—circumoral and extremities; hyperlipidemia, especially hypertriglyceridemia; hepatitis; asthenia; taste perversion; hyperglycemia; fat maldistribution; possible increased bleeding in patients with hemophilia. Lower doses used as a booster
Saquinavir (SQV) *Invirase*		GI intolerance; nausea; diarrhea; abdominal pain and dyspepsia; headache; hyperlipidemia; elevated transaminase enzymes; hyperglycemia; fat maldistribution; possible increased bleeding episodes in patients with hemophilia. Take with RTV as booster, if prescribed.
Tipranavir (TPV) *Aptivus*	Take with food	Serious liver problems, bleeding on the brain, rash, increased cholesterol and triglyceride levels, and changes in body fat; women taking birth control pills that contain estrogen may be more likely to develop a rash. Individuals with hemophilia may have increased bleeding. Take with RTV, if prescribed.
Darunavir *Prezista*		Diarrhea; nausea; headache; and coldlike symptoms, including runny nose or sore throat; inflammation of the liver; abnormal liver function tests; severe skin rash; fever; and abnormally high cholesterol and triglyceride levels have been reported. Take with RTV.
Fusion Inhibitors		
Enfuvirtide (T-20) *Fuzeon*	Injected subcutaneously, so meals are not an issue	Local injection site reactions—almost 100% of patients (pain, erythema, induration, nodules and cysts, pruritus, ecchymosis); increased rate of bacterial pneumonia; hypersensitivity reaction—symptoms may include rash, fever, nausea, vomiting, chills, rigors, hypotension, or elevated serum transaminases; may recur on challenge
Maraviroc *Selzentry*	Taken with or without food; requires CCR5 tropism blood test before starting	Cough, fever, dizziness, headache, lowered blood pressure, nausea, and bladder irritation; possible liver problems and cardiac events; an increased risk for some infections; a slight increase in cholesterol levels
Integrase Strand Transfer Inhibitor		
Raltegravir *Isentress*	No food restrictions identified	Diarrhea, nausea, headache, and fever have been reported.
Multiclass Combination Products		
Efavirenz, emtricitabine, and tenofovir *Atripla*		

*This information changes often. Check the U.S. Food and Drug Administration Web site (www.fda.gov/oashi/aids/virals.html) and www.aidsinfo.nih.gov/DrugsNew/Default.aspx?MenuItem=Drugs for current information when caring for people with HIV/AIDS.

treatment regimen adherence. Every health care encounter should be used as an opportunity to briefly review the treatment regimen, identify any new issues, and reinforce successful behaviors.

Results of therapy are evaluated with viral load tests (Guidelines, 2008). Viral load levels should be measured immediately before initiation of antiretroviral therapy and again after 2 to 8 weeks, because in most patients adherence to a regimen of potent antiretroviral agents should result in a large decrease in the viral load by 2 to 8 weeks. The viral load should continue to decline over the following weeks, and in most individuals it will drop below detectable levels (currently defined as less than 50 RNA copies/mL) by 16 to 20 weeks. The rate of viral load decline toward unde-

tectable levels is affected by the baseline T-cell count, the initial viral load, the potency of the medication, adherence to the medication regimen, prior exposure to antiretroviral agents, and the presence of any opportunistic infections. The confirmed absence of a viral load response should prompt the health care team to reevaluate the regimen. The CD4+ count should increase by 100 to 150 cells/mm^3 per year, with an accelerated response in the first 3 months of treatment (Guidelines, 2008).

Adverse effects associated with all HIV treatment regimens include hepatotoxicity, nephrotoxicity, and osteopenia, along with increased risk of cardiovascular disease and myocardial infarction (Moyle, et al., 2008) (see Table 52-3). Many of the antiretroviral agents that prolong life may simultaneously cause fat redistribution syndrome and metabolic alterations such as dyslipidemia and insulin resistance, which put the patient at risk for early-onset heart disease and diabetes (Calza, Manfredi, Pocaterra, et al., 2008). The fat redistribution syndrome consists of lipoatrophy (localized subcutaneous fat loss in the face, arms, legs, and buttocks) and lipohypertrophy (central visceral fat [lipomata] accumulation in the abdomen, although possibly in the breasts, dorsocervical region [buffalo hump], and within the muscle and liver) (Calza, et al., 2008). These changes can be very disturbing to the body image of people living with HIV/AIDS and may be a reason that they decline treatment, especially with regimens that include a PI.

Facial wasting, characterized as a sinking of the cheeks, eyes, and temples caused by the loss of fat tissue under the skin, may be treated by injectable fillers such as poly-L-lactic acid (Sculptra) (Fig. 52-2). Hepatotoxicity associated with certain protease inhibitors may limit the use of these agents, especially in patients with underlying liver dysfunction (Guidelines, 2008).

Drug Resistance

Drug resistance can be broadly defined as the ability of pathogens to withstand the effects of medications that are intended to be toxic to them. There are two major components of antiretroviral drug resistance: (1) transmission of drug-resistant HIV at the time of initial infection and (2) selective drug resistance in patients who are receiving nonsuppressive regimens (Kuritzkes, 2008). Factors associated with the development of drug resistance include monother-

apy (taking one medication), difficulty with adherence to complex and toxic regimens, and initiation of therapy late in the course of HIV/AIDS.

Resistance testing has a number of limitations and is more helpful in determining which antiretroviral agents should be eliminated rather than which ones should be used. Genotypic testing determines the sequence of viral RNA encoding relevant genes, which allows detection of amino acid mutations that are either proven or suspected to

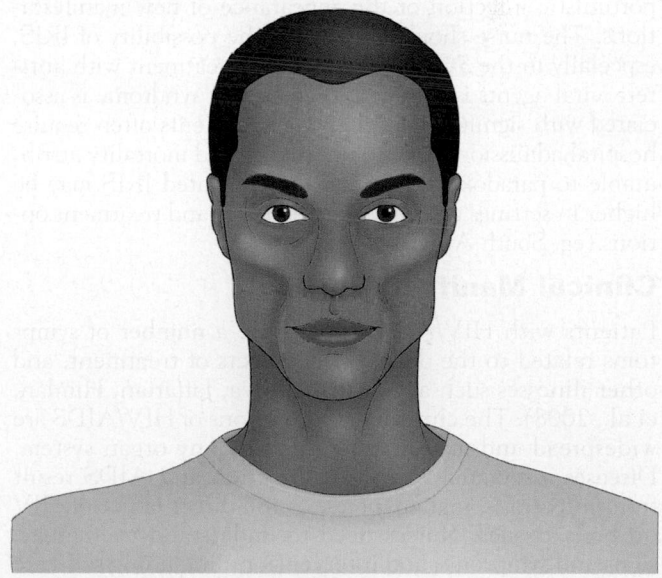

Figure 52-2 Facial lipoatrophy.

be associated with phenotypic resistance. Phenotypic testing determines the drug concentration needed to inhibit replication of a recombinant virus by 50% of a patient's isolate, when compared with a susceptible reference. Resistance testing is of greatest value when it is performed before drugs are discontinued or immediately afterward (within 4 weeks). Drug resistance testing is not advised for patients with a viral load of less than 1000 copies/mL, because the amount of the virus in the blood is too small to ensure reliable results (Guidelines, 2008).

In addition to resistance testing, several factors must be considered in choosing medications for a new regimen, once the prior regimen has failed. These factors include the patient's past treatment history, viral load, and medication tolerance; the likelihood of the patient's adhering to the medication regimen; and concomitant medical conditions or medications.

Treatment Interruption

Discontinuation of antiretroviral therapy may result in viral rebound, immune decompensation, and clinical progression. Unplanned interruption of antiretroviral therapy may become necessary because of severe drug toxicity, intervening illness, surgery that precludes oral therapy, pregnancy, or unavailability of antiretroviral medications. Planned treatment interruption, outside of clinical research trials, is not recommended (Guidelines, 2008).

Immune Reconstitution Inflammatory Syndrome

Immune reconstitution inflammatory syndrome (IRIS) results from rapid restoration of pathogen-specific immune responses to opportunistic infections that cause either the deterioration of a treated infection or new presentation of a subclinical infection. This syndrome typically occurs during the initial months after beginning antiretroviral treatment and is associated with a wide spectrum of pathogens, most commonly mycobacteria, herpes viruses, and deep fungal infections (Meintjes, Lawn, Scano, et al., 2008). IRIS is characterized by fever, respiratory and/or abdominal symptoms, and worsening of the clinical manifestations of an opportunistic infection or the appearance of new manifestations. The nurse should be alert to the possibility of IRIS, especially in the 3-month period after treatment with antiretroviral agents is initiated, because this syndrome is associated with significant morbidity and patients often require hospital admission. Rates of morbidity and mortality attributable to paradoxical tuberculosis-associated IRIS may be higher in settings with limited diagnostic and treatment options (eg, South Africa).

Clinical Manifestations

Patients with HIV/AIDS experience a number of symptoms related to the disease, side effects of treatment, and other illnesses such as hepatitis (Bova, Jaffarian, Himlan, et al., 2008). The clinical manifestations of HIV/AIDS are widespread and may involve virtually any organ system. Diseases associated with HIV infection and AIDS result from infections, malignancies, or the direct effect of HIV on body tissues. Nurses need to understand the causes, signs and symptoms, and interventions, including self-care strategies, that can enhance the quality of life for patients

throughout the illness. Symptom assessment tools can be used to assess patients' symptom intensity and severity. People with HIV/AIDS use a variety of self-care strategies to minimize common symptoms, which can arise from HIV disease, comorbidities, or the effects of medications used to treat HIV and opportunistic infections.

Fatigue is frequently cited by people living with HIV/AIDS as one of the most bothersome symptoms. It has a multifactorial etiology. For more information about fatigue in HIV, see Chart 52-8.

Respiratory Manifestations

Shortness of breath, dyspnea (labored breathing), cough, chest pain, and fever are associated with various opportunistic infections, such as those caused by *P. jiroveci*, *Mycobacterium avium-intracellulare*, CMV, and *Legionella* species.

Pneumocystis Pneumonia

The most common infection in people with AIDS is ***Pneumocystis* pneumonia (PCP),** which is caused by *P. jiroveci*. It is the most common opportunistic infection associated with AIDS. Without prophylactic therapy (discussed later), 80% of all people infected with HIV will develop PCP.

The clinical presentation of PCP in HIV infection is generally less acute than in people who are immunosuppressed as a result of other conditions. The time between the onset of symptoms and the actual documentation of disease may be weeks to months. Patients with AIDS initially develop nonspecific signs and symptoms, such as nonproductive cough, fever, chills, shortness of breath, dyspnea, and occasionally chest pain. PCP may be present despite the absence of crackles. Arterial oxygen concentrations in patients who are breathing room air may be mildly decreased, indicating minimal hypoxemia.

If left untreated, PCP eventually progresses and causes significant pulmonary impairment and, ultimately, respiratory failure. A few patients have a dramatic onset and a fulminating course involving severe hypoxemia, cyanosis, tachypnea, and altered mental status. Respiratory failure can develop within 2 to 3 days after the initial appearance of symptoms.

PCP can be diagnosed definitively by identifying the organism in lung tissue or bronchial secretions. This is accomplished by such procedures as sputum induction, bronchial-alveolar lavage, and transbronchial biopsy (by fiberoptic bronchoscopy).

Mycobacterium avium Complex

***Mycobacterium avium* complex (MAC)** disease is a common opportunistic infection in people with AIDS. MAC comprises a group of acid-fast bacilli (mycobacteria) that includes *M. avium*, *M. intracellulare*, and *M. scrofulaceum*. MAC usually causes respiratory infection but is also commonly found in the gastrointestinal tract, lymph nodes, and bone marrow. Most patients with AIDS who have T-cell counts lower than 100 cells/mm^3 have widespread disease at diagnosis and are debilitated. MAC infections are associated with rising mortality rates.

Tuberculosis

In HIV-negative people with latent tuberculosis (TB) infection, the *lifetime* risk of developing active TB disease is

| CHART 52-8 | NURSING RESEARCH PROFILE
HIV-Related Fatigue |

Barroso, J., Pence, B., Salahuddin, N., et al. (2008). Physiological correlates of HIV-related fatigue. *Clinical Nursing Research, 17*(1), 5–19.

Purpose

Symptom management in people with HIV infection is an increasingly pressing concern. The most frequent and debilitating symptom of HIV is fatigue, which has been defined as "awareness of a decreased capacity for physical and/or mental activity due to an imbalance in the availability, utilization, and/or restoration of resources needed to perform activity" (p. 6).

Design

This study used a longitudinal, repeated-measures design over a 3-year period with a total of seven study visits. The researchers investigated the cross-sectional relationship between fatigue and a wide range of physiologic characteristics in a sample of 128 HIV-positive individuals. Participants completed the HIV-related Fatigue Scale (HRFS), which consists of two subscales: (1) fatigue intensity and (2) impact of fatigue on daily functioning. After completion of the HRFS, blood was drawn to measure hepatic function, thyroid function, HIV viral load, immunologic function, gonadal function, hematologic function, and cellular injury.

Findings

None of the physiologic variables was significantly correlated with the HRFS scales in multivariate linear regression after controlling for income and years since HIV diagnosis. Income and years of HIV infection were more correlated with fatigue than any of the physiologic measures. Most of the participants had moderate fatigue.

Nursing Implications

Although fatigue is a common symptom that affects daily functioning and quality of life, and it was expected that physiologic variables such as viral load, liver function, and thyroid levels would be associated with fatigue, no statistically significant relationship was found. Fatigue affects the patient's ability to participate in activities of daily living such as grocery shopping and house cleaning and affects the patient's ability to maintain social relationships. Less income for people with HIV often means there are fewer choices and more energy is required to meet basic needs. The relationship between the length of time that patients have been HIV positive and have had fatigue might be a result of patients simply growing tired of living with the day-to-day challenges of HIV infection.

Until a better cause of fatigue is identified and treatments are developed, nurses need to help patients cope with this feeling of profound exhaustion. Nurses need to assist patients to create daily schedules around their periods of maximum energy and to assure them that fatigue is not necessarily associated with getting sicker. Nurses can support patients in accessing resources and also provide the emotional support needed to cope with an unpredictable chronic illness.

5% to 10%, whereas in HIV-positive people with latent TB, the *annual* risk is 10%. TB can develop in the lungs as well as in extrapulmonary sites such as the central nervous system (CNS), bone, pericardium, stomach, peritoneum, and scrotum. The CD4 T-cell count influences both the frequency and clinical picture of active TB disease. Important issues in the use of antiretroviral therapy in patients with active TB disease are (1) the sequencing of treatments, (2) the value of directly observed therapy, (3) risk of significant drug interactions with rifamycins, (4) the additive risk of hepatotoxicity and neuropathy associated with agents used to treat HIV and TB, (5) development of IRIS with TB after initiation of antiretroviral therapy, (6) the effect of antiretroviral therapy on results of tuberculin skin testing, and (7) the need for integration of therapy for HIV and TB (Guidelines, 2008).

Gastrointestinal Manifestations

The gastrointestinal manifestations of AIDS include loss of appetite, nausea, vomiting, oral and esophageal candidiasis, and chronic diarrhea. Diarrhea is a problem in 50% to 90% of all AIDS patients. Gastrointestinal symptoms may be related to the direct effect of HIV on the cells lining the intestines. Some of the enteric pathogens that occur most frequently, identified by stool cultures or intestinal biopsy, are *Cryptosporidium muris, Salmonella* species, *Isospora belli, Giardia lamblia,* CMV, *Clostridium difficile,* and M. *avium-intracellulare.* In patients with AIDS, the effects of diarrhea can be devastating in terms of profound weight loss (more than 10% of body weight), fluid and electrolyte imbalances, perianal skin excoriation, weakness, and inability to perform the usual activities of daily living.

Oral Candidiasis

Candidiasis, a fungal infection, occurs in almost all patients with AIDS and AIDS-related conditions. Commonly preceding other life-threatening infections, it is characterized by creamy-white patches in the oral cavity. If left untreated, oral candidiasis progresses to involve the esophagus and stomach. Associated signs and symptoms include difficult and painful swallowing and retrosternal pain. Some patients also develop ulcerating oral lesions and are particularly susceptible to dissemination of candidiasis to other body systems.

Wasting Syndrome

Wasting syndrome is part of the category C case definition for AIDS. Diagnostic criteria include profound involuntary weight loss exceeding 10% of baseline body weight and either chronic diarrhea for more than 30 days or chronic weakness and documented intermittent or constant fever in the absence of any concurrent illness that could explain these findings. This protein–energy malnutrition is multifactorial. In some AIDS-associated illnesses, patients experience a hypermetabolic state in which excessive calories are burned and lean body mass is lost. This state is similar to that seen in sepsis or trauma and can lead to organ failure. The distinction between cachexia (wasting) and malnutrition, or between cachexia and simple weight loss, is important, because the metabolic derangement seen in wasting syndrome may not be modified by nutritional support alone.

Anorexia, diarrhea, gastrointestinal malabsorption, and lack of nutrition in chronic disease all contribute to wasting syndrome. Progressive tissue wasting, however, may occur with only modest gastrointestinal involvement and without diarrhea. TNF and IL-1 are cytokines that play important roles in AIDS-related wasting syndrome. Both act directly on the hypothalamus to cause anorexia. Cytokine-induced fever accelerates the body's metabolism by 14% for every 1°F increase in temperature. TNF causes inefficient use of lipids by reducing enzymes that are needed for fat metabolism, whereas IL-1 triggers the release of amino acids from muscle tissue. People with AIDS generally experience increased protein metabolism in relation to fat metabolism, which results in significant decreases in lean body mass due to muscle and protein breakdown.

Hypertriglyceridemia, seen in people with AIDS and attributed to chronically elevated cytokine levels, can persist for months without tissue wasting and loss of lean body mass. It is believed that infections and sepsis lead to transient increases in TNF, IL-1, and other cell mediators above the chronically elevated levels that are often seen with AIDS. These transient increases in TNF and IL-1 trigger muscle wasting.

Oncologic Manifestations

Certain types of cancer occur often in people with AIDS. As a result, these cancers are considered AIDS-defining conditions; that is, their presence in a person infected with HIV is a clear sign that AIDS has developed. These AIDS-related cancers include Kaposi's sarcoma, lymphoma (especially non-Hodgkin lymphoma and primary central nervous system lymphoma), and invasive cervical cancer. With HAART, the incidence of both Kaposi's sarcoma and non-Hodgkin lymphoma has decreased considerably (Levine, 2008). Kaposi's sarcoma and lymphoma are discussed below. Cervical carcinoma is described later in Gynecologic Manifestations.

Kaposi's Sarcoma

Kaposi's sarcoma (KS), the most common HIV-related malignancy, is a disease that involves the endothelial layer of blood and lymphatic vessels. In people with AIDS, epidemic KS is most often seen among male homosexuals and bisexuals. AIDS-related KS exhibits a variable and aggressive course, ranging from localized cutaneous lesions to disseminated disease involving multiple organ systems. Cutaneous signs may be the first manifestation of HIV, appearing in more than 90% of HIV-infected patients as immune functions deteriorate. These skin signs correlate to low CD4+ counts. They can appear anywhere on the body and are usually brownish pink to deep purple. They may be flat or raised and surrounded by ecchymoses (hemorrhagic patches) and edema (Fig. 52-3). Rapid development of lesions involving large areas of skin is associated with extensive disfigurement. The location and size of some lesions can lead to venous stasis, lymphedema, and pain. Ulcerative lesions disrupt skin integrity and increase discomfort and

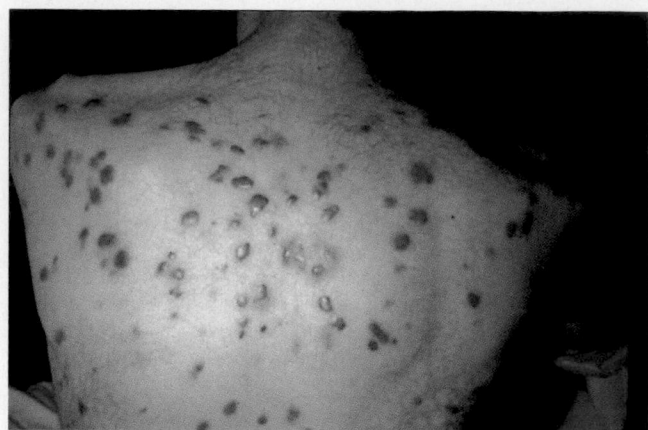

Figure 52-3 Lesions of the AIDS-related Kaposi's sarcoma. Whereas some patients may have lesions that remain flat, others experience extensively disseminated, raised lesions with edema. From DeVita Jr., V. T., Hellman, S. & Rosenberg, S. (Eds.). (1993). *AIDS: Etiology, diagnosis, treatment, and prevention* (4th ed.). Philadelphia: Lippincott Williams & Wilkins.

susceptibility to infection. The most common sites of visceral involvement are the lymph nodes, gastrointestinal tract, and lungs. Involvement of internal organs may eventually lead to organ failure, hemorrhage, infection, and death.

Diagnosis of KS is confirmed by biopsy of suspected lesions. Prognosis depends on the extent of the tumor, the presence of other symptoms of HIV infection, and the CD4+ count. Death may result from tumor progression. More often, however, it results from other complications of HIV infection.

B-Cell Lymphomas

B-cell lymphomas are the second most common malignancy occurring in people with AIDS. Lymphomas associated with AIDS usually differ from those occurring in the general population. Patients with AIDS are typically much younger than the usual population affected by non-Hodgkin lymphoma. In addition, AIDS-related lymphomas tend to develop outside the lymph nodes, most commonly in the brain, bone marrow, and gastrointestinal tract. These types of lymphomas are characteristically of a higher grade, indicating aggressive growth and resistance to treatment. The course of AIDS-related lymphomas includes multiple sites of organ involvement and complications related to opportunistic infections. Although aggressive combination chemotherapy is frequently successful in the treatment of non-Hodgkin lymphoma that is not associated with HIV infection, treatment is less successful in people with AIDS because of severe hematologic toxicity and complications of opportunistic infections that can occur from treatment.

Neurologic Manifestations

The advent of HAART greatly lowered the incidence of HIV dementia and increased the survival of people with HIV-associated neurocognitive disorders (McArthur, 2008). These disorders consist of cognitive impairment that is often accompanied by motor dysfunction and behavioral change. Neurologic dysfunction results from direct effects of

HIV on nervous system tissue, opportunistic infections, primary or metastatic neoplasms, cerebrovascular changes, metabolic encephalopathies, or complications secondary to therapy. Immune system response to HIV infection in the CNS includes inflammation, atrophy, demyelination, degeneration, and necrosis.

Peripheral Neuropathy

HIV-associated **peripheral neuropathy** is common across the trajectory of HIV disease and may occur in a variety of patterns, with distal sensory polyneuropathy (DSPN) or distal symmetric polyneuropathy the most frequently occurring type. DSPN occurs in advanced HIV disease as a result of immunosuppression, antiretroviral drug toxicity, and/or mitochondrial toxicity. It can lead to significant pain and decreased function (Nicholas, Voss, Corless, et al., 2007).

HIV Encephalopathy

HIV encephalopathy was formerly referred to as AIDS dementia complex (Chart 52-9). It is a clinical syndrome that is characterized by a progressive decline in cognitive, behavioral, and motor functions. Substantial evidence exists that HIV encephalopathy is a direct result of HIV infection. HIV has been found in the brain and cerebrospinal fluid (CSF) of patients with HIV encephalopathy. The brain cells infected by HIV are predominantly the CD4+ cells of monocyte-**macrophage** lineage. HIV infection is thought to trigger the release of toxins or lymphokines that result in cellular dysfunction or interference with neurotransmitter function rather than cellular damage.

Signs and symptoms may be subtle and difficult to distinguish from fatigue, depression, or the adverse effects of treatment for infections and malignancies. Early manifestations include memory deficits, headache, difficulty concentrating, progressive confusion, psychomotor slowing, apathy, and ataxia. Later stages include global cognitive impairments, delay in verbal responses, a vacant stare, spastic paraparesis, hyperreflexia, psychosis, hallucinations, tremor, incontinence, seizures, mutism, and death.

Confirming the diagnosis of HIV encephalopathy can be difficult. Extensive neurologic evaluation includes a computed tomography scan, which may indicate diffuse cerebral atrophy and ventricular enlargement. Other tests that may detect abnormalities include magnetic resonance imaging, analysis of CSF through lumbar puncture, and brain biopsy.

Cryptococcus neoformans

A fungal infection, *C. neoformans* is another common opportunistic infection among patients with AIDS, and it causes neurologic disease. Cryptococcal meningitis is characterized by symptoms such as fever, headache, malaise, stiff neck, nausea, vomiting, mental status changes, and seizures. Diagnosis is confirmed by CSF analysis.

Chart 52-9 • *Care of the Patient With HIV Encephalopathy*

Disturbed Thought Processes

- Assess mental status and neurologic functioning.
- Monitor for medication interactions, infections, electrolyte imbalance, and depression.
- Frequently orient the patient to time, place, person, reality, and the environment.
- Use simple explanations.
- Teach the patient to perform tasks in incremental steps.
- Provide memory aids (clocks and calendars).
- Provide memory aids for medication administration.
- Post activity schedule.
- Give positive feedback for appropriate behavior.
- Teach caretakers how to orient patient to time, place, person, reality, and the environment.
- Encourage the patient to designate a responsible person to assume power of attorney.

Disturbed Sensory Perception

- Assess sensory impairment.
- Decrease amount of stimuli in the patient's environment.
- Correct inaccurate perceptions.
- Provide reassurance and safety if the patient displays fear.
- Provide a secure and stable environment.
- Teach caregivers how to recognize inaccurate sensory perceptions.
- Teach caregivers techniques to correct inaccurate perceptions.
- Teach the patient and caregivers to report any changes in the patient's vision to the patient's health care provider.

Risk for Injury

- Assess the patient's level of anxiety, confusion, or disorientation.
- Assess the patient for delusions or hallucinations.
- Remove potentially dangerous objects from the patient's environment.
- Structure the environment for safety (ensure adequate lighting, avoid clutter, provide bed rails if needed).
- Supervise smoking.
- Do not let the patient drive a car if confusion is present.
- Instruct the patient and caregiver in home safety.
- Provide assistance as needed for ambulation and in getting in and out of bed.
- Pad headboard and side rails if the patient has seizures.

Self-Care Deficits

- Encourage activities of daily living within the patient's level of ability.
- Encourage independence but assist if the patient cannot perform an activity.
- Demonstrate any activity that the patient is having difficulty accomplishing.
- Monitor food and fluid intake.
- Weigh patient weekly.
- Encourage the patient to eat, and offer nutritious meals, snacks, and adequate fluids.
- If patient is incontinent, establish a routine toileting schedule.
- Teach caregivers how to meet the patient's self-care needs.

Progressive Multifocal Leukoencephalopathy

Progressive multifocal leukoencephalopathy (PML) is a demyelinating CNS disorder that affects the oligodendroglia. Clinical manifestations often begin with mental confusion and rapidly progress to include blindness, aphasia, muscle weakness, paresis (partial or complete paralysis), and death. Treatments have greatly reduced the threat of mortality associated with this disorder.

Other Neurologic Disorders

Other common infections involving the nervous system include *Toxoplasma gondii*, CMV, and *Mycobacterium tuberculosis* infections. Additional neurologic manifestations include both central and peripheral neuropathies. Vascular myelopathy is a degenerative disorder that affects the lateral and posterior columns of the spinal cord, resulting in progressive spastic paraparesis, ataxia, and incontinence.

Depressive Manifestations

The prevalence of depression among people with HIV infection is unknown. The causes of depression are multifactorial and may include a history of preexisting mental illness, neuropsychiatric disturbances, and psychosocial factors. Depression also occurs in people with HIV infection in response to the physical symptoms, including pain and weight loss, and the lack of someone to talk with about their concerns. People with HIV/AIDS who are depressed may experience irrational guilt and shame, loss of self-esteem, feelings of helplessness and worthlessness, and suicidal ideation.

Integumentary Manifestations

Cutaneous manifestations are associated with HIV infection and the accompanying opportunistic infections and malignancies. KS (described earlier) and opportunistic infections such as herpes zoster and herpes simplex are associated with painful vesicles that disrupt skin integrity. Molluscum contagiosum is a viral infection characterized by deforming plaque formation. Seborrheic dermatitis is associated with an indurated, diffuse, scaly rash involving the scalp and face. Patients with AIDS may also exhibit a generalized folliculitis associated with dry, flaking skin or atopic dermatitis, such as eczema or psoriasis. Up to 60% of patients treated with the antibacterial agent trimethoprim-sulfamethoxazole (TMP-SMZ) develop a drug-related rash that is pruritic with pinkish-red macules and papules. Patients with any of these rashes experience discomfort and are at increased risk for infection from disrupted skin integrity.

Endocrine Manifestations

The endocrine manifestations of HIV infection are not completely understood. At autopsy, endocrine glands show infiltration and destruction from opportunistic infections or neoplasms. Endocrine function may also be affected by therapeutic agents.

Gynecologic Manifestations

Persistent, recurrent vaginal candidiasis may be the first sign of HIV infection in women. Past or present genital ulcers are a risk factor for the transmission of HIV infection. Women with HIV infection are more susceptible to genital ulcers and venereal warts and have increased rates of incidence and recurrence of these conditions. Ulcerative sexually transmitted diseases (STDs) such as chancroid, syphilis, and herpes are more severe in women with HIV infection. **Human papillomavirus (HPV)** causes venereal warts and is a risk factor for cervical intraepithelial neoplasia, a cellular change that is frequently a precursor to cervical cancer. Women with HIV are 10 times more likely to develop cervical intraepithelial neoplasia than those not infected with HIV. There is a strong association between abnormal Papanicolaou (Pap) smears and HIV seropositivity. HIV-seropositive women with cervical carcinoma present at a more advanced stage of disease and have more persistent and recurrent disease and a shorter interval to recurrence and death than women without HIV infection.

A significant percentage of women who require hospitalization for pelvic inflammatory disease have HIV infection. Women with HIV are at increased risk for pelvic inflammatory disease, and the associated inflammation may potentiate the transmission of HIV infection. Moreover, women with HIV infection appear to have a higher incidence of menstrual abnormalities, including amenorrhea or bleeding between periods, than do women without HIV infection. The failure of health care providers to consider HIV infection in women may lead to a later diagnosis, thereby denying these patients appropriate treatment.

Medical Management

Treatment of Opportunistic Infections

Guidelines for the treatment of opportunistic infections should be consulted for the most current recommendations (Guidelines for Prevention and Treatment of Opportunistic Infections in HIV-Infected Adults and Adolescents [OI Guidelines], 2009). Despite the availability of antiretroviral medications, opportunistic infections (OIs) continue to cause considerable morbidity and mortality for three main reasons: (1) many patients are unaware of their HIV infection and present with an OI as the initial indicator of their disease, (2) some patients are aware of their HIV infection but do not take antiretroviral agents because of psychosocial or economic factors, and (3) others receive prescriptions for antiretroviral medications but fail to attain adequate virologic and immunologic response as a result of issues related to adherence, pharmacokinetics, or unexplained biologic factors (OI Guidelines, 2009).

Immune function should improve with initiation of HAART, resulting in faster resolution of the OI. This has been most clearly shown for OIs for which effective therapy does not exist, such as cryptosporidiosis, microsporidiosis, and PML. These conditions may resolve or at least stabilize after the institution of antiretroviral therapy as well as resolution of lesions of KS (OI Guidelines, 2009).

Pneumocystis Pneumonia

TMP-SMZ is the treatment of choice for PCP; it is as effective as parenteral pentamidine and more effective than other regimens. Oral outpatient therapy using TMP-SMZ is highly effective among patients with mild t-moderate PCP. Adjunctive corticosteroids should be started as early as possible and certainly within 72 hours after starting specific

PCP therapy. Alternative therapeutic regimens for patients with mild to moderate disease include (1) dapsone and TMP, (2) primaquine plus clindamycin, and (3) atovaquone suspension. Alternatives for patients with moderate to severe disease include (1) primaquine plus clindamycin or (2) IV pentamidine (generally the drug of second choice for severe disease; it can cause severe hypotension if it is administered too rapidly). Aerosolized pentamidine should not be used for the treatment of PCP because of limited efficacy and more frequent relapse. The recommended duration of therapy for PCP is 21 days (OI Guidelines, 2009). Adverse effects, in addition to hypotension, include impaired glucose metabolism leading to the development of diabetes mellitus from damage to the pancreas, renal damage, hepatic dysfunction, and neutropenia.

Mycobacterium Avium Complex

HIV-infected adults and adolescents should receive chemoprophylaxis against disseminated MAC disease if they have a CD4+ count less than 50 cells/μL. Azithromycin (Zithromax) or clarithromycin (Biaxin) are the preferred prophylactic agents. If azithromycin or clarithromycin cannot be tolerated, rifabutin is an alternative prophylactic agent for MAC disease, although drug interactions may make this agent difficult to use (OI Guidelines, 2009). Secondary prophylaxis for disseminated MAC may be discontinued in patients who have sustained increases in CD4 counts (greater than 100 cells/mm³; longer than 3 months) in response to HAART, have completed 12 months of MAC therapy, and have no signs or symptoms attributable to MAC.

Cryptococcal Meningitis

Cryptococcosis among patients with HIV infection most commonly occurs as a subacute meningitis or meningoencephalitis with fever, malaise, and headache. Current primary therapy for cryptococcal meningitis is IV amphotericin B with or without oral flucytosine (5-FC, Ancobon) or fluconazole (Diflucan). Serious potential adverse effects of amphotericin B include anaphylaxis, renal and hepatic impairment, electrolyte imbalances, anemia, fever, and severe chills (OI Guidelines, 2009).

Cytomegalovirus Retinitis

Retinitis caused by CMV is a leading cause of blindness in patients with AIDS. Oral valganciclovir, IV ganciclovir, IV ganciclovir followed by oral valganciclovir, IV foscarnet, IV cidofovir, and the ganciclovir intraocular implant coupled with valganciclovir are all effective treatments for CMV retinitis (OI Guidelines, 2009). A common adverse reaction to ganciclovir is severe neutropenia, which limits the concomitant use of zidovudine (AZT, Compound S, Retrovir). Common adverse reactions to foscarnet are nephrotoxicity, including acute renal failure, and electrolyte imbalances, including hypocalcemia, hyperphosphatemia, and hypomagnesemia, which can be life-threatening. Other common adverse effects include seizures, gastrointestinal disturbances, anemia, phlebitis at the infusion site, and low back pain. Possible bone marrow suppression (producing a decrease in white blood cell and platelet counts), oral candidiasis, and liver and renal impairments require close monitoring.

Other Infections

Oral acyclovir, famciclovir, or valacyclovir may be used to treat infections caused by herpes simplex or herpes zoster. Esophageal or oral candidiasis is treated topically with clotrimazole (Mycelex) oral troches or nystatin suspension. Chronic refractory infection with candidiasis (thrush) or esophageal involvement is treated with ketoconazole (Nizoral) or fluconazole (Diflucan).

Prevention of Opportunistic Infections

TMP-SMZ (Bactrim, Cotrim, Septra) is an antibacterial agent used to treat various organisms causing infection. It also confers cross-protection against toxoplasmosis and some common respiratory bacterial infections. People with HIV infection who have a T-cell count of less than 200 cells/mm³ should receive chemoprophylaxis with TMP-SMZ to prevent PCP. PCP prophylaxis can be safely discontinued in patients who are responding to HAART with a sustained increase in T lymphocytes.

Antidiarrheal Therapy

Although many forms of diarrhea respond to treatment, it is not unusual for this condition to recur and become a chronic problem for the patient with HIV infection. Therapy with octreotide acetate (Sandostatin), a synthetic analogue of somatostatin, has been shown to be effective in managing chronic severe diarrhea. High concentrations of somatostatin receptors have been found in the gastrointestinal tract and in other tissues. Somatostatin inhibits many physiologic functions, including gastrointestinal motility and intestinal secretion of water and electrolytes.

Chemotherapy

Kaposi's Sarcoma

Management of KS is usually difficult because of the variability of symptoms and the organ systems involved. KS is rarely life-threatening except when there is pulmonary or gastrointestinal involvement. The treatment goals are to reduce symptoms by decreasing the size of the skin lesions, to reduce discomfort associated with edema and ulcerations, and to control symptoms associated with mucosal or visceral involvement. No one treatment has been shown to increase survival. Radiation therapy is effective as a palliative measure to relieve localized pain due to tumor mass (especially in the legs) and for KS lesions that are in sites such as the oral mucosa, conjunctiva, face, and soles of the feet.

Interferon is known for its antiviral and antitumor effects. Patients with cutaneous KS treated with **alpha-interferon** have experienced tumor regression and improved immune system function. Alpha-interferon is administered by the IV, intramuscular, or subcutaneous route. Patients may self-administer interferon at home or receive interferon in an outpatient setting.

Lymphoma

Successful treatment of AIDS-related lymphomas has been limited because of the rapid progression of these malignancies. Combination chemotherapy and radiation therapy regimens may produce an initial response, but it is usually short-lived. Because standard regimens for non-AIDS lymphomas have been ineffective, many clinicians suggest that AIDS-related lymphomas should be studied as a separate group in clinical trials.

Antidepressant Therapy

Treatment for depression in people with HIV infection involves psychotherapy integrated with pharmacotherapy. If depressive symptoms are severe and of sufficient duration, treatment with antidepressants may be initiated. Antidepressants such as imipramine (Tofranil), desipramine (Norpramin), and fluoxetine (Prozac) may be used, because these medications also alleviate the fatigue and lethargy that are associated with depression. A psychostimulant such as methylphenidate (Ritalin) may be used in low doses in patients with neuropsychiatric impairment. Electroconvulsive therapy may be an option for patients with severe depression who do not respond to pharmacologic interventions.

Nutrition Therapy

Malnutrition increases the risk of infection and the incidence of opportunistic infections. Nutrition therapy should be part of the overall management plan and should be tailored to meet the nutritional needs of the patient, whether by oral diet, enteral tube feedings, or parenteral nutritional support, if needed. As with all patients, a healthy diet is essential for the patient with HIV infection. For patients with diarrhea, a diet low in fat, lactose, insoluble fiber, and caffeine and high in soluble fiber is helpful (Anastasi, Capili, Kim, et al., 2006). For all patients with AIDS who experience unexplained weight loss, calorie counts should be obtained to evaluate nutritional status and initiate appropriate therapy. The goal is to maintain the ideal weight and, when necessary, to increase weight.

Appetite stimulants have been successfully used in patients with AIDS-related anorexia. Megestrol acetate (Megace), a synthetic oral progesterone preparation, promotes significant weight gain and inhibits cytokine IL-1 synthesis. In patients with HIV infection, it increases body weight primarily by increasing body fat stores. Dronabinol (Marinol), which is a synthetic tetrahydrocannabinol (THC), the active ingredient in marijuana, has been used to relieve nausea and vomiting associated with cancer chemotherapy. After beginning dronabinol therapy, almost all patients with HIV infection experience a modest weight gain. The effects on body composition are unknown.

Oral supplements may be used to supplement diets that are deficient in calories and protein. Ideally, oral supplements should be lactose-free (many people with HIV infection are intolerant to lactose), high in calories and easily digestible protein, low in fat with the fat easily digestible, palatable, inexpensive, and tolerated without causing diarrhea. Advera is a nutritional supplement that has been developed specifically for people with HIV infection and AIDS. Parenteral nutrition is the final option because of its prohibitive cost and associated risks, including risk of infections.

Complementary and Alternative Modalities

Traditional Western medicine focuses on the treatment of disease. These treatments or interventions are taught in medical schools and are used by physicians in the care of patients. Complementary and alternative medicine (CAM) is often viewed as consisting of unconventional and unorthodox treatments or interventions that are not traditionally taught in medical schools. These modalities and therapies stress the need to treat the whole person, recognizing the interaction of the body, mind, and spirit. What is considered to be CAM in one culture may actually be a traditional therapy in another. People with HIV infection report substantial use of CAM for symptom management (Andrade & Anderson, 2008). The use of CAM in HIV infection and AIDS often results because of disillusionment with standard medical treatment, which to date has provided no cure. Combined with traditional therapies, CAM may improve the patient's overall well-being. However, there can be adverse drug–drug interactions between certain CAM therapies (eg, St. John's wort) and some antiretroviral medications.

CAM can be divided into four categories:

- Spiritual or psychological therapies may include humor, hypnosis, faith healing, guided imagery, and positive affirmations.
- Nutritional therapies may include vegetarian or macrobiotic diets, vitamin C or beta-carotene supplements, and turmeric, which contains curcumin, a food spice supplement. Chinese herbs, such as traditional herbal mixtures, are also used, in addition to compound Q (a Chinese cucumber extract) and *Momordica charantia* (bitter melon), which is given as an enema.
- Drug and biologic therapies include medications and other substances not approved by the FDA. Examples are N-acetylcysteine, pentoxifylline (Trental), and 1-chloro-2, 4-dinitrobenzene. Also included in this category are oxygen therapy, ozone therapy, and urine therapy.
- Treatment with physical forces and devices may include acupuncture, acupressure, massage therapy, reflexology, therapeutic touch, yoga, and crystals.

Although there is insufficient research on the effects of CAM, there is a growing body of literature reporting benefits for modalities involving nutrition, exercise, psychosocial treatment, and Chinese medicine.

Many patients who use these therapies do not report use of CAM to their health care providers. To obtain a complete health history, the nurse should ask about the patient's use of alternative therapies. Patients may need to be encouraged to report their use of CAM to their primary health care provider. Problems may arise, for example, when patients are using CAM while participating in clinical drug trials; alternative therapies can have significant adverse side effects, making it difficult to assess the effects of the medications in the clinical trial. The nurse needs to become familiar with the potential adverse side effects of these therapies. The nurse who suspects that CAM is causing a side effect needs to discuss this with the patient, the alternative therapy provider, and the primary health care provider. It is important for the nurse to view CAM with an open mind and to try to understand the importance of this treatment to the patient. This approach will improve communication with the patient and reduce conflict.

Supportive Care

Patients who are weak and debilitated as a result of chronic illness associated with HIV infection typically require many kinds of supportive care. Nutritional support may be as simple as providing assistance in obtaining or preparing meals. For patients with more advanced nutritional impairment resulting from decreased intake, wasting syndrome, or gastrointestinal malabsorption associated with diarrhea, parenteral feedings may be required. Imbalances that result from nausea, vomiting, and profuse diarrhea often necessitate IV fluid and electrolyte replacement.

Management of skin breakdown associated with KS, perianal skin excoriation, or immobility entails thorough and meticulous skin care that involves regular turning, cleansing, and applications of medicated ointments and dressings. To combat pain associated with skin breakdown, abdominal cramping, peripheral neuropathy, or KS, it is necessary to administer analgesic agents at regular intervals around the clock. Relaxation and guided imagery may be helpful in reducing pain and anxiety.

Pulmonary symptoms, such as dyspnea and shortness of breath, may be related to infection, KS, or fatigue. For patients with these symptoms, oxygen therapy, relaxation training, and energy conservation techniques may be effective. Patients with severe respiratory dysfunction may require mechanical ventilation. Before mechanical ventilation is instituted, the procedure is explained to the patient and the caregiver. If the patient decides to forgo mechanical ventilation, his or her wishes should be followed. Ideally, the patient has prepared an advance directive identifying preferences for treatments and end-of-life care, including hospice care. If the patient has not identified preferences in advance, treatment options are described so that the patient can make informed decisions and have those wishes respected.

NURSING PROCESS

THE PATIENT WITH HIV/AIDS

The nursing care of patients with AIDS is challenging because of the potential for any organ system to be the target of infections or cancer. In addition, this disease is complicated by many emotional, social, and ethical issues. The plan of care for the patient with AIDS (Chart 52-10) is individualized to meet the needs of the patient.

The scope and standards of HIV/AIDS nursing developed by the Association of Nurses in AIDS Care (2007) guide nursing practice. Care includes many of the interventions and concerns cited in the section on supportive care.

Assessment

Nursing assessment includes identification of potential risk factors, including a history of risky sexual practices or IV/injection drug use. The patient's physical status and psychological status are assessed. All factors affecting immune system functioning are thoroughly explored.

Nutritional Status

Nutritional status is assessed by obtaining a dietary history and identifying factors that may interfere with oral intake, such as anorexia, nausea, vomiting, oral pain, or difficulty swallowing. In addition, the patient's ability to purchase and prepare food is assessed. Weight history (ie, changes over time); anthropometric measurements; and blood urea nitrogen (BUN), serum protein, albumin, and transferrin levels provide objective measurements of nutritional status.

Skin Integrity

The skin and mucous membranes are inspected daily for evidence of breakdown, ulceration, or infection. The oral cavity is monitored for redness, ulcerations, and the presence of creamy-white patches indicative of candidiasis. Assessment of the perianal area for excoriation and infection in patients with profuse diarrhea is important. Wounds are cultured to identify infectious organisms.

Respiratory Status

Respiratory status is assessed by monitoring the patient for cough, sputum production (ie, amount and color), shortness of breath, orthopnea, tachypnea, and chest pain. The presence and quality of breath sounds are investigated. Other measures of pulmonary function include chest x-ray results, arterial blood gas values, pulse oximetry, and pulmonary function test results.

Neurologic Status

Neurologic status is determined by assessing level of consciousness; orientation to person, place, and time; and memory lapses. Mental status is assessed as early as possible to provide a baseline. The patient is also assessed for sensory deficits (visual changes, headache, or numbness and tingling in the extremities), motor involvement (altered gait, paresis, or paralysis), and seizure activity.

Fluid and Electrolyte Balance

Fluid and electrolyte status is assessed by examining the skin and mucous membranes for turgor and dryness. Dehydration may be indicated by increased thirst, decreased urine output, postural hypotension, weak and rapid pulse, and urine specific gravity of 1.025 or more. Electrolyte imbalances, such as decreased serum sodium, potassium, calcium, magnesium, and chloride, typically result from profuse diarrhea. The patient is assessed for signs and symptoms of electrolyte deficits, including decreased mental status, muscle twitching, muscle cramps, irregular pulse, nausea and vomiting, and shallow respirations.

Knowledge Level

The patient's level of knowledge about the disease and the modes of disease transmission is evaluated. In addition, the level of knowledge of family and friends is assessed. The patient's psychological reaction to the diagnosis of HIV infection or AIDS is important to explore. Reactions vary among patients and may include denial, anger, fear, shame, withdrawal from social interactions, and depression. It is often helpful to gain an understanding of how the patient has dealt with illness and major life stresses in the past. The patient's resources for support are also identified.

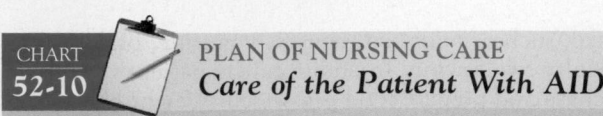

CHART
52-10

PLAN OF NURSING CARE
Care of the Patient With AIDS

NURSING DIAGNOSIS: Diarrhea related to enteric pathogens or HIV infection
GOAL: Resumption of usual bowel habits

Nursing Interventions	Rationale	Expected Outcomes
1. Assess patient's normal bowel habits.	1. Provides baseline for evaluation	• Exhibits return to normal bowel patterns
2. Assess for diarrhea: frequent, loose stools; abdominal pain or cramping, volume of liquid stools, and exacerbating and alleviating factors.	2. Detects changes in status, quantifies loss of fluid, and provides basis for nursing measures	• Reports decreasing episodes of diarrhea and abdominal cramping
3. Obtain stool cultures and administer antimicrobial therapy as prescribed.	3. Identifies pathogenic organism; therapy targets specific organism	• Identifies and avoids foods that irritate the gastrointestinal tract
4. Initiate measures to reduce hyperactivity of bowel:	4. Promotes bowel rest, which may decrease acute episodes	• Appropriate therapy is initiated as prescribed
a. Maintain food and fluid restrictions as prescribed. Suggest BRAT diet (*b*ananas, *r*ice, *a*pplesauce, *t*ea and *t*oast).	a. Reduces stimulation of bowel	• Exhibits normal stool cultures
b. Discourage smoking.	b. Eliminates nicotine, which acts as bowel stimulant	• Maintains adequate fluid intake
c. Avoid bowel irritants such as fatty or fried foods, raw vegetables, and nuts. Offer small, frequent meals.	c. Prevents stimulation of bowel and abdominal distention and promotes adequate nutrition	• Maintains body weight and reports no additional weight loss • States rationale for avoiding smoking • Enrolls in program to stop smoking • Uses medication as prescribed
5. Administer anticholinergic antispasmodics and opioids or other medications as prescribed.	5. Decreases intestinal spasms and motility	• Maintains adequate fluid status
6. Maintain fluid intake of at least 3 L/day unless contraindicated.	6. Prevents hypovolemia	• Exhibits normal skin turgor, moist mucous membranes, adequate urine output, and absence of excessive thirst

NURSING DIAGNOSIS: Risk for infection related to immunodeficiency
GOAL: Absence of infection

Nursing Interventions	Rationale	Expected Outcomes
1. Monitor for infection: fever, chills, and diaphoresis; cough; shortness of breath; oral pain or painful swallowing; creamy-white patches in oral cavity; urinary frequency, urgency, or dysuria; redness, swelling, or drainage from wounds; vesicular lesions on face, lips, or perianal area.	1. Allows for early detection of infection, essential for prompt initiation of treatment. Repeated and prolonged infections contribute to patient's debilitation.	• Identifies reportable signs and symptoms of infection
2. Teach patient or caregiver about need to report possible infection.	2. Allows early detection of infection	• Reports signs and symptoms of infection if present • Exhibits and reports absence of fever, chills, and diaphoresis
3. Monitor white blood cell count and differential.	3. Identifies elevated WBC possibly associated with infection	• Exhibits normal (clear) breath sounds without adventitious breath sounds
4. Obtain cultures of wound drainage, skin lesions, urine, stool, sputum, mouth, and blood as prescribed. Administer antimicrobial therapy as prescribed.	4. Assists in determining offending organism to initiate appropriate treatment	• Maintains weight • Reports adequate energy level without excessive fatigue • Reports absence of shortness of breath and cough
5. Instruct patient in ways to prevent infection:	5. Minimizes exposure to infection and transmission of HIV infection to others	• Exhibits pink, moist oral mucous membranes without fissures or lesions
a. Clean kitchen and bathroom surfaces with disinfectants.		• Takes appropriate therapy as prescribed
b. Clean hands thoroughly after exposure to body fluids.		• Experiences no infection
c. Avoid exposure to others' body fluids or sharing eating utensils.		• States rationale for strategies to avoid infection • Modifies activities to reduce exposure to infection or infectious persons
d. Turn, cough, and deep breathe, especially when activity is decreased.		• Practices "safer sex" • Avoids sharing eating utensils and toothbrush • Exhibits normal body temperature

Continued

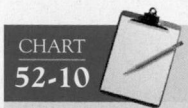

CHART 52-10

PLAN OF NURSING CARE
Care of the Patient With AIDS (Continued)

Nursing Interventions	Rationale	Expected Outcomes
e. Maintain cleanliness of perianal area. f. Avoid handling pet excreta or cleaning litter boxes, bird cages, or aquariums. g. Cook meat and eggs thoroughly. 6. Maintain aseptic technique when performing invasive procedures such as venipunctures, bladder catheterizations, and injections.	6. Prevents hospital-acquired infections	• Uses recommended techniques to maintain cleanliness of skin, skin lesions, and perianal area • Has others handle pet excreta and cleanup • Uses recommended cooking techniques

NURSING DIAGNOSIS: Ineffective airway clearance related to *Pneumocystis* pneumonia, increased bronchial secretions, and decreased ability to cough related to weakness and fatigue
GOAL: Improved airway clearance

Nursing Interventions	Rationale	Expected Outcomes

1. Assess and report signs and symptoms of altered respiratory status, tachypnea, use of accessory muscles, cough, color and amount of sputum, abnormal breath sounds, dusky or cyanotic skin color, restlessness, confusion, or somnolence.
2. Obtain sputum sample for culture prescribed. Administer antimicrobial therapy as prescribed.
3. Provide pulmonary care (cough, deep breathing, postural drainage, and vibration) every 2 to 4 hours.
4. Assist patient in attaining semi- or high Fowler's position.
5. Encourage adequate rest periods.
 	
6. Initiate measures to decrease viscosity of secretions:
  a. Maintain fluid intake of at least 3 L/day unless contraindicated.
  b. Humidify inspired air as prescribed.
  c. Consult with physician concerning use of mucolytic agents delivered through nebulizer or IPPB treatment.
7. Perform tracheal suctioning as needed.
8. Administer oxygen therapy as prescribed.
9. Assist with endotracheal intubation; maintain ventilator settings as prescribed.
	1. Indicates abnormal respiratory function
	
	2. Aids in identification of pathogenic organisms
	
	3. Prevents stasis of secretions and promotes airway clearance
	
	4. Facilities breathing and airway clearance
	5. Maximizes energy expenditure and prevents excessive fatigue
	6. Facilitates expectoration of secretions; prevents stasis of secretions
	
	7. Removes secretions if patient is unable to do so
	8. Increases availability of oxygen
	9. Maintains ventilation
		• Maintains normal airway clearance: Respiratory rate <20 breaths/min Unlabored breathing without use of accessory muscles and flaring nares (nostrils) Skin color pink (without cyanosis) Alert and aware of surroundings Arterial blood gas values normal Normal breath sounds without adventitious breath sounds
		• Begins appropriate therapy
		• Takes medication as prescribed
		• Reports improved breathing
		• Maintains clear airway
		• Coughs and takes deep breaths every 2–4 hours as recommended
		• Demonstrates appropriate positions and practices postural drainage every 2–4 hours
		• Reports reduced breathing difficulty when in semi- or high Fowler's position
		• Practices energy-conserving strategies and alternates rest with activity
		• Demonstrates reduction in thickness (viscosity) of pulmonary secretions
		• Reports increased ease in coughing up sputum
		• Uses humidified air or oxygen as prescribed and indicated
		• Indicates need for assistance with removal of pulmonary secretions
		• Understands need for and cooperates with endotracheal intubation and use of a mechanical ventilator
		• Verbalizes concerns about respiratory difficulty, intubation, and mechanical ventilation

NURSING DIAGNOSIS: Imbalanced nutrition, less than body requirements, related to decreased oral intake
GOAL: Improvement of nutritional status

Nursing Interventions	Rationale	Expected Outcomes
1. Assess for malnutrition with height, weight, age, BUN, serum protein, albumin, and transferrin levels, hemoglobin, hematocrit, and cutaneous anergy.	1. Provides objective measurement of nutritional status	• Identifies factors limiting oral intake and uses resources to promote adequate dietary intake

Continued on following page

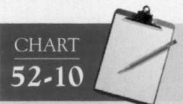

CHART 52-10

PLAN OF NURSING CARE
Care of the Patient With AIDS (Continued)

Nursing Interventions	Rationale	Expected Outcomes
2. Obtain dietary history, including likes and dislikes and food intolerances.	2. Defines need for nutritional education; helps individualize interventions	• Reports increased appetite
3. Assess factors that interfere with oral intake.	3. Provides basis and directions for interventions	• States understanding of nutritional needs
4. Consult with dietitian to determine patient's nutritional needs.	4. Facilitates meal planning	• Identifies ways to reduce factors that limit oral intake
5. Reduce factors limiting oral intake:	5. Addresses factors limiting intake:	• Rests before meals
a. Encourage patient to rest before meals.	a. Minimizes fatigue, which can decrease appetite	• Eats in pleasant, odor-free environment
b. Plan meals so that they do not occur immediately after painful or unpleasant procedures.	b. Decreases noxious stimuli	• Arranges meals to coincide with visitors' visits
c. Encourage patient to eat meals with visitors or others when possible.	c. Limits social isolation	• Reports increased dietary intake
		• Uses oral hygiene before meals
d. Encourage patient to prepare simple meals or to obtain assistance with meal preparation if possible.	d. Limits energy expenditure	• Takes analgesic agents before meals as prescribed
e. Serve small, frequent meals: 6 per day.	e. Prevents overwhelming patient	• Identifies ways to increase protein and caloric intake
f. Limit fluids 1 hour before meals and with meals.	f. Reduces satiety	• Identifies foods high in protein and calories
6. Instruct patient in ways to supplement nutrition: consume protein-rich foods (meat, poultry, fish) and carbohydrates (pasta, fruit, breads).	6. Provides additional proteins and calories	• Consumes foods high in protein and calories
		• Reports decreased rate of weight loss
7. Consult with physician and dietitian about alternative feeding (enteral or parenteral nutrition).	7. Provides nutritional support if patient is unable to take sufficient amounts by mouth	• Maintains adequate intake
		• States rationale for enteral or parenteral nutrition if needed
8. Consult with social worker or community liaison about financial assistance if patient cannot afford food.	8. Increases availability of resources and nutrition	• Demonstrates skill in preparing alternate sources of nutrition

NURSING DIAGNOSIS: Deficient knowledge related to means of preventing HIV transmission
GOAL: Increased knowledge concerning means of preventing disease transmission

Nursing Interventions	Rationale	Expected Outcomes
1. Instruct patient, family, and friends about routes of transmission of HIV.	1. Knowledge about disease transmission can help prevent spread of disease; may also alleviate fears.	• Patient, family, and friends state means of transmission.
2. Instruct patient, family, and friends about means of preventing transmission of HIV:	2. Reduces transmission risk	• Reports and demonstrates practices to reduce exposure of others to HIV
		• Demonstrates knowledge of safer sexual practices
a. Avoid sexual contact with multiple partners, and use precautions if sexual partner's HIV status is not certain.	a. The risk of infection increases with the number of sexual partners, male or female, and sexual contact with those who engage in high-risk behaviors.	• Identifies means of preventing disease transmission
		• States that sexual partners are informed about patient's positive HIV status in blood
b. Use condoms during sexual intercourse (vaginal, anal, oral–genital); avoid mouth contact with the penis, vagina, or rectum; avoid sexual practices that can cause cuts or tears in the lining of the rectum, vagina, or penis.	b. Risk of HIV transmission is reduced.	• Avoids IV/injection drug use and sharing of drug equipment with others
c. Avoid sex with sex workers and others at high risk.	c. Many sex workers are infected with HIV through sexual contact with multiple partners or IV/injection drug use.	

Continued

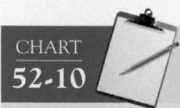

CHART 52-10	PLAN OF NURSING CARE

Care of the Patient With AIDS (Continued)

Nursing Interventions	Rationale	Expected Outcomes
d. Do not use IV/injection drugs; if addicted and unable or unwilling to change behavior, use clean needles and syringes. e. Women who may have been exposed to HIV through sexual or drug practices should consult with a physician before becoming pregnant; consider use of antiretroviral agents if pregnant.	d. Clean needles and syringes are the only way to prevent HIV transmission for those who continue to use drugs. Taking precautions is important for those who are antibody positive to prevent transmitting HIV. e. HIV can be transmitted from mother to child in utero; use of antiretroviral agents during pregnancy significantly reduces perinatal transmission of HIV.	

NURSING DIAGNOSIS: Social isolation related to stigma of the disease, withdrawal of support systems, isolation procedures, and fear of infecting others

GOAL: Decreased sense of social isolation

Nursing Interventions	Rationale	Expected Outcomes
1. Assess patient's usual patterns of social interaction. 2. Observe for behaviors indicative of social isolation, such as decreased interaction with others, hostility, noncompliance, sad affect, and stated feelings of rejection or loneliness. 3. Provide instruction concerning modes of transmission of HIV. 4. Assist patient to identify and explore resources for support and positive mechanisms for coping (eg, contact with family, friends, AIDS task force). 5. Allow time to be with patient other than for medications and procedures. 6. Encourage participation in diversional activities such as reading, television, or hand crafts.	1. Establishes basis for individualized interventions 2. Promotes early detection of social isolation, which may be manifested in several ways 3. Provides accurate information, corrects misconceptions, and alleviates anxiety 4. Enables mobilization of resources and supports 5. Promotes feelings of self-worth and provides social interaction 6. Provides distraction	• Shares with others the need for valued social interaction • Demonstrates interest in events, activities, and communication • Verbalizes feelings and reactions to diagnosis, prognosis, and life changes • Identifies modes of transmission of HIV • States ways of preventing transmission of AIDS virus to others while maintaining contact with valued friends and relatives • Reveals AIDS diagnosis to others when appropriate • Identifies resources (ie, family, friends, and support groups) • Uses resources when appropriate • Accepts offers of assistance and support • Reports decreased sense of isolation • Maintains contacts with those of importance to him or her • Develops or continues hobbies that effectively serve as diversion or distraction

COLLABORATIVE PROBLEMS: Opportunistic infections; impaired breathing; wasting syndrome and fluid and electrolyte imbalances; adverse reaction to medications

GOAL: Absence of complications

Nursing Interventions	Rationale	Expected Outcomes
Opportunistic Infections 1. Monitor vital signs. 2. Obtain laboratory specimens and monitor test results.	1. Changes in vital signs such as increases in pulse rate, respirations, blood pressure, and temperature may indicate infection. 2. Smears and cultures can identify causative agents such as bacteria, fungi, and protozoa, and sensitivity studies can identify antibiotics or other medications effective against the causative agent.	• Exhibits stable vital signs • Experiences control of infection • Identifies signs and symptoms correctly and experiences no complications • Identifies signs and symptoms that are reportable to the physician • Takes medications as prescribed

Continued on following page

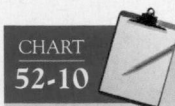

CHART 52-10

PLAN OF NURSING CARE
Care of the Patient With AIDS (*Continued*)

Nursing Interventions	Rationale	Expected Outcomes
3. Instruct the patient and caregiver about signs and symptoms of infection and the need to report them early.	3. Early recognition of symptoms facilitates prompt treatment and avoids extra complications.	
Impaired Breathing		
1. Monitor respiratory rate and pattern.	1. Rapid shallow breathing, diminished breath sounds, and shortness of breath may indicate respiratory failure resulting in hypoxia.	• Maintains stable respiratory rate and pattern within the normal limits
2. Auscultate the chest for breath sounds and abnormal lung sounds.	2. Crackles and wheezes may indicate fluid in the lungs, which disrupts respiratory function and alters the blood's oxygen-carrying capacity.	• Exhibits no adventitious lung sounds; normal breath sounds
3. Monitor pulse rate, blood pressure, and oxygen saturation levels.	3. Changes in pulse rate, blood pressure, and oxygen levels may indicate the development of respiratory or cardiac failure.	• Has stable pulse rate and blood pressure within normal limits, and exhibits no evidence of hypoxia
		• Oxygen saturation levels within acceptable range
Wasting Syndrome and Fluid and Electrolyte Disturbances		
1. Monitor weight and laboratory values for nutritional status.	1. Weight loss, malnutrition, and anemia are common in HIV infection and increase risk for superinfection.	• Maintains stable weight
		• Eats a nutritious diet
2. Monitor intake and output and laboratory values for fluid and electrolyte imbalance (potassium, sodium, calcium, phosphorus, magnesium, and zinc).	2. Chronic diarrhea, inadequate oral intake, vomiting, and profuse sweating deplete electrolytes. Small intestine inflammation may impair the absorption of fluids and electrolytes.	• Attains and maintains hemoglobin, hematocrit, and ferritin levels within normal limits
		• Sustains fluid and electrolyte balance within normal limits
3. Monitor for and report signs and symptoms of dehydration.	3. Fluid loss results in decreased circulating volume leading to tachycardia, dry skin and mucous membranes, poor skin turgor, elevated urine specific gravity, and thirst. Early detection allows early treatment.	• Exhibits no signs and symptoms of dehydration
Reactions to Medications		
1. Monitor for medication interactions.	1. People with HIV infection receive many medications for HIV and for disease complications. Early detection of medication interactions is necessary to prevent complications.	• Experiences no serious side effects or complications from medications
		• Correctly describes medication regimen and complies with therapy, including adaptations in eating routines and type of food used with prescribed medications
2. Monitor for and promptly report side effects from antiretroviral agents.	2. Side effects from antiretroviral agents can be life-threatening. Serious side effects include anemia, pancreatitis, peripheral neuropathy, mental confusion, and persistent nausea and vomiting. Corrective measures need to be instituted.	
3. Instruct the patient and caregiver in the medication regimen.	3. Knowledge of the medication purpose, correct administration, side effects, and strategies to manage or prevent side effects promote safety and greater compliance with treatment.	

Diagnosis

Nursing Diagnoses

The list of potential nursing diagnoses is extensive because of the complex nature of this disease. However, based on assessment data, major nursing diagnoses for the patient may include the following:

• Impaired skin integrity related to cutaneous manifestations of HIV infection, excoriation, and diarrhea
• Diarrhea related to enteric pathogens or HIV infection
• Risk for infection related to immunodeficiency
• Activity intolerance related to weakness, fatigue, malnutrition, impaired fluid and electrolyte balance, and hypoxia associated with pulmonary infections

- Disturbed thought processes related to shortened attention span, impaired memory, confusion, and disorientation associated with HIV encephalopathy
- Ineffective airway clearance related to PCP, increased bronchial secretions, and decreased ability to cough related to weakness and fatigue
- Pain related to impaired perianal skin integrity secondary to diarrhea, KS, and peripheral neuropathy
- Imbalanced nutrition, less than body requirements, related to decreased oral intake
- Social isolation related to stigma of the disease, withdrawal of support systems, isolation procedures, and fear of infecting others
- Anticipatory grieving related to changes in lifestyle and roles and unfavorable prognosis
- Deficient knowledge related to HIV infection, means of preventing HIV transmission, and self-care

Collaborative Problems/Potential Complications

Based on the assessment data, possible complications may include the following:
- Opportunistic infections
- Impaired breathing or respiratory failure
- Wasting syndrome and fluid and electrolyte imbalance
- Adverse reaction to medications

Planning and Goals

Goals for the patient may include achievement and maintenance of skin integrity, resumption of usual bowel patterns, absence of infection, improved activity tolerance, improved thought processes, improved airway clearance, increased comfort, improved nutritional status, increased socialization, expression of grief, increased knowledge regarding disease prevention and self-care, and absence of complications.

Nursing Interventions

Promoting Skin Integrity

The skin and oral mucosa are assessed routinely for changes in appearance, location and size of lesions, and evidence of infection and breakdown. The patient is encouraged to maintain a balance between rest and mobility whenever possible. Patients who are immobile are assisted to change position every 2 hours. Devices such as alternating-pressure mattresses and low-air-loss beds are used to prevent skin breakdown. Patients are encouraged to avoid scratching; to use nonabrasive, nondrying soaps; and to apply nonperfumed skin moisturizers to dry skin. Regular oral care is also encouraged.

Medicated lotions, ointments, and dressings are applied to affected skin surfaces as prescribed. Adhesive tape is avoided. Skin surfaces are protected from friction and rubbing by keeping bed linens free of wrinkles and avoiding tight or restrictive clothing. Patients with foot lesions are advised to wear cotton socks and shoes that do not cause the feet to perspire. Antipruritic, antibiotic, and analgesic agents are administered as prescribed.

The perianal region is assessed frequently for impairment of skin integrity and infection. The patient is instructed to keep the area as clean as possible. The perianal area is cleaned after each bowel movement with nonabrasive soap and water to prevent further excoriation and breakdown of the skin and infection. If the area is very painful, soft cloths or cotton sponges may be less irritating than washcloths. In addition, sitz baths or gentle irrigation may facilitate cleaning and promote comfort. The area is dried thoroughly after cleaning. Topical lotions or ointments may be prescribed to promote healing. Wounds are cultured if infection is suspected, so that the appropriate antimicrobial treatment can be initiated. Debilitated patients may require assistance in maintaining hygienic practices.

Promoting Usual Bowel Patterns

Bowel patterns are assessed for diarrhea. The nurse monitors the frequency and consistency of stools and the patient's reports of abdominal pain or cramping associated with bowel movements. Factors that exacerbate frequent diarrhea are also assessed. The quantity and volume of liquid stools are measured to document fluid volume losses. Stool cultures are obtained to identify pathogenic organisms.

The patient is counseled about ways to decrease diarrhea. The physician may recommend restriction of oral intake to rest the bowel during periods of acute inflammation associated with severe enteric infections. As the patient's dietary intake is increased, foods that act as bowel irritants, such as raw fruits and vegetables, popcorn, carbonated beverages, spicy foods, and foods of extreme temperatures, should be avoided. Small, frequent meals help to prevent abdominal distention. Medications, such as anticholinergic agents, antispasmodic, agents, or opioids, can be prescribed to decrease diarrhea by decreasing intestinal spasms and motility. Administering antidiarrheal agents on a regular schedule may be more beneficial than administering them on an as-needed basis. Antibiotics and antifungal agents may also be prescribed to combat pathogens identified by stool cultures. Assessment of self-care strategies being used is essential.

Preventing Infection

The patient and caregivers are instructed to monitor for signs and symptoms of infection: fever; chills; night sweats; cough with or without sputum production; shortness of breath; difficulty breathing; oral pain or difficulty swallowing; creamy-white patches in the oral cavity; unexplained weight loss; swollen lymph nodes; nausea; vomiting; persistent diarrhea; frequency, urgency, or pain on urination; headache; visual changes or memory lapses; redness, swelling, or drainage from skin wounds; and vesicular lesions on the face, lips, or perianal area. The nurse also monitors laboratory test results that indicate infection, such as the white blood cell count and differential. Cultures of specimens from wound drainage, skin lesions, urine, stool, sputum, mouth, and blood are obtained to identify pathogenic organisms and the most appropriate antimicrobial therapy. The patient is instructed to avoid others with active infections such as upper respiratory infections.

Improving Activity Tolerance

Activity tolerance is assessed by monitoring the patient's ability to ambulate and perform activities of daily living. Patients may be unable to maintain their usual levels of activity because of weakness, fatigue, shortness of breath, dizziness, and neurologic involvement. Assistance in planning daily routines that maintain a balance between activity and rest may be necessary. In addition, patients benefit from instructions about energy conservation techniques, such as sitting while washing or while preparing meals. Personal items that are frequently used should be kept within the patient's reach. Measures such as relaxation and guided imagery may be beneficial because they decrease anxiety, which contributes to weakness and fatigue.

Collaboration with other members of the health care team may uncover other factors associated with increasing fatigue and strategies to address them. For example, if fatigue is related to anemia, administering epoetin alfa (Epogen) as prescribed may relieve fatigue and increase activity tolerance.

Maintaining Thought Processes

The patient is assessed for alterations in mental status that may be related to neurologic involvement, metabolic abnormalities, infection, side effects of treatment, and coping mechanisms. Manifestations of neurologic impairment may be difficult to distinguish from psychological reactions to HIV infection, such as anger and depression.

If the patient experiences altered mental or cognitive status, family and support network members are instructed to speak to the patient in simple, clear language and give the patient sufficient time to respond to questions. The patient's support network is encouraged to orient the patient to the daily routine by talking about what is taking place during daily activities and encouraged to provide the patient with a regular daily schedule for medication administration, grooming, meal times, bedtimes, and awakening times. Posting the schedule in a prominent area (eg, on the refrigerator), providing night lights for the bedroom and bathroom, and planning safe leisure activities allow the patient to maintain a regular routine in a safe manner. Activities that the patient previously enjoyed are encouraged. These should be easy to accomplish and fairly short in duration. The nurse encourages the social support network to remain calm and not to argue with the patient while protecting the patient from injury. Around-the-clock supervision may be necessary, and strategies can be implemented to prevent the patient from engaging in potentially dangerous activities, such as driving, using the stove, or mowing the lawn. Strategies for improving or maintaining functional abilities and for providing a safe environment are used for patients with HIV encephalopathy (see Chart 52-9).

Improving Airway Clearance

Respiratory status, including rate, rhythm, use of accessory muscles, and breath sounds; mental status; and skin color must be assessed at least daily. Any cough and the quantity and characteristics of sputum are documented. Sputum specimens are analyzed for infectious organisms. Pulmonary therapy (coughing, deep breathing, postural drainage, percussion, and vibration) is provided as often as every 2 hours to prevent stasis of secretions and to promote airway clearance. Because of weakness and fatigue, many patients require assistance in attaining a position (such as a high Fowler's or semi-Fowler's position) that facilitates breathing

and airway clearance. Adequate rest is essential to minimize energy expenditure and prevent excessive fatigue. The fluid volume status is evaluated so that adequate hydration can be maintained. Unless contraindicated because of renal or cardiac disease, daily intake of 3 L of fluid is encouraged. Humidified oxygen may be prescribed, and nasopharyngeal or tracheal suctioning, intubation, and mechanical ventilation may be necessary to maintain adequate ventilation.

Relieving Pain and Discomfort

The patient is assessed for the quality and severity of pain associated with impaired perianal skin integrity, the lesions of KS, and peripheral neuropathy. In addition, the effects of pain on elimination, nutrition, sleep, affect, and communication are explored, along with exacerbating and relieving factors. Cleaning the perianal area, as previously described, can promote comfort. Topical anesthetic medications or ointments may be prescribed. Use of soft cushions or foam pads may increase comfort while sitting. The patient is instructed to avoid foods that act as bowel irritants. Antispasmodic and antidiarrheal medications may be prescribed to reduce the discomfort and frequency of bowel movements. If necessary, systemic analgesic agents may also be prescribed. Pain from KS is frequently described as a sharp, throbbing pressure, and heaviness, if lymphedema is present. Pain management may include use of nonsteroidal anti-inflammatory drugs (NSAIDs) and opioids plus nonpharmacologic approaches such as relaxation techniques. When NSAIDs are administered to patients who are receiving zidovudine, hepatic and hematologic status must be monitored.

The patient with pain related to peripheral neuropathy frequently describes it as burning, numbness, and "pins and needles." Pain management approaches may include opioids, tricyclic antidepressants, and anti-embolism stockings to equalize pressure. Tricyclic antidepressants have been found to be helpful in controlling the symptoms of neuropathic pain. They also potentiate the actions of opioids and can be used to relieve pain without increasing the dose of the opioid.

Improving Nutritional Status

Nutritional status is assessed by monitoring weight, dietary intake, and serum albumin, BUN, protein, and transferrin levels. The patient is also assessed for factors that interfere with oral intake, such as anorexia, oral and esophageal candidal infection, nausea, pain, weakness, fatigue, and lactose intolerance (Dudek, 2006). Based on the results of assessment, the nurse can implement specific measures to facilitate oral intake. The dietitian is consulted to determine the patient's nutritional requirements.

Control of nausea and vomiting with antiemetic medications administered on a regular basis may increase the patient's dietary intake. Inadequate food intake resulting from pain caused by oral lesions or a sore throat may be managed by administering prescribed opioids and viscous lidocaine (the patient is instructed to rinse the mouth and swallow). Additionally, the patient is encouraged to eat foods that are easy to swallow and to avoid rough, spicy, or sticky food items and foods that are excessively hot or cold. Oral hygiene before and after meals is encouraged. If fatigue and weakness interfere with intake, the nurse encourages the patient to rest before meals. If the patient is hospitalized, meals should be scheduled so that they do not occur immediately after painful or unpleasant procedures. The patient with diarrhea and abdominal cramping is encouraged to avoid foods that stimulate intestinal motility and abdominal distention, such as fiber-rich foods or lactose, if the patient is intolerant to lactose. The patient is instructed about ways to enhance the nutritional value of meals. Adding eggs, butter, or fortified milk (milk to which powdered skim milk has been added to increase the caloric content) to gravies, soups, or milkshakes can provide additional calories and protein. Supplements such as puddings, powders, milkshakes, and Advera (previously described) may also be useful (Dudek, 2006). Patients who cannot maintain their nutritional status through oral intake may require enteral feedings or parenteral nutrition.

Decreasing the Sense of Isolation

People with AIDS are at risk for double stigmatization. They have what society refers to as a "dreaded disease," and they may have a lifestyle that differs from what is considered acceptable by many people. Many people with AIDS are young adults at a developmental stage that is usually associated with establishing intimate relationships, personal goals, and career goals, as well as having and raising children. Their focus changes as they are faced with a disease that threatens their life expectancy with no cure. In addition, they may be forced to reveal hidden lifestyles or behaviors to family, friends, coworkers, and health care providers. As a result, people with HIV infection may be overwhelmed with emotions such as anxiety, guilt, shame, and fear. They also may be faced with multiple losses, such as loss of financial security; normal roles and functions; self-esteem; privacy; ability to control bodily functions; ability to interact meaningfully with the environment; and sexual functioning, as well as rejection by sexual partners, family, and friends. Some patients may harbor feelings of guilt because of their lifestyle or because they may have infected others in current or previous relationships. Other patients may feel anger toward sexual partners who transmitted the virus to them. Infection control measures used in the hospital or at home may further contribute to the patient's emotional isolation. Any or all of these stressors may cause the patient with AIDS to withdraw both physically and emotionally from social contact.

Nurses are in a key position to provide an atmosphere of acceptance and understanding for people with AIDS and their families and partners. The patient's usual level of social interaction is assessed as early as possible to provide a baseline for monitoring changes in behaviors that suggest social isolation (eg, decreased interaction with staff or family, hostility, nonadherence). Patients are encouraged to express feelings of isolation and loneliness, with the assurance that these feelings are not unique or abnormal.

Providing information about how to protect themselves and others may help patients avoid social isolation. Patients, family, and friends must be reassured that AIDS is not spread through casual contact. Education of ancillary personnel, nurses, and physicians helps reduce factors that might contribute to patients' feelings of isolation. Patient care conferences that address the psychosocial issues associated with AIDS may help sensitize the health care team to patients' needs.

Coping With Grief

The nurse can help the patient verbalize feelings and explore and identify resources for support and mechanisms for coping, especially when the patient is grieving anticipated losses. The patient is encouraged to maintain contact with family, friends, and coworkers and to use local or national AIDS support groups and hotlines. If possible, losses are identified and addressed. The patient is encouraged to continue usual activities whenever possible. Consultations with mental health counselors are useful for many patients.

Monitoring and Managing Potential Complications

OPPORTUNISTIC INFECTIONS. Patients who are immunosuppressed are at risk for opportunistic infections. Therefore, anti-infective agents may be prescribed and laboratory tests obtained to monitor their effect. Signs and symptoms of opportunistic infections, including fever, malaise, difficulty breathing, nausea or vomiting, diarrhea, difficulty swallowing, and any occurrences of swelling or discharge, should be reported as treated as indicated.

RESPIRATORY FAILURE. Impaired breathing is a major complication that increases the patient's discomfort and anxiety and may lead to respiratory and cardiac failure. The respiratory rate and pattern are monitored, and the lungs are auscultated for abnormal breath sounds. The patient is instructed to report shortness of breath and increasing difficulty in carrying out usual activities. Pulse rate and rhythm, blood pressure, and oxygen saturation are monitored. Suctioning and oxygen therapy may be prescribed to ensure an adequate airway and to prevent hypoxia. Mechanical ventilation may be necessary for the patient who cannot maintain adequate ventilation as a result of pulmonary infection, fluid and electrolyte imbalance, or respiratory muscle weakness. Arterial blood gas values are used to guide ventilator settings. If the patient is intubated, methods must be established to allow communication with the nurse and others. Attention must be given to assisting the patient receiving mechanical ventilation to cope with the stress associated with intubation and ventilator assistance. The possible need for mechanical ventilation in the future should be discussed early in the course of the disease, when the patient is able to make known his or her preferences about treatment. The use of mechanical ventilation should be consistent with the patient's decisions about end-of-life treatment. (Further discussion of end-of-life care can be found in Chapter 17.)

CACHEXIA AND WASTING. Wasting syndrome and fluid and electrolyte disturbances, including dehydration, are common complications of HIV infection and AIDS. The patient's nutritional and electrolyte status is evaluated by monitoring weight gains or losses, skin turgor, ferritin levels, hemoglobin and hematocrit values, and electrolyte levels. Fluid and electrolyte status is monitored on an ongoing basis; fluid intake and output and urine specific gravity may be monitored daily if the patient is hospitalized with complications. The skin is assessed for dryness and adequate turgor. Vital signs are monitored for decreased systolic blood pressure or increased pulse rate on sitting or standing. Signs and symptoms of electrolyte disturbances, such as muscle cramping, weakness, irregular pulse, decreased mental status, nausea, and vomiting, are documented and reported to the physician. Serum electrolyte values are monitored, and abnormalities are reported.

The nurse helps the patient select foods that will replenish electrolytes, such as oranges and bananas (potassium) and cheese and soups (sodium) (Dudek, 2006). A fluid intake of 3 L or more per day, unless contraindicated, is encouraged to replace fluid lost with diarrhea, and measures to control diarrhea are initiated. If fluid and electrolyte imbalances persist, the nurse administers IV fluids and electrolytes as prescribed. Effects of parenteral therapy are monitored.

SIDE EFFECTS OF MEDICATIONS. Adverse reactions are of concern in patients who receive many medications to treat HIV infection or its complications. Many medications can cause severe toxic effects. Information about the purpose of the medications, their correct administration, side effects, and strategies to manage or prevent side effects is provided. Patients and their caregivers need to know which signs and symptoms of side effects should be reported immediately to their primary health care provider (see Table 52-3).

In addition to medications used to treat HIV infection, other medications that may be required include opioids, tricyclic antidepressants, and NSAIDs for pain relief; medications for treatment of opportunistic infections; antihistamines (diphenhydramine [Benadryl]) for relief of pruritus; acetaminophen (Tylenol) or aspirin for management of fever; and antiemetic agents for control of nausea and vomiting. Concurrent use of these medications can cause many drug interactions, resulting in hepatic and hematologic abnormalities. Therefore, careful monitoring of laboratory test results is essential.

During each contact with the patient, it is important for the nurse to ask not only about side effects but also about how well the patient is managing the medication regimen. The nurse may be able to assist the patient in organizing and planning the medication schedule to promote adherence to the treatment regimen.

Promoting Home and Community-Based Care

TEACHING PATIENTS SELF-CARE. Patients, families, and friends are instructed about the routes of transmission of HIV. As discussed earlier, the nurse discusses precautions the patient can use to avoid transmitting HIV sexually (see Charts 52-2 and 52-3) or through sharing of body fluids. Patients and their families or caregivers must receive instructions about how to prevent disease transmission, including handwashing techniques and methods for safely handling and disposing of items soiled with body fluids. Clear guidelines about avoiding and controlling infection, regular health care appointments, symptom management, nutrition, rest, and exercise are necessary. The importance of personal and environmental hygiene is emphasized. Caregivers are taught many of the guidelines (standard precautions) described in Chart 52-4. Kitchen and bathroom surfaces should be cleaned regularly with disinfectants to prevent growth of fungi and bacteria. Patients with pets are encouraged to have another person clean areas soiled by animals, such as bird cages and litter boxes. If this is not possible, patients should use gloves and should wash their hands after they clean the area. Patients are advised to avoid exposure to others who are sick or who have been recently vaccinated. The importance of avoiding smoking, excessive alcohol, and over-the-counter and street drugs is emphasized. Patients who are HIV positive or who inject drugs are instructed not to donate blood. IV/injection drug users who are unwilling to stop using drugs are advised to avoid sharing drug equipment with others.

Caregivers in the home are taught how to administer medications, including IV preparations. The medication regimens used for patients with HIV infection and AIDS are often complex and expensive. Patients receiving combination therapies for treatment of HIV infection and its complications require careful teaching about the importance of taking medications as prescribed and explanations and assistance in fitting the medication regimen into their lives (see Chart 52-7). If the patient requires enteral or parenteral nutrition, instruction is provided to the patient and family about how to administer nutritional therapies at home. Home care nurses provide ongoing teaching and support for the patient and family.

CONTINUING CARE. Many people with AIDS remain in their community and continue their usual daily activities, whereas others can no longer work or maintain their independence. Families or caregivers may need assistance in providing supportive care. There are many community-based organizations that provide a variety of services for people living with HIV infection and AIDS; nurses can help identify these services.

Community health nurses, home care nurses, and hospice nurses are in an excellent position to provide the support and guidance so often needed in the home setting. As hospital costs continue to rise and insurance coverage continues to decline, the complexity of home care increases. Home care nurses are key to the safe and effective administration of parenteral antibiotics, chemotherapy, and nutrition in the home.

During home visits, the nurse assesses the patient's physical and emotional status and home environment. The patient's adherence to the therapeutic regimen is assessed, and strategies are suggested to assist with adherence. The patient is assessed for progression of disease and for adverse side effects of medications. Previous teaching is reinforced, and the importance of keeping follow-up appointments is stressed.

Complex wound care or respiratory care may be required in the home. Patients and families are often unable to meet these skilled care needs without assistance. Nurses may refer patients to community programs that offer a range of services for patients, friends, and families, including help with housekeeping, hygiene, and meals; transportation and shopping; individual and group therapy; support for caregivers; telephone networks for the homebound; and legal and financial assistance. These services are typically provided by both professionals and nonprofessional volunteers. A social worker may be consulted to identify sources of financial support, if needed.

Home care and hospice nurses are increasingly called on to provide physical and emotional support to patients and families as patients with AIDS enter the terminal stages of disease. This support takes on special meaning when people with AIDS lose friends and when family members fear the disease or feel anger concerning the patient's lifestyle. The nurse encourages the patient and family to discuss end-of-life decisions and to ensure that care is consistent with those decisions, all comfort measures are employed, and the patient is treated with dignity at all times.

Evaluation

Expected Patient Outcomes

Expected patient outcomes may include:

1. Maintains skin integrity
2. Resumes usual bowel habits
3. Experiences no infections
4. Maintains adequate level of activity tolerance
5. Maintains usual level of thought processes
6. Maintains effective airway clearance
7. Experiences increased sense of comfort and less pain
8. Maintains adequate nutritional status
9. Experiences decreased sense of social isolation
10. Progresses through grieving process
11. Reports increased understanding of AIDS and participates in self-care activities as possible
12. Remains free of complications

Detailed outcomes are included in the plan of nursing care for a patient with AIDS (see Chart 52-10).

EMOTIONAL AND ETHICAL CONCERNS

Nurses in all settings are called on to provide care for patients with HIV infection. In doing so, they encounter not only the physical challenges of this epidemic but also emotional and ethical concerns. The concerns raised by health care professionals involve issues such as fear of infection, responsibility for giving care, values clarification, confidentiality, developmental stages of patients and caregivers, and poor prognostic outcomes.

Many patients with HIV infection have engaged in "stigmatized" behaviors. Because these behaviors challenge some traditional religious and moral values, nurses may feel reluctant to care for these patients. In addition, health care providers may still have fear and anxiety about disease transmission despite education concerning infection control and the low incidence of transmission to health care providers (see Chart 52-5). Nurses are encouraged to examine their personal beliefs and to use the process of values clarification to approach controversial issues. The American Nurses Association's Code of Ethics for Nurses (2008) can also be used to help resolve ethical dilemmas that might affect the quality of care given to patients with HIV infection and AIDS.

Nurses are responsible for protecting the patient's right to privacy by safeguarding confidential information. Inad-

vertent disclosure of confidential patient information may result in personal, financial, and emotional hardships for the patient. The controversy surrounding confidentiality concerns the circumstances in which information may be disclosed to others. Health care team members need accurate patient information to conduct assessment, planning, implementation, and evaluation of patient care. Failure to disclose HIV status could compromise the quality of patient care. Sexual partners of HIV-infected patients should know about the potential for infection and the need to engage in safer sex practices, as well as the possible need for testing and health care. Nurses are advised to discuss concerns about confidentiality with nurse administrators and to consult professional nursing organizations such as the Association of Nurses in AIDS Care and legal experts in their state to identify the most appropriate course of action. Chart 52-11 explores issues related to revealing one's HIV status.

AIDS has had a high mortality rate, but advances in antiretroviral and multidrug therapy have demonstrated promise in slowing or controlling disease progression. It is not known whether current treatment regimens will remain effective, because viral drug resistance has developed with

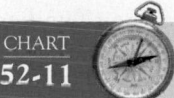

CHART 52-11 — Ethics and Related Issues: Revealing One's HIV Status

Should All People Who Are Infected With HIV Be Required to Reveal This Status to All Their Sexual and Drug-Sharing Contacts?

Situation

The human immunodeficiency virus (HIV) causes HIV infection, which progresses to AIDS. Because sexual contacts and needle-sharing partners are at risk for developing the disease, would a policy that requires notification of contacts infringe on the liberty and privacy of the known HIV-infected person?

Dilemma

The person's right to privacy conflicts with notifying all people who are contacts either through sexual or needle-sharing behavior (autonomy versus justice). The person's right to privacy conflicts with society's need to contain the deadly virus and stem a deadly epidemic (autonomy versus justice).

Discussion

1. What arguments would you offer in favor of notifying all the person's contacts?
2. What arguments would you offer against notifying all or some of the person's contacts?
3. Each state has various laws that pertain to whether contacts can be notified and who is responsible for notifying contacts. Is there a law for contact notification in the state in which you live? If there is such a law in your state, who is responsible for contact notification?
4. What would you do if the person responsible for contact notification refuses to do so based on his or her own beliefs for confidentiality of HIV infection status?
5. How would you respond if the HIV-positive person said that he or she is afraid to notify his or her contact because of fear of a violent response?

most previous medications. Most nurses in the United States have never faced an epidemic in which so many young and middle-aged adults experience serious illness and may die during the usual course of the disease process. Nurses may struggle with the value and meaning of their professional roles as they witness repeated instances of deterioration. Exposure to so many deaths among patients at the same developmental stage as many nurses can create stress. Contributing to this stress are personal fears of contagion or disapproval of the patient's lifestyle and behaviors. Unlike cancer or other diseases, AIDS is associated with controversies challenging our legal and political systems as well as religious and personal beliefs. Nurses who feel stressed and overburdened may experience physical and mental distress in the form of fatigue, headache, changes in appetite and sleep patterns, helplessness, irritability, apathy, negativity, and anger.

Many strategies have been used by nurses to cope with the stress associated with caring for AIDS patients. Education and provision of up-to-date information help to alleviate apprehension and prepare nurses to deliver safe, high-quality patient care. Interdisciplinary meetings allow participants to support one another and provide comprehensive patient care. Staff support groups give nurses an opportunity to solve problems and explore values and feelings about caring for AIDS patients and their families; they also provide a forum for grieving. Other sources of support include nursing administrators, peers, and spiritual advisors.

CRITICAL THINKING EXERCISES

EBP **1** A 43-year-old woman who has been using IV/injection drugs regularly for 20 years says that she is not going to stop using drugs but wants to reduce her risk of HIV infection. How would you counsel her? What is the evidence base on safer sex and strategies to reduce risk from use of IV/injection drugs? Is there evidence about the effectiveness of needle exchange programs? How would you determine the strength of the evidence and how would you present information to her?

2 During a code response in the intensive care unit (ICU), a nursing student is inadvertently stuck with a needle used on a patient with AIDS who has a high viral load. The student is apprehensive. What should the clinical instructor, in consultation with the nurse manager of the ICU, do? What reporting and documentation are needed (be sure to consider the student's health record)? What testing, treatment, and counseling are indicated for the student? Who should pay for the treatment?

EBP **3** During a home visit to a family in which two adolescents are HIV positive through vertical transmission, you are instructing the adolescents, their siblings, and their adult caregivers about strategies to protect the teens from other infections and to protect other family members from HIV transmission. What is the evidence for strategies that you plan to discuss with the adolescents

and their family members? What is the strength of that evidence, and what criteria would you use to evaluate the strength of the evidence?

4 A 48-year-old man who is bleeding from several stab wounds presents to the emergency department. He is intoxicated and combative. An OraQuick Rapid HIV-1 Antibody Test is performed as part of routine health care. What are the implications of this test? How would care in the emergency department be modified because of a positive test result? What are the ethical and legal ramifications of obtaining this test if the patient's ability to consent to testing is questioned?

5 You are making a home visit to a patient with AIDS who is exhibiting early signs of dementia and encephalopathy. Describe the aspects of the home environment that you would assess to ensure safety and adequate care. How would you modify your assessment if the patient lived alone in a third-floor apartment without an elevator? If the patient lived in a rural setting? If the patient had a physical disability that limited his ability to leave his apartment?

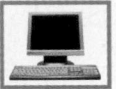 The Smeltzer suite offers these additional resources to enhance learning and facilitate understanding of this chapter:
- thePoint online resource, thepoint.lww.com/Smeltzer12E
- Student CD-ROM included with the book
- *Study Guide to Accompany Brunner & Suddarth's Textbook of Medical-Surgical Nursing*
- *Handbook for Brunner & Suddarth's Textbook of Medical-Surgical Nursing*

REFERENCES AND SELECTED READINGS

Asterisk indicates nursing research.
**Double asterisk indicates classic reference.*

Books

American Nurses Association. (2008). *Guide to the Code of Ethics for Nurses: Interpretation and application.* Silver Spring, MD: Author.

Association of Nurses in AIDS Care. (2007). *HIV/AIDS nursing: Scope and standards of practice.* Silver Springs, MD: American Nurses Association.

**Devita Jr., V. T., Hellman, S & Rosenberg, S. (Eds.). *AIDS: Etiology, diagnosis, treatment, and prevention* (4th ed.). Philadelphia: Lippincott Williams & Wilkins.

Dudek, S. G. (2006). *Nutrition essentials for nursing practice.* Philadelphia: Lippincott Williams & Wilkins.

Heckman, T., Kochman, A. & Sikkema, K. (2004). Depressive symptoms in older adults living with HIV disease: Application of the Chronic Illness Quality of Life model. In Emlet, C. (Ed.). *HIV/AIDS and older adults: Challenges for individuals, families, and communities.* New York: Springer.

Porth, C. M. & Matfin, G. (2009). *Pathophysiology: Concepts of altered health states* (8th ed.). Philadelphia: Lippincott Williams & Wilkins.

Journals and Electronic Documents

*Anastasi, J., Capili, B., Kim, G., et al. (2006). Symptom management of HIV-related diarrhea by using normal foods: A randomized controlled clinical trial. *Journal of the Association of Nurses in AIDS Care,* 17(2), 47–57.

*Andrade, S. & Anderson, E. (2008). The lived experience of a mind-body intervention for people living with HIV. *Journal of the Association of Nurses in AIDS Care,* 19(3), 192–199.

*Bova, C., Jaffarian, C., Himlan, P., et al. (2008). The symptom experience of HIV/HCV-coinfected adults. *Journal of the Association of Nurses in AIDS Care,* 19(3), 170–180.

Calza, L., Manfredi, R., Pocaterrra, D., et al. (2008). Risk of premature athero-sclerosis and ischemic heart disease associated with HIV infection and anti-retroviral therapy. *Journal of Infection, 57*(1), 16–32.

Centers for Disease Control and Prevention. (2005). Updated U.S. Public Health Service guidelines for the management of occupational exposures to HIV and recommendations for Postexposure Prophylaxis. *MMWR–Morbidity and Mortality Weekly Report, 54*(RR-9), 1–17.

Centers for Disease Control and Prevention. (2006). Revised recommendations for HIV testing of adults, adolescents, and pregnant women in health-care settings. *MMWR–Morbidity and Mortality Weekly Report, 55*(RR-14), 1–17.

Centers for Disease Control and Prevention. (2008). Estimates of new HIV in-fections in the United States. *CDC HIV/AIDS Facts.* www.cdc.gov/hiv/topics/surveillance/resources/factsheets/pdf/incidence.pdf

Centers for Disease Control, U.S. Department of Health and Human Services (1992). 1993 revised classification system for HIV infection and expanded surveillance case definition for AIDS among adolescents and adults. *MMWR–Morbidity and Mortality Weekly Report, 41*(RR-17), 1–19.

Coates, T. (2008). The US HIV epidemic: Why is prevention failing? HIV/AIDS annual update 2008. Postgraduate Institute for Medicine. *Clinical Care Options HIV.* www.clinicaloptions.com/ccohiv2008, 179–198.

Cooper, D., Steigbiegel, R., Gatell, J., et al. (2008). Subgroup and resistance analyses of raltegravir for resistant HIV-1 infection. *New England Journal of Medicine, 359*(4), 355–365.

Guidelines for Prevention and Treatment of Opportunistic Infections in HIV-infected Adults and Adolescents (2009). Recommendations of the National Institutes of Health (NIH), the Centers for Disease Control and Prevention (CDC), and the HIV Medicine Association of the Infectious Diseases Soci-ety of America (HIVMA/IDSA). *MMWR–Morbidity and Mortality Weekly Report. 58*(RR-4). 1–207 Available from http://AIDSinfo.nih.gov.

Hall, H. I., Song, R., Rhodes, P., et al. (2008). Estimation of HIV incidence in the United States. *Journal of the American Medical Association, 300*(5), 520–529.

Horton, R. & Das, P. (2008). Putting prevention at the forefront of HIV/AIDS. *Lancet, 372*(9637), 421–422.

Institute for Medicine. *Clinical care options HIV.* www.clinicaloptions.com/ccohiv2008, 49–84.

Kuritzkes, D. (2008) New findings on resistance to NRTIs, NNRTIs, and PIs. HIV/AIDS annual update 2008. Postgraduate Institute for Medicine. *Clini-cal Care Options HIV.* www.clinicaloptions.com/ccohiv2008, 33–47.

Levine, A. (2008). Non-AIDS defining cancers in the era of HAART. HIV/AIDS annual update 2008. Postgraduate Institute for Medicine. *Clini-cal Care Options HIV.* www.clinicaloptions.com/ccohiv2008, 113–142.

McArthur, J. (2008). Neurologic aspects of HIV infection and its therapy. HIV/AIDS annual update 2008. Postgraduate Institute for Medicine. *Clini-cal Care Options HIV.* www.clinicaloptions.com/ccohiv2008, 143–158.

McConnell, J. (2008). Leading edge: Does HIV/AIDS still require an excep-tional response? *Lancet Infectious Diseases, 8*(8), 457.

Meintjes, G., Lawn, S., Scano, F., et al. (2008). Tuberculosis-associated immune reconstitution inflammatory syndrome: Case definitions for use in resource-limited settings. *Lancet Infectious Diseases, 8*(8), 516–523.

Merson, M. H. (2006). The HIV-AIDS pandemic at 25: The global response. *New England Journal of Medicine, 354*(23), 2414–2417.

Merson, M., O'Malley, J., Serwadda, D., et al. (2008). The history and challenge of HIV prevention. *Lancet Infectious Diseases, 8*(8), 7–20.

Moyle, G., Gatell, J., Perno, C., et al. (2008). Potential for new antiretroviral to address unmet needs in the management of HIV infection. *AIDS Patient Care and STDs, 22*(6), 459–471.

National Institutes of Health, Centers for Disease Control and Prevention, and HIV Medicine Association of the Infectious Diseases Society of America. (June 18, 2008). *Guidelines for prevention and treatment of opportunistic infections in HIV-infected adults and adolescents* http://aidsinfo.nih.gov/contentfiles/Adult_OI.pdf

*Nicholas, P., Voss, J., Corless, I., et al. (2007). Unhealthy behaviors for self-management of HIV-related peripheral neuropathy. *AIDS Care, 19*(10), 1266–1273.

*Nokes, K., Rivero-Mendez, M., Valencia, C., et al. (2006). Socio-demographic and other characteristics in persons 50 years and older with HIV/AIDS in five countries. *Global Ageing: Issues and Action, 4*(2), 5–13.

Padian, N., Buve, A., Balkus, J., et al. (2008). Biomedical interventions to pre-vent HIV infection: Evidence, challenges, and way forward. *Lancet, 372*(9638), 585–599.

Panel of Antiretroviral Guidelines for Adults and Adolescents (Guidelines). Guidelines for the use of antiretroviral agents on HIV-1-infected adults and adolescents. Department of Health and Human Services. January 29, 2008;1–128. Available at http://www.aidsinfo.nih.gov/ContentFiles/AdultandAdolescentGL.pdf.

Senior, K. (2008). Back to basics for HIV vaccine research. *Lancet Infectious Dis-eases, 8*(8), 467.

Shippy, A. & Karpiak, S. (2005). Perceptions of support among older adults with HIV. *Research on Aging, 27*(3), 290–306.

Siegel, J. D, Rhinehart, E., Jackson, M., et al. (2007). *Guideline for isolation pre-cautions: Preventing transmission of infectious agents in healthcare settings.* http://www.cdc.gov/ncidod/dhqp/gl_isolation.html

UNAIDS (The Joint United Nations Programme on HIV/AIDS). (2008). *Report on the global AIDS epidemic 2008: Executive summary* (pp. 1–31). Geneva, Switzerland: Author. www.unaids.org

Zack, J. & Park, S. (2008). Eradication of HIV: Possible or still a pipe dream? HIV/AIDS annual update 2008. Postgraduate Institute for Medi-cine. *Clinical Care Options HIV.* www.clinicaloptions.com/ccohiv2008, 17–32.

RESOURCES

AIDS Action, www.aidsaction.org

AIDS Community Research Initiative of America, www.acria.org

AIDS Education and Training Centers (ETCs) Program (regional, national, and international training opportunities), www.aidsetc.org

American Red Cross, www.redcross.org

Antiretroviral medication information Web sites: www.AIDSmeds.com; www.projectinform.org; www.sfaf.org; http://hivinsite.ucsf.edu; www.amfAR.org; www.natap.org; www.thebody.com (many of these sites are coordinated by people living with HIV/AIDS

Centers for Disease Control and Prevention (2008): HIV/AIDS Prevention Research Synthesis Project, www.cdc.gov/hiv/topics/research/prs/evidence-based-interventions.htm; www.cdc.gov

Gay Men's Health Crisis Network, www.gmhc.org

Hemophilia and AIDS/HIV Network for the Dissemination of Information, www.hemophilia.org

HIV/AIDS Treatment, Prevention, and Research, ContactUs@aidsinfo.nih.gov, www.aidsinfo.nih.gov

HRSA National Clinician's Postexposure Prophylaxis hotline (health care providers only): 888-HIV-4911

HRSA National HIV Telephone Consultation Service, 800-933-3413

International AIDS Vaccine Initiative, www.iavi.org; e-mail: pubs@iavi.org

International Partnership for Microbicides, www.ipm-microbicides.org

Living with HIV/AIDS: Centers for Disease Control and Prevention, www.cdc.gov/hiv/pubs/brochure/livingwithhiv.htm

National Association of People with AIDS, www.napwa.org

National Pediatric and Family HIV Resource Center, www.womenchildrenhiv.org

Office of Minority Health Resource Center, www.omhrc.gov.

POZ, Health, Life, & HIV. Published by Smart+Strong, 500 Fifth Ave., Suite 320, New York, NY 10110

Pharmaceutical Research and Manufacturers of America, www.phrma.orgx

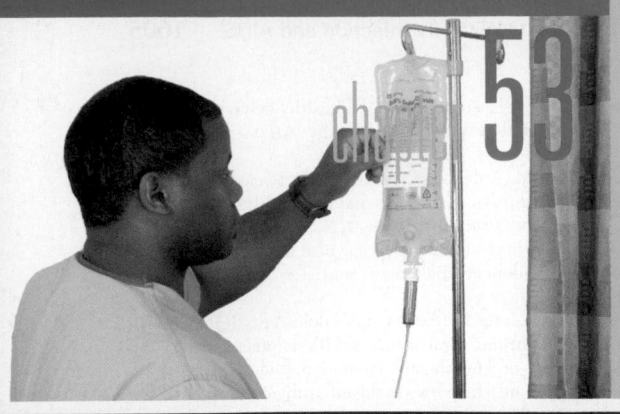

53

Assessment and Management of Patients With Allergic Disorders

LEARNING OBJECTIVES

On completion of this chapter, the learner will be able to:

1 Explain the physiologic events involved with allergic reactions.

2 Describe the types of hypersensitivity.

3 Describe the management of patients with allergic disorders.

4 Describe measures to prevent and manage anaphylaxis.

5 Use the nursing process as a framework for care of the patient with allergic rhinitis.

6 Discuss the different allergic disorders according to type.

GLOSSARY

allergen: substance that causes manifestations of allergy

allergy: inappropriate and often harmful immune system response to substances that are normally harmless

anaphylaxis: clinical response to an immediate immunologic reaction between a specific antigen and antibody

angioneurotic edema: condition characterized by urticaria and diffuse swelling of the deeper layers of the skin

antibody: protein substance developed by the body in response to and interacting with a specific antigen

antigen: substance that induces the production of antibodies

antihistamine: medication that opposes the action of histamine

atopic dermatitis: type I hypersensitivity involving inflammation of the skin evidenced by itching, redness, and a variety of skin lesions

atopy: term often used to describe immunoglobulin E–mediated diseases (ie, atopic dermatitis, asthma, and allergic rhinitis) with a genetic component

B lymphocytes: cells that are important in producing circulating antibodies

bradykinin: a substance that stimulates nerve fibers and causes pain

eosinophil: granular leukocyte

erythema: diffuse redness of the skin

hapten: incomplete antigen

histamine: substance in the body that causes increased gastric secretion, dilation of capillaries, and constriction of the bronchial smooth muscle

hypersensitivity: abnormal heightened reaction to a stimulus of any kind

immunoglobulins: a family of closely related proteins capable of acting as antibodies

leukotrienes: a group of chemical mediators that initiate the inflammatory response

mast cells: connective tissue cells that contain heparin and histamine in their granules

prostaglandins: unsaturated fatty acids that have a wide assortment of biologic activity

rhinitis: inflammation of the nasal mucosa

serotonin: chemical mediator that acts as a potent vasoconstrictor and bronchoconstrictor

T lymphocytes: cells that can cause graft rejection, kill foreign cells, or suppress production of antibodies

urticaria: hives

The human body is menaced by a host of potential invaders—allergens as well as microbial organisms—that constantly threaten its defenses. After penetrating those defenses, these allergens and organisms, if allowed to continue unimpeded, disrupt the body's enzyme systems and destroy its vital tissues. To protect against these agents, the body is equipped with an elaborate defense system.

The epithelial cells that coat the skin and make up the lining of the respiratory, gastrointestinal, and genitourinary tracts provide the first line of defense against microbial invaders. The structure and continuity of these surfaces and their resistance to penetration are initial deterrents to invaders.

One of the most effective defense mechanisms is the body's capacity to equip itself rapidly with weapons (antibodies) individually designed to meet each new invader, namely, specific protein antigens. Antibodies react with antigens in a variety of ways: (1) by coating the antigens' surfaces if they are particular substances, (2) by neutralizing the antigens if they are toxins, and (3) by precipitating the antigens out of solution if they are dissolved. The antibodies prepare the antigens so that the phagocytic cells of the blood and the tissues can dispose of them. However, although this system is normally protective, in some cases the body produces inappropriate or exaggerated responses to specific antigens, and the result is an allergic or hypersensitivity disorder.

ALLERGIC ASSESSMENT

Physiologic Overview

An allergic reaction is a manifestation of tissue injury resulting from interaction between an antigen and an **antibody.** **Allergy** is an inappropriate and often harmful response of the immune system to normally harmless substances, called **allergens** (eg, dust, weeds, pollen, dander). Chemical mediators released in allergic reactions may produce symptoms that range from mild to life-threatening.

In allergic reactions, the body encounters **antigens,** usually proteins that the body's defenses recognize as foreign, and a series of events occurs in an attempt to render the invaders harmless, destroy them, and remove them from the body. When lymphocytes respond to the antigens, **antibodies** (protein substances that protect against antigens) are produced.

Antibodies combine with antigens in a special way, which has been likened to keys fitting into a lock. Antigens (the keys) fit only certain antibodies (the locks). Hence, the term *specificity* refers to the specific reaction of an antibody to an antigen. There are many variations and complexities in these patterns.

Function of Immunoglobulins

Antibodies that are formed by lymphocytes and plasma cells in response to an immunogenic stimulus constitute a group of serum proteins called **immunoglobulins.** Grouped into five classes (IgE, IgD, IgG, IgM, and IgA), immunoglobulins can be found in the lymph nodes, tonsils, appendix, and Peyer's patches of the intestinal tract or circulating in the blood and lymph. These antibodies are capable of binding with a wide variety of antigens. Immunoglobulins of the IgE class are involved in allergic disorders and some parasitic infections. IgE-producing cells are located in the respiratory and intestinal mucosa. Two or more IgE molecules bind together to an allergen and trigger **mast cells** or basophils to release chemical mediators, such as histamine, serotonin, kinins, slow-reacting substances of anaphylaxis, and the neutrophil factor, which produces allergic skin reactions, asthma, and hay fever. **Atopy** refers to IgE-mediated diseases such as allergic rhinitis that have a genetic component.

Role of B Cells

B cells, or **B lymphocytes,** are programmed to produce one specific antibody. On encountering a specific antigen, B cells stimulate production of plasma cells, the site of antibody production. The result is the outpouring of antibodies for the purpose of destroying and removing the antigens.

Role of T Cells

T cells, or **T lymphocytes,** assist the B cells in producing antibodies. T cells secrete substances that direct the flow of cell activity, destroy target cells, and stimulate the macrophages. The macrophages present the antigens to the T cells and initiate the immune response. They also digest antigens and assist in removing cells and other debris. Unlike a specific antibody, a T cell does not bind free antigens.

Function of Antigens

Antigens are divided into two groups: complete protein antigens and low-molecular-weight substances. Complete protein antigens, such as animal dander, pollen, and horse serum, stimulate a complete humoral response. (See Chapter 50 for a discussion of humoral immunity.) Low-molecular-weight substances, such as medications, function as **haptens** (incomplete antigens), binding to tissue or serum proteins to produce a carrier complex that initiates an antibody response. In an allergic reaction, the production of antibodies requires active communication between cells. When the allergen is absorbed through the respiratory tract, gastrointestinal tract, or skin, allergen sensitization occurs. Macrophages process the antigen and present it to the appropriate cells. These cells mature into allergen-specific secreting plasma cells that synthesize and secrete antigen-specific antibodies.

Function of Chemical Mediators

Mast cells, which are located in the skin and mucous membranes, play a major role in IgE-mediated immediate hypersensitivity. When mast cells are stimulated by antigens, powerful chemical mediators are released, causing a sequence of physiologic events that results in symptoms of immediate hypersensitivity (Fig. 53-1). There are two types of chemical mediators: primary and secondary. Primary mediators are preformed and are found in mast cells or basophils. Secondary mediators are inactive precursors that are formed or released in response to primary mediators. Table 53-1 summarizes the actions of primary and secondary chemical mediators.

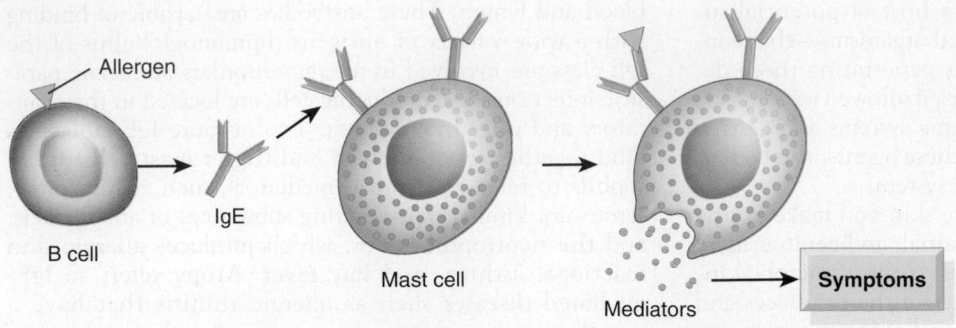

Allergen

IgE

B cell

Mast cell

Mediators → Symptoms

Figure 53-1 Allergen triggers the B cell to make IgE antibody, which attaches to the mast cell. When that allergen reappears, it binds to the IgE and triggers the mast cell to release its chemicals. Courtesy of U.S. Department of Health and Human Services, National Institutes of Health.

Primary Mediators

Histamine

Histamine, which is released by mast cells, plays an important role in the immune response. Its effects, which are greatest within about 15 minutes after antigen contact, include erythema; localized edema in the form of wheals; pruritus; contraction of bronchial smooth muscle, resulting in wheezing and bronchospasm; dilation of small venules and constriction of larger vessels; and increased secretion of gastric and mucosal cells, resulting in diarrhea. Histamine action results from stimulation of histamine-1 (H_1) and histamine-2 (H_2) receptors. H_1 receptors are found predominantly on bronchiolar and vascular smooth muscle cells; H_2 receptors are found on gastric parietal cells.

Certain medications are categorized by their action at these receptors. Diphenhydramine (Benadryl) is an example of an **antihistamine,** a medication that displays an affinity for H_1 receptors. Cimetidine (Tagamet) and ranitidine (Zantac) target H_2 receptors to inhibit gastric secretions in peptic ulcer disease.

Eosinophil Chemotactic Factor of Anaphylaxis

Eosinophil chemotactic factor of anaphylaxis affects movement of **eosinophils** (granular leukocytes) to the site of allergens. It is preformed in the mast cells and is released from disrupted mast cells.

Platelet-Activating Factor

Platelet-activating factor is responsible for initiating platelet aggregation and leukocyte infiltration at sites of immediate hypersensitivity reactions. It also causes bronchoconstriction and increased vascular permeability (Porth & Matfin, 2009).

Prostaglandins

Prostaglandins produce smooth muscle contraction as well as vasodilation and increased capillary permeability (Porth, 2009). The fever and pain that occur with inflammation in allergic responses are caused in part by the prostaglandins.

Secondary Mediators

Leukotrienes

Leukotrienes are chemical mediators that initiate the inflammatory response. Many manifestations of inflammation can be attributed in part to leukotrienes. In addition, leukotrienes cause smooth muscle contraction, bronchial constriction, mucus secretion in the airways, and the typical wheal-and-flare reactions of the skin. Compared with

Table 53-1 **CHEMICAL MEDIATORS OF HYPERSENSITIVITY**	
Mediators	**Action**
Primary Mediators *Preformed and Found in Mast Cells or Basophils*	
Histamine (preformed in mast cells)	Vasodilation
	Smooth muscle contraction, increased vascular permeability, increased mucus secretions
Eosinophil chemotactic factor of anaphylaxis (ECF-A) (preformed in mast cells)	Attracts eosinophils
Platelet-activating factor (PAF) (requires synthesis by mast cells, neutrophils, and macrophages)	Smooth muscle contraction
	Incites platelets to aggregate and release serotonin and histamine
Prostaglandins (chemically derived from arachidonic acid; require synthesis by cells)	D and F series → bronchoconstriction
	E series → bronchodilation
	D, E, and F series → vasodilation
Basophil kallikrein (preformed in mast cells)	Frees bradykinin, which causes bronchoconstriction, vasodilation, and nerve stimulation
Secondary Mediators *Inactive Precursors Formed or Released in Response to Primary Mediators*	
Bradykinin (derived from precursor kininogen)	Smooth muscle contraction, increased vascular permeability, stimulates pain receptors, increased mucus production
Serotonin (preformed in platelets)	Smooth muscle contraction, increased vascular permeability
Heparin (preformed in mast cells)	Anticoagulant
Leukotrienes (derived from arachidonic acid and activated by mast cell degranulation) C, D, and E or slow-reacting substance of anaphylaxis (SRS-A)	Smooth muscle contraction, increased vascular permeability

histamine, leukotrienes are 100 to 1000 times more potent in causing bronchospasm.

Bradykinin

Bradykinin is a substance that has the ability to cause increased vascular permeability, vasodilation, hypotension, and contraction of many types of smooth muscle, such as the bronchi. Increased permeability of the capillaries results in edema. Bradykinin stimulates nerve cell fibers and produces pain.

Serotonin

Serotonin acts as a potent vasoconstrictor and causes contraction of bronchial smooth muscle.

Hypersensitivity

Although the immune system defends the host against infections and foreign antigens, immune responses can themselves cause tissue injury and disease. **Hypersensitivity** is a reflection of excessive or aberrant immune response to any type of stimulus (Abbas & Lichtman, 2008). It usually does not occur with the first exposure to an allergen. Rather, the reaction follows a re-exposure after sensitization, or buildup of antibodies, in a predisposed person. To promote understanding of the immunopathogenesis of disease, hypersensitivity reactions have been classified into four specific types of reactions (Fig. 53-2). Most allergic reactions are either type I or type IV hypersensitivity reactions.

Anaphylactic (Type I) Hypersensitivity

The most severe hypersensitivity reaction is **anaphylaxis.** An unanticipated severe allergic reaction that is often explosive in onset, anaphylaxis is characterized by edema in many tissues, including the larynx, and is often accompanied by hypotension, bronchospasm, and cardiovascular collapse in severe cases. Type I or anaphylactic hypersensitivity is an immediate reaction beginning within minutes of exposure to an antigen. Primary chemical mediators are responsible for the symptoms of type I hypersensitivity because of their effects on the skin, lungs, and gastrointestinal tract. If chemical mediators continue to be released, a delayed reaction may occur and may last for up to 24 hours.

Clinical symptoms are determined by the amount of the allergen, the amount of mediator released, the sensitivity of the target organ, and the route of allergen entry. Type I hypersensitivity reactions may include both local and systemic anaphylaxis. Examples include allergic rhinitis, asthma, and severe allergic response in people sensitized to penicillin or latex.

Cytotoxic (Type II) Hypersensitivity

Type II, or cytotoxic, hypersensitivity occurs when the system mistakenly identifies a normal constituent of the body as foreign. This reaction may be the result of a cross-reacting antibody, possibly leading to cell and tissue damage.

Type II hypersensitivity reactions are associated with several disorders. For example, in myasthenia gravis, the body mistakenly generates antibodies against normal nerve ending receptors. In Goodpasture syndrome, it generates antibodies against lung and renal tissue, producing lung damage and renal failure. A type II hypersensitivity reaction resulting in red blood cell destruction is associated with drug-induced immune hemolytic anemia, Rh-hemolytic disease of the newborn, and incompatibility reactions in blood transfusions (see Chapter 33).

Immune Complex (Type III) Hypersensitivity

Type III, or immune complex, hypersensitivity involves immune complexes that are formed when antigens bind to antibodies. These complexes are cleared from the circulation by phagocytic action. If these type III complexes are deposited in tissues or vascular endothelium, two factors contribute to injury: the increased amount of circulating complexes and the presence of vasoactive amines. As a result, there is an increase in vascular permeability and tissue injury.

The joints and kidneys are particularly susceptible to this type of injury. Type III hypersensitivity is associated with systemic lupus erythematosus, rheumatoid arthritis, certain types of nephritis, and some types of bacterial endocarditis. These are discussed elsewhere in this text.

Delayed-Type (Type IV) Hypersensitivity

Type IV, or delayed-type, hypersensitivity, also known as cellular hypersensitivity, occurs 24 to 72 hours after exposure to an allergen. It is mediated by sensitized T cells and macrophages rather than antibodies.

An example of a type IV hypersensitivity reaction is contact dermatitis resulting from exposure to allergens such as cosmetics, adhesive tape, topical agents (eg, povidone-iodine), medication additives, and plant toxins. Symptoms include itching, erythema, and raised lesions.

Assessment

Health History

A comprehensive allergy history and a thorough physical examination provide useful data for the diagnosis and management of allergic disorders. An assessment form is useful for obtaining and organizing this information (Chart 53-1).

The degree of difficulty and discomfort experienced by the patient because of allergic symptoms and the degree of improvement in those symptoms with and without treatment are assessed and documented. The relationship of symptoms to exposure to possible allergens is noted.

Diagnostic Evaluation

Diagnostic evaluation of the patient with allergic disorders commonly includes blood tests, smears of body secretions, skin tests, and the radioallergosorbent test (RAST). Results of laboratory blood studies provide supportive data for various diagnostic possibilities; however, they are not the major criteria for the diagnosis of allergic disease.

Complete Blood Count With Differential

The white blood cell (WBC) count is usually normal except with infection. Eosinophils, which are granular leukocytes, normally make up 1% to 3% of the total number of

Type I

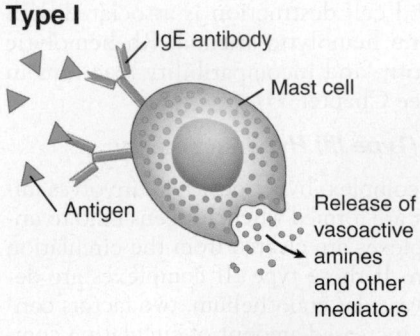

Type I. An anaphylactic reaction is characterized by vasodilation, increased capillary permeability, smooth muscle contraction, and eosinophilia. Systemic reactions may involve laryngeal stridor, angioedema, hypotension, and bronchial, GI, or uterine spasm; local reactions are characterized by hives. Examples of type I reactions include extrinsic asthma, allergic rhinitis, systemic anaphylaxis, and reactions to insect stings.

Type II

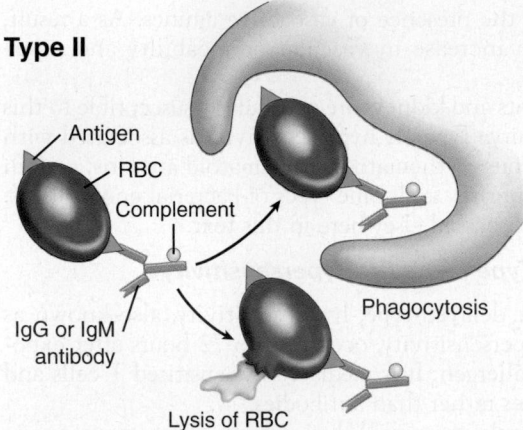

Type II. A cytotoxic reaction, which involves binding either the IgG or IgM antibody to a cell-bound antigen, may lead to eventual cell and tissue damage. The reaction is the result of mistaken identity when the system identifies a normal constituent of the body as foreign and activates the complement cascade. Examples of type II reactions are myasthenia gravis, Goodpasture's syndrome, pernicious anemia, hemolytic disease of the newborn, transfusion reaction, and thrombocytopenia.

Type III

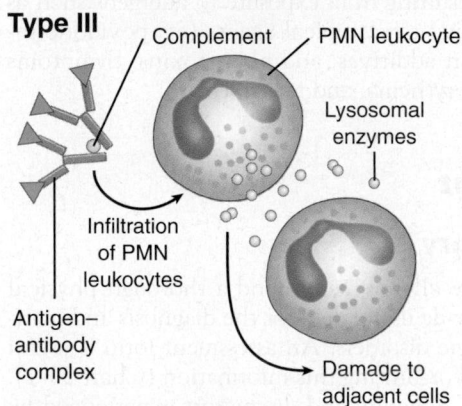

Type III. An immune complex reaction is marked by acute inflammation resulting from formation and deposition of immune complexes. The joints and kidneys are particularly susceptible to this kind of reaction, which is associated with systemic lupus erythematosus, serum sickness, nephritis, and rheumatoid arthritis. Some signs and symptoms include urticaria, joint pain, fever, rash, and adenopathy (swollen glands).

Type IV

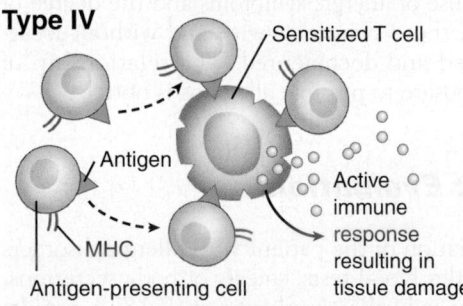

Type IV. A delayed, or cellular, reaction occurs 1 to 3 days after exposure to an antigen. The reaction, which results in tissue damage, involves activity by lymphokines, macrophages, and lysozymes. Erythema and itching are common; a few examples include contact dermatitis, graft-versus-host disease, Hashimoto's thyroiditis, and sarcoidosis.

Figure 53-2 Four types of hypersensitivity reactions. (Ig, immunoglobulin; PMN, polymorphonuclear; RBC, red blood cell.)

WBCs. A level between 5% and 15% is nonspecific but does suggest allergic reaction. Higher percentages of eosinophils are considered to represent moderate to severe eosinophilia. Moderate eosinophilia is defined as 15% to 40% eosinophils and may be found in patients with allergic disorders.

Eosinophil Count

An actual count of eosinophils can be obtained from blood samples or smears of secretions. During symptomatic episodes, smears obtained from nasal secretions, conjunctival secretions, and sputum of allergic patients usually reveal eosinophils, indicating an active allergic response.

CHART
53-1

Allergy Assessment Form

Name _____ Age _____ Sex _____ Date _____

I. Chief complaint: _____

II. Present illness: _____

III. Collateral allergic symptoms: _____

Eyes: Pruritus _____ Burning _____ Lacrimation _____
           Swelling _____ Injection _____ Discharge _____

Ears: Pruritus _____ Fullness _____ Popping _____
          Frequent infections _____

Nose: Sneezing _____ Rhinorrhea _____ Obstruction _____
         Pruritus _____ Mouth-breathing _____
         Purulent discharge _____

Throat: Soreness _____ Postnasal discharge _____
        Palatal pruritus _____ Mucus in the morning _____

Chest: Cough _____   Pain _____   Wheezing _____
         Sputum _____   Dyspnea _____
         Color _____   Rest _ _____
         Amount _____   Exertion _____

Skin: Dermatitis _____   Eczema _____   Urticaria _____

IV. Family allergies

V. Previous allergic treatment or testing: _____

Prior skin testing: _____

Medications: Antihistamines   Improved _____   Unimproved _____
             Bronchodilators   Improved _____   Unimproved _____
             Nose drops   Improved _____   Unimproved _____
             Hyposensitization Improved _____   Unimproved _____
                Duration _____
                Antigens _____
                Reactions _____
             Antibiotics   Improved _____   Unimproved _____
             Corticosteroids   Improved _____   Unimproved _____

VI. Physical agents and habits: _____

Bothered by:

Tobacco for _____ years   Alcohol _____   Air conditioning _____
Cigarettes ____ packs/day   Heat _____   Muggy weather _____
Cigars _____ per day   Cold _____   Weather changes _____
Pipes _____ per day   Perfumes _____   Chemicals _____
Never smoked _____   Paints _____   Hair spray _____
Bothered by smoke _____ Insecticides _____ Newspapers _____
                            Cosmetics _____   Latex _____

VII. When symptoms occur: _____

Time and circumstances of 1st episode: _____

Prior health: _____

Course of illness over decades: progressing _____ regressing _____

Time of year: _____ Exact dates: _____

    Perennial _____

    Seasonal _____

    Seasonally exacerbated _____

Monthly variations (menses, occupation): _____

Time of week (weekends vs. weekdays): _____

Time of day or night: _____

After insect stings: _____

VIII. Where symptoms occur: _____

Living where at onset: _____

Living where since onset: _____

Effect of vacation or major geographic change: _____

Symptoms better indoors or outdoors: _____

Effect of school or work: _____

Effect of staying elsewhere nearby: _____

Effect of hospitalization: _____

Effect of specific environments: _____

Continued on following page

CHART
53-1

Allergy Assessment Form (*Continued*)

Do symptoms occur around: _____
    old leaves _____ hay _____ lakeside _____ barns _____
    summer homes _____ damp basement _____ dry attic _____
    lawnmowing _____ animals _____ other _____
Do symptoms occur after eating:
    cheese _____ mushrooms _____ beer _____ melons _____
    bananas _____ fish _____ nuts _____ citrus fruits _____
    other foods (list)_____
Home: city _____ rural _____
         house _____ age _____
         apartment _____ basement _____ damp _____ dry _____
         heating system _____
         pets (how long) _____ dog _____ cat _____ other _____

Bedroom:	Type	Age	*Living room:*	Type	Age
Pillow	____	____	Rug	____	____
Mattress	____	____	Matting	____	____
Blankets	____	____	Furniture	____	____
Quilts	____	____			
Furniture	____	____			

    Anywhere in home symptoms are worse: _____
IX. What does patient think makes symptoms worse? _____
X. Under what circumstances is patient free of symptoms? _____
XI. Summary and additional comments: _____

Total Serum Immunoglobulin E Levels

High total serum IgE levels support the diagnosis of allergic disease. However, a normal IgE level does not exclude the diagnosis of an allergic disorder. IgE levels are not as sensitive as the paper radioimmunosorbent test (PRIST) or the enzyme-linked immunosorbent assay (ELISA), also referred to as enzyme immunoessay (EIA).

Skin Tests

Skin testing entails the intradermal injection or superficial application (epicutaneous) of solutions at several sites. Depending on the suspected cause of allergic signs and symptoms, several different solutions may be applied at separate sites. These solutions contain individual antigens representing an assortment of allergens most likely to be implicated in the patient's disease. Positive (wheal-and-flare) reactions are clinically significant when correlated with the history, physical findings, and results of other laboratory tests.

The results of skin tests complement the data obtained from the history. They indicate which of several antigens are most likely to provoke symptoms and provide some clue to the intensity of the patient's sensitization. The dosage of the antigen (allergen) injected is also important. Most patients are hypersensitive to more than one allergen. Under testing conditions, they may not react (although they usually do) to the specific allergens that induce their attacks.

In cases of doubt about the validity of the skin tests, a RAST or a provocative challenge test may be performed. If a skin test is indicated, there is a reasonable suspicion that a specific allergen is producing symptoms in an allergic patient. However, several precautionary steps must be observed before skin testing with allergens is performed:

- Testing is not performed during periods of bronchospasm.

- Epicutaneous tests (scratch or prick tests) are performed before other testing methods, in an effort to minimize the risk of systemic reaction.
- Emergency equipment must be readily available to treat anaphylaxis.

Types of Skin Tests

The methods of skin testing include prick skin tests, scratch tests, and intradermal skin testing (Fig. 53-3). After negative prick or scratch tests, intradermal skin testing is

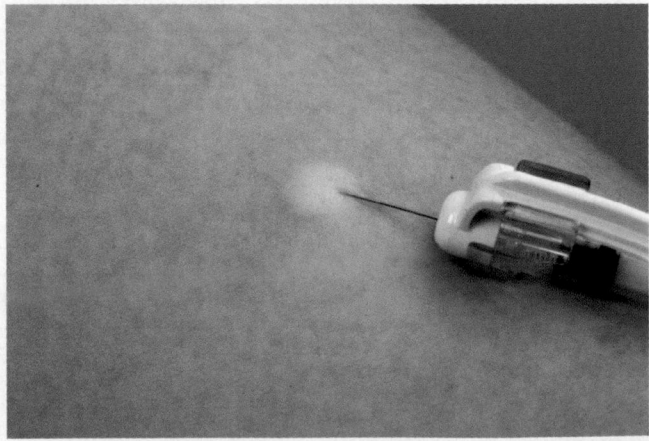

Figure 53-3 Intradermal testing. A 0.5-mL or 1-mL sterile syringe with a 26/27-gauge intradermal needle is used to inject 0.02 to 0.03 mL of intradermal allergen. The needle is inserted with the bevel facing upward and the syringe parallel to the skin. The skin is penetrated superficially, and a small amount of the allergen solution is injected to create a bleb (raised area) approximately 5 mm in diameter. A separate sterile syringe and needle are used for each injection. From Taylor, C., Lillis C. & LeMone, P. (2005). *Fundamentals of nursing: The art and science of nursing care* (5th ed.). Philadelphia: Lippincott Williams & Wilkins.

performed with allergens that are suggested by the patient's history to be problematic. The back is the most suitable area of the body for skin testing because it permits the performance of many tests. A multitest applicator with multiple test heads is commercially available for simultaneous administration of antigens by multiple punctures at different sites. A negative response on a skin test cannot be interpreted as an absence of sensitivity to an allergen. Such a response may occur with insufficient sensitivity of the test or with use of an inappropriate allergen in testing. Therefore, it is essential to observe the patient undergoing skin testing for an allergic reaction even if the previous response was negative.

Interpretation of Skin Test Results

Familiarity with and consistent use of a grading system are essential. The grading system used should be identified on a skin test record for later interpretation. A positive reaction, evidenced by the appearance of an urticarial wheal (round, reddened skin elevation) (Fig. 53-4), localized **erythema** (diffuse redness) in the area of inoculation or contact, or pseudopodia (irregular projection at the end of a wheal) with associated erythema is considered indicative of sensitivity to the corresponding antigen. False-positive results may occur because of improper preparation or administration of allergen solutions.

> ⚑ **NURSING ALERT**
>
> Corticosteroids and antihistamines, including over-the-counter allergy medications, suppress skin test reactivity and should be stopped 48 to 96 hours before testing, depending on the duration of their activity. False-positive results may occur because of improper preparation or administration of allergen solutions.

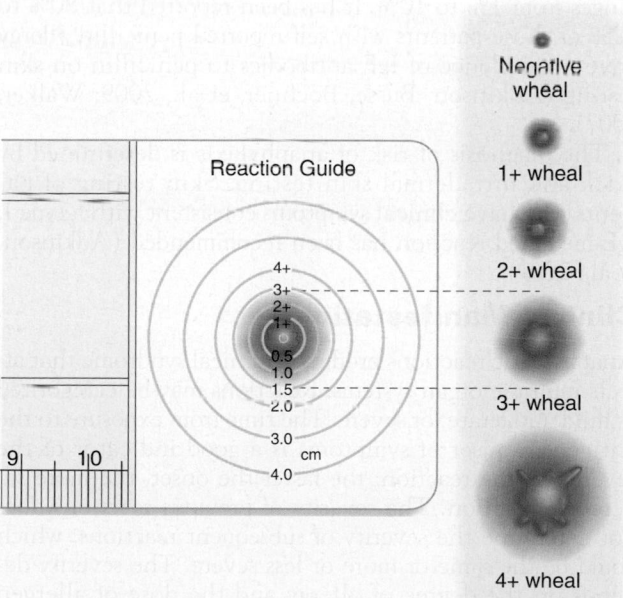

Figure 53-4 Interpretation of reactions: Negative = wheal soft with minimal erythema. 1+ = wheal present (5 to 8 mm) with associated erythema. 2+ = wheal (7 to 10 mm) with associated erythema. 3+ = wheal (9 to 15 mm), slight pseudopodia possible with associated erythema. 4+ = wheal (12 mm+) with pseudopodia and diffuse erythema.

Interpretation of positive or negative skin tests must be based on the history, physical examination, and other laboratory test results. The following guidelines are used for the interpretation of skin test results:

- Skin tests are more reliable for diagnosing atopic sensitivity in patients with allergic rhinoconjunctivitis than in patients with asthma.
- Positive skin tests correlate highly with food allergy.
- The use of skin tests to diagnose immediate hypersensitivity to medications is limited, because metabolites of medications, not the medications themselves, are usually responsible for causing hypersensitivity.

Provocative Testing

Provocative testing involves the direct administration of the suspected allergen to the sensitive tissue, such as the conjunctiva, nasal or bronchial mucosa, or gastrointestinal tract (by ingestion of the allergen), with observation of target organ response. This type of testing is helpful in identifying clinically significant allergens in patients who have a large number of positive tests. Major disadvantages of this type of testing are the limitation of one antigen per session and the risk of producing severe symptoms, particularly bronchospasm, in patients with asthma.

Radioallergosorbent Test

RAST is a radioimmunoassay that measures allergen-specific IgE. A sample of the patient's serum is exposed to a variety of suspected allergen particle complexes. If antibodies are present, they will combine with radiolabeled allergens. Test results are then compared with control values. In addition to detecting an allergen, RAST indicates the quantity of allergen necessary to evoke an allergic reaction. Values are reported on a scale from 0 to 5. Values of 2 or greater are considered significant. The major advantages of RAST over other tests include decreased risk of systemic reaction, stability of antigens, and lack of dependence on skin reactivity modified by medications. The major disadvantages include limited allergen selection and reduced sensitivity compared with intradermal skin tests, lack of immediate results, and higher cost.

ALLERGIC DISORDERS

There are two types of IgE-mediated allergic reactions: atopic and nonatopic disorders. Although the underlying immunologic reactions of the two types of disorders are the same, the predisposing factors and manifestations are different. The atopic disorders are characterized by a hereditary predisposition and production of a local reaction to IgE antibodies, which manifests in one or more of the following three atopic disorders: allergic rhinitis, asthma, and atopic dermatitis/eczema. The nonatopic disorders lack the genetic component and organ specificity of the atopic disorders (Porth & Matfin, 2009). Latex allergy (see later discussion) may be a type I or type IV hypersensitivity reaction, although true latex allergy is considered to be a type I hypersensitivity reaction (Rolland & O'Hehir, 2008). Contact dermatitis is considered to be a type IV hypersensitivity reaction.

Anaphylaxis

Anaphylaxis is a clinical response to an immediate (type I hypersensitivity) immunologic reaction between a specific antigen and an antibody. The reaction results from a rapid release of IgE-mediated chemicals, which can induce a severe, life-threatening allergic reaction. It is estimated that between 3.3 and 43 million people in the United States are at risk for anaphylaxis (Lieberman, 2006; Porth & Matfin, 2009).

Pathophysiology

Anaphylaxis is caused by the interaction of a foreign antigen with specific IgE antibodies found on the surface membrane of mast cells and peripheral blood basophils. The subsequent release of histamine and other bioactive mediators causes activation of platelets, eosinophils, and neutrophils. Histamine, prostaglandins, and inflammatory leukotrienes are potent vasoactive mediators that are implicated in the vascular permeability changes, flushing, urticaria, angioedema, hypotension, and bronchoconstriction that characterize anaphylaxis. Smooth muscle spasm, bronchospasm, mucosal edema and inflammation, and increased capillary permeability result. These systemic changes characteristically produce clinical manifestations within seconds or minutes after antigen exposure (Lieberman, 2006; Porth & Matfin, 2009). Closely related to anaphylaxis is a nonallergenic anaphylaxis (anaphylactoid) reaction, which is described in Chart 53-2.

Substances that most commonly cause anaphylaxis include foods, medications, insect stings, and latex (Chart 53-3). Foods that are common causes of anaphylaxis include peanuts, tree nuts, shellfish, fish, milk, eggs, soy, and wheat. Many medications have been implicated in anaphylaxis. Those that are most frequently reported include antibiotics (eg, penicillin), radiocontrast agents, intravenous (IV)

Chart 53-2 • Nonallergenic Anaphylaxis (Anaphylactoid Reaction)

Closely resembling anaphylaxis is an anaphylactoid reaction, which is caused by the release of mast cell and basophil mediators triggered by non–IgE-mediated events. This non-allergenic anaphylaxis reaction may occur with medications, food, exercise, or cytotoxic antibody transfusions. The reaction may be local or systemic. Local reactions usually involve urticaria and angioedema at the site of the antigen exposure. Although possibly severe, nonallergenic anaphylaxis reactions are rarely fatal. Systemic reactions occur within about 30 minutes after exposure and involve cardiovascular, respiratory, gastrointestinal, and integumentary organ systems. For the most part, the treatment of nonallergenic anaphylaxis reaction is identical to that of anaphylaxis (Johansson, Hourihane, Bousquet, et al., 2005).

Chart 53-3 • Common Causes of Anaphylaxis

Foods

Peanuts, tree nuts (eg, walnuts, pecans, cashews, almonds), shellfish (eg, shrimp, lobster, crab), fish, milk, eggs, soy, wheat

Medications

Antibiotics, especially penicillin and sulfa antibiotics, allopurinol, radiocontrast agents, anesthetic agents (lidocaine, procaine), vaccines, hormones (insulin, vasopressin, adrenocorticotropic hormone [ACTH]), aspirin, nonsteroidal anti-inflammatory drugs (NSAIDs)

Other Pharmaceutical/Biologic Agents

Animal serums (tetanus antitoxin, snake venom antitoxin, rabies antitoxin), antigens used in skin testing

Insect Stings

Bees, wasps, hornets, yellow jackets, ants, including fire ants

Latex

Medical and nonmedical products containing latex

anesthetic agents, aspirin and other nonsteroidal anti-inflammatory drugs (NSAIDs), and opioids. Antibiotics and radiocontrast agents cause the most serious anaphylactic reactions, producing reactions in about 1 of every 5000 exposures. Penicillin is the most common cause of anaphylaxis and accounts for about 75% of fatal anaphylactic reactions in the United States each year. The actual prevalence of penicillin allergy in the general population is unknown; however, the incidence of self-reported penicillin allergy ranges from 1% to 10%. It has been reported that 80% to 90% of those patients with self-reported penicillin allergy have no evidence of IgE antibodies to penicillin on skin testing (Adkinson, Busse, Bochner, et al., 2009; Walker, 2007).

The diagnosis of risk of anaphylaxis is determined by prick and intradermal skin testing. Skin testing of patients who have clinical symptoms consistent with a type I, IgE-mediated reaction has been recommended (Adkinson, et al., 2009).

Clinical Manifestations

Anaphylactic reactions produce a clinical syndrome that affects multiple organ systems. Reactions may be categorized as mild, moderate, or severe. The time from exposure to the antigen to onset of symptoms is a good indicator of the severity of the reaction: the faster the onset, the more severe the reaction. The severity of previous reactions does not determine the severity of subsequent reactions, which could be the same or more or less severe. The severity depends on the degree of allergy and the dose of allergen (Virella, 2007).

Mild systemic reactions consist of peripheral tingling and a sensation of warmth, possibly accompanied by a sensation of fullness in the mouth and throat. Nasal congestion, periorbital swelling, pruritus, sneezing, and tearing of the eyes can also be expected. Onset of symptoms begins within the first 2 hours after exposure.

Moderate systemic reactions may include flushing, warmth, anxiety, and itching in addition to any of the milder symptoms. More serious reactions include bronchospasm and edema of the airways or larynx with dyspnea, cough, and wheezing. The onset of symptoms is the same as for a mild reaction.

Severe systemic reactions have an abrupt onset with the same signs and symptoms described previously. These symptoms progress rapidly to bronchospasm, laryngeal edema, severe dyspnea, cyanosis, and hypotension. Dysphagia (difficulty swallowing), abdominal cramping, vomiting, diarrhea, and seizures can also occur. Cardiac arrest and coma may follow.

Prevention

Strict avoidance of potential allergens is an important preventive measure for the patient at risk for anaphylaxis. Patients at risk for anaphylaxis from insect stings should avoid areas populated by insects and should use appropriate clothing, insect repellent, and caution to avoid further stings.

If avoidance of exposure to allergens is impossible, the patient should be instructed to carry and administer epinephrine to prevent an anaphylactic reaction in the event of exposure to the allergen. People who are sensitive to insect bites and stings, those who have experienced food or medication reactions, and those who have experienced idiopathic or exercise-induced anaphylactic reactions should always carry an emergency kit that contains epinephrine. The EpiPen from Dey Pharmaceuticals (Napa, CA) is a commercially available first-aid device that delivers premeasured doses of 0.3 mg (EpiPen) or 0.15 mg (EpiPen Jr.) of epinephrine (Fig. 53-5). The autoinjection system requires no preparation, and the self-administration technique is not complicated. The patient must be given an opportunity to demonstrate the correct technique for use; an EpiPen training device can be used for teaching correct technique. Verbal and written information about the emergency kit, as well as strategies to avoid exposure to threatening allergens, must also be provided.

Screening for allergies before a medication is prescribed or first administered is an important preventive measure. A careful history of any sensitivity to suspected antigens must be obtained before administering any medication, particularly in parenteral form, because this route is associated with the most severe anaphylaxis. Nurses caring for patients in any setting (hospital, home, outpatient diagnostic testing sites, long-term care facilities) must assess patients' risks for anaphylactic reactions. Patients are asked about previous exposure to contrast agents used for diagnostic tests and any allergic reactions, as well as reactions to any medications, foods, insect stings, and latex. People who are predisposed

to anaphylaxis should wear some form of identification, such as a MedicAlert bracelet, which names allergies to medications, food, and other substances.

People who are allergic to insect venom may require venom immunotherapy, which is used as a control measure and not a cure. Immunotherapy administered after an insect sting is very effective in reducing the risk of anaphylaxis from future stings (Douglass & O'Hehir, 2006; Walker, 2007). Insulin-allergic patients with diabetes and those who are allergic to penicillin may require desensitization. Desensitization is based on controlled anaphylaxis, with a gradual release of mediators. Patients who undergo desensitization are cautioned that there should be no lapses in therapy, because this may lead to the reappearance of the allergic reaction when the use of the medication is resumed.

Medical Management

Management depends on the severity of the reaction. Initially, respiratory and cardiovascular functions are evaluated. If the patient is in cardiac arrest, cardiopulmonary resuscitation is instituted. Oxygen is provided in high concentrations during cardiopulmonary resuscitation or if the patient is cyanotic, dyspneic, or wheezing. Epinephrine, in a 1:1000 dilution, is administered subcutaneously in the upper extremity or thigh and may be followed by a continuous IV infusion. Most adverse events associated with administration of epinephrine (ie, adrenaline) occur when the dose is excessive or it is given intravenously. Patients at risk for adverse effects include elderly patients and those with hypertension, arteriopathies, or known ischemic heart disease.

Antihistamines and corticosteroids may also be administered to prevent recurrences of the reaction (Goroll & Mulley, 2006) and to treat urticaria and angioedema. IV fluids (eg, normal saline solution), volume expanders, and vasopressor agents are administered to maintain blood pressure and normal hemodynamic status. In patients with episodes of bronchospasm or a history of bronchial asthma or chronic obstructive pulmonary disease, aminophylline and corticosteroids may also be administered to improve airway patency and function. If hypotension is unresponsive to vasopressors, glucagon may be administered intravenously for its acute inotropic and chronotropic effects.

Patients who have experienced anaphylactic reactions and received epinephrine should be transported to the local emergency department for observation and monitoring because of the risk for a "rebound" reaction 4 to 10 hours after the initial allergic reaction. Patients with severe reactions are monitored closely for 12 to 14 hours in a facility that can provide emergency care, if needed. Because of the potential for recurrence, patients with even mild reactions must be informed about this risk (Goroll & Mulley, 2006; Lieberman, 2006).

Nursing Management

If a patient is experiencing an allergic response, the nurse's initial action is to assess the patient for signs and symptoms of anaphylaxis. The nurse assesses the airway, breathing pattern, and vital signs. The patient is observed for signs of increasing edema and respiratory distress. Prompt notification of the physician and preparation for initiation of emergency measures (intubation, administration of emergency medications, insertion of IV lines, fluid administration, oxygen

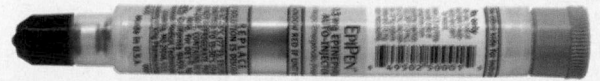

Figure 53-5 The EpiPen. Autoinjectors are commercially available first-aid devices that administer premeasured doses of epinephrine. An EpiPen training device is available for patients to practice correct self-injection technique. Courtesy of Dey, L. P., Napa, CA.

administration) are important to reduce the severity of the reaction and to restore cardiovascular function. The nurse documents the interventions used and the patient's vital signs and response to treatment.

The patient who has recovered from anaphylaxis needs an explanation of what occurred and instruction about avoiding future exposure to antigens and how to administer emergency medications to treat anaphylaxis. The patient must be instructed about antigens that should be avoided and about other strategies to prevent recurrence of anaphylaxis. All patients who have experienced an anaphylactic reaction should receive a prescription for preloaded syringes of epinephrine. The nurse instructs the patient and family in their use and has the patient and family demonstrate correct administration (Chart 53-4).

Allergic Rhinitis

Allergic **rhinitis** (hay fever, seasonal allergic rhinitis) is the most common form of respiratory allergy presumed to be mediated by an immediate (type I hypersensitivity) immunologic reaction, and it is among the top 10 reasons for visits to primary care physicians (Ferguson, 2008; Quillen & Feller, 2006). It affects about 10% to 25% of the U.S. population

(Nathan, 2008). The symptoms are similar to those of viral rhinitis (see Chapter 22) but are usually more persistent and demonstrate seasonal variation; rhinitis is considered to be the allergic form if the symptoms are caused by an allergen-specific IgE-mediated immunologic response. However, a sizable proportion of patients with rhinitis have mixed rhinitis, or coexisting allergic and nonallergic rhinitis (Nathan, 2008). The proportion of patients with the allergic form of rhinitis increases with age. It often occurs with other conditions, such as allergic conjunctivitis, sinusitis, and asthma. If symptoms are severe, allergic rhinitis may interfere with sleep, leisure, and school or work activities (Quillen & Feller, 2006). If left untreated, many complications may result, such as allergic asthma, chronic nasal obstruction, chronic otitis media with hearing loss, anosmia (absence of the sense of smell), and, in children, orofacial dental deformities. Early diagnosis and adequate treatment are essential to reduce complications and relieve symptoms.

Because allergic rhinitis is induced by airborne pollens or molds, it is characterized by the following seasonal occurrences:

- Early spring—tree pollen (oak, elm, poplar)
- Early summer—rose pollen (rose fever), grass pollen (Timothy, red-top)
- Early fall—weed pollen (ragweed)

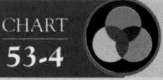

CHART 53-4

PATIENT EDUCATION
Self-Administration of Epinephrine

1. After removing the EpiPen autoinjector from its carrying tube, grasp the unit with the black tip (injecting end) pointing downward. Form fist around the unit with the black tip down and with your other hand, remove the gray safety release cap.

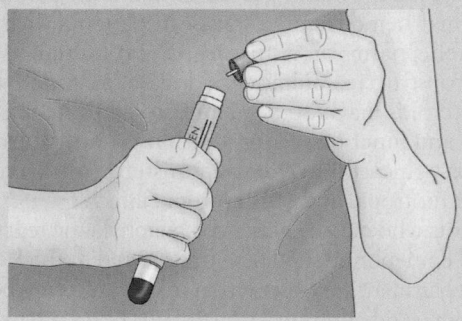

2. Hold black tip near outer thigh. Swing and **jab firmly** into outer thigh until a click is heard with the device perpendicular (90-degree angle) to the thigh.

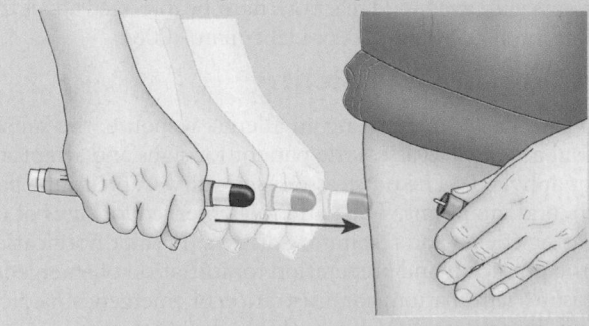

3. Hold firmly against the thigh for approximately 10 seconds. Remove the unit from the thigh and massage injection area for 10 seconds. Call 911 and seek immediate medical attention. Carefully place the used EpiPen, needle-end first, into the device storage tube without bending the needle. Screw on the storage tube completely, and take with you to the hospital emergency room.

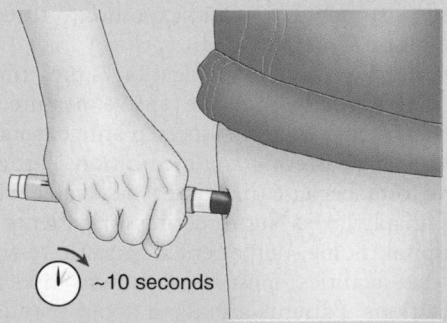

~10 seconds

Each year attacks begin and end at about the same time. Airborne mold spores require warm, damp weather. Although there is no rigid seasonal pattern, these spores appear in early spring, are rampant during the summer, then taper off and disappear by the first frost in areas that experience dramatic seasonal temperature variation. In temperate areas that do not experience freezing temperatures, these allergens, especially mold, can persist throughout the year.

Pathophysiology

Sensitization begins by ingestion or inhalation of an antigen. On re-exposure, the nasal mucosa reacts by the slowing of ciliary action, edema formation, and leukocyte (primarily eosinophil) infiltration. Histamine is the major mediator of allergic reactions in the nasal mucosa. Tissue edema results from vasodilation and increased capillary permeability.

Clinical Manifestations

Typical signs and symptoms of allergic rhinitis include sneezing and nasal congestion; clear, watery nasal discharge; and nasal itching. Itching of the throat and soft palate is common. Drainage of nasal mucus into the pharynx results in multiple attempts to clear the throat and results in a dry cough or hoarseness. Headache, pain over the paranasal sinuses, and epistaxis can accompany allergic rhinitis. The symptoms of this chronic condition depend on environmental exposure and intrinsic host responsiveness. Allergic rhinitis can affect quality of life by also producing fatigue, loss of sleep, and poor concentration (Nathan, 2008).

Assessment and Diagnostic Findings

Diagnosis of seasonal allergic rhinitis is based on history, physical examination, and diagnostic test results. Diagnostic tests include nasal smears, peripheral blood counts, total serum IgE, epicutaneous and intradermal testing, RAST, food elimination and challenge, and nasal provocation tests. Results indicative of allergy as the cause of rhinitis include increased IgE and eosinophil levels and positive reactions on allergen testing. False-positive and false-negative responses to these tests, particularly skin testing and provocation tests, may occur.

Medical Management

The goal of therapy is to provide relief from symptoms. Therapy may include one or all of the following interventions: avoidance therapy, pharmacotherapy, and immunotherapy. Verbal instructions must be reinforced by written information. Knowledge of general concepts regarding assessment and therapy in allergic diseases is important so that the patient can learn to manage certain conditions as well as prevent severe reactions and illnesses.

Avoidance Therapy

In avoidance therapy, every attempt is made to remove the allergens that act as precipitating factors. Simple measures and environmental controls are often effective in decreasing symptoms. Examples include use of air conditioners, air cleaners, humidifiers, and dehumidifiers; removal of dust-catching furnishings, carpets, and window coverings; removal of pets from the home or bedroom; use of pillow and mattress covers that are impermeable to dust mites; and a smoke-free environment (Nathan, 2008; Quillen & Feller, 2006). Because multiple allergens are often implicated, multiple measures to avoid exposure to allergens are often necessary (Nathan, 2008; Platts-Mills, Leung & Schatz, 2007). High-efficiency particulate air (HEPA) purifiers and vacuum cleaner filters may also be used to reduce allergens in the environment. Research has shown that multiple avoidance strategies tailored to a person's risk factors can reduce the severity of symptoms, the number of work or school days missed because of symptoms, and the number of unscheduled health care visits for treatment (Ferguson, 2008). In many cases, it is impossible to avoid exposure to all environmental allergens, so pharmacologic therapy or immunotherapy is needed.

Pharmacologic Therapy

Antihistamines

Antihistamines, now classified as H_1 receptor antagonists (or H_1-blockers), are used in the management of mild allergic disorders. H_1 blockers bind selectively to H_1 receptors, preventing the actions of histamines at these sites. They do not prevent the release of histamine from mast cells or basophils. The H_1 antagonists have no effect on H_2 receptors, but they do have the ability to bind to nonhistaminic receptors. The ability of certain antihistamines to bind to and block muscarinic receptors underlies several of the prominent anticholinergic side effects of these medications.

Oral antihistamines, which are readily absorbed, are most effective when given at the first occurrence of symptoms, because they prevent the development of new symptoms. The effectiveness of these medications is limited to certain patients with hay fever, vasomotor rhinitis, **urticaria** (hives), and mild asthma. They are rarely effective in other conditions or in any severe conditions.

Antihistamines are the major class of medications prescribed for the symptomatic relief of allergic rhinitis. The major side effect is sedation, although H_1 antagonists are less sedating than earlier antihistamines (Arcangelo & Peterson, 2005; Karch, 2008). Additional side effects include nervousness, tremors, dizziness, dry mouth, palpitations, anorexia, nausea, and vomiting. Antihistamines are contraindicated during the third trimester of pregnancy; in nursing mothers and newborns; in children and elderly people; and in patients whose conditions may be aggravated by muscarinic blockade (eg, asthma, urinary retention, open-angle glaucoma, hypertension, prostatic hyperplasia).

Newer antihistamines are called second-generation or nonsedating H_1 receptor antagonists. Unlike first-generation H_1 receptor antagonists, they do not cross the blood–brain barrier and do not bind to cholinergic, serotoninergic, or alpha-adrenergic receptors (Karch, 2008). They bind to peripheral rather than central nervous system H_1 receptors, causing less sedation. Examples of these medications are loratadine (Claritin), cetirizine (Zyrtec), and fexofenadine (Allegra). These are summarized in Table 53-2.

Antihistamines may also be combined with decongestants to reduce the nasal congestion associated with allergies. Some of these combination products are available as over-the-counter (nonprescription) medications; examples are desloratadine/pseudoephedrine (Claritin-D) and

Table 53-2 **SELECTED H₁ ANTIHISTAMINES**

H₁ Antihistamine	Contraindications	Major Side Effects	Nursing Implications and Patient Teaching
First-Generation H₁ Antihistamines (Sedating)			
Diphenhydramine (Benadryl)	Allergy to any antihistamines Third trimester of pregnancy Lactation Use cautiously with narrow-angle glaucoma, asthma, stenosing peptic ulcer, BPH or bladder neck obstruction, pregnancy, elderly patients, hypertension	Drowsiness, confusion, dizziness, dry mouth, nausea, vomiting, photosensitivity, urinary retention	Administer with food if gastrointestinal upset occurs. Caution patients to avoid alcohol, driving, or engaging in any hazardous activities until CNS response to medication is stabilized. Suggest sucking on sugarless lozenges or ice chips for relief of dry mouth. Encourage use of sunscreen and hat while outdoors. Assess for urinary retention; monitor urinary output.
Chlorpheniramine (Chlor-Trimeton)	Allergy to any antihistamines Third trimester of pregnancy Lactation Use cautiously with narrow-angle glaucoma, asthma, stenosing peptic ulcer, BPH or bladder neck obstruction, pregnancy, elderly patients, hypertension	Drowsiness, sedation, and dizziness, although less than other sedating agents; confusion, dry mouth, nausea, vomiting, urinary retention, epigastric distress, thickening of bronchial secretions	Caution patients to avoid alcohol, driving, or engaging in any hazardous activities until CNS response to medication is stabilized. Suggest sucking on sugarless lozenges or ice chips for relief of dry mouth. Recommend use of humidifier.
Hydroxyzine (Atarax)	Allergy to hydroxyzine or cetirizine (Zyrtec), pregnancy, lactation, hypertension	Drowsiness, dry mouth, involuntary motor activity, including tremor and seizures	Caution patients to avoid alcohol, driving, or engaging in any hazardous activities until CNS response to medication is stabilized. Suggest sucking on sugarless lozenges or ice chips for relief of dry mouth. Instruct patients to report tremors.
Second-Generation H₁ Antihistamines (Nonsedating)			
Cetirizine (Zyrtec)	Allergy to any antihistamines Narrow-angle glaucoma Asthma Stenosing peptic ulcer BPH or bladder neck obstruction Lactation Hypertension	Dry nasal mucosa, thickening of bronchial secretions	Can be taken without regard to meals. Instruct patients to use caution if driving or performing tasks that require alertness. Recommend use of humidifier.
Desloratadine (Clarinex)	Allergy to loratadine (Alavert, Claritin) Lactation Use cautiously with renal or hepatic impairment pregnancy, hypertension	Somnolence, nervousness, dizziness, fatigue, dry mouth	Can be taken without regard to meals. Suggest sucking on sugarless lozenges or ice chips for relief of dry mouth. Recommend use of humidifier.
Loratadine (Alavert, Claritin)	Allergy to any antihistamines Narrow-angle glaucoma Asthma Stenosing peptic ulcer BPH or bladder neck obstruction, hypertension	Headache, nervousness, dizziness, depression, edema, increased appetite	Instruct patients to take on empty stomach (1 h before or 2 h after meals or food). Instruct patients to avoid alcohol and to use caution if driving or performing tasks that require alertness. Suggest sucking on sugarless lozenges or ice chips for relief of dry mouth. Recommend use of humidifier.
Fexofenadine (Allegra)	Allergy to any antihistamines Pregnancy Lactation Use with caution with hepatic or renal impairment, in elderly patients, and with hypertension	Fatigue, drowsiness, GI upset	Should not be administered within 15 min of ingestion of antacids. Instruct patients to use caution if driving or performing tasks that require alertness. Recommend use of humidifier.

BPH = benign prostatic hyperplasia; CNS = central nervous system.

cetirizine/pseudoephedrine (Zyrtec-D). Decongestants can cause an increase in blood pressure; therefore, patients with a history of hypertension should be cautioned about long-term use of any medication containing decongestants.

Adrenergic Agents

Adrenergic agents, vasoconstrictors of mucosal vessels, are used topically (nasal and ophthalmic formulations) in addition to the oral route. The topical route (drops and sprays) causes fewer side effects than oral administration; however, the use of drops and sprays should be limited to a few days to avoid rebound congestion. Adrenergic nasal decongestants are applied topically to the nasal mucosa for the relief of nasal congestion. They activate the alpha-adrenergic receptor sites on the smooth muscle of the nasal mucosal blood vessels, reducing local blood flow, fluid exudation, and mucosal edema. Topical ophthalmic drops are used for symptomatic relief of eye irritations caused by allergies. Potential side effects include hypertension, dysrhythmias, palpitations, central nervous system stimulation, irritability, tremor, and tachyphylaxis (acceleration of hemodynamic status).

Mast Cell Stabilizers

Intranasal cromolyn sodium (NasalCrom) is a spray that acts by stabilizing the mast cell membrane, thus reducing the release of histamine and other mediators of the allergic response. In addition, it inhibits macrophages, eosinophils, monocytes, and platelets involved in the immune response

(Arcangelo & Peterson, 2005). Cromolyn interrupts the physiologic response to nasal antigens, and it is used prophylactically (before exposure to allergens) to prevent the onset of symptoms and to treat symptoms once they occur. It is also used therapeutically in chronic allergic rhinitis. This spray is as effective as antihistamines but is less effective than intranasal corticosteroids in the treatment of seasonal allergic rhinitis. The patient must be informed that the beneficial effects of the medication may take a week or so to manifest. The medication is of no benefit in the treatment of nonallergic rhinitis. Adverse effects (eg, sneezing, local stinging and burning sensations) are usually mild.

Corticosteroids

Intranasal corticosteroids are indicated in more severe cases of allergic and perennial rhinitis that cannot be controlled by more conventional medications such as decongestants, antihistamines, and intranasal cromolyn. Examples of these medications include beclomethasone (Beconase, Vancenase), budesonide (Rhinocort), dexamethasone (Decadron Phosphate Turbinaire), flunisolide (Nasalide), fluticasone (Cutivate, Flonase), and triamcinolone (Nasacort).

Because of their anti-inflammatory actions, corticosteroids are equally effective in preventing or suppressing the major symptoms of allergic rhinitis. These medications are administered by metered-spray devices. If the nasal passages are blocked, a topical decongestant may be used to clear the passages before the administration of the intranasal corticosteroid. Patients must be aware that full benefit may not be achieved for several days to 2 weeks. Adverse effects of intranasal corticosteroids are mild and include drying of the nasal mucosa and burning and itching sensations caused by the vehicle used to administer the medication. Systemic effects are more likely with dexamethasone. Recommended use of this medication is limited to 30 days. Beclomethasone, budesonide, flunisolide, fluticasone, and triamcinolone are deactivated rapidly after absorption, so they do not achieve significant blood levels. Because corticosteroids suppress host defenses, they must be used with caution in patients with tuberculosis or untreated bacterial infections of the lungs. Patients taking corticosteroids are at risk for infection and suppression of typical manifestations of inflammation, because host defenses are compromised. Inhaled corticosteroids do not affect the immune system to the same degree as systemic corticosteroids (ie, oral corticosteroids). Because corticosteroids are inhaled into the upper respiratory tract, tuberculosis or untreated bacterial infections of the lungs may become apparent and progress. Whenever possible, patients with tuberculosis or other bacterial infections of the lungs should avoid inhaled corticosteroids.

Oral and parenteral corticosteroids are used when conventional therapy has failed and symptoms are severe and of short duration. They can control symptoms of allergic reactions such as hay fever, medication-induced allergies, and allergic reactions to insect stings. Because the response to corticosteroids is delayed, these agents have little or no value in acute therapy for severe reactions such as anaphylaxis. Patients who receive corticosteroids must be cautioned not to stop taking the medication suddenly or without specific instructions from the physician. The patient is also instructed about side effects, which include fluid retention, weight gain, hypertension, gastric irritation, glucose intolerance, and adrenal suppression. Further discussion of corticosteroids is provided in Chapter 42.

Leukotriene Modifiers

As previously discussed, leukotrienes have many effects on the inflammatory cycle. Leukotriene modifiers, such as zileuton (Zyflo), zafirlukast (Accolate), and montelukast (Singulair), block the synthesis or action of leukotrienes and prevent the signs and symptoms associated with asthma (Table 53-3).

Leukotriene modifiers are for long-term use, and patients should be advised to take their medication daily. Patients take appropriate "rescue" medications for symptom exacerbation but continue to take the leukotriene modifier on a daily basis. The 2007 National Asthma Education and Prevention Program (NAEPP) suggests using a leukotriene modifier in conjunction with an inhaled corticosteroid for mild persistent asthma.

Immunotherapy

Allergen desensitization (allergen immunotherapy, hyposensitization) is primarily used to treat IgE-mediated diseases by injections of allergen extracts. Immunotherapy, also referred to as allergy vaccine therapy, involves the administration of gradually increasing quantities of specific allergens to the patient until a dose is reached that is effective in reducing disease severity from natural exposure (Stokes, 2008). This type of therapy provides an adjunct to symptomatic pharmacologic therapy and can be used when avoidance of allergens is not possible. Specific immunotherapy has been used in the treatment of allergic disorders for about 100 years. Goals of immunotherapy include reducing the level of circulating IgE, increasing the level of blocking antibody IgG, and reducing mediator cell sensitivity. Immunotherapy has been most effective for ragweed pollen;

Table 53-3	LEUKOTRIENE MODIFIERS		
Leukotriene Modifier	**Available Formulations**		**Frequency of Dosing**
Leukotriene-Receptor Antagonists (LTRAs)			
Zafirlukast (Accolate)	Tablets: 10 mg; 20 mg		Taken twice a day
Montelukast (Singulair)	Tablets: 10 mg		Taken once a day
	Chewable tablets: 4 mg; 5 mg		in PM
	Granules: 4 mg/packet		
Leukotriene-Receptor Inhibitors (LTRIs)			
Zileuton (Zyflo CR)	Tables: 600 mg extended release		Taken twice a day within 1 h after morning and evening meals

Chart 53-5 • *Immunotherapy: Indications and Contraindications*

Indications

- Allergic rhinitis, conjunctivitis, or allergic asthma
- History of a systemic reaction to Hymenoptera and specific IgE antibodies to Hymenoptera venom
- Desire to avoid the long-term use, potential adverse effects, or costs of medications
- Lack of control of symptoms by avoidance measures or use of medications

Contraindications

- Use of beta-blocker or angiotensin-converting enzyme (ACE) inhibitor therapy, which may mask early signs of anaphylaxis
- Presence of significant pulmonary or cardiac disease or organ failure
- Inability of the patient to recognize or report signs and symptoms of a systemic reaction
- Nonadherence of the patient to other therapeutic regimens and nonlikelihood that the patient will adhere to the immunization schedule (often weekly for an indefinite period)
- Inability to monitor the patient for at least 30 minutes after administration of immunotherapy
- Absence of equipment or adequate personnel to respond to allergic reaction if one occurs

however, treatment for grass, tree pollen, cat dander, and house dust mite allergens has also been effective. Indications and contraindications for immunotherapy are presented in Chart 53-5.

Correlation of a positive skin test with a positive allergy history is an indication for immunotherapy if the allergen cannot be avoided. The benefit of immunotherapy has been fairly well established in instances of allergic rhinitis and bronchial asthma that are clearly due to sensitivity to one of the common pollens, molds, or household dust. Unlike antiallergy medication, allergen immunotherapy has the potential to alter the allergic disease course after 3 to 5 years of therapy. Because it may prevent progression or development of asthma or multiple or additional allergies, it is also considered to be a potential preventive measure (Stokes, 2008). The patient must understand what to expect and the importance of continuing therapy for several years before immunotherapy is accomplished. When skin tests are performed, the results are correlated with symptoms; treatment is based on the patient's needs rather than on the results of skin tests.

The most common method of treatment is the serial injection of one or more antigens that are selected in each particular case on the basis of skin testing. This method provides a simple and efficient technique for identifying IgE antibodies to specific antigens. Specific treatment consists of injecting extracts of the allergens that cause symptoms in a particular patient. Injections begin with very small amounts and are gradually increased, usually at weekly intervals, until a maximum tolerated dose is attained. Maintenance booster injections are administered at 2- to 4-week intervals, frequently for a period of several years, before maximum benefit is achieved, although some patients will

note early improvement in their symptoms. Long-term benefit seems to be related to the cumulative dose of vaccine given over time (Stokes, 2008). Immunotherapy should not be initiated during pregnancy; for patients who have been receiving immunotherapy before pregnancy, the dosage should not be increased during pregnancy.

Although severe systemic reactions are rare, the risk of systemic and potentially fatal anaphylaxis exists. It tends to occur most frequently at the induction or "up-dosing" phase. Therefore, the patient must be monitored after administration of immunotherapy. Because of the risk of anaphylaxis, injections should not be administered by a lay person or by the patient. The patient must remain in the office or clinic for at least 30 minutes after the injection and is observed for possible systemic symptoms. If a large, local swelling develops at the injection site, the next dose should not be increased, because this may be a warning sign of a possible systemic reaction.

 NURSING ALERT

Because the injection of an allergen may induce systemic reactions, such injections are administered only in a setting (ie, physician's office, clinic) where epinephrine is immediately available.

Therapeutic failure is evident when a patient does not experience a decrease of symptoms within 12 to 24 months, fails to develop increased tolerance to known allergens, and cannot decrease the use of medications to reduce symptoms. Potential causes of treatment failure include misdiagnosis of allergies, inadequate doses of allergen, newly developed allergies, and inadequate environmental controls.

NURSING PROCESS

THE PATIENT WITH ALLERGIC RHINITIS

Assessment

The examination and history of the patient reveal sneezing, often in paroxysms; thin and watery nasal discharge; itching eyes and nose; lacrimation; and occasionally headache. The health history includes a personal or family history of allergy. The allergy assessment identifies the nature of antigens, seasonal changes in symptoms, and medication history. The nurse also obtains subjective data about how the patient feels just before symptoms become obvious, such as the occurrence of pruritus, breathing problems, and tingling sensations. In addition to these symptoms, hoarseness, wheezing, hives, rash, erythema, and edema are noted. Any relationship between emotional problems or stress and the triggering of allergy symptoms is assessed.

Diagnosis

Nursing Diagnoses

Based on the assessment data, the patient's major nursing diagnoses may include the following:

- Ineffective breathing pattern related to allergic reaction

- Deficient knowledge about allergy and the recommended modifications in lifestyle and self-care practices
- Ineffective individual coping with chronicity of condition and need for environmental modifications

Collaborative Problems/Potential Complications

Based on assessment data, potential complications may include the following:

- Anaphylaxis
- Impaired breathing
- Nonadherence to the therapeutic regimen

Planning and Goals

The goals for the patient may include restoration of normal breathing pattern, increased knowledge about the causes and control of allergic symptoms, improved coping with alterations and modifications, and absence of complications.

Nursing Interventions

Improving Breathing Pattern

The patient is instructed and assisted to modify the environment to reduce the severity of allergic symptoms or to prevent their occurrence. The patient is instructed to reduce exposure to people with upper respiratory tract infections. If an upper respiratory infection occurs, the patient is encouraged to take deep breaths and to cough frequently to ensure adequate gas exchange and prevent atelectasis. The patient is instructed to seek medical attention, because the presence of allergy symptoms along with an upper respiratory tract infection may compromise adequate lung function. Adherence to medication schedules and other treatment regimens is encouraged and reinforced.

Promoting Understanding of Allergy and Allergy Control

Instruction includes strategies to minimize exposure to allergens and explanation about desensitization procedures and correct use of medications. The nurse informs and reminds the patient of the importance of keeping appointments for desensitization procedures, because dosages are usually adjusted on a weekly basis, and missed appointments may interfere with the dosage adjustment.

Patients also need to understand that medications for allergy control should be used only when the allergy is apparent. This is usually on a seasonal basis. Continued use of medications when not required can cause an increased tolerance to the medication, with the result that the medication will not be effective when needed.

Coping With a Chronic Disorder

Although allergic reactions are infrequently life-threatening, they require constant vigilance to avoid allergens and modification of the lifestyle or environment to prevent recurrence of symptoms. Allergic symptoms are often present year-round and create discomfort and inconvenience for the patient. Although patients may not feel ill during allergy seasons, they often do not feel well, either. The need to be alert for possible allergens in the environment may be tiresome, placing a burden on the patient's ability to lead a normal life. Stress related to these difficulties may in turn increase the frequency or severity of symptoms.

To assist the patient in adjusting to these modifications, the nurse must have an appreciation of the difficulties encountered by the patient. The patient is encouraged to verbalize feelings and concerns in a supportive environment and to identify strategies to deal with them effectively.

Monitoring and Managing Potential Complications

ANAPHYLAXIS AND IMPAIRED BREATHING. Respiratory and cardiovascular functioning can be significantly altered during allergic reactions by the reaction itself or by the medications used to treat reactions. The respiratory status is evaluated by monitoring the respiratory rate and pattern and by assessing for breathing difficulties or abnormal lung sounds. The pulse rate and rhythm and blood pressure are monitored to assess cardiovascular status regularly or any time the patient reports symptoms such as itching or difficulty breathing. In the event of signs and symptoms suggestive of anaphylaxis, emergency medications and equipment must be available for immediate use.

NONADHERENCE TO THE THERAPEUTIC REGIMEN. Knowing about the treatment regimen does not ensure adherence. Having the patient identify potential barriers and explore acceptable solutions for effective management of the condition (eg, installing tile floors rather than carpet, not gardening in the spring) can increase adherence to the treatment regimen.

Promoting Home and Community-Based Care

TEACHING PATIENTS SELF-CARE. The patient is instructed about strategies to minimize exposure to allergens, the actions and adverse effects of medications, and the correct use of medications. The patient should know the name, dose, frequency, actions, and side effects of all medications taken.

Instruction about strategies to control allergic symptoms is based on the needs of the patient as determined by the results of tests, the severity of symptoms, and the motivation of the patient and family to deal with the condition. Suggestions for patients who are sensitive to dust and mold in the home are given in Chart 53-6. Additional nursing interventions for allergy management are presented in Chart 53-7.

If the patient is to undergo immunotherapy, the nurse reinforces the physician's explanation regarding the purpose and procedure. Instructions are given regarding the series of injections, which usually are administered initially every week and then at 2- to 4-week intervals. These instructions include remaining in the physician's office or the clinic for at least 30 minutes after the injection so that emergency treatment can be given if the patient has a reaction; avoiding rubbing or scratching the injection site; and continuing with the series for the period of time required. In addition, the patient and family are instructed about emergency treatment of severe allergic symptoms.

Because antihistamines may produce drowsiness, the patient is cautioned about this and other side effects of the particular medication. Operating machinery, driving a car, and performing activities that require intense concentration should be postponed. The patient is also informed about the dangers of drinking alcohol when taking these medications, because they tend to exaggerate the effects of alcohol.

CHART 53-6

HOME CARE CHECKLIST
Allergy Management

At the completion of the home care instruction, the patient or caregiver will be able to:	PATIENT	CAREGIVER
• Verbalize how to maintain a dust-free environment by removing drapes, curtains, and venetian blinds and replacing them with pull shades; covering the mattress with a hypoallergenic cover that can be zipped; and removing rugs and replacing them with wood flooring or linoleum.	✔	✔
• Identify rationale for washing the floor and dusting and vacuuming daily.	✔	✔
• Identify rationale for replacing stuffed furniture with wood pieces that can easily be dusted.	✔	✔
• State rationale for wearing a mask whenever cleaning is being done.	✔	✔
• Identify rationale for avoiding use of tufted bedspreads, stuffed toys, and feather pillows and replacing them with washable cotton material.	✔	✔
• State rationale for avoiding the use of any clothing that causes itching.	✔	✔
• Verbalize ways to reduce dust in the house as a whole by using steam or hot water for heating rather than air and using air filters or air conditioning.	✔	✔
• Verbalize ways to reduce exposure to pollens or molds by identifying seasons of the year when pollen counts are high; wearing a mask at times of increased exposure (windy days and when grass is being cut); and avoiding contact with weeds, dry leaves, and freshly cut grass.	✔	✔
• State rationale for seeking air-conditioned areas at the height of the allergy season.	✔	✔
• State rationale for avoiding sprays and perfumes.	✔	✔
• State rationale for use of hypoallergenic cosmetics.		
• State rationale for taking prescribed medications as ordered.	✔	✔
• Identify specific foods that may cause allergic symptoms. (Examples of foods that can cause allergic reactions are fish, nuts, eggs, and chocolate.)	✔	✔
• Develop a list of foods to avoid.	✔	✔

Chart 53-7 • *Selected Nursing Strategies for Allergy Management*

- Identify the patient's known allergens (eg, medications, foods, insects, environmental allergens).
- Describe the patient's typical allergic reaction and its severity.
- Document the patient's allergies (eg, medications, foods, insects, environmental allergens) in the patient's medical record.
- Post allergy alerts appropriately.
- Encourage the patient to wear a medical alert band and to carry information about allergies at all times.
- Monitor the patient closely after administration of new medications and exposure to new foods, contrast agents, latex, and other allergens.
- Investigate potential for allergic reactions with all new medications through consultation with the pharmacist.
- Instruct the patient to question all medications and new foods.
- Identify early manifestations of allergic reactions.
- Administer emergency treatment for allergic reactions.
- Monitor the patient's response and status for 12–14 hours after a severe allergic reaction.
- Instruct the patient and family about emergency home management of allergic reaction.
- Instruct the patient and family about avoidance measures to reduce risk of exposure to allergens.

The patient must be aware of the effects caused by overuse of the sympathomimetic agents in nose drops or sprays. A condition referred to as rhinitis medicamentosa may result (Fig. 53-6). After topical application of the medication, a rebound period occurs in which the nasal mucous membranes become more edematous and congested than they were before the medication was used. Such a reaction encourages the use of more medication, and a cyclic pattern results. The topical agent must be discontinued immediately and completely to correct this problem.

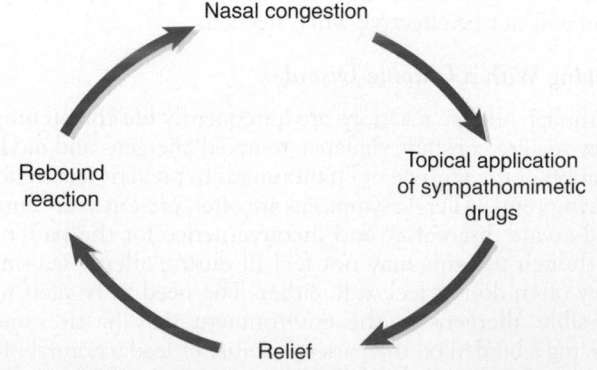

Figure 53-6 Rhinitis medicamentosa. This cyclic pattern results from overuse of sympathomimetic nose drops or sprays.

CONTINUING CARE. Follow-up telephone calls to the patient are often reassuring to the patient and family and provide an opportunity for the nurse to answer any questions. The patient is reminded to keep follow-up appointments and is informed about the importance of continuing with treatment. The importance of participating in health promotion activities and health screening is also emphasized.

Evaluation

Expected Patient Outcomes

Expected patient outcomes may include the following:

1. Exhibits normal breathing patterns
   a. Demonstrates lungs clear on auscultation
   b. Exhibits absence of adventitious breath sounds (crackles, rhonchi, wheezing)
   c. Has a normal respiratory rate and pattern
   d. Reports no complaints of respiratory distress (shortness of breath, difficulty on inspiration or expiration)
2. Demonstrates knowledge about allergy and strategies to control symptoms
   a. Identifies causative allergens, if known
   b. States methods of avoiding allergens and controlling indoor and outdoor precipitating factors
   c. Removes from the environment items that retain dust
   d. Wears a dampened mask if dust or mold may be a problem
   e. Avoids smoke-filled rooms and dust-filled or freshly sprayed areas
   f. Uses air conditioning for a major part of the day when allergens are high
   g. Takes antihistamines as prescribed; participates in hyposensitization program, if applicable
   h. Describes name, purpose, side effects, and method of administration of prescribed medications
   i. Identifies when to seek immediate medical attention for severe allergic responses
   j. Describes activities that are possible, including ways to participate in activities without activating the allergies
3. Experiences relief of discomfort while adapting to the inconveniences of an allergy
   a. Relates the emotional aspects of the allergic response
   b. Demonstrates use of measures to cope positively with allergy
4. Demonstrates absence of complications
   a. Exhibits vital signs within normal limits
   b. Reports no symptoms or episodes of anaphylaxis (urticaria, itching, peripheral tingling, fullness in the mouth and throat, flushing, difficulty swallowing, coughing, wheezing, or difficulty breathing)
   c. Demonstrates correct procedure to self-administer emergency medications to treat severe allergic reaction
   d. Correctly states medication names, dose and frequency of administration, and medication actions
   e. Correctly identifies side effects and untoward signs and symptoms to report to physician
   f. Discusses acceptable lifestyle changes and solutions for identified potential barriers to adherence to treatment and medication regimen

Contact Dermatitis

Contact dermatitis, a type IV delayed hypersensitivity reaction, is an acute or chronic skin inflammation that results from direct skin contact with chemicals or allergens. There are four basic types: allergic, irritant, phototoxic, and photoallergic (Table 53-4). Eighty percent of cases are caused by excessive exposure to or additive effects of irritants (eg, soaps, detergents, organic solvents). Skin sensitivity may develop after brief or prolonged periods of exposure, and the clinical picture may appear hours or weeks after the sensitized skin has been exposed.

Clinical Manifestations

Symptoms include itching, burning, erythema, skin lesions (vesicles), and edema, followed by weeping, crusting, and finally drying and peeling of the skin. In severe responses, hemorrhagic bullae may develop. Repeated reactions may be accompanied by thickening of the skin and pigmentary changes. Secondary invasion by bacteria may develop in skin that is abraded by rubbing or scratching. Usually, there are no systemic symptoms unless the eruption is widespread.

Assessment and Diagnostic Findings

The location of the skin eruption and the history of exposure aid in determining the condition. However, in cases of obscure irritants or an unobservant patient, the diagnosis can be extremely difficult, often involving many trial-and-error procedures before the cause is determined. Patch tests on the skin with suspected offending agents may clarify the diagnosis. The patch test most commonly used is the Thin-layer Rapid Use Epicutaneous (TRUE) test.

Atopic Dermatitis

Atopic dermatitis is a type I immediate hypersensitivity disorder characterized by inflammation and hyperreactivity of the skin. Other terms used to describe this skin disorder include atopic eczema, atopic dermatitis/eczema, and atopic dermatitis/eczema syndrome (AEDS). In a revised classification system developed to clarify terminology, AEDS includes both allergic and nonallergic disorders. The term *atopic dermatitis* is currently the most commonly used of these terms and is used in the following discussion.

Atopic dermatitis affects 15% to 20% of children and 1% to 3% of adults in developed countries (Bieber, 2008). Most patients have significant elevations of serum IgE and peripheral eosinophilia. Pruritus and hyperirritability of the skin are the most consistent features of atopic dermatitis and are related to large amounts of histamine in the skin. Excessive dryness of the skin with resultant itching is related to changes

Table 53-4	TYPES, TESTING, AND TREATMENT OF CONTACT DERMATITIS			
Type	**Etiology**	**Clinical Presentation**	**Diagnostic Testing**	**Treatment**
Allergic	Results from contact of skin and allergenic substance. Has a sensitization period of 10–14 days.	Vasodilation and perivascular infiltrates on the dermis Intracellular edema Usually seen on dorsal aspects of hand	Patch testing (contraindicated in acute, widespread dermatitis)	Avoidance of offending material Burow's solution or cool water compress Systemic corticosteroids (prednisone) for 7–10 days Topical corticosteroids for mild cases Oral antihistamines to relieve pruritus
Irritant	Results from contact with a substance that chemically or physically damages the skin on a nonimmunologic basis. Occurs after first exposure to irritant or repeated exposures to milder irritants over an extended time.	Dryness lasting days to months Vesication, fissures, cracks Hands and lower arms most common areas	Clinical picture Appropriate negative patch tests	Identification and removal of source of irritation Application of hydrophilic cream or petrolatum to soothe and protect Topical corticosteroids and compresses for weeping lesions Antibiotics for infection and oral antihistamines for pruritus
Phototoxic	Resembles the irritant type but requires sun and a chemical in combination to damage the epidermis.	Similar to irritant dermatitis	Photopatch test	Same as for allergic and irritant dermatitis
Photoallergic	Resembles allergic dermatitis but requires light exposure in addition to allergen contact to produce immunologic reactivity.	Similar to allergic dermatitis	Photopatch test	Same as for allergic and irritant dermatitis

in lipid content, sebaceous gland activity, and sweating. In response to stroking of the skin, immediate redness appears on the skin. Pallor follows in 15 to 30 seconds and persists for 1 to 3 minutes. Lesions develop secondary to the trauma of scratching and appear in areas of increased sweating and hypervascularity. Atopic dermatitis is chronic, with remissions and exacerbations. This condition has a tendency to recur, with remission from adolescence to 20 years of age.

It is important to note that atopic dermatitis is often the first step in a process that leads to asthma and allergic rhinitis. It is the result of interactions between susceptibility genes, the environment, defective function of the skin barrier, and immunologic responses.

Medical Management

Treatment of patients with atopic dermatitis must be individualized. Guidelines for treatment include decreasing itching and scratching by wearing cotton fabrics, washing with a mild detergent, humidifying dry heat in winter, maintaining room temperature at 20°C to 22.2°C (68°F to 72°F), using antihistamines such as diphenhydramine (Benadryl), and avoiding animals, dust, sprays, and perfumes. Keeping the skin moisturized with daily baths to hydrate the skin and the use of topical skin moisturizers is encouraged. Topical corticosteroids are used to prevent inflammation, and any infection is treated with antibiotics to eliminate *Staphylococcus aureus* when indicated. Use of immunosuppressive agents, such as cyclosporine (Neoral, Sandimmune), tacrolimus (Prograf, Protopic), and pimecrolimus (Elidel), may be effective in inhibiting T cells and mast cells involved in atopic dermatitis (Novak, 2007). Research to assess the effectiveness and the adverse side effects of medications used to treat atopic dermatitis is needed.

Nursing Management

Patients who experience atopic dermatitis and their families require assistance and support from the nurse to cope with the disorder. The symptoms are often disturbing to the patient and disruptive to the family. The appearance of the skin may affect the patient's self-esteem and his or her willingness to interact with others. Instructions and counseling about strategies to incorporate preventive measures and treatments into the lifestyle of the family may be helpful.

The patient and family need to be aware of signs of secondary infection and of the need to seek treatment if infection occurs. The nurse also teaches the patient and family about the side effects of medications used in treatment.

Dermatitis Medicamentosa (Drug Reactions)

Dermatitis medicamentosa, a type I hypersensitivity disorder, is the term applied to skin rashes associated with certain medications. Although people react differently to each medication, certain medications tend to induce eruptions of similar types. Rashes are among the most common adverse reactions to medications and occur in approximately 2% to 3% of hospitalized patients.

In general, drug reactions appear suddenly, have a particularly vivid color, manifest with characteristics that are more intense than the somewhat similar eruptions of infectious origin, and, with the exception of bromide and the iodide rashes, disappear rapidly after the medication is withdrawn. Rashes may be accompanied by systemic or generalized symptoms. On discovery of a medication allergy, patients are warned that they have a hypersensitivity to a particular medication and are advised not to take it again. Patients should carry information identifying the hypersensitivity with them at all times.

Skin eruptions related to medication therapy suggest more serious hypersensitivities. Frequent assessment and prompt reporting of the appearance of any eruptions are important so that early treatment can be initiated. Some cutaneous drug reactions may be associated with a clinical complex that involves other organs. These are known as complex drug reactions. Patients who suspect that a new rash may be caused by a drug allergy (newly prescribed medications, especially antibiotics such as penicillin or sulfa medications) should stop taking the medication immediately and contact their prescribing clinician, who will determine whether the medication and the rash are related.

Urticaria and Angioneurotic Edema

Urticaria (hives) is a type I hypersensitive allergic reaction of the skin characterized by the sudden appearance of pinkish, edematous elevations that vary in size and shape, itch, and cause local discomfort. They may involve any part of the body, including the mucous membranes (especially those of the mouth), the larynx (occasionally with serious respiratory complications), and the gastrointestinal tract.

Each hive remains for a few minutes to several hours before disappearing. For hours or days, clusters of these lesions may come, go, and return episodically. If this sequence continues for longer than 6 weeks, the condition is called chronic urticaria.

Angioneurotic edema involves the deeper layers of the skin, resulting in more diffuse swelling rather than the discrete lesions characteristic of hives. On occasion, this reaction covers the entire back. The skin over the reaction may appear normal but often has a reddish hue. The skin does not pit on pressure, as ordinary edema does. The regions most often involved are the lips, eyelids, cheeks, hands, feet, genitalia, and tongue; the mucous membranes of the larynx, the bronchi, and the gastrointestinal canal may also be affected, particularly in the hereditary type (see discussion in the following section). Swellings may appear suddenly, in a few seconds or minutes, or slowly, in 1 or 2 hours. In the latter case, their appearance is often preceded by itching or burning sensations. Seldom does more than a single swelling appear at one time, although one may develop while another is disappearing. Infrequently, swelling recurs in the same region. Individual lesions usually last 24 to 36 hours. On rare occasions, swelling may recur with remarkable regularity at intervals of 3 to 4 weeks.

Several frequently prescribed medications, such as angiotensin-converting enzyme (ACE) inhibitors and penicillin, may cause angioedema. The nurse needs to be aware of all medications the patient is taking and be alert to the potential of angioedema as a side effect.

Hereditary Angioedema

Hereditary angioedema, although not an immunologic disorder in the usual sense, is included because of its resemblance to allergic angioedema and because of the potential seriousness of the condition. Symptoms are caused by edema of the skin, the respiratory tract, or the digestive tract. Attacks may be precipitated by trauma, or they may seem to occur spontaneously.

Clinical Manifestations

When skin is involved, the swelling usually is diffuse, does not itch, and usually is not accompanied by urticaria. Gastrointestinal edema may cause abdominal pain severe enough to suggest the need for surgery. Typically, attacks last 1 to 4 days and are harmless; however, attacks can occasionally affect the subcutaneous and submucosal tissues in the region of the upper airway and can be associated with respiratory obstruction and asphyxiation. This disorder is inherited as an autosomal dominant trait. Approximately 85% of patients with this disorder have one nonproductive gene, and the remaining 15% have a gene mutation (Virella, 2007).

Medical Management

Attacks usually subside within 3 to 4 days, but during this time the patient should be observed carefully for signs of laryngeal obstruction, which may necessitate tracheostomy as a life-saving measure. Epinephrine, antihistamines, and corticosteroids are usually used in treatment, but their success is limited.

Food Allergy

IgE-mediated food allergy, a type I hypersensitivity reaction, occurs in 6% to 8% of children and about 2% of the adult population; it is thought to occur in people who have a genetic predisposition combined with exposure to allergens early in life through the gastrointestinal or respiratory tract or nasal mucosa (Bush, 2008). Researchers have also identified a second type of food allergy, a non-IgE–mediated food allergy syndrome in which T cells play a major role (Cappellano, 2008).

Almost any food can cause allergic symptoms. Any food can contain an allergen that results in anaphylaxis. The most common offenders are seafood (lobster, shrimp, crab, clams, fish), legumes (peanuts, peas, beans, licorice), seeds (sesame, cottonseed, caraway, mustard, flaxseed, sunflower seeds), tree nuts, berries, egg white, buckwheat, milk, and chocolate. Peanut and tree nut (eg, cashew, walnut) allergies are responsible for most severe food allergy reactions. In more than 70% of children with peanut allergy, symptoms develop at their first known exposure, suggesting unknown exposure through breast milk or another source (Burks, 2008; Bush, 2008). Pregnant and breast-feeding women who are aware of a family history of allergy (mother, father, or a sibling of the unborn infant with asthma, eczema, hay fever, or other allergy) should avoid peanuts and peanut-containing foods during pregnancy as a precaution (Burks, 2008; Cappellano, 2008).

One of the dangers of food allergens is that they may be hidden in other foods and not apparent to people who are susceptible to the allergen. For example, peanuts and peanut butter are often used in salad dressings and Asian, African, and Mexican cooking and may result in severe allergic reactions, including anaphylaxis. Previous contamination of equipment with allergens (eg, peanuts) during preparation of another food product (eg, chocolate cake) is enough to produce anaphylaxis in people with severe allergy.

Clinical Manifestations

The clinical symptoms are classic allergic symptoms (urticaria, dermatitis, wheezing, cough, laryngeal edema, angioedema) and gastrointestinal symptoms (itching; swelling of lips, tongue, and palate; abdominal pain; nausea; cramps; vomiting; and diarrhea).

Assessment and Diagnostic Findings

A careful diagnostic workup is required in any patient with a suspected food hypersensitivity. Included are a detailed allergy history, a physical examination, and pertinent diagnostic tests. Skin testing is used to identify the source of symptoms and is useful in identifying specific foods as causative agents.

Medical Management

Therapy for food hypersensitivity includes elimination of the food responsible for the hypersensitivity (Chart 53-8). Pharmacologic therapy is necessary for patients who cannot avoid exposure to offending foods and for patients with multiple food sensitivities not responsive to avoidance measures. Medication therapy involves the use of H_1 blockers, antihistamines, adrenergic agents, corticosteroids, and cromolyn sodium. Another essential aspect of management is teaching patients and family members how to recognize and manage the early stages of an acute anaphylactic reaction. Many food allergies disappear with time, particularly in children. About one third of proven allergies disappear in 1 to 2 years if the patient carefully avoids the offending food. However, peanut allergy has been reported to persist throughout adulthood in some people (Burks, 2008).

Nursing Management

In addition to participating in management of the allergic reaction, the nurse focuses on preventing future exposure of the patient to the food allergen. If a severe allergic or anaphylactic reaction to food allergens has occurred, the nurse must instruct the patient and family about strategies to prevent its recurrence. The patient is instructed about the importance of carefully assessing foods prepared by others for obvious as well as hidden sources of food allergens and of avoiding locations and facilities where those allergens are likely to be present. This includes careful reading of food labels and monitoring the preparation of food by others to be sure that exposure to even minute amounts of allergenic foods is avoided. The patient and family must be knowledgeable about early signs and symptoms of allergic reactions and must be proficient in emergency administration of epinephrine if a reaction occurs. The nurse also advises the patient to wear a medical alert bracelet or to carry identification and emergency equipment at all times. Patients' food allergies should be noted on their medical records, because there may be risk of allergic reactions not only to food but also to some medications containing similar substances (Bush, 2008). Pregnant women and those who are breastfeeding are instructed to avoid eating peanuts or food containing peanuts to minimize the risk of peanut allergy in their children.

Latex Allergy

Latex allergy, the allergic reaction to natural rubber proteins, has been implicated in rhinitis, conjunctivitis, contact dermatitis, urticaria, asthma, and anaphylaxis. Shortly after 1987, when hospitals and outpatient facilities mandated the use of powdered latex gloves to prevent transmission of infections, some health care workers began to experience numerous adverse reactions (Bernstein, 2006). From 1989 until the mid-1990s, the number of cases steadily increased. However, since that time, the prevalence has been steadily declining, possibly because of the use of nonpowdered latex and latex-free gloves (Rolland & O'Hehir, 2008).

Natural rubber latex is derived from the sap of the rubber tree (*Hevea brasiliensis*). The conversion of the liquid rubber latex into a finished product entails the addition of more than 200 chemicals. The proteins in the natural rubber latex (Hevea proteins) or the various chemicals that are used in the manufacturing process are thought to be the source of the allergic reactions. Not all objects composed of latex have the same ability to stimulate an allergic response. For example, the antigenicity of latex gloves can vary widely depending on the manufacturing method used.

CHART 53-8	HOME CARE CHECKLIST *Managing Food Allergies*		
At the completion of the home care instruction, the patient or caregiver will be able to:		**PATIENT**	**CAREGIVER**
• Verbalize understanding of the need to maintain an allergen-free diet.		✔	✔
• Demonstrate reading of food labels to identify hidden allergens in food.		✔	✔
• Identify ways to manage an allergen-free diet when eating away from home.		✔	✔
• State the need to wear a medical alert medallion or bracelet.		✔	✔
• List symptoms of food allergy.		✔	✔
• Demonstrate emergency administration of epinephrine.		✔	✔
• State the importance of replacing epinephrine when outdated.		✔	✔
• State the importance of prompt treatment of allergic reactions and health care follow-up.		✔	✔

Table 53-5 SELECTED PRODUCTS CONTAINING NATURAL RUBBER LATEX AND LATEX-FREE ALTERNATIVES

Products Containing Latex	Examples of Latex-Safe Alternatives*
Hospital Environment	
Ace bandage (brown)	Ace bandage, white all cotton
Adhesive bandages, Band-Aid dressing, Telfa	Cotton pads and plastic or silk tape, Active Strip (3M), Duoderm
Anesthesia equipment	Neoprene anesthesia kit (King)
Blood pressure cuff, tubing, and bladder	Clean Cuff, single-use nylon or vinyl blood pressure cuffs or wrap with stockinette or apply over clothing
Catheters	All-silicone or vinyl catheters
Catheter leg bag straps	Velcro straps
Crutch axillary pads and hand grips, tips	Cover with cloth, tape
ECG pads	Baxter, Red Dot 3M ECG pads
Elastic compression stockings	Kendall SCD stockings with stockinette
Gloves	Dermaprene, Neoprene, polymer, or vinyl gloves
IV catheters	Jelko, Deseret IV catheters
IV rubber injection ports	Cover Y-sites and ports; do not puncture. Use three-way stopcocks on plastic tubing
Levin tube	Salem sump tube
Medication vials	Remove rubber stopper
Penrose drains	Jackson-Pratt, Zimmer hemovac drains
Prepackaged enema kits	Theravac, Fleet Ready-to-use
Pulse oximeters	Nonin oximeters
Resuscitation bags	Laerdal, Puritan Bennett, *certain* Ambu
Stethoscope tubing	PVC tubing; cover with latex-free stockinette
Syringes—single use (Monoject, B & D)	Terumo syringes, Abbott PCA Abboject
Suction tubing	PVC (Davol, Laerdal)
Tapes	Dermicel, Micropore
Thermometer probes	Diatec probe covers
Tourniquets	X-Tourn straps (Avcor)
Theraband	New Thera-band Exercisers, plastic tubing
Home Environment	
Balloons	Mylar balloons
Diapers, incontinence pads	Huggies, Always, *some* Attends
Condoms, diaphragms	Polyurethane products, Durex/Avanti and Reality products (female condom)
Feminine hygiene pad	Kimberly-Clark products
Wheelchair cushions	ROHO cushions, Sof Care bed/chair cushions

*Confirmation is essential to verify that all items are latex-free before using, especially if risk of latex allergy is present.

Populations at risk include health care workers, patients with atopic allergies or multiple surgeries, people working in factories that manufacture latex products, females, and patients with spina bifida. Because more food handlers, hairdressers, automobile mechanics, and police often wear latex gloves, they may also be at risk for latex allergy. It is estimated that 1% to 3% of the general population have an allergy to latex and that as many as 10% to 20% of health care workers are sensitized (Rolland & O'Hehir, 2008). Patients are at risk for anaphylactic reactions as a result of contact with latex during medical treatments, especially surgical procedures.

Food that has been handled by people wearing latex gloves may stimulate an allergic response. Cross-reactions have been reported in people who are allergic to certain food products, such as kiwis, bananas, pineapples, mangos, passion fruit, avocados, and chestnuts (Bernstein, 2006).

Routes of exposure to latex products can be cutaneous, percutaneous, mucosal, parenteral, or aerosol. Allergic reactions are more likely with parenteral or mucous membrane exposure but can also occur with cutaneous contact or inhalation (Rolland & O'Hehir, 2008). The most frequent source of exposure is cutaneous, which usually involves the wearing of natural latex gloves. The powder used to facilitate putting on latex gloves can become a carrier of latex proteins from the gloves; when the gloves are put on or removed, the particles become airborne and can be inhaled or settle on skin, mucous membranes, or clothing. Mucosal exposure can occur from the use of latex condoms, catheters, airways, and nipples. Parenteral exposure can occur from IV lines or hemodialysis equipment. In addition to latex-derived medical devices, many household items also contain latex. Examples of medical and household items containing latex and a list of alternative products are found in Table 53-5. It is estimated that more than 40,000 medical devices and nonmedical products contain latex. Even chemical additives used in the manufacture of nonlatex gloves and other items have been associated with allergic symptoms, although these items otherwise have a low potential to stimulate an allergic response (Bernstein, 2006).

Clinical Manifestations

Several different types of reactions to latex are possible (Table 53-6). Irritant contact dermatitis, a nonimmunologic response, may be caused by mechanical skin irritation or an alkaline pH associated with latex gloves. Common symptoms of irritant dermatitis include erythema and pruritus. These symptoms can be eliminated by changing glove brands or by using powder-free gloves. Use of hand lotion before donning latex gloves can worsen the symptoms, because lotions may leach latex proteins from the gloves, increasing skin exposure and the risk of developing true allergic reactions (Bernstein, 2006).

Delayed hypersensitivity to latex, a type IV reaction mediated by T cells in the immune system, is localized to the area of exposure and is characterized by symptoms of

Table 53-6	**TYPES OF REACTIONS TO LATEX**		
Type of Reaction	**Cause**	**Signs/Symptoms**	**Treatment**
Irritant contact dermatitis	Damage to skin because of irritation and loss of epidermoid skin layer; not an allergic reaction. Can be caused by excessive use of soaps and cleansers, multiple handwashings, inadequate hand drying, mechanical irritation (eg, sweating, rubbing inside powdered gloves), exposure to chemicals added during the manufacturing of gloves, and alkaline pH of powdered gloves. Reaction may occur with first exposure, is usually benign, and is not life-threatening.	Acute: redness, edema, burning, discomfort, itching Chronic: dry, thickened, cracked skin	Referral for diagnostic testing Avoidance of exposure to irritant Thorough washing and drying of hands Use of powder-free gloves with more frequent changes of gloves Changing glove types Use of water- or silicone-based moisturizing creams, lotions, or topical barrier agents Avoidance of oil- or petroleum-based skin agents with latex products, because they cause breakdown of the latex product
Allergic contact dermatitis	Delayed hypersensitivity (type IV) reaction. Usually affects only area in contact with latex; reaction is usually to chemical additives used in the manufacturing process rather than to latex itself. Cause of reaction is T cell–mediated sensitization to additives of latex. Reaction is not life-threatening and is far more common than a type I reaction. Slow onset; occurs 18–24 h after exposure. Resolves within 3–4 days after exposure. More severe reactions may occur with subsequent exposures.	Pruritus, erythema, swelling, crusty thickened skin, blisters, other skin lesions	Referral for diagnosis (patch tests) and treatment Thorough washing and drying of hands Use of water- or silicone-based moisturizing creams, lotions, or topical barrier agents Avoidance of oil- or petroleum-based products unless they are latex compatible Avoidance of identified causative agent, because continued exposure to latex products in presence of breaks in skin may contribute to latex protein sensitization
Latex allergy	Type I IgE-mediated immediate hypersensitivity to plant proteins in natural rubber latex. In sensitized people, antilatex IgE antibody stimulates mast cell proliferation and basophil histamine release. Exposure can be through contact with the skin, mucous membranes, or internal tissues, or through inhalation of traces of powder from latex gloves. Severe reactions usually occur shortly after parenteral or mucous membrane exposure. People with any type I reaction to latex are at high risk for anaphylaxis. Local swelling, redness, edema, itching, and systemic reactions, including anaphylaxis, occur within minutes after exposure.	Rhinitis, flushing, conjunctivitis, urticaria, laryngeal edema, bronchospasm, asthma, severe vasodilation angioedema, anaphylaxis, cardiovascular collapse, death	Immediate treatment of reaction with epinephrine, fluids, vasopressors, and corticosteroids, and airway and ventilator support, with close monitoring for recurrence for next 12–14 h Prompt referral for diagnostic evaluation Treatment and diagnostic evaluation in latex-free environment Assessment of all patients for symptoms of latex allergy Teaching of patients and family members about the disorder and about the importance of preventing future reactions by avoiding latex (eg, wearing medical alert bracelet, carrying EpiPen)

contact dermatitis, including vesicular skin lesions, papules, pruritus, edema, erythema, and crusting and thickening of the skin. These symptoms usually appear on the back of the hands. This reaction is thought to be caused by chemicals that are used in the manufacturing of latex products. It is the most common allergic reaction to latex. Although not usually life-threatening, delayed hypersensitivity reactions often require major changes in the patient's home and work environment to avoid further exposure. People who are sensitized to latex are at increased risk for development of type I allergic reactions (Bernstein, 2006).

Immediate hypersensitivity, a type I allergic reaction, is mediated by the IgE mast cell system. Symptoms can include rhinitis, conjunctivitis, asthma, and anaphylaxis. The term *latex allergy* is usually used to describe the type I reaction. Clinical manifestations have a rapid onset and can include urticaria, wheezing, dyspnea, laryngeal edema, bronchospasm, tachycardia, angioedema, hypotension, and cardiac arrest.

Localized itching, erythema, or local urticaria within minutes after exposure to latex is often the initial symptom. Symptoms of subsequent reactions can include generalized urticaria, angioedema, rhinitis, conjunctivitis, asthma, and anaphylactic shock minutes after dermal or mucosal exposure to latex. An increasing number of people who are allergic to latex experience severe reactions characterized by generalized urticaria, bronchospasm, and hypotension.

Assessment and Diagnostic Findings

The diagnosis of latex allergy is based on the history and diagnostic test results (Rolland & O'Hehir, 2008). Sensitization is detected by skin testing, RAST, ELISA or level of Hevea latex-specific IgE antibody in the serum. Testing for the chemicals found in the rubber production that makes latex is performed using the patch test. Skin patch testing is the preferred method for patients with contact allergies. The TRUE test and other skin tests should be performed only by clinicians who have expertise in their administration and interpretation and who have the necessary equipment available to treat local or systemic allergic reactions to the reagent. Nasal challenge and dipstick tests may be useful in the future as screening tests for latex allergy.

Medical Management

The best treatment available for latex allergy is the avoidance of latex-based products, but this is often difficult because of their widespread use. Patients who have experienced an anaphylactic reaction to latex should be instructed to wear medical identification. Antihistamines and an emergency kit containing epinephrine should be provided to these patients, along with instructions about emergency management of latex allergy symptoms. Patients should be counseled to notify all health care workers as well as local paramedic and ambulance companies about their allergy. Warning labels can be attached to car windows to alert police and paramedics about the driver's or passenger's latex allergy in case of a motor vehicle crash. People with latex allergy should be provided with a list of alternative products and referred to local support groups; they are also urged to carry their own supply of nonlatex gloves.

People with type I latex sensitivity may be unable to continue to work if a latex-free work environment is not possible. This may occur with surgeons, dentists, operating room personnel, or intensive care nurses. Occupational implications for employees with type IV latex sensitivity are usually easier to manage by changing to nonlatex gloves and avoiding direct contact with latex-based medical equipment. Although latex-specific immunotherapy has been attempted, this method of treatment remains experimental.

Nursing Management

The nurse can assume a pivotal role in the management of latex allergies in both patients and staff. All patients should be asked about latex allergy, although special attention should be given to those at particularly high risk (eg, patients with spina bifida, patients who have undergone multiple surgical procedures). Every time an invasive procedure must be performed, the nurse should consider the possibility of latex allergies. Nurses working in operating rooms, intensive care units, short procedure units, and emergency departments need to pay particular attention to latex allergy. See Chapter 18 for a latex allergy screening form.

Although the type I reaction is the most significant of the reactions to latex, care must be taken in the presence of irritant contact dermatitis and delayed hypersensitivity reaction to avoid further exposure of the person to latex. Patients with latex allergy are advised to notify their health care providers and to wear a medical information bracelet. Patients must become knowledgeable about what products contain latex and what products are safe, nonlatex alternatives. They must also become knowledgeable about signs and symptoms of latex allergy and emergency treatment and self-injection of epinephrine in case of allergic reaction.

Nurses can be instrumental in establishing and participating in multidisciplinary committees to address latex allergy and to promote a latex-free environment. Latex allergy protocols and education of staff about latex allergy and precautions are important strategies to reduce this growing problem and to ensure assessment and prompt treatment of affected people.

CRITICAL THINKING EXERCISES

1 A 23-year-old college student has developed symptoms of severe seafood allergy. She is to receive instructions about self-administration of epinephrine if she experiences anaphylaxis. Develop a teaching plan for her and identify outcomes to measure the effectiveness of your teaching. Given her allergy to seafood, what other teaching or counseling is needed?

EBP **2** A 35-year-old woman has developed symptoms of asthma thought to be an allergic response to the two dogs and two cats her new roommate has brought with her into the apartment. Develop an evidence-based plan for strategies to reduce or eliminate the patient's allergen exposure. Describe the strength of the evidence and criteria used to assess its strength. What instructional strategies and outcome measures will you use to educate her about avoidance strategies and to assess the effectiveness of their use?

3 An 18-year-old man is scheduled for removal of his wisdom teeth in the dentist's office. He reports that he has severe seasonal and bee sting allergies. He also experienced an episode of hives and itching during a dental procedure in the past. He reports that he has had to use emergency epinephrine on several occasions in the past because of severe allergic reactions caused by bee stings. What precautions are needed preprocedure, during the procedure, and postprocedure for this patient to prevent the potential occurrence of a severe allergic reaction? What interventions and nursing management would be indicated if he developed a severe allergic reaction?

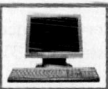 The Smeltzer suite offers these additional resources to enhance learning and facilitate understanding of this chapter:
- thePoint online resource, thepoint.lww.com/Smeltzer12E
- Student CD-ROM included with the book
- *Study Guide to Accompany Brunner & Suddarth's Textbook of Medical-Surgical Nursing*
- *Handbook for Brunner & Suddarth's Textbook of Medical-Surgical Nursing*

REFERENCES AND SELECTED READINGS

Books

Abbas, A. K. & Lichtman, A. H. (2008). *Basic immunology: Functions and disorders of the immune system.* Philadelphia: W. B. Saunders.

Adkinson, N. F., Busse, W. W., Bochner, B. S., et al. (Eds.). (2009). *Middleton's allergy: Principles and practice* (7th ed.). Philadelphia: Elsevier.

Arcangelo, V. P. & Peterson, A. (2005). *Pharmacotherapeutics for advanced practice: A practical approach.* Philadelphia: Lippincott Williams & Wilkins.

Buttaro, T. M., Trybulski, J., Bailey, P. P., et al. (2007). *Primary care: A collaborative practice.* St. Louis: Mosby.

Doan, T., Melvold, R., Waltenbaugh, C., et al. (2007). *Immunology.* Philadelphia: Lippincott Williams & Wilkins.

Dochterman, J. M. & Bulechek, G. M. (2007). *Nursing interventions and classification (NIC).* St. Louis: Mosby.

Goroll, A. G. & Mulley, A. G. (2006). *Primary care medicine: Office evaluation and management of the adult patient.* Philadelphia: Lippincott Williams & Wilkins.

Holgate, S. T., Lichtenstein, L. M. & Church, M. K. (2006). *Allergy*. Philadelphia: Elsevier Health Sciences.

Karch, A. M. (2008). *2008 Lippincott's nursing drug guide*. Philadelphia: Lippincott Williams & Wilkins.

Lieberman, P. (2007). *Anaphylaxis: An issue of immunology and allergy clinics*. Philadelphia: Elsevier.

Nurse Practitioners' Prescribing Reference. (2008). New York: Prescribing Reference, Inc.

Porth, C. M. & Matfin G. (2009). *Pathophysiology: Concepts of altered health states* (8th ed.). Philadelphia: Lippincott Williams & Wilkins.

Schwarzenberger, K., Werchniak, A. & Ko, C. (2009). *General dermatology*. Philadelphia: Elsevier-Saunders.

U.S. Department of Health and Human Services. (2007). *Food allergy: An overview*. NIH Publication No. 07-5518. Bethesda, MD: Author.

Virella, G. (2007). *Medical immunology*. Boca Raton, FL: CRC Press.

Wynne, A. L., Woo, T. M. & Olyaei, A. J. (2007). *Pharmacotherapeutics for nurse practitioner prescribers*. Philadelphia: F. A. Davis.

Journals & Electronic Documents

Bernstein, J. (2006). Allergic occupational disease among healthcare workers: Latex allergy and beyond. American Academy of Allergy, Asthma and Immunology 62nd Annual Meeting: March 3–7, 2006. Miami, FL. www.medscape.com/viewarticle/530091

Bernstein, I. L., Li, J. T., Bernstein, D. I., et al. (2008). Allergy diagnostic testing: An updated practice parameter. *Annals of Allergy, Asthma and Immunology, 100*(Suppl 3), S1–S148.

Bieber, T. (2008). Atopic dermatitis. *New England Journal of Medicine, 358*(14), 1483–1494.

Bonds, R. S., Midoro-Horiuti, T. & Goldblum, R. (2008). A structural basis for food allergy: The role of cross-reactivity. *Current Opinion in Allergy and Clinical Immunology, 8*(1), 82–86.

Bousquet, J., Flahault, A., Vandenplas, O., et al. (2006). Natural rubber latex allergy among healthcare workers: A systematic review of the evidence. *Journal of Allergy and Clinical Immunology, 118*(2), 447–454.

Buckingham, S. & Mardon, J. (2008). Allergy: A modern epidemic. *Health & Homeopathy*, Spring, 21–23.

Burks, A. (2008). Peanut allergy. *Lancet, 371*(3), 1538–1546.

Bush, R. K. (2008). Approach to patients with symptoms of food allergy. *American Journal of Medicine, 121*(5), 376–378.

Cappellano, K. L. (2008). Food allergy and intolerances: The nuts and bolts of detection and management. *Nutrition Today, 43*(1), 11–14.

Chacko, T. (2008). Are we following the practice parameter guidelines on allergen immunotherapy? *Annals of Allergy, Asthma, and Immunology, 100*(2), 178–180.

Chambers, C. (2006). Safety of asthma and allergy medications in pregnancy. *Immunology and Allergy Clinics of North America, 26*(1), 13–28.

Choo-Kang, L. R. (2006). Specific IgE testing: Objective laboratory evidence supports allergy diagnosis and treatment. *Medical Laboratory Observer, 38*(3), 10-2, 14, 17.

Cunha, B. (2006). Antibiotic selection in the penicillin-allergic patient. *Medical Clinics of North America, 90*(6), 1257–1264.

Dedlow, E. R. & Cohen, P. R. (2007). Incidence of latex allergy decreasing. *Clinical Advisor for Nurse Practitioners, 10*(7), 99.

Douglass, J. A. & O'Hehir, R. E. (2006). Diagnosis, treatment and prevention of allergic disease: The basics. *Medical Journal of Australia, 185*(4), 228–233.

Ferguson, B. J. (2008). Environmental controls of allergies. *Otolaryngologic Clinics of North America, 41*(2), 411–417.

Gruchalla, R. S. & Pirmohamed, M. (2006). Clinical practice: Antibiotic allergy. *New England Journal of Medicine, 354*(6), 601–609.

Guo, R., Pittler, M. H. & Ernst, E. (2007). Herbal medicines for the treatment of allergic rhinitis: A systematic review. *Annals of Allergy, Asthma & Immunology, 99*(6), 483–495.

Hovanec-Burns, D. (2008). Accuracy of IgE antibody laboratory results. *Annals of Allergy, Asthma & Immunology, 100*(2), 178–179.

Ilardi, D. (2006). Asthma and allergy watch: School guidelines for managing students with food allergies. *School Nurse News, 23*(3), 13–14.

Jacob, S. E. & Steele, T. (2006). Allergic contact dermatitis: Early recognition and diagnosis of important allergens. *Dermatology Nursing, 18*(5), 433–439, 446.

James, J. M. (2007). Allergic reactions to foods by inhalation. *Current Allergy Asthma Report, 7*(3), 167–174.

Johansson, S. G. O., Hourihane, J. O'B., Bousquet, J., et al. (2005). Revised nomenclature for allergy for global use. Report of the Nomenclature Review Committee of the World Allergy Organization, October 2003. *Allergy and Clinical Immunology International—Journal of the World Allergy Organization, 17*(1), 4–8.

Krouse, H. J. (2007). Diagnostic testing for inhalant allergies. *ORL-Head & Neck Nursing, 25*(2), 9–14.

Lieberman, P. (2006). Anaphylaxis. *Medical Clinics of North America, 90*(1), 77–95.

Nathan, R. A. (2008). The pathophysiology, clinical impact, and management of nasal congestion in allergic rhinitis. *Clinical Therapeutics, 30*(4), 573–586.

National Institute of Allergy and Infectious Diseases. (2006). *Report of the NIH Expert Panel on Food Allergy Research*. www3.niaid.nih.gov/topics/food Allergy/research/ReportFoodAllergy.htm

Noonan, A. & Mignon, M. (2005). Nurses and occupational contact dermatitis. *Australian Nursing Journal, 12*(11), S1–S3.

Novak, N. (2007). Allergen specific immunotherapy for atopic dermatitis. *Current Opinions in Allergy and Clinical Immunology, 7*(6), 542–546.

Ortiz, G. (2006). What you need to know about hives. *Clinical Advisor for Nurse Practitioners, 9*(10), 41–42, 46–47.

Ozol, D. & Mete, E. (2008). Asthma and food allergy. *Current Opinion in Pulmonary Medicine, 14*(1), 9–12.

Platts-Mills, T., Leung, D. Y. & Schatz, M. (2007). The role of allergens in asthma. *American Family Physician, 76*(5), 675–680.

Quillen, D. M. & Feller, D. B. (2006). Diagnosing rhinitis: Allergic vs. nonallergic. *American Family Physician, 73*(9), 1583–1590.

Rank, M. A. & Li, J. T. (2007). Allergen immunotherapy. *Mayo Clinic Proceedings, 82*(9), 1119–1123.

Roberts, J., Huissoon, A., Dretzke, J., et al. (2008). A systematic review of the clinical effectiveness of acupuncture for allergic rhinitis. *BMC Complementary Alternative Medicine, 8*, 13–22.

Rolland, J. M. & O'Hehir, R. E. (2008). Latex allergy: A model for therapy. *Clinical and Experimental Allergy, 38*(6), 898–912.

Romano, A. & Demoly, P. (2007). Recent advances in the diagnosis of drug allergy. *Current Opinion in Allergy & Clinical Immunology, 7*(4), 299–303.

Simons, E. E., Frew, A. J., Ansotegui, I. J., et al. (2007). Risk assessment in anaphylaxis: Current and future approaches. *Journal of Clinical Immunology, 120*, S2–S24.

Stokes, J. R. (2008). Allergy immunotherapy: Indications, efficacy, and safety. *Journal of Respiratory Diseases, 29*(3), 136–141.

U.S. Department of Health and Human Services. (2003). *Airborne allergens: Something in the air*. NIH Publication No. 03-7045. Bethesda, MD: Author. www.niaid.nih.gov/publications/allergens/airborne_allergens.pdf

Uter, W., Johansen, J. D., Orton, D. I., et al. (2005). Clinical update on contact allergy. *Current Opinion in Allergy and Clinical Immunology, 5*(5), 429–436.

Van Hoecke, H., Vandenbulcke, L. & Van Cauwenberge, P. (2007). Histamine and leukotriene receptor antagonism in the treatment of allergic rhinitis: An update. *Drugs, 67*(18), 2717–2726.

Walker, S. (2007). Treating anaphylaxis in primary care. *Practice Nurse, 33*(5), 50–52, 54–55.

Weinbaum, H. (2007). Strategies for managing students with food allergies. *School Nurse News, 24*(3), 10.

Wilbanks, S. (2008). Test your knowledge. Allergic rhinitis. *Journal for Nurse Practitioners, 4*(7), 559–559.

RESOURCES

American Academy of Allergy, Asthma and Immunology, www.aaaai.org
American College of Allergy, Asthma and Immunology, www.acaai.org
Asthma and Allergy Foundation of America, www.aafa.org
Centers for Disease Control and Prevention, www.cdc.gov
Food Allergy and Anaphylaxis Network, www.foodallergy.org
National Institute of Allergy and Infectious Disease, www3.niaid.nih.gov

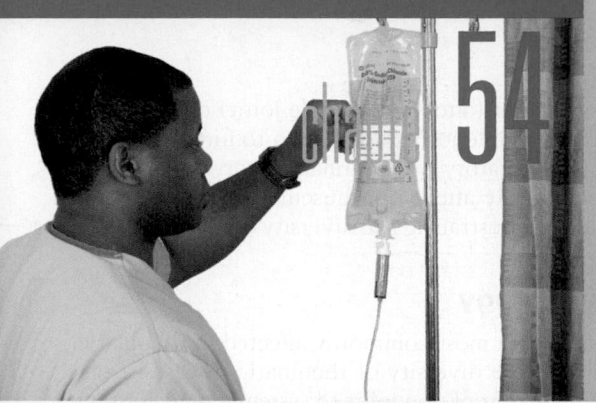

Assessment and Management of Patients With Rheumatic Disorders

LEARNING OBJECTIVES

On completion of this chapter, the learner will be able to:

1 Explain the pathophysiology of rheumatic diseases.

2 Describe the assessment and diagnostic findings seen in patients with a suspected diagnosis of rheumatic disease or disorder.

3 Discuss appropriate nursing interventions based on nursing diagnoses and collaborative problems that commonly occur with rheumatic disorders.

4 Describe the systemic effects of a connective tissue disease.

5 Devise a teaching plan for the patient with newly diagnosed rheumatic disease.

6 Identify modifications in interventions to accommodate changes in patients' functional ability that may occur with disease progression.

GLOSSARY

ankylosis: fixation or immobility of a joint

arthritis: inflammation of a joint

arthroplasty: replacement of a joint

osteoarthritis: degenerative joint disease

osteophyte: a bony outgrowth or protuberance; bone spur

pannus: proliferation of newly formed synovial tissue infiltrated with inflammatory cells

rheumatic diseases: numerous disorders affecting skeletal muscles, bones, cartilage, ligaments, tendons, and joints

rheumatoid arthritis: autoimmune disease of unknown origin

subchondral bone: bony plate that supports the articular cartilage

tophi: accumulation of crystalline deposits in articular surfaces, bones, soft tissue, and cartilage

Rheumatic diseases include common disorders such as osteoarthritis (OA) and less common conditions such as systemic lupus erythematosus (SLE) and scleroderma. These conditions can be life-threatening, or they can be minor illnesses. The problems caused by the rheumatic diseases include not only the obvious limitations in mobility and activities of daily living but also the more subtle systemic effects that can lead to organ failure and death or result in problems such as pain, fatigue, altered self-image, and sleep disturbances. The rheumatic disease may be the patient's primary health problem or a secondary diagnosis. An understanding of rheumatic diseases and their effects on a patient's function and well-being is essential to developing an appropriate plan of nursing care.

Rheumatic Diseases

Commonly called **arthritis** (inflammation of a joint) and thought of as one condition, the **rheumatic diseases** are more than 100 different types of disorders that primarily affect skeletal muscles, bones, cartilage, ligaments, tendons, and joints in males and females of all ages (Porth & Matfin, 2009). Some disorders are more likely to occur at a particular time of life or to affect one gender more than the other. The onset of these conditions may be acute or insidious, with a course possibly marked by periods of remission (a period when disease symptoms are reduced or absent) and exacerbation (a period when symptoms occur or increase). Treatment can be simple, aimed at localized relief, or it can be complex, directed toward relief of systemic effects. Permanent changes and disability may result from these disorders.

Nurses need to understand the classification of rheumatic diseases. One basic system is to classify disease as either monoarticular (affecting a single joint) or polyarticular (affecting multiple joints), and then to further classify it as either inflammatory or noninflammatory. Conditions that may secondarily affect the musculoskeletal structure are also included, illustrating the diversity of the rheumatic diseases.

Pathophysiology

The joint is the area most commonly affected in rheumatic diseases. Despite the diversity of rheumatic diseases, from localized involvement of one joint to systemic, multisystem disorders, they all involve some degree of inflammation and degeneration, which may occur simultaneously. Inflammation is manifested in the joints as synovitis. In inflammatory rheumatic diseases, the primary process is inflammation caused by the immune response. Degeneration occurs as a secondary process, resulting from the effect of **pannus** (proliferation of newly formed synovial tissue infiltrated with inflammatory cells). Conversely, in degenerative rheumatic diseases, inflammation occurs as a secondary process. This synovitis is usually milder, is more likely to be seen in advanced disease, and represents a reactive process.

Inflammation

Inflammation is a series of related steps. In response to the triggering event, (eg, trauma, increased stress), the antigen stimulus activates monocytes and T lymphocytes (also called T cells). Next, the immunoglobulin antibodies form immune complexes with antigens. Phagocytosis of the immune complexes is initiated, generating an inflammatory reaction (joint effusion, pain, and edema) (Fig. 54-1). During the next step, the immune response deviates from normal. Phagocytosis produces chemicals such as leukotrienes and prostaglandins. Leukotrienes contribute to the inflam-

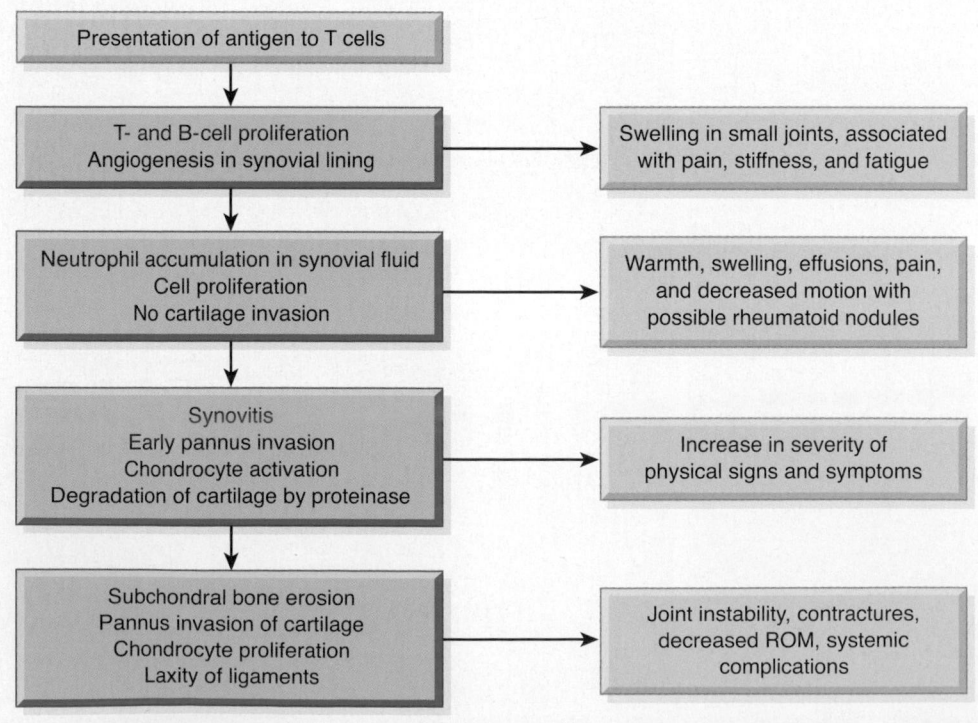

Figure 54-1 Pathophysiology and associated physical signs of rheumatoid arthritis. ROM, range of motion.

matory process by attracting other white blood cells to the area. Prostaglandins act as modifiers to inflammation. In some cases, they increase inflammation; in other cases, they decrease it. Leukotrienes and prostaglandins produce enzymes such as collagenase that break down collagen, a vital part of a normal joint. The release of these enzymes in the joint causes edema, proliferation of synovial membrane and pannus formation, destruction of cartilage, and erosion of bone.

The immunologic inflammatory process begins when antigens are presented to T lymphocytes, leading to a proliferation of T and B cells. B cells are a source of antibody-forming cells, or plasma cells. In response to specific antigens, plasma cells produce and release antibodies. Antibodies combine with corresponding antigens to form pairs, or immune complexes. The immune complexes build up and are deposited in synovial tissue or other organs in the body, triggering the inflammatory reaction that can ultimately damage the involved tissue.

The systemic nature of the rheumatic diseases is reflected in the resultant widespread inflammatory process. Although focused in the joints, inflammation also involves other areas. The blood vessels (vasculitis and arteritis), lungs, heart, and kidneys may also be affected by the inflammation. In the joints, this inflammatory response is manifested as pannus extending throughout the joint space and, if persistent, eroding the articular cartilage, causing secondary degenerative changes to the joint.

Degeneration

Although the cause of degeneration of the articular cartilage is poorly understood, the process is known to be metabolically active and therefore is more accurately called "degradation." One theory of degradation is that genetic or hormonal influences, mechanical factors, and prior joint damage cause cartilage failure. Degradation of cartilage ensues, and increased mechanical stress on bone ends causes stiffening of bone tissue. Another theory is that bone stiffening occurs and results in increased mechanical stress on cartilage, which in turn initiates the processes of degradation. (See Chapter 66 for more information on the structure and function of the articular system.)

Clinical Manifestations

The most common symptom in the rheumatic diseases that causes a person to seek medical attention is pain. Other common symptoms include joint swelling, limited movement, stiffness, weakness, and fatigue.

Assessment and Diagnostic Findings

Assessment begins with a general health history, which includes the onset of symptoms and how they evolved, family history, past health history, and any other contributing factors. Because many of the rheumatic diseases are chronic conditions, the health history should also include information about the patient's perception of the problem, previous treatments and their effectiveness, the patient's support systems, and the patient's current knowledge base and the source of that information. A complete health history is followed by a complete physical assessment (see Chapter 5).

Assessment for rheumatic diseases combines the physical examination with a functional assessment. Inspection of the patient's general appearance occurs during initial contact. Gait, posture, and general musculoskeletal size and structure are observed. Gross deformities and abnormalities in movement are noted. The symmetry, size, and contour of other connective tissues, such as the skin and adipose tissue, are also noted and recorded. Chart 54-1 outlines the important areas for consideration during the physical assessment. The functional assessment is a combination of history (what the patient reports that he or she can and cannot do) and examination (observation of activities: the patient demonstrates what he or she can and cannot do, such as dressing and getting in and out of a chair). Observation also includes the adaptations and adjustments the patient may have made (sometimes without awareness); for example, with shoulder or elbow involvement, the person may bend over to reach a fork, rather than raising the fork to the mouth.

The history and physical assessment data are supplemented by supportive or confirming diagnostic test findings. In some instances, tests are used to monitor the course of the disease. For example, the erythrocyte sedimentation rate (ESR) reflects inflammatory activity and, indirectly, the progression or remission of disease.

Laboratory Studies

Some of the most common laboratory studies are listed with their corresponding normal ranges and primary indications in Table 54-1. Many of the tests require special laboratory techniques and may not be performed in every health care facility. The primary health care provider determines which tests are necessary based on symptoms, stage of disease, cost, and likely benefit.

Other Diagnostic Studies

Imaging studies commonly used for patients with rheumatic diseases include x-ray studies, computed tomography (CT) scans and magnetic resonance imaging (MRI) scans, and arthrography. See Chapter 66 for further information about these and other diagnostic studies.

 Gerontologic Considerations

Although people of all ages, from infancy through childhood, adolescence, and adulthood, may be affected, rheumatic disease is commonly thought of by the patient, family, and society as a whole as an inevitable consequence of aging. Many older people expect and accept the immobility and self-care problems related to the rheumatic diseases and do not seek help, thinking that nothing can be done. Careful diagnosis and appropriate treatment can improve the quality of life for older people (Schmajuk, Schneeweiss, Katz, et al., 2007).

In elderly patients, other medical conditions may take precedence over the rheumatic disease, which commonly becomes a secondary diagnosis and concern. Identifying the effects of the rheumatic disease on the patient's lifestyle, independence, and other chronic or acute conditions is important.

The frequency, pattern of onset, clinical features, severity, and effects on function of the rheumatic disease in

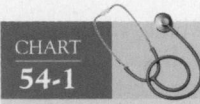

CHART
54-1

Assessing for Rheumatic Disorders

In addition to the head-to-toe assessment or systems review, the following are important areas of consideration to be noted when performing the complete physical assessment of a patient with a known or suspected rheumatic disorder.

Manifestation	Significance
Skin (inquire and inspect)	
Rash, lesions	Associated with lupus erythematosus (LE), vasculitis, adverse effect of medication
Increased bruising	Associated with several rheumatic diseases and adverse effect of medication
Erythema	Sign of inflammation
Thinning	Adverse effect of medication
Warmth	Sign of inflammation
Photosensitivity	Associated with systemic lupus erythematosus (SLE), dermatomyositis, adverse effect of medication
Hair (inquire and inspect)	
Alopecia or thinning	Associated with rheumatic diseases or adverse effect of medication
Eye (inquire and inspect)	
Dryness, grittiness	Associated with Sjögren's syndrome (commonly occurring with rheumatoid arthritis [RA] and LE)
Decreased acuity or blindness	Associated with temporal arteritis, medication complications
Cataracts	Adverse effect of medication
Decreased peripheral vision	Adverse effect of medication
Conjunctivitis, uveitis	Associated with ankylosing spondylitis and Reiter's syndrome
Ear (inquire)	
Tinnitus	Adverse effect of medication
Decreased acuity	Adverse effect of medication
Mouth (inquire and inspect)	
Buccal, sublingual lesions	Associated with vasculitis, dermatomyositis, adverse effect of medication
Altered sense of taste	Adverse effect of medication
Dryness	Associated with Sjögren's syndrome
Dysphagia	Associated with myositis
Difficulty chewing	Associated with decreased range of motion of jaw
Chest (inspect and inquire)	
Pleuritic pain	Associated with RA and SLE
Decreased chest expansion	Associated with ankylosing spondylitis
Activity intolerance (dyspnea)	Associated with pulmonary hypertension in scleroderma
Cardiovascular system (inquire, inspect, palpate)	
Blanching of fingers on exposure to cold	Associated with Raynaud's phenomenon
Peripheral pulses	Deficit may indicate vascular involvement or edema associated with medication effect or rheumatic diseases, especially SLE or scleroderma
Abdomen (inquire and palpate)	
Altered bowel habits	Associated with scleroderma, spondylosis, ulcerative colitis, decreased physical mobility, medication effect
Nausea, vomiting, bloating, and pain	Adverse effect of medication
Weight change (measure)	Associated with RA (decreased), adverse effect of medication (increased or decreased)
Genitalia (inquire and inspect)	
Dryness, itching	Associated with Sjögren's syndrome
Abnormal menses	Adverse effect of medication
Altered sexual performance	Fear of pain (or of pain caused by partner) and limitation of motion may affect sexual mobility.
Hygiene	Poor hygiene may be related to limitations in activities of daily living.
Urethritis, dysuria	Associated with ankylosing spondylitis and Reiter's syndrome
Lesions	Associated with vasculitis

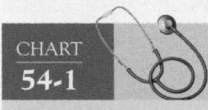

CHART 54-1	*Assessing for Rheumatic Disorders* (*Continued*)

Manifestation	**Significance**
Neurologic (inquire and inspect)	
Paresthesias of extremities; abnormal reflex pattern	Nerve compressions associated with carpal tunnel syndrome, spinal stenosis, etc.
Headaches	Associated with temporal arteritis, adverse effect of medication
Musculoskeletal (inspect and palpate)	
Joint redness, warmth, swelling, tenderness, deformity—location of first joint involved, pattern of progression, symmetry, acute versus chronic nature	Signs of inflammation
Joint range of motion	Decreased range of motion may indicate severity or progression of disease.
Surrounding tissue findings	
Muscle atrophy, subcutaneous nodules, popliteal cyst	Extra-articular manifestations
Muscle strength (grip)	Muscle strength decreases with increased disease activity.

elderly patients may be different in very old patients. One disease, OA, is the leading cause of disability and pain in the elderly (Porth & Matfin, 2009). OA may account for more total disability among elderly patients than many diseases (eg, stroke or cancer).

In some instances, the age of the patient and coexisting health problems make diagnosis difficult. A missed diagnosis is not unusual, because it is assumed that older people with joint problems have OA. In addition, it may be difficult to differentiate problems associated with aging from those caused by a rheumatic disease. For example, rheumatoid arthritis (RA), an autoimmune disorder that begins in the later years, has been shown to differ prognostically and therapeutically from RA that begins in childhood or early adulthood. In the older patient with early RA, the onset is more likely to be abrupt, but the clinical course does not appear to differ from that of RA with an insidious onset.

For the elderly person who has had a diffuse connective tissue disease, the risk of osteoporosis is increased. Pain, loss of mobility, diminished self-image, and increasing morbidity can result from progressive osteoporosis. Therefore, diagnosis and treatment of osteoporosis should not be overlooked in this population. Pharmacologic therapy including analgesic agents, exercise, postural assistance, modification of activities of daily living, and psychological support can be useful.

Other conditions (eg, soft tissue problems such as bursitis) usually are not problematic by themselves. However, when combined with other health problems and the normal physiologic processes of aging, these conditions may significantly affect the patient's quality of life. In fact, the effects of most forms of rheumatic disease may lead to considerable changes in the patient's lifestyle, possibly threatening his or her independence. Decreased vision and altered balance, often present in elderly people, may be problematic if rheumatic disease in the lower extremities affects locomotion. Also, the combination of decreased hearing and visual acuity, memory loss, and depression contributes to failure to follow the treatment regimen in elderly patients. Special techniques for promoting patient safety, self-management, and strategies such as memory aids for medications may be necessary.

Partly because of the more frequent contact of older adults with health care providers for a variety of health issues, overtreatment or inappropriate treatment is possible. Complaints of pain may be met with a prescription for an opioid analgesic agent rather than instructions for rest, use of an assistive device, and local comfort measures such as heat or cold. Acetaminophen may be appropriate and worth trying before other medications that pose a greater chance of side effects. Intra-articular corticosteroid injections, with their usually rapid relief of symptoms, may be requested by the patient who is unaware of the consequences of too-frequent use of this treatment. In addition, exercise programs may not be instituted or may be ineffective because the patient expects results to occur quickly or fails to appreciate the effectiveness of a program of exercise.

Pharmacologic treatment of rheumatic disease in older patients is more difficult than it is in younger patients. If therapeutic medications have an effect on the senses (hearing, cognition), this effect is intensified in the elderly. The cumulative effect of these medications is accentuated because of the physiologic changes of aging. For example, decreased renal function in the elderly alters the metabolism of certain medications, such as nonsteroidal anti-inflammatory drugs (NSAIDs). Older adults are more prone to side effects associated with the use of multiple-drug therapy for various disorders (Miller, 2009).

Elderly patients with rheumatic disease may unnecessarily accept or endure pain, loss of ambulation, and difficulty with activities of daily living. The need to view oneself as capable of managing life independently despite increasing age may take considerable energy. The body image and self-esteem of the elderly person with rheumatic disease, combined with underlying depression, may interfere with the use of assistive devices such as canes. Use of adaptive equipment such as long-handled reachers or tongs may be viewed as evidence of aging rather than as a means of increasing independence.

The elderly person usually has a lifelong pattern of dealing with the stresses of daily life. Depending on the success of that pattern, the elderly person can often maintain a

Table 54-1   COMMON BLOOD STUDIES FOR RHEUMATIC DISEASES

Test	Normal Value	Significance
Serum		
Creatinine		
Metabolic waste excreted through the kidneys	0.6–1.2 mg/dL (50–110 μmol/L)	Increase may indicate renal damage in SLE, scleroderma, and polyarteritis.
Erythrocyte Sedimentation Rate (ESR)		
Measures the rate at which red blood cells settle out of unclotted blood in 1 h	Westergren = Men, 0–15 mm/h, Women, 0–25 mm/h Wintrobe = Men, 0–9 mm/h, Women 0–15 mm/h	Increase is usually seen in inflammatory connective tissue diseases. An increase indicates rising inflammation, resulting in clustering of RBCs, which makes them heavier than normal. The higher the ESR, the greater the inflammatory activity.
Hematocrit		
Measures the size, capacity, and number of cells present in blood	Men: 42–52% Women: 35–47%	Decrease can be seen in chronic inflammation (anemia of chronic disease); also, blood loss through bowel due to medication.
Red Blood Cell Count		
Measures circulating erythrocytes	Men: Average 4.8 million/μL Women: Average 4.3 million/μL	Decrease can be seen in RA, SLE.
White Blood Cell Count		
Measures circulating leukocytes	5000–10,000 cells/mm³	Decrease may be seen in SLE.
VDRL (Venereal Disease Research Laboratory)		
Measures antibody to syphilis	Nonreactive	False-positive results are sometimes found with SLE.
Uric Acid		
Measures level of uric acid in serum	2.5–8 mg/dL (0.15–0.5 mmol/L)	Increase is seen with gout.
Serum Immunology		
Antinuclear Antibody (ANA)		
Measures antibodies that react with a variety of nuclear antigens If antibodies are present, further testing determines the type of ANA circulating in the blood (anti-DNA, anti-RNP).	Negative A few healthy adults have a positive ANA.	Positive test is associated with SLE, RA, scleroderma, Raynaud's disease, Sjögren's syndrome, necrotizing arteritis. The higher the titer, the greater the inflammation. The pattern of immunofluorescence (speckled, homogeneous, or nucleolar) helps determine the diagnosis.
Anti-DNA, DNA Binding		
Titer measurement of antibody to double-stranded DNA	Negative	High titer is seen in SLE; increases in titer may indicate increase in disease activity.
Complement Levels—C3, C4		
Complement is a protein substance that binds with antigen–antibody complexes for the purpose of lysis. When the number of complexes increases markedly, complement is used for lysis, thus depleting the amount available in the blood.	C3: 55–120 mg/dL (550–1200 mg/L) C4: 11–40 mg/dL (110–400 mg/L)	Decrease may be seen in RA and SLE. Decrease indicates autoimmune and inflammatory activity.
C-Reactive Protein Test (CRP)		
Shows presence of abnormal glycoprotein due to inflammatory process	<1 mg/dL (<10 mg/L)	A positive reading indicates active inflammation. Often is positive for RA and SLE
Immunoglobulin Electrophoresis		
Measures the values of immunoglobulins	IgA 80–400 mg/dL (0.8–4.0 g/L) IgG 600–1800 mg/dL (6.0–18.0 g/L) IgM 55–250 mg/dL (0.55–2.5 g/L)	Increased levels are found in people who have autoimmune disorders.
Rheumatoid Factor (RF)		
Determines the presence of abnormal antibodies seen in connective tissue disease	Negative	Positive titer >1:80 Present in 80% of those with RA Positive RF may also suggest SLE, Sjögren's syndrome, or mixed connective tissue disease. The higher the titer (number at right of colon), the greater the inflammation.
Tissue Typing		
HLA-B27 Antigen		
Measures presence of HLA antigens, which are used for tissue recognition	Negative	Found in 80–90% of those with ankylosing spondylitis and Reiter's syndrome.

DNA, deoxyribonucleic acid; HLA, human leukocyte antigen; RA, rheumatoid arthritis; RBCs, red blood cells; RNP, ribonucleoprotein; SLE, system lupus erythematosus.

positive attitude and self-esteem when faced with a rheumatic disease, especially if support is available. Previous stress management strategies are assessed. If these strategies have been effective, the patient is encouraged and supported in their use. If they were ineffective, the nurse assists the patient in identifying alternative strategies, encourages use of new strategies, and assesses their effectiveness.

Medical Management

A treatment program involving an interdisciplinary team, including the patient, is the basis for managing the rheumatic diseases. The chronic nature of most of these diseases mandates that the patient understand the disease, have the information necessary to make good self-management decisions, and be presented with a therapeutic program that is compatible with his or her lifestyle. Table 54-2 outlines goals and strategies for care of the patient with rheumatic diseases.

Pharmacologic Therapy

Medications are used with the rheumatic diseases to manage symptoms, to control inflammation, and, in some instances, to modify the disease. Useful medications include the salicylates, NSAIDs, and disease-modifying antirheumatic drugs (DMARDs). Table 54-3 reviews the medications commonly used.

Controlling the inflammation related to the disease process helps manage pain, but this is often a delayed response. Nonopioid medications are often used for pain management, especially early in the treatment program, until other measures can be instituted. Short-term use of low-dose antidepressant medications, such as amitriptyline (Elavil), may be prescribed to reestablish adequate sleep patterns and improve pain management (Karch, 2008).

Nonpharmacologic Pain Management

Nonpharmacologic methods of pain management are important. Heat applications are also helpful in relieving pain, stiffness, and muscle spasm (Robinson, Brosseau, Casimiro, et al., 2006). Superficial heat may be applied in the form of warm tub baths or showers and warm moist compresses. Paraffin baths (dips), which offer concentrated heat, are helpful to patients with wrist and small-joint involvement. Maximum benefit is achieved within 20 minutes after application. More frequent use for shorter lengths of time is most beneficial. Therapeutic exercises can be carried out more comfortably and effectively after heat has been applied.

Devices such as braces, splints, and assistive devices for ambulation (eg, canes, crutches, walkers) ease pain by limiting movement or stress from putting weight on painful joints. Acutely inflamed joints can be rested by applying splints to limit motion. Splints also support the joint to relieve spasm. Canes and crutches can relieve stress from inflamed and painful weight-bearing joints while promoting safe ambulation. Cervical collars may be used to support the weight of the head and limit cervical motion. A metatarsal bar or special pads may be put into the patient's shoes if foot pain or deformity is present (Egan, Brosseau, Farmer, et al., 2006). A combination of methods may be required, because different methods often work better at different times.

Exercise and Activity

The ongoing nature of most rheumatic diseases makes it important to maintain and, when possible, improve joint mobility and overall functional status. An individualized exercise program is crucial to movement. Table 54-4 summarizes the exercises appropriate for patients with rheumatic diseases. Appropriate programs of exercise have been shown to decrease pain and improve function (Miller, 2009). A mild analgesic agent may be suggested before exercise for a patient starting a program of exercise. Other strategies for decreasing pain include muscle relaxation techniques, imagery, self-hypnosis, and distraction, but acute or prolonged pain associated with exercise should be reported to a health care provider for evaluation. A weight reduction program may be recommended to relieve stress on painful joints.

The major challenge for the patient and the health care provider is the need to adjust all aspects of treatment according to the activity of the disease. Especially for the patient with an active diffuse connective tissue disease, such as RA or SLE, activity levels may vary from day to day and even within a single day.

Sleep

It is important to help the patient obtain restful sleep so he or she can cope with pain, minimize physical fatigue, and deal with the changes related to having a chronic disease. In patients with acute disease, sleep time is frequently reduced and fragmented by prolonged awakenings. Stiffness, depression, and medications may also compromise the quality of sleep and increase daytime fatigue. A sleep-inducing routine, medication, and comfort measures may help improve the quality of sleep.

Teaching sleep hygiene strategies may be helpful in promoting restorative sleep. These strategies include establishing a set time to sleep and a regular wake-up time, creating a quiet sleep environment with a comfortable room temperature,

Table 54-2	**MANAGEMENT GOALS AND STRATEGIES FOR RHEUMATIC DISEASES**
Goals	**Management Strategies**
Suppress inflammation and the autoimmune response	Optimize pharmacologic therapy (anti-inflammatory and disease-modifying agents)
Control pain	Protect joints; ease pain with splints, thermal modalities, relaxation techniques
Maintain or improve joint mobility	Implement exercise programs for joint motion and muscle strengthening and overall health
Maintain or improve functional status	Make use of adaptive devices and techniques
Increase patient's knowledge of disease process	Provide and reinforce patient teaching
Promote self-management by patient compliance with the therapeutic regimen	Emphasize compatibility of therapeutic regimen and lifestyle

Table 54-3 **MEDICATIONS USED IN RHEUMATIC DISEASES**

Medication	Action, Use, and Indication	Nursing Considerations
Salicylates *Acetylated:* aspirin *Nonacetylated:* choline salicylate (Arthropan, Trilisate), salsalate (Disalcid), sodium salicylate	*Action:* anti-inflammatory, analgesic, antipyretic Acetylated salicylates are platelet aggregation inhibitors. Anti-inflammatory doses will produce blood salicylate levels of 20–30 mg/dL.	Administer with meals to prevent gastric irritation. Assess for tinnitus, gastric intolerance, GI bleeding, and purpura. Monitor for possible confusion in the elderly.
Nonsteroidal Anti-inflammatory Drugs (NSAIDs) diclofenac (Voltaren), diflunisal (Dolobid), etodolac (Lodine), flurbiprofen (Ansaid), ibuprofen (Motrin), indomethacin (Indocin), ketoprofen (Orudis, Oruvail), meclofenamate (Meclomen), meloxicam (Mobic), nabumetone (Relafen), naproxen (Naprosyn), oxaprozin (Daypro), piroxicam (Feldene), sulindac (Clinoril), tolmetin sodium (Tolectin) COX-2 enzyme blockers: celecoxib (Celebrex)	*Action:* anti-inflammatory, analgesic, antipyretic, platelet aggregation inhibitor Anti-inflammatory effect occurs 2–4 weeks after initiation. All NSAIDs are useful for short-term treatment of acute gout attack. NSAIDs are alternative to salicylates for first-line therapy in several rheumatic diseases. *Action:* Inhibit only cyclo-oxygenase-2 (COX-2) enzymes, which are produced during inflammation, and spare COX-1 enzymes, which can be protective to the stomach	Administer NSAIDs with food. Monitor for GI, CNS, cardiovascular, renal, hematologic, and dermatologic adverse effects. Avoid salicylates; use acetaminophen for additional analgesia. Watch for possible confusion in older adults. Monitoring the same as for other NSAIDs Increased risk of cardiovascular events, including myocardial infarction and stroke Appropriate for the elderly and patients who are at high risk for gastric ulcers
Disease-Modifying Antirheumatic Drugs (DMARDs) Antimalarials: hydroxychloroquine (Plaquenil), chloroquine (Aralen)	*Action:* Anti-inflammatory, inhibits lysosomal enzymes Slow-acting, onset may take 2–4 mo Useful in RA and SLE	Administer concurrently with NSAIDs. Assess for visual changes, GI upset, skin rash, headaches, photosensitivity, bleaching of hair. Emphasize need for ophthalmologic examinations (every 6–12 mo).
Gold-containing compounds: aurothioglucose (Solganal), gold sodium thiomalate (Myochrysine), auranofin (Ridaura)	*Action:* Inhibits T- and B-cell activity, suppresses synovitis during active stage of rheumatoid disease Slow-acting, onset may take 3–6 mo IM preparations are given weekly for about 6 mo, then every 2–4 weeks	Administer concurrently with NSAIDs. Assess for stomatitis, diarrhea, dermatitis, proteinuria, hematuria, bone marrow suppression (decreased WBCs and/or platelets), CBC, and urinalysis with every other injection.
sulfasalazine (Azulfidine)	*Action:* Anti-inflammatory, reduces lymphocyte response, inhibits angiogenesis Useful in RA, seronegative spondyloarthropathies	Administer concurrently with NSAIDs. Do not use in patients with allergy to sulfa medications or salicylates. Emphasize adequate fluid intake. Assess for GI upset, skin rash, headache, liver abnormalities, anemia.
penicillamine (Cuprimine, Depen)	*Action:* Anti-inflammatory, inhibits T-cell function, impairs antigen presentation Slow-acting, onset may take 2–3 mo Useful in RA and systemic sclerosis	Administer concurrently with NSAIDs. Assess for GI irritation, decreased taste, skin rash or itching, bone marrow suppression, proteinuria with CBC, and urinalysis every 2–4 weeks.
Immunosuppressives: methotrexate (Rheumatrex), azathioprine (Imuran), cyclophosphamide (Cytoxan)	*Action:* Immune suppression, affect DNA synthesis and other cellular effects Have teratogenic potential; azathioprine and cyclophosphamide reserved for more aggressive or unresponsive disease Methotrexate is "gold standard" for RA treatment; also useful in SLE.	Assess for bone marrow suppression, GI ulcerations, skin rashes, alopecia, bladder toxicity, increased infections. Monitor CBC, liver enzymes, creatinine every 2–4 weeks. Advise patient of contraceptive measures because of teratogenicity.
Cyclosporine (Neoral)	*Action:* Immune suppression by inhibiting T lymphocytes Used for severe, progressive RA, unresponsive to other DMARDs Used in combination with methotrexate	Assess slow dose titration upward until response noted or toxicity occurs. Assess for toxic effects: bleeding gums, fluid retention, hair growth, tremors. Monitor blood pressure and creatinine every 2 weeks until stable.
Immunomodulators Pyrimidine synthesis inhibitor: leflunomide (Arava)	*Action:* Has antiproliferative and anti-inflammatory effects. Used in moderate to severe RA May be used alone or in combination with other DMARDs (except methotrexate)	Long half-life; requires loading dose followed by daily administration. Assess for diarrhea, hair loss, skin rash, mouth sores. Monitor liver function tests. Contraindicated in pregnancy and breastfeeding Administered orally

Continued

Table 54-3	MEDICATIONS USED IN RHEUMATIC DISEASES (Continued)	
Medication	**Action, Use, and Indication**	**Nursing Considerations**
TNF blocking agents: adalimumab (Humira), etanercept (Enbrel), infliximab (Remicade), golimumab (Simponi)	*Action:* Biologic response modifier that binds to TNF, a cytokine involved in inflammatory and immune responses. Used in moderate to severe RA unresponsive to methotrexate. Can be used alone or with methotrexate or other DMARDs. Humira is administered every 1–2 weeks, and Enbrel is administered twice a week.	Patient should be tested for tuberculosis before beginning this medication. Teach patient subcutaneous self-injection of adalimumab (Humira) or etanercept (Enbrel). Infliximab (Remicade) is administered by IV line over 2 h or more. Medication must be refrigerated. Monitor for injection site reactions. Educate patient about increased risk for infection and to withhold medication if fever occurs.
Interleukin-1 receptor antagonist: anakinra (Kineret)	*Action:* Human interleukin-1 (IL-1) receptor antagonist; blocks IL-1 receptors, decreasing inflammatory and immunologic responses. Used in moderate to severe RA unresponsive to methotrexate. Can be used alone or with methotrexate or DMARDs other than TNF blocking agents	Administered daily by subcutaneous injection. Teach patient subcutaneous self-injection to be administered daily. Medication must be refrigerated. Monitor for injection site reactions. Educate patient about increased risk of infection and to withhold medication if fever occurs.
Corticosteroids: prednisone, prednisolone, hydrocortisone	*Action:* Anti-inflammatory Used for shortest duration and at lowest dose possible to minimize adverse effects Useful for unremitting RA, SLE, polymyalgia rheumatica, myositis, arteritis Fast-acting; onset in days Intra-articular injections useful for joints unresponsive to NSAIDs	Assess for toxicity: cataracts, GI irritation, hyperglycemia, hypertension, fractures, avascular necrosis, hirsutism, psychosis. Joints most amenable to injections include ankles, knees, hips, shoulders, and hands. Repeated injections can cause joint damage.
Topical Analgesics capsaicin (Zostrix)	*Action:* analgesic	Teach patient to apply sparingly, avoid areas of open skin, avoid contact with eyes and mucous membranes. Wash hands carefully after application. Assess for local skin irritation.

CBC, complete blood count; CNS, central nervous system; GI, gastrointestinal; RA, rheumatoid arthritis; TNF, tumor necrosis factor; SLE, systemic lupus erythematosus; WBCs, white blood cells.

avoiding factors that interfere with sleep (eg, use of alcohol and caffeine), using relaxation exercises, and getting out of bed and engaging in another activity (eg, reading) if unable to sleep (Bulechek, Butcher & Dochterman, 2008).

Nursing Management

The plan of nursing care in Chart 54-2 details the nursing diagnoses, interventions, and expected outcomes for the patient with a rheumatic disorder.

Table 54-4	EXERCISE TO PROMOTE MOBILITY		
Type of Exercise	**Purpose**	**Recommended Performance**	**Precautions**
Range of motion	Maintain flexibility and joint motion	Active or active/self-assisted at least daily	Reduce number of repetitions when inflammation is present.
Isometric exercise	Improve muscle tone, static endurance, and strength; prepare for dynamic and weight-bearing exercises	Perform at 70% of maximal voluntary contraction daily.	Monitor blood pressure: isometric exercises may increase blood pressure and decrease blood flow to muscles.
Dynamic exercise	Maintain or increase dynamic strength and endurance; increase muscle power; enhance synovial blood flow; promote strength of bone and cartilage	Start with repetitions against gravity and add progressive resistance; perform 2–3 days per week.	May increase biomechanical stress on unstable or misaligned joints
Aerobic exercise	Improve cardiovascular fitness and endurance	Perform 3–5 days per week for 20–30 min of moderate-intensity exercise.	Progress slowly as activity tolerance and fitness improve.
Pool exercise	Water supports or resists movement; warm water may provide muscle relaxation.	Provides buoyant medium for performance of dynamic or aerobic exercise	Heated swimming pool; deep water to minimize joint compression; nonslip footwear for safety and comfort; receive appropriate instruction in a program designed for people with arthritis

Adapted from Firestein, G. S., Panayi, G. S. & Willheim, F. A. (2006). *Rheumatoid arthritis.* Oxford, UK: Oxford University Press.

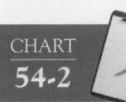

PLAN OF NURSING CARE
Care of the Patient With a Rheumatic Disorder

CHART 54-2

NURSING DIAGNOSIS: Acute and chronic pain related to inflammation and increased disease activity, tissue damage, fatigue, or lowered tolerance level
GOAL: Improvement in comfort level; incorporation of pain management techniques into daily life

Nursing Interventions	Rationale	Expected Outcomes

1. Provide variety of comfort measures
  a. Application of heat or cold
  b. Massage, position changes, rest
  c. Foam mattress, supportive pillow, splints
  d. Relaxation techniques, diversional activities
	1. Pain may respond to nonpharmacologic interventions such as joint protection, exercise, relaxation, and thermal modalities.	• Identifies factors that exacerbate or influence pain response
		• Identifies and uses pain management strategies
		• Verbalizes decrease in pain
		• Reports signs and symptoms of side effects in timely manner to prevent additional problems
		• Verbalizes that pain is characteristic of rheumatic disease
		• Establishes realistic pain relief goals
		• Verbalizes that pain often leads to the use of nontraditional and unproven self-treatment methods
		• Identifies changes in quality or intensity of pain

2. Administer anti-inflammatory, analgesic, and slow-acting antirheumatic medications as prescribed.	2. Pain of rheumatic disease responds to individual or combination medication regimens.	
3. Individualize medication schedule to meet patient's need for pain management.	3. Previous pain experiences and management strategies may be different from those needed for persistent pain.	
4. Encourage verbalization of feelings about pain and chronicity of disease.	4. Verbalization promotes coping.	
5. Teach pathophysiology of pain and rheumatic disease, and assist patient to recognize that pain often leads to unproven treatment methods.	5. Knowledge of rheumatic pain and appropriate treatment may help patient avoid unsafe, ineffective therapies.	
6. Assist in identification of pain that leads to use of unproven methods of treatment.	6. The impact of pain on an individual's life often leads to misconceptions about pain and pain management techniques.	
7. Assess for subjective changes in pain.	7. The individual's description of pain is a more reliable indicator than objective measurements such as change in vital signs, body movement, and facial expression.	

NURSING DIAGNOSIS: Fatigue related to increased disease activity, pain, inadequate sleep/rest, deconditioning, inadequate nutrition, and emotional stress/depression
GOAL: Incorporates as part of daily activities strategies necessary to modify fatigue

Nursing Interventions	Rationale	Expected Outcomes

1. Provide instruction about fatigue.
 	
  a. Describe relationship of disease activity to fatigue.
 	
  b. Describe comfort measures while providing them.
  c. Develop and encourage a sleep routine (warm bath and relaxation techniques that promote sleep).
  d. Explain importance of rest for relieving systematic, articular, and emotional stress.
  e. Explain how to use energy conservation techniques (pacing, delegating, setting priorities).
  f. Identify physical and emotional factors that can cause fatigue.
 	
2. Facilitate development of appropriate activity/rest schedule.
	1. The patient's understanding of fatigue will affect his or her actions.
	  a. The amount of fatigue is directly related to the activity of the disease.
	  b. Relief of discomfort can relieve fatigue.
	  c. Effective bedtime routine promotes restorative sleep.
	
	  d. Different kinds of rest are needed to relieve fatigue and are based on patient need and response.
	  e. A variety of measures can be used to conserve energy.
	
	  f. Awareness of the various causes of fatigue provides the basis for measures to modify the fatigue.
	2. Alternating rest and activity conserves energy while allowing most productivity.
		• Self-evaluates and monitors fatigue pattern
		• Verbalizes the relationship of fatigue to disease activity
		• Uses comfort measures as appropriate
		• Practices effective sleep hygiene and routine
		• Makes use of various assistive devices (splints, canes) and strategies (bed rest, relaxation techniques) to ease different kinds of fatigue
		• Incorporates time management strategies in daily activities
		• Uses appropriate measures to prevent physical and emotional fatigue
		• Has an established plan to ensure well-paced, therapeutic activity schedule
		• Adheres to therapeutic program
		• Follows a planned conditioning program

Continued

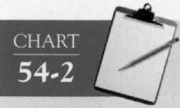

CHART 54-2

PLAN OF NURSING CARE

Care of the Patient With a Rheumatic Disorder (Continued)

Nursing Interventions	Rationale	Expected Outcomes
3. Encourage adherence to the treatment program. 4. Refer to and encourage a conditioning program. 5. Encourage adequate nutrition, including source of iron from food and supplements.	3. Overall control of disease activity can decrease the amount of fatigue. 4. Deconditioning resulting from lack of mobility, understanding, and disease activity contributes to fatigue. 5. A nutritious diet can help counteract fatigue.	• Consumes a nutritious diet consisting of appropriate food groups and recommended daily allowance of vitamins and minerals

NURSING DIAGNOSIS: Impaired physical mobility related to decreased range of motion, muscle weakness, pain on movement, limited endurance, lack of or improper use of ambulatory devices
GOAL: Attains and maintains optimal functional mobility

Nursing Interventions	Rationale	Expected Outcomes

1. Encourage verbalization regarding limitations in mobility.
 	
2. Assess need for occupational or physical therapy consultation:
  a. Emphasize range of motion of affected joints.
  b. Promote use of assistive ambulatory devices.
  c. Explain use of safe footwear.
  d. Use individual appropriate positioning/posture.
3. Assist to identify environmental barriers.
4. Encourage independence in mobility and assist as needed.
  a. Allow ample time for activity.
  b. Provide rest period after activity.
  c. Reinforce principles of joint protection and work simplification.
5. Initiate referral to community health agency.
	1. Mobility is not necessarily related to deformity. Pain, stiffness, and fatigue may temporarily limit mobility. The degree of mobility is not synonymous with the degree of independence. Decreased mobility may influence a person's self-concept and lead to social isolation.
	2. Therapeutic exercises, proper footwear, and/or assistive equipment may improve mobility. Correct posture and positioning are necessary for maintaining optimal mobility.
	
	3. Furniture and architectural adaptations may enhance mobility.
	4. Changes in mobility may lead to a decrease in personal safety.
	
	5. The degree of mobility may be slow to improve or may not improve with intervention.
		• Identifies factors that interfere with mobility
		• Describes and uses measures to prevent loss of motion
		• Identifies environmental (home, school, work, community) barriers to optimal mobility
		• Uses appropriate techniques and/or assistive equipment to aid mobility
		• Identifies community resources available to assist in managing decreased mobility

NURSING DIAGNOSIS: Self-care deficits related to contractures, fatigue, or loss of motion
GOAL: Achieves self-care independently or with the use of resources

Nursing Interventions	Rationale	Expected Outcomes

1. Assist patient to identify self-care deficits and factors that interfere with ability to perform self-care activities.
 	
2. Develop a plan based on the patient's perceptions and priorities on how to establish and achieve goals to meet self-care needs, incorporating joint protection, energy conservation, and work simplification concepts.
  a. Provide appropriate assistive devices.
  b. Reinforce correct and safe use of assistive devices.
	1. The ability to perform self-care activities is influenced by the disease activity and the accompanying pain, stiffness, fatigue, muscle weakness, loss of motion, and depression.
	2. Assistive devices may enhance self-care abilities. Effective planning for changes must include the patient, who must accept and adopt the plan.
		• Identifies factors that interfere with the ability to perform self-care activities
		• Identifies alternative methods for meeting self-care needs
		• Uses alternative methods for meeting self-care needs
		• Identifies and uses other health care resources for meeting self-care needs

Continued on following page

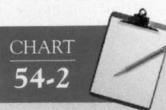

CHART
54-2

PLAN OF NURSING CARE
Care of the Patient With a Rheumatic Disorder (Continued)

Nursing Interventions	Rationale	Expected Outcomes
c. Allow patient to control timing of self-care activities. d. Explore with the patient different ways to perform difficult tasks or ways to enlist the help of someone else. 3. Consult with community health care agencies when individuals have attained a maximum level of self-care yet still have some deficits, especially regarding safety.	3. Individuals differ in ability and willingness to perform self-care activities. Changes in ability to care for self may lead to a decrease in personal safety.	

NURSING DIAGNOSIS: Disturbed body image related to physical and psychological changes and dependency imposed by chronic illness
GOAL: Adapts to physical and psychological changes imposed by the rheumatic disease

Nursing Interventions	Rationale	Expected Outcomes
1. Help patient identify elements of control over disease symptoms and treatment. 2. Encourage patient's verbalization of feelings, perceptions, and fears. a. Help to assess present situation and identify problems. b. Assist to identify past coping mechanisms. c. Assist to identify effective coping mechanisms.	1. The individual's self-concept may be altered by the disease or its treatment. 2. The individual's coping strategies reflect the strength of his or her self-concept.	• Verbalizes an awareness that changes taking place in self-concept are normal responses to rheumatic disease and other chronic illnesses • Identifies strategies to cope with altered self-concept

NURSING DIAGNOSIS: Ineffective coping related to actual or perceived lifestyle or role changes
GOAL: Use of effective coping behaviors for dealing with actual or perceived limitations and role changes

Nursing Interventions	Rationale	Expected Outcomes
1. Identify areas of life affected by disease. Answer questions and dispel possible myths. 2. Develop plan for managing symptoms and enlisting support of family and friends to promote daily function.	1. The effects of disease may be more or less manageable once identified and explored reasonably. 2. By taking action and involving others appropriately, patient develops or draws on coping skills and community support.	• Names functions and roles affected and not affected by disease process • Describes therapeutic regimen and states actions to take to improve, change, or accept a particular situation, function, or role

COLLABORATIVE PROBLEMS: Complications secondary to effects of medications
GOAL: Absence or resolution of complications

Nursing Interventions	Rationale	Expected Outcomes
1. Perform periodic clinical assessment and laboratory evaluation. 2. Instruct in correct self-administration, potential side effects, and importance of monitoring. 3. Counsel regarding methods to reduce side effects and manage symptoms. 4. Administer medications in modified doses as prescribed if complications occur.	1. Skillful assessment helps detect early symptoms of side effects of medications. 2. The patient needs accurate information about medications and potential side effects to avoid or manage them. 3. Appropriate identification and early intervention may minimize complications. 4. Modifications may help minimize side effects or other complications.	• Complies with monitoring procedures and experiences minimal side effects • Takes medication as prescribed and lists potential side effects • Identifies strategies to reduce or manage side effects • Reports that side effects or complications have subsided

Diffuse Connective Tissue Diseases

Diffuse connective tissue disease refers to a group of systematic disorders that are chronic in nature and are characterized by diffuse inflammation and degeneration in the connective tissues. These disorders share similar clinical features and may affect some of the same organs. The characteristic clinical course is one of exacerbations and remissions. Although the diffuse connective tissue diseases have unknown causes, they are thought to be the result of immunologic abnormalities. They include **rheumatoid arthritis** (RA), SLE, scleroderma, polymyositis, and polymyalgia rheumatica.

RHEUMATOID ARTHRITIS

RA is an autoimmune disease of unknown origin that affects 1% of the population worldwide, with a female-to-male ratio between 2:1 and 4:1 (Khanna, Arnold, Pencharz, et al., 2006).

Pathophysiology

In RA, the autoimmune reaction (Fig. 54-1) primarily occurs in the synovial tissue. Phagocytosis produces enzymes within the joint. The enzymes break down collagen, causing edema, proliferation of the synovial membrane, and ultimately pannus formation. Pannus destroys cartilage and erodes the bone. The consequence is loss of articular surfaces and joint motion. Muscle fibers undergo degenerative changes. Tendon and ligament elasticity and contractile power are lost.

Clinical Manifestations

Clinical manifestations of RA vary, usually reflecting the stage and severity of the disease. Joint pain, swelling, warmth, erythema, and lack of function are classic symptoms. Palpation of the joints reveals spongy or boggy tissue. Often fluid can be aspirated from the inflamed joint. Characteristically, the pattern of joint involvement begins in the small joints of the hands, wrists, and feet (Bickley, 2007). As the disease progresses, the knees, shoulders, hips, elbows, ankles, cervical spine, and temporomandibular joints are affected. The onset of symptoms is usually acute. Symptoms are usually bilateral and symmetric. In addition to joint pain and swelling, another classic sign of RA is joint stiffness in the morning.

In the early stages of disease, even before bony changes occur, limitation in function can occur when there is active inflammation in the joints. Joints that are hot, swollen, and painful are not easily moved. The patient tends to guard or protect these joints by immobilizing them. Immobilization for extended periods can lead to contractures, creating soft tissue deformity.

Deformities of the hands and feet are common in RA (see Chapter 66, Fig. 66-6). The deformity may be caused by misalignment resulting from swelling, progressive joint destruction, or the subluxation (partial dislocation) that occurs when one bone slips over another and eliminates the joint space.

RA is a systemic disease with multiple extra-articular features. Most common are fever, weight loss, fatigue, anemia, lymph node enlargement, and Raynaud's phenomenon (cold- and stress-induced vasospasm causing episodes of digital blanching or cyanosis). Rheumatoid nodules may be noted in patients with more advanced RA, and they develop at some time in the course of the disease in about 25% of patients. These nodules are usually nontender and movable in the subcutaneous tissue. They usually appear over bony prominences such as the elbow, are varied in size, and can disappear spontaneously. Nodules occur only in people who have rheumatoid factor. The nodules often are associated with rapidly progressive and destructive disease. Other extra-articular features include arteritis, neuropathy, scleritis, pericarditis, splenomegaly, and Sjögren's syndrome (dry eyes and dry mucous membranes).

Assessment and Diagnostic Findings

Several factors can contribute to a diagnosis of RA: rheumatoid nodules, joint inflammation detected on palpation, and laboratory findings. The history and physical examination address manifestations such as bilateral and symmetric stiffness, tenderness, swelling, and temperature changes in the joints. The patient is also assessed for extra-articular changes; these often include weight loss, sensory changes, lymph node enlargement, and fatigue. Rheumatoid factor is present in about three fourths of patients with RA, but its presence alone is not diagnostic of RA, and its absence does not rule out the diagnosis. The ESR is significantly elevated in RA. The red blood cell count and C4 complement component are decreased. C-reactive protein and antinuclear antibody (ANA) test results may also be positive (Karpoff & Labus, 2008) (Chart 54-3). Arthrocentesis shows synovial fluid that is cloudy, milky, or dark yellow and contains numerous inflammatory components, such as leukocytes and complement.

X-rays show bony erosions and narrowed joint spaces. X-rays of the hands and feet should be performed at baseline to help establish the diagnosis of RA and then every 3 years to monitor the progression of the disease (Khanna, et al., 2006).

Medical Management

Early Rheumatoid Arthritis

Patients with RA should receive aggressive and early treatment (Khanna, et al., 2006). Treatment includes education, a balance of rest and exercise, and referral to appropriate community agencies (such as the Arthritis Foundation) for support. Medical management begins with therapeutic doses of salicylates or NSAIDs. When used in full therapeutic dosages, these medications provide both anti-inflammatory and analgesic effects.

Several cyclo-oxygenase 2 (COX-2) enzyme blockers, another class of NSAIDs, have been approved for treatment of RA. Cyclo-oxygenase is an enzyme that is involved in the inflammatory process. COX-2 medications block the enzyme involved in inflammation (COX-2) while leaving intact the enzyme involved in protecting the stomach lining (COX-1). As a result, COX-2 enzyme blockers are less likely to cause gastric irritation and ulceration than other

CHART 54-3	NURSING RESEARCH PROFILE

Managing Symptoms in Rheumatoid Arthritis

Sousa, K. H., Ryu, E., Kwok, O., et al. (2007). Development of a model to measure symptom status in persons living with rheumatoid arthritis. *Nursing Research, 56*(6), 434–440.

Purpose

Rheumatoid arthritis (RA) is a chronic, progressive, inflammatory disease of unknown etiology that causes disability as well as morbidity and mortality. RA has a constellation of symptoms (eg, blurred vision, pain, dizziness) that affect quality of life. The purpose of this study was to develop and validate a structured model to measure symptom status in patients with RA.

Design

This study was a secondary analysis of symptom checklists available from 901 women enrolled in the Arthritis, Rheumatism, and Aging Medical Information System. The symptom checklists contained a list of 31 symptoms, and participants were asked to check off all symptoms they had experienced in the previous 6 months. Factor analysis was used to develop the model to measure symptoms.

Findings

Results of the factor analysis supported a two-factor model for the measurement of symptom status. The factors were (1) RA pain symptoms and (2) general symptoms. The two factors were found to be significantly different from each other, and the RA pain symptoms factor had a stronger impact on functional health than general symptoms.

Nursing Implications

The first aspect of effective symptom management for patients with RA is nursing assessment. This study provides a model and validated structure for such an assessment. For example, the symptoms that form the RA pain cluster could serve as a baseline assessment for nurses to identify goals and interventions to help improve the functional health and quality of life of patients with RA.

NSAIDs; however, they are associated with increased risk of cardiovascular disease and must be used with caution (Karch, 2008).

A window of opportunity for symptom control and improved disease management occurs within the first 2 years after disease onset. Therefore, it is recommended that treatment with the DMARDs (antimalarials, gold, penicillamine, or sulfasalazine) begin within 3 months of disease onset. If symptoms are aggressive (ie, early bony erosions as seen on x-rays), methotrexate may be considered. Methotrexate (Rheumatrex) is currently the standard treatment of RA because of its success in preventing both joint destruction and long-term disability (Schmajuk, et al., 2007).

An alternative treatment approach for RA has emerged in the area of biologic therapies. Biologic response modifiers are a group of agents that consist of molecules produced by cells of the immune system or by cells that participate in the inflammatory reactions. Research (Voulgari, Alamanos, Nikas, et al., 2005) using tumor necrosis factor-alpha (TNF-α) inhibitors in combination with other medications has shown that patients demonstrate significant improvement. Examples of biologic response modifiers that are currently available are etanercept (Enbrel), infliximab (Remicade), adalimumab (Humira), golimumab (Simponi), and anakinra (Kineret). Etanercept, infliximab, adalimumab, and golimumab inhibit the function of TNF-α, a key cytokine known to play a role in the disease process in RA (Porth & Matfin, 2009), whereas anakinra inhibits the function of interleukin-1, another cytokine that contributes to the destruction of the joint. Research in this area is ongoing.

Additional analgesia may be prescribed for periods of extreme pain. Opioid analgesic agents are avoided because of the potential for continuing need for pain relief. Nonpharmacologic pain management techniques (eg, relaxation techniques, heat and cold applications) are taught.

Moderate, Erosive Rheumatoid Arthritis

For moderate, erosive RA, a formal program with occupational and physical therapy is prescribed to educate the patient about principles of joint protection, pacing activities, work simplification, range of motion, and muscle-strengthening exercises. The patient is encouraged to participate actively in the management program. The medication program is reevaluated periodically, and appropriate changes are made if indicated. Cyclosporine (Neoral), an immunosuppressant, may be added to enhance the disease-modifying effect of methotrexate.

Persistent, Erosive Rheumatoid Arthritis

For persistent, erosive RA, reconstructive surgery and corticosteroids are often used. Reconstructive surgery is indicated when pain cannot be relieved by conservative measures and the threat of loss of independence is eminent. Surgical procedures include synovectomy (excision of the synovial membrane), tenorrhaphy (suturing of a tendon), arthrodesis (surgical fusion of the joint), and **arthroplasty** (surgical repair and replacement of the joint). Surgery is not performed during disease flares.

Systemic corticosteroids are used when the patient has unremitting inflammation and pain or needs a "bridging" medication while waiting for the slower DMARDs (eg, methotrexate) to begin taking effect. Low-dose corticosteroid therapy is prescribed for the shortest time necessary to minimize side effects (Khanna, et al., 2006). Single large joints that are severely inflamed and fail to respond promptly to the measures outlined previously may be treated by local injection of a corticosteroid.

Advanced, Unremitting Rheumatoid Arthritis

For advanced, unremitting RA, immunosuppressive agents are prescribed because of their ability to affect the production of antibodies at the cellular level. These include high-dose methotrexate (Rheumatrex), cyclophosphamide (Cytoxan), azathioprine (Imuran), and leflunomide (Arava). However, these medications are highly toxic and can produce bone marrow suppression, anemia, gastrointestinal disturbances, and rashes.

For most patients with RA, depression and sleep deprivation may require the short-term use of low-dose antidepressant medications, such as amitriptyline (Elavil), paroxetine (Paxil), or sertraline (Zoloft), to reestablish an adequate sleep pattern and to manage chronic pain.

The U.S. Food and Drug Administration (FDA) has approved a medical device for use in treating patients with more severe and long-standing RA who have had no response to or are intolerant of DMARDs. The device, a protein A immunoadsorption column (Prosorba), is used in 12 weekly 2-hour apheresis treatments to bind immunoglobulin G (IgG) (ie, circulating immune complex). In this unique population of patients, a significant improvement using the American College of Rheumatology criteria for improvement has been demonstrated (Eustice & Eustice, 2008).

Nutrition Therapy

Patients with RA frequently experience anorexia, weight loss, and anemia. A dietary history identifies usual eating habits and food preferences. Food selection should include the daily requirements from the basic food groups, with emphasis on foods high in vitamins, protein, and iron for tissue building and repair. For the patient who is extremely anorexic, small, frequent feedings with increased protein supplements may be prescribed. Supplemental vitamins and minerals may also be prescribed as needed (Klippel, Stone, Crofford, et al., 2008). Certain medications (ie, oral corticosteroids) used in RA treatment stimulate the appetite and, when combined with decreased activity, may lead to weight gain. Therefore, patients may need to be counseled about eating a healthy, calorie-restricted diet.

Nursing Management

Nursing care of the patient with RA follows the basic plan of care presented earlier (see Chart 54-2). The most common issues for the patient with RA include pain, sleep disturbance, fatigue, altered mood, and limited mobility (Sousa, Ryu, Kwok, et al., 2007). The patient with newly diagnosed RA needs information about the disease to make daily self-management decisions and to cope with having a chronic disease.

Monitoring and Managing Potential Complications

Medications used for treating RA may cause serious and adverse effects. These medication-induced complications may include bone marrow suppression, anemia, gastrointestinal disturbances, and rashes. The primary health care provider bases the prescribed medication regimen on clinical findings and past medical history, and then with the help of the nurse, monitors for side effects using periodic clinical assessments and laboratory testing. The nurse, who can be available for consultation between physician visits, works to help the patient recognize and deal with these side effects (see Table 54-3). The medication may need to be stopped or the dose reduced. If the patient experiences an increase in symptoms while the complication is being resolved or a new medication is being initiated, the nurse's counseling regarding symptom management may relieve potential anxiety and distress.

Promoting Home and Community-Based Care

Teaching Patients Self-Care

Patient teaching is an essential aspect of nursing care of the patient with RA to enable the patient to maintain as much independence as possible, to take medications accurately and safely, and to use adaptive devices correctly. Patient teaching focuses on the disorder itself, the possible changes related to the disorder, the therapeutic regimen prescribed to treat it, the potential side effects of medications, strategies to maintain independence and function, and patient safety in the home (Chart 54-4).

CHART 54-4

HOME CARE CHECKLIST
The Patient With Rheumatoid Arthritis

At the completion of the home care instruction, the patient or caregiver will be able to:	PATIENT	CAREGIVER
• Explain the nature of the disease and principles of disease management.	✔	✔
• Describe the medication regimen (name of medications, dosage, schedule of administration, precautions, potential side effects, and desired effects).	✔	✔
• Identify monitoring procedures and strategies that should be implemented.	✔	✔
• Identify sources of additional information, if necessary.	✔	✔
• Demonstrate accurate and safe self-administration of medications.	✔	✔
• Describe and demonstrate use of pain management techniques.	✔	✔
• Demonstrate use of joint protection techniques in activities of daily living (ADLs).	✔	✔
• Demonstrate ability to perform self-care activities independently or with assistive devices.	✔	
• Demonstrate a safe exercise program.	✔	
• Demonstrate a relaxation technique.	✔	

The patient and family are encouraged to verbalize their concerns and ask questions. Because RA commonly affects young women, major concerns may be related to the effects of the disease on childbearing potential, caring for family, or work responsibilities. The patient with a chronic illness may seek a "cure" or have questions about alternative therapies. One alternative therapy, an expensive one, used by many patients with RA is elk antler velvet. The velvet from elk antlers is harvested, ground, and put into capsules. In one randomized clinical trial of 168 patients with early stages of RA, researchers found that elk velvet has no clinical efficacy in the symptom management of the disease (Allen, Oberle, Grace, et al., 2008).

Pain, fatigue, and depression can interfere with the patient's ability to learn and should be addressed before teaching is initiated. Various educational strategies may then be used, depending on the patient's previous knowledge base, interest level, degree of comfort, social or cultural influences, and readiness to learn. The nurse instructs the patient about basic disease management and necessary adaptations in lifestyle. Because suppression of inflammation and autoimmune responses requires the use of anti-inflammatory, disease-modifying antirheumatic, and immunosuppressive agents, the patient is taught about prescribed medications, including type, dosage, rationale, potential side effects, self-administration, and required monitoring procedures. If hospitalized, the patient is encouraged to practice new self-management skills with support from caregivers and significant others. The nurse then reinforces disease management skills during each patient contact. Barriers to compliance are assessed, and measures are taken to promote adherence to medications and the treatment program.

Continuing Care

Depending on the severity of the disorder and the patient's resources and supports, referral for home care may or may not be warranted. However, the patient who is elderly or frail, has RA that limits function significantly, and lives alone may need referral for home care.

The impact of RA on everyday life is not always evident when the patient is seen in the hospital or in an ambulatory care setting. The increased frequency with which nurses see patients in the home provides opportunities for recognizing problems and implementing interventions aimed at improving the quality of life of patients with RA.

During home visits, the nurse has the opportunity to assess the home environment and its adequacy for patient safety and management of the disorder. Adherence to the treatment program can be more easily monitored in the home setting, where physical and social barriers to adherence are more readily identified. For example, a patient who also has diabetes and requires insulin may be unable to fill the syringe accurately or unable to administer the insulin because of impaired joint mobility. Appropriate adaptive equipment needed for increased independence is often identified more readily when the nurse sees how the patient functions in the home. Any barriers to adherence are identified, and appropriate referrals are made.

For patients at risk for impaired skin integrity, the home care nurse can closely monitor skin status and also instruct, provide, or supervise the patient and family in preventive skin care measures. The nurse also assesses the patient's need for assistance in the home and supervises home health aides who may meet many of the needs of the patient with RA. Referrals to physical and occupational therapists may be made as problems are identified and limitations increase. A home care nurse may visit the home to make sure the patient can function as independently as possible despite mobility problems and can safely manage treatments, including pharmacotherapy. The patient and family should be informed about support services such as Meals on Wheels and local Arthritis Foundation chapters.

Because many of the medications used to suppress inflammation are injectable, the nurse may administer the medication to the patient or teach self-injection. These frequent contacts allow the nurse to reinforce other disease management techniques.

The nurse also assesses the patient's physical and psychological status, adequacy of symptom management, and adherence to the management plan. Patients should know which type of rheumatic disease they have, not just that they have "arthritis" or "arthritis of the knee." The importance of attending follow-up appointments is emphasized to the patient and family, and they should be reminded about the importance of participating in other health promotion activities and health screening. Patients with chronic disorders such as RA often focus on the chronic disease and neglect general health issues.

SYSTEMIC LUPUS ERYTHEMATOSUS

The overall prevalence of SLE is estimated to be 1 per 2500 persons. It occurs 10 times more frequently in women than in men and approximately three times more frequently in African Americans than in Caucasians (Wandstrat, Carr-Johnson, Branch, et al., 2006).

Pathophysiology

SLE is a result of disturbed immune regulation that causes an exaggerated production of autoantibodies. This immunoregulatory disturbance is brought about by some combination of genetic factors, hormonal factors (as evidenced by the usual onset during the childbearing years), and environmental factors (eg, sunlight, thermal burns). Certain medications, such as hydralazine (Apresoline), procainamide (Pronestyl), isoniazid (INH), chlorpromazine (Thorazine), and some antiseizure medications, have been implicated in chemical or drug-induced SLE.

Specifically, B cells and T cells both contribute to the immune response in SLE (Croker & Kimberly, 2005). B cells are instrumental in promoting the onset and flares of the disease (Tieng & Peeva, 2008).

Clinical Manifestations

SLE is an autoimmune systemic disease that can affect any body system. Involvement of the musculoskeletal system, with arthralgias and arthritis (synovitis), is a common presenting feature of SLE. Joint swelling, tenderness, and pain on movement are also common. Frequently, these are accompanied by morning stiffness. The onset of disease may be insidious or acute.

Several different types of skin manifestations may occur in patients with SLE, including subacute cutaneous lupus erythematosus, which involves papulosquamous or annular polycyclic lesions, and discoid lupus erythematosus, which is a chronic rash that has erythematous papules or plaques and scaling and can cause scarring and pigmentation changes. The most familiar skin manifestation (occurring in more than 50% of patients with SLE) is an acute cutaneous lesion consisting of a butterfly-shaped rash across the bridge of the nose and cheeks (Bickley, 2007) (Fig. 54-2). In some cases of discoid lupus erythematosus, only skin involvement occurs. In some patients with SLE, the initial skin involvement is the precursor to more systemic involvement. The lesions often worsen during exacerbations (flares) of the systemic disease and possibly are provoked by sunlight or artificial ultraviolet light. Oral ulcers, which may accompany skin lesions, may involve the buccal mucosa or the hard palate, occur in crops, and are often associated with exacerbations.

Pericarditis is the most common cardiac manifestation. Women who have SLE are also at risk for early atherosclerosis.

Serum creatinine levels and urinalysis are used in screening for renal involvement. Early detection allows for prompt treatment so that renal damage can be prevented. Renal involvement may lead to hypertension, which also requires careful monitoring and management (see Chapter 32).

Central nervous system involvement is widespread, encompassing the entire range of neurologic disease. The varied and frequent neuropsychiatric presentations of SLE are now widely recognized. These are generally demonstrated by subtle changes in behavior patterns or cognitive ability.

Assessment and Diagnostic Findings

Diagnosis of SLE is based on a complete history, physical examination, and blood tests. Typically, assessment reveals classic symptoms, including fever, fatigue, weight loss, and possibly arthritis, pleurisy, and pericarditis. Interactions with the patient and family may provide further evidence of systemic involvement.

In addition to the general assessment performed for any patient with a rheumatic disease, assessment for known or suspected SLE has special features. The skin is inspected for erythematous rashes. Cutaneous erythematous plaques with an adherent scale may be observed on the scalp, face, or neck. Areas of hyperpigmentation or depigmentation may be noted, depending on the phase and type of the disease. The patient should be questioned about skin changes (because these may be transitory) and specifically about sensitivity to sunlight or artificial ultraviolet light. The scalp should be inspected for alopecia and the mouth and throat for ulcerations reflecting gastrointestinal involvement.

Cardiovascular assessment includes auscultation for pericardial friction rub, possibly associated with myocarditis and accompanying pleural effusions. The pleural effusions and infiltrations, which reflect respiratory insufficiency, are demonstrated by abnormal lung sounds. Papular, erythematous, and purpuric lesions developing on the fingertips, elbows, toes, and extensor surfaces of the forearms or lateral sides of the hand that may become necrotic suggest vascular involvement.

Joint swelling, tenderness, warmth, pain on movement, stiffness, and edema may be detected on physical examination. The joint involvement is often symmetric and similar to that found in RA.

The neurologic assessment is directed at identifying and describing any central nervous system changes. The patient and family members are asked about any behavioral changes, including manifestations of neurosis or psychosis. Signs of depression are noted, as are reports of seizures, chorea, or other central nervous system manifestations.

No single laboratory test confirms SLE; rather, blood testing reveals moderate to severe anemia, thrombocytopenia, leukocytosis, or leukopenia and positive ANAs (Wandstrat, et al., 2006). Other diagnostic immunologic tests support but do not confirm the diagnosis.

Medical Management

Treatment of SLE includes management of acute and chronic disease. Although SLE can be life-threatening, advances in its treatment have led to improved survival and reduced morbidity. Acute disease requires interventions directed at controlling increased disease activity or exacerbations that can involve any organ system. Disease activity is a composite of clinical and laboratory features that reflect active inflammation secondary to SLE. Management of the

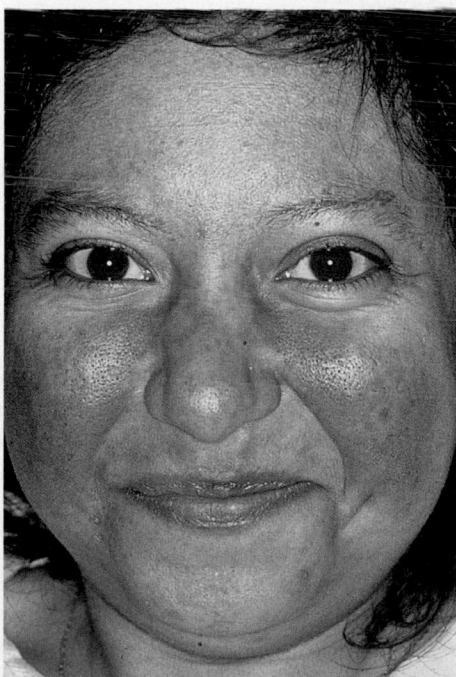

Figure 54-2 The characteristic butterfly rash of systemic lupus erythematosus.

more chronic condition involves periodic monitoring and recognition of meaningful clinical changes requiring adjustments in therapy.

The goals of treatment include preventing progressive loss of organ function, reducing the likelihood of acute disease, minimizing disease-related disabilities, and preventing complications from therapy. Management of SLE involves regular monitoring to assess disease activity and therapeutic effectiveness.

Pharmacologic Therapy

Medication therapy for SLE is based on the concept that local tissue inflammation is mediated by exaggerated or heightened immune responses, which can vary widely in intensity and require different therapies at different times. Corticosteroids are the single most important medication available for treatment. They are used topically for cutaneous manifestations, in low oral doses for minor disease activity, and in high doses for major disease activity. Intravenous (IV) administration of corticosteroids is an alternative to traditional high-dose oral use. Antimalarial medications are effective for managing cutaneous, musculoskeletal, and mild systemic features of SLE. The NSAIDs used for minor clinical manifestations are often used along with corticosteroids in an effort to minimize corticosteroid requirements.

Immunosuppressive agents (alkylating agents and purine analogues) are used because of their effect on immune function. These medications are generally reserved for patients who have serious forms of SLE that have not responded to conservative therapies. B-cell depleting therapies are the newest treatment for SLE. Monoclonal antibodies, rituximab (Rituxan), and epratuzumab (humanized anit-CD22 antibody) have shown good therapeutic results in clinical trials (Tieng & Peeva, 2008).

Nursing Management

Nursing care of the patient with SLE is based on the fundamental plan presented earlier in the chapter (see Chart 54-2). The most common nursing diagnoses include fatigue, impaired skin integrity, body image disturbance, and lack of knowledge for self-management decisions. The disease or its treatment may produce dramatic changes in appearance and considerable distress for the patient. The changes and the unpredictable course of SLE necessitate expert assessment skills and nursing care with sensitivity to the psychological reactions of the patient. The patient may benefit from participation in support groups, which can provide disease information, daily management tips, and social support. Because sun and ultraviolet light exposure can increase disease activity or cause an exacerbation, patients should be taught to avoid exposure or to protect themselves with sunscreen and clothing.

Because of the increased risk of involvement of multiple organ systems, patients should understand the need for routine periodic screenings as well as health promotion activities. A dietary consultation may be indicated to ensure that the patient is knowledgeable about dietary recommendations, given the increased risk of cardiovascular disease, including hypertension and atherosclerosis. The nurse instructs the patient about the importance of continuing prescribed medications and addresses the changes and potential side effects that are likely to occur with their use. The patient is reminded of the importance of monitoring because of the increased risk of systemic involvement, including renal and cardiovascular effects.

SCLERODERMA

Scleroderma ("hard skin") is a relatively rare disease that is poorly understood; the cause is unknown. The incidence of scleroderma (also known as systemic sclerosis) is 18 to 20 cases per million per year (Seibold, 2005). Like other diffuse connective tissue diseases, it has a variable course with remissions and exacerbations. Its prognosis is not as optimistic as that of SLE.

Pathophysiology

Scleroderma commonly begins with skin involvement. Mononuclear cells cluster on the skin and stimulate lymphokines to stimulate procollagen. Insoluble collagen is formed and accumulates excessively in the tissues. Initially, the inflammatory response causes edema formation, with a resulting taut, smooth, and shiny skin appearance. The skin then undergoes fibrotic changes, leading to loss of elasticity and movement. Eventually, the tissue degenerates and becomes nonfunctional. This chain of events, from inflammation to degeneration, also occurs in blood vessels, major organs, and body systems (Klippel, et al., 2008).

Clinical Manifestations

Scleroderma starts insidiously with Raynaud's phenomenon and swelling in the hands. The skin and the subcutaneous tissues become increasingly hard and rigid and cannot be pinched up from the underlying structures. Wrinkles and lines are obliterated. The skin is dry because sweat secretion over the involved region is suppressed. The extremities stiffen and lose mobility. The condition spreads slowly; for years, these changes may remain localized in the hands and the feet. The face appears masklike, immobile, and expressionless, and the mouth becomes rigid.

The changes within the body, although not visible directly, are vastly more important than the visible changes. The left ventricle of the heart is involved, resulting in heart failure. The esophagus hardens, interfering with swallowing. The lungs become scarred, impeding respiration. Digestive disturbances occur because of hardening (sclerosing) of the intestinal mucosa. Progressive renal failure may occur.

The patient may manifest a variety of symptoms referred to as the CREST syndrome. CREST stands for calcinosis (calcium deposits in the tissues), Raynaud's phenomenon, esophageal hardening and dysfunction, sclerodactyly (scleroderma of the digits), and telangiectasia (capillary dilation that forms a vascular lesion).

Assessment and Diagnostic Findings

Assessment focuses on the sclerotic changes in the skin, contractures in the fingers, and color changes or lesions in the fingertips. Assessment of systemic involvement requires a systems review with special attention to gastrointestinal, pulmonary, renal, and cardiac symptoms. Limitations in mobility and self-care activities should be assessed, along with the impact the disease has had (or will have) on body image.

There is no one conclusive test to diagnose scleroderma. A skin biopsy is performed to identify cellular changes specific to scleroderma. Pulmonary studies show ventilation–perfusion abnormalities. Echocardiography identifies pericardial effusion (often present with cardiac involvement). Esophageal studies demonstrate decreased motility in most patients with scleroderma. Blood tests may detect ANAs, indicating a connective tissue disorder and possibly distinguishing the subgroup (diffuse or limited) of scleroderma. A positive ANA test result is common in patients with scleroderma.

Medical Management

Treatment of scleroderma depends on the clinical manifestations. All patients require counseling, during which realistic individual goals may be determined. Support measures include strategies to decrease pain and limit disability. A moderate exercise program is encouraged to prevent joint contractures. Patients are advised to avoid extreme temperatures and to use lotion to minimize skin dryness.

Pharmacologic Therapy

No medication regimen has proved effective in modifying the disease process in scleroderma, but various medications are used to treat organ system involvement. Calcium channel blockers and other antihypertensive agents may provide improvement in symptoms of Raynaud's phenomenon. Anti-inflammatory medications can be used to control arthralgia, stiffness, and general musculoskeletal discomfort (Seibold, 2005).

Nursing Management

The nursing care of the patient with scleroderma is based on the fundamental plan of nursing care presented earlier (see Chart 54-2). The most common nursing diagnoses of the patient with scleroderma are impaired skin integrity; self-care deficits; imbalanced nutrition, less than body requirements; and disturbed body image. The patient with advanced disease may also have impaired gas exchange, decreased cardiac output, impaired swallowing, and constipation.

Providing meticulous skin care and preventing the effects of Raynaud's phenomenon are major nursing challenges. Patient teaching must include the importance of avoiding cold and protecting the fingers with mittens in cold weather and when shopping in the frozen-food section of the grocery store. Warm socks and properly fitting shoes are helpful in preventing ulcers. Careful, frequent inspection for early ulcers is important. Smoking cessation is critical.

POLYMYOSITIS

Polymyositis is a group of diseases that are termed idiopathic inflammatory myopathies (Klippel, et al., 2008). They are rare conditions, with an incidence estimated at 5 to 10 cases per million adults per year.

Pathophysiology

Polymyositis is classified as autoimmune because autoantibodies are present. However, these antibodies do not cause damage to muscle cells, indicating only an indirect role in tissue damage. The pathogenesis is multifactorial, and a genetic predisposition is likely. Drug-induced disease is rare. Some evidence suggests a viral link.

Clinical Manifestations

The onset ranges from sudden with rapid progression to very slow and insidious. Proximal muscle weakness is typically a first symptom. Muscle weakness is usually symmetric and diffuse. Dermatomyositis, a related condition, is most commonly identified by an erythematous smooth or scaly lesion found over the joint surface.

Assessment and Diagnostic Findings

A complete history and physical examination help exclude other muscle-related disorders. As with other diffuse connective tissue disorders, no single test confirms polymyositis. An electromyogram is performed to rule out degenerative muscle disease. A muscle biopsy may reveal inflammatory infiltrate in the tissue. Serum studies indicate increased muscle enzyme activity.

Medical Management

Management involves high-dose corticosteroid therapy initially, followed by a gradual dosage reduction over several months as muscle enzyme activity decreases. Patients who do not respond to corticosteroids require the addition of an immunosuppressive agent. Plasmapheresis, lymphapheresis, and total-body irradiation have been used if there is no response to corticosteroids and immunosuppressive medications. The antimalarial agent hydroxychloroquine (Plaquenil) may be effective for skin rashes. Physical therapy is initiated slowly, with range-of-motion exercises to maintain joint mobility, followed by gradual strengthening exercises (Klippel, et al., 2008).

Nursing Management

Nursing care is based on the fundamental plan of nursing care presented earlier (see Chart 54-2). The most frequent nursing diagnoses for the patient with polymyositis are impaired physical mobility, fatigue, self-care deficit, and insufficient knowledge of self-management techniques.

Patients with polymyositis may have symptoms similar to those of other inflammatory diseases. However, proximal muscle weakness is characteristic, making activities such as combing the hair, reaching overhead, and using stairs difficult. Therefore, use of assistive devices may be recommended, and referral to occupational or physical therapy may be warranted.

POLYMYALGIA RHEUMATICA

Pathophysiology

The underlying mechanism involved with polymyalgia rheumatica is unknown. This disease occurs predominately in Caucasians and often in first-degree relatives. An association with the genetic marker HLA-DR4 suggests a familial predisposition. Immunoglobulin deposits in the walls of inflamed temporal arteries also suggest an autoimmune process.

Polymyalgia rheumatica and giant cell arteritis are found almost exclusively in people older than 50 years of age. Polymyalgia rheumatica has an annual incidence rate of 52 cases per 100,000 people older than 50 years. Giant cell arteritis varies by geographic location and has the highest incidence in Scandinavian countries (Klippel, et al., 2008).

Clinical Manifestations

Polymyalgia rheumatica is characterized by severe proximal muscle discomfort with mild joint swelling. Severe aching in the neck, shoulder, and pelvic muscles is common. Stiffness is noticeable most often in the morning and after periods of inactivity. Systemic features include low-grade fever, weight loss, malaise, anorexia, and depression. Because polymyalgia rheumatica usually occurs in people 50 years of age and older, it may be confused with, or dismissed as, an inevitable consequence of aging.

Giant cell arteritis, sometimes associated with polymyalgia rheumatica, may cause headaches, changes in vision, and jaw claudication. These symptoms should be evaluated immediately because of the potential for a sudden and permanent loss of vision if the condition is left untreated. Polymyalgia rheumatica and giant cell arteritis typically have a self-limited course, lasting several months to several years (Klippel, et al., 2008).

Assessment and Diagnostic Findings

Assessment focuses on musculoskeletal tenderness, weakness, and decreased function. Careful attention should be directed toward assessing the head (for changes in vision, headaches, and jaw claudication).

Often, diagnosis is difficult because of the lack of specificity of tests. A markedly high ESR is a screening test but is not definitive. Diagnosis is more likely to be made by eliminating other potential diagnoses, but this is highly dependent on the skills and experience of the diagnostician. The dramatic and immediate response to treatment with corticosteroids is considered by some to be diagnostic.

Medical Management

The treatment for patients with polymyalgia rheumatica (without giant cell arteritis) is moderate doses of corticosteroids (Klippel, et al., 2008). NSAIDs are sometimes used for mild disease. The treatment for patients with giant cell arteritis is rapid initiation of and strict adherence to a regimen of corticosteroids. This is essential to avoid the complication of blindness. Aspirin is a useful adjunctive treatment that also helps reduce the risk of visual loss (Klippel, et al., 2008).

Nursing Management

Nursing care of the patient with polymyalgia rheumatica is based on the fundamental plan of nursing care presented earlier (see Chart 54-2). The most common nursing diagnoses are pain and insufficient knowledge of the medication regimen.

A management concern is that the patient will take the prescribed medication, frequently corticosteroids, until symptoms improve and then discontinue the medication. The decision to discontinue the medication should be based on clinical and laboratory findings and the physician's prescription. Nursing implications are related to helping the patient prevent and monitor side effects of medications (eg, infections, diabetes mellitus, gastrointestinal problems, and depression) and adjust to those side effects that cannot be prevented (eg, increased appetite and altered body image).

> ▶ **NURSING ALERT**
>
> The nurse must emphasize to the patient the need for continued adherence to the prescribed medication regimen to avoid complications of giant cell arteritis, such as blindness.

The loss of bone mass with corticosteroid use increases the risk of osteoporosis in this already at-risk population. Interventions to promote bone health, such as adequate dietary calcium and vitamin D, measurement of bone mineral density, weight-bearing exercise, smoking cessation, and reduction of alcohol consumption if indicated, should be emphasized.

Degenerative Joint Disease (Osteoarthritis)

Osteoarthritis, also known as degenerative joint disease or osteoarthrosis (even though inflammation may be present), is the most common and most frequently disabling of the joint disorders. OA is both overdiagnosed and trivialized; it is frequently overtreated or undertreated. The functional impact of OA on quality of life, especially for elderly patients, is often ignored.

OA has been classified as primary (idiopathic), with no prior event or disease related to the OA, and secondary, resulting from previous joint injury or inflammatory disease. The distinction between primary and secondary OA is not always clear.

Increasing age directly relates to the degenerative process in the joint, because the ability of the articular cartilage to resist microfracture with repetitive low loads diminishes with age. OA often begins in the third decade of life and peaks between the fifth and sixth decades. By 40 years of age, 90% of the population have degenerative joint changes in their weight-bearing joints, even though clinical symptoms are usually absent. Prevalence of OA is between 50% and 80% in the elderly (Ganz, Chang, Roth, et al., 2006).

Pathophysiology

OA may be thought of as the end result of many factors that, when combined, predispose the patient to the disease. OA affects the articular cartilage, **subchondral bone** (the bony plate that supports the articular cartilage), and synovium. A combination of cartilage degradation, bone stiffening, and reactive inflammation of the synovium occurs. Understanding of OA has been greatly expanded beyond what previously was thought of as simply "wear and tear" related to aging. The basic degenerative process in the joint exemplified in OA is presented in Figure 54-3.

Congenital and developmental disorders of the hip are well known for predisposing a person to OA of the hip. These include congenital subluxation–dislocation of the hip, acetabular dysplasia, Legg-Calvé-Perthes disease, and slipped capital femoral epiphysis.

Risk factors for OA include increased age, obesity, previous joint damage, repetitive use (occupational or recreational), anatomic deformity, and genetic susceptibility. Being overweight or obese also increases symptoms associated with the disease (Klippel, et al., 2008). Research has shown that a weight loss of 10% improves function by 28% in people with OA affecting the knee (Christensen, Astrup & Bliddal, 2005).

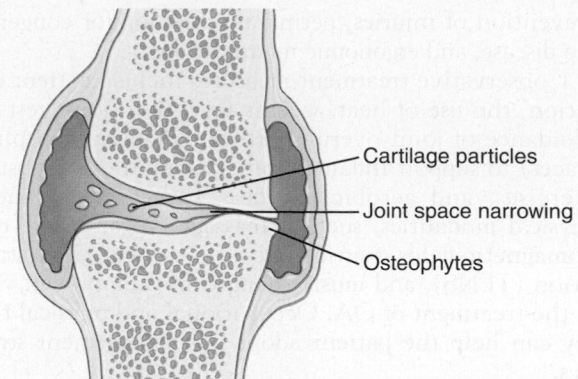

Figure 54-4 Joint space narrowing and osteophytes (bone spurs) are characteristic of degenerative changes in joints.

Clinical Manifestations

The primary clinical manifestations of OA are pain, stiffness, and functional impairment. The pain is caused by an inflamed synovium, stretching of the joint capsule or ligaments, irritation of nerve endings in the periosteum over **osteophytes** (bone spurs), trabecular microfracture, intraosseous hypertension, bursitis, tendinitis, and muscle spasm (Fig 54-4). Stiffness, which is most commonly experienced in the morning or after awakening, usually lasts less than 30 minutes and decreases with movement. Functional impairment results from pain on movement and limited motion caused by structural changes in the joints.

Although OA occurs most often in weight-bearing joints (hips, knees, cervical and lumbar spine), the proximal and distal finger joints are also often involved. Characteristic bony nodes may be present; on inspection and palpation, these are usually painless, unless inflammation is present.

Assessment and Diagnostic Findings

Diagnosis of OA is complicated because only 30% of patients with changes seen on x-ray report symptoms. Physical assessment of the musculoskeletal system reveals tender and enlarged joints. Inflammation, when present, is not the destructive type seen in the connective tissue diseases such as RA. OA is characterized by a progressive loss of the joint cartilage, which appears on x-ray as a narrowing of the joint space. In addition, reactive changes occur at the joint margins and on the subchondral bone in the form of osteophytes as the cartilage attempts to regenerate. Neither the presence of osteophytes nor joint space narrowing alone is specific for OA; however, when combined, these are sensitive and specific findings. In early or mild OA, there is only a weak correlation between joint pain and synovitis. Blood tests are not useful in the diagnosis of OA.

Medical Management

Although no treatment halts the degenerative process, certain preventive measures can slow the progress if undertaken early enough. These include weight reduction,

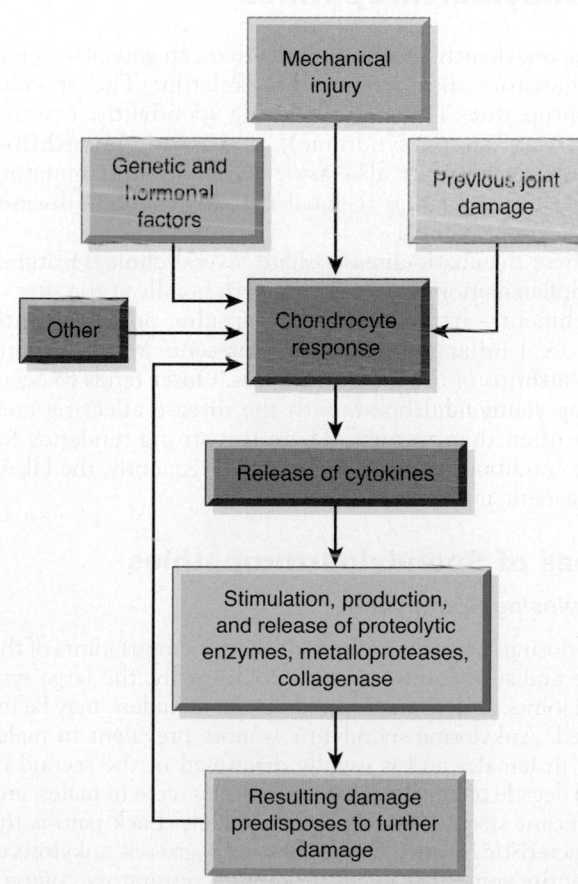

Figure 54-3 Pathophysiology of osteoarthritis.

prevention of injuries, perinatal screening for congenital hip disease, and ergonomic modifications.

Conservative treatment measures include patient education, the use of heat, weight reduction, joint rest and avoidance of joint overuse, orthotic devices (eg, splints, braces) to support inflamed joints, isometric and postural exercises, and aerobic exercise. Other miscellaneous physical modalities, such as massage, yoga, pulsed electromagnetic fields, transcutaneous electrical nerve stimulation (TENS), and music therapy, have unproven value in the treatment of OA. Occupational and physical therapy can help the patient adopt self-management strategies.

Patients with arthritis often use complementary and alternative therapies, many of which are not traditionally taught in American medical schools and are not traditionally available in American hospitals. These may include herbal and dietary supplements, other special diets, acupuncture, acupressure, wearing copper bracelets or magnets, and participation in T'ai chi. Research is under way to determine the effectiveness of many of these treatments (Little, Parsons & Logan, 2006).

Pharmacologic Therapy

Pharmacologic management of OA is directed toward symptom management and pain control. Selection of medication is based on the patient's needs, the stage of disease, and the risk of side effects. Medications are used in conjunction with nonpharmacologic strategies. In most patients with OA, the initial analgesic therapy is acetaminophen. Some patients respond to the nonselective NSAIDs, and patients who are at increased risk for gastrointestinal complications, especially gastrointestinal bleeding, have been managed effectively with COX-2 enzyme blockers. However, COX-2 enzyme blockers must be used with caution because of the associated risk of cardiovascular disease. Other medications that may be considered are the opioids and intra-articular corticosteroids. Topical analgesic agents such as capsaicin (Capsin, Zostrix) and methylsalicylate are also used (Klippel, et al., 2008).

Other therapeutic approaches include glucosamine and chondroitin. Although it has been suggested that these substances modify cartilage structure, studies have not shown them to be effective (Towheed, Maxwell, Anastassiades, et al., 2006). Viscosupplementation, the injection of gel-like substances (hyaluronates), into a joint (intra-articular) is thought to supplement the viscous properties of synovial fluid. Five hyaluronates are currently approved by the FDA for joint injection in OA (Eustice & Eustice, 2006).

Surgical Management

In moderate to severe OA, when pain is severe or because of loss of function, surgical intervention may be used. The procedures most commonly used are osteotomy (to alter the distribution of weight within the joint) and arthroplasty. In arthroplasty, diseased joint components are replaced (see Chapter 67).

Nursing Management

Nursing management of the patient with OA includes both pharmacologic and nonpharmacologic approaches. Nonpharmacologic interventions are used first and continued with pharmacologic agents. Pain management and optimal functional ability are major goals of nursing intervention. The patient's understanding of the disease process and symptom pattern is critical to a plan of care. Because patients with OA usually are older, they may have other health problems. Commonly they are overweight, and they may have a sedentary lifestyle. Weight loss and exercise are important approaches to pain and disability improvement (Christensen, et al., 2005; Klippel, et al., 2008). A referral for physical therapy or to an exercise program for people with similar problems can be very helpful. Canes or other assistive devices for ambulation should be considered. Exercises such as walking should be begun in moderation and increased gradually. Patients should plan their daily exercise for a time when the pain is least severe or plan to use an analgesic agent, if appropriate, before exercising. Adequate pain management is important for the success of an exercise program. Open discussion regarding the use of complementary and alternative therapies is important to maintain safe and effective practices for patients looking for a "cure."

Spondyloarthropathies

The spondyloarthropathies are another category of systemic inflammatory disorders of the skeleton. The spondyloarthropathies include ankylosing spondylitis, reactive arthritis (Reiter's syndrome), and psoriatic arthritis. Spondyloarthritis is also associated with inflammatory bowel diseases such as regional enteritis (Crohn's disease) and ulcerative colitis.

These rheumatic diseases share several clinical features. The inflammation tends to occur peripherally at the sites of attachment—at tendons, joint capsules, and ligaments. Periosteal inflammation may be present. Many patients have arthritis of the sacroiliac joints. Onset tends to occur during young adulthood, with the disease affecting men more often than women. There is a strong tendency for these conditions to occur in families. Frequently, the HLA-B27 genetic marker is found.

Types of Spondyloarthropathies

Ankylosing Spondylitis

Ankylosing spondylitis affects the cartilaginous joints of the spine and surrounding tissues. Occasionally, the large synovial joints, such as the hips, knees, or shoulders, may be involved. Ankylosing spondylitis is more prevalent in males than in females and is usually diagnosed in the second or third decade of life. The disease is more severe in males, and significant systemic involvement is likely. Back pain is the characteristic feature. As the disease progresses, ankylosis of the entire spine may occur, leading to respiratory compromise and complications.

Reactive Arthritis (Reiter's Syndrome)

The disease process involved in Reiter's syndrome is called reactive because the arthritis occurs after an infection. It mostly affects young adult males and is characterized primarily by urethritis, arthritis, and conjunctivitis. Dermatitis and ulcerations of the mouth and penis may also be present. Low back pain is common.

Psoriatic Arthritis

Psoriatic arthritis is characterized by synovitis, polyarthritis, and spondylitis. Both psoriasis and arthritis are common conditions, and one theory suggests that the overlap of the two conditions is a chance occurrence. However, epidemiologic data suggest that the prevalence of arthritis in patients with psoriasis is 15% to 25%, exceeding the rate in the general population. Similarly, the prevalence of psoriasis in persons with arthritis is 2.6% to 7.0%, compared with 0.1% to 2.8% in the general population, supporting the theory that these two processes occur together in a unique disease process (Klippel, et al., 2008).

Medical Management

Medical management of spondyloarthropathies focuses on treating pain and maintaining mobility by suppressing inflammation. For the patient with ankylosing spondylitis, good body positioning and posture are essential, so that if **ankylosis** (fixation) does occur, the patient is in the most functional position. Maintaining range of motion with a regular exercise and muscle-strengthening program is especially important.

Pharmacologic Management

NSAIDs and corticosteroids often produce marked improvement in back, skin, and joint symptoms. Sulfasalazine (Azulfidine) and methotrexate (Rheumatrex) may help with peripheral joint disease. Methotrexate is also used to control psoriasis. More recently, anti-TNF therapy is under investigation for treatment of the spondyloarthropathies (Klippel, et al., 2008).

Surgical Management

Surgical management may include total joint replacement (see Chapter 67).

Nursing Management

Major nursing interventions in the spondyloarthropathies are related to symptom management and maintenance of optimal functioning. Affected patients are primarily young men. Their major concerns are often related to prognosis and job modification, especially among those who perform physical work. Patients may also express concerns about leisure and recreational activities.

Metabolic and Endocrine Diseases Associated With Rheumatic Disorders

Metabolic and endocrine diseases may be associated with rheumatic disorders. These include biochemical abnormalities (amyloidosis and scurvy), endocrine diseases (diabetes mellitus and acromegaly), immunodeficiency diseases (human immunodeficiency virus [HIV] infection, acquired immunodeficiency syndrome [AIDS]), and some inherited disorders (hypermobility syndromes). However, the most common conditions are the crystal-induced arthropathies, in which crystals such as monosodium urate (gout) or calcium pyrophosphate (calcium pyrophosphate dihydrate disease [CPPD] or pseudogout) are deposited within joints and other tissues.

GOUT

Gout is a heterogeneous group of conditions related to a genetic defect of purine metabolism that results in hyperuricemia. Oversecretion of uric acid or a renal defect resulting in decreased excretion of uric acid, or a combination of both, occurs. The prevalence is reported to be about 2% and appears to be on the rise. The incidence of gout increases with age and body mass index, and the disorder occurs more commonly in males than in females (Singh, Hodges, Toscano, et al., 2007).

In primary hyperuricemia, elevated serum urate levels or manifestations of urate deposition appear to be consequences of faulty uric acid metabolism. Primary hyperuricemia may be caused by severe dieting or starvation, excessive intake of foods that are high in purines (shellfish, organ meats), or heredity. In secondary hyperuricemia, gout is a clinical feature secondary to any of a number of genetic or acquired processes, including conditions in which there is an increase in cell turnover (leukemia, multiple myeloma, some types of anemias, psoriasis) and an increase in cell breakdown. Altered renal tubular function, either as a major action or as an unintended side effect of certain pharmacologic agents (eg, diuretics such as thiazides and furosemide), low-dose salicylates, or ethanol, can contribute to uric acid underexcretion.

Pathophysiology

Hyperuricemia (serum concentration greater than 7 mg/dL) can, but does not always, cause urate crystal deposition (Karpoff & Labus, 2008). However, as uric acid levels increase, the risk becomes greater. Attacks of gout appear to be related to sudden increases or decreases of serum uric acid levels. When the urate crystals precipitate within a joint, an inflammatory response occurs, and an attack of gout begins. With repeated attacks, accumulations of sodium urate crystals, called **tophi,** are deposited in peripheral areas of the body, such as the great toe, the hands, and the ear. Renal urate lithiasis (kidney stones), with chronic renal disease secondary to urate deposition, may develop.

The finding of urate crystals in the synovial fluid of asymptomatic joints suggests that factors other than crystals may be related to the inflammatory reaction. Recovered monosodium urate crystals are coated with immunoglobulins that are mainly IgG. IgG enhances crystal phagocytosis, thereby demonstrating immunologic activity (Klippel, et al., 2008).

Clinical Manifestations

Manifestations of the gout syndrome include acute gouty arthritis (recurrent attacks of severe articular and periarticular inflammation), tophi (crystalline deposits accumulating in articular tissue, osseous tissue, soft tissue, and cartilage), gouty nephropathy (renal impairment), and uric acid urinary calculi. Four stages of gout can be identified: asymptomatic hyperuricemia, acute gouty arthritis, intercritical gout, and chronic tophaceous gout. The subsequent development of gout is directly related to the duration and magnitude of the hyperuricemia. Therefore, the commitment to lifelong pharmacologic treatment of hyperuricemia is deferred until there is an initial attack of gout.

For hyperuricemic people who are going to develop gout, acute arthritis is the most common early clinical manifestation. The metatarsophalangeal joint of the big toe is the most commonly affected joint (90% of patients) (Porth & Matfin, 2009). The tarsal area, ankle, or knee may also be affected. Less commonly, the wrists, fingers, and elbows may be affected. Trauma, alcohol ingestion, dieting, medications, surgical stress, or illness may trigger the acute attack. The abrupt onset often occurs at night, awakening the patient with severe pain, redness, swelling, and warmth of the affected joint. Early attacks tend to subside spontaneously over 3 to 10 days even without treatment. The attack is followed by a symptom-free period (the intercritical stage) until the next attack, which may not come for months or years. However, with time, attacks tend to occur more frequently, to involve more joints, and to last longer.

Tophi are generally associated with more frequent and severe inflammatory episodes. Higher serum concentrations of uric acid are also associated with more extensive tophus formation. Tophi most commonly occur in the synovium, olecranon bursa, subchondral bone, infrapatellar and Achilles tendons, and subcutaneous tissue on the extensor surface of the forearms and overlying joints. They have also been found in the aortic walls, heart valves, nasal and ear cartilage, eyelids, cornea, and sclerae. Joint enlargement may cause a loss of joint motion. Uric acid deposits may cause renal stones and kidney damage.

Medical Management

A definitive diagnosis of gouty arthritis is established by polarized light microscopy of the synovial fluid of the involved joint. Uric acid crystals are seen within the polymorphonuclear leukocytes in the fluid. Colchicine (oral or parenteral), an NSAID such as indomethacin, or a corticosteroid is prescribed to relieve an acute attack of gout. Management of hyperuricemia, tophi, joint destruction, and renal disorders is usually initiated after the acute inflammatory process has subsided. Uricosuric agents, such as probenecid (Benemid), correct hyperuricemia and dissolve deposited urate. When reduction of the serum urate level is indicated, uricosuric agents are the medications of choice. If the patient has, or is at risk for, renal insufficiency or renal calculi (kidney stones), allopurinol, a xanthine oxidase inhibitor, is recommended (Singh, et al., 2007). A new medication, febuxostat (Uloric), was approved by the FDA in 2009 for the treatment of gout that does not respond to usual treatment. Corticosteroids may also be used in patients who have no response to other therapy. If the patient experiences several acute episodes or there is evidence of tophi formation, prophylactic treatment is considered. Specific treatment is based on the serum uric acid level, 24-hour urinary uric acid excretion, and renal function (Table 54-5).

Nursing Management

Historically, gouty arthritis was thought to be a condition of royalty and the very rich, with the disease attributed to "high living." This has not been shown to be entirely true. Although severe dietary restriction is not necessary, the nurse should encourage the patient to restrict consumption of foods high in purines, especially organ meats, and to limit alcohol intake. Maintenance of normal body weight should be encouraged. In an acute episode of gouty arthritis, pain management with prescribed medications is essential, along with avoidance of factors that increase pain and inflammation, such as trauma, stress, and alcohol. Between acute episodes, the patient feels well and may abandon preventive behaviors, which may result in an acute attack. Acute attacks are most effectively treated if therapy is begun early in the course.

Fibromyalgia

Fibromyalgia is a chronic pain syndrome that involves chronic fatigue, generalized muscle aching, and stiffness. Two percent of the United States population is affected by this syndrome, with a prevalence rate of 4% in women and 0.5% in men (Klippel, et al., 2008). See Chapter 13.

Table 54-5	MEDICATIONS USED TO TREAT GOUT	
Medication	**Actions and Use**	**Nursing Implications**
colchicine	Lowers the deposition of uric acid and interferes with leukocyte infiltration, thus reducing inflammation; does not alter serum or urine levels of uric acid; used in acute and chronic management	*Acute management:* Administer when attack begins; dosage increased until pain is relieved or diarrhea develops *Chronic management:* Causes GI upset in most patients
probenecid (Benemid)	Uricosuric agent; inhibits renal reabsorption of urates and increases the urinary excretion of uric acid; prevents tophi formation	Be alert for nausea and rash.
allopurinol (Zyloprim) febuxostat (Uloric)	Xanthine oxidase inhibitors; interrupt the breakdown of purines before uric acid is formed; inhibits xanthinoxidase because it blocks uric acid formation	Monitor for side effects, including bone marrow depression, vomiting, and abdominal pain.

Medical Management

Treatment consists of attention to the specific symptoms reported by the patient. NSAIDs may be used to treat the diffuse muscle aching and stiffness. Tricyclic antidepressants are used to improve or restore normal sleep patterns. In addition, selective serotonin reuptake inhibitors and anticonvulsants have been effective in preliminary reports (Klippel, et al., 2008). Individualized programs of exercise are used to decrease muscle weakness and discomfort and to improve the general deconditioning that occurs in affected patients.

Nursing Management

Typically, patients with fibromyalgia have endured their symptoms for a long period of time. They may feel as if their symptoms have not been taken seriously. Nurses need to pay special attention to supporting these patients and providing encouragement as they begin their program of therapy. Patient support groups may be helpful. Careful listening to patients' descriptions of their concerns and symptoms is essential to help them make the changes that are necessary to improve their quality of life (Schaefer, 2005).

Arthritis Associated With Infectious Organisms

Arthritis, tenosynovitis, and bursitis can be associated with infectious organisms. Some inflammation of joints, tendons, and bursae is directly related to infection caused by bacterial, viral, fungal, or parasitic agents. Bacterial arthritis is the most rapidly destructive form of infectious arthritis. There are two major classes of bacterial arthritis: that caused by *Neisseria gonorrhoeae* and that caused by a nongonococcal bacterium. The most prevalent of the nongonococcal organisms include *Staphylococcus aureus* and the various streptococcal variants. Less common pathogens are related to syphilis, tuberculosis, leprosy, fungi (particularly coccidioidomycosis), mycoplasmas, and viral agents such as rubella, parvovirus, and hepatitis B.

Clinical Manifestations

The characteristic symptom is acute onset of a warm, swollen joint. Culture of the bacterium from the synovial fluid confirms the diagnosis. The patient often immobilizes the joint and elevates the affected extremity because of pain and swelling. Fever may be high, or it may be absent. Signs of systemic infection may be absent in elderly patients, in those with diabetes, and in those with suppressed immune systems. Diagnosis and treatment may be delayed by patients with preexisting arthritic conditions if they attribute the symptoms to a flare-up of arthritis.

Management

This condition is a medical emergency necessitating early diagnosis and appropriate treatment to eliminate the causative organism; otherwise, the joint may be destroyed relatively quickly. Treatment consists of parenteral antibiotics and drainage of the joint. The results of cultures are used to determine the appropriate antibiotic therapy. Immobilization of the joint and repeated joint aspirations may be necessary along with IV antibiotics. Nursing management focuses on providing pain relief, administering antibiotics, and assisting the patient with self-care activities. If the patient is sent home on IV antibiotic therapy, the nurse arranges for home care and instructs the patient and care providers in safe administration of the drug and changes that should be reported to a health care provider.

Neoplasms and Neurovascular, Bone, and Extra-Articular Disorders

Primary neoplasms of joints, tendon sheaths, and bursae are rare. Most neoplasms are benign, arising from the synovium. These benign tumors include lipoma, hemangioma, fibroma, and tumorlike lesions such as ganglion, bursitis, and synovial cyst. Malignant tumors include primary tumors, such as synovial and bone sarcomas, and secondary involvement as manifestations of joint invasion by leukemia, lymphoma, myeloma, or metastasis. Neoplasms may manifest as back or neck pain.

Neurovascular disorders include the compression syndromes, such as those with peripheral entrapment (eg, carpal tunnel syndrome), radiculopathy, and spinal stenosis. Raynaud's phenomenon and erythromelalgia (throbbing and burning pain often affecting the hands and feet) are also included in this category.

Bone and cartilage disorders include osteoporosis, osteomalacia, hypertrophic osteoarthropathy, diffuse idiopathic skeletal hyperostosis, Paget's disease, osteonecrosis, avascular necrosis, costochondritis, osteolysis or chondrolysis, and biomechanical or anatomic abnormalities. Notably, these conditions involve resorption, destruction, infection, or remodeling of bone.

Extra-articular rheumatism is a descriptive term for a group of conditions that affect structures other than the joints. Included are general and regional pain syndromes, low back pain and intervertebral disk disorders, tendonitis and bursitis, and ganglion cysts.

Miscellaneous Disorders

The last category in the classification of the rheumatic diseases is aptly labeled miscellaneous disorders because it contains a mix of disorders that are frequently associated with arthritis and other conditions. These include the direct consequences of trauma (including internal derangement and loose bodies of joints), pancreatic disease (related to avascular necrosis or osteonecrosis), sarcoidosis (a multisystem disorder particularly of the lymph nodes and lungs), and palindromic rheumatism (an uncommon variety of recurring and acute arthritis and periarthritis that in some may progress to RA but is characterized by symptom-free periods of days to months). Other conditions include villonodular synovitis, chronic active hepatitis, and drug-related rheumatic syndromes. The nursing interventions related to these varied conditions are specific to the multisystemic problems experienced by the patient. However, the musculoskeletal components should not be neglected or overlooked. Further information about these rare disorders can be found in specialty references.

CRITICAL THINKING EXERCISES

1 Your patient with a rheumatic disorder has NSAIDs, corticosteroids, and a biologic response modifier prescribed. How do the actions, uses, and indications of these medications differ? What instructions and recommendations would you give to the patient to ensure their safe administration?

EBP **2** A 30-year-old woman with a recent diagnosis of RA states she is having joint pain, stiffness, and swelling, especially in her hands and wrists. What resources would you use to identify the current guidelines for treatment of patients with RA? What is the evidence base for these treatment practices? Identify the criteria used to evaluate the strength of the evidence for these practices.

3 A 79-year-old woman with a 10-year history of OA of the right knee complains of pain every day and difficulty walking. She is taking multiple medications and currently she uses a walker to ambulate but needs to stop and rest every so often because of the pain. Describe the pharmacologic treatment and nursing measures that are indicated for this patient. What teaching is important for the patient? How would you modify your teaching if the patient understands little English?

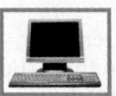 The Smeltzer suite offers these additional resources to enhance learning and facilitate understanding of this chapter:
- thePoint online resource, thepoint.lww.com/ Smeltzer12E
- Student CD-ROM included with the book
- *Study Guide to Accompany Brunner & Suddarth's Textbook of Medical-Surgical Nursing*
- *Handbook for Brunner & Suddarth's Textbook of Medical-Surgical Nursing*

REFERENCES

*Asterisk indicates nursing research.
**Double asterisk indicates classic reference.

Books

Bickley, L. S. (2007). *Bates' guide to physical examination and history taking* (9th ed.). Philadelphia: Lippincott Williams & Wilkins.
Bulechek, G. M., Butcher, H. K. & Dochterman, J. M. (2008). *Nursing interventions classification (NIC)* (5th ed.). St. Louis: Mosby.
Firestein, G .S., Panayi, G. S. & Willheim, F. A. (2006). *Rheumatoid arthritis.* Oxford, UK: Oxford University Press.
Karch, A. (2008). *Lippincott's nursing drug guide.* Philadelphia: Lippincott Williams & Wilkins.
Karpoff, S. & Labus, D. M. (2008). *Portable diagnostic tests.* Philadelphia: Lippincott Williams & Wilkins.

Klippel, J. H., Stone, J. H., Crofford, L. J., et al. (2008). *Primer on the rheumatic diseases* (13th ed.). New York: Springer.
Miller, C. A. (2009). *Nursing for wellness in older adults* (5th ed.). Philadelphia: Lippincott Williams & Wilkins.
Porth, C. M. & Matfin, G. (2009). *Pathophysiology: Concepts of altered health status* (8th ed.). Philadelphia: Lippincott Williams & Wilkins.
Seibold, J. R. (2005). Scleroderma. In Harris, E. D., Budd, R. C., Genovese, M. C., et al. (Eds.). *Kelley's textbook of rheumatology* (7th ed.). Philadelphia: Elsevier Saunders.

Journals and Electronic Documents

General

Fontaine, K. R., Bartlett, S. J. & Heo, M. (2005). Are health care professionals advising adults with arthritis to become more physically active? *Arthritis Care and Research, 53*(2), 279–283.
Singh, J. A., Hodges, J. S., Toscano, J. P., et al. (2007). Quality of care for gout in the U.S. needs improvement. *Arthritis and Rheumatism, 57*(5), 822–829.

Rheumatoid Arthritis

*Allen, M., Oberle, K., Grace, M., et al. (2008). A randomized clinical trial of elk velvet antler in rheumatoid arthritis. *Biological Research for Nursing, 9*(3), 254–261.
Egan, M., Brosseau, L., Farmer, M., et al. (2006). Splints and orthosis for treating rheumatoid arthritis. *The Cochrane Library, 1*, CD004018.
Eustice, C. & Eustice, R. (2008). *Which rheumatoid arthritis patients are good candidates for the Prosorba column?* Available at: http://arthritis.about.com/od/arthqa/f/prosorba.htm
Khanna, D., Arnold, E. L., Pencharz, J. N., et al. (2006). Measuring process of arthritis care: The arthritis foundation's quality indicator set for rheumatoid arthritis. *Seminars in Arthritis and Rheumatism, 35*(4), 211–237.
Little, C. V. & Parsons, T. (2006). Herbal therapy for treating rheumatoid arthritis. *The Cochrane Library, 1*, CD002948.
Robinson, V. A., Brosseau, L., Casimiro, L., et al. (2006). Thermotherapy for treating rheumatoid arthritis. *The Cochrane Library, 1*, CD002826.
Schmajuk, G., Schneeweiss, S., Katz, J. N., et al. (2007). Treatment of older adult patients diagnosed with rheumatoid arthritis: Improved but not optimal. *Arthritis and Rheumatism, 57*(6), 928–934.
*Sousa, K. H., Ryu, E., Kwok, O., et al. (2007). Development of a model to measure symptom status in persons living with rheumatoid arthritis. *Nursing Research, 56*(6), 434–440.
Steultjens, E. E. M., Bouter, L. L. M., Dekker, J. J., et al. (2006). Occupational therapy for rheumatoid arthritis. *The Cochrane Library, 1*, CD003114.
Voulgari, P. V., Alamanos, Y., Nikas, S. N., et al. (2005). Infliximab therapy in established rheumatoid arthritis: An observational study. *American Journal of Medicine, 118*(5), 515–520.

Osteoarthritis

Christensen, R., Astrup, A. & Bliddal, H. (2005). Weight loss: The treatment of choice for knee osteoarthritis? *OsteoArthritis and Cartilage, 13*(1), 20–27.
Eustice, C. & Eustice, G. (2006). *What is viscosupplementation?* Available at: http://arthritis.about.com/od/kneetreatments/g/viscosupplement.htm
Ganz, D. A., Chang, J. T., Roth, C. P., et al. (2006). Quality of osteoarthritis care for community-dwelling older adults. *Arthritis and Rheumatism, 55*(2), 241–247.
Little, C. V., Parsons, T. & Logan, S. (2006). Herbal therapy for treating osteoarthritis. *The Cochrane Library, 1*, CD002947.
Towheed, T. E., Maxwell, L., Anastassiades, T. P., et al. (2006). Glucosamine therapy for treating osteoarthritis. *The Cochrane Library, 1*, CD002946.

Systemic Lupus Erythematosus

Croker, J. A. & Kimberly, R. P. (2005). SLE: Challenges and candidates in human disease. *Trends in Immunology, 26*(11), 580–586.
Tieng, A. T. & Peeva, E. (2008). B-cell directed therapies in systemic lupus erythematosus. *Seminars in Arthritis & Rheumatology, 38*(2), 218–227.
Wandstrat, A. E., Carr-Johnson, F., Branch, V., et al. (2006). Autoantibody profiling to identify individuals at risk for systemic lupus erythematosus. *Journal of Autoimmunity, 27*(1), 153–160.

Other Rheumatic Diseases

Diep, J. T. & Gorevic, P. D. (2005). Geriatric autoimmune diseases: Systemic lupus erythematosus, Sjögren's syndrome, and myositis. *Geriatrics, 60*(5), 32–38.

*Schaefer, K. M. (2005). The lived experience of fibromyalgia in African American women. *Holistic Nursing Practice, 19*(1), 17–25.

**Wolfe, F., Smythe, H. A., Yunus, M. B., et al. (1990). The American College of Rheumatology 1990 criteria for the classification of fibromyalgia: Report of the multicenter criteria committee. *Arthritis and Rheumatism, 33*(2), 160–172.

RESOURCES

American College of Rheumatology and Association of Rheumatology Health Professionals, www.rheumatology.org

American Fibromyalgia Syndrome Association, Inc., www.afsafund.org

Arthritis Foundation, www.arthritis.org

Centers for Disease Control & Prevention, www.cdc.gov

Lupus Foundation of America, Inc., www.lupus.org

National Institute of Arthritis and Musculoskeletal and Skin Diseases, National Institutes of Health, www.niams.nih.gov

Scleroderma Foundation, www.scleroderma.org

Sjögren's Syndrome Foundation, www.sjogrens.org

Spondylitis Association of America, www.spondylitis.org

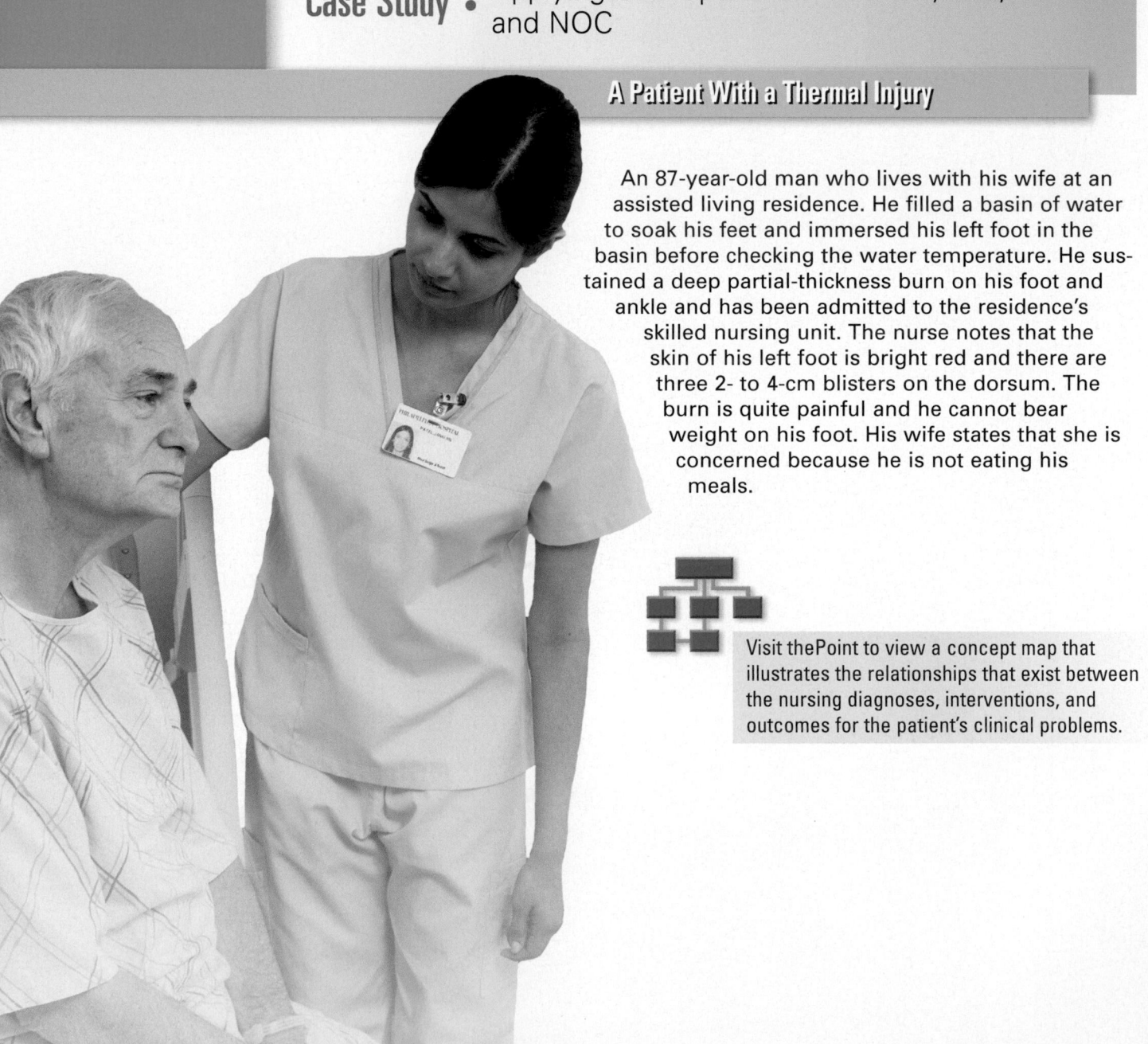

unit
12

Integumentary Function

Case Study • Applying Concepts From NANDA, NIC, and NOC

A Patient With a Thermal Injury

An 87-year-old man who lives with his wife at an assisted living residence. He filled a basin of water to soak his feet and immersed his left foot in the basin before checking the water temperature. He sustained a deep partial-thickness burn on his foot and ankle and has been admitted to the residence's skilled nursing unit. The nurse notes that the skin of his left foot is bright red and there are three 2- to 4-cm blisters on the dorsum. The burn is quite painful and he cannot bear weight on his foot. His wife states that she is concerned because he is not eating his meals.

Visit thePoint to view a concept map that illustrates the relationships that exist between the nursing diagnoses, interventions, and outcomes for the patient's clinical problems.

Nursing Classifications and Languages

NANDA NURSING DIAGNOSES	NIC NURSING INTERVENTIONS	NOC NURSING OUTCOMES
		Return to functional baseline status, stabilization of, or improvement in:
IMPAIRED SKIN INTEGRITY—Altered epidermis and/or dermis	**SKIN CARE: TOPICAL TREATMENTS**—Application of topical substances or manipulation of devices to promote skin integrity and minimize skin breakdown	**WOUND HEALING: SECONDARY INTENTION**—Extent of regeneration of cells and tissues in an open wound
ACUTE PAIN—Unpleasant sensory and emotional experience arising from actual or potential tissue damage or described in terms of such damage; sudden or slow onset of any intensity from mild to severe with an anticipated or predictable end and a duration of less than 6 months	**WOUND CARE**—Prevention of wound complications and promotion of wound healing	**PAIN CONTROL**—Personal actions to control pain
RISK FOR INFECTION—At increased risk for being invaded by pathogenic organisms	**PAIN MANAGEMENT**—Alleviation of pain or reduction in pain to a level of comfort that is acceptable to the patient	**INFECTION SEVERITY**—Severity of infection and associated symptoms
RISK FOR IMBALANCED NUTRITION: LESS THAN BODY REQUIREMENTS—At risk for intake of nutrients insufficient to meet metabolic needs	**INFECTION PROTECTION**—Prevention and early detection of infection in a patient at risk	**NUTRITIONAL STATUS**—Extent to which nutrients are available to meet metabolic needs
	NUTRITION MANAGEMENT—Assisting with or providing a balanced dietary intake of foods and fluids	

Bulechek, G. M., Butcher, H. K., & Dochterman, J. M. (2008). *Nursing interventions classification (NIC)* (5th ed.). St. Louis: Mosby.
Johnson, M., Bulechek, G., Butcher, H. K., et al. (2006). *NANDA, NOC, and NIC linkages* (2nd ed.). St. Louis: Mosby.
Moorhead, S., Johnson, M., Mass, M. L., et al. (2008). *Nursing outcomes classification (NOC)* (4th ed.). St. Louis: Mosby.
NANDA International. (2007). *Nursing diagnoses: Definitions & classification 2007–2008.* Philadelphia: North American Nursing Diagnosis Association.

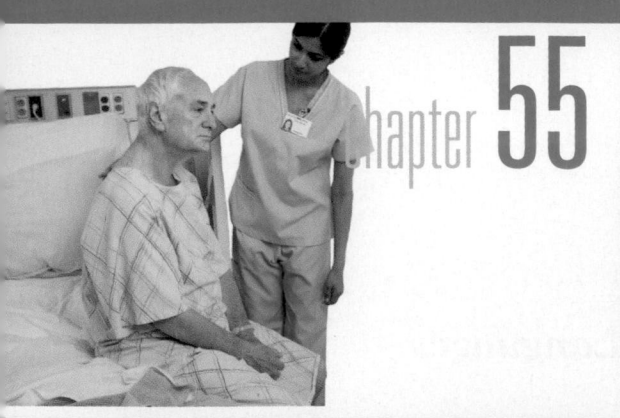

Chapter 55

Assessment of Integumentary Function

On completion of this chapter, the learner will be able to:

1 Identify the structures and functions of the skin.

2 Differentiate the composition and function of each skin layer: epidermis, dermis, and subcutaneous tissue.

3 Describe the normal aging process of the skin and skin changes common in elderly patients.

4 List appropriate questions that help elicit information during an assessment of the skin.

5 Describe the components of physical assessment that are most useful when examining the skin, hair, and nails.

6 Identify and describe primary and secondary skin lesions and their pattern and distribution.

7 Recognize common skin eruptions and manifestations associated with systemic disease.

8 Discuss common skin tests and procedures used in diagnosing skin and related disorders.

GLOSSARY

alopecia: loss of hair from any cause

dermatosis: any abnormal skin condition

erythema: redness of the skin caused by congestion of the capillaries

hirsutism: the condition of having excessive hair growth

hyperpigmentation: increase in the melanin of the skin, resulting in an increase in pigmentation

hypopigmentation: decrease in the melanin of the skin, resulting in a loss of pigmentation

keratin: an insoluble, fibrous protein that forms the outer layer of skin

Langerhans cells: dendritic clear cells in the epidermis that carry surface receptors for immunoglobulin and complement and that are active participants in delayed hypersensitivity of the skin

melanin: the substance responsible for coloration of the skin

melanocytes: cells of the skin that produce melanin

Merkel cells: cells of the epidermis that play a role in transmission of sensory messages

petechiae: pinpoint red spots that appear on the skin as a result of blood leakage into the skin

rete ridges: undulations and furrows that appear at the dermis–epidermis junction and are responsible for cementing together the two layers

sebaceous glands: glands that exist within the epidermis and secrete sebum to keep the skin soft and pliable

sebum: fatty secretion of the sebaceous glands

telangiectases: red marks on the skin caused by distention of the superficial blood vessels

vitiligo: a localized or widespread condition characterized by destruction of the melanocytes in circumscribed areas of the skin, resulting in white patches

Wood's light: a blue light used for diagnosing skin conditions

Skin disorders are encountered frequently in nursing practice. Skin-related disorders account for up to 10% of all ambulatory patient visits in the United States. Because the skin mirrors the general condition of the patient, many systemic conditions may be accompanied by dermatologic manifestations.

The psychological stress of illness or various personal and family problems is commonly exhibited outwardly as dermatologic problems. Any hospitalized patient may suddenly develop itching and a rash from the treatment regimen. In certain systemic conditions, such as hepatitis and some cancers, dermatologic manifestations may be the first sign of the disorder and the primary reason that a patient seeks health care.

Anatomic and Physiologic Overview

The largest organ system of the body, the skin, is essential for human life. It forms a barrier between the internal organs and the external environment and participates in many vital body functions. The skin is contiguous with the mucous membrane at the external openings of the digestive, respiratory, and urogenital systems.

Anatomy of the Skin, Hair, Nails, and Glands of the Skin

Skin

The skin is composed of three layers: epidermis, dermis, and subcutaneous tissue (Fig. 55-1). The epidermis is an outermost layer of stratified epithelial cells composed predominantly of keratinocytes. It ranges in thickness from about 0.1 mm on the eyelids to about 1 mm on the palms of the hands and soles of the feet. Four distinct layers compose the epidermis; from innermost to outermost they are the stratum germinativum, stratum granulosum, stratum lucidum, and stratum corneum. Each layer becomes more differentiated (ie, mature and with more specific functions) as it rises from the basal stratum germinativum layer to the outermost stratum corneum layer.

Epidermis

The epidermis, which is contiguous with the mucous membranes and the lining of the ear canals, consists of live, continuously dividing cells covered on the surface by dead cells that were originally deeper in the dermis but were pushed upward by the newly developing, more differentiated cells underneath. This external layer is almost completely replaced every 3 to 4 weeks. The dead cells contain large amounts of **keratin,** an insoluble, fibrous protein that forms the outer barrier of the skin and has the capacity to repel pathogens and prevent excessive fluid loss from the body. Keratin is the principal hardening ingredient of the hair and nails.

Melanocytes are the special cells of the epidermis that are primarily involved in producing the pigment **melanin,** which colors the skin and hair. Skin color darkens as melanin content increases. Most of the skin of dark-skinned people and the darker areas of the skin on light-skinned people (eg, the nipple) contain larger amounts of this pigment. Normal skin color depends on race and varies from pale, almost ivory, to deep brown, almost pure black. Systemic disease affects skin color as well. For example, the skin appears bluish when there is insufficient oxygenation of the blood, yellow-green in people with jaundice, or red or flushed when there is inflammation or fever.

Production of melanin is controlled by a hormone secreted from the hypothalamus of the brain called melanocyte-stimulating hormone. It is believed that melanin can absorb ultraviolet light in sunlight.

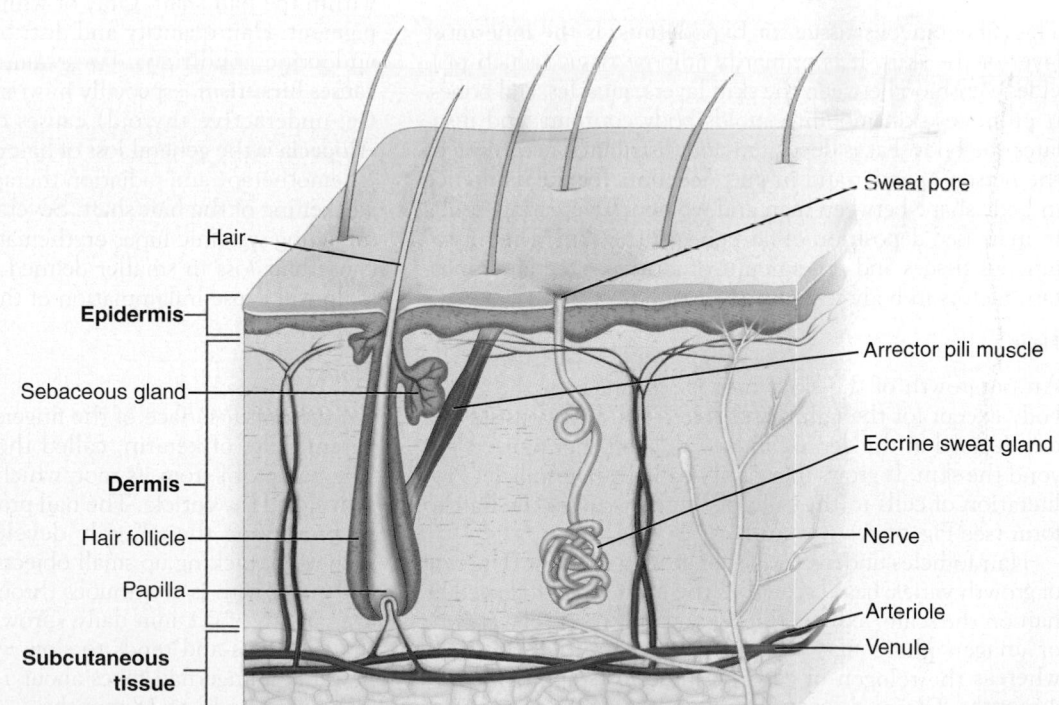

Figure 55-1 Anatomic structures of the skin.

Hair

Epidermis

Sebaceous gland

Dermis

Hair follicle

Papilla

Subcutaneous tissue

Sweat pore

Arrector pili muscle

Eccrine sweat gland

Nerve

Arteriole

Venule

Two other types of cells are common to the epidermis: Merkel and Langerhans cells. **Merkel cells** are receptors that transmit stimuli to the axon through a chemical synapse. **Langerhans cells** are believed to play a significant role in cutaneous immune system reactions. These accessory cells of the afferent immune system process invading antigens and transport the antigens to the lymph system to activate the T lymphocytes.

The characteristics of the epidermis vary in different areas of the body. It is thickest over the palms of the hands and soles of the feet and contains increased amounts of keratin. The thickness of the epidermis can increase with use and can result in calluses forming on the hands or corns forming on the feet.

The junction of the epidermis and dermis is an area of many undulations and furrows called **rete ridges.** This junction anchors the epidermis to the dermis and permits the free exchange of essential nutrients between the two layers. This interlocking between the dermis and epidermis produces ripples on the surface of the skin. On the fingertips, these ripples are called fingerprints. They are a person's most individual physical characteristic, and they rarely change.

Dermis

The dermis makes up the largest portion of the skin, providing strength and structure. It is composed of two layers: papillary and reticular. The papillary dermis lies directly beneath the epidermis and is composed primarily of fibroblast cells capable of producing one form of collagen, a component of connective tissue. The reticular layer lies beneath the papillary layer and also produces collagen and elastic bundles. The dermis is also made up of blood and lymph vessels, nerves, sweat and sebaceous glands, and hair roots. The dermis is often referred to as the "true skin."

Subcutaneous Tissue

The subcutaneous tissue, or hypodermis, is the innermost layer of the skin. It is primarily adipose tissue, which provides a cushion between the skin layers, muscles, and bones. It promotes skin mobility, molds body contours, and insulates the body. Fat is deposited and distributed according to the person's gender and in part accounts for the difference in body shape between men and women. Overeating results in increased deposition of fat beneath the skin. The subcutaneous tissues and the amount of fat deposited are important factors in body temperature regulation.

Hair

An outgrowth of the skin, hair is present over the entire body except for the palms and soles. The hair consists of a root formed in the dermis and a hair shaft that projects beyond the skin. It grows in a cavity called a hair follicle. Proliferation of cells in the bulb of the hair causes the hair to form (see Fig. 55-1).

Hair follicles undergo cycles of growth and rest. The rate of growth varies; beard growth is the most rapid, followed by hair on the scalp, axillae, thighs, and eyebrows. The growth or anagen phase may last up to 6 years for scalp hair, whereas the telogen or resting phase lasts approximately 4 months. During telogen, hair is shed from the body. The hair follicle recycles into the growing phase spontaneously, or it can be induced by plucking hairs. Growing and resting hairs can be found side by side on all parts of the body. About 90% of the 100,000 hair follicles on a normal scalp are in the growing phase at any one time, and 50 to 100 scalp hairs are shed each day.

There is a small bulge on the side of the hair follicle that houses the stem cells that migrate down to the follicle root and begin the cycle of reproducing the hair shaft. These bulges also contain the stem cells that migrate upward to reproduce skin. The location of these cells on the side of the hair shaft, rather than at the base, is a factor in hair loss. In conditions in which inflammation causes damage to the root of the hair, regrowth is possible. However, if inflammation causes damage to the side of the hair follicle, stem cells are destroyed and the hair does not grow.

In certain locations on the body, hair growth is controlled by sex hormones. The most obvious example is the growth of hair on the face (ie, beard and mustache), chest, and back, which is controlled by the male hormones known as androgens. Some women with higher levels of testosterone have hair in the areas generally thought of as masculine, such as the face, chest, and lower abdomen. This is often a normal genetic variation, but if it appears along with irregular menses and weight changes, it may indicate a hormonal imbalance.

Hair in different parts of the body serves different functions. The hairs of the eyes (ie, eyebrows and lashes), nose, and ears filter out dust, bugs, and airborne debris. The hair of the skin provides thermal insulation in mammals with hair or fur. This function is enhanced during cold or fright by piloerection (ie, hairs standing on end), caused by contraction of the tiny erector muscles attached to the hair follicle. The piloerector response that occurs in humans is probably vestigial (ie, rudimentary).

Hair color is supplied by various amounts of melanin within the hair shaft. Gray or white hair reflects the loss of pigment. Hair quantity and distribution can be affected by endocrine conditions. For example, Cushing's syndrome causes **hirsutism,** especially in women, and hypothyroidism (ie, underactive thyroid) causes changes in hair texture. **Alopecia** is the general loss of hair caused by various factors. Chemotherapy and radiation therapy cause hair thinning or weakening of the hair shaft. Several autoimmune disorders, including systemic lupus erythematosis and alopecia areata, cause hair loss in smaller defined areas. Folliculitis of the scalp will cause inflammation of the hair roots and scarring alopecia.

Nails

On the dorsal surface of the fingers and toes, a hard, transparent plate of keratin, called the nail, overlies the skin. The nail grows from its root, which lies under a thin fold of skin called the cuticle. The nail protects the fingers and toes by preserving their highly developed sensory functions, such as for picking up small objects.

Nail growth is continuous throughout life, with an average growth of 0.1 mm daily. Growth is faster in fingernails than toenails and tends to slow with aging. Complete renewal of a fingernail takes about 170 days, whereas toenail renewal takes 12 to 18 months.

Glands of the Skin

There are two types of skin glands: sebaceous glands and sweat glands (see Fig. 55-1). The **sebaceous glands** are associated with hair follicles. The ducts of the sebaceous glands empty **sebum** onto the space between the hair follicle and the hair shaft, thus lubricating the hair and rendering the skin soft and pliable.

Sweat glands are found in the skin over most of the body surface, but they are most heavily concentrated in the palms of the hands and soles of the feet. Only the glans penis, the margins of the lips, the external ear, and the nail bed are devoid of sweat glands. Sweat glands are subclassified into two categories: eccrine and apocrine.

The eccrine sweat glands are found in all areas of the skin. Their ducts open directly onto the skin surface. The thin, watery secretion called sweat is produced in the basal coiled portion of the eccrine gland and is released into its narrow duct. Sweat is composed predominantly of water and contains about half of the salt content of blood plasma. Sweat is released from eccrine glands in response to elevated ambient temperature and elevated body temperature. The rate of sweat secretion is under the control of the sympathetic nervous system. Excessive sweating of the palms and soles, axillae, forehead, and other areas may occur in response to pain and stress.

The apocrine sweat glands are larger than eccrine sweat glands and are located in the axillae, anal region, scrotum, and labia majora. Their ducts generally open onto hair follicles. The apocrine glands become active at puberty. In women, they enlarge and recede with each menstrual cycle. Apocrine glands produce a milky sweat that is sometimes broken down by bacteria to produce the characteristic underarm odor. Specialized apocrine glands called ceruminous glands are found in the external ear, where they produce cerumen (ie, wax).

Functions of the Skin

Protection

The skin covering most of the body is no more than 1 mm thick, but it provides very effective protection against invasion by bacteria and other foreign matter. The thickened skin of the palms and soles protects against the effects of the constant trauma that occurs in these areas.

The stratum corneum, the outer layer of the epidermis, provides the most effective barrier to epidermal water loss and penetration of environmental factors such as chemicals, microbes, and insect bites.

Various lipids are synthesized in the stratum corneum and are the basis for the barrier function of this layer. These are long-chain lipids that are better suited than phospholipids for water resistance. The presence of these lipids in the stratum corneum creates a relatively impermeable barrier for water loss and for the entry of toxins, microbes, and other substances that come in contact with the surface of the skin.

Some substances do penetrate the skin but meet resistance in trying to move through the channels between the cell layers of the stratum corneum. Microbes and fungi, which are part of the body's normal flora, cannot penetrate unless there is a break in the skin barrier.

The dermis–epidermis junction is the basal layer, which is composed of collagen. The basal layer serves four functions. It acts as a scaffold for tissue organization and a template for regeneration; it provides selective permeability for filtration of serum; it is a physical barrier between different types of cells; and it binds the epithelium to underlying cell layers.

Sensation

The receptor endings of nerves in the skin allow the body to constantly monitor the conditions of the immediate environment. The primary functions of the receptors in the skin are to sense temperature, pain, light touch, and pressure (or heavy touch). Different nerve endings respond to each of the different stimuli. Although the nerve endings are distributed over the entire body, they are more concentrated in some areas than in others. For example, the fingertips are more densely innervated than the skin on the back.

Fluid Balance

The stratum corneum, the outermost layer of the epidermis, has the capacity to absorb water, thereby preventing an excessive loss of water and electrolytes from the internal body and retaining moisture in the subcutaneous tissues. When skin is damaged, as occurs with a severe burn, large quantities of fluids and electrolytes may be lost rapidly, possibly leading to circulatory collapse, shock, and death.

The skin is not completely impermeable to water. Small amounts of water continuously evaporate from the skin surface. This evaporation, called insensible perspiration, amounts to approximately 600 mL daily in a normal adult. Insensible water loss varies with the body and ambient temperature. In a person with a fever, the loss can increase. During immersion in water, the skin can accumulate water up to three or four times its normal weight, such as the swelling of the skin that occurs after prolonged bathing.

Temperature Regulation

The body continuously produces heat as a result of the metabolism of food, which produces energy. This heat is dissipated primarily through the skin. Three major physical processes are involved in loss of heat from the body to the environment. The first process, radiation, is the transfer of heat to another object of lower temperature situated at a distance. The second process, conduction, is the transfer of heat from the body to a cooler object in contact with it. The third process, convection, which consists of movement of warm air molecules away from the body, is the transfer of heat by conduction to the air surrounding the body.

Evaporation from the skin aids heat loss by conduction. Heat is conducted through the skin into water molecules on its surface, causing the water to evaporate. The water on the skin surface may be from insensible perspiration, sweat, or the environment.

Normally, all of these mechanisms for heat loss are used. However, when the ambient temperature is very high, radiation and convection are ineffective, and evaporation becomes the only means of heat loss.

Under normal conditions, metabolic heat production is balanced by heat loss, and the internal temperature of the body is maintained constant at approximately 37°C (98.6°F). The rate of heat loss depends primarily on the surface temperature of the skin, which is a function of the skin blood flow. Under normal conditions, the total blood circulated through the skin is approximately 450 mL/min, or 10 to 20 times the amount of blood required to provide necessary metabolites and oxygen. Blood flow through these skin vessels is controlled primarily by the sympathetic nervous system. Increased blood flow to the skin results in more heat delivered to the skin and a greater rate of heat loss from the body. In contrast, decreased skin blood flow decreases the skin temperature and helps conserve heat for the body. When the temperature of the body begins to fall, as occurs on a cold day, the blood vessels of the skin constrict, thereby reducing heat loss from the body.

Sweating is another process by which the body can regulate the rate of heat loss. Sweating does not occur until the core body temperature exceeds 37°C, regardless of skin temperature. In extremely hot environments, the rate of sweat production may be as high as 1 L/h. Under some circumstances (eg, emotional stress), sweating may occur as a reflex and may be unrelated to the need to lose heat from the body.

Vitamin Production

Skin exposed to ultraviolet light can convert substances necessary for synthesizing vitamin D (cholecalciferol). Vitamin D is essential for preventing osteoporosis and rickets, a condition that causes bone deformities and results from a deficiency of vitamin D, calcium, and phosphorus.

Immune Response Function

Research has confirmed a definite action of Langerhans cells in facilitating the uptake of immunoglobulin E (IgE)-associated allergens. This action plays a pivotal role in the pathogenesis of atopic dermatitis and other allergic diseases such as asthma and allergic rhinitis. These findings support the concept of a systemic regulatory mechanism as a trigger for allergic diseases and suggest that this trigger can be aggravated by local inflammation of atopic eczema (Porth & Matfin, 2009).

 Gerontologic Considerations

The skin undergoes many physiologic changes associated with normal aging. A lifetime of excessive sun exposure, systemic diseases, and poor nutrition can increase the range of skin conditions and the rapidity with which they appear. In addition, certain medications (eg, antihistamines, antibiotics, diuretics) are photosensitizing and increase the damage that results from sun exposure. The outcome is an increasing vulnerability to injury and to certain diseases. Therefore, skin conditions are common among older people.

The major changes in the skin of older people include dryness, wrinkling, uneven pigmentation, and various proliferative lesions. Cellular changes associated with aging include a thinning at the junction of the dermis and epidermis. The result of this thinning is fewer anchoring sites between the two skin layers, which means that even minor injury or stress to the epidermis can cause it to shear away from the dermis. This phenomenon may account for the increased

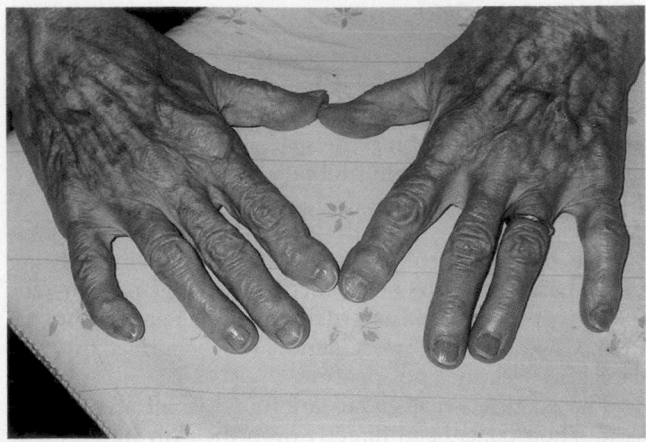

Figure 55-2 Hands with and overlapping folds common to aging skin.

vulnerability of aged skin to trauma. With increasing age, the epidermis and dermis thin and flatten, causing wrinkles, sags, and overlapping skin folds (Fig. 55-2).

Loss of the subcutaneous tissue substances of elastin, collagen, and fat diminishes the protection and cushioning of underlying tissues and organs, decreases muscle tone, and results in the loss of the insulating properties of fat.

Cellular replacement slows as a result of aging. As the dermal layers thin, the skin becomes fragile and transparent. The blood supply to the skin also changes with age. Vessels, especially the capillary loops, decrease in number and size. These vascular changes contribute to the delayed wound healing commonly seen in the elderly patient. Sweat and sebaceous glands decrease in number and functional capacity, leading to dry and scaly skin. Reduced hormonal levels of androgens are thought to contribute to declining sebaceous gland function.

Hair growth gradually diminishes, especially over the lower legs and dorsum of the feet. Thinning is common in the scalp, axilla, and pubic areas. Other functions affected by normal aging include the barrier function of skin, sensory perception, and thermoregulation.

Photoaging, or damage from excessive sun exposure, has detrimental effects on the normal aging of skin. A lifetime of outdoor work or outdoor activities (eg, construction work, lifeguarding, sunbathing) without prudent use of sunscreens can lead to profound wrinkling; increased loss of elasticity; mottled, pigmented areas; cutaneous atrophy; and benign or malignant lesions.

Many skin lesions are part of normal aging. Recognizing these lesions enables the examiner to assist the patient to feel less anxious about changes in skin. Chart 55-1 summarizes some skin lesions that are expected to appear as the skin ages. These are normal and require no special attention unless the skin becomes infected or irritated.

Assessment

When caring for patients with dermatologic disorders, the nurse obtains important information through the health history and direct observations. The nurse's skill in physical

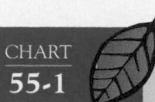

Benign Changes in Elderly Skin

CHART 55-1

- Cherry angiomas (bright red "moles")
- Diminished hair, especially on scalp and pubic area
- Dyschromias (color variations)
    - Solar lentigo (liver spots)
    - Melasma (dark discoloration of the skin)
    - Lentigines (freckles)
- Neurodermatitis (itchy spots)
- Seborrheic keratoses (crusty brown "stuck-on" patches)
- Spider angiomas
- Telangiectasias (red marks on skin caused by stretching of the superficial blood vessels)
- Wrinkles
- Xerosis (dryness)
- Xanthelasma (yellowish waxy deposits on upper and lower eyelids)

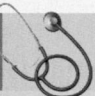

Assessing for Skin Disorders

CHART 55-2

Patient history relevant to skin disorders may be obtained by asking the following questions:
- When did you first notice this skin problem? (Also investigate duration and intensity.)
- Has it occurred previously?
- Are there any other symptoms?
- What site was first affected?
- What did the rash or lesion look like when it first appeared?
- Where and how fast did it spread?
- Do you have any itching, burning, tingling, or crawling sensations?
- Is there any loss of sensation?
- Is the problem worse at a particular time or season?
- How do you think it started?
- Do you have a history of hay fever, asthma, hives, eczema, or allergies?
- Who in your family has skin problems or rashes?
- Did the eruptions appear after certain foods were eaten? Which foods?
- When the problem occurred, had you recently consumed alcohol?
- What relation do you think there may be between a specific event and the outbreak of the rash or lesion?
- What medications are you taking?
- What topical medication (ointment, cream, salve) have you put on the lesion (including over-the-counter medications)?
- What skin products or cosmetics do you use?
- What is your occupation?
- What in your immediate environment (plants, animals, chemicals, infections) might be precipitating this disorder? Is there anything new, or are there any changes in the environment?
- Does anything touching your skin cause a rash?
- How has this affected you (or your life)?
- Is there anything else you wish to talk about in regard to this disorder?

assessment and an understanding of the anatomy and function of the skin can ensure that deviations from normal are recognized, reported, and documented.

Health History

During the health history interview, the nurse asks about any family and personal history of skin allergies; allergic reactions to food, medications, and chemicals; previous skin conditions; and skin cancer. The names of cosmetics, soaps, shampoos, and other personal hygiene products are obtained if there have been any recent skin conditions noticed with the use of these products. If suspicious areas are noted, the patient is questioned about nonprescription or herbal preparations that are being used. The health history addresses the onset, signs and symptoms, location, and duration of any pain, itching, rash, or other discomfort experienced by the patient. Chart 55-2 lists selected questions useful in obtaining appropriate information and Chart 55-3 provides genetic factors influencing skin conditions.

Physical Assessment

Assessment of the skin involves the entire skin area, including the mucous membranes, scalp, hair, and nails. The skin is a reflection of a person's overall health, and alterations commonly correspond to disease in other organ systems. Inspection and palpation are techniques commonly used in examining the skin. The room must be well lighted and warm. A penlight may be used to highlight lesions. The patient completely disrobes and is adequately draped. Gloves are worn during skin examination if a rash or lesions are to be palpated. However, it is important to avoid making the patient feel as if he or she cannot be touched.

The general appearance of the skin is assessed by observing color, temperature, moisture or dryness, skin texture (rough or smooth), lesions, vascularity, mobility, and the condition of the hair and nails. Skin turgor, possible edema, and elasticity are assessed by palpation.

Assessing Skin Color

The color gradations that occur in people with dark skin are largely determined by genetics; they may be described as light, medium, or dark. In people with dark skin, melanin is produced at a faster rate and in larger quantities than in people with light skin. Healthy dark skin has a reddish base or undertone. The buccal mucosa, tongue, lips, and nails normally are pink. The skin of exposed portions of the body, especially in sunny, warm climates, tends to be more pigmented than the rest of the body. Almost every process that occurs on the skin causes some color change. For example, **hypopigmentation** may be caused by a fungal infection, eczema, or **vitiligo; hyperpigmentation** can occur after sun injury or as a result of aging. Dark pigment responds with discoloration after injury or inflammation, and patients with dark skin more often experience postinflammatory hyperpigmentation than those with lighter skin. The hyperpigmentation eventually fades but may require months to a year to do so.

Changes in skin color in people with dark skin are more noticeable and may cause more concern because the discoloration is more readily visible. Because of the increased number of melanocytes in darker skin, pigment changes can become quite obvious and cause great psychological discomfort. Some variation in skin pigment levels is considered normal. Examples include the pigmented crease across

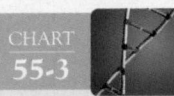

GENETICS IN NURSING PRACTICE
Integumentary Conditions

CHART
55-3

Integumentary conditions influenced by genetic factors include the following:

- Albinism
- Eczema
- Hypohidrotic ectodermal dysplasia
- Incontinentia pigmenti
- Neurofibromatosis type 1
- Pseudoxanthoma elasticum
- Psoriasis

Nursing Assessments

Family History Assessment

- Assess for other closely related family members with integumentary impairment or abnormalities.
- Inquire about the nature and type of skin lesions and age at onset (eg, skin involvement with incontinentia pigmenti occurs in the first few weeks of life with blistering of the skin, whereas lesions of neurofibromatosis type 1 may appear in early childhood through adulthood).
- Note gender of affected individuals (eg, mostly females with incontinentia pigmenti, mostly males with hypohidrotic ectodermal dysplasia).
- Inquire about the presence of other clinical features, such as unusual hair, teeth, or nails; thrombocytopenia; recurrent infections.

Patient Assessment

- Assess for related clinical features, such as sparse eyebrows and eyelashes, abnormally shaped teeth, alopecia, nail abnormalities (eg, hypohidrotic ectodermal dysplasia).
- Assess for related alterations in vision, such as nystagmus or strabismus; albinism; retinal abnormalities (eg, pseudox-

anthoma elasticum); Lisch nodules and/or optic glioma (neurofibromatosis type 1).

Management Issues Specific to Genetics

- Inquire whether DNA mutation or other genetics testing has been performed on affected family members.
- If indicated, refer for further genetics counseling and evaluation so that family members can discuss inheritance, risk to other family members, availability of genetics testing, and gene-based interventions.
- Offer appropriate genetics information and resources.
- Assess patient's understanding of genetics information.
- Provide support to families with newly diagnosed genetics-related integumentary conditions.
- Participate in management and coordination of care for patients with genetic conditions and for individuals predisposed to develop or pass on a genetic condition.

Genetics Resources

Genetic Alliance—a directory of support groups for patients and families with genetic conditions; www.geneticalliance. org

Gene Clinics—a listing of common genetic disorders with clinical summaries and genetic counseling and testing information; www.geneclinics.org

National Organization of Rare Disorders—a directory of support groups and information for patients and families with rare genetic disorders;www.rarediseases.org

Online Mendelian Inheritance in Man (OMIM)—a complete listing of inherited genetic conditions; www.ncbi.nlm.nih. gov/omim/stats/html

the bridge of the nose, pigmented streaks in the nails, and pigmented spots on the sclera of the eye.

Table 55-1 provides an overview of color changes in light-skinned and dark-skinned people.

Cyanosis

Cyanosis is the bluish discoloration that results from a lack of oxygen in the blood (Fig. 55-3). It appears with shock or with respiratory or circulatory compromise. In people with light skin, cyanosis manifests as a bluish hue to the lips, fingertips, and nail beds. Other indications of decreased tissue perfusion include cold, clammy skin; a rapid, thready pulse; and rapid, shallow respirations. The conjunctivae of the eyelids are examined for pallor and **petechiae.**

In a person with dark skin, the skin usually assumes a grayish cast. To detect cyanosis, the areas around the mouth and lips and over the cheekbones and earlobes should be observed.

Erythema

Erythema is redness of the skin caused by the congestion of capillaries. In light-skinned people, it is easily observable. To determine possible inflammation, the skin is palpated for increased warmth and for smoothness (ie, edema) or hardness (ie, intracellular infiltration). Because dark skin tends to assume a purple-gray cast when an inflammatory process is present, it may be difficult to detect erythema.

Jaundice

Jaundice, a yellowing of the skin, is directly related to elevations in serum bilirubin and is often first observed in the sclerae and mucous membranes (see Fig. 55-3).

Assessing Rash

In instances of pruritus (ie, itching) the patient is asked to indicate which areas of the body are involved. The skin is then stretched gently to decrease the reddish tone and make the rash more visible. Pointing a penlight laterally across the skin may highlight the rash, making it easier to observe. The differences in skin texture are then assessed by running the tips of the fingers lightly over the skin. The borders of the rash may be palpable. The patient's mouth and ears are included in the examination (rubeola, or measles, causes a red cast to appear on the ears, and skin cancers are quite common on the crest of the ears). The patient's temperature is assessed, and the lymph nodes are palpated especially in the axilla, inguinal fold, and behind the knees (popliteal area).

Assessing Skin Lesions

Skin lesions are the most prominent characteristics of dermatologic conditions. They vary in size, shape, and cause and are classified according to their appearance and origin.

Table 55-1 COLOR CHANGES IN LIGHT AND DARK SKIN

Etiology	Light Skin	Dark Skin
Pallor		
Anemia—decreased hematocrit	Generalized pallor	Brown skin appears yellow-brown, dull; black skin
Shock—decreased perfusion, vasoconstriction		appears ashen gray, dull. (Observe areas with least pigmentation: conjunctivae, mucous membranes.)
Local arterial insufficiency	Marked localized pallor (lower extremities, especially when elevated)	Ashen gray, dull; cool to palpation
Albinism—total absence of pigment melanin	Whitish pink	Tan, cream, white
Vitiligo—a condition characterized by destruction of the melanocytes in circumscribed areas of the skin (may be localized or widespread)	Patchy, milky white spots, often symmetric bilaterally	Same
Cyanosis		
Increased amount of unoxygenated hemoglobin:	Dusky blue	Dark but dull, lifeless; only severe cyanosis is apparent in skin. (Observe conjunctivae, oral mucosa, nail beds.)
Central—chronic heart and lung diseases cause arterial desaturation	Nail beds dusky	
Peripheral—exposure to cold, anxiety		
Erythema		
Hyperemia—increased blood flow through engorged arterial vessels, as in inflammation, fever, alcohol intake, blushing	Red, bright pink	Purplish tinge, but difficult to see. (Palpate for increased warmth with inflammation, taut skin, and hardening of deep tissues.)
Polycythemia—increased red blood cells, capillary stasis	Ruddy blue in face, oral mucosa, conjunctivae, hands and feet	Well concealed by pigment. (Observe for redness in lips.)
Carbon monoxide poisoning	Bright, cherry red in face and upper torso	Cherry red nail beds, lips, and oral mucosa
Venous stasis—decreased blood flow from area, engorged venules	Dusky rubor of dependent extremities (a prelude to necrosis with pressure ulcer)	Easily masked. (Use palpation to identify warmth or edema.)
Jaundice		
Increased serum bilirubin concentration (>2–3 mg/100 mL) due to liver dysfunction or hemolysis, as after severe burns or some infections	Yellow first in sclerae, hard palate, and mucous membranes; then over skin	Check sclerae for yellow near limbus; do not mistake normal yellowish fatty deposits in the periphery under eyelids for jaundice. (Jaundice is best noted at junction of hard and soft palate, on palms.)
Carotenemia—increased level of serum carotene from ingestion of large amounts of carotene-rich foods	Yellow-orange tinge in forehead, palms and soles, and nasolabial folds, but no yellowing in sclerae or mucous membranes	Yellow-orange tinge in palms and soles
Uremia—renal failure causes retained urochrome pigments in the blood	Orange-green or gray overlying pallor of anemia; may also have ecchymoses and purpura	Easily masked. (Rely on laboratory and clinical findings.)
Brown-Tan		
Addison's disease—cortisol deficiency stimulates increased melanin production	Bronzed appearance, an "external tan"; most apparent around nipples, perineum, genitalia, and pressure points (inner thighs, buttocks, elbows, axillae)	Easily masked. (Rely on laboratory and clinical findings.)
Café-au-lait spots—caused by increased melanin pigment in basal cell layer	Tan to light brown, irregularly shaped, oval patch with well-defined borders often not visible in the very dark skinned person	

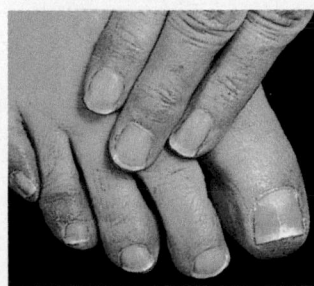
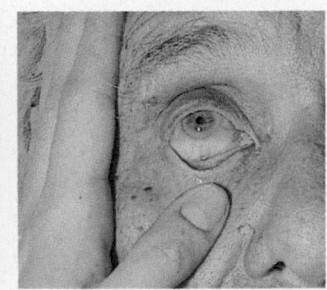

Figure 55-3 Examples of skin color changes: the bluish tint of cyanosis (*left*) and the yellow hue of jaundice (*right*).

Skin lesions can be described as primary or secondary. Primary lesions are the initial lesions and are characteristic of the disease itself. Secondary lesions result from changes in primary lesions resulting from external causes, such as scratching, trauma, infections, or changes caused by wound healing. Depending on the stage of development, skin lesions are further categorized by type and appearance (Table 55-2).

A preliminary assessment of the eruption or lesion helps identify the type of **dermatosis** and indicates whether the lesion is primary or secondary. At the same time, the anatomic distribution of the eruption or lesion

Table 55-2	PRIMARY AND SECONDARY SKIN LESIONS	
Lesion	**Description**	**Examples**
Primary Lesions		
MACULE, PATCH Macule Patch	Flat, nonpalpable skin color change (color may be brown, white, tan, purple, red) • *Macule:* less than 1 cm, circumscribed border • *Patch:* greater than 1 cm, may have irregular border	Freckles, flat moles, petechia, rubella, vitiligo, port wine stains, ecchymosis
PAPULE, PLAQUE Papule Plaque	Elevated, palpable, solid mass with a circumscribed border Plaque may be coalesced papules with flat top • *Papule:* less than 0.5 cm • *Plaque:* greater than 0.5 cm	*Papules:* Elevated nevi, warts, lichen planus *Plaques:* Psoriasis, actinic keratosis
NODULE, TUMOR Tumor	Elevated, palpable, solid mass that extends deeper into the dermis than a papule • *Nodule:* 0.5–2 cm; circumscribed • *Tumor:* greater than 1–2 cm; tumors do not always have sharp borders	*Nodules:* Lipoma, squamous cell carcinoma, poorly absorbed injection, dermatofibroma *Tumors:* Larger lipoma, carcinoma
VESICLE, BULLA Bulla Vesicle	Circumscribed, elevated, palpable mass containing serous fluid • *Vesicle:* less than 0.5 cm • *Bulla:* greater than 0.5 cm	*Vesicles:* Herpes simplex/zoster, chickenpox, poison ivy, second-degree burn (blister) *Bulla:* Pemphigus, contact dermatitis, large burn blisters, poison ivy, bullous impetigo
WHEAL Wheal	Elevated mass with transient borders; often irregular; size and color vary Caused by movement of serous fluid into the dermis; does not contain free fluid in a cavity (as, for example, a vesicle does)	Urticaria (hives), insect bites
PUSTULE Pustule	Pus-filled vesicle or bulla	Acne, impetigo, furuncles, carbuncles

Table 55-2   PRIMARY AND SECONDARY SKIN LESIONS (Continued)

Lesion	Description	Examples
CYST Cyst	Encapsulated fluid-filled or semisolid mass in the subcutaneous tissue or dermis	Sebaceous cyst, epidermoid cysts

Secondary Lesions

Lesion	Description	Examples
EROSION Erosion	Loss of superficial epidermis that does not extend to dermis; depressed, moist area	Ruptured vesicles, scratch marks
ULCER Ulcer	Skin loss extending past epidermis; necrotic tissue loss; bleeding and scarring possible	Stasis ulcer of venous insufficiency, pressure ulcer
FISSURE Fissure	Linear crack in the skin that may extend to dermis	Chapped lips or hands, athlete's foot
SCALES Scales	Flakes secondary to desquamated, dead epithelium that may adhere to skin surface; color varies (silvery, white); texture varies (thick, fine)	Dandruff, psoriasis, dry skin, pityriasis rosea
CRUST Crust	Dried residue of serum, blood, or pus on skin surface Large, adherent crust is a scab	Residue left after vesicle rupture: impetigo, herpes, eczema

Continued on following page

Table 55-2   PRIMARY AND SECONDARY SKIN LESIONS (Continued)

Lesion	Description	Examples
SCAR (CICATRIX) Scar	Skin mark left after healing of a wound or lesion; represents replacement by connective tissue of the injured tissue • *Young scars:* red or purple • *Mature scars:* white or glistening	Healed wound or surgical incision
KELOID Keloid	Hypertrophied scar tissue secondary to excessive collagen formation during healing; elevated, irregular, red Greater incidence among African Americans	Keloid of ear piercing or surgical incision
ATROPHY Atrophy	Thin, dry, transparent appearance of epidermis; loss of surface markings; secondary to loss of collagen and elastin; underlying vessels may be visible	Aged skin, arterial insufficiency
LICHENIFICATION Lichenification	Thickening and roughening of the skin or accentuated skin markings that may be secondary to repeated rubbing, irritation, scratching	Contact dermatitis

should be observed because certain diseases affect certain sites of the body and are distributed in characteristic patterns and shapes (Figs. 55-4 and 55-5). To determine the extent of the regional distribution, the left and right sides of the body should be compared while the color and shape of the lesions are assessed. The degree of pigmentation of the patient's skin may affect the appearance of a lesion. Lesions may be black, purple, or gray on dark skin and tan or red in patients with light skin. A metric ruler is used to measure the size of the lesions so that any further extension can be compared with this baseline measurement. After observation, the lesions are palpated to determine their texture, shape, and border and to see if they are soft and filled with fluid or hard and fixed to the surrounding tissue.

Skin lesions are described clearly and in detail on the patient's health record, using precise terminology:

- Color of the lesion
- Any redness, heat, pain, or swelling
- Size and location of the involved area
- Pattern of eruption (eg, macular, papular, scaling, oozing, discrete, confluent)
- Distribution of the lesion (eg, bilateral, symmetric, linear, circular)

If acute open wounds or lesions are found on inspection of the skin, a comprehensive assessment should be made and documented. This assessment should address the following issues:

- Wound bed: Inspect for necrotic and granulation tissue, epithelium, exudate, color, and odor
- Wound edges and margins: Observe for undermining (ie, extension of the wound under the surface skin), and evaluate for condition
- Wound size: Measure in millimeters or centimeters, as appropriate, to determine diameter and depth of the wound and surrounding erythema
- Surrounding skin: Assess for color, suppleness and moisture, irritation, and scaling

Assessing Vascularity and Hydration

After the color of the skin has been evaluated and lesions have been inspected, an assessment of vascular changes in the skin is performed. A description of vascular changes includes location, distribution, color, size, and the presence of

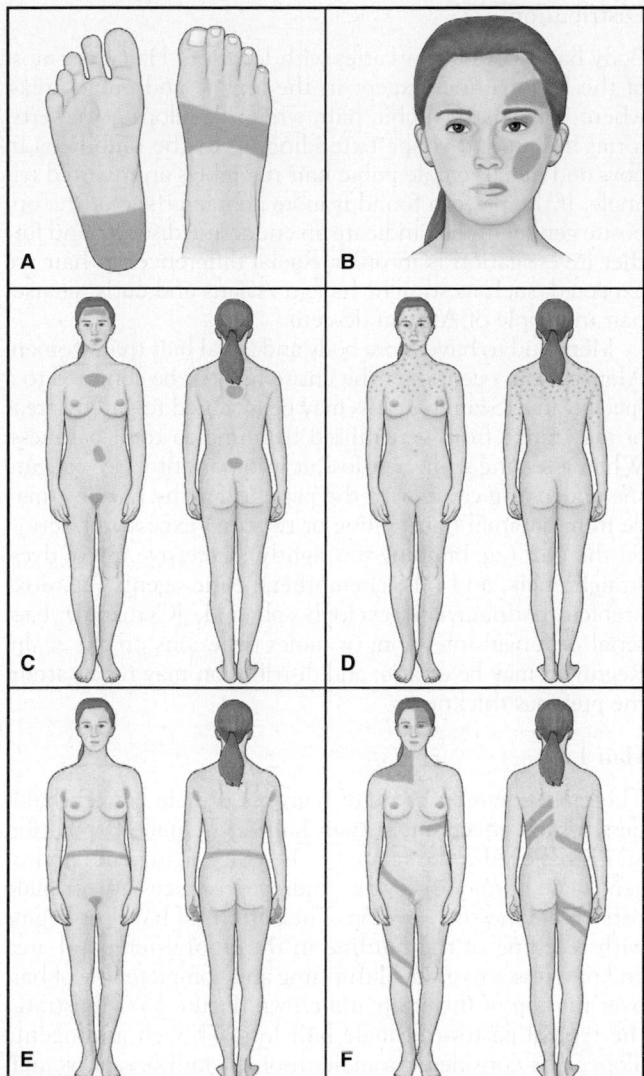

Figure 55-4 Anatomic distribution of common skin disorders. **A,** Contact dermatitis (shoes). **B,** Contact dermatitis (cosmetics, perfumes, earrings). **C,** Seborrheic dermatitis. **D,** Acne. **E,** Scabies. **F,** Herpes zoster (shingles).

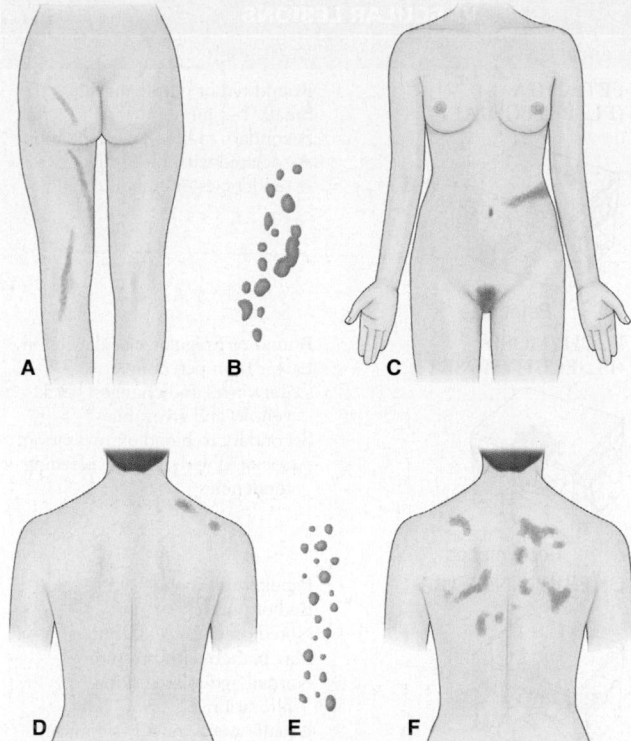

Figure 55-5 Skin lesion configurations. **A,** Linear (in a line). **B,** Annular and arciform (circular or arcing). **C,** Zosteriform (linear along a nerve route). **D,** Grouped (clustered). **E,** Discrete (separate and distinct). **F,** Confluent (merged).

pulsations. Common vascular changes include petechiae, ecchymoses, **telangiectases** (venous stars), and angiomas, (Table 55-3).

Skin moisture, temperature, and texture are assessed primarily by palpation. The turgor (ie, elasticity) of the skin, which decreases in normal aging, may be a factor in assessing the hydration status of a patient.

Assessing the Nails

A brief inspection of the nails includes observation of configuration, color, and consistency. Many alterations in the nail or nail bed reflect local or systemic abnormalities in progress or resulting from past events (Fig. 55-6). Transverse depressions known as Beau's lines in the nails may reflect retarded growth of the nail matrix because of severe illness or, more commonly, local trauma. Ridging, hypertrophy, and other changes may also be visible because of local trauma.

Paronychia, an inflammation of the skin around the nail, is usually accompanied by tenderness and erythema. Pitted surface of the nails is a definite indication of psoriasis. Spoon-shape nails can indicate a severe iron deficiency anemia. The angle between the normal nail and its base is 160 degrees. When palpated, the nail base is usually firm. Clubbing of the nails, which can occur from hypoxia, is manifested by a straightening of the normal angle (180 degrees or greater) and softening of the nail base. The softened area feels spongelike when palpated.

Assessing the Hair

The hair assessment is carried out by inspection and palpation. Gloves are worn by the examiner, and the examination room should be well lighted. Separating the hair so that the condition of the skin underneath can be easily seen, the nurse assesses color, texture, and distribution. The wooden end of a cotton swab can be used to make small parts in the hair so that the scalp can be inspected. Any abnormal lesions, evidence of itching, inflammation, scaling, or signs of infestation (ie, lice or mites) are documented.

Color and Texture

Natural hair color ranges from white to black. Hair begins to turn gray with age, initially during the third decade of life, when the loss of melanin begins to become apparent. However, it is not unusual for the hair of younger people to turn gray as a result of hereditary traits. The person with albinism (ie, partial or complete absence of pigmentation)

Table 55-3	VASCULAR LESIONS
Lesion	**Description**
PETECHIA (PL. PETECHIAE) Petechiae	Round red or purple macule Small: 1–2 mm Secondary to blood extravasation Associated with bleeding tendencies or emboli to skin
ECCHYMOSIS (PL. ECCHYMOSES) Ecchymoses	Round or irregular macular lesion Larger than petechia Color varies and changes: black, yellow, and green hues Secondary to blood extravasation Associated with trauma, bleeding tendencies
CHERRY ANGIOMA Cherry angioma	Papular and round Red or purple Noted on trunk, extremities May blanch with pressure Normal age-related skin alteration Usually not clinically significant
SPIDER ANGIOMA Spider angioma	Red, arteriole lesion Central body with radiating branches Noted on face, neck, arms, trunk Rare below the waist May blanch with pressure Associated with liver disease, pregnancy, vitamin B deficiency
TELANGIECTASIA (VENOUS STAR) Telangiectasia	Shape varies: spider-like or linear Color bluish or red Does not blanch when pressure is applied Noted on legs, anterior chest Secondary to superficial dilation of venous vessels and capillaries Associated with increased venous pressure states (varicosities)

has a genetic predisposition to white hair from birth. The natural state of the hair can be altered by using hair dyes, bleaches, and curling or relaxing products. The types of products used are identified in the assessment.

The texture of scalp hair ranges from fine to coarse, silky to brittle, oily to dry, and shiny to dull, and hair can be straight, curly, or kinky. Dry, brittle hair may result from overuse of hair dyes, hair dryers, and curling irons or from endocrine disorders, such as thyroid dysfunction. Oily hair is usually caused by increased secretion from the sebaceous glands close to the scalp. If the patient reports a recent change in hair texture, the underlying reason is pursued; the alteration may arise simply from the overuse of commercial hair products or from changing to a new shampoo.

Distribution

Body hair distribution varies with location. Hair over most of the body is fine, except in the axillae and pubic areas, where it is coarse. Pubic hair, which develops at puberty, forms a diamond shape extending up to the umbilicus in boys and men. Female pubic hair resembles an inverted triangle. If the pattern found is more characteristic of the opposite gender, it may indicate an endocrine disorder and further investigation is in order. Racial differences in hair are expected, such as straight hair in Asians and curly, coarser hair in people of African descent.

Men tend to have more body and facial hair than women. Alopecia can occur over the entire body or be confined to a specific area. Scalp hair loss may be localized to patchy areas or may range from generalized thinning to total baldness. When assessing scalp hair loss, it is important to investigate the underlying cause with the patient. Patchy hair loss may be from habitual hair pulling or twisting; excessive traction on the hair (eg, braiding too tightly); excessive use of dyes, straighteners, and oils; chemotherapeutic agents (eg, doxorubicin [Adriamycin], cyclophosphamide [Cytoxan]); bacterial or fungal infection; or moles or lesions on the scalp. Regrowth may be erratic, and distribution may never attain the previous thickness.

Hair Loss

The most common cause of hair loss is male pattern baldness, which affects more than half of the male population and is believed to be related to heredity, aging, and androgen (male hormone) levels. Androgen is necessary for male pattern baldness to develop. The pattern of hair loss begins with receding of the hairline in the frontal-temporal area and progresses to gradual thinning and complete loss of hair over the top of the scalp and crown. Figure 55-7 illustrates the typical pattern of male hair loss. Though androgenic alopecia is considered a male disorder, millions of women also experience it. Women tend to retain some of the hair on the crown of the scalp and never go completely bald.

Other Changes

Male pattern hair distribution may be seen in some women at the time of menopause, when the hormone estrogen is no longer produced by the ovaries. In women with hirsutism, excessive hair may grow on the face, chest, shoulders, and pubic area. If menopause is ruled out as the underlying cause, other hormonal changes related to pituitary or adrenal dysfunction must be investigated.

Because patients with skin conditions may be viewed negatively by others, these patients may become distraught and avoid interaction with people. Skin conditions can lead to disfigurement, isolation, job loss, and economic hardship.

Some conditions may lead to feelings of depression, frustration, self-consciousness, poor self-image, and rejection. Itching and skin irritation, features of many skin diseases, may be constant annoyances. These discomforts may result in loss of sleep, anxiety, and depression, all of which reinforce the general distress and fatigue that frequently accompany skin disorders.

For patients experiencing physical and psychological discomforts, the nurse needs to provide understanding,

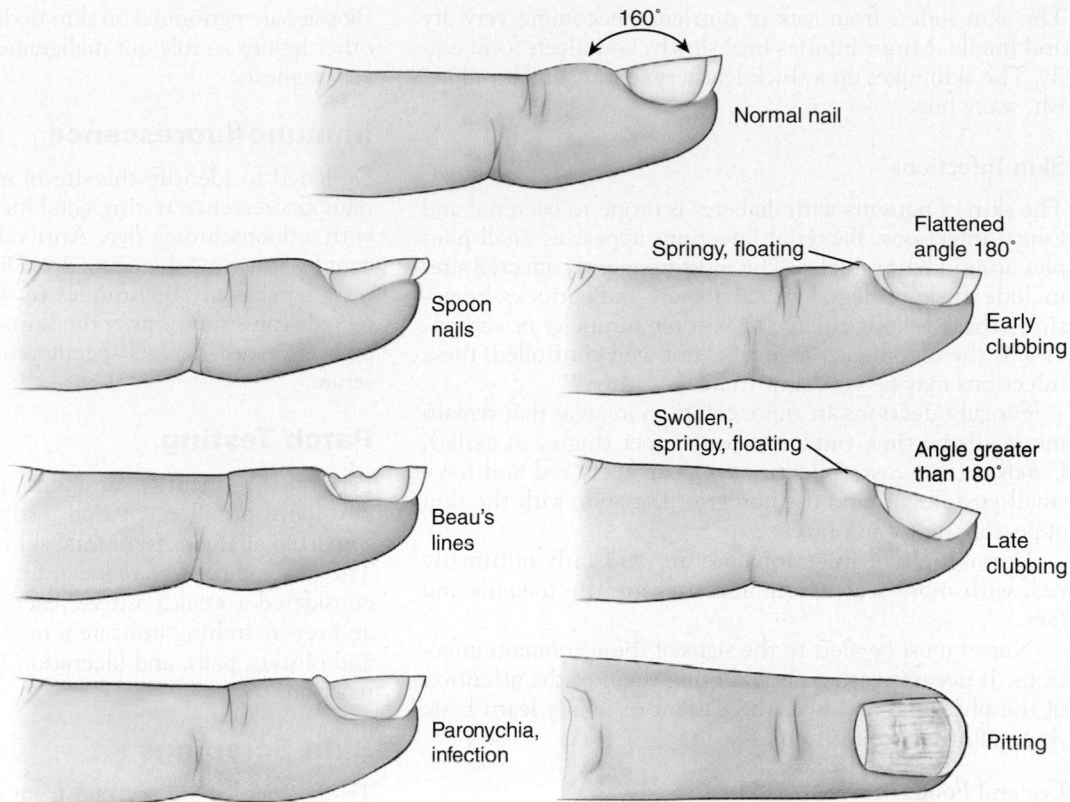

Figure 55-6 Common nail disorders.

explanations of the problem, appropriate instructions related to treatment, nursing support, and encouragement. It is imperative to overcome any aversion that may be felt when caring for patients with unattractive skin disorders. The nurse should show no sign of hesitancy when approaching patients with skin disorders. Such hesitancy only reinforces the psychological trauma of the disorder.

Skin Consequences of Selected Systemic Diseases

Diabetes Mellitus

Because diabetes causes changes in circulation and cell nutrition, it can have a great impact on skin status. Some of the more common skin conditions encountered in diabetes are discussed in this section. Further information can be found in Chapter 41.

Diabetic Dermopathy

Diabetic dermopathy (shin spots) occurs in about 50% of peoples with diabetes. These lesions are found on the lower anterior legs, forearms, and thighs and over other bony prominences. They are caused by breakdown of the small vessels that supply the skin. Each spot starts as a dull red bump, smaller than a pencil eraser. It slowly spreads to about one inch (the size of a quarter), becomes increasingly scaly, and eventually leaves a brownish scar on the skin. The lesions are usually bilateral and occur in linear clusters.

Stasis Dermatitis

Stasis dermatitis is not unique to diabetes, but because of the blood vessel damage that results from diabetes, it is very common in patients with diabetes. Large vessels are damaged, compromising circulation to the lower arms and legs.

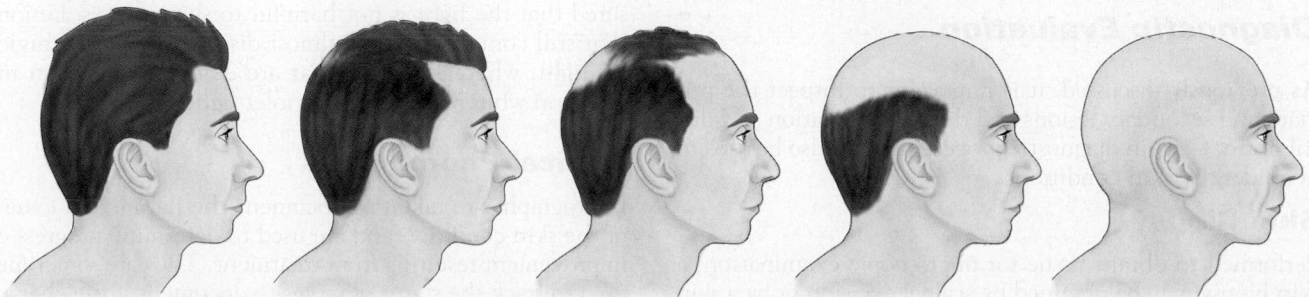

Figure 55-7 The progression of male pattern baldness.

The skin suffers from lack of nutrients, becoming very dry and fragile. Minor injuries heal slowly, and ulcers form easily. The skin takes on a thick leathery texture and a yellowish, waxy hue.

Skin Infections

The skin of patients with diabetes is prone to bacterial and fungal infections. Bacterial infections appear as small pimples around hair follicles. The most frequently affected sites include the lower legs, lower abdomen, and buttocks. Sometimes these lesions enlarge to become furuncles or carbuncles. If the blood glucose level is not well controlled, these infections may be very slow to heal.

Fungal infections are quite common in areas that remain moist all the time (under breasts, upper thighs, in axilla). *Candida* (ie, yeast) infections appear beefy red and have small pustules around the border of the area, with the skin appearing moist and raw.

Dermatophyte infections are dry and only minimally red, with more scale. Common sites are the toenails and feet.

Nurses must be alert to the signs of these common infections. If necessary, they should bring them to the attention of the physician and help the patient or family learn basic skin maintenance techniques.

Leg and Foot Ulcers

Because of changes in peripheral nerves, patients with diabetes do not always sense minor injuries to the lower legs and feet. Infections begin and if left untreated may lead to ulcerations. Ulcerations are often not noticed and become quite large before being treated. Ulcerations unresponsive to treatment are a leading cause of diabetic foot and leg amputations.

Human Immunodeficiency Virus Disease

Cutaneous signs may be the first manifestation of human immunodeficiency virus (HIV), appearing in more than 90% of HIV-infected people as immune function deteriorates. These skin signs correlate with low CD4 counts and may become very atypical in immunocompromised people. Some disorders such as Kaposi's sarcoma, oral hairy leukoplakia, facial molluscum contagiosum, and oral candidiasis may suggest that CD4 counts are less than 200 to 300 cell/μL. Being sensitive to these changes can alert the nurse so that early intervention can be initiated (Freytes, Arroyo-Novoa, Figueroa-Ramos, et al., 2007).

Diagnostic Evaluation

As previously discussed, it is important to inspect the primary and secondary lesions and their configuration and distribution. Certain diagnostic procedures may also be used to help identify skin conditions.

Skin Biopsy

Performed to obtain tissue for microscopic examination, a skin biopsy may be obtained by scalpel excision or by a skin punch instrument that removes a small core of tissue. Biopsies are performed on skin nodules, plaques, blisters, and other lesions to rule out malignancy and to establish an exact diagnosis.

Immunofluorescence

Designed to identify the site of an immune reaction, immunofluorescence testing combines an antigen or antibody with a fluorochrome dye. Antibodies can be made fluorescent by attaching them to a dye. Direct immunofluorescence tests on skin are techniques to detect autoantibodies directed against portions of the skin. The indirect immunofluorescence test detects specific antibodies in the patient's serum.

Patch Testing

Performed to identify substances to which the patient has developed an allergy, patch testing involves applying the suspected allergens to normal skin under occlusive patches. The development of redness, fine elevations, or itching is considered a weak positive reaction; fine blisters, papules, and severe itching indicate a moderately positive reaction; and blisters, pain, and ulceration indicate a strong positive reaction.

Skin Scrapings

Tissue samples are scraped from suspected fungal lesions with a scalpel blade moistened with oil so that the scraped skin adheres to the blade. The scraped material is transferred to a glass slide, covered with a coverslip, and examined microscopically. The spores and hyphae of dermatophyte infections, as well as infestations such as scabies, can be visualized.

Tzanck Smear

The Tzanck smear is a test used to examine cells from blistering skin conditions, such as herpes zoster, varicella, herpes simplex, and all forms of pemphigus. The secretions from a suspected lesion are applied to a glass slide, stained, and examined.

Wood's Light Examination

Wood's light is a special lamp that produces long-wave ultraviolet rays, which result in a characteristic dark purple fluorescence. The color of the fluorescent light is best seen in a darkened room, where it is possible to differentiate epidermal from dermal lesions and hypopigmented and hyperpigmented lesions from normal skin. The patient is reassured that the light is not harmful to skin or eyes. Lesions that still contain melanin almost disappear under ultraviolet light, whereas lesions that are devoid of melanin increase in whiteness with ultraviolet light.

Clinical Photographs

Photographs are taken to document the nature and extent of the skin condition and are used to determine progress or improvement resulting from treatment. They are sometimes used to track the status of moles to document if the characteristics of the mole are changing.

CRITICAL THINKING EXERCISE

EBP   You are volunteering at the skin cancer screening booth at a community health fair. A college student approaches you and asks about risk factors for skin cancer. He states that he lifeguards at a pool every summer and that he is on his school's golf team and plays golf year round. Identify the evidence to support the use of protection from the sun, including sunscreens, to prevent skin cancer. Discuss the strength of the evidence that supports the use of sunscreens. Identify the criteria used to evaluate the strength of the evidence for this practice.

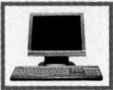   The Smeltzer suite offers these additional resources to enhance learning and facilitate understanding of this chapter:
- thePoint online resource, thepoint.lww.com /Smeltzer12E
- Student CD-ROM included with the book
- *Study Guide to Accompany Brunner & Suddarth's Text-book of Medical-Surgical Nursing*

REFERENCES AND SELECTED READINGS

*Asterisk indicates nursing research.

Books

Bickley, L. S. (2007). *Bates' guide to physical examination and history taking* (9th ed.). Philadelphia: Lippincott Williams & Williams.

James, W. D., Elston, D. & Berger, T. G. (2005). *Andrews' diseases of the skin* (10th ed.). Philadelphia: W. B. Saunders.

Johnson, R. A., Suurmond, R. & Wolff, K. (2005). *Color atlas & synopsis of clinical dermatology* (5th ed.). New York: McGraw-Hill.

Porth, C. M. & Matfin, G. (2009). *Pathophysiology. Concepts of altered health states* (8th ed.). Philadelphia: Lippincott Williams & Wilkins.

Weber, J. W. & Kelley, J. (2007). *Health assessment in nursing* (3rd ed.). Philadelphia: Lippincott Williams & Wilkins.

Wolff, K., Goldsmith, L., Katz, S. I., et al. (2007). *Fitzpatrick's dermatology in general medicine* (6th ed.). New York: McGraw-Hill.

Journals and Electronic Documents

Anderson, J., Langemo, D., Hanson, D., et al. (2007). What you can learn from a comprehensive skin assessment. *Nursing, 37*(4), 65–66.

Cokkinides, V., Weinstock, M., Glanz, K., et al. (2006). Trends in sunburns, sun protection practices, and attitudes toward sun exposure protection and tanning among U.S. adolescents, 1998–2004. *Pediatrics, 118*(3), 853–864.

Dobbinson, S. J., Wakefield, M. A., Jamsen, K. M., et al. (2008). Weekend sun protection and sunburn in Australia trends. *American Journal of Preventive Medicine, 34*(2), 171–172.

Draelos, Z. D. (1997). Understanding African-American hair. *Dermatology Nursing, 9*(4), 227–231.

*Freytes, D. M., Arroyo-Novoa, C. M., Figueroa-Ramos, M. I., et al. (2007). Skin disease in HIV-positive persons living in Puerto Rico. *Advanced Skin Wound Care, 20*(3), 149–150.

Hayden, M. L. (2005). Did that medication cause this rash? *Nursing, 35*(9), 62–64.

RESOURCES

American Academy of Dermatology, www.aad.org

Dermatology Online Atlas, a cooperation between the Department of Clinical Social Medicine (University of Heidelberg) and the Department of Dermatology (University of Erlangen), www.dermis.net

New Zealand Dermatology Society, www.dermnetnz.org

Skin Cancer Foundation (lists approved sunscreens and other sun protection products), www.skincancer.org

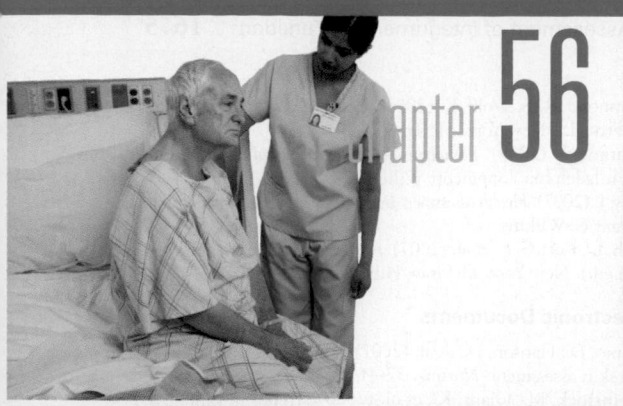

Chapter 56

Management of Patients With Dermatologic Problems

LEARNING OBJECTIVES

On completion of this chapter, the learner will be able to:

1 Describe the general management of the patient with an abnormal skin condition.

2 Describe the health education needs of the patient with infections of the skin and parasitic skin diseases.

3 Describe the management and nursing care of the patient with psoriasis.

4 Use the nursing process as a framework for care of patients with blistering disorders.

5 Use the nursing process as a framework for care of patients with toxic epidermal necrolysis and Stevens-Johnson syndrome.

6 Describe the management and nursing care of the patient with skin cancer.

7 Use the nursing process as a framework for care of the patient with malignant melanoma.

8 Describe characteristics of the various types of Kaposi's sarcoma.

9 Compare the various types of dermatologic and plastic reconstructive procedures.

10 Describe the nursing care of patients undergoing dermatologic and plastic reconstructive procedures.

GLOSSARY

acantholysis: separation of epidermal cells from each other due to damage or abnormality of the intracellular substance

balneotherapy: a bath with therapeutic additives

carbuncle: localized skin infection involving several hair follicles

cheilitis: inflammation of the lips (when dry, cracking, inflamed skin occurs at the corners of the mouth it is called angular cheilitis; when caused by sun exposure it is called solar cheilitis)

comedones: the primary lesions of acne, caused by sebum blockage in the hair follicle

cytotoxic: destructive of cells

débridement: removal of necrotic or dead tissue by mechanical, surgical, or autolytic means

dermatitis: any inflammation of the skin

dermatosis: any abnormal skin lesion

epidermopoiesis: development of epidermal cells

fibrinolytic: a substance that acts to break up fibrin, the fine filaments of blood clots

furuncle: localized skin infection of a single hair follicle

hydrophilic: a material that absorbs moisture

hydrophobic: a material that repels moisture

hygroscopic: a material that absorbs moisture from the air

lichenification: thickening of the horny layer of the skin

liniments: lotions with added oil for increased softening of the skin

mitogenic: a substance that stimulates mitosis or cell division and reproduction

plasmapheresis: removal of whole blood from the body, separation of its cellular elements by centrifugation, and reinfusion of them suspended in saline or some other plasma substitute, thereby depleting the body's own plasma without depleting its cells

pyodermas: bacterial skin infections

striae: bandlike streaks on the skin, distinguished by color, texture, depression, or elevation from the tissue in which they are found; usually purplish or white

suspensions: liquid preparations in which powder is suspended, requiring shaking before use

tinea: a superficial fungal infection on the skin or scalp

xerosis: overly dry skin

Nursing care for patients with dermatologic problems includes administering topical and systemic medications, managing wet dressings and other special dressings, and providing therapeutic baths. The four major objectives of therapy are to prevent additional damage, prevent secondary infection, reverse the inflammatory process, and relieve the symptoms.

SKIN CARE FOR PATIENTS WITH SKIN CONDITIONS

Some skin problems are markedly aggravated by soap and water, and bathing routines are modified according to the condition. Denuded skin, whether the area of desquamation is large or small, is excessively prone to damage by chemicals and trauma. The friction of a towel, if applied with vigor, is sufficient to produce a brisk inflammatory response that causes any existing lesion to flare up and extend.

Protecting the Skin

Basic skin care in bathing a patient with skin problems is as follows:
- A mild, lipid-free soap or soap substitute is used.
- The area is rinsed completely and blotted dry with a soft cloth.
- Deodorant soaps and laundry detergents are avoided.

Special care is necessary when changing dressings. Use of pledgets saturated with oil, sterile saline, or another prescribed solution helps loosen crusts, remove exudates, or free an adherent dry dressing.

Preventing Secondary Infection

Skin lesions should be regarded as potentially infectious, and proper precautions should be observed until the diagnosis is established. Most lesions with purulent drainage contain infectious material. The nurse and physician must adhere to standard precautions and wear gloves when inspecting the skin or changing a dressing. Use of standard precautions and proper disposal of any contaminated dressing is carried out according to the Occupational Safety and Health Administration (OSHA) regulations.

Reversing the Inflammatory Process

The type of skin lesion (eg, oozing, infected, or dry) usually determines the type of local medication or treatment that is prescribed. As a rule, if the skin is acutely inflamed (ie, hot, red, and swollen) and oozing, it is best to apply wet dressings and soothing lotions. For chronic conditions in which the skin surface is dry and scaly, water-soluble emulsions, creams, ointments, and pastes are used. The therapy is modified as the responses of the skin indicate. The patient and the nurse should note whether the medication or dressings seem to irritate the skin. The success or failure of therapy usually depends on adequate instruction and motivation of the patient and family, and the support of health care personnel promotes adherence to instructions.

WOUND CARE FOR SKIN CONDITIONS

There are three types of wound dressings: passive, interactive, and active. *Passive* dressings have only a protective function and maintain a moist environment for natural healing. They include those that just cover the area (eg, DuoDERM, Tegaderm) and may remain in place for several days. *Interactive* dressings are capable of absorbing wound exudate while (1) maintaining a moist environment in the area of the wound and (2) allowing the surrounding skin to remain dry. They include hydrocolloids, alginates, and hydrogels. It is thought that interactive dressings are able to modify the physiology of the wound environment by modulating and stimulating cellular activity and by releasing growth factor (Fonder, Lazarus, Cowan, et al., 2008). *Active* dressings improve the healing process and decrease healing time. They include skin grafts and biologic skin substitutes. Both interactive and active dressings create a moist environment at the interface of the wound with the dressing.

Because so many wound care products are available, it is often difficult to select the most appropriate product for a specific wound. Selection of products should be made carefully because of their expense. Both clinical efficacy and health-related outcomes (eg, decreased pain, increased mobility) should be used to measure the success of a product for a wound. Even with the availability of a large variety of dressings, an appropriate selection can be made if certain principles are maintained. These principles are referred to as the five rules of wound care (Krasner, Rodeheaver & Sibbald, 2007):

- *Rule 1: Categorization.* The nurse learns about dressings by generic category and compares new products with those that already make up the category. The nurse becomes familiar with indications, contraindications, and side effects. The best dressing may be created by combining products in different categories to achieve several goals at the same time. These categories are discussed in subsequent sections.
- *Rule 2: Selection.* The nurse selects the safest and most effective, easy-to-use, and cost-effective dressing possible. In many cases, nurses carry out the physician's prescriptions for dressings, but they must be prepared to give the physician feedback about the dressing's effect on the wound, ease of use for the patient, and other considerations when applicable.
- *Rule 3: Change.* The nurse changes dressings based on patient, wound, and dressing assessments, not on standardized routines.

⚑ NURSING ALERT

The natural wound-healing process should not be disrupted. Unless the wound is infected or has a heavy discharge, it is common to leave chronic wounds covered for 48 to 72 hours and acute wounds for 24 hours.

- *Rule 4: Evolution.* As the wound progresses through the phases of wound healing, the dressing protocol is altered to optimize wound healing. It is rare, especially in cases of chronic wounds, that the same dressing material is appropriate throughout the healing process. The nurse teaches the patient or family caregiver about wound care and ensures that the family has access to appropriate dressing choices.

- *Rule 5: Practice.* Practice with dressing material is required for the nurse to learn the performance parameters of the particular dressing. Refining the skills of applying appropriate dressings correctly and learning about new dressing products are essential nursing responsibilities. Dressing changes should not be delegated to unlicensed personnel; these techniques require the knowledge base and assessment skills of professional nurses.

Autolytic Débridement

Autolytic **débridement** is a process that uses the body's own digestive enzymes to break down necrotic tissue. The wound is kept moist with occlusive dressings. Eschar and necrotic debris are softened, liquefied, and separated from the bed of the wound.

Several commercially available products contain the same enzymes that the body produces naturally. These are called enzymatic débriding agents; examples include Accu-Zyme, collagenase (Santyl), Granulex, and Zymase. Application of these products speeds the rate at which necrotic tissue is removed. This method, although slower than surgical débridement, is more discriminating for tissue removal and does not damage healthy tissue surrounding the wound. When enzymatic débridement is being used under an occlusive dressing, a foul odor is produced by the breakdown of cellular debris. This odor does not indicate that the wound is infected. The nurse should expect this reaction and help the patient and family understand the reason for the odor.

Categories of Dressings

Table 56-1 is a guide to wound dressing functions and categories.

Occlusive Dressings

Occlusive dressings may be commercially produced or made inexpensively from sterile or nonsterile gauze squares or wrap. Occlusive dressings cover topical medication that is applied to a skin lesion. The area is kept airtight by using plastic film (eg, plastic wrap). Plastic film is thin and readily adapts to all sizes, body shapes, and skin surfaces. Generally, plastic wrap should be used no more than 12 hours each day. Plastic surgical tape containing a corticosteroid in the adhesive layer can be cut to size and applied to individual lesions.

Wet Dressings

Wet dressings (wet compresses applied to the skin) were traditionally used for acute, weeping, inflammatory lesions. They have become almost obsolete because of the many newer products available for wound care.

Table 56-1	QUICK GUIDE TO FUNCTION AND ACTION OF WOUND DRESSINGS	
Function	**Action**	**Example**
Absorption	Absorbs exudate	Alginates, composite dressings, foams, gauze, hydrocolloids, hydrogels
Cleansing	Removes purulent drainage, foreign debris, and devitalized tissue	Wound cleansers
Débridement	*Autolytic;* covers a wound and allows enzymes to self-digest sloughed skin	Absorption beads, pastes, powders; alginates; composite dressings; foams; hydrate gauze; hydrogels; hydrocolloids; transparent films; wound care systems
	Chemical or enzymatic; applied topically to break down devitalized tissue	Enzymatic débridement agents
	Mechanical; removes devitalized tissue with mechanical force	Wound cleansers, gauze (wet to dry), whirlpool
Diathermy	Produces electrical current to promote warmth and new tissue growth	
Hydration	Adds moisture to a wound	Gauze (saturated with saline) solution, hydrogels, wound care systems
Maintain moist environment	Manages moisture levels in a wound and maintains a moist environment	Composites, contact layers, foams, gauze (impregnated or saturated), hydrogels, hydrocolloids, transparent films, wound care systems
Manage high-output wounds	Manages excessive quantities of exudate	Pouching systems
Pack or fill dead space	Prevents premature wound closure or fills shallow areas and provides absorption	Absorbent beads, powders, pastes; alginates, composites, foams, gauze (impregnated and nonimpregnated)
Protect and cover wound	Provides protection from the external environment	Composites, compression bandages/wraps, foams, gauze dressings, hydrogels, hydrocolloids, transparent film dressings
Protect periwound skin	Prevents moisture and mechanical trauma from damaging delicate tissue around wound	Composites, foams, hydrocolloids, pouching systems, skin sealants, transparent film dressings
Provide therapeutic compression	Provides appropriate levels of support to the lower extremities in venous stasis disease	Compression bandages, wraps, graduated compression stockings

Moisture-Retentive Dressings

Commercially produced moisture-retentive dressings can perform the same functions as wet dressings but are more efficient at removing exudate because of their higher moisture-vapor transmission rate; some have reservoirs that can hold excessive exudate. A number of moisture-retentive dressings are already impregnated with saline solution, petrolatum, zinc-saline solution, hydrogel, or antimicrobial agents, thereby eliminating the need to coat the skin to avoid maceration. The main advantages of moisture-retentive dressings over wet dressings are improved fibrinolysis, accelerated epidermal resurfacing, reduced pain, fewer infections, less scar tissue, gentle autolytic débridement, and decreased frequency of dressing changes. Depending on the product used and the type of dermatologic conditions encountered, most moisture-retentive dressings may remain in place from 12 to 24 hours; some can remain in place as long as a week.

Hydrogels

Hydrogels are polymers with 90% to 95% water content. They are available in impregnated sheets or as gel in a tube. Their high moisture content makes them ideal for autolytic débridement of wounds. They are semitransparent, allowing for wound inspection without dressing removal. They are comfortable and soothing for the painful wound. They require a secondary dressing to keep them in place. Hydrogels are appropriate for superficial wounds with high serous output, such as abrasions, skin graft sites, and draining venous ulcers.

Hydrocolloids

Hydrocolloids are composed of a water-impermeable, polyurethane outer covering separated from the wound by a hydrocolloid material. They are adherent and nonpermeable to water vapor and oxygen. As water evaporates over the wound, it is absorbed into the dressing, which softens and discolors with the increased water content. The dressing can be removed without damage to the wound. As the dressing absorbs water, it produces a foul-smelling, yellowish covering over the wound. This is a normal chemical interaction between the dressing and wound exudate and should not be confused with purulent drainage from the wound. Unfortunately, most of the hydrocolloid dressings are opaque, preventing inspection of the wound without removal of the dressing.

Available in sheets and in gels, hydrocolloids are a good choice for exudative wounds and for acute wounds. Easy to use and comfortable, hydrocolloid dressings promote débridement and formation of granulation tissue. Most can be left in place for as long as 7 days and can be submerged in water for bathing or showering. A recent consensus statement of wound experts suggested that hydrocolloid dressings are better than saline gauze or paraffin gauze dressings for complete healing of chronic wounds (Vaneau, Chaby, Guillot, et al., 2007).

Foam Dressings

Foam dressings consist of microporous polyurethane with an absorptive **hydrophilic** (water-absorbing) surface that covers the wound and a **hydrophobic** (water-resistant) backing to block leakage of exudate. They are nonadherent and require a secondary dressing to keep them in place. Moisture is absorbed into the foam layer, decreasing maceration of surrounding tissue. A moist environment is maintained, and removal of the dressing does not damage the wound. The foams are opaque and must be removed for wound inspection. Foams are a good choice for exudative wounds. They are especially helpful over bony prominences because they provide contoured cushioning.

Calcium Alginates

Calcium alginates are derived from seaweed and consist of very absorbent calcium alginate fibers. They are hemostatic and bioabsorbable and can be used as sheets or mats of absorbent material. As the exudate is absorbed, the fibers turn into a viscous hydrogel. They are useful in areas where the tissue is more irritated or macerated. The alginate dressing forms a moist pocket over the wound while the surrounding skin stays dry. The dressing also reacts with wound fluid, which forms a foul-smelling coating. Alginates work well when packed into a deep cavity, wound, or sinus tract with heavy drainage (Krasner, et al., 2007). They are nonadherent and require a secondary dressing. A recent consensus statement of wound experts suggests that alginates are superior to other modern dressings for débriding necrotic wounds (Vaneau, et al., 2007).

Advances in Wound Treatment

Increasing understanding of how skin heals has led to several advances in therapy. Growth factors are cytokines or proteins that have potent **mitogenic** activity (Vaneau, et al., 2007). Low levels of cytokines circulate in the blood continuously and control key factors involved in wound healing. Many investigators believe that a deficit of cytokines contributes to poor wound healing. Regranex gel, which contains becaplermin, a recombinant human platelet-derived growth factor, promotes chemotactic recruitment and proliferation of the cells involved in wound healing (Fonder, et al., 2008).

Bioengineered skin substitutes have emerged in the past 25 years as the most effective method for management of chronic wounds. Most of these skin substitutes are cultures of keratinocytes delivered on a petrolatum gauze. They work by maintaining wound moisture, providing a structure for regeneration of cells, and supplying beneficial cytokines. These substitutes include AlloDerm, Apligraf, Dermagraf, Epicel, and Laserskin.

Some oral medications are being investigated for their benefits in healing chronic venous ulcers of the lower legs. Pentoxifylline (Trental) increases peripheral blood flow by decreasing the viscosity of blood. It has some **fibrinolytic** action and decreases leukocyte adhesion to the wall of the blood vessels. Enteric-coated aspirin was thought to be of value, but a more recent study suggests that aspirin inhibits the tensile strength of skin and prolongs the healing time (Fonder, et al., 2008).

A recent study (Jones, Fennie & Lenihan, 2007) found several surprising results related to healing of chronic wounds:

- Mechanical débridement is contraindicated because it may increase the possibility of infection and because there may be inadvertent damage to healthy tissue.
- The use of a commercial cleansing agent rather than water, normal saline, or povidone-iodine is related to faster healing.

- Initial selection of the dressing type to be used is critical to success. Wounds heal faster when the type of dressing is not changed during treatment. If the type of dressing was changed four or five times, healing times were more likely to be prolonged.
- Documenting the presence of bacteria is critical. Bacteria slow healing time. However, antibiotics are often overused; thus, it is important to check for the presence of bacteria before initiating antibiotic therapy.

Medical Management

Therapeutic Baths (Balneotherapy)

Baths or soaks, known as **balneotherapy,** are useful when large areas of skin are affected. The baths remove crusts, scales, and previously applied topical medications and relieve the inflammation and pruritus (itching) that accompany acute dermatoses. Additional information about therapeutic baths is given in Chart 56-1.

Pharmacologic Therapy

Because skin is easily accessible, topical medications are often used. High concentrations of some medications can be applied directly to the affected site with little systemic absorption and therefore with few systemic side effects. However, some medications are readily absorbed through the skin and can produce systemic effects. Because topical preparations may induce allergic contact **dermatitis** in sensitive patients, any untoward response should be reported immediately and the medication discontinued.

Chart 56-1 • *Therapeutic Baths*

Types of Therapeutic Baths

Bath Solution	Effects and Uses
Water	Same effect as wet dressings
Saline	Used for widely disseminated lesions
Colloidal (Aveeno, oatmeal)	Antipruritic, soothing
Sodium bicarbonate (baking soda)	Cooling
Starch	Soothing
Medicated tars	Psoriasis and chronic eczema
Bath oils	Antipruritic and emollient action; acute and subacute generalized eczematous eruptions

Nursing Interventions

- Fill the tub half full.
- Keep the water at a comfortable temperature.
- Do not allow the water to cool excessively.
- Use a bath mat, because *medications added to the bath can cause the tub to be slippery.*
- Apply an emollient cream to damp skin after the bath if lubrication is desired.
- Because tars are volatile, the bath area should be well ventilated.
- Maintain a constant room temperature without drafts.
- Encourage the patient to wear light, loose clothing after the bath.

Medicated lotions, creams, ointments, and powders are frequently used to treat skin lesions. In general, moisture-retentive dressings, with or without medication, are used in the acute stage; lotions and creams are reserved for the subacute stage; and ointments are used when inflammation has become chronic and the skin is dry with scaling or **lichenification.**

With all types of topical medication, the patient is taught to apply the medication gently but thoroughly and, when necessary, to cover the medication with a dressing to protect clothing. Table 56-2 lists commonly used topical preparations.

Lotions

Lotions are frequently used to replenish lost skin oils or to relieve pruritus. They are usually applied directly to the skin, but a dressing soaked in the lotion can be placed on the affected area. Lotions must be applied every 3 or 4 hours for sustained therapeutic effect. If left in place for a longer period, they may crust and cake on the skin.

Lotions are of two types: suspensions and liniments. **Suspensions,** consist of a powder in water that requires shaking before application, and clear solutions, contain completely dissolved active ingredients. A suspension such as calamine lotion provides a rapid cooling and drying effect as it evaporates, leaving a thin, medicinal layer of powder on the affected skin. **Liniments** are lotions with oil added to prevent crusting. Because lotions are easy to use, therapeutic compliance is generally high.

Powders

Powders usually have a talc, zinc oxide, bentonite, or cornstarch base and are dusted on the skin with a shaker or with cotton sponges. Although their therapeutic action is brief, powders act as **hygroscopic** agents that absorb and retain moisture from the air and reduce friction between skin surfaces and clothing or bedding.

Creams

Creams may be suspensions of oil in water or emulsions of water in oil, with additional ingredients to prevent bacterial and fungal growth. Both may cause an allergic reaction such as contact dermatitis. Oil-in-water creams are easily applied and usually are the most cosmetically acceptable to the patient. Although they can be used on the face, they tend to have a drying effect. Water-in-oil emulsions are greasier and are preferred for drying and flaking dermatoses. Creams usually are rubbed into the skin by hand. They are used for their moisturizing and emollient effects.

Gels

Gels are semisolid emulsions that become liquid when applied to the skin or scalp. They are cosmetically acceptable to the patient because they are not visible after application, and they are greaseless and nonstaining. The newer water-based gels appear to penetrate the skin more effectively and cause less stinging on application. They are especially useful for acute dermatitis in which there is weeping exudate (eg, poison ivy).

Pastes

Pastes are mixtures of powders and ointments and are used in inflammatory blistering conditions. They adhere to the

Table 56-2	COMMON TOPICAL PREPARATIONS AND MEDICATIONS
Preparation	**Product Name**
Bath preparations	
With tar	Balnetar, Doak Oil, Lavatar
With colloidal oatmeal	Aveeno Oilated Bath Powder
With oatmeal and mineral oil	Aveeno Bath Oil, Nutra Soothe
With mineral oil	Nutraderm Bath Oil, Lubath, Alpha-Keri Bath Oil
Moisturizer creams	Acid Mantle Cream, Curel Cream, Dermasil, Eucerin, Lubriderm, Noxzema Skin Cream
Moisturizer ointments	Aquaphor Ointment, Eutra Swiss Skin Cream, Vaseline Ointment
Topical anesthetics	lidocaine (Xylocaine) of various strengths in the form of spray, ointment, gel; EMLA cream (lidocaine 2.5% and prilocaine 2.5%)
Topical antibiotics	bacitracin, Polysporin (bacitracin and polymixin B), Bactroban ointment or cream (mupirocin 2%), erythromycin 2% (Emgel, Eryderm Solution), clindamycin phosphate 1% (Cleocin cream, gel, solution), gentamicin sulfate 1% (Garamycin cream or ointment), 1% silver sulfadiazine cream (Silvadene)

skin and may be difficult to remove without using an oil (eg, olive oil, mineral oil). Pastes are applied with a wooden tongue depressor or gloved hand.

Ointments

Ointments retard water loss and lubricate and protect the skin. They are the preferred vehicle for delivering medication to chronic or localized dry skin conditions, such as eczema or psoriasis. Ointments are applied with a wooden tongue depressor or gloved hand.

Sprays and Aerosols

Spray and aerosol preparations may be used on any widespread dermatologic condition. They evaporate on contact and are used infrequently.

Corticosteroids

Corticosteroids are widely used in treating dermatologic conditions to provide anti-inflammatory, antipruritic, and vasoconstrictive effects. The patient is taught to apply this medication according to strict guidelines, using it sparingly but rubbing it into the prescribed area thoroughly. Absorption of topical corticosteroids is enhanced when the skin is hydrated or the affected area is covered by an occlusive or moisture-retentive dressing. Inappropriate use of topical corticosteroids can result in local and systemic side effects, especially when the medication is absorbed through inflamed and excoriated skin, is used under occlusive dressings, or is used for long periods on sensitive areas. Local side effects may include skin atrophy and thinning, **striae** (bandlike streaks), and telangiectasia (small, red lesions caused by dilation of blood vessels). Thinning of the skin results from the ability of corticosteroids to inhibit skin collagen synthesis. The thinning process can be reversed by discontinuing the medication, but striae and telangiectasia are permanent. Systemic side effects may include hyperglycemia and symptoms of Cushing's syndrome. Caution is required when applying corticosteroids around the eyes for two reasons: (1) long-term use may cause glaucoma or

cataracts, and (2) the anti-inflammatory effect of corticosteroids may mask existing viral or fungal infections.

Concentrated (fluorinated) corticosteroids are never applied on the face or intertriginous areas (ie, axilla and groin) because these areas have a thinner stratum corneum and absorb the medication much more quickly than areas such as the forearm or legs. Persistent use of concentrated topical corticosteroids in any location may produce acnelike dermatitis, known as steroid-induced acne, and hypertrichosis (excessive hair growth). Because some topical corticosteroid preparations are available without prescription, patients should be cautioned about prolonged and inappropriate use. Table 56-3 lists topical corticosteroid preparations according to potency.

Intralesional Therapy

Intralesional therapy consists of injecting a sterile suspension of medication (usually a corticosteroid) into or just below a lesion. Although this treatment may have an anti-inflammatory effect, local atrophy may result if the medication is injected into subcutaneous fat. Skin lesions treated with intralesional therapy include psoriasis, keloids, and cystic acne. Occasionally, immunotherapeutic and antifungal agents are administered as intralesional therapy.

Systemic Medications

Systemic medications are also prescribed for skin conditions. These include corticosteroids for short-term therapy for contact dermatitis or for long-term treatment of a chronic **dermatosis,** such as pemphigus vulgaris. Other frequently used systemic medications include antibiotics, antifungals, antihistamines, sedatives, tranquilizers, analgesics, and **cytotoxic** (destructive of cells) agents.

Nursing Management

Management begins with a health history, direct observation, and a complete physical examination. (Chapter 55 provides a description of integumentary assessment.) Because of its visibility, a skin condition is usually difficult to ignore or conceal from others and may therefore cause the patient

Table 56-3	POTENCY: TOPICAL CORTICOSTEROIDS	
Potency	**Topical Corticosteroid**	**Preparations**
OTC	0.5–1.0% hydrocortisone	cr, lot, oint
Lowest	dexamethasone 0.1% (Decaderm)	cr, oint, aerosol, gel
	alclometasone 0.05% (Aclovate)	cr, oint
	hydrocortisone 2.5% (Hytone)	cr, lot, oint
Low–medium	desonide 0.05% (DesOwen, Tridesilon)	cr, lot, oint
	fluocinolone acetonide 0.025% (Synalar)	cr, solution
	hydrocortisone valerate 0.2% (Westcort)	cr, solution
	betamethasone valerate 0.1% (Valisone)	cr, oint
	fluticasonepropionate 0.05% (Cutivate)	cr, oint
Medium–high	triamcinolone acetonide 0.1–0.5% (Aristocort)	cr, oint, lot
	fluocinonide 0.05% (Lidex)	cr, oint, gel
	desoximetasone 0.05–0.25% (Topicort)	cr, oint, gel
	fluocinolone 0.2% (Synalar)	cr, oint
	diflorasone diacetate 0.05% (Psorcon)	cr, oint
Very high	clobetasol propionate 0.05% (Temovate)	cr, oint, gel
	betamethasone dipropionate 0.05% (Diprolene)	cr, oint, gel
	halobetasole propionate 0.05% (Ultravate)	cr, oint

cr, cream; lot, lotion; oint, ointment; OTC, over the counter.

emotional distress. The major goals for the patient may include maintenance of skin integrity, relief of discomfort, promotion of restful sleep, self-acceptance, knowledge about skin care, and avoidance of complications.

Nursing management for patients who must perform self-care for skin problems, such as applying medications and dressings, focuses mainly on teaching the patient how to wash the affected area and pat it dry, apply medication to the lesion while the skin is moist, cover the area with plastic (eg, Telfa pads, plastic wrap, vinyl gloves, plastic bag) if recommended, and cover it with an elastic bandage, dressing, or paper tape to seal the edges. Dressings that contain or cover a topical corticosteroid should be removed for 12 of every 24 hours to prevent skin thinning, striae, and telangiectasia.

Other forms of dressings, such as those used to cover topical medications, include soft cotton cloth and stretchable cotton dressings (eg, Surgitube, TubeGauz) that can be used for fingers, toes, hands, and feet. The hands can be covered with disposable polyethylene or vinyl gloves sealed at the wrists; the feet can be wrapped in plastic bags covered by cotton socks. Gloves and socks that are already impregnated with emollients, making application to the hands and feet more convenient, are also available. When large areas of the body must be covered, cotton cloth topped by an expandable stockinette can be used. Disposable diapers or cloths folded in diaper fashion are useful for dressing the groin and the perineal areas. Axillary dressings can be made of cotton cloth, or a commercially prepared dressing may be used and taped in place or held by dress shields. A turban or plastic shower cap is useful for holding dressings on the scalp. A face mask, made from gauze with holes cut out for the eyes, nose, and mouth, may be held in place with gauze ties looped through holes cut in the four corners of the mask.

PRURITUS

General Pruritus

Pruritus (itching) is one of the most common symptoms of patients with dermatologic disorders. Itch receptors are unmyelinated, penicillate (brushlike) nerve endings that are found exclusively in the skin, mucous membranes, and cornea. Although pruritus is usually caused by primary skin disease with resultant rash or lesions, it may occur without a rash or lesion. This is referred to as essential pruritus, which generally has a rapid onset, may be severe, and interferes with normal daily activities.

Pruritus may be the first indication of a systemic internal disease such as diabetes mellitus, blood disorders, or cancer (occult malignancy of the breast or colon; lymphoma). It may also accompany renal, hepatic, and thyroid diseases (Chart 56-2). Some common oral medications such as aspirin, antibiotics, hormones (ie, estrogens, testosterone, or oral contraceptives), and opioids (ie, morphine or cocaine) may cause pruritus directly or by increasing sensitivity to ultraviolet light. Certain soaps and chemicals, radiation therapy, prickly heat (miliaria), and contact with woolen garments are also associated with pruritus. Pruritus may also be

Chart 56-2 • Systemic Disorders Associated With Generalized Pruritus

Chronic renal disease
Obstructive biliary disease (primary biliary cirrhosis, extrahepatic biliary obstruction, drug-induced cholestasis)
Endocrine disease (thyrotoxicosis, hypothyroidism, diabetes mellitus)
Psychiatric disorders (emotional stress, anxiety, neurosis, phobias)
Malignancies (polycythemia vera, Hodgkin's lymphoma, lymphoma, leukemia, multiple myeloma, mycosis fungoides, and cancers of the lung, breast, central nervous system, and gastrointestinal tract)
Neurologic disorders (multiple sclerosis, brain abscess, brain tumor)
Infestations (scabies, lice, other insects)
Pruritus of pregnancy (pruritic urticarial papules of pregnancy [PUPP], cholestasis of pregnancy, pemphigoid of pregnancy)
Folliculitis (bacterial, candidiasis, dermatophyte)
Skin conditions (seborrheic dermatitis, folliculitis, iron deficiency anemia, atopic dermatitis)

caused by psychological factors, such as excessive stress in family or work situations.

 Gerontologic Considerations

Pruritus occurs frequently in elderly people as a result of dry skin. Elderly people are also more likely to have a systemic illness that triggers pruritus, are at higher risk for occult malignancy, and are more likely to be taking multiple medications than younger people. All of these factors increase the incidence of pruritus in elderly people.

Pathophysiology

Scratching the pruritic area causes the inflamed cells and nerve endings to release histamine, which produces more pruritus, generating a vicious itch–scratch cycle. If the patient responds to an itch by scratching, the integrity of the skin may be altered, and excoriation, redness, raised areas (ie, wheals), infection, or changes in pigmentation may result. Pruritus usually is more severe at night and is less frequently reported during waking hours, probably because the person is distracted by daily activities. At night, when there are fewer distractions, the slightest pruritus cannot be easily ignored. Severe itching can be debilitating.

Medical Management

A thorough history and physical examination usually provide clues to the underlying cause of the pruritus, such as hay fever, allergy, recent administration of a new medication, or a change of cosmetics or soaps. After the cause has been identified, treatment of the condition should relieve the pruritus. Signs of infection and environmental clues, such as warm, dry air or irritating bed linens, should be identified. In general, washing with soap and hot water is avoided. Bath oils containing a surfactant that allows the oil to mix with bath water (eg, Lubath, Alpha-Keri) may be sufficient for cleaning. However, an elderly patient or a patient with unsteady balance should avoid adding oil because it increases the danger of slipping in the bathtub. A warm bath with a mild soap followed by application of a bland emollient to moist skin can control **xerosis** (dry skin). Applying a cold compress, ice cube, or cool agents that contain menthol and camphor (which constrict blood vessels) may also help relieve pruritus.

Pharmacologic Therapy

Topical corticosteroids may be beneficial as anti-inflammatory agents to decrease itching. Oral antihistamines are even more effective because they can overcome the effects of histamine release from damaged mast cells. An antihistamine, such as diphenhydramine (Benadryl) or hydroxyzine (Atarax), prescribed in a sedative dose at bedtime is often effective in producing a restful and comfortable sleep. Nonsedating antihistamine medications such as fexofenadine (Allegra) are more appropriate to relieve daytime pruritus. Tricyclic antidepressants, such as doxepin (Sinequan), may be prescribed for pruritus of neuropsychogenic origin. If pruritus continues, further investigation of a systemic problem is advised.

Nursing Management

The nurse reinforces the reasons for the prescribed therapeutic regimen and counsels the patient on specific points of care. If baths have been prescribed, the patient is reminded to use tepid (not hot) water and to shake off the excess water and blot between intertriginous areas (body folds) with a towel. Rubbing vigorously with the towel is avoided because this overstimulates the skin and causes more itching. It also removes water from the stratum corneum. Immediately after bathing, the skin should be lubricated with an emollient to trap moisture.

The patient is instructed to avoid situations that cause vasodilation. Examples include exposure to an overly warm environment and ingestion of alcohol or hot foods and liquids. All can induce or intensify pruritus. Using a humidifier is helpful if environmental air is dry. Activities that result in perspiration should be limited because perspiration may irritate and promote pruritus. If the patient is troubled at night with itching that interferes with sleep, the nurse can advise wearing cotton clothing next to the skin rather than synthetic materials. The room should be kept cool and humidified. Vigorous scratching should be avoided and nails kept trimmed to prevent skin damage and infection. When the underlying cause of pruritus is unknown and further testing is required, the nurse explains each test and the expected outcome.

Perineal and Perianal Pruritus

Pruritus of the genital and anal regions may be caused by small particles of fecal material lodged in the perianal crevices or attached to anal hairs. Alternatively, it may result from perianal skin damage caused by scratching, moisture, and decreased skin resistance as a result of corticosteroid or antibiotic therapy. Other possible causes of perianal itching include local irritants such as scabies and lice, local lesions such as hemorrhoids, fungal or yeast infections, and pinworm infestation. Conditions such as diabetes mellitus, anemia, hyperthyroidism, and pregnancy may also result in pruritus. Occasionally, no cause can be identified.

Management

The patient is instructed to follow proper hygiene measures and to discontinue home and over-the-counter remedies. The perineal or anal area should be rinsed with lukewarm water and blotted dry with cotton balls. Premoistened tissues may be used after defecation. Cornstarch can be applied in the skinfold areas to absorb perspiration.

As part of health teaching, the nurse instructs the patient to avoid bathing in water that is too hot and to avoid using bubble baths, sodium bicarbonate, and detergent soaps, all of which aggravate dryness. To keep the perineal or perianal skin as dry as possible, patients should avoid wearing underwear made of synthetic fabrics. Local anesthetic agents should not be used because of possible allergic effects. The patient should also avoid vasodilating agents or stimulants (eg, alcohol, caffeine) and mechanical irritants such as rough or woolen clothing. A diet that includes adequate fiber may help maintain soft stools and prevent minor trauma to the anal mucosa.

SECRETORY DISORDERS

The main secretory function of the skin is performed by the sweat glands, which help regulate body temperature. These glands excrete perspiration that evaporates, thereby cooling the body. The sweat glands are located in various parts of the body and respond to different stimuli. Those on the trunk generally respond to thermal stimulation; those on the palms and soles respond to nervous stimulation; and those in the axillae and on the forehead respond to both kinds of stimulation. Normal perspiration has no odor. Body odor is produced by the increase in bacteria on the skin and the interaction of bacterial waste products with the chemicals of perspiration. As a rule, moist skin is warm, and dry skin is cool, but this is not always true. It is not unusual to observe warm, dry skin in a dehydrated patient and very hot, dry skin in some febrile states.

Normally, sweat can be controlled with the use of antiperspirants and deodorants. Most antiperspirants are aluminum salts that block the opening to the sweat duct. Pure deodorants inhibit bacterial growth and block the metabolism of sweat; they have no antiperspirant effect. Fragrance-free deodorants are available for those with sensitive skin.

Hidradenitis Suppurativa

Hidradenitis suppurativa is a chronic suppurative folliculitis of the perianal, axillary, and genital areas or under the breasts. It develops after puberty and can produce abscesses or sinuses with scarring. The cause is unknown, but it appears to have a genetic basis.

Pathophysiology

Abnormal blockage of the sweat glands causes recurring inflammation, nodules, and draining sinus tracts. Eventually, hypertrophic bands of scar tissue form in the area of the sweat glands.

Clinical Manifestations

The condition occurs more frequently in the axilla but also appears in inguinal folds, on the mons pubis, and around the buttocks. The patient can be extremely uncomfortable with multiple suppurative lesions within a small area.

Management

Management is often difficult. Hot compresses and oral antibiotics are used frequently. Isotretinoin (Accutane, Sotret) or acitretin (Soriatane) can be tried; careful monitoring for side effects is important. Incision and drainage of large suppurating areas with gauze packs inserted to facilitate drainage are often necessary. Rarely, the entire area is excised, removing the scar tissue and any infection. This surgery is drastic and performed only as a last resort.

Seborrheic Dermatoses

Seborrhea is excessive production of sebum (secretion of sebaceous glands) in areas where sebaceous glands are normally found in large numbers, such as the face, scalp, eyebrows, eyelids, sides of the nose and upper lip, malar regions (cheeks), ears, axillae, under the breasts, groin, and gluteal crease of the buttocks. Seborrheic dermatitis is a chronic inflammatory disease of the skin with a predilection for areas that are well supplied with sebaceous glands or lie between skin folds, where the bacteria count is high.

Clinical Manifestations

Two forms of seborrheic dermatoses can occur: an oily form and a dry form. Either form may start in childhood and continue throughout life. The oily form appears moist or greasy. There may be patches of sallow, greasy skin, with or without scaling, and slight erythema, predominantly on the forehead, nasolabial fold, beard area, scalp, and between adjacent skin surfaces in the regions of the axillae, groin, and breasts. Small pustules or papulopustules resembling acne may appear on the trunk. The dry form, consisting of flaky desquamation of the scalp with a profuse amount of fine, powdery scales, is commonly called dandruff. The mild forms of the disease are asymptomatic. When scaling occurs, it is often accompanied by pruritus, which may lead to scratching and secondary infections and excoriation.

Seborrheic dermatitis has a genetic predisposition. Hormones, nutritional status, infection, and emotional stress influence its course. The remissions and exacerbations of this condition should be explained to the patient. If a person has not previously been diagnosed with this condition and suddenly appears with a severe outbreak, a complete history and physical examination should be conducted.

Medical Management

Because there is no known cure for seborrhea, the objectives of therapy are to control the disorder and allow the skin to repair itself. Seborrheic dermatitis of the body and face may respond to a topically applied corticosteroid cream, which allays the secondary inflammatory response. However, this medication should be used with caution near the eyelids because it can lead to glaucoma and cataracts. Patients with seborrheic dermatitis may develop a secondary candidal (yeast) infection in body creases or folds. To avoid this, patients should be advised to ensure maximum aeration of the skin and to clean areas where there are creases or folds in the skin carefully. Patients with persistent candidiasis should be evaluated for diabetes.

The mainstay of dandruff treatment is proper, frequent shampooing (at least three times weekly) with medicated shampoos. Two or three different types of shampoo should be used in rotation to prevent the seborrhea from becoming resistant to a particular shampoo. The shampoo is left on at least 5 to 10 minutes. As the condition of the scalp improves, the treatment can be less frequent. Antiseborrheic shampoos include those containing selenium sulfide suspension, zinc pyrithione, salicylic acid or sulfur compounds, and tar shampoo that contains sulfur or salicylic acid.

Nursing Management

A person with seborrheic dermatitis is advised to avoid external irritants, excessive heat, and perspiration; rubbing and scratching prolong the disorder. To avoid secondary infection, the patient should air the skin and keep skin folds clean and dry.

Instructions for using medicated shampoos are reinforced for people with dandruff who require treatment. Frequent shampooing is contrary to some cultural practices; the nurse should be sensitive to these differences when teaching the patient about home care.

The patient is cautioned that seborrheic dermatitis is a chronic condition that tends to reappear. The goal is to keep it under control. Patients need to be encouraged to adhere to the treatment program. Those who become discouraged and disheartened by the effect on body image should be treated with sensitivity and encouraged to express their feelings.

Acne Vulgaris

Acne vulgaris is a common disorder affecting susceptible hair follicles, most commonly on the face, neck, and upper trunk. It is characterized by **comedones** (primary acne lesions), both closed and open, and by papules, pustules, nodules, and cysts.

Acne is the most commonly encountered skin condition in adolescents and young adults between 12 and 35 years. It accounts for at least 15% of all dermatology visits. Both males and females are affected equally, although onset is slightly earlier in females, because they reach puberty at a younger age than males. Acne becomes more marked during adolescence because the endocrine glands that influence the secretions of the sebaceous glands are functioning at peak activity. Acne appears to stem from an interplay of genetic, hormonal, and bacterial factors. In most cases, there is a family history of acne.

Pathophysiology

During puberty, androgens stimulate the sebaceous glands, causing them to enlarge and secrete a natural oil, sebum, which rises to the top of the hair follicle and flows out onto the skin surface. In adolescents who develop acne, androgenic stimulation produces a heightened response in the sebaceous glands so that acne occurs when accumulated sebum plugs the pilosebaceous ducts.

Clinical Manifestations

The primary lesions of acne are comedones. Closed comedones (whiteheads) form from impacted lipids or oils and keratin that plug the dilated follicle. Closed comedones may evolve into open comedones, in which the contents of the ducts are in open communication with the external environment. The color of open comedones (blackheads) results from an accumulation of lipid, bacterial, and epithelial debris. Some closed comedones may rupture, resulting in an inflammatory reaction caused by leakage of follicular contents (eg, sebum, keratin, bacteria) into the dermis. The resultant inflammation is seen clinically as erythematous papules, inflammatory pustules, and inflammatory cysts. Mild papules and cysts drain and heal without treatment. Deeper papules and cysts cause scarring of the skin. Acne is usually graded as mild, moderate, or severe based on the number and type of lesions.

Assessment and Diagnostic Findings

The diagnosis of acne is based on the history and physical examination, evidence of lesions characteristic of acne, and age. Women may report a history of flare-ups a few days before

menses. The presence of the typical comedones along with excessively oily skin is characteristic. Oiliness is more prominent in the midfacial area; other parts of the face may appear dry. When there are numerous lesions, some of which are open, the person may exude a distinct sebaceous odor. Biopsy of lesions is seldom necessary for a definitive diagnosis.

Medical Management

The goals of management are to reduce bacterial colonies, decrease sebaceous gland activity, prevent the follicles from becoming plugged, reduce inflammation, combat secondary infection, minimize scarring, and eliminate factors that predispose the person to acne. The therapeutic regimen depends on the type of lesion (eg, comedones, papule, pustule, cyst). The duration of treatment depends on the extent and severity of the acne. In severe cases, treatment may extend over years.

There is no predictable cure for the disease, but combinations of therapies are available that can effectively control its activity. Table 56-4 summarizes the treatment modalities for acne vulgaris.

Nutrition and Hygiene Therapy

Diet is not believed to play a major role in therapy. However, the elimination of a specific food or food product

Table 56-4	TYPE OF TREATMENTS COMMONLY USED FOR ACNE VULGARIS
Type of Therapy	**Prescribed Treatment Agent**
Topical	benzoyl peroxide wash, gel
	benzoyl peroxide and erythromycin (Benzamycin gel)
	benzoyl peroxide and sulfur (Benzulfoid cream)
	resorcinol (as ingredient in other preparations)
	salicylic acid (as ingredient in other preparations)
	sulfur (as ingredient in other preparations)
	tretinoin (Retin A, Avita)
	other comedogenics (adapalene [Differin], azelaic acid [Azelex], tazorotene [Tazorac])
	topical antibiotics
Systemic	oral antibiotics (erythromycin, tetracycline, clindamycin, doxycycline, minocin, penicillins)
	isotretinoin (Accutane)
	hormones:
	corticosteroids
	high dose for anti-nflammatory action
	low dose to suppress androgenic action
	intralesional for anti-inflammatory action
	antiandrogens
	oral contraceptives (women only)
Surgical	extraction of comedo contents
	drainage of pustules and cysts
	excision of sinus tracts and cysts
	intralesional corticosteroids for anti-inflammatory action
	cryotherapy
	dermabrasion for scars
	laser resurfacing of scars

Treatments listed are common but do not include all available forms of therapy.

associated with a flare-up of acne, such as chocolate, cola, fried foods, or milk products, should be promoted. Maintenance of good nutrition equips the immune system for effective action against bacteria and infection.

For mild cases of acne, washing twice each day with a cleansing soap may be all that is required. Oil-free cosmetics and creams should be chosen. These products are usually designated as useful for acne-prone skin.

Pharmacologic Therapy

Topical Therapy

Over-the-counter acne medications contain either salicylic acid or benzoyl peroxide, both of which are very effective at removing the sebaceous follicular plugs. However, the skin of some people is sensitive to these products, which can cause irritation or excessive dryness, especially when used with some prescribed topical medications. The patient should be instructed to discontinue use of the product if severe irritation occurs.

Benzoyl peroxide preparations are widely used because they produce a rapid and sustained reduction of inflammatory lesions. They depress sebum production and promote breakdown of comedo plugs and have an antibacterial effect. Initially, benzoyl peroxide causes redness and scaling, but the skin usually adjusts quickly to its use. Typically, the patient applies a gel of benzoyl peroxide once daily. In many instances, this is the only treatment needed. Benzoyl peroxide, benzoyl erythromycin (Benzamycin), and benzoyl sulfur (Sulfoxyl) are available over the counter and by prescription.

Vitamin A acid (tretinoin) applied topically is used to clear the keratin plugs from the pilosebaceous ducts. The patient should be informed that symptoms may worsen during early weeks of therapy because inflammation, erythema, and peeling may occur. The patient is cautioned against sun exposure while using this topical medication because it may cause an exaggerated sunburn. Package insert directions should be followed carefully. Improvement may take 8 to 12 weeks.

Topical antibiotic treatment for acne is common. Topical antibiotics suppress bacterial growth; reduce superficial free fatty acid levels; decrease comedones, papules, and pustules; and produce no systemic side effects.

Systemic Therapy

Oral antibiotics administered in small doses over a long period are very effective in treating moderate and severe acne, especially when the acne is inflammatory and results in pustules, abscesses, and scarring. Therapy may continue for months to years. The tetracycline family of antibiotics is contraindicated in children younger than 12 years and in pregnant women. Administration during pregnancy can affect the development of teeth, causing enamel hypoplasia and permanent discoloration of teeth in infants. Side effects of tetracyclines include photosensitivity, nausea, diarrhea, cutaneous infection in either gender, and vaginitis in women. In some women, broad-spectrum antibiotics may suppress normal vaginal bacteria and predispose the patient to candidiasis, a fungal infection.

Synthetic vitamin A compounds (ie, retinoids) are used with dramatic results in patients with nodular cystic acne unresponsive to conventional therapy. One compound is isotretinoin, which is used for active inflammatory papular pustular acne that has a tendency to scar. Isotretinoin reduces sebaceous gland size and inhibits sebum production. It also causes the epidermis to shed (epidermal desquamation), thereby unseating and expelling existing comedones.

The most common side effect, experienced by almost all patients, is **cheilitis** (inflammation of the lips). Dry and chafed skin and mucous membranes are frequent side effects. These changes are reversible with the withdrawal of the medication. Most important, isotretinoin, like other vitamin A metabolites, is teratogenic in humans, meaning that it can have an adverse effect on a fetus. Effective contraceptive measures for women of childbearing age are mandatory during treatment and for about 4 to 8 weeks thereafter. To avoid additive toxic effects, patients are cautioned not to take vitamin A supplements while taking isotretinoin.

Estrogen therapy (including progesterone–estrogen preparations) suppresses sebum production and reduces skin oiliness. It is usually reserved for young women when the acne begins somewhat later than usual and tends to flare up at certain times in the menstrual cycle. Estrogen-dominant oral contraceptive compounds may be administered on a prescribed cyclic regimen. Estrogen is not administered to male patients because of undesirable side effects such as enlargement of the breasts and decrease in body hair.

Surgical Management

Treatment includes comedo extraction, injections of corticosteroids into the inflamed lesions, and incision and drainage of large, fluctuant (moving in palpable waves), nodular cystic lesions. Cryosurgery (freezing with liquid nitrogen) may be used for nodular and cystic forms of acne. Patients with deep scars may be treated with deep abrasive therapy (dermabrasion), in which the epidermis and some superficial dermis are removed down to the level of the scars.

Comedones may be removed with a comedo extractor. The site is first cleaned with alcohol. The opening of the extractor is then placed over the lesion, and direct pressure is applied to cause extrusion of the plug through the extractor. Removal of comedones leads to erythema, which may take several weeks to subside. Recurrence of comedones after extraction is common.

Nursing Management

Nursing care of patients with acne consists largely of monitoring and managing potential complications of skin treatments. Major nursing activities include patient education, particularly in proper skin care techniques, and managing potential problems related to the skin disorder or therapy. Providing positive reassurance, listening attentively, and being sensitive to the feelings of the patient with acne are essential for the patient's psychological well-being and understanding of the disease and treatment plan.

Preventing Scarring

Prevention of scarring is the ultimate goal of therapy. The chance of scarring increases with the severity of the grade of acne. Severe acne (25 to more than 50 comedones, papules, or pustules) usually requires longer-term therapy with systemic antibiotics or isotretinoin. Patients should be warned that discontinuing these medications can lead to more flare-ups and increase the chance of deep scarring. Furthermore, manipulation of the comedones, papules, and pustules increases the potential for scarring.

When acne surgery is prescribed to extract deep-seated comedones or inflamed lesions or to incise and drain cystic lesions, the intervention itself may result in further scarring. Dermabrasion, which levels existing scar tissue, can also increase scar formation. Hyperpigmentation or hypopigmentation also may affect the tissue involved. The patient should be informed of these potential outcomes before choosing surgical intervention for acne.

Promoting Home and Community-Based Care

Teaching Patients Self-Care

In addition to instructions for taking prescribed medications, patients are instructed to wash the face and other affected areas with mild soap and water twice each day to remove surface oils and prevent obstruction of the oil glands. Mild abrasive soaps and drying agents are prescribed to eliminate the oily feeling that troubles many patients. At the same time, patients are cautioned to avoid excessive abrasion because it makes acne worse.

All forms of friction and trauma are avoided, including propping the hands against the face, rubbing the face, and wearing tight collars and helmets. Patients are instructed to avoid manipulation of pimples or blackheads. Squeezing merely worsens the problem, because a portion of the blackhead is pushed down into the skin, which may cause the follicle to rupture. Because cosmetics, shaving creams, and lotions can aggravate acne, these substances are best avoided unless the patient is advised otherwise.

INFECTIOUS DERMATOSES

Bacterial Skin Infections

Also called **pyodermas,** pus-forming bacterial infections of the skin may be primary or secondary. Primary skin infections originate in previously normal-appearing skin and are usually caused by a single organism. Secondary skin infections arise from a preexisting skin disorder or from disruption of the skin integrity from injury or surgery. In either case, several microorganisms may be implicated (eg, *Staphylococcus aureus*, group A streptococci). The most common primary bacterial skin infections are impetigo and folliculitis. Folliculitis may lead to furuncles or carbuncles.

IMPETIGO

Impetigo is a superficial infection of the skin caused by staphylococci, streptococci, or multiple bacteria. Bullous impetigo, a more deep-seated infection of the skin caused by *S. aureus*, is characterized by the formation of bullae (large, fluid-filled blisters) from original vesicles. The bullae rupture, leaving raw, red areas.

The exposed areas of the body, face, hands, neck, and extremities are most frequently involved. Impetigo is contagious and may spread to other parts of the patient's skin or to other members of the family who touch the patient or use towels or combs that are soiled with the exudate of the lesions.

Impetigo is seen in people of all ages. It is particularly common in children living in poor hygienic conditions. It often follows pediculosis capitis (head lice), scabies (itch mites), herpes simplex, insect bites, poison ivy, or eczema. Chronic health problems, poor hygiene, and malnutrition may predispose an adult to impetigo. There is some indication that excessive use of antibacterial soaps may create resistant bacteria and contribute to the problem.

Clinical Manifestations

The lesions of impetigo begin as small, red macules, which quickly become discrete, thin-walled vesicles that rupture and become covered with a loosely adherent honey-yellow crust (Fig. 56-1). These crusts are easily removed to reveal smooth, red, moist surfaces on which new crusts soon develop. If the scalp is involved, the hair is matted, which distinguishes the condition from ringworm.

Medical Management

Systemic antibiotic therapy is the usual treatment. It reduces contagious spread, treats deep infection, and prevents acute glomerulonephritis (kidney infection), which may occur as a consequence of streptococcal skin diseases. In non-bullous impetigo, benzathine penicillin or oral penicillin may be prescribed. In bullous impetigo, a penicillinase-resistant penicillin (eg, cloxacillin [Cloxapen], dicloxacillin [Dycill]) may be used. In penicillin-allergic patients, erythromycin is an effective alternative.

Topical antibacterial therapy (eg, mupirocin [Bactroban]) may be prescribed when the disease is limited to a small area. The medication must be applied to the lesions several times daily for a week; this treatment regimen may be impossible for some patients or their caregivers to follow. Topical antibiotics generally are not as effective as systemic therapy in eradicating or preventing the spread of streptococci from the respiratory tract, thereby increasing the risk of developing glomerulonephritis.

When topical therapy is prescribed, lesions are soaked or washed with soap solution to remove the central site of bacterial growth, giving the topical antibiotic an opportunity to reach the infected site. After the crusts are removed, a topical antibiotic cream is applied. Gloves are worn when providing patient care. An antiseptic solution, such as povidone iodine (Betadine), may be used to clean the skin,

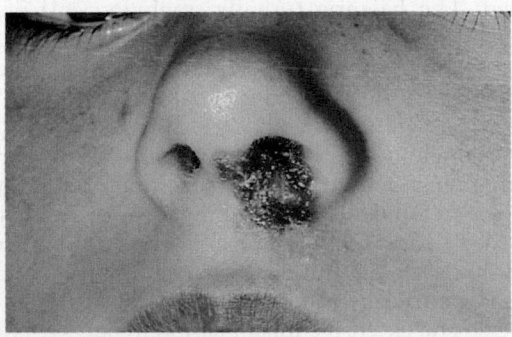

Figure 56-1 Impetigo of the nostril.

reduce bacterial content in the infected area, and prevent spread.

Nursing Management

The nurse instructs the patient and family members to bathe at least once daily with bactericidal soap. Cleanliness and good hygiene practices help prevent the spread of the lesions from one skin area to another and from one person to another. Each person should have a separate towel and washcloth. Because impetigo is a contagious disorder, infected people should avoid contact with other people until the lesions heal.

FOLLICULITIS, FURUNCLES, AND CARBUNCLES

Folliculitis is an infection of bacterial or fungal origin that arises within the hair follicles. Lesions may be superficial or deep. Single or multiple papules or pustules appear close to the hair follicles. Folliculitis commonly affects the beard area of men who shave, as well as women's legs, if they shave. Other areas include the axillae, trunk, and buttocks. Follicular disorders are usually caused by staphylococci, although if the immune system is impaired, the causative organisms may be gram-negative bacilli.

Pseudofolliculitis barbae (shaving bumps) occur predominately on the faces of African American and other curly haired men as a result of shaving. The sharp ingrowing hairs have a curved root that grows at a more acute angle and pierces the skin, provoking an irritative reaction. The only entirely effective treatment is to avoid shaving. Other treatments include using special lotions or antibiotics or using a hand brush to dislodge the hairs mechanically. If the patient must remove facial hair, a depilatory cream or electric razor may be used.

A **furuncle** (boil) is an acute inflammation arising deep in one or more hair follicles and spreading into the surrounding dermis. This inflammation is a deep form of folliculitis. Furunculosis refers to multiple or recurrent lesions. Furuncles may occur anywhere on the body but are more prevalent in areas subjected to irritation, pressure, friction, and excessive perspiration, such as the back of the neck, the axillae, and the buttocks.

A furuncle may start as a small, red, raised, painful pimple. Frequently, the infection progresses and involves the skin and subcutaneous fatty tissue, causing tenderness, pain, and surrounding cellulitis. The area of redness and induration represents an effort of the body to keep the infection localized. The bacteria (usually staphylococci) produce necrosis of the invaded tissue. The characteristic pointing of a boil follows in a few days. When this occurs, the center becomes yellow or black, and the boil is said to have "come to a head."

A **carbuncle** is an abscess of the skin and subcutaneous tissue that represents an extension of a furuncle that has invaded several follicles and is large and deep seated. It is usually caused by a staphylococcal infection. Carbuncles appear most commonly in areas where the skin is thick and inelastic; the back of the neck and the buttocks are common sites. The extensive inflammation frequently prevents a complete walling off of the infection; purulent material

may be absorbed, resulting in high fever, pain, leukocytosis, and even extension of the infection to the bloodstream.

Furuncles and carbuncles are more likely to occur in patients with underlying systemic diseases, such as diabetes or hematologic malignancies, and in those receiving immunosuppressive therapy for other diseases. Both are more prevalent in hot climates, especially on skin beneath occlusive clothing.

Medical Management

In treating staphylococcal infections, it is important not to rupture or destroy the protective wall of induration that localizes the infection. The boil or pimple should never be squeezed. Systemic antibiotic therapy, selected by culture and sensitivity study, is generally indicated. Oral cloxacillin and dicloxacillin are first-line medications. Cephalosporins and erythromycin are also effective. To promote comfort, bed rest is advised for patients who have boils on the perineum or in the anal region, and a course of systemic antibiotic therapy is indicated to prevent the spread of the infection.

When the pus has localized and is fluctuant, a small incision with a scalpel can speed resolution by relieving the tension and ensuring direct evacuation of the pus and debris. The patient is instructed to keep the draining lesion covered with a dressing.

Nursing Management

Intravenous (IV) fluids, fever reduction, and other supportive treatments are indicated for patients who are acutely ill from infection. Warm, moist compresses hasten resolution of the furuncle or carbuncle. The surrounding skin may be cleaned gently with antibacterial soap, and an antibacterial ointment may be applied. Soiled dressings are handled according to standard precautions. Nursing personnel should carefully follow standard precautions to avoid becoming carriers of staphylococci. Disposable gloves are worn when caring for these patients.

 NURSING ALERT

Nurses must take special precautions in caring for boils on the face because the skin area drains directly into the cranial venous sinuses. Sinus thrombosis with fatal pyemia can develop after manipulating a boil in this location. The infection can travel through the sinus tract and penetrate the brain cavity, causing a brain abscess.

Promoting Home And Community-Based Care

Teaching Patients Self-Care

To prevent and control staphylococcal skin infections such as boils and carbuncles, the staphylococcal pathogen must be eliminated from the skin and environment. Efforts must be made to increase the patient's resistance and provide a hygienic environment. If lesions are actively draining, the mattress and pillow should be covered with plastic material and wiped with disinfectant daily; the bed linens, towels, and clothing should be laundered after each use; and the patient should use an antibacterial soap and shampoo for an indefinite period, often several months.

Recurrent infection is prevented with the use of long-term antibiotic therapy (longer than about 3 months). The patient must take the full dose for the time prescribed. The purulent exudate is a source of reinfection or transmission of infection to caregivers. If the patient has a history of recurrent infections, a carrier state may exist, which should be investigated and treated with an antibacterial cream such as mupirocin (Bactroban).

Viral Skin Infections

HERPES ZOSTER

Herpes zoster, also called shingles, is an infection caused by the varicella-zoster viruses (VZVs), members of a group of DNA viruses. The viruses that cause chickenpox (varicella) and herpes zoster are indistinguishable, hence the two-part name. The disease is characterized by a painful vesicular eruption along the area of distribution of the sensory nerves from one or more posterior ganglia. After a case of chickenpox runs its course, the VZV responsible for the outbreak lies dormant inside nerve cells near the brain and spinal cord. Later, when these latent viruses are reactivated because of declining cellular immunity, they travel by way of the peripheral nerves to the skin, where the viruses multiply and create a red rash of small, fluid-filled blisters.

It is thought that during the aging process, natural immunity to the varicella wanes, allowing the virus to reactivate and maintaining it in the population. Herpes zoster develops in about 10% of adults during their lifetimes, usually after 50 years of age; the disease develops in as many as 50% of people by 85 years of age. These episodes tend to be localized and have few sequelae. Compared with Caucasians, African Americans are affected by herpes zoster much less frequently; however, if they do develop the disease, they often have it at a younger age. There is an increased frequency of herpes zoster infections in patients with weakened immune systems, including those with human immunodeficiency virus (HIV) infection and in those with cancer. In these patients, the infection can become widespread and cause significant complications.

Clinical Manifestations

The eruption is usually accompanied or preceded by pain, which may radiate over the entire region supplied by the affected nerves. The pain may be burning, lancinating (tearing or sharply cutting), stabbing, or aching. Some patients have no pain, but itching and tenderness may occur over the area. Malaise and gastrointestinal disturbances may precede the eruption. The patches of grouped vesicles appear on the red and swollen skin. The early vesicles, which contain serum, later may become purulent, rupture, and form crusts. The inflammation is usually unilateral, involving the thoracic, cervical, or cranial nerves in a bandlike configuration. The blisters are usually confined to a narrow region of the face or trunk (Fig. 56-2). The clinical course varies from 1 to 3 weeks. If an ophthalmic nerve is involved, the patient may have eye pain. Inflammation and a rash on the trunk

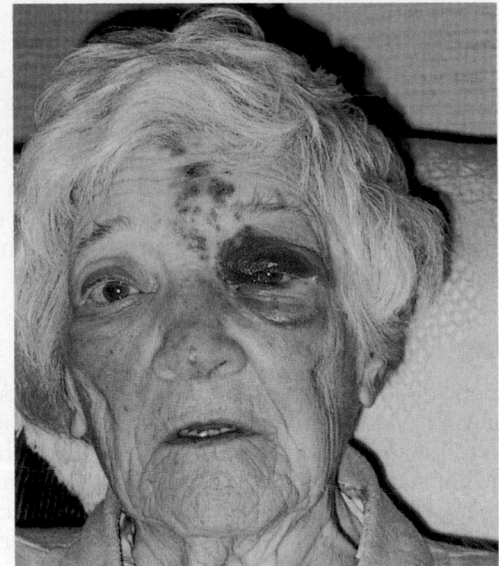

Figure 56-2 Herpes zoster (shingles).

may cause pain with the slightest touch. The healing time varies from 7 to 26 days.

The most common complication of herpes zoster is postherpetic neuralgia, which occurs in approximately 20% of cases, becoming more common in the elderly. Fifty percent of patients older than 60 years of age have persistent pain that lasts longer than 6 months (High, 2005).

Medical Management

Herpes zoster infection can be arrested if oral antiviral agents such as acyclovir (Zovirax), valacyclovir (Valtrex), or famciclovir (Famvir) are administered within 24 hours of the initial eruption. IV acyclovir, if started early, is effective in significantly reducing the pain and halting the progression of the disease. In older patients, the pain from herpes zoster may persist as postherpetic neuralgia for months after the skin lesions disappear.

The goals of herpes zoster management are to relieve the pain and to reduce or avoid complications, which include infection, scarring, and postherpetic neuralgia and eye complications. Pain is controlled with analgesics because adequate pain control during the acute phase helps prevent persistent pain patterns. Systemic corticosteroids may be prescribed for patients older than 50 years of age to reduce the incidence and duration of postherpetic neuralgia (persistent pain of the affected nerve after healing). Healing usually occurs more quickly in those who have been treated with corticosteroids. Triamcinolone (Aristocort, Kenacort, Kenalog) injected subcutaneously under painful areas is effective as an anti-inflammatory agent.

Ophthalmic herpes zoster occurs when an eye is involved. This is considered an ophthalmic emergency, and the patient should be referred to an ophthalmologist immediately to prevent the possible sequelae of keratitis, uveitis, ulceration, and blindness.

People who have been exposed to varicella by primary infection or by vaccination are not at risk for infection after exposure to patients with herpes zoster.

A vaccination for childhood varicella developed in the 1970s has been used successfully to decrease the incidence of childhood disease. A more potent formulation of the vaccine was developed to boost VZV cellular immunity in people older than 55 years of age. Studies have shown favorable results with very few side effects. One large study by the Veterans Administration showed a reduction in incidence of VZV infections by almost 50% in 60- to 69-year-old participants. This vaccination is now being recommended as part of prevention strategies in older adults (High, 2005).

Nursing Management

The patient and family members are instructed about the importance of taking antiviral agents as prescribed and in keeping follow-up appointments with the health care provider. The nurse assesses the patient's discomfort and response to medication and collaborates with the physician to make necessary adjustments to the treatment regimen. The patient is taught how to apply wet dressings or medication to the lesions and to follow proper hand hygiene techniques to avoid spreading the virus.

Diversionary activities and relaxation techniques are encouraged to ensure restful sleep and to alleviate discomfort. A caregiver may be required to assist with dressings, particularly if the patient is elderly and unable to apply them. Food preparation for patients who cannot care for themselves or prepare nourishing meals must be arranged.

HERPES SIMPLEX

Herpes simplex is a common skin infection. There are two types of the causative virus, which are identified by viral typing. Generally, herpes simplex type 1 occurs on the mouth and type 2 occurs in the genital area, but both viral types can be found in both locations. About 85% of adults worldwide are seropositive for herpes type 1. The prevalence of type 2 is lower; type 2 usually appears at the onset of sexual activity. Serologic testing shows that many more people are infected than have a history of clinical disease.

Herpes simplex is classified as a true primary infection, a nonprimary initial episode, or a recurrent episode. True primary infection is the initial exposure to the virus. A nonprimary initial episode is the initial episode of either type 1 or type 2 in a person previously infected with the other type. Recurrent episodes are subsequent episodes of the same viral type.

Types of Herpes Simplex

Orolabial Herpes

Orolabial herpes, also called fever blisters or cold sores, consists of erythematous-based clusters of grouped vesicles on the lips. A prodrome of tingling or burning with pain may precede the appearance of the vesicles by up to 24 hours. Certain triggers, such as sunlight exposure or increased stress, may cause recurrent episodes. Fewer than 1% of people with primary orolabial herpes infections develop herpetic gingivostomatitis. This complication occurs more often in children and young adults than in people of other ages. The onset is often accompanied by high fever, regional lymphadenopathy, and generalized malaise. Another com-

plication of orolabial herpes is the development of erythema multiforme, an acute inflammation of the skin and mucous membranes with characteristic lesions that have the appearance of targets (ie, concentric red rings with white bands between the red rings).

Genital Herpes

Genital herpes, or type 2 herpes simplex, manifests with a broad spectrum of clinical signs. Minor infections may produce no symptoms at all; severe primary infections with type 1 can cause systemic flulike illness. Lesions appear as grouped vesicles on an erythematous base initially involving the vagina, rectum, or penis. New lesions can continue to appear for 7 to 14 days. Lesions are symmetric and usually cause regional lymphadenopathy. Fever and flulike symptoms are common. Typical recurrences begin with a prodrome of burning, tingling, or itching about 24 hours before the vesicles appear. As the vesicles rupture, erosions and ulcerations begin to appear. Severe infections can cause extensive erosions of the vaginal or anal canal. For further information, see Chapter 47.

Assessment and Diagnostic Findings

Herpes simplex infections are confirmed in several ways. Generally, the appearance of the skin eruption is strongly suggestive. Viral cultures and rapid assays are available, and the type of test used depends on lesion morphology. Acute vesicular lesions are more likely to react positively to the rapid assay, whereas older, crusted patches are better diagnosed with viral culture. In all cases, it is imperative to obtain enough viral cells for testing, and careful collection methods are therefore important. All crusts should be gently removed or vesicles gently unroofed. A sterile cotton swab premoistened in viral culture preservative is used to swab the base of the vesicle to obtain a specimen for analysis.

Complications

Eczema herpeticum is a condition in which patients with eczema contract herpes that spreads throughout the eczematous areas. The same type of spread of herpes can occur in severe seborrhea, scabies, and other chronic skin conditions. Eczema herpeticum is managed with oral or IV acyclovir.

Herpetic whitlow is an infection of the pulp of a fingertip with herpes type 1 or 2. There is tenderness and erythema of the cuticle. Deep-seated vesicles appear within 24 hours.

In mothers who have primary infections during pregnancy, intrauterine neonatal infections can occur. Most cases of neonatal infection with herpes occur during delivery by contact of the infant with the mother's active ulcerations. Fetal anomalies include skin lesions, microcephaly, encephalitis, and intracerebral calcifications.

Medical Management

In many patients, recurrent orolabial herpes represents more of a nuisance than a disease. Because sun exposure is a common trigger, people with recurrent orolabial herpes should use a sunscreen liberally on the lips and face. Topical treatment with drying agents may accelerate healing. In more severe outbreaks or in patients with identified triggers, intermittent treatment with 200 mg acyclovir administered five times each day for 5 days is often started as soon as the earliest symptoms occur.

Treatment of genital herpes depends on the severity, the frequency, and the psychological impact of recurrences and on the infectious status of the sexual partner. For people who have mild or rare outbreaks, no treatment may be required. For those who have more severe outbreaks, but for whom outbreaks are still infrequent, intermittent treatment as described for oral lesions can be used. Use of intermittent oral medication has been shown to reduce the duration of herpes genital infections by only 24 to 36 hours. If a patient is using intermittent treatment for infrequent episodes, the medication should be initiated within the first 24 hours after the infection is identified.

Patients who have more than six recurrences per year may benefit from suppressive therapy. Use of acyclovir, valacyclovir, or famciclovir suppresses 85% of recurrences, and 20% of patients are free of recurrences during suppressive therapy. Suppressive therapy also reduces viral shedding by almost 95%, making the person less contagious. Treatment with suppressive doses of oral antiviral medications prevents recurrent erythema multiforme (acute eruption of macules, papules, and vesicles with a multiform appearance).

Management of genital herpes in pregnancy differs among clinicians. Routine prenatal cultures do not predict shedding at the time of delivery. The use of scalp electrodes during delivery should be avoided because they increase the risk of infection in the newborn. Because the risk of neonatal herpes is greater in women with their initial episode during pregnancy, suppression therapy should be started in affected women to reduce outbreaks during the third trimester. All women with active lesions at the time of delivery undergo cesarean section.

In immunocompromised patients, suppression therapy should be considered. In severe infections of hospitalized patients, IV acyclovir is prescribed.

Fungal (Mycotic) Skin Infections

Fungi, tiny members of a subdivision of the plant kingdom that thrive on organic matter, cause various common skin infections. In some cases, they affect only the skin and its appendages (hair and nails). In other cases, internal organs are involved, and the diseases may be life-threatening. However, superficial infections rarely cause even temporary disability and respond readily to treatment. Secondary infection with bacteria, *Candida*, or both organisms may occur.

The most common fungal skin infection is **tinea,** which is also called ringworm because of its characteristic appearance of a ring or rounded tunnel under the skin. Tinea infections affect the head, body, groin, feet, and nails. Table 56-5 summarizes the tinea infections.

To obtain a specimen for diagnosis, the lesion is cleaned and a scalpel or glass slide is used to remove scales from the margin of the lesion. The scales are dropped onto a slide to which potassium hydroxide has been added. The diagnosis is made by examination of the infected scales microscopically for spores and hyphae or by isolating the organism in

Table 56-5 TINEA (RINGWORM) INFECTIONS		
Type and Location	**Clinical Manifestations**	**Treatment**
Tinea capitis (head) Contagious fungal infection of the hair shaft	• Common in children • Oval, scaling, erythematous patches • Small papules or pustules on the scalp • Brittle hair that breaks easily	• Griseofulvin for 6 weeks • Shampoo hair two or three times with Nizoral or selenium sulfide shampoo
Tinea corporis (body)	• Begins with red macule, which spreads to a ring of papules or vesicles with central clearing • Lesions found in clusters • Many spread to the hair, scalp, or nails • Very pruritic • An infected pet may be the source	• Mild conditions: topical antifungal creams • Severe conditions: griseofulvin or terbinafine
Tinea cruris (groin area; "jock itch")	• Begins with small, red scaling patches, which spread to form circular elevated plaques • Very pruritic • Clusters of pustules may be seen around borders	• Mild conditions: topical antifungal creams • Severe conditions: griseofulvin or terbinafine
Tinea pedis (foot; "athlete's foot")	• Soles of one or both feet have scaling and mild redness with maceration in the toe webs • More acute infections may have clusters of clear vesicles on dusky base	• Soak feet in vinegar and water solution • Resistant infections: griseofulvin or terbinafine • Terbinafine (Lamisil) daily for 3 months
Tinea ungum (toenails; affects about 50% of adults)	• Nails thicken, crumble easily, and lack luster • Whole nail may be destroyed	• Itraconazole (Sporanox) in pulses of 1 week a month for 3 months in cases of terbinafine failure

culture. Under Wood's light, a specimen of infected hair appears fluorescent; this may be helpful in diagnosing some cases of tinea capitis.

Parasitic Skin Infestations

These conditions include infestations of the skin by lice (pediculosis) and the itch mite (scabies).

PEDICULOSIS: LICE INFESTATION

Lice infestation affects people of all ages. Three varieties of lice infest humans: *Pediculus humanus capitis* (head louse), *Pediculus humanus corporis* (body louse), and *Phthirus pubis* (pubic louse or crab louse). Lice are called ectoparasites because they live on the outside of the host's body. They depend on the host for their nourishment, feeding on human blood approximately five times each day. They inject their digestive juices and excrement into the skin, which causes severe itching.

Types of Pediculosis

Pediculosis Capitis

Pediculosis capitis is an infestation of the scalp by the head louse. The female louse lays her eggs (nits) close to the scalp. The nits become firmly attached to the hair shafts with a tenacious substance. The young lice hatch in about 10 days and reach maturity in 2 weeks. Head lice may be transmitted directly by physical contact or indirectly by infested combs, brushes, wigs, hats, and bedding.

Pediculosis Corporis and Pubis

Pediculosis corporis is an infestation of the body by the body louse. This is a disease of unwashed people or those who live in close quarters and do not change their clothing (eg, survivors of natural disasters such as hurricanes, floods, and earthquakes who must live with others in temporary housing without access to running water and clean clothes). Pediculosis pubis is extremely common. The infestation is generally localized in the genital region and is transmitted chiefly by sexual contact.

Clinical Manifestations

Head lice are found most commonly along the back of the head and behind the ears. To the naked eye, the eggs look like silvery, glistening oval bodies. The bite of the insect causes intense pruritus, and the resultant scratching often leads to secondary bacterial infection, such as impetigo or furunculosis. The infestation is more common in children and people with long hair.

With body lice, the areas of the skin that come in closest contact with the underclothing (ie, neck, trunk, and thighs) are chiefly involved. The body louse lives primarily in the seams of underwear and clothing, to which it clings as it pierces the skin with its proboscis. Its bites cause characteristic minute hemorrhagic points. Widespread excoriation may appear as a result of intense pruritus and scratching, especially on the trunk and neck. Among the secondary lesions produced are parallel linear scratches and a slight degree of eczema. In long-standing cases, the skin may become thick, dry, and scaly, with dark pigmented areas.

Pruritus, particularly at night, is the most common symptom of pediculosis pubis. Reddish-brown dust (ie, excretions of the insects) may be found in the patient's underclothing. The pubic area should be examined with a magnifying glass for lice crawling down a hair shaft or nits cemented to the hair or at the junction with the skin. Infestation by pubic lice may coexist with sexually transmitted diseases such as gonorrhea, herpes, or syphilis. There may also be infestation of the hairs of the chest, axillae, beard, and eyelashes. Gray-blue macules may sometimes be seen on the trunk, thighs, and axillae as a result of either the reaction of the insects' saliva with bilirubin (converting it to biliverdin) or an excretion produced by the salivary glands of the louse.

Medical Management

Treatment of head lice involves washing the hair with a shampoo containing lindane (Kwell) or pyrethrin compounds with piperonyl butoxide (RID or R&C Shampoo). The patient is instructed to shampoo the scalp and hair according to the product directions. After the hair is rinsed thoroughly, it is combed with a fine-toothed comb dipped in vinegar to remove any remaining nits or nit shells freed from the hair shafts. They are extremely difficult to remove and may have to be picked off one by one.

All articles, clothing, towels, and bedding that may have lice or nits should be washed in hot water—at least 54°C (130°F)—or dry cleaned to prevent reinfestation. Upholstered furniture, rugs, and floors should be vacuumed frequently. Combs and brushes are also disinfected with the shampoo. All family members and close contacts are treated. Complications such as severe pruritus, pyoderma, and dermatitis are treated with antipruritics, systemic antibiotics, and topical corticosteroids.

The patient with body lice is instructed to bathe with soap and water, after which a prescription scabicide (lindane or 5% permethrin [Elimite]) is applied to affected areas of the skin and to hairy areas, according to the product directions. An alternative topical therapy is an over-the-counter strength of permethrin (1% Nix). If the eyelashes are involved, petrolatum may be thickly applied twice daily for 8 days, followed by mechanical removal of any remaining nits.

Complications, such as severe pruritus, pyoderma, and dermatitis, are treated with antipruritics, systemic antibiotics, and topical corticosteroids. Body lice can transmit epidemic rickettsial disease (eg, epidemic typhus, relapsing fever, and trench fever) to humans. The causative organism may be in the gastrointestinal tract of the insect and may be excreted on the skin surface of the infested person.

Nursing Management

The nurse informs the patient that head lice may infest anyone and are not a sign of uncleanliness. Because the condition spreads rapidly, treatment must be started immediately. School epidemics may be managed by having all of the students shampoo their hair on the same night. Students should be warned not to share combs, brushes, and hats. Each family member should be inspected for head lice daily for at least 2 weeks. The patient should be instructed that lindane may be toxic to the central nervous system when used more frequently or for longer periods of time than specified in the package insert.

Treatment is necessary for all family members and sexual contacts of patients with body and/or pubic lice. The nurse instructs them about personal hygiene and methods to prevent or control infestation. The patient and partner must also be scheduled for a diagnostic workup for coexisting sexually transmitted disease.

SCABIES

Scabies is an infestation of the skin by the itch mite *Sarcoptes scabiei*. The disease may be found in people living in substandard hygienic conditions, but it can occur in anyone. Infestations may or may not be associated with sexual activity. The mites frequently involve the fingers, and hand contact may produce infection. In children, overnight stays with friends or the exchange of clothes may be a source of infection. Health care personnel who have prolonged hands-on physical contact with an infected patient may become infected.

Clinical Manifestations

It takes approximately 4 weeks from the time of contact for the patient's symptoms to appear. The patient complains of severe itching caused by a delayed type of immunologic reaction to the mite or its fecal pellets. During examination, the patient is asked where the pruritus is most severe. A magnifying glass and a penlight are held at an oblique angle to the skin while a search is made for the small, raised burrows created by the mites. The burrows may be multiple, straight or wavy, brown or black, threadlike lesions, most commonly observed between the fingers and on the wrists. Other sites are the extensor surfaces of the elbows, the knees, the edges of the feet, the points of the elbows, around the nipples, in the axillary folds, under pendulous breasts, and in or near the groin or gluteal fold, penis, or scrotum. Red, pruritic eruptions usually appear between adjacent skin areas. However, the burrow is not always visible. Any patient with a rash may have scabies.

One classic sign of scabies is the increased itching that occurs during the overnight hours, perhaps because the increased warmth of the skin has a stimulating effect on the parasite. Hypersensitivity to the organism and its products of excretion also may contribute to the pruritus. If the infection has spread, other members of the family and close friends also complain of pruritus about 1 month later.

Secondary lesions are quite common and include vesicles, papules, excoriations, and crusts. Bacterial superinfection may result from constant excoriation of the burrows and papules.

 ### Gerontologic Considerations

Elderly patients living in long-term care facilities are susceptible to outbreaks of scabies because of close living quarters, poor hygiene due to limited physical ability, and the potential for incidental spread of the organisms by staff members. Although pruritus may be severe in the older patient, the vivid inflammatory reaction seen in younger people seldom occurs. Scabies may not be recognized in the elderly person; the pruritus may erroneously be attributed to the dry skin of old age or to anxiety.

Health care personnel in extended-care facilities should wear gloves when providing hands-on care for a patient suspected of having scabies until the diagnosis is confirmed and treatment completed. It is advisable to treat all residents, staff, and families of patients at the same time to prevent reinfection. Because geriatric patients may be more sensitive to side effects of the scabicides, they should be closely observed for reactions.

Assessment and Diagnostic Findings

The diagnosis is confirmed by recovering *S. scabiei* or the mites' byproducts from the skin. A sample of superficial epidermis is scraped from the top of the burrows or papules with a small scalpel blade. The scrapings are placed on a microscope slide and examined through a microscope at low power to demonstrate evidence of the mite.

Medical Management

The patient is instructed to take a warm, soapy bath or shower to remove the scaling debris from the crusts and then to dry thoroughly and allow the skin to cool. A prescription scabicide, such as lindane, crotamiton (Eurax), or 5% permethrin, is applied thinly to the entire skin from the neck down, sparing only the face and scalp (which are not affected in scabies). The medication is left on for 12 to 24 hours, after which the patient is instructed to wash thoroughly. One application may be curative, but it is advisable to repeat the treatment in 1 week.

 NURSING ALERT

The patient must understand medication instructions because application of a scabicide immediately after bathing and before the skin dries and cools increases percutaneous absorption of the scabicide and the potential for central nervous system abnormalities such as seizures.

Nursing Management

The patient should wear clean clothing and sleep between freshly laundered bed linens. All bedding and clothing should be washed in hot water and dried on the hot dryer cycle. If bed linens or clothing cannot be washed in hot water, dry cleaning is advised.

After treatment is completed, the patient should apply an ointment, such as a topical corticosteroid, to skin lesions because the scabicide may irritate the skin. The patient's hypersensitivity does not cease on destruction of the mites. Pruritus may continue for several weeks as a manifestation of hypersensitivity, particularly in atopic (allergic) people. This is not a sign that the treatment has failed. The patient is instructed (1) not to apply more scabicide, because it will cause more irritation and increased itching, and (2) not to take frequent hot showers, because they can dry the skin and produce pruritus. Oral antihistamines such as diphenhydramine or hydroxyzine can help control the pruritus.

All family members and close contacts should be treated simultaneously to eliminate the mites. Some scabicides are approved for use in infants and pregnant women. If scabies is sexually transmitted, the patient may require treatment for coexisting sexually transmitted disease. Scabies may also coexist with pediculosis.

CONTACT DERMATITIS

Contact dermatitis is an inflammatory reaction of the skin to physical, chemical, or biologic agents. The epidermis is damaged by repeated physical and chemical irritations. Contact dermatitis may be of the primary irritant type, in which a nonallergic reaction results from exposure to an irritating substance, or it may be an allergic reaction resulting from exposure of sensitized people to contact allergens. Allergic dermatoses are discussed in Chapter 53. Common causes of irritant dermatitis are soaps, detergents, scouring compounds, and industrial chemicals. Predisposing factors include extremes of heat and cold, frequent contact with soap and water, and a preexisting skin disease (Chart 56-3).

Clinical Manifestations

The eruptions begin when the causative agent contacts the skin. The first reactions include pruritus, burning, and erythema, followed closely by edema, papules, vesicles, and oozing or weeping. In the subacute phase, these vesicular changes are less marked, and they alternate with crusting, drying, fissuring, and peeling. If repeated reactions occur or if the patient continually scratches the skin, lichenification and pigmentation occur. Secondary bacterial invasion may follow.

Medical Management

The objectives of management are to soothe and heal the involved skin and protect it from further damage. The distribution pattern of the reaction is identified to differentiate between allergic and irritant contact dermatitis. A detailed history is obtained. If possible, the offending irritant is removed. Local irritation should be avoided, and soap is not generally used until healing occurs.

Many preparations are advocated for relieving dermatitis. In general, a bland, unmedicated lotion is used for small patches of erythema. Cool, wet dressings also are applied over small areas of vesicular dermatitis. Finely cracked ice added to the water often enhances its antipruritic effect.

Wet dressings usually help clear the oozing eczematous lesions. A thin layer of cream or ointment containing a corticosteroid then may be used. Medicated baths at room temperature are prescribed for larger areas of dermatitis. For severe, widespread conditions, a short course of systemic corticosteroids may be prescribed.

NONINFECTIOUS INFLAMMATORY DERMATOSES

Psoriasis

Considered one of the most common skin diseases, psoriasis affects approximately 2% of the population, appearing more often in people of European ancestry. It is thought that this chronic disease stems from a hereditary defect that causes overproduction of keratin. Onset may occur at any age, but psoriasis is most common in people between 15 and 35 years of age. Psoriasis has a tendency to improve and then recur periodically throughout life (Porth & Matfin, 2009).

Pathophysiology

Current evidence supports an immunologic basis for psoriasis (Porth & Matfin, 2009). Periods of emotional stress and anxiety aggravate the condition, and trauma, infections, and seasonal and hormonal changes also are trigger factors.

In this disease, the cells in the basal layer of the skin divide too quickly, and the newly formed cells move so rapidly to the skin surface that they become evident as profuse scales or plaques of epidermal tissue. As a result of the increased number of basal cells and rapid cell passage, the normal events of cell maturation and growth cannot occur, which prevent formation of the normal protective layers of the skin.

Clinical Manifestations

Psoriasis may range in severity from a cosmetic source of annoyance to a physically disabling and disfiguring disorder. Lesions appear as red, raised patches of skin covered with silvery scales. The scaly patches are formed by the buildup of living and dead skin (Fig. 56-3). If the scales are scraped away, the dark-red base of the lesion is exposed, producing multiple bleeding points. The patches are not moist and may be pruritic. In approximately one fourth to one half of patients, the nails are also involved, with pitting, discoloration, crumbling beneath the free edges, and separation of the nail plate.

Bilateral symmetry is a feature of psoriasis. Particular sites of the body affected most by this condition include the scalp, the extensor surface of the elbows and knees, the lower part of the back, and the genitalia, as well as the nails.

Complications

Asymmetric rheumatoid factor–negative arthritis of multiple joints occurs in about 5% of people with psoriasis, before or after the skin lesions appear. Psoriatic arthritis is discussed in more detail later in this chapter.

Erythrodermic psoriasis, an exfoliative psoriatic state, involves disease progression that involves the total body

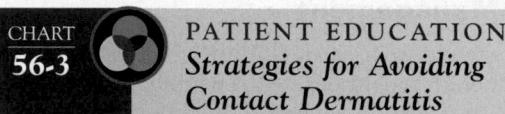

CHART 56-3

PATIENT EDUCATION
Strategies for Avoiding Contact Dermatitis

The following precautions may help prevent repeated cases of contact dermatitis. Follow these instructions for at least 4 months after your skin appears to be completely healed.

- Study the pattern and location of your dermatitis and think about which things have touched your skin and which things may have caused the problem.
- Try to avoid contact with these materials.
- Avoid heat, soap, and rubbing, all of which are external irritants.
- Choose bath soaps, laundry detergents, and cosmetics that do not contain fragrance.
- Avoid using a fabric softener dryer sheet (Bounce, Cling Free). Fabric softeners that are added to the washer may be used.
- Avoid topical medications, lotions, or ointments, except those specifically prescribed for your condition.
- Wash your skin thoroughly immediately after exposure to possible irritants.
- When wearing gloves (for example, for washing dishes or general cleaning), be sure they are cotton-lined. Do not wear them more than 15 or 20 minutes at a time.

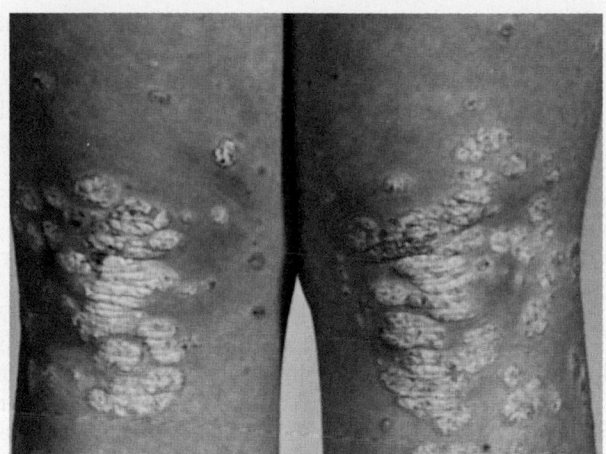

Figure 56-3 Psoriasis. Courtesy of Roche Laboratories.

surface. The patient is acutely ill. Erythrodermic psoriasis often appears in people with chronic psoriasis after infections, after exposure to certain medications, or following withdrawal of systemic corticosteroids.

Assessment and Diagnostic Findings

The presence of the classic plaque-type lesions generally confirms the diagnosis of psoriasis. If in doubt, the health care provider should assess for signs of nail and scalp involvement and for a positive family history. Biopsy of the skin is of little diagnostic value.

Medical Management

The goals of management are to slow the rapid turnover of epidermis, to promote resolution of the psoriatic lesions, and to control the natural cycles of the disease. There is no known cure.

The therapeutic approach should be one that the patient understands; it should be cosmetically acceptable and minimally disruptive of lifestyle. Treatment involves the commitment of time and effort by the patient and possibly the family. Any precipitating or aggravating factors are addressed. An assessment is made of lifestyle because psoriasis is significantly affected by stress. Management of emotional factors should be addressed as part of the overall treatment of psoriasis. Disruption of self-image and depression have been reported in up to 50% of patients with severe psoriasis. The patient is informed that treatment of severe psoriasis can be time-consuming, expensive, and aesthetically unappealing at times. More than 50% of patients report difficulty complying with treatment plans, either for time reasons or lack of response to the treatment.

The most important principle of psoriasis treatment is gentle removal of scales. This can be accomplished with baths. Oils (eg, olive oil, mineral oil, Aveeno Oilated Oatmeal Bath) or coal tar preparations (eg, Balnetar) can be added to the bath water and a soft brush used to scrub the psoriatic plaques gently. After bathing, the application of emollient creams containing alpha-hydroxy acids (eg, Lac-Hydrin, Penederm) or salicylic acid continues to soften thick scales. The patient and family should be encouraged to establish a regular skin care routine that can be maintained even when the psoriasis is not in an acute stage.

Pharmacologic Therapy

With the recent addition of biologic medications, three types of therapy are now commonly used: topical, systemic, and phototherapy (Table 56-6).

Topical Agents

Topically applied agents are used to slow the overactive epidermis. Topical corticosteroids may be applied for their

Table 56-6	CURRENT PHARMACOLOGIC TREATMENT FOR PSORIASIS	
Topical Agents	**Use**	**Selected Agents**
Biologicals	Moderate to severe lesions	Cyclosporine (Neoral), alefacept (Amevive), etanercept (Enbrel), infliximab (Remicade)
Topical corticosteroids	Mild to moderate lesions	Triamcinolone acetonide (Aristocort, Kenalog), bethamethasone valerate (Valisone, Diprosone)
	Moderate to severe lesions	Fluocinonide (Lidex)
	Severe lesions	Clobetasol (Temovate), betamethasone dipropionate (Diprolene), halobetasol (Ultravate)
	Lesions on face and groin	Alclometasome (Aclovate), desonide (DesOwen), hydrocortisone (Hytone 2.5%)
Topical nonsteroidals	Mild to severe	Retinoids such as tazarotene (Tazorac)
		Vitamin D₃ derivative calcipotriene (Dovonex)
Coal tar products	Mild to moderate lesions	Coal tar and salicylic acid ointment (Aquatar, Estar gel, Fototar, Zetar); anthralin (AnthraDerm, Dritho-Cream); Neutrogena T-Derm, Psori Gel
Medicated shampoos	Scalp lesions	Neutrogena T-Gel, T-Sal, Zetar, Head & Shoulders, Desenex, Selsun Blue, Bakers P&S (emulsifying agent with phenol, saline solution, and mineral oil)
Intralesional therapy	Thick plaques and nails	Kenalog, Cordran-impregnated tape, Fluoroplex
Systemic therapy	Extensive lesions and nails	Methotrexate (Folex, Mexate); hydrourea (Hydrea); retinoic acid (Tegison) (not to be used in women of childbearing age)
	Psoriatic arthritis	Oral gold (auranofin), etrentinate, methotrexate
Photochemotherapy	Moderate to severe lesions	UVA or UVB light with or without topical medications
		PUVA (combines UVA light with oral psoralens, or topical tripsoralen)

anti-inflammatory effect. Choosing the correct strength of corticosteroid for the involved site and choosing the most effective vehicle base are important aspects of topical treatment. In general, high-potency topical corticosteroids should not be used on the face and intertriginous areas, and their use on other areas should be limited to a 4-week course of twice-daily applications. A 2-week break should be taken before repeating treatment with the high-potency corticosteroids. For long-term therapy, moderate-potency corticosteroids are used. On the face and intertriginous areas, only low-potency corticosteroids are appropriate for long-term use (see Table 56-3).

Occlusive dressings may be applied to increase the effectiveness of the corticosteroid. Large plastic bags may be used—one for the upper body with openings cut for the head and arms and one for the lower body with openings for the legs. Large rolls of tubular plastic can be used to cover the arms and legs. Another option is a vinyl jogging suit. The medication is applied, and the suit is put on over it. The hands can be wrapped in gloves, the feet in plastic bags, and the head in a shower cap. Occlusive dressings should not remain in place longer than 8 hours. The skin should be inspected carefully for the appearance of atrophy, hypopigmentation, striae, and telangiectasias, all side effects of corticosteroids.

> ◣ **NURSING ALERT**
>
> **When plastic substances are used, the nurse needs to check for flammability. Some thin plastic films burn slowly (if touched by a lighted cigarette), whereas others burst rapidly into flame. The patient should be cautioned not to smoke while wrapped in a plastic dressing.**

When psoriasis involves large areas of the body, topical corticosteroid treatment can be expensive and involve some systemic risk. The more potent corticosteroids, when applied to large areas of the body, have the potential to cause adrenal suppression through percutaneous absorption of the medication. In this event, other treatment modalities (eg, nonsteroidal topical medications, ultraviolet light) may be used instead or in combination to decrease the need for corticosteroids.

Two relatively new topical nonsteroidal treatments are calcipotriene (Dovonex) and tazarotene (Tazorac). Treatment with these agents tends to suppress **epidermopoiesis** (ie, development of epidermal cells) and cause sloughing of the rapidly growing epidermal cells. Calcipotriene 0.05% is a derivative of vitamin D_2. It works by decreasing the mitotic turnover of the psoriatic plaques. Its most common side effect is local irritation. The intertriginous areas and face should be avoided when using this medication. The patient should be monitored for symptoms of hypercalcemia. Calcipotriene is available as a cream for use on the body and a solution for the scalp. It is not recommended for use by elderly patients because of their more fragile skin or by pregnant or lactating women.

Tazarotene, a retinoid, causes sloughing of the scales covering psoriatic plaques. As with other retinoids, it causes increased sensitivity to sunlight by loss of the outermost layer of skin, so the patient should be cautioned to use an effective

sunscreen and avoid other photosensitizers (eg, tetracycline, antihistamines). Tazarotene is listed as a Category X drug in pregnancy; reports indicate evidence of fetal risk, and the risk of use in pregnant women clearly outweighs any possible benefits. A negative result on a pregnancy test should be obtained before initiating this medication in women of childbearing age, and an effective contraceptive should be continued during treatment. Side effects include burning, erythema, or irritation at the site of application and worsening of psoriasis.

Intralesional injections of the corticosteroid triamcinolone acetonide (Aristocort, Kenalog-10, Trymex) can be administered directly into highly visible or isolated patches of psoriasis that are resistant to other forms of therapy. Care must be taken to ensure that the medication is not injected into normal skin.

Systemic Agents

Although systemic corticosteroids may cause rapid improvement of psoriasis, the usual risks and the possibility of triggering a severe flare-up on withdrawal limit their use. Systemic cytotoxic preparations, such as methotrexate, have been used in treating extensive psoriasis that fails to respond to other forms of therapy.

Biological Agents. The newest line of treatments for psoriasis includes a group called biologics because of their derivation from immunomodulators and bioengineered proteins (such as antibodies or recombinant cytokines) and their targeted action directly on the T cells. These agents act by inhibiting activation and migration, eliminating the T cells completely, slowing postsecretory cytokines or inducing immune deviation. Five biologics are approved by the U.S. Food and Drug Administration (FDA) for treatment of moderate to severe psoriasis with or without psoriatic arthritis. They are administered either intravenously or subcutaneously, and patients must have the ability and motivation to self-administer injections.

Because of suppressed immune status, live vaccines could trigger full-blown disease in susceptible patients. Discussion with an infectious disease specialist is recommended. Some biological agents are designated as pregnancy Category B; all are secreted in breast milk (Pirzada, Tomi & Gulliver, 2007).

Infliximab (Remicade) is a monoclonal antibody that binds to tumor necrosis factor-α (TNF-α) and can only be administered by IV infusion. Etanercept (Enbrel) is a fusion protein that binds to soluble TNF-α and blocks its interaction with cell surface receptors. Efalizumab (Raptiva) is a murine antibody that inhibits T-cell activation and adherence to keratinocytes. Alefacept (Amevive) is a fusion protein that inhibits T-cell proliferation. Adalimumab (Humira) is a recombinant human immunoglobulin G1 (IgG1) monoclonal antibody against TNF-α. These biological agents have significant side effects, making close monitoring essential.

Oral Agents. Methotrexate appears to inhibit DNA synthesis in epidermal cells, thereby reducing the turnover time of the psoriatic epidermis. However, the medication can be toxic, especially to the liver, kidneys, and bone marrow. Laboratory studies must be monitored to ensure that the hepatic, hematopoietic, and renal systems are functioning adequately. The patient should avoid drinking alcohol while taking methotrexate because alcohol ingestion increases the possibility of liver damage. The medication is teratogenic (produces physical defects in the fetus) and thus should not be administered to pregnant women.

Cyclosporine A, a cyclic peptide used to prevent rejection of transplanted organs, has shown some success in treatment of severe, therapy-resistant cases of psoriasis. However, its use is limited by side effects such as hypertension and nephrotoxicity.

Oral retinoids (ie, synthetic derivatives of vitamin A and its metabolite, vitamin A acid) modulate the growth and differentiation of epithelial tissue. Etretinate (Tegison, Tigason) is especially useful for severe pustular or erythrodermic psoriasis. Etretinate is a teratogen with a very long half-life; it cannot be used in women with childbearing potential.

Photochemotherapy

When psoriasis becomes widespread (defined as too many plaques to count or as involving more than 50% of the body surface), another treatment option involves combining a photosensitizing oral medication with exposure to ultraviolet-A light (PUVA). The patient takes a photosensitizing medication (usually 8-methoxypsoralen [8-mop, Houva-caps, meladinine, meloxine]) in a standard dose and is subsequently exposed to long-wave ultraviolet light as the medication plasma levels peak. It is thought that when psoralen-treated skin is exposed to UVA light, the psoralen binds with DNA and decreases cellular proliferation. PUVA has been associated with long-term risks of skin cancer, cataracts, and premature aging of the skin (Porth & Matfin, 2009).

The patient is usually treated two or three times each week until the psoriasis clears. An interim period of 48 hours between treatments is necessary to allow any burns resulting from PUVA therapy to become evident. After the psoriasis clears, the patient begins a maintenance program. Once little or no disease is active, less potent therapies are used to keep minor flare-ups under control.

Very often, phototherapy in the ultraviolet-B (UVB) spectrum is used as a single therapy modality. Research has shown that the most effective UVB range for therapeutic response is the range of 310 to 312 nm; therapy in this range precludes many of the negative side effects that can be experienced with broader range light. UVB is used alone or in combination with topical coal tar, emollients, and mild topical corticosteroids. Side effects are similar to those of PUVA therapy. A new therapy unit provides UVB in the narrow range of 311 to 312 nm, which decreases the harmful effects of UVB while providing more intense therapy. Response to treatment can be improved if narrow-band UVB is combined with the topical cream, calcipotriol (Dovonex). This cream induces synthesis of vitamin D in the skin and decreases the need for ultraviolet exposure (Lui & Mamelak, 2007).

If access to a light treatment unit is not feasible, the patient can expose himself or herself to sunlight. The risks of all light treatments are similar and include acute sunburn; exacerbation of photosensitive disorders such as lupus and rosacea; as well as other skin changes such as increased wrinkles, thickening, and an increased risk for skin cancer.

Excimer lasers have come into use in treating psoriasis. These lasers function at 308 nm. Studies show that medium-size psoriatic plaques clear in four to six treatments and remain clear for up to 9 months. A laser can be more effective on the scalp or on other hard-to-treat areas because it can be aimed very specifically on the plaque (Taibjee, 2005).

Nursing Management

Assessment

The nursing assessment focuses on the appearance of the normal skin, the appearance of the skin lesions, and how the patient is coping with the psoriatic skin condition. It is important to examine the areas especially prone to psoriasis: elbows, knees, scalp, gluteal cleft, and all nails (for small pits).

Psoriasis may cause despair and frustration for the patient; observers may stare, comment, ask embarrassing questions, or even avoid the person. The disease can eventually exhaust the patient's resources, interfere with his or her job, and negatively affect many aspects of life. Teenagers are especially vulnerable to the psychological effects of this disorder.

The nurse assesses the impact of the disease on the patient and the coping strategies used for conducting normal activities and interactions with family and friends. Many patients need reassurance that the condition is not infectious, is not a reflection of poor personal hygiene, and is not skin cancer. The nurse can create an environment in which the patient feels comfortable discussing important quality-of-life issues related to his or her psychosocial and physical response to this chronic illness.

Nursing Interventions

Promoting Understanding

The nurse explains with sensitivity that although there is no cure for psoriasis and lifetime management is necessary, the condition can usually be controlled. The pathophysiology of psoriasis is reviewed, as are the factors that provoke it—irritation or injury to the skin (eg, cut, abrasion, sunburn), current illness (eg, pharyngeal streptococcal infection), and emotional stress. It is emphasized that repeated trauma to the skin and an unfavorable environment (eg, cold) or a specific medication (eg, lithium, beta-blockers, indomethacin [Indocin]) may exacerbate psoriasis. The patient is cautioned about taking any nonprescription medications because some may aggravate mild psoriasis.

Reviewing and explaining the treatment regimen are essential to ensure compliance. For example, if the patient has a mild condition confined to localized areas, such as the elbows or knees, application of an emollient to maintain softness and minimize scaling may be all that is required. Most patients need a comprehensive plan of care that ranges from using topical medications and shampoos to more complex and lengthy treatment with systemic medications and photochemotherapy, such as PUVA therapy. Patient education materials that include a description of the therapy and specific guidelines are helpful but cannot replace face-to-face discussions of the treatment plan.

Increasing Skin Integrity

To avoid injuring the skin, the patient is advised not to pick at or scratch the affected areas. Measures to prevent dry skin are encouraged because dry skin worsens psoriasis. Too-frequent washing produces more soreness and scaling. Water should be warm, not hot, and the skin should be dried by patting with a towel rather than by rubbing. Emollients have a moisturizing effect, providing an occlusive film on the skin surface so that normal water loss through the skin is halted and allowing the trapped water to hydrate the stratum corneum. A bath oil or emollient cleansing agent can comfort sore and scaling skin. Softening the skin can prevent fissures.

Improving Self-Concept and Body Image

A therapeutic relationship between health care professionals and the patient with psoriasis includes education and support. Introducing the patient to successful coping strategies used by others with psoriasis and making suggestions for reducing or coping with stressful situations at home, school, and work can facilitate a more positive outlook and acceptance of the chronicity of the disease.

Monitoring and Managing Potential Complications

The diagnosis of psoriasis, especially when it is accompanied by the complication of arthritis, is usually difficult to make. Psoriatic arthritis involving the sacroiliac and distal joints of the fingers may be overlooked, especially if the patient has the typical psoriatic lesions. However, patients who complain of mild joint discomfort and some pitting of the fingernails may not be diagnosed with psoriasis until the more obvious cutaneous lesions appear. The patient requires education about the care and treatment of the involved joints and the need for compliance with therapy. However, when the psoriasis is extensive and a family history of inflammatory arthritis is elicited, the chance that the patient will develop psoriatic arthritis increases substantially. It is recommended that a rheumatologist be consulted to assist in the diagnosis and treatment of the arthropathy.

Promoting Home and Community-Based Care

Teaching Patients Self-Care. Printed patient education materials may be provided to reinforce face-to-face discussions about treatment guidelines and other considerations.

Patients using topical corticosteroid preparations repeatedly on the face and around the eyes should be aware that cataract development is possible. Strict guidelines for applying these medications should be emphasized because overuse can result in skin atrophy, striae, and medication resistance.

PUVA, which is reserved for moderate to severe psoriasis, produces photosensitization. If exposure to the sun is unavoidable, the skin must be protected with sunscreen and clothing. Gray-tinted or green-tinted wraparound sunglasses should be worn to protect the eyes during and after treatment, and ophthalmologic examinations should be performed on a regular basis. Contraceptives should be used by sexually active women of reproductive age because the teratogenic effect of PUVA has not been determined.

If indicated, referral may be made to a mental health professional who can help to ease emotional strain and give support. Belonging to a support group may also help patients recognize that they are not alone in experiencing life adjustments in response to a visible, chronic disease. The National Psoriasis Foundation publishes periodic bulletins and reports about new and relevant developments in this condition.

Chart 56-4 is a Home Care Checklist for the patient with psoriasis.

Exfoliative Dermatitis

Exfoliative dermatitis is a serious condition characterized by progressive inflammation in which generalized erythema and scaling occur. It may be associated with chills, fever, prostration, severe toxicity, and a pruritic scaling of the skin. There is a profound loss of stratum corneum (ie, outermost layer of the skin), which causes capillary leakage, hypoproteinemia, and negative nitrogen balance. Because of widespread dilation of cutaneous vessels, large amounts of body heat are lost, and exfoliative dermatitis has a marked effect on the entire body.

Exfoliative dermatitis has a variety of causes. It is considered to be a secondary or reactive process to an underlying skin or systemic disease. It may appear as a part of the lymphoma group of diseases and may precede the clinical manifestations of lymphoma. Preexisting skin disorders

---

CHART 56-4	HOME CARE CHECKLIST *The Patient With Psoriasis*		
At the completion of the home care instruction, the patient or caregiver will be able to:		**PATIENT**	**CAREGIVER**
• Describe the etiology of psoriasis.		✔	✔
• Describe optimal skin maintenance practices to maintain moisture of skin and prevent infection.		✔	✔
• Demonstrate correct application of prescribed topical medications.		✔	✔
• Describe common side effects of oral medication, if prescribed.		✔	✔
• Demonstrate appropriate therapeutic bath technique, if prescribed.		✔	✔
• Verbalize optimism about condition.		✔	
• Identify a support person with whom to discuss feelings and concerns.		✔	

that have been implicated include psoriasis, atopic dermatitis, and contact dermatitis. It also appears as a severe reaction to many medications, including penicillin and phenylbutazone (Butazolidin). The cause is unknown in approximately 25% of cases (James, Berger & Elston, 2005).

Clinical Manifestations

This condition starts acutely as a patchy or generalized erythematous eruption accompanied by fever, malaise, and occasionally gastrointestinal symptoms. The skin color changes from pink to dark red. After a week, the characteristic exfoliation (ie, scaling) begins, usually in the form of thin flakes that leave the underlying skin smooth and red, with new scales forming as the older ones come off. Hair loss may accompany this disorder. Relapses are common. The systemic effects include high-output heart failure, other gastrointestinal disturbances, breast enlargement, elevated levels of uric acid in the blood (ie, hyperuricemia), and temperature disturbances.

Medical Management

The objectives of management are to maintain fluid and electrolyte balance and to prevent infection. The treatment is individualized and supportive and should be initiated as soon as the condition is diagnosed.

The patient may be hospitalized and placed on bed rest. All medications that may be implicated are discontinued. A comfortable room temperature should be maintained because the patient does not have normal thermoregulatory control as a result of temperature fluctuations caused by vasodilation and evaporative water loss. Fluid and electrolyte balance must be maintained because there is considerable water and protein loss from the skin surface. Administration of plasma volume expanders may be indicated.

Nursing Management

Continual nursing assessment is carried out to detect infection. The disrupted, erythematous, moist skin is susceptible to infection and becomes colonized with pathogenic organisms, which produce more inflammation. Antibiotics, which are prescribed if infection is present, are selected on the basis of culture and sensitivity.

> ⚑ **NURSING ALERT**
>
> The nurse observes the patient for signs and symptoms of heart failure because hyperemia and increased cutaneous blood flow can produce high-output cardiac failure.

Hypothermia may occur because increased blood flow in the skin, coupled with increased water loss through the skin, leads to heat loss by radiation, conduction, and evaporation. Changes in vital signs are closely monitored and reported.

Topical therapy is used to provide symptomatic relief. Soothing baths, compresses, and lubrication with emollients are used to treat the extensive dermatitis. The patient is likely to be extremely irritable because of the severe pruritus. Oral or parenteral corticosteroids may be prescribed

when the disease is not controlled by more conservative therapy. When a specific cause is known, more specific therapy may be used. The patient is advised to avoid all irritants in the future, particularly medications that are known to cause the disease.

BLISTERING DISEASES

Blisters of the skin have many origins, including bacterial, fungal, or viral infections; allergic contact reactions; burns; metabolic disorders; and immunologically mediated reactions. Some of these have been discussed previously (eg, herpes simplex and zoster infections, contact dermatitis). Immunologically mediated diseases are autoimmune reactions and represent a defect of IgM, IgE, IgG, and complement, C3. Some of these conditions are life-threatening; others become chronic.

The diagnosis is always made by histologic examination of a biopsy specimen, usually by a dermatopathologist. A specimen from the blister and surrounding skin demonstrates **acantholysis** (separation of epidermal cells from each other because of damage to or an abnormality of the intracellular substance). Circulating antibodies may be detected by immunofluorescent studies of the patient's serum.

Pemphigus

Pemphigus is a group of serious diseases of the skin characterized by the appearance of bullae (blisters) of various sizes on apparently normal skin (Fig. 56-4) and mucous membranes. Pemphigus is an autoimmune disease involving IgG. It is thought that the pemphigus antibody is directed against a specific cell-surface antigen in epidermal cells. A blister forms from the antigen–antibody reaction. The level of serum antibody is predictive of disease severity. Genetic factors may also have a role in its development, with the highest incidence in people of Jewish or Mediterranean descent. This disorder usually occurs in men and women in middle and late adulthood. The condition may be associated with penicillins and captopril (Capoten) and with myasthenia gravis.

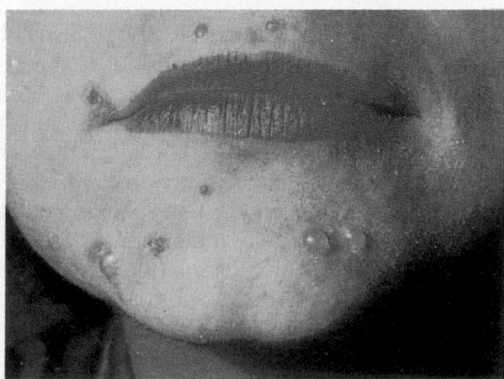

Figure 56-4 Vesicles on the chin (in pemphigus). From Hall, J. C. (2006). *Sauer's manual of skin diseases*. Philadelphia: Lippincott Williams & Wilkins.

Clinical Manifestations

Most patients present with oral lesions appearing as irregularly shaped erosions that are painful, bleed easily, and heal slowly. The skin bullae enlarge, rupture, and leave large, painful eroded areas that are accompanied by crusting and oozing. A characteristic odor emanates from the bullae and the exuding serum. There is blistering or sloughing of uninvolved skin when minimal pressure is applied (Nikolsky's sign). The eroded skin heals slowly, and large areas of the body eventually are involved. Bacterial superinfection is common.

Complications

The most common complications arise when the disease process is widespread. Before the advent of corticosteroid and immunosuppressive therapy, patients were very susceptible to secondary bacterial infection. Skin bacteria have relatively easy access to the bullae as they ooze, rupture, and leave denuded areas exposed to the environment. Fluid and electrolyte imbalance results from fluid and protein loss as the bullae rupture. Hypoalbuminemia is common when the disease process includes extensive areas of the body skin surface and mucous membranes.

Management

The goals of therapy are to bring the disease under control as rapidly as possible, to prevent loss of serum and the development of secondary infection, and to promote re-epithelization (ie, renewal of epithelial tissue).

Corticosteroids are administered in high doses to control the disease and keep the skin free of blisters. The high dosage level is maintained until remission is apparent. In some cases, corticosteroid therapy must be maintained for life. High-dose corticosteroid therapy has serious toxic effects (see Chapter 42).

Immunosuppressive agents (eg, azathioprine [Azasan], cyclophosphamide [Cytoxan], gold [Aurasol]) may be prescribed to help control the disease and reduce the corticosteroid dose. **Plasmapheresis** temporarily decreases the serum antibody level and has been used with variable success, although it is generally reserved for life-threatening cases.

Bullous Pemphigoid

Bullous pemphigoid is an acquired disease of flaccid blisters appearing on normal or erythematous skin. It appears more often on the flexor surfaces of the arms, legs, axilla, and groin. Oral lesions, if present, are usually transient and minimal. When the blisters break, the skin has shallow erosions that heal fairly quickly. Pruritus can be intense, even before the appearance of the blisters. Bullous pemphigoid is common in the elderly, with a peak incidence at about 60 years of age. There is no gender or racial predilection, and the disease can be found throughout the world.

Management

Medical treatment includes topical corticosteroids for localized eruptions and systemic corticosteroids for widespread involvement. Systemic corticosteroids (eg, prednisone [Delta-

sone]) may be continued for months, in alternate-day doses. The patient needs to understand the implications of long-term corticosteroid therapy (see Chapter 42).

Dermatitis Herpetiformis

Dermatitis herpetiformis is an intensely pruritic, chronic disease that manifests with small, tense blisters that are distributed symmetrically over the elbows, knees, buttocks, and nape of the neck. It most commonly occurs between 20 and 40 years of age but can appear at any age. Most patients with dermatitis herpetiformis have a subclinical defect in gluten metabolism.

Management

Most patients respond to Dapsone and to a gluten-free diet. All patients should be screened for glucose-6-phosphate dehydrogenase (G6PD) deficiency because dapsone can induce severe hemolysis in those with this deficiency. Patients benefit from dietary counseling because the dietary restrictions are lifelong, and a gluten-free diet is often difficult to follow. They need emotional support as they deal with the process of learning new habits and accepting major changes in their lives.

NURSING PROCESS

CARE OF THE PATIENT WITH BLISTERING DISEASES

Assessment

Patients with blistering disorders may experience significant disability. There is constant itching and possible pain in the denuded areas of skin. There may be drainage from the denuded areas, which may be malodorous. Effective assessment and nursing management become a challenge.

Disease activity is monitored clinically by examining the skin for the appearance of new blisters. Areas where healing has occurred may show signs of hyperpigmentation. Particular attention is given to assessing for signs and symptoms of infection.

Diagnosis

Nursing Diagnoses

Based on nursing assessment data, the patient's major nursing diagnoses may include the following:

- Acute pain of skin and oral cavity related to blistering and erosions
- Impaired skin integrity related to ruptured bullae and denuded areas of the skin
- Anxiety and ineffective coping related to the appearance of the skin and no hope of a cure
- Deficient knowledge about medications and side effects

Collaborative Problems/Potential Complications

Based on the assessment data, potential complications include the following:

- Infection and sepsis related to loss of protective barrier of skin and mucous membranes
- Fluid volume deficit and electrolyte imbalance related to loss of tissue fluids

Planning and Goals

The major goals for the patient may include relief of discomfort from lesions, skin healing, reduced anxiety and improved coping capacity, and absence of complications.

Nursing Interventions

Relieving Oral Discomfort

The patient's entire oral cavity may be affected with erosions and denuded surfaces. Necrotic tissue may develop over these areas, adding to the patient's discomfort and interfering with eating. Weight loss and hypoproteinemia may result. Meticulous oral hygiene is important to keep the oral mucosa clean and allow the epithelium to regenerate. Frequent rinsing of the mouth with a solution of salt and baking soda is prescribed to rid the mouth of debris and to soothe ulcerated areas. Commercial mouthwashes are avoided. The lips are kept moist with lanolin, petrolatum, or lip balm. Cool mist therapy helps humidify environmental air.

Enhancing Skin Integrity and Relieving Discomfort

Cool, wet dressings or baths are protective and soothing. The patient with painful and extensive lesions should be premedicated with analgesics before skin care is initiated. Patients with large areas of blistering have a characteristic odor that decreases when secondary infection is controlled. After the patient's skin is bathed, it is dried carefully and dusted liberally with nonirritating powder (eg, cornstarch), which enables the patient to move about freely in bed. Fairly large amounts are necessary to keep the patient's skin from adhering to the sheets. Tape should never be used because it may produce more blisters. Hypothermia is common, and measures to keep the patient warm and comfortable are priority nursing activities. The nursing management of patients with bullous skin conditions is similar to that for patients with extensive burns (see Chapter 57).

Reducing Anxiety

Attention to the psychological needs of the patient requires listening to the patient, being available, providing expert nursing care, and educating the patient and the family. The patient is encouraged to express anxieties, discomfort, and feelings of hopelessness. Arranging for a family member or a close friend to spend more time with the patient can be supportive. When patients receive information about the disease and its treatment, uncertainty and anxiety often decrease, and the patient's capacity to act on his or her own behalf is enhanced. Psychological counseling may assist the patient in dealing with fears, anxiety, and depression.

Monitoring and Managing Potential Complications

INFECTION AND SEPSIS. The patient is susceptible to infection because the barrier function of the skin is compromised. Bullae are also susceptible to infection, and sepsis may follow. The skin is cleaned to remove debris and dead skin and to prevent infection.

Secondary infection may be accompanied by an unpleasant odor from skin or oral lesions. *C. albicans* of the mouth (ie, thrush) commonly affects patients receiving high-dose corticosteroid therapy. The oral cavity is inspected daily, and any changes are reported. Oral lesions are slow to heal.

Infection is the leading cause of death in patients with blistering diseases. Particular attention is given to assessment for signs and symptoms of local and systemic infection. Seemingly trivial complaints or minimal changes are investigated because corticosteroids can mask or alter typical signs and symptoms of infection. The patient's vital signs are monitored, and temperature fluctuations are documented. The patient is observed for chills, and all secretions and excretions are monitored for changes suggesting infection. Results of culture and sensitivity tests are monitored. Antimicrobial agents are administered as prescribed, and response to treatment is assessed. Health care personnel must perform effective hand hygiene and wear gloves.

In hospitalized patients, environmental contamination is reduced as much as possible. Protective isolation measures and standard precautions are warranted.

FLUID AND ELECTROLYTE IMBALANCE. Extensive denudation of the skin leads to fluid and electrolyte imbalance because of significant loss of fluids and sodium chloride from the skin. This sodium chloride loss is responsible for many of the systemic symptoms associated with the disease and is treated by IV administration of saline solution.

A large amount of protein and blood is also lost from the denuded skin areas. Blood component therapy may be prescribed to maintain the blood volume, hemoglobin level, and plasma protein concentration. Serum albumin, protein, hemoglobin, and hematocrit values are monitored.

The patient is encouraged to maintain adequate oral fluid intake. Cool, nonirritating fluids are encouraged to maintain hydration. Small, frequent meals or snacks of high-protein, high-calorie foods (eg, oral nutritional supplements, eggnog, milk shakes) help maintain nutritional status. Parenteral nutrition is considered if the patient cannot eat an adequate diet.

Evaluation

Expected Patient Outcomes

Expected patient outcomes may include the following:

1. Reports relief from pain of oral lesions
   a. Identifies therapies that reduce pain
   b. Uses mouthwashes and anesthetic or antiseptic aerosol mouth spray
   c. Drinks chilled fluids at 2-hour intervals
2. Achieves skin healing
   a. States purpose of therapeutic regimen
   b. Cooperates with soaks and bath regimen
   c. Reminds caregivers to use liberal amounts of nonirritating powder on bed linens
3. Reports that anxiety and ability to cope with the condition have improved
   a. Verbalizes concerns about condition, self, and relationships with others

b. Participates in self-care
4. Experiences no complications
   a. Has cultures from bullae, skin, and orifices that are negative for pathogenic organisms
   b. Has no purulent drainage
   c. Shows signs that skin is clearing
   d. Has normal body temperature
   e. Keeps intake record to ensure adequate fluid intake and normal fluid and electrolyte balance
   f. Verbalizes the rationale for IV infusion therapy
   g. Has urine output within normal limits
   h. Has serum chemistry and hemoglobin and hematocrit values within normal limits

Toxic Epidermal Necrolysis and Stevens-Johnson Syndrome

Toxic epidermal necrolysis (TEN) and Stevens-Johnson syndrome (SJS) are potentially fatal skin disorders and the most severe forms of erythema multiforme. These diseases are mucocutaneous reactions that constitute a spectrum of reactions, with TEN being the most severe. The mortality rate from TEN is 30% to 35%. TEN and SJS are triggered by a reaction to medications. Antibiotics, especially sulfonamides, antiseizure agents, nonsteroidal anti-inflammatory drugs (NSAIDs), and sulfonamides are the most frequent medications implicated (Porth & Maffin, 2009).

TEN and SJS occur in all ages and both genders. The incidence is increased in older people because of their use of many medications. People who are immunosuppressed, including those with HIV infection and acquired immunodeficiency syndrome (AIDS), have a high risk of TEN and SJS. Although the incidence of these diseases in the general population is about two to three cases per 1 million people in the United States, the risk associated with sulfonamides in HIV-positive people may approach 1 case per 1000 (Porth & Maffin, 2009). Most patients with TEN have an abnormal metabolism of the medication; the mechanism leading to TEN seems to be a cell-mediated cytotoxic reaction.

Clinical Manifestations

TEN and SJS are characterized initially by conjunctival burning or itching, cutaneous tenderness, fever, cough, sore throat, headache, extreme malaise, and myalgias (ie, aches and pains). These signs are followed by a rapid onset of erythema involving much of the skin surface and mucous membranes, including the oral mucosa, conjunctiva, and genitalia. In severe cases of mucosal involvement, there may be danger of damage to the larynx, bronchi, and esophagus from ulcerations. Large, flaccid bullae develop in some areas; in other areas, large sheets of epidermis are shed, exposing the underlying dermis. Fingernails, toenails, eyebrows, and eyelashes may be shed along with the surrounding epidermis. The skin is excruciatingly tender, and the loss of skin leaves a weeping surface similar to that of a total-body, partial-thickness burn; hence, the condition is also referred to as "scalded skin syndrome."

Complications

Sepsis and keratoconjunctivitis are complications of TEN and SJS. Unrecognized and untreated sepsis can be life-threatening. Keratoconjunctivitis can impair vision and result in conjunctival retraction, scarring, and corneal lesions.

Assessment and Diagnostic Findings

Histologic studies of frozen skin cells from a fresh lesion and cytodiagnosis of collections of cellular material from a freshly denuded area are conducted. A history of use of medications known to precipitate TEN or SJS may confirm medication reaction as the underlying cause.

Immunofluorescent studies may be performed to detect atypical epidermal autoantibodies. A genetic predisposition to erythema multiforme has been suggested but has not been confirmed in all cases.

Medical Management

The goals of treatment include control of fluid and electrolyte balance, prevention of sepsis, and prevention of ophthalmic complications. Supportive care is the mainstay of treatment.

All nonessential medications are discontinued immediately. If possible, the patient is treated in a regional burn center because aggressive treatment similar to that for severe burns is required. Skin loss may approach 100% of the total body surface area. Surgical débridement or hydrotherapy in a Hubbard tank (large steel tub) may be performed to remove involved skin.

Tissue samples from the nasopharynx, eyes, ears, blood, urine, skin, and unruptured blisters are obtained for culture to identify pathogenic organisms. IV fluids are prescribed to maintain fluid and electrolyte balance, especially in the patient who has severe mucosal involvement and who cannot easily take oral nourishment. Because an indwelling IV catheter may be a site of infection, fluid replacement is carried out by nasogastric tube and then orally as soon as possible.

Initial treatment with systemic corticosteroids is controversial. Some experts argue for early high-dose corticosteroid treatment. However, in most cases, the risk of infection, fluid and electrolyte imbalance, delayed healing, and difficulty in initiating oral corticosteroids early in the course of the disease outweigh its benefits. In patients with TEN thought to be due to a medication reaction, corticosteroids may be administered; however, the patient should be closely monitored for adverse effects.

Administration of IV immunoglobulin (IVIG) may provide rapid improvement and skin healing. This response is dramatically better than that obtained with immunosuppressives, and IVIG may become the treatment of choice (Mittmann, Chan, Knowles, et al., 2007).

Protecting the skin with topical agents is crucial. Various topical antibacterial and anesthetic agents are used to prevent wound sepsis and to assist with pain management. Systemic antibiotic therapy is used with extreme caution. Temporary biologic dressings (eg, pigskin, amniotic membrane) or plastic semipermeable dressings (eg, Vigilon) may be used to reduce pain, decrease evaporation, and prevent secondary infection until the epithelium regenerates. Meticulous oropharyngeal and eye care is essential when there is involvement of the mucous membranes and the eyes.

NURSING PROCESS

CARE OF THE PATIENT WITH TOXIC EPIDERMAL NECROLYSIS OR STEVENS-JOHNSON SYNDROME

Assessment

A careful inspection of the skin is made, including its appearance and the extent of involvement. The normal skin is closely observed to determine if new areas of blisters are developing. Drainage from blisters is monitored for amount, color, and odor. The oral cavity is inspected daily for blistering and erosive lesions; the patient is assessed daily for itching, burning, and dryness of the eyes. The patient's ability to swallow and drink fluids, as well as speak normally, is determined.

The patient's vital signs are monitored, and special attention is given to the presence and character of fever and the respiratory rate, depth, rhythm, and cough. The characteristics and amount of respiratory secretions are observed. Assessment for high fever, tachycardia, and extreme weakness and fatigue is essential because these factors indicate the process of epidermal necrosis, increased metabolic needs, and possible gastrointestinal and respiratory mucosal sloughing. Urine volume, specific gravity, and color are monitored. The insertion sites of IV lines are inspected for signs of local infection. Body weight is recorded daily.

The patient is asked to describe fatigue and pain levels. An attempt is made to evaluate the patient's level of anxiety. The patient's basic coping mechanisms are assessed, and effective coping strategies are identified.

Diagnosis

Nursing Diagnoses

Based on the assessment data, the patient's major nursing diagnoses may include the following:

- Impaired tissue integrity (ie, oral, eye, and skin) related to epidermal shedding
- Deficient fluid volume and electrolyte losses related to loss of fluids from denuded skin
- Risk for imbalanced body temperature (ie, hypothermia) related to heat loss secondary to skin loss
- Acute pain related to denuded skin, oral lesions, and possible infection
- Anxiety related to the physical appearance of the skin and prognosis

Collaborative Problems/Potential Complications

Based on the assessment data, potential complications include the following:

- Sepsis
- Conjunctival retraction, scars, and corneal lesions

Planning and Goals

The major goals for the patient may include skin and oral tissue healing, fluid balance, prevention of heat loss, relief of pain, reduced anxiety, and absence of complications.

Nursing Interventions

Maintaining Skin and Mucous Membrane Integrity

The local care of the skin is an important area of nursing management. The skin denudes easily, especially when the patient is lifted and turned. The nursing staff must take special care to avoid friction involving the skin when moving the patient in bed. The skin should be checked after each position change to ensure that no new denuded areas have appeared. The nurse applies the prescribed topical agents to reduce the bacterial population of the wound surface. Warm compresses, if prescribed, should be applied gently to denuded areas. The topical antibacterial agent may be used in conjunction with hydrotherapy in a tank, bathtub, or shower. The nurse monitors the patient's condition during the treatment and encourages the patient to exercise the extremities during hydrotherapy.

The painful oral lesions make oral hygiene difficult. Careful oral hygiene is performed to keep the oral mucosa clean. Prescribed mouthwashes, anesthetics, or coating agents are used frequently to rid the mouth of debris, soothe ulcerative areas, and control foul mouth odor. The oral cavity is inspected several times each day, and any changes are documented and reported. Petrolatum or a prescribed ointment is applied to the lips.

Attaining Fluid Balance

The vital signs, urine output, and sensorium are observed for indications of hypovolemia. Mental changes from fluid and electrolyte imbalance, sensory overload, or sensory deprivation may occur. Laboratory test results are evaluated, and abnormal results are reported. The patient is weighed daily (with a bed scale if necessary).

Oral lesions may result in dysphagia, making tube feeding or parenteral nutrition necessary until oral ingestion can be tolerated. A daily calorie count and accurate recording of all intake and output are essential.

Preventing Hypothermia

The patient with TEN is prone to chilling. Dehydration may be made worse by exposing the denuded skin to a continuous current of warm air. The patient is usually sensitive to changes in room temperature. Measures similar to those implemented for a burn patient, such as cotton blankets, ceiling-mounted heat lamps, and heat shields, are useful in maintaining body temperature. To minimize shivering and heat loss, the nurse should work rapidly and efficiently when large wounds are exposed for wound care. The patient's temperature is monitored frequently.

Relieving Pain

The nurse assesses the patient's pain, its characteristics, factors that influence the pain, and the patient's behavioral responses. Prescribed analgesics are administered on a regular schedule, and the nurse documents pain relief and any side effects. Analgesics are administered before painful treatments are performed. Providing thorough explanations and speaking calmly to the patient during treatments can allay the anxiety that may intensify pain. Offering emotional support and reassurance and implementing measures that promote rest and sleep are basic in achieving pain control. As the pain diminishes and the patient has more physical and emotional energy, self-management techniques for pain relief, such as progressive muscle relaxation and imagery, may be taught.

Reducing Anxiety

Because the lifestyle of the patient with TEN has been abruptly changed to one of complete dependence, an assessment of his or her emotional state may reveal anxiety, depression, and fear of dying. The patient can be reassured that these reactions are normal. The patient also needs nursing support, honest communication, and hope that the situation can improve. The patient is encouraged to express his or her feelings. Listening to the patient's concerns and being readily available with skillful and compassionate care are important anxiety-relieving interventions. Emotional support by a psychiatric nurse, spiritual advisor, psychologist, or psychiatrist may be helpful to promote coping during the long recovery period.

Monitoring and Managing Potential Complications

SEPSIS. The major cause of death from TEN is infection, and the most common sites of infection are the skin and mucosal surfaces, lungs, and blood. The organisms most often involved are *S. aureus, Pseudomonas, Klebsiella, Escherichia coli, Serratia,* and *Candida.* Monitoring vital signs closely and noticing changes in respiratory, renal, and gastrointestinal function may quickly detect the beginning of an infection. Strict asepsis is always maintained during routine skin care measures. Hand hygiene and wearing sterile gloves when carrying out procedures are essential. When the condition involves a large portion of the body, the patient should be in a private room to prevent possible cross-infection from other patients. Visitors should wear protective garments and wash their hands before and after coming into contact with the patient. People with any infections or infectious disease should not visit the patient until they are no longer a danger to the patient. The nurse is critical in identifying early signs and symptoms of infection and notifying the physician. Antibiotics are not generally begun until there is indication for their use.

CONJUNCTIVAL RETRACTION, SCARS, AND CORNEAL LESIONS. The eyes are inspected daily for signs of pruritus, burning, and dryness, which may indicate progression to keratoconjunctivitis, the principal eye complication. Applying a cool, damp cloth over the eyes may relieve burning sensations. The eyes are kept clean and observed for signs of discharge or discomfort, and the progression of symptoms is documented and reported. Administering an eye lubricant, when prescribed, may alleviate dryness and prevent corneal abrasion. Using eye patches or reminding the patient to blink periodically may also counteract dryness. The patient is instructed to avoid rubbing the eyes or putting any medication into the eyes that has not been prescribed or approved by the physician.

Promoting Home and Community-Based Care

TEACHING PATIENTS SELF-CARE. Patients with TEN or SJS with involvement of large areas of the skin require care that is similar to that of patients with thermal burns. As the patient completes the acute inpatient stage of illness, the focus is directed toward rehabilitation and outpatient care or care in a rehabilitation center. Throughout this care, the patient and family members are involved in the care and are instructed in the procedures, such as wound care and dressing changes, that will need to be continued at home. The patient and family members are assisted in acquiring dressing supplies that will be needed at home.

The patient and family members are also provided with instructions about pain management, nutrition, measures to increase mobility, and prevention of complications, including prevention of infection. They are taught the signs and symptoms of complications and instructed when to notify the health care provider. When appropriate, instructions are provided in writing to the patient and family so they can refer to these instructions when necessary at later times.

CONTINUING CARE. Interdisciplinary follow-up care is imperative to ensure that the patient's progress continues. Some patients will require care in a rehabilitation center before returning home. Others will require outpatient physical and occupational therapy for an extended period. When the patient returns home, the home care nurse coordinates the care provided by the various members of the health care team (eg, physician, physical therapist, occupational therapist, dietician). The nurse also monitors the patient's progress, provides ongoing assessment to identify complications, and monitors the patient's adherence to the plan of care. The patient's adaptation to the home care environment and the patient's and family's needs for support and assistance are also assessed. Referrals to community agencies are made as appropriate.

Evaluation

Expected Patient Outcomes

Expected patient outcomes may include the following:

1. Achieves increasing skin and oral tissue healing
   a. Demonstrates areas of healing skin
   b. Swallows fluids and speaks clearly
2. Attains fluid balance
   a. Demonstrates laboratory values within normal ranges
   b. Maintains urine volume and specific gravity within acceptable range
   c. Shows stable vital signs
   d. Increases intake of oral fluids without discomfort
   e. Maintains weight or gains weight, if appropriate
3. Attains thermoregulation
   a. Registers body temperature within normal range
   b. Reports no chills
4. Achieves pain relief
   a. Uses analgesics as prescribed
   b. Uses self-management techniques for relief of pain
5. Appears less anxious
   a. Discusses concerns freely
   b. Sleeps for progressively longer periods

6. Absence of complications, such as sepsis and impaired vision
    a. Has body temperature within normal range
    b. Laboratory values within normal ranges
    c. Has no abnormal discharges or signs of infection
    d. Continues to see objects at baseline acuity level
    e. Shows no signs of keratoconjunctivitis

ULCERATIONS

Superficial loss of surface tissue as a result of death of cells is called an ulceration. A simple ulcer, such as the kind found in a small, superficial, partial-thickness burn, tends to heal by granulation if kept clean and protected from injury. If exposed to the air, the serum that escapes dries and forms a scab, under which the epithelial cells grow and cover the surface completely. Certain diseases cause characteristic ulcers (eg, tuberculous ulcers, syphilitic ulcers).

Ulcers related to problems with arterial circulation are seen in patients with peripheral vascular disease, arteriosclerosis, Raynaud's disease, and frostbite. In these patients, treatment of the ulcers is concurrent with treatment of the arterial disease (see Chapter 31). Nursing management includes the use of the dressings discussed at the beginning of this chapter. If nursing interventions are instituted early in the progression of an ulcer, the condition can often be effectively improved. Surgical amputation of an affected limb is a last resort.

Pressure ulcers involve breakdown of the skin due to prolonged pressure, friction and shear forces, and insufficient blood supply, usually at bony prominences. Information about these ulcers is presented in Chapter 11.

SKIN TUMORS

Benign Skin Tumors

Cysts

Cysts of the skin are epithelium-lined cavities that contain fluid or solid material. Epidermal cysts (epidermoid cysts) occur frequently and may be described as slow-growing, firm, elevated tumors found most frequently on the face, neck, upper chest, and back. Removal of the cysts provides a cure.

Pilar cysts (trichilemmal cysts), formerly called sebaceous cysts, are most frequently found on the scalp. They originate from the middle portion of the hair follicle and from the cells of the outer hair root sheath. Treatment is surgical removal.

Seborrheic and Actinic Keratoses

Seborrheic keratoses are benign, wartlike lesions of various sizes and colors, ranging from light tan to black. They are usually located on the face, shoulders, chest, and back and are the most common skin tumors seen in middle-age and elderly people. They may be cosmetically unacceptable to the patient. A black keratosis may be erroneously diagnosed as malignant melanoma. Treatment is removal of the tumor

tissue by excision, electrodesiccation (destruction of the skin lesions by monopolar high-frequency electric current) and curettage, or application of carbon dioxide or liquid nitrogen. However, there is no harm in allowing these growths to remain because there is no medical significance to their presence.

Actinic keratoses are premalignant skin lesions that develop in chronically sun-exposed areas of the body. They appear as rough, scaly patches with underlying erythema. A small percentage of these lesions gradually transform into cutaneous squamous cell carcinoma; they are usually removed by cryotherapy or shave excision.

Verrucae: Warts

Warts are common, benign skin tumors caused by infection with the human papillomavirus, which belongs to the DNA virus group. People of all ages may be affected, but the warts occur most frequently between the ages of 12 and 16 years. There are many types of warts.

As a rule, warts are asymptomatic, except when they occur on weight-bearing areas, such as the soles of the feet. They may be treated with locally applied laser therapy, liquid nitrogen, salicylic acid plasters, or electrodesiccation.

Warts occurring on the genitalia and perianal areas are known as condylomata acuminata. They may be transmitted sexually and are treated with liquid nitrogen, cryosurgery, electrosurgery, topically applied trichloroacetic acid, and curettage. Condylomata that affect the uterine cervix predispose the patient to cervical cancer (see Chapter 47).

Angiomas

Angiomas are benign vascular tumors that involve the skin and the subcutaneous tissues. They are present at birth and may occur as flat, violet-red patches (port-wine angiomas) or as raised, bright-red, nodular lesions (strawberry angiomas). The latter tend to involute spontaneously within the first few years of life, but port-wine angiomas usually persist indefinitely. Most patients use masking cosmetics (ie, Covermark or Dermablend) to camouflage the lesions. The argon laser is being used on various angiomas with some success. Treatment of strawberry angiomas is more successful if undertaken as soon after birth as possible.

Pigmented Nevi: Moles

Moles are common skin tumors of various sizes and shades, ranging from yellowish brown to black. They may be flat, macular lesions or elevated papules or nodules that occasionally contain hair. Most pigmented nevi are harmless lesions. However, in rare cases, malignant changes occur, and a melanoma develops at the site of the nevus. Some authorities believe that all congenital moles should be removed because they may have a higher incidence of malignant change. However, depending on the quantity and location, this may be impractical. Nevi that show a change in color or size, become symptomatic (eg, itch), or develop irregular borders should be removed to determine if malignant changes have occurred. Moles that occur in unusual places should be examined carefully for any irregularity and for notching of the border and variation in color. Early melanomas may display some redness and irritation and areas of bluish pigmentation where the pigment-containing cells have spread deeper into the skin. Late melanomas have areas of paler color, where pigment cells have stopped producing melanin. Nevi larger than 1 cm should be examined carefully. Excised nevi should be examined histologically.

Keloids

Keloids are benign overgrowths of fibrous tissue at the site of a scar or trauma. They appear to be more common among dark-skinned people. Keloids are asymptomatic but may cause disfigurement and cosmetic concern. The treatment, which is not always satisfactory, consists of surgical excision, intralesional corticosteroid therapy, and radiation.

Dermatofibroma

A dermatofibroma is a common, benign tumor of connective tissue that occurs predominantly on the extremities. It is a firm, dome-shaped papule or nodule that may be skin-colored or pinkish brown. Excisional biopsy is the recommended method of treatment.

Neurofibromatosis: Von Recklinghausen's Disease

Neurofibromatosis is a hereditary condition manifested by pigmented patches (*café-au-lait* macules), axillary freckling, and cutaneous neurofibromas that vary in size. Developmental changes may occur in the nervous system, muscles, and bone. Malignant degeneration of the neurofibromas occurs in some patients.

Malignant Skin Tumors

Skin cancer is the most common cancer in the United States. If the incidence continues at the present rate, an estimated one of eight fair-skinned Americans will eventually develop skin cancer, especially basal cell carcinoma (Chart 56-5). Because the skin is easily inspected, skin cancer is readily seen and detected and is the most successfully treated type of cancer (Neville, Welch & Leffell, 2007).

Exposure to the sun is the leading cause of skin cancer; incidence is related to the total amount of exposure to the sun. Sun damage is cumulative, and harmful effects may be severe by 20 years of age. The increase in skin cancer probably reflects changing lifestyles and the emphasis on sunbathing and related activities in light of changes in the environment, such as holes in the earth's ozone layer. Protective measures should be used throughout life, and nurses should inform patients about risk factors associated with skin cancer.

BASAL CELL AND SQUAMOUS CELL CARCINOMA

The most common types of skin cancer are basal cell carcinoma (BCC) and squamous cell (epidermoid) carcinoma (SCC). The third most common type, malignant melanoma, is discussed separately. Skin cancer is diagnosed by biopsy and histologic evaluation.

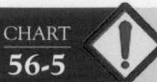

CHART 56-5 *Risk Factors for Skin Cancer*

Changes in the ozone layer from the effects of worldwide industrial air pollutants, such as chlorofluorocarbons, have prompted concern that the incidence of skin cancers, especially malignant melanoma, will increase. The ozone layer, a stratospheric blanket of bluish, explosive gas formed by the sun's ultraviolet radiation, varies in depth with the seasons and is thickest at the North and South Poles and thinnest at the equator. Scientists believe that it helps protect the earth from the effects of solar ultraviolet radiation. Proponents of this theory predict an increase in skin cancers as a consequence of changes in the ozone layer. Other skin cancer risk factors follow:

- Fair-skinned, fair-haired, blue-eyed people, particularly those of Celtic origin, with insufficient skin pigmentation to protect underlying tissues
- People who sustain sunburn and who do not tan
- Chronic sun exposure (certain occupations, such as farming, construction work)
- Exposure to chemical pollutants (industrial workers in arsenic, nitrates, coal, tar and pitch, oils and paraffins)
- Sun-damaged skin (elderly people)
- History of x-ray therapy for acne or benign lesions
- Scars from severe burns
- Chronic skin irritations
- Immunosuppression
- Genetic factors

Clinical Manifestations

BCC is the most common type of skin cancer. It generally appears on sun-exposed areas of the body and is more prevalent in regions where the population is subjected to intense and extensive exposure to the sun. The incidence is proportional to the age of the patient (average: 60 years) and the total amount of sun exposure, and it is inversely proportional to the amount of melanin in the skin.

BCC usually begins as a small, waxy nodule with rolled, translucent, pearly borders; telangiectatic vessels may be present. As it grows, it undergoes central ulceration and sometimes crusting (Fig. 56-5). The tumors appear most

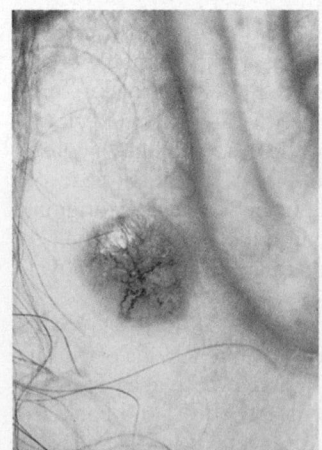
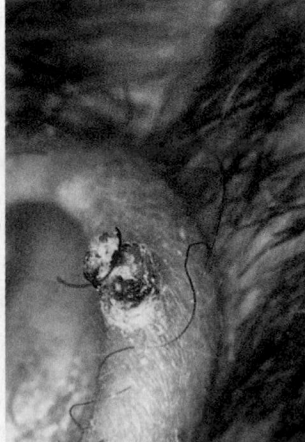

Figure 56-5 Basal cell carcinoma (*left*) and squamous cell carcinoma (*right*). Reprinted by permission from *New England Journal of Medicine, 326,* 169–170, 1992.

frequently on the face. BCC is characterized by invasion and erosion of contiguous (adjoining) tissues. It rarely metastasizes, but recurrence is common. However, a neglected lesion can result in the loss of a nose, an ear, or a lip. Other variants of BCC may appear as shiny, flat, gray or yellowish plaques.

SCC is a malignant proliferation arising from the epidermis. Although it usually appears on sun-damaged skin, it may arise from normal skin or from preexisting skin lesions. It is of greater concern than BCC because it is a truly invasive carcinoma, metastasizing by the blood or lymphatic system.

Metastases account for 75% of deaths from SCC. The lesions may be primary, arising on the skin and mucous membranes, or they may develop from a precancerous condition, such as actinic keratosis (lesions occurring in sun-exposed areas), leukoplakia (premalignant lesion of the mucous membrane), or scarred or ulcerated lesions. SCC appears as a rough, thickened, scaly tumor that may be asymptomatic or may involve bleeding (see Fig. 56-5). The border of an SCC lesion may be wider, more infiltrated, and more inflammatory than that of a BCC lesion. Secondary infection can occur. Exposed areas, especially of the upper extremities and of the face, lower lip, ears, nose, and forehead, are common sites.

The incidence of BCC and SCC is increased in all immunocompromised people, including those infected with HIV. Clinically, the tumors have the same appearance as in non–HIV-infected people; however, in HIV-positive people, the tumors may grow more rapidly and recur more frequently. These tumors are managed the same as those for the general population. Frequent follow-up (every 4 to 6 months) is recommended to monitor for recurrence.

Prognosis

The prognosis for BCC is usually good because tumors remain localized. Although some require wide excision with resultant disfigurement, the risk of death from BCC is low. The prognosis for SCC depends on the incidence of metastases, which is related to the histologic type and the level or depth of invasion. Usually, SCC arising in sun-damaged areas is less invasive and rarely causes death, whereas SCC that arises without a history of sun or arsenic exposure or scar formation appears to have a greater chance of spread. Regional lymph nodes should be evaluated for metastases.

Medical Management

The goal of treatment is to eradicate the tumor. The treatment method depends on the tumor location; the cell type, location, and depth; the cosmetic desires of the patient; the history of previous treatment; whether the tumor is invasive; and whether metastatic nodes are present. The management of BCC and SCC includes surgical excision, Mohs' micrographic surgery, electrosurgery, cryosurgery, and radiation therapy.

Surgical Management

The primary goal is to remove the tumor entirely. The best way to maintain cosmetic appearance is to place the incision properly along natural skin tension lines and natural anatomic body lines. In this way, scars are less noticeable.

The size of the incision depends on the tumor size and location but usually involves a length-to-width ratio of 3:1.

The adequacy of the surgical excision is verified by microscopic evaluation of sections of the specimen. When the tumor is large, reconstructive surgery with use of a skin flap or skin grafting may be required. The incision is closed in layers to enhance cosmetic effect. A pressure dressing applied over the wound provides support. Infection after a simple excision is uncommon if proper surgical asepsis is maintained.

Mohs' Micrographic Surgery

This technique is the most accurate surgical technique and best conserves normal tissue. The procedure removes the tumor layer by layer. The first layer excised includes all evident tumor and a small margin of normal-appearing tissue. The specimen is frozen and analyzed by section to determine if all the tumor has been removed. If not, additional layers of tissue are shaved and examined until all tissue margins are tumor free. In this manner, only the tumor and a safe, normal-tissue margin are removed. Mohs' surgery is the recommended tissue-sparing procedure, with extremely high cure rates for BCC and SCC. It is the treatment of choice and the most effective for tumors around the eyes, nose, upper lip, and auricular and periauricular areas (Bowen, White & Gerwels, 2005).

Electrosurgery

Electrosurgery is the destruction or removal of tissue by electrical energy. The current is converted to heat, which then passes to the tissue from a cold electrode. Electrosurgery may be preceded by curettage (excising the skin tumor by scraping its surface with a curette). Electrodesiccation is then implemented to achieve hemostasis and to destroy any viable malignant cells at the base of the wound or along its edges. Electrodesiccation is useful for lesions smaller than 1 to 2 cm (0.4 to 0.8 in) in diameter.

This method takes advantage of the fact that the tumor is softer than surrounding skin and therefore can be outlined by a curette, which "feels" the extent of the tumor. The tumor is removed and the base cauterized. The process is repeated twice. Usually, healing occurs within 1 month.

Cryosurgery

Cryosurgery destroys the tumor by deep freezing the tissue. A thermocouple needle apparatus is inserted into the skin, and liquid nitrogen is directed to the center of the tumor until the tumor base is –40°C to –60°C (–40°F to –76°F). Liquid nitrogen has the lowest boiling point of all cryogens, is inexpensive, and is easy to obtain. The tumor tissue is frozen, allowed to thaw, and then refrozen. The site thaws naturally and then becomes gelatinous and heals spontaneously. Swelling and edema follow the freezing. The appearance of the lesion varies. Normal healing, which may take 4 to 6 weeks, occurs faster in areas with a good blood supply.

Radiation Therapy

Radiation therapy is frequently performed for cancer of the eyelid, the tip of the nose, and areas in or near vital structures (eg, facial nerve). It is reserved for older patients, because x-ray changes may be seen after 5 to 10 years, and malignant changes in scars may be induced by irradiation 15 to 30 years later.

The patient should be informed that the skin may become red and blistered. A bland skin ointment prescribed by the physician may be applied to relieve discomfort. The patient should also be cautioned to avoid exposure to the sun.

Nursing Management

Because many skin cancers are removed by excision, patients are usually treated in outpatient surgical units. The role of the nurse is to teach the patient about prevention of skin cancer and about self-care after treatment (Chart 56-6).

Promoting Home and Community-Based Care

Teaching Patients Self-Care

The wound is usually covered with a dressing to protect the site from physical trauma, external irritants, and contaminants. The patient is advised when to report for a dressing change or is given written and verbal information on how to change dressings, including the type of dressing to purchase, how to remove dressings and apply fresh ones, and the importance of hand hygiene before and after the procedure.

The patient is advised to watch for excessive bleeding and tight dressings that compromise circulation. If the lesion is in the perioral area, the patient is instructed to drink liquids through a straw and limit talking and facial movement. Dental work should be avoided until the area is completely healed.

After the sutures are removed, an emollient cream may be used to help reduce dryness. Applying a sunscreen over the wound is advised to prevent postoperative hyperpigmentation if the patient spends time outdoors.

Follow-up examinations should be at regular intervals, usually every 3 months for a year, and should include palpation of the adjacent lymph nodes. The patient should also

be instructed to seek treatment for any moles that are subject to repeated friction and irritation and to watch for indications of potential malignancy in moles as described previously. The importance of lifelong follow-up evaluations is emphasized.

Teaching About Prevention

Studies show that regular daily use of a sunscreen with a sun protection factor (SPF) of at least 15 can reduce the recurrence of skin cancer by as much as 40%. The sunscreen should be applied to head, neck, arms, and hands every morning at least 30 minutes before leaving the house and reapplied every 4 hours if the skin perspires. Intermittent application of sunscreen only when exposure is anticipated has been shown to be less effective than daily use. Research has shown that daily use of sunscreen on the hands and face reduces the total incidence of solar keratoses (Barclay, 2007), which are precursors of SCC, but has no effect on the overall incidence of BCC. These data are inconsistent, but one theory is that people have a false sense of security when wearing sunscreen and tend to stay out in the sun for longer periods. This longer exposure is believed to contribute to the increasing incidence of melanoma. Although the evidence is insufficient, nurses should discuss the issues with patients who are at high risk of skin cancer.

MALIGNANT MELANOMA

A malignant melanoma is a cancerous neoplasm in which atypical melanocytes are present in the epidermis and the dermis (and sometimes the subcutaneous cells). It is the most lethal of all the skin cancers and is responsible for about 3% of all cancer deaths (Porth & Maffin, 2009).

Malignant melanoma can occur in one of several forms: superficial spreading melanoma, lentigo-maligna melanoma, nodular melanoma, and acral-lentiginous melanoma. These types have specific clinical and histologic features as well as different biologic behaviors. Most melanomas arise from

---

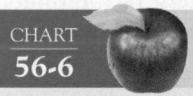

CHART 56-6	HEALTH PROMOTION

Preventing Skin Cancer

- Teach patients that sunscreens are rated in strength from 4 (weakest) to 50 (strongest). The solar protection factor, or SPF, indicates how much longer a person can stay in the sun before the skin begins to redden. For example, if the person can normally stay in the sun for 10 minutes before reddening begins, an SPF of 4 will protect the person from reddening for about 40 minutes.
- Remind patients that up to 50% of ultraviolet rays can penetrate loosely woven clothing.
- Remind patients that ultraviolet light can penetrate cloud cover, and a sunburn can still occur.
- Teach children to avoid all but modest sun exposure and to use a sunscreen regularly for lifelong protection.
- Advise patients to:
  - Avoid tanning if their skin burns easily, never tans, or tans poorly.
  - Avoid unnecessary exposure to the sun, especially during the time of day when ultraviolet radiation (sunlight) is most intense (10 AM to 3 PM).

- Avoid sunburns.
- Apply a sunscreen daily to block harmful sun rays.
- Use a sunscreen with an SPF of 15 or higher that protects against both ultraviolet-A (UVA) and ultraviolet-B (UVB) light.
- Reapply water-resistant sunscreens after swimming, if heavily sweating, and every 2 to 3 hours during prolonged periods of sun exposure.
- Avoid applying oils before or during sun exposure (oils do not protect against sunlight or sun damage).
- Use a lip balm that contains a sunscreen with an SPF of 15 or higher.
- Wear protective clothing, such as a broad-brimmed hat and long sleeves.
- Avoid using sun lamps for indoor tanning, and avoid commercial tanning booths.

cutaneous epidermal melanocytes, but some appear in pre-existing nevi (ie, moles) in the skin or develop in the uveal tract of the eye. Melanomas occasionally appear simultaneously with cancer of other organs.

The worldwide incidence of cutaneous melanoma continues to rise faster than any other malignancy in the Caucasian population. Despite better understanding of prevention and several new treatment options, mortality rates continue to climb. The highest incidence of the disease occurs in men, probably because of increased recreational sun exposure and decreasing ozone levels. In 2007, approximately 108,000 people in the United States were diagnosed with melanoma, and about 8,000 of these will die of the disease. Any short-term decrease in mortality will be related to improved detection and treatment. The impact of primary preventive measures will not be noticeable for several decades (American Melanoma Foundation, 2007).

Risk Factors

The cause of malignant melanoma is unknown, but ultraviolet rays are strongly suspected, based on indirect evidence such as the increased incidence of melanoma in countries near the equator and in people younger than 30 years of age who have used a tanning bed more than 10 times per year. One in 100 Caucasians develops melanoma each year. As many as 10% of patients with melanoma are members of melanoma-prone families who have multiple changing moles (dysplastic nevi) that are susceptible to malignant transformation. Patients with dysplastic nevus syndrome have been found to have unusual moles, larger and more numerous moles, lesions with irregular outlines, and pigmentation located all over the skin. Microscopic examination of dysplastic moles shows disordered, faulty growth (Sekulic, Haluska, Miller, et al., 2008). Chart 56-7 lists risk factors for malignant melanoma.

Research has identified a gene that resides on chromosome 9p, the absence of which increases the likelihood that potentially mutagenic DNA damage will escape repair before cell division. The absence of this gene can be identified in melanoma-prone families (Price, Herlyn, Dent, et al., 2005).

Patients who have the melanoma gene, those who have a larger number of pigmented lesions (more than 100), and those with a strong family history of melanoma can benefit from total body digital photography. This procedure is increasingly being offered at research facilities and large teaching facilities as a way to document lesion status. It is intended to decrease the number of unnecessary skin biopsies; it targets only lesions that show change over time, usually 3 to 6 months. Although the use of this photographic method has not reduced the number of skin biopsies in the short term, most practitioners who specialize in the treatment of pigmented lesions believe that the diagnostic value of this procedure will be realized in the next several decades. Some patients with high risk of melanoma would also benefit from "mole mapping" to track changes in individual lesions (Risser, Pressley, Veledar, et al., 2007).

Clinical Manifestations

Superficial Spreading Melanoma

Superficial spreading melanoma occurs anywhere on the body and is the most common form of melanoma. It usually affects middle-age people and occurs most frequently on the trunk and lower extremities. The lesion tends to be circular, with irregular outer portions. The margins of the lesion may be flat or elevated and palpable (Fig. 56-6). This type of melanoma may appear in a combination of colors, with hues of tan, brown, and black mixed with gray, blue-black, or white. Sometimes a dull pink rose color can be seen in a small area within the lesion.

Lentigo-Maligna Melanoma

Lentigo-maligna melanoma is a slowly evolving, pigmented lesion that occurs on exposed skin areas, especially the dorsum of the hand, the head, and the neck in elderly people. Often, the lesion is present for many years before it is examined by a physician. It first appears as a tan, flat lesion, but in time it undergoes changes in size and color.

Nodular Melanomas

Nodular melanoma is a spherical, blueberry-like nodule with a relatively smooth surface and a relatively uniform, blue-black color (see Fig. 56-6). It may be dome shaped with a smooth surface. It may have other shadings of red, gray, or purple. Sometimes, nodular melanomas appear as irregularly shaped plaques. The patient may describe this as a blood blister that fails to resolve. A nodular melanoma directly invades the adjacent dermis (ie, vertical growth) and therefore has a poorer prognosis.

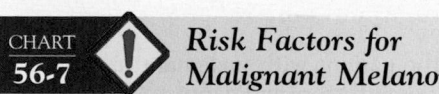

CHART
56-7

Risk Factors for Malignant Melanoma

- Fair-skinned or freckled, blue-eyed, light-haired people of Celtic or Scandinavian origin
- People who burn and do not tan or who have a significant history of severe sunburn
- Environmental exposure to intense sunlight (older Americans retiring to the southwestern United States appear to have a higher incidence)
- History of melanoma (personal or family)
- Skin with giant congenital nevi

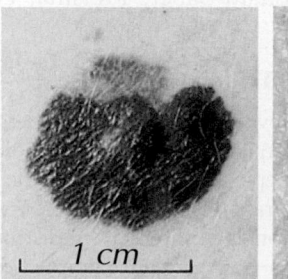
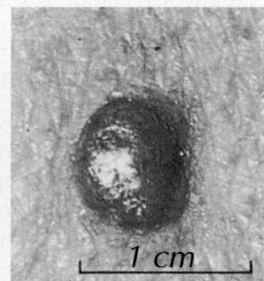

Figure 56-6 Two forms of malignant melanoma: superficial spreading (*left*) and nodular (*right*). From Bickley, L. S. (2009). *Bates' guide to physical examination* (10th ed.). Philadelphia: Lippincott Williams & Wilkins.

Acral-Lentiginous Melanoma

Acral-lentiginous melanoma occurs in areas not excessively exposed to sunlight and where hair follicles are absent. It is found on the palms of the hands, on the soles, in the nail beds, and in the mucous membranes in dark-skinned people. These melanomas appear as irregular, pigmented macules that develop nodules. They may become invasive early.

Assessment and Diagnostic Findings

Biopsy results confirm the diagnosis of melanoma. An excisional biopsy specimen provides information on the type, level of invasion, and thickness of the lesion. An excisional biopsy specimen that includes a 1-cm margin of normal tissue and a portion of underlying subcutaneous fatty tissue is sufficient for staging a melanoma in situ or an early, noninvasive melanoma. Incisional biopsy should be performed when the suspicious lesion is too large to be removed safely without extensive scarring. Biopsy specimens obtained by shaving, curettage, or needle aspiration are not considered reliable histologic proof of disease.

A thorough history and physical examination should include a meticulous skin examination and palpation of regional lymph nodes that drain the lesional area. Because melanoma occurs in families, a positive family history of melanoma is investigated so that first-degree relatives, who may be at high risk for melanoma, can be evaluated for atypical lesions. After the diagnosis of melanoma has been confirmed, a chest x-ray, complete blood cell count, liver function tests, and radionuclide or computed tomography scans are usually performed to stage the extent of disease.

Prognosis

The prognosis for long-term (5-year) survival is considered poor when the lesion is more than 1.5 mm thick or there is regional lymph node involvement. A person with a thin lesion and no lymph node involvement has a 3% chance of developing metastases and a 95% chance of surviving 5 years. If regional lymph nodes are involved, there is a 20% to 50% chance of surviving 5 years. Patients with melanoma on the hand, foot, or scalp have a better prognosis; those with lesions on the torso have an increased chance of metastases to the bone, liver, lungs, spleen, and central nervous system. Men and elderly patients also have poor prognoses (Jade, Kashani-Sabet, Messina, et al., 2005).

Medical Management

Treatment depends on the level of invasion and the depth of the lesion. Surgical excision is the treatment of choice for small, superficial lesions. Deeper lesions require wide local excision, after which skin grafting may be necessary. Regional lymph node dissection is commonly performed to rule out metastasis, although new surgical approaches call for only sentinel node biopsy. This technique is used to sample the nodes nearest the tumor and to spare the patient the long-term sequelae of extensive removal of lymph nodes if the sample nodes are negative.

Despite many years of investigation, no dependable systemic treatment for melanoma has been identified. Recently, greater understanding of the stem cells of melanoma indicates that effective therapies will have to be individualized for each patient. Clinical observations suggest that very few single-agent therapies provide significant clinical benefits because of the complex molecular nature of melanoma and the need to further define individual cell variations (Sekulic, et al., 2008).

Current treatments for metastatic melanoma, rarely, if ever, produce a satisfactory outcome. Further surgical intervention may be performed to debulk the tumor or to remove part of the organ involved (eg, lung, liver, or colon). However, the rationale for more extensive surgery is for relief of symptoms, not for cure. Chemotherapy for metastatic melanoma may be used; however, only a few agents (eg, dacarbazine [DTIC-Dome], nitrosoureas, cisplatin [Platinol]) have been effective in controlling the disease. When the melanoma is located in an extremity, regional perfusion may be used; the chemotherapeutic agent is perfused directly into the area that contains the melanoma. This approach delivers a high concentration of cytotoxic agents while avoiding systemic, toxic side effects. The limb is perfused for 1 hour with high concentrations of the medication at temperatures of 39°C to 40°C (102.2°F to 104°F) with a perfusion pump. Inducing hyperthermia enhances the effect of the chemotherapy so that a smaller total dose can be used. The goal of regional perfusion is control of the metastasis, especially if it is used in combination with surgical excision of the primary lesion and with regional lymph node dissection.

Investigators are exploring the potential for the use of lipid-lowering medications to prevent melanoma. A 2008 review concluded that there was a reduction in the incidence of melanoma in patients taking statins and fibrates, but the results were not highly significant. More research is needed before conclusions can be drawn (Dellavalle, Drake, Graber, et al., 2005). Several other studies continue to explore the potential for vaccine therapy, but none has yet identified an effective agent (Russo, Maccalli, Pilla, et al., 2008).

NURSING PROCESS

CARE OF THE PATIENT WITH MALIGNANT MELANOMA

Assessment

Assessment of the patient with malignant melanoma is based on the patient's history and symptoms. The patient is asked specifically about pruritus, tenderness, and pain, which are not features of a benign nevus. The patient is also questioned about changes in preexisting moles or the development of new, pigmented lesions. People at risk are assessed carefully.

A magnifying lens and good lighting are needed for inspecting the skin for irregularity and changes in the mole. Signs that suggest malignant changes are referred to as the ABCDs of moles (Chart 56-8).

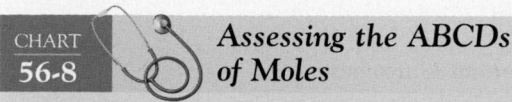

CHART
56-8

Assessing the ABCDs of Moles

A for Asymmetry

- The lesion does not appear balanced on both sides. If an imaginary line were drawn down the middle, the two halves would not look alike.
- The lesion has an irregular surface with uneven elevations (irregular topography) either palpable or visible. A change in the surface may be noted from smooth to scaly.
- Some nodular melanomas have a smooth surface.

B for Irregular Border

- Angular indentations or multiple notches appear in the border.
- The border is fuzzy or indistinct, as if rubbed with an eraser.

C for Variegated Color

- Normal moles are usually a uniform light to medium brown. Darker coloration indicates that the melanocytes have penetrated to a deeper layer of the dermis.
- Colors that may indicate malignancy if found together within a single lesion are shades of red, white, and blue; shades of blue are ominous.
- White areas within a pigmented lesion are suspicious.
- Some malignant melanomas, however, are not variegated but are uniformly colored (bluish-black, bluish-gray, bluish-red).

D for Diameter

- A diameter exceeding 6 mm (about the size of a pencil eraser) is considered more suspicious, although this finding without other signs is not significant. Many benign skin growths are larger than 6 mm, whereas some early melanomas may be smaller.

Common sites of melanomas are the skin of the back, the legs (especially in women), between the toes, and on the feet, face, scalp, fingernails, and backs of hands. In dark-skinned people, melanomas are most likely to occur in less pigmented sites: palms, soles, subungual areas, and mucous membranes. Satellite lesions (ie, those situated near the mole) are inspected.

Diagnosis

Nursing Diagnoses

Based on the nursing assessment data, the patient's major nursing diagnoses may include the following:

- Acute pain related to surgical excision and grafting
- Anxiety and depression related to possible life-threatening consequences of melanoma and disfigurement
- Deficient knowledge about early signs of melanoma

Collaborative Problems/Potential Complications

Based on the assessment data, potential complications include the following:

- Metastasis
- Infection of the surgical site

Planning and Goals

The major goals for the patient may include relief of pain and discomfort, reduced anxiety and depression, increased knowledge of early signs of melanoma, and absence of complications.

Nursing Interventions

Relieving Pain and Discomfort

Surgical removal of melanoma in different locations presents different challenges, taking into consideration the removal of the primary melanoma, the intervening lymphatic vessels, and the lymph nodes to which metastases may spread. Nursing management of the patient having surgery in these regions is discussed in the appropriate chapters.

Nursing interventions after surgery for a malignant melanoma center on promoting comfort, because wide excision surgery may be necessary. A split-thickness or full-thickness skin graft may be necessary when large defects are created by surgical removal of a melanoma. Anticipating the need for and administration of appropriate analgesic medications is important.

Reducing Anxiety and Depression

Psychological support is essential when disfiguring surgery is performed. Support includes allowing the patient to express feelings about the seriousness of the cutaneous neoplasm, understanding the patient's anxiety and depression, and conveying understanding of these feelings. During the diagnostic workup and staging of the depth, type, and extent of the tumor, the nurse answers questions, clarifies information, and helps clarify misconceptions. Learning that he or she has a melanoma can cause the patient considerable fear and anguish. Pointing out the patient's resources, past effective coping mechanisms, and social support systems helps the patient cope with the diagnosis and need for treatment and continuing follow-up. Family members should be included in all discussions to enable them to clarify information, ask questions that the patient might be reluctant to ask, and provide emotional support to the patient.

Monitoring and Managing Potential Complications

Metastasis of malignant melanoma is closely related to prognosis: the deeper and thicker (more than 4 mm) the melanoma, the greater is the likelihood of metastasis. If the melanoma is growing radially (ie, horizontally) and is characterized by peripheral growth with minimal or no dermal invasion, the prognosis is favorable. When the melanoma invades the dermal layer, the prognosis is poor. Lesions with ulceration have a poor prognosis. Melanomas of the trunk appear to have a poorer prognosis than those of other sites, perhaps because the network of lymphatics in the trunk permits metastasis to regional lymph nodes.

The role of the nurse in caring for the patient with metastatic disease is to provide holistic care. The nurse must be knowledgeable about the most effective current therapies and must deliver supportive care, provide and clarify information about the therapy and the rationale for its use, identify potential side effects of therapy and ways to manage them, and instruct the patient and family about the expected outcomes of treatment. The nurse monitors and documents symptoms that may indicate metastasis: lung (eg, difficulty breathing, shortness of breath, increasing cough), bone (eg, pain, decreased mobility and function, pathologic fractures), and liver (eg, change in liver enzyme levels, pain, jaundice). Nursing care is based on the patient's symptoms and emotional needs.

Although the chance of a cure for malignant melanoma that has metastasized is poor, the nurse encourages hope while maintaining a realistic perspective about the disease and ultimate outcome. Furthermore, the nurse provides time for the patient to express fears and concerns regarding future activities and relationships, offers information about support groups and contact people, and arranges palliative and hospice care if appropriate (see Chapter 17).

Promoting Home and Community-Based Care

TEACHING PATIENTS SELF-CARE. The best hope of decreasing the incidence of skin cancer lies in educating patients about the early signs. Patients at risk are taught to examine their skin and scalp monthly in a systematic manner and to seek prompt medical attention if changes are detected (Chart 56-9). The nurse also points out that a key factor in the development of melanoma is exposure to sunlight. Because melanoma is thought to be genetically linked, the family as well as the patient should be taught sun-avoiding measures and the importance of annual assessment by a health care provider.

Evaluation

Expected Patient Outcomes

Expected patient outcomes may include the following:

1. Experiences relief of pain and discomfort
   a. States pain is diminishing
   b. Exhibits healing of surgical scar without heat, redness, or swelling
2. Is less anxious
   a. Expresses fears and fantasies
   b. Asks questions about medical condition
   c. Requests facts about melanoma
   d. Identifies support and comfort provided by family member or significant other
3. Demonstrates understanding of the means for detecting and preventing melanoma
   a. Demonstrates how to conduct self-examination of skin on a monthly basis
   b. Verbalizes the following danger signals of melanoma: change in size, color, shape, or outline of mole, mole surface, or skin around mole
   c. Identifies measures to protect self from exposure to sunlight
4. Experiences absence of complications
   a. Recognizes abnormal signs and symptoms that should be reported to physician
   b. Complies with recommended follow-up procedures and prevention strategies

---

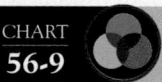

CHART 56-9

PATIENT EDUCATION
Periodic Self-Examination

Prevention of melanoma/skin cancer is the best weapon against these diseases, but if a melanoma should develop, it is almost always curable if caught in the early stages. Practice periodic self-examination to aid in early recognition of any new or developing lesion. The following is one way of self-examination that will ensure that no area of the body is neglected. To perform your self-examination, you will need a full-length mirror, a hand mirror, and a brightly lit room.

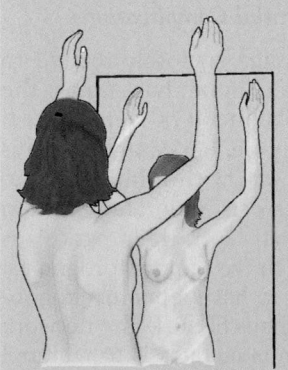 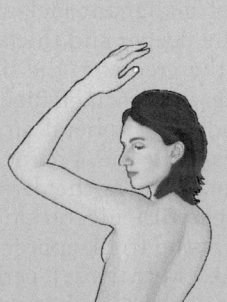 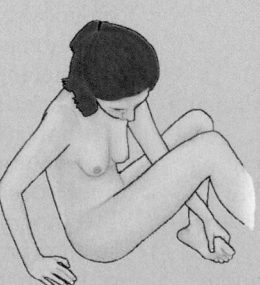 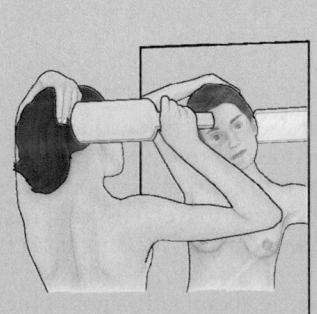 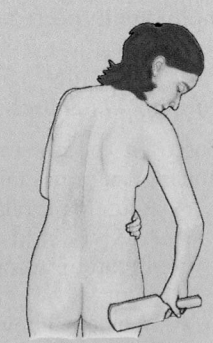

1. Examine the body front and back in the mirror, then the right and left sides, with the arms raised.

2. Bend the elbows, looking carefully at the forearms, back of the upper arms, and palms

3. Next, look at the back of the legs and feet, the spaces between the toes, and the soles of the feet.

4. Examine the back of the neck and the scalp with a hand-held mirror. Part the hair to lift.

5. Finally, check the back and buttocks with a hand mirror.

Metastatic Skin Tumors

The skin is an important, although not a common, site of metastatic cancer. All types of cancer may metastasize to the skin, but carcinoma of the breast is the primary source of cutaneous metastases in women. Other sources include cancer of the large intestine, ovaries, and lungs. In men, the most common primary sites are the lungs, large intestine, oral cavity, kidneys, or stomach. Skin metastases from melanomas are found in both genders. The clinical appearance of metastatic skin lesions is not distinctive, except perhaps in some cases of breast cancer in which diffuse, brawny hardening of the skin of the involved breast is seen. In most instances, metastatic lesions occur as multiple cutaneous or subcutaneous nodules of various sizes that may be skin colored or different shades of red.

Kaposi's Sarcoma

Kaposi's sarcoma (KS) is a malignancy of endothelial cells that line the small blood vessels. KS is manifested clinically by lesions of the skin, oral cavity, gastrointestinal tract, and lungs. The skin lesions consist of reddish-purple to dark-blue macules, plaques, or nodules. KS is subdivided into three categories:

- *Classic KS* occurs predominantly in men of Mediterranean or Jewish ancestry between 40 and 70 years of age. Most patients have nodules or plaques on the lower extremities that rarely metastasize beyond this area. Classic KS is chronic, relatively benign, and rarely fatal.
- *Endemic (African) KS* affects people predominantly in the eastern half of Africa near the equator. Men are affected more often than women, and children can be affected as well. The disease may resemble classic KS or it may infiltrate and progress to lymphadenopathic forms.
- *Immunosuppression-associated KS* occurs in transplant recipients and people with AIDS. This form of KS is characterized by local skin lesions and disseminated visceral and mucocutaneous diseases. The greater the degree of immunosuppression, the higher the incidence of KS. Immunosuppression-related KS that results from AIDS is an aggressive tumor that involves multiple body organs. Its presentation resembles that of KS associated with immunosuppressive therapy. Most patients are between 20 and 40 years of age. More information on AIDS-related KS can be found in Chapter 52.

DERMATOLOGIC AND PLASTIC RECONSTRUCTIVE PROCEDURES

The word *plastic* comes from a Greek word meaning *to form*. Plastic or reconstructive procedures are performed to reconstruct or alter congenital or acquired defects to restore or improve the body's form and function. Often the terms "plastic" and "reconstructive" are used interchangeably. This type of surgery includes closure of wounds, removal of skin tumors, repair of soft tissue injuries or burns, correction of deformities, and repair of cosmetic defects. Plastic surgery can be used to repair many parts of the body and numerous structures, such as bone, cartilage, fat, fascia, mucous membrane, muscle, nerve, and cutaneous structures. Bone inlays and transplants for deformities and nonunion can be performed, muscle can be transferred, nerves can be reconstructed and spliced, and cartilage can be replaced. As important as any of these measures is the reconstruction of the cutaneous tissues around the neck and the face; this is usually referred to as aesthetic or cosmetic surgery.

Cosmetic procedures are generally considered to be ones that correct defects that are not life-threatening or caused by disease. An example would be removal of a benign mole or sebaceous cyst from the face. Most health insurance plans do not cover procedures deemed to be cosmetic, and these procedures can be expensive. Procedures that are performed to correct a surgical defect, such as removal of a skin cancer or correction of a significant congenital defect such as a cleft lip, are generally covered by insurance, but this should be confirmed before surgery is scheduled.

Wound Coverage: Grafts and Flaps

Various surgical techniques, including skin grafts and flaps, are used to cover skin wounds.

Skin Grafts

Skin grafting is a technique in which a section of skin is detached from its own blood supply and transferred as free tissue to a distant (recipient) site. Skin grafting can be used to repair almost any type of wound and is the most common form of reconstructive surgery.

Skin grafts are commonly used to repair surgical defects such as those that result from excision of skin tumors, to cover areas denuded of skin (eg, burns), and to cover wounds in which insufficient skin is available to permit wound closure. They are also used when primary closure of the wound increases the risk of complications or when primary wound closure would interfere with function.

Skin grafts may be classified as autografts, allografts, or xenografts. An autograft is tissue obtained from the patient's own skin. An allograft is tissue obtained from a donor of the same species. These grafts are also called allogeneic or homograft. A xenograft or heterograft is tissue obtained from another species. A common xenograft for human skin is the pig.

Grafts are also referred to by their thickness. A skin graft may be a split-thickness (ie, thin, intermediate, or thick) or a full-thickness graft, depending on the amount of dermis included in the specimen. A split-thickness graft can be cut at various thicknesses and is commonly used to cover large wounds or defects for which a full-thickness graft or flap is impractical (Fig. 56-7). A full-thickness graft consists of epidermis and the entire dermis without the underlying fat. It is used to cover wounds that are too large to be closed directly.

Site Selection

The site where the intact skin is harvested is called the donor site. Selection of the donor site is made to match the

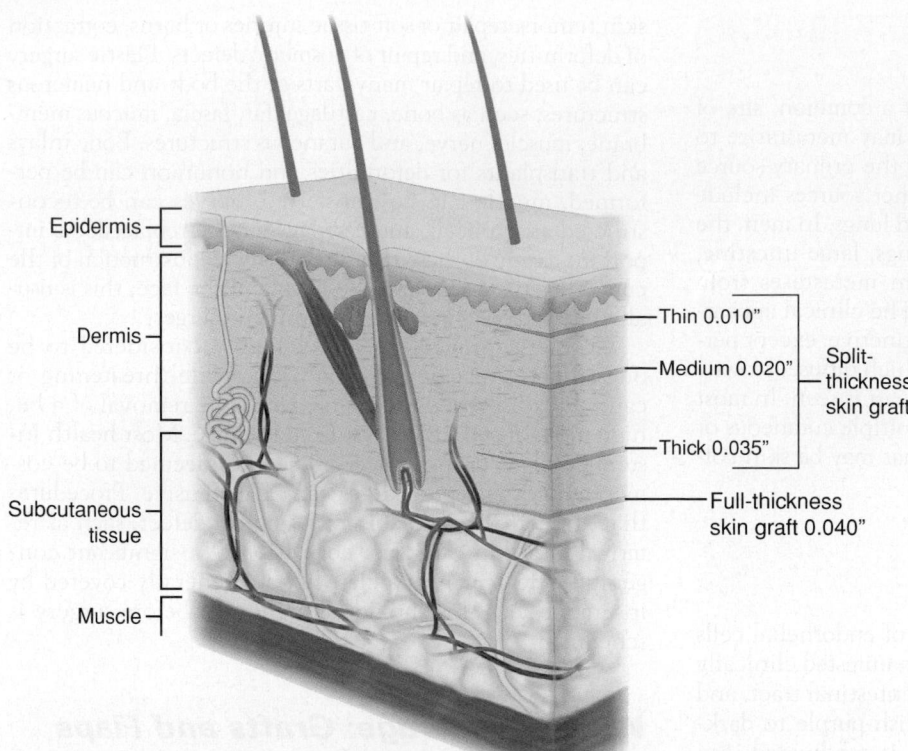

Epidermis

Dermis

Subcutaneous tissue

Muscle

Thin 0.010"

Medium 0.020"

Thick 0.035"

Split-thickness skin graft

Full-thickness skin graft 0.040"

Figure 56-7 Layers of skin appropriate for split-thickness and full-thickness graft.

color and texture of skin at the surgical site and to leave as little scarring as possible.

Graft Application

The skin graft is taken from the donor or host site and applied to the desired site, called the recipient site or graft bed.

For a graft to survive and be effective, certain conditions must be met:

- The recipient site must have an adequate blood supply so that normal physiologic function can resume.
- The graft must be in close contact with its bed to avoid accumulation of blood or fluid between the graft and the recipient site.
- The graft must be fixed firmly (immobilized) so that it remains in place on the recipient site.
- The area must be free of infection.

The graft, when applied to the recipient site, may be sutured in place; alternatively, it may be slit and spread apart to cover a greater area. The process of revascularization (establishing the blood supply) and reattachment of a skin graft to a recipient bed is referred to as a "take." After a skin graft is put in place, it may be left exposed (in areas that are impossible to immobilize) or covered with a light dressing or a pressure dressing, depending on the area of the body.

Nursing Interventions

The nurse must ensure that both the surgical and the donor sites receive proper postoperative care. The surgical site is covered by the harvested skin, and the donor site heals by re-epithelization of the raw, exposed dermis. Both sites are

protected by dressings as they heal. Prevention of infection is essential as with all surgical sites. Both sites can be kept soft and pliable with cream (eg, lanolin). Both the donor site and the grafted area must be protected from exposure to extremes in temperature, external trauma, and sunlight because these areas are sensitive, especially to thermal injuries.

Flaps

Another form of wound coverage is provided by flaps. A flap is a segment of tissue that remains attached at one end (ie, a base or pedicle) while the other end is moved to a recipient area. Its survival depends on functioning arterial and venous blood supplies and lymphatic drainage in its pedicle or base. A flap differs from a graft in that a portion of the tissue is attached to its original site and retains its blood supply. An exception is the free flap, which is described below.

Flaps may consist of skin, mucosa, muscle, adipose tissue, omentum, and bone. They are used for wound coverage and provide bulk, especially when bone, tendon, blood vessels, or nerve tissue is exposed. Flaps are used to repair defects caused by congenital deformity, trauma, or tumor ablation (removal, usually by excision) in an adjacent part of the body.

Flaps offer an aesthetic solution because a flap retains the color and texture of the donor area, is more likely to survive than a graft, and can be used to cover nerves, tendons, and blood vessels. However, several surgical procedures are usually required to advance a flap. The major complication is necrosis of the pedicle or base as a result of failure of the blood supply.

Free Flaps

A striking advance in reconstructive surgery is the use of free flaps or free-tissue transfer achieved by microvascular techniques. A free flap is completely severed from the body and transferred to another site. A free flap receives early vascular supply from microvascular anastomosis with vessels at the recipient site. The procedure usually is completed in one step, eliminating the need for a series of surgical procedures to move the flap. Microvascular surgery allows surgeons to use a variety of donor sites for tissue reconstruction.

Cosmetic Procedures

Chemical Face Peeling

Chemical face peeling involves application of a chemical mixture to the face for superficial destruction of the epidermis and the upper layers of the dermis to treat fine wrinkles, keratoses, and pigment problems. It is especially useful for wrinkles at the upper and lower lip, forehead, and periorbital areas. The type of chemical used depends on the planned depth of the peel. The conscious patient feels a burning sensation that continues for 12 to 24 hours. Frequent small doses of analgesics and tranquilizers are prescribed to keep the patient comfortable. The most common complications include discoloration of the skin, infection of the burned area, persistent sensory changes or itching, and occasionally permanent scarring of the skin.

Dermabrasion

Dermabrasion is a form of skin abrasion used to treat acne scarring, aging, and sun-damaged skin. A special instrument (ie, motor-driven wire brush, diamond-impregnated disk, or serrated wheel) is used. The epidermis and some superficial dermis are removed by a sanding-like action, and enough of the dermis is preserved to allow re-epithelization of the treated areas. Results are best in the face because it is rich in intradermal epithelial elements.

The primary reason for undergoing dermabrasion is to improve appearance.

Facial Reconstructive Surgery

Reconstructive procedures on the face are individualized to the patient's needs and desired outcomes. They are performed to repair deformities or restore normal function. They may vary from closure of small defects to complicated procedures involving implantation of prosthetic devices to conceal a large defect or reconstruct a lost part of the face (eg, nose, ear, jaw). Each surgical procedure is customized and involves a variety of incisions, flaps, and grafts. Multiple surgical procedures may be required.

The process of facial reconstruction is often slow and tedious. Because a person's facial appearance affects self-esteem so greatly, this type of reconstruction is often a very emotional experience for the patient.

Face Lift

Rhytidectomy (face lift) is a surgical procedure that removes soft tissue folds and minimizes cutaneous wrinkles on the face.

It is performed to create a more youthful appearance. Psychological preparation requires that the patient recognize the limitations of surgery and the fact that miraculous rejuvenation will not occur. The patient is informed that the face may appear bruised and swollen after the dressings are removed and that several weeks may pass before the edema subsides.

LASER TREATMENT OF CUTANEOUS LESIONS

Lasers are devices that amplify or generate highly specialized light energy. They can mobilize immense heat and power when focused at close range and are valuable tools in surgical procedures. The argon laser, carbon dioxide (CO_2) laser, and tunable pulse-dye laser are used in dermatologic surgery. Each type of laser emits its own wavelength within the color spectrum.

Argon Laser

The argon laser is useful in treating vascular lesions: port-wine stains, telangiectases, vascular tumors, and pigmented lesions. The argon beam can penetrate approximately 1 mm of skin and reach the pigmented layer, causing protein coagulation in this area. An immediate effect is that tiny blood vessels under the skin coagulate, causing the area to turn a much lighter color. A crust forms within a few days.

Carbon Dioxide Laser

The CO_2 laser is a precise surgical instrument that vaporizes and excises tissue with minimal damage. Because the beam can seal blood and lymphatic vessels, it creates a dry surgical field that makes many procedures easier and quicker. Therefore, it is safe to use on patients with bleeding disorders or those receiving anticoagulant therapy. It is useful for removing epidermal nevi, tattoos, certain warts, skin cancer, ingrown toenails, and keloids. Incisions made with the laser beam heal and scar much like those made by a scalpel.

Pulse-Dye Laser

The tunable pulse-dye laser is especially useful in treating cutaneous vascular lesions such as port-wine stains and telangiectasia. The procedure is generally painless. For procedures requiring anesthesia, lidocaine without epinephrine is sufficient because local vasoconstriction (which epinephrine induces) is unnecessary.

Nursing Management

The majority of dermatologic and reconstructive procedures are performed in the physician's office or in an outpatient surgical department; therefore, most care takes place in the home. Most procedures, except very extensive reconstruction, are performed under local anesthesia or moderate sedation, therefore requiring a very short recovery time. Unless there are complications, the patient does not need hospitalization. It is important for the nurse to prepare both the patient and family for what to expect during the postoperative recovery time. Table 56-7 lists a few of the nursing considerations that must be reviewed in educating the patient and family.

Table 56–7   NURSING CONSIDERATIONS IN COSMETIC PROCEDURES

Nursing Consideration	Interventions and Patient Education
Maintaining airway and pulmonary function	Cosmetic surgeries involving the face and neck can cause considerable swelling; bandages can restrict breathing or eating. Check dressings frequently and ensure that no constriction occurs as swelling develops.
Relieving pain and achieving comfort	Procedures that involve a large surface area will cause considerable pain. Cool compresses or ice packs will relieve the burning of dermabrasion or chemical peels. Oral analgesics should be administered regularly to control pain.
Maintaining adequate nutrition	When the face is involved, the patient may be unable to fully open the mouth, and chewing may be painful. Provide soft or liquid diet that is high in protein to assist with healing.
Enhancing communication	Depending on the type of cosmetic procedure, a nonverbal method of communication might be necessary until pain and swelling have subsided.
Improving self-concept	Recovery time from cosmetic procedures is slow. Expected results will take weeks to become apparent. Persons of color will experience increased pigmentation long after the initial wounds have healed. Helping patients to understand postoperative expectations will allow them to feel more comfortable with the healing process.
Promoting family coping	Most cosmetic procedures are performed in an outpatient facility; therefore, family members are integral to postoperative care. They should understand what to expect as the patient emerges from the procedure room: the type of dressings that will be in place, the skin care plan that is prescribed, and how to cope with the patient's pain.
Monitoring and managing potential complications	Infection is the most common complication, but excessive pain, nerve damage, and emotional distress about appearance are also common. If opioids are used, there may be gastrointestinal upset, mental status changes, or allergic reaction to the medication. Alert the caregiver to signs of these complications and how and when to report changes in status.

CRITICAL THINKING EXERCISES

EBP **1** You are caring for a middle-age woman who has diabetes and peripheral vascular disease. She has now developed a venous stasis ulcer on her lower leg just above the ankle. Her physician has prescribed a moisture-retentive dressing that is impregnated with hydrogel. The dressing is to be changed every 3 days, and the patient asks you why the dressing is not changed every day. How would you explain to the patient the purpose of the dressing? Identify the evidence that supports the use of moisture-retentive dressings for venous ulcers. Discuss the strength of the evidence regarding their effectiveness in the promotion of wound healing. What other teaching would you provide to this patient about care of her skin?

2 A 35-year-old woman, who has two small children at home and is in the middle of a divorce, is admitted to your nursing unit for treatment of an acute flare of psoriasis. Her skin is covered with bright red, dry scaling plaques, involving 60% of her body surface. Additionally, she has distortions of her fingers and pitted nail plates, and she reports bilateral ankle pain on awakening each day. She has been admitted for twice-daily bath treatments and to initiate an injectable biologic for management of her condition. What should be included in the admission nursing assessment? What should be included in the teaching plan? List some of the possible psychosocial issues that that may arise as you care for this patient.

3 A 50-year-old professional golfer is having a routine physical examination. He states that his mother had malignant melanoma and that he is concerned about several lesions on his arms and neck. He asks about the risk factors for melanoma and about total body digital photography that a colleague had recently had. How would you explain the purpose of this photographic method? Identify the evidence and the strength of the evidence that supports the diagnostic value of this procedure. What teaching would you provide to this patient about prevention of melanoma and self-examination of the skin?

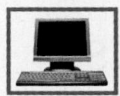 The Smeltzer suite offers these additional resources to enhance learning and facilitate understanding of this chapter:

• thePoint online resource, thepoint.lww.com/Smeltzer12E
• Student CD-ROM included with the book
• *Study Guide to Accompany Brunner & Suddarth's Textbook of Medical-Surgical Nursing*
• *Handbook for Brunner & Suddarth's Textbook of Medical-Surgical Nursing*

REFERENCES AND SELECTED READINGS

Asterisk indicates nursing research.

Books

American Cancer Society. (2009). *Cancer facts and figures.* Atlanta, GA: Author.

Baran, R. & Maibach, H. I. (2005). *Textbook of cosmetic dermatology* (3rd ed.). New York: Taylor & Francis Group.

Goldman, M. P. (2005). *Principles and practices in cutaneous laser surgery.* Philadelphia: Mosby.

Hall, J. C. (2006). *Sauer's manual of skin diseases* (9th ed.). Philadelphia: Lippincott Williams & Wilkins.

Harahap, M. & Abadir, A. D. (2008). *Anesthesia and analgesia in dermatologic surgery.* London: CRC Press.

James, W. D., Berger, T. & Elston, D. (2005). *Andrews' diseases of the skin: Clinical dermatology.* Philadelphia: Saunders.

Krasner, D., Rodeheaver, G. & Sibbald, G. (2007). *Chronic wound care: A clinical source book for healthcare professionals.* Malvern, PA: HMP Communications.

Murphy, J. L. (2007). *Nurse practitioners' prescribing reference.* New York: Prescribing Reference.

Porth, C. M. & Matfin, G. (2009). *Pathophysiology. Concepts of altered health states* (8th ed.). Philadelphia: Lippincott Williams & Wilkins.

Scher, R. K. & Daniel, C. R. (2005). *Nails—Diagnosis, therapy, surgery* (3rd ed.). Philadelphia: Saunders.

Wolff, K., Goldsmith, L., Katz, S. I., et al. (2007). *Fitzpatrick's dermatology in general medicine* (6th ed.). New York: McGraw-Hill.

Wolff, K., Johnson, R. A., & Suurmond, D. (2005). *Color atlas and synopsis of clinical dermatology* (5th ed.). New York: McGraw-Hill.

Journals and Electronic Documents

American Melanoma Foundation. (2007). Skin cancer fact sheet. www.melanomafoundation.org/facts/statistics.htm

Barclay, L. (2007). Behavioral strategies recommended to reduce risk for skin cancer. *Medscape Medical News.* http://cme.medscape.com/viewarticle/556250

*Beitz, J. M. & Goldberg, E. (2005). The lived experience of having a chronic wound: A phenomenologic study. *MedSurg Nursing, 14*(1), 51–62.

Black J, Baharestani, M., Cuddigan, J., et al. (2007). National Pressure Ulcer Advisory Panel's updated pressure ulcer staging system. *Dermatology Nursing, 19*(4), 343–349.

Bowen, G. M., White, G. L. & Gerwels, J. W. (2005). Mohs micrographic surgery. *American Family Physician, 72*(5), 845–848.

Busti, A. J., Hooper, J. S., Amaya, C. J., et al. (2005). Effects of perioperative antiinflamatory and immunomodulating therapy on surgical wound healing *Pharmacotherapy, 25*(11), 1566–1591.

Chaby, G., Senet, P., Vaneau, M., et al. (2007). Dressings for acute and chronic wounds: A systematic review. *Archives of Dermatology, 143*(10), 1297–1304.

Davis, M. D., Scalf, L. A. & Yiannias, J. (2008). Changing trends and allergens in the patch test standard series: A Mayo Clinic 5-year retrospective review, January 1, 2001, through December 31, 2005. *Archives of Dermatology, 144*(1), 67–72.

Dellavalle, R. P., Drake, A., Graber, M., et al. (2005). Statins and fibrates for preventing melanoma. *Cochrane Database of Systematic Reviews, 4*, CD003697.

Dente, K. M. (2007). Alternative treatments for wounds: Leeches, maggots and bees. *Medscape General Surgery.* www.medscape.com/viewarticle/563656

Fonder, M. A., Lazarus, G. S., Cowan, D., et al. (2008). Treating the chronic wound: A practical approach to the care of nonhealing wounds and wound care dressings. *Journal of American Academy of Dermatology, 58*(2), 185–206.

Giblin, A. V. & Thomas, J. M. (2007). Incidence, mortality and survival in cutaneous melanoma. *Journal of Plastic, Reconstructive & Aesthetic Surgery, 60*(1), 32–40.

High, K. (2005). Reducing the public health burden of herpes zoster and postherpetic neuralgia. http://cme.medscape.com/viewarticle/513508_4

Hillhouse, J, Turrisi, R. & Shields, A. L. (2007). Patterns of indoor tanning use: Implications for clinical interventions. *Archives of Dermatology, 143*(12), 1530–1535.

Holcomb, S. S. (2007). Dodging the bullae: Stevens-Johnson syndrome. *Nursing, 37*(4), 64CC1–64CC3.

Jade, H., Kashani-Sabet, M., Messina, J. L., et al. (2005). Cutaneous melanoma: Prognostic factors. *Cancer Control, 12*(4), 223–229.

*Jones K. R., Fennie K. & Lenihan, A. (2007). Chronic wounds: Factors influencing healing within 3 months, and nonhealing after 6 months. *Wounds, 19*(3), 51–63.

Lui, H. & Mamelak, A. J. (2007). Psoriasis, plaque. www.emedicine.com/DERM/topic365.htm

Milne, C. (2008). Wound healing in older adults. *Advance for Nurse Practitioners, 16*(7), 53.

Mittmann, N., Chan, B. C., Knowles, S., et al. (2007). IVIG for the treatment of toxic epidermal necrolysis. *Skin Therapy Letter, 12*(1), 1–8.

Neville, J. A., Welch, E. & Leffell, D. J. (2007) Management of nonmelanoma skin cancer in 2007. *National Clinical Practice of Oncology, 4*(8), 432–469.

Pipkin, C. A. & Lio, P. A. (2008). Cutaneous manifestations of internal malignancies: An overview. *Dermatologic Clinics, 26*(1), 1–15.

Pirzada, S., Tomi, Z. & Gulliver, W. (2007). A review of biologic treatment for psoriasis with emphasis on infliximab. *Skin Therapy Letter, 12*(3), 1–4.

Price, K. L., Herlyn, M., Dent, C. L., et al. (2005). The prevalence of interferon-alpha transcription deficits in malignant melanoma. *Melanoma Research, 15*(2), 91–98.

Risser J., Pressley Z., Veledar E., et al. (2007). The impact of total body photography on biopsy rate in patients from a pigmented lesion clinic. *Journal of American Academy of Dermatology, 57*, 428–434.

Russo, V., Maccali, C., Pilla, L., et al. (2008). Update on vaccines for melanoma patients. *Expert Review of Dermatology, 3*(2), 195–207.

Sekulic, A., Haluska, P., Miller, A. J., et al. (2008). For the Melanoma Study Group of the Mayo Clinic Cancer Center. Malignant melanoma in the 21st century: The emerging molecular landscape. *Mayo Clinic Proceedings, 83*(7), 825–846.

Shaw R. J., Dayal, S., Good, J., et al. (2007). Psychiatric medications for the treatment of pruritus. *Psychosomatic Medicine, 69*(9), 970–978.

Singh, M., Lin J., Hocker T. L., et al. (2008). Genetics of melanoma tumorigenesis. *British Journal of Dermatology, 158*(1), 15–21.

Taibjee, S. M. (2005). Controlled study of excimer and pulse dye lasers in the treatment of psoriasis. *British Journal of Dermatology, 153*, 960–966.

Vaneau, M., Chaby, G., Guillot, B., et al. (2007). Consensus panel recommendations for chronic and acute wound dressings. *Archives of Dermatology, 143*(10), 1291–1294.

Wurster, J. (2007). What role can nurses play in reducing the incidence of pressure sores? *Nursing Economics, 25*(5), 267–269.

RESOURCES

Dermatology online atlas, a cooperation between the Department of Clinical Social Medicine (University of Heidelberg) and the Department of Dermatology (University of Erlangen), www.dermis.net

Foundation for Ichthyosis and Related Skin Types, www.scalyskin.org

Lupus Foundation, www.lupus.org

National Alopecia Areata Foundation (NAAF), www.naaf.org

National Eczema Association for Science and Education, www.nationaleczema.org

National Organization for Albinism and Hypopigmentation, www.albinism.org

National Pressure Ulcer Advisory Panel, www.npuap.org

National Psoriasis Foundation (USA), www.psoriasis.org

National Rosacea Society, www.rosacea.org

National Vitiligo Foundation, www.nvfi.org

New Zealand Dermatology Society, www.dermnetnz.org

Skin Cancer Foundation, www.skincancer.org

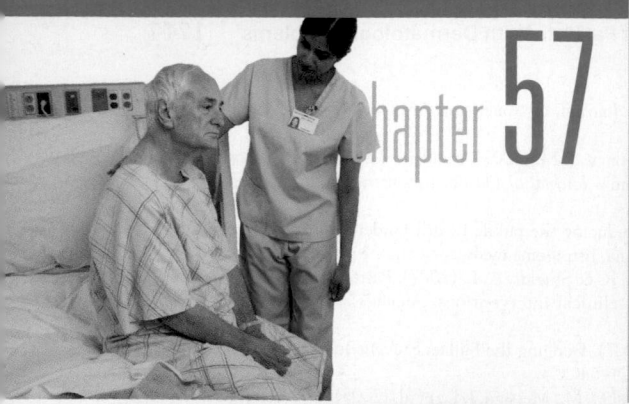

chapter 57

Management of Patients With Burn Injury

GLOSSARY

AlloDerm: processed dermis from human cadaver skin; can be used as dermal layer for skin grafts

autograft: a graft derived from one part of a patient's body and used on another part of that same patient's body

Biobrane: synthetic dressing composed of a nylon, Silastic membrane combined with a collagen derivative

carboxyhemoglobin: a compound of carbon monoxide and hemoglobin, formed in the blood with exposure to carbon monoxide

collagen: a protein present in skin, tendon, bone, cartilage, and connective tissue

contracture: shrinkage of burn scar through collagen maturation

cultured epithelial autograft (CEA): autologous epidermal cells that proliferate in culture and then are regrafted onto the patient

débridement: removal of foreign material and devitalized tissue until surrounding healthy tissue is exposed

donor site: the area from which skin is taken to provide a skin graft for another part of the body

eschar: devitalized tissue resulting from a burn

escharotomy: a linear excision made through eschar to release constriction of underlying tissue

excision: surgical removal of tissue

fasciotomy: an incision made through the fascia to release constriction of underlying muscle

heterograft: graft (ie, pigskin) obtained from an animal of a species other than that of the recipient; also called a xenograft

homograft: a graft transferred from one human (living or cadaveric) to another human; also called allograft

hydrotherapy: cleansing of wounds through use of bath, shower, shower cart table, or immersion

hypertrophic scar: excessive scar formation that rises above the level of the skin

Integra: synthetic dermal substitute

rule of nines: method for calculating body surface area burned by dividing the body into multiples of nine

The nurse who cares for a patient with a burn injury requires a high level of knowledge about the physiologic changes that occur after a burn, as well as astute assessment skills to detect subtle changes in the patient's condition. The patient's health history affects burn care. This makes each burn patient very unique and provides a variety of challenges to the patient's plan of care. In addition, the nurse provides sensitive, compassionate care to patients who are critically ill and initiates rehabilitation early in the course of care. The nurse must also be able to communicate effectively with patients who have burn injuries, family members in crisis, and members of the entire interdisciplinary burn management team. Care of the patient with a burn requires knowledge and skill throughout the care continuum from injury to recovery. This ensures quality care, improved patient outcomes, and optimal quality of life.

Overview of Burn Injury

Incidence

A burn injury can affect people of all age groups, in all socioeconomic groups. An estimated 500,000 people are treated for minor burn injury annually (Pitts, Niska, Xu, et al., 2008). The number of patients who are hospitalized each year with burn injuries is more than 40,000. This includes approximately 25,000 people who require hospitalization in specialized burn centers across the country. As emergency transportation and awareness of burn specialized hospitals has increased, the number of patients referred to these centers has risen. The remaining 5,000 hospitals see an average of three burns per year. Of those people admitted to burn centers, 47% of their injuries occurred at home, 27% on the road, 8% are occupational, 5% are recreational, and the remaining 13% from other sources. Forty percent of these injuries were flame related, 30% scald injuries, 4% electrical, 3% chemical, with the remaining unspecified (Miller, Bessey, Lentz, et al., 2008).

Males have greater then twice the chance of burn injury than women, and the most frequent age group for contact burns is between 20 to 40 years of age (Miller, et al., 2008). The National Fire Protection Association reports 4,000 fire and burn deaths each year. Of these, 3,500 deaths occur from residential fires and the remaining 500 from other sources such as motor vehicle crashes, scalds, or electrical and chemical sources. The overall mortality rate, for all ages and for total body surface area (TBSA) burned is 4.9% (Miller, et al., 2008).

Gerontologic Considerations

Reduced mobility, coordination, strength, and sensation and changes in vision place elderly people at higher risk for burn injury. Difficulties cooking and bathing and other activities of daily living are associated with flame and scald injury in this age group. These changes also place older people at risk for severe burn because they have difficulty in extinguishing the fire and removing themselves from the burn source (Sheridan, 2007a).

Morbidity and mortality rates associated with burns are greater in elderly patients than in younger patients when comparing injuries with similar severity. In 2007 patients over the age of 60 who had a 60% TBSA or greater had an overall mortality rate of 96% (Sheridan, 2007a). Predisposing factors and the health history in the older adult influence the complexity of care for the patient. Pulmonary function is limited in the older adult, therefore, airway exchange, lung elasticity, and ventilation can be affected. This can be further affected by a history of smoking. Decreased cardiac function and coronary artery disease increase the risk of complications in elderly patients with burn injuries. Malnutrition and presence of diabetes mellitus or other endocrine disorders present nutritional challenges and require close monitoring. Varying degrees of orientation may present themselves on admission or through the course of care, making assessment of pain and anxiety a challenge for the burn team. The skin of the elderly is thinner and less elastic, which affects the depth of injury and its ability to heal (Sheridan, 2007a).

An important goal of nurses in community and home settings is to provide education on the prevention of burn injury, especially among the elderly (Chart 57-1). Nurses

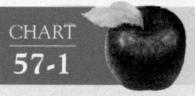

CHART 57-1	HEALTH PROMOTION *Burn Prevention*

- Advise that matches and lighters be kept out of the reach of children.
- Emphasize the importance of never leaving children unattended around fire or in bathroom/bathtub.
- Advise the installation and maintenance of smoke detectors on every level of the home, changing batteries annually on birthday.
- Recommend the development and practice of a home exit fire drill with all members of the household.
- Advise setting the water heater temperature no higher than 120°F.
- Caution against smoking in bed, while using home oxygen, or against falling asleep while smoking.
- Caution against throwing flammable liquids onto an already burning fire.

- Caution against using flammable liquids to start fires.
- Caution against removing the radiator cap from a hot car engine.
- Recommend avoidance of overhead electrical wires and underground wires when working outside.
- Advise that hot irons and curling irons be kept out of the reach of children.
- Caution against running electric cords under carpets or rugs.
- Recommend storage of flammable liquids well away from a fire source, such as a pilot light.
- Advocate caution when cooking, being aware of loose clothing hanging over the stove top.
- Recommend having a working fire extinguisher in the home and knowing how to use it.

need to assess an elderly patient's ability to safely perform activities of daily living, assist elderly patients and families to modify their environment to ensure safety, and make referrals as needed.

Outlook for Survival and Recovery

The National Center for Injury Prevention and Control of the Centers for Disease Control and Prevention (CDC) identifies fire or burn injury as the fifth most common cause of death from unintentional injury in the United States and the third leading cause of death in the home from injury (CDC, 2008).

Great strides in research have helped to increase the survival rate of patients with burn injuries. Mortality has fallen to levels never thought possible. Long-term outcomes can now be explored because patients with very large burns are surviving their injuries. Research in areas such as fluid resuscitation, emergency burn treatment, inhalation injury and management, nutritional needs and changes in wound care practice with early excision, skin grafting, and use of skin substitutes have contributed greatly to the decrease in burn deaths. Continued research and advances in the areas of critical care, rehabilitation, psychosocial, and scar management are essential for continued progress in burn care.

Severity

The severity of each burn injury is determined by multiple factors that when assessed help the burn team estimate the likelihood that a patient will survive and plan for the care for each patient. These factors include age of the patient; depth of the burn; amount of surface area of the body that is burned; the presence of inhalation injury; presence of other injuries; location of the injury in special care areas such as the face, the perineum, hands, or feet; and the presence of a past medical history.

Age

Young children and the elderly continue to have increased morbidity and mortality when compared to other age groups with similar injuries and present a challenge for burn care. This is an important factor when determining the severity of injury and possible outcome for the patient.

Burn Depth

Burns are classified according to the depth of tissue destruction as superficial partial-thickness injuries, deep partial-thickness injuries, or full-thickness injuries (Table 57-1). These three categories are similar to, but not the same as, first-, second-, and third-degree burn classifications. Although the term fourth-degree burn is not used universally, it occurs with prolonged flame contact or high-voltage injury that destroys all layers of the skin and damages tendons and muscles.

In a superficial partial-thickness burn, the epidermis is destroyed or injured and a portion of the dermis may be injured. A deep partial-thickness burn involves destruction of the epidermis and upper layers of the dermis and injury to deeper portions of the dermis. Capillary refill follows tissue blanching. Hair follicles remain intact. A full-thickness burn involves total destruction of epidermis and dermis and, in some cases, destruction of underlying tissue, muscle, and bone. Wound color ranges widely from pale white to red, brown, or charred black. The burned area is painless and lacks sensation because nerve fibers are destroyed. The wound appears leathery; hair follicles and sweat glands are destroyed (Fig. 57-1). The severity of this burn is often deceiving to patients because they have no pain in the injury area. These wounds require skin grafting for healing.

Burn depth determines whether epithelialization will occur. Determining burn depth can be difficult even for the experienced burn care provider. The following factors are

Table 57-1	CHARACTERISTICS OF BURNS ACCORDING TO DEPTH			
Depth of Burn and Causes	**Skin Involvement**	**Symptoms**	**Wound Appearance**	**Recuperative Course**
Superficial Partial-Thickness (Similar to First Degree)				
Sunburn Low-intensity flash	Epidermis; possibly a portion of dermis	Tingling Hyperesthesia (supersensitivity) Pain that is soothed by cooling	Reddened; blanches with pressure; dry Minimal or no edema Possible blisters	Complete recovery within a week; no scarring Peeling
Deep Partial-Thickness (Similar to Second Degree)				
Scalds Flash flame Contact	Epidermis, upper dermis, portion of deeper dermis	Pain Hyperesthesia Sensitive to cold air	Blistered, mottled red base; broken epidermis; weeping surface Edema	Recovery in 2 to 4 weeks Some scarring and depigmentation contractures Infection may convert it to full thickness
Full-Thickness (Similar to Third Degree)				
Flame Prolonged exposure to hot liquids Electric current Chemical Contact	Epidermis, entire dermis, and sometimes subcutaneous tissue; may involve connective tissue, muscle, and bone	Pain free Shock Hematuria (blood in the urine) and possibly hemolysis (blood cell destruction) Possible entrance and exit wounds (electrical burn)	Dry; pale white, leathery, or charred Broken skin with fat exposed Edema	Eschar sloughs Grafting necessary Scarring and loss of contour and function; contractures Loss of digits or extremity possible

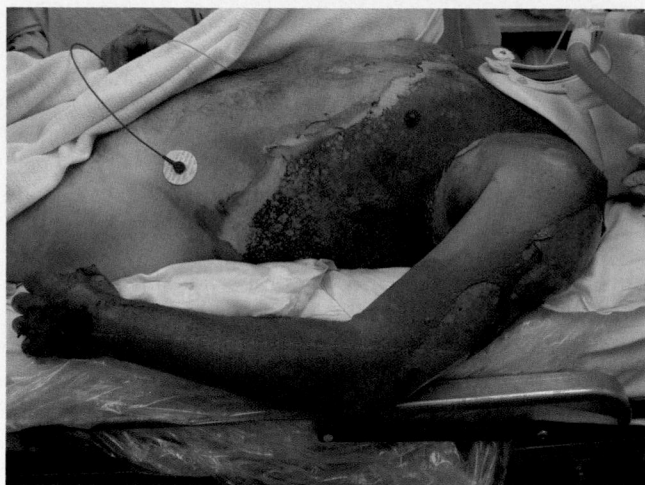

Figure 57-1 Full-thickness injury to chest and upper extremity. Epidermis, varying levels of the dermis and subcutaneous tissue is injured. Used with permission. Lehigh Valley Health Network, Allentown, PA.

considered in determining the depth of a burn: how the injury occurred, causative agent (such as flame or scalding liquid), temperature of the burning agent, duration of contact with the agent, and thickness of the skin.

Extent of Body Surface Area Injured

Various methods are used to estimate the TBSA affected by burns; among them are the rule of nines, the Lund and Browder method, and the palmer method. These methods assist the burn team in making decisions about treatment and transfer of the patient to a burn center.

Rule of Nines

A common method, the **rule of nines** (Fig. 57-2), is a quick way to estimate the extent of burns in adults. The system divides the body into multiples of nine. The sum total of these parts equals the total body surface area and is an important measurement in the severity of injury (Shukla & Sheridan, 2008).

Lund and Browder Method

A more precise method of estimating the extent of a burn is the Lund and Browder method, which recognizes the percentage of surface area of various anatomic parts, especially the head and legs, as it relates to the age of the patient. By dividing the body into very small areas and providing an estimate of the proportion of TBSA accounted for by each body part, one can obtain a reliable estimate of TBSA burned. The initial evaluation is made on arrival of the patient at the hospital and is revised within the first 72 hours because demarcation of the wound and its depth presents itself more clearly by this time.

Palmer Method

In patients with scattered burns, or for a quick prehospital assessment, the palmer method may be used to estimate the extent of the burns. The size of the patient's palm, not including the surface area of the digits, is approximately 1% of the TBSA. The patient's palm without the fingers is equiv-

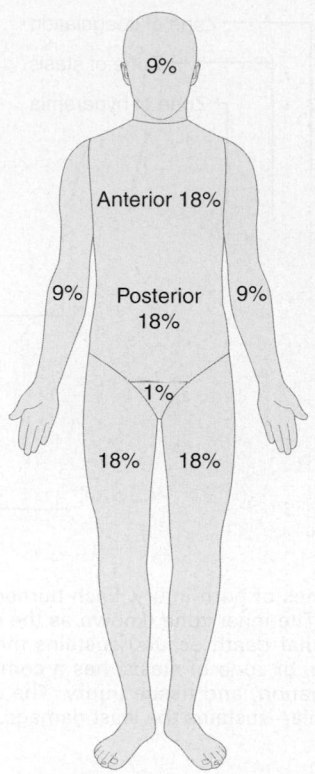

Figure 57-2 The rule of nines: Estimated percentage of total body surface area (TBSA) in the adult is arrived at by sectioning the body surface into areas with a numerical value related to nine. (Note: The anterior and posterior head total 9% of TBSA.)

alent to 0.5% TBSA and serves as a general measurement for all age groups (Shukla & Sheridan, 2008).

Pathophysiology

Burn injury is a result of heat transfer from one site to another. Tissue destruction results from coagulation, protein denaturation, or ionization of cellular contents (Fig. 57-3). The skin and the mucosa of the upper airways are sites of tissue destruction. Deep tissues, including the viscera, can be damaged by electrical burns (Chart 57-2) or by prolonged contact with a heat source. Disruption of the skin can lead to increased fluid loss, infection, hypothermia, scarring, compromised immunity, and changes in function, appearance, and body image.

The depth of the injury depends on the temperature of the burning agent and the duration of contact with the agent. For example, in the case of scald burns in adults, 1 second of contact with hot tap water at 68.9°C (156°F) may result in a burn that destroys both the epidermis and the dermis, causing a full-thickness (third-degree) injury. Fifteen seconds of exposure to hot water at 56.1°C (133°F) results in a similar full-thickness injury. Temperatures less than 44°C (111°F) can be tolerated for long periods without injury.

Burns that do not exceed 20% TBSA produce a primarily local response. Burns that exceed 20% TBSA may produce both a local and a systemic response and are considered major burn injuries. The systemic response is caused by

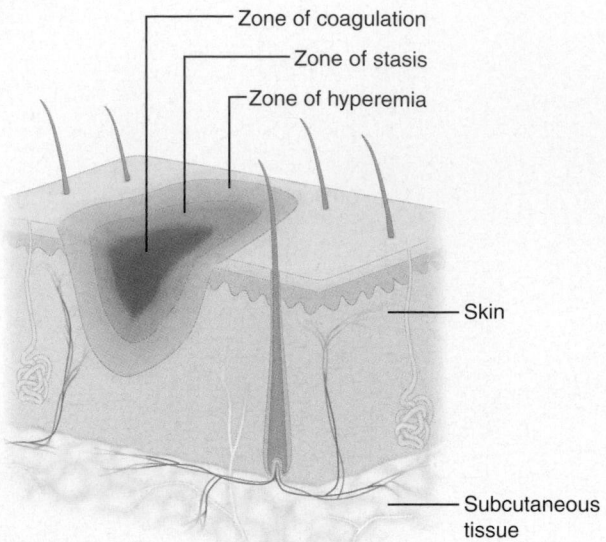

Figure 57-3 Zones of burn injury. Each burned area has three zones of injury. The inner zone (known as the area of coagulation, where cellular death occurs) sustains the most damage. The middle area, or zone of stasis, has a compromised blood supply, inflammation, and tissue injury. The outer zone—the zone of hyperemia—sustains the least damage.

the release of cytokines and other mediators into the systemic circulation. The release of local mediators and changes in blood flow, tissue edema, and infection can cause progression of the burn injury.

Pathophysiologic changes resulting from major burns during the initial burn-shock period include tissue hypoperfusion and organ hypofunction secondary to decreased cardiac output, followed by hyperdynamic and hypermetabolic phases. The incidence, magnitude, and duration of pathophysiologic changes in burns are proportional to the extent of burn injury, with a maximal response seen in burns covering 60% or more TBSA.

The initial systemic event after a major burn injury is hemodynamic instability, which results from loss of capillary integrity and a subsequent shift of fluid, sodium, and protein from the intravascular space into the interstitial spaces. Hemodynamic instability involves cardiovascular, fluid and electrolyte, blood volume, pulmonary, and other mechanisms.

Cardiovascular Alterations

Hypovolemia is the immediate consequence of fluid loss and results in decreased perfusion and oxygen delivery. Cardiac output decreases before any significant change in blood volume is evident. As fluid loss continues and vascular

Chart 57-2 • *Electrical Burns*

Electrical injury accounts for a small percentage of burn unit admissions each year, yet it is one of the most destructive types of burn injuries that can be sustained. The devastating effects of an electrical injury can cause lifelong neurovascular problems. Low-voltage injury (ie, less than 500 V exposure) generally does not cause significant damage or medical problems. Midrange exposure (ie, 200–1000 V) can cause local destruction to the tissue. High-voltage exposure (ie, greater than 1000 V) can cause loss of consciousness, fractures, compartment syndrome, arrhythmias, and is often associated with falls (Shukla & Sheridan, 2008).

Tissue and bone destruction often results in amputations and possible loss of life as the result of cardiac and respiratory abnormalities. A true electrical injury results when a current of electricity travels through the body and exits to the ground, causing internal damage to tissue and organs. Such an injury results in an entrance wound, which is the patient's point of contact with the source. The exit wound has a blow-out appearance, causing extensive damage to the surrounding tissue and structures. The amount of damage depends on the strength of the current and the length of the duration of contact with the source. An arc injury is the result of the electricity's traveling on the outside of the body or arcing around it. There is usually also a thermal injury due to clothing catching on fire. The surface injury from an electrical source is usually small compared with the damage under the surface of the skin. Electricity travels through areas of least resistance, nerves and blood vessels, to the most resistant, bone. The most severe damage occurs beneath the skin surface and is difficult to determine without surgical intervention (Shukla & Sheridan, 2008).

Once the patient is out of the path of the electricity, emergency care can safely be provided. The ABCs of emergency care are always followed. An electrical current immediately contracts muscles as it travels through the body, and cardiac dysrhythmias and spinal injuries often result from the

muscular contraction. Cardiac dysrhythmias can occur in both low-voltage and high-voltage injury and therefore require electrocardiogram evaluation and monitoring. Those patients with loss of consciousness, dysrhythmias, or ST changes on ECG must be admitted and cardiac monitoring should occur (Arnoldo, Klein & Gibran, 2006). Until it is known that the patient has no fractures, it is imperative that a neck collar remain in place and that the patient is log-rolled to eliminate the chance of further spinal cord injury. With high-voltage electrical injuries, cervical spine immobilization is a priority until cervical spine injury is ruled out.

Prompt administration of intravenous (IV) fluids and monitoring of urine output are critical components of care. Patients with electrical burns are prone to acute renal failure because of the release of myoglobin resulting from the destruction of muscle and tissue. Myoglobin can constrict renal arteries and block urine flow through the kidneys. Patients can have gross hematuria on admission to the hospital. Administration of large amounts of IV fluids helps maintain the flow of urine. It is difficult to assess the amount of fluid a patient will require because the electrical injury creates such extensive internal damage. The nurse should expect 75 to 100 mL/h of urine output for a patient who is receiving fluid resuscitation. Creatine kinase (CK) is released by damaged muscle cells and it is measured during the early phases of care to assist in determining the degree of muscle injury.

In patients with electrical injuries, neurovascular checks of affected extremities are very important. Assessment of color, temperature, and sensation in the extremity as well as the monitoring of palpable or Doppler pulses should be done to assess adequate blood flow to the extremity. If indicated by clinical assessment, the measurement of compartment syndrome to determine deep tissue injury can be performed. Compartment pressures greater than 30 mm Hg can indicate poor tissue perfusion and the need for surgical decompression (Arnoldo, et al., 2006).

volume decreases, cardiac output continues to decrease and the blood pressure drops. This is the onset of burn shock. In response, the sympathetic nervous system releases catecholamines, resulting in an increase in peripheral resistance (vasoconstriction) and an increase in pulse rate. Peripheral vasoconstriction further decreases cardiac output.

Prompt fluid resuscitation maintains the blood pressure in the low to normal range and improves cardiac output. Despite adequate fluid resuscitation, cardiac filling pressures (central venous pressure, pulmonary artery pressure, and pulmonary artery wedge pressure) remain low during the burn-shock period. If inadequate fluid resuscitation occurs, distributive shock occurs (see Chapter 15).

Generally the greatest volume of fluid leak occurs in the first 24 to 36 hours after the burn, peaking by 6 to 8 hours. As the capillaries begin to regain their integrity, burn shock resolves and fluid returns to the vascular compartment. As fluid is reabsorbed from the interstitial tissue into the vascular compartment, blood volume increases. If renal and cardiac function is adequate, urinary output increases. Diuresis continues for several days to 2 weeks.

At the time of burn injury, some red blood cells may be destroyed and others damaged, resulting in anemia. Despite this, the hematocrit may be elevated due to plasma loss. Blood losses sustained during surgical procedures, wound care, and diagnostic studies and ongoing hemolysis further contribute to anemia. Blood transfusions are required periodically to maintain adequate hemoglobin levels for oxygen delivery. Abnormalities in coagulation, including a decrease in platelets (thrombocytopenia) and prolonged clotting and prothrombin times, also occur with burn injury.

Fluid and Electrolyte Alterations

Edema forms rapidly after a burn injury. A superficial burn will cause edema to form within 4 hours after injury, while a deeper burn will continue to form over a longer period of time up to 18 hours postinjury. This is caused by increased perfusion to the injured area and is reflective of the amount of vascular and lymphatic damage to the tissue. There is loss of capillary integrity, and fluid is localized to the burn itself, resulting in blister formation and edema only in the area of injury. Patients with more severe burns develop massive systemic edema (Greenhalgh, 2007). Reabsorption begins at about 4 hours and is complete by 4 days postburn injury. However, the reabsorption is dependent on the depth of injury to the tissue. Partial-thickness injury resolves more quickly due to a more functioning lymphatic system and increased perfusion when compared to the full-thickness injury (Greenhalgh, 2007). Edema in burn wounds can be reduced by avoiding excessive fluid administration during the early postburn period. Excessive fluid administration increases edema formation in both burned and nonburned tissue.

As the taut, burned tissue becomes unyielding to the edema underneath its surface, it begins to act like a tourniquet, especially if the burn is circumferential. As edema increases, pressure on small blood vessels and nerves in the distal extremities causes an obstruction of blood flow and consequent ischemia. This complication is similar to a compartment syndrome. The physician may need to perform an **escharotomy,** a surgical incision into the **eschar** (devitalized tissue resulting from a burn) to relieve the constricting effect of the burned tissue (Demling, 2005a).

Circulating blood volume decreases dramatically during burn shock. In addition, evaporative fluid loss through the burn wound may reach 3 to 5 L or more over a 24-hour period until the burn surfaces are covered.

During burn shock, serum sodium levels vary in response to fluid resuscitation. Usually, hyponatremia (sodium depletion) is present. Hyponatremia is also common during the first week of the acute phase, as water shifts from the interstitial space to the vascular space.

Immediately after burn injury, hyperkalemia (excessive potassium) results from massive cell destruction. Hypokalemia (potassium depletion) may occur later with fluid shifts and inadequate potassium replacement.

Pulmonary Alterations

Approximately 10% to 20% of patients admitted to burn centers have an inhalation injury. The presence of this injury increases the hospital length of stay, is a determinant of the severity of injury, and increases mortality and morbidity (Palmieri, 2007). An inhalation injury occurs when a person is trapped inside a burning structure or involved in an explosion that leads to the inhalation of superheated air and noxious gas (McCall & Cahill, 2005).

Deterioration in severely burned patients can occur without obvious evidence of a smoke inhalation injury. Bronchoconstriction (caused by release of histamine, serotonin, and thromboxane, a powerful vasoconstrictor) and chest constriction secondary to circumferential full-thickness chest burns cause this deterioration. Even without pulmonary injury, hypoxia (oxygen starvation) may be present. Early in the postburn period, catecholamine release in response to the stress of the burn injury alters peripheral blood flow, thereby reducing oxygen delivery to the periphery. Later, hypermetabolism and continued catecholamine release lead to increased tissue oxygen consumption, which can lead to hypoxia. To ensure that adequate oxygen is available to the tissues, supplemental oxygen may be needed.

Pulmonary injuries are categorized as upper airway injury or inhalation injury below the glottis. Upper airway injury results from inhalation of direct heat greater then 150°C (302°F) to the epithelium. This damage results in severe upper airway edema, which can cause obstruction of the upper airway, including the pharynx and larynx, in the early hours postburn (Palmieri, 2007). Because of the cooling effect of rapid vaporization in the pulmonary tract, direct heat injury does not normally occur below the level of the bronchus. Upper airway injury is treated by early nasotracheal or endotracheal intubation.

Inhalation injury below the glottis results from inhaling the products of incomplete combustion or noxious gases. Inhalation of noxious gases is often the source of death at the scene of a fire. These products include carbon monoxide, cyanide, ammonia, aldehydes, acrolein, sulfur dioxide, and isocyanates (Barillo, 2009; Kealey, 2009; Palmieri, 2007). Tissue hypoxia is the result of carbon monoxide inhalation. It combines with hemoglobin to form **carboxyhemoglobin.** The affinity of hemoglobin for carbon monoxide is 250 times greater than that for oxygen. This injury results directly from chemical irritation of the pulmonary tissues at the alveolar level. Inhalation injuries below the glottis cause loss of ciliary action, hypersecretion, severe mucosal edema, and possibly bronchospasm. The pulmonary surfactant is reduced, resulting in atelectasis (collapse of alveoli). Expectoration of carbon particles in the sputum is the cardinal sign of this injury.

Treatment usually consists of early intubation and mechanical ventilation with 100% oxygen, which reduces the half-life of carboxyhemoglobin from 4 hours to 45 minutes (Kealey, 2009; Pham & Gibran, 2007). However, some patients require only oxygen therapy, depending on the extent of pulmonary injury and edema.

Restrictive pulmonary excursion may occur with full-thickness burns encircling the neck and thorax. Chest excursion may be greatly restricted, resulting in decreased tidal volume. In such situations, escharotomy is necessary.

Pulmonary abnormalities are not always immediately apparent. More than half of all patients with burn injuries with pulmonary involvement do not initially demonstrate pulmonary signs and symptoms. Any patient with possible inhalation injury must be observed for at least 24 hours for respiratory complications. Airway obstruction may occur very rapidly or develop in hours, even while fluid resuscitation is under way. Decreased lung compliance, decreased arterial oxygen levels, and respiratory acidosis may occur gradually over the first 5 days after a burn.

Indicators of possible upper airway injury include (1) injury occurring in an enclosed space; (2) burns of the face or neck; (3) singed nasal hair; (4) hoarseness, high-pitched voice change, dry cough, stridor; (5) sooty or bloody sputum; (6) labored breathing or tachypnea (rapid breathing) and other signs of reduced oxygen levels (hypoxemia); and (7) erythema and blistering of the oral or pharyngeal mucosa.

Diagnosis of lower airway inhalation injury includes monitoring of arterial blood gases and carboxyhemoglobin levels and direct observation of the airway by fiberoptic bronchoscopy to confirm the clinical diagnosis. Findings on bronchoscopy include airway edema, inflammation, necrosis, and soot in the airway (Edelman, White, Tyburski, et al., 2006). Less frequently, xenon scan and computed tomography scans can be used to aid diagnosis but are of questionable value (Pham & Gibran, 2007).

Pulmonary complications secondary to inhalation injuries include sloughing of the airway, increased secretions and inflammation, atelectasis, airway obstruction and ulceration, pulmonary edema, and tissue hypoxia. As a result, respiratory failure and acute respiratory distress syndrome (ARDS) and pneumonia can develop (Edelman, et al., 2006). Respiratory failure and ARDS are discussed in Chapter 23.

Renal Alterations

Renal function may be altered as a result of decreased blood volume. Destruction of red blood cells at the injury site results in free hemoglobin in the urine. If muscle damage occurs (eg, from electrical burns), myoglobin is released from the muscle cells and excreted by the kidneys. Adequate fluid volume replacement restores renal blood flow, increasing the glomerular filtration rate and urine volume. If there is inadequate blood flow through the kidneys, the hemoglobin and myoglobin occlude the renal tubules, resulting in acute tubular necrosis and renal failure (see Chapter 44).

Immunologic Alterations

The immunologic defenses of the body are greatly altered by a burn injury. Patients with burn injury are at high risk for infection and sepsis. The skin is the largest barrier to infection, and when it is compromised, the patient is continually exposed to the environment. The loss of skin integrity is compounded by the release of abnormal inflammatory factors, altered levels of immunoglobulins and serum complement, impaired neutrophil function, and a reduction in lymphocytes (lymphocytopenia). These alterations result in immunosuppression and increase the risk for sepsis. As a result, the major cause of death in the burn patient who survives after 24 hours is multiple organ dysfunction syndrome (MODS) (Greenhalgh, 2007). Most burn centers are specifically designed to provide an infection-controlled environment to protect the patient and minimize exposure to potentially harmful organisms.

Thermoregulatory Alterations

Loss of skin also results in an inability to regulate body temperature. Patients with burn injuries may therefore exhibit low body temperatures in the early hours after injury. Then, as hypermetabolism resets core temperature, the patient becomes hyperthermic for much of the postburn period, even in the absence of infection. Most burn centers have heat panels at the bedside and additional heating sources to help maintain the patient's body temperature.

Gastrointestinal Alterations

Two potential gastrointestinal (GI) complications may occur: paralytic ileus (absence of intestinal peristalsis) and Curling's ulcer. Decreased peristalsis and bowel sounds are manifestations of paralytic ileus resulting from burn trauma. Gastric distention and nausea may lead to vomiting unless gastric decompression is initiated. Gastric bleeding secondary to massive physiologic stress may be signaled by occult blood in the stool, regurgitation of "coffee ground" material from the stomach, or bloody vomitus. These signs suggest gastric or duodenal erosion (Curling's ulcer).

Other alterations affect the GI tract after burn injury: the mucosal barrier becomes permeable, the permeability allows for overgrowth of GI bacteria, and the bacteria translocate to other organs, causing infection. Patients are unable to defend against their own bacteria due to immunosuppression. In addition, alcohol ingestion, which is common in the burn population, affects GI integrity and immune response, further increasing the risk of infection and possible bleeding complications (Gosain & Gamelli, 2005a).

Patients with large TBSA burns are also at risk for abdominal compartment syndrome (ACS). During resuscitation, fluid shifts into the abdominal cavity, causing increased abdominal distention, decreased urine output, hypotension, and respiratory insufficiency. The development of ACS is related to the volume of fluids administered. Factors such as the presence of inhalation injury, deep thermal injury, glucosuria, delayed or inadequate resuscitation, and hemoglobinuria may necessitate additional fluids that may not be calculated by formulas. Bladder pressure is measured to determine the need for invasive intervention to treat increasing abdominal pressure. Bladder pressures greater than 25 mm Hg over time indicate increasing abdominal pressure. Although the prevention of this complication is not always possible, cautious and continuous measurement of fluids administered and urine output is essential (Hershberger, Hunt, Arnoldo, et al., 2007).

Management of Burn Injury

Burn care is typically categorized into three phases of care: emergent/resuscitative phase, acute/intermediate phase, and rehabilitation phase. Although priorities exist for each of the phases, the phases overlap, assessment, and management of specific problems and complications are not limited to these phases but take place throughout burn care. The three phases and the priorities for care are summarized in Table 57-2.

EMERGENT/RESUSCITATIVE PHASE

On-the-Scene Care

Preventing injury to the rescuer is the first priority of on-the-scene care. If needed, fire and emergency medical services should be requested at the first opportunity. Usually, rescue workers cover the wound, establish an airway, supply oxygen, and insert at least one large-bore intravenous (IV) line. Chart 57-3 describes the procedures and care required at the burn scene.

The burned person's appearance can be frightening at first. Although the local effects of a burn are the most evident, the systemic effects pose greater threats to life. A primary survey of the patient is carried out to assess the airway (A), gas exchange or breathing (B), and circulatory status (C) as well as the need for cervical spine immobilization and cardiac monitoring for patients with high-voltage electrical injuries. The circulatory system must be assessed quickly. Apical pulse and blood pressure are monitored frequently. Tachycardia (abnormally rapid heart rate) and slight hypotension are expected soon after the burn. In the patient with extensive burns, neurologic status is assessed quickly. Often the patient is awake and alert initially, and vital information can be obtained at that time.

NURSING ALERT

Breathing must be assessed and a patent airway established immediately during the initial minutes of emergency care. Immediate therapy is directed toward establishing an airway and administering humidified 100% oxygen. If such a high concentration of oxygen is not available under emergency conditions, oxygen by mask or nasal cannula is given initially. If qualified personnel and equipment are available and the victim has severe respiratory distress or airway edema, the rescuers can insert an endotracheal tube and initiate manual ventilation.

NURSING ALERT

No food or fluid is given by mouth, and the patient is placed in a position that will prevent aspiration of vomitus, because nausea and vomiting typically occur due to paralytic ileus resulting from the stress of injury.

The secondary survey focuses on the completion of the total body system assessment, including the mechanism of injury, inhalation injury, and presence of corneal injury. A secondary head-to-toe survey of the patient is carried out to identify other potentially life-threatening injuries (Shukla & Sheridan, 2008).

Medical Management

The patient is transported to the nearest emergency department (ED). The hospital and physician are alerted that the patient is en route so that life-saving measures can be initiated immediately by a trained team and plans for referral to a burn center can be made.

Initial priorities in the ED remain airway, breathing, and circulation. For mild pulmonary injury, 100% humidified

Table 57-2	**PHASES OF BURN CARE**	
Phase	**Duration**	**Priorities**
Emergent/resuscitative	From onset of injury to completion of fluid resuscitation	• First aid • Prevention of shock • Prevention of respiratory distress • Detection and treatment of concomitant injuries • Wound assessment and initial care
Acute/intermediate	From beginning of diuresis to near completion of wound closure	• Wound care and closure • Prevention or treatment of complications, including infection • Nutritional support
Rehabilitation	From major wound closure to return to individual's optimal level of physical and psychosocial adjustment	• Prevention of scars and contractures • Physical, occupational, and vocational rehabilitation • Functional and cosmetic reconstruction • Psychosocial counseling

Chart 57-3 • *Emergency Procedures at the Burn Scene*

- **Extinguish the flames.** When clothes catch fire, the flames can be extinguished if the person falls to the floor or ground and rolls ("stop, drop, and roll"); anything available to smother the flames, such as a blanket, rug, or coat, may be used. Standing still forces the person to breathe flames and smoke, and running fans the flames. If the burn source is electrical, the electrical source must be disconnected safely.
- **Cool the burn.** After the flames are extinguished, the burned area and adherent clothing are soaked with *cool* water, briefly, to cool the wound and halt the burning process. Once a burn has been sustained, the application of cool water is the best first-aid measure. However, *never* apply ice directly to the burn, *never* wrap the person in ice, and *never* use cold soaks or dressings for longer than several minutes; such procedures may worsen the tissue damage and lead to hypothermia in people with large burns.
- **Remove restrictive objects.** If possible, remove clothing immediately. Adherent clothing may be left in place once cooled. Other clothing and all jewelry, including all piercings, should be removed to allow for assessment and

to prevent constriction secondary to rapidly developing edema.
- **Cover the wound.** The burn should be covered as quickly as possible to minimize bacterial contamination, to maintain body temperature, and decrease pain by preventing air from coming in contact with the injured surface. Sterile dressings are best, but any clean, dry cloth can be used as an emergency dressing. Ointments and salves should *not* be used. Other than the dressing, no medication or material should be applied to the burn wound.
- **Irrigate chemical burns.** Chemical burns resulting from contact with a corrosive material are irrigated immediately. Most chemical laboratories have a high-pressure shower for such emergencies. If such an injury occurs at home, brush off the chemical agent, remove clothes immediately, and rinse all areas of the body that have come in contact with the chemical. Rinsing can occur in the shower or any other source of continuous running water. If a chemical gets in or near the eyes, the eyes should be flushed with cool, clean water immediately. Outcomes for the patient with chemical burns are significantly improved by rapid, sustained flushing of the injury at the scene.

oxygen is administered and the patient is encouraged to cough so that secretions can be removed by suctioning. For more severe situations, it is necessary to remove secretions by bronchial suctioning and to administer bronchodilators and mucolytic agents. If edema of the airway develops, endotracheal intubation may be necessary. Continuous positive airway pressure and mechanical ventilation may also be required to achieve adequate oxygenation.

After adequate respiratory function and circulatory status have been established, the patient is assessed for cervical spinal injuries or head injury if he or she was involved in an explosion, a fall, a jump, or an electrical injury. Once the patient's condition is stable, attention is directed to the burn wound itself. All clothing and jewelry are removed. For chemical burns, flushing of the exposed areas is continued. The patient is checked for contact lenses. These are removed immediately if chemicals have contacted the eyes or if facial burns have occurred.

It is important to validate an account of the burn scenario provided by the patient, witnesses at the scene, and paramedics. Information needs to include the time of the burn injury, the source of the burn, the place where the burn occurred, how long the patient was in the burning structure, how the burn was treated at the scene, and any history of falling or jumping at the scene. A history of preexisting diseases, allergies, medications, and the use of drugs, alcohol, and tobacco is obtained at this point to aid in planning the patient's care. A large-bore (16- or 18-gauge) IV catheter should be inserted in a nonburned area (if not inserted earlier). Most patients will have a central venous catheter inserted so that large amounts of IV fluids can be administered quickly and central venous pressures can be monitored.

If the burn exceeds 20% to 25% TBSA, a nasogastric tube is inserted and connected to low intermittent suction.

Often, patients with large burns become nauseated as a result of the GI effects of the burn injury, such as paralytic ileus, and the effects of medication, such as opioids. All patients who are intubated should have a nasogastric tube inserted to decompress the stomach and prevent vomiting.

The physician evaluates the patient's general condition, assesses the burn, determines the priorities of care, and directs the individualized plan of treatment, which is divided into systemic management and local care of the burned area. Nonsterile gloves, caps, masks and cover gowns are worn by personnel while assessing the exposed burned areas. Clean technique is maintained while assessing and treating the burn wounds.

Assessment of both the TBSA burned and the depth of the burn are completed after soot and debris have been gently cleansed from the burn wound. Careful attention is paid to keeping the patient warm during wound assessment and cleansing. Assessment is repeated frequently throughout burn wound care. Photographs may be taken of the burn areas initially and periodically throughout treatment; in this way, the initial injury and burn wound can be documented. Such documentation is invaluable for insurance and legal claims.

Clean sheets are placed under and over the patient to protect the burn wound from contamination, maintain body temperature, and reduce pain caused by air currents passing over exposed nerve endings. An indwelling urinary catheter is inserted to permit more accurate monitoring of urine output and renal function for patients with moderate to severe burns. Baseline height, weight, arterial blood gases, hematocrit, electrolyte values, blood alcohol level, drug panel, urinalysis, and chest x-rays are obtained. If the patient is elderly or has an electrical burn, a baseline electrocardiogram (ECG) is obtained. Because burns are contaminated wounds, tetanus prophylaxis is administered if the patient's immunization status is not current or is unknown.

NURSING ALERT

If necessary, a blood pressure cuff can be placed around a patient's burned extremity. The cuff must be of the correct size with accommodations made for bulky dressings.

Although the major focus of care during the emergent phase is physical stabilization, the nurse must also attend to the patient's and family's psychological needs. Burn injury is a crisis, one that causes varying emotional responses. The patient's and family's coping abilities and available supports are assessed. Circumstances surrounding the burn injury should be considered when providing care. Individualized psychosocial support must be given to the patient and family. Because the patient is usually anxious and in pain, nurses should provide reassurance and support, explanations of procedures, and adequate pain relief. Because poor tissue perfusion accompanies burn injuries, only IV analgesia (usually morphine) is administered, titrated for the individual patient. If the patient wishes to see a spiritual advisor or counselor, one is notified.

Transfer to a Burn Center

Patients with the following types of injuries are referred to a burn center for evaluation and care: burns with partial-thickness injury greater than 10% or full-thickness burns in any age group; a burn in an area of the body that requires special attention, such as the face, hands, feet, genitalia, perineum, and over joints; and chemical, electrical, or inhalation burns. Patients with preexisting medical problems or who may have additional trauma that could complicate care should be referred. Children with burns are transferred if they cannot be managed by the available pediatric team. Lastly, any burn injury that carries special social, emotional, or rehabilitative need should be referred to a burn center where these needs are addressed more readily (Guidelines for the Operation of Burn Centers, 2007).

If the patient is to be transported to a burn center, the following measures, listed in order of importance, are instituted before transfer:
- A patent airway is ensured.
- Adequate peripheral circulation is established in any burned extremity.
- A secure IV catheter is inserted with lactated Ringer's solution infusing at the rate required to maintain a urine output of at least 30 mL per hour.
- An indwelling urinary catheter is inserted.
- Adequate pain relief is attained.
- Wounds are covered with a clean, dry sheet, and the patient is kept comfortably warm.

All assessments and treatments are documented, and this information is provided to the burn center personnel. The transferring facility must relay accurate vital signs, temperature, and intake and output totals to burn center personnel so that adequate fluid resuscitation measures will continue.

Management of Fluid Loss and Shock

Next to managing respiratory difficulties, the most urgent need is preventing irreversible shock by replacing lost fluids and electrolytes. As stated previously, survival of the patient with burn injury depends on adequate fluid resuscitation. Table 57-3 describes the fluid changes that occur in the emergent/resuscitative phase of care. Baseline weight and laboratory test results are obtained, and these parameters must be monitored closely in the immediate postburn (resuscitation) period. Both underresuscitation and overresuscitation are associated with poor outcome, and the optimal formula has not been identified; however, regardless of rate and composition of the fluids and colloids administered, diligent monitoring through the first 72 hours is critical to ensure optimal management (Pham, Cancio & Gilbran, 2008).

Fluid Replacement Therapy

The total volume and rate of IV fluid replacement are gauged by the patient's response and guided by the resuscitation formula. The adequacy of fluid resuscitation is determined by monitoring urine output totals, an index of renal

Table 57-3 **FLUID AND ELECTROLYTE CHANGES IN THE EMERGENT/RESUSCITATIVE PHASE**	
Fluid accumulation phase (shock phase)	
Plasma → interstitial fluid (edema at burn site)	
Observation	**Explanation**
Generalized dehydration	Plasma leaks through damaged capillaries
Reduction of blood volume	Secondary to plasma loss, fall of blood pressure, and diminished cardiac output
Decreased urinary output	Secondary to:
	Fluid loss
	Decreased renal blood flow
	Sodium and water retention caused by increased adrenocortical activity
	Hemolysis of red blood cells, causing hemoglobinuria and myonecrosis or myoglobinuria
Potassium (K^+) excess	Massive cellular trauma causes release of K^+ into extracellular fluid (ordinarily, most K^+ is intracellular)
Sodium (Na^+) deficit	Large amount of Na^+ is lost in trapped edema fluid and exudate and by shift into cells as K^+ is released from cells (ordinarily most Na^+ is extracellular)
Metabolic acidosis (base-bicarbonate deficit)	Loss of bicarbonate ions accompanies sodium loss
Hemoconcentration (elevated hematocrit)	Liquid blood component is lost into extravascular space

perfusion. Urine output totals of 0.5 to 1.0 mL/kg/h for adults have been used as resuscitation goals (Pham, et al., 2008).

NURSING ALERT

Clinical parameters are far more important in resuscitation than any formula. Indeed, the patient's individual response is the key to assessing the adequacy of fluid resuscitation.

Additional gauges of fluid requirements and response to fluid resuscitation include hematocrit and hemoglobin and serum sodium levels. Within the first 24 hours after injury, if the hematocrit and the hemoglobin levels decrease or if the urinary output exceeds 50 mL/h, the rate of IV fluid administration may be decreased. One goal is to maintain serum sodium levels in the normal range during fluid replacement.

Appropriate resuscitation endpoints for patients with burn injuries remain unresolved, although some studies have examined hemodynamic and oxygen transport as resuscitation endpoints. Successful resuscitation is associated with increased delivery of oxygen and consumption of oxygen with declining serum lactate levels (Demling, 2005a). Factors associated with increased fluid requirements include delayed resuscitation, full-thickness injury, and presence of inhalation injuries. A State-of-the-Science in Burn Care conference was held in 2006 to identify the focus of research in the next decade. Overresuscitation was identified as a high-priority topic along with a need to identify endpoints for resuscitation (Pham, et al., 2008).

Fluid Requirements

The projected fluid requirements for the first 24 hours are calculated by the clinician based on the extent of the burn injury. Some combination of fluid categories may be used, including colloids (whole blood, plasma, and plasma expanders) and crystalloids/electrolytes (physiologic sodium chloride or lactated Ringer's solution). Adequate fluid resuscitation results in slightly decreased blood volume levels during the first 24 postburn hours and restoration of plasma levels to normal by the end of 48 hours. Formulas have been developed for estimating fluid loss based on the estimated percentage of burned TBSA and the weight of the patient. TBSA greater than 20% to 25% is associated with increased capillary permeability and intravascular fluid shifts that are most profound in the first 24 hours postburn (Pham, et al., 2008).

Oral and enteral resuscitation can be successful in adults with less than 20% TBSA burned (Atiyeh, Gunn & Hayek, 2005). Intravenous resuscitation is recommended when burn TBSA is greater then 20% (Pham, et al., 2008).

Although there is no consensus on the formulas for resuscitation, currently the most popular formula provides for the volume of an isotonic solution to be administered during the first 24 hours in a range of 2 to 4 mL/kg per percentage of TBSA burned. As with the other formulas, half of the calculated total should be given over the first

8 postburn hours, and the other half should be given over the next 16 hours. The hourly rate and volume of the infusion are modified based on the patient's response (Pham, et al., 2008). Clinicians should take note that the resuscitation formulas serve only as guidelines, and the patient's response to fluid therapy is the best parameter to use (Atiyeh, et al., 2005).

With large burns, there is a failure of the sodium–potassium pump (a physiologic mechanism involved in fluid–electrolyte balance) at the cellular level. Therefore, patients with very large burns may need proportionately more milliliters of fluid per percentage of burn than those with smaller burns. Also, patients with electrical injury, inhalation injury, or delayed fluid resuscitation and those who were burned while intoxicated may need additional fluids.

The following example illustrates the use of the consensus formula in a 70-kg (154-lb) patient with a 50% TBSA burn:

1. Formula: 2 to 4 mL/kg/% TBSA
2. 2 mL × 70 kg × 50 TBSA = 7000 mL/24 h
3. Plan to administer: first 8 hours = 3500 mL, or 437 mL/h; next 16 hours = 3500 mL, or 219 mL/h

Most fluid replacement formulas use isotonic electrolyte solutions. Regardless of which standard replacement formula is used, the patient receives approximately the same fluid volume and sodium replacement during the first 48 hours.

Another fluid replacement method requires hypertonic electrolyte solutions. The goal is to deliver smaller amounts of fluid and maintain the same urine output. Hypertonic resuscitation increases the osmolarity of the blood and encourages a shift of fluid into the intravascular space from the interstitial space. Careful monitoring of serum sodium level is required to prevent hypernatremia and acute renal failure (Pham, et al., 2008).

The use of colloids during resuscitation has been the subject of much controversy. Administration of large volumes of crystalloid during resuscitation decreases the protein content in the blood. Proteins help to prevent the movement of fluid and decrease edema. The purpose of adding colloid to the formula is to decrease the amount of fluid needed and also prevent massive edema formation. In contrast, some clinicians believe that after 24 hours the integrity of the capillaries begins to be restored and the use of colloids during that time would not be advantageous. These theories require further study (Pham, et al., 2008).

NURSING ALERT

Formulas are only a guide. The patient's response, evidenced by heart rate, blood pressure, and urine output, is the primary determinant of actual fluid therapy and must be assessed at least hourly. Patient outcomes are improved by optimal fluid resuscitation.

Nursing Management

Nursing assessment in the emergent phase of burn injury focuses on the major priorities for any trauma patient; the burn wound is a secondary consideration. Aseptic management of the burn wounds and invasive lines continues.

The nurse monitors vital signs frequently. Respiratory status is monitored closely, and apical, carotid, and femoral pulses are evaluated particularly in areas of circumferential burn injury to an extremity. Cardiac monitoring is indicated initially or if the patient has a history of cardiac disease, electrical injury, or respiratory conditions.

If all extremities are burned, determining blood pressure may be difficult. A sterile dressing applied under the blood pressure cuff protects the wound from contamination. Because increasing edema makes blood pressure difficult to auscultate, a Doppler (ultrasound) device or a noninvasive electronic blood pressure device may be helpful. In patients with severe burns, an arterial catheter is used for blood pressure measurement and for collecting blood specimens. Peripheral pulses of burned extremities are checked hourly; the Doppler device is useful for this. Elevation of burned upper extremities above the level of the heart is crucial to decrease edema. Elevation of the lower extremities on pillows and of the upper extremities on pillows or by suspension using IV poles may be helpful.

Large-bore IV catheters and an indwelling urinary catheter are inserted, if not already in place, and the nurse's assessment includes monitoring of fluid intake and output. Urine output, an indicator of renal perfusion, is monitored carefully and measured hourly. The amount of urine first obtained when the urinary catheter was inserted is recorded. This may assist in determining the extent of preburn renal function and fluid status.

Burgundy-colored urine suggests the presence of hemochromogen and myoglobin resulting from muscle damage. This is associated with deep burns caused by electrical injury or prolonged contact with flames. Glycosuria, a common finding in the early postburn hours, results from the release of stored glucose from the liver in response to stress.

Although not responsible for prescribing the fluids the nurse should be able to calculate the patient's expected fluid requirements. Infusion pumps are used to deliver a complex regimen of IV fluids prescribed. Administering and monitoring IV therapy are major nursing responsibilities. Strict monitoring of fluid intake and output is essential during the resuscitative phase along with reporting laboratory values and reporting patient responses to the physician.

Body temperature, body weight, preburn weight, and history of allergies, tetanus immunization, past medical and surgical disorders, current illnesses, and a list of current medications are essential to help guide medication needs for the patient. A head-to-toe assessment is performed, focusing on signs and symptoms of concomitant illness, associated injury, or developing complications. If the patient has facial burns, his or her eyes should be examined for injury to the corneas. An ophthalmologist is consulted for complete assessment via fluorescent staining.

Assessing the extent of the burn wound continues and is facilitated with anatomic diagrams (described previously). In addition, the nurse works with the physician to assess the depth of the wound and areas of full-thickness and partial-thickness injury. Assessment of the circumstances surrounding the injury is important. Obtaining a history of the burn injury can help in planning the care for the patient. Assessment should include the time of injury, mechanism of burn, whether the burn occurred in a closed space, the possibility of inhalation of noxious chemicals, and any related trauma. The neurologic assessment focuses on the patient's level of consciousness, psychological status, pain and anxiety levels, and behavior.

The patient's and family's understanding of the injury and treatment is assessed as well. A family meeting upon admission is helpful to explain the detail of the patient's injuries and the course of treatment. Ethical dilemmas, such as those discussed in Chart 57-4, may also occur during hospitalization.

Nursing care of the patient during the emergent/resuscitative phase of burn injury is detailed in the plan of nursing care in Chart 57-5.

 Gerontologic Considerations

Comorbid conditions coupled with the burn injury contribute to the high mortality rates of patients 65 years and older. Demling (2005b) reported that more than 60% of elderly patients with burn injuries admitted to the hospital had moderate to severe protein–energy malnutrition, which contributed to an increase in infection compared with well-nourished elderly burn patients. Decreased function of the cardiovascular, renal, and pulmonary systems increases the need for close observation of elderly patients with even relatively minor burns during the emergent and acute phases. Acute renal failure is much more common in elderly patients than in those younger than 40 years of age. The margin of difference between hypovolemia and fluid overload is very small. Suppressed immunologic response, a high incidence of malnutrition, and an inability to withstand metabolic stressors (eg, a cold environment) further compromise the elderly person's ability to heal. As a result of these issues in elderly patients who sustain burn injury, close monitoring and prompt treatment of complications are mandatory.

ACUTE/INTERMEDIATE PHASE

The acute/intermediate phase of burn care follows the emergent/resuscitative phase and begins 48 to 72 hours after the burn injury. During this phase, attention is directed toward continued assessment and maintenance of respiratory and circulatory status, fluid and electrolyte balance, and GI function. Infection prevention, burn wound care (ie, wound cleaning, topical antibacterial therapy, wound dressing, dressing changes, wound débridement, and wound grafting), pain management, and nutritional support are priorities at this stage and are discussed in detail in the following sections.

Medical Management

Airway obstruction caused by upper airway edema can take as long as 48 hours to develop. Changes detected by x-ray and arterial blood gas analysis may occur as the effects of resuscitative fluid and the chemical reactions of smoke ingredients with lung tissues become apparent. Pulmonary complications are not unusual in burn injury. Those with ventilator-associated pneumonia (VAP) have a 40% mortality rate, increasing to 60% to 77% for VAP with an inhalation injury. Bronchial washing or bronchioalveolar lavage can assist in the diagnosis and treatment of pneumonia (Wahl, Ahrns, Brandt, et al., 2005). Ideally, the best practice

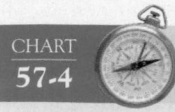

CHART 57-4 · *Ethics and Related Issues*

How Much Is Enough and What Is Comfort Care?

Situation

A 71-year-old woman was flown to the nearest burn center. She lives alone and was cooking on top of a gas stove. She reached over the burner and caught her robe on fire. The flame consumed most of her upper body. She sustained a full-thickness burn to 42% of her body (face, neck, both arms, and chest). In addition, she turned to remove herself from the room quickly, slipped, and fell, fracturing two ribs and spraining her right ankle. Due to the nature of the fire she was enclosed in a burning area so she also sustained an upper airway inhalation injury. She was awake and alert at the scene and indicated a past medical history of diabetes, hypertension, and renal disease. She was in little pain at the time due to the depth of the burn injury; however, she was asking the team questions related to the survivability of her injury, "Am I going to die?"

Upon admission she was intubated to treat her upper airway edema and suspected inhalation injury. Family arrived and the burn surgeon explained the extent of injury. A decision was made to proceed with care and assess her progress postresuscitation. They were prepared for a future decision regarding withdrawal of care if survival becomes futile.

Dilemma

Initial resuscitation has occurred and approximately 4 days postburn the patient begins to show signs of renal failure. She has had one surgical procedure for débridement and grafting to her chest, and although grafts are intact, they do not look healthy. She is showing increased signs of discomfort and pain due to the operative procedure and the addition of another wound (the new donor site). The family decides in a team meeting that they do not want to initiate hemodialysis and therefore place the patient on comfort measures. Approximately 3 days later she remains on comfort care and

has increased signs of restlessness and pain. The nurse caring for the patient requests an order from the physician for an increase in pain medication from 5 mg morphine to 10 mg IV. Within 2 hours after administration the patient expired without discomfort. Six months later the facility is contacted by an attorney and informed that the family is taking legal action against the nurse and physician for performing euthanasia on their mother.

Discussion

The burn team is faced with these types of ethical dilemmas on a regular basis. Whenever possible the team should attempt to elicit the patient's wishes as early as possible, including any advanced directives. This should be considered again prior to intubation unless it is an emergency situation. The problem in this case is that due to absence of pain it is often difficult for a patient to understand the severity of his or her burn injury. The patient begins to experience increased pain as care progresses and increased medication is expected. Once the patient is unable to make decisions for herself, family members assume this responsibility. Clear and documented discussions with the family are essential for communication. Decision makers should always make decisions based on what the patient would want them to do, not their individual concerns. They often have difficulty making comfort care decisions; not all family members always agree. If death does not occur rapidly after a decision, they have feelings of remorse and guilt.

Discussion Questions

1. As a member of the team when the patient arrived at your facility, what would you have done differently?
2. Do you believe this was a survivable injury?
3. Given the failing renal status of the patient, do you believe additional medication should have been administered?
4. Do you believe there is reason for the family to seek legal action for their mother's death?

---

is to remove the endotracheal tube as soon as possible so that a route for pathogens is not accessible to the lungs. The arterial blood gas values and other parameters determine the need for intubation and mechanical ventilation.

As capillaries regain integrity, 48 or more hours after the burn, fluid moves from the interstitial to the intravascular compartment and diuresis begins (Table 57-4). If cardiac or renal function is inadequate, for example in an elderly patient or in a patient with preexisting cardiac disease, fluid overload occurs and symptoms of congestive heart failure may result (see Chapter 30).

Cautious administration of fluids and electrolytes continues during this phase of burn care because of the shifts in fluid from the interstitial to the intravascular compartment, losses of fluid from large burn wounds, and the patient's physiologic responses to the burn injury. Blood components are administered as needed to treat blood loss and anemia.

Fever is common in patients after burn shock resolves. A resetting of the core body temperature in severely burned patients results in a body temperature a few degrees higher than normal for several weeks after the burn. Bacteremia and septicemia also cause fever in many patients. Acetaminophen (Tylenol) and hypothermia blankets and

Table 57-4 FLUID AND ELECTROLYTE CHANGES IN THE ACUTE PHASE

Fluid remobilization phase (state of diuresis)
Interstitial fluid → plasma

Observation	Explanation
Hemodilution (decreased hematocrit)	Blood cell concentration is diluted as fluid enters the intravascular compartment; loss of red blood cells destroyed at burn site.
Increased urinary output	Fluid shift into intravascular compartment increases renal blood flow and causes increased urine formation.
Sodium (Na^+) deficit	With diuresis, sodium is lost with water; existing serum sodium is diluted by water influx.
Potassium (K^+) deficit (occurs occasionally in this phase)	Beginning on the fourth or fifth postburn day, K^+ shifts from extracellular fluid into cells.
Metabolic acidosis	Loss of sodium depletes fixed base; relative carbon dioxide content increases.

ancillary heating devices may be required to maintain body temperature in a range of 37.2°C to 38.3°C (99°F to 101°F) so as to reduce metabolic stress and tissue oxygen demand.

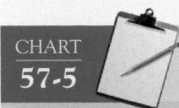

CHART 57-5

PLAN OF NURSING CARE
Care of the Patient During the Emergent/Resuscitative Phase of Burn Injury

NURSING DIAGNOSIS: Impaired gas exchange related to carbon monoxide poisoning, smoke inhalation, and upper airway obstruction
GOAL: Maintenance of adequate tissue oxygenation

Nursing Interventions	Rationale	Expected Outcomes
1. Provide humidified oxygen.	1. Humidified oxygen provides moisture to injured tissues; supplemental oxygen increases alveolar oxygenation.	• Absence of dyspnea • Respiratory rate between 12 and 20 breaths/min • Lungs clear on auscultation • Arterial oxygen saturation greater than 96% by pulse oximetry • Arterial blood gas levels within normal limits
2. Assess breath sounds, and respiratory rate, rhythm, depth, and symmetry. Monitor patient for signs of hypoxia.	2. These factors provide baseline data for further assessment and evidence of increasing respiratory compromise.	

3. Observe for the following:
  a. Erythema or blistering of lips or buccal mucosa
  b. Singed nostrils
  c. Burns of face, neck, or chest
  d. Increasing hoarseness
  e. Soot in sputum or tracheal tissue in respiratory secretions
	3. These signs indicate possible inhalation injury and risk of respiratory dysfunction.	

4. Monitor arterial blood gas values, pulse oximetry readings, and carboxyhemoglobin levels.	4. Increasing $PaCO_2$ and decreasing PaO_2 and O_2 saturation may indicate need for mechanical ventilation.	
5. Report labored respirations, decreased depth of respirations, or signs of hypoxia to physician immediately.	5. Immediate intervention is indicated for respiratory difficulty.	
6. Prepare to assist with intubation and escharotomies.	6. Intubation allows mechanical ventilation. Escharotomy enables chest excursion in circumferential chest burns.	
7. Monitor mechanically ventilated patient closely.	7. Monitoring allows early detection of decreasing respiratory status or complications of mechanical ventilation.	

NURSING DIAGNOSIS: Ineffective airway clearance related to edema and effects of smoke inhalation
GOAL: Maintain patent airway and adequate airway clearance

Nursing Interventions	Rationale	Expected Outcomes
1. Maintain patent airway through proper patient positioning, removal of secretions, and artificial airway if needed.	1. A patent airway is crucial to respiration.	• Patent airway • Respiratory secretions are minimal, colorless, and thin • Respiratory rate, pattern, and breath sounds normal
2. Provide humidified oxygen.	2. Humidity liquefies secretions and facilitates expectoration.	
3. Encourage patient to turn, cough, and deep breathe. Encourage patient to use incentive spirometry. Suction as needed.	3. These activities promote mobilization and removal of secretions.	

NURSING DIAGNOSIS: Fluid volume deficit related to increased capillary permeability and evaporative losses from the burn wound
GOAL: Restoration of optimal fluid and electrolyte balance and perfusion of vital organs

Nursing Interventions	Rationale	Expected Outcomes
1. Observe vital signs (including central venous pressure or pulmonary artery pressure, if indicated) and urine output, and be alert for signs of hypovolemia or fluid overload.	1. Hypovolemia is a major risk immediately after the burn injury. Overresuscitation might cause fluid overload.	• Serum electrolytes within normal limits • Urine output between 0.5 and 1.0 mL/kg/h • Blood pressure higher than 90/60 mm Hg • Heart rate less than 120 beats/min • Exhibits clear sensorium • Voids clear yellow urine with specific gravity within normal limits
2. Monitor urine output at least hourly and weigh patient daily.	2. Output and weight provide information about renal perfusion, adequacy of fluid replacement, and fluid requirement and fluid status.	

Continued on following page

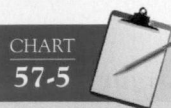

CHART 57-5

PLAN OF NURSING CARE
Care of the Patient During the Emergent/Resuscitative Phase of Burn Injury (Continued)

Nursing Interventions	Rationale	Expected Outcomes
3. Maintain IV lines and regulate fluids at appropriate rates, as prescribed.	3. Adequate fluids are necessary to maintain fluid and electrolyte balance and perfusion of vital organs.	
4. Observe for symptoms of deficiency or excess of serum sodium, potassium, calcium, phosphorus, and bicarbonate.	4. Rapid shifts in fluid and electrolyte status are possible in the postburn period.	
5. Elevate head of patient's bed and elevate burned extremities.	5. Elevation promotes venous return.	
6. Notify physician immediately of decreased urine output, blood pressure, central venous, pulmonary artery, or pulmonary artery wedge pressures, or increased pulse rate.	6. Because of the rapid fluid shifts in burn shock, fluid deficit must be detected early so that distributive shock does not occur.	

NURSING DIAGNOSIS: Hypothermia related to loss of skin microcirculation and open wounds
GOAL: Maintenance of adequate body temperature

Nursing Interventions	Rationale	Expected Outcomes
1. Provide a warm environment through use of heat shield, space blanket, heat lights, or blankets.	1. A stable environment minimizes evaporative heat loss.	• Body temperature remains 36.1°C to 38.3°C (97°F to 101°F) • Absence of chills or shivering
2. Work quickly when wounds must be exposed.	2. Minimal exposure minimizes heat loss from wound.	
3. Assess core body temperature frequently.	3. Frequent temperature assessments help detect developing hypothermia.	

NURSING DIAGNOSIS: Pain related to tissue and nerve injury and emotional impact of injury
GOAL: Control of pain

Nursing Interventions	Rationale	Expected Outcomes
1. Use pain intensity scale to assess pain level (ie, 1 to 10). Differentiate restlessness due to pain from restlessness due to hypoxia.	1. Pain level provides baseline for evaluating effectiveness of pain relief measures. Hypoxia can cause similar signs and must be ruled out before analgesic medication is administered.	• States pain level is decreased • Absence of nonverbal cues of pain
2. Administer intravenous opioid analgesics as prescribed. Observe for respiratory depression in the patient who is not mechanically ventilated. Assess response to analgesic.	2. Intravenous administration is necessary because of altered tissue perfusion from burn injury.	
3. Provide emotional support and reassurance.	3. Emotional support is essential to reduce fear and anxiety resulting from burn injury. Fear and anxiety increase the perception of pain.	

NURSING DIAGNOSIS: Anxiety related to fear and the emotional impact of burn injury
GOAL: Minimization of patient's and family's anxiety

Nursing Interventions	Rationale	Expected Outcomes
1. Assess patient's and family's understanding of burn injury, coping skills, and family dynamics.	1. Previous successful coping strategies can be fostered for use in the present crisis. Assessment allows planning of individualized interventions.	• Patient and family verbalize understanding of emergent burn care • Able to answer simple questions
2. Individualize responses to the patient's and family's coping level.	2. Reactions to burn injury are extremely variable. Interventions must be appropriate to the patient's and family's present level of coping.	

Continued

CHART 57-5

PLAN OF NURSING CARE
Care of the Patient During the Emergent/Resuscitative Phase of Burn Injury (Continued)

Nursing Interventions	Rationale	Expected Outcomes
3. Explain all procedures to the patient and the family in clear, simple terms.	3. Increased understanding alleviates fear of the unknown. High levels of anxiety may interfere with understanding of complex explanations.	
4. Maintain adequate pain relief.	4. Pain increases anxiety.	
5. Consider administering prescribed antianxiety medications if the patient remains extremely anxious despite nonpharmacologic interventions.	5. Anxiety levels during the emergent phase may exceed the patient's coping abilities. Medication decreases physiologic and psychological anxiety responses.	

COLLABORATIVE PROBLEMS: Acute respiratory failure, distributive shock, acute renal failure, compartment syndrome, paralytic ileus, Curling's ulcer

GOAL: Absence of complications

Nursing Interventions	Rationale	Expected Outcomes
Acute Respiratory Failure		
1. Assess for increasing dyspnea, stridor, changes in respiratory patterns.	1. Such signs reflect deteriorating respiratory status.	• Arterial blood gas values within acceptable limits: PaO_2 greater than 80 mm Hg, $PaCO_2$ less than 50 mm Hg
2. Monitor pulse oximetry, arterial blood gas values for decreasing PaO_2 and oxygen saturation, and increasing $PaCO_2$.	2. Such signs reflect decreased oxygenation status.	• Breathes spontaneously with adequate tidal volume
3. Monitor chest x-ray results.	3. X-ray may disclose pulmonary injury.	• Chest x-ray findings normal
4. Assess for restlessness, confusion, difficulty attending to questions, or decreasing level of consciousness.	4. Such manifestations may indicate cerebral hypoxia.	• Absence of cerebral signs of hypoxia
5. Report deteriorating respiratory status immediately to physician.	5. Acute respiratory failure is life-threatening, and immediate intervention is required.	
6. Prepare to assist with intubation or escharotomies as indicated.	6. Intubation allows mechanical ventilation. Escharotomies allow improved chest excursion with respirations.	
Distributive Shock		
1. Assess for decreasing urine output and blood pressure as well as increasing pulse rate. (If hemodynamic monitoring is used, assess for decreasing pulmonary artery and pulmonary artery wedge pressures and cardiac output.)	1. Such signs and symptoms may indicate distributive shock and inadequate intravascular volume.	• Urine output between 0.5 and 1.0 mL/kg/h • Blood pressure within patient's normal range (usually greater than 90/60 mm Hg) • Heart rate within patient's normal range (usually less than 110/min) • Pressures and cardiac output remain within normal limits
2. Assess for progressive edema as fluid shifts occur.	2. As fluid shifts into the interstitial spaces in burn shock, edema occurs and may compromise tissue perfusion.	
3. Adjust fluid resuscitation in collaboration with the physician in response to physiologic findings.	3. Optimal fluid resuscitation prevents distributive shock and improves patient outcomes.	
Acute Renal Failure		
1. Monitor urine output and blood urea nitrogen (BUN) and serum creatinine levels.	1. These values reflect renal function.	• Adequate urine output • BUN and serum creatinine values remain normal
2. Report decreased urine output or increased BUN and creatinine values to physician.	2. These laboratory values indicate possible renal failure.	
3. Assess urine for hemoglobin or myoglobin.	3. Hemoglobin or myoglobin in the urine points to an increased risk of renal failure.	

Continued on following page

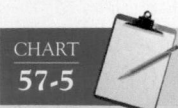

CHART
57-5

PLAN OF NURSING CARE
Care of the Patient During the Emergent/Resuscitative Phase of Burn Injury (Continued)

Nursing Interventions	Rationale	Expected Outcomes
4. Administer increased fluids as prescribed.	4. Fluids help to flush hemoglobin and myoglobin from renal tubules, decreasing the potential for renal failure.	
Compartment Syndrome		
1. Assess peripheral pulses hourly with Doppler ultrasound device.	1. Assessment with Doppler device substitutes for auscultation and indicates characteristics of arterial blood flow.	• Absence of paresthesias or symptoms of ischemia of nerves and muscles • Peripheral pulses detectable by Doppler
2. Assess warmth, capillary refill, sensation, and movement of extremity hourly. Compare affected with unaffected extremity.	2. These assessments indicate characteristics of peripheral perfusion.	
3. Remove blood pressure cuff after each reading.	3. Cuff may act as a tourniquet as extremities swell.	
4. Elevate burned extremities.	4. Elevation reduces edema formation.	
5. Report loss of pulse or sensation or presence of pain to physician immediately.	5. These signs and symptoms may indicate inadequate tissue perfusion.	
6. Prepare to assist with escharotomies.	6. Escharotomies relieve the constriction caused by swelling under circumferential burns and improve tissue perfusion.	
Paralytic Ileus		
1. Maintain nasogastric tube on low intermittent suction until bowel sounds resume.	1. This measure relieves gastric and abdominal distention, also prevents vomiting.	• Absence of abdominal distention • Normal bowel sounds within 48 hours
2. Auscultate for bowel sounds, abdominal distention.	2. As bowel sounds resume, feeding may be slowly initiated. Abdominal distention reflects inadequate decompression.	
Curling's Ulcer		
1. Assess gastric aspirate for pH and blood.	1. Acidic pH indicates need for antacids or histamine blockers. Blood indicates possible gastric bleeding.	• Absence of abdominal distention • Normal bowel sounds within 48 hours • Gastric aspirate and stools do not contain blood
2. Assess stools for occult blood.	2. Blood in stools may indicate gastric or duodenal ulcer.	
3. Administer histamine blockers and antacids as prescribed.	3. Such medications reduce gastric acidity and risk of ulceration.	

Central venous, peripheral arterial, or pulmonary artery thermodilution catheters may be required for monitoring venous and arterial pressures, pulmonary artery pressures, pulmonary capillary wedge pressures, or cardiac output. It is not uncommon for patients with major burns to have multiple invasive line sites due to the amount and frequency of fluid and medication that need to be administered. Whenever possible, burned areas of the body are avoided as sites for insertion of invasive lines.

Infection Prevention

Infection progressing to sepsis is the major cause of death in patients who have survived the first few days after a major burn. Burn patients are at risk for infection for a few reasons. The loss of skin removes their ability to protect themselves from the environment. The longer length of stay in the hospital predisposes them to hospital-associated infections. The number and frequency of invasive procedures, both in the patient room and in the operating room, increase the risk of infection. Lastly, immunosuppression that accompanies extensive burn injury places patients at high risk. The nursing goal is to provide protection and safety in the patients' environment to ultimately prevent or control infection in the burn population (Hodle, Richter & Thompson, 2006).

The burn wound is an excellent medium for bacterial growth and proliferation. The burn eschar is nonviable tissue and has no blood supply; therefore, neither leukocytes or antibodies nor systemic antibiotics can reach the area. More than 1 billion bacteria per gram of tissue may be present and subsequently spread to the bloodstream or release their toxins, which reach distant sites. *Pseudomonas* is the major challenge in 44% of burn centers. Other common organisms are methicillin-resistant *Staphylococcus aureus* (MRSA) and *Acinetobacter*. Important but somewhat less common are *Staphylococcus* and vancomycin-resistant enterococci (VRE) (Hodle, et al., 2006). *Staphylococcus* and *Enterococci* are responsible for more than 50% of nosocomial bloodstream infections in patients with burn injuries. Other bacteria that are important in burn care include *Proteus*, *Escherichia coli*, and *Klebsiella*. Bloodstream infections are confirmed if two positive blood cultures are obtained or if one positive culture is obtained in the presence of clinical signs of sepsis (Greenhalgh, 2007). Fungi such as *Candida albicans* also grow easily in burn wounds.

Infection impedes burn wound healing by promoting excessive inflammation and damaging tissue. When the burn wound is healing through spontaneous reepithelialization or is being prepared for skin grafting, it must be protected from sepsis. Characteristics of burn wound sepsis are 10^5 bacteria per gram of tissue, inflammation or destruction of unburned skin, and invasive infection with or without signs of sepsis (Greenhalgh, 2007).

A primary source of bacterial infection is the patient's intestinal tract, the source of most microbes. The intestinal mucosa normally serves as a barrier to keep the internal environment free from a variety of pathogens. After a severe burn injury, the intestinal mucosa becomes markedly permeable (Gosain & Gamelli, 2005b), allowing microbial flora and endotoxins to pass freely into the systemic circulation and causing infection. Early enteral feeding is one strategy to help avoid increased intestinal permeability and prevent early endotoxin translocation (De-Souza & Greene, 2005).

A major secondary source of pathogenic microbes is the environment. Compliance with infection-control policies has been identified as the single greatest challenge along with the abundance of resistant organisms (Hodle, et al., 2006). Burn centers are designed with specific measures to reduce the risk of infection: private rooms and bathrooms; increased airflow within patient rooms to create a more positive airflow; low humidification to prevent bacterial growth; limited use of cloth (eg, patient privacy curtains, window treatments); accessibility of proper protective equipment such as caps, masks, gowns and gloves; convenient and available hand washing/hand hygiene areas; and room design with antidust and dirt collection areas.

Use of cap, gown, mask, and gloves is essential while caring for the patient with open burn wounds. Aseptic technique is used when caring directly for burn wounds. Gowns and gloves are worn by all caregivers and visitors; hand hygiene is used before and after leaving the patient room. Special instruction is given to all visitors with the goal of preventing the spread of infection because of the immunosuppression experienced by patients with burns.

Bacteria are found on all skin surfaces; by itself, their presence does not determine burn infection. Constant monitoring and observation of the wound (eg, changes in the wound, presence of purulent drainage, pain, and increasing depth of burn wound) are needed to detect wound infection. Tissue specimens may be obtained for culture to monitor colonization (Greenhalgh, 2007). Antibiotics are seldom prescribed prophylactically because of the risk of promoting resistant strains of bacteria. Systemic antibiotics are administered when there is documented burn wound sepsis or other positive cultures such as urine, sputum, or blood. Sensitivity of the organisms to the prescribed antibiotics should be determined before administration. Careful attention is paid to antibiotic use in the burn unit because inappropriate use of antibiotics significantly affects the microbial flora present in the burn unit and increases the risk of drug resistance.

Wound Cleaning

Various measures are used to clean the burn wound, such as **hydrotherapy.** If the patient is ambulatory, the wounds can be cleansed in a shower. The wounds of nonambulatory patients can be cleansed using shower carts—mobile stretchers made with removable sides, drainage holes, and positioning capabilities. Retractable shower hoses suspended from walls and ceilings provide the nurse with easy access to a water source for washing the wounds. Unstable patients may have their wounds washed at the bedside. Total immersion hydrotherapy is rarely performed. Because of the high risk for infection and sepsis, the use of plastic liners, water filters, and thorough decontamination of hydrotherapy equipment and wound care areas is required to prevent cross-contamination. The temperature of the water is maintained at 37.8°C (100°F), and the temperature of the room should be maintained between 26.6°C and 29.4°C (80°F to 85°F). The duration of wound cleansing and dressing change is determined by the patient's ability to tolerate the treatment and to maintain a satisfactory body temperature.

During the bath, the patient is encouraged to be as active as possible. Hydrotherapy provides an excellent opportunity for exercising the extremities and cleaning the entire body. When the patient is removed, any residue adhering to the body is washed away with a clear water spray or shower. Unburned areas, including the hair, must be washed regularly as well. At the time of wound cleaning, all skin is inspected for any hints of redness, breakdown, or local infection. Hair in and around the burn area, except the eyebrows, should be clipped short or shaved. Intact blisters should be left alone and débrided only if they rupture or break.

Conscientious management of the burn wound is essential. When nonviable loose skin is removed, aseptic conditions must be established. Wound cleansing is usually performed daily in wound areas that are not undergoing surgical intervention. Mechanical débridement can be performed to remove loose nonviable tissue. However, surgical removal as soon as possible is preferred.

After the burn wounds are cleaned, they are gently patted dry, and the prescribed method of wound care is performed. Whatever the method is used, the goal is to protect the wound from overwhelming proliferation of pathogenic organisms and invasion of deeper tissues until either spontaneous healing or skin grafting can be achieved.

Patient comfort and ability to participate in the prescribed treatment are also important considerations. During the treatment, the patient is assessed for signs of chilling, fatigue, changes in hemodynamic status, and pain unrelieved by analgesic medications or relaxation techniques.

Topical Antibacterial Therapy

Variations in topical wound care for nonsurgical burn wounds exist among burn centers across the country and choices are made based on the individualized needs of each patient. There is general agreement that some form of antimicrobial therapy applied to the burn wound is an acceptable method of local care in extensive burn injury. Silver sulfadiazine is considered the gold standard for protecting wounds from infection (Caruso, Foster, Blome-Eberwein, et al., 2006). Topical antibacterial therapy becomes more important in the deep dermal and full-thickness injury because they are more prone to infection. Silver has been introduced into a variety of topical treatments because of its broad spectrum effectiveness against *Staphylococcus aureus* and *Pseudomonas aeruginosa* (Pham & Gibran, 2007). The goal of topical therapy is to provide a dressing that

- Is effective against gram-positive and gram-negative organisms and fungi,
- Penetrates the eschar but is not systemically toxic,

- Does not lose effectiveness or allow another infection to develop,
- Is cost-effective, available, and acceptable to the patient,
- Is easy to apply and remove, and decreases the frequency of dressing changes, decreases pain, and minimizes nursing time.

Table 57-5 describes three commonly used topical agents, silver sulfadiazine (Silvadene), silver nitrate, and mafenide acetate (Sulfamylon), two of which contain silver. Many other topical agents are available, including povidone–iodine ointment 10% (Betadine), gentamicin sulfate, nitrofurazone (Furacin), Dakin's solution, acetic acid, and antifungal agents (miconazole, clotrimazole, and mupirocin [Bactroban]). Bacitracin or a triple antibiotic agent may be used for facial burns or on skin grafts initially.

No single topical medication is universally effective, and use of different agents at different times in the postburn period may be necessary. Prudent use and alternation of antimicrobial agents result in less-resistant strains of bacteria, greater effectiveness of the agents, and a decreased risk of sepsis.

Table 57-5	OVERVIEW OF SELECTED TOPICAL ANTIBACTERIAL AGENTS USED FOR BURN WOUNDS		
Agent	**Indication/Comment**	**Application**	**Nursing Implications**
Silver sulfadiazine 1% (Silvadene) water-soluble cream	• Most bactericidal agent • Minimal penetration of eschar	Apply 1/16-inch layer of cream with a sterile glove 1–3 times daily.	• Watch for leukopenia 2–3 days after initiation of therapy. (Leukopenia usually resolves within 2–3 days.) • Anticipate formation of pseudo-eschar (proteinaceous gel), which is removed easily after 72 hours.
Mafenide acetate 5% to 10% (Sulfamylon) hydrophilic-based cream	• Effective against gram-negative and gram-positive organisms • Diffuses rapidly through eschar • In 10% strength, it is the agent of choice for electrical burns because of its ability to penetrate thick eschar	Apply thin layer with sterile glove twice a day and leave open as prescribed; if the wound is dressed, change the dressing every 6 hours as prescribed.	• Monitor arterial blood gas levels and discontinue as prescribed, if acidosis occurs. Mafenide acetate is a strong carbonic anhydrase inhibitor that may reduce renal buffering and cause metabolic acidosis. • Premedicate the patient with an analgesic before applying mafenide acetate because this agent causes severe burning pain for up to 20 minutes after application.
Silver nitrate 0.5% aqueous solution	• Bacteriostatic and fungicidal • Does not penetrate eschar	Apply solution to gauze dressing and place over wound. Keep the dressing wet but covered with dry gauze and dry blankets to decrease vaporization. Remoisten every 2 hours, and redress wound twice a day.	• Monitor serum sodium (Na$^+$) and potassium (K$^+$) levels and replace as prescribed. Silver nitrate solution is hypotonic and acts as wick for sodium and potassium. • Protect bed linen and clothing from contact with silver nitrate, which stains everything it touches black.
Acticoat	• Effective against gram-negative and gram-positive organisms and some yeasts and molds • Delivers a uniform, antimicrobial concentration of silver to the burn wound	Moisten with sterile water only (never use normal saline). Apply directly to wound. Cover with absorbent secondary dressing. Remoisten every 3–4 hours with sterile water.	• Do not use oil-based products or topical antimicrobials with Acticoat burn dressing. Keep Acticoat moist, not saturated. May produce a "pseudo-eschar" from silver after application. • Can be left in place for 3–5 days. Also available in Acticoat 7, which can be left in place for up to 7 days without the need to change the dressing.

Wound Dressing

After wound cleaning, the burned areas are patted dry and the prescribed topical agent is applied; the wound is then covered with several layers of dressings. A light dressing is used over joint areas to allow for motion (unless the particular area has a graft and motion is contraindicated). A light dressing is also applied over areas for which a splint has been designed to conform to the body contour for proper positioning. Circumferential dressings should be applied distally to proximally. If the hand or foot is burned, the fingers and toes should be wrapped individually to promote adequate healing.

Burns to the face may be left open to air once they have been cleaned and the topical agent has been applied. Careful attention must be given to ensure that the topical agent does not interfere with the eyes or mouth. A light dressing can be applied to the face to absorb excess exudates that might run into the eyes, causing irritation.

Occlusive dressings may be used over areas with new skin grafts to protect the graft and promote an optimal condition for its adherence to the recipient site. An occlusive dressing is a thin gauze that is impregnated with a topical antimicrobial agent or is applied after application of a topical antimicrobial agent. Ideally, these dressings remain in place for 3 to 5 days, at which time they are removed for examination of the graft. When occlusive dressings are applied, precautions are taken to prevent two body surfaces from touching, such as fingers or toes, ear and scalp, the areas under the breasts, any point of flexion, or between the genital folds. Functional body alignment positions are maintained by using splints or by regular repositioning of the patient.

NURSING ALERT

Dressings impede circulation if they are too tightly wrapped. The peripheral pulses must be checked frequently and burned extremities elevated on two pillows. Extremities are always wrapped from distal to proximal to the heart. If the patient's pulse is diminished, this is a critical situation and must be addressed immediately.

Dressings that adhere to the wound can be removed more comfortably and without damaging healing tissue by moistening the wound with tap water. The remaining dressings are carefully and gently removed. The patient may participate in removing the dressings, providing some degree of control over this painful procedure. The wounds are then cleaned and débrided to remove any remaining topical agent, exudate, and dead skin. Sterile scissors and forceps may be used to trim loose eschar and encourage separation of devitalized skin. During this procedure, the wound and surrounding skin are carefully inspected. The color, odor, size, exudate, signs of reepithelialization, and other characteristics of the wound and the eschar and any changes from the previous dressing change are noted.

Wound Débridement

The goals of, **débridement,** the removal of devitalized tissue, are:
- Removal of tissue contaminated by bacteria and foreign bodies, thereby protecting the patient from invasion of bacteria

- Removal of devitalized tissue or burn eschar in preparation for grafting and wound healing

There are three types of débridement—natural, mechanical, and surgical.

Natural Débridement

With natural débridement, the dead tissue separates from the underlying viable tissue spontaneously. Bacteria that are present at the interface of the burned tissue and the viable tissue underneath gradually liquefy the fibrils of **collagen** that hold the eschar in place for the first or second postburn weeks. Proteolytic and other natural enzymes cause this phenomenon. However, use of antibacterial topical agents tends to slow this natural process of eschar separation and slows the healing process.

Mechanical Débridement

Mechanical débridement involves the use of surgical scissors, scalpels, and forceps to separate and remove the eschar. This technique can be performed by skilled physicians, nurses, or physical therapists and is usually done with daily dressing changes. If bleeding occurs, hemostatic agents or pressure can be used to stop the bleeding from small vessels. Wet-to-dry dressings are not advocated in burn care because of the chance of removing viable cells along with necrotic tissue. Dressing changes alone aid the removal of wound debris.

Chemical Débridement

Topical enzymatic débridement agents are available to promote débridement of the burn wounds. Because such agents usually do not have antimicrobial properties, they should be used together with topical antibacterial therapy to protect the patient from bacterial invasion. Heavy metals such as silver deactivate the débriding agent; therefore, caution is necessary to ensure that the débriding agent does not interfere with the topical antimicrobial agent. Separate dressings are used to prevent this from occurring.

Surgical Débridement

Early surgical excision to remove devitalized tissue along with early burn wound closure is now recognized as one of the most important factors contributing to survival in a patient with a major burn injury. Aggressive surgical wound closure has reduced the incidence of burn wound sepsis, thus improving survival rates (Burke, 2005). Early excision is carried out before the natural separation of eschar is allowed to occur.

Surgical débridement is an operative procedure involving either primary **excision** (surgical removal of tissue) of the full thickness of the skin down to the fascia (tangential excision) or shaving of the burned skin layers gradually down to freely bleeding, viable tissue. Surgical excision is initiated early in burn wound management. This may be performed within the first few days after the burn or as soon as the patient is hemodynamically stable and edema has decreased. Ideally, the wound is then covered immediately with a skin graft, if needed, and an occlusive dressing. If the wound bed is not ready for a skin graft at the time of excision, a temporary biologic dressing may be used until a skin graft can be applied during subsequent surgery.

The use of surgical excision carries with it risks and complications, especially with large burns. The procedure creates a high risk of extensive blood loss (as much as 100 to 125 mL of blood per percentage of body surface excised) and lengthy operating and anesthesia times. However, when conducted in a timely and efficient manner, surgical excision results in shorter hospital stays and possibly a decreased risk of complications from invasive burn wound sepsis.

 Gerontologic Considerations

Eschar separation in full-thickness burns is typically delayed in elderly patients, and older patients are frequently poor risks for surgical excision. For these reasons, prolonged hospitalization, immobilization, and associated problems are common. If the elderly patient can tolerate surgery, early excision with skin grafting is the treatment of choice because it decreases the mortality rate in this population. If the patient is not a surgical candidate, chemical débridement is often chosen to enhance the removal of eschar over time. Prevention of complications of prolonged hospitalization, immobility, and surgery is essential in the care of the elderly burn patient.

Wound Grafting

The patient with deep partial-thickness or full-thickness burns may be a candidate for skin grafting. If so, temporary coverage of the burn wound is necessary until coverage with a graft of the patient's own skin (**autograft**) is possible. The purposes of wound coverage are to decrease the risk of infection; prevent further loss of protein, fluid, and electrolytes through the wound; and minimize heat loss through evaporation. Several methods of wound coverage are available; some are temporary until grafting with permanent coverage is possible. Wound coverage may consist of biologic, biosynthetic, synthetic, and autologous methods or a combination of these approaches.

The main areas for skin grafting include the face (for cosmetic and psychological reasons); functional areas, such as the hands and feet; and areas that involve joints. Grafting permits earlier functional ability and reduces wound **contractures.** When burns are very extensive, the order in which areas are grafted is chosen based on the ability to achieve wound closure as soon as possible, and, therefore, the chest and abdomen or back may be grafted first to reduce the burn surface.

Granulation tissue fills the space created by the wound, creates a barrier to bacteria, and serves as a bed for epithelial cell growth. Richly vascular granulation tissue is pink, firm, shiny, and free of exudate and debris. It should have a bacterial count of less than 100,000/g of tissue to optimize graft success. If the wound is not ready for skin grafting, the burn wound is excised and allowed to granulate. Once the wound is excised, a wound covering is applied to keep the wound bed moist and promote the granulation process.

Biologic Dressings (Homografts and Heterografts)

Biologic dressings have several uses. In extensive burns, they provide temporary wound coverage and protect the granulation tissue until autografting is possible. Biologic dressings are commonly used in patients with large areas of burn and little remaining normal skin for donor sites. They can be used as a test graft in preparation for the patient's own skin graft to determine if the bed will accept the graft.

Once the biologic dressing appears to be "taking," or adhering to the granulating surface with minimal underlying exudation, the patient is ready for an autologous skin graft.

Biologic dressings also provide temporary immediate coverage for clean, superficial burns and decrease the wound's evaporative water and protein loss. They decrease pain by protecting nerve endings and are an effective barrier against water loss and entry of bacteria. When applied to superficial partial-thickness wounds, they seem to speed healing. Biologic materials can be left open or covered. They stay in place for varying lengths of time but are removed in instances of infection or rejection. Another advantage for the patient is that these dressings often require fewer dressing changes, therefore, decreasing pain. They can also be used in the outpatient environment.

Biologic dressings consist of **homografts** (or allografts) and **heterografts** (or xenografts). Homografts are skin obtained from living or recently deceased humans. Heterografts consist of skin taken from animals (usually pigs). Most biologic dressings are used as temporary coverings of burn wounds and are eventually rejected because of the body's immune reaction to them as foreign.

Homografts tend to be the most expensive biologic dressings. They are available from skin banks in fresh and cryopreserved (frozen) forms. Homografts are thought to provide the best infection control of all the biologic or biosynthetic dressings available. Revascularization occurs within 48 hours, and the graft may be left in place for several weeks.

Pigskin is available from commercial suppliers. It is available fresh, frozen, or lyophilized (freeze dried) for longer shelf life. Pigskin is used for temporary covering of clean wounds such as superficial partial-thickness wounds and donor sites. Although pigskin does not vascularize, it does adhere to clean superficial wounds and provides excellent pain control while the underlying wound epithelializes (Atiyeh, et al., 2005).

Biosynthetic and Synthetic Dressings

Problems with availability, sterility, and cost have prompted the search for biosynthetic and synthetic skin substitutes, which may eventually replace biologic dressings as temporary wound coverings. A widely used synthetic dressing is **Biobrane,** which is composed of a nylon, silastic membrane combined with a collagen derivative. The material is semitransparent and sterile. It has an indefinite shelf life and is less costly than homograft or pigskin. Like biologic dressings, Biobrane protects the wound from fluid loss and bacterial invasion (Fig. 57-4).

Biobrane adheres to the wound fibrin, which binds to the nylon–collagen material. Within 5 days, cells migrate into the nylon mesh. In general, adherence to the wound surface correlates directly with low bacterial counts. When the Biobrane dressing adheres to the wound, the wound remains stable. Biobrane can remain in place until spontaneous epithelialization and wound healing occur. It can be laid on top of a wide-meshed autograft to protect the wound until the autograft epithelium grows out to close the interstices. As the Biobrane gradually separates, it is trimmed, leaving a healed wound.

Another temporary wound covering is BCG Matrix. This dressing combines beta-glucan, a complex carbohydrate, with collagen in a meshed reinforced wound dressing. Beta-glucan is known to stimulate macrophages, which are vital in the inflammatory process of healing. BCG Matrix is

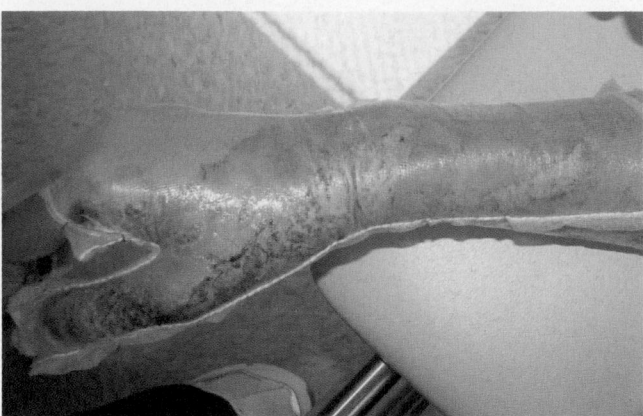

Figure 57-4 Biobrane dressing for partial-thickness burn wound. Biobrane dressing applied to a clean wound bed on the hand. Used with permission. Lehigh Valley Health Network, Allentown, PA.

a temporary wound covering intended for use with partial-thickness burns and donor sites. It is applied immediately after cleaning and débridement. If the burn wound surface remains free of infection, BCG Matrix can be left in place until healing is complete (Atiyeh, et al., 2005).

Several other synthetic dressings are available for burn wound care. Op Site, a thin, transparent, polyurethane elastic film, can be used to cover clean partial-thickness wounds and donor sites. This dressing is occlusive and waterproof but permeable to water vapor and air; this permeability not only provides protection from microbial contamination but also allows for the exchange of gases, which occurs much more quickly in a moist environment. Other synthetic dressings used for burn wounds include Tegaderm, N-Terface, and DuoDerm.

Skin Substitutes

In an attempt to develop the ideal burn wound covering product, skin substitutes have been created that surgically replace the epidermis and the dermis. It is believed that skin substitutes enhance the healing process of an open wound when autologous skin is unavailable or limited for use. These products are often the choice when donor sites are inadequate or unavailable.

A **cultured epithelial autograft (CEA)** provides permanent coverage of large wounds when harvesting of skin for autografting is not an option. This involves a biopsy of the patient's skin in an unburned area. Keratinocytes are isolated, and epithelial cells are cultured in a laboratory. The original epithelial cell reproduces multiple plated sheets of CEA to cover an already surgically excised wound. These cells are then attached to the burn wound surface, and extreme care is taken until they have adhered to the wound surface. Varying degrees of success have been reported and results are encouraging. However, the disadvantages of the CEA are that the grafts are thin and fragile and can shear easily. Patients have longer hospital stays and higher hospital costs and require more surgical procedures than those treated by traditional methods. In addition, patients require more reconstructive procedures in the first 1 to 2 years after injury. Therefore, CEA use is very limited and is reserved for burn patients whose donor sites are limited (Pham & Gibran, 2007).

Two dermal substitutes are **Integra** Artificial Skin and **AlloDerm**. Artificial skin (Integra) is the newest type of dermal substitute (Fig. 57-5). A dermal analogue, Integra is

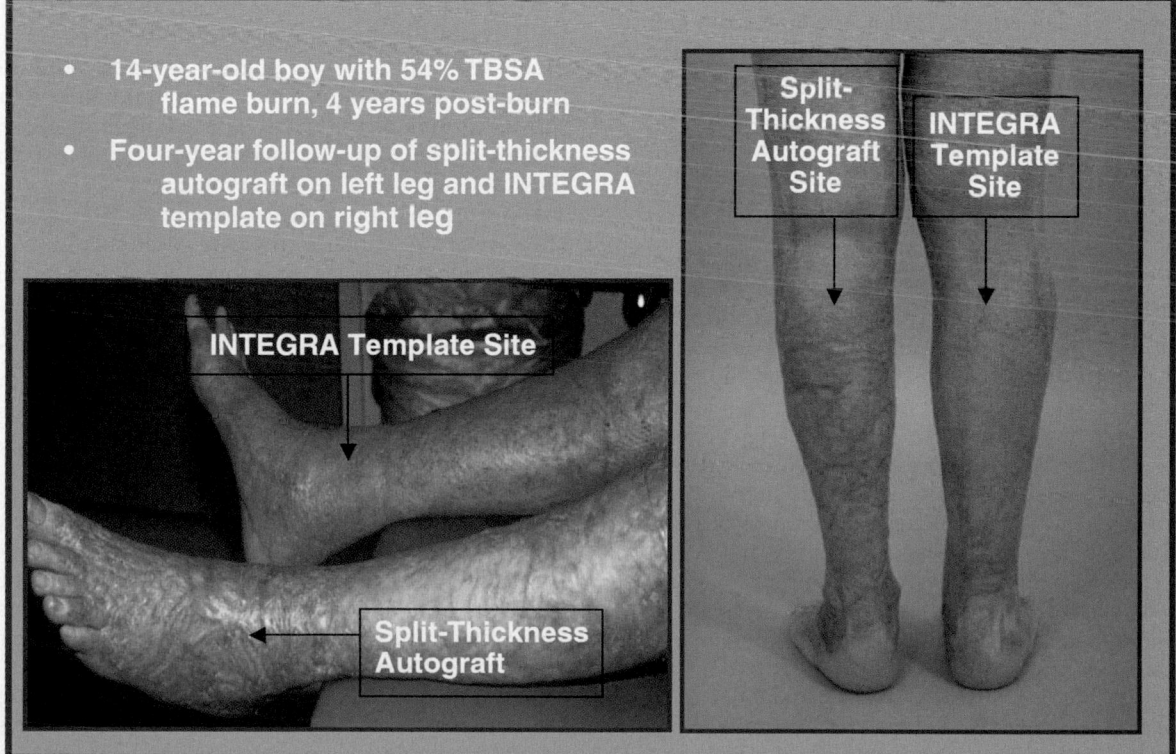

- 14-year-old boy with 54% TBSA flame burn, 4 years post-burn
- Four-year follow-up of split-thickness autograft on left leg and INTEGRA template on right leg

INTEGRA Template Site

Split-Thickness Autograft

Split-Thickness Autograft Site

INTEGRA Template Site

Figure 57-5 Comparison of Integra template site (*right leg*) to split-thickness autograft site (*left leg*). Used with permission from Glenn Warden, MD.

composed of two main layers. The epidermal layer, consisting of silicone, acts as a bacterial barrier and prevents water loss from the dermis. The dermal layer is composed of animal collagen. It interfaces with the open wound surface and allows migration of fibroblasts and capillaries into the material. This "neodermis" becomes a permanent structure. The artificial dermis is biodegraded and reabsorbed. The outer silicone membrane is removed 2 weeks after application and is replaced with the patient's own skin in the form of a thin epidermal skin graft. When a thinner autologous donor graft is used, donor site healing is quicker. Long-term effects of Integra include minimal contracture formation. The graft site is very pliable, almost eliminating the need for repeated cosmetic surgery. Most important, Integra has resulted in less hypertrophic scarring, thus reducing the need for compression devices once the burn wound has healed. Because Integra allows for earlier excision and coverage of the burn wound, metabolic demands of the patient are reduced. Integra allows for the increased survivability of patients with large burn injuries and improves the functional and cosmetic qualities of the healed burns. The combination of Integra with cultured skin substitutes has demonstrated promise in burn management (Pham & Gibran, 2007).

Another promising dermal substitute is AlloDerm. It is processed dermis from human cadaver skin, which can be used as the dermal layer for skin grafts. When a **donor site** (the area from which skin is taken to provide a skin graft for another part of the body) is harvested for an autologous skin graft, both the epidermal and the dermal layers of skin are removed from the donor site. AlloDerm provides a permanent dermal layer replacement. Its use allows the burn surgeon to harvest a thinner skin graft, consisting of the epidermal layer only. The patient's epidermal layer is placed directly over the dermal base (AlloDerm). The new graft is then treated according to the burn unit's protocol. Use of AlloDerm has also resulted in less scarring and contractures with healed grafts; donor sites heal more quickly than conventional donor sites because only the epidermal layer has been harvested. This is important when donor sites are limited because of extensive burns (Boyce, Greenhalgh, Palmieri, et al., 2006; Pham & Gibran, 2007).

Autografts

Autografts remain the preferred material for definitive burn wound closure after excision. Autografts are the ideal means of covering burn wounds because the grafts are the patient's own skin and therefore are not rejected by the patient's immune system. They can be split-thickness (Fig. 57-6), full-thickness, pedicle flaps, or epithelial grafts. Full-thickness autografts and pedicle flaps are commonly used for reconstructive surgery, which may take place months or years after the initial injury.

Split-thickness autografts can be applied in sheets or they can be expanded by meshing so that they cover 1.5 to 9 times more than a given donor site area. Skin meshers enable the surgeon to cut tiny slits into a sheet of donor skin, making it possible to cover large areas with smaller amounts of donor skin. These expanded grafts adhere to the recipient site more easily than sheet grafts and prevent the accumulation of blood, serum, air, or purulent material under

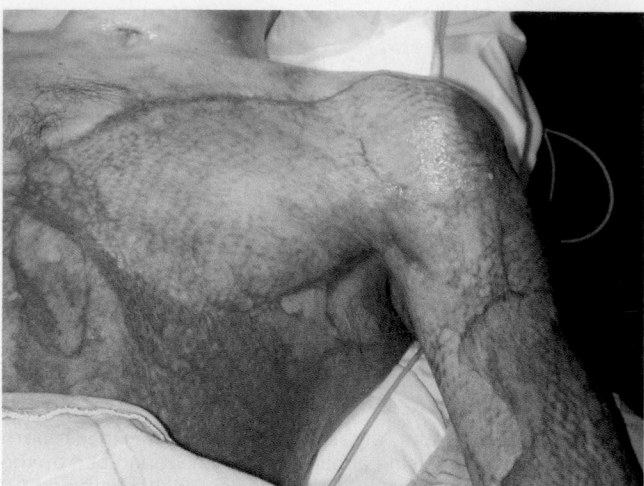

Figure 57-6 Healed split-thickness skin graft to the chest and upper extremity. Used with permission. Lehigh Valley Health Network, Allentown, PA.

the graft. However, any kind of graft other than a sheet graft contributes to scar formation as it heals. Use of expanded grafts may be necessary in large wounds but should be viewed as a compromise in terms of cosmesis.

If blood, serum, air, fat, or necrotic tissue lies between the recipient site and the graft, there may be partial or total loss of the graft. Infection or mishandling of the graft and trauma during dressing changes account for most other instances of graft loss. Use of split-thickness grafts allows the remaining donor site to retain sweat glands and hair follicles and minimizes donor site healing time.

Care of the Graft Site. Protection is the key goal of caring for skin grafts postoperatively. Occlusive dressings are commonly used initially after grafting to immobilize the graft. Occupational therapists may be helpful in constructing splints to immobilize newly grafted areas to prevent dislodging of the graft. Homografts, heterografts, or synthetic dressings may also be used to protect grafts.

The first dressing change is usually performed 2 to 5 days after surgery, or earlier in the case of clinical signs of infection, purulent drainage, or a foul odor. Infection, bleeding beneath the graft, and shearing force are the most common reasons for graft loss in the early postoperative period.

The patient is positioned and turned carefully to avoid disturbing the graft or putting pressure on the graft site. If an extremity has been grafted, it is elevated to minimize edema. The patient begins exercising the grafted area 5 to 7 days after grafting.

Care of the Donor Site. Donor sites are clean new wounds that are usually very painful. Caregivers need to recognize this additional source of pain and possible site of infection. Since the donor site is a clean wound created in a surgical environment, it should heal easily unless other complications exist. A moist gauze dressing is applied at the time of surgery to maintain pressure and to stop any oozing. After the donor skin is excised, a thrombostatic agent such as thrombin or epinephrine may be applied directly to the site. The donor site may be covered in several ways, from single-layer gauze impregnated with petrolatum, scarlet red, or bismuth to new biosynthetic dressings such as Biobrane or BCG Matrix. Acticoat can also be used as a dressing on donor sites. With all types of covering, donor sites must remain clean, dry, and free from pressure. Because a donor site is a partial-thickness wound, it is very painful and will heal spontaneously within 7 to 14 days with proper care.

Pain Management

The ability to quantify pain may be difficult in any patient; however, the patient who has experienced a burn has many additional challenges. A burn injury is considered one of the most painful types of trauma that a patient can endure. The nature of the injury requires multiple procedures, débridement, surgery and treatments. All of these experiences vary in length and intensity, therefore creating variations in sensation. Additional pain occurs with each skin graft because a new painful donor site is created. In addition, moving, changing position, and receiving occupational and physical therapy cause addition discomfort. This is a constantly changing source of pain throughout the entire healing process, and to the patient it appears to be never ending. Therefore, the pain management plan for any patient needs to be flexible, evaluated regularly using standardized scales, and individualized to meet the patient's needs (Faucher & Furukawa, 2006, Connor-Ballard, 2009a, 2009b).

The American Burn Association's guidelines for pain management are: there must be an organized approach to pain management that addresses background, procedural, and breakthrough pain; the goal should be for patients to be comfortable and alert; and pain needs to be differentiated from anxiety (Faucher & Furukawa, 2006).

Background pain is a continuous level of discomfort even when the patient is inactive or not undergoing any procedures. The goal of treatment is to provide a long-acting analgesic that will provide even coverage for this long-term discomfort. It is helpful to use escalating doses when initiating the medication to reach the level of pain control that is acceptable to the patient. The use of patient-controlled analgesia (PCA) gives control to the patient and achieves this goal. Breakthrough pain is described as acute, intense, and episodic pain. It is generally related to an activity or movement of the affected area. Short-acting agents are used to achieve pain control in addition to the baseline treatment the patient receives for background pain. Procedural pain is discomfort that occurs with procedures such as daily wound treatments, invasive line insertions, physical and occupational therapy. The goal is to plan proper sedation that will place the patient in a state of comfort throughout the procedure. Depending on the agent, an anesthesia provider can be helpful in achievement of pain relief (Faucher & Furukawa, 2006).

Most severe burns are a combination of partial-thickness and full-thickness burns and the depth influences the amount of pain the patient experiences. Superficial and deep partial-thickness burns are very painful because the nerve endings are exposed, resulting in excruciating pain with exposure to temperature, pressure, and movement. In a full-thickness burn the nerve endings are destroyed, and upon admission there is numbness and decreased sensation to the area. Thus, severe injuries are often underestimated

by the patient because the pain at that time is minimal. Educating patients and their families about burn pain and its relationship to the depth of injury as well as the pain management plan is an important priority for the nurse.

The pharmacologic treatment for the management of burn pain includes the use of opioids, nonsteroidal anti-inflammatory drugs (NASIDs), anxiolytics, and anesthetic agents. These and other pain management strategies are discussed in Chapter 13. Treatment of anxiety with benzodiazepines is used along with opioids to achieve both a pain-free and anxiety-free experience. The use of anesthetics in a nonoperative setting (ie, moderate sedation) requires administration by qualified personnel. Recent advances include the use of agents with rapid onset and short duration, which have been very effective in pain control during a planned procedure (Faucher & Furukawa, 2006).

Nonpharmacologic pain control can be achieved by using relaxation techniques, distraction, guided imagery, hypnosis, therapeutic touch, humor, music therapy, and more recently virtual reality techniques (see Chapter 13). These techniques can be used either alone or in conjunction with medications to achieve an acceptable level of comfort for the burn patient (Hansen, Gauld, Wathen, et al., 2008).

Nutritional Support

Burn injuries produce profound metabolic abnormalities fueled by the exaggerated stress response to the injury. The body's response has been classified as hyperdynamic, hypermetabolic, and hypercatabolic. Hypermetabolism can affect morbidity and mortality by increasing the risk for infection and slowing the healing rate. Patients' metabolic demands vary with the extent of the burn injury and age (Demling, 2005b). Hypermetabolism is evident immediately after a burn injury. The degree of the response depends on the size of the burn and the patient's age, body composition, size, and genetic response to insult (Jeschke, Chinkes, Finnerty, et al., 2008). Persistent hypermetabolism may last up to 1 year after burn injury.

Major metabolic abnormalities after a burn injury include increased catabolic hormones (cortisol and catechols); decreased anabolic hormones (human growth factor and testosterone); a marked increase in the metabolic rate; a sustained increase in body temperature; a marked increase in glucose demands; rapid skeletal muscle breakdown with amino acids serving as the energy source; lack of ketosis, indicating that fat is not a major source of calories; and catabolism that does not respond to nutrient intake (Pereira, Murphy & Herndon, 2005). Therefore, it is essential to control the stress response by increasing the anabolic process through adequate nutrition and increased muscle activity, decreasing heat loss from wounds, and maintaining a warm environment. Controlling secondary stressors, such as pain and anxiety, also helps control the stress response.

The most important nutritional intervention is to provide energy and nutrients for prevention of infection and promotion of wound healing (Wolfe, 2007). Healing of the burn wound consumes large quantities of energy. Patients with burns greater than 40% TBSA have resting metabolic rates twice that of normal (Pereira, et al., 2005). Effective nutrition management depends on how well the energy expenditure due to the burn injury can be estimated and matched with appropriate amounts of micronutrients, carbohydrates, lipids, and protein. The nutritional support required is based on the patient's preburn status and the TBSA burned.

Several formulas exist for estimating the daily metabolic expenditure and caloric requirements of patients with burn injuries. The most commonly used formulas are the Harris-Benedict equation, which determines basal energy requirements based on activity and burn size, Ireton-Jones formula, and the Modified Schoefield (Masters & Wood, 2008). Protein requirements may range from 2.0 to 3.0 g of protein per kilogram of body weight every 24 hours, which is 15% to 25% of the caloric intake. Although variation exists, most burn centers use a low fat and high carbohydrate enteral feeding, approximately 55% to 85% carbohydrate and 3% to 20% fat. Carbohydrates are included to meet caloric requirements and to spare protein, which is essential for wound healing. The patient may also receive added vitamins and minerals in excess of the normal requirements (Masters & Wood, 2008).

Feeding usually begins immediately or at least within 24 to 72 hours postburn injury. Nutrition can be administered either by the enteral or parenteral route, or a combination of both. The goal is to reach the patient's nutritional needs, which are usually in proportion to the burn size. These feedings are continued until the patient can adequately consume the recommended daily requirements by mouth (Wolfe, 2007). When the oral route is used, high-protein, high-calorie meals and supplements are given. Dietary consultations are useful in helping patients meet their nutritional needs. Daily calorie counts aid in assessing the adequacy of nutritional intake.

Patients lose a great deal of weight during recovery from severe burns. Reserve fat deposits are catabolized, fluids are lost, and caloric intake may be limited. Because a burn injury decreases the patient's resistance to infection and disease, the nutritional status must be improved and maintained even though the patient has a poor appetite and is weak. One goal of nutrition management is to decrease or stop the catabolic process and promote protein anabolism.

In addition, research is focused on aggressive alteration of the hyperglycemic response and administration of insulin therapy to promote wound healing. Other treatment modalities include early excision and skin grafting of the burn wound, aggressive prevention or treatment of infections, and adequate exercise with physical therapy to lessen muscle wasting and increase strength. Additional pharmacologic modalities used to alter the hypermetabolic state of burn injury include the use of oxandrolone (Oxandrin), an anabolic steroid; an adrenergic antagonist (propranolol [Indural]); and the anabolic protein, recombinant human growth hormone (Pereira, et al., 2005).

Indications for parenteral nutrition include weight loss greater than 10% of normal body weight, inadequate intake of enteral nutrition due to clinical status, prolonged wound exposure, and malnutrition or debilitated condition before injury. The risk of infection at the site of the central venous catheter required for parenteral nutrition must be considered.

Nursing Management

Continued assessment of the patient during the early weeks after the burn injury focuses on hemodynamic alterations, wound healing, pain and psychosocial responses, and early detection of complications. Assessment of respiratory and fluid status remains the highest priority for detection of potential complications.

The nurse assesses vital signs frequently. Continued assessment of peripheral pulses is essential for the first few postburn days while edema continues to increase, potentially damaging peripheral nerves and restricting blood flow. Close observation of the hourly fluid intake and urinary output as well as blood pressure and cardiac rhythm is essential during this phase and changes should be reported to the burn surgeon promptly.

The patient with an inhalation injury will require regular monitoring of level of consciousness, pulmonary function, and ability to ventilate. When inadequate ventilation and airway edema require the patient to be intubated and placed on a ventilator, frequent suctioning and assessment of the airway are priorities.

Restoring Normal Fluid Balance

To reduce the risk of fluid overload and consequent heart failure and pulmonary edema, the nurse closely monitors IV and oral fluid intake, using IV infusion pumps to minimize the risk of rapid fluid infusion. To monitor changes in fluid status, careful intake and output and daily weights are obtained. Changes, including those of blood pressure and pulse rate, are reported to the physician (invasive hemodynamic monitoring is avoided because of the high risk of infection).

Preventing Infection

A major part of the nurse's role during the acute phase of burn care is detection and prevention of infection. The nurse is responsible for providing a clean and safe environment and for closely scrutinizing the burn wound to detect early signs of infection. Culture results and white blood cell counts are monitored.

Aseptic technique is used for wound care procedures. Sterile technique is used for any invasive procedures, such as insertion of IV lines and urinary catheters or tracheal suctioning. Meticulous hand hygiene before and after each patient contact is also an essential component of preventing infection, even though gloves are worn to provide care.

The nurse protects the patient from sources of contamination, including other patients, staff members, visitors, and equipment. Invasive lines and tubing must be routinely changed according to recommendations of the CDC. Tube feeding reservoirs, ventilator circuits, and drainage containers are replaced regularly. Fresh flowers, plants, and fresh fruit baskets are not permitted in the patient's room because of the risk of microorganism growth. Visitors are screened to avoid exposure of the immunocompromised patient to pathogens.

Patients can inadvertently promote migration of microorganisms from one burned area to another by touching their wounds or dressings. Bed linens also can spread infection through either colonization with wound microorganisms or fecal contamination. Regular bathing of unburned areas and changing of linens can help prevent infection.

Maintaining Adequate Nutrition

Oral fluids should be initiated slowly after bowel sounds resume. The patient's tolerance is recorded. If vomiting and distention do not occur, fluids may be increased gradually and the patient may be advanced to a normal diet or to tube feedings.

The nurse collaborates with the dietitian or nutrition support team to plan a protein- and calorie-rich diet that is acceptable to the patient. Family members may be encouraged to bring nutritious and favorite foods to the hospital. High-calorie nutritional supplements such as Ensure and Resource may be provided. Caloric intake must be documented. Vitamin and mineral supplements may be prescribed.

If caloric goals cannot be met by oral feeding, a feeding tube is inserted and used for continuous or bolus feedings of specific formulas. The volume of residual gastric secretions should be checked to ensure absorption.

The patient should be weighed each day and the results graphed. The patient can use this information to set goals for nutritional intake and to monitor weight loss and gain. Ideally, the patient will lose no more than 5% of preburn weight if aggressive nutritional management is implemented.

Promoting Skin Integrity

Wound care is usually the single most time-consuming element of burn care after the emergent phase. The physician prescribes the desired topical antibacterial agents and specific biologic, biosynthetic, or synthetic wound coverings and plans for surgical excision and grafting. The nurse needs to make astute assessments of wound status, use creative approaches to wound dressing, and support the patient during the emotionally distressing and very painful experience of wound care.

Assessment of the burn wound requires an experienced eye, hand, and sense of smell. Important wound assessment features include size, color, odor, eschar, exudate, epithelial buds (small pearl-like clusters of cells on the wound surface), bleeding, granulation tissue, the status of graft take, healing of the donor site, and the condition of the surrounding skin. Any significant changes in the wound are reported to the physician because they usually indicate burn infection and require immediate intervention.

A diagram, updated daily by the nurse responsible for the patient's care, helps inform all those concerned about the latest wound care procedures in use for the patient.

The nurse also assists the patient and family by providing instruction, support, and encouragement to take an active part in dressing changes and wound care when appropriate. Discharge planning needs for wound care are anticipated early in the course of burn management, and the strengths of the patient and family are assessed and used in preparing for the patient's eventual discharge and home care.

Relieving Pain and Discomfort

Pain measures are continued during the acute phase of burn recovery. Analgesic agents and anxiolytic medications are administered as prescribed. Frequent assessment of pain and discomfort is essential. To increase its effectiveness, analgesic medication is provided before the pain becomes severe.

Nursing interventions such as teaching the patient relaxation techniques, giving the patient some control over wound care and analgesia, and providing frequent reassurance are helpful. Guided imagery and distraction (eg, video programs or video games) can be used to alter the patient's perceptions of and responses to pain. Other pain-relieving approaches include hypnosis, music therapy, and virtual reality.

The nurse assesses the patient's sleep patterns daily. Lack of sleep and rest interferes with healing, comfort, and restoration of energy. If necessary, sedatives are prescribed on a regular basis in addition to analgesics and anxiolytics.

The nurse works quickly to complete treatments and dressing changes to reduce pain and discomfort. The patient is encouraged to take analgesic medications before painful procedures. The patient's response to the medication and other interventions is assessed and documented.

Healing burn wounds are typically described by patients as itchy and tight. Oral antipruritic agents, a cool environment, frequent lubrication of the skin with water or a silica-based lotion, exercise and splinting to prevent skin contracture, and diversional activities all help promote comfort in this phase.

Promoting Physical Mobility

An early priority is to prevent complications of immobility. Deep breathing, turning, and proper positioning are essential nursing practices that prevent atelectasis and pneumonia, control edema, and prevent pressure ulcers and contractures. These interventions are modified to meet the patient's needs. Low-air-loss and rotation beds may be useful, and early sitting and ambulation are encouraged. If the lower extremities are burned, elastic pressure bandages should be applied before the patient is placed in an upright position. These bandages promote venous return and minimize edema formation. Prevention of deep vein thrombosis (DVT) is an important factor in care. Patients with burn injuries are at high risk because of their hypercoagulability, loss of vascular integrity, immobility, multiple invasive lines and need for other operative procedures. In fact, there is a 1% to 23% incidence of DVT in burn patients documented. There is cautious use of heparin due to the bleeding potential; however, most burn centers use prophylactic therapy including sequential graduated compression devices in the high-risk groups (Faucher & Conlon, 2007).

The burn wound is in a dynamic state for at least 1 year after wound closure. During this time, aggressive efforts must be made to prevent contracture and hypertrophic scarring. Both passive and active range-of-motion exercises are initiated from the day of admission and are continued after grafting, within prescribed limitations. Splints or functional devices may be applied to the extremities for contracture control. The nurse monitors the splinted areas for signs of vascular insufficiency, nerve compression, and skin breakdown. Occupational and physical therapists are consulted to develop a patient-specific plan of care throughout hospitalization and recovery.

Strengthening Coping Strategies

In the acute phase of burn care, the patient is facing the reality of the burn injury and is grieving over obvious losses. Depression, anger, regression, and manipulative behavior are common responses of patients who have burn injuries. Withdrawal from participation in required treatments and regression must be viewed with an understanding that such behavior may help the patient cope with an enormously stressful event. Although most patients recover emotionally from a burn injury, some have more difficult psychological reactions to the injury and its outcomes (Kildal, Willebrand, Andersson, et al., 2004). There is evidence that psychological distress and depression are common in people who have experienced burns; however, more studies are needed in this area (Fauerbach, Pruzinsky & Saxe, 2007).

Difficulty coping along with other psychological stressors often limits the patient's physical and psychological recovery (Fauerbach, Lezotte, Hills, et al., 2005). Patients who experience a burn injury tend to have high rates of involvement in risky behaviors (eg, alcohol and substance abuse, depression) before the injury (Appleby, 2005). Intrusive thoughts of the burn event and reliving it over and over may also occur and can indicate posttraumatic stress disorder (PTSD).

Much of the patient's energy goes into maintaining vital physical functions and wound healing in the early postburn weeks, leaving little emotional energy for coping in a more effective manner. The nurse can assist the patient to develop effective coping strategies by setting specific expectations for behavior, promoting truthful communication to build trust, helping the patient practice appropriate strategies, and giving positive reinforcement when appropriate.

The patient frequently vents feelings of anger. At times the anger may be directed inward because of a sense of guilt, perhaps for causing the fire or even for surviving when loved ones perished. The anger may be directed outward toward those who escaped unharmed or toward those who are now providing care. One way to help the patient handle these emotions is to enlist someone to whom the patient can vent feelings without fear of retaliation. A nurse, social worker, psychiatric liaison nurse, or spiritual advisor or counselor who is not involved in direct care activities may fill this role successfully.

Patients with burn injuries are very dependent on health care team members during the long period of treatment and recovery. However, even when physically unable to contribute much to self-care, they should be included in decisions regarding care and encouraged to assert their individuality in terms of preferences and recognition of their unique identities. As the patient improves in mobility and strength, the nurse works with the patient to set realistic expectations for self-care, including self-feeding, assistance with wound care procedures, exercise, and planning for the future. Many patients respond positively to the use of contractual agreements and other strategies that recognize their independence and their specific role as part of the health care team moving toward the goal of self-care. Consultation with psychiatric/mental health care providers may be helpful to assist the patient in developing effective coping strategies.

Supporting Patient and Family Processes

Family functioning is disrupted with burn injury. One of the nurse's responsibilities is to support the patient and family and to address their spoken and unspoken concerns. Family members need to be instructed about ways that they can support the patient as adaptation to burn trauma occurs.

The family also needs support from the health care team. The burn injury has tremendous psychological, economic, and practical impact on the patient and family. Referrals for social services or psychological counseling should be made as appropriate. This support continues into the rehabilitation phase. Some burn centers offer a peer support program that involves a burn survivor visiting the patient while hospitalized to provide support. Many survivors enjoy the opportunity to help others through this experience.

Patients who experience major burns are commonly sent to burn centers far from home. Because burn injuries are sudden and unexpected, family roles are disrupted. Therefore, both the patient and the family need thorough information about the patient's burn care and expected course of treatment. Patient and family education begins at the initiation of burn management. Barriers to learning are assessed and considered in teaching. The preferred learning styles of both the patient and family are assessed. This information is used to tailor teaching activities. The nurse assesses the ability of the patient and family to grasp and cope with the information. Verbal information is supplemented with videos, models, or printed materials if available. Patient and family education is a priority in the acute and rehabilitation phases.

Nurses must remain sensitive to the possibility of changing family dynamics. It is not unusual for the provider in the family to be the one who is injured. Roles begin to change, which adds more stress to the family. In addition, families are often relocated due to loss of property from the fire. Social services play an integral part in providing support at this time.

Monitoring and Managing Potential Complications

Heart Failure and Pulmonary Edema

The patient is assessed for fluid overload, which may occur as fluid is mobilized from the interstitial compartment back into the intravascular compartment. If the cardiac and renal systems cannot compensate for the excess vascular volume, heart failure and pulmonary edema may result. The patient is assessed for signs of heart failure, including decreased cardiac output, oliguria, jugular vein distention, edema, and the onset of an S_3 or S_4 heart sound. If invasive hemodynamic monitoring is used, increasing central venous, pulmonary artery, and wedge pressures indicate increased fluid volume.

Crackles in the lungs and increased difficulty with respiration may indicate a fluid buildup in the lungs, which is reported promptly to the physician. In the meantime, the patient is positioned comfortably, with the head of the bed raised (if not contraindicated because of other treatments or injuries) to promote lung expansion and gas exchange. Management of this complication includes providing supplemental oxygen, administering IV diuretic agents, carefully assessing the patient's response, and providing vasoactive medications, if indicated.

Sepsis

The signs of early systemic sepsis are subtle and require a high index of suspicion and very close monitoring of changes in the patient's status. Early signs of sepsis may include increased temperature, increased pulse rate, widened pulse pressure, and flushed dry skin in unburned areas. As with many observations of the patient with a burn injury, one needs to look for patterns or trends in the data. (See Chapter 15 for a more detailed discussion of septic shock.)

Wound and blood cultures are performed as prescribed, and results are reported to the physician immediately. The nurse also observes for and reports early signs of sepsis and promptly intervenes, administering prescribed IV fluids and antibiotics to prevent septic shock, a complication with a high mortality rate. Antibiotics must be administered as scheduled to maintain proper blood concentrations. Serum antibiotic levels are monitored for evidence of maximal effectiveness, and the patient is monitored for toxic side effects.

Acute Respiratory Failure and Acute Respiratory Distress Syndrome

The patient's respiratory status is monitored closely for increased difficulty in breathing, change in respiratory pattern, or onset of adventitious (abnormal) sounds. Typically, at this stage, signs and symptoms of injury to the respiratory tract become apparent. Respiratory failure may follow. As described previously, signs of hypoxia (decreased oxygen to the tissues), decreased breath sounds, wheezing, tachypnea, stridor, and sputum tinged with soot (or in some cases containing sloughed tracheal tissue) are among the many possible findings. Patients receiving mechanical ventilation must be assessed for a decrease in tidal volume and lung compliance. The key sign of the onset of ARDS is hypoxemia while receiving 100% oxygen, with decreased lung compliance and significant shunting. The physician should be notified immediately of deteriorating respiratory status.

Medical management of the patient with acute respiratory failure requires intubation and mechanical ventilation (if not already in use). If ARDS has developed, higher oxygen levels, positive end-expiratory pressure, and pressure support are used with mechanical ventilation to promote gas exchange across the alveolar–capillary membrane (see Chapter 25).

Visceral Damage. The nurse must be alert to signs of necrosis of visceral organs due to electrical injury. Tissues affected are usually located between the entrance and exit wounds of the electrical burn. All patients with electrical burns should undergo cardiac monitoring, with dysrhythmias being reported to the physician. Careful attention must also be paid to signs or reports of pain related to deep muscle ischemia. To minimize the severity of complications, visceral ischemia must be detected as early as possible. In the operating room, the burn surgeon may perform **fasciotomies** to relieve the swelling and ischemia in the muscles and fascia and to promote oxygenation of the injured tissues. Because of the deep incisions involved with fasciotomies, the patient must be monitored carefully for signs of excessive blood loss and hypovolemia.

 ### Gerontologic Considerations

In elderly patients, a careful history of preburn medications and preexisting illnesses is essential. Nursing assessment of the elderly patient with burns should include particular attention to pulmonary function, response to fluid resuscitation, and signs of mental confusion or disorientation. Fever may be absent in the presence of complications such as sepsis. Therefore, surveillance for other signs of infection becomes even more important. Nursing care of the elderly patient with burn injuries promotes early mobilization, aggressive pulmonary care, and attention to preventing complications.

REHABILITATION PHASE

Rehabilitation begins immediately after the burn has occurred and often extends for years after injury. The emphasis on early rehabilitation cannot be overestimated. In this final phase of care, the focus becomes rehabilitation, reconstruction, and reintegration of the burn survivor (Sheridan, 2007b). In addition, the burn team focuses on late complications (Table 57-6).

Burn rehabilitation is time-consuming and challenging and is very specific to the severity and location of injury as well as the patient's needs and goals. These goals vary based on phase of care and need to be addressed frequently to ensure constant progress. During hospitalization the goals include maintaining range of motion (ROM), preventing contractures through splinting techniques, decreasing edema, and the preventing skin breakdown through proper positioning. As the acute phase comes to a close, patients become more aware of their injuries and the challenges they face. The goals are functional and aimed at activities of daily living such as ambulation and participation in self-care as well as scar management and returning to work or school (Chart 57-6). Occupational and physical therapists are essential to optimizing patient goals and outcomes (Sheridan, 2007b).

Psychological Support

A patient's outlook, motivation, and support system are important to his or her overall well-being and ability to progress through the rehabilitation phase. There are three basic phases of psychological recovery from a burn injury. During the critical phase, patients often are confused from medication they are taking, but they have an underlying sense of fear, anxiety, and pain. In the acute phase, patients recognize that survival is expected. They have periods of depression due to their awareness of the functional and body image challenges ahead and can recognize all they have lost. Thirty percent of burn patients develop some form of PTSD. The symptoms and psychological responses to traumatic events including PTSD are discussed further in Chapter 7.

The final stage of psychological recovery occurs within 1 to 2 years following discharge. This is an emotional time as the patient and family begin to live with new physical limitations and challenges in relationships. The role of various team members and the support from peer burn survivors during this time cannot be understated (Sheridan, 2007b).

Psychological treatment plans should include a full assessment of these issues and a targeted plan with the appropriate resources to promote the patient's social and vocational reintegration and improved quality of life (Wallis, Renneberg, Ripper, et al., 2006). Burn injuries can have a major impact

Table 57-6 COMPLICATIONS IN REHABILITATION PHASE OF BURN CARE		
Complications	**Contributing Factors**	**Interventions**
Neuropathies, peripheral neuropathies, mononeuropathies, multimononeuropathies, nerve entrapment	Electrical injury, large deep burns, improper positioning, edema, scar tissue	Assess peripheral pulses and sensation (neurovascular checks). Prevent edema and pressure by elevation, positioning, and prevention of constricting dressings. Assess splints for proper fit and application. Consult occupational therapy (OT) and physical therapy (PT) for positioning.
Heterotopic ossification (abnormal formation of bone in response to soft tissue trauma)	Prolonged immobility	Perform gentle range-of-motion exercises.
Hypertrophic scarring	Partial-thickness and full-thickness burns	Keep skin pliable and soft. Apply pressure garments as prescribed. Massage.
Contractures	Partial-thickness and full-thickness burns	Maintain position of joints in alignment. Perform gentle range of motion exercises. Consult OT and PT for exercises and positioning recommendations.
Wound breakdown	Shearing, pressure, inadequate nutrition	Teach patient about importance of good nutrition. Protect wound from pressure and shearing forces.
Gait deviations	Pain, burn wound, donor site, scarring of joints, electrical injury of the brain	Provide adequate pain management. Consult OT and PT. Promote ambulation and mobility training.
Complex regional pain syndrome (previous reflex sympathetic dystrophy [RSD])	Trauma and burns	Provide adequate pain management. Consult OT and PT for exercises. Promote gentle motion of affected extremities.
Joint instability	Burn wound, burn scar and contractures	Maintain joint through appropriate application of splints. Monitor joint pinning if indicated. Consult OT and PT.

on quality of life. Changes in physical activity as well as social and psychological adjustments, such as returning to school and employment status, may be challenging. It is important throughout this process to assess and address the family needs. When one member of a family sustains a major burn injury, the entire family is affected. Separation, feelings of helplessness, loss, and psychological dysfunction may be experienced in varying degrees. Family and friends need support, education, and guidance in assisting the patient to return to their optimal health (Ceranoglu & Stern, 2006).

CHART 57-6 **NURSING RESEARCH PROFILE**
Life After Burn Injury

Moi, A. L. & Gjengedal, E. (2008). Life after burn injury: Striving for regained freedom. *Qualitative Health Research*, *18*(12), 1621–1630.

Purpose

Second only to the patient's survival, the priority of burn care today is optimal quality of life of survivors. The purpose of this study was to identify and describe the meaning of the experience of life after major burn injury.

Design

This qualitative study used a phenomenological perspective to describe and explore the meaning that 14 people who survived severe burn injury attributed to the experience. They were recruited from an outpatient clinic at a burn center in Norway. The researchers intentionally recruited participants of both genders (men = 11, women = 4), across a wide age range (19 to 74, with mean age of 46 years), who had experienced different types of burns (flames = 9, electrical injury = 3, scalding = 2), and received different treatments of their burns. In-depth unstructured interviews were conducted 10 to 35 months after the burn injury; the interviews were audiotaped, transcribed, and analyzed using Giorgi's phenomenological method.

Findings

The major finding was the effort on the part of participants to regain freedom that included reduced or absent bodily or social restrictions and a meaningful life that was the same as or better than before the injury occurred. The experiences described as supporting this goal included (1) facing the extreme and trying to restore order and minimize damage, (2) having a disrupted life history with the loss of memory that occurred during the immediate postburn period, (3) accepting the unchangeable, and (4) changing what could be changed. Some participants indicated that experiencing and surviving their injury gave them a new view of life and made their lives richer.

Nursing Implications

The experience of surviving a severe burn injury is life-altering. The researchers suggest that patients should be given the opportunity to tell their stories and to express their views. Positive feelings and growth on the part of patients should be recognized by burn-care staff, particularly during the later phases of burn care. Patients should be encouraged to share their experiences and views. The researchers also suggest that patients and families be provided with information about what to expect as they move through the phases of burn care.

Abnormal Wound Healing

Partial-thickness wounds involving the epidermis and superficial dermis tend to heal without scarring. However, deep partial-thickness and full-thickness wounds involving the dermis and subcutaneous tissue heal with varying degrees of scarring due to abnormal healing (Arnt, Dover & Alam, 2006).

Normal scarring occurs in a superficial tissue injury and begins forming within 7 to 10 days postinjury and progresses over the next 6 to 12 months. Abnormal scarring occurs after a longer period of wound healing and forms either hypertrophic or keloid scars.

Hypertrophic and Keloid Scars

Hypertrophic scars form within the boundaries of the initial wound and push outward on the perimeter of the wound. They are common in areas over joints and in the younger population. These scars may be hypopigmented or hyperpigmented (Arnt, et al., 2006).

The scar becomes red (because of its hypervascular nature), raised, and hard. A keloid is an irregularly formed scar that extends beyond the margins of the original wound. They are large, nodular, and ropelike, often causing itching and tenderness. They are more common in dark pigmented skin, uncommon in children and the elderly, and have familial tendencies. Scars occur in all forms and arise in different areas, making some more undesirable than others. Therefore, prevention and treatment is individualized to the patient's needs (Arnt, et al., 2006).

Prevention and Treatment of Scars

Treatment modalities that are theoretically based on wound healing and scar formation are used to prevent scar contractures and excess hypertrophic tissue. Compression is introduced early in burn wound treatment. Elastic bandage wraps are used initially to help promote adequate circulation, but they can also be used as the first form of compression followed by elasticized tubular bandage until the patient can be measured for a customized garment (Fig. 57-7). Tools of therapy include pressure, use of topical silicone, scar massage, and steroid injections (Sheridan, 2007b). Application of elastic pressure garments loosens collagen bundles and encourages parallel orientation of the collagen to the skin surface. As pressure continues over time, there is a restructuring of the collagen and a decrease in vascularity and cellularity. Although this therapy is somewhat controversial, pressure has shown to be beneficial in controlling scar formation over time. Garments are worn continuously (ie, 23 hours a day). Many areas of the body are difficult to compress due to the contours or location of the injury. Silicone sheets are helpful for these small troublesome areas and are placed beneath the garment to enhance scar compression. Gentle superficial scar massage can be performed with a moisturizer several times a day. This is helpful in smaller areas and is convenient for the patient. The use of steroid injections into the scar may be helpful in areas of scar development, but they are difficult and painful. Pruritus is a common discomfort in the healed burn wound and can last up to 6 months after healing has occurred. It is treated with moisturizers, massage, oral and topical antihis-

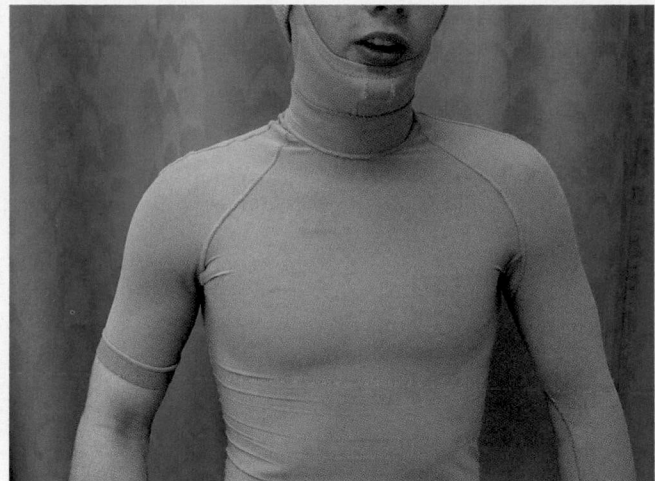

Figure 57-7 Pressure garments. Application of pressure garments helps prevent hypertrophic burn scarring. Used with permission of Jobst Institute, Inc., Toledo, OH.

tamines, and topical compresses or baths. This is a troublesome part of recovery and requires further research (Sheridan, 2007b).

Burn reconstruction is a treatment option after all scars have matured and is discussed within the first few years after injury. This decision requires individualized planning, realistic expectations, and patience. The procedures utilized by the surgeon include contracture release and skin grafting, use of tissue expansion, and skin flaps to cover or reconstruct the defect area (Sheridan, 2007b).

NURSING PROCESS

CARE OF THE PATIENT DURING THE REHABILITATION PHASE

Assessment

The nurse obtains information about the patient's education level, occupation, leisure activities, cultural background, religion, and family interactions early. The patient's self-concept, mental status, emotional response to the injury and hospitalization, level of intellectual functioning, previous hospitalizations, response to pain and pain relief measures, and sleep pattern are also essential components of a comprehensive assessment. Information about the patient's general self-concept, self-esteem, and coping strategies in the past are valuable in addressing emotional needs.

Ongoing physical assessments related to rehabilitation goals include range of motion of affected joints, functional abilities in activities of daily living, early signs of skin breakdown from splints or positioning devices, evidence of neuropathies (neurologic damage), activity tolerance, and quality or condition of healing skin. The patient's participation in care and ability to demonstrate self-care in such areas as ambulation, eating, wound cleaning, and applying pressure wraps are documented on a regular basis. In addition to these assessment parameters, specific complications and treatments require additional specific assessments; for example, the patient undergoing primary excision requires postoperative assessment.

Diagnosis

Nursing Diagnoses

Based on the assessment data, priority nursing diagnoses in the long-term rehabilitation phase of burn care may include the following:

- Activity intolerance related to pain on exercise, limited joint mobility, muscle wasting, and limited endurance
- Disturbed body image related to altered physical appearance and self-concept
- Deficient knowledge about postdischarge home care and recovery needs

Collaborative Problems/Potential Complications

Based on the assessment data, potential complications that may develop in the rehabilitation phase include:

- Contractures
- Inadequate psychological adaptation to burn injury

Planning and Goals

The major goals for the patient include increased participation in activities of daily living; increased understanding of the injury, treatment, and planned follow-up care; adaptation and adjustment to alterations in body image, self-concept, and lifestyle; and absence of complications.

Nursing Interventions

Promoting Activity Tolerance

Nursing interventions that must be carried out according to a strict regimen and the pain that accompanies movement take their toll on the patient. The patient may become confused and disoriented and lack the energy or motivation to participate optimally in care. The nurse must schedule care in such a way that the patient has periods of uninterrupted sleep. A good time for planned patient rest is after the stress of dressing changes and exercise, while pain interventions and sedatives are still effective. This plan must be communicated to family members and other care providers.

The patient may have insomnia related to frequent nightmares about the burn injury or to other fears and anxieties about the outcome of the injury. The nurse listens to and reassures the patient and administers hypnotic agents, as prescribed, to promote sleep.

Reducing metabolic stress by relieving pain, preventing chilling or fever, and promoting the physical integrity of all body systems help the patient conserve energy for therapeutic activities and wound healing.

The nurse incorporates physical therapy exercises in the patient's care to prevent muscle atrophy and to maintain the mobility required for daily activities. The patient's activity tolerance, strength, and endurance gradually increase if activity occurs over increasingly longer periods. Fatigue, fever, and pain tolerance are monitored and used to determine the amount of activity to be encouraged on a daily basis. Activities such as family visits and recreational or play therapy (eg, video games, radio, television) can provide diversion, improve the patient's outlook, and increase tolerance for physical activity. In elderly patients and those with chronic illnesses and disabilities, rehabilitation must take into account preexisting functional abilities and limitations.

Improving Body Image and Self-Concept

Patients who have survived burn injuries frequently suffer profound losses. These include not only a loss of body image due to disfigurement but also losses of personal property, homes, loved ones, and ability to work. They lack the benefit of anticipatory grief often seen in a patient who is approaching surgery or dealing with the terminal illness of a loved one.

As care progresses, the patient who is recovering from burns becomes aware of daily improvement and begins to exhibit basic concerns: Will I be disfigured or be disabled? How long will I be in the hospital? What about my job and family? Will I ever be independent again? How can I pay for my care? Was my burn the result of my carelessness?

As the patient expresses such concerns, the nurse must take time to listen and to provide realistic support. The nurse can refer the patient to a support group, such as those usually available at regional burn centers or through organizations such as the Phoenix Society (see Resources at the end of the chapter). Through participation in such groups, the patient will meet others with similar experiences and learn coping strategies to help him or her deal with losses. Interaction with other burn survivors allows the patient to see that adaptation to the burn injury is possible. If a support group is not available, visits from other survivors of burn injuries can be helpful to the patient coping with such a traumatic injury.

A major responsibility of the nurse is to constantly assess the patient's psychosocial reactions. Questions to consider include the following: What are the patient's fears and concerns? Does the patient fear loss of control of care, independence, or sanity itself? Is the patient afraid of rejection by family and loved ones? Does he or she fear being unable to cope with pain or physical appearance? Does the patient have concerns about sexuality, including sexual function? Being aware of these anxieties and understanding the basis of the patient's fears enable the nurse to provide support and to cooperate with other members of the health care team in developing a plan to help the patient deal with these feelings. Journaling can be helpful for patients to express themselves and track their progress with psychological healing.

When caring for a patient with a burn injury, the nurse needs to be aware that there are prejudices and misunderstandings in society about those who are viewed as different. Opportunities and accommodations available to others are often denied those who are disfigured. These include social participation, employment, prestige, various roles, and status. The health care team must actively promote a healthy body image and self-concept in patients with burn injuries so that they can accept or challenge others' perceptions of those who are disfigured or disabled. Survivors themselves must show others who they are, how they function, and how they want to be treated.

The nurse can help patients practice their responses to people who may stare or inquire about their injury once they are discharged from the hospital. The nurse can help patients build self-esteem by recognizing their uniqueness—for example, with small gestures such as providing a birthday cake, combing the patient's hair before visiting hours, giving information about the availability of a cosmetician to enhance appearance, and teaching the patient ways to direct attention away from a disfigured body to the self within. Consultants such as psychologists, social workers, vocational counselors, and teachers are valuable participants in assisting burn patients to regain their self-esteem.

Monitoring and Managing Potential Complications

CONTRACTURES. With early and aggressive physical and occupational therapy, contractures are rarely a long-term complication. However, surgical intervention is indicated if a full range of motion in the burn patient is not achieved. (See Chapter 11 for a discussion of prevention of contractures.)

IMPAIRED PSYCHOLOGICAL ADAPTATION TO THE BURN INJURY. Some patients, particularly those with limited coping skills or psychological function or a history of psychiatric problems before the burn injury, may not achieve adequate psychological adaptation to the burn injury. Psychological counseling or psychiatric referral may be made to assess the patient's emotional status, to help the patient develop coping skills, and to intervene if major psychological issues or ineffective coping is identified.

Promoting Home and Community-Based Care

TEACHING PATIENTS SELF-CARE. As the inpatient phase of recovery becomes shorter, the focus of rehabilitative interventions is directed toward outpatient care, home care, or care in a rehabilitation center. Throughout the phases of burn care, efforts are made to prepare the patient and family for the care that will continue at home. They are instructed about the measures and procedures that they will need to perform. For example, patients commonly have small areas of clean, open wounds that are healing slowly. They are instructed to wash these areas daily with mild soap and water and to apply the prescribed topical agent or dressing.

In addition to instructions about wound care, patients and families require careful written and verbal instructions about pain management, nutrition, and prevention of complications. Information about specific exercises and use of pressure garments and splints is reviewed with both the patient and the family, and written instructions are provided for their use at home. The patient and family are taught to recognize abnormal signs and report them to the physician. The patient and family are assisted in planning for the patient's continued care by identifying and acquiring supplies and equipment that are needed at home (Chart 57-7).

CONTINUING CARE. Follow-up care after discharge by the multidisciplinary team is necessary. Patients who receive care in a burn center usually return to the burn clinic or center periodically for evaluation by the burn team, modification of home care instructions, and planning for reconstructive surgery. Other patients receive ongoing care from the burn surgeon who cared for them during the acute phase of their management. Still other patients require the services of a rehabilitation center and may be transferred to such a center for aggressive rehabilitation before going home. Many patients require outpatient physical or occupational therapy, often several times weekly. It is often the nurse who is responsible for coordinating all aspects of care and ensuring that the patient's needs are met. Such coordination is an important aspect of assisting the patient to achieve independence.

Patients who return home after a severe burn injury, those who cannot manage their own burn care, and those with inadequate support systems need referral for home care. During visits to the patient at home, the home care nurse assesses the patient's physical and psychological status as well as the adequacy of the home setting for safe and adequate care. The nurse monitors the patient's progress and adherence to the plan of care and notes any problems that interfere with the patient's ability to carry out the care. During the visit, the nurse assists the patient and family with wound care and exercises. Patients with severe or persistent depression or difficulty adjusting to changes in their social or occupational roles are identified and referred to the burn team for possible referral to a psychologist, psychiatrist, or vocational counselor.

The burn team or home care nurse identifies community resources that may be helpful for the patient and family. Several burn patient support groups and other organizations throughout the United States offer services for burn survivors. They provide contact with caring people (often people who have themselves recovered from burn injuries) who can visit the patient in the hospital or home or telephone the patient and family periodically to provide support and counseling about skin care, cosmetics, and problems related to psychosocial adjustment. Such organizations, and many regional burn centers, sponsor group meetings and social functions at which outpatients are welcome. Some also provide reentry programs or burn retreats and are active in burn prevention activities.

Evaluation

Expected Patient Outcomes

Expected patient outcomes may include the following:

1. Demonstrates activity tolerance required for desired daily activities
   a. Obtains adequate sleep daily
   b. Reports absence of nightmares or sleep disturbances
   c. Shows gradually increasing tolerance and endurance in physical activities
   d. Can concentrate during conversations
   e. Has energy available to sustain desired daily activities
2. Adapts to altered body image
   a. Verbalizes accurate description of alterations in body image and accepts physical appearance
   b. Demonstrates interest in resources that may improve body appearance and function
   c. Uses cosmetics, wigs, and prostheses as desired to achieve acceptable appearance
   d. Socializes with significant others, peers, and usual social group

CHART 57-7	HOME CARE CHECKLIST *The Patient With a Burn Injury*		
At the completion of the home care instruction, the patient or caregiver will be able to:		**PATIENT**	**CAREGIVER**

Mental Health

Identify strategies to promote own mental health; for example:

	PATIENT	CAREGIVER
• Remember that changes in lifestyle take time.	✔	✔
• Resume previous interests and activities gradually.	✔	
• Take one day at a time to regain physical and mental strength.	✔	
• Be aware of own feelings and fears and discuss them with selected others.	✔	✔
• Expect concerns, frustrations, and depression about changes in appearance.	✔	✔
• Be honest with self, family, and friends about needs, hopes, and fears.	✔	✔
• Realize that emotional adjustment to the burn injury will occur with time.	✔	✔

Burn Skin Precautions and Wound Care

Identify the following skin precautions and wound care:

	PATIENT	CAREGIVER
• Wear sun block with the highest SPF possible to protect burned skin from the sun.	✔	
• Avoid further trauma to burned skin; leave unbroken blisters that may form.	✔	✔
• Lubricate healed burned skin with mild lotion (as prescribed); avoid scratching.	✔	
• Wear wide-brimmed hats if face has been burned to protect the area from the sun.	✔	
• Use only mild soap and lotion (ie, products without perfume) on burned areas.	✔	✔

Exercise

Describe the following guidelines for exercise:

	PATIENT	CAREGIVER
• Do as much for self as possible.	✔	
• Adhere to the exercise regimen given by the therapist.	✔	
• Participate in exercise every day, several times a day, even when "not feeling like it."	✔	

Nutrition

Identify the following guidelines for nutrition:

	PATIENT	CAREGIVER
• Eat a diet high in calories and protein.	✔	
• Drink adequate volume of fluids to prevent constipation associated with use of analgesic medications.	✔	

Pain Management

Describe the following steps for managing pain:

	PATIENT	CAREGIVER
• Avoid situations that require alertness (analgesic agents may produce drowsiness).	✔	
• Take analgesic medication as prescribed (30 minutes before painful procedures such as dressing changes).	✔	
• Use relaxation and distraction to relieve pain and discomfort.	✔	

Thermoregulation

Identify strategies to compensate for inability to regulate body temperature:

	PATIENT	CAREGIVER
• Dress to accommodate cold and hot weather or environment.	✔	
• Avoid extremes of temperature.	✔	

CHART 57-7	HOME CARE CHECKLIST *The Patient With a Burn Injury (Continued)*		
		PATIENT	**CAREGIVER**
Clothing Considerations			
State the following strategies in selection of clothing to wear:			
• Avoid tight clothing over burned areas.		✔	
• Select white cotton, loose-fitting clothing so that dyes in colored clothes do not irritate healing skin.		✔	
• Wear clothing and gloves to protect healing skin from unnecessary bruises, bumps, and scratches.		✔	
Management of Burn Scar			
Describe the following strategies to manage burn scar:			
• Massage and stretch skin to maintain/increase its elasticity.		✔	✔
• Use lotion for massage as recommended by therapist.		✔	✔
• Wear compression garments 23 hours a day.		✔	
Resumption of Sexual Relations			
Identify the following guidelines regarding resumption of sexual relationships:			
• Realize that resumption of sexual relationships is the rule rather than the exception.		✔	✔
• Expect sensitivity of and around the genital area for several months if these areas were burned.		✔	
• Resume sexual activity slowly; endurance will increase with time.		✔	

Adapted with permission from Orlando Regional Medical Center Burn Unit's Personal Guide to Burn Care.

e. Seeks and achieves return to role in family, school, and community as a contributing member
3. Demonstrates knowledge of required self-care and follow-up care
   a. Describes surgical procedures and treatments accurately
   b. Verbalizes detailed plan for follow-up care
   c. Demonstrates ability to perform wound care and prescribed exercises
   d. Returns for follow-up appointments as scheduled
   e. Identifies resource people and agencies to contact for specific problems
4. Exhibits no complications
   a. Demonstrates full range of motion
   b. Shows no signs of withdrawal or depression
   c. Displays no psychotic behaviors

Outpatient Burn Care

Increasing numbers of patients receive treatment of burns in outpatient settings in an effort to coordinate specific burn care needs and to decrease healthcare costs and length of hospitalization. The increased availability of outpatient surgery and access to expert burn care in outpatient settings make this option possible for the treatment of minor burn care as well as a destination for the discharged burn patient.

The goals for treatment in an outpatient setting may include burn wound management, pain management, scar and reconstructive care, and rehabilitation. However, a number of factors must be considered in determining if outpatient care is appropriate for the patient: age, past medical history, the extent and depth of the burn, location of the burn wounds, the availability of family support systems and community resources, the patient's compliance and the distance from home, and availability of transportation from home to the outpatient setting.

The frequency of follow-up visits is individualized and based on these factors. The initial outpatient visit for a discharged burn patient is usually scheduled within 2 or 3 days after hospital discharge and then biweekly until there is evidence of a successful outcome. After healing has occurred, appointments are monthly and eventually every 4 to 6 weeks for continued assessment of pain, physical limitations, and scar maturation. Patient and family education is very important and should include verbal and written instructions as well as return demonstration of the burn or scar care required. These include the wound treatment, pain management, treatment for itching, provision of adequate nutrition, and promotion of exercise and rest. Instruction is also provided about the signs and symptoms of infection that should be reported to the burn team. The importance of notifying the outpatient setting about early complications and of keeping follow-up appointments is emphasized to the patient and family. Physical therapy and occupational therapy are often provided in the outpatient burn setting. The rehabilitation goals are to increase range of motion and to strengthen and build the patient's endurance. This is accomplished with a specific plan of care and includes routine visits for up to 2 years following the injury. Adaptation to lifestyle changes and emotional status should be assessed during the outpatient visits and proper referrals made for counseling services. These assessments are difficult to recognize due to the infrequent nature of the visits, and, therefore, it is helpful to incorporate family response and interactions into the assessment. The health care team must also be alert to issues of substance abuse, safety concerns, suicidal thoughts, depression, and PTSD.

CRITICAL THINKING EXERCISES

1 A 35-year-old woman was scalded in the bathtub, where she sustained 40% full-thickness burns to her lower legs, right arm, and back. It is not known how long the woman was in the tub. She apparently had a seizure while showering and fell onto the hot water faucet. On admission to the emergency department, the woman's temperature is 35.5°C (94°F) and her weight is 111 lb (50 kg). She has diabetes as well as a history of uncontrolled seizure activity. What are the priorities in her medical and nursing care during the emergent phase of burn care? What assessment parameters would you monitor closely?

2 An 82-year-old man who is wheelchair dependent and has a history of chronic obstructive pulmonary disease was smoking while using oxygen at home. He sustained superficial partial-thickness burns to his face, including his nose, lips, and chin. This is his second admission for the same type of injury in less than 1 year. His pulse oximetry is 91% and his vital signs are stable. Before he is intubated in the emergency room, he asks for a cigarette and states he wants to go home. What are this patient's immediate care needs? What referrals for inpatient services should be arranged before his discharge? What important factors need to be addressed as part of his discharge plan?

3 A 19-year-old, 233 lb (105 kg) man sustained partial-thickness and full-thickness burn injuries to his face, neck, and both hands and forearms circumferentially that occurred while he was working on his car while smoking a cigarette. Using the rule of nines, estimate the percentage of TBSA burned and estimate his fluid resuscitation needs. What immediate concerns would you have for his airway? How would you handle the care of the circumferential injury of his forearms?

EBP **4** A 52-year-old man suffered an electrical burn when he touched a high-voltage wire inside a closet while on the job. There was an explosion and he was thrown backward. The current entered his right hand and exited his left knee, leaving a large deficit in his knee. He also sustained a 45% TBSA flame burn when his clothing ignited. When asked to rate the intensity of his pain, he reports a "10" on a 10-point pain scale. What immediate concerns would

you have related to his cardiopulmonary and neurological status? What strategies would you use to relieve his pain? What is the evidence that supports the pain relief strategies that you identified and the strength of that evidence?

5 A 28-year-old woman involved in a house fire is brought to the emergency department by her boyfriend. There is no information from the scene. She is complaining of severe pain in her neck and back. She sustained a full-thickness burn of her lower extremities and her lower back. She is asking about the status of her two children who perished in the fire. What would you be concerned about related to her complaints that requires action from the burn team? What are the psychological and emotional issues that need to be addressed? Who might you consult to assist in the psychological management of this patient?

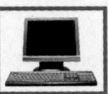 The Smeltzer suite offers these additional resources to enhance learning and facilitate understanding of this chapter:
- thePoint online resource, thepoint.lww.com/Smeltzer12E
- Student CD-ROM included with the book
- *Study Guide to Accompany Brunner & Suddarth's Textbook of Medical-Surgical Nursing*
- *Handbook for Brunner & Suddarth's Textbook of Medical-Surgical Nursing*

REFERENCES AND SELECTED READINGS

Asterisk indicates nursing research.

Books

Arnt, K., Dover, J. & Alam, M. (2006). *Procedures in cosmetic dermatology*. Philadelphia: Elsevier Saunders.

Appleby, T. (2005). Burns. In Morton, P. G., Fontaine, D. K., Hudak, C. M., et al. *Critical care nursing: A holistic approach*. Philadelphia: Lippincott Williams & Wilkins.

Dudek, S. G. (2006). *Nutrition essentials for nursing practice* (5th ed.). Philadelphia: Lippincott Williams & Wilkins.

Hall, J. R. (2005). *Children playing with fire*. Quincy, MA: National Fire Protection Association.

Journals and Electronic Sources

Acton, A. R., Mounsey, E. & Gilyard, C. (2007). The burn survivor perspective. *Journal of Burn Care & Research, 28*(4), 615–620.

American Burn Association. (2007). Burn incidence and treatment in the U.S.: 2007 fact sheet. www.ameriburn.org/resources_factsheet.php

Arnoldo, B., Klein, M. & Gibran, N. (2006). Practice guidelines for the management of electrical injuries. *Journal of Burn Care & Research, 27*(4), 439–447.

Atiyeh, B. S., Gunn, S. W. & Hayek, S. N. (2005). State of the art in burn treatment. *World Journal of Surgery, 29*(2), 131–148.

Barillo, D. J. (2009). Diagnosis and treatment of cyanide toxicity. *Journal of Burn Care & Research, 30*(1), 148–152

Boyce, S. T., Greenhalgh, D. G., Palmieri, T. L., et al. (2006). Autologous cultured skin substitutes reduce requirements for split-thickness skin autograft in treatment of excised, full-thickness burns. *Journal of Burn Care & Research, 27*(2), S59.

Burke, J. F. (2005). Burn treatment's evolution in the 20th century. *Journal of the American College of Surgeons, 200*(2), 152–153.

Caruso, D. M., Foster, K. N, Blome-Eberwein, S. A., et al. (2006). Randomized clinical study of hydrofiber dressing with silver or silver sulfadiazine in the management of partial-thickness burns. *Journal of Burn Care & Research, 27*(3), 298–309.

Centers for Disease Control and Prevention (CDC), National Center for Injury Prevention and Control. (2008). Fire deaths and injuries: Fact sheet. www.cdc.gov/ncipc/factsheets/fire.htm

Ceranoglu, T. A. & Stern, T. A. (2006). Posttraumatic stress disorder in the child of an adult burn victim: A case report and review of the literature. *Journal of Intensive Care Medicine, 21*(5), 316–319.

Cone, J. B. (2005). What's new in general surgery: Burns and metabolism. *Journal of the American College of Surgeons, 200*(4), 607–615.

Connor-Ballard, P. A. (2009a). Understanding and managing burn pain: Part 1. *American Journal of Nursing, 109*(4), 48–56.

Connor-Ballard, P. A. (2009b). Understanding and managing burn pain: Part 2. *American Journal of Nursing, 109*(5), 54–62.

Demling, R. H. (2005a). The burn edema process: Current concepts. *Journal of Burn Care and Rehabilitation, 26*(3), 207–228.

Demling, R. H. (2005b). The incidence and impact of pre-existing protein energy malnutrition on outcomes in the elderly burn patient population. *Journal of Burn Care and Rehabilitation, 26*(1), 94–100.

De-Souza, D. A. & Greene, L. J. (2005). Intestinal permeability and systemic infection in critically ill patients: Effect of glutamine. *Critical Care Medicine, 33*(5), 1125–1135.

DuBose, C., Groher, M. G., Mann, G. C., et al. (2005). Pattern of dysphasia recovery after thermal burn injury. *Journal of Burn Care and Rehabilitation, 26*(3), 233–237.

Edelman, D. A., White, M. T., Tyburski, J. G., et al. (2006). Factors affecting prognosis of inhalation injury. *Journal of Burn Care & Research, 27*(6), 848–853.

Faucher, L. & Furukawa, K. (2006). Practice guidelines for the management of pain. *Journal of Burn Care & Research, 27*(5), 659–668.

Faucher, L. D. & Conlon, K. M. (2007). Practice guidelines for deep venous thrombosis prophylaxis in burns. *Journal of Burn Care & Research, 28*(8), 661–663.

Fauerbach, J. A., Lezotte, D., Hills, R. A., et al. (2005). Burden of burn: A norm-based inquiry into the influence of burn size and distress on recovery of physical and psychosocial function. *Journal of Burn Care and Rehabilitation, 26*(1), 21–32.

Fauerbach, J. A., Pruzinsky, T. & Saxe, G. N. (2007). Psychological health and function after burn injury: Setting research priorities. *Journal of Burn Care & Research, 28*(4), 587–592.

Flynn, M. B. (2004). Nutritional support for the burn-injured patient. *Critical Care Nursing Clinics of North America, 16*(1), 139–144.

*Fry, C., Edelman, L. S. & Cochran, A. (2009). Response to a nursing-driven protocol for sedation and analgesia in a burn-trauma ICU. *Journal of Burn Care & Research, 30*(1), 112–118.

Gibran, N. S. (2006). Practice guidelines for burn care, 2006. *Journal of Burn Care & Research, 27*(4), 437–438.

Gosain, A. & Gamelli, R. (2005a). Role of the gastrointestinal tract in burn sepsis. *Journal of Burn Care and Rehabilitation, 26*(1), 85–91.

Gosain, A. & Gamelli, R. (2005b). A primer in cytokines. *Journal of Burn Care and Rehabilitation, 26*(1), 7–12.

Greenhalgh, D. G. (2007). Burn resuscitation. *Journal of Burn Care & Research, 28*(4), 1–10.

Guidelines for the operation of burn centers. Special report. (2007). *Journal of Burn Care & Research, 28*(1), 134–141.

Hansen, M., Gauld, M., Wathen, C., et al. (2008). Nonpharmacological interventions for acute wound care distress in pediatric patients with a burn injury. *Journal of Burn Care & Research, 29*(5), 730–741.

Heggers, J., Goodheart, R., Washington, J., et al. (2005). Therapeutic efficacy of three silver dressings in an infected animal model. *Journal of Burn Care and Rehabilitation, 26*(1), 53–56.

Hershberger, R. C., Hunt, J. L., Arnoldo, B. D., et al. (2007). Abdominal compartment syndrome in the severely burned patient. *Journal of Burn Care & Research, 28*(5), 708–714.

Hodle, A. E., Richter, K. P. & Thompson, R. M. (2006). Infection control practices in U.S. burn units. *Journal of Burn Care & Research, 27*(2), 142–151.

Jeschke, M. G., Chinkes, D. L., Finnerty, C. C., et al. (2008). Pathophysiologic response to severe burn injury. *Annals of Surgery, 248*(3), 387–401.

Kealey, G. P. (2009). Carbon monoxide toxicity. *Journal of Burn Care & Research, 30*(1), 146–147.

Kildal, M., Willebrand, M., Andersson, G., et al. (2004). Personality characteristics and perceived health problems after burn injury. *Journal of Burn Care and Rehabilitation, 25*(3), 228–235.

Masters, B. & Wood, F. (2008). Nutrition support in burns—Is there consistency in practice? *Journal of Burn Care & Research, 29*(4), 561–571.

McCall, J. & Cahill, T. (2005). Respiratory care of the burn patient. *Journal of Burn Care and Rehabilitation, 26*(3), 200–206.

Miller, S. F., Bessey, P., Lentz, C. W., et al. (2008). National Burn Repository 2007 report: A synopsis of the 2007 call for data. *Journal of Burn Care & Research, 29*(6), 862–870,

Palmieri, T. L. (2007). Inhalation injuries: Research progress and needs. *Journal of Burn Care & Research, 28*(4), 549–554.

Palmieri, T. L. (2009). Long term outcomes after inhalation injury. *Journal of Burn Care & Research, 30*(1), 201–203.

Palmieri, T. L. & Klein, M. B. (2007). Burn research state of the science: Introduction. *Journal of Burn Care & Research, 28*(4), 544–545.

Pereira, C., Murphy, K. & Herndon, D. (2005). Altering metabolism. *Journal of Burn Care and Rehabilitation, 26*(3), 194–199.

Pham, T. N. & Gibran, N. S. (2007). Thermal and electrical injuries. *Surgical Clinics of North America, 87*(1), 1–18.

Pham, T. N., Cancio, L. C. & Gibran, N. S. (2008). American Burn Association practice guidelines burn shock resuscitation. *Journal of Burn Care & Research, 29*(1), 257–266.

Pitts, S. R., Niska, R. W., Xu, J., et al. (2008). National Hospital Ambulatory Medical Care Survey: 2006 emergency department summary. *National Health Statistics Reports, 7.* Hyattsville, MD: National Center for Health Statistics.

Shankar, R., Melstrom, K. A. Jr. & Gamelli, R. L. (2007). Inflammation and sepsis: Past, present, and the future. *Journal of Burn Care & Research, 28*(4), 566–571.

Sheridan, R. L. (2007a). Burns at the extremes of age. *Journal of Burn Care and Rehabilitation, 28*(4), 580–585.

Sheridan, R. L. (2007b). Burn rehabilitation. *eMedicine.* http://emedicine.medscape.com/article/318436-overview

Shukla, P. C. & Sheridan, R. L. (2008). Initial evaluation and management of the burn patient. *eMedicine.* http://emedicine.medscape.com/article/435402-overview

Snedeker, A. A., Yowler, C. J. & Fratianne, R. B. (2006). The impact of guided imagery on pain and anxiety levels of burn patients. *Journal of Burn Care & Research, 27*(2), 151.

Van Twillert, B., Bremer, M. & Faber, A. W. (2007). Computer generated virtual reality to control pain and anxiety in pediatric and adult burn patients. *Journal of Burn Care & Research, 28*(5), 694–702.

Wahl, W. L., Ahrns, K. S., Brandt, M. M., et al. (2005). Bronchoalveolar lavage in diagnosis of ventilator-associated pneumonia in patients with burns. *Journal of Burn Care & Research, 26*(1), 57–61.

Wallis, H., Renneberg, B., Ripper, S., et al. (2006). Emotional distress and psychosocial resources in patients recovering from severe burn injury. *Journal of Burn Care & Research, 27*(5), 734–741.

*Wikehult, B., Hedlund, M., Marsenic, M., et al. (2008). Evaluation of negative emotional care experiences in burn care. *Journal of Clinical Nursing, 17*(14), 1923–1929.

Williams, C. (2008). Fluid resuscitation in burn patients 2: Nursing care. *Nursing Times, 104*(15), 24–25.

Wolfe, S. (2007). Nutrition and metabolism in burns: State of the science, 2007. *Journal of Burn Care & Research, 28*(4), 572–576.

Woodson, L. C. (2009). Diagnosis and grading of inhalation injury. *Journal of Burn Care & Research, 28*(4), 143–145.

RESOURCES

Alisa Ann Ruch Burn Foundation, www.aarbf.org
American Burn Association, www.ameriburn.org
American Red Cross, www.redcross.org
Burn Children Recovery Foundation, www.burnchildrenrecovery.org
Burn Foundation, www.burnfoundation.org/
Burn Institute, www.burninstitute.org
Burn Prevention, www.burnprevention.org
Chemical Educational Foundation, www.chemed.org
Firefighters Pacific Burn Institute, www.ffburn.org
Integra Life Sciences Corporation, www.integra-ls.com
International Association of Fire Fighters Burn Foundation, www.iaff.org
International Medical Education Foundation. www.burnsurgery.org
International Society for Burn Injuries, www.worldburn.org
National Burn Center Reporting System Report Form, U.S. Consumer Product Safety Commission, www.cpsc.gov/burnctr.html
National Fire Protection Association Fire, www.nfpa.org
Phoenix Society for Burn Survivors, Inc., www.phoenix-society.org
United States Fire Administration, www.usfa.dh.gov

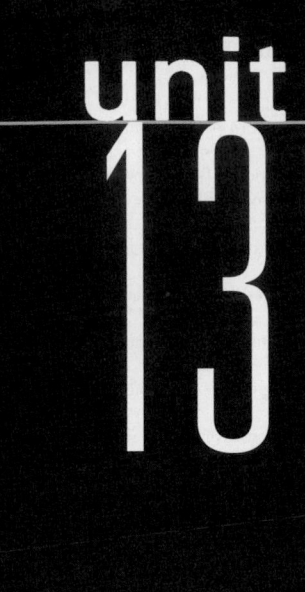

unit 13

Sensorineural Function

Case Study • Applying Concepts From NANDA, NIC, and NOC

A Patient With Impaired Vision and Decreased Attention to One Side of the Body

Mr. Martin is a 60-year-old man who has had several strokes. Ophthalmologic testing reveals that he has homonymous hemianopsia of the left visual field and visual spatial neglect; as a result, he has limited vision in the left visual fields of both eyes. He has difficulty in many areas, such as bumping into objects and ignoring the left side of his body.

Visit thePoint to view a concept map that illustrates the relationships that exist between the nursing diagnoses, interventions, and outcomes for the patient's clinical problems.

Nursing Classifications and Languages

NANDA NURSING DIAGNOSES	NIC NURSING INTERVENTIONS	NOC NURSING OUTCOMES
		Return to functional baseline status, stabilization of, or improvement in:
DISTURBED SENSORY PERCEPTION: VISUAL—Change in the amount or patterning of incoming stimuli accompanied by a diminished, exaggerated, distorted, or impaired response to such stimuli	**COMMUNICATION ENHANCEMENT: VISUAL DEFICIT**—Assistance in accepting and learning alternative methods for living with diminished vision	**VISION COMPENSATION BEHAVIOR**—Personal actions to compensate for visual impairment
UNILATERAL NEGLECT—Lack of awareness and attention to one side of the body	**UNILATERAL NEGLECT MANAGEMENT**—Protecting and safely reintegrating the affected part of the body while helping the patient adapt to disturbed perceptual abilities	**SAFE HOME ENVIRONMENT**—Physical arrangements to minimize environmental factors that might cause physical harm or injury in the home
RISK FOR INJURY—At risk for injury as a result of environmental conditions interacting with the individual's adaptive and defensive resources	**POSITIONING**—Deliberative placement of the patient or a body part to promote physiological and/or psychological well-being	**PHYSICAL INJURY SEVERITY**—Severity of injuries from trauma

Bulechek, G. M., Butcher, H. K., & Dochterman, J. M. (2008). *Nursing interventions classification (NIC)* (5th ed.). St. Louis: Mosby.
Johnson, M., Bulechek, G., Butcher, H. K., et al. (2006). *NANDA, NOC, and NIC linkages* (2nd ed.). St. Louis: Mosby.
Moorhead, S., Johnson, M., Mass, M. L., et al. (2008). *Nursing outcomes classification (NOC)* (4th ed.). St. Louis: Mosby.
NANDA International. (2007). *Nursing diagnoses: Definitions & classification 2007–2008*. Philadelphia: North American Nursing Diagnosis Association.

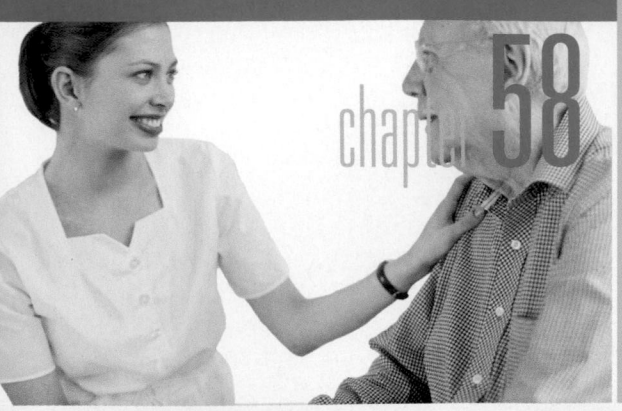

chapter 58

Assessment and Management of Patients With Eye and Vision Disorders

LEARNING OBJECTIVES

On completion of this chapter, the learner will be able to:

1 Identify significant eye structures and describe their functions.

2 Identify diagnostic tests for assessment of vision and evaluation of visual disabilities.

3 Discuss clinical features, diagnostic assessment and examinations, medical or surgical management, and nursing management of ocular disorders.

4 Describe therapeutic effects of ophthalmic medications.

5 Define low vision and blindness and differentiate between functional and visual impairment.

6 List and describe assessment and management strategies for low vision.

7 Demonstrate orientation and mobility techniques for patients with low vision in a hospital setting.

8 Demonstrate installation of eye drops and ointment.

9 Discuss general discharge instructions for patients after ocular surgery.

10 Discuss strategies for patient safety in ophthalmology.

GLOSSARY

accommodation: process by which the eye adjusts for near distance (eg, reading) by changing the curvature of the lens to focus a clear image on the retina

anterior chamber: space in the eye bordered anteriorly by the cornea and posteriorly by the iris and pupil

aphakia: absence of the natural lens

aqueous humor: watery fluid that fills the anterior and posterior chambers of the eye

astigmatism: refractive error in which light rays are spread over a diffuse area rather than sharply focused on the retina, a condition caused by differences in the curvature of the cornea and lens

binocular vision: normal ability of both eyes to focus on one object and fuse the two images into one

blindness: inability to see, usually defined as corrected visual acuity of 20/400 or less, or a visual field of no more than 20 degrees in the better eye

bullous keratopathy: corneal edema with painful blisters in the epithelium due to excessive corneal hydration

chemosis: edema of the conjunctiva

cones: retinal photoreceptor cells essential for visual acuity and color discrimination

GLOSSARY *(Continued)*

diplopia: seeing one object as two; double vision

emmetropia: absence of refractive error

enucleation: complete removal of the eyeball and part of the optic nerve

evisceration: removal of the intraocular contents through a corneal or scleral incision; the optic nerve, sclera, extraocular muscles, and sometimes, the cornea are left intact

exenteration: surgical removal of the entire contents of the orbit, including the eyeball and lids

hyperemia: "red eye" resulting from dilation of the vasculature of the conjunctiva

hyperopia: farsightedness; a refractive error in which the focus of light rays from a distant object is behind the retina

hyphema: blood in the anterior chamber

hypopyon: collection of inflammatory cells that has the appearance of a pale layer in the inferior anterior chamber of the eye

injection: congestion of blood vessels

keratoconus: cone-shaped deformity of the cornea

limbus: junction of the cornea and sclera

miotics: medications that cause pupillary constriction

mydriatics: medications that cause pupillary dilation

myopia: nearsightedness; a refractive error in which the focus of light rays from a distant object is anterior to the retina

neovascularization: growth of abnormal new blood vessels

nystagmus: involuntary oscillation of the eyeball

papilledema: swelling of the optic disc due to increased intracranial pressure

photophobia: ocular pain on exposure to light

posterior chamber: space between the iris and vitreous

proptosis: downward displacement of the eyeball resulting from an inflammatory condition of the orbit or a mass within the orbital cavity

ptosis: drooping eyelid

refraction: determination of the refractive errors of the eye and correction by lenses

rods: retinal photoreceptor cells essential for bright and dim light

scotomas: blind or partially blind areas in the visual field

strabismus: a condition in which there is deviation from perfect ocular alignment

sympathetic ophthalmia: an inflammatory condition created in the fellow eye by the affected eye (without useful vision); the condition may become chronic and result in blindness (of the fellow eye)

trachoma: a bilateral chronic follicular conjunctivitis of childhood that leads to blindness during adulthood, if left untreated

vitreous humor: gelatinous material (transparent and colorless) that fills the eyeball behind the lens

Note: Common abbreviations related to vision and eye health are OD (oculus dexter, right eye), OS (oculus sinister, left eye), and OU (oculus uterque, both eyes).

The ability to see the world clearly can easily be taken for granted. The eye is a sensitive, highly specialized sense organ subject to various disorders, many of which lead to impaired vision. Impaired vision may affect a person's independence in self-care, work and lifestyle choices, sense of self-esteem, safety, ability to interact with society and the environment, and overall quality of life. Many of the leading causes of visual impairment are associated with aging (eg, cataracts, glaucoma, macular degeneration). Careful fitting with corrective lenses could help more than 80% of the 14 million Americans who are visually impaired (Bressler, Quigley & Schein, 2008). Two thirds of the population with impaired vision is older than 65 years of age. Younger people are also at risk for eye disorders, particularly traumatic injuries. The rapidly changing technological advances of ophthalmic surgery affect all age groups. These include refractive procedures as well as implantation of intraocular lenses and telescopic devices.

Although most people with eye disorders are treated in an ambulatory care setting, many patients receiving health care have an eye disorder as a comorbid condition. In addition to understanding the prevention, treatment, and consequences of eye disorders, nurses in all settings assess visual acuity in patients at risk (eg, those who are elderly, those with diabetes or acquired immunodeficiency syndrome [AIDS]), refer patients to eye care specialists as appropriate, implement measures to prevent further visual loss, and help patients adapt to impaired vision.

ASSESSMENT OF THE EYE

Anatomic and Physiologic Overview

Unlike most organs of the body, the eye is available for external examination, and its anatomy is more easily assessed than many other body parts (Fig. 58-1). The eyeball, or globe, sits in a protective bony structure known as the orbit.

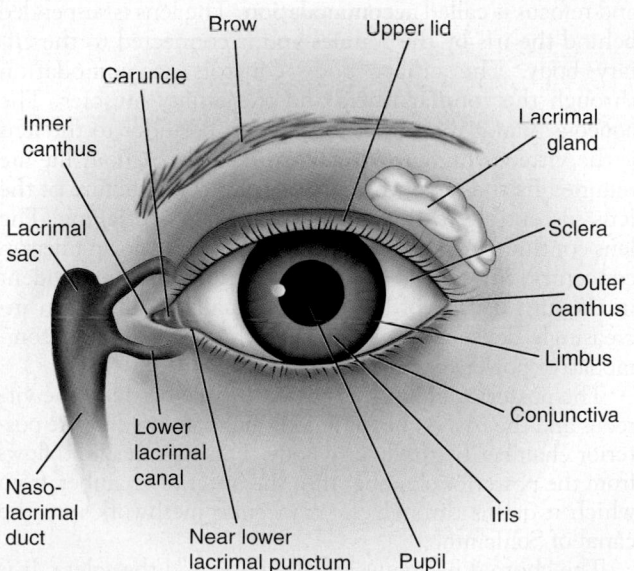

Figure 58-1 External structures of the eye and position of the lacrimal structures.

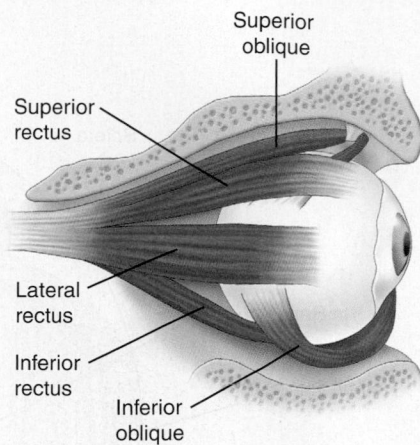

Figure 58-2 The extraocular muscles responsible for eye movement. The medial rectus muscle (not shown) is responsible for opposing the movement of the lateral rectus muscle.

Lined with muscle and connective and adipose tissues, the orbit is about 4-cm high, wide, and deep, and it is shaped roughly like a four-sided pyramid, surrounded on three sides by the sinuses: ethmoid (medially), frontal (superiorly), and maxillary (inferiorly). The optic nerve and the ophthalmic artery enter the orbit at its apex through the optic foramen. The eyeball is moved through all fields of gaze by the extraocular muscles. The four rectus muscles and two oblique muscles (Fig. 58-2) are innervated by cranial nerves (CN) III, IV, and VI. Normally, the movements of the two eyes are coordinated, and the brain perceives a single image.

The eyelids, composed of thin elastic skin that covers striated and smooth muscles, protect the anterior portion of the eye. The eyelids contain multiple glands, including sebaceous, sweat, and accessory lacrimal glands, and they are lined with conjunctival material. The upper lid normally covers the uppermost portion of the iris and is innervated by the oculomotor nerve (CN III). The lid margins contain meibomian glands, the inferior and superior puncta, and the eyelashes. The triangular spaces formed by the junction of the eyelids are known as the inner or medial canthus and the outer or lateral canthus. With every blink of the eyes, the lids wash the cornea and conjunctiva with tears.

Tears are vital to eye health. They are formed by the lacrimal gland and the accessory lacrimal glands. A healthy tear is composed of three layers: lipoid, aqueous, and mucoid. If there is a defect in the composition of any of these layers, the integrity of the cornea may be compromised. Tears are secreted in response to reflex or emotional stimuli.

The conjunctiva, a mucous membrane, provides a barrier to the external environment and nourishes the eye. The goblet cells of the conjunctiva secrete lubricating mucus. The bulbar conjunctiva covers the sclera, whereas the palpebral conjunctiva lines the inner surface of the upper and lower eyelids. The junction of the two portions is known as the fornix.

The sclera, commonly known as the white of the eye, is a dense, fibrous structure that makes up the posterior five sixths of the eye (Fig. 58-3). The sclera helps maintain the shape of the eyeball and protects the intraocular contents from trauma. The sclera may have a slightly bluish tinge in young children, a dull white color in adults, and a slightly

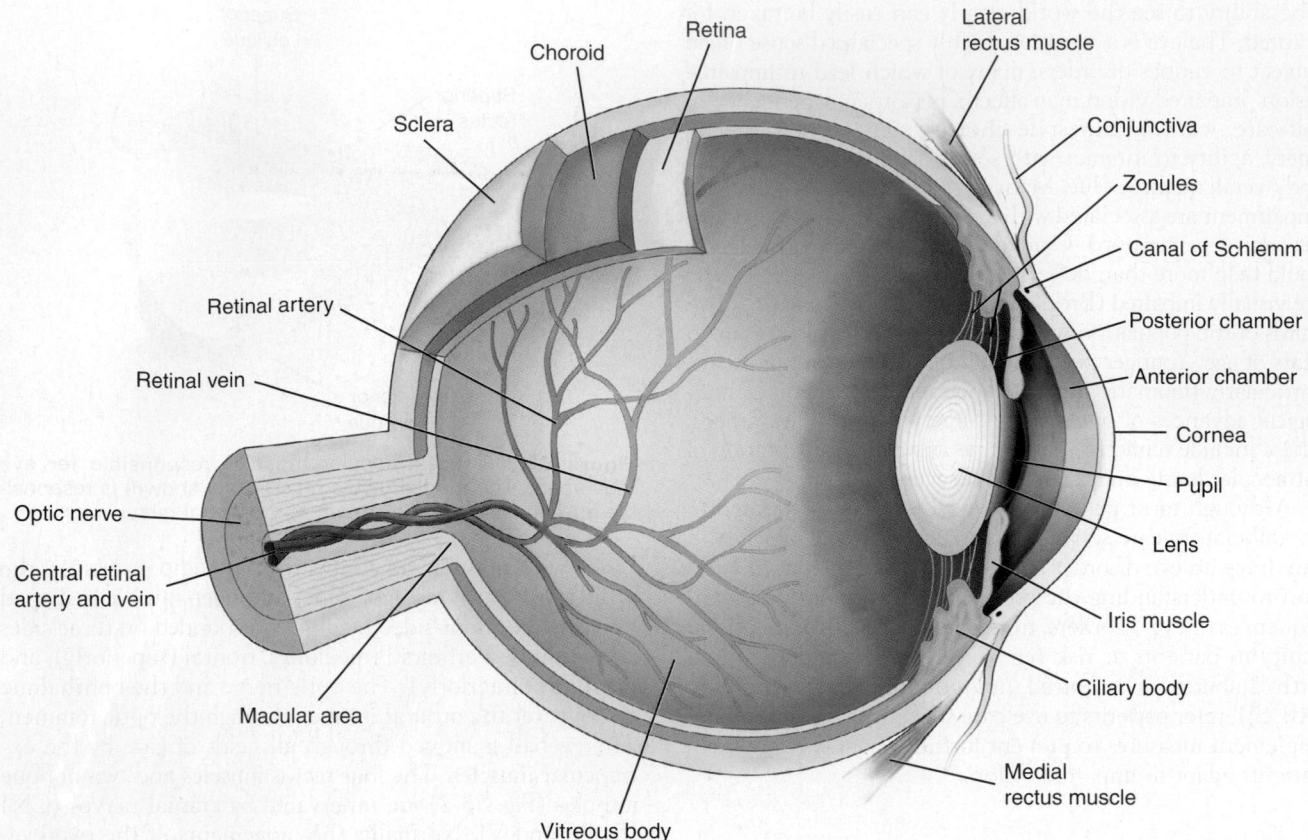

Figure 58-3 Three-dimensional cross-section of the eye.

yellowish color in the elderly. Externally, it is overlaid with conjunctiva, which is a thin, transparent, mucous membrane that contains fine blood vessels. The conjunctiva meets the cornea at the **limbus** on the outermost edge of the iris.

The cornea (Fig. 58-4), a transparent, avascular, domelike structure, forms the most anterior portion of the eyeball and is the main refracting surface of the eye. It is composed of five layers: epithelium, Bowman's membrane, stroma, Descemet's membrane, and endothelium. The epithelial cells are capable of rapid replication and are completely replaced every 7 days.

Behind the cornea lies the **anterior chamber,** filled with a continually replenished supply of clear aqueous humor, which nourishes the cornea. The **aqueous humor** is produced by the ciliary body, and its production is related to the intraocular pressure (IOP). Normal IOP is 10 to 21 mm Hg.

The uvea consists of the iris, the ciliary body, and the choroid. The iris, or colored part of the eye, is a highly vascularized, pigmented collection of fibers surrounding the pupil. The pupil is a space that dilates and constricts in response to light. Normal pupils are round and constrict symmetrically when a bright light shines on them. About 20% of the population have pupils that are slightly unequal in size but that respond equally to light. Dilation and constriction are controlled by the sphincter and dilator pupillae muscles. The dilator muscles are controlled by the sympathetic nervous system, whereas the sphincter muscles are controlled by the parasympathetic nervous system.

Directly behind the pupil and iris lies the lens, a colorless and almost completely transparent, biconvex structure held in position by zonular fibers. It is avascular and has no nerve or pain fibers. The lens enables focusing for near vision and refocusing for distance vision. The ability to focus and refocus is called **accommodation.** The lens is suspended behind the iris by the zonules and is connected to the ciliary body. The ciliary body controls accommodation through the zonular fibers and the ciliary muscles. The aqueous humor is anterior to the lens; posterior to the lens is the vitreous humor. All cells formed throughout life are retained by the lens, which makes the cell structure of the lens susceptible to the degenerative effects of aging. The lens continues to grow throughout life, laying down fibers in concentric rings. This gradual thickening becomes evident in the fifth decade of life and eventually results in an increasingly dense core or nucleus, which can limit accommodative powers.

The **posterior chamber** is a small space between the vitreous and the iris. Aqueous fluid is manufactured in the posterior chamber by the ciliary body. This aqueous fluid flows from the posterior chamber into the anterior chamber, from which it drains through the trabecular meshwork into the canal of Schlemm.

The choroid lies between the retina and the sclera. It is avascular tissue, supplying blood to the portion of the sensory retina closest to it.

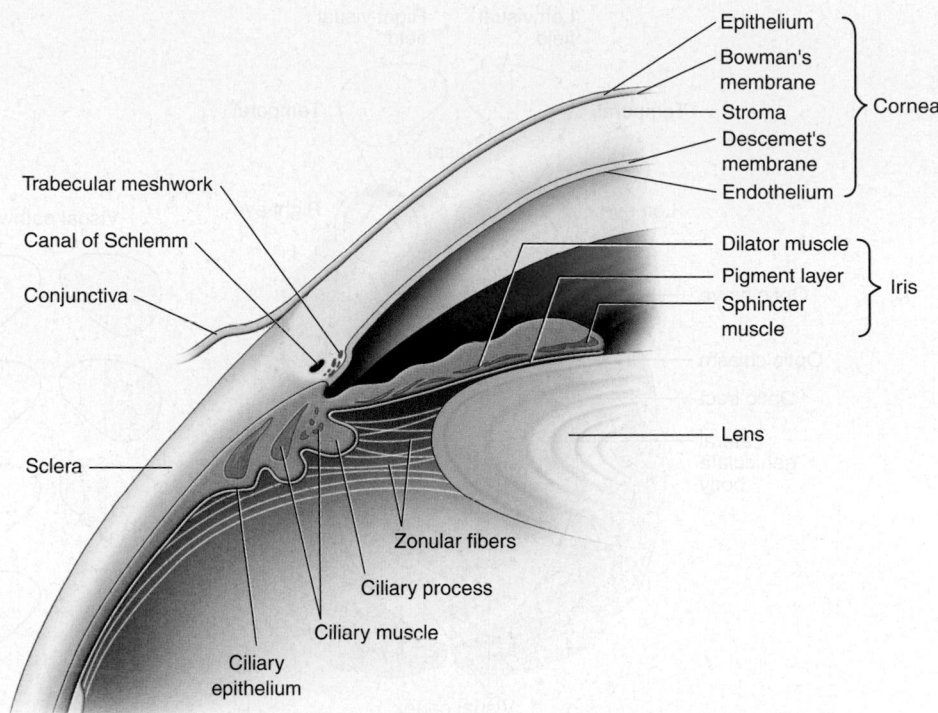

Figure 58-4 Internal structures of the eye. From American Society of Ophthalmic Registered Nurses. (2008). *Core curriculum for ophthalmic nursing* (3rd ed.) Dubuque, IA: Kendall/Hunt Publishing.

The ocular fundus is the largest chamber of the eye and contains the **vitreous humor,** a clear, gelatinous substance, composed mostly of water and encapsulated by a hyaloid membrane. The vitreous humor occupies about two thirds of the eye's volume and helps maintain the shape of the eye. As the body ages, the gel-like characteristics are gradually lost, and various cells and fibers cast shadows that the patient perceives as "floaters." The vitreous is in continuous contact with the retina and is attached to the retina by scattered collagenous filaments. The vitreous shrinks and shifts with age.

The innermost surface of the fundus is the retina. The retina is composed of 10 microscopic layers and has the consistency of wet tissue paper. It is neural tissue, an extension of the optic nerve. Viewed through the pupil, the landmarks of the retina are the optic disc, the retinal vessels, and the macula. The point of entrance of the optic nerve into the retina is the optic disc. The optic disc is pink; it is oval or circular and has sharp margins. In the disc, a physiologic depression or cup is present centrally, with the retinal blood vessels emerging from it. The retinal tissues arise from the optic disc and line the inner surface of the vitreous chamber. The retinal vessels also enter the eye through the optic disc, branching out through the retina and forming superior and inferior branches. The macula is the area of the retina responsible for central vision. The rest of the retina is responsible for peripheral vision. In the center of the macula is the most sensitive area, the fovea, which is avascular and surrounded by the superior and inferior vascular arcades. Two important layers of the retina are the retinal pigment epithelium (RPE) and the sensory retina. A single layer of cells constitutes the RPE, and these cells have numerous functions, including the absorption of light. The sensory retina contains the photoreceptor cells: **rods** and **cones.** The rods are mainly responsible for night vision or vision in low light, whereas the cones provide the best vision for bright light, color vision, and fine detail. Cones are distributed throughout the retina, with their greatest concentration in the fovea. Rods are absent in the fovea.

Visual acuity depends on a healthy, functioning eyeball and an intact visual pathway (Fig. 58-5). This pathway is made up of the retina, optic nerve, optic chiasm, optic tracks, lateral geniculate bodies, and optic radiations, and the visual cortex area of the brain. The pathway is an extension of the central nervous system.

The optic nerve is also known as the second cranial nerve (CN II). Its purpose is to transmit impulses from the retina to the occipital lobe of the brain. The optic nerve head, or optic disc, is the physiologic blind spot in each eye. The optic nerve leaves the eye and then meets the optic nerve from the other eye at the optic chiasm. The chiasm is the anatomic point at which the nasal fibers from the nasal retina of each eye cross to the opposite side of the brain. The nerve fibers from the temporal retina of each eye remain uncrossed. Fibers from the right half of each eye, which would be the left visual field, carry impulses to the right occipital lobe. Fibers from the left half of each eye, or the right visual field, carry impulses to the left occipital lobe. Beyond the chiasm, these fibers are known as the optic tract. The optic tract continues on to the lateral geniculate body. The lateral geniculate body leads to the optic radiations and then to the cortex of the occipital lobe of the brain.

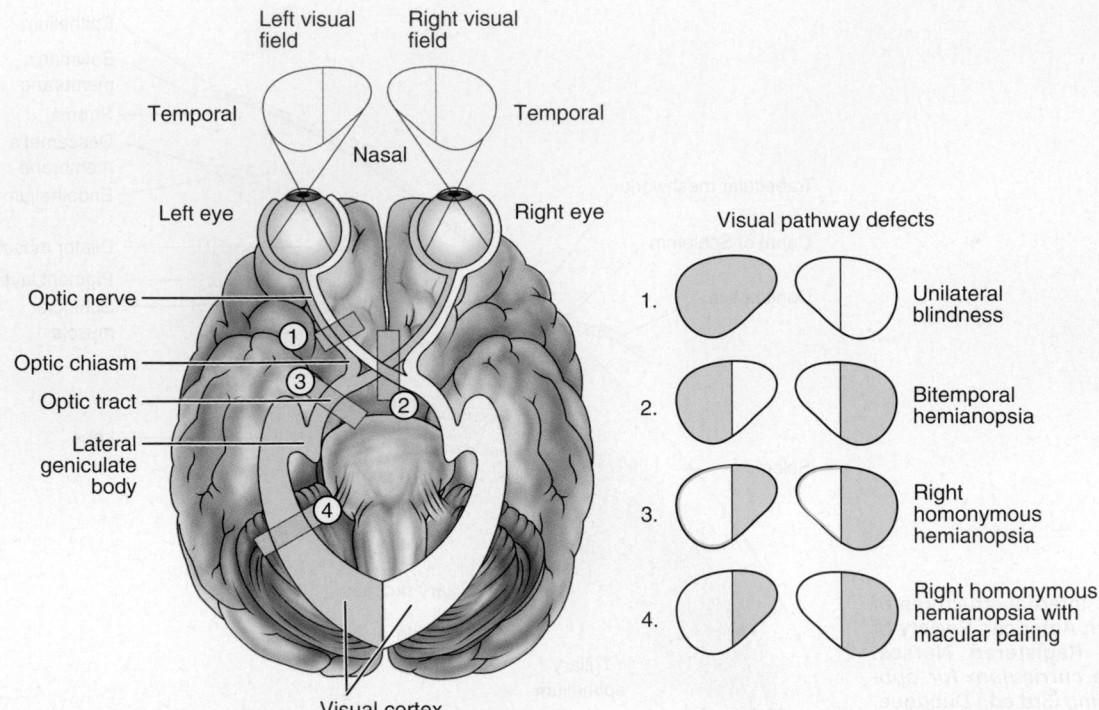

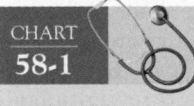

Figure 58-5 The visual pathway. From Fuller, J. & Schaller-Ayers, J. (2000). *Health assessment: A nursing approach* (3rd ed.). Philadelphia: Lippincott Williams & Wilkins.

Assessment

Ocular History

The nurse, through careful questioning, elicits the necessary information that can assist in diagnosis of an ophthalmic condition. Pertinent questions to ask during the interview are presented in Chart 58-1. Genetics plays a role in many eye and vision problems; for more information, see Chart 58-2.

Visual Acuity

Following the health history, the patient's visual acuity is assessed. This is an essential part of the eye examination and a measure against which all therapeutic outcomes are based.

The Snellen chart, which is composed of a series of progressively smaller rows of letters, is used to test distance vision. The fraction 20/20 is considered the standard of normal vision. Most people can see the letters on the line designated as 20/20 from a distance of 20 feet. A person whose vision is 20/200 can see an object from 20 feet away that a person with 20/20 vision can see from 200 feet away. The patient is positioned at the prescribed distance, usually 20 feet, from the chart and is asked to read the smallest line that he or she can see. The patient should wear distance correction (eyeglasses or contact lenses) if required, and each eye should be tested separately. If the patient cannot read the 20/20 line, he or she is given a pinhole occluder and asked to read again using the eye in question. A makeshift occluder may be created by making a pinhole in an index card and asking the patient to look through the pinhole. Squinting produces the same effect. Patients should be encouraged to read more letters and to guess, if

necessary. Often, patients avoid guessing and prefer not to try at all rather than to make a mistake. The patient should be encouraged to read every letter possible.

CHART 58-1

Taking an Ocular History

- What does the patient perceive to be the problem?
- Is visual acuity diminished?
- Does the patient experience blurred, double, or distorted vision?
- Is there pain; is it sharp or dull; is it worse when blinking?
- Is the discomfort an itching sensation or more of a foreign body sensation?
- Are both eyes affected?
- Is there a history of discharge? If so, inquire about color, consistency, odor.
- Describe the onset of the problem (sudden, gradual). Is it worsening?
- What is the duration of the problem?
- Is this a recurrence of a previous condition?
- How has the patient self-treated?
- What makes the symptoms improve or worsen?
- Has the condition affected performance of activities of daily living (ADLs)?
- Are there any systemic diseases? What medications are used in their treatment?
- What concurrent ophthalmic conditions does the patient have?
- Is there a history of ophthalmic surgery?
- Have other family members had the same symptoms or condition?

> **CHART 58-2**
>
> ## GENETICS IN NURSING PRACTICE
> ### Eye and Vision Disorders
>
> Several eye and vision disorders are associated with genetic abnormalities. Some examples are:
> - Albinism
> - Aniridia
> - Color blindness
> - Glaucoma
> - Homocystinuria
> - Isolated familial congenital cataracts
> - Leber hereditary optic neuropathy
> - Leber congenital amaurosis
> - Marfan syndrome
> - Retinitis pigmentosa
>
> ### Nursing Assessments
>
> #### Family History Assessment
> - Assess history of family members with glaucoma, cataracts, night blindness (retinitis pigmentosa), color blindness, or other vision impairment.
> - Inquire about the age of onset of symptoms (the onset of Leber congenital amaurosis is in childhood, while the onset of Leber hereditary optic neuropathy is in young adulthood).
> - Inquire about family members with other disorders that may include visual impairment, such as cutaneous, metabolic, or connective tissue disorders and hearing loss.
>
> #### Patient Assessment
> - Assess for other systemic and/or clinical features such as cutaneous or skeletal conditions, or hearing loss.
>
> ### Management Issues Specific to Genetics
> - Inquire whether DNA gene mutation or other genetics testing has been performed on any affected family members.
> - If indicated, refer for further genetics counseling and evaluation so that family members can discuss inheritance, risk to other family members, availability of genetics testing, and gene-based interventions.
> - Offer appropriate genetics information and resources.
> - Assess patient's understanding of genetics information.
> - Provide support to families with newly diagnosed genetic-related sensorineural disorders.
> - Participate in management and coordination of care of patients with genetic conditions and individuals pre-disposed to develop or pass on a genetic condition
>
> ### Genetics Resources
>
> **Genetic Alliance**—a directory of support groups for patients and families with genetic conditions, www.geneticalliance.org
>
> **Gene Clinics**—a listing of common genetic disorders with up-to-date clinical summaries, genetic counseling and testing information, www.geneclinics.org
>
> **National Organization of Rare Disorders**—a directory of support groups and information for patients and families with rare genetic disorders, www.rarediseases.org
>
> **OMIM: Online Mendelian Inheritance in Man**—a complete listing of inherited genetic conditions, www.ncbi.nlm.nih.gov/omim/stats/html

Visual acuity is then recorded. If the patient reads all five letters from the 20/20 line with the right eye (OD) and three of the five letters on the 20/15 line with the left eye (OS), the examiner writes OD 20/20, OS 20/15-2.

If the patient cannot read the largest letter on the chart (the 20/200 line), the patient should be moved toward the chart or the chart moved toward the patient until the patient can identify the largest letter on the chart. If the patient can recognize only the letter E on the top line at a distance of 10 feet, the visual acuity would be recorded as 10'/200. If the patient cannot see the letter E at any distance, the examiner should determine if the patient can count fingers (CF). The examiner holds up a random number of fingers and asks the patient to count the number he or she sees. If the patient correctly identifies the number of fingers at 3 feet, the examiner would record CF/3'.

If the patient cannot count fingers, the examiner raises one hand up and down or moves it side to side and asks in which direction the hand is moving. This level of vision is known as hand motion (HM). A patient who can perceive only light is described as having light perception (LP). The vision of a patient who cannot perceive light is described as no light perception (NLP).

External Eye Examination

After the visual acuity has been recorded, an external eye examination is performed. The position of the eyelids is noted. Commonly, the upper 2 mm of the iris are covered by the upper lid. The patient is examined for **ptosis** (drooping eyelid) and for lid retraction (too much of the eye exposed). Sometimes, the upper or lower lid turns out, affecting closure. The lid margins and lashes should have no edema, erythema, or lesions. The examiner looks for scaling or crusting, and the sclera is inspected. A normal sclera is opaque and white. Lesions on the conjunctiva, discharge, and tearing or blinking are noted.

The room should be darkened so that the pupils can be examined. The pupillary response is checked with a penlight to determine if the pupils are equally reactive and regular. A normal pupil is black. An irregular pupil may result from trauma, previous surgery, or a disease process.

The patient's eyes are observed in primary or direct gaze, and any head tilt is noted. A tilt may indicate cranial nerve palsy. The patient is asked to stare at a target; each eye is covered and uncovered quickly while the examiner looks for any shift in gaze. The examiner observes for **nystagmus** (ie, oscillating movement of the eyeball). The extraocular movements of the eyes are tested by having the patient follow the examiner's finger, pencil, or a hand light through the six cardinal directions of gaze (ie, up, down, right, left, and both diagonals). This is especially important when screening patients for ocular trauma or for neurologic disorders.

Diagnostic Evaluation

Direct Ophthalmoscopy

A direct ophthalmoscope is a hand-held instrument with various plus and minus lenses. The lenses can be rotated into place, enabling the examiner to bring the cornea, lens, and retina into focus sequentially. The examiner holds the ophthalmoscope in the right hand and uses the right eye to examine the patient's right eye. The examiner switches to the left hand and left eye when examining the patient's left eye. During this examination, the room should be darkened, and the patient's eye should be on the same level as the examiner's eye. The patient and the examiner should be comfortable, and both should breathe normally. The patient is given a target to gaze at and is encouraged to keep both eyes open and steady.

When the fundus is examined, the vasculature comes into focus first. The veins are larger in diameter than the arteries. The examiner focuses on a large vessel and then follows it toward the midline of the body, which leads to the optic nerve. The central depression in the disc is known as the cup. The normal cup is about one-third the size of the diameter of the disc. The size of the physiologic optic cup should be estimated and the disc margins described as sharp or blurred. A silvery or coppery appearance, which indicates arteriolosclerosis, should be noted. The periphery of the retina is examined by having the patient shift his or her gaze. The last area of the fundus to be examined is the macula, because this area is the most sensitive to light. The retina of a young person often has a glistening effect, sometimes referred to as a cellophane reflex.

The healthy fundus should be free of any lesions. The examiner looks for intraretinal hemorrhages, which may appear as red smudges, and, if the patient has hypertension, they may be somewhat flame shaped. Lipid may be present in the retina of patients with hypercholesterolemia or diabetes. This lipid has a yellowish appearance. Soft exudates that have a fuzzy, white appearance (cotton-wool spots) should be noted. The examiner looks for microaneurysms, which look like little red dots, and nevi. Drusen (small, hyaline, globular deposits), commonly found in macular degeneration, appear as yellowish areas with indistinct edges. Small drusen have a more distinct edge. The examiner should sketch the fundus and document any abnormalities.

Indirect Ophthalmoscopy

The indirect ophthalmoscope is an instrument commonly used by the ophthalmologist to see larger areas of the retina, although in an unmagnified state. It produces a bright and intense light. The light source is affixed with a pair of binocular lenses mounted on the examiner's head. The ophthalmoscope is used with a hand-held, 20-diopter lens.

Slit-Lamp Examination

The slit lamp is a binocular microscope mounted on a table. This instrument enables the user to examine the eye with magnification of 10 to 40 times the real image. The illumination can be varied from a broad to a narrow beam of light for different parts of the eye. For example, by varying the width and intensity of the light, the anterior chamber can be examined for signs of inflammation. Cataracts may be evaluated by changing the angle of the light. When a hand-held contact lens, such as a three-mirror lens, is used with the slit lamp, the angle of the anterior chamber may be examined, as may the ocular fundus.

Color Vision Testing

The ability to differentiate colors has a dramatic effect on the activities of daily living (ADLs). For example, the inability to differentiate between red and green can compromise traffic safety. Some careers (eg, commercial artist, [color] photographer, airline pilot, electrician) may be closed to people with significant color deficiencies. The photoreceptor cells responsible for color vision are the cones, and the greatest area of color sensitivity is in the macula, the area of densest cone concentration.

A screening test, such as the polychromatic plates discussed in the next paragraph, can be used to establish whether a person's color vision is within normal range. Color vision deficits can be inherited. For example, red–green color deficiencies are inherited in an X-linked manner, affecting approximately 8% of men and 0.4% of women. Acquired color vision losses may be caused by medications (eg, digitalis) or pathology (eg, cataracts). A simple test, such as asking a patient if the red top on a bottle of eye drops appears redder to one eye than the other, can be an effective tool. A difference in the perception of the intensity of the color red between the two eyes can be a symptom of a neurologic problem and may provide information about the location of the lesion.

Because alteration in color vision sometimes indicates conditions of the optic nerve, color vision testing is often performed in a neuro-ophthalmologic workup. The most common color vision test is performed using Ishihara polychromatic plates. These plates are bound together in a booklet. On each plate of this booklet are dots of primary colors that are integrated into a background of secondary colors. The dots are arranged in simple patterns, such as numbers or geometric shapes. Patients with diminished color vision may be unable to identify the hidden shapes. Patients with central vision conditions (eg, macular degeneration) have more difficulty identifying colors than those with peripheral vision conditions (eg, glaucoma) because central vision identifies color.

Amsler Grid

The Amsler grid is a test often used for patients with macular problems, such as macular degeneration. It consists of a geometric grid of identical squares with a central fixation point. The grid should be viewed by the patient wearing normal reading glasses. Each eye is tested separately. The patient is instructed to stare at the central fixation spot on the grid and report any distortion in the squares of the grid itself. For patients with macular problems, some of the squares may look faded, or the lines may be wavy. Patients with age-related macular degeneration are commonly given these Amsler grids to take home. The patient is encouraged to check them frequently, as often as daily, to detect any early signs of distortion that may indicate the development of a neovascular choroidal membrane, an advanced stage of macular degeneration characterized by the growth of abnormal choroidal vessels.

Ultrasonography

Lesions in the globe or the orbit may not be directly visible and are evaluated by ultrasonography. Ultrasonography is a valuable diagnostic technique, especially when the view of the retina is obscured by opaque media such as cataract or hemorrhage. Ultrasonography can be used to identify orbital tumors, retinal detachment, vitreous hemorrhage, and changes in tissue composition with minimal discomfort for the patient.

Optical Coherence Tomography

Optical coherence tomography is a technology that involves low-coherence interferometry. Light is used to evaluate retinal and macular diseases as well as anterior segment conditions. This method is noninvasive and involves no physical contact with the eye.

Color Fundus Photography

Fundus photography is used to detect and document retinal lesions. The patient's pupils are widely dilated before the procedure. The resulting fundus photographs can be viewed stereoscopically so that elevations such as macular edema can be identified. Visual acuity is diminished for about 30 minutes as a result of retinal "bleaching" by the intense flashing lights.

Fluorescein Angiography

Fluorescein angiography evaluates clinically significant macular edema, documents macular capillary nonperfusion, and identifies retinal and choroidal **neovascularization** (growth of abnormal new blood vessels) in age-related macular degeneration. It is an invasive procedure in which fluorescein dye is injected, usually into an antecubital vein. Within 10 to 15 seconds, this dye can be seen coursing through the retinal vessels. Over a 10-minute period, serial black-and-white photographs are taken of the retinal vasculature. The dye may impart a gold tone to the skin of some patients, and urine may turn deep yellow or orange. This discoloration usually disappears in 24 hours.

Indocyanine Green Angiography

Indocyanine green angiography is used to evaluate abnormalities in the choroidal vasculature, conditions often seen in macular degeneration. Indocyanine green dye is injected intravenously, and multiple images are captured using digital videoangiography over a period of 30 seconds to 20 minutes. The dye is generally well tolerated, but some patients experience nausea and vomiting. Allergic reactions are rare; however, indocyanine green angiography is contraindicated in patients with a history of iodide reactions.

Tonometry

Tonometry measures IOP by determining the pressure necessary to indent or flatten (applanate) a small anterior area of the globe of the eye. Pressure is measured in millimeters of mercury (mm Hg). High readings indicate high pressure; low readings indicate low pressure. The procedure is noninvasive and usually painless. A topical anesthetic eye drop is instilled in the lower conjunctival sac, and the tonometer is then used to measure the IOP.

Perimetry Testing

Perimetry testing evaluates the field of vision. A visual field is the area or extent of physical space visible to an eye in a given position. Its average extent is 65 degrees upward, 75 degrees downward, 60 degrees inward, and 95 degrees outward when the eye is in the primary gaze (ie, looking directly forward). Visual field testing (ie, perimetry) helps identify which parts of the patient's central and peripheral visual fields have useful vision. It is most helpful in detecting central **scotomas** (blind areas in the visual field) in macular degeneration and the peripheral field defects in glaucoma and retinitis pigmentosa.

IMPAIRED VISION

Refractive Errors

In refractive errors, vision is impaired because a shortened or elongated eyeball prevents light rays from focusing sharply on the retina. Blurred vision from refractive error can be corrected with eyeglasses or contact lenses. The appropriate eyeglass or contact lens is determined by **refraction.** Ophthalmic refraction consists of placing various types of lenses in front of the patient's eyes to determine which lens best improves the patient's vision.

The depth of the eyeball is important in determining refractive error (Fig. 58-6). Patients for whom the visual image focuses precisely on the macula and who do not need

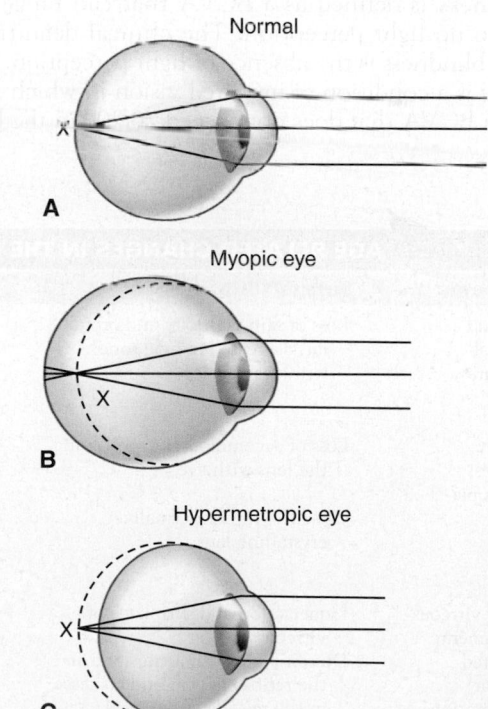

Figure 58-6 Eyeball shape determines visual acuity in refractive errors. **A,** Normal eye. **B,** Myopic eye. **C,** Hypermetropic eye.

eyeglasses or contact lenses are said to have **emmetropia** (normal vision). Some people have deeper eyeballs; thus, the distant visual image focuses in front of, or short of, the retina. They have **myopia,** are said to be nearsighted, and have blurred distance vision. Other people have shallower eyeballs; thus, the visual image focuses beyond the retina. They have **hyperopia,** are said to be farsighted, and have excellent distance vision but blurry near vision.

Another important cause of refractive error is **astigmatism,** an irregularity in the curve of the cornea. Because astigmatism causes a distortion of the visual image, acuity of distance and near vision can be decreased. Hard contact lenses, which by means of their tear film correct astigmatic errors, or soft toric contact lenses with a cylinder correction may be used in place of eyeglasses for patients with astigmatism.

Ophthalmology has entered the era of customized vision correction in its desire to achieve "super-normal vision." Wavefront technology to measure unique refractive imperfections of the cornea or higher aberrations (ie, myopia, hyperopia, astigmatism) is currently used to customize laser-assisted in situ keratomileusis (LASIK) procedures. To customize the corneal flaps during LASIK, a newer procedure uses a femtosecond (ultrashort-pulse) laser (Slade, 2007).

Low Vision and Blindness

Low vision is a general term describing visual impairment that requires patients to use devices and strategies in addition to corrective lenses to perform visual tasks. Low vision is defined as a best corrected visual acuity (BCVA) of 20/70 to 20/200.

Blindness is defined as a BCVA that can range from 20/400 to no light perception. The clinical definition of absolute blindness is the absence of light perception. Legal blindness is a condition of impaired vision in which a person has a BCVA that does not exceed 20/200 in the better eye or whose widest visual field diameter is 20 degrees or less. This definition neither equates with functional ability nor classifies the degrees of visual impairment. Legal blindness ranges from an inability to perceive light to having some vision remaining. A person who meets the criteria for legal blindness may be eligible for government financial assistance.

Impaired vision is often accompanied by difficulty in performing functional activities. People with visual acuity of 20/80 to 20/100 with a visual field restriction of 60 degrees to greater than 20 degrees can read at a nearly normal level with optical aids. Their visual orientation is near normal but requires increased scanning of the environment (ie, systematic use of head and eye movements). In a visual acuity range of 20/200 to 20/400 with a 20-degree to greater than 10-degree visual field restriction, the person can read slowly with optical aids. His or her visual orientation is slow, with constant scanning of the environment. People in this category may have the ability to negotiate their environment without auxiliary aids. This ability is termed "travel vision." People with HM vision or no vision may benefit from the use of mobility devices (eg, cane, guide dog) and should be encouraged to learn Braille and to use computer aids.

The most common causes of blindness and visual impairment among adults 40 years of age or older are diabetic retinopathy, macular degeneration, glaucoma, and cataracts (Prevent Blindness America, 2008). Macular degeneration is more prevalent among Caucasians, whereas glaucoma is more prevalent among African Americans. Age-related changes in the eye are summarized in Table 58-1.

Assessment and Diagnostic Testing

The assessment of low vision includes a thorough history and the examination of distance and near visual acuity, visual field, contrast sensitivity, glare, color perception, and refraction. Specially designed, low-vision visual acuity charts are used to evaluate patients.

Table 58-1   AGE-RELATED CHANGES IN THE EYE

The External Eye	Structural Change	Functional Change	History & Physical Findings
Eyelids and lacrimal structures	Loss of skin elasticity and orbital fat, decreased muscle tone; wrinkles develop	Lid margins turn in, causing lashes to irritate cornea and conjunctiva (entropian); or lid margins may turn out, resulting in increased corneal exposure (ectropian).	Reports of burning, foreign body sensation, increased tearing (epiphoria); injection, inflammation, and ulceration may occur
Refractive changes; presbyopia	Loss of accommodative power in the lens with age	Reading materials must be held at increasing distance in order to focus.	Patient reports, "Arms are too short!"; need for increased light; reading glasses or bifocals needed
Cataract	Opacities in the normally crystalline lens	Interference with the focus of a sharp image on the retina	Patients report increased glare, decreased vision, changes in color values (blue and yellow especially affected)
Posterior vitreous detachment	Liquefaction and shrinkage of vitreous body	May lead to retinal tears and detachment	Reports light flashes, cobwebs, floaters
Age-related macular degeneration (AMD)	Drusen (yellowish aging spots in the retina) appear and coalesce in the macula. Abnormal choroidal blood vessels may lead to formation of fibrotic disciform scars in the macula.	Central vision is affected; onset is more gradual in dry AMD, more rapid in wet AMD; distortion and loss of central vision may occur.	Reading vision is affected; words may be missing letters, faded areas appear on the page, straight lines may appear wavy; drusen, pigmentary changes in retina; abnormal submacular choroidal vessels

Table 58-2 ACTIVITIES AFFECTED BY VISUAL IMPAIRMENT AND SUGGESTIONS FOR LOW-VISION AIDS

Activity	Optical Aids	Nonoptical Aids
Shopping	Hand magnifier	Lighting, color cues
Fixing a snack	Bifocals	Color cues; consistent food storage plan
Eating out	Hand magnifier	Flashlight, portable lamp
Identifying money	Bifocals, hand magnifier	Arrange paper money in wallet compartments
Reading print	High-power spectacle, bifocals, hand magnifier, stand magnifier, closed-circuit television	Lighting, high-contrast print, large print, reading slit
Writing	Hand magnifier,	Lighting, bold-tip pen, black ink
Using a telephone	Hand magnifier	Large print dial or touch tone buttons, hand-printed directory
Crossing streets	Lightweight hand held monoscopes/telescopes	Cane, ask directions
Finding taxis and bus signs	Lightweight hand held monoscopes/telescopes	Ask for assistance
Reading medication labels	Hand magnifier	Color codes, large print
Reading stove dials	Hand magnifier	Color codes, raised dots
Adjusting the thermostat	Hand magnifier	Enlarged print model
Using a computer	Spectacles	High-contrast color, large-print program
Reading signs	Spectacles	Move closer
Watching sporting event	Lightweight hand held monoscopes/telescopes	Sit in front rows

Adapted from Riordan-Eva, P. & Whitcher, J. P. (2008). *Vaughn and Asbury's general ophthalmology.* New York: McGraw-Hill.

Patient Interview

During history taking, the cause and duration of the patient's visual impairment are identified. Patients with retinitis pigmentosa, for example, have a genetic abnormality. Patients with diabetic macular edema typically have fluctuating visual acuity. Patients with macular degeneration have central acuity problems, which cause difficulty in performing activities that require finer vision, such as reading. People with peripheral field defects have more difficulties with mobility. The patient's customary ADLs, medication regimen, habits (eg, smoking), acceptance of the physical limitations brought about by the visual impairment, and realistic expectations of low-vision aids are identified and included in the plan of care, including provision of guidelines for safety and referrals to social services.

Contrast-Sensitivity Testing and Glare Testing

Contrast-sensitivity testing measures visual acuity in different degrees of contrast. The initial test may take the form of simply turning on the lights while testing the distance acuity. If the patient can read better with the lights on, the patient can benefit from magnification. Glare testing enables the examiner to obtain a more realistic evaluation of the patient's ability to function in his or her environment. Glare can reduce a person's ability to see, especially in patients with cataracts. Devices that test glare, such as the Brightness Acuity Tester, produce three degrees of bright light to create a dazzle effect while the patient is viewing a target, such as Snellen letters on the wall. The lights have been calibrated to imitate certain objects that create glare, such as a car's headlights at night.

Medical Management

Managing low vision involves magnification and image enhancement through the use of low-vision aids and strategies and referrals to social services and community agencies serving those with visual impairment. The goals are to optimize the patient's remaining vision, whether central or peripheral, and assist the patient to perform customary activities. Low-vision aids include optical and nonoptical devices (Table 58-2) The optical devices include convex lens aids, such as magnifiers and spectacles; telescopic devices; antireflective lenses that diminish glare; and electronic reading systems, such as closed-circuit television and computers with large print. Continuing advances in computer software provide very useful products for patients with low vision. Scanners and the appropriate software enable the user to scan printed material and have it read by computer voice or enlarge the print for reading. Magnifiers can be hand-held or attached to a stand with or without illumination. Telescopic devices can be spectacle telescopes or clip-on or hand-held loupes.

A telephone system has been developed that allows access to the Internet and e-mail using voice commands (Chart 58-3). A mobile telephone-based communication support system allows people with poor eyesight to communicate by mobile phone. The system consists of a low-power mobile phone (personal handyphone system; PHS) and a large screen. When the person telephones, a registered support personnel picture is displayed on the screen and the PHS telephone dials that person automatically (Ogawa, Yonezawa, Maki, et al., 2007).

Referrals to community agencies may be necessary for patients with low vision who live alone and cannot self-administer their medications. Community agencies, such as the Lighthouse National Center for Vision and Aging, offer services to patients with low vision that include training in independent living skills and the provision of occupational and recreational activities and a wide variety of assistive devices for vision enhancement and orientation and mobility.

Ophthalmologists have worked for years toward visual restoration for people who are blind. Retinal implants for those whose optic nerves are functional as well as cortical implants for those whose optic nerves are diseased are being developed but are still experimental (Zaqloul & Boahen, 2006). The rapid changes in technology and miniaturization of computer chips may enable dramatic advances in synthetic vision in the future.

Chart 58-3 • *Web Access for the Visually Impaired*

People with impaired vision need not be left behind in the computer age. Various technologies are available. A list of general equipment needs follows:
- Computer: software specifically developed for people with visual impairment.
- Internet service provider (eg, AOL, Netscape, Earthlink, Comcast)
- Screen-reader program: converts text on the computer screen to synthesized speech (eg, JAWS for Windows, Windows Eyes, Slimware Window Bridge, ProTalk 32, Hal Screen Reader, WinVision, WYNN, outSPOKEN for Windows)
- Browser program to navigate the World Wide Web (eg, Microsoft Internet Explorer, IBM Home Page Reader)

The following Web sites provide extensive information about low vision resources for people with vision loss, vision impairment, and blindness:
- www.lowvision.org
- www.magnifiers.org

Researchers are developing graphic tactile displays that provide information for people with visual impairment using the sense of touch. Efficient, low-cost tactile displays are not yet available. At this time, most of these devices are research prototypes (Vidal-Verdu & Hafez, 2007).

Nursing Management

Coping with blindness involves three types of adaptation: emotional, physical, and social. The emotional adjustment to blindness or severe visual impairment determines the success of the physical and social adjustments of the patient. Successful emotional adjustment means acceptance of blindness or severe visual impairment.

Promoting Coping Efforts

Effective coping may not occur until the patient recognizes the permanence of the low vision or blindness. Clinging to false hopes of regaining vision hampers effective adaptation to blindness. A patient who is newly visually impaired and his or her family members (especially those who live with the patient) undergo the various steps of grieving: denial and shock, anger and protest, restitution, loss resolution, and acceptance. The ability to accept the changes that must come with visual loss and willingness to adapt to those changes influence the successful rehabilitation of the patient who is blind. Additional aspects to consider are value changes, independence–dependence conflicts, coping with stigma, and learning to function in social settings without visual cues and landmarks.

Promoting Spatial Orientation and Mobility

A person who is blind or severely visually impaired requires strategies for adapting to the environment. ADLs, such as walking to a chair from a bed, require spatial concepts. The person needs to know where he or she is in relation to the rest of the room, to understand the changes that may occur, and to know how to approach the desired location safely. This requires a collaborative effort between the patient and the responsible adult who serves as the sighted guide.

A patient whose visual impairment results from a chronic progressive eye disorder, such as glaucoma, has better cognitive mapping skills than the patient who loses vision suddenly. Patients with progressive eye disorders develop the use of spatial and topographic concepts early and gradually; hence, remembering a room layout is easier for them. Patients who lose vision suddenly have more difficulty in adjusting, and emotional and behavioral issues of coping with loss of vision may hinder their learning. These patients require intensive emotional support. The nurse must assess the degree of physical assistance the person with vision loss requires and communicate this to other health care personnel.

In the hospital, the bedside table and the call button must always be within reach. The parts of the call button are explained, and the patient is taught to touch and press the buttons or dials until the activity is mastered. The patient must be familiarized with the location of the telephone, water pitcher, and other objects on the bedside table. The food tray's composition is likened to the face of a clock; for example, the main plate may be described as being at 12 o'clock or the coffee cup at 3 o'clock. All articles and furniture must remain in the same positions throughout the patient's hospitalization. The nurse should introduce himself or herself on entering a patient's room and alert the patient to his or her departure. Such behaviors are always polite and help in the care of a patient with vision loss.

The nurse should be aware of the importance of techniques in providing physical assistance, encouraging independence, and ensuring safety. Specific guidelines for interacting with the patient with vision loss are presented in Chart 58-4. The readiness of the patient and his or her family to learn must be assessed before initiating orientation and mobility training.

Promoting Home and Community-Based Care

The nurse, social worker, family, and others collaborate to assess the patient's home condition and support system. If available, a low-vision specialist or occupational therapist should be consulted, particularly for patients for whom identifying and administering medications pose problems. The level of visual acuity and patient preference help determine appropriate interventions. Some private and nonprofit services are identified in the Resources section at the end of this chapter.

Other interventions that are appropriate for some people with low vision or blindness include Braille and service animals. Recent rapid advances in technology have led to the erroneous conclusion by some that Braille is an outmoded communication tool. There has been an ever-increasing reliance on print magnification technology as well as computer-assisted speech output. However, although the use of Braille may be less important for adults who have already learned language and grammar skills, educators and low-vision specialists have continued to advocate that children who are legally blind be given the opportunity to learn Braille.

Guide dogs, also known as seeing-eye dogs or service dogs, are dogs that are specially bred, raised, and rigorously trained to assist people who are blind. The guide dog is a constant companion to the person who is blind (also

Chart 58-4 • *Guidelines for Interacting With People Who Are Blind Or Have Low Vision*

- Remember that the only difference between you and people who are blind or have low vision is that they are not able to see through their eyes what you are able to see through yours.
- Do not be uncomfortable when in the company of a person who is blind or has low vision. Talk with the person as you would talk with any other individual, honestly and without pity; do not be concerned about using words like "see" and "look." There is no need to raise your voice unless the person asks you to do so.
- Identify yourself as you approach the person and before you make physical contact. Tell the person your name and your role. If another person approaches, introduce him or her. When you leave the room, be sure to tell the person that you are leaving and if anyone else remains in the room.
- It is often appropriate to touch the person's hand or arm lightly to indicate that you are about to speak.
- When talking, face the person and speak directly to him or her using a normal tone of voice.
- Be specific when communicating direction. Mention a specific distance or use clock cues when possible (eg, walk left about 2 yards; walk about 20 feet to the right; the telephone is at 2 o'clock). Avoid using phrases such as "over there."
- When you offer to assist someone, allow the person to hold on to your arm just above the elbow and to walk a half-step behind you.
- When offering the person a seat, place the person's hand on the back or the arm of the seat.
- When you are about to go up or down a flight of stairs, tell the person and place his or her hand on the banister.
- Make sure that the environment is free of obstacles; close doors and cabinets so they are not in the path.
- Offer to read written information, such as a menu.
- If you serve food to the person, use clock cues to specify where everything is on the plate.
- When the person who is blind or who has low vision is a patient in a health care facility:
  - Make sure all objects the person will need are close at hand.
  - Identify the location of objects that the person may need (eg, "The call light is near your right hand"; "The telephone is on the table on the left side of your bed.")
  - Remove obstacles that may be in the person's pathway and could cause a fall.
  - Place all assistive devices the person uses close at hand; let the person feel the devices so that he or she knows their location.
- Do not distract the service animal unless the owner has given permission.
- Ask the person, "How can I help you?" At some times the person needs help, but at other times help may not be needed.

This material is adapted from and based in part on *Achieving Physical and Communication Accessibility,* a publication of the National Center for Access Unlimited; *Community Access Facts,* an Adaptive Environments Center publication; and *The Ten Commandments of Interacting with People with Mental Health Disabilities,* a publication of The Ability Center of Greater Toledo.

referred to as the animal's handler) and is allowed on airplanes and in restaurants, stores, hotels, and other public places. With the assistance of the guide dog, the person who is blind can be extremely mobile and accomplish normal activities both within and outside of the home and workplace. A dog in harness is a working dog, not a pet. The dog should not be distracted from his job by well-intentioned strangers who want to pet, feed, or play with the animal. The dog's handler should always be consulted before approaching the working guide dog. Most health care facilities have a service animal policy that outlines the responsibilities of the handler with regard to the care of the animal.

Glaucoma

The term *glaucoma* is used to refer to a group of ocular conditions characterized by optic nerve damage. In the past, glaucoma was seen more as a condition of elevated IOP than of optic neuropathy. Increasingly, that is no longer the case. There is no doubt that increased IOP damages the optic nerve and nerve fiber layer, but the degree of harm is highly variable (McKinnon, Goldberg, Peeples, et al., 2008). The optic nerve damage is related to the IOP caused by congestion of aqueous humor in the eye. A range of IOPs are considered "normal," but these may be associated with vision loss in some patients.

Glaucoma is the second leading cause of blindness in adults in the United States. It is estimated that at least 2.2 million Americans have glaucoma and that 3 to 6 million more are at risk for the disease (Bressler, et al., 2008). Glaucoma is more prevalent in people older than 40 years of age, and it is the third most common age-related eye disease in the United States. It also occurs more frequently in African Americans than Caucasians (Chart 58-5). There is no cure for glaucoma, but the disease can be controlled (Sharts-Hopko & Glynn-Milley, 2009).

Physiology

Aqueous humor flows between the iris and the lens, nourishing the cornea and lens. Most (90%) of the fluid then flows out of the anterior chamber, draining through the spongy trabecular meshwork into the canal of Schlemm and

CHART 58-5 ⚠️ *Risk Factors for Glaucoma*

- Family history of glaucoma
- Thin cornea
- African American race
- Older age
- Diabetes mellitus
- Cardiovascular disease
- Migraine syndromes
- Nearsightedness (myopia)
- Eye trauma
- Prolonged use of topical or systemic corticosteroids

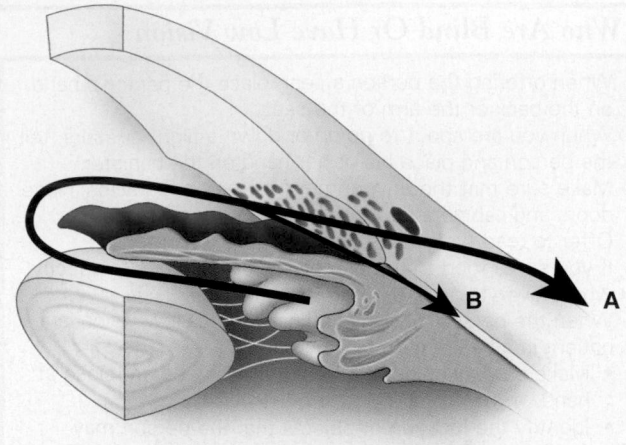

Figure 58-7 Normal outflow of aqueous humor. **A,** Trabecular meshwork. **B,** Uveoscleral route. From Kanski, J. J. (2007). *Clinical ophthalmology.* Oxford: Butterworth-Heinemann.

the episcleral veins (Fig. 58-7). About 10% of the aqueous fluid exits through the ciliary body into the suprachoroidal space and then drains into the venous circulation of the ciliary body, choroid, and sclera. Unimpeded outflow of aqueous fluid depends on an intact drainage system and an open angle (about 45 degrees) between the iris and the cornea. A narrower angle places the iris closer to the trabecular meshwork, diminishing the angle. The amount of aqueous humor produced tends to decrease with age, in systemic diseases such as diabetes, and in ocular inflammatory conditions.

IOP is determined by the rate of aqueous production, the resistance encountered by the aqueous humor as it flows out of the passages, and the venous pressure of the episcleral veins that drain into the anterior ciliary vein. When aqueous fluid production and drainage are in balance, the IOP is between 10 and 21 mm Hg. When aqueous fluid is inhibited from flowing out, pressure builds up within the eye. Fluctuations in IOP occur with time of day, exertion, diet, and medications. IOP tends to increase with blinking, tight lid squeezing, and upward gazing. Systemic conditions such as diabetes and intraocular conditions such as uveitis and retinal detachment have been associated with elevated IOP. Glaucoma may not be recognized in people with thin corneas because measurement of the IOP may be falsely low as a result of this thinness (Bressler, et al., 2008).

Pathophysiology

There are two accepted theories regarding how increased IOP damages the optic nerve in glaucoma. The direct mechanical theory suggests that high IOP damages the retinal layer as it passes through the optic nerve head. The indirect ischemic theory suggests that high IOP compresses the microcirculation in the optic nerve head, resulting in cell injury and death. Some glaucomas appear as exclusively mechanical, and some are exclusively ischemic types. Typically, most cases are a combination of both. Regardless of the cause of damage, glaucomatous changes typically evolve through clearly discernible stages (Chart 58-6).

Chart 58-6 • *Stages of Glaucoma*

1. **Initiating events.** Precipitating factors include illness, emotional stress, congenital narrow angles, long-term use of corticosteroids, and use of mydriatics (ie, medications causing pupillary dilation). These events may lead to the second stage.
2. **Structural alterations in the aqueous outflow system.** Tissue and cellular changes caused by factors that affect aqueous humor dynamics lead to structural alterations and may lead to the third stage.
3. **Functional alterations.** Conditions such as increased intraocular pressure or impaired blood flow create functional changes that may lead to the fourth stage.
4. **Optic nerve damage.** Atrophy of the optic nerve is characterized by loss of nerve fibers and blood supply. This fourth stage inevitably progresses to the fifth stage.
5. **Visual loss.** Progressive loss of vision is characterized by visual field defects.

Classification of Glaucoma

There are several types of glaucoma. Although glaucoma classification is changing as knowledge increases, current clinical forms of glaucoma are identified as open-angle glaucoma, angle-closure glaucoma (also called pupillary block), congenital glaucoma, and glaucoma associated with other conditions, such as developmental anomalies or corticosteroid use. Glaucoma can be primary or secondary, depending on whether associated factors contribute to the rise in IOP. The two common clinical forms of glaucoma encountered in adults are primary open-angle glaucoma (POAG) and angle-closure glaucoma, which are differentiated by the mechanisms that cause impaired aqueous outflow. Table 58-3 summarizes the characteristics of the different types of open-angle and angle-closure glaucoma.

Clinical Manifestations

Glaucoma is often called the "silent thief of sight" because most patients are unaware that they have the disease until they have experienced visual changes and vision loss. The patient may not seek health care until he or she experiences blurred vision or "halos" around lights, difficulty focusing, difficulty adjusting eyes in low lighting, loss of peripheral vision, aching or discomfort around the eyes, and headache.

Assessment and Diagnostic Findings

The purpose of a glaucoma workup is to establish the diagnostic category, assess the optic nerve damage, and formulate a treatment plan. The patient's ocular and medical history must be detailed to investigate the history of predisposing factors. Four major types of examinations are used in glaucoma evaluation, diagnosis, and management: tonometry to measure the IOP, ophthalmoscopy to inspect the optic nerve, gonioscopy to examine the filtration angle of the anterior chamber, and perimetry to assess the visual fields.

The changes in the optic nerve related to glaucoma are pallor and cupping of the optic nerve disc. The pallor of the optic nerve is caused by a lack of blood supply that results from cellular destruction. Cupping is characterized by exaggerated bending of the blood vessels as they cross the optic

Table 58-3	GLAUCOMA TYPES, CLINICAL MANIFESTATION, AND TREATMENT	
Types of Glaucoma	**Clinical Manifestations**	**Treatment**
Open-Angle Glaucoma		
Usually bilateral, but one eye may be more severely affected than the other. In all three types of open-angle glaucoma, the anterior chamber angle is open and appears normal.		
Primary open-angle glaucoma (POAG)	Optic nerve damage, visual field defects, IOP >21 mm Hg. May have fluctuating IOPs. Usually no symptoms but possible ocular pain, headache, and halos.	Decrease IOP 20% to 50%. Additional topical and oral agents added as necessary. If medical treatment is unsuccessful, laser trabeculoplasty (LT) can decrease intraocular pressure by 20%. Glaucoma filtering surgery if continued optic nerve damage despite medication therapy and LT.
Normal tension glaucoma	IOP ≤21 mm Hg. Optic nerve damage, visual field defects.	Treatment similar to POAG, however, the best management for normal tension glaucoma management is yet to be established. Goal is to lower the IOP by at least 30%.
Ocular hypertension	Elevated IOP. Possible ocular pain or headache.	Decrease IOP by at least 20%.
Angle-Closure (Pupillary Block) Glaucoma		
Obstruction in aqueous humor outflow due to the complete or partial closure of the angle from the forward shift of the peripheral iris to the trabecula. The obstruction results in an increased IOP.		
Acute angle-closure glaucoma (AACG)	Rapidly progressive visual impairment, periocular pain, conjunctival hyperemia, and congestion. Pain may be associated with nausea, vomiting, bradycardia, and profuse sweating. Reduced central visual acuity, severely elevated IOP, corneal edema. Pupil is vertically oval, fixed in a semidilated position, and unreactive to light and accommodation.	Ocular emergency; administration of hyperosmotics, azetazolamide, and topical ocular hypotensive agents, such as pilocarpine and beta-blockers (betaxolol). Possible laser incision in the iris (iridotomy) to release blocked aqueous and reduce IOP. Other eye is also treated with pilocarpine eye drops and/or surgical management to avoid a similar spontaneous attack.
Subacute angle-closure glaucoma	Transient blurring of vision, halos around lights; temporal headaches and/or ocular pain; pupil may be semidilated.	Prophylactic peripheral laser iridotomy. Can lead to acute or chronic angle-closure glaucoma if untreated.
Chronic angle-closure glaucoma	Progression of glaucomatous cupping and significant visual field loss; IOP may be normal or elevated; ocular pain and headache.	Management similar to that for POAG: includes laser iridotomy and medications.

IOP, intraocular pressure.

disc, resulting in an enlarged optic cup that appears more basinlike compared with a normal cup. The progression of cupping in glaucoma is caused by the gradual loss of retinal nerve fibers accompanied by the loss of blood supply, resulting in increased pallor of the optic disc.

As the optic nerve damage increases, visual perception in the area is lost. The localized areas of visual loss (ie, scotomas) represent loss of retinal sensitivity and nerve fiber damage and are measured and mapped by perimetry. The results are mapped on a graph. In patients with glaucoma, the graph has a distinct pattern that is different from other ocular diseases and is useful in establishing the diagnosis. Figure 58-8 shows the progression of visual field defects caused by glaucoma.

Medical Management

The aim of all glaucoma treatment is prevention of optic nerve damage. Lifelong therapy is almost always necessary because glaucoma cannot be cured. Treatment focuses on pharmacologic therapy, laser procedures, surgery, or a combination of these approaches, all of which have potential complications and side effects. The object is to achieve the greatest benefit at the least risk, cost, and inconvenience to the patient. Although treatment cannot reverse optic nerve damage, further damage can be controlled. The goal is to maintain an IOP within a range unlikely to cause further damage.

The initial target for IOP among patients with elevated IOP and those with low-tension glaucoma with progressive visual field loss is typically set at 30% lower than the current pressure. The patient is monitored for changes in the appearance of the optic nerve. If there is evidence of progressive damage, the target IOP is again lowered until the optic nerve shows stability.

Pharmacologic Therapy

Medical management of glaucoma relies on systemic and topical ocular medications that lower IOP. Periodic follow-up examinations are essential to monitor IOP, the appearance of the optic nerve, the visual fields, and side effects of medications. Therapy takes into account the patient's health and stage of glaucoma. Comfort, affordability, convenience, lifestyle, and personality are factors to consider in the patient's adherence to the medical regimen.

The patient is usually started on the lowest dose of topical medication and then advanced to increased concentrations until the desired IOP level is reached and maintained. Because of their efficacy, minimal dosing (can be used once each day), and low cost, beta-blockers are the preferred initial topical medications. One eye is treated first, with the other eye used as a control in determining the efficacy of the medication; once efficacy has been established, treatment of

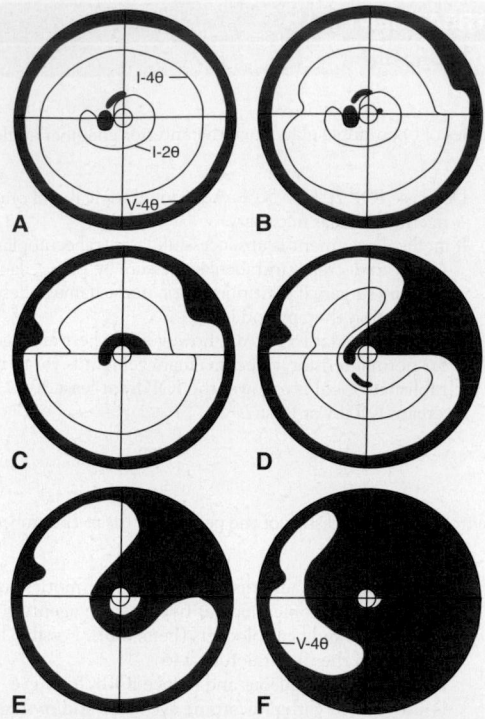

Figure 58-8 Progression of glaucomatous visual field defects. A central scotoma at 10 to 20 degrees of fixation near the blind spot is the initial significant finding **(A, B)**. As the glaucoma progresses, the scotomas enlarge and deepen, resulting in peripheral vision loss. **C,** Defect within 5 degrees of fixation point nasally. **D,** Peripheral involvement enlarges. **E,** Ringlike scotoma. **F,** Eventually, vision is lost. The resulting "island of vision" becomes the characteristic visual field appearance of glaucoma and correlates with the "tunnel vision," in which peripheral vision is lost. From Kanski, J. J. (2007). *Clinical ophthalmology.* Oxford: Butterworth-Heinemann.

the other eye is started. If the IOP is elevated in both eyes, both are treated. When results are not satisfactory, a new medication is substituted. The main markers of the efficacy of the medication in glaucoma control are lowering of the IOP to the target pressure, appearance of the optic nerve head, and the visual field.

Several types of ocular medications are used to treat glaucoma (Table 58-4), including **miotics** (medications that cause pupillary constriction), adrenergic agonists (ie, sympathomimetic agents), beta-blockers, alpha$_2$-agonists (ie, adrenergic agents), carbonic anhydrase inhibitors, and prostaglandins. Cholinergics (ie, miotics) increase the outflow of the aqueous humor by affecting ciliary muscle contraction and pupil constriction, allowing flow through a larger opening between the iris and the trabecular meshwork. Adrenergic agonists increase aqueous outflow but primarily decrease aqueous production with an action similar to beta-blockers and carbonic anhydrase inhibitors. Prostaglandin analogues reduce IOP by increasing aqueous humor outflow. They can be used once daily and do not affect pupil size.

Surgical Management

In *laser trabeculoplasty* for glaucoma, laser burns are applied to the inner surface of the trabecular meshwork to open the intratrabecular spaces and widen the canal of Schlemm, thereby promoting outflow of aqueous humor and decreasing IOP. The procedure is indicated when IOP is inadequately controlled by medications, and it is contraindicated when the trabecular meshwork cannot be fully visualized because of narrow angles. A serious complication of this procedure is a transient increase in IOP (usually 2 hours after surgery) that may become persistent. IOP assessment in the immediate postoperative period is essential.

In *laser iridotomy* for pupillary block glaucoma, an opening is made in the iris to eliminate the pupillary block. Laser iridotomy is contraindicated in patients with corneal edema, which interferes with laser targeting and strength. Potential complications are burns to the cornea, lens, or retina; transient elevated IOP; closure of the iridotomy; uveitis; and blurring. Pilocarpine (Pilocar) is usually prescribed to prevent closure of the iridotomy.

Filtering procedures for chronic glaucoma are used to create an opening or fistula in the trabecular meshwork to drain aqueous humor from the anterior chamber to the subconjunctival space into a bleb (fluid collection on the outside of the eye), thereby bypassing the usual drainage structures. This allows the aqueous humor to flow and exit by different routes (ie, absorption by the conjunctival vessels or mixing with tears). *Trabeculectomy* is the standard filtering technique used to remove part of the trabecular meshwork. Complications include hemorrhage, an extremely low (hypotony) or extremely elevated IOP, uveitis, cataracts, bleb failure, bleb leak, and endophthalmitis. Unlike other surgical procedures, the goal of the filtering procedure is to achieve incomplete healing of the surgical wound. The outflow of aqueous humor in a newly created drainage fistula is circumvented by the granulation of fibrovascular tissue or scar tissue formation on the surgical site. Scarring is inhibited by using antifibrosis agents such as the antimetabolites fluorouracil (Efudex) and mitomycin (Mutamycin). Like all antineoplastic agents, they require special handling procedures before, during, and after the procedure. Fluorouracil can be administered intraoperatively and by subconjunctival injection during follow-up; mitomycin is much more potent and is administered only intraoperatively.

Drainage implants or *shunts* are open tubes implanted in the anterior chamber to shunt aqueous humor to the episcleral plate in the conjunctival space. These implants are used when failure has occurred with one or more trabeculectomies in which antifibrotic agents were used. A fibrous capsule develops around the episcleral plate and filters the aqueous humor, thereby regulating the outflow and controlling IOP.

Trabectome surgery is reserved for patients in whom pharmacologic treatment and/or laser trabeculoplasty do not control the IOP sufficiently (Filippopoulos & Rhee, 2008). This minimally invasive procedure is specifically designed to improve fluid drainage from the eye to balance IOP. By restoring the eye's natural fluid balance, trabectome surgery stabilizes the optic nerve and minimizes further visual field damage. The surgery is performed through a small incision and does not require creation of a permanent hole in the eye wall or an external filtering bleb or an implant.

	MEDICATIONS USED IN THE MANAGEMENT OF GLAUCOMA		
Medication	**Action**	**Side Effects**	**Nursing Implications**
Cholinergics (miotics) (pilocarpine, carbachol)	Increases aqueous fluid outflow by contracting the ciliary muscle and causing miosis (constriction of the pupil) and opening of trabecular meshwork	Periorbital pain, blurry vision, difficulty seeing in the dark	Caution patients about diminished vision in dimly lit areas.
Adrenergic agonists (dipivefrin, epinephrine)	Reduces production of aqueous humor and increases outflow	Eye redness and burning; can have systemic effects, including palpitations, elevated blood pressure, tremor, headaches, and anxiety	Teach patients punctal occlusion to limit systemic effects (described in Chart 58-13).
Beta-blockers (betaxolol, timolol)	Decreases aqueous humor production	Can have systemic effects, including bradycardia, exacerbation of pulmonary disease, and hypotension	Contraindicated in patients with asthma, chronic obstructive pulmonary disease, second- or third-degree heart block, bradycardia, or cardiac failure; teach patients punctal occlusion to limit systemic effects.
Alpha-adrenergic agonists (apraclonidine, brimonidine)	Decreases aqueous humor production	Eye redness, dry mouth and nasal passages	Teach patients punctal occlusion to limit systemic effects.
Carbonic anhydrase inhibitors (acetazolamide, methazolamide, dorzolamide)	Decreases aqueous humor production	Oral medications (acetazolamide and methazolamide) associated with serious side effects, including anaphylactic reactions, electrolyte loss, depression, lethargy, gastrointestinal upset, impotence, and weight loss; side effects of topical form (dorzolamide) include topical allergy	Do not administer to patients with sulfa allergies; monitor electrolyte levels.
Prostaglandin analogs (latanoprost, bimatoprost)	Increases uveoscleral outflow	Darkening of the iris, conjunctival redness, possible rash	Instruct patients to report any side effects.

Nursing Management

Promoting Home and Community-Based Care

Teaching Patients Self-Care

The medical and surgical management of glaucoma slows the progression of glaucoma but does not cure it. The life-long therapeutic regimen mandates patient education. The nature of the disease and the importance of strict adherence to the medication regimen must be included in a teaching plan to help ensure compliance. A thorough discussion of the medication program, particularly the interactions of glaucoma-control medications with other medications, is essential. For example, the diuretic effect of acetazolamide (Diamox) has an additive effect on the diuretic effects of other antihypertensive medications and can result in hypokalemia. The effects of glaucoma-control medications on vision must also be explained. Miotics and sympathomimetics result in altered focus; therefore, patients need to be cautious in navigating their surroundings. Information about instilling ocular medication and preventing systemic absorption with punctal occlusion is given in the section of this chapter on ophthalmic medications.

Nurses in all settings encounter patients with glaucoma. Even patients with long-standing disease and those with glaucoma as a secondary diagnosis should be assessed for knowledge level and compliance with the therapeutic regimen. Chart 58-7 contains points to review with patients with glaucoma.

CHART 58-7 PATIENT EDUCATION
Managing Glaucoma

- Know your intraocular pressure (IOP) measurement and the desired range.
- Be informed about the extent of your vision loss and optic nerve damage.
- Keep a record of your eye pressure measurements and visual field test results to monitor your own progress.
- Review all your medications (including over-the-counter and herbal medications) with your ophthalmologist, and mention any side effects each time you visit.
- Ask about potential side effects and drug interactions of your eye medications.
- Ask whether generic or less costly forms of your eye medications are available.
- Review the dosing schedule with your ophthalmologist and inform him or her if you have trouble following the schedule.
- Participate in the decision-making process. Let your doctor know what dosing schedule works for you and other preferences regarding your eye care.
- Have the nurse observe you instilling eye medication to determine whether you are administering it properly.
- Be aware that glaucoma medications can cause adverse effects if used inappropriately. Eye drops are to be administered as prescribed, not when eyes feel irritated.
- Ask your ophthalmologist to send a report to your doctor after each appointment.
- Keep all follow-up appointments.

Continuing Care

For the patient with severe glaucoma and impaired function, referral to services that assist the patient in performing ADLs may be needed. The loss of peripheral vision impairs mobility the most. These patients need to be referred for low vision and rehabilitation services. Patients who meet the criteria for legal blindness should be offered referrals to agencies that can assist them in obtaining federal assistance.

Reassurance and emotional support are important aspects of care. A lifelong disease involving possible loss of sight has psychological, physical, social, and vocational ramifications. The family must be integrated into the plan of care, and because the disease has a familial tendency, family members should be encouraged to undergo examinations at least once every 2 years to detect glaucoma early.

Cataracts

A cataract is a lens opacity or cloudiness (Fig. 58-9). Cataracts rank behind only arthritis and heart disease as a leading cause of disability in older adults. Cataracts affect nearly 20.5 million Americans who are 40 years of age or older, or about one in six people in this age range. By 80 years of age, more than half of all Americans have cataracts. According to the World Health Organization, cataract is the leading cause of blindness in the world (Prevent Blindness America, 2008).

Pathophysiology

Cataracts can develop in one or both eyes at any age as a result of a variety of causes (Chart 58-8). Cigarette smoking, long-term use of corticosteroids, especially at high doses, sunlight and ionizing radiation, diabetes, obesity, and eye

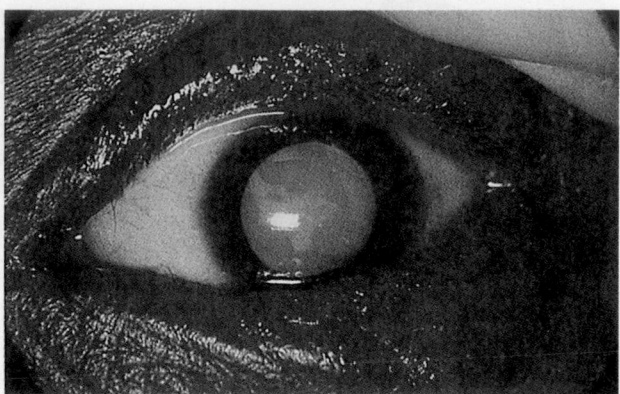

Figure 58-9 A cataract is a cloudy or opaque lens. On visual inspection, the lens appears gray or milky. From Rubin, E., Gorstein, F., Rubin, R., et al. (2005). *Pathology* (4th ed.). Philadelphia: Lippincott Williams & Wilkins.

injuries can increase the risk of cataracts. Recent studies have linked cataract risk to lower income and educational level, smoking for 35 or more pack-years, and high triglyceride levels in men (Klein, Klein, Lee, et al., 2003). The three most common types of senile (age-related) cataracts are defined by their location in the lens: nuclear, cortical, and posterior subcapsular. The extent of visual impairment depends on their size, density, and location in the lens. More than one type can be present in one eye.

A nuclear cataract is caused by central opacity in the lens and has a substantial genetic component. It is associated with myopia (ie, nearsightedness), which worsens when the cataract progresses. If dense, the cataract severely blurs vision. Periodic changes in prescription eyeglasses help manage this condition.

CHART 58-8   Risk Factors for Cataract Formation

Aging

- Loss of lens transparency
- Clumping or aggregation of lens protein (which leads to light scattering)
- Accumulation of a yellow-brown pigment due to the breakdown of lens protein
- Decreased oxygen uptake
- Increase in sodium and calcium
- Decrease in levels of vitamin C, protein, and glutathione (an antioxidant)

Associated Ocular Conditions

- Retinitis pigmentosa
- Myopia
- Retinal detachment and retinal surgery
- Infection (eg, herpes zoster, uveitis)

Toxic Factors

- Corticosteroids, especially at high doses and in long-term use
- Alkaline chemical eye burns, poisoning
- Cigarette smoking

- Calcium, copper, iron, gold, silver, and mercury, which tend to deposit in the pupillary area of the lens

Nutritional Factors

- Reduced levels of antioxidants
- Poor nutrition
- Obesity

Physical Factors

- Dehydration associated with chronic diarrhea, use of purgatives in anorexia nervosa, and use of hyperbaric oxygenation
- Blunt trauma, perforation of the lens with a sharp object or foreign body, electric shock
- Ultraviolet radiation in sunlight and x-ray

Systemic Diseases and Syndromes

- Diabetes mellitus
- Down syndrome
- Disorders related to lipid metabolism
- Renal disorders
- Musculoskeletal disorders

A cortical cataract involves the anterior, posterior, or equatorial cortex of the lens. A cataract in the equator or periphery of the cortex does not interfere with the passage of light through the center of the lens and has little effect on vision. Cortical cataracts progress at a highly variable rate. Vision is worse in very bright light. People with the highest levels of sunlight exposure have twice the risk of developing cortical cataracts as those with low-level sunlight exposure.

Posterior subcapsular cataracts occur in front of the posterior capsule. This type typically develops in younger people and, in some cases, is associated with prolonged corticosteroid use, diabetes, or ocular trauma. Near vision is diminished, and the eye is increasingly sensitive to glare from bright light (eg, sunlight, headlights). Caucasians are more likely to develop nuclear and posterior subcapsular cataracts, whereas cortical cataracts are more prevalent among African Americans.

Clinical Manifestations

Painless, blurry vision is characteristic of cataracts. The person perceives that surroundings are dimmer, as if his or her glasses need cleaning. Light scattering is common, and the person experiences reduced contrast sensitivity, sensitivity to glare, and reduced visual acuity. Other effects include myopic shift (return of ability to do close work [eg, reading fine print] without eyeglasses), astigmatism, monocular **diplopia** (double vision), color shift (the aging lens become progressively more absorbent at the blue end of the spectrum), brunescens (color values shift to yellow-brown), and reduced light transmission.

Assessment and Diagnostic Findings

Decreased visual acuity is directly proportionate to cataract density. The Snellen visual acuity test, ophthalmoscopy, and slit-lamp biomicroscopic examination are used to establish the degree of cataract formation. The degree of lens opacity does not always correlate with the patient's functional status. Some patients can perform normal activities despite clinically significant cataracts. Others with less lens opacification have a disproportionate decrease in visual acuity; hence, visual acuity is an imperfect measure of visual impairment.

Medical Management

No nonsurgical (medications, eyedrops, eyeglasses) treatment cures cataracts or prevents age-related cataracts. Results from the Age-Related Eye Disease Study Research Group (2001b), a randomized, placebo-controlled trial, found no benefit from antioxidant supplements, vitamins C and E, beta-carotene, and selenium. Results of studies that have attempted to determine the possible benefit of a once-a-day multivitamin supplement to prevent or delay the onset of cataracts have been mixed. (Clinical Trial of Nutritional Supplements and Age-Related Cataract Study Group, 2008). In the early stages of cataract development, glasses, contact lenses, strong bifocals, or magnifying lenses may improve vision.

Surgical Management

In general, if reduced vision from cataract does not interfere with normal activities, surgery may not be needed. In deciding when cataract surgery is to be performed, the patient's functional and visual status should be a primary consideration. Surgery is performed on an outpatient basis and usually takes less than 1 hour, with the patient being discharged in 30 minutes or less afterward. Although complications from cataract surgery are uncommon, they can have significant effects on vision (Table 58-5). Restoration of visual function through a safe and minimally invasive procedure is the surgical goal, which is achieved with advances in topical anesthesia, smaller wound incision (ie, clear cornea incision), and lens design (ie, foldable and more accurate intraocular lens measurements).

Injection-free topical and intraocular anesthesia, such as 1% lidocaine gel applied to the surface of the eye, eliminates the hazards of regional (retrobulbar and peribulbar) anesthesia, such as ocular perforation, retrobulbar hemorrhage, optic injuries, diplopia, and ptosis, and is ideal for patients receiving anticoagulants. Furthermore, patients can communicate and cooperate during surgery. Intravenous (IV) moderate sedation may be used to minimize anxiety and discomfort.

When both eyes have cataracts, one eye is treated first, with at least several weeks, preferably months, separating the two procedures. Because cataract surgery is performed to improve visual functioning, the delay for the other eye gives time for the patient and the surgeon to evaluate whether the results from the first surgery are adequate to preclude the need for a second operation. The delay also provides time for the first eye to recover; if there are any complications, the surgeon may decide to perform the second procedure differently.

Phacoemulsification

In this method of extracapsular cataract surgery, a portion of the anterior capsule is removed, allowing extraction of the lens nucleus and cortex while the posterior capsule and zonular support are left intact. An ultrasonic device is used to liquefy the nucleus and cortex, which are then suctioned out through a tube. An intact zonular–capsular diaphragm provides the needed safe anchor for the posterior chamber intraocular lens (IOL). After the pupil has been dilated and the surgeon has made a small incision on the upper edge of the cornea, a viscoelastic substance (clear gel) is injected into the space between the cornea and the lens. This prevents the space from collapsing and facilitates insertion of the IOL. Because the incision is smaller than the manual extracapsular cataract extraction, the wound heals more rapidly, and there is early stabilization of refractive error and less astigmatism. New phaco needles that are used to cut and aspirate the cataract permit safe and efficient removal of nearly all cataracts through a clear cornea incision (Hoffman, Fine & Packer, 2005). With increasing frequency, self-sealing (sutureless) clear corneal incisions in the temporal part of the cornea are performed with phacoemulsification, minimizing postoperative astigmatism and thus decreasing bleeding and subconjunctival hemorrhage while speeding recovery of visual acuity.

Lens Replacement

After removal of the crystalline lens, the patient is referred to as *aphakic* (ie, without lens). The lens, which focuses light on the retina, must be replaced for the patient to see clearly. There are three lens replacement options: aphakic eyeglasses, contact lenses, and IOL implants.

Aphakic glasses, although effective, are rarely used. Objects are magnified by 25%, making them appear closer than

Table 58-5   POTENTIAL COMPLICATIONS OF CATARACT SURGERY

Complication	Effects	Management and Outcome
Immediate Preoperative		
Retrobulbar hemorrhage: can result from retrobulbar infiltration of anesthetic agents if the short ciliary artery is located by the injectia	Increased IOP, proptosis, lid tightness, and subconjunctival hemorrhage with or without edema	Emergent lateral canthotomy (slitting of the canthus) is performed to stop central retinal perfusion when the IOP is dangerously elevated. If this procedure fails to reduce IOP, a puncture of the anterior chamber with removal of fluid is considered. The patient must be closely monitored for at least a few hours. Postponement of cataract surgery for 2 to 4 weeks is advised. Complications such as iris prolapse, vitreous loss, and choroidal hemorrhage could result in a catastrophic visual outcome.
Intraoperative Complications		
Rupture of the posterior capsule	May result in loss of vitreous	Anterior vitrectomy is required if vitreous loss occurs.
Suprachoroidal (expulsive) hemorrhage: profuse bleeding into the suprachoroidal space	Extrusion of intraocular contents from the eye or opposition of retinal surfaces	Closure of the incision and administration of a hyperosmotic agent to reduce IOP or corticosteroids to reduce intraocular inflammation. Vitrectomy is performed 1 to 2 weeks later. Visual prognosis is poor; some useful vision may be salvaged on rare occasions.
Early Postoperative Complications		
Acute bacterial endophthalmitis: devastating complication that occurs in about 1 in 1000 cases; the most common causative organisms are *Staphylococcus epidermidis*, *S. aureus*, *Pseudomonas* and *Proteus* species	Characterized by marked visual loss, pain, lid edema, hypopyon, corneal haze, and chemosis	Managed by aggressive antibiotic therapy. Broad-spectrum antibiotics are administered while awaiting culture and sensitivity results. Once results are obtained, the appropriate antibiotics are administered via intravitreal injection. Corticosteroid therapy is also administered.
Toxic anterior segment syndrome: non-infectious inflammation that is a complication of anterior chamber surgery; caused by a toxic agent such as an agent used to sterilize surgical instruments	Corneal edema occurs less than 24 hours after surgery; symptoms include reduced visual acuity and pain	If there is no growth of microorganisms, the treatment is topical steroids alone.
Late Postoperative Complications		
Suture-related problems	Toxic reactions or mechanical injury from broken or loose sutures	Suture removal relieves the symptoms. Topical corticosteroids are used when the incision is not healed and sutures cannot be removed.
Malposition of the IOL	Results in astigmatism, sensitivity to glare, or appearance of halos	Miotics are used for mild cases, whereas IOL removal and replacement is necessary for severe cases.
Chronic endophthalmitis	Persistent, low-grade inflammation and granuloma	Corticosteroids and antibiotics are administered systemically. If the condition persists, removal of the IOL and capsular bag, vitrectomy, and intravitreal injection of antibiotics are required.
Opacification of the posterior capsule (most common late complication of extracapsular cataract extraction)	Visual acuity is diminished	YAG laser is used to create a hole in the posterior capsule. Blurred vision is cleared immediately.

IOL, intraocular lens; IOP, intraocular pressure.

they actually are. This magnification creates distortion. Peripheral vision is also limited, and **binocular vision** (ie, ability of both eyes to focus on one object and fuse the two images into one) is impossible if the other eye is phakic (normal).

Contact lenses provide patients with almost normal vision, but because contact lenses need to be removed occasionally, the patient also needs a pair of aphakic glasses. Contact lenses are not advised for patients who have difficulty inserting, removing, and cleaning them. Frequent handling and improper disinfection increase the risk of infection.

Insertion of IOLs during cataract surgery is the usual approach to lens replacement. After cataract extraction, or phacoemulsification, the surgeon implants an IOL. Cataract extraction and posterior chamber IOLs are associated with a relatively low incidence of complications (eg, hyphema, macular edema, secondary glaucoma, damage to the corneal endothelium). IOL implantation is contraindicated in patients with recurrent uveitis, proliferative diabetic retinopathy, neovascular glaucoma, or rubeosis iridis.

The most common IOL is the single-focus lens or mono-focal IOL. Eyeglasses are still needed for distant or close vision, because the single-focus lens, unlike the natural lens of the eye, cannot alter its shape to bring objects at different distances into focus. Multifocal IOLs reduce the need for eyeglasses (near, intermediate, or far vision). Accommodative IOLs mimic the accommodative response of the youthful, phakic eye and are also known as presbyopia-correcting IOLs (Fong, 2007). A combined surgical approach using customized IOLs and refractive surgery for a customized vision correction is now proving beneficial for elderly patients (Fine, Hoffman & Packer, 2007).

Toxic Anterior Segment Syndrome

Toxic anterior segment syndrome (TASS), which is also known as toxic endothelial cell destruction or sterile endophthalmitis, is a noninfectious anterior segment inflammation caused by a toxic agent within days of an uncomplicated and uneventful cataract surgery. In recent years, TASS has emerged as a complication of increasing frequency. Investigations have shown that it may be caused by toxins from improperly rinsed surgical instruments soaked in enzymatic detergents, residue from instruments sterilized with plasma gas, abnormalities in the pH or ionic composition of irrigation solutions, ophthalmic viscoelastic devices, intraocular medications, or even the finish of the IOL (Mamalis, Edelhauser, Dawson, et al., 2006). Specific intraoperative causes have been identified such as endotoxin contamination of balanced salt solution and antibiotic ointment penetrating the anterior chamber (Holland, Morck & Lee, 2007). Decontamination and cleaning of ophthalmic instruments should follow recommended procedures, in particular use of enzymatic solutions and rinsing with copious amounts of deionized or distilled water.

TASS is characterized by corneal edema that occurs less than 24 hours after surgery, compared with classic endophthalmitis, which appears 48 to 72 hours after surgery and is bacterial in nature. Like classic endophthalmitis, the symptoms include reduction in visual acuity and pain. In the absence of micro-organism growth, improvement has occurred with topical steroid treatment alone.

Nursing Management

The patient with cataracts should receive the usual preoperative care for ambulatory surgical patients undergoing eye surgery. The standard battery of preoperative tests (eg, complete blood count, electrocardiogram, urinalysis) that were once required in all cases are prescribed only if they are indicated by the patient's medical history.

Providing Preoperative Care

It has been common practice to withhold any anticoagulant therapy (eg, aspirin, warfarin [Coumadin]) to reduce the risk of retrobulbar hemorrhage (after retrobulbar injection) for 5 to 7 days before surgery. However, a recent study showed that the risk of adverse events for patients who continued anticoagulant therapy before cataract surgery was very low (0.1% to 0.8%). The researchers speculated that regular users of aspirin or warfarin are already at higher risk for transient ischemic attacks or angina and suggest that patients may not need to discontinue these medications prior to surgery (Katz, Feldman, Bass, et al., 2003).

Dilating drops are administered every 10 minutes for four doses at least 1 hour before surgery. Additional dilating drops may be administered in the operating room (immediately before surgery). Antibiotic, corticosteroid, and anti-inflammatory drops may be administered prophylactically to prevent postoperative infection and inflammation.

Providing Postoperative Care

Before discharge, the patient receives verbal and written instructions about how to protect the eye, administer medications, recognize signs of complications, and obtain emergency care. Activities to be avoided are identified in Chart 58-9. The nurse also explains that there should be minimal discomfort after surgery and instructs the patient to take a mild analgesic agent, such as acetaminophen, as needed. Antibiotic, anti-inflammatory, and corticosteroid eye drops or ointments are prescribed postoperatively. A clinical pathway for the care of patients undergoing ambulatory cataract surgery is presented in Appendix B at the end of this textbook.

Promoting Home and Community-Based Care

Teaching Patients Self-Care

To prevent accidental rubbing or poking of the eye, the patient wears a protective eye patch for 24 hours after surgery, followed by eyeglasses worn during the day and a metal shield worn at night for 1 to 4 weeks. The nurse instructs the patient and family in applying and caring for the eye shield. Sunglasses should be worn while outdoors during the day because the eye is sensitive to light.

Slight morning discharge, some redness, and a scratchy feeling may be expected for a few days. A clean, damp washcloth may be used to remove slight morning eye discharge. Because cataract surgery increases the risk of retinal detachment, the patient must know to notify the surgeon if new floaters (dots) in vision, flashing lights, decrease in vision, pain, or increase in redness occurs.

Continuing Care

The eye patch is removed after the first follow-up appointment. The patient may experience blurring of vision for several days to weeks. Sutures, if used, are left in the eye but alter the curvature of the cornea, resulting in temporary blurring and some astigmatism. Vision gradually improves as the eye heals. Patients with IOL implants have functional vision on the first day after surgery. Vision is stabilized when the eye is completely healed, usually within 6 to 12 weeks, when final corrective prescription is completed. Visual correction may still be needed for any remaining refractive errors. Patients who choose multifocal IOLs should be aware that there may be increased night glare and contrast sensitivity.

CORNEAL DISORDERS

Corneal Dystrophies

Corneal dystrophies are inherited as autosomal dominant traits and manifest when the person is about 20 years of age. They are characterized by deposits in the corneal layers. Decreased vision is caused by the irregular corneal surface and

CHART
58-9

HOME CARE CHECKLIST
Intraocular Lens Implant

At the completion of the home care instruction, the patient or caregiver will be able to:	PATIENT	CAREGIVER
• Wear glasses or metal eye shield at all times following surgery as instructed by the physician.	✔	
• Always wash hands before touching or cleaning the postoperative eye.	✔	✔
• Clean postoperative eye with a clean tissue; wipe the closed eye with a single gesture from the inner canthus outward.	✔	✔
• Bathe or shower; shampoo hair cautiously or seek assistance.	✔	
• Avoid lying on the side of the affected eye the night after surgery.	✔	
• Keep activity light (eg, walking, reading, watching television). Resume the following activities only as directed by the physician: driving, sexual activity, unusually strenuous activity.	✔	
• Avoid lifting, pushing, or pulling objects heavier than 15 lb.	✔	
• Avoid bending or stooping for an extended period.	✔	
• Be careful when climbing or descending stairs.	✔	
• Know when to contact the physician.*	✔	✔

*Contact the physician immediately if any of the following problems occur before the next physician's appointment: (1) vision changes; (2) continuous flashing lights appear to the affected eye; (3) redness, swelling, or pain increase in the eye; (4) the amount or type of eye drainage changes; (5) the eye is injured in any way; (6) significant pain is not relieved by acetaminophen.

corneal deposits. Corneal endothelial decompensation leads to corneal edema and blurring of vision. Persistent edema leads to **bullous keratopathy** (formation of blisters that cause pain and discomfort on rupturing). This condition is usually associated with primary open-angle glaucoma.

A bandage contact lens is used to flatten the bullae, protect the exposed corneal nerve endings, and relieve discomfort. Symptomatic treatments, such as hypertonic drops or ointment (5% sodium chloride), may reduce epithelial edema; lowering the IOP also reduces stromal edema.

Keratoconus

Keratoconus is a condition characterized by a conical protuberance of the cornea with progressive thinning on protrusion and irregular astigmatism. This hereditary condition has a higher incidence among women. Onset occurs at puberty; the condition may progress for more than 20 years and is bilateral. Corneal scarring occurs in severe cases. Blurred vision is a prominent symptom. Rigid, gas-permeable contact lenses correct irregular astigmatism and improve vision. Advances in contact lens design have reduced the need for surgery. Penetrating keratoplasty is indicated when contact lens correction is no longer effective.

Corneal Surgeries

Among the surgical procedures used to treat diseased corneal tissue are phototherapeutic keratectomy, penetrating keratoplasty and corneal endothelial transplantation, and Descemet's stripping endothelial keratoplasty.

Phototherapeutic Keratectomy

Phototherapeutic keratectomy (PTK) is a laser procedure that is used to treat diseased corneal tissue by removing or reducing corneal opacities and smoothing the anterior corneal surface to improve functional vision. PTK is a safer, more effective (when indicated) alternative than penetrating or lamellar keratoplasty. PTK is contraindicated in patients with active herpetic keratitis because the ultraviolet rays may reactivate latent virus. Common side effects are induced hyperopia and stromal haze. Complications are delayed reepithelization (particularly in patients with diabetes) and bacterial keratitis. Postoperative management consists of oral analgesics for eye pain. Reepithelization is promoted with a pressure patch or therapeutic soft contact lens. Antibiotic and corticosteroid ointments and nonsteroidal anti-inflammatory agents (NSAIDs) are prescribed postoperatively. Follow-up examinations are required for up to 2 years.

Penetrating Keratoplasty

Penetrating keratoplasty (PKP; corneal transplantation or corneal grafting) involves replacing abnormal host tissue with healthy donor (cadaver) corneal tissue. Common indications are keratoconus, corneal dystrophy, corneal scarring from herpes simplex keratitis, and chemical burns.

Several factors affect the success of the graft: the condition of the ocular structures (eg, lids, conjunctiva), quality of the tears, adequacy of blinking, and viability of the donor endothelium. Tissue that is typically not used for grafting (Chart 58-10) includes tissue that may be the source of disease transmission from donor to recipient; corneas with functionally compromised endothelium; and corneas from donors who have undergone LASIK, because the cornea is no longer intact. Conditions such as glaucoma, retinal

Chart 58-10 • *Contraindications to the Use of Donor Tissue for Corneal Transplantation: Donor Characteristics*

Systemic Disorders

- Death from unknown cause
- Creutzfeldt-Jacob disease
- AIDS or high risk for HIV infection
- Hepatitis
- Eye infection, systemic infection

Intrinsic Eye Disease

- Retinoblastoma
- Ocular inflammation
- Malignant tumors of anterior segment
- Disorders of the conjunctiva or corneal surface involving the optical zone of the cornea

Other

- History of eye trauma
- Corneal scars
- Previous surgical procedure
- Corneal graft
- LASIK eye surgery

disease, and **strabismus** (deviation in ocular alignment) can negatively affect the outcome.

In PKP, the surgeon determines the graft size before the procedure, and the appropriate size is marked on the surface of the cornea. The surgeon prepares the donor cornea and the recipient bed, removes the diseased cornea, places the donor cornea on the recipient bed, and sutures it in place. Sutures remain in place for 12 to 18 months and are then removed. Potential complications include early graft failure due to poor quality of donor tissue, surgical trauma, acute infection, and persistently increased IOP and late graft failure due to rejection.

Postoperatively, the patient receives **mydriatics** (medications causing pupillary dilation) for 2 weeks and topical corticosteroids for 12 months (daily doses for 6 months and tapered doses thereafter). These mydriatics and corticosteroid drops should be preservative free to prevent a reactive inflammation. Patients typically describe a sensation of postoperative eye discomfort rather than acute pain.

Descemet's Stripping Endothelial Keratoplasty

For the past 50 years, PKP has been the standard of care for patients with corneal endothelial failure but with poor refractive results. Recently, a technique known as Descemet's stripping endothelial keratoplasty (DSEK) has been developed. Layers of the cornea are dissected and selectively replaced by donor cornea tissue. DSEK offers several advantages such as less postoperative astigmatism, faster visual recovery, and stronger wound integrity. Theoretically, the risk of rejection is less because less of the patient's tissue is replaced.

Nursing Management

For corneal surgeries, the nurse reinforces the surgeon's recommendations and instructions regarding visual rehabilitation and visual improvement. A technically successful graft may initially produce disappointing results because the procedure has produced a new optical surface. Only after several months do patients start seeing the natural and true colors of their environment. Correction of a resultant refractive error with eyeglasses or contact lenses determines the final visual outcome. The nurse assesses the patient's support system and his or her ability to comply with long-term follow-up, which includes frequent clinic visits for several months for tapering of topical corticosteroid therapy, selective suture removal, and ongoing evaluation of the graft site and visual acuity. The nurse also initiates appropriate referrals to community services when indicated.

Because graft failure is an ophthalmic emergency that can occur at any time, the primary goal of nursing care is to teach the patient to identify signs and symptoms of graft failure. The early symptoms are blurred vision, discomfort, tearing, or redness of the eye. Decreased vision results after graft destruction. The patient must contact the ophthalmologist as soon as symptoms occur. Treatment of graft rejection involves prompt administration of hourly topical corticosteroids and periocular corticosteroid injections. Systemic immunosuppressive agents may be necessary for severe, resistant cases.

In DSEK, the nurse keeps the patient in a supine position postoperatively for 1 hour and instructs the patient to remain supine until the first postoperative day (Pramanik, Goins & Sutphin, 2007). Patients are maintained on low-dose topical corticosteroids indefinitely (Price & Price, 2007).

Refractive Surgeries

Refractive surgeries are cosmetic, elective procedures performed to recontour corneal tissue and correct refractive errors so that eyeglasses or contact lenses are no longer needed. Both photorefractive keratectomy (PRK) and LASIK use an excimer laser (193-nm wavelength argon fluoride laser), which can evaporate corneal tissue very cleanly with almost no damage to the epithelial cells. Newer excimer lasers have a smaller spot size, a robust tracking system for eye movements, and wavefront custom ablation technology. These advances have minimized or eliminated aberrations induced by conventional laser vision correction as well as preexisting aberrations; they have improved treatment accuracy and therefore have provided for better vision, including the reduction of postoperative night vision problems.

Laser vision correction alters the major optical function of the eye and thereby carries certain surgical risks. The patient must fully understand the benefits, potential risks and complications, common side effects, and limitations of the procedure. Refractive surgery does not alter the normal aging process of the eye. If the reason for the procedure is to meet vision requirements for the patient's occupation, the results must satisfy both the patient and the employer. Precise visual outcome cannot be guaranteed. Typically, patients must be at least 18 years of age.

The corneal structure must be normal and the refractive error must be stable. The patient is required to discontinue using contact lenses for a period before the procedure (2 to 3 weeks for soft lenses and 4 weeks for hard lenses). Patients with conditions that are likely to adversely affect corneal wound healing (eg, corticosteroid use, immunosuppression, elevated IOP) are not good candidates for the procedure.

Any superficial eye disease must be diagnosed and fully treated before a refractive procedure.

Patient satisfaction is the ultimate goal; therefore, patient education and counseling about potential risks, complications, and postoperative follow-up are critical. Minimal postoperative care includes topical corticosteroid or NSAID and antibiotic drops.

Laser Vision Correction Photorefractive Keratectomy

PRK is used to treat myopia and hyperopia with or without astigmatism. The excimer laser is applied directly to the cornea according to carefully calculated measurements. For myopia, the relative curvature is decreased; for hyperopia, the relative curvature is increased. A bandage contact lens is placed over the cornea to promote epithelial healing and reduce pain, which is similar to that of a severe corneal abrasion. The major limitations of this procedure are postoperative pain, corneal haze, and prolonged recovery of vision.

Laser-Assisted In Situ Keratomileusis

An improvement over PRK, particularly for correcting high (severe) myopia, LASIK involves flattening the anterior curvature of the cornea by removing a stromal lamella or layer. The surgeon creates a corneal flap with a microkeratome, which is an automatic corneal shaper similar to a carpenter's plane. The surgeon retracts a flap of corneal tissue less than one-third the thickness of a human hair to access the corneal stroma and then uses the excimer laser on the stromal bed to reshape the cornea according to calculated measurements (Fig. 58-10). LASIK causes less postoperative discomfort, has fewer side effects, and is safer than PRK. The patient has no corneal haze and requires less postoperative care. However, with LASIK, the cornea has been invaded at a deeper level, and any complications are more significant than those that can occur with PRK. With the increasing success and popularity of LASIK, PRK is now reserved for patients who are unsuitable for LASIK, such as people with very thin corneas.

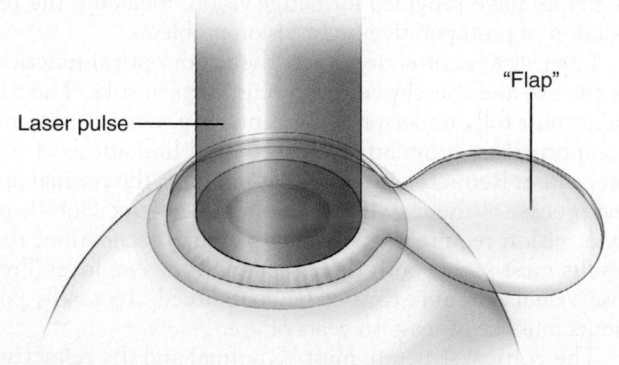

Laser pulse

"Flap"

Figure 58-10 LASIK combines delicate surgical procedures and laser treatment. A flap is surgically created and lifted to one side. A laser is then applied to the cornea to reshape it. With permission from The Wilmer Laser Vision Center, Lutherville, MD.

Perioperative Complications

Surgically Induced Abnormalities

Corneal surface irregularities can occur after LASIK treatment. These include central islands (central areas of stiffness or elevation), decentered ablations resulting from misalignment of the laser treatment or from involuntary eye movement during laser treatment, and forms of irregular astigmatism. Symptoms of central islands and decentered ablations include monocular diplopia or ghost images, halos, glare, and decreased visual acuity.

Diffuse Lamellar Keratitis

As LASIK is performed more frequently, the vision-threatening complication known as diffuse lamellar keratitis (DLK) is reported more often. DLK is a peculiar, noninfectious, inflammatory reaction in the lamellar interface after LASIK. DLK seems to be strongly associated with a decrease of contrast sensitivity up to 6 months postoperatively (Han, Wee, Lee, et al., 2007). Depending on the severity of the condition, treatment methods range from administering corticosteroid drops to intervening surgically.

Phakic Intraocular Lenses

Because the results of refractive surgery on high (severe) myopia, hyperopia, and astigmatism are less predictable, there has been increasing interest in the use of phakic IOL implantation in patients who retain their natural lens. These phakic IOLs may be used in either the anterior or posterior chamber. The implantation of such devices is reversible because the natural lens is left in place and the normal architecture of the cornea is preserved. This procedure may provide more predictable refractive results than procedures that alter the corneal curvature. Potential complications include cataract, iritis or uveitis, endothelial cell loss, and increased IOP.

Although phakic IOL implantation provides a more predictable alternative to corneal refractive surgery, more controlled, longitudinal multicenter trials are needed to evaluate its long-term safety. The design of phakic IOLs continues to improve.

Conductive Keratoplasty

A recent innovation in refractive surgery for the correction of low to mild hyperopia uses the principles of thermal keratoplasty by applying radiofrequency current to the peripheral cornea using a thin, hand-held probe. It does not involve the removal of cornea tissue. Clinical trials have shown that postprocedure visual acuity, predictability, and stability are as good as, if not better than, with other refractive procedures (Du, Fan & Asbell, 2007).

RETINAL DISORDERS

Although the retina is composed of multiple microscopic layers, the two innermost layers, the sensory retina and the retinal pigment epithelium (RPE), are the most relevant to common retinal disorders. Just as the film in a camera captures an image, so does the retina, the neural tissue of the eye. The rods and cones, the photoreceptor cells, are found

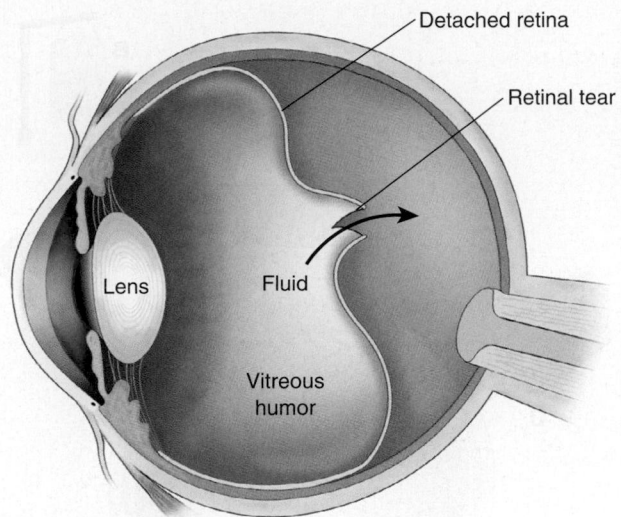

Figure 58-11 Retinal detachment.

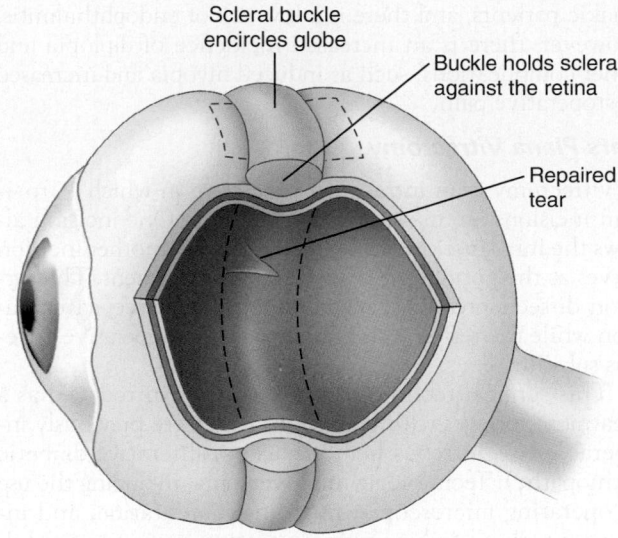

Figure 58-12 Scleral buckle.

in the sensory layer of the retina. Beneath the sensory layer lies the RPE, the pigmented layer. When the rods and cones are stimulated by light, an electrical impulse is generated, and the image is transmitted to the brain.

Retinal Detachment

Retinal detachment refers to the separation of the RPE from the sensory layer. The four types of retinal detachment are rhegmatogenous, traction, a combination of rhegmatogenous and traction, and exudative. *Rhegmatogenous detachment* is the most common form. In this condition, a hole or tear develops in the sensory retina, allowing some of the liquid vitreous to seep through the sensory retina and detach it from the RPE (Fig. 58-11). People at risk for this type of detachment include those with high myopia or **aphakia** after cataract surgery. Trauma may also play a role in rhegmatogenous retinal detachment. Between 5% and 10% of all rhegmatogenous retinal detachments are associated with proliferative retinopathy, a retinopathy associated with diabetic neovascularization (see Chapter 41).

Tension, or a pulling force, is responsible for *traction retinal detachment*. An ophthalmologist must ascertain all of the areas of retinal break and identify and release the scars or bands of fibrous material providing traction on the retina. Generally, patients with this condition have developed fibrous scar tissue from conditions such as diabetic retinopathy, vitreous hemorrhage, or the retinopathy of prematurity. The hemorrhages and fibrous proliferation associated with these conditions exert a pulling force on the delicate retina.

Patients can have both rhegmatogenous and traction retinal detachment. *Exudative retinal detachments* are the result of the production of a serous fluid under the retina from the choroid. Conditions such as uveitis and macular degeneration may cause the production of this serous fluid.

Clinical Manifestations

Patients may report the sensation of a shade or curtain coming across the vision of one eye, cobwebs, bright flashing lights, or the sudden onset of a great number of floaters. Patients do not complain of pain.

Assessment and Diagnostic Findings

After visual acuity is determined, the patient must have a dilated fundus examination using an indirect ophthalmoscope as well as slit-lamp biomicroscopy. Stereo fundus photography and fluorescein angiography are commonly used during the evaluation.

Increasingly, optical coherence tomography and ultrasound are used for the complete retinal assessment, especially if the view is obscured by a dense cataract or vitreal hemorrhage. All retinal breaks, all fibrous bands that may be causing traction on the retina, and all degenerative changes must be identified.

Surgical Management

In rhegmatogenous detachment, an attempt is made to surgically reattach the sensory retina to the RPE. In traction detachment, the source of traction must be removed and the sensory retina reattached. New surgical techniques as well as advances in instrumentation have led to an increased rate of success of surgical reattachment and better visual outcomes. The most commonly used surgical interventions are the scleral buckle, the pars plana vitrectomy, and pneumatic retinopexy. A recently developed procedure is the 25-gauge transconjunctival sutureless vitrectomy.

Scleral Buckle

The retinal surgeon compresses the sclera (often with a scleral buckle or a silicone band; Fig. 58-12) to indent the scleral wall from the outside of the eye and bring the two retinal layers in contact with each other. This type of surgery has a high success rate in the hands of experienced retinal surgeons. It causes less damage to the lens of the eye in phakic patients, and there is a low risk of endophthalmitis. However, there is an increased incidence of diplopia and other complications, such as induced myopia and increased postoperative pain.

Pars Plana Vitrectomy

A vitrectomy is an intraocular procedure in which 1- to 4-mm incisions are made at the pars plana. One incision allows the introduction of a light source, and another incision serves as the portal for the vitrectomy instrument. The surgeon dissects preretinal membranes under direct visualization while the retina is stabilized by an intraoperative vitreous substitute.

This surgical technique was originally introduced as a treatment for eyes with conditions that were previously inoperable (eg, vitreous hemorrhage, proliferative diabetic retinopathy). Technologic improvements, including the use of operating microscopes, microinstrumentation, and instruments that combine vitreous cutting, aspiration, and illumination capabilities in one device, have advanced vitreoretinal surgery. The techniques of vitreoretinal surgery can be used in various procedures, including the removal of foreign bodies, vitreous opacities such as blood, and dislocated lenses. Traction on the retina may be relieved through vitrectomy and may be combined with scleral buckling to repair retinal breaks. Treatment of macular holes includes vitrectomy, laser photocoagulation, air-fluid-gas exchanges, and the use of growth factor.

Pneumatic Retinopexy

This technique is used for the repair of a rhegmatogenous retinal detachment. It is the least invasive of the three procedures described. A gas bubble, silicone oil, or perfluorocarbon and liquids may be injected into the vitreous cavity to help push the sensory retina up against the RPE Argon laser photocoagulation or cryotherapy is also used to "spotweld" small holes.

Transconjunctival Sutureless Vitrectomy

The 25-gauge transconjunctival sutureless vitrectomy is a significant advancement in vitreoretinal surgery. Replacement of the larger 20-gauge approach with the less invasive 25-gauge technique allows for self-sealing transconjunctival pars plana sclerotomies. As a result, postoperative inflammation is decreased, thus promoting rapid wound healing and patient recovery. The 25-gauge microcannula maintains the alignment between the entry site of the conjunctiva and the sclera (Chen, 2007) (Fig. 58-13).

Complications such as hypotony and endophthalmitis may be related to the unsutured sclerotomy. However, clinical experience has shown that this sutureless system is both safe and effective with decreased surgical times, reduced postoperative inflammation, and more rapid recovery (Chen, 2007).

Nursing Management

For the most part, nursing interventions consist of educating the patient and providing supportive care. For pneumatic retinopexy, postoperative positioning of the patient is critical because the injected bubble must float into a position overlying the area of detachment, providing consistent

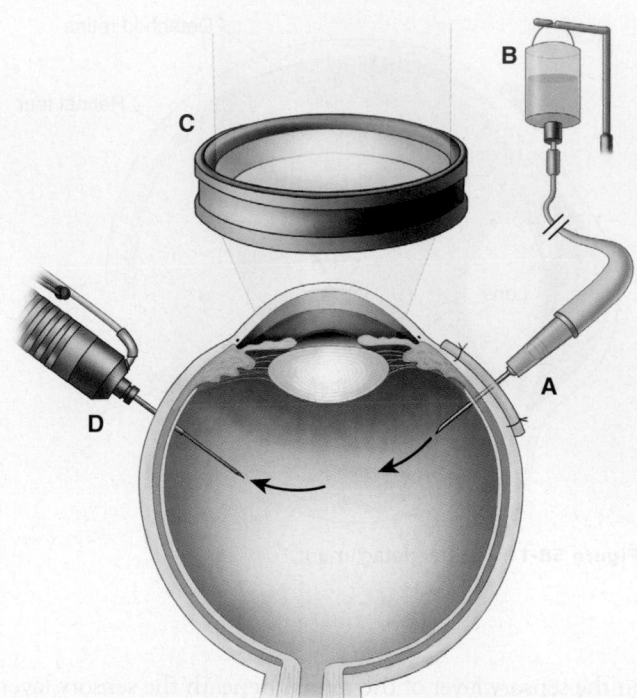

Figure 58-13 25-gauge transconjunctival sutureless vitrectomy with simultaneous suction and infusion. **A,** Infusion of fluid through a 25-gauge needle secured by passing through a block of plastic sutured to the eye. **B,** Balanced salt solution is fed into the eye by gravity. **C,** Illumination and observation are provided with the indirect ophthalmoscope. **D,** The vitreous is aspirated into the port of the sharp-tipped vitreous cutter.

pressure to reattach the sensory retina. The patient must maintain a prone position that would allow the gas bubble to act as a tamponade for the retinal break (Ross & Lavina, 2008). Patients and family members should be made aware of these special needs beforehand so that the patient can be made as comfortable as possible.

Teaching About Complications

In many cases, vitreoretinal procedures are performed on an outpatient basis, and the patient is seen the next day for a follow-up examination and closely monitored thereafter as required. Postoperative complications may include increased IOP, endophthalmitis, development of other retinal detachments, development of cataracts, and loss of turgor of the eye. Patients must be taught the signs and symptoms of complications, particularly of increasing IOP and postoperative infection. Patients should be provided with telephone numbers of members of the ophthalmic team and encouraged to call immediately if discomfort escalates.

Retinal Vascular Disorders

Loss of vision can occur from occlusion of a retinal artery or vein. Such occlusions may result from atherosclerosis, cardiac valvular disease, venous stasis, hypertension, or increased blood viscosity. Associated risk factors include diabetes mellitus, glaucoma, and aging.

Central Retinal Vein Occlusion

Blood supply to and from the ocular fundus is provided by the central retinal artery and vein. Central retinal vein occlusions (CRVOs) are relatively common and found most often in people older than 50 years of age. Patients who have suffered a CRVO report decreased visual acuity, which may range from mild blurring to vision that is severely limited.

Direct ophthalmoscopy of the retina shows optic disc swelling, venous dilation and tortuousness, retinal hemorrhages, cotton-wool spots, and a "blood and thunder" (extremely bloody) appearance of the retina. The better the initial visual acuity, the better the general prognosis.

Fluorescein angiography may show extensive areas of capillary closure. The patient should be monitored carefully over the ensuing several months for signs of neovascularization and neovascular glaucoma. Laser panretinal photocoagulation may be necessary to treat the abnormal neovascularization. Neovascularization of the iris may cause neovascular glaucoma, which may be difficult to control. Macular edema, macular nonperfusion, and vitreous hemorrhage from the neovascularization are among the potential complications of CRVO. In addition, CRVO is a significant cause of vision loss (Mohamed, McIntosh, Seang, et al., 2007).

Branch Retinal Vein Occlusion

Some patients with branch retinal vein occlusion (BRVO) are symptom free, whereas others complain of a sudden loss of vision if the macular area is involved. A more gradual loss of vision may occur if macular edema associated with BRVO develops. Studies have shown that a gridlike pattern of laser burns reduces macular edema and improves visual acuity by two or more lines on the Snellen chart (Esrick, Subramanian, Heier, et al., 2005).

On examination, the ocular fundus appears similar to that found in CRVO; however, only those portions of the retina affected by the obstructive veins have what is known as a "blood and thunder" appearance. The occlusions generally occur at the arteriovenous crossings. The diagnostic evaluation and follow-up assessments are the same as for CRVO. Potential complications are similar. Associated conditions include glaucoma, systemic hypertension, diabetes mellitus, hyperlipidemia, and hyperviscosity syndrome.

Central Retinal Artery Occlusion

Patients with central retinal artery occlusion, a relatively rare disorder that accounts for approximately 1 in 10,000 ophthalmologic visits, present with a sudden loss of vision. Visual acuity is reduced to being able to count the examiner's fingers, or the field of vision is tremendously restricted. A relative afferent pupillary defect is present. Examination of the ocular fundus reveals a pale retina with a cherry-red spot at the fovea. The retinal arteries are thin, and emboli are occasionally seen in the central retinal artery or its branches. Central retinal artery occlusion is a true ocular emergency. Various treatments are used: ocular massage, anterior chamber paracentesis, IV administration of hyperosmotic agents such as acetazolamide (Diamox), and high concentrations of oxygen. An aggressive stepwise approach may be beneficial, depending on the underlying cause of the occlusion and the amount of time from onset of occlusion to treatment. Most visual loss associated with central retinal artery occlusion is severe and permanent.

Age-Related Macular Degeneration

Age-related macular degeneration (AMD) is the most common cause of visual loss in people older than 60 years of age in developed countries (Seddon & Chen, 2004). In the United States alone, the number of cases is expected to reach almost 3 million by the year 2020 (Bressler, et al., 2008). AMD is characterized by tiny, yellowish spots called drusen (Fig. 58-14) beneath the retina. Most people older than 60 years of age have at least a few small drusen. These drusen are small clusters of debris or waste material that lie deep within the RPE. When these drusen are located in the macular area, they can affect vision. Patients with AMD have a wide range of visual loss, but most do not experience total blindness. Central vision is generally the most affected, with most patients retaining peripheral vision (Fig. 58-15). There are two types of AMD, commonly known as the dry type and wet type.

Between 85% and 90% of people with AMD have the dry (nonneovascular, nonexudative) type of the condition, in which the outer layers of the retina slowly break down (Fig. 58-16). With this breakdown comes the appearance of drusen. When the drusen occur outside of the macular area, patients generally have no symptoms. When the drusen occur within the macula, however, there is a gradual blurring of vision that patients may notice when they try to read.

The second type of AMD, the wet (neovascular, exudative) type, may have an abrupt onset. Patients report that straight lines appear crooked and distorted or that letters in words appear broken. This effect results from proliferation of abnormal blood vessels growing under the retina, within the choroid layer of the eye, a condition known as choroidal neovascularization. The affected vessels can leak fluid and blood, elevating the retina. Some patients can be treated with the argon laser to stop the leakage from these vessels. However, this treatment is not ideal because vision may be affected by the laser treatment and abnormal vessels often grow back after treatment.

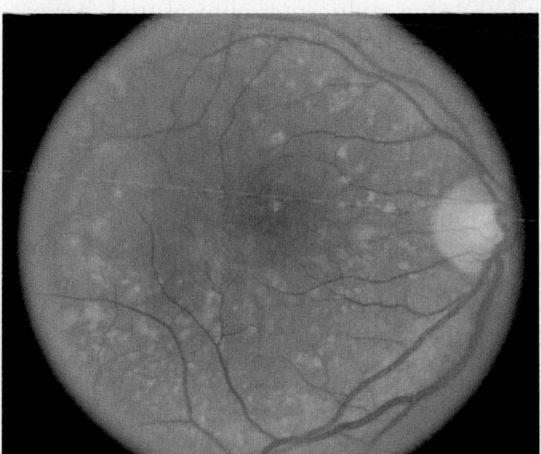

Figure 58-14 Retina showing drusen and age-related macular degeneration (AMD).

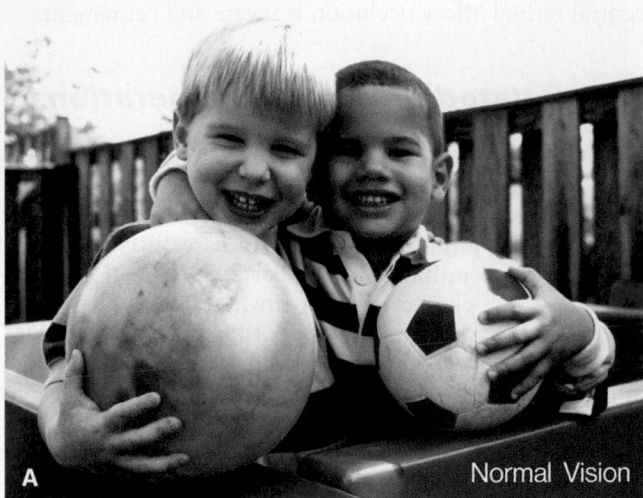

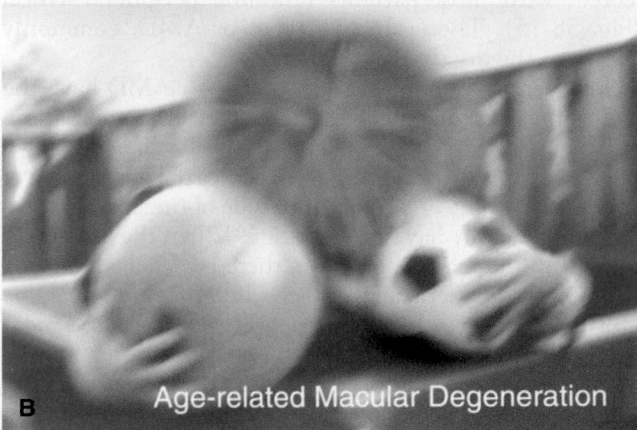

Figure 58-15 Visual loss associated with macular degeneration. **(A)** Normal vision. **(B)** Visual changes resulting from age-related macular degeneration. Photos courtesy of the National Eye Institute/National Institutes of Health.

Medical Management

There is no known cure for the dry (nonexudative, nonneovascular) type of AMD. The Age-Related Eye Disease Study (2001a), a multicenter clinical trial, has provided promising information about the prevention and treatment of AMD. The study was designed to determine whether large doses of macronutrients are effective in preventing or slowing the course of the disease. The study revealed that use of antioxidants (vitamin C, vitamin E, and beta-carotene) and minerals (zinc oxide) in megadoses can slow the progression of AMD and vision loss for people at high risk for developing advanced AMD. Research continues; the National Eye Institute (NEI) is sponsoring an ongoing clinical trial, Age-Related Eye Disease Study II (AREDS II), to study the effect of lutein and zeaxanthin (carotenoids) or fish oils in protecting the macula and preventing the progression of AMD (NEI, 2008).

Antiangiogenic Therapy

An important component of treatment of neovascular (wet, exudative) AMD targets development and progression of angiogenesis (abnormal blood vessel formation). Studies continue toward identification of agents that can be used to inhibit angiogenesis. This has implications for ocular neovascularization (Andreoli & Miller, 2007).

Vasoproliferation in exudative AMD is believed to be caused by an underlying angiogenic stimulus known as vascular endothelial growth factor (VEGF). Research has resulted in the development of agents that inhibit the development of VEGF and therefore angiogenesis. Pegaptanib sodium (Macugen), a VEGF antagonist, is designed to inhibit the ability of VEGF to bind to cellular receptors. This agent is no longer widely used because visual acuity has improved in only a limited number of patients as a result of this treatment (Jager, Mieler & Miller, 2008). Ranibizumab (Lucentis) is designed to bind and inactivate all isoforms of VEGF. Approved in 2006, it is administered by intravitreal injection once a month. Studies have shown that, on average, patients may gain one to two lines of vision on the Snellen chart after a year of treatment (Bressler, et al., 2008). This is a dramatic positive step; in the early days of photocoagulation therapy, the best that could be achieved was a slowing of visual loss that was accompanied by a treatment-related scotoma.

The monoclonal antibody bevacizumab (Avastin) has been found to be helpful in the treatment of neovascular AMD. Originally developed for the treatment of colon cancer, it has been used "off-label" by many ophthalmologists for AMD, with results that rival those of the more expensive ranibizumab.

Nursing Management

Amsler grids are given to patients to use in their homes to monitor for a sudden onset or distortion of vision. These may provide the earliest sign that macular degeneration is getting worse. Patients should be encouraged to look at these grids, one eye at a time, several times each week with glasses on. If there is a change in the grid (eg, if the lines or squares appear distorted or faded), the patient should notify the ophthalmologist immediately and should arrange to be seen promptly.

ORBITAL AND OCULAR TRAUMA

Whether affecting the eye or the orbit, trauma to the eye and surrounding structures may have devastating consequences for vision. It is preferable to prevent injury rather than treat it. Chart 58-11 details safety measures to prevent orbital and ocular trauma.

Orbital Trauma

Injury to the orbit is usually associated with a head injury; hence, the patient's general medical condition must first be stabilized before conducting an ocular examination. Only then is the globe assessed for soft tissue injury. During inspection, the face is meticulously assessed for underlying fractures, which should always be suspected in cases of blunt trauma. To establish the extent of ocular injury, visual acuity is assessed as soon as possible, even if it is only a rough

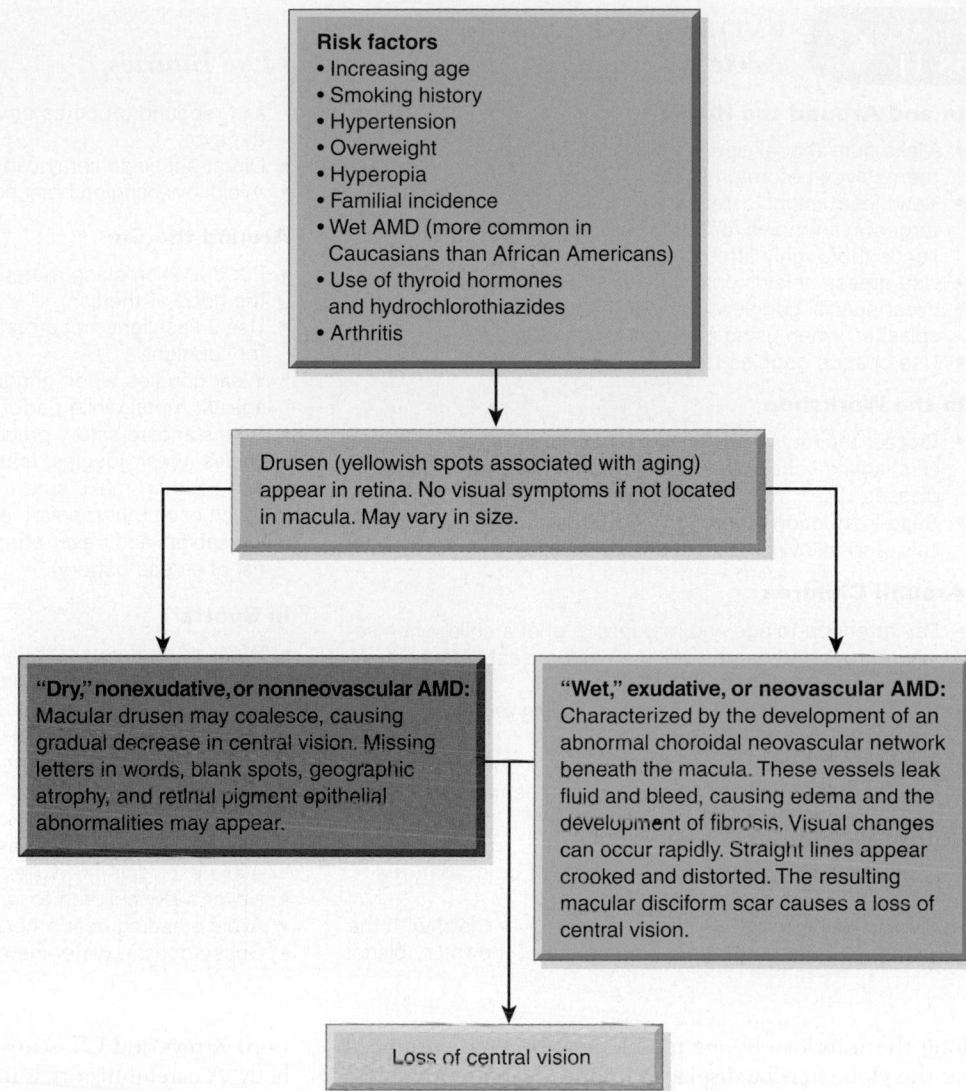

Risk factors
- Increasing age
- Smoking history
- Hypertension
- Overweight
- Hyperopia
- Familial incidence
- Wet AMD (more common in Caucasians than African Americans)
- Use of thyroid hormones and hydrochlorothiazides
- Arthritis

Drusen (yellowish spots associated with aging) appear in retina. No visual symptoms if not located in macula. May vary in size.

"Dry," nonexudative, or nonneovascular AMD: Macular drusen may coalesce, causing gradual decrease in central vision. Missing letters in words, blank spots, geographic atrophy, and retinal pigment epithelial abnormalities may appear.

"Wet," exudative, or neovascular AMD: Characterized by the development of an abnormal choroidal neovascular network beneath the macula. These vessels leak fluid and bleed, causing edema and the development of fibrosis. Visual changes can occur rapidly. Straight lines appear crooked and distorted. The resulting macular disciform scar causes a loss of central vision.

Loss of central vision

Figure 58-16 Progression of age-related macular degeneration (AMD): pathways to vision loss.

estimate. Soft tissue orbital injuries often result in damage to the optic nerve. Major ocular injuries indicated by a soft globe, prolapsing tissue, ruptured globe, and hemorrhage require immediate surgical attention.

Soft Tissue Injury and Hemorrhage

The signs and symptoms of soft tissue injury from blunt or penetrating trauma include tenderness, ecchymosis, lid swelling, **proptosis** (ie, downward displacement of the eyeball), and hemorrhage. Closed injuries lead to contusions with subconjunctival hemorrhage, commonly known as a *black eye*. Blood accumulates in the tissues of the conjunctiva. Hemorrhage may be caused by a soft tissue injury to the eyelid or by an underlying fracture.

Management of soft tissue hemorrhage that does not threaten vision is usually conservative and consists of thorough inspection, cleansing, and repair of wounds. Cold compresses are used in the early phase, followed by warm compresses. Hematomas that appear as swollen, fluctuating areas may be surgically drained or aspirated; if they are

causing significant orbital pressure, they may be surgically evacuated.

Penetrating injuries or a severe blow to the head can result in severe optic nerve damage. Visual loss can be sudden or delayed and progressive. Immediate loss of vision after an ocular injury is usually irreversible. Delayed visual loss has a better prognosis. Corticosteroid therapy is indicated to reduce optic nerve swelling. Surgery, such as optic nerve decompression, may be performed.

Orbital Fractures

Orbital fractures are detected by facial x-rays. Depending on the orbital structures involved, orbital fractures can be classified as blowout, zygomatic or tripod, maxillary, midfacial, orbital apex, and orbital roof fractures. Blowout fractures result from compression of soft tissue and the sudden increase in orbital pressure when the force is transmitted to the orbital floor, the area of least resistance.

The inferior rectus and inferior oblique muscles, with their fat and fascial attachments, or the nerve that courses

---

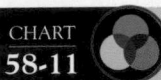

CHART 58-11

PATIENT EDUCATION
Advice for Patients About Preventing Eye Injuries

In and Around the House

- Make sure that all spray nozzles are directed away from themselves before pressing down on the handle.
- Read instructions carefully before using cleaning fluids, detergents, ammonia, or harsh chemicals, and to wash hands thoroughly after use.
- Use grease shields on frying pans to decrease spattering.
- Wear special goggles to shield their eyes from fumes and splashes when using powerful chemicals.
- Use opaque goggles to avoid burns from sunlamps.

In the Workshop

- Protect their eyes from flying fragments, fumes, dust particles, sparks, and splashed chemicals by wearing safety glasses.
- Read instructions thoroughly before using tools and chemicals, and follow precautions for their use.

Around Children

- Pay attention to age and maturity level of a child when selecting toys and games, and to avoid projectile toys, such as darts and pellet guns.
- Supervise children when they are playing with toys or games that can be dangerous.
- Teach children the correct way to handle potentially dangerous items, such as scissors and pencils.

In the Garden

- Avoid letting anyone stand at the side of or in front of a moving lawn mower.
- Pick up rocks and stones before going over them with the lawn mower (stones can be hurled out of the rotary blades and rebound off curbs or walls, causing severe injury to the eye).
- Direct pesticide spray can nozzles away from the face.
- Avoid low-hanging branches.

Around the Car

- Put out all smoking materials and matches before opening the hood of the car.
- Use a flashlight, not a match or lighter, to look at the battery at night.
- Wear goggles when grinding metal or striking metal against metal while performing auto body repair.
- Take standard safety precautions when using jumper cables (wear goggles; make sure the cars are not touching one another; make sure the jumper cable clamps never touch each other; never lean over the battery when attaching cables; and never attach a cable to the negative terminal of a dead battery).

In Sports

- Wear protective safety glasses, especially for sports such as racquetball, squash, tennis, baseball, and basketball.
- Wear protective caps, helmets, or face protectors when appropriate, especially for sports such as ice hockey.

Around Fireworks

- Wear eye glasses or safety goggles.
- Avoid explosive fireworks.
- Never allow children to ignite fireworks.
- Avoid standing near others when lighting fireworks.
- Douse duds in water instead of attempting to relight them.

---

along the inferior oblique muscle may become entrapped, and the globe may be displaced inward (ie, enophthalmos). Computed tomography (CT) can identify the muscle and its auxiliary structures that are entrapped. These fractures are usually caused by blunt small objects, such as a fist, knee, elbow, or tennis or golf ball.

Orbital roof fractures are dangerous because of potential complications to the brain. Surgical management of these fractures requires a neurosurgeon and an ophthalmologist. The most common indications for surgical intervention are displacement of bone fragments disfiguring the normal facial contours, interference with normal binocular vision caused by extraocular muscle entrapment, interference with mastication in zygomatic fracture, and obstruction of the nasolacrimal duct. Surgery is usually nonemergent, and a period of 10 to 14 days gives the ophthalmologist time to assess ocular function, especially the extraocular muscles and the nasolacrimal duct. Emergency surgical repair is usually not performed unless the globe is displaced into the maxillary sinus. Surgical repair is primarily directed at freeing the entrapped ocular structures and restoring the integrity of the orbital floor.

Foreign Bodies

Foreign bodies that enter the orbit are usually tolerated, except for copper, iron, and vegetable materials such as those from plants or trees, which may cause purulent infection. X-rays and CT scans are used to identify the foreign body. A careful history is important, especially if the foreign body has been in the orbit for a period of time and the incident forgotten. It is important to identify metallic foreign bodies because they prohibit the use of magnetic resonance imaging (MRI) as a diagnostic tool.

After the extent of the orbital damage is assessed, the decision to use conservative treatment or surgical removal is made. In general, orbital foreign bodies are removed if they are superficial and anterior in location; have sharp edges that may affect adjacent orbital structures; or are composed of copper, iron, or vegetable material. Surgical intervention is directed at preventing further ocular injury and maintaining the integrity of the affected areas. Cultures are usually obtained, and the patient is placed on prophylactic IV antibiotics that are later changed to oral antibiotics.

Ocular Trauma

Ocular trauma is the leading cause of blindness among children and young adults, especially male trauma victims. The most common circumstances of ocular trauma are occupational injuries (eg, construction industry), sports (eg, baseball, basketball, racquet sports, boxing), weapons (eg, air guns, BB guns), assault, motor vehicle

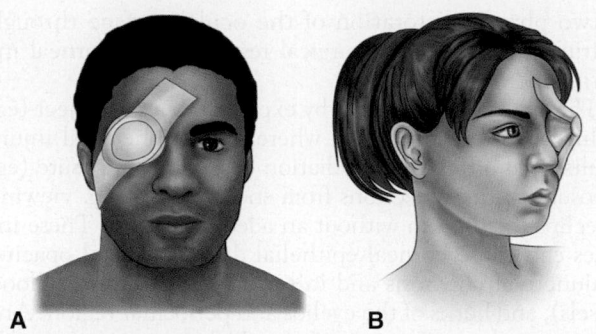

Figure 58-17 Two kinds of eye patches. **A,** Aluminum shield. **B,** Stiff paper cup shield (innovative substitute when aluminum shield is unavailable).

crashes (eg, broken windshields), and explosions (eg, blast fragments).

There are two types of ocular trauma in which the first response is critical: chemical burn and foreign object in the eye. With a chemical burn, the eye should be immediately irrigated with tap water or normal saline. With a foreign body, no attempt should be made to remove the foreign object. The object should be protected from jarring or movement to prevent further ocular damage. No pressure or patch should be applied to the affected eye. All traumatic eye injuries should be protected using a metal shield if available or a stiff paper cup until medical treatment can be obtained (Fig. 58-17).

Assessment and Diagnostic Findings

A thorough history is obtained, particularly assessing the patient's ocular history, such as preinjury vision in the affected eye or past ocular surgery. Details related to the injury that help in the diagnosis and assessment of need for further tests include the nature of the ocular injury (ie, blunt or penetrating trauma); the type of activity that caused the injury to determine the nature of the force striking the eye; and whether onset of vision loss was sudden, slow, or progressive. For chemical eye burns, the chemical agent must be identified and tested for pH if the agent is available. The corneal surface is examined for foreign bodies, wounds, and abrasions, after which the other external structures of the eye are examined. Pupillary size, shape, and light reaction of the pupil of the affected eye are compared with the other eye. Ocular motility (ability of the eyes to move synchronously up, down, right, and left) is also assessed.

Medical Management

Splash Injuries

Splash injuries are irrigated with normal saline solution before further evaluation occurs. In cases of a ruptured globe, cycloplegic agents (agents that paralyze the ciliary muscle) or topical antibiotics must be deferred because of potential toxicity to exposed intraocular tissues. Further manipulation of the eye must be avoided until the patient is under general anesthesia. Parenteral, broad-spectrum antibiotics are initiated. Tetanus antitoxin is administered, if indicated, as well as analgesics. (Tetanus prophylaxis is recommended for full-thickness ocular and skin wounds.) Any topical ophthalmic medication (eg, anesthetic, dyes) must be sterile.

Foreign Bodies and Corneal Abrasions

After removal of a foreign body from the surface of the eye, an antibiotic ointment is applied and the eye is patched. The eye is examined daily for evidence of infection until the wound is completely healed.

Contact lens wear is a common cause of corneal abrasion. The patient experiences severe pain and **photophobia** (ocular pain on exposure to light). Corneal epithelial defects are treated with antibiotic ointment and a pressure patch to immobilize the eyelids. Topical anesthetic eye drops must not be given to the patient to take home for repeated use after corneal injury because their effects mask further damage, delay healing, and can lead to permanent corneal scarring. Corticosteroids are avoided while the epithelial defect exists.

Penetrating Injuries and Contusions of the Eyeball

Sharp penetrating injury or blunt contusion force can rupture the eyeball. When the globe, cornea, and sclera rupture, rapid decompression or herniation of the orbital contents into adjacent sinuses can occur. In general, blunt traumatic injuries (with an increased incidence of retinal detachment, intraocular tissue avulsion, and herniation) have a worse prognosis than penetrating injuries. Most penetrating injuries result in marked loss of vision with the following signs: hemorrhagic **chemosis** (edema of the conjunctiva), conjunctival laceration, shallow anterior chamber with or without an eccentrically placed pupil, **hyphema** (hemorrhage within the chamber), or vitreous hemorrhage.

Hyphema is caused by contusion forces that tear the vessels of the iris and damage the anterior chamber angle. Preventing rebleeding and prolonged increased IOP are the goals of treatment for hyphema. In severe cases, the patient is hospitalized with moderate activity restriction. An eye shield is applied. Topical corticosteroids are prescribed to reduce inflammation. An antifibrinolytic agent, aminocaproic acid (Amicar), stabilizes clot formation at the site of hemorrhage. Aspirin is contraindicated.

A ruptured globe and severe injuries with intraocular hemorrhage require surgical intervention. Vitrectomy is performed for traumatic retinal detachments. Primary **enucleation** (complete removal of the eyeball and part of the optic nerve) is considered only if the globe is irreparable and has no light perception. It is a general rule that enucleation is performed within 2 weeks of the initial injury (in an eye that has no useful vision after sustaining penetrating injury) to prevent the risk of **sympathetic ophthalmia** (an inflammation created in the uninjured eye by the affected eye that can result in blindness of the uninjured eye).

Intraocular Foreign Bodies

A patient who complains of blurred vision and discomfort should be questioned carefully about recent injuries and exposures. Patients may be injured in a number of different situations and experience an intraocular foreign body (IOFB). Precipitating circumstances can include working in construction; striking metal against metal; being involved in a motor vehicle crash with facial injury; a gunshot wound; grinding-wheel work; and an explosion.

IOFB is diagnosed and localized by slit-lamp biomicroscopy and indirect ophthalmoscopy, as well as CT or ultrasonography. MRI is contraindicated because most foreign bodies are metallic and magnetic. It is important to determine the composition, size, and location of the IOFB and affected eye structures. Every effort should be made to identify the type of IOFB and whether it is magnetic. Iron, steel, copper, and vegetable matter cause intense inflammatory reactions. The incidence of endophthalmitis is also high. If the cornea is perforated, tetanus prophylaxis and IV antibiotics are administered. The extraction route (ie, surgical incision) of the foreign body depends on its location and composition and associated ocular injuries. Specially designed IOFB forceps and magnets are used to grasp and remove the foreign body. Any damaged area of the retina is treated to prevent retinal detachment.

Ocular Burns

Alkali, acid, and other chemically active organic substances, such as Mace and tear gas, cause chemical burns. Alkali burns (eg, lye, ammonia) result in the most severe injury because they penetrate the ocular tissues rapidly and continue to cause damage long after the initial injury is sustained. They also cause an immediate rise in IOP. Acids (eg, bleach, car batteries, refrigerant) generally cause less damage because the precipitated necrotic tissue proteins form a barrier to further penetration and damage. Chemical burns may appear as superficial punctate keratopathy (ie, spotty damage to the cornea), subconjunctival hemorrhage, or complete marbleizing of the cornea.

In treating chemical burns, every minute counts. Immediate tap-water irrigation should be started on site before transport of the patient to an emergency department. Only a brief history and examination are performed. Critical information, if available, is the name of the substance that went into the eye (the actual container is best). Material Safety Data Sheets (MSDS) should be accessed for reference. The corneal surfaces and conjunctival fornices are immediately and copiously irrigated with normal saline or any neutral solution. A local anesthetic is instilled, and a lid speculum is applied to overcome blepharospasm (ie, spasms of the eyelid muscles that result in closure of the lids). Particulate matter must be removed from the fornices using moistened, cotton-tipped applicators and minimal pressure on the globe. Irrigation continues until the conjunctival pH normalizes (between 7.3 and 7.6). The pH of the corneal surface is checked by placing a pH paper strip in the fornix. Antibiotics are instilled, and the eye is patched.

The goal of intermediate treatment is to prevent tissue ulceration and promote reepithelization. Intense lubrication using nonpreserved (ie, without preservatives to avoid allergic reactions) artificial tears is essential. Reepithelization is promoted with patching or therapeutic soft lenses, both of which act to keep the eye quiet by preventing blinking, thus retarding replication of corneal cells. The patient is usually monitored daily for several days. Prognosis depends on the type of injury and adequacy of the irrigation immediately after exposure. Long-term treatment consists

of two phases: restoration of the ocular surface through grafting procedures and surgical restoration of corneal integrity and optical clarity.

Thermal injury is caused by exposure to a hot object (eg, curling iron, tobacco, ash), whereas photochemical injury results from ultraviolet irradiation or infrared exposure (eg, exposure to the reflections from snow, sun gazing, viewing an eclipse of the sun without an adequate filter). These injuries can cause corneal epithelial defect, corneal opacity, conjunctival chemosis and **injection** (congestion of blood vessels), and burns of the eyelids and periocular region. Antibiotics and a pressure patch for 24 hours constitute the treatment of mild injuries. Scarring of the eyelids may require oculoplastic surgery, whereas corneal scarring may require corneal surgery.

INFECTIOUS AND INFLAMMATORY CONDITIONS

Inflammation and infections of eye structures are common. Eye infection is a leading cause of blindness worldwide. Table 58-6 summarizes selected common infections and their treatment.

Dry Eye Syndrome

Dry eye syndrome, or keratoconjunctivitis sicca, is a deficiency in the production of any of the aqueous, mucin, or lipid tear film components; lid surface abnormalities; or epithelial abnormalities related to systemic diseases or conditions (eg, thyroid disorders, Parkinson's disease), menopause, infection, injury, or complications of medications (eg, antihistamines, oral contraceptives, phenothiazines).

Clinical Manifestations

The most common complaint in dry eye syndrome is a scratchy or foreign body sensation. Other symptoms include itching, excessive mucus secretion, inability to produce tears, a burning sensation, redness, pain, and difficulty moving the lids.

Assessment and Diagnostic Findings

Slit-lamp examination shows an absent or interrupted tear meniscus at the lower lid margin, and the conjunctiva is thickened, edematous, and hyperemic and has lost its luster. A tear meniscus is the crescent-shaped edge of the tear film in the lower lid margin. Chronic dry eyes may result in chronic conjunctival and corneal irritation that can lead to corneal erosion, scarring, ulceration, thinning, or perforation that can seriously threaten vision. Secondary bacterial infection can occur.

Management

Management of dry eye syndrome requires the complete cooperation of the patient with a regimen that needs to be followed at home for a long period; otherwise, complete relief of symptoms is unlikely. Instillation of artificial tears during the day and an ointment at night is the usual regimen to

Table 58-6	COMMON INFECTIONS AND INFLAMMATORY DISORDERS OF EYE STRUCTURES	
Disorder	**Description**	**Management**
Hordeolum (stye)	Acute suppurative infection of the glands of the eyelids caused by *Staphylococcus aureus*. The lid is red and edematous with a small collection of pus in the form of an abscess. There is considerable discomfort.	Warm compresses are applied directly to the affected lid area three to four times a day for 10–15 minutes. If the condition is not improved after 48 hours, incision and drainage may be indicated. Application of topical antibiotics may be prescribed thereafter.
Chalazion	Sterile inflammatory process involving chronic granulomatous inflammation of the meibomian glands; can appear as a single granuloma or multiple granulomas in the upper or lower eyelids.	Warm compresses applied three to four times a day for 10–15 minutes may resolve the inflammation in the early stages. Most often, however, surgical excision is indicated. Corticosteroid injection to the chalazion lesion may be used for smaller lesions.
Blepharitis	Chronic bilateral inflammation of the eyelid margins. There are two types: staphylococcal and seborrheic. Staphylococcal blepharitis is usually ulcerative and is more serious due to the involvement of the base of hair follicles. Permanent scarring can result.	The seborrheic type is chronic and is usually resistant to treatment, but the milder cases may respond to lid hygiene. Staphylococcal blepharitis requires topical antibiotic treatment. Instructions on lid hygiene (to keep the lid margins clean and free of exudates) are given to the patient.
Bacterial keratitis	Infection of the cornea by *Staphylococcus aureus*, *Streptococcus pneumoniae*, and *Pseudomonas aeruginosa*.	Fortified (high-concentration) antibiotic eyedrops are administered every 30 minutes around the clock for the first few days, then every 1–2 hours. Systemic antibiotics may be administered. Cycloplegics are administered to reduce pain caused by ciliary spasm. Corticosteroid therapy and subconjunctival injections of antibiotics are controversial.
Herpes simplex keratitis	Leading cause of corneal blindness in the United States. Symptoms are severe pain, tearing, and photophobia. The dendritic ulcer has a branching, linear pattern with feathery edges and terminal bulbs at its ends. Herpes simplex keratitis can lead to recurrent stromal keratitis and persist to 12 months with residual corneal scarring.	Many lesions heal without treatment and residual effects. The treatment goal is to minimize the damaging effect of the inflammatory response and eliminate viral replication within the cornea. Penetrating keratoplasty is indicated for corneal scarring and must be performed when the herpetic disease has been inactive for many months.

hydrate and lubricate the eye and preserve a moist ocular surface. Cyclosporine ophthalmic emulsion (Restasis) is an effective agent that increases tear production and is used once daily. Anti-inflammatory medications are also used, and moisture chambers (eg, moisture chamber spectacles, swim goggles) may provide additional relief.

Patients may become hypersensitive to chemical preservatives such as benzalkonium chloride and thimerosal. For these patients, preservative-free ophthalmic solutions are used. Management of the dry eye syndrome also includes the concurrent treatment of infections, such as chronic blepharitis and acne rosacea, and treating the underlying systemic disease, such as Sjögren syndrome (an autoimmune disease).

In advanced cases of dry eye syndrome, surgical treatment that includes punctal occlusion, grafting procedures, and lateral tarsorrhaphy (uniting the edges of the lids) are options. Punctal plugs are made of silicone material for the temporary or permanent occlusion of the puncta. This helps preserve the natural tears and prolongs the effects of artificial tears. Short-term occlusion is performed by inserting punctal or silicone rods in all four puncta. If tearing is induced by the occlusion, the upper plugs are removed, and the remaining lower plugs are removed in another week. Permanent occlusion is performed only in severe cases in adults who do not develop tearing after partial occlusion and who have results on a repeated Schirmer's test of 2 mm or less (filter paper is used to measure tear production).

Conjunctivitis

Conjunctivitis (inflammation of the conjunctiva) is the most common ocular disease worldwide. It is characterized by a pink appearance (hence the common term *pink eye*) because of subconjunctival blood vessel congestion.

Clinical Manifestations

General symptoms include foreign body sensation, scratching or burning sensation, itching, and photophobia. Conjunctivitis may be unilateral or bilateral, but the infection usually starts in one eye and then spreads to the other eye by hand contact.

Assessment and Diagnostic Findings

The four main clinical features important to evaluate are the type of discharge (watery, mucoid, purulent, or mucopurulent), type of conjunctival reaction (follicular or papillary), presence of pseudomembranes or true membranes, and presence or absence of lymphadenopathy (enlargement of the preauricular and submandibular lymph nodes where the eyelids drain). Pseudomembranes consist of coagulated exudate that adheres to the surface of the inflamed conjunctiva. True membranes form when the exudate adheres to the superficial layer of the conjunctiva, and removal results in bleeding. Follicles are multiple, slightly elevated lesions encircled by tiny blood vessels; they look like grains of rice. Papillae are hyperplastic conjunctival epithelium in numerous projections that are usually seen as a fine mosaic pattern under slit-lamp examination. Diagnosis is based on the distinctive characteristics of ocular signs, acute or chronic presentation, and identification of any precipitating events. Positive results of swab smear preparations and cultures confirm the diagnosis.

Types of Conjunctivitis

Conjunctivitis is classified according to its cause. The major causes are microbial infection, allergy, and irritating toxic stimuli. A wide spectrum of organisms can cause conjunctivitis, including bacteria (eg, *Chlamydia*), viruses, fungus, and parasites. Conjunctivitis can also result from an existing ocular infection or can be a manifestation of a systemic disease.

Microbial Conjunctivitis

Bacterial Conjunctivitis

Bacterial conjunctivitis can be acute or chronic. The acute type can develop into a chronic condition. Signs and symptoms can vary from mild to severe. Chronic bacterial conjunctivitis is usually seen in patients with lacrimal duct obstruction, chronic dacryocystitis, and chronic blepharitis. The most common causative microorganisms are *Streptococcus pneumoniae*, *Haemophilus influenzae*, and *Staphylococcus aureus*.

Bacterial conjunctivitis manifests with an acute onset of redness, burning, and discharge. There is papillary formation, conjunctival irritation, and injection in the fornices. The exudates are variable but are usually present on waking in the morning. The eyes may be difficult to open because of adhesions caused by the exudate. Purulent discharge occurs in severe acute bacterial infections, whereas mucopurulent discharge appears in mild cases. In gonococcal conjunctivitis, the symptoms are more acute. The exudate is profuse and purulent, and there is lymphadenopathy. Pseudomembranes may be present.

Chlamydial conjunctivitis includes **trachoma** (a bilateral chronic follicular conjunctivitis of childhood that leads to blindness during adulthood if left untreated) and inclusion conjunctivitis. Trachoma is an ancient disease and is the leading cause of preventable blindness in the world. It is prevalent in areas with hot, dry, and dusty climates and in areas with poor living conditions. It is spread by direct contact or fomites, and the vectors can be insects such as flies and gnats. The onset of trachoma in children is usually insidious, but it can be acute or subacute in adults. The initial symptoms include red inflamed eyes, tearing, photophobia, ocular pain, purulent exudates, preauricular lymphadenopathy, and lid edema. Initial ocular signs include follicular and papillary formations. At the middle stage of the disease, there is an acute inflammation with papillary hypertrophy and follicular necrosis, after which trichiasis (turning inward of hair follicles) and entropion begin to develop. The lashes that are turned in rub against the cornea and, after prolonged irritation, cause corneal erosion and ulceration. The late stage of the disease is characterized by scarred conjunctiva, subepithelial keratitis, abnormal vascularization of the cornea (pannus), and residual scars from the follicles that look like depressions in the conjunctiva (Herbert's

pits). Severe corneal ulceration can lead to perforation and blindness.

Inclusion conjunctivitis affects sexually active people who have genital chlamydial infection. Transmission is by oral–genital sex or hand-to-eye transmission. Indirect transmission can occur in inadequately chlorinated swimming pools. The eye lesions usually appear a week after exposure and may be associated with a nonspecific urethritis or cervicitis. The discharge is mucopurulent, follicles are present, and there is lymphadenopathy.

Viral Conjunctivitis

Viral conjunctivitis can be acute and chronic. The discharge is watery, and follicles are prominent. Severe cases include pseudomembranes. The common causative organisms are adenovirus and herpes simplex virus. Conjunctivitis caused by adenovirus is highly contagious. The condition is usually preceded by symptoms of upper respiratory infection. Corneal involvement causes extreme photophobia. Symptoms include extreme tearing, redness, and foreign body sensation that can involve one or both eyes. There is lid edema, ptosis, and conjunctival **hyperemia** (dilation of the conjunctival blood vessels) (Fig. 58-18). These signs and symptoms vary from mild to severe and may last for 2 weeks. Viral conjunctivitis, although self-limited, tends to last longer than bacterial conjunctivitis.

Epidemic keratoconjunctivitis (EKC) is a highly contagious viral conjunctivitis that is easily transmitted from one person to another among household members, schoolchildren, and health care workers. The outbreak of epidemics is seasonal, especially during the summer when people use swimming pools. EKC is most often accompanied by preauricular lymphadenopathy and occasionally periorbital pain. There are marked follicular and papillary formations. This type of conjunctivitis can lead to keratopathy.

Allergic Conjunctivitis

Immunologic or allergic conjunctivitis is a hypersensitivity reaction that occurs as part of allergic rhinitis (hay fever), or it can be an independent allergic reaction. The patient usually has a history of an allergy to pollens and other environmental allergens. There is extreme pruritus, epiphora (ie, excessive secretion of tears), injection, and usually severe

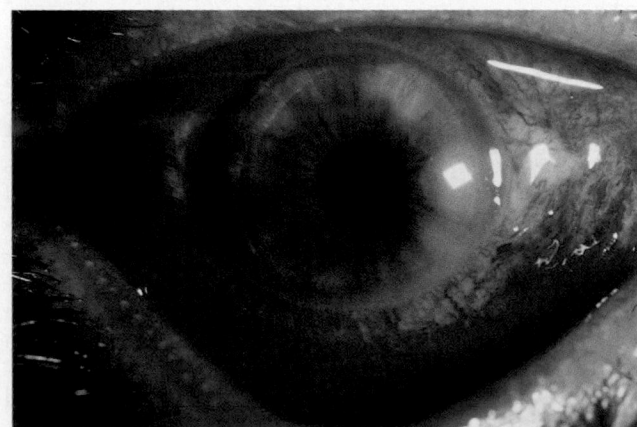

Figure 58-18 Conjunctival hyperemia in viral conjunctivitis.

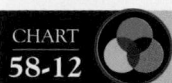

PATIENT EDUCATION
Instructions for Patients With Viral Conjunctivitis

CHART 58-12

Viral conjunctivitis is a highly contagious eye infection. It can easily spread from one person to another. The symptoms can be alarming, but they are not serious. The following information will help you understand this eye condition and how to take care of yourself and/or your family member at home.

- Your eyes will look red and will have watery discharge, and your lids will be swollen for about a week.
- You will experience eye pain, a sandy sensation in your eye, and sensitivity to light.
- Symptoms will resolve after about 1 week.
- You may use light cold compresses over your eyes for about 10 minutes four to five times a day to soothe the pain.
- You may use artificial tears for the sandy sensation in your eye and mild pain medications such as acetaminophen (Tylenol).
- You need to stay at home. Children must not play outside. You may return to work or school after 7 days when the

redness and discharge have cleared. You may obtain a doctor's note to return to work or school.
- Do not share towels, linens, makeup, or toys.
- Wash your hands thoroughly with soap and water frequently, including and before and after you apply artificial tears or cold compresses.
- Use a new tissue every time you wipe the discharge from your eye. You may dampen the tissue with clean water to clean the outside of the eye.
- You may wash your face and take a shower as you normally do.
- Discard all of your makeup articles. You must not apply makeup until the infection has resolved.
- Wear dark glasses if bright lights bother you.
- If the discharge from your eye turns yellowish and puslike or you experience changes in your vision, you need to return to the health care provider for an examination.

photophobia. The stringlike mucoid discharge is usually associated with rubbing the eyes because of severe pruritus. Vernal conjunctivitis is also known as seasonal conjunctivitis because it appears mostly during warm weather. There may be large formations of papillae that have a cobblestone appearance. It is more common in children and young adults. Most affected people have a history of asthma or eczema.

Toxic Conjunctivitis

Chemical conjunctivitis can be the result of medications; chlorine from swimming pools; exposure to toxic fumes among industrial workers; or exposure to other irritants such as smoke, hair sprays, acids, and alkalis.

Management

The management of conjunctivitis depends on the type. Most types of mild and viral conjunctivitis are self-limiting, benign conditions that may not require treatment and laboratory procedures. For more severe cases, topical antibiotics, eye drops, or ointments are prescribed. Patients with gonococcal conjunctivitis require urgent antibiotic therapy. If left untreated, this ocular disease can lead to corneal perforation and blindness. The systemic complications can include meningitis and generalized septicemia.

Bacterial Conjunctivitis

Acute bacterial conjunctivitis is almost always self-limiting, lasting 2 weeks if left untreated. If treated with antibiotics, it may last a few days, except for gonococcal and staphylococcal conjunctivitis.

For trachoma, usually broad-spectrum antibiotics are administered topically and systemically. Surgical management includes the correction of trichiasis (eyelashes growing inward toward the conjunctiva and cornea) to prevent conjunctival scarring.

Adult inclusion conjunctivitis requires 1 week of antibiotics. Prevention of reinfection is important, and affected people and their sexual partners must seek treatment for sexually transmitted disease, if indicated.

Viral Conjunctivitis

Viral conjunctivitis is not responsive to any treatment. Cold compresses may alleviate some symptoms. It is extremely important to remember that viral conjunctivitis, especially epidemic keratoconjunctivitis, is highly contagious. Patients must be made aware of the contagious nature of the disease, and adequate instructions must be given (Chart 58-12). These instructions should include an emphasis on hand hygiene and avoiding sharing of hand towels, face cloths, and eye drops. Tissues should be directly discarded into a covered trash can.

Proper steps must be taken to avoid nosocomial infections. Frequent hand hygiene and procedures for environmental cleaning and disinfection of equipment used for eye examination must be strictly followed at all times. To prevent spread during outbreaks of conjunctivitis caused by adenovirus, health care facilities must set aside specified areas for treating patients with or suspected of having conjunctivitis caused by adenovirus to prevent spread. All forms of tonometry must be avoided unless medically indicated. All multidose ophthalmic medications must be discarded at the end of each day or when contaminated. Infected employees and others must not be allowed to work or attend school until symptoms have resolved, which can take 3 to 7 days.

Allergic Conjunctivitis

Patients with allergic conjunctivitis, especially recurrent vernal or seasonal conjunctivitis, are usually given corticosteroids in ophthalmic preparations. Depending on the severity of the disease, they may be given oral preparations. Use of vasoconstrictors, such as topical epinephrine solution, cold compresses, ice packs, and cool ventilation usually provide comfort by decreasing swelling.

Toxic Conjunctivitis

For conjunctivitis caused by chemical irritants, the eye must be irrigated immediately and profusely with saline or sterile water.

Uveitis

Inflammation of the uveal tract (uveitis) can affect the iris, the ciliary body, or the choroid. There are two types of uveitis: nongranulomatous and granulomatous.

The more common type of uveitis is the nongranulomatous type, which manifests as an acute condition with pain, photophobia, and a pattern of conjunctival injection, especially around the cornea. The pupil is small or irregular, and vision is blurred. There may be small, fine precipitates on the posterior corneal surface and cells in the aqueous humor (ie, cell and flare). If the uveitis is severe, a **hypopyon** (accumulation of pus in the anterior chamber) may develop. The condition may be unilateral or bilateral and may be recurrent. Repeated attacks of nongranulomatous anterior uveitis can cause anterior synechiae (peripheral iris adheres to the cornea and impedes outflow of aqueous humor). Posterior synechiae (adherence of the iris and lens) block aqueous outflow from the posterior chamber. Secondary glaucoma can result from either anterior or posterior synechiae. Cataracts may also occur as a sequela to uveitis.

Granulomatous uveitis can have a more insidious onset and can involve any portion of the uveal tract. It tends to be chronic. Symptoms such as photophobia and pain may be minimal. Vision is markedly and adversely affected. Conjunctival injection is diffuse, and there may be vitreous clouding. In a severe posterior uveitis, such as chorioretinitis, there may be retinal and choroidal hemorrhages.

Management

Because photophobia is a common symptom, patients should wear dark glasses outdoors. Ciliary spasm and synechia are best avoided through mydriasis; cyclopentolate (Cyclogyl) and atropine are commonly used. Local corticosteroid drops, such as Pred Forte 1% and Flarex 0.1%, instilled four to six times a day are also used to decrease inflammation. In very severe cases, systemic corticosteroids, as well as intravitreal corticosteroids, may be used. Daclizumab (Zenapax), a monoclonal antibody, is designed to prevent a specific chemical interaction needed by immune cells, such as lymphocytes, to produce inflammation. The National Eye Institute of the National Institutes of Health has conducted a preliminary clinical trial to examine the safety and effectiveness of treating uveitis with daclizumab with positive results. Larger-scale trials are planned (Yeh, Wroblewski, Buggage, et al., 2008).

If the uveitis is recurrent, a careful history should be initiated to discover any underlying causes. This evaluation should include a complete history, physical examination, and diagnostic tests, including a complete blood cell count, erythrocyte sedimentation rate, antinuclear antibodies, and Venereal Disease Research Laboratory (VDRL) and Lyme disease titers. Underlying causes include autoimmune disorders such as ankylosing spondylitis and sarcoidosis as well as toxoplasmosis, herpes zoster virus, ocular candidiasis, histoplasmosis, herpes simplex virus, tuberculosis, and syphilis.

Orbital Cellulitis

Orbital cellulitis is inflammation of the tissues surrounding the eye and may result from bacterial, fungal, or viral inflammatory conditions of contiguous structures, such as the face, oropharynx, dental structures, or intracranial structures. It can also result from foreign bodies and from a preexisting ocular infection, such as dacryocystitis and panophthalmitis, or from generalized septicemia. Infection of the sinuses is the most frequent cause. Infection originating in the sinuses can spread easily to the orbit through the thin bony walls and foramina or by means of the interconnecting venous system of the orbit and sinuses. The most common causative organisms are staphylococci and streptococci in adults and H. influenzae in children. The symptoms include pain, lid swelling, conjunctival edema, proptosis, and decreased ocular motility. With such edema, optic nerve compression can occur and IOP may increase.

The severe intraorbital tension caused by abscess formation and the impairment of optic nerve function in orbital cellulitis can result in permanent visual loss. Because of the orbit's proximity to the brain, orbital cellulitis can lead to life-threatening complications, such as intracranial abscess and cavernous sinus thrombosis.

Management

Immediate administration of high-dose, broad-spectrum, systemic antibiotics is indicated. Cultures and Gram-stained smears are obtained. Monitoring changes in visual acuity, degree of proptosis, central nervous system function (eg, nausea, vomiting, fever, cognitive changes), displacement of the globe, extraocular movements, pupillary signs, and the fundus is extremely important. Consultation with an otolaryngologist is necessary, especially when rhinosinusitis is suspected. In the event of abscess formation or progressive loss of vision, surgical drainage of the abscess or sinus is performed. Sinusotomy and antibiotic irrigation are also performed.

ORBITAL AND OCULAR TUMORS

Benign Tumors of the Orbit

Benign tumors can develop from infancy and grow rapidly or slowly and present in later life. Some benign tumors are superficial and are easily identifiable by external presentation, palpation, and x-rays, but some are deep and may require a CT scan for a more thorough and precise diagnosis. There can be a significant proptosis, and visual function may be jeopardized. Benign tumors are masses characterized by the lack of infiltration in the surrounding tissues. Examples are cystic dermoid cysts and mucocele, hemangiomas, lymphangiomas, lacrimal tumors, and neurofibromas.

To prevent recurrence, benign masses are excised completely when possible. Sometimes, excision is difficult because of the involvement of some portions of the orbital bones, such as deep dermoid cysts, in which dissection of the bone is required. Subtotal resection may be indicated in deep benign tumors that intertwine with other orbital structures, such as optic nerve meningiomas. Complete removal of the tumor may endanger visual function.

Benign Tumors of the Eyelids

Benign tumors include a wide variety of neoplasms and increase in frequency with age. Nevi may be unpigmented at birth and may enlarge and darken in adolescence or may never acquire any pigment at all. Hemangiomas are vascular capillary tumors that may be bright, superficial, strawberry-red lesions (ie, strawberry nevus) or bluish and purplish deeper lesions. Milia are small, white, slightly elevated cysts of the eyelid that may occur in multiples. Xanthelasma are yellowish, lipoid deposits on both lids near the inner angle of the eye that commonly appear as a result of the aging of the skin or a lipid disorder. Molluscum contagiosum lesions are flat, symmetric growths along the lid margin caused by a virus that can result in conjunctivitis and keratitis if debris gets into the conjunctival sac.

Treatment of benign congenital lid lesions is rarely indicated, except when visual function is affected. Corticosteroid injection to the hemangioma lesion is usually effective, but surgical excision may be performed. Benign lid lesions usually present aesthetic problems rather than visual function problems. Surgical excision, or electrocautery, is primarily performed for cosmetic reasons, except for cases of molluscum contagiosum, for which surgical intervention is performed to prevent an infectious process that may ensue.

Benign Tumors of the Conjunctiva

Conjunctival nevus, a congenital, benign neoplasm, is a flat, slightly elevated, brown spot that becomes pigmented during late childhood or adolescence. This should be differentiated from the pigmented lesion melanosis acquired at middle age, which tends to wax and wane and become malignant melanoma. Keratin- and sebum-containing dermoid cysts are congenital and can be found in the conjunctiva. Dermolipoma is a congenital tumor that manifests as a smooth, rounded growth in the conjunctiva near the lateral canthus. Papillomas are usually soft with irregular surfaces and appear on the lid margins. Treatment consists of surgical excision.

Malignant Tumors of the Orbit

Rhabdomyosarcoma is the most common malignant primary orbital tumor in childhood, but it can also develop in elderly people. The symptoms of rhabdomyosarcoma include sudden painless proptosis of one eye followed by lid swelling, conjunctival chemosis, and impairment of ocular motility. Imaging of these tumors establishes the size, configuration, location, and stage of the disease; delineates the degree of bone destruction; and is useful in estimating the field for radiation therapy, if needed. The most common site of metastasis is the lung.

Management of these primary malignant orbital tumors involves three major therapeutic modalities: surgery, radiation therapy, and adjuvant chemotherapy. The degree of orbital destruction is important in planning the surgical approach. Resection often involves removal of the eyeball. The psychological needs of the patient and family are paramount in planning the management approach.

Malignant Tumors of the Eyelid

Basal cell carcinoma is the most common malignant tumor of the eyelid. Squamous cell carcinoma occurs less frequently but is considered the second most common malignant tumor. Malignant melanoma is rare. Malignant eyelid tumors occur more frequently among people with a fair complexion who have a history of chronic exposure to the sun.

Basal cell carcinoma appears as a painless nodule that may ulcerate. The lesion is invasive, spreads to the surrounding tissues, and grows slowly but does not metastasize. It usually appears on the lower lid margin near the inner canthus with a pearly white margin. Squamous cell carcinoma of the eyelids may resemble basal cell carcinoma initially because it also grows slowly and painlessly. It tends to ulcerate and invade the surrounding tissues, but it can metastasize to the regional lymph nodes. Malignant melanoma may not be pigmented and can arise from nevi. It spreads to the surrounding tissues and metastasizes to other organs.

Complete excision of these carcinomas is followed by reconstruction with skin grafting if the surgical excision is extensive. The ocular postoperative site and the graft donor site are monitored for bleeding. Donor graft sites may include the buccal mucosa, the thigh, or the abdomen. The patient is referred to an oncologist for evaluation of the need for radiation therapy and monitoring for metastasis. Early diagnosis and surgical management are the basis of a good prognosis. These conditions have life-threatening consequences, and surgical excisions may result in facial disfigurement. Emotional support is an extremely important aspect of nursing management.

Malignant Tumors of the Conjunctiva

Conjunctival carcinoma most often grows in the exposed areas of the conjunctiva. The typical lesions are usually gelatinous and whitish due to keratin formation. They grow gradually, and deep invasion and metastasis are rare. Malignant melanoma is rare but may arise from a preexisting nevus or acquired melanosis during middle age. Squamous cell carcinoma is also rare but invasive.

The management is surgical incision. Some benign tumors and most malignant tumors recur. To avoid recurrences, patients usually undergo radiation therapy and cryotherapy after the excision of malignant tumors. Cosmetic disfigurement may result from extensive excision when deep invasion by the malignant tumor is involved.

Malignant Tumors of the Globe

Retinoblastoma, a malignant tumor of the retina, occurs in childhood and is hereditary, found in 1 of 15,000 live births. It is hereditary in 30% to 40% of cases. All bilateral cases are hereditary. The retinoblastoma gene is found on chromosome 13, region q14. If this gene is inhibited, the growth in retinal cells is unchecked and the retinoblastoma results. Signs and symptoms include an initial leukocoria or "white" pupil with a peculiar light reflection and possible strabismus as well. Less frequent signs are uveitis, glaucoma, hyphema, nystagmus, and periorbital cellulitis. Treatment for this life-threatening tumor is enucleation, if the tumor is large and unilateral. If the eye is removed before cancer spreads to the optic nerve, the cure rate is greater than 90%.

Ocular melanoma, another cancer, primarily occurs in adults. This rare, malignant choroidal tumor is often discovered on a retinal examination. In its early stages, it could be mistaken for a nevus. Many ophthalmologists may practice for decades and never encounter this lesion. For this reason, any patient who is suspected of having ocular melanoma should be immediately referred to an ocular oncologist with experience in this disease.

Although many patients do not have symptoms in the early stages, some patients complain of blurred vision or a change in eye color. A number of such tumors have been found in people with blindness who have painful eyes. In addition to a complete physical examination to discover any evidence of metastasis (to the liver, lung, and breast), retinal fundus photography, fluorescein angiography, and ultrasonography are performed. The diagnosis is confirmed at biopsy after enucleation.

Tumors are classified according to boundary lines (apical height and basal diameter) as small, medium, or large. Small tumors are generally monitored, whereas medium and large tumors require treatment. Treatment consists of radiation, enucleation, or both. Radiation therapy may be achieved by external beam performed in repeated episodes over several days or through the implantation of a small plaque that contains radioactive iodine (I-125) pellets over the tumor.

SURGICAL PROCEDURES AND ENUCLEATION

Orbital Surgeries

Orbital surgeries may be performed to repair fractures, remove a foreign body, or remove benign or malignant growths. Surgical procedures involving the orbit and lids affect facial appearance (cosmesis). The goals are to recover and preserve visual function and to maintain the anatomic relationship of the ocular structures to achieve cosmesis. During the repair of orbital fractures, the orbital bones are realigned to follow the anatomic positions of facial structures.

Orbital surgical procedures involve working around delicate structures of the eye, such as the optic nerve, retinal blood vessels, and ocular muscles. Complications of orbital surgical procedures may include blindness as a result of damage to the optic nerve and its blood supply. Sudden pain and loss of vision may indicate intraorbital hemorrhage or compression of the optic nerve. Ptosis and diplopia may result from trauma to the extraocular muscles during the surgical

procedure, but these conditions typically resolve after a few weeks.

Prophylaxis with IV antibiotics is the usual postoperative regimen after orbital surgery, especially with repair of orbital fractures and intraorbital foreign body removal. IV corticosteroids are used if there is a concern about optic nerve swelling. Topical ocular antibiotics are typically instilled, and antibiotic ointments are applied externally to the skin suture sites.

For the first 24 to 48 hours postoperatively, ice compresses are applied over the periocular area to decrease periorbital swelling, facial swelling, and hematoma. The head of the patient's bed should be elevated to a comfortable position (30 to 45 degrees).

Discharge teaching should include medication instructions for oral antibiotics, instillation of ophthalmic medications, and application of ocular compresses.

Enucleation

Enucleation is the removal of the entire eye and part of the optic nerve. It may be performed for the following conditions:
- Severe injury resulting in prolapse of uveal tissue or loss of light projection (the ability to identify the direction of the light source) or perception
- An irritated, blind, painful, deformed, or disfigured eye, usually caused by glaucoma, retinal detachment, or chronic inflammation
- An eye without useful vision that is producing or has produced sympathetic ophthalmia in the other eye
- Intraocular tumors that are untreatable by other means

The procedure for enucleation involves the separation and cutting of each of the ocular muscles, dissection of the Tenon's capsule (fibrous membrane covering the sclera), and cutting of the optic nerve from the eyeball. The insertion of an orbital implant typically follows, and the conjunctiva is closed. A large pressure dressing is applied over the area.

Evisceration involves the surgical removal of the intraocular contents through an incision or opening in the cornea or sclera. Evisceration may be performed to treat severe ocular trauma with ruptured globe, severe ocular inflammation, or severe ocular infection. The optic nerve, sclera, extraocular muscles, and sometimes the cornea are left intact. The main advantage of evisceration over enucleation is that the final cosmetic result and motility after fitting the ocular prosthesis are enhanced. This procedure would be more acceptable to a patient whose body image is severely threatened. The main disadvantage is the high risk of sympathetic ophthalmia.

Exenteration is the removal of the eyelids, the eye, and various amounts of orbital contents. It is indicated in malignancies in the orbit that are life-threatening or when more conservative modalities of treatment have failed or are inappropriate. An example is squamous cell carcinoma of the paranasal sinuses, skin, and conjunctiva with deep orbital involvement. In its most extensive form, exenteration may include the removal of all orbital tissues and resection of the orbital bones.

Ocular Prostheses

Orbital implants and conformers (ocular prostheses usually made of silicone rubber) maintain the shape of the eye after enucleation or evisceration to prevent a contracted, sunken appearance. The temporary conformer is placed over the conjunctival closure after the implantation of an orbital implant. A conformer is placed after the enucleation or evisceration procedure to protect the suture line, maintain the fornices, prevent contracture of the socket in preparation for the ocular prosthesis, and promote the integrity of the eyelids.

All ocular prosthetics have limitations in their motility. There are two designs of eye prostheses. The anophthalmic ocular prostheses are used in the absence of the globe. Scleral shells look just like the anophthalmic prosthesis (Fig. 58-19) but are thinner and fit over a globe with intact corneal sensation. An eye prosthesis usually lasts about 6 years, depending on the quality of fit, comfort, and cosmetic appearance. When the anophthalmic socket is completely healed, conformers are replaced with prosthetic eyes.

An ocularist is a specially trained and skilled professional who makes prosthetic eyes. After the ophthalmologist is satisfied that the anophthalmic socket is completely healed and is ready for prosthetic fitting, the patient is referred to an ocularist. The healing period is usually 6 to 8 weeks. It is advisable for the patient to have a consultation with the ocularist before the fitting. Obtaining accurate information and verbalizing concerns can lessen anxiety about wearing an ocular prosthesis.

Medical Management

Removal of an eye has physical, social, and psychological ramifications for any person. The significance of loss of the eye and vision must be addressed in the plan of care. The patient's preparation should include information about the surgical procedure and placement of orbital implants and conformers and the availability of ocular prosthetics to enhance cosmetic appearance. In some cases, patients may choose to see an ocularist before the surgery to discuss ocular prosthetics.

Nursing Management

Teaching About Postsurgical and Prosthetic Care

Patients who undergo eye removal need to know that they will usually have a large ocular pressure dressing, which is

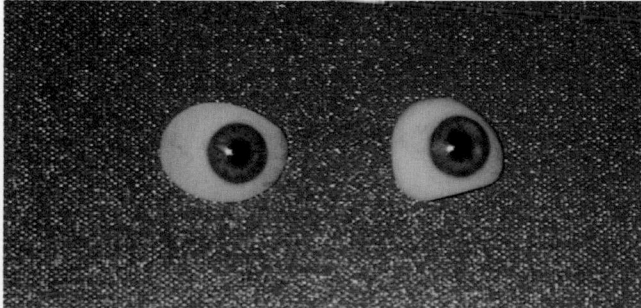

Figure 58-19 Eye prostheses. (*Left*) Anophthalmic ocular prosthesis. (*Right*) Scleral shell.

typically removed after a week, and that an ophthalmic topical antibiotic ointment is applied in the socket three times daily.

After the removal of an eye, there is a loss of depth perception. Patients must be advised to take extra caution in their ambulation and movement to avoid miscalculations that may result in injury. It may take some time to adjust to monocular vision.

The patient must be advised that conformers may accidentally fall out of the socket. If this happens, the conformer must be washed, wiped dry, and placed back in the socket.

When surgical eye removal is unexpected, such as in severe ocular trauma, leaving no time for the patient and family to prepare for the loss, the nurse's role in providing emotional support is crucial.

Promoting Home and Community-Based Care

Teaching Patients Self-Care

Patients need to be taught how to insert, remove, and care for the prosthetic eye. Proper hand hygiene must be observed before inserting and removing an ocular prosthesis. A suction cup may be used if there are problems with manual dexterity. Precautions, such as draping a towel over the sink and closing the sink drain, must be taken to avoid loss of the prosthesis. When instructing patients or family members, a return demonstration is important to assess the level of understanding and ability to perform the procedure.

Before insertion, the inner punctal or outer lateral aspects and the superior and inferior aspects of the prosthesis must be identified by locating the identifying marks, such as a reddish color in the inner punctal area. For people with low vision, other forms of identifying markers, such as dots or notches, are used. The upper lid is raised high enough to create a space; then the patient learns to slide the prosthesis up, underneath, and behind the upper eyelid. Meanwhile, the patient pulls the lower eyelid down to help put the prosthesis in place and to have its inferior edge fall back gradually to the lower eyelid. The lower eyelid is checked for correct positioning.

To remove the prosthesis, the patient cups one hand on the cheek to catch the prosthesis, places the forefinger of the free hand against the midportion of the lower eyelid, and gazes upward. Gazing upward brings the inferior edge of the prosthesis nearer the inferior eyelid margin. With the finger pushing inward, downward, and laterally against the lower eyelid, the prosthesis slides out into the cupped hand.

Continuing Care

An eye prosthesis can be worn and left in place for several months. Hygiene and comfort are usually maintained with daily irrigation of the prosthesis in place with normal saline solution, hard contact lens solution, or artificial tears. In the case of dry eye symptoms, the use of ophthalmic ointment lubricants or oil-based drops, such as vitamin E and mineral oil, can be helpful. Removing crusting and mucous discharge that accumulate overnight is performed with the prosthesis in place. Malpositions may occur when wiping or rubbing the prosthesis in the socket. The prosthesis can be repositioned with the use of clean fingers. Proper wiping of the prosthesis should be a gentle temporal-to-nasal motion to avoid malpositions.

The prosthesis needs to be removed and cleaned when it becomes uncomfortable and when there is increased mucous discharge. The socket should also be rendered free of mucus and inspected for any signs of infection. Any unusual discomfort, irritation, or redness of the globe or eyelids may indicate excessive wear, debris under the shell, or lack of proper hygiene. Any infection or irritation that does not resolve needs medical attention.

OCULAR CONSEQUENCES OF SYSTEMIC DISEASE

Diabetic Retinopathy

Of all of the medical disorders that the nurse encounters, diabetes mellitus is one of the most common. One of the most serious complications of diabetes is retinopathy. In the United States today, diabetes is the leading cause of new cases of blindness in people between 20 and 74 years of age (Prevent Blindness America, 2008). Before the discovery of insulin in the 1920s, diabetic retinopathy was relatively rare because most people with diabetes did not survive for more than 1 or 2 years. However, with the many advancements in the treatment of diabetes, more and more patients are able to survive and enjoy relatively normal lifespans, but they are also confronted with the complications of long-term diabetes. With the rate of obesity in the United States rising, type 2 diabetes has become epidemic, and the incidence of diabetic retinopathy may be expected to increase. Chapter 41 provides a detailed discussion of diabetic retinopathy.

Cytomegalovirus Retinitis

Many ophthalmic complications have been associated with AIDS. Cytomegalovirus (CMV) is the most common cause of retinal inflammation in patients with AIDS. Early symptoms of CMV retinitis vary from patient to patient. Some patients complain of floaters or a decrease in peripheral vision. Some have a paracentral or central scotoma, whereas others have fluctuations in vision from macular edema. The retina often becomes thin and atrophic and susceptible to retinal tears and breaks.

CMV retinitis generally takes one of three forms: hemorrhagic, brushfire, or granular. In the hemorrhagic type, large areas of white, necrotic retina may be associated with retinal hemorrhage. In the brushfire type, a yellow-white margin begins at the edge of burned-out atrophic retina. This retinitis expands and, if untreated, involves the entire retina. In the granular type, white granular lesions in the periphery of the retina gradually expand. The white, feathery infiltration of the retina destroys sensory retina and leads to necrosis, optic atrophy, and retinal detachment.

Medical Management

Pharmacologic Therapy

Pharmacologic agents available for treatment of CMV retinitis include ganciclovir (Cytovene), foscarnet (Foscavir), and cidofovir (Vistide).

Ganciclovir is administered intravenously, orally, or intravitreously in the acute stage of CMV retinitis. The intravitreous form is available as a 4-mm intraocular implant or insert containing the medication embedded in a polymer-based system that slowly releases the medication. The insert is surgically placed in the posterior segment of the eye, and the medication diffuses locally to the site of the infection over a period of 5 to 8 months before the insert must be replaced. When administered systemically, ganciclovir is a very potent medication; it can cause neutropenia, thrombocytopenia, anemia, and elevated serum creatinine levels. The surgically implanted sustained-release insert enables higher concentrations of ganciclovir to reach the CMV retinitis, but there are risks and complications associated with the inserts, including endophthalmitis, retinal detachment, and hypotony.

Foscarnet inhibits viral DNA replication. It may be the medication of choice when ganciclovir is ineffective. It may be administered by IV or intravitreal injections. The combination of foscarnet and ganciclovir has been more effective than either medication alone. Nephrotoxicity may occur with systemic foscarnet, and renal function must be monitored carefully.

Cidofovir impedes CMV replication and is administered by IV. Cidofovir has been shown to delay the progression of CMV retinitis significantly. Nephrotoxicity, proteinuria, and increased serum creatinine levels are significant side effects.

In the late 1990s, the routine management of patients with AIDS, including those with CMV retinitis, changed with the introduction of highly active antiretroviral therapy (HAART). HAART is a combination of two or three medications of different categories. For example, a nucleoside analogue such as zidovudine (Retrovir) administered in combination with one or more protease inhibitors such as ritonavir (Norvir) has led to a suppression of human immunodeficiency virus (HIV) replication for sustained periods. The immune system can then recover to a functional level. Several patients who had been treated for CMV retinitis have been able to discontinue treatment for CMV retinitis as their immune systems rebounded. However, some patients develop immune recovery uveitis, characterized by intraocular inflammation, cystoid macular edema, and the formation of epiretinal membranes. Immune recovery uveitis is managed by corticosteroids or by injection of corticosteroids into the sub-Tenon's area of the eye.

Hypertension-Related Eye Changes

Hypertension can shorten the lifespan by as many as 20 years and affects the eye as well as the heart, brain, and kidneys. Long-standing hypertension goes hand in hand with atherosclerosis, and the associated retinal changes are evidenced by the development of retinal arteriolar changes, such as tortuousness, narrowing, and a change in light reflex. Funduscopic examination reveals a copper or silver coloration of the arterioles and venous compression (arteriovenous nicking) at the arteriolar and venous crossings. Intraretinal hemorrhages from hypertension appear flame-shaped because they occur in the nerve fiber layer of the retina.

Hypertension can also occur as an acute consequence of conditions such as pheochromocytoma, acute renal failure, and pregnancy-induced hypertension. The retinopathy associated with these crisis states is extensive, and the manifestations include cotton-wool spots, retinal hemorrhages, retinal edema, and retinal exudates, often clustered around the macula.

The choroid is also affected by the profound and abrupt rise in blood pressure and resulting vasoconstriction, and ischemia may result in serous retinal detachments and infarction of the RPE. Ischemic optic neuropathy and **papilledema** (swelling of the optic disc due to increased IOP) may also result. Blood pressure in these more severe stages should be lowered in a controlled gradual fashion to avoid ischemia of the optic nerve and brain secondary to a too-rapid fall in blood pressure. For further information about hypertension, see Chapter 32.

CONCEPTS IN OCULAR MEDICATION ADMINISTRATION

The main objective of ocular medication delivery is to maximize the amount of medication that reaches the ocular site of action in sufficient concentration to produce a beneficial therapeutic effect. This is determined by the dynamics of ocular pharmacokinetics: absorption, distribution, metabolism, and excretion.

Topical administration of ocular medications results in only a 1% to 7% absorption rate by the ocular tissues. Ocular absorption involves the entry of a medication into the aqueous humor through the different routes of ocular medication administration. The rate and extent of aqueous humor absorption are determined by the characteristics of the medication and the anatomy and physiology of the eye. Natural barriers of absorption that diminish the efficacy of ocular medications include the following:

- *Limited size of the conjunctival sac.* The conjunctival sac can hold only 50 µL, and any excess is wasted. The volume of one eye drop from commercial topical ocular solutions typically ranges from 20 to 35 µL.
- *Corneal membrane barriers.* The epithelial, stromal, and endothelial layers are barriers to absorption.
- *Blood–ocular barriers.* Blood–ocular barriers prevent high ocular tissue concentration of most ophthalmic medications because they separate the bloodstream from the ocular tissues and keep foreign substances from entering the eye, thereby limiting a medication's efficacy.
- *Tearing, blinking, and drainage.* Increased tear production and drainage due to ocular irritation or an ocular

condition may dilute or wash out an instilled eye drop; blinking expels an instilled eye drop from the conjunctival sac.

Distribution of an ocular medication into the various ocular tissues varies by tissue type; the various tissues (eg, conjunctiva, cornea, lens, iris, ciliary body, choroids) absorb medications to varying degrees. Medications penetrate the corneal epithelium by diffusion by passing through the cells (intracellular) or by passing between the cells (intercellular). Water-soluble (hydrophilic) medications diffuse through the intracellular route, and fat-soluble (lipophilic) medications diffuse through the intercellular route. Topical administration usually does not reach the retina in significant concentrations. Because the space between the ciliary process and the lens is small, medication diffusion in the vitreous is slow. When high concentrations of medication in the vitreous are required, intraocular injection is often chosen to bypass the natural ocular anatomic and physiologic barriers.

Aqueous solutions are most commonly used for the eye. They are the least expensive medications and interfere least with vision. However, corneal contact time is brief because tears dilute the medication. Ophthalmic ointments have extended retention time in the conjunctival sac and provide a higher concentration than eye drops. The major disadvantage of ointments is the blurred vision that results after application. In general, eyelids and eyelid margins are best treated with ointments. The conjunctiva, limbus, cornea, and anterior chamber are treated most effectively with instilled solutions or suspensions. Subconjunctival injection may be necessary for better absorption in the anterior chamber. If high medication concentrations are required in the posterior chamber, intravitreal injections or systemically absorbed medications are considered. Contact lenses and collagen shields soaked in antibiotics are alternative delivery methods for treating corneal infections.

Of all these delivery methods, the topical route of administration—instilled eye drops and applied ointments—remains the most common. Topical instillation, which is the least invasive method, permits self-administration of medication and produces fewer side effects.

Preservatives are commonly used in ocular medications. Benzalkonium chloride, for example, prevents the growth of organisms and enhances the corneal permeability of most medications; however, some patients are allergic to this preservative. This may be suspected even if the patient had never before experienced an allergic reaction to systemic use of the medication in question. Eye drops without preservatives can be prepared by pharmacists.

Commonly Used Ocular Medications

Common ocular medications include topical anesthetic, mydriatic, and cycloplegic agents that reduce IOP; anti-infective medications; corticosteroids; NSAIDs; antiallergy medications; eye irrigants; and lubricants.

Topical Anesthetics

One or two drops of proparacaine hydrochloride (Ophthaine 0.5%) and tetracaine hydrochloride (Pontocaine 0.5%) are instilled before diagnostic procedures such as tonometry and gonioscopy and in minor ocular procedures such as removal of sutures or conjunctival or corneal scrapings. Topical anesthetics are also used for severe eye pain to allow the patient to open his or her eyes for examination or treatment (eg, eye irrigation for chemical burns). Anesthesia occurs within 20 seconds to 1 minute and lasts 10 to 20 minutes. The nurse must instruct the patient not to rub his or her eyes while anesthetized because this may result in corneal damage.

Most patients are not allowed to take topical anesthetics home because of the risk of overuse. Patients with corneal abrasions and erosions experience severe pain and are often tempted to overuse topical anesthetic eye drops. Overuse of these drops results in softening of the cornea. Prolonged use of anesthetic drops can delay wound healing and can lead to permanent corneal opacification and scarring, resulting in visual loss.

Mydriatics and Cycloplegics

Mydriasis, or pupil dilation, is the main objective of the administration of mydriatic and cycloplegic agents (Table 58-7). These two types of medications function differently and are used in combination to achieve the maximal dilation that is needed during surgery and fundus examinations to give the ophthalmologist a better view of the internal eye structures. Mydriatics potentiate alpha-adrenergic sympathetic effects that result in the relaxation of the ciliary muscle. This causes the pupil to dilate. However, this sympathetic action alone is not enough to sustain mydriasis because of its short duration of action. The strong light used during an eye examination also stimulates miosis (ie, pupillary contraction). Cycloplegic medications are administered to paralyze the iris sphincter.

The patient is instructed about the temporary effects of mydriasis on vision, such as glare and the inability to focus properly. The patient may have difficulty reading. The effects of the various mydriatics and cycloplegics can last 3 hours to several days. The patient is advised to wear sunglasses (most eye clinics provide protective sunglasses). The ability to drive is dependent on the person's age, vision, and comfort level. Some patients can drive safely with the use of sunglasses, whereas others may need to be driven home.

Mydriatic and cycloplegic agents affect the central nervous system. Their effects are most prominent in children and elderly patients; these patients must be assessed closely for symptoms, such as increased blood pressure, tachycardia, dizziness, ataxia, confusion, disorientation, incoherent speech, and hallucination. These medications are contraindicated in patients with narrow angles or shallow anterior chambers and in patients taking monoamine oxidase inhibitors or tricyclic antidepressants.

Medications Used to Treat Glaucoma

Therapeutic medications for glaucoma are used to lower IOP by decreasing aqueous production or increasing aqueous outflow. Because glaucoma calls for lifetime therapy, the patient must be instructed regarding both the ocular and systemic side effects of the medications.

Most antiglaucoma medications affect the accommodation of the lens and limit light entry through a constricted pupil. Visual acuity and the ability to focus may be affected. Some drops (eg, prostaglandin analogues) may cause iris color change as well as eyelash hypertrichosis (excessive growth of hair). Factors to consider in selecting glaucoma medications are efficacy, systemic and ocular side effects, convenience, and cost.

Table 58-7		MYDRIATICS AND CYCLOPLEGICS				
	Available Preparation/		Peak		Recovery Time	
Medication	Concentration	Indication/Dosage	Mydriasis	Cycloplegia	Mydriasis	Cycloplegia
phenylephrine (Neo-Synephrine)	Solutions (2.5%, 10%)	Administered with cycloplegics in pupillary dilation for ophthalmoscopy and surgical procedures every 5–10 min × 3 or until the pupils are fully dilated	10–60 min	—	3–6 h	—
atropine (Atropine Ophthalmic)	Ointment (0.5%–2%) Solutions (0.5%–3%)	In glaucoma, uveitis, or after surgery, 2× to 4× daily	30–40 min	60–180 min	7–10 d	6–12 d
scopolamine (Isopto Hyoscine Ophthalmic)	Solution (0.25%)	Same as atropine	20–30 min	30–60 min	3–7 d	3–7 d
homatropine (Homatropine HBR)	Solution (5%–2.5%)	Same as atropine and scopolamine	40–60 min	30–60 min	1–3 d	1–3 d
cyclopentolate (AK-Pentolate)	Solution (0.5%–2%)	Administered with mydriatics every 5–10 min × 3 or until the pupils are fully dilated for ophthalmoscopy and surgical procedures	30–60 min	25–75 min	1 d	6–24 h
tropicamide (Mydriacyl)	Solution (0.25%–1%)		20–40 min	20–35 min	6 h	<6 h

Data on peak and recovery time from *Ophthalmic drug facts by facts and comparisons* (2008), pp. 45 and 49.
Copyright 2008 by Facts and Comparisons, a Wolters Kluwer Company. Adapted with permission.

Anti-Infective Medications

Anti-infective medications include antibiotic, antifungal, and antiviral agents. Most are available as drops, ointments, or subconjunctival or intravitreal injections. Antibiotics include penicillin, cephalosporins, aminoglycosides, and fluoroquinolones. The main antifungal agent is amphotericin B. Side effects of amphotericin are serious and include severe pain, conjunctival necrosis, iritis, and retinal toxicity. Antiviral medications include acyclovir (Zovirax) and ganciclovir. They are used to treat ocular infections associated with herpesvirus and CMV. Patients receiving ocular anti-infective agents are subject to the same side effects and adverse reactions as those receiving oral or parenteral medications.

Corticosteroids and Nonsteroidal Anti-Inflammatory Drugs

The topical preparations of corticosteroids are commonly used in inflammatory conditions of the eyelids, conjunctiva, cornea, anterior chamber, lens, and uvea. In posterior segment diseases that involve the posterior sclera, retina, and optic nerve, the topical agents are less effective, and parenteral and oral routes are preferred. Because these topical eye drop preparations are suspensions, the patient is instructed to shake the bottle several times to promote mixture of the medication and maximize its therapeutic effect. The most common ocular side effects of long-term topical corticosteroid administration are glaucoma, cataracts, susceptibility to infection, impaired wound healing, mydriasis, and ptosis. High IOP may develop, which is reversible after corticosteroid use is discontinued. To avoid the side effects of corticosteroids, NSAIDs are used as an alternative in controlling inflammatory eye conditions and postoperatively to reduce inflammation. NSAID therapy in combination with topical and oral preparations is an important adjunct therapy in managing uveitis.

Antiallergy Medications

Ocular hypersensitivity reactions, such as allergic conjunctivitis, are extremely common. These conditions result primarily from responses to environmental allergens. Most allergens are airborne or carried to the eye by the hand or by other means, although allergic reactions may also be drug induced. Corticosteroids are commonly used as anti-inflammatory and immunosuppressive agents to control ocular hypersensitivity reactions.

Ocular Irrigants and Lubricants

Most irrigating solutions are used to cleanse the external lids to maintain lid hygiene, to irrigate the external corneal surface to regain normal pH (eg, in chemical burns), to irrigate the corneal surface to eliminate debris, or to inflate the globe intraoperatively. These solutions have various compositions that include sodium, potassium, magnesium, calcium, bicarbonate, glucose, and glutathione (ie, substance found in the aqueous humor). Sterile irrigating solutions, such as Dacriose, for lid hygiene are available. Irrigating solutions are safe to use with an intact corneal surface; however, the corneal surface should not be irrigated in cases of threatened corneal perforation. For patients with severe corneal ulcer, specific orders must be obtained regarding whether it is safe to irrigate the corneal surface or just to cleanse the external lids. Although it is good practice to promote hygiene, prevention of complications must be the primary concern. Normal saline solutions are commonly used to irrigate the corneal surface when chemical burns occur.

Lubricants, such as artificial tears, help alleviate corneal irritation, such as dry eye syndrome. Artificial tears are topical preparations of methyl or hydroxypropyl cellulose that are prepared as eye drop solutions, ointments, or ocular inserts (inserted at the lower conjunctival cul-de-sac once each day). The eye drops can be instilled as often as every hour, depending on the severity of symptoms.

Nursing Management

The objectives in administering ocular medications are to ensure proper administration to maximize the therapeutic effects and to ensure the safety of the patient by monitoring for systemic and local side effects. Absorption of eye drops by the nasolacrimal duct is undesirable because of the potential systemic side effects of ocular medications. To diminish systemic absorption and minimize the side effects, it is important to occlude the puncta (Chart 58-13). This is especially important for patients who are most vulnerable to medication overdose, including elderly people, children, infants, women who are lactating or are pregnant, and patients with cardiac, pulmonary, hepatic, or renal disease. A 1-minute interval between instillation of different types of ocular drops is recommended.

Before the administration of ocular medications, the nurse warns the patient that blurred vision, stinging, and a burning sensation are symptoms that ordinarily occur after instillation and are temporary. Risk for interactions of the ocular medication with other ocular and systemic medications must be emphasized; therefore, a careful patient interview regarding the medications being taken must be obtained.

Emphasis must be placed on hand hygiene techniques before and after medication instillation. The tip of the eye drop bottle or the ointment tube must never touch any part of the eye. The medication must be recapped immediately after each use. If a patient who instills his or her own medications cannot feel the eye drops when they are instilled, the eye medication may be refrigerated, because a cold drop is easier to detect. A 5-minute interval between successive administrations allows adequate drug retention and absorption. The patient or the caregiver at home should be asked to demonstrate actual eye drop or ointment instillation and punctal occlusion.

ISSUES IN OPHTHALMOLOGY

The well-being of the patient physically, emotionally, financially, socially, and spiritually can be at risk when vision is threatened. Patients with a deteriorating eye condition often worry about the impact that visual loss will have on their lives. As they experience visual

CHART 58-13	**PATIENT EDUCATION** *Instilling Eye Medications*

- Shake suspensions or "milky" solutions to obtain the desired medication level.
- Wash hands thoroughly before and after the procedure.
- Ensure adequate lighting.
- Read the label of the eye medication to make sure it is the correct medication.
- Assume a comfortable position.
- Do not touch the tip of the medication container to any part of the eye or face.
- Hold the lower lid down; do not press on the eyeball. Apply gentle pressure to the cheek bone to anchor the finger holding the lid.

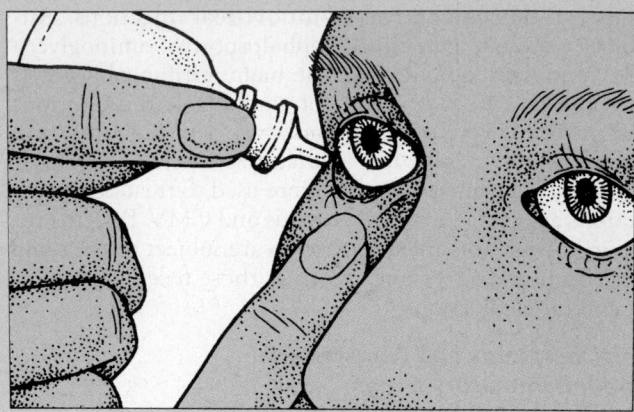

- Instill eye drops before applying ointments.
- Apply a ½-inch ribbon of ointment to the lower conjunctival sac.

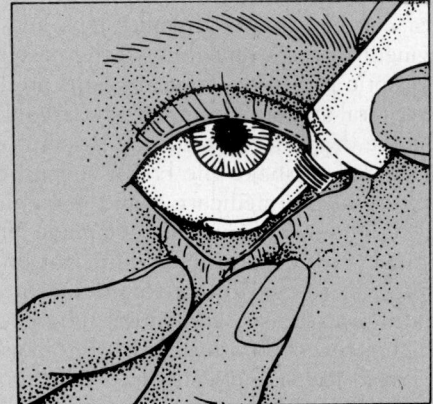

- Keep the eyelids closed, and apply gentle pressure on the inner canthus (punctal occlusion) near the bridge of the nose for 1 or 2 minutes immediately after instilling eyedrops.
- Using a clean tissue, gently pat skin to absorb excess eyedrops that run onto the cheeks.
- Wait 5 to 10 minutes before instilling another eye medication.

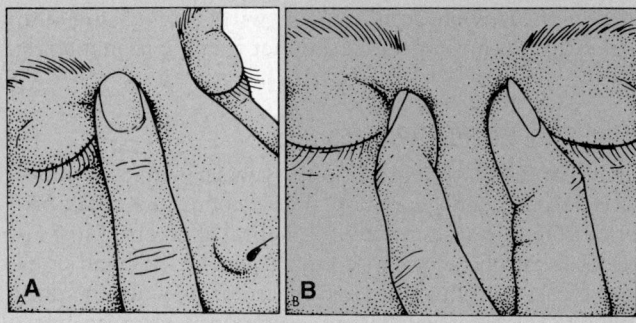

distortions, scotomas, or gradual visual loss, what was a vague worry can become a consuming preoccupation. The patient may equate a decrease in visual acuity with a loss of independence. The loss of a driver's license may force a patient to relocate or give up or change careers.

Vision Loss

Major goals should include the preservation of vision and the prevention of further visual loss in patients who have already experienced some degree of loss. Aging itself is a risk factor for many conditions such as cataracts, glaucoma, and AMD, which may lead to visual loss. Therefore, people older than 50 years of age should have regular examinations by an eye care specialist to help detect problems at their earliest stages, when there may be more treatment options. Those with diabetes or other systemic conditions should also be proactive in obtaining regular ophthalmic care.

For patients with visual impairment, effective communication is essential to promote rehabilitation. The nurse together with the patient should establish goals. The nurse listens to the patient, tries to determine his or her level of health care need, and makes suggestions and recommendations.

Patient Safety

With the advent of the 2000 report from the Institute of Medicine on medical errors and the subsequent report of the Institute's Committee on Identifying and Preventing Medication Errors (Aspden, Wolcott, Bootman, et al., 2007), the nurse must be aware of patient safety practices unique to ophthalmology and must be an active participant in the development of a culture of safety. High-volume, efficient, fast-paced procedures characterize ophthalmic practice. This means that patient identification is critical. Active identification (asking the patient his or her name) and a second identifier (birth date, history, hospital number) must be verified before any procedure. As with other organs involving laterality, the correct eye must be verified before medication administration and surgery. Verification of the correct eye before surgery with the involvement of the patient or caregiver (for pediatric patients and adults with cognitive impairment) must be done before initiating any procedure or transferring the patient to another unit. Marking of the operative eye by the surgeon and a final verification of the correct eye by the surgeon, anesthesiologist, and nurse immediately before incision must be performed in all cases.

Cataract surgery with an IOL implant is one of the most frequently performed surgeries. Each facility must have a policy for multiple checks and verification of the IOL type, power, and diopter, as well as the operative eye. The surgeon, scrub nurse or technician, and circulating nurse should each verify the correct IOL measurements, the correct patient, and the patient's chart.

CRITICAL THINKING EXERCISES

1   An ophthalmic surgeon calls a meeting with the operating room (OR) nurse manager and you, the charge nurse of the OR where he performs surgeries. Five of 15 postoperative cataract patients in the past week have complained of blurred vision and eye pain 1 to 5 days postoperatively. The operative eye showed corneal edema and inflammation of the anterior chamber. The patients were placed on topical nonsteroidal anti-inflammatory agents and were showing some improvement. Is there a need to be alarmed? Identify the steps you plan to take to investigate what is causing the postoperative problems. What initial measures are you planning?

2   You are working in a medical unit of a community hospital. An 86-year-old woman, a cardiac patient who has previously been diagnosed with dry age-related macular degeneration, is worried about some changes in her vision that she has noticed. When checking her vision with her glasses on, you are relieved to find that her vision for distance seems satisfactory. However, the patient complains that when she reads the menu, some of the letters on some lines seem to be missing. In addition, she seems to have some visual distortion; she cannot tell the letter D from the letter O. The patient has a follow-up appointment scheduled with her ophthalmologist in 4 months. Should she be seen sooner? What additional tests do you think will be necessary? What could be the etiol-ogy of her complaints? How can you make this patient's environment safer?

EBP   **3**   You are working the evening shift in the operating room and an environmental services' employee runs to you stating that he accidently splashed his eyes with a cleaning solution. He is holding the bottle that has no label but still has some solution left in it. He has a lot of eye pain, and his vision is extremely blurred. What should you do immediately? What is the evidence base that supports the treatment of chemical burns to the eyes? What is the strength of this evidence? What critical information do you need to provide to the emergency physician? What environmental safety measures do you need to put in place?

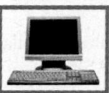

The Smeltzer suite offers these additional resources to enhance learning and facilitate understanding of this chapter:
- thePoint online resource, thepoint.lww.com/Smeltzer12E
- Student CD-ROM included with the book
- *Study Guide to Accompany Brunner & Suddarth's Textbook of Medical-Surgical Nursing*
- *Handbook for Brunner & Suddarth's Textbook of Medical-Surgical Nursing*

REFERENCES AND SELECTED READINGS

Books

American Society of Ophthalmic Registered Nurses. (2006). *Care and handling of ophthalmic microsurgical instruments*, Dubuque, IA: Kendall/Hunt Publishing Company.

Aspden, P., Wolcott, J., Bootman, J. L., et al. (2007). *Preventing medication errors: Quality chasm series*. Washington, DC: National Academy Press.

Bartlett, J. D., Bennett, E. S. & Fiscella, R. G. (Eds.). (2008). *Ophthalmic drug facts, 2008*. St. Louis: Facts & Comparisons.

Bickley, L. S. (2007), *Bates' guide to physical examination* (9th ed.). Philadelphia: Lippincott Williams & Wilkins.

Bressler, S. B., Quigley, H. A. & Schein, O. D. (2008). *Vision: The Johns Hopkins white papers*. New York: Medletter Associates.

Ehlers, J. P. & Shah, C. P. (Eds.). (2008). *The Wills eye manual: Office and emergency room diagnosis and treatment of eye disease* (5th ed.). Philadelphia: Lippincott Williams & Wilkins.

Kanski, J. J. (2007). *Clinical ophthalmology: A systematic approach* (6th ed.). Oxford: Butterworth-Heinemann.

Prevent Blindness America. (2008). *Vision problems in the U.S. Update to the fourth edition*. Schaumberg, IL: Prevent Blindness America/National Eye Institute.

Riordan-Eva, P. & Whitcher, J. P. (2008). *Vaughn & Asbury's general ophthalmology* (17th ed.). New York McGraw-Hill.

Shields, M. B. (2005). *Textbook of glaucoma* (5th ed.). Philadelphia: Lippincott Williams & Wilkins.

Sinha, A. & Ayyala, R. (2008). Conjunctivitis. In R. Rakel & E. T. Bope (Eds.). *Conn's current therapy* (60th ed.). Philadelphia: Saunders Elsevier.

Tipperman, R. (2007). Cataract surgery 2007. In C. J. Rapuano (Ed.). *Yearbook of ophthalmology 2007*. Philadelphia: Elsevier Mosby.

Whitcher, J. (2008). Blindness. In Riordan-Eva, P. & Whitcher, J. P. *Vaughn & Asbury's general ophthalmology*. New York: McGraw-Hill.

Yanoff, M. & Duker, J. (2009). *Ophthalmology*. St. Louis: Mosby.

Journals and Electronic Documents

Age-Related Eye Disease Study Research Group. (2001a). Risk factors associated with age-related macular degeneration. *Ophthalmology, 107*(12), 2224–2232.

Age-Related Eye Disease Study Research Group. (2001b). A randomized, placebo-controlled clinical trial of high-dose supplementation with vitamins

C and E, beta-carotene, and zinc for age-related macular degeneration and vision loss. *Archives of Ophthalmology, 119*(10), 1439–1452.

Andreoli, C. M. & Miller, J. W. (2007). Anti-vascular endothelial growth factor therapy for ocular neovascular disease. *Current Opinion in Ophthalmology, 18*(6), 502–508.

Bulgarelli, E. (2009). Retinal tear. *Nursing, 39*(4), 72.

Chen, E. (2007). 25-Gauge transconjunctival sutureless vitrectomy. *Current Opinion in Ophthalmology, 18*(3), 188–193.

Clinical Trial of Nutritional Supplements and Age-Related Cataract Study Group. (2008). A randomized, double-masked, placebo-controlled clinical trial of multivitamin supplementation for age-related lens opacities. *Ophthalmology, 115*(4), 599–607.

Du, T. T., Fan, V. C. & Asbell, P. A. (2007). Conductive keratoplasty. *Current Opinion in Ophthalmology, 18*(4), 334–337.

Esrick, E., Subramanian, M. L., Heier, J. S., et al. (2005). Multiple laser treatments for macular edema attributable to branch retinal vein occlusion. *American Journal of Ophthalmology, 139*(4), 653–657.

Filippopoulos, T. & Rhee, D. J. (2008). Novel surgical procedures in glaucoma: Advances in penetrating glaucoma surgery. *Current Opinion in Ophthalmolog, 19*(2), 149–154.

Fine, I. H., Hoffman, R. S. & Packer, M. (2007). Editorial review: The new challenge for cataract surgeons. *Current Opinion in Ophthalmology, 18*(1), 1–3.

Fong, C. S. (2007). Refractive surgery: The future of perfect vision? *Singapore Medical Journal, 48*(8), 709–719.

Han, E. S., Wee, W. R., Lee, J. H., et al. (2007). The effect of diffuse lamellar keratitis on visual acuity and contrast sensitivity following LASIK. *Korean Journal of Ophthalmology, 21*(1), 6–10.

Hoffman, R., Fine, I. H. & Packer, M. (2005). New phacoemulsification technology. *Current Opinion in Ophthalmology, 16*(1), 38–43.

Holland, S. P., Morck, D. W. & Lee, T. L. (2007). Update on toxic anterior segment syndrome. *Current Opinion in Ophthalmology, 18*(1), 4–8.

Jager, R. D., Mieler, W. G. & Miller, J. W. (2008). Medical progress. Age-related macular degeneration. *New England Journal of Medicine, 358*(24), 2606–2617.

Johnston, J. (2006). Home study program: Toxic anterior segment syndrome—More than sterility meets the eye. *AORN Journal, 84*(6), 967–984.

Katz, J., Feldman, M. A., Bass, E. B., et al. (2003). Study of Medical Testing for Cataract Surgery Team. Risks and benefits of anticoagulant and antiplatelet medication use before cataract surgery. *Ophthalmology, 110*(9), 1784–1788.

Klein, B. E. K., Klein, R., Lee, K. E., et al. (2003). Socioeconomic and lifestyle factors and the 10-year incidence of age-related cataracts. *American Journal of Ophthalmology, 136*(3), 506–512.

Lalwani, G. A., Flynn, H. W. Jr., Scott, I. U., et al. (2008). Acute-onset endophthalmitis after clear corneal cataract surgery (1996–2005). *Ophthalmology, 115*(3), 473–476.

Mamalis, N., Edelhauser, H. F., Dawson, D. G., et al. (2006). Toxic anterior segment syndrome. *Journal of Cataract and Refractive Surgery, 32*(2), 324–333.

McKinnon, S. J., Goldberg, L. D., Peeples, P., et al. (2008). Current management of glaucoma and the need for complete therapy. *American Journal of Managed Care, 14*(Suppl 1), S20–S27.

Mohamed, Q., McIntosh, R. L., Seang, M. S., et al. (2007) Interventions for central retinal vein occlusion: An evidence-based systemic review. *Ophthalmology, 114*(3), 507–519.

National Eye Institute (NEI). (2008). Age-Related Eye Disease Study 2 (AREDS2). www.nei.nih.gov/neitrials/viewStudyWeb.aspx?id=120

Ogawa, H., Yonezawa, Y., Maki, H., et al. (2007). A mobile phone-based communication support system for elderly persons. Conference Proceedings:Annual International Conference of the IEE. *Engineering in Medicine & Biology Society*, 3798–3801.

Pramanik, S., Goins, K. M. & Sutphin, J. E. (2007). Corneal endothelial transplantation: Descemet's stripping endothelial keratoplasty (DSEK). Eyerounds.org. http://webeye.ophth.uiowa.edu/eyeforum/cases/54-Descemets-Stripping-Endothelial-Keratoplasty-DSEK.htm

Price, M. O. & Price, F. W. (2007). Descemet's stripping endothelial keratoplasty. *Current Opinion in Ophthalmology, 18*(4), 290–294.

Ross, W. H. & Lavina, A. (2008). Pneumatic retinopexy, scleral buckling, and vitrectomy surgery in the management of pseudophakic retinal detachments. *Canadian Journal of Ophthalmology, 43*(1), 65–72.

Seddon, J. M. & Chen, C. A. (2004). The epidemiology of age-related macular degeneration. *International Ophthalmology Clinics, 44*(4), 17–39.

Sharts-Hopko, N. C. & Glynn-Milley, C. (2009). Primary open-angle glaucoma. Catching and treating the "sneak thief of sight." *American Journal of Nursing, 109*(2), 40–48.

Slade, S. G. (2007). The use of femtosecond laser in the customization of corneal flaps in laser in situ keratomileusis. *Current Opinion in Ophthalmology, 18*(4), 314–317.

Taban, M., Behrens, A., Newcomb, R. I., et al. (2005). Acute endophthalmitis following cataract surgery: A systematic review of the literature. *Archives of Ophthalmology, 123*(5), 613–620.

Vidal-Verdu, F. & Hafez, M. (2007). Graphical tactile displays for visually-impaired people. *IEEE Transactions of Neural Systems and Rehabilitation Engineering, 15*(1), 119–130.

Yeh, S., Wroblewski, K., Buggage, R., et al. (2008). High-dose humanized anti-IL-2 receptor alpha antibody (daclizumab) for the treatment of active, noninfectious uveitis. *Journal of Autoimmunity, 31*(2), 91–97.

Zaqloul, K. A. & Boahen, K. (2006). A silicone retina that reproduces in the optic nerve. *Journal of Neural Engineering, 3*(4), 257–267.

RESOURCES

American Academy of Ophthalmology www.aao.org

American Council of the Blind, www.acb.org

American Society of Ophthalmic Registered Nurses, http://webeye.ophth.uiowa.edu/ASORN

Association for Macular Diseases, Inc., www.macular.org

Foundation Fighting Blindness, www.blindness.org

Glaucoma Research Foundation, www.glaucoma.org

Lighthouse National Center for Vision and Aging, www.lighthouse.org

Macular Degeneration Foundation, www.eyesight.org

National Association for Visually Handicapped, www.navh.org

National Eye Institute Information Office, www.nei.nih.gov

Prevent Blindness America, www.preventblindness.org

Research to Prevent Blindness, www.rpbusa.org

VISION Community Services, www.mablind.org

Vision World Wide, Inc., www.visionww.org

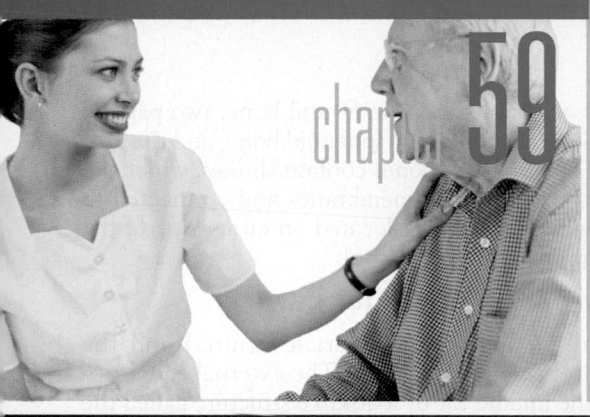

chapter**59**

Assessment and Management of Patients With Hearing and Balance Disorders

On completion of this chapter, the learner will be able to:

1 Describe methods used to assess hearing and to diagnose hearing and balance disorders.

2 List the manifestations that may be exhibited by a person with a hearing disorder.

3 Identify ways to communicate effectively with a person with a hearing disorder.

4 Differentiate problems of the external ear from those of the middle ear and inner ear.

5 Compare the various types of surgical procedures used for managing middle ear disorders and appropriate nursing care.

6 Describe the teaching topics that need to be addressed for patients undergoing middle ear and mastoid surgery.

7 Describe the different types of inner ear disorders, including the clinical manifestations, diagnosis, and management.

acute otitis media: inflammation in the middle ear lasting less than 6 weeks

cholesteatoma: tumor of the middle ear or mastoid, or both, that can destroy structures of the temporal bone

chronic otitis media: repeated episodes of acute otitis media causing irreversible tissue damage and persistent tympanic membrane perforation

conductive hearing loss: loss of hearing in which efficient sound transmission to the inner ear is interrupted by some obstruction or disease process

deafness: partial or complete loss of the ability to hear

dizziness: altered sensation of orientation in space

endolymphatic hydrops: dilation of the endolymphatic space of the inner ear; the pathologic correlate of Ménière's disease

exostoses: small, hard, bony protrusions in the lower posterior bony portion of the ear canal

labyrinthitis: inflammation of the labyrinth of the inner ear

Ménière's disease: condition of the inner ear characterized by a triad of symptoms: episodic vertigo, tinnitus, and fluctuating sensorineural hearing loss

middle ear effusion: fluid in the middle ear without evidence of infection

myringotomy (ie, tympanotomy): incision in the tympanic membrane

nystagmus: involuntary rhythmic eye movement

ossiculoplasty: surgical reconstruction of the middle ear bones to restore hearing

otalgia: sensation of fullness or pain in the ear

otitis externa (ie, external otitis): inflammation of the external auditory canal

otorrhea: drainage from the ear

otosclerosis: a condition characterized by abnormal spongy bone formation around the stapes

presbycusis: progressive hearing loss associated with aging

rhinorrhea: drainage from the nose

sensorineural hearing loss: loss of hearing related to damage of the end organ for hearing or cranial nerve VIII, or both

tinnitus: subjective perception of sound with internal origin; unwanted noises in the head or ear

tympanoplasty: surgical repair of the tympanic membrane

vertigo: illusion of movement in which the individual or the surroundings are sensed as moving

The ear is a sensory organ with dual functions—hearing and balance. The sense of hearing is essential for normal development and maintenance of speech as well as the ability to communicate with others. Balance, or equilibrium, is essential for maintaining body movement, position, and coordination.

The delicate structure and function of the ear make early detection and accurate diagnosis of disorders necessary for preservation of normal hearing and balance. The diagnosis and treatment of these disorders requires skilled health care professionals such as otolaryngologists, internists, and nurses. Nurses can become certified in the specialty of otolaryngology.

This chapter addresses the assessment and management of hearing and balance disorders common to adults. The pediatric otolaryngology literature provides information about otologic disorders that pertain to children.

ASSESSMENT OF THE EAR
Anatomic and Physiologic Overview

The cranium encloses and protects the brain and surrounding structures, providing attachment for various muscles that control head and jaw movements. Eight bones form the

cranium: the occipital bone, the frontal bone, two parietal bones, two temporal bones, the sphenoid bone, and the ethmoid bone. Some of these bones contain sinuses, which are cavities lined with mucous membranes and connected to the nasal cavity. The ears are located on either side of the cranium at approximately eye level.

Anatomy of the External Ear

The external ear includes the auricle (pinna) and the external auditory canal (Fig. 59-1). The external ear is separated from the middle ear by a disklike structure called the tympanic membrane (eardrum).

Auricle

The auricle, attached to the side of the head by skin, is composed mainly of cartilage, except for the fat and subcutaneous tissue in the earlobe. The auricle collects the sound waves and directs vibrations into the external auditory canal.

External Auditory Canal

The external auditory canal is approximately 2.5 cm long. The lateral third is an elastic cartilaginous and dense fibrous framework to which thin skin is attached. The medial two thirds is bone lined with thin skin. The external auditory canal ends at the tympanic membrane.

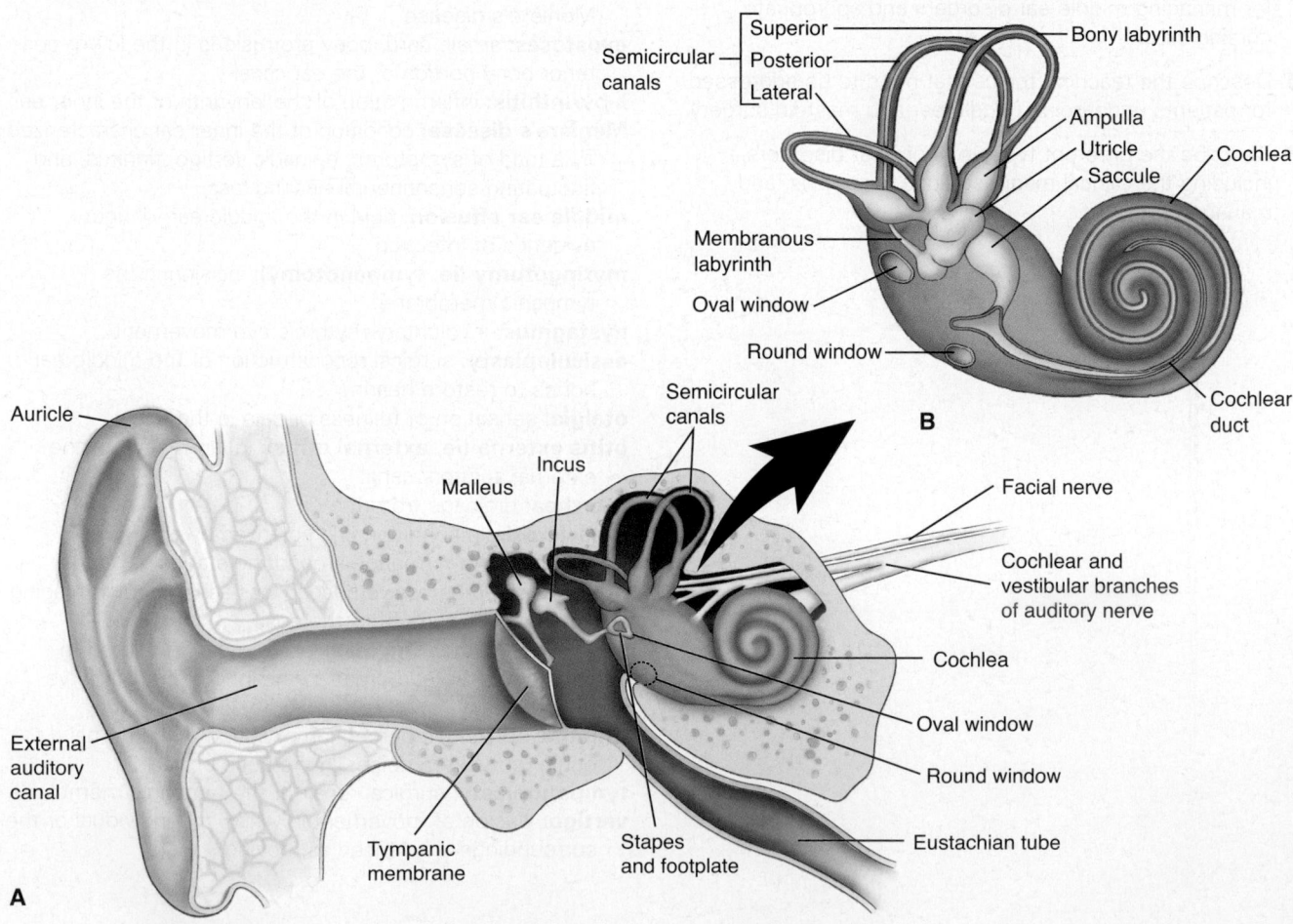

Figure 59-1 A, Anatomy of the ear. **B,** The inner ear.

The skin of the canal contains hair, sebaceous glands, and ceruminous glands, which secrete a brown, waxlike substance called cerumen (ear wax). The ear's self-cleaning mechanism moves old skin cells and cerumen to the outer part of the ear.

Just anterior to the external auditory canal is the temporomandibular joint. The head of the mandible can be felt by placing a fingertip in the external auditory canal while the patient opens and closes the mouth.

Anatomy of the Middle Ear

The middle ear, an air-filled cavity, includes the tympanic membrane laterally and the otic capsule medially. The middle ear cleft lies between the two. The middle ear is connected to the nasopharynx by the eustachian tube and is continuous with air-filled cells in the adjacent mastoid portion of the temporal bone.

The eustachian tube, which is approximately 1 mm wide and 35 mm long, connects the middle ear to the nasopharynx. Normally, the eustachian tube is closed, but it opens by action of the tensor veli palatini muscle when the person performs a Valsalva maneuver, yawns, or swallows. It drains normal and abnormal secretions of the middle ear and equalizes pressure in the middle ear with that of the atmosphere.

Tympanic Membrane

The tympanic membrane (eardrum), about 1 cm in diameter and very thin, is normally pearly gray and translucent. It consists of three layers of tissue: an outer layer, continuous with the skin of the ear canal; a fibrous middle layer; and an inner mucosal layer, continuous with the lining of the middle ear cavity. Approximately 80% of the tympanic membrane is composed of all three layers and is called the pars tensa. The remaining 20% lacks the middle layer and is called the pars flaccida. The absence of this fibrous middle layer makes the pars flaccida more vulnerable to pathologic disorders than the pars tensa. Distinguishing landmarks

include the annulus, the fibrous border that attaches the eardrum to the temporal bone; the short process of the malleus; the long process of the malleus; the umbo of the malleus, which attaches to the tympanic membrane in the center; the pars flaccida; and the pars tensa (Fig. 59-2).

The tympanic membrane protects the middle ear and conducts sound vibrations from the external canal to the ossicles. The sound pressure is magnified 22 times as a result of transmission from a larger area to a smaller one.

Ossicles

The middle ear contains the three smallest bones (the ossicles) of the body: the malleus, the incus, and the stapes. The ossicles, which are held in place by joints, muscles, and ligaments, assist in the transmission of sound. Two small fenestrae (oval and round windows), located in the medial wall of the middle ear, separate the middle ear from the inner ear. The footplate of the stapes sits in the oval window, secured by a fibrous annulus (ring-shaped structure). The footplate transmits sound to the inner ear. The round window, covered by a thin membrane, provides an exit for sound vibrations (see Fig. 59-1).

Anatomy of the Inner Ear

The inner ear is housed deep within the temporal bone. The organs for hearing (cochlea) and balance (semicircular canals), as well as cranial nerves VII (facial nerve) and VIII (vestibulocochlear nerve), are all part of this complex anatomy (see Fig. 59-1). The cochlea and semicircular canals are housed in the bony labyrinth. The bony labyrinth surrounds and protects the membranous labyrinth, which is bathed in a fluid called perilymph.

Membranous Labyrinth

The membranous labyrinth is composed of the utricle, the saccule, the cochlear duct, the semicircular canals, and the organ of Corti, all of which are surrounded by a fluid called

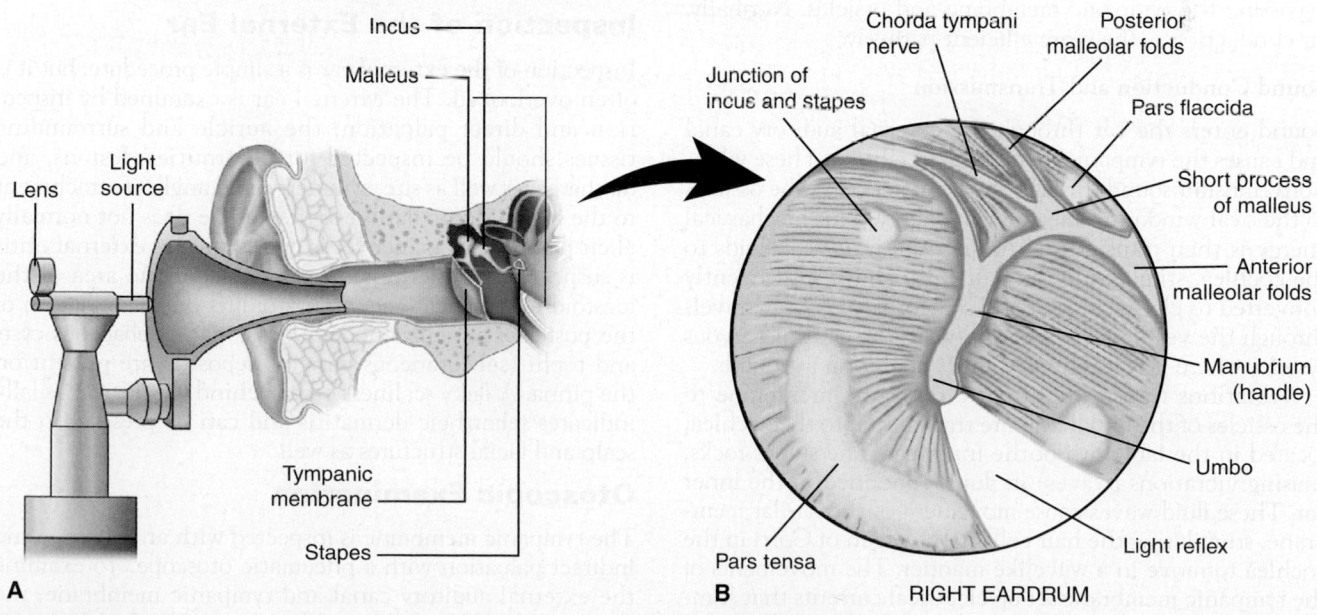

Figure 59-2 Technique for using the otoscope **(A)** to see the tympanic membrane **(B)**.

endolymph. The three semicircular canals—posterior, superior, and lateral, which lie at 90-degree angles to one another—contain sensory receptor organs, arranged to detect rotational movement. These receptor end organs are stimulated by changes in the rate or direction of a person's movement. The utricle and saccule are involved with linear movements.

Organ of Corti

The organ of Corti is housed in the cochlea, a snail-shaped, bony tube about 3.5 cm long with two and a half spiral turns. Membranes separate the cochlear duct (scala media) from the scala vestibuli and the scala tympani from the basilar membrane. The organ of Corti is located on the basilar membrane that stretches from the base to the apex of the cochlea. As sound vibrations enter the perilymph at the oval window and travel along the scala vestibuli, they pass through the scala tympani, enter the cochlear duct, and cause movement of the basilar membrane. The organ of Corti, also called the end organ for hearing, transforms mechanical energy into neural activity and separates sounds into different frequencies. This electrochemical impulse travels through the acoustic nerve to the temporal cortex of the brain to be interpreted as meaningful sound. In the internal auditory canal, the cochlear (acoustic) nerve, arising from the cochlea, joins the vestibular nerve, arising from the semicircular canals, utricle, and saccule, to become the vestibulocochlear nerve (cranial nerve VIII). This canal also houses the facial nerve and the blood supply from the ear to the brain.

Function of the Ears

Hearing

Hearing is conducted over two pathways: air and bone. Sounds transmitted by air conduction travel over the air-filled external and middle ear through vibration of the tympanic membrane and ossicles. Sounds transmitted by bone conduction travel directly through bone to the inner ear, bypassing the tympanic membrane and ossicles. Normally, air conduction is the more efficient pathway.

Sound Conduction and Transmission

Sound enters the ear through the external auditory canal and causes the tympanic membrane to vibrate. These vibrations transmit sound through the lever action of the ossicles to the oval window as mechanical energy. This mechanical energy is then transmitted through the inner ear fluids to the cochlea, stimulating the hair cells, and is subsequently converted to electrical energy. The electrical energy travels through the vestibulocochlear nerve to the central nervous system, where it is interpreted in its final form as sound.

Vibrations transmitted by the tympanic membrane to the ossicles of the middle ear are transmitted to the cochlea, located in the labyrinth of the inner ear. The stapes rocks, causing vibrations (waves) in fluids contained in the inner ear. These fluid waves cause movement of the basilar membrane, stimulating the hair cells of the organ of Corti in the cochlea to move in a wavelike manner. The movements of the tympanic membrane set up electrical currents that stimulate the various areas of the cochlea. The hair cells set up

neural impulses that are encoded and then transferred to the auditory cortex in the brain, where they are decoded into a sound message.

The footplate of the stapes receives impulses transmitted by the incus and the malleus from the tympanic membrane. The round window, which opens on the opposite side of the cochlear duct, is protected from sound waves by the intact tympanic membrane, permitting motion of the inner ear fluids by sound wave stimulation. For example, in the normally intact tympanic membrane, sound waves stimulate the oval window first, and a lag occurs before the terminal effect of the stimulus reaches the round window. However, this lag phase is changed when a perforation of the tympanic membrane allows sound waves to impinge on the oval and round windows simultaneously. This effect cancels the lag and prevents the maximal effect of inner ear fluid motility and its subsequent effect in stimulating the hair cells in the organ of Corti. The result is a reduction in hearing ability (Fig. 59-3).

Balance and Equilibrium

Body balance is maintained by the cooperation of the muscles and joints of the body (proprioceptive system), the eyes (visual system), and the labyrinth (vestibular system). These areas send their information about equilibrium, or balance, to the brain (cerebellar system) for coordination and perception in the cerebral cortex. The brain obtains its blood supply from the heart and arterial system. A problem in any of these areas, such as arteriosclerosis or impaired vision, can cause a disturbance of balance. The vestibular apparatus of the inner ear provides feedback regarding the movements and the position of the head and body in space.

Assessment

Assessment of hearing and balance involves inspection of the external, middle, and inner ear. Evaluation of gross hearing acuity also is included in every physical examination.

Inspection of the External Ear

Inspection of the external ear is a simple procedure, but it is often overlooked. The external ear is examined by inspection and direct palpation; the auricle and surrounding tissues should be inspected for deformities, lesions, and discharge, as well as size, symmetry, and angle of attachment to the head. Manipulation of the auricle does not normally elicit pain. If this maneuver is painful, acute external otitis is suspected. Tenderness on palpation in the area of the mastoid may indicate acute mastoiditis or inflammation of the posterior auricular node. Occasionally, sebaceous cysts and tophi (subcutaneous mineral deposits) are present on the pinna. A flaky scaliness on or behind the auricle usually indicates seborrheic dermatitis and can be present on the scalp and facial structures as well.

Otoscopic Examination

The tympanic membrane is inspected with an otoscope and indirect palpation with a pneumatic otoscope. To examine the external auditory canal and tympanic membrane, the otoscope should be held in the examiner's right hand, in a

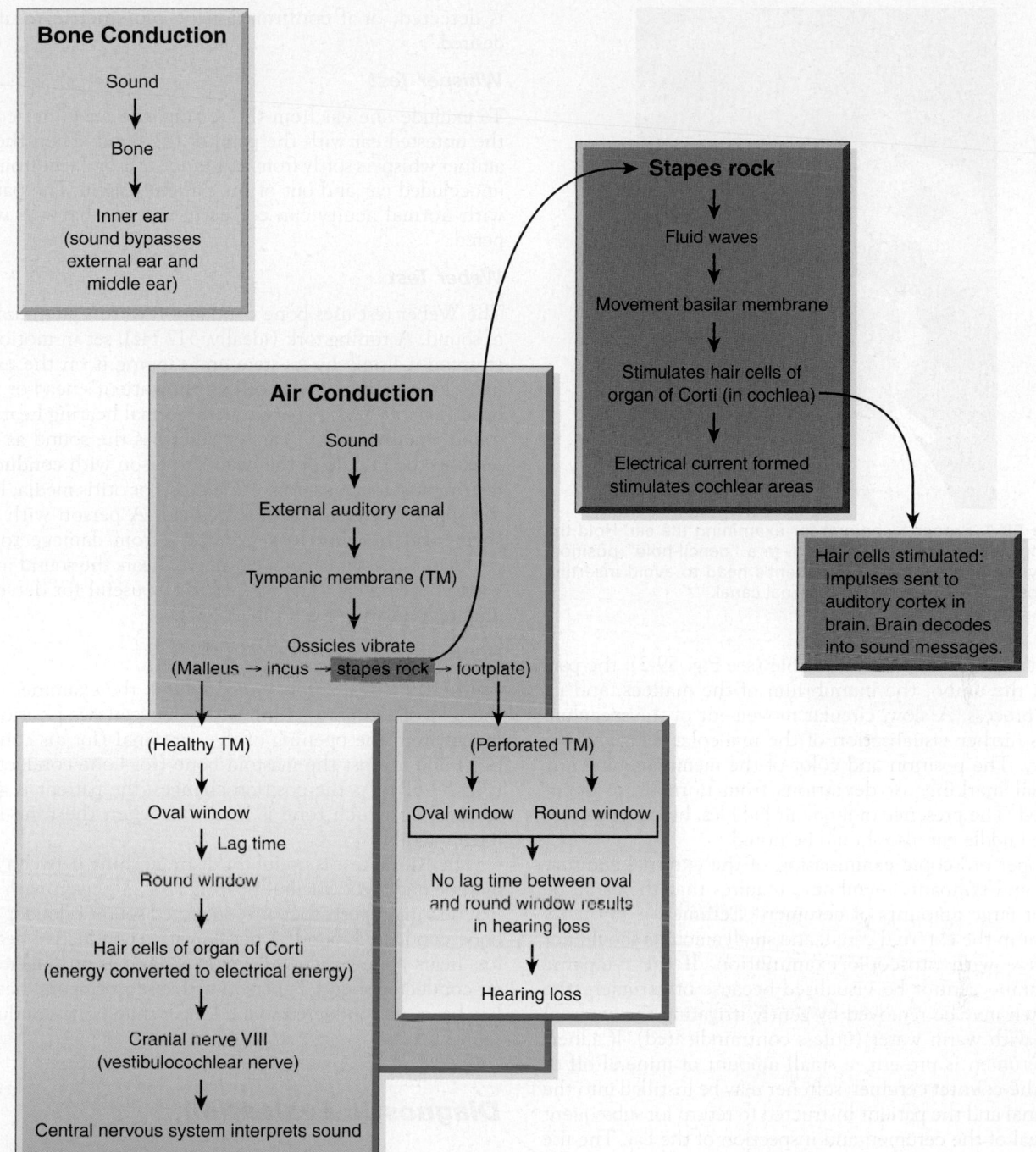

Figure 59-3 Bone conduction compared to air conduction.

pencil-hold position, with the examiner's hand braced against the patient's face (Fig. 59-4). This position prevents the examiner from inserting the otoscope too far into the external canal. Using the opposite hand, the auricle is grasped and gently pulled back to straighten the canal in the adult. If the canal is not straightened with this technique, the tympanic membrane is more difficult to visualize because the canal obstructs the view.

The speculum is slowly inserted into the ear canal, with the examiner's eye held close to the magnifying lens of the otoscope to visualize the canal and tympanic membrane. The largest speculum that the canal can accommodate (usually 5 mm in an adult) is guided gently down into the canal and slightly forward. Because the distal portion of the canal is bony and covered by a sensitive layer of epithelium, only light pressure can be used without causing pain. The external auditory canal is examined for discharge, inflammation, or a foreign body.

The healthy tympanic membrane is pearly gray and is positioned obliquely at the base of the canal. The following

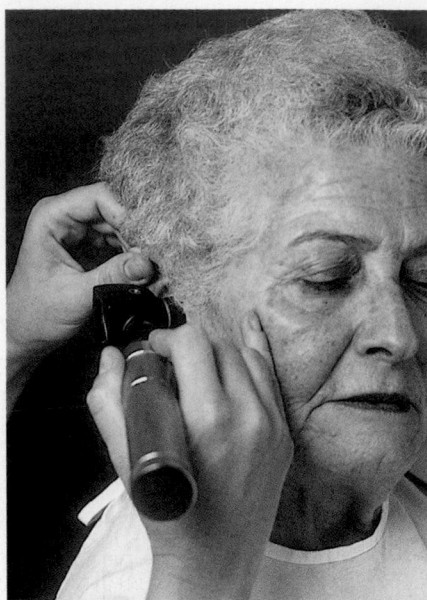

Figure 59-4 Proper technique for examining the ear. Hold the otoscope in the right or left hand, in a "pencil-hold" position. Steady the hand against the patient's head to avoid inserting the otoscope too far into the external canal.

landmarks are identified, if visible (see Fig. 59-2): the pars tensa, the umbo, the manubrium of the malleus, and its short process. A slow, circular movement of the speculum allows further visualization of the malleolar folds and periphery. The position and color of the membrane and any unusual markings or deviations from normal are documented. The presence of fluid, air bubbles, blood, or masses in the middle ear also should be noted.

Proper otoscopic examination of the external auditory canal and tympanic membrane requires that the canal be free of large amounts of cerumen. Cerumen is normally present in the external canal, and small amounts should not interfere with otoscopic examination. If the tympanic membrane cannot be visualized because of cerumen, the cerumen may be removed by gently irrigating the external canal with warm water (unless contraindicated). If adherent cerumen is present, a small amount of mineral oil or over-the-counter cerumen softener may be instilled into the ear canal and the patient instructed to return for subsequent removal of the cerumen and inspection of the ear. The use of instruments such as a cerumen curette for cerumen removal is reserved for otolaryngologists and nurses with specialized training because of the danger of perforating the tympanic membrane or excoriating the external auditory canal. Cerumen buildup is a common cause of hearing loss and local irritation.

Evaluation of Gross Auditory Acuity

A general estimate of hearing can be made by assessing the patient's ability to hear a whispered phrase or a ticking watch, testing one ear at a time. The Weber and Rinne tests may be used to distinguish conductive loss from sensorineural loss when hearing is impaired. These tests are part of the usual screening physical examination and are useful if a more specific assessment is needed, if hearing loss

is detected, or if confirmation of audiometric results is desired.

Whisper Test

To exclude one ear from the testing, the examiner covers the untested ear with the palm of the hand. Then the examiner whispers softly from a distance of 1 or 2 feet from the unoccluded ear and out of the patient's sight. The patient with normal acuity can correctly repeat what was whispered.

Weber Test

The Weber test uses bone conduction to test lateralization of sound. A tuning fork (ideally, 512 Hz), set in motion by grasping it firmly by its stem and tapping it on the examiner's knee or hand, is placed on the patient's head or forehead (Fig. 59-5A). A person with normal hearing hears the sound equally in both ears or describes the sound as centered in the middle of the head. A person with **conductive hearing loss,** such as from otosclerosis or otitis media, hears the sound better in the affected ear. A person with **sensorineural hearing loss,** resulting from damage to the cochlear or vestibulocochlear nerve, hears the sound in the better-hearing ear. The Weber test is useful for detecting unilateral hearing loss (Table 59-1).

Rinne Test

In the Rinne test (pronounced *rin-ay*), the examiner shifts the stem of a vibrating tuning fork between two positions: 2 inches from the opening of the ear canal (for air conduction) and against the mastoid bone (for bone conduction) (Fig. 59-5B). As the position changes, the patient is asked to indicate which tone is louder or when the tone is no longer audible.

The Rinne test is useful for distinguishing between conductive and sensorineural hearing loss. A person with normal hearing reports that air-conducted sound is louder than bone-conducted sound. A person with a conductive hearing loss hears bone-conducted sound as long as or longer than air-conducted sound. A person with a sensorineural hearing loss hears air-conducted sound longer than bone-conducted sound.

Diagnostic Evaluation

Many diagnostic procedures are available to measure the auditory and vestibular systems indirectly. These tests are usually performed by an audiologist who is certified by the American Speech-Language-Hearing Association. Prior to each of the following tests, the nurse explains the procedure to the patient.

Audiometry

In detecting hearing loss, audiometry is the single most important diagnostic instrument. Audiometric testing is of two kinds: pure-tone audiometry, in which the sound stimulus consists of a pure or musical tone (the louder the tone before the patient perceives it, the greater the hearing loss), and speech audiometry, in which the spoken word is used to determine the ability to hear and discriminate sounds and words.

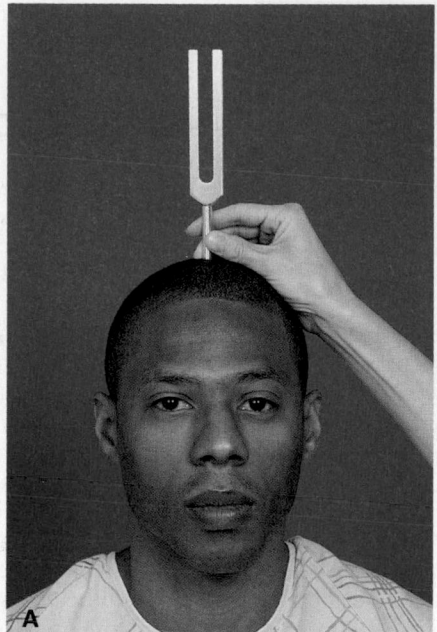
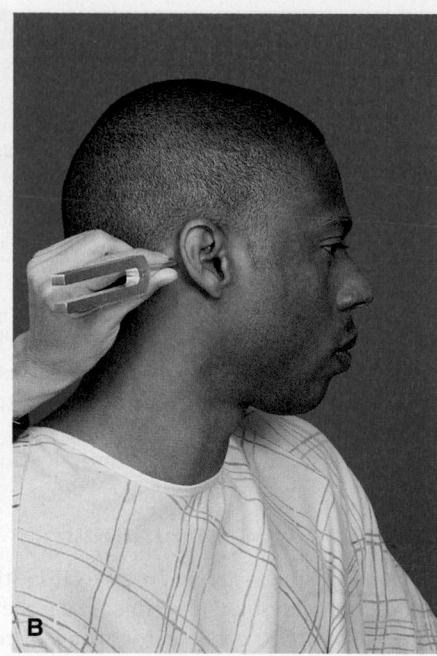

Figure 59-5 A, The Weber test assesses bone conduction of sound. **B,** The Rinne test assesses both air and bone conduction of sound.

When evaluating hearing, three characteristics are important: frequency, pitch, and intensity. *Frequency* refers to the number of sound waves emanating from a source per second, measured as cycles per second, or Hertz (Hz). The normal human ear perceives sounds ranging in frequency from 20 to 20,000 Hz. The frequencies from 500 to 2000 Hz are important in understanding everyday speech and are referred to as the speech range or speech frequencies. *Pitch* is the term used to describe frequency; a tone with 100 Hz is considered of low pitch, and a tone of 10,000 Hz is considered of high pitch.

The unit for measuring loudness (*intensity* of sound) is the decibel (dB), the pressure exerted by sound. Hearing loss is measured in decibels, a logarithmic function of intensity that is not easily converted into a percentage. The critical level of loudness is approximately 30 dB. The shuffling of papers in quiet surroundings is about 15 dB; a low conversation, 40 dB; and a jet plane 100 feet away, about 150 dB. Sound louder than 80 dB is perceived by the human ear to be harsh and can be damaging to the inner ear. Table 59-2 classifies hearing loss based on decibel level. In surgical treatment of patients with hearing loss, the aim is to improve the hearing level to 30 dB or better within the speech frequencies.

With audiometry, the patient wears earphones and signals to the audiologist when a tone is heard. When the tone is applied directly over the external auditory canal, air conduction is measured. When the stimulus is applied to the mastoid bone, bypassing the conductive mechanism (ie, the ossicles), nerve conduction is tested. For accuracy, testing is performed in a soundproof room. Responses are plotted on a graph known as an audiogram, which differentiates conductive from sensorineural hearing loss.

Tympanogram

A tympanogram, or impedance audiometry, measures middle ear muscle reflex to sound stimulation and compliance of the tympanic membrane by changing the air pressure in a sealed ear canal. Compliance is impaired with middle ear disease.

Auditory Brain Stem Response

The auditory brain stem response is a detectable electrical potential from cranial nerve VIII and the ascending auditory pathways of the brain stem in response to sound stimulation. Electrodes are placed on the patient's forehead. Acoustic stimuli (eg, clicks) are made in the ear. The resulting electrophysiologic measurements can determine at which decibel level a patient hears and whether there are any impairments along the nerve pathways (eg, tumor on cranial nerve VIII).

Electronystagmography

Electronystagmography is the measurement and graphic recording of the changes in electrical potentials created by eye movements during spontaneous, positional, or calorically evoked nystagmus. It is also used to assess the

Table 59-1	COMPARISON OF WEBER AND RINNE TESTS	
Hearing Status	**Weber**	**Rinne**
Normal hearing	Sound is heard equally in both ears.	Air conduction is audible longer than bone conduction.
Conductive hearing loss	Sound is heard best in affected ear (hearing loss).	Sound is heard as long or longer in affected ear (hearing loss).
Sensorineural hearing loss	Sound is heard best in normal hearing ear.	Air conduction is audible longer than bone conduction in affected ear.

Table 59-2	SEVERITY OF HEARING LOSS
Loss in Decibels	**Interpretation**
0–15	Normal hearing
>15–25	Slight hearing loss
>25–40	Mild hearing loss
>40–55	Moderate hearing loss
>55–70	Moderate to severe hearing loss
>70–90	Severe hearing loss
>90	Profound hearing loss

oculomotor and vestibular systems and their corresponding interaction. It helps diagnose conditions such as Ménière's disease and tumors of the internal auditory canal or posterior fossa. Any vestibular suppressants, such as sedatives, tranquilizers, antihistamines, and alcohol, are withheld for 24 hours before testing.

Platform Posturography

Platform posturography is used to investigate postural control capabilities such as vertigo. It can be used to evaluate if a person's vertigo is becoming worse or to evaluate the person's response to treatment. The integration of visual, vestibular, and proprioceptive cues (ie, sensory integration) with motor response output and coordination of the lower limbs is tested. The patient stands on a platform, surrounded by a screen, and different conditions such as a moving platform with a moving screen or a stationary platform with a moving screen are presented. The responses from the patient on six different conditions are measured and indicate which of the anatomic systems may be impaired. Preparation for the testing is the same as for electronystagmography.

Sinusoidal Harmonic Acceleration

Sinusoidal harmonic acceleration, or a rotary chair, is used to assess the vestibulo-ocular system by analyzing compensatory eye movements in response to the clockwise and counterclockwise rotation of the chair. Although such testing cannot identify the side of the lesion in unilateral disease, it helps identify disease (eg, Ménière's disease and tumors of the auditory canal) and evaluate the course of recovery. The same patient preparation is required as for electronystagmography.

Middle Ear Endoscopy

With endoscopes with very small diameters and acute angles, the ear can be examined by an endoscopist specializing in otolaryngology. Middle ear endoscopy is performed safely and effectively as an office procedure to evaluate suspected perilymphatic fistula and new-onset conductive hearing loss, the anatomy of the round window before transtympanic treatment of Ménière's disease, and the tympanic cavity before ear surgery to treat chronic middle ear and mastoid infections.

The tympanic membrane is anesthetized topically for about 10 minutes before the procedure. Then, the external auditory canal is irrigated with sterile normal saline solution. With the aid of a microscope, a tympanotomy is created with a laser beam or a myringotomy knife, so that the endoscope can be inserted into the middle ear cavity. Video and photo documentation can be accomplished through the scope.

HEARING LOSS

Hearing impairment has been reported to occur in 3 of every 1000 births, and approximately one half of the time it is related to genetic factors (U.S. Department of Health and Human Services [USDHHS], 2007). Chart 59-1 contains more information about hearing disorders that have a genetic cause. It has been reported that approximately 73% of hospitals or birthing centers are now offering universal hearing screenings for all newborns after birth and prior to discharge.

Hearing loss is greater in men than in women. By the year 2050, about one of every five people in the United States, or almost 58 million people, will be 55 years of age or older. Of this population, almost half can expect to have a hearing impairment (USDHHS, 2007). Hearing loss is an important health issue, and as people age, hearing screening and treatment are indicated.

Approximately 10 million people in the United States have irreversible hearing loss (Mitchell, 2006). It is estimated that more than 30 million people are exposed on a daily basis to noise levels that produce hearing loss. Occupations such as carpentry, plumbing, and coal mining have the highest risk of noise-induced hearing loss. Wise Ears was developed in 1999 by the National Institute on Deafness and Other Communication Disorders (NIDCD) and the National Institute for Occupational Safety and Health. It aims to educate the public about noise-induced hearing loss and ways to prevent this hearing loss (NIDCD, 2008)

Conductive hearing loss usually results from an external ear disorder, such as impacted cerumen, or a middle ear disorder, such as otitis media or otosclerosis. In such instances, the efficient transmission of sound by air to the inner ear is interrupted. A sensorineural loss involves damage to the cochlea or vestibulocochlear nerve.

Mixed hearing loss and functional hearing loss also may occur. Patients with mixed hearing loss have conductive loss and sensorineural loss, resulting from dysfunction of air and bone conduction. A functional (or psychogenic) hearing loss is nonorganic and unrelated to detectable structural changes in the hearing mechanisms; it is usually a manifestation of an emotional disturbance.

Clinical Manifestations

Early manifestations of hearing impairment and loss may include tinnitus, increasing inability to hear when in a group, and a need to turn up the volume of the television. Hearing impairment can also trigger changes in attitude, the ability to communicate, the awareness of surroundings, and even the ability to protect oneself, affecting a person's quality of life. In a classroom, a student with impaired hearing may be uninterested and inattentive and have failing grades. A person at home may feel isolated because of an inability to hear the clock chime or to hear the telephone. A pedestrian who is hearing-impaired may attempt to cross the street and fail to hear an approaching car. People with impaired hearing may miss parts of a conversation. Many people are unaware

CHART 59-1

GENETICS IN NURSING PRACTICE
Hearing Disorders

Selected Hearing Disorders Influenced by Genetic Factors

- Autosomal dominant hearing loss
- Autosomal recessive hearing loss (eg, connexin 26 gene)
- Otosclerosis
- Pendred syndrome
- Usher syndrome
- Waardenburg syndrome

Nursing Assessments

Family History Assessment

- Assess for other family members in several generations with hearing loss (autosomal dominant hearing loss)
- Inquire about genetic relatedness (eg, individuals who are related, such as first cousins, have a higher chance to share the same recessive genes—autosomal recessive hearing loss)
- Inquire about age at onset of hearing loss

Patient Assessment

- Assess for related genetic conditions, such as vision impairment (eg, retinitis pigmentosa in Usher syndrome; thyroid disorder in Pendred syndrome)
- Assess for iris, pigment, and hair alterations (white forelock) seen in Waardenburg syndrome

Management Issues Specific to Genetics

- Inquire whether DNA gene mutation or other genetic testing has been performed on affected family members.
- If indicated, refer for further genetic counseling and evaluation so that family members can discuss inheritance, risk to other family members, availability of genetic testing, and gene-based interventions.
- Offer appropriate genetic information and resources.
- Assess patient's understanding of genetic information.
- Provide support to families with newly diagnosed genetic-related sensorineural disorders.
- Participate in management and coordination of care of patients with genetic conditions, and individuals predisposed to develop or pass on a genetic condition.

Genetics Resources

Genetic Alliance—a directory of support groups for patients and families with genetic conditions; www.geneticalliance.org

Gene Clinics—a listing of common genetic disorders with up-to-date clinical summaries, genetic counseling and testing information; www.geneclinics.org

National Organization of Rare Disorders—a directory of support groups and information for patients and families with rare genetic disorders; www.rarediseases.org

OMIM: Online Mendelian Inheritance in Man—a complete listing of inherited genetic conditions; www.ncbi.nlm.nih.gov/omim/stats/html

---

of their gradual hearing impairment. Often, it is not the person with the hearing loss but the people with whom he or she is communicating who recognizes the impairment first (Chart 59-2).

For various reasons, some people with hearing loss refuse to seek medical attention or wear a hearing aid. They may feel self-conscious wearing a hearing aid. Other more insightful people generally ask those with whom they are trying to communicate to let them know whether difficulties in communication exist. The attitudes and behaviors of patients who need hearing assistance should be taken into account when counseling them. The decision to wear a hearing aid is a personal one that is affected by these attitudes and behaviors.

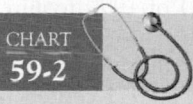

CHART 59-2

Assessing for Hearing Loss

Be alert for the following:

Speech deterioration: The person who slurs words or drops word endings, or produces flat-sounding speech, may not be hearing correctly. The ears guide the voice, both in loudness and in pronunciation.

Fatigue: If a person tires easily when listening to conversation or to a speech, fatigue may be the result of straining to hear. Under these circumstances, the person may become irritable very easily.

Indifference: It is easy for the person who cannot hear what others say to become depressed and disinterested in life in general.

Social withdrawal: Not being able to hear what is going on causes the hearing-impaired person to withdraw from situations that might prove embarrassing.

Insecurity: Lack of self-confidence and fear of mistakes create a feeling of insecurity in many hearing-impaired people. No one likes to say the wrong thing or do anything that might appear foolish.

Indecision and procrastination: Loss of self-confidence makes it increasingly difficult for a hearing-impaired person to make decisions.

Suspiciousness: The hearing-impaired person, who often hears only part of what is being said, may suspect that others are talking about him or her, or that portions of the conversation are deliberately spoken softly so that he or she will not hear them.

False pride: The hearing-impaired person wants to conceal the hearing loss and thus often pretends to be hearing when he or she actually is not.

Loneliness and unhappiness: Although everyone wishes for quiet now and then, *enforced* silence can be boring and even somewhat frightening. People with a hearing loss often feel isolated.

Tendency to dominate the conversation: Many hearing-impaired people tend to dominate the conversation, knowing that as long as it is centered on them and they can control it, they are not so likely to be embarrassed by some mistake.

Prevention

Many environmental factors have an adverse effect on the auditory system and, with time, result in permanent sensorineural hearing loss. The most common is noise. Noise (unwanted and unavoidable sound) has been identified as one of today's environmental hazards. The volume of noise that surrounds us daily has increased into a potentially dangerous source of physical and psychological damage.

Loud, persistent noise has been found to cause constriction of peripheral blood vessels, increased blood pressure and heart rate (because of increased secretion of adrenalin), and increased gastrointestinal activity. Although research is needed to address the overall effects of noise on the human body, a quiet environment is more conducive to peace of mind. A person who is ill feels more at ease when noise is kept to a minimum.

Numerous factors contribute to hearing loss (Chart 59-3). *Noise-induced hearing loss* refers to hearing loss that follows a long period of exposure to loud noise (eg, heavy machinery, engines, artillery, rock-band music). *Acoustic trauma* refers to hearing loss caused by a single exposure to an extremely intense noise, such as an explosion. Usually, noise-induced hearing loss occurs at a high frequency (about 4000 Hz). However, with continued noise exposure, the hearing loss can become more severe and include adjacent frequencies. The minimum noise level known to cause noise-induced hearing loss, regardless of duration, is about 85 to 90 dB.

Noise exposure is inherent in many jobs (eg, mechanics, printers, pilots, flight attendants, musicians) and in hobbies such as woodworking and hunting. Noise level regulations are based on the amount of noise a person is exposed to, with the maximum legal amount being exposure to noise over an average working day or week of 80 dB, with a peak sound pressure of 135 dB (Health and Safety Executive, 2008). The Occupational Safety and Health Administration requires that workers wear ear protection to prevent noise-induced hearing loss when exposed to noise above the legal limits. Ear protection against noise is the most effective preventive measure available. Hearing loss due to noise is permanent because the hair cells in the organ of Corti are destroyed.

 ### Gerontologic Considerations

Approximately half of all people with hearing loss or **deafness** are 65 years of age or older. The cause is unknown; linkages to diet, metabolism, arteriosclerosis, stress, and heredity have been inconsistent (Mitchell, 2006).

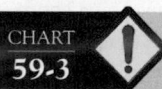

CHART 59-3 **! Risk Factors for Hearing Loss**

- Family history of sensorineural impairment
- Congenital malformations of the cranial structure (ear)
- Low birth weight (<1500 g)
- Use of ototoxic medications (eg, gentamycin, loop diuretics)
- Recurrent ear infections
- Bacterial meningitis
- Chronic exposure to loud noises
- Perforation of the tympanic membrane

With aging, changes occur in the ear that may eventually lead to hearing deficits. Although few changes occur in the external ear, cerumen tends to become harder and drier, posing a greater chance of impaction. In the middle ear, the tympanic membrane may atrophy or become sclerotic. In the inner ear, cells at the base of the cochlea degenerate. A familial predisposition to sensorineural hearing loss is also seen, manifested by inability to hear high-frequency sounds, followed in time by the loss of middle and lower frequencies. The term **presbycusis** is used to describe this progressive hearing loss.

In addition to age-related changes, other factors can affect hearing in the elderly population, such as lifelong exposure to loud noises. Certain medications, such as aminoglycosides and aspirin, have ototoxic effects when renal changes (eg, in the older person) result in delayed medication excretion and increased levels of the medications in the blood. Many older people have taken quinine for treatment of leg cramps; this medication also can contribute to hearing loss. Psychogenic factors and other disease processes (eg, diabetes) also may be partially responsible for sensorineural hearing loss.

When hearing loss occurs, proper evaluation and treatment are warranted. *Healthy People 2010* identifies eight objectives for decreasing the problems caused by hearing loss. One of these objectives is for people diagnosed with hearing loss or deafness to use rehabilitation services and supplemental devices to improve communication with other people. Resources are available in workplaces and in schools. The Individuals with Disabilities Education Act (IDEA) was developed to ensure that children and adults, including elderly adults, receive the same opportunities in the educational system as those without hearing impairment (U.S. Department of Education, 2008).

Even with the best health care, people with hearing loss must learn to adjust to it. Care of elderly patients includes recognizing emotional reactions related to hearing loss, such as suspicion of others because of an inability to hear adequately; frustration and anger, with repeated statements such as, "I didn't hear what you said"; and feelings of insecurity because of the inability to hear the telephone or alarms. The Americans with Disabilities Act (ADA) of 1990 requires that all emergency services are accessible to people who have text message telephones (TTYs). In addition, in 1998, the Department of Justice mandated that all 911 centers in the United States be accessible to people with TTYs.

Medical Management

If a hearing loss is permanent or untreatable or if the patient elects not to be treated, aural rehabilitation (discussed at the end of the chapter) may be beneficial.

Nursing Management

Nurses who understand the different types of hearing loss are more successful in adopting a communication style to fit the needs and preferences of each patient. Trying to speak in a loud voice to a person who cannot hear high-frequency sounds only makes understanding more difficult. However, strategies such as talking into the less-impaired ear and using gestures and facial expressions can help (Chart 59-4).

A major issue for many people who are deaf or hearing-impaired is that they have other health problems that often do not receive attention, in large part because of

Chart 59-4 • *Communicating With People Who Are Hearing-Impaired*

For the Person Who is Hearing-impaired Whose Speech is Difficult to Understand:

- Determine how the person prefers to communicate with others. Do not assume that writing, gestures, or other means are the best or preferred technique.
- Consider if the person uses sign language. Interpreters are available from the American Sign Language, Inc., Interpreting Service (ASLI). These specialists provide the best means of communication, providing accurate, professional services.
- Devote full attention to what the person is saying. Look and listen—do not try to attend to another task while listening.
- Engage the speaker in conversation when it is possible for you to anticipate the replies. This enables you to become accustomed to any peculiarities in speech patterns.
- Try to determine the essential context of what is being said; you can often fill in the details from context.
- Do not try to appear as if you understand if you do not.
- If you cannot understand at all or have serious doubt about your ability to understand what is being said, have the person write the message rather than risk misunderstanding. Having the person repeat the message in speech, after you know its content, also aids you in becoming accustomed to the person's pattern of speech.

- Written communication is an excellent resource. Written material should be written at a third-grade level so that the majority of people can understand it.

For the Person Who is Hearing-impaired Who Speech Reads:

- When speaking, always face the person as directly as possible.
- Make sure your face is as clearly visible as possible. Locate yourself so that your face is well lighted; avoid being silhouetted against strong light. Do not obscure the person's view of your mouth in any way; avoid talking with any object held in your mouth.
- Be sure that the patient knows the topic or subject before going ahead with what you plan to say. This enables the person to use contextual clues in speech reading.
- Speak slowly and distinctly, pausing more frequently than you would normally.
- If you question whether some important direction or instruction has been understood, check to be certain that the patient has the full meaning of your message.
- If for any reason your mouth must be covered (as with a mask) and you must direct or instruct the patient, write the message.

communication barriers with their health care practitioners. To meet the health care needs of these patients, practitioners are legally obligated to make accommodations for a patient's inability to hear. Providing interpreters for those who can communicate through sign language is essential in many situations so that the practitioner can effectively communicate with the patient.

During health care and screening procedures, the practitioner (eg, dentist, physician, nurse) must be aware that patients who are deaf or hearing-impaired are unable to read lips, see a signer, or read written materials in the dark rooms required during some diagnostic tests. The same situation exists if the practitioner is wearing a mask or is not in sight (eg, x-ray studies, magnetic resonance imaging [MRI], colonoscopy).

Nurses and other health care practitioners must work with patients who are deaf or hearing-impaired and their families to identify practical and effective means of communication. Nurses can serve as catalysts throughout the health care system to ensure that accommodations are made to meet the communication needs of these patients.

CONDITIONS OF THE EXTERNAL EAR

Cerumen Impaction

Cerumen normally accumulates in the external canal in various amounts and colors. Although wax does not usually need to be removed, impaction occasionally occurs, causing **otalgia,** a sensation of fullness or pain in the ear, with or without a hearing loss. Accumulation of cerumen as a cause of hearing loss is especially significant in the elderly population. Attempts to clear the external auditory canal with matches, hairpins, and other implements are dangerous

because trauma to the skin, infection, and damage to the tympanic membrane can occur.

Management

Cerumen can be removed by irrigation, suction, or instrumentation. Unless the patient has a perforated eardrum or an inflamed external ear (ie, otitis externa), gentle irrigation usually helps remove impacted cerumen, particularly if it is not tightly packed in the external auditory canal. For successful removal, the water stream must flow behind the obstructing cerumen to move it first laterally and then out of the canal. To prevent injury, the lowest effective pressure should be used. However, if the eardrum behind the impaction is perforated, water can enter the middle ear, producing acute vertigo and infection. If irrigation is unsuccessful, direct visual, mechanical removal can be performed on a cooperative patient by a trained health care provider.

Instilling a few drops of warmed glycerin, mineral oil, or half-strength hydrogen peroxide into the ear canal for 30 minutes can soften cerumen before its removal. Ceruminolytic agents, such as peroxide in glyceryl (Debrox), are available; however, these compounds may cause an allergic dermatitis reaction. Using any softening solution two or three times a day for several days is generally sufficient. If the cerumen cannot be dislodged by these methods, instruments, such as a cerumen curette, aural suction, and a binocular microscope for magnification, can be used.

Foreign Bodies

Some objects are inserted intentionally into the ear by adults who may have been trying to clean the external canal or relieve itching or by children who introduce peas, beans, pebbles, toys, and beads. Insects may also enter the ear canal. In either case, the effects may range from no symptoms to profound pain and decreased hearing.

Management

Removing a foreign body from the external auditory canal can be quite challenging. The three standard methods for removing foreign bodies are the same as those for removing cerumen: irrigation, suction, and instrumentation. The contraindications for irrigation are also the same. Foreign vegetable bodies and insects tend to swell; thus, irrigation is contraindicated. Usually, an insect can be dislodged by instilling mineral oil, which will kill the insect and allow it to be removed.

Attempts to remove a foreign body from the external canal may be dangerous in unskilled hands. The object may be pushed completely into the bony portion of the canal, lacerating the skin and perforating the tympanic membrane. In rare circumstances, the foreign body may have to be extracted in the operating room with the patient under general anesthesia.

External Otitis (Otitis Externa)

External otitis, or **otitis externa,** refers to an inflammation of the external auditory canal. Causes include water in the ear canal (swimmer's ear); trauma to the skin of the ear canal, permitting entrance of organisms into the tissues; and systemic conditions, such as vitamin deficiency and endocrine disorders. Bacterial or fungal infections are most frequently encountered. The most common bacterial pathogens associated with external otitis are *Staphylococcus aureus* and *Pseudomonas* species. The most common fungus isolated in both normal and infected ears is *Aspergillus*. External otitis is often caused by a dermatosis such as psoriasis, eczema, or seborrheic dermatitis. Even allergic reactions to hair spray, hair dye, and permanent wave lotions can cause dermatitis, which clears when the offending agent is removed.

Clinical Manifestations

Patients usually report pain, discharge from the external auditory canal, aural tenderness (usually not present in middle ear infections), and occasionally fever, cellulitis, and lymphadenopathy. Other symptoms may include pruritus and hearing loss or a feeling of fullness. On otoscopic examination, the ear canal is erythematous and edematous. Discharge may be yellow or green and foul-smelling. In fungal infections, hairlike black spores may even be visible.

Medical Management

The principles of therapy are aimed at relieving the discomfort, reducing the swelling of the ear canal, and eradicating the infection. Patients may require analgesic medications for the first 48 to 92 hours. If the tissues of the external canal are edematous, a wick should be inserted to keep the canal open so that liquid medications (eg, Burow's solution, antibiotic otic preparations) can be introduced. These medications may be administered by dropper at room temperature. Such medications usually combine

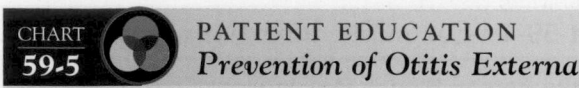

CHART 59-5

PATIENT EDUCATION
Prevention of Otitis Externa

- Protect the external canal when swimming, showering, or washing hair. Ear plugs or a swim cap should be worn. Drying the external canal afterward with a hair dryer on low heat may be suggested.
- Alcohol drops may be placed in the external canal to act as an astringent to help prevent infection after water exposure.
- Prevent trauma to the external canal. Procedures, foreign objects (eg, bobby pin), scratching, or any other trauma to the canal that breaks the skin integrity may cause infection.
- If otitis externa is diagnosed, refrain from any water sport activity for approximately 7 to 10 days to allow the canal to heal completely. Recurrence is highly likely unless you allow the external canal to heal completely.

antibiotic and corticosteroid agents to soothe the inflamed tissues. For cellulitis or fever, systemic antibiotics may be prescribed. For fungal disorders, antifungal agents are prescribed.

Nursing Management

Nurses should instruct patients not to clean the external auditory canal with cotton-tipped applicators and to avoid events that traumatize the external canal such as scratching the canal with the fingernail or other objects. Trauma may lead to infection of the canal. Patients should also avoid getting the canal wet when swimming or shampooing the hair. A cotton ball can be covered in a water-insoluble gel such as petroleum jelly and placed in the ear as a barrier to water contamination. Infection can be prevented by using antiseptic otic preparations after swimming (eg, Swim Ear, Ear Dry), unless there is a history of tympanic membrane perforation or a current ear infection (Chart 59-5).

Malignant External Otitis

A more serious, although rare, external ear infection is malignant external otitis (temporal bone osteomyelitis). This is a progressive, debilitating, and occasionally fatal infection of the external auditory canal, the surrounding tissue, and the base of the skull. *Pseudomonas aeruginosa* is usually the infecting organism in patients with low resistance to infection (eg, patients with diabetes). Successful treatment includes control of the diabetes, administration of antibiotics (usually intravenously), and aggressive local wound care. Standard parenteral antibiotic treatment includes the combination of an antipseudomonal agent and an aminoglycoside, both of which have potentially serious side effects. Because aminoglycosides are nephrotoxic and ototoxic, serum aminoglycoside levels and renal and auditory function must be monitored during therapy. Local wound care includes limited débridement of the infected tissue, including bone and cartilage, depending on the extent of the infection.

Masses of the External Ear

Exostoses are small, hard, bony protrusions found in the lower posterior bony portion of the ear canal; they usually occur bilaterally. The skin covering the exostosis is normal. It is believed that exostoses are caused by an exposure to cold water, as in scuba diving or surfing. The usual treatment, if any, is surgical excision.

Malignant tumors also may occur in the external ear. Most common are basal cell carcinomas on the pinna and squamous cell carcinomas in the ear canal. If untreated, squamous cell carcinoma may spread through the temporal bone, causing facial nerve paralysis and hearing loss. Carcinomas must be treated surgically.

Gapping Earring Puncture

Gapping earring puncture results from wearing heavy pierced earrings for a long time or after an infection, or as a reaction from the earring or impurities in the earring. This deformity can only be corrected surgically.

CONDITIONS OF THE MIDDLE EAR

Tympanic Membrane Perforation

Perforation of the tympanic membrane is usually caused by infection or trauma. Sources of trauma include skull fracture, explosive injury, or a severe blow to the ear. Less frequently, perforation is caused by foreign objects (eg, cotton-tipped applicators, bobby pins, keys) that have been pushed too far into the external auditory canal. In addition to tympanic membrane perforation, injury to the ossicles and even the inner ear may result from this type of trauma. Attempts by patients to clear the external auditory canal should be discouraged. During infection, the tympanic membrane can rupture if the pressure in the middle ear exceeds the atmospheric pressure in the external auditory canal.

Medical Management

Although most tympanic membrane perforations heal spontaneously within weeks after rupture, some may take several months to heal. Some perforations persist because scar tissue grows over the edges of the perforation, preventing extension of the epithelial cells across the margins and final healing. In the case of a head injury or temporal bone fracture, a patient is observed for evidence of cerebrospinal fluid

otorrhea or rhinorrhea—a clear, watery drainage from the ear or nose, respectively. While healing, the ear must be protected from water.

Surgical Management

Perforations that do not heal on their own may require surgery. The decision to perform a **tympanoplasty** (surgical repair of the tympanic membrane) is usually based on the need to prevent potential infection from water entering the ear or the desire to improve the patient's hearing. Performed on an outpatient basis, tympanoplasty may involve a variety of surgical techniques. In all techniques, tissue (commonly from the temporalis fascia) is placed across the perforation to allow healing. Surgery is usually successful in closing the perforation permanently and improving hearing.

Acute Otitis Media

Ear infections can occur at any age; however, they are most commonly seen in children. **Acute otitis media (AOM)** is an acute infection of the middle ear, usually lasting less than 6 weeks. The pathogens that cause acute otitis media are usually *Streptococcus pneumoniae*, *Haemophilus influenzae*, and *Moraxella catarrhalis*, which enter the middle ear after eustachian tube dysfunction caused by obstruction related to upper respiratory infections, inflammation of surrounding structures (eg, rhinosinusitis, adenoid hypertrophy), or allergic reactions (eg, allergic rhinitis). Bacteria can enter the eustachian tube from contaminated secretions in the nasopharynx and the middle ear from a tympanic membrane perforation. A purulent exudate is usually present in the middle ear, resulting in a conductive hearing loss.

Clinical Manifestations

The symptoms of otitis media vary with the severity of the infection. The condition, usually unilateral in adults, may be accompanied by otalgia. The pain is relieved after spontaneous perforation or therapeutic incision of the tympanic membrane. Other symptoms may include drainage from the ear, fever, and hearing loss. On otoscopic examination, the external auditory canal appears normal. The tympanic membrane is erythematous and often bulging. Patients report no pain with movement of the auricle. Table 59-3 differentiates acute external otitis from AOM. Risk factors for AOM include age (younger than 12 months), chronic upper respiratory infections, medical conditions that predispose to ear infections (Down syndrome, cystic fibrosis, cleft palate), and chronic exposure to secondhand cigarette smoke.

Table 59-3	CLINICAL FEATURES OF OTITIS	
Feature	**Acute Otitis Externa**	**Acute Otitis Media**
Otorrhea	May or may not be present	Present if tympanic membrane perforates; discharge is profuse
Otalgia	Persistent, may awaken patient at night	Relieved if tympanic membrane ruptures
Aural tenderness	Present on palpation of auricle	Usually absent
Systemic symptoms	Absent	Fever, upper respiratory infection, rhinitis
Edema of external auditory canal	Present	Absent
Tympanic membrane	May appear normal	Erythema, bulging, may be perforated
Hearing loss	Conductive type	Conductive type

Medical Management

The outcome of AOM depends on the efficacy of therapy (the prescribed dose of an oral antibiotic and the duration of therapy), the virulence of the bacteria, and the physical status of the patient. With early and appropriate broad-spectrum antibiotic therapy, otitis media may resolve with no serious sequelae. If drainage occurs, an antibiotic otic preparation is usually prescribed. The condition may become subacute (lasting 3 weeks to 3 months), with persistent purulent discharge from the ear. Rarely does permanent hearing loss occur. Secondary complications involving the mastoid and other serious intracranial complications, such as meningitis or brain abscess, although rare, can occur.

Surgical Management

An incision in the tympanic membrane is known as **myringotomy** (ie, **tympanotomy**). The tympanic membrane is numbed with a local anesthetic agent such as phenol or by iontophoresis (ie, electrical current flows through a lidocaine-and-epinephrine solution to numb the ear canal and tympanic membrane). The procedure is painless and takes less than 15 minutes. Under microscopic guidance, an incision is made through the tympanic membrane to relieve pressure and to drain serous or purulent fluid from the middle ear.

Normally, this procedure is unnecessary for treating AOM, but it may be performed if pain persists. Myringotomy also allows the drainage to be analyzed (by culture and sensitivity testing) so that the infecting organism can be identified and appropriate antibiotic therapy prescribed. The incision heals within 24 to 72 hours.

If AOM recurs and there is no contraindication, a ventilating, or pressure-equalizing, tube may be inserted. The ventilating tube, which temporarily takes the place of the eustachian tube in equalizing pressure, is retained for 6 to 18 months. The ventilating tube is then extruded with normal skin migration of the tympanic membrane, with the hole healing in nearly every case. Ventilating tubes are used to treat recurrent episodes of AOM.

Serous Otitis Media

Serous otitis media (**middle ear effusion**) involves fluid, without evidence of active infection, in the middle ear. In theory, this fluid results from a negative pressure in the middle ear caused by eustachian tube obstruction. When this condition occurs in adults, an underlying cause for the eustachian tube dysfunction must be sought. Middle ear effusion is frequently seen in patients after radiation therapy or barotrauma and in patients with eustachian tube dysfunction from a concurrent upper respiratory infection or allergy. Barotrauma results from sudden pressure changes in the middle ear caused by changes in barometric pressure, as in scuba diving or airplane descent. A carcinoma (eg, nasopharyngeal cancer) obstructing the eustachian tube should be ruled out in adults with persistent unilateral serous otitis media.

Clinical Manifestations

Patients may complain of hearing loss, fullness in the ear or a sensation of congestion, or popping and crackling noises that occur as the eustachian tube attempts to open. The tympanic membrane appears dull on otoscopy, and air bubbles may be visualized in the middle ear. Usually, the audiogram shows a conductive hearing loss.

Management

Serous otitis media need not be treated medically unless infection (ie, AOM) occurs. If the hearing loss associated with middle ear effusion is significant, a myringotomy can be performed, and a tube may be placed to keep the middle ear ventilated. Corticosteroids in small doses may decrease the edema of the eustachian tube in cases of barotrauma. Decongestants have not proved effective. A Valsalva maneuver, which forcibly opens the eustachian tube by increasing nasopharyngeal pressure, may be cautiously performed; this maneuver may cause worsening pain or perforation of the tympanic membrane.

Chronic Otitis Media

Chronic otitis media is the result of recurrent AOM causing irreversible tissue pathology and persistent perforation of the tympanic membrane. Chronic infections of the middle ear damage the tympanic membrane, destroy the ossicles, and involve the mastoid. Before the discovery of antibiotics, infections of the mastoid were life-threatening. Today, acute mastoiditis is rare in developed countries.

Clinical Manifestations

Symptoms may be minimal, with varying degrees of hearing loss and a persistent or intermittent, foul-smelling otorrhea. Pain is not usually experienced, except in cases of acute mastoiditis, when the postauricular area is tender and may be erythematous and edematous. Otoscopic examination may show a perforation, and cholesteatoma can be identified as a white mass behind the tympanic membrane or coming through to the external canal from a perforation.

Cholesteatoma is an ingrowth of the skin of the external layer of the eardrum into the middle ear. It is generally caused by a chronic retraction pocket of the tympanic membrane, creating a persistently high negative pressure of the middle ear. The skin forms a sac that fills with degenerated skin and sebaceous materials. The sac can attach to the structures of the middle ear or mastoid, or both.

Chronic otitis media can cause chronic mastoiditis and lead to the formation of cholesteatoma. It can occur in the middle ear, mastoid cavity, or both, often dictating the type of surgery to be performed. If untreated, cholesteatoma will continue to enlarge, possibly causing damage to the facial nerve and horizontal canal and destruction of other surrounding structures.

Cholesteatomas are common benign tumors of the inner ear (Semaan & Megerian, 2006). They usually do not cause pain; however, if treatment or surgery is delayed, they may destroy structures of the temporal bone. These fast-growing tumors may cause severe sequelae such as hearing loss or neurologic disorders. Congenital cholesteatomas are usually found in children and may cause severe bone loss of the incus. Cholesteatomas found in elderly patients generally develop in the external canal.

Cholesteatomas may be asymptomatic or they may cause hearing loss, facial pain and paralysis, tinnitus, or vertigo. Audiometric tests often show a conductive or mixed hearing loss. Based on presenting symptoms, diagnosis may be made by visual examination or by computed tomography (CT) or MRI. Therapy includes treatment of the acute infection and surgical removal of the mass to restore hearing.

Medical Management

Local treatment of chronic otitis media consists of careful suctioning of the ear under otoscopic guidance. Instillation of antibiotic drops or application of antibiotic powder is used to treat purulent discharge. Systemic antibiotics are prescribed only in cases of acute infection.

Surgical Management

Surgical procedures, including tympanoplasty, ossiculoplasty, and mastoidectomy, are used if medical treatments are ineffective.

Tympanoplasty

The most common surgical procedure for chronic otitis media is a tympanoplasty, or surgical reconstruction of the tympanic membrane. Reconstruction of the ossicles may also be required. The purposes of a tympanoplasty are to reestablish middle ear function, close the perforation, prevent recurrent infection, and improve hearing.

There are five types of tympanoplasties. The simplest surgical procedure, type I (myringoplasty), is designed to close a perforation in the tympanic membrane. The other procedures, types II through V, involve more extensive repair of middle ear structures. The structures and the degree of involvement can differ, but all tympanoplasty procedures include restoring the continuity of the sound conduction mechanism.

Tympanoplasty is performed through the external auditory canal with a transcanal approach or through a postauricular incision. The contents of the middle ear are carefully inspected, and the ossicular chain (malleus and incus unit) is evaluated. Ossicular interruption is most frequent in chronic otitis media, but problems of reconstruction can also occur with malformations of the middle ear and ossicular dislocations due to head injuries. Dramatic improvement in hearing can result from closure of a perforation and reestablishment of the ossicles. Surgery is usually performed in an outpatient facility under moderate sedation or general anesthesia.

Ossiculoplasty

Ossiculoplasty is the surgical reconstruction of the middle ear bones to restore hearing. Prostheses made of materials such as Teflon, stainless steel, and hydroxyapatite are used to reconnect the ossicles, thereby reestablishing the sound conduction mechanism. However, the greater the damage, the lower the success rate for restoring normal hearing.

Mastoidectomy

The objectives of mastoid surgery are to remove the cholesteatoma, gain access to diseased structures, and create a dry (noninfected) and healthy ear. If possible, the ossicles are reconstructed during the initial surgical procedure. Occasionally, extensive disease or damage dictates that this be performed as part of a two-stage operation.

A mastoidectomy is usually performed through a postauricular incision. Infection is eliminated by removing the mastoid air cells. A second mastoidectomy may be necessary to check for recurrent or residual cholesteatoma. The hearing mechanism may be reconstructed at this time. The success rate for correcting this conductive hearing loss is approximately 75%. Surgery is usually performed in an outpatient setting. The patient has a mastoid pressure dressing, which can be removed 24 to 48 hours after surgery. Although infrequently injured, the facial nerve, which runs through the middle ear and mastoid, is at some risk for injury during mastoid surgery. As the patient awakens from anesthesia, any evidence of facial paresis should be reported to the physician.

NURSING PROCESS

The Patient Undergoing Mastoid Surgery

Although several otologic surgical procedures are performed under moderate sedation, mastoid surgery is performed using general anesthesia.

Assessment

The health history includes a complete description of the ear disorder, including infection, otalgia, otorrhea, hearing loss, and vertigo. Data are collected about the duration and intensity of the disorder, its causes, and previous treatments. Information is obtained about other health problems and all medications that the patient is taking. Medication allergies and family history of ear disease also should be obtained.

Physical assessment addresses erythema, edema, otorrhea, lesions, and characteristics such as odor and color of discharge. The results of the audiogram are reviewed.

Nursing Diagnoses

Based on the assessment data, the major nursing diagnoses may include the following:

- Anxiety related to surgical procedure, potential loss of hearing, potential taste disturbance, and potential loss of facial movement
- Acute pain related to mastoid surgery
- Risk for infection related to mastoidectomy; placement of grafts, prostheses, and electrodes; and surgical trauma to surrounding tissues and structures
- Disturbed auditory sensory perception related to ear disorder, surgery, or packing
- Risk for trauma related to impaired balance or vertigo during the immediate postoperative period or from dislodgment of the graft or prosthesis
- Disturbed sensory perception related to potential damage to facial nerve (cranial nerve VII) and chorda tympani nerve
- Deficient knowledge about mastoid disease, surgical procedure, and postoperative care and expectations

Planning and Goals

The major goals of caring for a patient undergoing mastoidectomy include reduction of anxiety; freedom from pain and discomfort; prevention of infection; stable or improved hearing and communication; absence of vertigo and related injury; absence of or adjustment to sensory or perceptual alterations; and increased knowledge regarding the disease, surgical procedure, and postoperative care.

Nursing Interventions

Reducing Anxiety

The nurse reinforces the information discussed by the otologic surgeon with the patient, including anesthesia, the location of the incision (postauricular), and expected surgical results (eg, hearing, balance, taste, facial movement). The patient also is encouraged to discuss any anxieties and concerns about the surgery.

Relieving Pain

Although most patients complain very little about incisional pain after mastoid surgery, they do have some ear discomfort. Aural fullness or pressure after surgery is caused by residual blood or fluid in the middle ear. The prescribed analgesic medication may be taken for the first 24 hours after surgery and then only as needed.

A wick or external auditory canal packing is used if a tympanoplasty was performed at the time of the mastoidectomy. For the next 2 to 3 weeks after surgery, the patient may experience sharp, shooting pains intermittently as the eustachian tube opens and allows air to enter the middle ear. Constant, throbbing pain accompanied by fever may indicate infection and should be reported to the physician.

Preventing Infection

Measures are initiated to prevent infection in the operated ear. The external auditory canal wick, or packing, may be impregnated with an antibiotic solution before instillation. Prophylactic antibiotics are administered as prescribed, and the patient is instructed to prevent water from entering the external auditory canal for 6 weeks. A cotton ball or lamb's wool covered with a water-insoluble substance (eg, petroleum jelly) and placed loosely in the ear canal usually prevents water contamination and should be used when the patient showers or washes his or her hair, or in any situations in which water may enter the ear. The postauricular incision should be kept dry for the first 2 days. Signs of infection such as an elevated temperature and purulent drainage should be reported. Some serosanguineous drainage from the external auditory canal is normal after surgery.

Improving Hearing and Communication

Hearing in the operated ear may be reduced for several weeks because of edema, accumulation of blood and tissue fluid in the middle ear, and dressings or packing. Measures are initiated to improve hearing and communication, such as reducing environmental noise, facing the patient when speaking, speaking clearly and distinctly without shouting, providing good lighting if the patient relies on speech reading, and using nonverbal clues (eg, facial expression, pointing, gestures)

and other forms of communication. Family members or significant others are instructed about effective ways to communicate with the patient. If the patient uses assistive hearing devices, one can be used in the unaffected ear.

Preventing Injury

Vertigo may occur after mastoid surgery if the semicircular canals or other areas of the inner ear are traumatized. Antiemetic or antivertiginous medications (eg, antihistamines) can be prescribed if a balance disturbance or vertigo occurs. Safety measures such as assisted ambulation are implemented to prevent falls and injury. The patient is instructed to avoid heavy lifting, straining, exertion, and nose blowing for 2 to 3 weeks after surgery to prevent dislodging the tympanic membrane graft or ossicular prosthesis.

Preventing Altered Sensory Perception

Facial nerve injury is a potential, although rare, complication of mastoid surgery. The patient is instructed to report immediately any evidence of facial nerve (cranial nerve VII) weakness, such as drooping of the mouth on the operated side, slurred speech, decreased sensation, and difficulty swallowing. A more frequent occurrence is a temporary disturbance in the chorda tympani nerve, a small branch of the facial nerve that runs through the middle ear. Patients experience a taste disturbance and dry mouth on the side of surgery for several months until the nerve regenerates.

Promoting Home and Community-Based Care

TEACHING PATIENTS SELF-CARE. Patients require instruction about medication therapy, such as analgesic and antivertiginous agents (eg, antihistamines) prescribed for balance disturbance. Teaching includes information about the expected effects and potential side effects of the medication. Patients also need instruction about any activity restrictions. Possible complications such as infection, facial nerve weakness, or taste disturbances, including the signs and symptoms to report immediately, should be addressed (Chart 59-6).

CONTINUING CARE. Some patients, particularly elderly patients, who have had mastoid surgery may require the services of a home care nurse for a few days after returning home. However, most people find that assistance from a family member or a friend is sufficient. The caregiver and patient are cautioned that the patient may experience some vertigo and will therefore require help with ambulation to avoid falling. Any symptoms of complications are to be reported promptly to the surgeon. The importance of scheduling and keeping follow-up appointments is also stressed.

Evaluation

Expected Patient Outcomes

Expected patient outcomes may include:

1. Demonstrates reduced anxiety about surgical procedure
   a. Verbalizes and exhibits less stress, tension, and irritability
   b. Verbalizes acceptance of the results of surgery and adjustment to possible hearing impairment

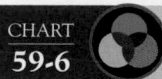
2. Remains free of discomfort or pain
   a. Exhibits no facial grimacing, moaning, or crying, and reports absence of pain
   b. Uses analgesic agents appropriately
3. Demonstrates no signs or symptoms of infection
   a. Has normal vital signs, including temperature
   b. Demonstrates absence of purulent drainage from the external auditory canal
   c. Describes method for preventing water from contaminating packing
4. Exhibits signs that hearing has stabilized or improved
   a. Describes surgical goal for hearing and judges whether the goal has been met
   b. Verbalizes that hearing has improved
5. Remains free of injury and trauma
   a. Reports absence of vertigo or balance disturbance
   b. Experiences no injury or fall
   c. Avoids activities that can cause dislodgement of graft or prosthesis
6. Adjusts to or remains free from altered sensory perception
   a. Reports no taste disturbance, mouth dryness, or facial weakness
7. Verbalizes the reasons for and methods of care and treatment
   a. Discusses the discharge plan formulated with the nurse with regard to rest periods, medication, and activities permitted and restricted
   b. Lists symptoms that should be reported to health care personnel
   c. Keeps follow-up appointments

Otosclerosis

Otosclerosis involves the stapes and is thought to result from the formation of new, abnormal spongy bone, especially around the oval window, with resulting fixation of the stapes. The efficient transmission of sound is prevented because the stapes cannot vibrate and carry the sound as conducted from the malleus and incus to the inner ear. Otosclerosis is more common in women and frequently hereditary, and pregnancy may worsen it.

Clinical Manifestations

Otosclerosis may involve one or both ears and manifests as a progressive conductive or mixed hearing loss. The patient may or may not complain of tinnitus. Otoscopic examination usually reveals a normal tympanic membrane. Bone conduction is better than air conduction on Rinne testing. The audiogram confirms conductive hearing loss or mixed loss, especially in the low frequencies.

Medical Management

There is no known nonsurgical treatment for otosclerosis. However, some physicians believe the use of sodium fluoride can mature the abnormal spongy bone growth and prevent the breakdown of the bone tissue. Amplification with a hearing aid also may help (Porth & Matfin, 2009).

Surgical Management

One of two surgical procedures may be performed, the stapedectomy or the stapedotomy. A stapedectomy involves removing the stapes superstructure and part of the footplate and inserting a tissue graft and a suitable prosthesis (Fig. 59-6). The surgeon drills a small hole into the footplate to hold a prosthesis. The prosthesis bridges the gap between the incus and the inner ear, providing better sound conduction. Approximately 95% of patients experience resolution of conductive hearing loss following stapes surgery. Balance disturbance or true vertigo may occur during the postoperative period for several days. Long-term balance disorders are rare.

Middle Ear Masses

Other than cholesteatoma, masses in the middle ear are rare. Glomus tympanicum is a tumor that arises from Jacobson's nerve (in the temporal bone of the skull) and remains limited to the middle ear. On otoscopy, a red blemish on or behind the tympanic membrane is seen. Glomus jugulare tumors are rarely malignant; however, because of their location, treatment may be necessary to relieve symptoms. The treatment is surgical excision, except in poor surgical candidates, in whom radiation therapy is used.

A facial nerve neuroma is a tumor on cranial nerve VII. These types of tumors are usually not visible on otoscopic

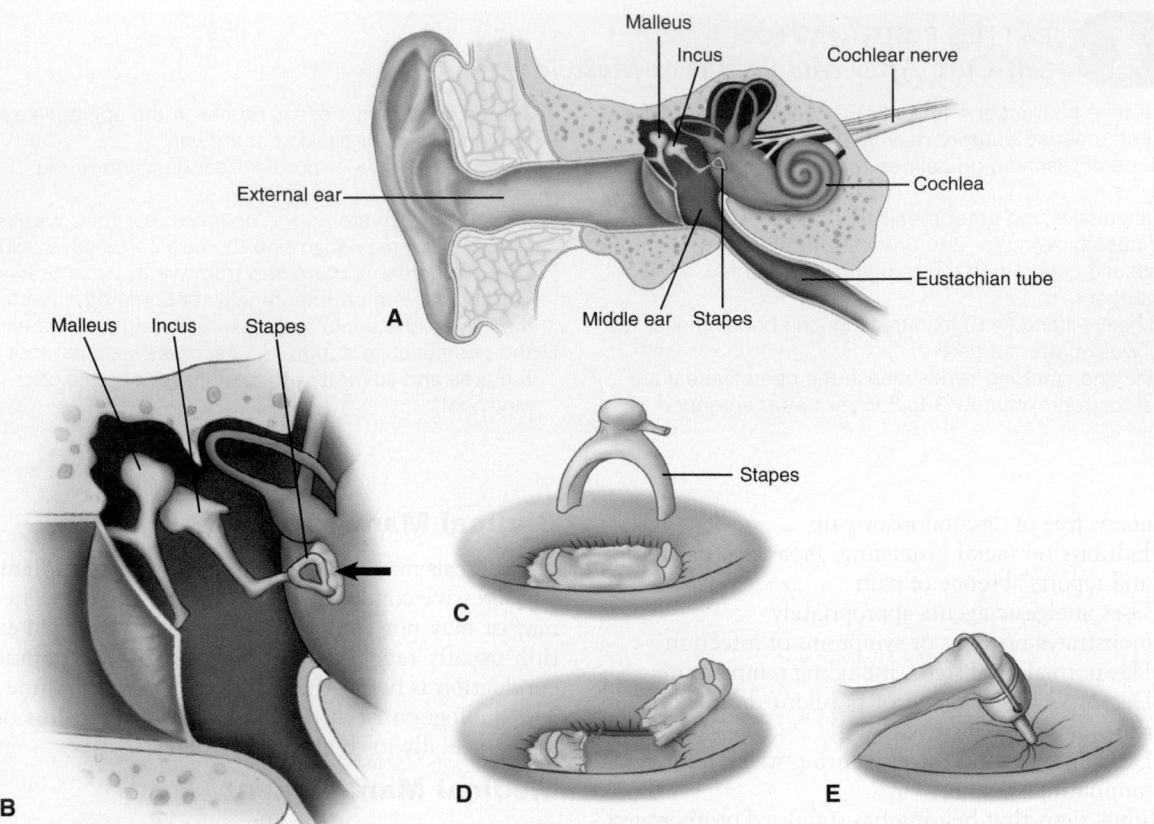

Figure 59-6 Stapedectomy for otosclerosis. **A,** Normal anatomy. **B,** Arrow points to sclerotic process at the foot of the stapes. **C,** Stapes broken away surgically from its diseased base. The hole in the footplate provides an area where an instrument can grasp the plate. **D,** The footplate is removed from its base. Some otosclerotic tissue may remain, and tissue is placed over it. **E,** Robinson stainless steel prosthesis in position.

examination but are suspected when a patient presents with a facial nerve paresis. X-ray evaluation is used to identify the site of the tumor along the facial nerve. The treatment is surgical removal.

CONDITIONS OF THE INNER EAR

Almost 8 million American adults are affected by a chronic problem with balance and an additional 2.4 million are affected by dizziness alone. Disorders of balance are a major cause of falls of elderly people (NIDCD, 2005).

The term **dizziness** is used frequently by patients and health care providers to describe any altered sensation of orientation in space. **Vertigo** is defined as the misperception or illusion of motion of the person or the surroundings. Most people with vertigo describe a spinning sensation or say they feel as though objects are moving around them. Ataxia is a failure of muscular coordination and may be present in patients with vestibular disease. Syncope, fainting, and loss of consciousness are not forms of vertigo and usually indicate disease in the cardiovascular system.

Nystagmus is an involuntary rhythmic movement of the eyes. Nystagmus occurs normally when a person watches a rapidly moving object (eg, through the side window of a moving car or train). However, pathologically it is an ocular disorder associated with vestibular dysfunction. Nystag-

mus can be horizontal, vertical, or rotary and can be caused by a disorder in the central or peripheral nervous system.

Motion Sickness

Motion sickness is a disturbance of equilibrium caused by constant motion. For example, it can occur aboard a ship, while riding on a merry-go-round or swing, or in a car.

Clinical Manifestations

The syndrome manifests itself in sweating, pallor, nausea, and vomiting caused by vestibular overstimulation. These manifestations may persist for several hours after the stimulation stops.

Management

Over-the-counter antihistamines such as dimenhydrinate (Dramamine) or meclizine hydrochloride (Antivert) may provide some relief of nausea and vomiting by blocking the conduction of the vestibular pathway of the inner ear. Anticholinergic medications, such as scopolamine patches, may also be effective because they antagonize the histamine response. These must be replaced every few days. Side effects such as dry mouth and drowsiness may occur. Potentially hazardous activities such as driving a car or operating heavy machinery should be avoided if drowsiness occurs.

Ménière's Disease

Ménière's disease is an abnormal inner ear fluid balance caused by a malabsorption in the endolymphatic sac or a blockage in the endolymphatic duct. **Endolymphatic hydrops,** a dilation in the endolymphatic space, develops, and either increased pressure in the system or rupture of the inner ear membrane occurs, producing symptoms of Ménière's disease.

Ménière's disease affects 15 to 50 people per 100,000 people in the United States (Kitahara, Kubo, Okumura, et al., 2008). More common in adults, it has an average age of onset in the 40s, with symptoms usually beginning between the ages of 20 and 60 years. Ménière's disease appears to be equally common in men and women, and it occurs bilaterally in about 20% of patients. About 50% of the patients who have Ménière's disease have a positive family history of the disease.

Clinical Manifestations

Symptoms of Ménière's disease include fluctuating, progressive sensorineural hearing loss; **tinnitus** or a roaring sound; a feeling of pressure or fullness in the ear; and episodic, incapacitating vertigo, often accompanied by nausea and vomiting. These symptoms range in severity from a minor nuisance to extreme disability, especially if the attacks of vertigo are severe. At the onset of the disease, perhaps only one or two of the symptoms are manifested.

Some clinicians believe that there are two subsets of the disease: cochlear and vestibular. Cochlear Ménière's disease is recognized as a fluctuating, progressive sensorineural hearing loss associated with tinnitus and aural pressure in the absence of vestibular symptoms or findings. Vestibular Ménière's disease is characterized as the occurrence of episodic vertigo associated with aural pressure but no cochlear symptoms. Patients may experience either cochlear or vestibular disease symptoms; however, eventually all of these symptoms develop.

Assessment and Diagnostic Findings

Vertigo is usually the most troublesome complaint related to Ménière's disease. A careful history is taken to determine the frequency, duration, severity, and character of the vertigo attacks. Vertigo may last minutes to hours, possibly accompanied by nausea or vomiting. Diaphoresis and a persistent feeling of imbalance or disequilibrium may waken patients at night. Some patients report that these feelings last for days. However, they usually feel well between attacks. Hearing loss may fluctuate, with tinnitus and aural pressure waxing and waning with changes in hearing. These feelings may occur during or before attacks, or they may be constant.

Physical examination findings are usually normal, with the exception of those of cranial nerve VIII. Sounds from a tuning fork (Weber test) may lateralize to the ear opposite the hearing loss, the one affected with Ménière's disease. An audiogram typically reveals a sensorineural hearing loss in the affected ear. This can be in the form of a "Pike's Peak" pattern, which looks like a hill or mountain. A sensorineural loss in the low frequencies occurs as the disease progresses. The electronystagmogram may be normal or may show reduced vestibular response.

Medical Management

Most patients with Ménière's disease can be successfully treated with diet and medication. Many patients can control their symptoms by adhering to a low-sodium (1000 to 1500 mg/day or less) diet. Chart 59-7 describes dietary guidelines that may be useful in Ménière's disease. The amount of sodium is one of many factors that regulate the balance of fluid within the body. Sodium and fluid retention disrupts the delicate balance between endolymph and perilymph in the inner ear. Psychological evaluation may be indicated if a patient is anxious, uncertain, fearful, or depressed.

Pharmacologic Therapy

Pharmacologic therapy for Ménière's disease consists of antihistamines, such as meclizine (Antivert), which suppress the vestibular system. Tranquilizers such as diazepam (Valium) may be used in acute instances to help control vertigo. Antiemetic agents such as promethazine (Phenergan) suppositories help control the nausea and vomiting and the vertigo because of their antihistamine effect. Diuretic therapy (eg, hydrochlorothiazide [Dyazide], triamterene [Dyrenium]) may relieve symptoms by lowering the pressure in the endolymphatic system. Intake of foods containing potassium (eg, bananas, tomatoes, oranges) is necessary if the patient takes a diuretic that causes potassium loss. There is no scientific basis for the use of vasodilators, such as papaverine hydrochloride (Pavabid) to alleviate the symptoms, but they are often used in conjunction with other therapies, such as methantheline bromide (Banthine).

In patients who may be noncompliant with the therapeutic regimen, intratympanic injection of gentamicin (Garamycin) is being used to cause ablation of the vestibular

---

CHART 59-7	PATIENT EDUCATION

Dietary Guidelines for Patients With Ménière's Disease

- Limit foods high in salt or sugar. Be aware of foods with hidden salts and sugars.
- Eat meals and snacks at regular intervals to stay hydrated. Missing meals or snacks may alter the fluid level in the inner ear.
- Eat fresh fruits, vegetables, and whole grains. Limit the amount of canned, frozen, or processed foods with high sodium content.
- Drink plenty of fluids daily. Water, milk, and low-sugar fruit juices are recommended. Limit intake of coffee, tea,

and soft drinks. Avoid caffeine because of its diuretic effect.
- Limit alcohol intake. Alcohol may change the volume and concentration of the inner ear fluid and may worsen symptoms.
- Avoid monosodium glutamate (MSG), which may increase symptoms.
- Avoid aspirin and aspirin-containing medications. Aspirin may increase tinnitus and dizziness.

hair cells. However, the risk of significant hearing loss is high (Swartz & Longwell, 2005).

Surgical Management

Although most patients respond well to conservative therapy, some continue to have disabling attacks of vertigo. If these attacks reduce their quality of life, patients may elect to undergo surgery for relief. Surgical procedures include endolymphatic sac procedures and vestibular nerve section. However, hearing loss, tinnitus, and aural fullness may continue, because the surgical treatment of Ménière's disease is aimed at eliminating the attacks of vertigo (Mayo Clinic, 2008).

Endolymphatic Sac Decompression

Endolymphatic sac decompression, or shunting, theoretically equalizes the pressure in the endolymphatic space. A shunt or drain is inserted in the endolymphatic sac through a postauricular incision. This procedure is favored by many otolaryngologists as a first-line surgical approach to treat the vertigo of Ménière's disease because it is relatively simple and safe and can be performed on an outpatient basis.

Vestibular Nerve Sectioning

Vestibular nerve sectioning provides the greatest success rate (approximately 98%) in eliminating the attacks of vertigo. It can be performed by a translabyrinthine approach (ie, through the hearing mechanism) or in a manner that can conserve hearing (ie, suboccipital or middle cranial fossa), depending on the degree of hearing loss. Most patients with incapacitating Ménière's disease have little or no effective hearing. Cutting the nerve prevents the brain from receiving input from the semicircular canals. This procedure may require a brief hospital stay. A plan of nursing care for the patient with vertigo is presented in Chart 59-8.

Benign Paroxysmal Positional Vertigo

Benign paroxysmal positional vertigo is a brief period of incapacitating vertigo that occurs when the position of the patient's head is changed with respect to gravity, typically by placing the head back with the affected ear turned down. The onset is sudden and followed by a predisposition for positional vertigo, usually for hours to weeks but occasionally for months or years.

Benign paroxysmal positional vertigo is thought to be due to the disruption of debris within the semicircular canal. This debris is formed from small crystals of calcium carbonate from the inner ear structure, the utricle. This is frequently stimulated by head trauma, infection, or other events. In severe cases, vertigo may easily be induced by any head movement. The vertigo is usually accompanied by nausea and vomiting; however, hearing impairment does not generally occur (Labuguen, 2006).

Bed rest is recommended for patients with acute symptoms. There are repositioning techniques that can be used to treat vertigo. The canalith repositioning procedure is commonly used. This noninvasive procedure, which involves quick movements of the body, rearranges the debris in the canal. The procedure is performed by placing the patient in a sitting position, turning the head to a 45-degree angle on the affected side, and then quickly moving the patient to the supine position. The procedure is safe, inexpensive, and easy to perform.

Patients with acute vertigo may be treated with meclizine for 1 to 2 weeks. After this time, the meclizine is stopped, and the patient is reassessed. Patients who continue to have severe positional vertigo may be premedicated with prochlorperazine (Compazine) 1 hour before the canalith repositioning procedure is performed.

Vestibular rehabilitation can be used in the management of vestibular disorders. This strategy promotes active use of the vestibular system through an interdisciplinary team approach, including medical and nursing care, stress management, biofeedback, vocational rehabilitation, and physical therapy. A physical therapist prescribes balance exercises that help the brain compensate for the impairment to the balance system (Swartz & Longwell, 2005).

Tinnitus

Tinnitus is a symptom of an underlying disorder of the ear that is associated with hearing loss. This condition affects approximately 37 million people in the United States, and it is most prevalent between 40 and 70 years of age (Porth & Matfin, 2009). The severity of tinnitus may range from mild to severe. Patients describe tinnitus as a roaring, buzzing, or hissing sound in one or both ears. Numerous factors may contribute to the development of tinnitus, including several ototoxic substances (Chart 59-9). Underlying disorders that contribute to tinnitus may include thyroid disease, hyperlipidemia, vitamin B_{12} deficiency, psychological disorders (eg, depression, anxiety), fibromyalgia, otologic disorders (Ménière's disease, acoustic neuroma), and neurologic disorders (head injury, multiple sclerosis).

A physical examination should be performed to determine the cause of tinnitus. Diagnostic testing determines if hearing loss is present. An audiograph speech discrimination test or a tympanogram may be used to help determine the cause. Some forms of tinnitus are irreversible; therefore, patients may need teaching and counseling about ways of adjusting to their treatment and dealing with tinnitus in the future.

Labyrinthitis

Labyrinthitis, an inflammation of the inner ear, can be bacterial or viral in origin. Bacterial labyrinthitis is rare because of antibiotic therapy, but it sometimes occurs as a complication of otitis media. The infection can spread to the inner ear by penetrating the membranes of the oval or round windows. Viral labyrinthitis is a common diagnosis, but little is known about this disorder, which affects hearing and balance. The most common viral causes are mumps, rubella, rubeola, and influenza. Viral illnesses of the upper respiratory tract and herpetiform disorders of the facial and acoustic nerves (ie, Ramsay Hunt syndrome) also cause labyrinthitis.

Clinical Manifestations

Labyrinthitis is characterized by a sudden onset of incapacitating vertigo, usually with nausea and vomiting, various degrees of hearing loss, and possibly tinnitus. The first

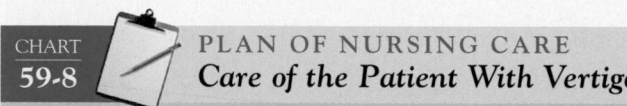

CHART 59-8

PLAN OF NURSING CARE
Care of the Patient With Vertigo

NURSING DIAGNOSIS: Risk for injury related to altered mobility because of gait disturbance and vertigo
GOAL: Remains free of any injuries associated with imbalance and/or falls

Nursing Interventions	Rationale	Expected Outcomes
1. Assess for vertigo, including history, onset, description of attacks, duration, frequency, and any associated ear symptoms (hearing loss, tinnitus, aural fullness).	1. History provides basis for interventions.	• Experiences no falls due to balance disturbance • Fear and anxiety are reduced. • Performs exercises as prescribed • Takes prescribed medications appropriately • Assumes safe position when vertigo is present • Keeps head still when vertigo is present • Identifies a characteristic fullness or sense of pressure in the ear as occurring before a full-blown attack • Reports measures that help reduce vertigo
2. Assess extent of disability in relation to activities of daily living.	2. Extent of disability indicates risk of falling.	
3. Teach or reinforce vestibular/balance therapy as prescribed.	3. Exercises hasten labyrinthine compensation, which may decrease vertigo and gait disturbance.	
4. Administer, or teach administration of, antivertiginous medications and/or vestibular sedation medication; instruct patient about side effects.	4. Alleviates acute symptoms of vertigo	
5. Encourage patient to sit down when dizzy.	5. Decreases possibility of falling and injury	
6. Place pillow on each side of head to restrict movement.	6. Movement aggravates vertigo.	
7. Assist patient in identifying aura that suggests an impending attack.	7. Recognition of aura may trigger the need to take medication before an attack occurs, thereby minimizing the severity of effects.	
8. Recommend that the patient keep eyes open and stare straight ahead when lying down and experiencing vertigo.	8. Sensation of vertigo decreases and motion decelerates if eyes are kept in a fixed position.	

NURSING DIAGNOSIS: Risk-prone health behavior related to disability requiring change in lifestyle due to unpredictability of vertigo
GOAL: Modifies lifestyle to decrease disability and exert maximum control and independence within limits posed by chronic vertigo

Nursing Interventions	Rationale	Expected Outcomes
1. Encourage patient to identify personal strengths and roles that can still be fulfilled.	1. Maximizes sense of regaining control and independence	• Exerts maximum control of environment and independence within limits imposed by vertigo • Is informed about condition • Family and significant others are included in rehabilitation process. • Uses strengths and potentials to engage in the most independent and constructive lifestyle
2. Provide information about vertigo and what to expect.	2. Reduces fear and anxiety	
3. Include family and significant others in rehabilitative process.	3. Perceived beliefs of significant others are important for patient's adherence to medical regimen.	
4. Encourage patient to maintain sense of control by making decisions and assuming more responsibility for care.	4. Reinforces positive psychological and social outcomes	

NURSING DIAGNOSIS: Risk for deficient fluid volume related to increased fluid output, altered intake, and medications
GOAL: Maintains normal fluid and electrolyte balance

Nursing Interventions	Rationale	Expected Outcomes
1. Assess, or have patient assess, intake and output (including emesis, liquid stools, urine, and diaphoresis). Monitor laboratory values.	1. Accurate records provide basis for fluid replacement.	• Laboratory values within normal limits • Alert and oriented; vital signs within normal limits, skin turgor normal; electrolytes normal

Continued on following page

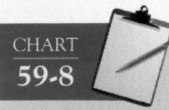

CHART 59-8

PLAN OF NURSING CARE
Care of the Patient With Vertigo (Continued)

Nursing Interventions	Rationale	Expected Outcomes
2. Assess indicators of dehydration, including blood pressure (orthostasis), pulse, skin turgor, mucous membranes, and level of consciousness. 3. Encourage oral fluids as tolerated; discourage beverages containing caffeine (a vestibular stimulant). 4. Administer, or teach administration of, antiemetic and antidiarrheal medications as prescribed and needed. Instruct patient in side effects.	2. Prompt recognition of dehydration allows early intervention. 3. Oral replacement is begun as soon as possible to replace losses. Caffeine may increase diarrhea. 4. Antiemetics medications reduce nausea and vomiting, reducing fluid losses and improving oral intake. Antidiarrheal medication reduces intestinal motility and fluid losses.	• Mucous membranes are moist. • Vomiting or diarrhea has stopped; usual oral intake resumed

NURSING DIAGNOSIS: Anxiety related to threat of, or change in, health status and disability effects of vertigo
GOAL: Experiences less or no anxiety

Nursing Interventions	Rationale	Expected Outcomes
1. Assess level of anxiety. Help patient identify coping skills used successfully in the past. 2. Provide information about vertigo and its treatment. 3. Encourage patient to discuss anxieties and explore concerns about vertigo attacks. 4. Teach patient stress management techniques or make appropriate referral. 5. Provide comfort measures and avoid stress-producing activities. 6. Instruct patient in aspects of treatment regimen.	1. Guides therapeutic interventions and participation in self-care. Past coping skills can relieve anxiety. 2. Increased knowledge helps to decrease anxiety. 3. Promotes awareness and understanding of relationship between anxiety level and behavior 4. Improved stress management can reduce the frequency and severity of some vertiginous attacks. 5. Stressful situations may exacerbate symptoms of the condition. 6. Patient knowledge helps to decrease anxiety.	• Fear and anxiety about attacks of vertigo reduced or eliminated • Acquires knowledge and skills to deal with vertigo • Feels less tension, apprehension, and uncertainty • Uses stress management techniques when needed • Avoids upsetting encounters • Repeats instructions given and verbalizes understanding of treatments

NURSING DIAGNOSIS: Risk for trauma related to impaired balance
GOAL: Reduces the risk of trauma by adapting the home environment and by using assistive devices as necessary

Nursing Interventions	Rationale	Expected Outcomes
1. Assess for balance disturbance and/or vertigo by taking history and by examination for nystagmus, positive Romberg, and inability to perform tandem Romberg. 2. Assist with ambulation when indicated. 3. Assess for visual acuity and proprioceptive deficits. 4. Encourage increased activity level with or without use of assistive devices. 5. Help identify hazards in home environment.	1. Peripheral vestibular disorders cause these signs and symptoms. 2. Abnormal gait can predispose patient to unsteadiness and falls. 3. Balance depends on visual, vestibular, and proprioceptive systems. 4. Increased activity may help retrain balance system. 5. Adaptation of home environment can reduce risk of falls during rehabilitative process.	• Has adapted home environment or uses rehabilitative devices to reduce risk of falling • Ambulates with needed assistance • Visual and proprioceptive risks identified • Activity level increased • Home environment free of hazards

NURSING DIAGNOSIS: Self-care deficit: feeding, bathing/hygiene, dressing/grooming, toileting, related to labyrinth dysfunction and episodes of vertigo
GOAL: Able to care for self

Nursing Interventions	Rationale	Expected Outcomes
1. Administer, or teach administration of, antiemetic and other prescribed medications to relieve nausea and vomiting associated with vertigo.	1. Antiemetic and sedative-type medications depress stimuli in the cerebellum.	• Carries out necessary functions during symptom-free periods. Takes medications to relieve nausea, vomiting, or vertigo

Continued

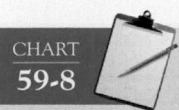

CHART 59-8

PLAN OF NURSING CARE
Care of the Patient With Vertigo *(Continued)*

Nursing Interventions	Rationale	Expected Outcomes
2. Encourage patient to perform self-care when free of vertigo. 3. Review diet with patient and caregivers. Offer fluids as necessary.	2. Spacing activities is important because episodes of vertigo vary in occurrence. 3. Sodium restriction helps improve an inner ear fluid imbalance in some patients, thereby decreasing vertigo. Fluids help prevent dehydration.	• Carries out daily activities • Accepts dietary plan and reports its effectiveness. • Drinks fluids in sufficient amounts

NURSING DIAGNOSIS: Powerlessness related to illness regimen and being helpless in certain situations due to vertigo/balance disturbance

GOAL: Experiences increased sense of control over life and activities despite vertigo/balance disturbance

Nursing Interventions	Rationale	Expected Outcomes
1. Assess patient's needs, values, attitudes, and readiness to initiate activities. 2. Provide opportunities for patient to express feelings about self and illness. 3. Help patient identify previous coping behaviors that were successful.	1. Involving patient in planning activities and care enhances potential for mastery. 2. Expressing feelings increases understanding of individual coping styles and defense mechanisms. 3. Awareness increases understanding of stressors that trigger feeling of powerlessness. Awareness of past successes enhances self-confidence.	• Does not restrict activities unnecessarily due to vertigo • Verbalizes positive feelings about own ability to achieve a sense of power and control • Identifies previous successful coping behaviors

episode is usually the worst; subsequent attacks, which usually occur over a period of several weeks to months, are less severe.

Management

Treatment of bacterial labyrinthitis includes IV antibiotic therapy, fluid replacement, and administration of an antihistamine (eg, meclizine [Antivert]) and antiemetic medications. Treatment of viral labyrinthitis is based on the patient's symptoms.

Otoxicity

A variety of medications may have adverse effects on the cochlea, vestibular apparatus, or cranial nerve VIII. All but a few, such as aspirin and quinine, cause irreversible hearing loss. At high doses, aspirin toxicity can produce bilateral tinnitus. IV medications, especially the aminoglycosides, are the most common cause of ototoxicity, and they destroy the hair cells in the organ of Corti (see Chart 59-9).

To prevent loss of hearing or balance, patients receiving potentially ototoxic medications should be counseled about the side effects of these medications. These medications should be used with caution in patients who are at high risk for complications, such as children, the elderly, pregnant patients, patients with kidney or liver problems, and patients with current hearing disorders. Blood levels of the medications should be monitored, and patients receiving long-term IV antibiotics should be monitored with an audiogram twice each week during therapy.

Acoustic Neuroma

Acoustic neuromas are slow-growing, benign tumors of cranial nerve VIII, usually arising from the Schwann cells of the vestibular portion of the nerve. Most acoustic tumors arise within the internal auditory canal and extend into the cerebellopontine angle to press on the brain stem, possibly destroying the vestibular nerve. Most acoustic neuromas are unilateral, except in von Recklinghausen's disease (neurofibromatosis type 2), in which bilateral tumors occur (Porth & Matfin, 2009).

Acoustic neuromas develop in 1 of every 10,000 people per year. These neuromas account for 5% to 10% of all intracranial tumors and seem to occur with equal frequency in men and women at any age, although most occur during middle age.

CHART 59-9

PHARMACOLOGY
Selected Otoxic Substances

- **Diuretics:** ethacrynic acid, furosemide, acetazolamide
- **Chemotherapeutic agents:** cisplatin, nitrogen mustard
- **Antimalarial agents:** quinine, chloroquine
- **Anti-inflammatory agents:** salicylates (aspirin), indomethacin
- **Chemicals:** alcohol, arsenic
- **Aminoglycoside antibiotics:** amikacin, gentamicin, kanamycin, netilmicin, neomycin, streptomycin, tobramycin
- **Other antibiotics:** erythromycin, minocycline, polymyxin B, vancomycin
- **Metals:** gold, mercury, lead

Assessment and Diagnostic Findings

The most common assessment findings of patients with acoustic neuromas are unilateral tinnitus and hearing loss with or without vertigo or balance disturbance. It is important to identify asymmetry in audiovestibular test results so that further workup can be performed to rule out an acoustic neuroma. MRI with a contrast agent (ie, gadolinium or Magnevist) is the imaging study of choice. If the patient is claustrophobic or cannot undergo an MRI for other reasons or if the scan is unavailable, a CT scan with contrast dye is performed. However, MRI is more sensitive than CT in delineating a small tumor.

Management

Surgical removal of acoustic tumors is the treatment of choice because these tumors do not respond well to radiation or chemotherapy. Because treatment of acoustic tumors crosses several specialties, the interdisciplinary treatment approach involves a neurologist and a neurosurgeon. The objective of the surgery is to remove the tumor while preserving facial nerve function. Most acoustic tumors have damaged the cochlear portion of cranial nerve VIII, and hearing is impaired. In these patients, the surgery is performed using a translabyrinthine approach, and the hearing mechanism is destroyed. If hearing is still good before surgery, a suboccipital or middle cranial fossa approach to removing the tumor may be used. This procedure exposes the lateral third of the internal auditory canal and preserves hearing.

Complications of surgery include facial nerve paralysis, cerebrospinal fluid leakage, meningitis, and cerebral edema. Death from acoustic neuroma surgery is rare.

AURAL REHABILITATION

If hearing loss is permanent or cannot be treated by medical or surgical means or if the patient elects not to undergo surgery, aural rehabilitation may be beneficial. The purpose of aural rehabilitation is to maximize the communication skills of the person with hearing impairment. Aural rehabilitation includes auditory training, speech reading, speech training, and the use of hearing aids and hearing guide dogs.

Auditory training emphasizes listening skills, so the person who is hearing-impaired concentrates on the speaker. Speech reading (also known as lip reading) can help fill the gaps left by missed or misheard words. The goals of speech training are to conserve, develop, and prevent deterioration of current communication skills.

It is important to identify the type of hearing impairment a person has so that rehabilitative efforts can be directed at his or her particular need. Surgical correction may be all that is necessary to treat and improve a conductive hearing loss by eliminating the cause of the hearing loss. With advances in hearing aid technology, amplification for patients with sensorineural hearing loss is more helpful than ever.

Hearing Aids

A hearing aid is a device through which speech and environmental sounds are received by a microphone, converted to electrical signals, amplified, and reconverted to acoustic

---

Chart 59-10 • *Hearing Aid Problems*

Whistling Noise

Loose ear mold
Improperly made
Improperly worn
Worn out

Improper Aid Selection

Too much power required in aid, with inadequate separation between microphone and receiver
Open mold used inappropriately

Inadequate Amplification

Dead batteries
Cerumen in ear
Cerumen or other material in mold
Wires or tubing disconnected from aid
Aid turned off or volume too low
Improper mold
Improper aid for degree of loss

Pain from Mold

Improperly fitted mold
Ear skin or cartilage infection
Middle ear infection
Ear tumor
Unrelated conditions of the temporomandibular joint, throat, or larynx

---

signals. Many aids available for sensorineural hearing loss depress the low frequencies, or tones, and enhance hearing for the high frequencies. A general guideline for assessing the patient's need for a hearing aid is a hearing loss exceeding 30 dB in the range of 500 to 2000 Hz in the better-hearing ear.

A hearing aid makes sounds louder, but it does not improve a patient's ability to discriminate words or understand speech. People who have low discrimination scores (ie, 20%) on audiograms may derive little benefit from a hearing aid. Hearing aids amplify all sounds, including background noise, which may be disturbing to the wearer. Chart 59-10 identifies additional problems associated with hearing aid use. Computerized hearing aids are available to compensate for background noise or allow amplification at certain programmed frequencies rather than at all frequencies. Occasionally, depending on the type of hearing loss, binaural aids (ie, one for each ear) may be indicated. Chart 59-11 provides tips for hearing aid care.

A hearing aid should be fitted according to the patient's needs (eg, type of hearing loss, manual dexterity, and preferences), rather than the brand name, by a certified audiologist licensed to dispense hearing aids. Many states have consumer protection laws that allow the hearing aid to be returned after a trial use if the patient is not completely satisfied. In addition, to protect the health and safety of people with hearing impairments, the U.S. Food and Drug Administration (FDA) has established certain regulations. A medical evaluation of the impairment by a physician must be obtained within 6 months before the purchase of a hearing aid. However, the written statement from a physician may be waived if the patient (a fully informed adult 18 years

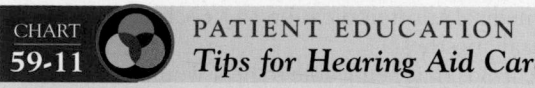

CHART 59-11 PATIENT EDUCATION
Tips for Hearing Aid Care

Cleaning

- The ear mold is the only part of the hearing aid that may be washed frequently.
- Wash ear mold daily with soap and water.
- Allow the ear mold to dry completely before it is snapped into the receiver.
- Clean the cannula with a small pipe cleaner–like device.
- Proper care of the ear device and keeping the ear canal clean and dry can prevent complications.

Malfunctioning

- Inadequate amplification, a whistling noise, or pain from the mold can occur when a hearing aid is not functioning properly.
- Check for malfunctions:
  - Is the switch on properly?
  - Are the batteries charged and positioned correctly?
- If the hearing aid is still not working properly, notify the hearing aid dealer.
- If the unit requires extended time for repair, the dealer may lend you a hearing aid until the repair can be accomplished.

Recognizing Complications

- Common medical complications include external otitis media and pressure ulcers in the external auditory canal. Signs and symptoms of these infections include painful ear, especially when the external ear is touched; canal swelling; redness; difficulty hearing; pain radiating to the jaw area; and fever.
- If any of these symptoms are present, notify your health care provider for evaluation. You may need medication to treat infection, pain, or both.

of age or older) signs a document to this effect. Health care professionals who dispense hearing aids are required to refer prospective users to a physician if any of the following otologic conditions are evident:

- Visible congenital or traumatic deformity of the ear
- Active drainage from the ear within the previous 90 days
- Sudden or rapidly progressive hearing loss within the previous 90 days
- Complaints of dizziness or tinnitus

- Unilateral hearing loss that occurred suddenly or within the previous 90 days
- Audiometric air–bone gap of 15 dB or more at 500, 1000, and 2000 Hz
- Significant accumulation of cerumen or a foreign body in the external auditory canal
- Pain or discomfort in the ear

A user instruction brochure is provided with every hearing aid device. In this brochure, the following information is presented:

- Notification that good health practice requires a medical evaluation before purchasing a hearing aid
- Notification that any of the eight otologic conditions previously listed should be investigated by a physician before purchase of a hearing aid
- Instructions for proper use, maintenance, and care of the hearing aid, as well as instructions for replacing or recharging the batteries
- Repair service information
- Description of avoidable conditions that could damage the hearing aid
- List of any known side effects that may warrant physician consultation (eg, skin irritation, accelerated cerumen accumulation)

The evolution in technology has led to the availability of many smaller and more effective hearing aids. It is estimated that 98% of all hearing aids sold today are behind-the-ear, in-the-ear, or in-the-canal types (Table 59-4). One of the newest in-the-ear models is the Lyric, and other new models are being developed. The Lyric is placed in the ear canal just 4 mm from the tympanic membrane. Its volume is controlled by a magnet, and when its batteries no longer function (1 to 4 months), a physician can remove it with the magnet and reinsert a new device. This device does not have many of the problems (eg, feedback noise, overamplification of background noise) associated with other hearing aids, and it does not involve the expense and uncertainty of surgical procedures. However, it is not an option for a person whose ear canal is too narrow to accommodate it.

Implanted Hearing Devices

Three types of implanted hearing devices are commercially available or in the investigational stage: the cochlear implant, the bone conduction device, and the semi-implantable

Table 59-4 HEARING AIDS		
Site (and Range of Hearing Loss)	**Advantages**	**Disadvantages**
Body, usually on the trunk (mild–profound)	Separation of receiver and microphone prevents acoustic feedback, allowing high amplification. Generally used in a school setting	Bulky; requires long wire, which may be cosmetically displeasing; some loss of high-frequency response
Behind the ear (mild–profound)	Economical; powerful, with no long wires; easily used by children—adapts easily as the child grows, with only the ear mold needing replacement	Large size
In the ear (mild–moderately severe)	One-piece custom fit to contour of ear; no tubes or cords; miniature microphone is located in the ear, which is a more natural placement; more cosmetically appealing due to easy concealment	Smaller size limits output; patients who have arthritis or cannot perform tasks requiring good manual dexterity may have difficulty with the small size of aid and/or battery; can require more repair than the behind-the-ear aid
In the canal (mild–moderately severe)	Same as in-the-ear aids; less visible, so more cosmetically pleasing	Even smaller than in-the-ear aids; requires good manual dexterity

hearing device. Cochlear implants are for patients with little or no hearing. Bone conduction devices, which transmit sound through the skull to the inner ear, are used in patients with a conductive hearing loss if a hearing aid is contraindicated (eg, those with chronic infection). The device is implanted postauricularly under the skin into the skull, and an external device—worn above the ear, not in the canal—transmits the sound through the skin. There are two types of implantable hearing aids. The bone anchored hearing aid (BAHA) is implanted behind the ear in the mastoid area. The middle ear implantation (MEI) is implanted in the middle ear cavity. The BAHA is used for conductive or mixed hearing loss, while the MEI is used for sensorineural hearing loss.

A cochlear implant is an auditory prosthesis used for people with profound sensorineural hearing loss bilaterally who do not benefit from conventional hearing aids. The hearing loss may be congenital or acquired. An implant does not restore normal hearing; rather, it helps the person detect medium to loud environmental sounds and conversation. The implant provides stimulation directly to the auditory nerve, bypassing the nonfunctioning hair cells of the inner ear. The microphone and signal processor, worn outside the body, transmit electrical stimuli to the implanted electrodes. The electrical signals stimulate the auditory nerve fibers and then the brain, where they are interpreted.

Worldwide, more than 112,000 people have received a cochlear implant. In the United States, more than 23,000 adults and 15,500 children have cochlear implants (NIDCD, 2007).

Candidates for a cochlear implant, who are usually at least 1 year of age, are selected after careful screening by otologic history, physical examination, audiologic testing, x-rays, and psychological testing. Criteria for choosing adults who may benefit from a cochlear implant include the following:

- Profound sensorineural hearing loss in both ears
- Inability to hear and recognize speech well with hearing aids
- No medical contraindication to a cochlear implant or general anesthesia
- Indications that being able to hear would enhance the patient's life

The surgery involves implanting a small receiver in the temporal bone through a postauricular incision and placing electrodes into the inner ear (Fig. 59-7). The microphone and transmitter are worn on an external unit. The patient undergoes extensive cochlear rehabilitation with the multidisciplinary team, which includes an audiologist and speech pathologist. Several months may be needed to learn to interpret the sounds heard. Children and adults who lost their hearing before they learned to speak take much longer to acquire speech. There are wide variations of success with cochlear implants, and there is also controversy about their use, especially among the deaf community. Patients who have had a cochlear implant are cautioned that an MRI will inactivate the implant; MRI should be used only when there is no other diagnostic option.

Hearing Guide Dogs

Specially trained dogs (service dogs) are available to assist the person with a hearing loss. People who live alone are eligible to apply for a dog trained by International Hearing Dog, Inc. The dog reacts to the sound of a telephone, a doorbell, an alarm clock, a baby's cry, a knock at the door, a smoke alarm, or an intruder. The dog alerts its master by physical contact; the dog then runs to the source of the noise. In public, the dog positions itself between the person with hearing impairment and any potential hazard that the person cannot hear, such as an oncoming vehicle or a loud, hostile person. In many states, a certified hearing guide dog is legally permitted access to public transportation, public eating places, and stores, including food markets.

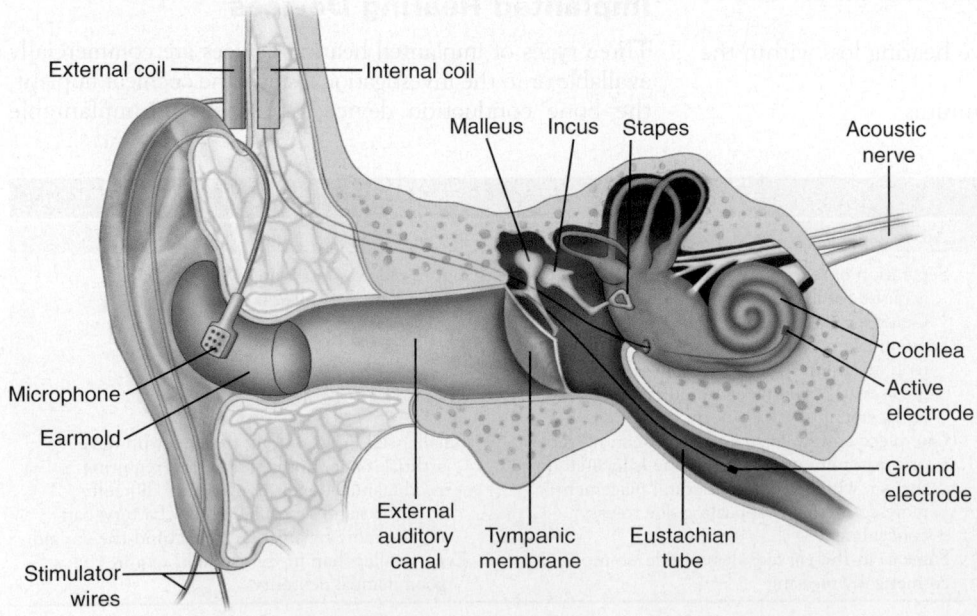

Figure 59-7 The cochlear implant. The internal coil has a stranded electrode lead. The electrode is inserted through the round window into the scala tympani of the cochlea. The external coil (the transmitter) is held in alignment with the internal coil (the receiver) by a magnet. The microphone receives the sound. The stimulator wire receives the signal after it has been filtered, adjusted, and modified so that the sound is at a comfortable level for the patient. Sound is passed by the external transmitter to the inner coil receiver by magnetic conduction and is then carried by the electrode to the cochlea.

CRITICAL THINKING EXERCISES

1 You are a new nurse in the outpatient clinic and you notice that many of the preoperative patients whom you interview have some type of hearing impairment. Discuss barriers for patients with hearing impairment and techniques you can use to assess hearing. List how you can improve your practice and communication techniques with patients who are hearing-impaired.

EBP **2** A 20-year-old man, a member of a college swim team, has recurrent external otitis—his third episode in the past 6 weeks. He is being treated at an ear-nose-throat clinic. Devise an evidence-based practice teaching plan for this patient.

3 A 44-year-old man has recently been diagnosed with Ménière's disease. Develop a teaching plan that focuses on control of the patient's symptoms. Provide rationale for each component of the teaching plan. Discuss the strength of the evidence that supports specific dietary strategies for controlling the symptoms of Ménière's disease.

4 A 50-year-old man is scheduled for coronary artery bypass graft surgery. He has been profoundly deaf since childhood. How should the preoperative and postoperative plans of nursing care be modified to meet this patient's communication needs? How would you modify discharge teaching for him?

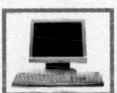
The Smeltzer suite offers these additional resources to enhance learning and facilitate understanding of this chapter:
* thePoint online resource, thepoint.lww.com/Smeltzer12E
* Student CD-ROM included with the book
* *Study Guide to Accompany Brunner & Suddarth's Textbook of Medical-Surgical Nursing*
* *Handbook for Brunner & Suddarth's Textbook of Medical-Surgical Nursing*

REFERENCES AND SELECTED READINGS

Books

Harris, L. L. & Huntoon, M. B. (2008). *Core curriculum for otorhinolaryngology and head/neck nursing* (2nd ed.). New Smyrna Beach, FL: Society of Otorhinolaryngology and Head & Neck Nurses.

McPhee, S. J., Papadakis, M. & Tierney, L. (2008). *Current 2008 medical diagnosis and treatment* (47th ed.). New York: McGraw-Hill.

Porth, C. M. & Matfin, G. (2009). *Pathophysiology. Concepts of altered health states* (8th ed.). Philadelphia: Lippincott Williams & Wilkins.

U.S. Department of Health and Human Services (USDHHS). (2007). *Healthy people 2010 Midcourse review*. Washington, DC: Author.

Journals & Electronic Documents

Chung, J. H., Des Roches, C. M., Meunier, J., et al. (2005). Evaluation of noise-induced hearing loss in young people using a web-based survey technique. *Pediatrics, 115*(4), 861–867.

Folmer, R. (2006). Noise-induced hearing loss in young people. *Pediatrics, 117*(1), 248–249.

Folmer, R. L., Martin, W. H. & Shi, Y. (2004). Tinnitus: Questions to reveal the cause, answers to provide relief. *Journal of Family Practice, 53*(7), 532–540.

Garcia-Berrocal, J. R., Ramirez-Camacho, R., Trinidad, A., et al. (2004). Controversies and criticisms on designs for experimental autoimmune labyrinthitis. *Annals of Otology, Rhinology & Laryngology, 113*(5), 404–410.

Haginomori, S., Takamaki, A., Nonaka, R., et al. (2008). Residual cholesteatoma: Incidence & localization in canal wall down tympanoplasty with soft-wall reconstruction. *Archives of Otolaryngology—Head & Neck Surgery, 134*(6), 652–657.

Health and Safety Executive. (2008). *Employers' responsibilities—legal duties*. www.hse.gov.uk/noise/employers.htm

Healthy People 2010. *Healthy hearing 2010*. www.nidcd.nih.gov/health/healthy-hearing

Holmes, A., Widen, S., Erlandsson, S., et al. (2007). Perceived hearing status & attitudes toward noise in young adults. *American Journal of Audiology, 16*, S182–S189.

Kacker, A. & Selesnick, S. (2008). External ear, infections. E-medicine. www.emedicine.com/ent/topic202.htm

Kitahara, T., Kondoh, K. & Morihana, T. (2004). Surgical management of special cases of intractable Ménière's disease: Unilateral cases with intact canals and bilateral cases. *Annals of Otorhinolaryngology, 113*(5), 339–403.

Kitahara, T., Kubo, T., Okumura, S., et al. (2008). Effects of endolymphatic sac drainage with steroids for intractable Ménière's disease: A long-term follow-up and randomized controlled study. *Laryngoscope, 118*(5), 854–861.

Kunst, S. J., Hol, M. K., Mylanus, E. A., et al. (2008). Subjective benefit after BAHA system application in patients with congenital unilateral conductive hearing impairment. *Otology & Neurotology, 29*(3), 353–358.

Labuguen, R. H. (2006). Initial evaluation of vertigo. *American Family Physician, 73*(2), 244–251.

MayoClinic.com Tools for healthier lives. (2008). Ménière's disease. www.mayoclinic.com/health/menieres-disease/DS00535/DSEC

Mitchell, R. E. (2006). How many deaf people are there in the United States? Estimates from the survey of income and program participation. *Journal of Deaf Studies and Deaf Education, 11*(1), 112–119.

National Institute on Deafness and Other Communication Disorders (NIDCD). (2008). Strategic plan. FY 2009–2011. www.nidcd.nih.gov/Static.Resources/about/plans/stategic/FY2009-2011NIDCDstrategicplan.pdf

National Institute on Deafness and Other Communication Disorders (NIDCD). (2007). *Cochlear implants*. www.nidcd.nih.gov/health/hearing/coch.asp

National Institute on Deafness and Other Communication Disorders (NIDCD). (2008). *Wise Ears®*. www.nidcd.nih.gov/health/wise

Osguthorpe, J. D. & Nielsen D. R. (2006). Otitis externa: Review and clinical update. *American Family Physician, 74*(9), 1510–1516.

Rovers, M., Schilder, A., Zielhuis, G., et al. (2004). Otitis media. *Lancet, 363*(9407), 465–473.

Semaan, M. T. & Megerian, C. A. (2006). The pathophysiology of cholesteatoma. *Otolaryngology Clinics of North America, 39*(6), 1143–1159.

Swartz, R. & Longwell, P. (2005). Treatment of vertigo. *American Family Physician, 71*(6), 1115–1122.

U.S. Department of Education. (2008). *Building the legacy: IDEA 2004*. http://idea.ed.gov/explore/home

RESOURCES

Acoustic Neuroma Association, www.anausa.org

Alexander Graham Bell Association for the Deaf and Hard of Hearing, www.agbell.org

American Academy of Audiology, www.audiology.org

American Academy of Facial Plastic and Reconstructive Surgery, www.aafprs.org

American Academy of Otolaryngology–Head & Neck Surgery, www.entnet.org

American Board of Facial Plastic and Reconstructive Surgery, www.abfprs.org

American Speech-Language-Hearing Association, www.asha.org

American Tinnitus Association, www.ata.org

International Hearing Dog, Inc., www.ihdi.org

National Institute on Deafness and Other Communication Disorders (NIDCD), National Institutes of Health, www.nidcd.nih.gov

Society of Otorhinolaryngology and Head-Neck Nurses, Inc., www.sohnnurse.com

Vestibular Disorders Association, www.vestibular.org

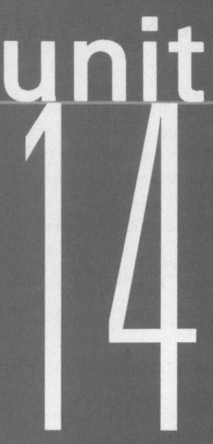

unit 14

Neurologic Function

Case Study • Applying Concepts From NANDA, NIC, and NOC

A Patient With Brain Injury and a History of Alcohol Abuse

Mr. Williams is a 36-year-old man with a history of alcohol abuse. On the evening before his admission to the hospital, Mr. Williams fell down a flight of stairs while intoxicated, hitting the front and left side of his head. He was admitted to the neurologic intensive care unit (NICU) and diagnosed with a traumatic brain injury. After several days in the NICU, Mr. Williams developed increased intracranial pressure (ICP) and is being treated for alcohol withdrawal. When family members come to visit, they admit to a significant history of alcoholism in the family.

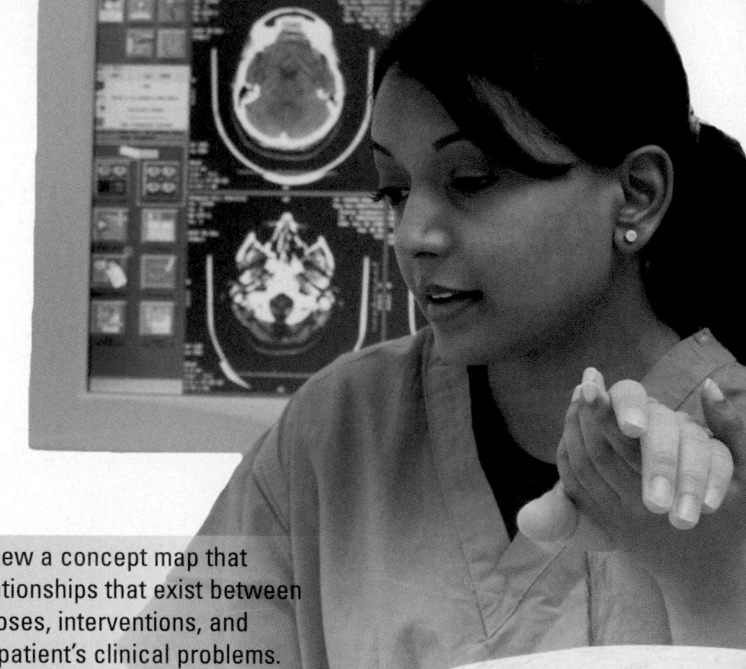

Visit thePoint to view a concept map that illustrates the relationships that exist between the nursing diagnoses, interventions, and outcomes for the patient's clinical problems.

Nursing Classifications and Languages

NANDA NURSING DIAGNOSES	NIC NURSING INTERVENTIONS	NOC NURSING OUTCOMES
		Return to functional baseline status, stabilization of, or improvement in:
DECREASED INTRACRANIAL ADAPTIVE CAPACITY—Intracranial fluid dynamic mechanisms that normally compensate for increases in intracranial volumes are compromised, resulting in repeated disproportionate increases in increased intracranial pressure (ICP) in response to a variety of noxious stimuli	**NEUROLOGIC MONITORING**—Collection and analysis of patient data to prevent or minimize neurologic complications	**NEUROLOGICAL STATUS**—Ability of the peripheral and central nervous system to receive, process, and respond to internal and external stimuli
RISK FOR INJURY—At risk of injury as a result of environmental conditions interacting with the individual's adaptive and defensive resources	**CEREBRAL EDEMA MANAGEMENT**—Limitation of secondary cerebral injury resulting from swelling of brain tissue	**SEIZURE CONTROL**—Personal actions to reduce or minimize the occurrence of seizure episodes
DYSFUNCTIONAL FAMILY PROCESSES: ALCOHOLISM—Psychosocial, spiritual, and physiological functions of the family unit are chronically disorganized, which leads to conflict, denial of problems, resistance to change, ineffective problem solving, and a series of self-perpetuating crises	**MEDICATION ADMINISTRATION**—Preparing, giving, and evaluating the effectiveness of prescription and nonprescription drugs	**PHYSICAL INJURY SEVERITY**—Severity of injuries from trauma
	SURVEILLANCE: SAFETY—Purposeful and ongoing collection and analysis of information about the patient and the environment for use in promoting and maintaining patient safety	**FAMILY COPING**—Family actions to manage stressors that tax family resources
	FAMILY SUPPORT—Promotion of family values, interests and goals	

Bulechek, G. M., Butcher, H. K., & Dochterman, J. M. (2008). *Nursing interventions classification (NIC)* (5th ed.). St. Louis: Mosby.
Johnson, M., Bulechek, G., Butcher, H. K., et al. (2006). *NANDA, NOC, and NIC linkages* (2nd ed.). St. Louis: Mosby.
Moorhead, S., Johnson, M., Mass, M. L., et al. (2008). *Nursing outcomes classification (NOC)* (4th ed.). St. Louis: Mosby.
NANDA International. (2007). *Nursing diagnoses: Definitions & classification 2007–2008.* Philadelphia: North American Nursing Diagnosis Association.

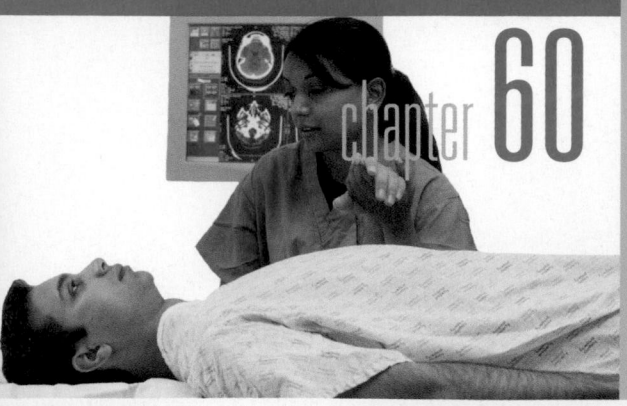

chapter 60

Assessment of Neurologic Function

Nurses in many practice settings encounter patients with altered neurologic function. Disorders of the nervous system can occur at any time during the lifespan and can vary from mild, self-limiting symptoms to devastating, life-threatening disorders. Nurses must be skilled in the general assessment of neurologic function and be able to focus on specific areas as needed. Assessment requires knowledge of the anatomy and physiology of the nervous system and an understanding of the array of tests and procedures used to diagnose neurologic disorders. Knowledge about the nursing implications and interventions related to assessment and diagnostic testing is also essential.

Anatomic and Physiologic Overview

The nervous system consists of two major parts: the central nervous system (CNS), including the brain and spinal cord, and the peripheral nervous system, which includes the cranial nerves, spinal nerves, and autonomic nervous system. The function of the nervous system is to control motor, sensory, autonomic, cognitive, and behavioral activities. The brain itself contains more than 100 billion cells that link the motor and sensory pathways, monitor the body's processes, respond to the internal and external environment, maintain homeostasis, and direct all psychological, biologic, and physical activity through complex chemical and electrical messages (Klein & Stewart-Amidei, 2009).

Cells of the Nervous System

The basic functional unit of the brain is the neuron (Fig. 60-1). It is composed of dendrites, a cell body, and an axon. The **dendrites** are branch-type structures for receiving electrochemical messages. The **axon** is a long projection that carries electrical impulses away from the cell body. Some neurons have a myelinated sheath that increases speed of conduction. Nerve cell bodies occurring in clusters are called ganglia or nuclei. A cluster of cell bodies with the same function is called a center (eg, the respiratory center). Neuroglial cells, 50 times greater in number than neurons, serve to support, protect, and nourish neurons (Hickey, 2009).

Neurotransmitters

Neurotransmitters communicate messages from one neuron to another or from a neuron to a specific target tissue. Neurotransmitters are manufactured and stored in synaptic vesicles. As an electrical action potential propagated along the axon reaches the nerve terminal, neurotransmitters are released into the synapse. The neurotransmitter diffuses or is transported across the synapse, binding to receptors in the postsynaptic cell membrane. A neurotransmitter potentiates, terminates, or modulates a specific action, and it can either excite or inhibit activity of the target cell. Usually, multiple neurotransmitters are at work in the neural synapse. The source and action of major neurotransmitters are described in Table 60-1. Once released, enzymes either destroy the neurotransmitter or reabsorb it into the cell for future use.

Many neurologic disorders are due, at least in part, to an imbalance in neurotransmitters. For example, Parkinson's disease develops from decreased availability of dopamine, while acetylcholine binding to muscle cells is impaired in myasthenia gravis (Porth & Matfin, 2009). All brain functions are modulated through neurotransmitter receptor site activity, including memory and other cognitive processes (Hickey, 2009).

Ongoing research is evaluating diagnostic tests that can detect abnormal levels of neurotransmitters in the brain. Positron emission tomography (PET), for example, can detect dopamine, serotonin, and acetylcholine. Single photon emission computed tomography (SPECT), similar to PET, can detect changes in some neurotransmitters such as dopamine in Parkinson's disease (Bremner, 2005). Both PET and SPECT are discussed in more detail later in this chapter.

The Central Nervous System

The Brain

The brain accounts for approximately 2% of the total body weight; in an average young adult, the brain weighs approximately 1400 g, whereas in an average elderly person, the brain weighs approximately 1200 g (Hickey, 2009). The brain is divided into three major areas: the cerebrum, the brain stem, and the cerebellum. The cerebrum is composed of two hemispheres, the thalamus, the hypothalamus, and the basal ganglia. The brain stem includes the midbrain, pons, and medulla. The cerebellum is located under the cerebrum and behind the brain stem (Fig. 60-2).

Cerebrum

The outside surface of the hemispheres has a wrinkled appearance that is the result of many folded layers or

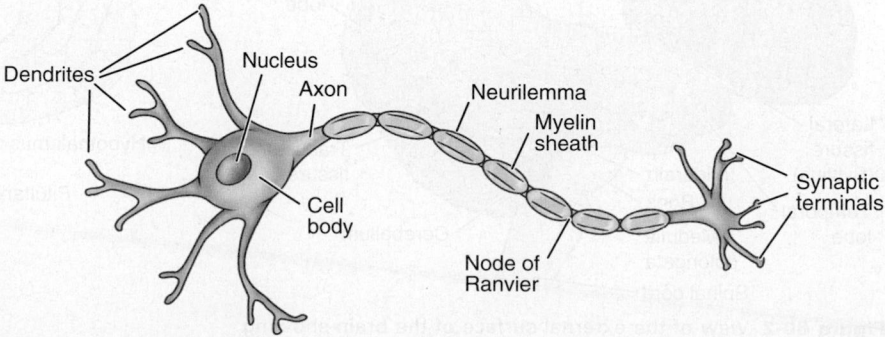

Figure 60-1 Neuron.

Table 60-1 MAJOR NEUROTRANSMITTERS

Neurotransmitter	Source	Action
Acetylcholine (major transmitter of the parasympathetic nervous system)	Many areas of the brain; autonomic nervous system	Usually excitatory; parasympathetic effects sometimes inhibitory (stimulation of heart by vagal nerve)
Serotonin	Brain stem, hypothalamus, dorsal horn of the spinal cord	Inhibitory, helps control mood and sleep, inhibits pain pathways
Dopamine	Substantia nigra and basal ganglia	Usually inhibits, affects behavior (attention, emotions) and fine movement
Norepinephrine (major transmitter of the sympathetic nervous system)	Brain stem, hypothalamus, postganglionic neurons of the sympathetic nervous system	Usually excitatory; affects mood and overall activity
Gamma-aminobutyric acid (GABA)	Spinal cord, cerebellum, basal ganglia, some cortical areas	Inhibitory
Enkephalin, endorphin	Nerve terminals in the spine, brain stem, thalamus and hypothalamus, pituitary gland	Excitatory; pleasurable sensation, inhibits pain transmission

convolutions called gyri, which increase the surface area of the brain, accounting for the high level of activity carried out by such a small-appearing organ. Between each gyrus is a sulcus or fissure that serves as an anatomic division. In between the cerebral hemispheres is the great longitudinal fissure that separates the cerebrum into the right and left hemispheres. The two hemispheres are joined at the lower portion of the fissure by the corpus callosum. The external or outer portion of the hemispheres (the cerebral cortex) is made up of gray matter approximately 2 to 5 mm in depth; it contains billions of neuron cell bodies, giving it a gray appearance. White matter makes up the innermost layer and is composed of myelinated nerve fibers and neuroglia cells that form tracts or pathways connecting various parts of the brain with one another. These pathways also connect the cortex with lower portions of the brain and spinal cord. The cerebral hemispheres are divided into pairs of lobes as follows (see Fig. 60-2):

- Frontal—the largest lobe, located in the front of the brain. The major functions of this lobe are concentration, abstract thought, information storage or memory, and motor function. It contains Broca's area, which is located in the left hemisphere and is critical for motor control of speech. The frontal lobe is also responsible in large part for a person's affect, judgment, personality, and inhibitions (Hickey, 2009).
- Parietal—a predominantly sensory lobe posterior to the frontal lobe. This lobe analyzes sensory information and relays the interpretation of this information to other cortical areas and is essential to a person's awareness of body position in space, size and shape discrimination, and right–left orientation (Hickey, 2009).
- Temporal—located inferior to the frontal and parietal lobes, this lobe contains the auditory receptive areas and plays a role in memory of sound and understanding of language and music.
- Occipital—located posterior to the parietal lobe, this lobe is responsible for visual interpretation and memory.

The corpus callosum (Fig. 60-3), a thick collection of nerve fibers that connects the two hemispheres of the brain, is responsible for the transmission of information from one side of the brain to the other. Information transferred includes sensation, memory, and learned discrimination. Right-handed people and some left-handed people have cerebral dominance on the left side of the brain for verbal, linguistic, arithmetic, calculation, and analytic functions.

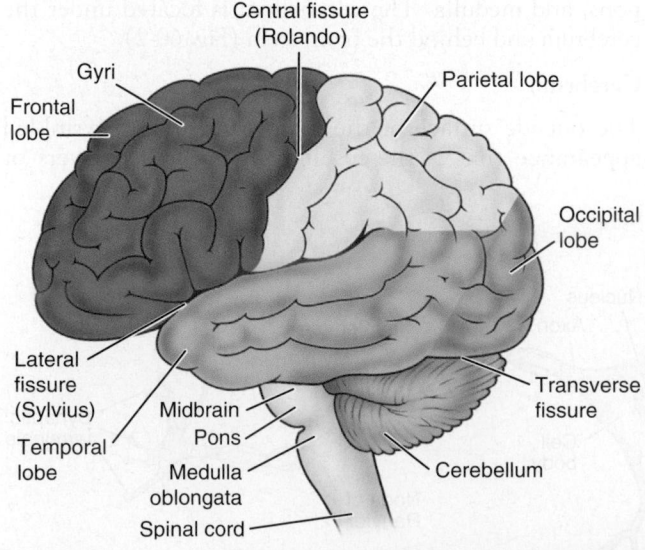

Figure 60-2 View of the external surface of the brain showing lobes, cerebellum, and brain stem.

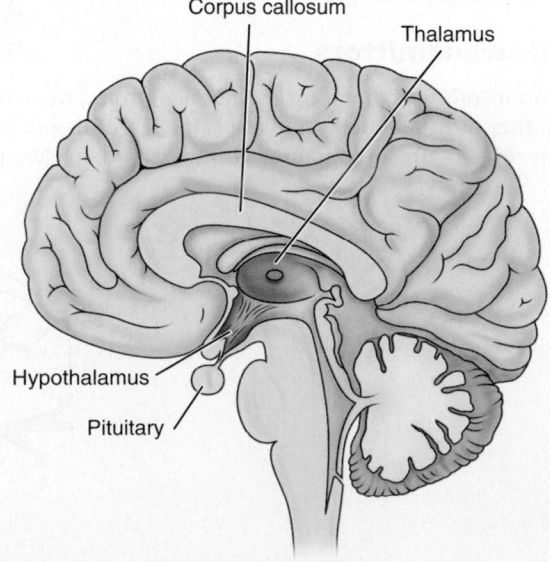

Figure 60-3 Medial view of the brain.

The nondominant hemisphere is responsible for geometric, spatial, visual, pattern, and musical functions. Nuclei for cranial nerves I and II are also located in the cerebrum.

The basal ganglia are masses of nuclei located deep in the cerebral hemispheres that are responsible for control of fine motor movements, including those of the hands and lower extremities.

The thalamus (see Fig. 60-3) lies on either side of the third ventricle and acts primarily as a relay station for all sensation except smell. All memory, sensation, and pain impulses pass through this section of the brain.

The hypothalamus (see Fig. 60-3) is located anterior and inferior to the thalamus, and beneath and lateral to the third ventricle. The infundibulum of the hypothalamus connects it to the posterior pituitary gland. The hypothalamus plays an important role in the endocrine system because it regulates the pituitary secretion of hormones that influence metabolism, reproduction, stress response, and urine production. It works with the pituitary to maintain fluid balance through hormonal release and maintains temperature regulation by promoting vasoconstriction or vasodilatation. In addition, the hypothalamus is the site of the hunger center and is involved in appetite control. It contains centers that regulate the sleep–wake cycle, blood pressure, aggressive and sexual behavior, and emotional responses (ie, blushing, rage, depression, panic, and fear). The hypothalamus also controls and regulates the autonomic nervous system. The optic chiasm (the point at which the two optic tracts cross) and the mamillary bodies (involved in olfactory reflexes and emotional response to odors) are also found in this area.

Brain Stem

The brain stem consists of the midbrain, pons, and medulla oblongata (see Fig. 60-2). The midbrain connects the pons and the cerebellum with the cerebral hemispheres; it contains sensory and motor pathways and serves as the center for auditory and visual reflexes. Cranial nerves III and IV originate in the midbrain. The pons is situated in front of the cerebellum between the midbrain and the medulla and is a bridge between the two halves of the cerebellum, and between the medulla and the midbrain. Cranial nerves V through VIII originate in the pons. The pons also contains motor and sensory pathways. Portions of the pons help regulate respiration.

Motor fibers from the brain to the spinal cord and sensory fibers from the spinal cord to the brain are located in the medulla. Most of these fibers cross, or decussate, at this level. Cranial nerves IX through XII originate in the medulla. Reflex centers for respiration, blood pressure, heart rate, coughing, vomiting, swallowing, and sneezing are located in the medulla as well. The reticular formation, responsible for arousal and the sleep–wake cycle, begins in the medulla and connects with numerous higher structures.

Cerebellum

The cerebellum is posterior to the midbrain and pons, and below the occipital lobe (see Fig. 60-2). The cerebellum integrates sensory information to provide smooth coordinated movement. It controls fine movement, balance, and **position (postural) sense** or proprioception (awareness of where each part of the body is).

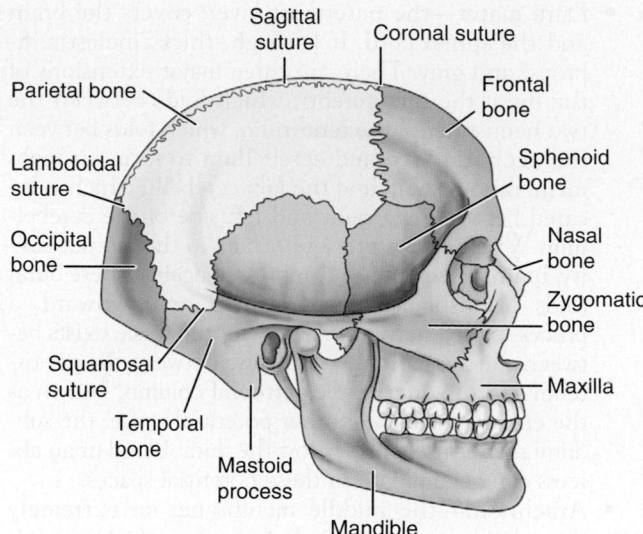

Figure 60-4 Bones and sutures of the skull.

Structures Protecting the Brain

The brain is contained in the rigid skull, which protects it from injury. The major bones of the skull are the frontal, temporal, parietal, occipital, and sphenoid bones. These bones join at the suture lines (Fig. 60-4) and form the base of the skull. Indentations in the skull base are known as fossae. The anterior fossa contains the frontal lobe, the middle fossa contains the temporal lobe, and the posterior fossa contains the cerebellum and brain stem.

The meninges, fibrous connective tissues that cover the brain and spinal cord, provide protection, support, and nourishment. The layers of the meninges are the dura mater, arachnoid, and pia mater (Fig. 60-5).

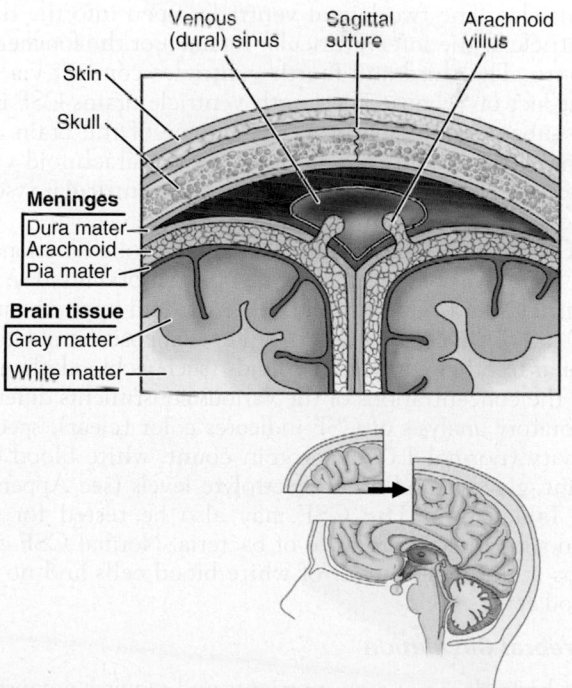

Figure 60-5 Meninges and related structures.

- Dura mater—the outermost layer; covers the brain and the spinal cord. It is tough, thick, inelastic, fibrous, and gray. There are three major extensions of the dura: the falx cerebri, which folds between the two hemispheres; the tentorium, which folds between the occipital lobe and cerebellum to form a tough, membranous shelf; and the falx cerebelli, which is located between the right and left side of the cerebellum. When excess pressure occurs in the cranial cavity, brain tissue may be compressed against these dural folds or displaced around them or downward, a process called herniation. A potential space exists between the dura and the skull, and between the periosteum and the dura in the vertebral column, known as the epidural space. Another potential space, the subdural space, also exists below the dura. Blood or an abscess can accumulate in these potential spaces.
- Arachnoid—the middle membrane; an extremely thin, delicate membrane that closely resembles a spider web (hence the name arachnoid). The arachnoid membrane has cerebrospinal fluid (CSF) in the space below it, called the subarachnoid space. This membrane has unique fingerlike projections, called arachnoid villi, that absorb CSF into the venous system. When blood or bacteria enter the subarachnoid space, the villi become obstructed and *communicating* hydrocephalus (increased size of ventricles) may result.
- Pia mater—the innermost, thin, transparent layer that hugs the brain closely and extends into every fold of the brain's surface.

Cerebrospinal Fluid

CSF is a clear and colorless fluid that is produced in the choroid plexus of the ventricles and circulates around the surface of the brain and the spinal cord. There are four ventricles: the right and left lateral and the third and fourth ventricles. The two lateral ventricles open into the third ventricle at the interventricular foramen or the foramen of Monro. The third and fourth ventricles connect via the aqueduct of Sylvius. The fourth ventricle drains CSF into the subarachnoid space on the surface of the brain and spinal cord, where it is absorbed by the arachnoid villi. Blockage of CSF flow anywhere in the ventricular system produces *obstructive* hydrocephalus.

CSF is important in immune and metabolic functions in the brain. It is produced at a rate of about 500 mL/day; the ventricles and subarachnoid space contain approximately 150 mL of fluid (Hickey, 2009). The composition of CSF is similar to other extracellular fluids (such as blood plasma), but the concentrations of the various constituents differ. A laboratory analysis of CSF indicates color (clear), specific gravity (normal 1.007), protein count, white blood cell count, glucose, and other electrolyte levels (see Appendix A, Table A-5). The CSF may also be tested for immunoglobulins or presence of bacteria. Normal CSF contains a minimal number of white blood cells and no red blood cells.

Cerebral Circulation

The brain does not store nutrients and requires a constant supply of oxygen. These needs are met through cerebral circulation; the brain receives approximately 15% of the cardiac output, or 750 mL per minute of blood flow. Brain circulation is unique in several aspects. First, arterial and venous circulation are not parallel as in other organs in the body; this is due in part to the role the venous system plays in CSF absorption. Second, the brain has collateral circulation through the circle of Willis, allowing blood flow to be redirected on demand. Third, blood vessels in the brain have two rather than three layers, which may make them more prone to rupture when weakened or under pressure.

Arteries

Arterial blood supply to the brain originates from the common carotid artery, the first bifurcation off the aorta. The internal carotid arteries arise at the bifurcation of the common carotid and supply much of the anterior circulation of the brain. Branches of the internal carotid arteries, anterior and middle cerebral arteries, along with their connections, anterior and posterior communicating arteries, form the circle of Willis (Fig. 60-6).

The vertebral arteries branch from the subclavian arteries to supply most of the posterior circulation of the brain. At the level of the brain stem, the vertebral arteries join to form the basilar artery. The basilar artery divides to form the two branches of the posterior cerebral arteries. Functionally, the posterior portion of the circulation and the anterior or carotid circulation usually remain separate. However, the circle of Willis can provide collateral circulation if one of the vessels supplying it becomes occluded or is ligated.

The bifurcations along the circle of Willis are frequent sites of aneurysm formation. Aneurysms are outpouchings of the blood vessel due to vessel wall weakness. Aneurysms can rupture and cause a hemorrhagic stroke. Aneurysms are discussed in more detail in Chapter 62.

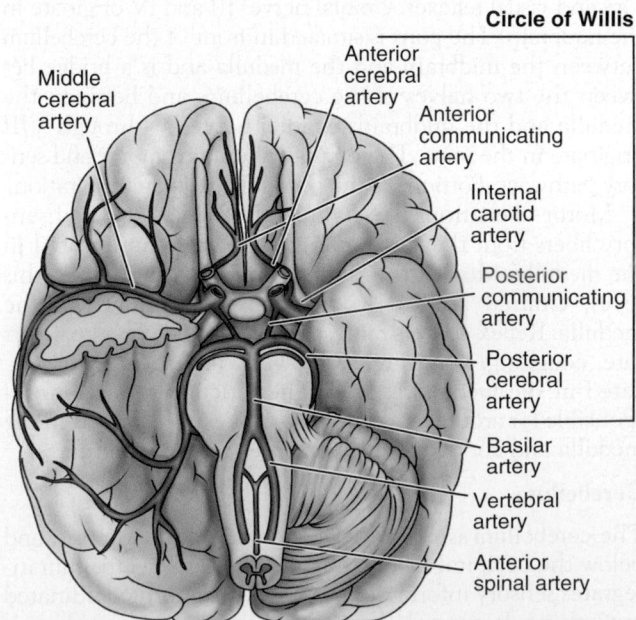

Figure 60-6 Arterial blood supply of the brain, including the circle of Willis, as viewed from the ventral surface.

Veins

Venous drainage for the brain does not follow the arterial circulation as in other body structures. The veins reach the brain's surface, join larger veins, then cross the subarachnoid space and empty into the dural sinuses, which are the vascular channels laying within the dura (see Fig. 60-5). The network of the sinuses carries venous outflow from the brain and empties into the internal jugular veins, returning the blood to the heart. Cerebral veins are unique because, unlike other veins in the body, they do not have valves to prevent blood from flowing backward and depend on both gravity and blood pressure for flow.

Blood–Brain Barrier

The CNS is inaccessible to many substances that circulate in the blood plasma (eg, dyes, medications, and antibiotics) because of the blood–brain barrier. This barrier is formed by the endothelial cells of the brain's capillaries, which form continuous tight junctions, creating a barrier to macromolecules and many compounds. All substances entering the CSF must filter through the capillary endothelial cells and astrocytes. The blood–brain barrier has a protective function but can be altered by trauma, cerebral edema, and cerebral hypoxemia; this has implications in the treatment and selection of medication for CNS disorders (Hickey, 2009).

The Spinal Cord

The spinal cord is continuous with the medulla, extending from the cerebral hemispheres and serving as the connection between the brain and the periphery. Approximately 45 cm (18 inches) long and about the thickness of a finger, it extends from the foramen magnum at the base of the skull to the lower border of the first lumbar vertebra, where it tapers to a fibrous band called the *conus medullaris*. Continuing below the second lumbar space are the nerve roots that extend beyond the conus, which are called the *cauda equina* because they resemble a horse's tail. Meninges surround the spinal cord.

In a cross-sectional view, the spinal cord has an H-shaped central core of nerve cell bodies (gray matter) surrounded by ascending and descending tracts (white matter) (Fig. 60-7). The lower portion of the H is broader than the upper portion and corresponds to the anterior horns. The anterior horns contain cells with fibers that form the anterior (motor) root and are essential for the voluntary and reflex activity of the muscles they innervate. The thinner posterior (upper horns) portion contains cells with fibers that enter over the posterior (sensory) root and thus serve as a relay station in the sensory/reflex pathway.

The thoracic region of the spinal cord has a projection from each side at the crossbar of the H-shaped structure of gray matter called the lateral horn. It contains the cells that give rise to the autonomic fibers of the sympathetic division. The fibers leave the spinal cord through the anterior roots in the thoracic and upper lumbar segments.

The Spinal Tracts

The white matter of the spinal cord is composed of myelinated and unmyelinated nerve fibers. The fast-conducting myelinated fibers form bundles that also contain glial cells. Fiber bundles with a common function are called tracts.

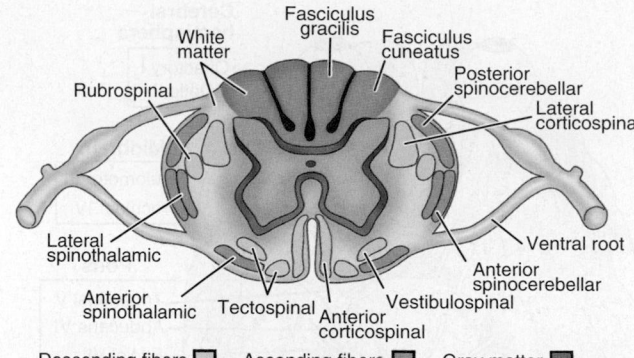

Figure 60-7 Cross-sectional diagram of the spinal cord showing major spinal tracts.

There are six ascending tracts. Two tracts, known as the fasciculus cuneatus and gracilis or the posterior columns, conduct sensations of deep touch, pressure, vibration, position, and passive motion from the same side of the body. Before reaching the cerebral cortex, these fibers cross to the opposite side in the medulla. The anterior and posterior spinocerebellar tracts conduct sensory impulses from muscle spindles, providing necessary input for coordinated muscle contraction. They ascend essentially uncrossed and terminate in the cerebellum. The anterior and lateral spinothalamic tracts are responsible for conduction of pain, temperature, proprioception, fine touch, and vibratory sense from the upper body to the brain. They cross to the opposite side of the cord, and then ascend to the brain, terminating in the thalamus (Klein & Stewart-Amidei, 2009).

There are eight descending tracts. The anterior and lateral corticospinal tracts conduct motor impulses to the anterior horn cells from the opposite side of the brain, cross in the medulla, and control voluntary muscle activity. The three vestibulospinal tracts descend uncrossed and are involved in some autonomic functions (sweating, pupil dilation, and circulation) and involuntary muscle control. The corticobulbar tract conducts impulses responsible for voluntary head and facial muscle movement and crosses at the level of the brain stem. The rubrospinal and reticulospinal tracts conduct impulses involved with involuntary muscle movement.

Vertebral Column

The bones of the vertebral column surround and protect the spinal cord and normally consist of 7 cervical, 12 thoracic, and 5 lumbar vertebrae, as well as the sacrum (a fused mass of 5 vertebrae), and terminate in the coccyx. Nerve roots exit from the vertebral column through the intervertebral foramina (openings). The vertebrae are separated by disks, except for the first and second cervical, the sacral, and the coccygeal vertebrae. Each vertebra has a ventral solid body and a dorsal segment or arch, which is posterior to the body. The arch is composed of two pedicles and two laminae supporting seven processes. The vertebral body, arch, pedicles, and laminae all encase and protect the spinal cord.

The Peripheral Nervous System

The peripheral nervous system includes the cranial nerves, the spinal nerves, and the autonomic nervous system.

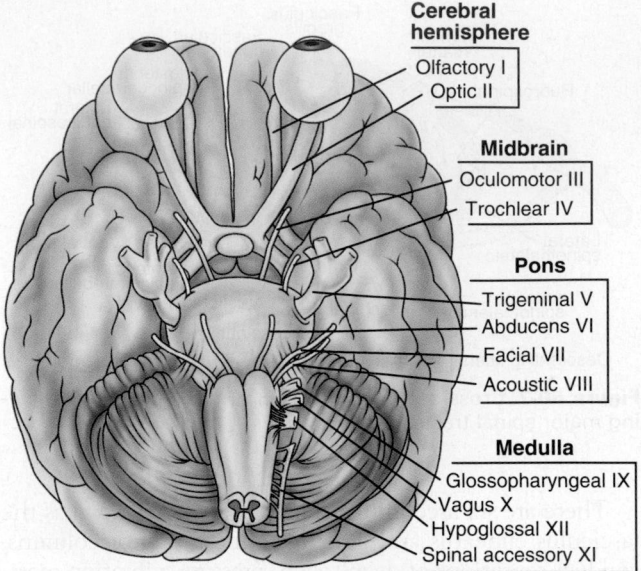

Olfactory I
Optic II
Cerebral hemisphere

Midbrain
Oculomotor III
Trochlear IV

Pons
Trigeminal V
Abducens VI
Facial VII
Acoustic VIII

Medulla
Glossopharyngeal IX
Vagus X
Hypoglossal XII
Spinal accessory XI

Figure 60-8 Diagram of the base of the brain showing entrance or exit of the cranial nerves. The right column shows the anatomic location of the connection of each cranial nerve to the central nervous system.

Cranial Nerves

Twelve pairs of cranial nerves emerge from the lower surface of the brain and pass through openings in the base of the skull. Three are entirely sensory (I, II, VIII), five are motor (III, IV, VI, XI, and XII), and four are mixed sensory and motor (V, VII, IX, and X). The cranial nerves are numbered in the order in which they arise from the brain (Fig. 60-8). The cranial nerves innervate the head, neck, and special sense structures. Table 60-2 identifies primary functions of the cranial nerves.

Spinal Nerves

The spinal cord is composed of 31 pairs of spinal nerves: 8 cervical, 12 thoracic, 5 lumbar, 5 sacral, and 1 coccygeal. Each spinal nerve has a ventral root and a dorsal root. The dorsal roots are sensory and transmit sensory impulses from specific areas of the body known as dermatomes (Fig. 60-9) to the dorsal horn ganglia. The sensory fiber may be somatic, carrying information about pain, temperature, touch, and position sense (proprioception) from the tendons, joints, and body surfaces; or visceral, carrying information from the internal organs.

The ventral roots are motor and transmit impulses from the spinal cord to the body, and these fibers are also either somatic or visceral. The visceral fibers include autonomic fibers that control the cardiac muscles and glandular secretions.

Autonomic Nervous System

The **autonomic nervous system** regulates the activities of internal organs such as the heart, lungs, blood vessels, digestive organs, and glands. Maintenance and restoration of internal homeostasis is largely the responsibility of the autonomic nervous system. There are two major divisions: the **sympathetic nervous system,** with predominantly excita-

Table 60-2	CRANIAL NERVES	
Cranial Nerve	**Type**	**Function**
I (olfactory)	Sensory	Sense of smell
II (optic)	Sensory	Visual acuity and visual fields
III (oculomotor)	Motor	Muscles that move the eye and lid, pupillary constriction, lens accommodation
IV (trochlear)	Motor	Muscles that move the eye
V (trigeminal)	Mixed	Facial sensation, corneal reflex, mastication
VI (abducens)	Motor	Muscles that move the eye
VII (facial)	Mixed	Facial expression and muscle movement, salivation and tearing, taste, sensation in the ear
VIII (acoustic)	Sensory	Hearing and equilibrium
IX (glossopharyngeal)	Mixed	Taste, sensation in pharynx and tongue, pharyngeal muscles, swallowing
X (vagus)	Mixed	Muscles of pharynx, larynx, and soft palate; sensation in external ear, pharynx, larynx, thoracic and abdominal viscera; parasympathetic innervation of thoracic and abdominal organs
XI (spinal accessory)	Motor	Sternocleidomastoid and trapezius muscles
XII (hypoglossal)	Motor	Movement of the tongue

tory responses, most notably the "fight-or-flight" response, and the **parasympathetic nervous system,** which controls mostly visceral functions.

The autonomic nervous system innervates most body organs. Although usually considered part of the peripheral nervous system, this system is regulated by centers in the spinal cord, brain stem, and hypothalamus. The autonomic nervous system has two neurons in a series extending between the centers in the CNS and the organs innervated. The first neuron, the preganglionic neuron, is located in the brain or spinal cord, and its axon extends to the autonomic ganglia. There, it synapses with the second neuron, the postganglionic neuron, located in the autonomic ganglia, and its axon synapses with the target tissue and innervates the effector organ. Its regulatory effects are exerted not on individual cells but on large expanses of tissue and on entire organs. The responses elicited do not occur instantaneously but after a lag period. These responses are sustained far longer than other neurogenic responses to ensure maximal functional efficiency on the part of receptor organs, such as blood vessels.

The hypothalamus is the major subcortical center for the regulation of visceral and somatic activities, serving an inhibitory–excitatory role in the autonomic nervous system. The hypothalamus has connections that link the autonomic system with the thalamus, the cortex, the olfactory apparatus, and the pituitary gland. Located here are the mechanisms for the control of visceral and somatic reactions that were originally important for defense or attack and are associated with emotional states (eg, fear, anger, anxiety); for the control of metabolic processes, including fat, carbohydrate, and water metabolism; for the regulation

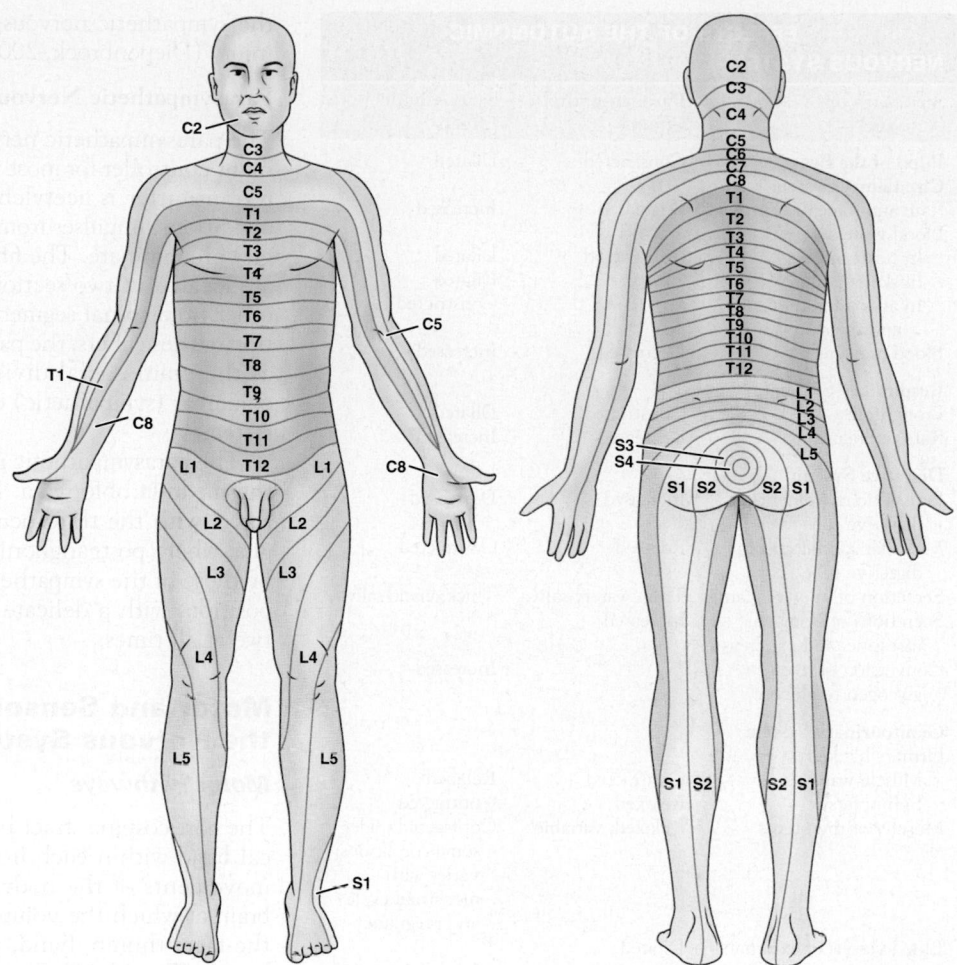

Figure 60-9 Dermatome distribution.

of body temperature, arterial pressure, and all muscular and glandular activities of the gastrointestinal tract; for control of genital functions; and for the sleep cycle.

The autonomic nervous system is separated into the anatomically and functionally distinct sympathetic and parasympathetic divisions. Most of the tissues and the organs under autonomic control are innervated by both systems. For example, the parasympathetic division causes contraction (stimulation) of the urinary bladder muscles and a decrease (inhibition) in heart rate, whereas the sympathetic division produces relaxation (inhibition) of the urinary bladder and an increase (stimulation) in the rate and force of the heartbeat. Table 60-3 compares the sympathetic and the parasympathetic effects on the different systems of the body.

Sympathetic Nervous System

The sympathetic division of the autonomic nervous system is best known for its role in the body's "fight-or-flight" response. Under stress from either physical or emotional causes, sympathetic impulses increase greatly. As a result, the bronchioles dilate for easier gas exchange; the heart's contractions are stronger and faster; the arteries to the heart and voluntary muscles dilate, carrying more blood to these organs; peripheral blood vessels constrict, making the skin feel cool but shunting blood to essential organs; the pupils dilate; the liver releases glucose for quick energy; peristalsis slows; hair stands on end; and perspiration increases. The main sympathetic neurotransmitter is norepinephrine (noradrenaline). A sympathetic discharge is the same as if the body has been given an injection of adrenalin—hence, the term *adrenergic* is often used to refer to this division.

Sympathetic neurons are located primarily in the thoracic and the lumbar segments of the spinal cord, and their axons, or the preganglionic fibers, emerge by way of anterior nerve roots from the eighth cervical or first thoracic segment to the second or third lumbar segment. A short distance from the cord, these fibers diverge to join a chain, composed of 22 linked ganglia, that extends the entire length of the spinal column, adjacent to the vertebral bodies on both sides. Some form multiple synapses with nerve cells within the chain. Others traverse the chain without making connections or losing continuity to join large "prevertebral" ganglia in the thorax, the abdomen, or the pelvis or one of the "terminal" ganglia in the vicinity of an organ, such as the bladder or the rectum (Fig. 60-10). Postganglionic nerve fibers originating in the sympathetic chain rejoin the spinal nerves that supply the extremities and are distributed to blood vessels, sweat glands, and smooth muscle tissue in the skin. Postganglionic fibers from the prevertebral plexuses

Table 60-3	EFFECTS OF THE AUTONOMIC NERVOUS SYSTEM	
Structure or Activity	**Parasympathetic Effects**	**Sympathetic Effects**
Pupil of the Eye	Constricted	Dilated
Circulatory System		
Rate and force of heartbeat	Decreased	Increased
Blood vessels		
In heart muscle	Constricted	Dilated
In skeletal muscle	*	Dilated
In abdominal viscera and the skin	*	Constricted
Blood pressure	Decreased	Increased
Respiratory System		
Bronchioles	Constricted	Dilated
Rate of breathing	Decreased	Increased
Digestive System		
Peristaltic movements of digestive tube	Increased	Decreased
Muscular sphincters of digestive tube	Relaxed	Contracted
Secretion of salivary glands	Thin, watery saliva	Thick, viscid saliva
Secretions of stomach, intestine, and pancreas	Increased	*
Conversion of liver glycogen to glucose	*	Increased
Genitourinary System		
Urinary bladder		
Muscle walls	Contracted	Relaxed
Sphincters	Relaxed	Contracted
Muscles of the uterus	Relaxed; variable	Contracted under some conditions; varies with menstrual cycle and pregnancy
Blood vessels of external genitalia	Dilated	*
Integumentary System		
Secretion of sweat	*	Increased
Pilomotor muscles	*	Contracted (goose-flesh)
Adrenal Medulla	*	Secretion of epinephrine and norepinephrine

*No direct effect.

From Hickey, J. (2009). *Clinical practice of neurological and neurosurgical nursing* (6th ed.). Philadelphia: Lippincott Williams & Wilkins.

(eg, the cardiac, pulmonary, splanchnic, and pelvic plexuses) supply structures in the head and neck, thorax, abdomen, and pelvis, respectively, having been joined in these plexuses by fibers from the parasympathetic division.

The adrenal glands, kidneys, liver, spleen, stomach, and duodenum are under the control of the giant celiac plexus, commonly known as the solar plexus. This receives its sympathetic nerve components by way of the three splanchnic nerves, composed of preganglionic fibers from nine segments of the spinal cord (T4 to L1), and is joined by the vagus nerve, representing the parasympathetic division. From the celiac plexus, fibers of both divisions travel along the course of blood vessels to their target organs.

Sympathetic Syndromes. Certain syndromes are distinctive to diseases of the sympathetic nerve trunks. For example, sympathetic storm is a syndrome associated with changes in level of consciousness, altered vital signs, diaphoresis, and agitation that may result from hypothalamic stimulation of the sympathetic nervous system following traumatic brain injury (Diepenbrock, 2007).

Parasympathetic Nervous System

The parasympathetic nervous system functions as the dominant controller for most visceral effectors; the primary neurotransmitter is acetylcholine. During quiet, nonstressful conditions, impulses from parasympathetic fibers (cholinergic) predominate. The fibers of the parasympathetic system are located in two sections, one in the brain stem and the other from spinal segments below L2. Because of the location of these fibers, the parasympathetic system is referred to as the craniosacral division, as distinct from the thoracolumbar (sympathetic) division of the autonomic nervous system.

The parasympathetic nerves arise from the midbrain and the medulla oblongata. Fibers from cells in the midbrain travel with the third oculomotor nerve to the ciliary ganglia, where postganglionic fibers of this division are joined by those of the sympathetic system, creating controlled opposition, with a delicate balance maintained between the two at all times.

Motor and Sensory Pathways of the Nervous System

Motor Pathways

The corticospinal tract begins in the motor cortex, a vertical band within each frontal lobe, and controls voluntary movements of the body. The exact locations within the brain at which the voluntary movements of the muscles of the face, thumb, hand, arm, trunk, and leg originate are known (Fig. 60-11). To initiate movement, these particular cells must send the stimulus along their fibers. Stimulation of these cells with an electric current also results in muscle contraction. En route to the pons, the motor fibers converge into a tight bundle known as the internal capsule. A comparatively small injury to the internal capsule results in a more severe paralysis than does a larger injury to the cortex itself.

At the medulla, the corticospinal tracts cross to the opposite side, continuing to the anterior horn of the spinal cord, in proximity to a motor nerve cell. Until this point, neurons are known as upper motor neurons. As they connect to motor fibers of the spinal nerves, they become lower motor neurons. The lower motor neurons receive the impulse in the posterior part of the cord and run to the myoneural junction located in the peripheral muscle.

Involuntary motor activity is also possible and is mediated through reflex arcs. Synaptic connections between anterior horn cells and sensory fibers that have entered adjacent or neighboring segments of the spinal cord serve as protective mechanisms. These connections are seen during deep tendon reflex testing.

Upper and Lower Motor Neurons

The voluntary motor system consists of two groups of neurons: upper motor neurons and lower motor neurons. Upper motor neurons originate in the cerebral cortex, the cerebellum, and the brain stem. Their fibers make up the descending motor pathways, are located entirely within the CNS,

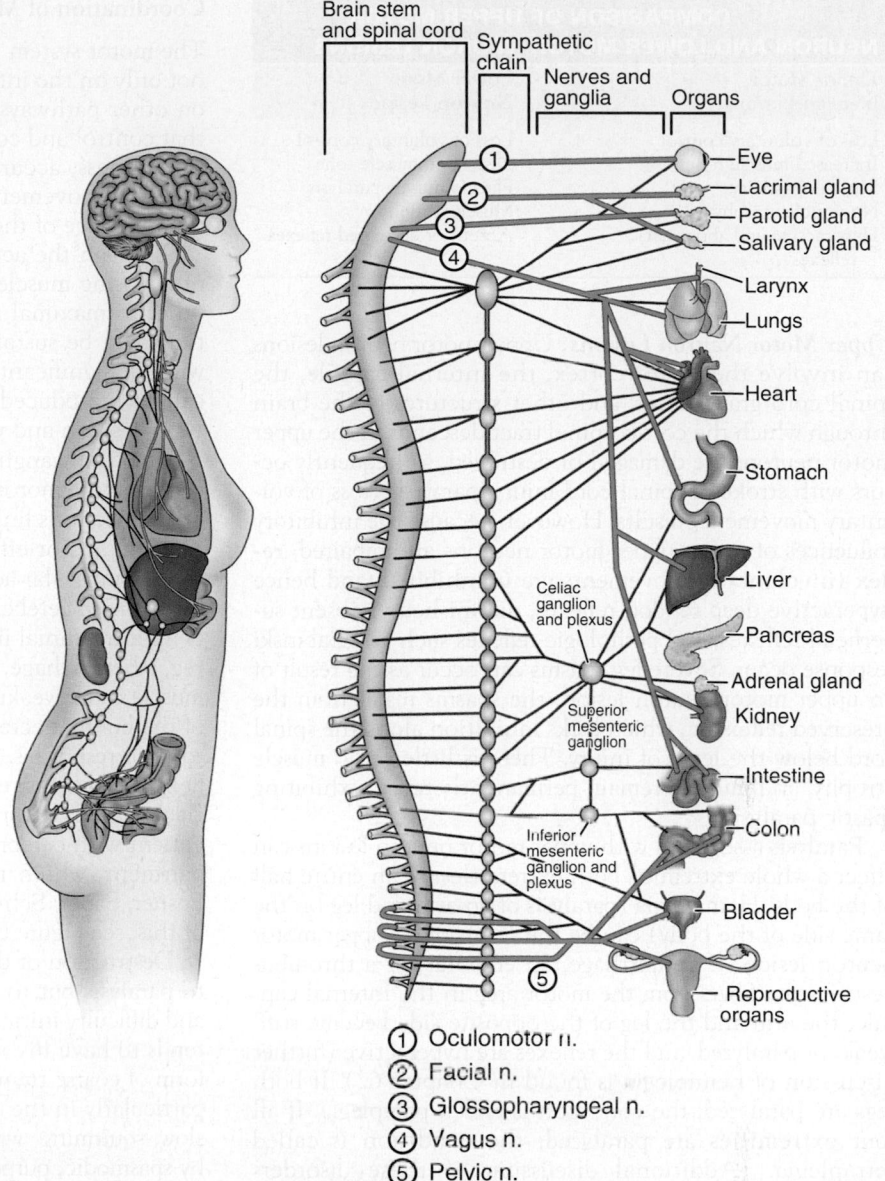

Figure 60-10 Anatomy of the autonomic nervous system.

① Oculomotor n.
② Facial n.
③ Glossopharyngeal n.
④ Vagus n.
⑤ Pelvic n.

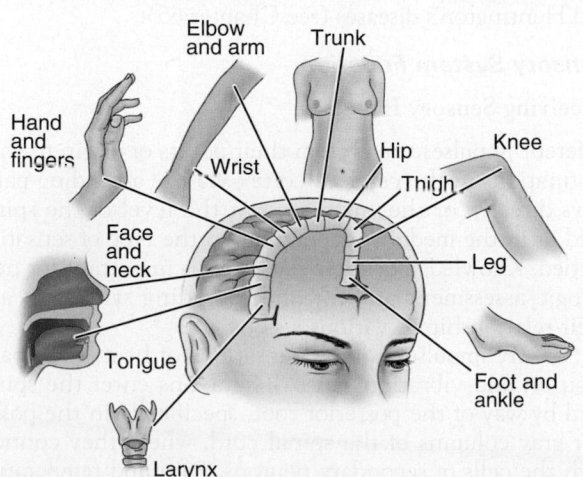

Figure 60-11 Diagrammatic representation of the cerebrum showing locations for control of motor movement of various parts of the body.

and modulate the activity of the lower motor neurons. Lower motor neurons are located either in the anterior horn of the spinal cord gray matter or within cranial nerve nuclei in the brain stem. Axons of lower motor neurons in both sites extend through peripheral nerves and terminate in skeletal muscle. Lower motor neurons are located in both the CNS and the peripheral nervous system.

The motor pathways from the brain to the spinal cord, as well as from the cerebrum to the brain stem, are formed by upper motor neurons. They begin in the cortex of one side of the brain, descend through the internal capsule, cross to the opposite side in the brain stem, descend through the corticospinal tract, and synapse with the lower motor neurons in the cord. The lower motor neurons receive the impulse in the posterior part of the cord and run to the myoneural junction located in the peripheral muscle. The clinical features of lesions of upper and lower motor neurons are discussed in the following sections and in Table 60-4.

Table 60-4 COMPARISON OF UPPER MOTOR NEURON AND LOWER MOTOR NEURON LESIONS	
Upper Motor Neuron Lesions	**Lower Motor Neuron Lesions**
Loss of voluntary control	Loss of voluntary control
Increased muscle tone	Decreased muscle tone
Muscle spasticity	Flaccid muscle paralysis
No muscle atrophy	Muscle atrophy
Hyperactive and abnormal reflexes	Absent or decreased reflexes

Upper Motor Neuron Lesions. Upper motor neuron lesions can involve the motor cortex, the internal capsule, the spinal cord gray matter, and other structures of the brain through which the corticospinal tract descends. If the upper motor neurons are damaged or destroyed, as frequently occurs with stroke or spinal cord injury, paralysis (loss of voluntary movement) results. However, because the inhibitory influences of intact upper motor neurons are impaired, **reflex** (involuntary) movements are uninhibited, and hence hyperactive deep tendon reflexes, diminished or absent superficial reflexes, and pathologic reflexes such as a Babinski response occur. Severe leg spasms can occur as the result of an upper motor neuron lesion; the spasms result from the preserved reflex arc, which lacks inhibition along the spinal cord below the level of injury. There is little or no muscle atrophy, and muscles remain permanently tense, exhibiting spastic paralysis.

Paralysis associated with upper motor neuron lesions can affect a whole extremity, both extremities, or an entire half of the body. Hemiplegia (paralysis of an arm and leg on the same side of the body) can be the result of an upper motor neuron lesion. If hemorrhage, an embolus, or a thrombus destroys the fibers from the motor area in the internal capsule, the arm and the leg of the opposite side become stiff, weak, or paralyzed, and the reflexes are hyperactive (further discussion of hemiplegia is found in Chapter 62). If both legs are paralyzed, the condition is called paraplegia. If all four extremities are paralyzed, the condition is called tetraplegia. (Additional discussion of these disorders appears in Chapter 63.)

Lower Motor Neuron Lesions. A patient is considered to have lower motor neuron damage if a motor nerve is damaged between the spinal cord and muscle. The result of lower motor neuron damage is muscle paralysis. Reflexes are lost, and the muscle becomes flaccid (limp) and atrophied from disuse. If the patient has injured the spinal trunk and it can heal, use of the muscles connected to that section of the spinal cord may be regained. However, if the anterior horn motor cells are destroyed, the nerves cannot regenerate and the muscles are never useful again.

Flaccid paralysis and atrophy of the affected muscles are the principal signs of lower motor neuron disease. Lower motor neuron lesions can be the result of trauma, infection (poliomyelitis), toxins, vascular disorders, congenital malformations, degenerative processes, and neoplasms. Compression of nerve roots by herniated intervertebral disks is a common cause of lower motor neuron dysfunction. The clinical features of lesions of upper and lower motor neurons are discussed in the following sections and in Table 60-4.

Coordination of Movement

The motor system is complex, and motor function depends not only on the integrity of the corticospinal tracts but also on other pathways from the basal ganglia and cerebellum that control and coordinate voluntary motor function. The smoothness, accuracy, and strength that characterize the muscular movements of a normal person are attributable to the influence of the cerebellum and the basal ganglia.

Through the action of the cerebellum, the contractions of opposing muscle groups are adjusted in relation to each other to maximal mechanical advantage; muscle contractions can be sustained evenly at the desired tension and without significant fluctuation, and reciprocal movements can be reproduced at high and constant speed, in stereotyped fashion and with relatively little effort.

The basal ganglia play an important role in planning and coordinating motor movements and posture. Complex neural connections link the basal ganglia with the cerebral cortex. The major effect of these structures is to inhibit unwanted muscular activity.

Impaired cerebellar function, which may occur as a result of an intracranial injury or some type of an expanding mass (eg, a hemorrhage, an abscess, or a tumor), results in loss of muscle tone, weakness, and fatigue. Depending on the area of the brain affected, the patient has different motor symptoms or responses. The patient may demonstrate abnormal flexion, abnormal extension, or flaccid posturing. **Flaccidity** (lack of muscle tone) preceded by abnormal posturing in a patient with cerebral injury indicates severe neurologic impairment, which may herald brain death (Peiffer, 2007; Posner, Saper, Schiff, et al., 2007). For further explanation of this, see Figure 61-1 in Chapter 61.

Destruction or dysfunction of the basal ganglia leads not to paralysis but to muscle rigidity, disturbances of posture, and difficulty initiating or changing movement. The patient tends to have involuntary movements. These may take the form of coarse tremors, most often in the upper extremities, particularly in the distal portions; athetosis, movement of a slow, squirming, writhing, twisting type; or chorea, marked by spasmodic, purposeless, irregular, uncoordinated motions of the trunk and the extremities, and facial grimacing. Disorders affecting basal ganglia activity include Parkinson's and Huntington's diseases (see Chapter 65).

Sensory System Function

Receiving Sensory Impulses

Afferent impulses travel from their points of origin to their destinations in the cerebral cortex via the ascending pathways directly, or they may cross at the level of the spinal cord or in the medulla, depending on the type of sensation carried. Knowledge of these pathways is important for neurologic assessment and for understanding symptoms and their relationship to various lesions.

Sensory impulses convey sensations of heat, cold, pain, position and vibration sense. The axons enter the spinal cord by way of the posterior root, specifically in the posterior gray columns of the spinal cord, where they connect with the cells of secondary neurons. Pain and temperature fibers (located in the spinothalamic tract) cross immediately to the opposite side of the cord and course upward to the thalamus. Fibers carrying sensations of touch, light pressure, and localization do not connect immediately with the second neuron but ascend the cord for a variable distance before entering the gray matter and completing this connection. The axon of the secondary neuron traverses the cord, crosses in the medulla, and proceeds upward to the thalamus.

Position and vibratory sensations are produced by stimuli arising from muscles, joints, and bones. These stimuli are conveyed, uncrossed, all the way to the brain stem by the axon of the primary neuron. In the medulla, synaptic connections are made with cells of the secondary neurons, whose axons cross to the opposite side and then proceed to the thalamus.

Integrating Sensory Impulses

The thalamus integrates all sensory impulses except olfaction. It plays a role in the conscious awareness of pain and the recognition of variation in temperature and touch. The thalamus is responsible for the sense of movement and position as well as the ability to recognize the size, shape, and quality of objects. Sensory information is relayed from the thalamus to the parietal lobe for interpretation.

Sensory Losses

Destruction of a sensory nerve results in total loss of sensation in its area of distribution (see Fig. 60-9). Lesions affecting the posterior spinal nerve roots may cause impairment of tactile sensation, including intermittent severe pain that is referred to their areas of distribution. Destruction of the spinal cord yields complete anesthesia below the level of injury. Selective destruction or degeneration of the posterior columns of the spinal cord is responsible for a loss of position and vibratory sense in segments distal to the lesion, without loss of touch, pain, or temperature perception. A cyst in the center of the spinal cord causes dissociation of sensation—loss of pain at the level of the lesion. This occurs because the fibers carrying pain and temperature cross within the cord immediately on entering; thus, any lesion that divides the cord longitudinally divides these fibers. Other sensory fibers ascend the cord for variable distances, some even to the medulla, before crossing, thereby bypassing the lesion and avoiding destruction. Lesions in the thalamus or parietal lobe result in impaired touch, pain, temperature, and proprioceptive sensations.

Assessment of the Nervous System

Health History

An important aspect of the neurologic assessment is the history of the present illness. The initial interview provides an excellent opportunity to systematically explore the patient's current condition and related events while simultaneously observing overall appearance, mental status, posture, movement, and affect. Depending on the patient's condition, the nurse may need to rely on yes-or-no answers to questions, a review of the medical record, input from witnesses or the family, or a combination of these.

Neurologic disease may be stable or progressive, characterized by symptom-free periods as well as fluctuations in symptoms. The health history therefore includes details about the onset, character, severity, location, duration, and frequency of symptoms and signs; associated complaints; precipitating, aggravating, and relieving factors; progression, remission, and exacerbation; and the presence or absence of similar symptoms among family members.

Common Symptoms

The symptoms of neurologic disorders are as varied as the disease processes themselves. Symptoms may be subtle or intense, fluctuating or permanent, inconvenient or devastating. This chapter discusses the most common signs and symptoms associated with neurologic disease; the relationship of specific signs and symptoms to a particular disorder is presented in later chapters in this unit.

Pain

Pain is considered an unpleasant sensory perception and emotional experience associated with actual or potential tissue damage or described in terms of such damage. Pain is therefore considered multidimensional and entirely subjective. Pain can be acute or chronic. In general, acute pain lasts for a relatively short period of time and remits as the pathology resolves. In neurologic disease, acute pain may be associated with brain hemorrhage, spinal disk disease (Jarvis, 2007), or trigeminal neuralgia. In contrast, chronic or persistent pain extends for long periods of time and may represent a broader pathology. This type of pain can occur with many degenerative and chronic neurologic conditions (eg, multiple sclerosis). See Chapter 13 for a more detailed discussion of pain.

Seizures

Seizures are the result of abnormal paroxysmal discharges in the cerebral cortex, which then manifest as an alteration in sensation, behavior, movement, perception, or consciousness. The alteration may be short, such as in a blank stare that lasts only a second, or of longer duration, such as a tonic–clonic grand mal seizure that can last several minutes. The seizure activity reflects the area of the brain affected. Seizures can occur as isolated events, such as when induced by a high fever, alcohol or drug withdrawal, or hypoglycemia. A seizure may also be the first obvious sign of a brain lesion (Hickey, 2009).

Dizziness and Vertigo

Dizziness is an abnormal sensation of imbalance or movement. It is fairly common in the elderly and one of the most common complaints encountered by health professionals (Jarvis, 2007). Dizziness can have a variety of causes, including viral syndromes, hot weather, roller coaster rides, and middle ear infections, to name a few. One difficulty confronting health care providers when assessing dizziness is the vague and varied terms patients use to describe the sensation.

About 50% of all patients with dizziness have **vertigo,** which is defined as an illusion of movement, usually rotation (Jarvis, 2007). Vertigo is usually a manifestation of vestibular dysfunction. It can be so severe as to result in spatial disorientation, lightheadedness, loss of equilibrium (staggering), and nausea and vomiting.

Visual Disturbances

Visual defects that cause people to seek health care can range from the decreased visual acuity associated with aging to sudden blindness caused by glaucoma. Normal vision depends on functioning visual pathways through the retina and optic chiasm and the radiations into the visual cortex in the occipital lobes. Lesions of the eye itself (eg, cataract), lesions along the pathway (eg, tumor), or lesions in the visual cortex (eg, stroke) interfere with normal visual acuity. Abnormalities of eye movement (as in the nystagmus associated with multiple sclerosis) can also compromise vision by causing diplopia or double vision. See Chapter 58 for a more detailed discussion of disorders that affect vision.

Muscle Weakness

Muscle weakness is a common manifestation of neurologic disease. It frequently coexists with other symptoms of disease and can affect a variety of muscles, causing a wide range of disability. Weakness can be sudden and permanent, as in stroke, or progressive, as in neuromuscular diseases such as amyotrophic lateral sclerosis. Any muscle group can be affected.

Abnormal Sensation

Abnormal sensation is a neurologic manifestation of both central and peripheral nervous system disease. Altered sensation can affect small or large areas of the body. It is frequently associated with weakness or pain and is potentially disabling. Lack of sensation places a person at risk for falls and injury.

Past Health, Family, and Social History

The nurse may inquire about any family history of genetic diseases (Chart 60-1). A review of the medical history, including a system-by-system evaluation, is part of the health history. The nurse should be aware of any history of trauma or falls that may have involved the head or spinal cord. Questions regarding the use of alcohol, medications, and illicit drugs are also relevant. The history-taking portion of the neurologic assessment is critical and, in many cases of neurologic disease, leads to an accurate diagnosis.

Physical Assessment

The neurologic examination is a systematic process that includes a variety of clinical tests, observations, and assessments designed to evaluate the neurologic status of a complex system. Many neurologic rating scales exist (Herndon, 2006), and some of the more common ones are discussed in this chapter.

The brain and spinal cord cannot be examined as directly as other systems of the body. Thus, much of the neurologic examination is an indirect evaluation that assesses

---

CHART 60-1 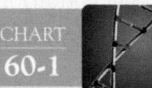 **GENETICS IN NURSING PRACTICE**
Neurologic Disorders

Diseases and Conditions Influenced by Genetic Factors

- Alzheimer's disease
- Amyotrophic lateral sclerosis (ALS)
- Duchenne muscular dystrophy
- Epilepsy
- Friedrich ataxia
- Huntington disease
- Myotonic dystrophy
- Neurofibromatosis type I
- Parkinson's disease
- Spina bifida
- Tourette syndrome

Nursing Assessments

Family History Assessment

- Assess for other similarly affected relatives with neurologic impairment.
- Inquire about age of onset (eg, present at birth—spina bifida; developed in childhood—Duchenne muscular dystrophy; developed in adulthood—Huntington disease, Alzheimer's disease, amyotrophic lateral sclerosis).
- Inquire about the presence of related conditions such as mental retardation and/or learning disabilities (neurofibromatosis type I).

Patient Assessment

- Assess for the presence of other physical features suggestive of an underlying genetic condition, such as skin lesions seen in neurofibromatosis type 1 (café-au-lait spots).
- Assess for other congenital abnormalities (eg, cardiac, ocular).

Management Specific to Genetics

- Inquire whether DNA mutation or other genetic testing has been performed on affected family members.
- If indicated, refer for further genetic counseling and evaluation so that family members can discuss inheritance, risk to other family members, availability of genetic testing, and gene-based interventions.
- Offer appropriate genetic information and resources.
- Assess patient's understanding of genetic information.
- Provide support to families with newly diagnosed genetic-related neurologic disorders.
- Participate in management and coordination of care of patients with genetic conditions and individuals predisposed to develop or pass on a genetic condition.

Genetics Resources for Nurses and Their Patients on the Web

Genetic Alliance—a directory of support groups for patients and families with genetic conditions, www.geneticalliance.org

Gene Clinics—a listing of common genetic disorders with up-to-date clinical summaries, genetic counseling, and testing information, www.geneclinics.org

National Organization of Rare Disorders—a directory of support groups and information for patients and families with rare genetic disorders, www.rarediseases.org

OMIM: Online Mendelian Inheritance in Man—a complete listing of inherited genetic conditions, www.nchi.nlm.nih.gov/omim/stats/html

the function of the specific body part or parts controlled by the nervous system. A neurologic assessment is divided into five components: consciousness and cognition, cranial nerves, motor system, sensory system, and reflexes. One or more components may become the priority assessment, depending on the patient's condition. For example, motor, sensory, and reflex assessments are the priority in patients with spinal injury, while in a comatose patient, the cranial nerves and level of consciousness become the priority.

Assessing Consciousness and Cognition

Cerebral abnormalities may cause disturbances in mental status, intellectual functioning, thought content, and emotional status. There may also be alterations in language abilities, as well as lifestyle. The examiner must also be aware of the patient's overall level of consciousness and any changes over time (Posner, et al., 2007).

The examiner records and reports specific observations regarding mental status, intellectual function, thought content, and emotional status, all of which permit comparison by others over time. Alterations should be described in specific and nonjudgmental terms. Use of terms such as "inappropriate" or "demented" are avoided as they often mean different things to different people and are therefore not useful when describing behavior. Analysis and the conclusions that may be drawn from these findings usually depend on the examiner's knowledge of neuroanatomy, neurophysiology, and neuropathology.

Mental Status

An assessment of mental status begins by observing the patient's appearance and behavior, noting dress, grooming, and personal hygiene. Posture, gestures, movements, and facial expressions often provide important information about the patient. Does the patient appear to be aware of and interact with the surroundings?

Assessing orientation to time, place, and person assists in evaluating mental status. Does the patient know what day it is, what year it is, and the name of the president of the United States? Is the patient aware of where he or she is? Is the patient aware of who the examiner is and of his or her purpose for being in the room? Assessment of immediate and remote memory is also important. Is the capacity for immediate memory intact? (See Chapter 12.)

Intellectual Function

A person with an average IQ can repeat seven digits without faltering and can recite five digits backward. The examiner might ask the patient to count backward from 100 or to subtract 7 from 100, then 7 from that, and so forth (called serial 7s). The capacity to interpret well-known proverbs tests abstract reasoning, which is a higher intellectual function; for example, does the patient know what is meant by "a stitch in time saves nine"? The intellectual function of patients with damage to the frontal cortex appears intact until one or more tests of intellectual capacity are performed. Questions designed to assess this capacity might include the ability to recognize similarities: for example, how are a mouse and dog or pen and pencil alike? Can the patient make judgments about situations: for example, if the patient arrived home without a house key, what alternatives are there?

Thought Content

During the interview, it is important to assess the patient's thought content. Are the patient's thoughts spontaneous, natural, clear, relevant, and coherent? Does the patient have any fixed ideas, illusions, or preoccupations? What are his or her insights into these thoughts? Preoccupation with death or morbid events, hallucinations, and paranoid ideation are examples of unusual thoughts or perceptions that require further evaluation.

Emotional Status

An assessment of consciousness and cognition also includes the patient's emotional status. Is the patient's affect (external manifestation of mood) natural and even, or irritable and angry, anxious, apathetic or flat, or euphoric? Does his or her mood fluctuate normally, or does the patient unpredictably swing from joy to sadness during the interview? Is affect appropriate to words and thought content? Are verbal communications consistent with nonverbal cues?

Language Ability

The person with normal neurologic function can understand and communicate in spoken and written language. Does the patient answer questions appropriately? Can he or she read a sentence from a newspaper and explain its meaning? Can the patient write his or her name or copy a simple figure that the examiner has drawn? A deficiency in language function is called aphasia. Different types of aphasia result from injury to different parts of the brain (Table 60-5). Aphasia is discussed in detail in Chapter 62.

Impact on Lifestyle

The nurse assesses the impact any impairment has on the patient's lifestyle. Issues to consider include the limitations imposed on the patient by any cognitive deficit and the patient's role in society, including family and community roles. The plan of care that the nurse develops needs to address and support adaptation to the neurologic deficit and continued function to the extent possible within the patient's support system.

Level of Consciousness

Consciousness is the patient's wakefulness and ability to respond to the environment. Level of consciousness is the most sensitive indicator of neurologic function. To assess level of consciousness, the examiner observes for alertness and ability to follow commands.

If the patient is not alert or able to follow commands, the examiner observes for eye opening; verbal response and motor response to stimuli, if any; and the type of stimuli needed to obtain a response. Noxious stimuli should be used first, then painful stimuli if no response is observed. In the

Table 60-5	TYPES OF APHASIA AND REGION OF BRAIN INVOLVED
Type of Aphasia	**Brain Area Involved**
Auditory-receptive	Temporal lobe
Visual-receptive	Parietal-occipital area
Expressive speaking	Inferior posterior frontal areas
Expressive writing	Posterior frontal area

CHART 60-2	NURSING RESEARCH PROFILE
	Early Identification of Vasospasm Following Subarachnoid Hemorrhage

Doerksen, K. & Naimark, B. (2006). Nonspecific behaviors as early indicators of cerebral vasospasm. *Journal of Neuroscience Nursing, 38*(6), 409–415.

Purpose

The significance of behavioral changes seen early after subarachnoid hemorrhage is not understood. The purpose of this study was to delineate nonspecific behaviors seen after subarachnoid hemorrhage and to determine the prevalence of those behaviors in patients with vasospasm (a complication of subarachnoid hemorrhage). If significant, such behaviors may be better early predictors of problems as compared to other assessment findings.

Design

This prospective study evaluated nursing documentation of nonspecific behaviors during the acute phase of care of 60 patients (39 female and 21 male) with subarachnoid hemorrhage. After record reviews, behavioral descriptors were quantified. The prevalence of the behavioral descriptors was determined in the 31 patients who developed vasospasm and compared to those who did not develop vasospasm.

Findings

Twenty-four of the 31 patients who developed vasospasm demonstrated nonspecific behaviors prior to development of the traditional signs and symptoms of vasospasm (decreased level of consciousness, focal deficits, or aphasia). The three primary nonspecific behaviors were acting restless, impulsive, or strange.

Nursing Implications

More research is needed but this study illustrates that nursing assessment can reveal nonspecific behaviors that are useful in the early identification of vasospasm after subarachnoid hemorrhage. Use of earlier identification may result in earlier intervention and prevention of brain ischemia.

---

patient with decreased level of consciousness, motor and cranial nerve function become the priority assessments, as abnormalities can indicate the area of involvement in the absence of responsiveness. Further discussion of changes in level of consciousness is found in Chapter 61. See Chart 60-2.

Examining the Cranial Nerves

Cranial nerves are assessed when level of consciousness is decreased, with brain stem pathology, or in the presence of peripheral nervous system disease. Chart 60-3 describes assessment of the cranial nerves and significant findings. Right and left cranial nerve functions are compared throughout the examination.

Examining the Motor System

Motor Ability

A thorough examination of the motor system includes an assessment of muscle size and tone as well as strength, coordination, and balance. The patient is instructed to walk across the room, if possible, while the examiner observes posture and gait. The muscles are inspected, and palpated if necessary, for their size and symmetry. Any evidence of atrophy or involuntary movements (tremors, tics) is noted. Muscle tone (the tension present in a muscle at rest) is evaluated by palpating various muscle groups at rest and during passive movement. Resistance to these movements is assessed and documented. Abnormalities in tone include **spasticity** (increased muscle tone), **rigidity** (resistance to passive stretch), and **flaccidity**.

Muscle Strength

Assessing the patient's ability to flex or extend the extremities against resistance tests muscle strength. The function of an individual muscle or group of muscles is evaluated by placing the muscle at a disadvantage. The quadriceps, for example, is a powerful muscle responsible for straightening the leg. Once the leg is straightened, it is exceedingly diffi-cult for the examiner to flex the knee. If the knee is flexed and the patient is asked to straighten the leg against resistance, weakness can be elicited. The evaluation of muscle strength compares the sides of the body to each other. For example, the right upper extremity is compared to the left upper extremity. Subtle differences in strength may be evaluated by testing for drift. For example, both arms are out in front of the patient with palms up; drift is seen as pronation of the palm, indicating a subtle weakness that may not have been detected on the resistance examination.

Clinicians use a 5-point scale to rate muscle strength. A 5 indicates full power of contraction against gravity and resistance or normal muscle strength; 4 indicates fair but not full strength against gravity and a moderate amount of resistance or slight weakness; 3 indicates just sufficient strength to overcome the force of gravity or moderate weakness; 2 indicates the ability to move but not to overcome the force of gravity or severe weakness; 1 indicates minimal contractile power (weak muscle contraction can be palpated but no movement is noted) or very severe weakness; and 0 indicates no movement (Jarvis, 2007). A stick figure may be used to record muscle strength and is a precise form of documenting findings. Distal and proximal strength in both upper and lower extremities is recorded using the 5-point scale (Fig. 60-12).

Assessment of muscle strength may be as detailed as necessary. One may quickly test the strength of the proximal muscles of the upper and lower extremities, always comparing both sides. The strength of the finer muscles that control the function of the hand (hand grasp) and the foot (dorsiflexion and plantar flexion) can then be assessed.

Balance and Coordination

Cerebellar and basal ganglia influence on the motor system is reflected in balance control and coordination. Coordination in the hands and upper extremities is tested by having the patient perform rapid, alternating movements and

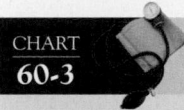

CHART 60-3   Guidelines for Assessing Cranial Nerve Function

Equipment

- Tongue depressor
- Flashlight
- Sugar and salt samples
- Watch
- Cotton-tipped swab
- Snellen chart
- Ophthalmoscope
- Samples of familiar odors
- Tuning fork

Implementation

Step	Rationale
1. Assess cranial nerve (CN) I (olfactory). With eyes closed, patient is asked to identify familiar odors (coffee, tobacco). Each nostril is tested separately.	The significant finding is loss of sense of smell (anosmia).
2. Assess CN II (optic). Assess vision using a Snellen eye chart. Assess visual fields. Perform ophthalmoscopic examination.	Significant findings include visual field defects (hemianopias) and decreased visual acuity or blindness.
3. Assess CN III (oculomotor). Test for eye movement toward the nose; inspect for conjugate movements and nystagmus. Evaluate papillary size and test for pupillary reactivity to light; inspect ability to open eyelids.	Significant findings include dysconjugate gaze; gaze weakness or paralysis; double vision; dilated pupil, with or without impaired pupillary reaction to light; and inability to open the affected eyelid.
4. Assess CN IV (trochlear). Test for upward eye movement; inspect for conjugate movements and nystagmus.	Significant findings include dysconjugate gaze, gaze weakness or paralysis, and double vision.
5. Assess CN V (trigeminal). Have patient close the eyes. Touch cotton to forehead, cheeks, and jaw. Sensitivity to superficial pain is tested in these same three areas by using the sharp and dull ends of a broken tongue blade. Alternate between the sharp point and the dull end. Patient reports "sharp" or "dull" with each movement. If responses are incorrect, test for temperature sensation. Test tubes of cold and hot water are used alternately. While patient looks up, *lightly* touch a wisp of cotton against the temporal surface of each cornea. A blink and tearing are normal responses. Have patient clench and move the jaw from side to side. Palpate the masseter and temporal muscles, noting strength and equality.	Significant findings include impaired or absent corneal reflex, facial numbness, and jaw weakness.
6. Assess CN VI (abducens). Test for lateral eye movement; inspect for conjugate movement.	Significant findings include dysconjugate gaze, gaze weakness or paralysis, and double vision.
7. Assess CN VII (facial). Observe for symmetry while patient performs facial movements: smiles, whistles, elevates eyebrows, frowns, tightly closes eyelids against resistance (examiner attempts to open them). Observe face for flaccid paralysis (shallow nasolabial folds). Have patient extend tongue. Test ability to discriminate between sugar and salt.	Significant findings include facial weakness, inability to completely close the eyelid, and impaired taste.
8. Assess CN VIII (acoustic). Perform whisper or watch-tick test. Test for lateralization (Weber test). Test for air and bone conduction (Rinne test). Assess standing balance with eyes closed (Romberg test).	Significant findings include decreased hearing or deafness and impaired balance.
9. Assess CN IX (glossopharyngeal). Assess patient's ability to swallow and discriminate between sugar and salt on posterior third of the tongue.	Significant findings include difficulty swallowing (dysphagia) and impaired taste.
10. Assess CN X (vagus). Depress a tongue blade on posterior tongue, or stimulate posterior pharynx to elicit gag reflex. Note any hoarseness in voice. Check ability to swallow. Have patient say "ah." Observe for symmetric rise of uvula and soft palate.	Significant findings include weak or absent gag reflex, difficulty swallowing, aspiration, hoarseness, and slurred speech (dysarthria).

Continued on following page

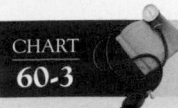

CHART 60-3 — Guidelines for Assessing Cranial Nerve Function (Continued)

11. Assess CN XI (spinal accessory). While patient shrugs shoulders against resistance, palpate and note strength of trapezius muscles. As patient turns head against opposing pressure of the examiner's hand, palpate and note strength of each sternocleidomastoid muscle.

Significant findings include weak or absent shoulder shrug and inability to turn the head to the side.

12. Assess CN XII (hypoglossal). While patient protrudes the tongue, note any deviation or tremors. Test the strength of the tongue by having patient move the protruded tongue from side to side against a tongue depressor.

Significant findings include difficulty swallowing and slurred speech.

point-to-point testing. First, the patient is instructed to pat his or her thigh as fast as possible with each hand separately. Then the patient is instructed to alternately pronate and supinate the hand as rapidly as possible. Last, the patient is asked to touch each of the fingers with the thumb in a consecutive motion. Speed, symmetry, and degree of difficulty are noted. Point-to-point testing is accomplished by having the patient touch the examiner's extended finger and then his or her own nose. This is repeated several times.

Coordination in the lower extremities is tested by having the patient run the heel down the anterior surface of the tibia of the other leg. Each leg is tested in turn. **Ataxia** is defined as incoordination of voluntary muscle action, particularly of the muscle groups used in activities such as walking or reaching for objects. Tremors (rhythmic, involuntary movements) noted at rest or during movement suggest a problem in the anatomic areas responsible for balance and coordination.

The **Romberg test** is a screening test for balance. The patient stands with feet together and arms at the side, first with eyes open and then with both eyes closed for 20 to 30 seconds. The examiner stands close to support the patient if he or she begins to fall. Slight swaying is normal, but a loss of balance is abnormal and is considered a positive Romberg test. Additional cerebellar tests for balance in the ambulatory patient include hopping in place, alternating knee bends, and heel-to-toe walking (both forward and backward).

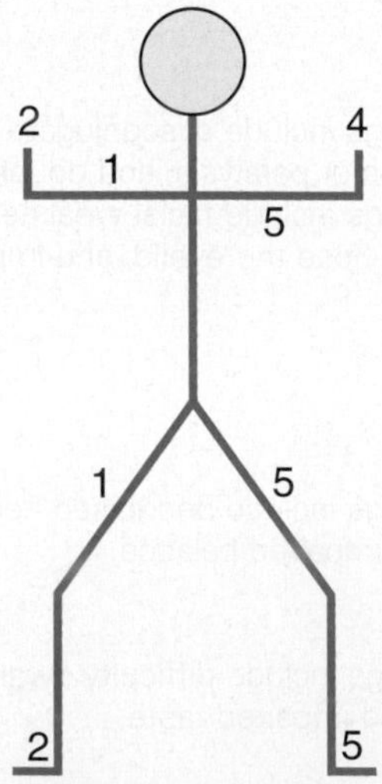

Examining the Sensory System

The sensory system is even more complex than the motor system, because sensory modalities are more widespread throughout the central and peripheral nervous systems. The sensory examination is largely subjective and requires the cooperation of the patient. The examiner should be familiar with dermatomes that represent the distribution of the peripheral nerves that arise from the spinal cord (see Fig. 60-9) (Bickley, 2009; Jarvis, 2007).

Assessment of the sensory system involves tests for tactile sensation, superficial pain, temperature, vibration, and position sense (proprioception). During the sensory assessment, the patient's eyes are closed. Simple directions and reassurance that the examiner will not hurt or startle the patient encourage the cooperation of the patient.

Tactile sensation is assessed by lightly touching a cotton wisp or fingertip to corresponding areas on each side of the body. The sensitivity of proximal parts of the extremities is compared with that of distal parts, and the right and left sides are compared.

Pain and temperature sensations are transmitted together in the lateral part of the spinal cord, so it is unnecessary to test for temperature sense in most circumstances. Determining the patient's sensitivity to a sharp object can assess superficial pain perception. However, pain sensation is usually reserved for patients who do not respond to or cannot discriminate touch stimulation. The patient is asked to differentiate between the sharp and dull ends of a broken wooden cotton swab or tongue blade; using a safety pin is inadvisable because it breaks the integrity of the skin. Both the sharp and dull sides of the object are applied with equal intensity at all times, and the two sides are compared.

Vibration and proprioception are transmitted together in the posterior part of the cord. Vibration may be evaluated through the use of a low-frequency (128- or 256-Hz) tuning fork. The handle of the vibrating fork is placed against a bony prominence, and the patient is asked if he or she feels a sensation and is instructed to signal the examiner when the sensation ceases. Common locations used to test for vibratory sense include the distal joint of the great toe and the

Figure 60-12 A stick figure may be used to record muscle strength as follows: 5, full range of motion against gravity and resistance; 4, full range of motion against gravity and a moderate amount of resistance; 3, full range of motion against gravity only; 2, full range of motion when gravity is eliminated; 1, a weak muscle contraction when muscle is palpated, but no movement; and 0, complete paralysis.

proximal thumb joint. If the patient does not perceive the vibrations at the distal bony prominences, the examiner progresses upward with the tuning fork until the patient perceives the vibrations. As with all measurements of sensation, a side-to-side comparison is made.

Position sense or proprioception may be determined by asking the patient to close both eyes and indicate, as the great toe or index finger is alternately moved up and down, in which direction movement has taken place. Vibration and position sense are often lost together, frequently in circumstances in which all other sensation remains intact.

Integration of sensation in the brain is evaluated by testing two-point discrimination. When the patient is touched with two sharp objects simultaneously, are they perceived as two or as one? If touched simultaneously on opposite sides of the body, the patient should normally report being touched in two places. If only one site is reported, the one not being recognized is said to demonstrate extinction. Another test of higher cortical sensory ability is tactile identification. The patient is instructed to close both eyes and identify an object (eg, key, coin) that is placed in one hand by the examiner; inability to identify an object by touch is known as tactile agnosia or astereognosis. **Agnosia** is the general loss of ability to recognize objects through a particular sensory system. The patient can also be shown a familiar object and asked to identify it by name; inability to identify a visualized object is known as visual agnosia. Each of these dysfunctions implicates a different part of the brain (Table 60-6).

Decreased or absent sensations occur with problems anywhere along the sensory pathway. Sensory deficits resulting from peripheral neuropathy or spinal cord injury follow anatomic dermatomes. Destructive lesions of the brain may affect sensation on an entire side of the body. Stroke affecting a portion of the sensory cortex will produce altered sensory discrimination.

Examining the Reflexes

Reflexes are involuntary contractions of muscles or muscle groups in response to a stimulus. Reflexes are classified as deep tendon, superficial, or pathologic. Testing reflexes enables the examiner to assess involuntary reflex arcs that depend on the presence of afferent stretch receptors, spinal or brain stem synapses, efferent motor fibers, and a variety of modifying influences from higher levels.

Deep Tendon Reflexes

A reflex hammer is used to elicit a deep tendon reflex. The handle of the hammer is held loosely between the thumb and index finger, allowing a full swinging motion. The wrist

Table 60-6	TYPES OF AGNOSIA AND CORRESPONDING SITES OF LESIONS
Type of Agnosia	**Affected Cerebral Area**
Visual	Occipital lobe
Auditory	Temporal lobe (lateral and superior portions)
Tactile	Parietal lobe
Body parts and relationships	Parietal lobe (posteroinferior regions)

motion is similar to that used during percussion. The extremity is positioned so that the tendon is slightly stretched. This requires a sound knowledge of the location of muscles and their tendon attachments. The tendon is then struck briskly (Fig. 60-13), and the response is compared with that on the opposite side of the body. A wide variation in reflex response may be considered normal; however, it is more important that the reflexes be symmetrically equivalent. When the comparison is made, both sides should be equivalently relaxed and each tendon struck with equal force.

Valid findings depend on several factors: proper use of the reflex hammer, proper positioning of the extremity, and a relaxed patient (Bickley, 2007; Jarvis, 2007). If the reflexes are symmetrically diminished or absent, the examiner may use isometric contraction of other muscle groups to increase reflex activity. For example, if lower extremity reflexes are diminished or absent, the patient is instructed to lock the fingers together and pull in opposite directions. Having the patient clench the jaw or press the heels against the floor or examining table may similarly elicit more reliable biceps, triceps, and brachioradialis reflexes.

The absence of reflexes is significant, although ankle jerks (Achilles reflex) may be normally absent in older people. Deep tendon reflex responses are often graded on a scale of 0 to 4+ (Chart 60-4). As stated previously, scale ratings are highly subjective. Findings can be recorded as a fraction, indicating the scale range (eg, 2/4). Some examiners prefer to use the terms *present, absent,* and *diminished* when describing reflexes. As with muscle strength recording, a stick figure may be used to record numerical findings.

Biceps Reflex. The biceps reflex is elicited by striking the biceps tendon over a slightly flexed elbow (see Fig. 60-13A). The examiner supports the forearm with one arm while placing the thumb against the tendon and striking the thumb with the reflex hammer. The normal response is flexion at the elbow and contraction of the biceps.

Triceps Reflex. To elicit a triceps reflex, the patient's arm is flexed at the elbow and positioned in front of the chest. The examiner supports the patient's arm and identifies the triceps tendon by palpating 2.5 to 5 cm (1 to 2 inches) above the elbow. A direct blow on the tendon (see Fig. 60-13B) normally produces contraction of the triceps muscle and extension of the elbow.

Brachioradialis Reflex. With the patient's forearm resting on the lap or across the abdomen, the brachioradialis reflex is assessed. A gentle strike of the hammer 2.5 to 5 cm (1 to 2 inches) above the wrist results in flexion and supination of the forearm (Weber & Kelley, 2007).

Patellar Reflex. The patellar reflex is elicited by striking the patellar tendon just below the patella. The patient may be in a sitting or a lying position. If the patient is supine, the examiner supports the legs to facilitate relaxation of the muscles (see Fig. 60-13C). Contractions of the quadriceps and knee extension are normal responses.

Achilles Reflex. To elicit an Achilles reflex, the foot is dorsiflexed at the ankle and the hammer strikes the stretched Achilles tendon (see Fig. 60-13D). This reflex normally produces plantar flexion. If the examiner cannot

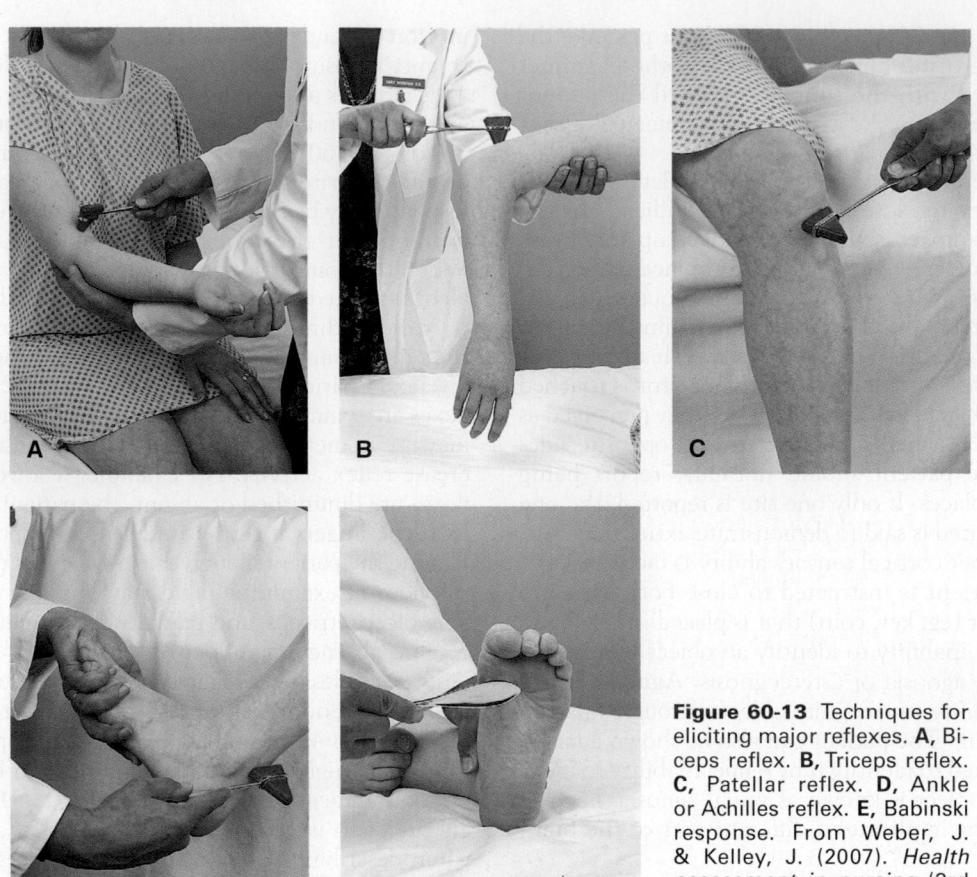

Figure 60-13 Techniques for eliciting major reflexes. **A,** Biceps reflex. **B,** Triceps reflex. **C,** Patellar reflex. **D,** Ankle or Achilles reflex. **E,** Babinski response. From Weber, J. & Kelley, J. (2007). *Health assessment in nursing* (3rd ed.). Philadelphia: Lippincott Williams & Wilkins. © B. Proud.

elicit the ankle reflex and suspects that the patient cannot relax, the patient is instructed to kneel on a chair or similar elevated, flat surface. This position places the ankles in dorsiflexion and reduces any muscle tension in the gastrocnemius. The Achilles tendons are struck in turn, and plantar flexion is usually demonstrated (Weber & Kelley, 2007).

Clonus. When reflexes are very hyperactive, a phenomenon called **clonus** may be elicited. If the foot is abruptly dorsiflexed, it may continue to "beat" two or three times before it settles into a position of rest. Occasionally with central nervous system disease this activity persists, and the foot does not come to rest while the tendon is being stretched but persists in repetitive activity. The unsustained clonus associated with normal but hyperactive reflexes is not considered pathologic. Sustained clonus always indicates the presence of central nervous system disease and requires further evaluation.

Chart 60-4 • *Documenting Reflexes*

Deep tendon reflexes are graded on a scale of 0 to 4:

0   No response
1+ Diminished (hypoactive)
2+ Normal
3+ Increased (may be interpreted as normal)
4+ Hyperactive (hyperreflexia)

The deep tendon responses and plantar reflexes are commonly recorded on stick figures. The arrow points downward if the plantar response is normal and upward if the response is abnormal.

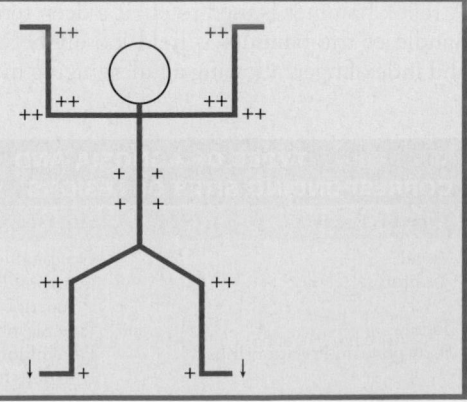

Superficial Reflexes

The major superficial reflexes include corneal, palpebral, gag, upper/lower abdominal, cremasteric (men only), plantar, and perianal. These reflexes are graded differently than the motor reflexes and are noted to be present (+) or absent (−). Of these, only the corneal, gag, and plantar reflexes are tested commonly.

The corneal reflex is tested carefully using a clean wisp of cotton and lightly touching the outer corner of each eye on the sclera. The reflex is present if the action elicits a blink. A stroke or brain injury might result in loss of this reflex, either unilaterally or bilaterally. Loss of this reflex indicates the need for eye protection and possible lubrication to prevent corneal damage.

The gag reflex is elicited by gently touching the back of the pharynx with a cotton-tipped applicator, first on one side of the uvula and then the other. Positive response is an equal elevation of the uvula and "gag" with stimulation. Absent response on one or both sides can be seen following a stroke and requires careful evaluation and treatment of the resultant swallowing dysfunction to prevent aspiration of food and fluids.

The plantar reflex is elicited by stroking the sole of the foot with a tongue blade or the handle of a reflex hammer. Stimulation normally causes toe flexion.

Pathologic Reflexes

Pathologic reflexes are seen in the presence of neurologic disease; they often represent emergence of earlier reflexes that disappeared with maturity of the nervous system. A well-known pathologic reflex indicative of central nervous system disease affecting the corticospinal tract is the **Babinski reflex.** In a person with an intact central nervous system, if the lateral aspect of the sole of the foot is stroked, the toes contract and draw together (see Fig. 60-13E). However, in a person who has central nervous system disease of the motor system, the toes fan out and draw back (Jarvis, 2007; Weber & Kelley, 2007). This is normal in newborns but represents a serious abnormality in adults. Several other pathologic reflexes convey similar information. Although many of them are interesting, they are not particularly informative.

 Gerontologic Considerations

During the normal aging process, the nervous system undergoes many changes, and is more vulnerable to illness. Changes throughout the nervous system that occur with age vary in degree. Nervous system changes due to aging must be distinguished from those due to disease; it is important for clinicians not to attribute abnormality or dysfunction to aging without appropriate investigation (Neal-Boylan, 2007). For example, while diminished strength and agility are a normal part of aging, localized weakness can only be attributed to disease.

Structural and Physiologic Changes

A number of alterations occur with increasing age. A loss of neurons occurs, leading to a decrease in the number of synapses and neurotransmitters. This results in slowed nerve conduction and response time. Brain weight is decreased and the ventricle size increases to maintain cranial volume. Cerebral blood flow and metabolism are reduced, leading to slower mental functions. Temperature regulation becomes less efficient. In the peripheral nervous system, myelin is lost, resulting in a decrease in conduction velocity in some nerves. Visual and auditory nerves degenerate, leading to loss of visual acuity and hearing. Taste buds atrophy and nerve cell fibers in the olfactory bulb degenerate (Jarvis, 2007). Nerve cells in the vestibular system of the inner ear, cerebellum, and proprioceptive pathways also degenerate, leading to balance difficulties. Deep tendon reflexes can be decreased or in some cases absent. Hypothalamic function is modified such that stage IV sleep is reduced. There is an overall slowing of autonomic nervous system responses. Pupillary responses are reduced or may not appear at all in the presence of cataracts.

Motor Alterations

Reduced nerve input into muscle contributes to an overall reduction in muscle bulk, with atrophy most easily noted in the hands. Changes in motor function often result in decreased strength and agility, with increased reaction time. Gait is often slowed and wide based. These changes can create difficulties in maintaining balance, predisposing the older person to falls.

Sensory Alterations

Tactile sensation is dulled in the elderly person due to a decrease in the number of sensory receptors. There may be difficulty in identifying objects by touch, because fewer tactile cues are received from the bottom of the feet and the person may become confused about body position and location (Wickremaratchi & Llewelyn, 2006).

Sensitivity to glare, decreased peripheral vision, and a constricted visual field occur due to degeneration of visual pathways, resulting in disorientation, especially at night when there is little or no light in the room. Because the elderly person takes longer to recover visual sensitivity when moving from a light to dark area, nightlights and a safe and familiar arrangement of furniture are essential.

Loss of hearing can contribute to confusion, anxiety, disorientation, misinterpretation of the environment, feelings of inadequacy, and social isolation. A decreased sense of taste and smell may contribute to weight loss and disinterest in food. A decreased sense of smell may present a safety hazard, because elderly people living alone may be unable to detect household gas leaks or fires. Smoke and carbon monoxide detectors, important for all, are critical for the elderly.

Temperature Regulation and Pain Perception

The elderly patient may feel cold more readily than heat and may require extra covering when in bed; a room temperature somewhat higher than usual may be desirable. Reaction to painful stimuli may be decreased with age. Because pain is an important warning signal, caution must be used when hot or cold packs are used. The older patient may be burned or suffer frostbite before being aware of any discomfort. Complaints of pain, such as abdominal discomfort or chest pain, may be more serious than the patient's perception might indicate and thus require careful evaluation (Neal-Boylan, 2007). Two pain syndromes that are common in the neurologic system in older adults are diabetic neuropathies and postherpetic neuropathies (Bickley, 2007).

Mental Status

Although mental processing time decreases with age, memory, language, and judgment capacities remain intact. Change in mental status should never be assumed to be a normal part of aging. **Delirium** (mental confusion, usually with delusions and hallucinations) is seen in elderly patients who have underlying central nervous system damage or are experiencing an acute condition such as infection, adverse medication reaction, or dehydration. Drug toxicity and depression may produce impairment of attention and memory, and should be evaluated as a possible cause of mental status change. Delirium must be differentiated from dementia, which is a chronic and irreversible deterioration of cognitive status. Chapter 12 contains further discussion of delirium and dementia.

Nursing Implications

Nursing care for patients with age-related changes to the nervous system and for patients with long-term neurologic disability who are aging should include the previously described modifications. In addition, the consequences of any neurologic deficit and its impact on overall function such as activities of daily living, use of assistive devices, and individual coping should be assessed and considered in planning patient care. Fall risk must be evaluated, and fall prevention measures instituted for the hospitalized patient as well as in the home.

The nurse must understand the altered responses and the changing needs of the elderly patient before providing education. Visual and hearing deficits require adaptations in activities such as preoperative teaching, diet therapy, and instruction about new medications. When using visual materials for teaching or menu selection, adequate lighting without glare, contrasting colors, and large print are used to offset visual difficulties caused by rigidity and opacity of the lens in the eye and slower pupillary reaction. Procedures and preparations needed for diagnostic tests are explained, taking into account the possibility of impaired hearing and slowed responses in the elderly. Even with hearing loss, the elderly patient often hears adequately if the speaker uses a low-pitched, clear voice; shouting only makes it harder for the patient to understand the speaker. Providing auditory and visual cues aids understanding; if the patient has a significant hearing or visual loss, assistive devices, a signer, an interpreter, or a translator may be needed.

Teaching at an unrushed pace and using reinforcement enhance learning and retention. Material should be short, concise, and concrete. Vocabulary is matched to the patient's ability, and terms are clearly defined. The elderly patient requires adequate time to receive and respond to stimuli, learn, and react. These measures allow comprehension, memory, and formation of association and concepts.

Diagnostic Evaluation

Computed Tomography Scanning

Computed tomography (CT) scanning uses a narrow x-ray beam to scan body parts in successive layers. The images provide cross-sectional views of the brain, distinguishing differences in tissue densities of the skull, cortex, subcortical structures, and ventricles. An intravenous (IV) contrast agent may be used to highlight differences further. The brightness of each slice of the brain in the final image is proportional to the degree to which it absorbs x-rays. The image is displayed on an oscilloscope or TV monitor and is photographed and stored digitally (Bremner, 2005). CT scanning is usually performed first without contrast material and then with IV contrast, if needed. The patient lies on an adjustable table with the head in a head rest while the scanning system rotates around the head and produces cross-sectional images. The patient must lie with the head held perfectly still without talking or moving the face, because head motion distorts the image. CT scanning is quick and painless and uses a small amount of radiation to produce images; it has a high degree of sensitivity for detecting lesions.

Brain lesions have a different tissue density from the surrounding normal brain tissue. Abnormalities detected on brain CT include tumor or other masses, infarction, hemorrhage, displacement of the ventricles, and cortical atrophy (Bremner, 2005). CT angiography allows visualization of blood vessels; in some situations this eliminates the need for formal angiography. Whole-body CT scanners allow cross-sections of the spinal cord to be visualized. The injection of a water-soluble iodinated contrast agent into the subarachnoid space through lumbar puncture improves the visualization of the spinal and intracranial contents on these images. The CT scan, along with magnetic resonance imaging (MRI), has largely replaced myelography as a diagnostic procedure for the diagnosis of herniated lumbar disks.

Nursing Interventions

Essential nursing interventions include preparation for the procedure and patient monitoring. Preparation includes teaching the patient about the need to lie quietly throughout the procedure. A review of relaxation techniques may be helpful for patients with claustrophobia. Sedation can be used if agitation, restlessness, or confusion interferes with a successful study. Ongoing patient monitoring during sedation is necessary. If a contrast agent is used, the patient must be assessed before the CT scan for an iodine/shellfish allergy, because the contrast agent used may be iodine based. Renal function must also be evaluated, as the contrast material is cleared through the kidneys. A suitable IV line for contrast injection and a period of fasting (usually 4 hours) are required prior to the study. Patients who receive an IV contrast agent are monitored during and after the procedure for allergic reactions and changes in kidney function (Karpoff & Labus, 2008).

Magnetic Resonance Imaging

MRI uses a powerful magnetic field to obtain images of different areas of the body. The magnetic field causes the hydrogen nuclei (protons) within the body to align like small magnets in a magnetic field. In combination with radiofrequency pulses, the protons emit signals, which are converted to images. An MRI scan can be performed with or without a contrast agent and can identify a cerebral abnormality earlier and more clearly than other diagnostic tests (Bremner, 2005). It can provide information about the chemical changes within cells, allowing the clinician to monitor a tumor's response to treatment. It is particularly useful in the diagnosis of brain tumor, stroke, and multiple sclerosis, and does not involve ionizing radiation. A complete MRI scan may take an hour or longer to complete, so use in emergency situations is limited.

Newer MRI applications allow imaging of brain blood flow and metabolism via special imaging techniques added to the MRI. Such techniques include diffusion-weighted imaging (DWI), perfusion-weighted imaging (PWI), magnetic resonance spectroscopy, and fluid attenuation inversion recovery (FLAIR) (Bremner, 2005). Magnetic resonance angiography (MRA) allows separate visualization of the cerebral vasculature without the administration of an arterial contrast agent. Both MRI and CT images are used as tools to plan and direct surgical intervention.

Nursing Interventions

Patient preparation includes teaching and obtaining an adequate history. Ferromagnetic substances in the body may become dislodged by the magnet, so history of working with metal fragments must be reviewed. The patient is questioned about any implants of any metal objects (eg, aneurysm clips, orthopedic hardware, pacemakers, artificial heart valves, intrauterine devices). These objects could malfunction, be dislodged, or heat up as they absorb energy. Cochlear implants will be inactivated by MRI; therefore, other imaging procedures are considered. A complete list of metal compatibility may be found on MRI manufacturers' Web sites contained in the resource section at the end of the chapter.

Before the patient enters the room where the MRI is to be performed, all metal objects and credit cards (the magnetic field can erase them) must be removed. This includes medication patches that have a metal backing and metallic lead wires; these can cause burns if not removed (Bremner, 2005). No metal objects may be brought into the room where the MRI is located; this includes oxygen tanks, IV poles, ventilators, or even stethoscopes. The magnetic field generated by the unit is so strong that any metal-containing items will be strongly attracted and literally can be pulled away with such force that they fly like projectiles toward the magnet. There is a risk of severe injury and death. Further, damage to expensive equipment may occur.

> ⚑ **NURSING ALERT**
>
> For patient safety, the nurse must make sure that no patient care equipment (eg, portable oxygen tanks) that contains metal or metal parts enters the room where the MRI is located. The patient must be assessed for the presence of medication patches with foil backing (such as nicotine) that may cause a burn.

For the MRI, the patient lies with the head in a frame on a flat platform that is moved into a tube housing the magnet (Fig. 60-14). The tube is narrow; persons with a wide girth may not fit into the scanner. Patients who are unable to lie flat will not be able to tolerate an MRI. The scanning process is painless, but the patient hears loud thumping of the magnetic coils as the magnetic field is being pulsed. Patients may experience claustrophobia while inside the narrow tube; sedation may be prescribed in these circumstances. Newer versions of MRI machines (open MRI) are

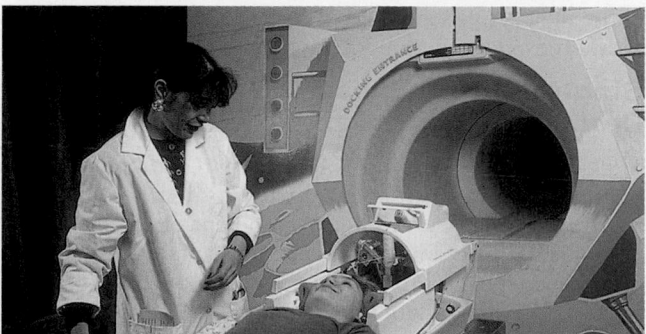

Figure 60-14 Technician explains what to expect during a magnetic resonance imaging procedure.

less claustrophobic than the earlier devices and are available in some locations. However, the images produced on these machines are often not as detailed, and traditional devices are preferable for accurate diagnosis. The patient may be taught to use relaxation techniques while in the scanner. The patient is informed that he or she will be able to talk to the staff during the scan through a microphone inside the scanner (Karpoff & Labus, 2008).

Positron Emission Tomography

PET is a computer-based nuclear imaging technique that produces images of actual organ functioning. The patient either inhales a radioactive gas or is injected with a radioactive substance that emits positively charged particles. When these positrons combine with negatively charged electrons (normally found in the body's cells), the resultant gamma rays can be detected by a scanning device that produces a series of two-dimensional views at various levels of the brain. This information is integrated by a computer and gives a composite picture of the brain at work.

PET permits the measurement of blood flow, tissue composition, and brain metabolism and thus indirectly evaluates brain function. The brain is one of the most metabolically active organs, consuming 80% of the glucose the body uses. PET measures this activity in specific areas of the brain and can detect changes in glucose use.

PET is useful in showing metabolic changes in the brain (Alzheimer's disease), locating lesions (brain tumor, epileptogenic lesions), identifying blood flow and oxygen metabolism in patients with strokes, distinguishing tumor from areas of necrosis, and revealing biochemical abnormalities associated with mental illness. The isotopes used have a very short half-life and are expensive to produce, requiring specialized equipment for production. PET scanning has been useful in research settings for the last 20 years and is becoming more available in clinical settings. Improvement in the scanning procedure and production of isotopes, as well as the advent of reimbursement by third-party payers, has increased the availability of PET studies.

Nursing Interventions

Key nursing interventions include patient preparation, which involves explaining the test and teaching the patient about inhalation techniques and the sensations (eg, dizziness, lightheadedness, and headache) that may occur. The IV injection of the radioactive substance produces similar side effects. Relaxation exercises may reduce anxiety during the test.

Single Photon Emission Computed Tomography

SPECT is a three-dimensional imaging technique that uses radionuclides and instruments to detect single photons. It is a perfusion study that captures a moment of cerebral blood flow at the time of injection of a radionuclide. Gamma photons are emitted from a radiopharmaceutical agent administered to the patient and are detected by a rotating gamma camera or cameras; the image is sent to a minicomputer. This approach allows areas behind overlying structures or background to be viewed, greatly increasing the contrast between normal and abnormal tissue. It is relatively inexpensive, and the duration is similar to that of a CT scan.

SPECT is useful in detecting the extent and location of abnormally perfused areas of the brain, thus allowing detection, localization, and sizing of stroke (before it is visible by CT scan); localization of seizure foci in epilepsy; detection of tumor progression (Bremner, 2005); and evaluation of perfusion before and after neurosurgical procedures. Pregnancy and breast-feeding are contraindications to SPECT.

Nursing Interventions

The nursing interventions for SPECT primarily include patient preparation and patient monitoring. Teaching about what to expect before the test can allay anxiety and ensure patient cooperation during the test. Premenopausal women are advised to practice effective contraception before and for several days after testing, and the woman who is breast-feeding is instructed to stop nursing for the time period recommended by the nuclear medicine department (Pagana & Pagana, 2006).

The nurse may need to accompany and monitor the patient during transport to the nuclear medicine department for the scan. Patients are monitored during and after the procedure for allergic reactions to the radiopharmaceutical agent.

Cerebral Angiography

Cerebral angiography is an x-ray study of the cerebral circulation with a contrast agent injected into a selected artery. A valuable tool in investigating vascular disease or anomalies, it is used to determine vessel patency, identify presence of collateral circulation, and provide detail on vascular anomalies that can be used in planning interventions. With the advent of additional imaging techniques, formal cerebral angiography is less frequently performed.

Cerebral angiograms are performed by threading a catheter through the femoral artery in the groin and up to the desired vessel. Alternatively, direct puncture of the carotid artery or retrograde injection of a contrast agent into the brachial artery may be performed. X-ray images are obtained as the contrast agent flows through the vessels; the carotid and vertebral arterial systems are visualized, as well as venous drainage. Arterial access may also be used for interventional procedures, such as placing coils in an aneurysm or arteriovenous malformation.

Nursing Interventions

Prior to the angiography, the patient's blood urea nitrogen and creatinine should be checked to ensure the kidneys will be able to clear the contrast agent. The patient should be well hydrated, and clear liquids are usually permitted up to the time of the test. The patient is instructed to void immediately before the test, and locations of the appropriate peripheral pulses are marked with a felt-tip pen. The patient is instructed to remain immobile during the angiogram process and is told to expect a brief feeling of warmth in the face, behind the eyes, or in the jaw, teeth, tongue, and lips, and a metallic taste when the contrast agent is injected.

After the groin is shaved and prepared, a local anesthetic agent is administered to minimize pain at the insertion site and to reduce arterial spasm. A catheter is introduced into the femoral artery, flushed with heparinized saline, and filled with contrast agent. Fluoroscopy is used to guide the catheter to the appropriate vessels. Neurologic assessment is conducted during and immediately following cerebral angiography to observe for embolism or arterial dissection that may occur during the test. Signs of these complications include new onset of alterations in the level of consciousness, weakness on one side of the body, motor or sensory deficits, and speech disturbances.

Nursing care after cerebral angiography includes observation of the injection site for bleeding or hematoma formation (a localized collection of blood). Because a hematoma at the puncture site or embolization to a distal artery affects the peripheral pulses, peripheral pulses that were marked prior to the test are monitored frequently. The color and temperature of the involved extremity are assessed to detect possible embolism (Karpoff & Labus, 2008).

Myelography

A myelogram is an x-ray of the spinal subarachnoid space taken after the injection of a contrast agent into the spinal subarachnoid space through a lumbar puncture. The water-based contrast agent disperses upward through the CSF to outline the spinal subarachnoid space and show any distortion of the spinal cord or spinal dural sac caused by tumors, cysts, herniated vertebral disks, or other lesions. Myelography is performed infrequently today because of the sensitivity of CT and MRI scanning (Bremner, 2005).

Nursing Interventions

Because many patients have misconceptions about myelography, the nurse clarifies the explanation given by the physician and answers questions. The patient is informed about what to expect during the procedure and made aware that changes in position may be made during the procedure. After myelography, the patient lies in bed with the head of the bed elevated 30 to 45 degrees. The patient is advised to remain in bed in the recommended position for 3 hours or as prescribed. Drinking liberal amounts of fluid for rehydration and replacement of CSF may decrease the incidence of post–lumbar puncture headache. The blood pressure, pulse, respiratory rate, and temperature are monitored, as well as the patient's ability to void. Untoward signs include headache, fever, stiff neck, **photophobia** (sensitivity to light), seizures, and signs of chemical or bacterial meningitis (Hickey, 2009).

Noninvasive Carotid Flow Studies

Noninvasive carotid flow studies use ultrasound imagery and Doppler measurements of arterial blood flow to evaluate carotid and deep orbital circulation. The graph produced indicates blood velocity. Increased blood velocity can indicate stenosis or partial obstruction. These tests are often obtained before more invasive tests such as arteriography, or used as screening tools. Carotid Doppler, carotid ultrasonography, oculoplethysmography, and ophthalmodynamometry are four common noninvasive vascular techniques that permit evaluation of arterial blood flow and detection of arterial stenosis, occlusion, and plaques. These vascular studies allow noninvasive imaging of extracranial and intracranial circulation (Diepenbrock, 2007).

Transcranial Doppler

Transcranial Doppler uses the same noninvasive techniques as carotid flow studies except that it records the blood flow velocities of the intracranial vessels. Arterial flow velocities can be measured through thin areas of the temporal and occipital bones of the skull. A handheld Doppler probe emits a pulsed beam; the signal is reflected by the moving red blood cells within the blood vessels. Transcranial Doppler is a noninvasive technique that is helpful in assessing vasospasm (a complication following subarachnoid hemorrhage), altered cerebral blood flow found in occlusive vascular disease, other cerebral pathology, and brain death.

Nursing Interventions

When a carotid flow study or transcranial Doppler is scheduled, the procedure is described to the patient. The patient is informed that this is a noninvasive test, that a handheld transducer will be placed over the neck and the orbits of the eyes, and that a water-soluble jelly is used on the transducer. Either one of these low-risk tests can be performed at the patient's bedside (Littlejohns & Bader, 2009).

Electroencephalography

An electroencephalogram (EEG) represents a record of the electrical activity generated in the brain (Hickey, 2009). It is obtained through electrodes applied on the scalp or through microelectrodes placed within the brain tissue. It provides an assessment of cerebral electrical activity. It is useful for diagnosing and evaluating seizure disorders, coma, or organic brain syndrome. Tumors, brain abscesses, blood clots, and infection may cause abnormal patterns in electrical activity. The EEG is also used in making a determination of brain death.

Electrodes are applied to the scalp to record the electrical activity in various regions of the brain. The amplified activity of the neurons between any two of these electrodes is recorded on continuously moving paper; this record is called the encephalogram.

For a baseline recording, the patient lies quietly with both eyes closed. The patient may be asked to hyperventilate for 3 to 4 minutes or to look at a bright, flashing light for photic stimulation. These activation procedures are performed to evoke abnormal electrical discharges, such as seizure potentials. A sleep EEG may be recorded after sedation because some abnormal brain waves are seen only when the patient is asleep. If the epileptogenic area is inaccessible to conventional scalp electrodes, nasopharyngeal electrodes may be used.

Depth recording of EEG is performed by introducing electrodes stereotactically (radiologically placed using instrumentation) into a target area of the brain, as indicated by the patient's seizure pattern and scalp EEG. It is used to identify patients who may benefit from surgical excision of epileptogenic foci. Special transsphenoidal, mandibular, and nasopharyngeal electrodes can be used, and video recording combined with EEG monitoring and telemetry is used in hospital settings to capture epileptiform abnormalities and their sequelae. Some epilepsy centers provide long-term ambulatory EEG monitoring with portable recording devices.

Nursing Interventions

To increase the chances of recording seizure activity, it is sometimes recommended that the patient be deprived of sleep on the night before the EEG. Antiseizure agents, tranquilizers, stimulants, and depressants should be withheld 24 to 48 hours before an EEG because these medications can alter the EEG wave patterns or mask the abnormal wave patterns of seizure disorders (Pagana & Pagana, 2006). Coffee, tea, chocolate, and cola drinks are omitted in the meal before the test because of their stimulating effect. However, the meal is not omitted, because an altered blood glucose level can cause changes in brain wave patterns.

The patient is informed that the standard EEG takes 45 to 60 minutes; a sleep EEG requires 12 hours. The patient is assured that the procedure does not cause an electric shock and that the EEG is a diagnostic test, not a form of treatment. An EEG requires the patient to lie quietly during the test. Sedation is not advisable, because it may lower the seizure threshold in patients with a seizure disorder and it alters brain wave activity in all patients. The nurse needs to check the physician's prescription regarding the administration of antiseizure medication prior to testing.

Routine EEGs use a water-soluble lubricant for electrode contact, which can be wiped off and removed by shampooing later. Sleep EEGs involve the use of collodion glue for electrode contact, which requires acetone for removal.

Electromyography

An electromyogram (EMG) is obtained by inserting needle electrodes into the skeletal muscles to measure changes in the electrical potential of the muscles (Pagana & Pagana, 2006). The electrical potentials are shown on an oscilloscope and amplified so that both the sound and appearance of the waves can be analyzed and compared simultaneously.

An EMG is useful in determining the presence of neuromuscular disorders and myopathies. It helps distinguish weakness due to neuropathy (functional or pathologic changes in the peripheral nervous system) from weakness resulting from other causes.

Nursing Interventions

The procedure is explained, and the patient is warned to expect a sensation similar to that of an intramuscular injection as the needle is inserted into the muscle. The muscles examined may ache for a short time after the procedure.

Nerve Conduction Studies

Nerve conduction studies are performed by stimulating a peripheral nerve at several points along its course and recording the muscle action potential or the sensory action potential that results. Surface or needle electrodes are placed on the skin over the nerve to stimulate the nerve fibers. This test is useful in the study of peripheral neuropathies and is often included as part of the EMG.

Evoked Potential Studies

Evoked potential studies involve application of an external stimulus to specific peripheral sensory receptors with subsequent measurement of the electrical potential generated. Electrical changes are detected with the aid of computerized devices that extract the signal, display it on an oscilloscope, and store the data on magnetic tape or disk. In neurologic diagnosis, they reflect nerve conduction times in the peripheral nervous system. In clinical practice, the visual, auditory, and somatosensory systems are most often tested.

In visual evoked responses, the patient looks at a visual stimulus (flashing lights, a checkerboard pattern on a screen). The average of several hundred stimuli is recorded by EEG leads placed over the occipital lobe. The transit time from the retina to the occipital area is measured using computer-averaging methods.

Brain stem auditory evoked responses (BAERs) are measured by applying an auditory stimulus (repetitive auditory click) and measuring the transit time via the brain stem into the cortex. Specific lesions in the auditory pathway modify or delay the response. BAERs may be used in the diagnosis of brain stem abnormalities and in determination of brain death.

In somatosensory evoked responses (SERs), the peripheral nerves are stimulated (electrical stimulation through skin electrodes) and the transit time along the spinal cord to the cortex is measured and recorded from scalp electrodes. SERs are used to detect deficits in spinal cord or peripheral nerve conduction and to monitor spinal cord function during surgical procedures. It is also useful in the diagnosis of demyelinating diseases, such as multiple sclerosis and polyneuropathies, where nerve conduction is slowed.

Nursing Interventions

The nurse explains the procedure and reassures the patient and encourages him or her to relax. The patient is advised to remain perfectly still throughout the recording to prevent artifacts (signals not generated by the brain) that interfere with the recording and interpretation of the test.

Lumbar Puncture and Examination of Cerebrospinal Fluid

A lumbar puncture (spinal tap) is carried out by inserting a needle into the lumbar subarachnoid space to withdraw CSF. The test may be performed to obtain CSF for examination, to measure and reduce CSF pressure, to determine the presence or absence of blood in the CSF, and to administer medications intrathecally (into the spinal canal).

The needle is usually inserted into the subarachnoid space between the third and fourth or fourth and fifth lumbar vertebrae. Because the spinal cord ends at the first lumbar vertebra, insertion of the needle below the level of the third lumbar vertebra prevents puncture of the spinal cord.

A successful lumbar puncture requires that the patient be relaxed; an anxious patient is tense, and this may increase the pressure reading. CSF pressure with the patient in a lateral recumbent position is normally 50 to 1800 mm H_2O (Karpoff & Labus, 2008).

A lumbar puncture may be risky in the presence of an intracranial mass lesion because intraspinal pressure is decreased by removal of CSF, and the brain may herniate downward through the foramen magnum. See Chart 60-5 for instructions for assisting with a lumbar puncture.

Cerebrospinal Fluid Analysis

The CSF should be clear and colorless. Pink, blood-tinged, or grossly bloody CSF may indicate a subarachnoid hemorrhage. The CSF may be bloody initially because of local trauma but becomes clearer as more fluid is drained. Specimens are obtained for cell count, culture, glucose, protein, and other tests as indicated. The specimens should be sent to the laboratory immediately because changes will take place and alter the result if the specimens are allowed to stand. (See Table A-5 in Appendix A for the normal values of CSF.)

Post–Lumbar Puncture Headache

A post–lumbar puncture headache, ranging from mild to severe, may occur a few hours to several days after the procedure. This complication occurs in 15% to 30% of patients. It is a throbbing bifrontal or occipital headache, dull and deep in character. It is particularly severe on sitting or standing but lessens or disappears when the patient lies down.

The headache is caused by CSF leakage at the puncture site. The fluid continues to escape into the tissues by way of the needle track from the spinal canal. As a result of a leak, the supply of CSF in the cranium is depleted to a point at which it is insufficient to maintain proper mechanical stabilization of the brain. When the patient assumes an upright position, tension and stretching of the venous sinuses and pain-sensitive structures occur.

Post–lumbar puncture headache may be avoided if a small-gauge needle is used and if the patient remains prone after the procedure. When more than 20 mL of CSF is removed, the patient is positioned supine for several hours. Keeping the patient flat overnight may reduce the incidence of headaches.

A postpuncture headache is usually managed by bed rest, analgesic agents, and hydration. Occasionally, if the headache persists, the epidural blood patch technique may be used. Blood is withdrawn from the antecubital vein and injected into the epidural space, usually at the site of the previous spinal puncture. The rationale is that the blood acts as a gelatinous plug to seal the hole in the dura, preventing further loss of CSF.

Other Complications of Lumbar Puncture

Herniation of the intracranial contents, spinal epidural abscess, spinal epidural hematoma, and meningitis are rare but serious complications of lumbar puncture. Other

Chart 60-5 • *Assisting With a Lumbar Puncture*

A needle is inserted into the subarachnoid space through the third and fourth or fourth and fifth lumbar interface to withdraw spinal fluid.

Preprocedure

1. Determine whether written consent for the procedure has been obtained.
2. Explain the procedure to the patient and describe sensations that are likely during the procedure (ie, a sensation of cold as the site is cleansed with solution, a needle prick when local anesthetic agent is injected).
3. Determine whether the patient has any questions or misconceptions about the procedure; reassure the patient that the needle will not enter the spinal cord or cause paralysis.
4. Instruct the patient to void before the procedure.

Procedure

1. The patient is positioned on one side at the edge of the bed or examining table with back toward the physician; the thighs and legs are flexed as much as possible to increase the space between the spinous processes of the vertebrae, for easier entry into the subarachnoid space.

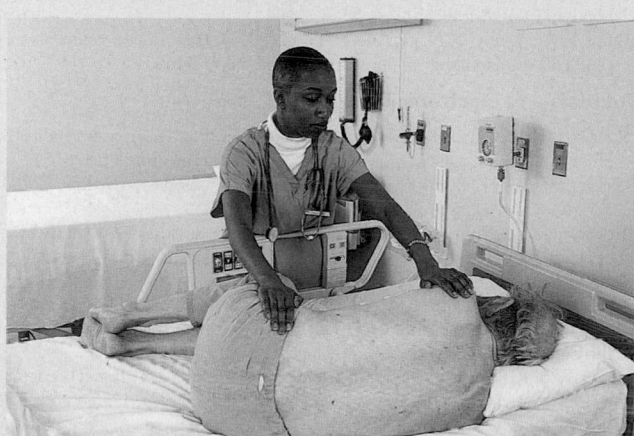

© B. Proud.

2. A small pillow may be placed under the patient's head to maintain the spine in a horizontal position; a pillow may be placed between the legs to prevent the upper leg from rolling forward.
3. The nurse assists the patient to maintain the position to avoid sudden movement, which can produce a traumatic (bloody) tap.
4. The patient is encouraged to relax and is instructed to breathe normally, because hyperventilation may lower an elevated pressure.

5. The nurse describes the procedure step by step to the patient as it proceeds.
6. The physician cleanses the puncture site with an antiseptic agent solution and drapes the site.
7. The physician injects local anesthetic agent to numb the puncture site, and then inserts a spinal needle into the subarachnoid space through the third and fourth or fourth and fifth lumbar interspace. A pressure reading may be obtained.
8. A specimen of CSF is removed and usually collected in three test tubes, labeled in order of collection. The needle is withdrawn.
9. The physician applies a small dressing to the puncture site.
10. The tubes of CSF are sent to the laboratory immediately.

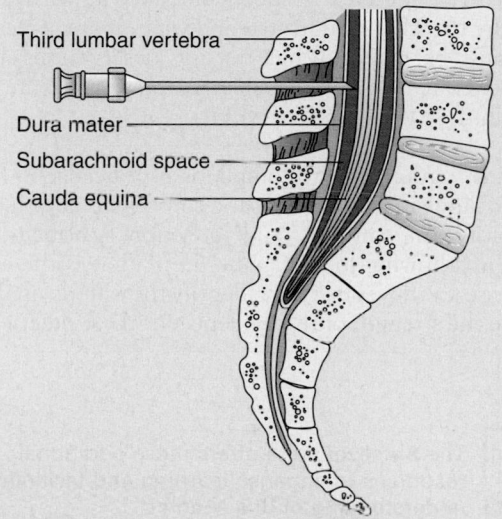

Third lumbar vertebra
Dura mater
Subarachnoid space
Cauda equina

Postprocedure

1. Instruct the patient to lie prone for 2 to 3 hours to separate the alignment of the dural and arachnoid needle punctures in the meninges, to reduce leakage of CSF.
2. Monitor the patient for complications of lumbar puncture; notify physician if complications occur.
3. Encourage increased fluid intake to reduce the risk of postprocedure headache.

---

complications include temporary voiding problems, slight elevation of temperature, backache or spasms, and stiffness of the neck.

Promoting Home and Community-Based Care

Teaching Patients Self-Care

Many diagnostic tests that were once performed as part of a hospital stay are now carried out in short-procedure units or outpatient testing settings or units. As a result, family members often provide the postprocedure care. Therefore, the patient and family must receive clear verbal and written instructions about precautions to take after the procedure, complications to watch for, and steps to take if complications occur. Because many patients undergoing neurologic diagnostic studies are elderly or have neurologic deficits, provisions must be made to ensure that transportation, postprocedure care, and appropriate monitoring are available.

Continuing Care

Contacting the patient and family after diagnostic testing enables the nurse to determine whether they have any questions about the procedure or whether the patient had any untoward results. Teaching is reinforced and the patient and family are reminded to make and keep follow-up appointments. Patients, family members, and health care providers are focused on the immediate needs, issues, or deficits that necessitated the diagnostic testing.

CRITICAL THINKING EXERCISES

1 A patient is admitted to your unit with lower extremity paralysis. What findings in your examination help distinguish between upper motor neuron and lower motor neuron causes for the paralysis? How do those findings affect your care?

2 A 78-year-old patient is scheduled for an MRI. Explain why the MRI is indicated and what, if any, precautions must be taken. What nursing observations and assessments are indicated? What safety precautions are essential in the MRI suite, and why?

EBP 3 Your patient complains of a headache following a lumbar puncture. What resources would you use to identify the current guidelines for treatment of headache following lumbar puncture? What is the evidence base for these practices? Identify the criteria used to evaluate the strength of the evidence for these practices.

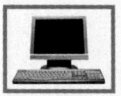

The Smeltzer suite offers these additional resources to enhance learning and facilitate understanding of this chapter:
- thePoint online resource, thepoint.lww.com/Smeltzer12E
- Student CD-ROM included with the book
- *Study Guide to Accompany Brunner & Suddarth's Textbook of Medical-Surgical Nursing*

REFERENCES AND SELECTED READINGS

Asterisk indicates nursing research.

Books

Bickley, L. S. (2007). *Bates' guide to physical examination and history taking* (9th ed.). Philadelphia: Lippincott Williams & Wilkins.

Bremner, J. D. (2005). *Brain imaging handbook*. New York: W. W. Norton.

Bulechek, G. M., Butcher, H. K. & Dochterman, J. M. (2008). *Nursing interventions classification* (NIC) (5th ed.). St. Louis: Mosby.

Diepenbrock, N. H. (2007). *Quick reference to critical care* (3rd ed.). Philadelphia: Lippincott Williams & Wilkins.

Fischbach, F. T. & Dunning, M. B. (2005). *Nurse's quick reference to common laboratory and diagnostic tests* (4th ed.). Philadelphia: Lippincott Williams & Wilkins.

Hickey, J. V. (2009). *The clinical practice of neurological & neurosurgical nursing* (6th ed.). Philadelphia: Lippincott Williams & Wilkins.

Herndon, R. M. (2006). *Handbook of neurologic rating scales* (2nd ed.). New York: Demos Medical Publishing.

Jarvis, C. (2007). *Physical examination and health assessment* (5th ed.). Philadelphia: Saunders.

Karpoff, S. & Labus, D. (2008). *Portable diagnostic tests*. Philadelphia: Lippincott Williams & Wilkins.

Klein, D. G. & Stewart-Amidei, C. (2009). Nervous system alterations. In Sole, M. L., Klein, D. G. & Moseley, M. J. (Eds.). *Introduction to critical care nursing* (5th ed.). St. Louis: Elsevier Saunders.

Johnson, M., Bulachek, G. M., Butcher, H. K., et al. (2006). *NANDA, NOC, and NIC linkages* (2nd ed.). St. Louis: Mosby.

Littlejohns, L. R. & Bader, M. K. (2009). *AACN-AANN protocols for practice: Monitoring technologies in critically ill neuroscience patients*. Sudbury, MA: Jones and Bartlett Publishers.

Pagana, K. D. & Pagana, T. J. (2006). *Manual of diagnostic and laboratory tests* (3rd ed.). St. Louis: Mosby Elsevier.

Porth, C. M. & Matfin, G. (2009). *Pathophysiology: Concepts of altered health states* (8th ed.). Philadelphia: Lippincott Williams & Wilkins.

Posner, J. B., Saper, C. B., Schiff, N. D., et al. (2007). *Plum and Posner's diagnosis of stupor and coma* (4th ed.). Oxford, UK: Oxford University Press.

Weber, J. & Kelley, J. (2007). *Health assessment in nursing* (3rd ed.). Philadelphia: Lippincott Williams & Wilkins.

Woodward, S. (2006). *Neuroscience nursing: Assessment and patient management*. London: Quay Books.

Young, P. A., Young, P. H. & Tolbert, D. L. (2007). *Basic clinical neuroanatomy* (2nd ed.). Philadelphia: Lippincott Williams & Wilkins.

Journals and Electronic Documents

Alverzo, J. P. (2006). A review of the literature on orientation as an indicator of level of consciousness. *Journal of Nursing Scholarship, 38*(2), 159–164.

Beattle, S. (2007). Bedside emergency: Unconscious patients. *RN, 70*(9), 32–37.

*Doerksen, K. & Naimark, B. (2006). Nonspecific behaviors as early indicators of cerebral vasospasm. *Journal of Neuroscience Nursing, 38*(6), 409–415.

Neal-Boylan, L. (2007). Assessing the very old person at home. *Home Healthcare Nurse, 25*(6), 388–400.

Olson, D. M. & Graffagnino, C. (2005). Consciousness, coma, and caring for the brain-injured patient. *AACN Clinical Issues, 16*(4), 441–455.

Palmer, R. & Knight, J. (2006). Consciousness. Assessment of altered conscious level in clinical practice. *British Journal of Nursing, 15*(22), 1255–1259.

Peiffer, K. M. Z. (2007). Brain death and organ procurement. *American Journal of Nursing, 107*(3), 58–68.

Tanenbaum, L. N. (2005). 3T MRI in clinical practice. *Applied Radiology, 35*(1), 8–17.

White, A. (2006). Neurologic assessment: Vital in prioritizing emergency department interventions. *American Journal for Nurse Practitioners, 10*(9), 60–67.

Wickremaratchi, M. M. & Llewelyn, J. G. (2006). Effects of aging on touch. *Postgraduate Medical Journal, 82*, 301–304.

RESOURCES

American Headache Society, www.ahsnet.org
Brain Injury Association, www.biausa.org
Brain Trauma Foundation, www.braintrauma.org
Epilepsy Foundation, www.epilepsyfoundation.org
Harvard Health Publications, HMS Office of Public Affairs, www.health.harvard.edu/diagnostic-tests/#brain
National Headache Foundation, www.headaches.org

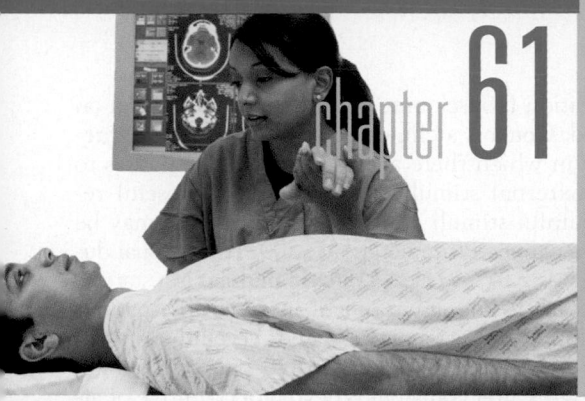

chapter 61

Management of Patients With Neurologic Dysfunction

On completion of this chapter, the learner will be able to:

1 Describe the nursing needs of patients with various neurologic dysfunctions.

2 Describe the multiple needs of the patient with altered level of consciousness.

3 Use the nursing process as a framework for care of the patient with altered level of consciousness.

4 Identify the early and late clinical manifestations of increased intracranial pressure.

5 Use the nursing process as a framework for care of the patient with increased intracranial pressure.

6 Describe the needs of the patient undergoing intracranial or transsphenoidal surgery.

7 Use the nursing process as a framework for care of the patient undergoing intracranial or transsphenoidal surgery.

8 Identify the various types and causes of seizures.

9 Use the nursing process to develop a plan of care for the patient experiencing seizures.

10 Identify the needs of the patient experiencing headaches.

GLOSSARY

akinetic mutism: unresponsiveness to the environment; the patient makes no movement or sound but sometimes opens the eyes

altered level of consciousness: condition of being less responsive to and aware of environmental stimuli

autoregulation: ability of cerebral blood vessels to dilate or constrict to maintain stable cerebral blood flow despite changes in systemic arterial blood pressure

brain death: irreversible loss of all functions of the entire brain, including the brain stem

coma: prolonged state of unconsciousness

craniectomy: a surgical procedure that involves removal of a portion of the skull

craniotomy: a surgical procedure that involves entry into the cranial vault

Cushing's response: the brain's attempt to restore blood flow by increasing arterial pressure to overcome the increased intracranial pressure

Cushing's triad: three classic signs—bradycardia, hypertension, and bradypnea—seen with pressure on the medulla as a result of brain stem herniation

GLOSSARY *(Continued)*

decerebration: an abnormal body posture associated with a severe brain injury, characterized by extreme extension of the upper and lower extremities

decortication: an abnormal posture associated with severe brain injury, characterized by abnormal flexion of the upper extremities and extension of the lower extremities

epidural monitor: a sensor placed between the skull and the dura to monitor intracranial pressure

epilepsy: a group of syndromes characterized by paroxysmal transient disturbances of brain function

fiberoptic monitor: a system that uses light refraction to determine intracranial pressure

herniation: abnormal protrusion of tissue through a defect or natural opening

intracranial pressure: pressure exerted by the volume of the intracranial contents within the cranial vault

locked-in syndrome: condition resulting from a lesion in the pons in which the patient lacks all distal motor activity (paralysis) but cognition is intact

microdialysis: procedure in which an intracranial catheter is inserted near an injured area of brain to measure lactate, pyruvate, glutamate, and glucose levels

migraine headache: a severe, unrelenting headache often accompanied by symptoms such as nausea, vomiting, and visual disturbances

Monro-Kellie hypothesis: theory that states that due to limited space for expansion within the skull, an increase in any one of the cranial contents—brain tissue, blood, or cerebrospinal fluid—causes a change in the volume of the others

persistent vegetative state: condition in which the patient is wakeful but devoid of conscious content, without cognitive or affective mental function

primary headache: a headache for which no specific organic cause can be found

secondary headache: headache identified as a symptom of another organic disorder (eg, brain tumor, hypertension)

seizures: paroxysmal transient disturbance of the brain resulting from a discharge of abnormal electrical activity

status epilepticus: episode in which the patient experiences multiple seizure bursts with no recovery time in between

subarachnoid screw or bolt: device placed into the subarachnoid space to measure intracranial pressure

transsphenoidal: surgical approach to the pituitary via the sphenoid sinuses

ventriculostomy: a catheter placed in one of the lateral ventricles of the brain to measure intracranial pressure and allow for drainage of fluid

This chapter presents an overview of care of the patient with an altered level of consciousness, the patient with increased **intracranial pressure (ICP),** and the patient who is undergoing neurosurgical procedures, experiencing seizures, or experiencing headaches. Some of the disorders in this chapter, such as headaches and seizures, may be symptoms of dysfunction in another body system. Alternatively, headaches and seizures can be symptoms of a disruption of the neurologic system. These disorders can also be diagnosed at times as "idiopathic," or without an identifiable cause. The commonalities of these disorders are often the behaviors and needs of the patient and the approaches nurses use to support the patient.

The central nervous system (CNS) contains a vast network of neurons that control the body's vital functions. Yet this system is vulnerable, and its optimal function depends on several key factors. First, the neurologic system relies on its structural integrity for support and homeostasis, but this integrity may be disrupted. Examples of structural disruption include head injury, brain tumor, intracranial hemorrhage, infection, and stroke. As brain tissue expands in the inflexible cranium, ICP rises, and cerebral perfusion is impaired. Further expansion places pressure on vital centers, which can cause permanent neurologic deficits or lead to brain death.

Second, the neurologic system relies on the body's ability to maintain a homeostatic environment. It requires the delivery of the essential elements of oxygen and glucose, as well as filtration of substrates that are toxic to the neurons. The functions of the neurologic system may be decreased or absent because of the effect of toxic substrates or the body's inability to provide essential substrates. Sepsis, hypovolemia, myocardial infarction, respiratory arrest, hypoglycemia, electrolyte imbalance, drug and/or alcohol overdose, encephalopathy, and ketoacidosis are all examples of such circumstances. Some conditions can be treated and reversed; others result in permanent neurologic deficits and disabilities.

Although the specialty of neuroscience nursing requires an understanding of neuroanatomy, neurophysiology, neurodiagnostic testing, critical care nursing, and rehabilitation nursing, nurses in all settings care for patients with neurologic disorders. Ongoing assessment of the patient's neurologic function and health needs, identification of problems, mutual goal setting, development and implementation of care plans (including teaching, counseling, and coordinating activities), and evaluation of the outcomes of care are nursing actions integral to the recovery of the patient. The nurse also collaborates with other members of the health care team to provide essential care, offer a variety of solutions to problems, help the patient and family gain control of their lives, and explore the educational and supportive resources available in the community. The goals are to achieve as high a level of function as possible and to enhance the quality of life for the patient with neurologic impairment and his or her family.

ALTERED LEVEL OF CONSCIOUSNESS

An **altered level of consciousness (LOC)** is apparent in the patient who is not oriented, does not follow commands, or needs persistent stimuli to achieve a state of alertness. LOC is gauged on a continuum, with a normal state of alertness and full cognition (consciousness) on one end and coma on the other end. **Coma** is a clinical state of unarousable unresponsiveness in which there are no purposeful responses to internal or external stimuli, although nonpurposeful responses to painful stimuli and brain stem reflexes may be present (Gusa, Miers, Pfrimmer, et al., 2007). The usual duration of coma is 2 to 4 weeks. **Akinetic mutism** is a state of unresponsiveness to the environment in which the patient makes no voluntary movement. **Persistent vegetative state** is a condition in which the unresponsive patient resumes sleep–wake cycles after coma but is devoid of cognitive or affective mental function. **Locked-in syndrome** results from a lesion affecting the pons and results in paralysis and the inability to speak, but vertical eye movements and lid elevation remain intact and are used to indicate responsiveness (Maurer, 2008). The level of responsiveness and consciousness is the most important indicator of the patient's condition.

Pathophysiology

Altered LOC is not a disorder itself; rather, it is a result of multiple pathophysiologic phenomena. The cause may be neurologic (head injury, stroke), toxicologic (drug overdose, alcohol intoxication), or metabolic (hepatic or renal failure, diabetic ketoacidosis).

The underlying cause of neurologic dysfunction is disruption in the cells of the nervous system, neurotransmitters, or brain anatomy (see Chapter 60). Disruptions result from cellular edema or other mechanisms, such as disruption of chemical transmission at receptor sites by antibodies.

Intact anatomic structures of the brain are needed for normal function. The two hemispheres of the cerebrum must communicate, via an intact corpus callosum, and the lobes of the brain (frontal, parietal, temporal, and occipital) must communicate and coordinate their specific functions (see Chapter 60). Other anatomic structures of importance are the cerebellum and the brain stem. The cerebellum has both excitatory and inhibitory actions and is largely responsible for coordination of movement. The brain stem contains areas that control the heart, respiration, and blood pressure. Disruptions in the anatomic structures result from trauma, edema, pressure from tumors, or other mechanisms, such as an increase or decrease in the circulation of blood or cerebrospinal fluid (CSF).

Clinical Manifestations

Alterations in LOC occur along a continuum, and the clinical manifestations depend on where the patient is on this continuum. As the patient's state of alertness and consciousness decreases, changes occur in the pupillary response, eye opening response, verbal response, and motor response. However, initial alterations in LOC may be reflected by subtle behavioral changes, such as restlessness or increased anxiety. The pupils, normally round and quickly reactive to light, become sluggish (response is slower); as the patient becomes comatose, the pupils become fixed (no response to light). The patient in a coma does not open the eyes, respond verbally, or move the extremities in response to a request to do so.

Assessment and Diagnostic Findings

The patient with an altered LOC is at risk for alterations in every body system. A complete assessment is performed, with particular attention to the neurologic system. The neurologic examination should be as complete as the LOC allows (American Association of Neuroscience Nurses [AANN], 2005). It includes an evaluation of mental status, cranial nerve function, cerebellar function (balance and co-ordination), reflexes, and motor and sensory function. LOC, a sensitive indicator of neurologic function, is assessed based on the criteria in the Glasgow Coma Scale: eye opening, verbal response, and motor response (Gusa, et al., 2007). The patient's responses are rated on a scale from 3 to 15. A score of 3 indicates severe impairment of neurologic function, brain death, or pharmacologic inhibition of the neurologic response. A score of 15 indicates that the patient is fully responsive (see Chapter 63).

If the patient is comatose and has localized signs such as abnormal pupillary and motor responses, it is assumed that neurologic disease is present until proven otherwise. If the patient is comatose but pupillary light reflexes are preserved, a toxic or metabolic disorder is suspected. Common diagnostic procedures used to identify the cause of unconsciousness include computed tomography (CT) scanning, magnetic resonance imaging (MRI), and electroencephalography (EEG). Less common procedures include positron emission tomography (PET) and single photon emission computed tomography (SPECT; see Chapter 60). Laboratory tests include analysis of blood glucose, electrolytes, serum ammonia, and liver function tests; blood urea nitrogen (BUN) levels; serum osmolality; calcium level; and partial thromboplastin and prothrombin times. Other studies may be used to evaluate serum ketones, alcohol and drug concentrations, and arterial blood gases.

Medical Management

The first priority of treatment for the patient with altered LOC is to obtain and maintain a patent airway. The patient may be orally or nasally intubated, or a tracheostomy may be performed. Until the ability of the patient to breathe is determined, a mechanical ventilator is used to maintain adequate oxygenation and ventilation. The circulatory status (blood pressure, heart rate) is monitored to ensure adequate perfusion to the body and brain. An intravenous (IV) catheter is inserted to provide access for IV fluids and medications. Neurologic care focuses on the specific neurologic pathology, if known. Nutritional support, via a feeding tube or a gastrostomy tube, is initiated as soon as possible. In addition to measures designed to determine and treat the underlying causes of altered LOC, other medical interventions are aimed at pharmacologic management and prevention of complications.

NURSING PROCESS

THE PATIENT WITH AN ALTERED LEVEL OF CONSCIOUSNESS

Assessment

Assessment of the patient with an altered LOC often starts with assessing the verbal response through determining the patient's orientation to time, person, and place. Patients are asked to identify the day, date, or season of the year and to identify where they are or to identify the clinicians, family members, or visitors present. Other

questions such as, "Who is the president?" or "What is the next holiday?" may be helpful in determining the patient's processing of information. (Verbal response cannot be evaluated if the patient is intubated or has a tracheostomy, and this should be clearly documented.)

Alertness is measured by the patient's ability to open the eyes spontaneously or in response to a vocal or noxious stimulus (pressure or pain). Patients with severe neurologic dysfunction cannot do this. The nurse assesses for periorbital edema (swelling around the eyes) or trauma, which may prevent the patient from opening the eyes, and documents any such condition that interferes with eye opening.

Motor response includes spontaneous, purposeful movement (eg, the awake patient can move all four extremities with equal strength on command), movement only in response to painful stimuli, or abnormal posturing (Olsen & Graffagnino, 2005). If the patient is not responding to commands, the motor response is tested by applying a painful stimulus (firm but gentle pressure) to the nail bed or by squeezing a muscle. If the patient attempts to push away or withdraw, the response is recorded as purposeful or appropriate ("patient withdraws to painful stimulus"). This response is considered purposeful if the patient can cross the midline from one side of the body to the other in response to a painful stimulus. An inappropriate or nonpurposeful response is random and aimless. Posturing may be decorticate or decerebrate (Fig. 61-1; see also Chapter 60). The most severe neurologic impairment results in flaccidity. The motor response cannot be elicited or assessed when the patient has been administered pharmacologic paralyzing agents.

In addition to LOC, the nurse monitors parameters such as respiratory status, eye signs, and reflexes on an ongoing basis. Table 61-1 summarizes the assessment and the clinical significance of the findings. Body functions (circulation, respiration, elimination, fluid and electrolyte balance) are examined in a systematic and ongoing manner.

Diagnosis

Nursing Diagnoses

Based on the assessment data, the major nursing diagnoses may include the following:

- Ineffective airway clearance related to altered LOC
- Risk of injury related to decreased LOC
- Deficient fluid volume related to inability to take fluids by mouth
- Impaired oral mucous membrane related to mouth breathing, absence of pharyngeal reflex, and altered fluid intake
- Risk for impaired skin integrity related to prolonged immobility
- Impaired tissue integrity of cornea related to diminished or absent corneal reflex
- Ineffective thermoregulation related to damage to hypothalamic center
- Impaired urinary elimination (incontinence or retention) related to impairment in neurologic sensing and control
- Bowel incontinence related to impairment in neurologic sensing and control and also related to changes in nutritional delivery methods

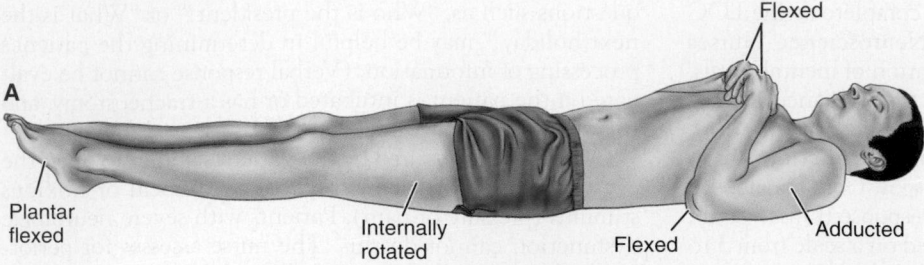

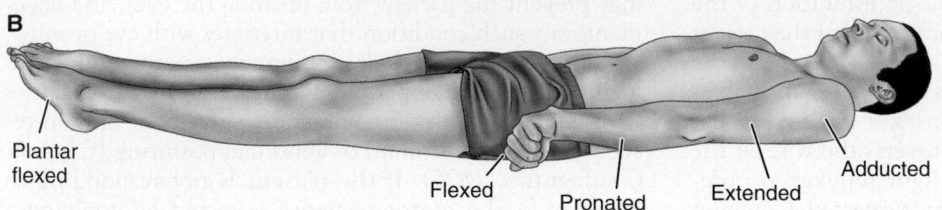

Figure 61-1 Abnormal posture response to stimuli. **A,** Decorticate posturing and flexion of the upper extremities, internal rotation of the lower extremities, and plantar flexion of the feet. **B,** Decerebrate posturing, involving extension and outward rotation of upper extremities and plantar flexion of the feet.

- Disturbed sensory perception related to neurologic impairment
- Interrupted family processes related to health crisis

Collaborative Problems/Potential Complications

Based on the assessment data, potential complications may include:
- Respiratory distress or failure
- Pneumonia
- Aspiration
- Pressure ulcer
- Deep vein thrombosis (DVT)
- Contractures

Planning and Goals

The patient with altered LOC is subject to all the complications associated with immobility. Therefore, the goals of care for the patient with altered LOC include maintenance of a clear airway, protection from injury, attainment of fluid volume balance, achievement of intact oral mucous membranes, maintenance of normal skin integrity, absence of corneal irritation, attainment of effective thermoregulation, and effective urinary elimination. Additional goals include bowel continence, accurate perception of environmental stimuli, maintenance of intact family or support system, and absence of complications.

Because the unconscious patient's protective reflexes are impaired, the quality of nursing care provided may mean the difference between life and death. The nurse must assume responsibility for the patient until the basic reflexes (coughing, blinking, and swallowing) return and the patient becomes conscious and oriented. Therefore, the major nursing goal is to compensate for the absence of these protective reflexes.

Nursing Interventions

Maintaining the Airway

The most important consideration in managing the patient with altered LOC is to establish an adequate airway and ensure ventilation. Obstruction of the airway is a risk because the epiglottis and tongue may relax, occluding the orophar-

ynx, or the patient may aspirate vomitus or nasopharyngeal secretions.

The accumulation of secretions in the pharynx presents a serious problem. Because the patient cannot swallow and lacks pharyngeal reflexes, these secretions must be removed to eliminate the danger of aspiration. Elevating the head of the bed to 30 degrees helps prevent aspiration. Positioning the patient in a lateral or semiprone position also helps, because it allows the jaw and tongue to fall forward, thus promoting drainage of secretions.

Positioning alone is not always adequate, however. Suctioning and oral hygiene may be required. Suctioning is performed to remove secretions from the posterior pharynx and upper trachea. Before and after suctioning, the patient is adequately ventilated to prevent hypoxia (Hickey, 2009). Chest physiotherapy and postural drainage may be initiated to promote pulmonary hygiene, unless contraindicated by the patient's underlying condition. The chest should be auscultated at least every 8 hours to detect adventitious breath sounds or absence of breath sounds.

Despite these measures, or because of the severity of impairment, the patient with altered LOC often requires intubation and mechanical ventilation. Nursing actions for the mechanically ventilated patient include maintaining the patency of the endotracheal tube or tracheostomy, providing frequent oral care, monitoring arterial blood gas measurements, and maintaining ventilator settings (see Chapter 25).

Protecting the Patient

For the protection of the patient, side rails are padded. Two rails are kept in the raised position during the day and three at night; however, raising all four side rails is considered a restraint by the Joint Commission if the intent is to limit the patient's mobility. Care should be taken to prevent injury from invasive lines and equipment, and other potential sources of injury should be identified, such as restraints, tight dressings, environmental irritants, damp bedding or dressings, and tubes and drains.

Protection also includes ensuring the patient's dignity during altered LOC. Simple measures such as providing privacy and speaking to the patient during nursing care

Table 61-1   NURSING ASSESSMENT OF THE UNCONSCIOUS PATIENT

Examination	Clinical Assessment	Clinical Significance
Level of responsiveness or consciousness	Eye opening; verbal and motor responses; pupils (size, equality, reaction to light)	Obeying commands is a favorable response and demonstrates a return to consciousness.
Pattern of respiration	Respiratory pattern	Disturbances of respiratory center of brain may result in various respiratory patterns.
	Cheyne-Stokes respiration	Suggests lesions deep in both hemispheres; area of basal ganglia and upper brain stem
	Hyperventilation	Suggests onset of metabolic problem or brain stem damage
	Ataxic respiration with irregularity in depth/rate	Ominous sign of damage to medullary center
Eyes Pupils (size, equality, reaction to light)	Equal, normally reactive pupils Equal or unequal diameter Progressive dilation Fixed dilated pupils	Suggests that coma is toxic or metabolic in origin Helps determine location of lesion Indicates increasing intracranial pressure Indicates injury at level of midbrain
Eye movements	Normally, eyes should move from side to side.	Functional and structural integrity of brain stem is assessed by inspection of extraocular movements; usually absent in deep coma.
Corneal reflex	When cornea is touched with a wisp of clean cotton, blink response is normal.	Tests cranial nerves V and VII; helps determine location of lesion if unilateral; absent in deep coma
Facial symmetry Swallowing reflex	Asymmetry (sagging, decrease in wrinkles) Drooling versus spontaneous swallowing	Sign of paralysis Absent in coma Paralysis of cranial nerves X and XII
Neck	Stiff neck Absence of spontaneous neck movement	Subarachnoid hemorrhage, meningitis Fracture or dislocation of cervical spine
Response of extremity to noxious stimuli	Firm pressure on a joint of the upper and lower extremity Observe spontaneous movements.	Asymmetric response in paralysis Absent in deep coma
Deep tendon reflexes	Tap patellar and biceps tendons.	Brisk response may have localizing value Asymmetric response in paralysis Absent in deep coma
Pathologic reflexes	Firm pressure with blunt object on sole of foot, moving along lateral margin and crossing to the ball of foot	Flexion of the toes, especially the great toe, is normal except in newborn. Dorsiflexion of toes (especially great toe) indicates contralateral pathology of corticospinal tract (Babinski reflex). Helps determine location of lesion in brain
Abnormal posture	Observation for posturing (spontaneous or in response to noxious stimuli) Flaccidity with absence of motor response Decorticate posture (flexion and internal rotation of forearms and hands) Decerebrate posture (extension and external rotation)	Deep extensive brain lesion Seen with cerebral hemisphere pathology and in metabolic depression of brain function Decerebrate posturing indicates deeper and more severe dysfunction than does decorticate posturing; implies brain pathology; poor prognostic sign.

activities preserve the patient's dignity. Not speaking negatively about the patient's condition or prognosis is also important, because patients in a light coma may be able to hear. The comatose patient has an increased need for advocacy, and the nurse is responsible for seeing that these advocacy needs are met.

 NURSING ALERT

> If the patient begins to emerge from unconsciousness, every measure that is available and appropriate for calming and quieting the patient should be used. Any form of restraint is likely to be countered with resistance, leading to self-injury or to a dangerous increase in ICP. Therefore, physical restraints should be avoided if possible; a written prescription must be obtained if their use is essential for the patient's well-being.

Maintaining Fluid Balance and Managing Nutritional Needs

Hydration status is assessed by examining tissue turgor and mucous membranes, assessing intake and output trends, and analyzing laboratory data. Fluid needs are met initially by administering the required IV fluids. However, IV solutions (and blood component therapy) for patients with intracranial conditions must be administered slowly. If they are administered too rapidly, they can increase ICP. The quantity of fluids administered may be restricted to minimize the possibility of cerebral edema.

If the patient does not recover quickly and sufficiently enough to take adequate fluids and calories by mouth, a feeding or gastrostomy tube will be inserted for the administration of fluids and enteral feedings (Dudek, 2006).

Providing Mouth Care

The mouth is inspected for dryness, inflammation, and crusting. The unconscious patient requires careful oral care, because there is a risk of parotitis if the mouth is not kept scrupulously clean. The mouth is cleansed and rinsed carefully to remove secretions and crusts and to keep the mucous membranes moist. A thin coating of petrolatum on the lips prevents drying, cracking, and encrustations. If the patient has an endotracheal tube, the tube should be moved to the opposite side of the mouth daily to prevent ulceration of the mouth and lips. If the patient is intubated and mechanically ventilated, good oral care is also necessary. Recent evidence shows that a routine of toothbrushing every 8 hours significantly decreases ventilator-associated pneumonia (Fields, 2008).

Maintaining Skin and Joint Integrity

Preventing skin breakdown requires continuing nursing assessment and intervention. Special attention is given to unconscious patients, because they cannot respond to external stimuli. Assessment includes a regular schedule of turning to avoid pressure, which can cause breakdown and necrosis of the skin. Turning also provides kinesthetic (sensation of movement), proprioceptive (awareness of position), and vestibular (equilibrium) stimulation. After turning, the patient is carefully repositioned to prevent ischemic necrosis over pressure areas. Dragging or pulling the patient up in bed must be avoided, because this creates a shearing force and friction on the skin surface (see Chapter 11).

Maintaining correct body position is important; equally important is passive exercise of the extremities to prevent contractures. The use of splints or foam boots aids in the prevention of foot drop and eliminates the pressure of bedding on the toes. The use of trochanter rolls to support the hip joints keeps the legs in proper alignment. The arms are in abduction, the fingers lightly flexed, and the hands in slight supination. The heels of the feet are assessed for pressure areas. Specialty beds, such as fluidized or low-air-loss beds, may be used to decrease pressure on bony prominences (Hickey, 2009).

Preserving Corneal Integrity

Some unconscious patients have their eyes open and have inadequate or absent corneal reflexes. The cornea may become irritated, dried out, or scratched, leading to ulceration. The eyes may be cleansed with cotton balls moistened with sterile normal saline to remove debris and discharge. If artificial tears are prescribed, they may be instilled every 2 hours. Periorbital edema (swelling around the eyes) often occurs after cranial surgery. If cold compresses are prescribed, care must be exerted to avoid contact with the cornea. Eye patches should be used cautiously because of the potential for corneal abrasion from contact with the patch.

Maintaining Body Temperature

High fever in the unconscious patient may be caused by infection of the respiratory or urinary tract, drug reactions, or damage to the hypothalamic temperature-regulating center. A slight elevation of temperature may be caused by dehydration. The environment can be adjusted, depending on the patient's condition, to promote a normal body temperature. If body temperature is elevated, a minimum amount of bedding is used. The room may be cooled to 18.3°C (65°F). However, if the patient is elderly and does not have an elevated temperature, a warmer environment is needed.

Because of damage to the temperature-regulating center in the brain or severe intracranial infection, unconscious patients often develop very high temperatures. Such temperature elevations must be controlled, because the increased metabolic demands of the brain can exceed cerebral circulation and oxygen delivery, potentially resulting in cerebral deterioration (Hickey, 2009). Studies suggest that hyperthermia may contribute to poor outcome after brain injury but not through a decreased brain oxygen level (Spiotta, Stiefel, Heuer, et al., 2008). Persistent hyperthermia with no identified clinical source of infection indicates brain stem damage and a poor prognosis.

 NURSING ALERT

> The body temperature of an unconscious patient is never taken by mouth. Rectal or tympanic (if not contraindicated) temperature measurement is preferred to the less accurate axillary temperature.

Strategies for reducing fever include:
- Removing all bedding over the patient (with the possible exception of a light sheet, towel, or small drape)

- Administering acetaminophen as prescribed
- Giving cool sponge baths and allowing an electric fan to blow over the patient to increase surface cooling
- Using a hypothermia blanket
- Frequent temperature monitoring to assess the patient's response to the therapy and to prevent an excessive decrease in temperature and shivering

Preventing Urinary Retention

The patient with an altered LOC is often incontinent or has urinary retention. The bladder is palpated or scanned at intervals to determine whether urinary retention is present, because a full bladder may be an overlooked cause of overflow incontinence. A portable bladder ultrasound instrument is a useful tool in bladder management and retraining programs (Wu & Baguley, 2005).

If the patient is not voiding, an indwelling urinary catheter is inserted and connected to a closed drainage system. A catheter may also be inserted during the acute phase of illness to monitor urinary output. Because catheters are a major cause of urinary tract infection, the patient is observed for fever and cloudy urine. The area around the urethral orifice is inspected for drainage. The urinary catheter is usually removed if the patient has a stable cardiovascular system and if no diuresis, sepsis, or voiding dysfunction existed before the onset of coma. Although many unconscious patients urinate spontaneously after catheter removal, the bladder should be palpated or scanned with a portable ultrasound device periodically for urinary retention (Wu & Baguley, 2005). An intermittent catheterization program may be initiated to ensure complete emptying of the bladder at intervals, if indicated.

An external catheter (condom catheter) for the male patient and absorbent pads for the female patient can be used for unconscious patients who can urinate spontaneously, although involuntarily. As soon as consciousness is regained, a bladder-training program is initiated (Hickey, 2009). The incontinent patient is monitored frequently for skin irritation and skin breakdown. Appropriate skin care is implemented to prevent these complications.

Promoting Bowel Function

The abdomen is assessed for distention by listening for bowel sounds and measuring the girth of the abdomen with a tape measure. There is a risk of diarrhea from infection, antibiotics, and hyperosmolar fluids. Frequent loose stools may also occur with fecal impaction. Commercial fecal collection bags are available for patients with fecal incontinence.

Immobility and lack of dietary fiber can cause constipation. The nurse monitors the number and consistency of bowel movements and performs a rectal examination for signs of fecal impaction. Stool softeners may be prescribed and can be administered with tube feedings. To facilitate bowel emptying, a glycerin suppository may be indicated. The patient may require an enema every other day to empty the lower colon.

Providing Sensory Stimulation

Once increased ICP is not a problem, sensory stimulation can help overcome the profound sensory deprivation of the unconscious patient. This involves using auditory, visual, olfactory, gustatory, tactile, and kinesthetic activities to stimulate the patient emerging from coma (Gerber, 2005). Efforts are made to restore the sense of daily rhythm by maintaining usual day and night patterns for activity and sleep. The nurse touches and talks to the patient and encourages family members and friends to do so. Communication is extremely important and includes touching the patient and spending enough time with the patient to become sensitive to his or her needs. It is also important to avoid making any negative comments about the patient's status or prognosis in the patient's presence.

The nurse orients the patient to time and place at least once every 8 hours. Sounds from the patient's usual environment may be introduced using a tape recorder. Family members can read to the patient from a favorite book and may suggest radio and television programs that the patient previously enjoyed as a means of enriching the environment and providing familiar input.

When arousing from coma, many patients experience a period of agitation, indicating that they are becoming more aware of their surroundings but still cannot react or communicate in an appropriate fashion. Although this is disturbing for many family members, it is actually a positive clinical sign. At this time, it is necessary to minimize stimulation by limiting background noises, having only one person speak to the patient at a time, giving the patient a longer period of time to respond, and allowing for frequent rest or quiet times. After the patient has regained consciousness, videotaped family or social events may assist the patient in recognizing family and friends and allow him or her to experience missed events.

Various programs of structured sensory stimulation for patients with brain injury have been developed to improve outcomes. Although these are controversial programs with inconsistent results, some research supports the concept of providing structured stimulation (Gerber, 2005).

Meeting the Family's Needs

The family of the patient with altered LOC may be thrown into a sudden state of crisis and go through the process of severe anxiety, denial, anger, remorse, grief, and reconciliation. Depending on the disorder that caused the altered LOC and the extent of the patient's recovery, the family may be unprepared for the changes in the cognitive and physical status of their loved one. If the patient has significant residual deficits, the family may require considerable time, assistance, and support to come to terms with these changes. To help family members mobilize resources and coping skills, the nurse reinforces and clarifies information about the patient's condition, permits the family to be involved in care, and listens to and encourages ventilation of feelings and concerns while supporting decision making about management and placement after hospitalization. Families may benefit from participation in support groups offered through the hospital, rehabilitation facility, or community organizations.

In some circumstances, the family may need to face the death of their loved one. The patient with a neurologic disorder is often pronounced brain dead before the heart stops beating. The term **brain death** describes irreversible loss of all functions of the entire brain, including the brain stem (Burck, Anderson-Shaw, Sheldon, et al., 2006). The term may be misleading to the family because, although brain function has ceased, the patient appears to be alive, with the heart rate and blood pressure sustained by vasoactive medications and breathing continued by mechanical ventilation. When discussing a patient who is brain dead with family members, it is important to provide accurate, timely, understandable, and consistent information (Peiffer, 2007). End-of-life care is discussed in Chapter 17.

Monitoring and Managing Potential Complications

Pneumonia, aspiration, and respiratory failure are potential complications in any patient who has a depressed LOC and who cannot protect the airway or turn, cough, and take deep breaths. The longer the period of unconsciousness, the greater the risk is of pulmonary complications.

Vital signs and respiratory function are monitored closely to detect any signs of respiratory failure or distress. Total blood count and arterial blood gas measurements are assessed to determine whether there are adequate red blood cells to carry oxygen and whether ventilation is effective. Chest physiotherapy and suctioning are initiated to prevent respiratory complications such as pneumonia. Oral care interventions are performed for patients receiving mechanical ventilation to decrease the incidence of pneumonia (Fields, 2008). If pneumonia develops, cultures are obtained to identify the organism so that appropriate antibiotics can be administered.

The patient with altered LOC is monitored closely for evidence of impaired skin integrity, and strategies to prevent skin breakdown and pressure ulcers are continued through all phases of care, including hospitalization, rehabilitation, and home care. Factors that contribute to impaired skin integrity (eg, incontinence, inadequate dietary intake, pressure on bony prominences, edema) are addressed. If pressure ulcers develop, strategies to promote healing are undertaken. Care is taken to prevent bacterial contamination of pressure ulcers, which may lead to sepsis and septic shock. Assessment and management of pressure ulcers are discussed in Chapter 11.

The patient should also be monitored for signs and symptoms of deep vein thrombosis (DVT). Patients who develop DVT are at risk for pulmonary embolism. Prophylaxis such as subcutaneous heparin or low-molecular-weight heparin (Fragmin, Orgaran) should be prescribed if not contraindicated (Vergouwen, Roos & Kamphuisen, 2008). Anti-embolism stockings or pneumatic compression devices should also be prescribed to reduce the risk of clot formation. The nurse observes for signs and symptoms of DVT.

Evaluation

Expected Patient Outcomes

Expected patient outcomes may include the following:

1. Maintains clear airway and demonstrates appropriate breath sounds
2. Experiences no injuries
3. Attains or maintains adequate fluid balance
   a. Has no clinical signs or symptoms of dehydration
   b. Demonstrates normal range of serum electrolytes
   c. Has no clinical signs or symptoms of overhydration

4. Achieves healthy oral mucous membranes
5. Maintains normal skin integrity
6. Has no corneal irritation
7. Attains or maintains thermoregulation
8. Has no urinary retention
9. Has no diarrhea or fecal impaction
10. Receives appropriate sensory stimulation
11. Has family members who cope with crisis
    a. Verbalize fears and concerns
    b. Participate in patient's care and provide sensory stimulation by talking and touching
12. Is free of complications
    a. Has arterial blood gas values or O_2 saturation levels within normal range
    b. Displays no signs or symptoms of pneumonia
    c. Exhibits intact skin over pressure areas
    d. Does not develop DVT or pulmonary embolism (PE)

INCREASED INTRACRANIAL PRESSURE

The rigid cranial vault contains brain tissue (1400 g), blood (75 mL), and CSF (75 mL). The volume and pressure of these three components are usually in a state of equilibrium and produce the ICP. ICP is usually measured in the lateral ventricles, with the normal pressure being 0 to 10 mm Hg, and 15 mm Hg being the upper limit of normal (Hickey, 2009).

The **Monro-Kellie hypothesis** states that, because of the limited space for expansion within the skull, an increase in any one of the components causes a change in the volume of the others. Because brain tissue has limited space to expand, compensation typically is accomplished by displacing or shifting CSF, increasing the absorption or diminishing the production of CSF, or decreasing cerebral blood volume. Without such changes, ICP begins to rise. Under normal circumstances, minor changes in blood volume and CSF volume occur constantly as a result of alterations in intrathoracic pressure (coughing, sneezing, straining), posture, blood pressure, and systemic oxygen and carbon dioxide levels (Hickey, 2009).

Pathophysiology

Increased ICP affects many patients with acute neurologic conditions because pathologic conditions alter the relationship between intracranial volume and ICP. Although elevated ICP is most commonly associated with head injury, it also may be seen as a secondary effect in other conditions, such as brain tumors, subarachnoid hemorrhage, and toxic and viral encephalopathies. Increased ICP from any cause decreases cerebral perfusion, stimulates further swelling (edema), and may shift brain tissue, resulting in **herniation,** a dire and frequently fatal event.

Decreased Cerebral Blood Flow

Increased ICP may reduce cerebral blood flow, resulting in ischemia and cell death. In the early stages of cerebral ischemia, the vasomotor centers are stimulated and the systemic pressure rises to maintain cerebral blood flow. Usually, this is accompanied by a slow bounding pulse and respiratory irregularities. These changes in blood pressure, pulse, and respiration are important clinically because they suggest increased ICP.

The concentration of carbon dioxide in the blood and in the brain tissue also plays a role in the regulation of cerebral blood flow. An increase in the arterial partial pressure of carbon dioxide ($PaCO_2$) causes cerebral vasodilation, leading to increased cerebral blood flow and increased ICP. A decrease in $PaCO_2$ has a vasoconstrictive effect, limiting blood flow to the brain. Decreased venous outflow may also increase cerebral blood volume, thus raising ICP.

Cerebral Edema

Cerebral edema or swelling is defined as an abnormal accumulation of water or fluid in the intracellular space, extracellular space, or both, associated with an increase in the volume of brain tissue. Edema can occur in the gray, white, or interstitial matter. As brain tissue swells within the rigid skull, several mechanisms attempt to compensate for the increasing ICP. These compensatory mechanisms include autoregulation as well as decreased production and flow of CSF. **Autoregulation** refers to the brain's ability to change the diameter of its blood vessels to maintain a constant cerebral blood flow during alterations in systemic blood pressure. This mechanism can be impaired in patients who are experiencing a pathologic and sustained increase in ICP.

Cerebral Response to Increased Intracranial Pressure

As ICP rises, compensatory mechanisms in the brain work to maintain blood flow and prevent tissue damage. The brain can maintain a steady perfusion pressure if the arterial systolic blood pressure is 50 to 150 mm Hg and the ICP is less than 40 mm Hg. Changes in ICP are closely linked with cerebral perfusion pressure (CPP). The CPP is calculated by subtracting the ICP from the mean arterial pressure (MAP). For example, if the MAP is 100 mm Hg and the ICP is 15 mm Hg, then the CPP is 85 mm Hg. The normal CPP is 70 to 100 mm Hg (Hickey, 2009). As ICP rises and the autoregulatory mechanism of the brain is overwhelmed, the CPP can increase to greater than 100 mm Hg or decrease to less than 50 mm Hg. Patients with a CPP of less than 50 mm Hg experience irreversible neurologic damage. Therefore, the CPP must be maintained at 70 to 80 mm Hg to ensure adequate blood flow to the brain. If ICP is equal to MAP, cerebral circulation ceases.

A clinical phenomenon known as the **Cushing's response** (or Cushing's reflex) is seen when cerebral blood flow decreases significantly. When ischemic, the vasomotor center triggers an increase in arterial pressure in an effort to overcome the increased ICP. A sympathetically mediated response causes an increase in the systolic blood pressure with a widening of the pulse pressure and cardiac slowing. This response is seen clinically as an increase in systolic blood pressure, widening of the pulse pressure, and reflex slowing of the heart rate. It is a late sign requiring immediate intervention; however, perfusion may be recoverable if the Cushing's response is treated rapidly.

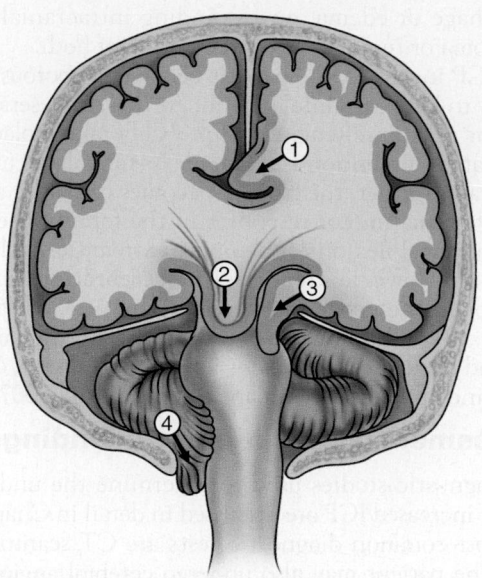

Figure 61-2 Brain with intracranial shifts from supratentorial lesions. *1,* Herniation of the cingulate gyrus under the falx cerebri. *2,* Central transtentorial herniation. *3,* Uncal herniation of the temporal lobe into the tentorial notch. *4,* Infratentorial herniation of the cerebral tonsils. Adapted from Porth, C. M. & Matfin, G. (2009). *Pathophysiology: Concepts of altered health states* (8th ed.). Philadelphia: Lippincott Williams & Wilkins.

At a certain point, the brain's ability to autoregulate becomes ineffective and decompensation (ischemia and infarction) begins. When this occurs, the patient exhibits significant changes in mental status and vital signs. The bradycardia, hypertension, and bradypnea associated with this deterioration are known as **Cushing's triad,** a grave sign. At this point, herniation of the brain stem and occlusion of the cerebral blood flow occur if therapeutic intervention is not initiated. Herniation refers to the shifting of brain tissue from an area of high pressure to an area of lower pressure (Fig. 61-2). The herniated tissue exerts pressure on the brain area into which it has shifted, which interferes with the blood supply in that area. Cessation of cerebral blood flow results in cerebral ischemia, infarction, and brain death.

Clinical Manifestations

If ICP increases to the point at which the brain's ability to adjust has reached its limits, neural function is impaired; this may be manifested at first by clinical changes in LOC and later by abnormal respiratory and vasomotor responses.

 NURSING ALERT

The earliest sign of increasing ICP is a change in LOC. Slowing of speech and delay in response to verbal suggestions are other early indicators.

Any sudden change in the patient's condition, such as restlessness (without apparent cause), confusion, or increasing drowsiness, has neurologic significance. These signs may result from compression of the brain due to swelling from hemorrhage or edema, an expanding intracranial lesion (hematoma or tumor), or a combination of both.

As ICP increases, the patient becomes stuporous, reacting only to loud or painful stimuli. At this stage, serious impairment of brain circulation is probably taking place, and immediate intervention is required. As neurologic function deteriorates further, the patient becomes comatose and exhibits abnormal motor responses in the form of **decortication** (abnormal flexion of the upper extremities and extension of the lower extremities), **decerebration** (extreme extension of the upper and lower extremities), or flaccidity (see Fig. 61-1). If the coma is profound, with the pupils dilated and fixed and respirations impaired or absent, death is usually inevitable (Posner, Saper, Schiff, et al., 2007).

Assessment and Diagnostic Findings

The diagnostic studies used to determine the underlying cause of increased ICP are discussed in detail in Chapter 60. The most common diagnostic tests are CT scanning and MRI. The patient may also undergo cerebral angiography, PET, or SPECT. Transcranial Doppler studies provide information about cerebral blood flow. The patient with increased ICP may also undergo electrophysiologic monitoring to observe cerebral blood flow indirectly. Evoked potential monitoring measures the electrical potentials produced by nerve tissue in response to external stimulation (auditory, visual, or sensory). Lumbar puncture is avoided in patients with increased ICP, because the sudden release of pressure in the lumbar area can cause the brain to herniate (Mazzoni, Pearson & Rowland, 2006). (See Chapter 60 for further discussion of lumbar puncture and other diagnostic tests.)

Complications

Complications of increased ICP include brain stem herniation, diabetes insipidus, and syndrome of inappropriate antidiuretic hormone (SIADH).

Brain stem herniation results from an excessive increase in ICP in which the pressure builds in the cranial vault and the brain tissue presses down on the brain stem. This increasing pressure on the brain stem results in cessation of blood flow to the brain, leading to irreversible brain anoxia and brain death.

Diabetes insipidus is the result of decreased secretion of antidiuretic hormone (ADH). The patient has excessive urine output, decreased urine osmolality, and serum hyperosmolarity (Porth & Matfin, 2009). Therapy consists of administration of fluids, electrolyte replacement, and vasopressin (desmopressin, [DDAVP]) therapy. Diabetes insipidus is discussed in Chapters 14 and 42.

SIADH is the result of increased secretion of ADH. The patient becomes volume overloaded, urine output diminishes, and serum sodium concentration becomes dilute. Treatment of SIADH includes fluid restriction (less than 800 mL/day with no free water), which is usually sufficient to correct the hyponatremia. In severe cases, careful administration of a 3% hypertonic saline solution may be therapeutic (Mortimer & Jancik, 2006). The change in serum sodium concentration should not exceed a correction rate of approximately 1.3 mEq/L/h. Further discussion of SIADH is presented in Chapters 14 and 42.

Medical Management

Increased ICP is a true emergency and must be treated promptly. Invasive monitoring of ICP is an important component of management. Immediate management to relieve increased ICP requires decreasing cerebral edema, lowering the volume of CSF, or decreasing cerebral blood volume while maintaining cerebral perfusion. These goals are accomplished by administering osmotic diuretics, restricting fluids, draining CSF, controlling fever, maintaining systemic blood pressure and oxygenation, and reducing cellular metabolic demands. Management of increased ICP is discussed in Chapter 63.

Monitoring Intracranial Pressure and Cerebral Oxygenation

The purposes of ICP monitoring are to identify increased pressure early in its course (before cerebral damage occurs), to quantify the degree of elevation, to initiate appropriate treatment, to provide access to CSF for sampling and drainage, and to evaluate the effectiveness of treatment. ICP can be monitored with the use of an intraventricular catheter (ventriculostomy), a subarachnoid bolt, an epidural or subdural catheter, or a fiberoptic transducer-tipped catheter placed in the subdural space or in the ventricle (Fig. 61-3).

When a **ventriculostomy** or ventricular catheter monitoring device is used for monitoring ICP, a fine-bore catheter is inserted into a lateral ventricle, preferably in the nondominant hemisphere of the brain (Hickey, 2009). The catheter is connected by a fluid-filled system to a transducer, which records the pressure in the form of an electrical impulse. In addition to obtaining continuous ICP recordings, the ventricular catheter allows CSF to drain, particularly during acute increases in pressure. The ventriculostomy can also be

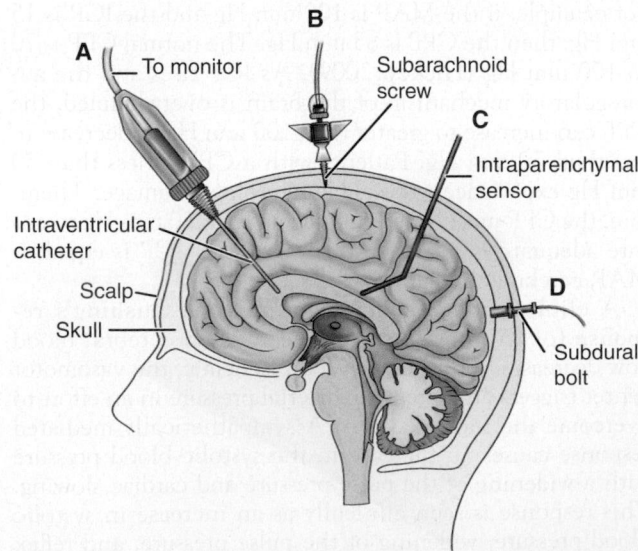

Figure 61-3 Intracranial pressure monitoring. A device may be placed in **(A)** the ventricle **(B)** the subarachnoid space **(C)** the intraparenchymal space or **(D)** the subdural space.

used to drain blood from the ventricle. Continuous drainage of CSF under pressure control is an effective method of treating intracranial hypertension. Another advantage of a ventricular catheter is access for the intraventricular administration of medications and the occasional instillation of air or a contrast agent for ventriculography. Complications associated with its use include infection, meningitis, ventricular collapse, occlusion of the catheter by brain tissue or blood, and problems with the monitoring system.

The **subarachnoid screw or bolt** is a hollow device that is inserted through the skull and dura mater into the cranial subarachnoid space (Hickey, 2009). It has the advantage of not requiring a ventricular puncture. The subarachnoid screw is attached to a pressure transducer, and the output is recorded on an oscilloscope. The hollow screw technique also has the advantage of avoiding complications from brain shift and small ventricle size. Complications include infection and blockage of the screw by clot or brain tissue, which leads to a loss of pressure tracing and a decrease in accuracy at high ICP readings.

An **epidural monitor** uses a pneumatic flow sensor to detect ICP. The epidural ICP monitoring system has a low incidence of infection and complications and appears to read pressures accurately. Calibration of the system is maintained automatically, and abnormal pressure waves trigger an alarm system. One disadvantage of the epidural catheter is the inability to withdraw CSF for analysis.

A **fiberoptic monitor,** or transducer-tipped catheter, is an alternative to other intraventricular, subarachnoid, and subdural systems (Haitsma & Maas, 2007). The miniature transducer reflects pressure changes, which are converted to electrical signals in an amplifier and displayed on a digital monitor. The catheter can be inserted into the ventricle, subarachnoid space, subdural space, or brain parenchyma or under a bone flap. If inserted into the ventricle, it can also be used in conjunction with a CSF drainage device.

Interpreting Intracranial Pressure Waveforms

Waves of high pressure and troughs of relatively normal pressure indicate changes in ICP. Waveforms are captured and recorded on an oscilloscope. These waves have been classified as A waves (plateau waves), B waves, and C waves (Fig. 61-4). The plateau waves (A waves) are transient, paroxysmal, recurring elevations of ICP that may last 5 to 20 minutes and range in amplitude from 50 to 100 mm Hg (AANN, 2005). Plateau waves have clinical significance and indicate changes in vascular volume within the intracranial compartment that are beginning to compromise cerebral perfusion. The A waves may increase in amplitude and frequency, reflecting cerebral ischemia and brain damage that can occur before overt signs and symptoms of raised ICP are seen clinically. B waves are shorter (30 seconds to 2 minutes) and have smaller amplitude (up to 50 mm Hg). They have less clinical significance, but if seen in a series in a patient with depressed consciousness, they may precede the appearance of A waves. B waves may be seen in patients with intracranial hypertension and decreased intracranial compliance. C waves are small, rhythmic oscillations with frequencies of approximately six per minute. They appear to be related to rhythmic variations of the systemic arterial blood pressure and respirations. The clinical significance of C waves is unknown (Littlejohns & Bader, 2009).

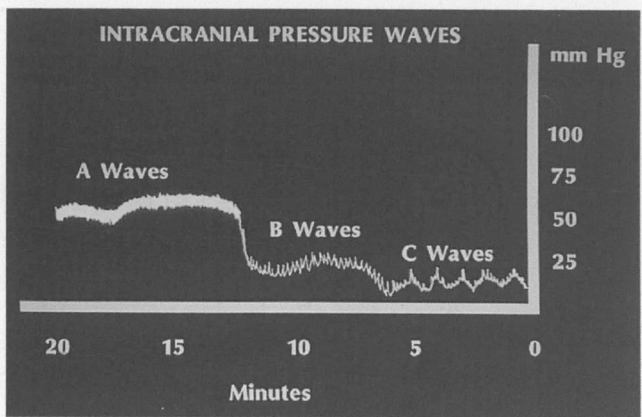

Figure 61-4 Intracranial pressure waves. Composite diagram of A (plateau) waves, which indicate cerebral ischemia; B waves, which indicate intracranial hypertension and variations in the respiratory cycle; and C waves, which relate to variations in systemic arterial pressure and respirations.

Other Neurologic Monitoring Systems

Additional trends in neurologic monitoring include **microdialysis** of the patient with a brain injury (McAdoo & Wu, 2008). Cortical probes are placed near the injured area and are used to measure levels of glutamate, lactate, pyruvate, and glucose, substances that reflect the metabolic function of the brain. Some researchers theorize that direct measurements of glucose and energy byproducts in the brain will lead to better management of these patients and, ultimately, to improved outcomes.

An additional trend is monitoring of cerebral oxygenation through monitoring of the oxygen saturation in the jugular venous bulb ($SjvO_2$) or via a catheter in the brain. Cerebral oxygenation is thought to be important because changes in cerebral perfusion may reflect an increase in ICP. Readings taken from a catheter residing in the jugular outflow tract allow for a comparison of arterial and venous oxygen saturation, and the balance of cerebral oxygen supply and demand is demonstrated. Venous jugular desaturations can reflect early cerebral ischemia, alerting the clinician before an increase in ICP occurs. Minimizing cerebral desaturations can potentially improve outcomes (Haitsma & Maas, 2007). This type of monitoring is now widely available and has been successfully used to identify secondary brain insults. A limiting factor is that this saturation reflects overall perfusion of the brain rather than that of a specific injured area (Lescot, Abdennour, Boch, et al., 2008).

Another method of measuring cerebral oxygenation and temperature is by inserting a fiberoptic catheter into the brain matter (Jaeger, Soehle & Meixensberger, 2005). The most common system is LICOX (manufactured by Integra NeuroSciences, Plainsboro, NJ; Fig. 61-5). The system includes a monitor with a screen for the display of oxygen and temperature values and cables that connect to the monitoring probes in the brain (Hickey, 2009).

Decreasing Cerebral Edema

Osmotic diuretics such as mannitol may be administered to dehydrate the brain tissue and reduce cerebral edema. They

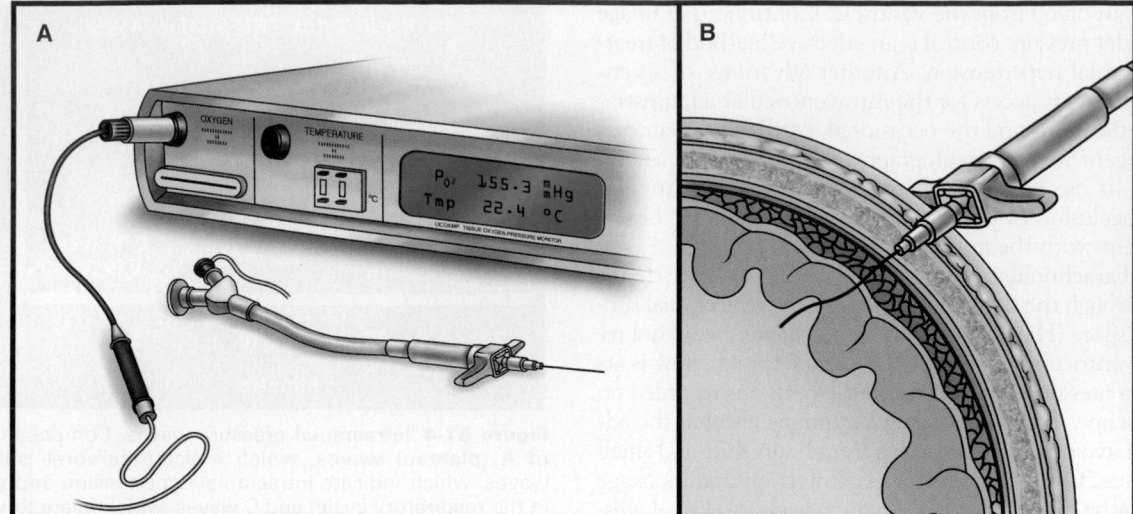

Figure 61-5 LICOX catheter system. **A,** The brain tissue oxygen catheter and monitor. **B,** Placement of the catheter in brain white matter. Redrawn with permission of Integra NeuroSciences, Plainsboro, NJ.

act by drawing water across intact membranes, thereby reducing the volume of the brain and extracellular fluid. An indwelling urinary catheter is usually inserted to monitor urinary output and to manage the resulting diuresis. If the patient is receiving osmotic diuretics, serum osmolality should be determined to assess hydration status. If a brain tumor is the cause of the increased ICP, corticosteroids (eg, dexamethasone) help reduce the edema surrounding the tumor.

Another method for decreasing cerebral edema is fluid restriction (Hickey, 2009). Limiting overall fluid intake leads to dehydration and hemoconcentration, which draws fluid across the osmotic gradient and decreases cerebral edema. Conversely, overhydration of the patient with increased ICP is avoided, because it increases cerebral edema.

Researchers have long hypothesized that lowering body temperature would decrease cerebral edema by reducing the oxygen and metabolic requirements of the brain, thus protecting the brain from continued ischemia. If body metabolism can be reduced by lowering the body temperature, the collateral circulation in the brain may be able to provide an adequate blood supply to the brain. The effect of hypothermia on ICP requires more study; thus far, induced hypothermia has not consistently been shown to be beneficial for patients with brain injury. Inducing and maintaining hypothermia is a major clinical treatment and requires knowledge and skilled nursing observation and management. The type and length of rewarming techniques after hypothermia may also be factors in the outcome of patients with neurologic injuries (Lescot, et al., 2008).

Maintaining Cerebral Perfusion

Cardiac output may be manipulated to provide adequate perfusion to the brain. Improvements in cardiac output are made using fluid volume and inotropic agents such as dobutamine (Dobutrex) and norepinephrine (Levophed). The effectiveness of the cardiac output is reflected in the CPP, which is maintained at greater than 70 mm Hg (Lescot,

et al., 2008). A lower CPP indicates that the cardiac output is insufficient to maintain adequate cerebral perfusion. $SjvO_2$ and LICOX, described earlier, assist in monitoring cerebral perfusion.

Reducing Cerebrospinal Fluid and Intracranial Blood Volume

CSF drainage is frequently performed, because the removal of CSF with a ventriculostomy drain can dramatically reduce ICP and restore CPP. Caution should be used in draining CSF, however, because excessive drainage may result in collapse of the ventricles and herniation. The reduction in $PaCO_2$ may result in hypoxia, ischemia, and an increase in cerebral lactate levels. Maintaining the $PaCO_2$ at greater than 30 mm Hg may prove beneficial (Hickey, 2009).

Controlling Fever

Preventing a temperature elevation is critical, because fever increases cerebral metabolism and the rate at which cerebral edema forms. Strategies to reduce body temperature include administration of antipyretic medications, as prescribed, and use of a hypothermia blanket. Additional strategies for reducing fever were previously discussed in the Nursing Process section on altered LOC. The patient's temperature is monitored closely, and the patient is observed for shivering, which should be avoided because it is associated with increased oxygen consumption, increased levels of circulating catecholamines, and increased vasoconstriction (Mcilvoy, 2007).

Maintaining Oxygenation and Reducing Metabolic Demands

Arterial blood gases and pulse oximetry are monitored to ensure that systemic oxygenation remains optimal. Metabolic demands may be reduced through the administration of high doses of barbiturates if the patient is unresponsive to conventional treatment. The mechanism by which barbiturates decrease ICP and protect the brain is uncertain, but the resultant comatose state is thought to reduce the metabolic requirements of the brain, thus providing cerebral protection (Bader, Arbour & Palmer, 2005).

Another method of reducing cellular metabolic demand and improving oxygenation is the administration of paralyzing medication such as propofol (Diprivan). The patient who receives these agents cannot move; this decreases the metabolic demands and results in a decrease in cerebral oxygen demand. Paralyzing agents do not produce either sedation or analgesia, which must be provided, because the patient cannot respond to or report pain. The most common agents used for barbiturate or paralytic therapy are pentobarbital (Nembutal), thiopental (Pentothal), and propofol (Bader, et al., 2005).

If barbiturates or paralyzing agents are used, the ability to perform serial neurologic assessments is lost. Therefore, other monitoring tools are needed to assess the patient's status and response to therapy. Important parameters that must be assessed include ICP, blood pressure, heart rate, respiratory rate, and the patient's response to ventilator therapy (eg, "bucking the ventilator"). The level of pharmacologic paralysis is adjusted based on serum levels of the medications administered and the assessed parameters. Potential complications include hypotension caused by decreased sympathetic tone and myocardial depression.

Patients receiving high doses of barbiturates or pharmacologic paralyzing agents require continuous cardiac monitoring, endotracheal intubation, mechanical ventilation, and arterial pressure monitoring, as well as ICP monitoring. In addition, serum barbiturate levels must be routinely monitored (Lescot, et al., 2008).

NURSING PROCESS

THE PATIENT WITH INCREASED INTRACRANIAL PRESSURE

Assessment

Initial assessment of the patient with increased ICP includes obtaining a history of events leading to the present illness and the pertinent past medical history. It is usually necessary to obtain this information from family or friends. The neurologic examination should be as complete as the patient's condition allows. It includes an evaluation of mental status, LOC, cranial nerve function, cerebellar function (balance and coordination), reflexes, and motor and sensory function. Because the patient is critically ill, ongoing assessment is more focused, including pupil checks, assessment of selected cranial nerves, frequent measurements of vital signs and ICP, and use of the Glasgow Coma Scale. Assessment of the patient with altered LOC is summarized in Table 61-1.

Diagnosis

Nursing Diagnoses

Based on the assessment data, the major nursing diagnoses for patients with increased ICP include the following:
- Ineffective airway clearance related to diminished protective reflexes (cough, gag)

- Ineffective breathing patterns related to neurologic dysfunction (brain stem compression, structural displacement)
- Ineffective cerebral tissue perfusion related to the effects of increased ICP
- Deficient fluid volume related to fluid restriction
- Risk for infection related to ICP monitoring system (fiberoptic or intraventricular catheter)

Other relevant nursing diagnoses are included in the section on altered LOC.

Collaborative Problems/Potential Complications

Based on the assessment data, potential complications include:
- Brain stem herniation
- Diabetes insipidus
- SIADH

Planning and Goals

The goals for the patient include maintenance of a patent airway, normalization of respiration, adequate cerebral tissue perfusion through reduction in ICP, restoration of fluid balance, absence of infection, and absence of complications.

Nursing Interventions

Maintaining a Patent Airway

The patency of the airway is assessed. Secretions that are obstructing the airway must be suctioned with care, because transient elevations of ICP occur with suctioning (Hickey, 2009). Hypoxia caused by poor oxygenation leads to cerebral ischemia and edema. Coughing is discouraged because it increases ICP. The lung fields are auscultated at least every 8 hours to determine the presence of adventitious sounds or any areas of congestion. Elevating the head of the bed may aid in clearing secretions and improve venous drainage of the brain.

Achieving an Adequate Breathing Pattern

The patient must be monitored constantly for respiratory irregularities. Increased pressure on the frontal lobes or deep midline structures may result in Cheyne-Stokes respirations, whereas pressure in the midbrain can cause hyperventilation. If the lower portion of the brain stem (the pons and medulla) is involved, respirations become irregular and eventually cease.

If hyperventilation therapy is deemed appropriate to reduce ICP (by causing cerebral vasoconstriction and a decrease in cerebral blood volume), the nurse collaborates with the respiratory therapist in monitoring the $PaCO_2$, which is usually maintained at less than 30 mm Hg (Hickey, 2009).

A neurologic observation record (Fig. 61-6) is maintained, and all observations are made in relation to the patient's baseline condition. Repeated assessments of the patient are made (sometimes minute by minute) so that improvement or deterioration may be noted immediately. If the patient's condition deteriorates, preparations are made for surgical intervention.

Optimizing Cerebral Tissue Perfusion

In addition to ongoing nursing assessment, strategies are initiated to reduce factors contributing to the elevation of ICP (Table 61-2).

NURSING NEUROLOGICAL CRITICAL CARE FLOWSHEET		ADDRESSOGRAPH														
	Date															
	Time															
	Initials															
Level of orientation (✓)	Person															
	Place															
	Date and time															
	No orientation															
Awakens to (✓)	Voice															
	Touch															
	Noxious stimuli															
	Painful stimuli															
	No response															
Best verbal response (✓)	Clear and appropriate															
	Clear and inappropriate															
	Difficulty speaking*															
	Perseveration															
	Aphasic expressive (non-fluent)															
	Aphasic receptive (fluent)															
	Sounds no speech															
	No verbal response															
	ETT/TRACH															
Best motor response (✓)	Moves all extremities purposefully															
	Withdraws and lifts to painful stimuli															
	Moves to painful stimuli															
	Decorticates (spinal reflex)															
	Decerebrates (spinal reflex)															
	No motor response															
Best motor strength upper extremities (✓)	No drifts (R/L)	R/L	R/L	R/L	R/L	R/L	R/L	R/L	R/L	R/L	R/L	R/L	R/L	R/L	R/L
	Drift (R/L)	R/L	R/L	R/L	R/L	R/L	R/L	R/L	R/L	R/L	R/L	R/L	R/L	R/L	R/L
	Can only lift forearm (R/L)	R/L	R/L	R/L	R/L	R/L	R/L	R/L	R/L	R/L	R/L	R/L	R/L	R/L	R/L
	Trace movement of hand or arm (R/L)	R/L	R/L	R/L	R/L	R/L	R/L	R/L	R/L	R/L	R/L	R/L	R/L	R/L	R/L
	Trace movement of fingers only (R/L)	R/L	R/L	R/L	R/L	R/L	R/L	R/L	R/L	R/L	R/L	R/L	R/L	R/L	R/L
	No motor response (R/L)	R/L	R/L	R/L	R/L	R/L	R/L	R/L	R/L	R/L	R/L	R/L	R/L	R/L	R/L
Best strength lower extremities (✓)	Raises leg off bed (R/L)	R/L	R/L	R/L	R/L	R/L	R/L	R/L	R/L	R/L	R/L	R/L	R/L	R/L	R/L
	Drags heel on bed and lifts knee (R/L)	R/L	R/L	R/L	R/L	R/L	R/L	R/L	R/L	R/L	R/L	R/L	R/L	R/L	R/L
	Trace movement of foot or leg (R/L)	R/L	R/L	R/L	R/L	R/L	R/L	R/L	R/L	R/L	R/L	R/L	R/L	R/L	R/L
	Trace movement of toes only (R/L)	R/L	R/L	R/L	R/L	R/L	R/L	R/L	R/L	R/L	R/L	R/L	R/L	R/L	R/L
	No response (R/L)	R/L	R/L	R/L	R/L	R/L	R/L	R/L	R/L	R/L	R/L	R/L	R/L	R/L	R/L
Seizure activity (✓)	No seizure activity															
	With loss of consciousness*															
	Without loss of consciousness*															
Ataxia (✓)	Gross ataxia															
	Fine motor ataxia															
	Does not apply															
ICP monitoring	Ventriculostomy mL															
	ICP mm Hg															
	Not applicable															

*= FURTHER DOCUMENTATION IS REQUIRED TO VALIDATE ASSESSMENT

Figure 61-6 A neurologic assessment flow chart.

PUPIL GAUGE (mm)

·	•	●	●	●
2	3	4	5	6

●	●	●
7	8	9

B=Brisk, S=Sluggish, F=Fixed

ADDRESSOGRAPH

		Date											
		Time											
		Initials											
Incision +/−	Dry and intact												
	Drainage												
Pupils: refer to above gauge (✓) (+)=Present (−)=Absent	Size (R/L)	R/L	R/L	R/L	R/L	R/L	R/L	R/L	R/L	R/L	R/L	R/L	R/L
	Regular (R/L)	R/L	R/L	R/L	R/L	R/L	R/L	R/L	R/L	R/L	R/L	R/L	R/L
	Irregular* (R/L)	R/L	R/L	R/L	R/L	R/L	R/L	R/L	R/L	R/L	R/L	R/L	R/L
	Reaction (R/L) (B) - (S) - (F)	R/L	R/L	R/L	R/L	R/L	R/L	R/L	R/L	R/L	R/L	R/L	R/L
	Ptosis (R/L) (+) (−)	R/L	R/L	R/L	R/L	R/L	R/L	R/L	R/L	R/L	R/L	R/L	R/L
	Gaze preference (R/L) (+)* (−)	R/L	R/L	R/L	R/L	R/L	R/L	R/L	R/L	R/L	R/L	R/L	R/L
Meningeal signs (+)=Present (−)=Absent	Headache												
	Nuchal rigidity												
	Photophobia												
Visual fields (+)=Present (−)=Absent* NA=Not applicable	Right upper outer												
	Right lower outer												
	Left upper outer												
	Left lower outer												
Nystagmus (+)=Present (−)=Absent	Lateral (R/L)	R/L	R/L	R/L	R/L	R/L	R/L	R/L	R/L	R/L	R/L	R/L	R/L
	Vertical (R/L)	R/L	R/L	R/L	R/L	R/L	R/L	R/L	R/L	R/L	R/L	R/L	R/L
Cranial nerves (+)=Present (−)=Absent	III, IV, VI, Extraocular movements												
	VII – Peripheral facial droop (R/L)	R/L	R/L	R/L	R/L	R/L	R/L	R/L	R/L	R/L	R/L	R/L	R/L
	XII – Tongue deviation (R/L)	R/L	R/L	R/L	R/L	R/L	R/L	R/L	R/L	R/L	R/L	R/L	R/L
	IX – Gag reflex												
	V, VII – Corneal reflex (R/L)	R/L	R/L	R/L	R/L	R/L	R/L	R/L	R/L	R/L	R/L	R/L	R/L
	X, IX – Cough reflex												
	Doll's eyes if appropriate												
Follows commands	Two step verbal command												
	One step verbal command												
	Unable to follow command												

*= FURTHER DOCUMENTATION IS REQUIRED TO VALIDATE ASSESSMENT

Initials	Signature	Title	Initials	Signature	Title

Figure 61-6 (*Continued*).

Table 61-2	INCREASED INTRACRANIAL PRESSURE AND INTERVENTIONS		
Factor	**Physiology**	**Interventions**	**Rationale**
Cerebral edema	Can be caused by contusion, tumor, or abscess; water intoxication (hypo-osmolality); alteration in the blood–brain barrier (protein leaks into the tissue, causing water to follow)	Administer osmotic diuretics as prescribed (monitor serum osmolality). Maintain head of bed elevated 30 degrees. Maintain alignment of the head.	Promotes venous return. Prevents impairment of venous return through the jugular veins
Hypoxia	A decrease in the PaO_2 causes cerebral vasodilation at <60 mm Hg.	Maintain PaO_2 >60 mm Hg. Maintain oxygen therapy. Monitor arterial blood gas values. Suction when needed. Maintain a patent airway.	Prevents hypoxia and vasodilation
Hypercapnia (elevated $PaCO_2$)	Causes vasodilation	Maintain $PaCO_2$ (normally 35–45 mm Hg) by establishing ventilation.	Normalizing $PaCO_2$ minimizes vasodilation and thus reduces the cerebral blood volume
Impaired venous return	Increases the cerebral blood volume	Maintain head alignment. Elevate head of bed 30 degrees.	Hyperextension, rotation, or hyper-flexion of the neck causes decreased venous return
Increase in intrathoracic or abdominal pressure	An increase in these presures due to coughing, PEEP, or Valsalva maneuver causes a decrease in venous return.	Monitor arterial blood gas values and keep PEEP as low as possible. Provide humidified oxygen. Administer stool softeners as prescribed.	To keep secretions loose and easy to suction or expectorate. Soft bowel movements will prevent straining or Valsalva maneuver

Proper positioning helps reduce ICP. The patient's head is kept in a neutral (midline) position, maintained with the use of a cervical collar if necessary, to promote venous drainage. Elevation of the head is maintained at 30 to 45 degrees unless contraindicated (Littlejohns & Bader, 2009). Extreme rotation of the neck and flexion of the neck are avoided, because compression or distortion of the jugular veins increases ICP. Extreme hip flexion is also avoided, because this position causes an increase in intra-abdominal and intrathoracic pressures, which can produce an increase in ICP. Relatively minor changes in position can significantly affect ICP. If monitoring reveals that turning the patient raises ICP, rotating beds, turning sheets, and holding the patient's head during turning may minimize the stimuli that increase ICP.

The Valsalva maneuver, which can be produced by straining at defecation or even moving in bed, raises ICP and is to be avoided. Stool softeners may be prescribed. If the patient is alert and able to eat, a diet high in fiber may be indicated. Abdominal distention, which increases intra-abdominal and intrathoracic pressure and ICP, should be noted. Enemas and cathartics are avoided if possible. When moving or being turned in bed, the patient can be instructed to exhale (which opens the glottis) to avoid the Valsalva maneuver.

Mechanical ventilation presents unique problems for the patient with increased ICP. Before suctioning, the patient should be preoxygenated and briefly hyperventilated using 100% oxygen on the ventilator. Suctioning should not last longer than 15 seconds. High levels of positive end-expiratory pressure (PEEP) are avoided, because they may decrease venous return to the heart and decrease venous drainage from the brain through increased intrathoracic pressure (Littlejohns & Bader, 2009).

Activities that increase ICP, as indicated by changes in waveforms, should be avoided if possible. Spacing of nursing interventions may prevent transient increases in ICP.

During nursing interventions, the ICP should not increase more than 25 mm Hg, and it should return to baseline levels within 5 minutes. Patients with increased ICP should not demonstrate a significant increase in pressure or change in the ICP waveform. Patients with the potential for a significant increase in ICP may need sedation and a paralytic agent before initiation of nursing activities (Olsen & Graffagnino, 2005).

Emotional stress and frequent arousal from sleep are avoided. A calm atmosphere is maintained. Environmental stimuli (eg, noise, conversation) should be minimal.

Maintaining Negative Fluid Balance

The administration of osmotic and loop diuretics is part of the treatment protocol to reduce ICP. Corticosteroids may be used to reduce cerebral edema (except when it results from trauma), and fluids may be restricted. All of these treatment modalities promote dehydration.

Skin turgor, mucous membranes, urine output, and serum and urine osmolality are monitored to assess fluid status. If IV fluids are prescribed, the nurse ensures that they are administered at a slow to moderate rate with an IV infusion pump, to prevent too-rapid administration and avoid overhydration. For the patient receiving mannitol, the nurse observes for the possible development of heart failure and pulmonary edema, because the intent of treatment is to promote a shift of fluid from the intracellular to the intravascular compartment, thus controlling cerebral edema.

For patients undergoing dehydrating procedures, vital signs, including blood pressure, must be monitored to assess fluid volume status. An indwelling urinary catheter is inserted to permit assessment of renal function and fluid status. During the acute phase, urine output is monitored hourly. An output greater than 200 mL/h for 2 consecutive hours may indicate the onset of diabetes insipidus (Hickey, 2009).

These patients need careful oral hygiene, because mouth dryness occurs with dehydration. Frequently rinsing the mouth with nondrying solutions, lubricating the lips, and removing encrustations relieve dryness and promote comfort.

Preventing Infection

The risk of infection is greatest when ICP is monitored with an intraventricular catheter and increases with the duration of the monitoring. Most health care facilities have written protocols for managing these systems and maintaining their sterility; strict adherence to the protocols is essential.

Aseptic technique must be used when managing the system and changing the ventricular drainage bag. The drainage system is also checked for loose connections, because they can cause leakage and contamination of the CSF as well as inaccurate readings of ICP. The nurse observes the character of the CSF drainage and reports increasing cloudiness or blood. The patient is monitored for signs and symptoms of meningitis: fever, chills, nuchal (neck) rigidity, and increasing or persistent headache. (See Chapter 64 for a discussion of meningitis.)

Monitoring and Managing Potential Complications

The primary complication of increased ICP is brain herniation resulting in death (see Fig. 61-2). Nursing management focuses on detecting early signs of increasing ICP, because medical interventions are usually ineffective once later signs develop. Frequent neurologic assessments and documentation and analysis of trends will reveal the subtle changes that may indicate increasing ICP.

DETECTING EARLY INDICATIONS OF INCREASING INTRACRANIAL PRESSURE. The nurse assesses for and immediately reports any of the following early signs or symptoms of increasing ICP:

- Disorientation, restlessness, increased respiratory effort, purposeless movements, and mental confusion; these are early clinical indications of increasing ICP because the brain cells responsible for cognition are extremely sensitive to decreased oxygenation
- Pupillary changes and impaired extraocular movements; these occur as the increasing pressure displaces the brain against the oculomotor and optic nerves (cranial nerves II, III, IV, and VI), which arise from the midbrain and brain stem (see Chapter 60)
- Weakness in one extremity or on one side of the body; this occurs as increasing ICP compresses the pyramidal tracts
- Headache that is constant, increasing in intensity, and aggravated by movement or straining; this occurs as increasing ICP causes pressure and stretching of venous and arterial vessels in the base of the brain

DETECTING LATER INDICATIONS OF INCREASING INTRACRANIAL PRESSURE. As ICP increases, the patient's condition worsens, as manifested by the following signs and symptoms:

- The LOC continues to deteriorate until the patient is comatose.
- The pulse rate and respiratory rate decrease or become erratic, and the blood pressure and temperature increase. The pulse pressure (the difference between the systolic and the diastolic pressures) widens. The pulse fluctuates rapidly, varying from bradycardia to tachycardia.
- Altered respiratory patterns develop, including Cheyne-Stokes breathing (rhythmic waxing and waning of rate and depth of respirations alternating with brief periods of apnea) and ataxic breathing (irregular breathing with a random sequence of deep and shallow breaths).
- Projectile vomiting may occur with increased pressure on the reflex center in the medulla.
- Hemiplegia or decorticate or decerebrate posturing may develop as pressure on the brain stem increases; bilateral flaccidity occurs before death.
- Loss of brain stem reflexes, including pupillary, corneal, gag, and swallowing reflexes, is an ominous sign of approaching death.

MONITORING INTRACRANIAL PRESSURE. Because clinical assessment is not always a reliable guide in recognizing increased ICP, especially in comatose patients, monitoring of ICP and cerebral oxygenation is an essential part of management. ICP is monitored closely for continuous elevation or significant increase over baseline. The trend of ICP measurements over time is an important indication of the patient's underlying status. Vital signs are assessed when an increase in ICP is noted.

Strict aseptic technique is used when handling any part of the monitoring system. The insertion site is inspected for signs of infection. Temperature, pulse, and respirations are closely monitored for systemic signs of infection. All connections and stopcocks are checked for leaks, because even small leaks can distort pressure readings and lead to infection (Littlejohns & Bader, 2009).

When ICP is monitored with a fluid system, the transducer is calibrated at a particular reference point, usually 2.5 cm (1 inch) above the ear with the patient in the supine position; this point corresponds to the level of the foramen of Monro (Fig. 61-7). CSF pressure readings depend on the patient's position. For subsequent pressure readings, the head should be in the same position relative to the transducer. Fiberoptic catheters are calibrated before insertion and do not require further referencing; they do not require the head of the bed to be at a specific position to obtain an accurate reading.

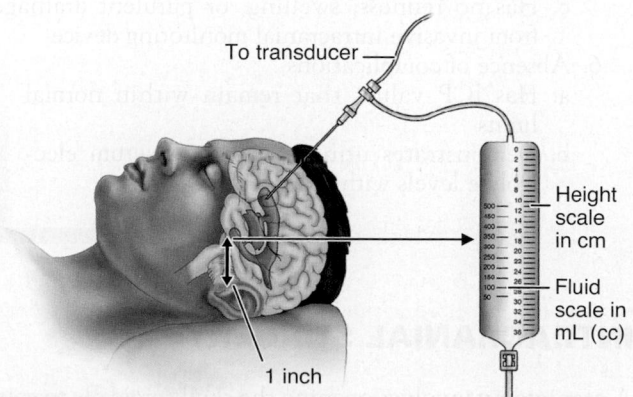

To transducer

Height scale in cm

Fluid scale in mL (cc)

1 inch

Figure 61-7 Location of the foramen of Monro for calibration of intracranial pressure monitoring system.

When technology is associated with patient management, the nurse must be certain that the technologic equipment is functioning properly. The most important concern must be the patient to whom equipment is attached. The patient and family must be informed about the technology and the goals of its use. The patient's response is monitored, and appropriate comfort measures are implemented to ensure that the patient's stress is minimized.

ICP measurement is only one parameter; repeated neurologic checks and clinical examinations remain important measures. Astute observation, comparison of findings with previous observations, and interventions can assist in preventing life-threatening ICP elevations.

MONITORING FOR SECONDARY COMPLICATIONS. The nurse also assesses for complications of increased ICP, including diabetes insipidus and SIADH (see Chapters 14 and 42). Urine output should be monitored closely. Diabetes insipidus requires fluid and electrolyte replacement, along with the administration of vasopressin, to replace and slow the urine output. Serum electrolyte levels are monitored for imbalances. SIADH requires fluid restriction and monitoring of serum electrolyte levels.

Evaluation

Expected Patient Outcomes

Expected patient outcomes may include the following:

1. Maintains patent airway
2. Attains optimal breathing pattern
   a. Breathes in a regular pattern
   b. Attains or maintains arterial blood gas values within acceptable range
3. Demonstrates optimal cerebral tissue perfusion
   a. Increasingly oriented to time, place, and person
   b. Follows verbal commands; answers questions correctly
4. Attains desired fluid balance
   a. Maintains fluid restriction
   b. Demonstrates serum and urine osmolality values within acceptable range
5. Has no signs or symptoms of infection
   a. Has no fever
   b. Shows no redness, swelling, or drainage at arterial, IV, and urinary catheter sites
   c. Has no redness, swelling, or purulent drainage from invasive intracranial monitoring device
6. Absence of complications
   a. Has ICP values that remain within normal limits
   b. Demonstrates urine output and serum electrolyte levels within acceptable limits

INTRACRANIAL SURGERY

A **craniotomy** involves opening the skull surgically to gain access to intracranial structures. This procedure is performed to remove a tumor, relieve elevated ICP, evacuate a

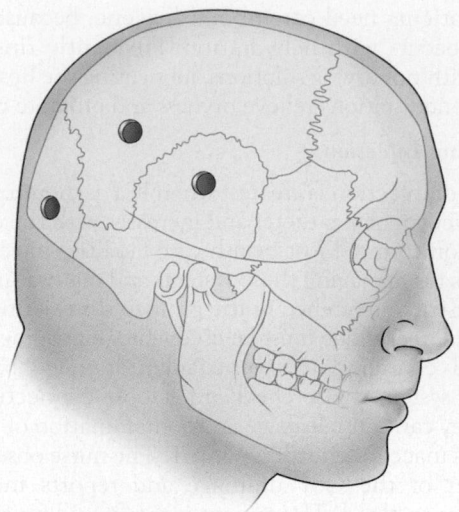

Figure 61-8 Burr holes may be used in neurosurgical procedures to make a bone flap in the skull, to aspirate a brain abscess, or to evacuate a hematoma.

blood clot, or control hemorrhage. The surgeon cuts the skull to create a bony flap, which can be repositioned after surgery and held in place by periosteal or wire sutures. One of two approaches through the skull is used: (1) above the tentorium (supratentorial craniotomy) into the supratentorial compartment, or (2) below the tentorium into the infratentorial (posterior fossa) compartment. A third approach, the **transsphenoidal** approach (through the mouth and nasal sinuses) is often used to gain access to the pituitary gland (Musleh, Sonabend & Lesniak, 2006). Table 61-3 compares the three different surgical approaches: supratentorial, infratentorial, and transsphenoidal.

Alternatively, intracranial structures may be approached through burr holes (Fig. 61-8), which are circular openings made in the skull by either a hand drill or an automatic craniotome (which has a self-controlled system to stop the drill when the bone is penetrated). Burr holes may be used to determine the presence of cerebral swelling and injury and the size and position of the ventricles. They are also a means of evacuating an intracranial hematoma or abscess and for making a bone flap in the skull that allows access to the ventricles for decompression, ventriculography, or shunting procedures. Other cranial procedures include **craniectomy** (excision of a portion of the skull) and cranioplasty (repair of a cranial defect using a plastic or metal plate).

Supratentorial and Infratentorial Approaches

PREOPERATIVE MANAGEMENT

Medical Management

Preoperative diagnostic procedures may include a CT scan to demonstrate the lesion and show the degree of surrounding brain edema, the ventricular size, and the displacement. An MRI scan provides information similar to that of a CT scan with improved tissue contrast, resolution,

Table 61-3   COMPARISON OF CRANIAL SURGICAL APPROACHES

Supratentorial	Infratentorial	Transsphenoidal

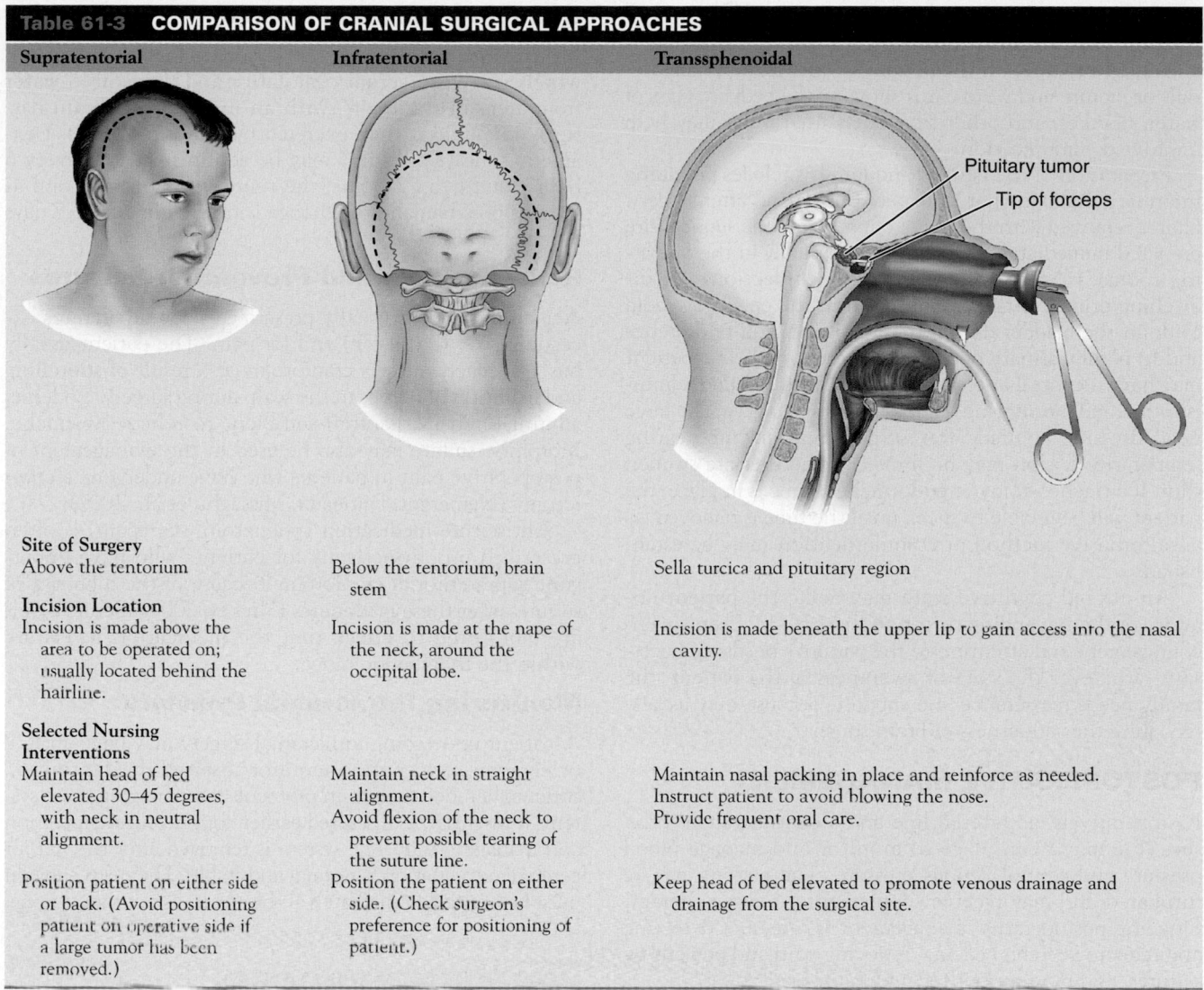

Pituitary tumor
Tip of forceps

Site of Surgery

Above the tentorium	Below the tentorium, brain stem	Sella turcica and pituitary region

Incision Location

Incision is made above the area to be operated on; usually located behind the hairline.	Incision is made at the nape of the neck, around the occipital lobe.	Incision is made beneath the upper lip to gain access into the nasal cavity.

Selected Nursing Interventions

Maintain head of bed elevated 30–45 degrees, with neck in neutral alignment.	Maintain neck in straight alignment. Avoid flexion of the neck to prevent possible tearing of the suture line.	Maintain nasal packing in place and reinforce as needed. Instruct patient to avoid blowing the nose. Provide frequent oral care.
Position patient on either side or back. (Avoid positioning patient on operative side if a large tumor has been removed.)	Position the patient on either side. (Check surgeon's preference for positioning of patient.)	Keep head of bed elevated to promote venous drainage and drainage from the surgical site.

and anatomic definition. Cerebral angiography may be used to study a tumor's blood supply or obtain information about vascular lesions. Transcranial Doppler flow studies are used to evaluate the blood flow within intracranial blood vessels.

Most patients are prescribed an antiseizure medication such as phenytoin (Dilantin) or a phenytoin metabolite (Cerebyx) before surgery to reduce the risk of postoperative **seizures** (paroxysmal transient disturbances of the brain resulting from a discharge of abnormal electrical activity) (Karch, 2008). Before surgery, corticosteroids such as dexamethasone (Decadron) may be administered to reduce cerebral edema if the patient has a brain tumor. Fluids may be restricted. A hyperosmotic agent (mannitol) and a diuretic agent such as furosemide (Lasix) may be administered IV immediately before and sometimes during surgery if the patient tends to retain fluid, as do many who have intracranial dysfunction. Antibiotics may be administered if there is a chance of cerebral contamination; diazepam (Valium) or lorazepam (Ativan) may be prescribed before surgery to allay anxiety.

Nursing Management

The preoperative assessment serves as a baseline against which postoperative status and recovery are compared. This assessment includes evaluating the LOC and responsiveness to stimuli and identifying any neurologic deficits, such as paralysis, visual dysfunction, alterations in personality or speech, and bladder and bowel disorders. Distal and proximal motor strength in both upper and lower extremities is recorded on a 5-point scale. Testing of motor function is discussed in Chapter 60.

The patient's and family's understanding of and reactions to the anticipated surgical procedure and its possible sequelae are assessed, as is the availability of support systems for the patient and family. Adequate preparation for surgery, with attention to the patient's physical and emotional status, can reduce the risk of anxiety, fear, and postoperative complications. The patient is assessed for neurologic deficits and their potential impact after surgery. For motor deficits or weakness or paralysis of the arms or legs, trochanter rolls are applied to the extremities, and the feet are positioned against a footboard or the ankles are supported in a neutral position with orthotic boots. A patient who can ambulate is encouraged to do so. If the patient is aphasic, writing materials or picture and word cards showing the bedpan, glass of water, blanket, and other frequently used items may help improve communication.

Preparation of the patient and family includes providing information about what to expect during and after surgery. Hair is removed with the use of clippers and the surgical site prepared immediately before surgery (usually in the operating room), to decrease the chance of infection. An indwelling urinary catheter is inserted in the operating room to drain the bladder during the administration of diuretics and to permit urinary output to be monitored. The patient may have a central and arterial line placed for fluid administration and monitoring of pressures after surgery. The large head dressing applied after surgery may impair hearing temporarily. Vision may be limited if the eyes are swollen shut. If a tracheostomy or endotracheal tube is in place, the patient will be unable to speak until the tube is removed, so an alternative method of communication must be established.

An altered cognitive state may make the patient unaware of the impending surgery (Chart 61-1). Even so, encouragement and attention to the patient's needs are necessary. Whatever the state of awareness of the patient, the family needs reassurance and support, because they usually recognize the seriousness of brain surgery.

POSTOPERATIVE MANAGEMENT

Postoperatively, an arterial line and a central venous pressure line may be in place to monitor and manage blood pressure and central venous pressure. The patient may be intubated and may receive supplemental oxygen therapy. Ongoing postoperative management is aimed at detecting and reducing cerebral edema, relieving pain and preventing seizures, and monitoring ICP and neurologic status.

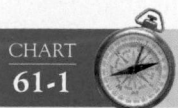

| CHART 61-1 | *Ethics and Related Issues* |

What Ethical Principles Are Involved With Surrogate Consent?

Situation

A 35-year-old woman has had a brain injury, is in and out of a comatose state, and needs a craniotomy for removal of an epidural hematoma. The health care provider determines that the patient is unable to give informed consent for the procedure, so consent is obtained from the next of kin.

Dilemma

The principle of autonomy for the patient conflicts with the principle of paternalism for the health care providers.

Discussion

1. What are the essential elements of informed consent pertinent to this situation?
2. What mechanisms can the nursing staff use to assist them in resolving any dilemma they have regarding the patient's right to autonomy?

Reducing Cerebral Edema

Medications to reduce cerebral edema include mannitol, which increases serum osmolality and draws free water from areas of the brain (with an intact blood–brain barrier). The fluid is then excreted by osmotic diuresis. Dexamethasone (Decadron) may be administered IV every 6 hours for 24 to 72 hours; the route is changed to oral as soon as possible, and the dosage is tapered over 5 to 7 days (Karch, 2008).

Relieving Pain and Preventing Seizures

Acetaminophen is usually prescribed for temperatures exceeding 37.5°C (99.6°F) and for pain. The patient usually has a headache after a craniotomy as a result of stretching and irritation of nerves in the scalp during surgery. Codeine, administered IV, is often sufficient to relieve headache. Morphine sulfate may also be used in the management of postoperative pain in patients who have undergone a craniotomy (Nemergut, Durieaux, Missaghi, et al., 2007).

Antiseizure medication (phenytoin, diazepam) is often prescribed prophylactically for patients who have undergone supratentorial craniotomy because of the high risk of seizures after these procedures (Hickey, 2009). Serum levels are monitored to check that the medication levels are within the therapeutic range.

Monitoring Intracranial Pressure

A patient undergoing intracranial surgery may have an ICP or cerebral oxygenation monitor inserted during surgery. Strict adherence to written protocols for managing these systems is essential, as discussed earlier, for preventing infection and managing ICP. The system is removed after the ICP or cerebral oxygenation is normal and stable. The neurosurgeon must be notified immediately if the system is not functioning.

NURSING PROCESS

THE PATIENT WHO HAS UNDERGONE INTRACRANIAL SURGERY

Assessment

After surgery, the frequency of postoperative monitoring is based on the patient's clinical status. Assessing respiratory function is essential, because even a small degree of hypoxia can increase cerebral ischemia. The respiratory rate and pattern are monitored, and arterial blood gas values are assessed frequently. Fluctuations in vital signs are carefully monitored and documented, because they may indicate increased ICP. The patient's temperature is measured to assess for hyperthermia secondary to infection or damage to the hypothalamus. Neurologic checks are made frequently to detect increased ICP resulting from cerebral edema or bleeding. A change in LOC or response to stimuli may be the first sign of increasing ICP.

The surgical dressing is inspected for evidence of bleeding and CSF drainage. The incision is monitored for redness, tenderness, bulging, separation, or foul odor. Sodium retention may occur in the immediate postoperative period. Serum and urine electrolytes, BUN, blood glucose, weight, and clinical status are monitored. Intake and output are measured in view of losses associated with fever, respiration, and CSF drainage. The nurse must be alert to the development of complications; all assessments are carried out with these problems in mind. Seizures are a potential complication, and any seizure activity is carefully recorded and reported. Restlessness may occur as the patient becomes more responsive, or restlessness may be caused by pain, confusion, hypoxia, or other stimuli.

Diagnosis

Nursing Diagnoses

Based on the assessment data, the patient's major nursing diagnoses after intracranial surgery may include the following:
- Ineffective cerebral tissue perfusion related to cerebral edema
- Risk for imbalanced body temperature related to damage to the hypothalamus, dehydration, and infection
- Potential for impaired gas exchange related to hypoventilation, aspiration, and immobility
- Disturbed sensory perception related to periorbital edema, head dressing, endotracheal tube, and effects of ICP
- Body image disturbance related to change in appearance or physical disabilities

Other nursing diagnoses may include impaired communication (aphasia) related to insult to brain tissue and high risk for impaired skin integrity related to immobility, pressure, and incontinence; impaired physical mobility related to a neurologic deficit secondary to the neurosurgical procedure or to the underlying disorder may also occur.

Collaborative Problems/Potential Complications

Potential complications include the following:
- Increased ICP
- Bleeding and hypovolemic shock
- Fluid and electrolyte disturbances
- Infection
- Seizures

Planning and Goals

The major goals for the patient include neurologic homeostasis to improve cerebral tissue perfusion, adequate thermoregulation, normal ventilation and gas exchange, ability to cope with sensory deprivation, adaptation to changes in body image, and absence of complications.

Nursing Interventions

Maintaining Cerebral Tissue Perfusion

Attention to the patient's respiratory status is essential, because even slight decreases in the oxygen level (hypoxia) or slight increases in the carbon dioxide level (hypercarbia) can affect cerebral perfusion, the clinical course, and the patient's outcome. The endotracheal tube is left in place until the patient shows signs of awakening and has adequate spontaneous ventilation, as evaluated clinically and by arterial blood gas analysis. Secondary brain damage can result from impaired cerebral oxygenation.

Some degree of cerebral edema occurs after brain surgery; it tends to peak 24 to 36 hours after surgery, producing decreased responsiveness on the second postoperative day. The control of cerebral edema was discussed earlier. Nursing strategies used to control factors that may raise ICP were presented in the previous Nursing Process section on increased ICP. Intraventricular drainage is carefully monitored, using strict asepsis when any part of the system is handled.

Vital signs and neurologic status (LOC and responsiveness, pupillary and motor responses) are assessed every 15 to 60 minutes. Extreme head rotation is avoided, because this raises ICP. After supratentorial surgery, the patient is placed on his or her back or side (on the unoperated side if a large lesion was removed) with one pillow under the head. The head of the bed may be elevated 30 degrees, depending on the level of the ICP and the neurosurgeon's preference. After posterior fossa (infratentorial) surgery, the patient is kept flat on one side (off the back) with the head on a small, firm pillow. The patient may be turned on either side, keeping the neck in a neutral position. When the patient is being turned, the body should be turned as a unit to prevent placing strain on the incision and possibly tearing the sutures. The head of the bed may be elevated slowly as tolerated by the patient.

The patient's position is changed every 2 hours, and skin care is given frequently. During position changes, care is taken to prevent disruption of the ICP monitoring system. A turning sheet placed under the patient's head to midthigh makes it easier to move and turn the patient safely.

Regulating Temperature

Moderate temperature elevation can be expected after intracranial surgery because of the reaction to blood at the operative site or in the subarachnoid space. Injury to the hypothalamic centers that regulate body temperature can occur during surgery. Fever is treated vigorously to combat the effect of an elevated temperature on brain metabolism and function.

Nursing interventions include monitoring the patient's temperature and using the following measures to reduce body temperature: removing blankets, applying ice bags to axilla and groin areas, using a hypothermia blanket as prescribed, and administering prescribed medications to reduce fever (Thompson, Kirkness, Mitchell, et al., 2007).

Conversely, hypothermia may be seen after lengthy neurosurgical procedures. Therefore, frequent measurements of rectal temperatures are necessary. Rewarming should occur slowly to prevent shivering, which increases cellular oxygen demands.

Improving Gas Exchange

The patient undergoing neurosurgery is at risk for impaired gas exchange and pulmonary infections due to immobility, immunosuppression, decreased LOC, and fluid restriction. Immobility compromises the respiratory system by causing pooling and stasis of secretions in dependent areas and the development of atelectasis. The patient whose fluid intake is restricted may be more vulnerable to atelectasis as a result of inability to expectorate thickened secretions. Pneumonia can develop due to aspiration and restricted mobility.

Repositioning the patient every 2 hours helps to mobilize pulmonary secretions and prevent stasis. After the patient regains consciousness, additional measures to expand collapsed alveoli can be instituted, such as yawning, sighing, deep breathing, incentive spirometry, and coughing (unless contraindicated). If necessary, the oropharynx and trachea are suctioned to remove secretions that cannot be raised by coughing; however, coughing and suctioning increase ICP. Therefore, suctioning should be used cautiously. Increasing the humidity in the oxygen delivery system may help to loosen secretions. The nurse and the respiratory therapist work together to monitor the effects of chest physical therapy.

Managing Sensory Deprivation

Periorbital edema is a common consequence of intracranial surgery, because fluid drains into the dependent periorbital areas when the patient has been positioned in a prone position during surgery. A hematoma may form under the scalp and spread down to the orbit, producing an area of ecchymosis (black eye).

Before surgery, the patient and family should be informed that one or both eyes may be edematous temporarily after surgery. After surgery, elevating the head of the bed (if not contraindicated) and applying cold compresses over the eyes will help reduce the edema. If periorbital edema increases significantly, the surgeon is notified, because this may indicate that a postoperative clot is developing or that there is increasing ICP and poor venous drainage. Health care personnel should announce their presence when entering the room to avoid startling the patient whose vision is impaired due to periorbital edema or neurologic deficits.

Additional factors that can affect sensation include a bulky head dressing, the presence of an endotracheal tube, and effects of increased ICP. The first postoperative dressing change is usually performed by the neurosurgeon. In the absence of bleeding or a CSF leak, every effort is made to minimize the size of the head dressing. If the patient requires an endotracheal tube for mechanical ventilation, every effort is made to extubate the patient as soon as clinical signs indicate it is possible. The patient is monitored closely for the effects of elevated ICP.

Enhancing Self-Image

The patient is encouraged to verbalize feelings and frustrations about any change in appearance. Nursing support is based on the patient's reactions and feelings. Factual information may need to be provided if the patient has misconceptions about puffiness about the face, periorbital bruising, and hair loss. Attention to grooming, the use of the patient's own clothing, and covering the head with a turban (and later a wig until hair growth occurs) are encouraged. Social interaction with close friends, family, and hospital personnel may increase the patient's sense of self-worth.

The family and social support system can be of assistance while the patient recovers from surgery.

Monitoring and Managing Potential Complications

The nurse must be vigilant for complications that may develop within hours of surgery and require close collaboration with the neurosurgeon. These include increased ICP, bleeding and hypovolemic shock, altered fluid and electrolyte balance (eg, water intoxication and diabetes insipidus), infection, and seizures.

MONITORING FOR INCREASED INTRACRANIAL PRESSURE AND BLEEDING. Increased ICP and bleeding are life-threatening to the patient who has undergone intracranial surgery. The following points must be kept in mind when caring for any patient who has undergone such surgery:

- An increase in blood pressure and decrease in pulse with respiratory failure may indicate increased ICP.
- An accumulation of blood under the bone flap (extradural, subdural, or intracerebral hematoma) may pose a threat to life. A clot must be suspected in any patient who does not awaken as expected or whose condition deteriorates. An intracranial hematoma is suspected if the patient has any new postoperative neurologic deficits (especially a dilated pupil on the operative side). In these circumstances, the patient is returned to the operating room immediately for evacuation of the clot if indicated.
- Cerebral edema, infarction, metabolic disturbances, and hydrocephalus are conditions that may mimic the clinical manifestations of a clot.

The patient is monitored closely for indicators of complications, and early signs and trends in clinical status are reported to the surgeon. Treatments are initiated promptly, and the nurse assists in evaluating the patient's response to treatment. The nurse also provides support to the patient and family.

If signs and symptoms of increased ICP occur, efforts to decrease the ICP are initiated: alignment of the head in a neutral position without flexion to promote venous drainage, elevation of the head of the bed to 30 degrees (when prescribed), administration of mannitol (an osmotic diuretic), and possible administration of pharmacologic paralyzing agents.

MANAGING FLUID AND ELECTROLYTE DISTURBANCES. Fluid and electrolyte imbalances may occur because of the patient's underlying condition and its management or as complications of surgery. These disturbances can contribute to the development of cerebral edema.

The postoperative fluid regimen depends on the type of neurosurgical procedure and is determined on an individual basis. The volume and composition of fluids are adjusted based on daily serum electrolyte values, along with fluid intake and output. Fluids may have to be restricted in patients with cerebral edema.

Oral fluids are usually resumed after the first 24 hours. The presence of gag and swallowing reflexes must be checked before initiation of oral fluids. Some patients with posterior fossa tumors have impaired swallowing, so fluids may need to be administered by alternative routes. The patient should be observed for signs and symptoms of nausea and vomiting as the diet is progressed (Hickey, 2009).

Patients undergoing surgery for brain tumors often receive large doses of corticosteroids and therefore tend to develop hyperglycemia. Serum glucose levels are measured every 4 to 6 hours. These patients are prone to stress ulcers, so histamine-2 receptor antagonists (H_2 blockers) are prescribed to suppress the secretion of gastric acid. Patients also are monitored for bleeding and assessed for gastric pain.

If the surgical site is near to (or causes edema to) the pituitary gland and hypothalamus, the patient may develop symptoms of diabetes insipidus, which is characterized by excessive urinary output, elevated serum osmolality, decreased urine osmolality, hypernatremia, and a low urine specific gravity. The urine specific gravity is measured hourly, and fluid intake and output are monitored. Fluid replacement must compensate for urine output, and serum potassium levels must be monitored.

SIADH, which results in water retention with hyponatremia and serum hypo-osmolality, occurs in a wide variety of central nervous system disorders (eg, brain tumor, head trauma) causing fluid disturbances. Nursing management includes careful intake and output measurements, specific gravity determinations of urine, and monitoring of serum and urine electrolyte levels while following directives for fluid restriction. SIADH is usually self-limited.

PREVENTING INFECTION. The patient undergoing neurosurgery is at risk for infection related to the neurosurgical procedure (brain exposure, bone exposure, wound hematomas) and the presence of IV and arterial lines for fluid administration and monitoring. Risk for infection is increased in patients who undergo lengthy intracranial operations, in those who have external ventricular drains in place longer than 5 days, and with those who have ventricular catheters placed outside of the operating room (March, 2005).

The dressing is often stained with blood in the immediate postoperative period. Because blood is an excellent culture medium for bacteria, the dressing is reinforced with sterile pads so that contamination and infection are avoided. A heavily stained or displaced dressing should be reported immediately. A drain is sometimes placed in the craniotomy incision to facilitate drainage.

After suboccipital surgical procedures, CSF may leak through the incision. This complication is dangerous because of the possibility of meningitis. Any sudden discharge of fluid from a cranial incision is reported at once, because a massive leak requires surgical repair. Attention should be paid to the patient who complains of a salty taste or "postnasal drip," because this can be caused by CSF trickling down the throat. After a craniotomy, the patient is instructed to avoid coughing, sneezing, or nose blowing, which can cause CSF leakage by creating pressure on the operative site.

Aseptic technique is used when handling dressings, drainage systems, and IV and arterial lines. The patient is monitored carefully for signs and symptoms of infection, and cultures are obtained if infection is suspected. Appropriate antibiotics are administered as prescribed. Other causes of infection in the patient undergoing intracranial surgery, such as pneumonia and urinary tract infections, are similar to those in other postoperative patients.

MONITORING FOR SEIZURE ACTIVITY. Seizures may occur as complications after any intracranial neurosurgical procedure. Preventing seizures is essential to avoid further cerebral edema. Administering the prescribed antiseizure medication before and after surgery may prevent the development of seizures in subsequent months and years. **Status epilepticus** (prolonged seizures without recovery of consciousness in the

intervals between seizures) may occur after craniotomy and also may be related to the development of complications (hematoma, ischemia). The management of status epilepticus is described later in this chapter.

MONITORING AND MANAGING OTHER COMPLICATIONS. Other complications may occur during the first 2 weeks or later and may compromise the patient's recovery. The most important of these are thromboembolic complications (DVT, pulmonary embolism), pulmonary and urinary tract infection, and pressure ulcers. Most of these complications may be avoided with frequent changes of position, adequate suctioning of secretions, thrombosis prophylaxis, early ambulation, and skin care.

Promoting Home and Community-Based Care

TEACHING PATIENTS SELF-CARE. The recovery of a neurosurgical patient at home depends on the extent of the surgical procedure and its success. The patient's strengths as well as limitations are assessed and explained to the family, along with the family's part in promoting recovery. Because administration of antiseizure medication is a priority, the patient and family are taught to use a check-off system, pill boxes, and alarms to ensure that the medication is taken as prescribed.

The patient and family are taught what to expect after surgery. Dietary restrictions usually are not required unless another health problem necessitates a special diet. Although showering or tub bathing is permitted, the scalp should be kept dry until all the sutures have been removed. A clean scarf or cap may be worn until a wig or hairpiece is purchased. If skull bone has been removed, the neurosurgeon may prescribe a protective helmet. After a craniotomy, the patient may require rehabilitation, depending on the postoperative level of function. The patient may require physical therapy for residual weakness and mobility issues. An occupational therapist is consulted to assist with self-care issues. If the patient is aphasic, speech therapy may be necessary.

CONTINUING CARE. Barring complications, patients are discharged from the hospital as soon as possible. Patients with severe motor deficits require extensive physical therapy and rehabilitation. Those with postoperative cognitive and speech impairments require psychological evaluation, speech therapy, and rehabilitation. The nurse collaborates with the physician and other health care professionals during hospitalization and home care to achieve as complete a rehabilitation as possible and to assist the patient in living with residual disability.

If tumor, injury, or disease makes the prognosis poor, care is directed toward making the patient as comfortable as possible. With return of the tumor or cerebral compression, the patient becomes less alert and aware. Other possible consequences include paralysis, blindness, and seizures. The home care nurse, hospice nurse, and social worker collaborate with the family to plan for additional home health care or hospice services or placement of the patient in an extended-care facility (see also the section on cerebral metastases in Chapter 65). The patient and family are encouraged to discuss end-of-life preferences for care; the patient's end-of-life preferences must be respected (see Chapter 17). The nurse involved in home and continuing care of patients after cranial surgery also needs to remind patients and family members of the need for health promotion and recommended health screening.

Evaluation

Expected Patient Outcomes

Expected patient outcomes may include the following:

1. Achieves optimal cerebral tissue perfusion
   a. Opens eyes on request; uses recognizable words, progressing to normal speech
   b. Obeys commands with appropriate motor responses
2. Maintains normal body temperature
   a. Registers normal body temperature
3. Has normal gas exchange
   a. Has arterial blood gas values within normal ranges
   b. Breathes easily; lung sounds are clear without adventitious sounds
   c. Takes deep breaths and changes position as directed
4. Copes with sensory deprivation
5. Demonstrates improving self-concept
   a. Pays attention to grooming
   b. Visits and interacts with others
6. Exhibits absence of complications
   a. Exhibits ICP within normal range
   b. Has minimal bleeding at surgical site; surgical incision is healing without evidence of infection
   c. Shows fluid balance and electrolyte levels within desired ranges
   d. Exhibits no evidence of seizures

Transsphenoidal Approach

Tumors within the sella turcica and small adenomas of the pituitary can be removed through a transsphenoidal approach: An incision is made beneath the upper lip, and entry is then gained successively into the nasal cavity, sphenoidal sinus, and sella turcica (see Table 61-3). Although an otorhinolaryngologist may make the initial opening, the neurosurgeon completes the opening into the sphenoidal sinus and exposes the floor of the sella. Microsurgical techniques provide improved illumination, magnification, and visualization so that nearby vital structures can be avoided.

The transsphenoidal approach offers direct access to the sella turcica with minimal risk of trauma and hemorrhage (Musleh, et al., 2006). It avoids many of the risks of craniotomy, and the postoperative discomfort is similar to that of other transnasal surgical procedures. It may also be used for pituitary ablation (destruction) in patients with disseminated breast or prostatic cancer.

Complications

Manipulation of the posterior pituitary gland during surgery may produce transient diabetes insipidus of several days' duration (Hickey, 2009). It is treated with vasopressin but occasionally persists. Other complications include CSF leakage, visual disturbances, postoperative meningitis, pneumocephalus (air in the intracranial cavity), and SIADH (see Chapter 42).

PREOPERATIVE MANAGEMENT

Medical Management

The preoperative workup includes a series of endocrine tests, rhinologic evaluation (to assess the status of the sinuses and nasal cavity), and neuroradiologic studies. Funduscopic examination and visual field determinations are performed, because the most serious effect of pituitary tumor is localized pressure on the optic nerve or chiasm. In addition, the nasopharyngeal secretions are cultured, because a sinus infection is a contraindication to an intracranial procedure using this approach. Corticosteroids may be administered before and after surgery, because the surgery involves removal of the pituitary, the source of adrenocorticotropic hormone (ACTH). Antibiotics may or may not be administered prophylactically.

Nursing Management

Deep breathing is taught before surgery. The patient is instructed that after the surgery he or she will need to avoid vigorous coughing, blowing the nose, sucking through a straw, or sneezing, because these actions may place increased pressure at the surgical site and cause a CSF leak (Hickey, 2009).

POSTOPERATIVE MANAGEMENT

Medical Management

Because the procedure disrupts the oral and nasal mucous membranes, management focuses on preventing infection and promoting healing. Medications include antimicrobial agents (which are continued until the nasal packing inserted at the time of surgery is removed), corticosteroids, analgesic agents for discomfort, and agents for the control of diabetes insipidus if necessary (Hickey, 2009).

Nursing Management

Vital signs are measured to monitor hemodynamic, cardiac, and ventilatory status. Because of the anatomic proximity of the pituitary gland to the optic chiasm, visual acuity and visual fields are assessed at regular intervals. One method is to ask the patient to count the number of fingers held up by the nurse. Evidence of decreasing visual acuity suggests an expanding hematoma.

The head of the bed is raised to decrease pressure on the sella turcica and to promote normal drainage. The patient is cautioned against blowing the nose or engaging in any activity that raises ICP, such as bending over or straining during urination or defecation.

Intake and output are measured as a guide to fluid and electrolyte replacement and to assess for diabetes insipidus. The urine specific gravity is measured after each voiding. Daily weight is monitored. Fluids are usually given after nausea ceases, and the patient then progresses to a regular diet.

The nasal packing inserted during surgery is checked frequently for blood or CSF drainage. The major discomfort is related to the nasal packing and to mouth dryness and thirst caused by mouth breathing. Oral care is provided every 4 hours or more frequently. Usually, the teeth are not brushed until the incision above the teeth has healed. Warm saline mouth rinses and the use of a cool mist vaporizer are helpful. Petrolatum is soothing when applied to the lips. A room humidifier assists in keeping the mucous membranes moist. The packing is removed in 3 to 4 days, and only then can the area around the nares be cleaned with the prescribed solution to remove crusted blood and moisten the mucous membranes (Hickey, 2009).

Home care considerations include advising the patient to use a room humidifier to keep the mucous membranes moist and to soothe irritation. The head of the bed is elevated for at least 2 weeks after surgery.

SEIZURE DISORDERS

Seizures are episodes of abnormal motor, sensory, autonomic, or psychic activity (or a combination of these) that result from sudden excessive discharge from cerebral neurons (Hickey, 2009). A part or all of the brain may be involved. The international classification of seizures differentiates between two main types: partial seizures that begin in one part of the brain, and generalized seizures that involve electrical discharges in the whole brain (Chart 61-2). In a simple partial seizure, consciousness remains intact,

---

Chart 61-2 • *International Classification of Seizures*

Partial Seizures (seizures beginning locally)

Simple Partial Seizures (with elementary symptoms, generally without Impairment of consciousness)
- With motor symptoms
- With special sensory or somatosensory symptoms
- With autonomic symptoms
- Compound forms

Complex Partial Seizures (with complex symptoms, generally with impairment of consciousness)
- With impairment of consciousness only
- With cognitive symptoms
- With affective symptoms
- With psychosensory symptoms
- With psychomotor symptoms (automatisms)
- Compound forms

Partial Seizures Secondarily Generalized

Generalized Seizures (convulsive or nonconvulsive, bilaterally symmetric, without local onset)

Tonic–clonic seizures
Tonic seizures
Clonic seizures
Absence (petit mal) seizures
Atonic seizures
Myoclonic seizures (bilaterally massive epileptic)
Unclassified seizures

---

whereas in a complex partial seizure, consciousness is impaired. Unclassified seizures are so termed because of incomplete data.

The underlying cause is an electrical disturbance (dysrhythmia) in the nerve cells in one section of the brain; these cells emit abnormal, recurring, uncontrolled electrical discharges. The characteristic seizure is a manifestation of this excessive neuronal discharge. Associated loss of consciousness, excess movement or loss of muscle tone or movement, and disturbances of behavior, mood, sensation, and perception may also occur.

The specific causes of seizures are varied and can be categorized as idiopathic (genetic, developmental defects) and acquired. Causes of acquired seizures include:
- Cerebrovascular disease
- Hypoxemia of any cause, including vascular insufficiency
- Fever (childhood)
- Head injury
- Hypertension
- Central nervous system infections
- Metabolic and toxic conditions (eg, renal failure, hyponatremia, hypocalcemia, hypoglycemia, pesticide exposure)
- Brain tumor
- Drug and alcohol withdrawal
- Allergies

Nursing Management

During a Seizure

A major responsibility of the nurse is to observe and record the sequence of signs. The nature of the seizure usually indicates the type of treatment that is required (AANN, 2007). Before and during a seizure, the patient is assessed and the following items are documented:
- The circumstances before the seizure (visual, auditory, or olfactory stimuli; tactile stimuli; emotional or psychological disturbances; sleep; hyperventilation) (Chart 61-3)
- The occurrence of an aura (a premonitory or warning sensation, which can be visual, auditory, or olfactory)
- The first thing the patient does in the seizure—where the movements or the stiffness begins, conjugate gaze position, and the position of the head at the beginning of the seizure. This information gives clues to the location of the seizure origin in the brain. (In recording, it is important to state whether the beginning of the seizure was observed.)
- The type of movements in the part of the body involved
- The areas of the body involved (turn back bedding to expose patient)
- The size of both pupils and whether the eyes are open
- Whether the eyes or head turned to one side
- The presence or absence of automatisms (involuntary motor activity, such as lip smacking or repeated swallowing)
- Incontinence of urine or stool
- Duration of each phase of the seizure
- Unconsciousness, if present, and its duration

NURSING RESEARCH PROFILE

CHART 61-3   *Seizure Events During Computer-Based Assessment*

DiIorio, C., Reisinger, E. L., Yeager, K., et al. (2008). A descriptive analysis of seizure events among adults who participated in a computer-based assessment. *Journal of Neuroscience Nursing, 40*(3), 134–141.

Purpose

It is known that seizures can be induced by visual stimuli such as television and video games in some people; therefore, it is important to understand how computer monitors affect people with epilepsy. This study both documented seizure events associated with a computer-based assessment and described contextual factors surrounding seizure episodes.

Design

This descriptive study was part of a larger, longitudinal study of self-management in adults with epilepsy. For this portion of the study, participants underwent three computer-based assessments at baseline, 3 months, and 6 months. Investigators collected data on demographic characteristics and seizure characteristics and used various psychosocial instruments to assess self-management practices.

Findings

A total of 14 seizure events occurred during the 896 computer-based assessments, which constituted 1.6% of the assessments and affected 4.4% of the participants. The mean age of people who experienced the seizure events was 41 years; 70% were female, and 70% were Caucasian. Contextual factors that could have precipitated seizure events included hunger, fatigue, stress, and medication changes. In two instances, participants indicated that the computer monitor could have triggered their seizure.

Nursing Implications

Although some seizures can be induced by visual stimuli, nurses working with people with epilepsy can be fairly confident that computer-based assessments pose minimal risks for inducing seizures. With increases in computer technology use in health care, these are reassuring findings for nurses and patients.

- Any obvious paralysis or weakness of arms or legs after the seizure
- Inability to speak after the seizure
- Movements at the end of the seizure
- Whether or not the patient sleeps afterward
- Cognitive status (confused or not confused) after the seizure

In addition to providing data about the seizure, nursing care is directed at preventing injury and supporting the patient, not only physically but also psychologically. Consequences such as anxiety, embarrassment, fatigue, and depression can be devastating to the patient.

After a Seizure

After a patient has a seizure, the nurse's role is to document the events leading to and occurring during and after the seizure and to prevent complications (eg, aspiration, injury). The patient is at risk for hypoxia, vomiting, and pulmonary aspiration. To prevent complications, the patient is placed in the side-lying position to facilitate drainage of oral secretions, and suctioning is performed, if needed, to maintain a patent airway and prevent aspiration (Chart 61-4). Seizure precautions are maintained, including having available functioning suction equipment with a suction catheter and oral airway. The bed is placed in a low position with two to three side rails up and padded, if necessary, to prevent injury to the patient. The patient may be drowsy and may wish to sleep after the seizure; he or she may not remember events leading up to the seizure and for a short time thereafter.

The Epilepsies

Epilepsy is a group of syndromes characterized by unprovoked, recurring seizures (AANN, 2007). Epileptic syndromes are classified by specific patterns of clinical features,

including age at onset, family history, and seizure type. Types of epilepsies are differentiated by how the seizure activity manifests (see Chart 61-3), the most common syndromes being those with generalized seizures and those with partial-onset seizures (Hickey, 2009). Epilepsy can be primary (idiopathic) or secondary (when the cause is known and the epilepsy is a symptom of another underlying condition, such as a brain tumor).

Epilepsy affects an estimated 3% of people during their lifetime, and most forms of epilepsy occur in childhood. The improved treatment of cerebrovascular disorders, head injuries, brain tumors, meningitis, and encephalitis has increased the number of patients at risk for seizures after recovery from these conditions. Also, advances in EEG have aided in the diagnosis of epilepsy. The general public has been educated about epilepsy, which has reduced the stigma associated with it; as a result, more people are willing to acknowledge that they have epilepsy.

Although some evidence suggests that susceptibility to some types of epilepsy may be inherited, the cause of seizures in many people is idiopathic (unknown). Epilepsy can follow birth trauma, asphyxia neonatorum, head injuries, some infectious diseases (bacterial, viral, parasitic), toxicity (carbon monoxide and lead poisoning), circulatory problems, fever, metabolic and nutritional disorders, or drug or alcohol intoxication. It is also associated with brain tumors, abscesses, and congenital malformations.

Pathophysiology

Messages from the body are carried by the neurons (nerve cells) of the brain by means of discharges of electrochemical energy that sweep along them. These impulses occur in bursts whenever a nerve cell has a task to perform. Sometimes, these cells or groups of cells continue firing after a task is finished. During the period of unwanted discharges,

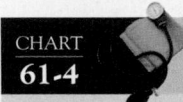

CHART 61-4   *Guidelines for Seizure Care*

Nursing Care During a Seizure

- Provide privacy and protect the patient from curious onlookers. (The patient who has an aura [warning of an impending seizure] may have time to seek a safe, private place.)
- Ease the patient to the floor, if possible.
- Protect the head with a pad to prevent injury (from striking a hard surface).
- Loosen constrictive clothing.
- Push aside any furniture that may injure the patient during the seizure.
- If the patient is in bed, remove pillows and raise side rails.
- If an aura precedes the seizure, insert an oral airway to reduce the possibility of the patient's biting the tongue or cheek.
- *Do not attempt to pry open jaws that are clenched in a spasm or to insert anything.* Broken teeth and injury to the lips and tongue may result from such an action.
- No attempt should be made to restrain the patient during the seizure, because muscular contractions are strong and restraint can produce injury.

- If possible, place the patient on one side with head flexed forward, which allows the tongue to fall forward and facilitates drainage of saliva and mucus. If suction is available, use it if necessary to clear secretions.

Nursing Care After the Seizure

- Keep the patient on one side to prevent aspiration. Make sure the airway is patent.
- There is usually a period of confusion after a grand mal seizure.
- A short apneic period may occur during or immediately after a generalized seizure.
- The patient, on awakening, should be reoriented to the environment.
- If the patient becomes agitated after a seizure (postictal), use persuasion and gentle restraint to assist him or her to stay calm.

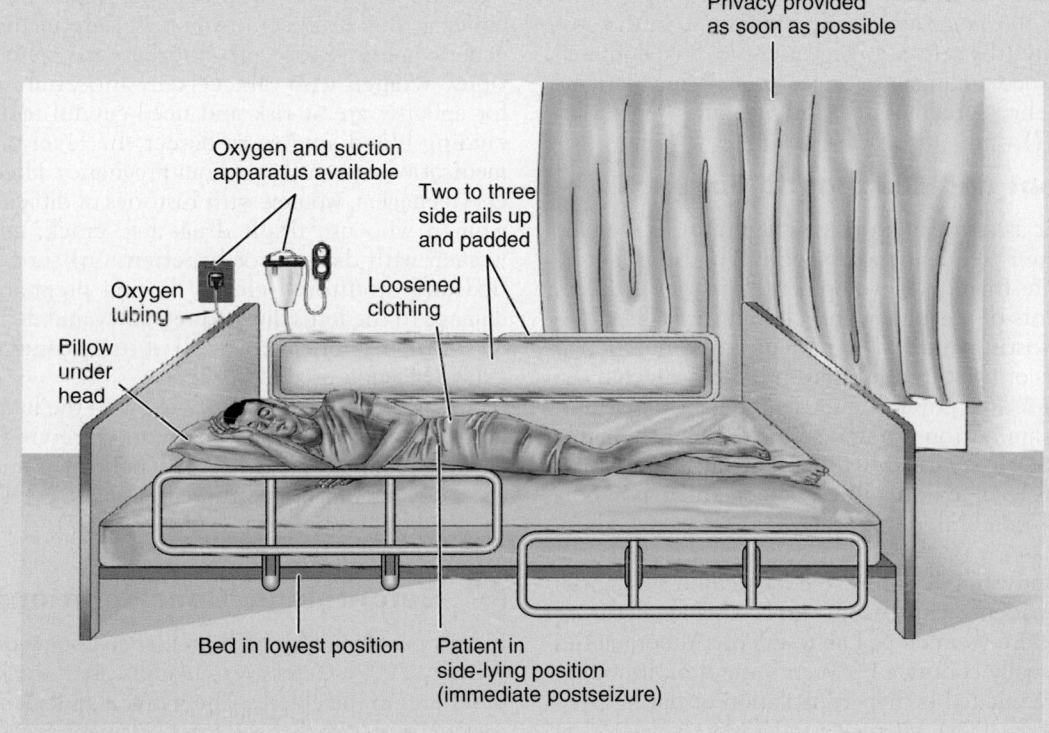

Privacy provided as soon as possible

Oxygen and suction apparatus available

Two to three side rails up and padded

Oxygen tubing

Loosened clothing

Pillow under head

Bed in lowest position

Patient in side-lying position (immediate postseizure)

parts of the body controlled by the errant cells may perform erratically. Resultant dysfunction ranges from mild to incapacitating and often causes loss of consciousness (Hickey, 2009). If these uncontrolled, abnormal discharges occur repeatedly, a person is said to have an epileptic syndrome. Epilepsy is not associated with intellectual level. People who have epilepsy without other brain or nervous system disabilities fall within the same intelligence ranges as the overall population. Epilepsy is not synonymous with mental retardation or illness. However, many people who have developmental disabilities because of serious neurologic damage also have epilepsy.

Clinical Manifestations

Depending on the location of the discharging neurons, seizures may range from a simple staring episode (absence seizure) to prolonged convulsive movements with loss of consciousness.

The initial pattern of the seizures indicates the region of the brain in which the seizure originates (see Chart 61-3). In simple partial seizures, only a finger or hand may shake, or the mouth may jerk uncontrollably. The person may talk unintelligibly; may be dizzy; and may experience unusual or unpleasant sights, sounds, odors, or tastes, but without loss of consciousness (Hickey, 2009).

In complex partial seizures, the person either remains motionless or moves automatically but inappropriately for time and place, or he or she may experience excessive emotions of fear, anger, elation, or irritability. Whatever the manifestations, the person does not remember the episode when it is over.

Generalized seizures, previously referred to as grand mal seizures, involve both hemispheres of the brain, causing both sides of the body to react (Hickey, 2009). Intense rigidity of the entire body may occur, followed by alternating muscle relaxation and contraction (generalized tonic–clonic contraction). The simultaneous contractions of the diaphragm and chest muscles may produce a characteristic epileptic cry. The tongue is often chewed, and the patient is incontinent of urine and feces. After 1 or 2 minutes, the convulsive movements begin to subside; the patient relaxes and lies in deep coma, breathing noisily. The respirations at this point are chiefly abdominal. In the postictal state (after the seizure), the patient is often confused and hard to arouse and may sleep for hours. Many patients report headache, sore muscles, fatigue, and depression (AANN, 2007).

Assessment and Diagnostic Findings

The diagnostic assessment is aimed at determining the type of seizures, their frequency and severity, and the factors that precipitate them. A developmental history is taken, including events of pregnancy and childbirth, to seek evidence of preexisting injury. The patient is also questioned about illnesses or head injuries that may have affected the brain. In addition to physical and neurologic evaluations, diagnostic examinations include biochemical, hematologic, and serologic studies. MRI is used to detect structural lesions such as focal abnormalities, cerebrovascular abnormalities, and cerebral degenerative changes (AANN, 2007).

The EEG furnishes diagnostic evidence for a substantial proportion of patients with epilepsy and assists in classifying the type of seizure (Karpoff & Labus, 2008). Abnormalities in the EEG usually continue between seizures or, if not apparent, may be elicited by hyperventilation or during sleep (Kotagal & Yardi, 2008). Microelectrodes (depth electrodes) can be inserted deep in the brain to probe the action of single brain cells. Some people with clinical seizures have normal EEGs, whereas others who have never had seizures have abnormal EEGs. Telemetry and computerized equipment are used to monitor electrical brain activity while the patient pursues his or her normal activities and to store the readings on computer tapes for analysis. Video recording of seizures taken simultaneously with EEG telemetry is useful in determining the type of seizure as well as its duration and magnitude. This type of intensive monitoring is changing the treatment of severe epilepsy (Dilorio, Reisinger, Yeager, et al., 2008).

SPECT is an additional tool that is sometimes used in the diagnostic workup. It is useful for identifying the epileptogenic zone so that the area in the brain giving rise to seizures can be removed surgically (AANN, 2007).

Epilepsy in Women

More than 1 million American women have epilepsy, and they face particular needs associated with the syndrome. Women with epilepsy often note an increase in seizure frequency during menses; this has been linked to the increase in sex hormones that alter the excitability of neurons in the cerebral cortex. The effectiveness of contraceptives is decreased by antiseizure medications. Therefore, patients should be encouraged to discuss family planning with their primary health care provider and to obtain preconception counseling if they are considering childbearing (Meador, Pennell, Harden, et al., 2008).

Women of childbearing age who have epilepsy require special care and guidance before, during, and after pregnancy. Many women note a change in the pattern of seizure activity during pregnancy. The risk of congenital fetal anomaly is two to three times higher in women with epilepsy. Maternal seizures, antiseizure medications, and genetic predisposition all contribute to possible malformations. Women who take certain antiseizure medications for epilepsy are at risk and need careful monitoring, including blood studies to detect the level of antiseizure medications taken throughout pregnancy. High-risk mothers (teenagers, women with histories of difficult deliveries, women who use illicit drugs [eg, crack, cocaine], and women with diabetes or hypertension) should be identified and monitored closely during pregnancy, because damage to the fetus during pregnancy and delivery can increase the risk of epilepsy. All of these issues need further study (Meador, et al., 2008).

Because of bone loss associated with the long-term use of antiseizure medications, patients receiving antiseizure agents should be assessed for low bone mass and osteoporosis. They should be instructed about strategies to reduce their risks of osteoporosis (AANN, 2007).

 Gerontologic Considerations

Elderly people have a high incidence of new-onset epilepsy (Hickey, 2009). Cerebrovascular disease is the leading cause of seizures in the elderly. The increased incidence is also associated with stroke, head injury, dementia, infection, alcoholism, and aging. Treatment depends on the underlying cause. Because many elderly people have chronic health problems, they may be taking other medications that can interact with medications prescribed for seizure control. In addition, the absorption, distribution, metabolism, and excretion of medications are altered in the elderly as a result of age-related changes in renal and liver function. Therefore, elderly patients must be monitored closely for adverse and toxic effects of antiseizure medications and for osteoporosis. The cost of antiseizure medications can lead to poor adherence to the prescribed regimen in elderly patients on fixed incomes.

Prevention

Society-wide efforts are the key to prevention of epilepsy. Head injury is one of the main causes of epilepsy that can be prevented. Through highway safety programs and occupational safety precautions, lives can be saved and epilepsy due to head injury prevented; these programs are discussed in Chapter 63.

Medical Management

The management of epilepsy is individualized to meet the needs of each patient and not just to manage and prevent seizures. Management differs from patient to patient, because some forms of epilepsy arise from brain damage and others result from altered brain chemistry.

Pharmacologic Therapy

Many medications are available to control seizures, although the exact mechanisms of action are unknown. The objective is to achieve seizure control with minimal side effects. Medication therapy controls rather than cures seizures. Medications are selected on the basis of the type of seizure being treated and the effectiveness and safety of the medications. If properly prescribed and taken, medications control seizures in 70% to 80% of patients with seizures. However, 20% of patients with generalized seizures and 30% of those with partial seizures do not demonstrate improvement with any prescribed medication or may be unable to tolerate the side effects of medications (AANN, 2007). Table 61-4 lists the medications in current use.

> ### ▶ NURSING ALERT
>
> Nurses must take care when administering lamotrigine (Lamictal), an antiseizure medication. The drug packaging was recently changed in an attempt to reduce medication errors, because this medication has been confused with terbinafine (Lamisil), labetalol hydrochloride (Trandate), lamivudine (Epivir), maprotiline (Ludiomil), and the combination of diphenoxylate and atropine (Lomotil). Patients with epilepsy are at risk for status epilepticus from having their medication regimen interrupted.

Treatment usually starts with a single medication. The starting dose and the rate at which the dosage is increased depend on the occurrence of side effects. The medication levels in the blood are monitored, because the rate of drug absorption varies among patients. Changing to another medication may be necessary if seizure control is not achieved or if toxicity makes it impossible to increase the dosage. The medication may need to be adjusted because of concurrent illness, weight changes, or increases in stress. Side effects of antiseizure medications may be divided into three groups: (1) idiosyncratic or allergic disorders, which manifest primarily as skin reactions; (2) acute toxicity, which may occur when the medication is initially prescribed; and (3) chronic toxicity, which occurs late in the course of therapy.

The manifestations of drug toxicity are variable, and any organ system may be involved. Gingival hyperplasia

Table 61-4	MAJOR ANTISEIZURE MEDICATIONS	
Medication	**Dose-Related Side Effects**	**Toxic Effects**
carbamazepine (Tegretol)	Dizziness, drowsiness, unsteadiness, nausea and vomiting, diplopia, mild leukopenia	Severe skin rash, blood dyscrasias, hepatitis
clonazepam (Klonopin)	Drowsiness, behavior changes, headache, hirsutism, alopecia, palpitations	Hepatotoxicity, thrombocytopenia, bone marrow failure, ataxia
ethosuximide (Zarontin)	Nausea and vomiting, headache, gastric distress	Skin rash, blood dyscrasias, hepatitis, systemic lupus erythematosus
felbamate (Felbatol)	Cognitive impairments, insomnia, nausea, headache, fatigue	Aplastic anemia, hepatotoxicity
gabapentin (Neurotonin)	Dizziness, drowsiness, somnolence, fatigue, ataxia, weight gain, nausea	Leukopenia, hepatotoxicity
lamotrigine (Lamictal)	Drowsiness, tremor, nausea, ataxia, dizziness, headache, weight gain	Severe rash (Stevens-Johnson syndrome)
levetiracetam (Keppra)	Somnolence, dizziness, fatigue	Unknown
oxacarbazepine (Trileptal)	Dizziness, somnolence, double vision, fatigue, nausea, vomiting, loss of coordination, abnormal vision, abdominal pain, tremor, abnormal gait	Hepatotoxicity
phenobarbital (Luminal)	Sedation, irritability, diplopia, ataxia	Skin rash, anemia
phenytoin (Dilantin)	Visual problems, hirsutism, gingival hyperplasia, dysrhythmias, dysarthria, nystagmus	Severe skin reaction, peripheral neuropathy, ataxia, drowsiness, blood dyscrasias
primidone (Mysoline)	Lethargy, irritability, diplopia, ataxia, impotence	Skin rash
tiagabine (Gabitril)	Dizziness, fatigue, nervousness, tremor, difficulty concentrating, dysarthria, weak or buckling knees, abdominal pain	Unknown
topiramate (Topamax)	Fatigue, somnolence, confusion, ataxia, anorexia, depression, weight loss	Nephrolithiasis
valproate (Depakote, Depakene)	Nausea and vomiting, weight gain, hair loss, tremor, menstrual irregularities	Hepatotoxicity, skin rash, blood dyscrasias, nephritis
zonisamide (Zonegran, Excegran)	Somnolence, dizziness, anorexia, headache, nausea, agitation, rash	Leukopenia, hepatotoxicity

(swollen and tender gums) can be associated with long-term use of phenytoin (Dilantin), for example (Karch, 2008). Periodic physical and dental examinations and laboratory tests are performed for patients receiving medications that are known to have hematopoietic, genitourinary, or hepatic effects.

Surgical Management

Surgery is indicated for patients whose epilepsy results from intracranial tumors, abscesses, cysts, or vascular anomalies. Some patients have intractable seizure disorders that do not respond to medication. A focal atrophic process may occur secondary to trauma, inflammation, stroke, or anoxia. If the seizures originate in a reasonably well-circumscribed area of the brain that can be excised without producing significant neurologic deficits, the removal of the area generating the seizures may produce long-term control and improvement (AANN, 2007).

This type of neurosurgery has been aided by several advances, including microsurgical techniques, EEGs with depth electrodes, improved illumination and hemostasis, and the introduction of neuroleptanalgesic agents (droperidol and fentanyl). These techniques, combined with use of local anesthetic agents, enable the neurosurgeon to perform surgery on an alert and cooperative patient. Using special testing devices, electrocortical mapping, and the patient's responses to stimulation, the boundaries of the epileptogenic focus (ie, abnormal area of the brain) are determined. Any abnormal epileptogenic focus is then excised (AANN, 2007). Resection surgery significantly reduces the incidence of seizures in patients with refractory epilepsy.

When seizures are refractory to medication in adolescents and adults with partial seizures, a generator may be implanted under the clavicle. The device is connected to the vagus nerve in the cervical area, where it delivers electrical signals to the brain to control and reduce seizure activity (AANN, 2007). An external programming system is used by the physician to change stimulator settings. Patients can turn the stimulator on and off with a magnet (Krapohl, Deutinger & Komurcu, 2007).

More research is needed to determine the effects of the various surgical approaches on complication rates, quality of life, anxiety, and depression, all of which are issues for patients with epilepsy.

NURSING PROCESS

THE PATIENT WITH EPILEPSY

Assessment

The nurse elicits information about the patient's seizure history. The patient is asked about the factors or events that may precipitate the seizures. Alcohol intake is documented. The nurse determines whether the patient has an aura before an epileptic seizure, which may indicate the origin of the seizure (eg, seeing a flashing light may indicate that the seizure originated in the occipital lobe). Observation and assessment during and after a seizure assist in identifying the type of seizure and its management.

The effects of epilepsy on the patient's lifestyle are assessed (AANN, 2007). What limitations are imposed by the seizure disorder? Does the patient participate in any recreational activities? Have any social contacts? Is the patient working, and is it a positive or stressful experience? What coping mechanisms are used?

Diagnosis

Nursing Diagnoses

Based on the assessment data, the patient's major nursing diagnoses may include the following:
- Risk for injury related to seizure activity
- Fear related to the possibility of seizures
- Ineffective individual coping related to stresses imposed by epilepsy
- Deficient knowledge related to epilepsy and its control

Collaborative Problems/Potential Complications

The major potential complications for patients with epilepsy are status epilepticus and medication side effects (toxicity).

Planning and Goals

The major goals for the patient may include prevention of injury, control of seizures, achievement of a satisfactory psychosocial adjustment, acquisition of knowledge and understanding about the condition, and absence of complications.

Nursing Interventions

Preventing Injury

Injury prevention for the patient with seizures is a priority. Patients for whom seizure precautions are instituted should have pads applied to the side rails while in bed. Steps to prevent or minimize injury are presented in Chart 61-4.

Reducing Fear of Seizures

Fear that a seizure may occur unexpectedly can be reduced by the patient's adherence to the prescribed treatment regimen. Cooperation of the patient and family and their trust in the prescribed regimen are essential for control of seizures. The nurse emphasizes that the prescribed antiseizure medication must be taken on a continuing basis and that drug dependence or addiction does not occur. Periodic monitoring is necessary to ensure the adequacy of the treatment regimen, to prevent side effects, and to monitor for drug resistance (Hickey, 2009).

In an effort to control seizures, factors that may precipitate them are identified, such as emotional disturbances, new environmental stressors, onset of menstruation in female patients, or fever (AANN, 2007). The patient is encouraged to follow a regular and moderate routine in lifestyle, diet (avoiding excessive stimulants), exercise, and rest (sleep deprivation may lower the seizure threshold). Moderate activity is therapeutic, but excessive exercise should be avoided. An additional dietary intervention, referred to as the ketogenic diet, may be helpful for control of seizures in some patients. This high-protein, low-carbohydrate, high-fat diet is most effective in children whose seizures have not been controlled with two antiepileptic medications, but it is sometimes used for adults who have had poor seizure control (Yudkoff, Daikhin, Melo, et al., 2007).

Photic stimulation (eg, bright flickering lights, television viewing) may precipitate seizures; wearing dark glasses or covering one eye may be preventive. Tension states (anxiety, frustration) induce seizures in some patients. Classes in stress management may be of value. Because seizures are known to occur with alcohol intake, alcoholic beverages should be avoided.

Improving Coping Mechanisms

The social, psychological, and behavioral problems that frequently accompany epilepsy can be more of a disability than the actual seizures. Epilepsy may be accompanied by feelings of stigmatization, alienation, depression, and uncertainty. The patient must cope with the constant fear of a seizure and the psychological consequences (AANN, 2007). Children with epilepsy may be ostracized and excluded from school and peer activities. These problems are compounded during adolescence and add to the challenges of dating, not being able to drive, and feeling different from other people. Adults face these problems in addition to the burden of finding employment, concerns about relationships and childbearing, insurance problems, and legal barriers. Alcohol abuse may complicate matters. Family reactions may vary from outright rejection of the person with epilepsy to overprotection.

Counseling assists the patient and family to understand the condition and the limitations it imposes. Social and recreational opportunities are necessary for good mental health. Nurses can improve the quality of life for patients with epilepsy by teaching them and their families about symptoms and their management (AANN, 2007) (see Chart 61-3).

Providing Patient and Family Education

Perhaps the most valuable facets of care contributed by the nurse to the person with epilepsy are education and efforts to modify the attitudes of the patient and family toward the disorder. The person who experiences seizures may consider every seizure a potential source of humiliation and shame. This may result in anxiety, depression, hostility, and secrecy on the part of the patient and family. Ongoing education and encouragement should be given to patients to enable them to overcome these reactions. The patient with epilepsy should carry an emergency medical identification card or wear a medical information bracelet. The patient and family need to be educated about medications as well as care during a seizure.

Monitoring and Managing Potential Complications

Status epilepticus, the major complication, is described later in this chapter. Another complication is the toxicity of medications. The patient and family are instructed about side effects and are given specific guidelines to assess and report signs and symptoms that indicate medication overdose. Antiseizure medications require careful monitoring for therapeutic levels. The patient should plan to have serum drug levels assessed at regular intervals. Many known drug interactions occur with antiseizure medications. A complete pharmacologic profile should be reviewed with the patient to avoid interactions that either potentiate or inhibit the effectiveness of the medications.

Promoting Home and Community-Based Care

TEACHING PATIENTS SELF-CARE. Thorough oral hygiene after each meal, gum massage, daily flossing, and regular dental care are essential to prevent or control gingival hyperplasia in patients receiving phenytoin (Dilantin). The patient is also instructed to inform all health care providers of the medication being taken, because of the possibility of drug interactions. An individualized comprehensive teaching plan is needed to assist the patient and family to adjust to this chronic disorder. Written patient education materials must be appropriate for the patient's reading level and must be provided in alternative formats if warranted. See Chart 61-5 for home care instruction points.

CONTINUING CARE. Because epilepsy is a long-term disorder, the use of costly medications can create a significant financial burden. The Epilepsy Foundation of America (EFA) offers a mail-order program to provide medications at minimal cost and access to life insurance. This organization also serves as a referral source for special services for people with epilepsy.

For many, overcoming employment problems is a challenge. State vocational rehabilitation agencies can provide information about job training. The EFA has a training and placement service. If seizures are not well controlled, information about sheltered workshops or home employment programs may be obtained. Federal and state agencies and federal legislation may be of assistance to people with epilepsy who experience job discrimination. As a result of the Americans with Disabilities Act, the number of employers who knowingly hire people with epilepsy is increasing, but barriers to employment still exist.

People who have uncontrollable seizures accompanied by psychological and social difficulties can be referred to comprehensive epilepsy centers where continuous audio-video and EEG monitoring, specialized treatment, and rehabilitation services are available (AANN, 2007). Patients and their families need to be reminded of the importance of following the prescribed treatment regimen and of keeping follow-up appointments. In addition, they are reminded of the importance of participating in health promotion activities and recommended health screenings to promote a healthy lifestyle. Genetic and preconception counseling is advised.

Evaluation

Expected Patient Outcomes

Expected patient outcomes may include the following:

1. Sustains no injury during seizure activity
   a. Complies with treatment regimen and identifies the hazards of stopping the medication
   b. Can identify appropriate care during seizure; caregivers can also do so
2. Indicates a decrease in fear
3. Displays effective individual coping
4. Exhibits knowledge and understanding of epilepsy
   a. Identifies the side effects of medications

CHART 61-5	HOME CARE CHECKLIST *The Patient With Epilepsy*		
At the completion of the home instruction, the patient and caregiver will be able to:		**PATIENT**	**CAREGIVER**
• Take medications daily as prescribed to keep the drug level constant to prevent seizures. The patient should never discontinue medications, even if there is no seizure activity.		✔	
• Keep a medication and seizure chart, noting when medications are taken and any seizure activity.		✔	✔
• Notify the patient's physician if patient cannot take medications due to illness.		✔	✔
• Have antiseizure medication serum levels checked regularly. When testing is prescribed, the patient should report to the laboratory for blood sampling before taking morning medication.		✔	
• Avoid activities that require alertness and coordination (driving, operating machinery) until after the effects of the medication have been evaluated.		✔	
• Report signs of toxicity so dosage can be adjusted. Common signs include drowsiness, lethargy, dizziness, difficulty walking, hyperactivity, confusion, inappropriate sleep, and visual disturbances.		✔	✔
• Avoid over-the-counter medications unless approved by the patient's physician.		✔	
• Carry a medical alert bracelet or identification card specifying the name of the patient's antiseizure medication and physician.		✔	
• Avoid seizure triggers, such as alcoholic beverages, electrical shocks, stress, caffeine, constipation, fever, hyperventilation, and hypoglycemia.		✔	
• Take showers rather than tub baths to avoid drowning if seizure occurs; never swim alone.		✔	
• Exercise in moderation in a temperature-controlled environment to avoid excessive heat.		✔	
• Develop regular sleep patterns to minimize fatigue and insomnia.		✔	✔
• Use the Epilepsy Foundation of America's special services, including help in obtaining medications, vocational rehabilitation, and coping with epilepsy.		✔	✔

    b. Avoids factors or situations that may precipitate seizures (eg, flickering lights, hyperventilation, alcohol)

    c. Follows a healthy lifestyle by getting adequate sleep and eating meals at regular times to avoid hypoglycemia

  5. Absence of complications

Status Epilepticus

Status epilepticus (acute prolonged seizure activity) is a series of generalized seizures that occur without full recovery of consciousness between attacks (Tocco, 2007). The term has been broadened to include continuous clinical or electrical seizures (on EEG) lasting at least 30 minutes, even without impairment of consciousness. It is considered a medical emergency. Status epilepticus produces cumulative effects. Vigorous muscular contractions impose a heavy metabolic demand and can interfere with respirations. Some respiratory arrest at the height of each seizure produces venous congestion and hypoxia of the brain. Repeated episodes of cerebral anoxia and edema may lead to irreversible and fatal brain damage. Factors that precipitate status epilepticus include withdrawal of antiseizure medication, fever, and concurrent infection.

Medical Management

The goals of treatment are to stop the seizures as quickly as possible, to ensure adequate cerebral oxygenation, and to maintain the patient in a seizure-free state. An airway and adequate oxygenation are established. If the patient remains unconscious and unresponsive, a cuffed endotracheal tube is inserted. IV diazepam (Valium), lorazepam (Ativan), or fosphenytoin (Cerebyx) is administered slowly in an attempt to halt seizures immediately. Other medications (phenytoin, phenobarbital) are administered later to maintain a seizure-free state.

An IV line is established, and blood samples are obtained to monitor serum electrolytes, glucose, and phenytoin levels. EEG monitoring may be useful in determining the nature of the seizure activity. Vital signs and neurologic signs are monitored on a continuing basis. An IV infusion of dextrose is administered if the seizure is caused by hypoglycemia. If initial treatment is unsuccessful, general anesthesia with a short-acting barbiturate may be used. The serum concentration of the antiseizure medication is measured, because a low level suggests that the patient was not taking the medication or that the dosage was too low. Cardiac involvement or respiratory depression may be life-threatening. The potential for postictal cerebral edema also exists.

Nursing Management

The nurse initiates ongoing assessment and monitoring of respiratory and cardiac function because of the risk for delayed depression of respiration and blood pressure secondary to administration of antiseizure medications and sedatives to halt the seizures. Nursing assessment also includes monitoring and documenting the seizure activity and the patient's responsiveness.

The patient is turned to a side-lying position, if possible, to assist in draining pharyngeal secretions. Suction equipment must be available because of the risk of aspiration. The IV line is closely monitored, because it may become dislodged during seizures.

A person who has received long-term antiseizure therapy has a significant risk for fractures resulting from bone disease (osteoporosis, osteomalacia, and hyperparathyroidism), a side effect of therapy. Therefore, during seizures, the patient is protected from injury with the use of seizure precautions and is monitored closely. The patient having seizures can inadvertently injure nearby people, so nurses should protect themselves. Additional nursing interventions for the person having seizures are presented in Chart 61-4.

HEADACHE

Headache, or cephalgia, is one of the most common of all human physical complaints. Headache is a symptom rather than a disease entity; it may indicate organic disease (neurologic or other disease), a stress response, vasodilation (migraine), skeletal muscle tension (tension headache), or a combination of factors. A **primary headache** is one for which no organic cause can be identified. These types of headache include migraine, tension-type, and cluster headaches (Hickey, 2009). Cranial arteritis is another common cause of headache. A classification of headaches was issued first by the Headache Classification Committee of the International Headache Society in 1988. The International Headache Society revised the headache classification in 2004; an abbreviated list is shown in Chart 61-6.

Chart 61-6 • *International Headache Society Classification of Headache*

1. Migraine
2. Tension-type headache
3. Cluster headache and other trigeminal-autonomic cephalalgias
4. Other primary headaches
5. Headache attributed to head and/or neck trauma
6. Headache attributed to cranial or cervical vascular disorder
7. Headache attributed to nonvascular intracranial disorder
8. Headache attributed to a substance or its withdrawal
9. Headache attributed to infection
10. Headache attributed to disorder of homeostasis
11. Headache or facial pain attributed to disorder of cranium, neck, eyes, ears, nose, sinuses, teeth, mouth, or other facial or cranial structures
12. Headache attributed to psychiatric disorder
13. Cranial neuralgias and central causes of facial pain
14. Other headache

From Headache Classification Subcommittee of the International Headache Society. (2004). International classification of headache disorders (2nd ed.). *Cephalalgia, 24*(Suppl 1), 1–150.

Migraine is a complex of symptoms characterized by periodic and recurrent attacks of severe headache lasting from 4 to 72 hours in adults. The cause of migraine has not been clearly demonstrated, but it is primarily a vascular disturbance that occurs more commonly in women and has a strong familial tendency. The typical time of onset is at puberty, and the incidence is 18% in women and 6% in men (Lipton, Bigal, Diamond, et al., 2007).

There are six subtypes of **migraine headache,** including migraine with and without aura. Most patients have migraine without an aura. *Tension-type headaches* tend to be chronic and less severe and are probably the most common type of headache. *Cluster headaches* are a severe form of vascular headache. They are seen five times more frequently in men than in women. Types of headaches not subsumed under these categories fall into the *Other Primary Headache* group and include headaches triggered by cough, exertion, and sexual activity.

Cranial arteritis is a cause of headache in the older population, reaching its greatest incidence in those older than 70 years of age. Inflammation of the cranial arteries is characterized by a severe headache localized in the region of the temporal arteries. The inflammation may be generalized (in which case cranial arteritis is part of a vascular disease) or focal (in which case only the cranial arteries are involved).

A **secondary headache** is a symptom associated with an organic cause, such as a brain tumor or an aneurysm. Although most headaches do not indicate serious disease, persistent headaches require further investigation. Serious disorders related to headache include brain tumors, subarachnoid hemorrhage, stroke, severe hypertension, meningitis, and head injuries.

Pathophysiology

The cerebral signs and symptoms of *migraine* result from dysfunction of the brain stem pathways that normally modulate sensory input. Abnormal metabolism of serotonin, a vasoactive neurotransmitter found in platelets and cells of the brain, plays a major role. The headache is preceded by a rise in plasma serotonin, which dilates the cerebral vessels, but migraines are more than just vascular headaches. The exact mechanism of pain in migraine is poorly understood but is thought to be related to the cranial blood vessels, the innervation of the vessels, and the reflex connections in the brain stem (Porth & Matfin, 2009).

Migraines can be triggered by menstrual cycles, bright lights, stress, depression, sleep deprivation, fatigue, overuse of certain medications, and certain foods containing tyramine, monosodium glutamate, nitrites, or milk products. Food triggers also include aged cheese and many processed foods. Use of oral contraceptives may be associated with increased frequency and severity of attacks in some women (Kelman, 2007).

Emotional or physical stress may cause contraction of the muscles in the neck and scalp, resulting in *tension* headache. The pathophysiology of *cluster* headache is not fully understood. One theory is that it is caused by dilation of orbital and nearby extracranial arteries. *Cranial arteritis* is thought to represent an immune vasculitis in which immune complexes are deposited within the walls of affected blood vessels, producing vascular injury and inflammation. A biopsy may be performed on the involved artery to make the diagnosis.

Clinical Manifestations

Migraine

The migraine with aura can be divided into four phases: prodrome, aura, the headache, and recovery (headache termination and postdrome).

Prodrome Phase

The prodrome phase is experienced by 60% of patients, with symptoms that occur hours to days before a migraine headache. Symptoms may include depression, irritability, feeling cold, food cravings, anorexia, change in activity level, increased urination, diarrhea, or constipation. Patients usually experience the same prodrome with each migraine headache.

Aura Phase

Aura occurs in a minority of patients who experience migraines (Cutrer & Heurter, 2007). The aura usually lasts less than 1 hour and may provide enough time for the patient to take the prescribed medication to avert an attack (see later discussion). This period is characterized by focal neurologic symptoms. Visual disturbances (ie, light flashes and bright spots) are most common and may be hemianopic (affecting only half of the visual field). Other symptoms that may follow include numbness and tingling of the lips, face, or hands; mild confusion; slight weakness of an extremity; drowsiness; and dizziness.

This period of aura corresponds to the phenomenon of cortical spreading depression that is associated with reduced metabolic demand in abnormally functioning neurons. This is associated with decreased blood flow that is the initial physiologic change characteristic of classic migraine (Cutrer & Heurter, 2007). Cerebral blood flow studies performed during migraine headaches demonstrate that during all phases of migraine, cerebral blood flow is reduced throughout the brain, with subsequent loss of autoregulation and impaired carbon dioxide responsiveness.

Headache Phase

As vasodilation and a decline in serotonin levels occur, a throbbing headache (unilateral in 60% of patients) intensifies over several hours. This headache is severe and incapacitating and is often associated with photophobia, nausea, and vomiting. Its duration varies, ranging from 4 to 72 hours (Hickey, 2009).

Recovery Phase

In the recovery phase (termination and postdrome), the pain gradually subsides. Muscle contraction in the neck and scalp is common, with associated muscle ache and localized tenderness, exhaustion, and mood changes. Any physical exertion exacerbates the headache pain. During this postheadache phase, patients may sleep for extended periods.

Other Headache Types

The *tension-type headache* is characterized by a steady, constant feeling of pressure that usually begins in the forehead, temple, or back of the neck. It is often bandlike or may be described as "a weight on top of my head."

Cluster headaches are unilateral and come in clusters of one to eight daily, with excruciating pain localized to the eye and orbit and radiating to the facial and temporal regions. The pain is accompanied by watering of the eye and nasal congestion. Each attack lasts 15 minutes to 3 hours and may have a crescendo–decrescendo pattern (Hickey, 2009). The headache is often described as penetrating.

Cranial arteritis often begins with general manifestations, such as fatigue, malaise, weight loss, and fever. Clinical manifestations associated with inflammation (heat, redness, swelling, tenderness, or pain over the involved artery) usually are present. Sometimes a tender, swollen, or nodular temporal artery is visible. Visual problems are caused by ischemia of the involved structures.

Assessment and Diagnostic Findings

The diagnostic evaluation includes a detailed history, a physical assessment of the head and neck, and a complete neurologic examination. Headaches may manifest differently in the same person over the course of a lifetime, and the same type of headache may manifest differently from patient to patient. The health history focuses on assessing the headache itself, with emphasis on the factors that precipitate or provoke it. The patient is asked to describe the headache in his or her own words.

Because headache is often the presenting symptom of various physiologic and psychological disturbances, a general health history is an essential component of the patient database. Headache may be a symptom of endocrine, hematologic, gastrointestinal, infectious, renal, cardiovascular, or psychiatric disease. Therefore, questions addressed in the health history should cover major medical and surgical illness as well as a body systems review.

The medication history can provide insight into the patient's overall health status and indicate medications that may be provoking headaches. Antihypertensive agents, diuretic medications, anti-inflammatory agents, and monoamine oxidase (MAO) inhibitors are a few of the categories of medications that can provoke headaches. Emotional factors can play a role in precipitating headaches. Stress is thought to be a major initiating factor in migraine headaches; therefore, sleep patterns, level of stress, recreational interests, appetite, emotional problems, and family stressors are relevant. There is a strong familial tendency for headache disorders, and a positive family history may help in making a diagnosis.

A direct relationship may exist between exposure to toxic substances and headache. Careful questioning may uncover chemicals to which a worker has been exposed. Under the Right to Know law, employees have access to the material safety data sheets (commonly referred to as MSDSs) for all the substances with which they come in contact in the workplace. The occupational history also includes assessment of the workplace as a possible source of stress and for a possible ergonomic basis of muscle strain and headache.

A complete description of the headache itself is crucial. The nurse reviews the age at onset of headache; the headache's frequency, location, and duration; the type of pain; factors that relieve and precipitate the event; and associated symptoms. The data obtained should include the patient's own words about the headache in response to the following questions:

- What is the location? Is it unilateral or bilateral? Does it radiate?
- What is the quality—dull, aching, steady, boring, burning, intermittent, continuous, paroxysmal?
- How many headaches occur during a given period of time?
- What are the precipitating factors, if any—environmental (eg, sunlight, weather change), foods, exertion, other?
- What makes the headache worse (eg, coughing, straining)?
- What time (day or night) does it occur?
- How long does a typical headache last?
- Are there any associated symptoms, such as facial pain, lacrimation (excessive tearing), or scotomas (blind spots in the field of vision)?
- What usually relieves the headache (aspirin, nonsteroidal anti-inflammatory drugs, ergot preparation, food, heat, rest, neck massage)?
- Does nausea, vomiting, weakness, or numbness in the extremities accompany the headache?
- Does the headache interfere with daily activities?
- Do you have any allergies?
- Do you have insomnia, poor appetite, loss of energy?
- Is there a family history of headache?
- What is the relationship of the headache to your lifestyle or physical or emotional stress?
- What medications are you taking?

Diagnostic testing often is not helpful in the investigation of headache, because often there are few objective findings. In patients who demonstrate abnormalities on the neurologic examination, CT, cerebral angiography, or MRI may be used to detect underlying causes, such as tumor or aneurysm. Electromyography (EMG) may reveal a sustained contraction of the neck, scalp, or facial muscles. Laboratory tests may include complete blood count, erythrocyte sedimentation rate, electrolytes, glucose, creatinine, and thyroid hormone levels.

Prevention

Prevention begins by having the patient avoid specific triggers that are known to initiate the headache syndrome. Preventive medical management of migraine involves the daily use of one or more agents that are thought to block the physiologic events leading to an attack. Treatment regimens vary greatly, as do patient responses; therefore, close monitoring is indicated.

Several widely used medications for the prevention of migraine are available. Two beta-blocking agents, propranolol (Inderal) and metoprolol (Lopressor), inhibit the action of beta-receptors—cells in the heart and brain that control the dilation of blood vessels. This is thought to be a major reason for their antimigraine action. Other medications that are prescribed for migraine prevention include amitriptyline hydrochloride (Elavil), divalproex (Valproate), flunarizine (Sibelium), and serotonin antagonists (Pizotyline) (Bigal & Lipton, 2007).

Calcium antagonists (eg, verapamil) are widely used but may require several weeks at a therapeutic dosage before improvement is noted. Calcium channel blockers are not as effective as beta-blockers for prevention but may be more appropriate for some patients, such as those with bradycardia, diabetes mellitus, or asthma (Bigal & Lipton, 2007).

Researchers are evaluating several antiseizure medications for migraine prevention. Topiramate (Topamax), the most extensively studied preventive agent, has been shown to be effective. Started at a low dose, topiramate is titrated to 100 to 200 mg/day in divided doses (Bigal & Lipton, 2007). Other research suggests that the use of topiramate and gabapentin (Neurontin), another antiseizure medication, for migraine prevention may impair cognitive ability (Salinsky, Storzbach, Spencer, et al., 2005).

Alcohol, nitrites, vasodilators, and histamines may precipitate cluster headaches. Elimination of these factors helps prevent the headaches. Other prophylactic medication therapy may include antiseizure medications, ergotamine tartrate (occasionally), lithium, naproxen (Naprosyn), and methysergide (Sansert) (Bigal & Lipton, 2007).

Medical Management

Therapy for migraine headache is divided into abortive (symptomatic) and preventive approaches. The abortive approach, best used in those patients who have less frequent attacks, is aimed at relieving or limiting a headache at the onset or while it is in progress. The preventive approach is used in patients who experience more frequent attacks at regular or predictable intervals and may have a medical condition that precludes the use of abortive therapies (Hickey, 2009).

The triptans, serotonin receptor agonists, are the most specific antimigraine agents available. These agents cause vasoconstriction, reduce inflammation, and may reduce pain transmission. The five triptans in routine clinical use include sumatriptan (Imitrex), naratriptan (Amerge), rizatriptan (Maxalt), zolmitriptan (Zomig), and almotriptan (Axert) (Mett & Tfelt-Hansen, 2008). Numerous serotonin receptor agonists are under study. Many of the triptan medications are available in a variety of formulations, such as nasal sprays, inhalers, suppositories, or injections. The nasal sprays are useful for patients experiencing nausea and vomiting (Hickey, 2009).

The most widely used triptan is sumatriptan succinate (Imitrex) and is effective for the treatment of acute migraine and cluster headaches in adults (Bigal & Lipton, 2007). The subcutaneous form usually relieves symptoms within 1 hour and is available in an autoinjector for immediate patient use, although this form is expensive. Sumatriptan has been found to be effective in relieving moderate to severe migraine headaches in a large number of adult patients. Sumatriptan can cause chest pain and is contraindicated in patients with ischemic heart disease. Careful administration and dosing instructions to patients are important to prevent adverse reactions such as increased blood pressure, drowsiness, muscle pain, sweating, and anxiety. Interactions are possible if the medication is taken in conjunction with St. John's wort (Karch, 2008).

Ergotamine preparations (taken orally, sublingually, subcutaneously, intramuscularly, by rectum, or by inhalation) may be effective in aborting the headache if taken early in the migraine process. They are low in cost. Ergotamine tartrate acts on smooth muscle, causing prolonged constriction of the cranial blood vessels. Each patient's dosage is based on individual needs. Side effects include aching muscles, paresthesias (numbness and tingling), nausea, and vomiting. Cafergot, a combination of ergotamine and caffeine, can arrest or reduce the severity of the headache if it is taken at the first sign of an attack (Karch, 2008). None of the triptan medications should be taken concurrently with medications containing ergotamine, because of the potential for a prolonged vasoactive reaction (Karch, 2008).

The medical management of an acute attack of cluster headaches may include 100% oxygen by face mask for 15 minutes, ergotamine tartrate, sumatriptan, corticosteroids, or a percutaneous sphenopalatine ganglion blockade (Hickey, 2009).

The medical management of cranial arteritis consists of early administration of a corticosteroid to prevent the possibility of loss of vision due to vascular occlusion or rupture of the involved artery. The patient is instructed not to stop the medication abruptly, because this can lead to relapse. Analgesic agents are prescribed for comfort.

Nursing Management

When migraine or the other types of headaches have been diagnosed, the goal of nursing management is to enhance pain relief. It is reasonable to try nonpharmacologic interventions first, but the use of medications should not be delayed. The goal is to treat the acute event of the headache and to prevent recurrent episodes. Prevention involves patient education regarding precipitating factors, possible lifestyle or habit changes that may be helpful, and pharmacologic measures.

Relieving Pain

Individualized treatment depends on the type of headache and differs for migraine, cluster headaches, cranial arteritis, and tension headache. Nursing care is directed toward treatment of the acute episode. A migraine or a cluster headache in the early phase requires abortive medication therapy instituted as soon as possible. Some headaches can be prevented if the appropriate medications are taken before the onset of pain. Nursing care during an attack includes comfort measures such as a quiet, dark environment; elevation of the head of the bed to 30 degrees; and symptomatic treatment (ie, administration of antiemetic medication) (Hickey, 2009).

Symptomatic pain relief for tension headache may be obtained by application of local heat or massage. Additional strategies may include administration of analgesic agents, antidepressant medications, and muscle relaxants.

Promoting Home and Community-Based Care

Teaching Patients Self-Care

Headaches, especially migraines, are more likely to occur when the patient is ill, overly tired, or stressed. Nonpharmacologic therapies are important and include patient education about the type of headache, its mechanism (if known), and appropriate changes in lifestyle to avoid triggers. Regular sleep, meals, exercise, relaxation, and avoidance of dietary triggers may be helpful in avoiding headaches (Hickey, 2009).

The patient with tension headaches needs teaching and reassurance that the headache is not the result of a brain tumor; this is a common unspoken fear. Stress reduction techniques, such as biofeedback, exercise programs, and meditation, are examples of nonpharmacologic therapies that may prove helpful. The patient and family need to be reminded of the importance of following the prescribed treatment regimen for headache and keeping follow-up appointments. In addition, the patient is reminded of the importance of participating in health promotion activities and recommended health screenings to promote a healthy lifestyle. Chart 61-7 presents a home care checklist for the patient with migraine headaches.

CHART 61-7 HOME CARE CHECKLIST
The Patient With Migraine Headaches

At the completion of the home instruction, the patient or caregiver will be able to:	PATIENT	CAREGIVER
• Define migraine headaches and describe characteristics and manifestations.	✔	✔
• Identify triggers of migraine headaches and how to avoid such triggers as:		
• Foods that contain tyramine, such as chocolate, cheese, coffee, dairy products	✔	✔
• Dietary habits that result in long periods between meals	✔	✔
• Menstruation and ovulation (caused by hormone fluctuation)	✔	✔
• Alcohol (causes vasodilation of blood vessels)	✔	✔
• Fatigue and fluctuations in sleep patterns	✔	✔
• State importance of developing and using a headache diary.	✔	✔
• State stress management and lifestyle changes to minimize the frequency of headaches.	✔	✔
• State pharmacologic management: acute therapy and prophylaxis, to include medication regimen and side effects.	✔	✔
• Identify comfort measures during headache attacks, such as resting in a quiet and dark environment, applying cold compresses to the painful area, and elevating the head.	✔	✔
• Identify resources for education and support, such as the National Headache Foundation.	✔	✔

Continuing Care

The National Headache Foundation (see Resources) provides a list of clinics in the United States and the names of physicians who specialize in headache and who are members of the American Association for the Study of Headache.

CRITICAL THINKING EXERCISES

EBP 1 Your 25-year-old patient with a brain injury has signs of ICP. Describe the nursing measures that are indicated. How would you determine whether your interventions were effective in alleviating the increased ICP? What is the evidence base for practices to decrease ICP? Identify the criteria used to evaluate the strength of the evidence for these practices.

2 A patient is admitted to your unit after undergoing transsphenoidal surgery for a pituitary tumor. Describe the major complications to assess for, along with the signs and symptoms of each. Describe the pharmacologic treatment and nursing measures that are indicated postoperatively. What patient and family teaching is important for the patient and family? How would you modify your teaching and discharge planning if the patient understands little English?

EBP 3 You are caring for a 35-year-old patient who is admitted to the hospital for evaluation of her seizures. What resources would you use to identify the current guidelines for classification and treatment of seizures? What is the evidence base for treatment practices? Identify the criteria used to evaluate the strength of the evidence for these practices.

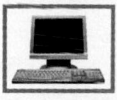

The Smeltzer suite offers these additional resources to enhance learning and facilitate understanding of this chapter:

- thePoint online resource, thepoint.lww.com/ Smeltzer12E
- Student CD-ROM included with the book
- *Study Guide to Accompany Brunner & Suddarth's Textbook of Medical-Surgical Nursing*
- *Handbook for Brunner & Suddarth's Textbook of Medical-Surgical Nursing*

REFERENCES AND SELECTED READINGS

*Asterisks indicate nursing research.
**Double asterisk indicates classic references.

Books

American Association of Neuroscience Nurses. (2005). *Guide to the care of the patient with intracranial pressure monitoring: AANN reference series for clinical practice.* Glenview, IL: Author.

American Association of Neuroscience Nurses. (2007). *Care of the patient with seizures. AANN clinical practice guidelines series.* Glenview, IL: Author

Brain Trauma Foundation. (2007). *Guidelines for the management of severe traumatic brain injury.* New York: Author.

Dudek, S. G. (2006). *Nutrition essentials for nursing practice* (5th ed.). Philadelphia: Lippincott Williams & Wilkins.

Hickey, J. V. (2009). *The clinical practice of neurological & neurosurgical nursing* (6th ed.). Philadelphia: Lippincott Williams & Wilkins.

Karch, A. (2008). *Lippincott's nursing drug guide.* Philadelphia: Lippincott Williams & Wilkins.

Karpoff, S. & Labus, D. M. (2008). *Portable diagnostic tests.* Philadelphia: Lippincott Williams & Wilkins.

Littlejohns, L. R. & Bader, M. K. (2009). *AACN-AANN protocols for practice: Monitoring technologies in critically ill neuroscience patients.* Sudbury, MA: Jones and Bartlett Publishers.

Mazzoni, P., Pearson, T. S. & Rowland, L. P. (2006). *Merritt's neurology handbook.* Philadelphia: Lippincott Williams & Wilkins.

Porth, C. M. & Matfin, C. (2009). *Pathophysiology: Concepts of altered health states* (8th ed.). Philadelphia: Lippincott Williams & Wilkins.

Posner, J. B., Saper, C. B., Schiff, N. D., et al. (2007). *Plum and Posner's diagnosis of stupor and coma* (4th ed.). Oxford, UK: Oxford University Press.

Journals and Electronic Documents

General

*Fields, L. B. (2008). Oral care interventions to reduce incidence of ventilator-associated pneumonia in the neurologic intensive care unit. *Journal of Neuroscience Nursing, 40*(5), 291–298.

Gusa, D., Miers, A., Pfrimmer, D., et al. (2007). Using the FOUR score scale to assess comatose patients. *American Nurse Today, 2*(6), 18–19.

Olsen, D. M. & Graffagnino, C. (2005). Consciousness, coma, and caring for the brain-injured patient. *AACN Clinical issues, 16*(4), 441–455.

Peiffer, K. M. Z. (2007). Brain death and organ procurement. *American Journal of Nursing, 107*(3), 58–68.

*Thompson, H., Kirkness, C., Mitchell, P., et al. (2007). Fever management practices of neuroscience nurses: National and regional perspectives. *Journal of Neuroscience Nursing, 39*(3), 151–162.

Wu, J. & Baguley, I. J. (2005). Urinary retention in a general rehabilitation unit: Prevalence, clinical outcome, and the role of screening. *Archives of Physical Medicine & Rehabilitation, 86*(9), 1772–1777.

Headache

Bigal, M. E. & Lipton, R. B. (2007). The preventive treatment of migraine. *The Neurologist, 12*(4), 204–213.

Cutrer, M. C. & Heurter, K. (2007). Migraine aura. *The Neurologist, 13*(3), 118–125.

**Headache Classification Subcommittee of the International Headache Society. (2004). International classification of headache disorders (2nd ed.). *Cephalalgia, 24*(Suppl. 1), 1–150.

Kelman, L. (2007). The triggers or precipitants of the acute migraine attack. *Cephalalgia, 27*(5), 394–402.

Lipton, R. B., Bigal, M. E., Diamond, M., et al. (2007). Migraine prevalence disease burden and the need for preventive therapy. *Neurology, 68*(4), 343–349.

Mett, A. & Tfelt-Hansen, P. (2008). Acute migraine therapy: Recent evidence from randomized comparative trials. *Current Opinions in Neurology, 21*(3), 331–341.

Salinsky, M. C., Storzbach, D., Spencer, D. C., et al. (2005). Effects of topiramate and gabapentin on cognitive abilities in healthy volunteers. *Neurology, 64*(3), 792–798.

Increased Intracranial Pressure

Bader, M. K., Arbour, R. & Palmer, S. (2005). Refractory increased intracranial pressure in severe traumatic brain injury: Barbiturate coma and bispectral index monitoring. *AACN Clinical Issues, 16*(4), 526–541.

Haitsma, I. K. & Maas, A. I. (2007). Monitoring cerebral oxygenation in traumatic brain injury. *Progress in Brain Research, 161*(8), 207–216.

Jaeger, M., Soehle, M. & Meixensberger, J. (2005). Brain tissue oxygenation (PtiO2): A clinical comparison of two monitoring devices. *Acta Neurochirurgica, 147*(1), 79–81.

Johnston, A., Steiner, L., Coles, J., et al. (2005). Effect of cerebral perfusion pressure augmentation on regional oxygenation and metabolism after head injury. *Critical Care Medicine, 33*(1), 198–195.

Lescot, T., Abdennour, L., Boch, A., et al. (2008). Treatment of intracranial hypertension. *Current Opinion in Critical Care, 14*(2), 129–134.

McAdoo, D. J. & Wu, P. (2008). Microdialysis in central nervous system disorders and their treatments. *Pharmacology, Biochemistry, and Behavior, 90*(2), 282–296.

*Mcilvoy, L. (2007). The impact of brain temperature and core temperature on intracranial pressure and cerebral perfusion pressure. *Journal of Neuroscience Nursing, 39*(6), 324–331.

Neurosurgical Care

March, K. (2005). Intracranial pressure monitoring: Why monitor? *AACN Clinical Issues*, 16(4), 456–475.

Mortimer, D. S. & Jancik, J. (2006). Administering hypertonic saline to patients with severe traumatic brain injury. *Journal of Neuroscience Nursing*, 38(3), 142–146.

Musleh, W., Sonabend, A. M. & Lesniak, M. S. (2006). Role of craniotomy in the management of pituitary adenomas and sellar/parasellar tumors. *Expert Review of Anticancer Therapy*, 6(Suppl. 9), 579–583.

Nemergut, F. C., Durieaux, M. E., Missaghi, N. B., et al. (2007). Pain management after craniotomy. *Best Practice & Research: Clinical Anesthesiology*, 21(4), 557–573.

Spiotta, A., Stiefel, M., Heuer, G., et al. (2008). Brain hyperthermia after traumatic brain injury does not reduce brain oxygen. *Neurosurgery*, 62(4), 664–872.

Stapelfeldt, C., Lobo, E., Brown, R., et al. (2005). Intraoperative clonidine administration to neurosurgical patients. *Anesthesia and Analgesia*, 100(1), 226–232.

Vergouwen, M. D., Roos, Y. B. & Kamphuisen, P. W. (2008). Venous thromboembolism prophylaxis and treatment in patients with acute stroke and traumatic brain injury. *Current Opinion in Critical Care*, 14, 149–155.

Seizures and Epilepsy

*Dilorio, C., Reisinger, E. L., Yeager, K., et al. (2008). A descriptive analysis of seizure events among adults who participated in a computer-based assessment. *Journal of Neuroscience Nursing*, 40(3), 134–141.

Kotagal, P. & Yardi, N. (2008). The relationship between sleep and epilepsy. *Seminars in Pediatric Neurology*, 15(2), 42–49.

Krapohl, B., Deutinger, M. & Komurcu, F. (2007). Vagus nerve stimulation: Treatment modality for epilepsy. *MedSurg Nursing*, 16(1), 39–45.

Meador, K. J., Pennell, P. B., Harden, C. L., et al. (2008). Pregnancy registries in epilepsy: A consensus statement on health outcomes. *Neurology*, 71(14), 1109–1117.

Tocco, S. B. (2007). Overcoming the fear of tonic-clonic seizures. *American Nurse Today*, 2(5), 10–12.

Yudkoff, M., Daikhin, Y., Melo, T. M., et al. (2007). The ketogenic diet and brain metabolism of amino acids: Relationship to the anticonvulsant effect. *Annual Review of Nutrition*, 27, 415–430.

Unconsciousness and Coma

Burck, R., Anderson-Shaw, L., Sheldon, M., et al. (2006). The clinical response to brain death: A policy proposal. *JONA's Healthcare Law, Ethics and Regulation*, 8(2), 53–59.

Gerber, C. S. (2005). Understanding and managing coma stimulation: Are we doing everything we can? *Critical care nursing Quarterly*, 28(2), 94–108.

Maurer, B. T. (2008). Locked-in syndrome. *American Journal of Hospice and Palliative Care*, 25(2), 151.

RESOURCES

American Headache Society, www.ahsnet.org
Brain Injury Association, www.biausa.org
Brain Trauma Foundation, www.braintrauma.org
Epilepsy Foundation, www.epilepsyfoundation.org
Hydrocephalus Association, hydroassoc@aol.com.
National Headache Foundation, www.headaches.org

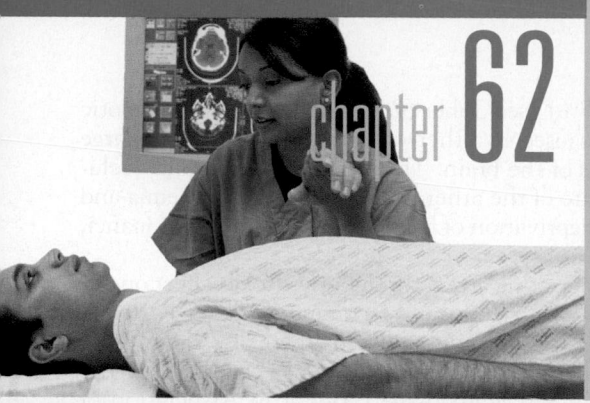

chapter 62

Management of Patients With Cerebrovascular Disorders

Cerebrovascular disorders is an umbrella term that refers to a functional abnormality of the central nervous system (CNS) that occurs when the normal blood supply to the brain is disrupted. Stroke is the primary cerebrovascular disorder in the United States, and it is the third leading cause of death after heart disease and cancer. Approximately 780,000 people experience a stroke each year in the United States. Approximately 600,000 of these are new strokes, and 180,000 are recurrent strokes (Rosamond, Flegal, Furie, et al., 2008). About 5.6 million noninstitutionalized stroke survivors are alive today; stroke is a leading cause of serious, long-term disability in the United States. The financial impact of stroke is profound, with estimated direct and indirect costs of $65.5 billion in 2008 (Rosamond, et al., 2008).

Strokes can be divided into two major categories: ischemic (85%), in which vascular occlusion and significant hypoperfusion occur, and hemorrhagic (15%), in which there is extravasation of blood into the brain or subarachnoid space (Hinkle & Guanci, 2007). Although there are some similarities between the two broad types of stroke, differences exist in etiology, pathophysiology, medical management, surgical management, and nursing care. Table 62-1 compares ischemic and hemorrhagic strokes.

Ischemic Stroke

An ischemic stroke, cerebrovascular accident (CVA), or "brain attack" is a sudden loss of function resulting from disruption of the blood supply to a part of the brain. The term *brain attack* is being used to suggest to health care practitioners and the public that a stroke is an urgent health care issue similar to a heart attack. With the approval of thrombolytic therapy for the treatment of acute ischemic stroke in 1996 came a revolution in the care of patients after a stroke. Early treatment with thrombolytic therapy for ischemic stroke results in fewer stroke symptoms and less loss of function (National Institute of Neurologic Disorders and Stroke [NINDS], 1995). Currently approved thrombolytic therapy has a treatment window of only 3 hours after the onset of a stroke. Urgency is needed on the part of the public and health care practitioners for rapid transport of the patient to a hospital for assessment and administration of the medication.

Ischemic strokes are subdivided into five different types based on the cause: large artery thrombotic strokes (20%), small penetrating artery thrombotic strokes (25%), cardiogenic embolic strokes (20%), cryptogenic strokes (30%),

and other (5%) (see Table 62-1). Large artery thrombotic strokes are caused by atherosclerotic plaques in the large blood vessels of the brain. Thrombus formation and occlusion at the site of the atherosclerosis result in ischemia and **infarction** (deprivation of blood supply) (Hinkle & Guanci, 2007).

Small penetrating artery thrombotic strokes affect one or more vessels and are the most common type of ischemic stroke. Small artery thrombotic strokes are also called lacunar strokes because of the cavity that is created after the death of infarcted brain tissue (American Association of Neuroscience Nurses [AANN], 2008).

Cardiogenic embolic strokes are associated with cardiac dysrhythmias, usually atrial fibrillation. Embolic strokes can also be associated with valvular heart disease and thrombi in the left ventricle. Emboli originate from the heart and circulate to the cerebral vasculature, most commonly the left middle cerebral artery, resulting in a stroke. Embolic strokes may be prevented by the use of anticoagulation therapy in patients with atrial fibrillation.

The last two classifications of ischemic strokes are cryptogenic strokes, which have no known cause, and strokes from other causes, such as illicit drug use, coagulopathies, migraine, and spontaneous dissection of the carotid or vertebral arteries.

Pathophysiology

In an ischemic brain attack, there is disruption of the cerebral blood flow due to obstruction of a blood vessel. This disruption in blood flow initiates a complex series of cellular metabolic events referred to as the ischemic cascade (Fig. 62-1).

The ischemic cascade begins when cerebral blood flow decreases to less than 25 mL per 100 g of blood per minute. At this point, neurons are no longer able to maintain aerobic respiration. The mitochondria must then switch to anaerobic respiration, which generates large amounts of lactic acid, causing a change in the pH. This switch to the less efficient anaerobic respiration also renders the neuron incapable of producing sufficient quantities of adenosine triphosphate (ATP) to fuel the depolarization processes. The membrane pumps that maintain electrolyte balances begin to fail, and the cells cease to function.

Early in the cascade, an area of low cerebral blood flow, referred to as the **penumbra region,** exists around the area of infarction. The penumbra region is ischemic brain tissue that may be salvaged with timely intervention. The ischemic cascade threatens cells in the penumbra because

Table 62-1	COMPARISON OF MAJOR TYPES OF STROKE	
Item	**Ischemic**	**Hemorrhagic**
Causes	Large artery thrombosis Small penetrating artery thrombosis Cardiogenic embolic Cryptogenic (no known cause) Other	Intracerebral hemorrhage Subarachnoid hemorrhage Cerebral aneurysm Arteriovenous malformation
Main presenting symptoms	Numbness or weakness of the face, arm, or leg, especially on one side of the body	"Exploding headache" Decreased level of consciousness
Functional recovery	Usually plateaus at 6 months	Slower, usually plateaus at about 18 months

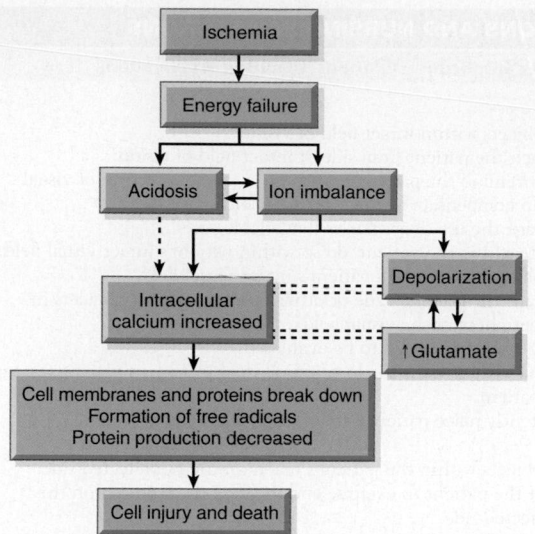

Figure 62-1 Processes contributing to ischemic brain cell injury. Courtesy of National Stroke Association, Englewood, Colorado.

membrane depolarization of the cell wall leads to an increase in intracellular calcium and the release of glutamate. The influx of calcium and the release of glutamate, if continued, activate a number of damaging pathways that result in the destruction of the cell membrane, the release of more calcium and glutamate, vasoconstriction, and the generation of free radicals. These processes enlarge the area of infarction into the penumbra, extending the stroke. A person experiencing a stroke typically loses 1.9 million neurons each minute that a stroke is not treated, and the ischemic brain ages 3.6 years each hour without treatment (Saver, 2006).

Each step in the ischemic cascade represents an opportunity for intervention to limit the extent of secondary brain damage caused by a stroke. The penumbra area may be revitalized by administration of tissue plasminogen activator (t-PA). Medications that protect the brain from secondary injury are called neuroprotectants. A number of ongoing clinical trials focus on neuroprotective medications and strategies to improve stroke recovery and survival (Lapchak & Araujo, 2007).

Clinical Manifestations

An ischemic stroke can cause a wide variety of neurologic deficits, depending on the location of the lesion (which vessels are obstructed), the size of the area of inadequate perfusion, and the amount of collateral (secondary or accessory) blood flow (see Chapter 60 for discussion of anatomy and brain blood supply). The patient may present with any of the following signs or symptoms:
- Numbness or weakness of the face, arm, or leg, especially on one side of the body
- Confusion or change in mental status
- Trouble speaking or understanding speech
- Visual disturbances
- Difficulty walking, dizziness, or loss of balance or coordination
- Sudden severe headache

Motor, sensory, cranial nerve, cognitive, and other functions may be disrupted. Table 62-2 reviews the neurologic deficits frequently seen in patients with strokes. Table 62-3 compares the symptoms and behaviors seen in right hemispheric stroke with those seen in left hemispheric stroke.

Motor Loss

A stroke is an upper motor neuron lesion and results in loss of voluntary control over motor movements. Because the upper motor neurons decussate (cross), a disturbance of voluntary motor control on one side of the body may reflect damage to the upper motor neurons on the opposite side of the brain. The most common motor dysfunction is **hemiplegia** (paralysis of one side of the body) caused by a lesion of the opposite side of the brain. **Hemiparesis,** or weakness of one side of the body, is another sign. The concept of upper and lower motor neuron lesions is described in more detail in Table 60-4 in Chapter 60.

In the early stage of stroke, the initial clinical features may be flaccid paralysis and loss of or decrease in the deep tendon reflexes. When these deep reflexes reappear (usually by 48 hours), increased tone is observed along with spasticity (abnormal increase in muscle tone) of the extremities on the affected side.

Communication Loss

Other brain functions affected by stroke are language and communication. In fact, stroke is the most common cause of aphasia. The following are dysfunctions of language and communication:
- **Dysarthria** (difficulty in speaking), caused by paralysis of the muscles responsible for producing speech
- Dysphasia (impaired speech) or **aphasia** (loss of speech), which can be **expressive aphasia, receptive aphasia,** or global (mixed) aphasia
- **Apraxia** (inability to perform a previously learned action), as may be seen when a patient makes verbal substitutions for desired syllables or words

Perceptual Disturbances

Perception is the ability to interpret sensation. Stroke can result in visual-perceptual dysfunctions, disturbances in visual-spatial relations, and sensory loss.

Visual-perceptual dysfunctions are caused by disturbances of the primary sensory pathways between the eye and visual cortex. Homonymous **hemianopsia** (loss of half of the visual field) may occur from stroke and may be temporary or permanent. The affected side of vision corresponds to the paralyzed side of the body.

Disturbances in visual-spatial relations (perceiving the relationship of two or more objects in spatial areas) are frequently seen in patients with right hemispheric damage.

Sensory Loss

The sensory losses from stroke may take the form of slight impairment of touch, or it may be more severe, with loss of proprioception (ability to perceive the position and motion of body parts) as well as difficulty in interpreting visual, tactile, and auditory stimuli. **Agnosias** are deficits in the ability to recognize previously familiar objects perceived by one or more of the senses.

Table 62-2	NEUROLOGIC DEFICITS OF STROKE: MANIFESTATIONS AND NURSING IMPLICATIONS	
Neurologic Deficit	**Manifestation**	**Nursing Implications/Patient Teaching Applications**
Visual Field Deficits		
Homonymous hemianopsia (loss of half of the visual field)	• Unaware of persons or objects on side of visual loss • Neglect of one side of the body • Difficulty judging distances	Place objects within intact field of vision. Approach the patient from side of intact field of vision. Instruct/remind the patient to turn head in the direction of visual loss to compensate for loss of visual field. Encourage the use of eyeglasses if available. When teaching the patient, do so within patient's intact visual field.
Loss of peripheral vision	• Difficulty seeing at night • Unaware of objects or the borders of objects	Place objects in center of patient's intact visual field. Encourage the use of a cane or other object to identify objects in the periphery of the visual field. Driving ability will need to be evaluated.
Diplopia	• Double vision	Explain to the patient the location of an object when placing it near the patient. Consistently place patient care items in the same location.
Motor Deficits		
Hemiparesis	• Weakness of the face, arm, and leg on the same side (due to a lesion in the opposite hemisphere)	Place objects within the patient's reach on the nonaffected side. Instruct the patient to exercise and increase the strength on the unaffected side.
Hemiplegia	• Paralysis of the face, arm, and leg on the same side (due to a lesion in the opposite hemisphere)	Encourage the patient to provide range-of-motion exercises to the affected side. Provide immobilization as needed to the affected side. Maintain body alignment in functional position. Exercise unaffected limb to increase mobility, strength, and use.
Ataxia	• Staggering, unsteady gait • Unable to keep feet together; needs a broad base to stand	Support patient during the initial ambulation phase. Provide supportive device for ambulation (walker, cane). Instruct the patient not to walk without assistance or supportive device.
Dysarthria	• Difficulty in forming words	Provide the patient with alternative methods of communicating. Allow the patient sufficient time to respond to verbal communication. Support patient and family to alleviate frustration related to difficulty in communicating.
Dysphagia	• Difficulty in swallowing	Test the patient's pharyngeal reflexes before offering food or fluids. Assist the patient with meals. Place food on the unaffected side of the mouth. Allow ample time to eat.
Sensory Deficits		
Paresthesia (occurs on the side opposite the lesion)	• Numbness and tingling of extremity • Difficulty with proprioception	Instruct patient that sensation may be altered. Provide range of motion to affected areas and apply corrective devices as needed.
Verbal Deficits		
Expressive aphasia	• Unable to form words that are understandable; may be able to speak in single-word responses	Encourage patient to repeat sounds of the alphabet. Explore the patient's ability to write as an alternative means of communication.
Receptive aphasia	• Unable to comprehend the spoken word; can speak but may not make sense	Speak slowly and clearly to assist the patient in forming the sounds. Explore the patient's ability to read as an alternative means of communication.
Global (mixed) aphasia	• Combination of both receptive and expressive aphasia	Speak clearly and in simple sentences; use gestures or pictures when able. Establish alternative means of communication.
Cognitive Deficits		
	• Short- and long-term memory loss • Decreased attention span • Impaired ability to concentrate • Poor abstract reasoning • Altered judgment	Reorient patient to time, place, and situation frequently. Use verbal and auditory cues to orient patient. Provide familiar objects (family photographs, favorite objects). Use noncomplicated language. Match visual tasks with a verbal cue; holding a toothbrush, simulate brushing of teeth while saying, "I would like you to brush your teeth now." Minimize distracting noises and views when teaching the patient. Repeat and reinforce instructions frequently.
Emotional Deficits		
	• Loss of self-control • Emotional lability	Support patient during uncontrollable outbursts. Discuss with the patient and family that the outbursts are due to the disease process.
	• Decreased tolerance to stressful situations • Depression • Withdrawal • Fear, hostility, and anger • Feelings of isolation	Encourage patient to participate in group activity. Provide stimulation for the patient. Control stressful situations, if possible. Provide a safe environment. Encourage patient to express feelings and frustrations related to disease process.

Table 62-3	COMPARISON OF LEFT AND RIGHT HEMISPHERIC STROKES
Left Hemispheric Stroke	**Right Hemispheric Stroke**
Paralysis or weakness on right side of body	Paralysis or weakness on left side of body
Right visual field deficit	Left visual field deficit
Aphasia (expressive, receptive, or global)	Spatial-perceptual deficits
Altered intellectual ability	Increased distractibility
	Impulsive behavior and poor judgment
Slow, cautious behavior	Lack of awareness of deficits

Adapted from Hickey, J. V. (2009). *The clinical practice of neurological and neurosurgical nursing* (6th ed., p. 600). Philadelphia: Lippincott Williams & Wilkins.

Cognitive Impairment and Psychological Effects

If damage has occurred to the frontal lobe, learning capacity, memory, or other higher cortical intellectual functions may be impaired. Such dysfunction may be reflected in a limited attention span, difficulties in comprehension, forgetfulness, and a lack of motivation. These changes can cause the patient to become easily frustrated during rehabilitation. Depression is common and may be exaggerated by the patient's natural response to this catastrophic event. Emotional lability, hostility, frustration, resentment, lack of cooperation, and other psychological problems may occur.

Assessment and Diagnostic Findings

Any patient with neurologic deficits needs a careful history and a complete physical and neurologic examination. Initial assessment focuses on airway patency, which may be compromised by loss of gag or cough reflexes and altered respiratory pattern; cardiovascular status (including blood pressure, cardiac rhythm and rate, carotid bruit); and gross neurologic deficits.

Patients may present to the acute care facility with temporary neurologic symptoms. A transient ischemic attack (TIA) is a neurologic deficit typically lasting less than 1 hour. A TIA is manifested by a sudden loss of motor, sensory, or visual function. The symptoms result from temporary ischemia (impairment of blood flow) to a specific region of the brain but when brain imaging is performed there is no evidence of ischemia. A TIA may serve as a warning of impending stroke. Lack of evaluation and treatment of a patient who has experienced previous TIAs may result in a stroke and irreversible deficits (Lewandowski, Rao & Silver, 2008).

The initial diagnostic test for a stroke is usually a noncontrast computed tomography (CT) scan performed emergently to determine if the event is ischemic or hemorrhagic (the category of stroke determines treatment). Further diagnostic workup for ischemic stroke involves attempting to identify the source of the thrombi or emboli. A 12-lead electrocardiogram (ECG) and a carotid ultrasound are standard tests. Other studies may include CT angiography or magnetic resonance imaging and angiography (MRI and MRA) of the brain and neck vessels; transcranial Doppler flow studies; transthoracic or transesophageal echocardiography; xenon-enhanced CT scan; and single photon emission CT (SPECT) scan (Adams, Zoppo, Alberts, et al., 2007).

Prevention

Primary prevention of ischemic stroke remains the best approach. Leading a healthy lifestyle, which includes not smoking, maintaining a healthy weight, following a healthy diet (including modest alcohol consumption), and daily exercise, can reduce the risk of having a stroke by about one half (Chiuve, Rexrode, Spiegelman, et al., 2008). The risk of coronary heart disease and stroke has decreased in women on the Dietary Approaches to Stop Hypertension (DASH) diet. The DASH diet is high in fruits and vegetables, moderate in low-fat dairy products, and low in animal protein (has a substantial amount of plant protein from legumes and nuts) (Fung, Chiuve, McCullough, et al., 2008). Stroke risk screenings are an ideal opportunity to lower stroke risk by identifying people or groups of people who are at high risk for stroke and by educating patients and the community about recognition and prevention of stroke. Research findings suggest that low-dose aspirin may lower the risk of stroke in women who are at risk (Ridker, Cook, Lee, et al., 2005).

Advanced age, gender, and race are well-known nonmodifiable risk factors for stroke. High-risk groups include people older than 55 years of age; the incidence of stroke more than doubles in each successive decade. Men have a higher rate of stroke than that of women. Another high-risk group is African Americans; the incidence of first stroke in African Americans is almost twice that in Caucasian Americans (Rosamond, et al., 2008).

Modifiable risk factors for ischemic stroke include hypertension, atrial fibrillation, hyperlipidemia, obesity, smoking, and diabetes (Chart 62-1). For people who are at high risk, interventions that alter modifiable factors, such as treating hypertension and hyperglycemia and stopping smoking, reduce stroke risk. Other treatable conditions that increase risk of stroke are asymptomatic carotid stenosis and valvular heart disease (eg, endocarditis, prosthetic heart valves). Periodontal disease has also been linked to stroke risk. The association between periodontal disease and stroke may result from the host inflammatory response and the chronic bacterial infection, but the exact mechanism is not fully understood. Periodontal disease is a treatable and preventable condition.

Several methods of preventing recurrent stroke have been identified for patients with TIAs or ischemic stroke. Patients with moderate to severe carotid stenosis are treated with carotid endarterectomy (Sacco, Adams, Albers, et al., 2006). In patients with atrial fibrillation, which increases the risk of emboli, administration of warfarin (Coumadin), an anticoagulant that inhibits clot formation, may prevent both thrombotic and embolic strokes.

CHART 62-1   *Modifiable Risk Factors for Ischemic Stroke*

- Hypertension (controlling hypertension, the major risk factor, is the key to preventing stroke)
- Atrial fibrillation
- Hyperlipidemia
- Diabetes mellitus (associated with accelerated atherogenesis)
- Smoking
- Asymptomatic carotid stenosis
- Obesity
- Excessive alcohol consumption

Medical Management

Patients who have experienced a TIA or stroke should have medical management for secondary prevention. Those with atrial fibrillation (or cardioembolic strokes) are treated with dose-adjusted warfarin (Coumadin) unless contraindicated. The international normalized ratio (INR) target is 2 to 3. If warfarin is contraindicated, aspirin is the best option, although other medications may be used if both are contraindicated (Karch, 2008).

Platelet-inhibiting medications, including aspirin, extended-release dipyridamole (Persantine) plus aspirin, clopidogrel (Plavix), and ticlopidine (Ticlid), decrease the incidence of cerebral infarction in patients who have experienced TIAs and stroke from suspected embolic or thrombotic causes. The specific medication that is used is based on the patient's health history.

Research has found that medications classified as 3-hydroxy-2-methyl-glutaryl-coenzyme A reductase inhibitors (also known as statins) reduce coronary events and strokes. Benefits were independent of cholesterol levels, and these medications are now widely used for stroke prevention. The U.S. Food and Drug Administration (FDA) has recently updated indications for a statin medication, such as simvastatin (Zocor), to include secondary stroke prevention (Nassief & Marsh, 2008). After the acute stroke period, antihypertensive medications are also used, if indicated, for secondary stroke prevention. Angiotensin-converting enzyme (ACE) inhibitors and thiazide diuretics may also have benefits in stroke prevention (Luders, 2007).

Ongoing research is focusing on several aspects of the medical management of acute ischemic stroke. The FDA has approved a clot retrieval device (shaped like a tiny corkscrew) that opens the blocked artery and restores blood flow to the brain (Felton, Ogden, Pena, et al., 2005). Other clot retrieval devices are under investigation, including catheters using vacuum and ultrasound techniques to assist in the removal of clots in the brain.

Thrombolytic Therapy

Thrombolytic agents are used to treat ischemic stroke by dissolving the blood clot that is blocking blood flow to the brain. Recombinant t-PA is a genetically engineered form of t-PA, a thrombolytic substance made naturally by the body. It works by binding to fibrin and converting plasminogen to plasmin, which stimulates fibrinolysis of the atherosclerotic lesion. Rapid diagnosis of stroke and initiation of thrombolytic therapy (within 3 hours) in patients with ischemic stroke leads to a decrease in the size of the stroke and an overall improvement in functional outcome after 3 months (Adams, et al., 2007; NINDS, 1995). Ongoing clinical trials continue to investigate other thrombolytic agents (Lapchak & Araujo, 2007).

To realize the full potential of thrombolytic therapy, community education directed at recognizing the symptoms of stroke and obtaining appropriate emergency care is necessary to ensure rapid transport to a hospital and initiation of therapy within the 3-hour period. Delays make the patient ineligible for thrombolytic therapy, because revascularization of necrotic tissue (which develops after 3 hours) increases the risk of cerebral edema and hemorrhage.

Enhancing Prompt Diagnosis

After being notified by emergency medical service personnel, the emergency department contacts the appropriate staff (neurologist, neuroradiologist, radiology department, nursing staff, ECG, and laboratory technicians) and informs them of the patient's imminent arrival at the hospital. Many institutions have acute stroke teams that respond rapidly, ensuring that treatment occurs within the allotted period (AANN, 2008).

Initial management requires the definitive diagnosis of an ischemic stroke by brain imaging and a careful history to determine whether the patient meets the criteria for t-PA therapy (Chart 62-2). Some of the absolute contraindications for thrombolytic therapy include symptom onset greater than 3 hours before admission, a patient who is anticoagulated (with an INR above 1.7), or a patient who has recently had any type of intracranial pathology (eg, previous stroke, head injury, trauma). Once it is determined that the patient is a candidate for t-PA therapy, no anticoagulants are administered for the next 24 hours.

Before receiving t-PA, the patient is assessed using the National Institutes of Health Stroke Scale (NIHSS), a standardized assessment tool that helps evaluate stroke severity (Table 62-4). Total NIHSS scores range from 0 (normal) to 42 (severe stroke) (Kasner, 2006). Certification in the administration of the scale is recommended and is available for nurses and other health care professionals.

Dosage and Administration

The patient is weighed to determine the dose of t-PA. The dosage for t-PA is 0.9 mg/kg, with a maximum dose of 90 mg. Ten percent of the calculated dose is administered as an intravenous (IV) bolus over 1 minute. The remaining dose (90%) is administered IV over 1 hour via an infusion pump.

The patient is admitted to the intensive care unit or an acute stroke unit, where continuous cardiac monitoring and frequent neurologic assessments are conducted. Vital signs are obtained frequently, with particular attention to blood

---

Chart 62-2 • *Eligibility Criteria for t-PA Administration*

- Age 18 years or older
- Clinical diagnosis of ischemic stroke
- Time of onset of stroke known and is 3 hours or less
- Systolic blood pressure ≤185 mm Hg; diastolic ≤110 mm Hg
- Not a minor stroke or rapidly resolving stroke
- No seizure at onset of stroke
- Not taking warfarin (Coumadin)
- Prothrombin time ≤15 seconds or INR ≤1.7
- Not receiving heparin during the past 48 hours with elevated partial thromboplastin time
- Platelet count ≥100,000/mm³
- No prior intracranial hemorrhage, neoplasm, arteriovenous malformation, or aneurysm
- No major surgical procedures within 14 days
- No stroke, serious head injury, or intracranial surgery within 3 months
- No gastrointestinal or urinary bleeding within 21 days

Table 62-4 SUMMARY OF NATIONAL INSTITUTES OF HEALTH STROKE SCALE (NIHSS)

Category	Description	Score
1a. Level of consciousness (LOC)	Alert	0
	Arousable by minor stimulation	1
	Obtunded, strong stimulation to attend	2
	Unresponsive, or reflexic responses only	3
1b. LOC questions (month, age)	Answers both correctly	0
	Answers one correctly	1
	Both incorrect	2
1c. LOC commands (open, close eyes; make fist, let go)	Obeys both correctly	0
	Obeys one correctly	1
	Both incorrect	2
2. Best gaze (eyes open—patient follows examiner's finger or face)	Normal	0
	Partial gaze palsy	1
	Forced deviation	2
3. Visual (introduce visual stimulus/threat to patient's visual field quadrants)	No visual loss	0
	Partial hemianopsia	1
	Complete hemianopsia	2
	Bilateral hemianopsia	3
4. Facial palsy (show teeth, raise eyebrows and squeeze eyes shut)	Normal	0
	Minor	1
	Partial	2
	Complete	3
5a. Motor; arm—left (elevate extremity to 90° and score drift/movement)	No drift	0
	Drift but maintains in air	1
	Unable to maintain in air	2
	No effort against gravity	3
	No movement	4
	Amputation, joint fusion (explain)	N/A
5b. Motor; arm—right (elevate extremity to 90° and score drift/movement)	No drift	0
	Drift but maintains in air	1
	Unable to maintain in air	2
	No effort against gravity	3
	No movement	4
	Amputation, joint fusion (explain)	N/A
6a. Motor; leg—left (elevate extremity to 30° and score drift/movement)	No drift	0
	Drift but maintains in air	1
	Unable to maintain in air	2
	No effort against gravity	3
	No movement	4
	Amputation, joint fusion (explain)	N/A
6b. Motor; leg—right (elevate extremity to 30° and score drift/movement)	No drift	0
	Drift but maintains in air	1
	Unable to maintain in air	2
	No effort against gravity	3
	No movement	4
	Amputation, joint fusion (explain)	N/A
7. Limb ataxia (finger-to-nose and heel-to-shin testing)	Absent	0
	Present in one limb	1
	Present in two limbs	2
8. Sensory (pinprick to face, arm, trunk, and leg—compare side to side)	Normal	0
	Mild to moderate loss	1
	Severe to total loss	2
9. Best language (name items, describe a picture and read sentences)	No aphasia	0
	Mild to moderate aphasia	1
	Severe aphasia	2
	Mute	3
10. Dysarthria (evaluate speech clarity by having patient repeat words)	Normal	0
	Mild to moderate dysarthria	1
	Severe dysarthria, mostly unintelligible or worse	2
	Intubated or other physical barrier	N/A
11. Extinction and inattention (use information from prior testing to score)	No abnormality	0
	Visual, tactile, auditory, or other extinction to bilateral simultaneous stimulation	1
	Profound hemiattention or extinction to more than one modality.	2
Total score		

Adapted from the version available at the National Institute of Neurological Disorders and Stroke, National Institutes of Health, Bethesda, MD 20892, www.ninds.nih.gov/doctors/NIH_Stroke_Scale.pdf. It is recommended that the full scale with all instructions be used.

pressure (with the goal of lowering the risk of intracranial hemorrhage). An example of a standard protocol would be to obtain vital signs every 15 minutes for the first 2 hours, every 30 minutes for the next 6 hours, then every hour until 24 hours after treatment. Blood pressure should be maintained with the systolic pressure less than 180 mm Hg and the diastolic pressure less than 105 mm Hg (Adams, et al., 2007). Airway management is instituted based on the patient's clinical condition and arterial blood gas values.

Side Effects

Bleeding is the most common side effect of t-PA administration, and the patient is closely monitored for any bleeding (IV insertion sites, urinary catheter site, endotracheal tube, nasogastric tube, urine, stool, emesis, other secretions). A 24-hour delay in placement of nasogastric tubes, urinary catheters, and intra-arterial pressure catheters is recommended. Intracranial bleeding is a major complication that occurred in approximately 6.4% of patients in the initial t-PA study (NINDS, 1995). A number of factors are associated with the occurrence of symptomatic intracranial bleeding: age greater than 70 years, baseline NIHSS score greater than 20, serum glucose concentration 300 mg/dL or higher, and edema or mass effect observed on the patient's initial CT scan.

Therapy for Patients With Ischemic Stroke Not Receiving t-PA

Not all patients are candidates for t-PA therapy. Other treatments may include anticoagulant administration (IV heparin or low-molecular-weight heparin). Because of the risks associated with anticoagulation, their general use is no longer recommended for patients with acute ischemic stroke, whether treated with t-PA or not (Adams, et al., 2007).

Careful maintenance of cerebral hemodynamics to maintain cerebral perfusion is extremely important after a stroke. Increased intracranial pressure (ICP) from brain edema, and associated complications, may occur after a large ischemic stroke. Interventions during this period include measures to reduce ICP, such as administering an osmotic diuretic (eg, mannitol), maintaining the partial pressure of carbon dioxide ($PaCO_2$) within the range of 30 to 35 mm Hg, and positioning to avoid hypoxia. Other treatment measures include the following:

- Elevation of the head of the bed to promote venous drainage and to lower increased ICP
- Possible hemicraniectomy for increased ICP from brain edema in a very large stroke
- Intubation with an endotracheal tube to establish a patent airway, if necessary
- Continuous hemodynamic monitoring (the goals for blood pressure remain controversial for a patient who has not received thrombolytic therapy; antihypertensive treatment may be withheld unless the systolic blood pressure exceeds 220 mm Hg or the diastolic blood pressure exceeds 120 mm Hg)
- Neurologic assessment to determine if the stroke is evolving and if other acute complications are developing; such complications may include seizures, bleeding from anticoagulation, or medication-

induced bradycardia, which can result in hypotension and subsequent decreases in cardiac output and cerebral perfusion pressure

An acute ischemic stroke clinical pathway is shown in Appendix B.

Managing Potential Complications

Adequate cerebral blood flow is essential for cerebral oxygenation. If cerebral blood flow is inadequate, the amount of oxygen supplied to the brain will decrease, and tissue ischemia will result. Adequate oxygenation begins with pulmonary care, maintenance of a patent airway, and administration of supplemental oxygen as needed. The importance of adequate gas exchange in these patients cannot be overemphasized as many are at risk for aspiration pneumonia.

Other potential complications after a stroke include urinary tract infections, cardiac dysrhythmias, and complications of immobility.

Surgical Prevention of Ischemic Stroke

The main surgical procedure for selected patients with TIAs and mild stroke is carotid endarterectomy, which is currently the most frequently performed noncardiac vascular procedure. A carotid endarterectomy is the removal of an atherosclerotic plaque or thrombus from the carotid artery to prevent stroke in patients with occlusive disease of the extracranial cerebral arteries (Fig. 62-2). This surgery is indicated for patients with symptoms of TIA or mild stroke found to be caused by severe (70% to 99%) carotid artery stenosis or moderate (50% to 69%) stenosis with other significant risk factors (Chaturvedi, Bruno, Feasby, et al., 2005).

Carotid stenting, with or without angioplasty, is a less invasive procedure that is used, at times, for severe stenosis. It is used for selected patients who are at high risk for surgery, and its efficacy continues to be investigated. In a recent

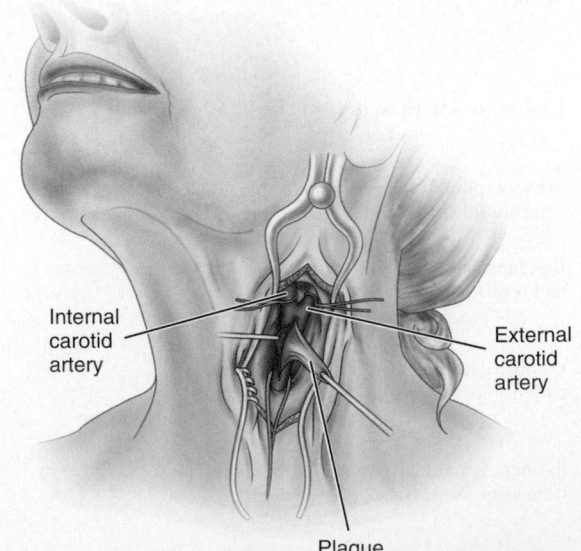

Internal carotid artery

External carotid artery

Plaque

Figure 62-2 Plaque, a potential source of emboli in transient ischemic attack and stroke, is surgically removed from the carotid artery.

Table 62-5	SELECTED COMPLICATIONS OF CAROTID ENDARTERECTOMY AND NURSING INTERVENTIONS	
Complication	**Characteristics**	**Nursing Interventions**
Incision hematoma	Occurs in 5.5% of patients. Large or rapidly expanding hematomas require emergency treatment. If the airway is obstructed by the hematoma, the incision may be opened at the bedside.	Monitor neck discomfort and wound expansion. Report swelling, subjective feelings of pressure in the neck, difficulty breathing.
Hypertension	Poorly controlled hypertension increases the risk of postoperative complications, including hematoma and hyperperfusion syndrome. There is an increased incidence of neurologic impairment and death due to intracerebral hemorrhage. May be related to surgically induced abnormalities of carotid baroreceptor sensitivity.	Risk is highest in the first 48 h after surgery. Check blood pressure frequently and report deviations from baseline. Observe for and report new onset of neurologic deficits.
Postoperative hypotension	Occurs in approximately 5% of patients. Treated with fluids and low-dose phenylephrine infusion. Usually resolves in 24–48 h. Patients with hypotension should have serial ECGs to rule out myocardial infarction.	Monitor blood pressure and observe for signs and symptoms of hypotension.
Hyperperfusion syndrome	Occurs when cerebral vessel autoregulation fails. Arteries accustomed to diminished blood flow may be permanently dilated; increased blood flow after endarterectomy coupled with insufficient vasoconstriction leads to capillary bed damage, edema, and hemorrhage.	Observe for severe unilateral headache improved by sitting upright or standing.
Intracerebral hemorrhage	Occurs infrequently, but is often fatal (60%) or results in serious neurologic impairment. Can occur secondary to hyperperfusion syndrome. Increased risk with advanced age, hypertension, presence of high-grade stenosis, poor collateral flow, and slow flow in the region of the middle cerebral artery.	Monitor neurologic status and report any changes in mental status or neurologic functioning immediately.

study, 334 patients with severe carotid artery stenosis and at high risk for surgery underwent stenting with the use of an emboli protection device or carotid endarterectomy. This study demonstrated that this procedure is not inferior to carotid endarterectomy as it resulted in similar long-term outcomes (Gurm, Yadav, Fayad, et al., 2008).

Nursing Management

The primary complications of carotid endarterectomy are stroke, cranial nerve injuries, infection or hematoma at the incision, and carotid artery disruption. It is important to maintain adequate blood pressure levels in the immediate postoperative period. Hypotension is avoided to prevent cerebral ischemia and thrombosis. Uncontrolled hypertension may precipitate cerebral hemorrhage, edema, hemorrhage at the surgical incision, or disruption of the arterial reconstruction. Medications are used to reduce the blood pressure to previous levels. Close cardiac monitoring is necessary, because these patients have a high incidence of coronary artery disease.

After carotid endarterectomy, a neurologic flow sheet is used to monitor and document assessment parameters for all body systems, with particular attention to neurologic status. The surgeon is notified immediately if a neurologic deficit develops. Formation of a thrombus at the site of the endarterectomy is suspected if there is a sudden increase in neurologic deficits, such as weakness on one side of the body. The patient should be prepared for repeat endarterectomy.

Difficulty in swallowing, hoarseness, or other signs of cranial nerve dysfunction must be assessed. The nurse focuses on assessment of the following cranial nerves: facial (VII), vagus (X), spinal accessory (XI), and hypoglossal (XII). Some edema in the neck after surgery is expected;

however, extensive edema and hematoma formation can obstruct the airway. Emergency airway supplies, including those needed for a tracheostomy, must be available. Table 62-5 provides more information about potential complications of carotid surgery.

NURSING PROCESS

THE PATIENT RECOVERING FROM AN ISCHEMIC STROKE

The acute phase of an ischemic stroke may last 1 to 3 days, but ongoing monitoring of all body systems is essential as long as the patient requires care. The patient who has had a stroke is at risk for multiple complications, including deconditioning and other musculoskeletal problems, swallowing difficulties, bowel and bladder dysfunction, inability to perform self-care, and skin breakdown. After the stroke is complete, management focuses on the prompt initiation of rehabilitation for any deficits.

Assessment

During the acute phase, a neurologic flow sheet is maintained to provide data about the following important measures of the patient's clinical status:

- Change in level of consciousness or responsiveness as evidenced by movement, resistance to changes of position, and response to stimulation; orientation to time, place, and person
- Presence or absence of voluntary or involuntary movements of the extremities; muscle tone; body posture; and position of the head

- Stiffness or flaccidity of the neck
- Eye opening, comparative size of pupils and pupillary reactions to light, and ocular position
- Color of the face and extremities; temperature and moisture of the skin
- Quality and rates of pulse and respiration; arterial blood gas values as indicated, body temperature, and arterial pressure
- Ability to speak
- Volume of fluids ingested or administered; volume of urine excreted each 24 hours
- Presence of bleeding
- Maintenance of blood pressure within the desired parameters

After the acute phase, the nurse assesses mental status (memory, attention span, perception, orientation, affect, speech/language), sensation/perception (usually the patient has decreased awareness of pain and temperature), motor control (upper and lower extremity movement), swallowing ability, nutritional and hydration status, skin integrity, activity tolerance, and bowel and bladder function. Ongoing nursing assessment continues to focus on any impairment of function in the patient's daily activities, because the quality of life after stroke is closely related to the patient's functional status.

Diagnosis

Nursing Diagnoses

Based on the assessment data, the major nursing diagnoses for a patient with a stroke may include the following:

- Impaired physical mobility related to hemiparesis, loss of balance and coordination, spasticity, and brain injury
- Acute pain (painful shoulder) related to hemiplegia and disuse
- Self-care deficits (bathing, hygiene, toileting, dressing, grooming, and feeding) related to stroke sequelae
- Disturbed sensory perception (kinesthetic, tactile or visual) related to altered sensory reception, transmission, and/or integration
- Impaired swallowing
- Impaired urinary elimination related to flaccid bladder, detrusor instability, confusion, or difficulty in communicating
- Disturbed thought processes related to brain damage
- Impaired verbal communication related to brain damage
- Risk for impaired skin integrity related to hemiparesis, hemiplegia, or decreased mobility
- Interrupted family processes related to catastrophic illness and caregiving burdens
- Sexual dysfunction related to neurologic deficits or fear of failure

Collaborative Problems/Potential Complications

Potential complications include:
- Decreased cerebral blood flow due to increased ICP
- Inadequate oxygen delivery to the brain
- Pneumonia

Planning and Goals

Although rehabilitation begins on the day the patient has the stroke, the process is intensified during convalescence and requires a coordinated team effort. It is helpful for the team to know what the patient was like before the stroke: his or her illnesses, abilities, mental and emotional state, behavioral characteristics, and activities of daily living (ADLs). It is also helpful for clinicians to be knowledgeable about the relative importance of predictors of stroke outcome (age, NIHSS score, and level of consciousness at time of admission) in order to provide stroke survivors and their families with realistic goals (Adams, et al., 2007).

The major goals for the patient (and family) may include improved mobility, avoidance of shoulder pain, achievement of self-care, relief of sensory and perceptual deprivation, prevention of aspiration, continence of bowel and bladder, improved thought processes, achieving a form of communication, maintaining skin integrity, restored family functioning, improved sexual function, and absence of complications.

Nursing Interventions

Nursing care has a significant impact on the patient's recovery. Often, many body systems are impaired as a result of the stroke, and conscientious care and timely interventions can prevent debilitating complications. During and after the acute phase, nursing interventions focus on the whole person. In addition to providing physical care, the nurse encourages and fosters recovery by listening to the patient and asking questions to elicit the meaning of the stroke experience.

Improving Mobility and Preventing Joint Deformities

A patient with hemiplegia has unilateral paralysis (paralysis on one side). When control of the voluntary muscles is lost, the strong flexor muscles exert control over the extensors. The arm tends to adduct (adductor muscles are stronger than abductors) and to rotate internally. The elbow and the wrist tend to flex, the affected leg tends to rotate externally at the hip joint and flex at the knee, and the foot at the ankle joint supinates and tends toward plantar flexion.

Correct positioning is important to prevent contractures; measures are used to relieve pressure, assist in maintaining good body alignment, and prevent compressive neuropathies, especially of the ulnar and peroneal nerves. Because flexor muscles are stronger than extensor muscles, a splint applied at night to the affected extremity may prevent flexion and maintain correct positioning during sleep. (See Chapter 11 for additional information.)

PREVENTING SHOULDER ADDUCTION. To prevent adduction of the affected shoulder while the patient is in bed, a pillow is placed in the axilla when there is limited external rotation; this keeps the arm away from the chest. A pillow is placed under the arm, and the arm is placed in a neutral (slightly flexed) position, with distal joints positioned higher than the more proximal joints (ie, the elbow is positioned higher than the shoulder and the wrist higher than the elbow). This helps to prevent edema and the resultant joint fibrosis that will limit range of motion if the patient regains control of the arm (Fig. 62-3).

POSITIONING THE HAND AND FINGERS. The fingers are positioned so that they are barely flexed. The hand is placed in slight supination (palm faces upward), which is its most functional position. If the upper extremity is flaccid, a splint can be used to support the wrist and hand in a functional

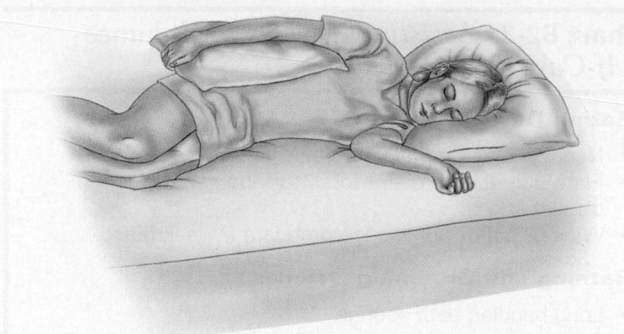

Figure 62-3 Correct positioning to prevent shoulder adduction.

position. If the upper extremity is spastic, a hand roll is not used, because it stimulates the grasp reflex. In this instance a dorsal wrist splint is useful in allowing the palm to be free of pressure. Every effort is made to prevent hand edema.

Spasticity, particularly in the hand, can be a disabling complication after stroke. Researchers have reported that repeated intramuscular injections of botulinum toxin type A into wrist and finger muscles reduced upper limb spasticity after stroke, resulting in significant and sustained improvements in muscle tone, lessened disability, and improved quality of life (Elovic, Brashear, Kaelin, et al., 2008). Other treatments for spasticity may include stretching and splinting.

CHANGING POSITIONS. The patient's position should be changed every 2 hours. To place a patient in a lateral (side-lying) position, a pillow is placed between the legs before the patient is turned. To promote venous return and prevent edema, the upper thigh should not be acutely flexed. The patient may be turned from side to side, but if sensation is impaired, the amount of time spent on the affected side should be limited.

If possible, the patient is placed in a prone position for 15 to 30 minutes several times a day. A small pillow or a support is placed under the pelvis, extending from the level of the umbilicus to the upper third of the thigh (Fig. 62-4). This position helps promote hyperextension of the hip joints, which is essential for normal gait and helps prevent knee and hip flexion contractures. The prone position also helps drain bronchial secretions and prevents contractural deformities of the shoulders and knees. During positioning, it is important to reduce pressure and change position frequently to prevent pressure ulcers.

ESTABLISHING AN EXERCISE PROGRAM. The affected extremities are exercised passively and put through a full range of motion four or five times a day to maintain joint mobility, regain motor control, prevent contractures in the

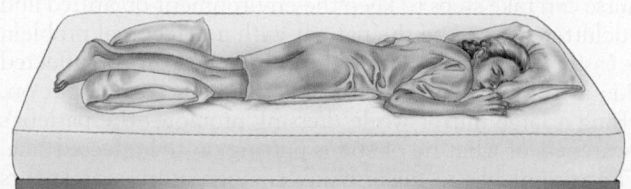

Figure 62-4 Prone position with pillow support helps prevent hip flexion.

paralyzed extremity, prevent further deterioration of the neuromuscular system, and enhance circulation. Exercise is helpful in preventing venous stasis, which may predispose the patient to thrombosis and pulmonary embolus.

Repetition of an activity forms new pathways in the CNS and therefore encourages new patterns of motion. At first, the extremities are usually flaccid. If tightness occurs in any area, the range-of-motion exercises should be performed more frequently (see Chapter 11).

The patient is observed for signs and symptoms that may indicate pulmonary embolus or excessive cardiac workload during exercise; these include shortness of breath, chest pain, cyanosis, and increasing pulse rate with exercise. Frequent short periods of exercise always are preferable to longer periods at infrequent intervals. Regularity in exercise is most important. Improvement in muscle strength and maintenance of range of motion can be achieved only through daily exercise.

The patient is encouraged and reminded to exercise the unaffected side at intervals throughout the day. It is helpful to develop a written schedule to remind the patient of the exercise activities. The nurse supervises and supports the patient during these activities. The patient can be taught to put the unaffected leg under the affected one to assist in moving it when turning and exercising. Flexibility, strengthening, coordination, endurance, and balancing exercises prepare the patient for ambulation. Quadriceps muscle setting and gluteal setting exercises are started early to improve the muscle strength needed for walking; these are performed at least five times daily for 10 minutes at a time.

PREPARING FOR AMBULATION. As soon as possible, the patient is assisted out of bed and an active rehabilitation program is started. The patient is first taught to maintain balance while sitting and then to learn to balance while standing. If the patient has difficulty in achieving standing balance, a tilt table, which slowly brings the patient to an upright position, can be used. Tilt tables are especially helpful for patients who have been on bed rest for prolonged periods and have orthostatic blood pressure changes.

If the patient needs a wheelchair, the folding type with hand brakes is the most practical because it allows the patient to manipulate the chair. The chair should be low enough to allow the patient to propel it with the uninvolved foot and narrow enough to permit it to be used in the home. When the patient is transferred from the wheelchair, the brakes must be applied and locked on both sides of the chair.

The patient is usually ready to walk as soon as standing balance is achieved. Parallel bars are useful in these first efforts. A chair or wheelchair should be readily available in case the patient suddenly becomes fatigued or feels dizzy.

The training periods for ambulation should be short and frequent. As the patient gains strength and confidence, an adjustable cane can be used for support. Generally, a three- or four-pronged cane provides a stable support in the early phases of rehabilitation.

Preventing Shoulder Pain

As many as 72% of patients who have had a stroke have pain in the shoulder (Duncan, Zorowitz, Bates, et al., 2005). That pain may prevent them from learning new skills and affect their quality of life (Chae, Mascarenhas, Yu, et al., 2007). Shoulder function is essential in achieving balance and performing transfers and self-care activities. Three problems can occur: painful shoulder, subluxation of the shoulder, and shoulder–hand syndrome.

A flaccid shoulder joint may be overstretched by the use of excessive force in turning the patient or from overstrenuous arm and shoulder movement. To prevent shoulder pain, the nurse should never lift the patient by the flaccid shoulder or pull on the affected arm or shoulder. Overhead pulleys should also be avoided. If the arm is paralyzed, subluxation (incomplete dislocation) at the shoulder can occur as a result of overstretching of the joint capsule and musculature by the force of gravity when the patient sits or stands in the early stages after a stroke. This results in severe pain. Shoulder–hand syndrome (painful shoulder and generalized swelling of the hand) can cause a frozen shoulder and ultimately atrophy of subcutaneous tissues. When a shoulder becomes stiff, it is usually painful.

Many shoulder problems can be prevented by proper patient movement and positioning. The flaccid arm is positioned on a table or with pillows while the patient is seated. Some clinicians advocate the use of a properly worn sling when the patient first becomes ambulatory, to prevent the paralyzed upper extremity from dangling without support. Range-of-motion exercises are important in preventing painful shoulder. Overstrenuous arm movements are avoided. The patient is instructed to interlace the fingers, place the palms together, and push the clasped hands slowly forward to bring the scapulae forward; he or she then raises both hands above the head. This is repeated throughout the day. The patient is instructed to flex the affected wrist at intervals and move all the joints of the affected fingers. The patient is encouraged to touch, stroke, rub, and look at both hands. Pushing the heel of the hand firmly down on a surface is useful. Elevation of the arm and hand is also important in preventing dependent edema of the hand. Patients with continuing pain after attempted movement and positioning may require the addition of analgesia to their treatment program. Other treatments may include injections to the shoulder joint with corticosteroid medications, electrical stimulation, heat or ice, and soft tissue massage (Duncan, et al., 2005).

Medications are helpful in the management of poststroke pain. Amitriptyline hydrochloride (Elavil) has been used, but it can cause cognitive problems, has a sedating effect, and is not effective in all patients. The antiseizure medications lamotrigine (Lamictal) and pregabalin (Lyrica) have been found to be effective for poststroke pain, and they may serve as alternatives for patients who cannot tolerate amitriptyline (Vranken, Dijkgraaf, Kruis, et al., 2008).

Enhancing Self-Care

As soon as the patient can sit up, personal hygiene activities are encouraged. The patient is helped to set realistic goals; if feasible, a new task is added daily. The first step is to carry out all self-care activities on the unaffected side. Such activities as combing the hair, brushing the teeth, shaving with an electric razor, bathing, and eating can be carried out with one hand and should be encouraged. Although the patient may feel awkward at first, these motor

---

Chart 62-3• Assistive Devices to Enhance Self-Care After Stroke

Eating Devices

- Nonskid mats to stabilize plates
- Plate guards to prevent food from being pushed off plate
- Wide-grip utensils to accommodate a weak grasp

Bathing and Grooming Devices

- Long-handled bath sponge
- Grab bars, nonskid mats, handheld shower heads
- Electric razors with head at 90 degrees to handle
- Shower and tub seats, stationary or on wheels

Toileting Aids

- Raised toilet seat
- Grab bars next to toilet

Dressing Aids

- Velcro closures
- Elastic shoelaces
- Long-handled shoe horn

Mobility Aids

- Canes, walkers, wheelchairs
- Transfer devices such as transfer boards and belts

---

skills can be learned by repetition, and the unaffected side will become stronger with use. The nurse must be sure that the patient does not neglect the affected side. Assistive devices will help make up for some of the patient's deficits (Chart 62-3). A small towel is easier to control while drying after bathing, and boxed paper tissues are easier to use than a roll of toilet tissue.

Return of functional ability is important to the patient recovering after a stroke. An early baseline assessment of functional ability with an instrument such as the Functional Independence Measure (FIM) is important in team planning and goal setting for the patient. The FIM is a widely used instrument in stroke rehabilitation and provides valuable information about motor, social, and cognitive function (Kasner, 2006). The patient's morale may improve if ambulatory activities are carried out in street clothes. The family is instructed to bring in clothing that is preferably a size larger than that normally worn. Clothing fitted with front or side fasteners or Velcro closures is the most suitable. The patient has better balance if most of the dressing activities are carried out while seated.

Perceptual problems may make it difficult for the patient to dress without assistance because of an inability to match the clothing to the body parts. To assist the patient, the nurse can take steps to keep the environment organized and uncluttered, because the patient with a perceptual problem is easily distracted. The clothing is placed on the affected side in the order in which the garments are to be put on. Using a large mirror while dressing promotes the patient's awareness of what he or she is putting on the affected side. The patient has to make many compensatory movements when dressing; these can produce fatigue and painful twisting of the intercostal muscles. Support and encouragement are provided to prevent the patient from becoming overly fatigued and discouraged. Even with intensive training, not all patients can achieve independence in dressing.

Managing Sensory-Perceptual Difficulties

Patients with a decreased field of vision should be approached on the side where visual perception is intact. All visual stimuli (eg, clock, calendar, television) should be placed on this side. The patient can be taught to turn the head in the direction of the defective visual field to compensate for this loss. The nurse should make eye contact with the patient and draw his or her attention to the affected side by encouraging the patient to move the head. The nurse may also want to stand at a position that encourages the patient to move or turn to visualize who is in the room. Increasing the natural or artificial lighting in the room and providing eyeglasses are important aids to increasing vision.

The patient with homonymous hemianopsia (loss of half of the visual field) turns away from the affected side of the body and tends to neglect that side and the space on that side; this is called amorphosynthesis. In such instances, the patient cannot see food on half of the tray, and only half of the room is visible. It is important for the nurse to constantly remind the patient of the other side of the body, to maintain alignment of the extremities, and, if possible, to place the extremities where the patient can see them.

Assisting With Nutrition

Stroke can result in swallowing problems (dysphagia) due to impaired function of the mouth, tongue, palate, larynx, pharynx, or upper esophagus. Patients must be observed for paroxysms of coughing, food dribbling out of or pooling in one side of the mouth, food retained for long periods in the mouth, or nasal regurgitation when swallowing liquids. Swallowing difficulties place the patient at risk for aspiration, pneumonia, dehydration, and malnutrition.

A speech therapist will evaluate the patient's swallowing ability. If swallowing function is partially impaired, it may return over time, or the patient may be taught alternative swallowing techniques, advised to take smaller boluses of food, and taught about types of foods that are easier to swallow. The patient may be started on a thick liquid or puréed diet, because these foods are easier to swallow than thin liquids. Having the patient sit upright, preferably out of bed in a chair, and instructing him or her to tuck the chin toward the chest as he or she swallows will help prevent aspiration. The diet may be advanced as the patient becomes more proficient at swallowing. If the patient cannot resume oral intake, a gastrointestinal feeding tube is placed for ongoing tube feedings and medication administration.

Enteral tubes can be either nasogastric (placed in the stomach) or nasoenteral (placed in the duodenum) to reduce the risk of aspiration. Nursing responsibilities in feeding include elevating the head of the bed at least 30 degrees to prevent aspiration, checking the position of the tube before feeding, ensuring that the cuff of the tracheostomy tube (if in place) is inflated, and giving the tube feeding slowly. The feeding tube is aspirated periodically to ensure that the feedings are passing through the gastrointestinal tract. Retained or residual feedings increase the risk of aspiration.

Patients with retained feedings may benefit from the placement of a gastrostomy tube or a percutaneous endoscopic gastrostomy tube. In a patient with a nasogastric tube, the feeding tube should be placed in the duodenum to reduce the risk of aspiration. For long-term feedings, a gastrostomy tube is preferred. Management of patients with tube feedings is discussed in Chapter 36.

Attaining Bowel and Bladder Control

After a stroke, the patient may have transient urinary incontinence due to confusion, inability to communicate needs, and inability to use the urinal or bedpan because of impaired motor and postural control. Occasionally after a stroke, the bladder becomes atonic, with impaired sensation in response to bladder filling. Sometimes control of the external urinary sphincter is lost or diminished. During this period, intermittent catheterization with sterile technique is carried out. After muscle tone increases and deep tendon reflexes return, bladder tone increases and spasticity of the bladder may develop. Because the patient's sense of awareness is clouded, persistent urinary incontinence or urinary retention may be symptomatic of bilateral brain damage. The voiding pattern is analyzed, and the urinal or bedpan is offered on this pattern or schedule. The upright posture and standing position are helpful for male patients during this aspect of rehabilitation.

Patients may have problems with bowel control, particularly constipation. Unless contraindicated, a high-fiber diet and adequate fluid intake (2 to 3 L/day) should be provided and a regular time (usually after breakfast) should be established for toileting. See Chapter 11 for additional information about bowel and bladder control.

Improving Thought Processes

After a stroke, the patient may have problems with cognitive, behavioral, and emotional deficits related to brain damage. However, in many instances, a considerable degree of function can be recovered, because not all areas of the brain are equally damaged; some remain more intact and functional than others.

After assessment that delineates the patient's deficits, the neuropsychologist, in collaboration with the primary care physician, psychiatrist, nurse, and other professionals, structures a training program using cognitive-perceptual retraining, visual imagery, reality orientation, and cueing procedures to compensate for losses.

The role of the nurse is supportive. The nurse reviews the results of neuropsychological testing, observes the patient's performance and progress, gives positive feedback, and, most importantly, conveys an attitude of confidence and hope. Interventions capitalize on the patient's strengths and remaining abilities while attempting to improve performance of affected functions. Other interventions are similar to those for improving cognitive functioning after a head injury (see Chapter 63).

Improving Communication

Aphasia, which impairs the patient's ability to express himself or herself and to understand what is being said, may become apparent in various ways. The cortical area that is responsible for integrating the myriad pathways required for the comprehension and formulation of language is called Broca's area. It is located in a convolution adjoining the middle cerebral artery. This area is responsible for control of the combinations of muscular movements needed to speak each word. Broca's area is so close to the left motor area that a disturbance in the motor area often affects the speech area. This is why so many patients who are paralyzed on the right side (due to damage or injury to the left side of the brain) cannot speak, whereas those paralyzed on the left side are less likely to have speech disturbances.

The speech therapist assesses the communication needs of the stroke patient, describes the precise deficit, and suggests the best overall method of communication. Most language intervention strategies can be tailored for the individual patient. The patient is expected to take an active part in establishing goals.

A person with aphasia may become depressed. The inability to talk on the telephone, answer a question, or participate in conversation often causes anger, frustration, fear of the future, and hopelessness. Nursing interventions include strategies to make the atmosphere conducive to communication. This includes being sensitive to the patient's reactions and needs and responding to them in an appropriate manner, while always treating the patient as an adult. The nurse provides strong emotional support and understanding to allay anxiety and frustration.

A common pitfall is for the nurse or other health care team member to complete the thoughts or sentences of the patient. This should be avoided, because it causes the patient to become more frustrated at not being allowed to speak and may deter efforts to practice putting thoughts together and completing sentences. A consistent schedule, routines, and repetition help the patient to function despite significant deficits. A written copy of the daily schedule, a folder of personal information (birth date, address, names of relatives), checklists, and an audiotaped list help improve the patient's memory and concentration. The patient may also benefit from a communication board, which has pictures of common needs and phrases. The board may be translated into any language.

When talking with the patient, it is important for the nurse to gain the patient's attention, speak slowly, and keep the language of instruction consistent. One instruction is given at a time, and time is allowed for the patient to process what has been said. The use of gestures may enhance comprehension. Speaking is thinking out loud, and the emphasis is on thinking. Listening and sorting out incoming messages requires mental effort; the patient must struggle against mental inertia and needs time to organize a response.

In working with the patient with aphasia, the nurse must remember to talk to the patient during care activities. This provides social contact for the patient. Chart 62-4 describes points to keep in mind when communicating with the patient with aphasia.

Maintaining Skin Integrity

The patient who has had a stroke may be at risk for skin and tissue breakdown because of altered sensation and inability to respond to pressure and discomfort by turning and moving. Preventing skin and tissue breakdown requires frequent

---

Chart 62-4 • *Communicating With the Patient With Aphasia*

- Face the patient and establish eye contact.
- Speak in a normal manner and tone.
- Use short phrases, and pause between phrases to allow the patient time to understand what is being said.
- Limit conversation to practical and concrete matters.
- Use gestures, pictures, objects, and writing.
- As the patient uses and handles an object, say what the object is. It helps to match the words with the object or action.
- Be consistent in using the same words and gestures each time you give instructions or ask a question.
- Keep extraneous noises and sounds to a minimum. Too much background noise can distract the patient or make it difficult to sort out the message being spoken.

---

assessment of the skin, with emphasis on bony areas and dependent parts of the body. During the acute phase, a specialty bed (eg, low-air-loss bed) may be used until the patient can move independently or assist in moving.

A regular turning schedule (eg, every 2 hours) is adhered to even if pressure-relieving devices are used to prevent tissue and skin breakdown. When the patient is positioned or turned, care must be used to minimize shear and friction forces, which cause damage to tissues and predispose the skin to breakdown.

The patient's skin must be kept clean and dry; gentle massage of healthy (nonreddened) skin and adequate nutrition are other factors that help to maintain normal skin and tissue integrity (see Chapter 11).

Improving Family Coping

Family members play an important role in the patient's recovery. Family members are encouraged to participate in counseling and to use support systems that will help with the emotional and physical stress of caring for the patient. Involving others in the patient's care and teaching stress management techniques and methods for maintaining personal health also facilitate family coping.

The family may have difficulty accepting the patient's disability and may be unrealistic in their expectations. They are given information about the expected outcomes and are counseled to avoid doing activities for the patient that he or she can do. They are assured that their love and interest are part of the patient's therapy.

The family needs to be informed that the rehabilitation of the hemiplegic patient requires many months and that progress may be slow. The gains made by the patient in the hospital or rehabilitation unit must be maintained. All caregivers should approach the patient with a supportive and optimistic attitude, focusing on the patient's remaining abilities. The rehabilitation team, the medical and nursing team, the patient, and the family must all be involved in developing attainable goals for the patient at home.

Most relatives of patients with stroke handle the physical changes better than the emotional aspects of care. The family should be prepared to expect occasional episodes of emotional lability. The patient may laugh or cry easily and may be irritable and demanding or depressed and confused. The nurse can explain to the family that the patient's laughter does not necessarily connote happiness, nor does crying reflect sadness, and that emotional lability usually improves with time.

Helping the Patient Cope With Sexual Dysfunction

Sexual functioning can be profoundly altered by stroke. Although research in this area of stroke management is limited, it appears that patients who have had a stroke consider sexual function important, and many have sexual dysfunction. Sexual dysfunction after stroke is multifactorial. There may be medical reasons for the dysfunction (neurologic and cognitive deficits, previous diseases, medications), as well as various psychosocial factors, including depression. A stroke is such a catastrophic illness that the patient experiences loss of self-esteem and value as a sexual being. These psychosocial factors play an important role in determining sexual drive, activity, and satisfaction after a stroke.

Nurses in the rehabilitation setting play a crucial role in beginning a dialogue between the patient and his or her partner about sexuality after a stroke. In-depth assessments to determine sexual history before and after the stroke should be followed by appropriate interventions. Interventions for the patient and partner focus on providing relevant information, education, reassurance, adjustment of medications, counseling regarding coping skills, suggestions for alternative sexual positions, and a means of sexual expression and satisfaction (Kautz, 2007).

Promoting Home and Community-Based Care

TEACHING PATIENTS SELF-CARE. Patient and family education is a fundamental component of rehabilitation. The nurse provides teaching about stroke, its causes and prevention, and the rehabilitation process. In both acute care and rehabilitation facilities, the focus is on teaching the patient to resume as much self-care as possible. This may entail using assistive devices or modifying the home environment to help the patient live with a disability.

An occupational therapist may be helpful in assessing the home environment and recommending modifications to help the patient become more independent. For example, a shower is more convenient than a tub for the patient with hemiplegia because most patients do not gain sufficient strength to get up and down from a tub. Sitting on a stool of medium height with rubber suction tips allows the patient to wash with greater ease. A long-handled bath brush with a soap container is helpful to the patient who has only one functional hand. If a shower is not available, a stool may be placed in the tub and a portable shower hose attached to the faucet. Handrails may be attached alongside the bathtub and the toilet. Other assistive devices include special utensils for eating, grooming, dressing, and writing (see Chart 62-3).

A program of physical therapy can be beneficial, whether it takes places in the home or in an outpatient program. Recent research has focused on techniques using robotics and constraint-induced movement therapy. Constraint-induced movement therapy involves constraint of the less affected upper limb with a mitt and intensely training the more affected limb. This technique has shown improved arm function in patients who had a stroke 3 to 9 months prior to receiving the treatment (Wolf, Winstein, Miller, et al., 2006). Robot-assisted therapy uses sensorimotor training of the upper limb. This method allows patients to train without the presence of a therapist.

CONTINUING CARE. The recovery and rehabilitation process after stroke may be prolonged and requires patience and perseverance on the part of both the patient and the family. Depending on the specific neurologic deficits resulting from the stroke, the patient at home may require the services of a number of health care professionals. The nurse often coordinates the care of the patient at home and considers the many educational needs of caregivers and patients. The family (often the spouse) requires education as well as assistance in planning and providing care.

The family is advised that the patient may tire easily, may become irritable and upset by small events, and may be less interested in events than expected. Emotional problems associated with stroke are often related to speech dysfunction and the frustrations of being unable to communicate. A speech therapist allows the family to be involved and gives the family practical instructions to help the patient between therapy sessions.

Depression is a common and serious problem in the patient who has had a stroke. Incidence of depression in patients who have had a stroke ranges from less than 10% to more than 50%. Risk factors include increased severity of stroke, a history of depression, and cognitive or physical impairment (Johnson, Minarik, Nyström, et al., 2006). Nurses should identify patients who may be at risk while they are in the hospital. In the home or in the rehabilitation setting, nurses may be involved in coordinating care and referring patients and family to appropriate resources. The family can help by continuing to support the patient and by giving positive reinforcement for the progress that is being made. Antidepressant therapy may help if depression dominates the patient's life.

Community-based stroke support groups may allow the patient and family to learn from others with similar problems and to share their experiences. Support groups take the form of in-person meetings as well as Internet-based support programs. The patient is encouraged to continue hobbies and recreational and leisure interests and to maintain contact with friends to prevent social isolation. All nurses coming in contact with the patient should encourage the patient to keep active, adhere to the exercise program, and remain as self-sufficient as possible.

The nurse should recognize the potential effects of caregiving on the family. Not all families have the adaptive coping skills and adequate psychological functioning necessary for the long-term care of another person. The patient's spouse may be elderly, with his or her own health concerns; in some instances, the patient may have been the provider of care to the spouse. A spouse may have to take on new roles and responsibilities in the relationship and around the home. He or she may also feel a sense of loss (of freedom and leisure time as well as of the marital relationship) (Chart 62-5).

Depression is common in caregivers of stroke survivors, and it may last 18 months or more (Berg, Palomäki,

NURSING RESEARCH PROFILE
Spouses Caring for Stroke Survivors

CHART 62-5

Coombs, U. (2007). Spousal caregiving for stroke survivors. *Journal of Neuroscience Nursing, 39*(2), 112–119.

Purpose

Survivors of a stroke may be discharged to an acute rehabilitation facility or skilled nursing facility. The ultimate goal after a stroke is to have survivors return home. A spouse plays an important role in caring for stroke survivors and also provides much-needed emotional support. The purpose of this study was to explore the phenomenon of spousal caregiving from the perspective of the spousal caregivers (the lived experience of spousal caregivers).

Design

This phenomenologic study was guided by the research question: What is it like for older caregivers to care for a spouse who has survived a stroke? This study used eight interviews from adults who were at least 50 years of age and were caring for a stroke survivor who was at least 1 year poststroke. Data were collected through taped interviews. Each participant had two separate interviews lasting 60 to 120 minutes using an interview guide containing five to six questions. Participants were asked to describe their caregiv-

ing experience, and the interview guide questions were used as prompts if needed.

Findings

Five females and three males participated, the mean age was 65 years, and all were married. The number of years caring for their spouses ranged from 1.5 to 5 years. The mean age of the stroke survivors was 68 years. Six themes emerged for this study: experiencing a profound sense of loss, adjusting to a new relationship with the spouse, taking on a new responsibility, feeling the demands of caregiving, having to depend on others, and maintaining hope and optimism.

Nursing Implications

The findings of this study may help nurses working in hospital, rehabilitation, community, or home health care settings understand the impact of caregiving on spouses. More attention should be given to the spouse in the acute care setting, and support resources should be provided. By being aware of the particular concerns of caregivers, nurses may anticipate problems and stresses that caregivers may encounter.

Lönnqvist, et al., 2005). Nurses should assess caregivers for signs of depression (Lightbody, Auton, Baldwin, et al., 2007). Caregivers who are depressed may be more likely to resort to physical or emotional abuse of the patient and to place the patient in a nursing home.

Caregivers may require reminders to attend to their own health concerns and well-being. Even healthy caregivers may find it difficult to maintain a schedule that includes being available around the clock. The nurse encourages the family to arrange for respite care services (planned short-term care to relieve the family from having to provide continuous 24-hour care), which may be available from an adult day care center. Some hospitals also offer weekend respite care that can provide caregivers with needed time for themselves. The nurse involved in home and continuing care also needs to remind the patient and family of the need for respite care as well as continuing health promotion and screening practices.

Evaluation

Expected Patient Outcomes

Expected patient outcomes may include the following:

1. Achieves improved mobility
   a. Avoids deformities (contractures and footdrop)
   b. Participates in prescribed exercise program
   c. Achieves sitting balance
   d. Uses unaffected side to compensate for loss of function of hemiplegic side
2. Reports absence of shoulder pain
   a. Demonstrates shoulder mobility; exercises shoulder
   b. Elevates arm and hand at intervals
3. Achieves self-care; performs hygiene care; uses adaptive equipment

4. Demonstrates techniques to compensate for altered sensory reception, such as turning the head to see people or objects
5. Demonstrates safe swallowing
6. Achieves normal bowel and bladder elimination
7. Participates in cognitive improvement program
8. Demonstrates improved communication
9. Maintains intact skin without breakdown
   a. Demonstrates normal skin turgor
   b. Participates in turning and positioning activities
10. Family members demonstrate a positive attitude and coping mechanisms
    a. Encourage patient in exercise program
    b. Take an active part in rehabilitation process
    c. Contact respite care programs or arrange for other family members to assume some responsibilities for care
11. Develops alternative approaches to sexual expression

Hemorrhagic Stroke

Hemorrhagic strokes account for 15% to 20% of cerebrovascular disorders and are primarily caused by intracranial or subarachnoid hemorrhage. Hemorrhagic strokes are caused by bleeding into the brain tissue, the ventricles, or the subarachnoid space. Primary intracerebral hemorrhage from a spontaneous rupture of small vessels accounts for approximately 80% of hemorrhagic strokes and is caused chiefly by uncontrolled hypertension. Subarachnoid hemorrhage results from a ruptured intracranial **aneurysm** (a weakening in the arterial wall) in about half the cases (Hickey, 2009).

Another common cause of intracerebral hemorrhage in the elderly is cerebral amyloid angiopathy, which involves damage caused by the deposit of beta-amyloid protein in the small and medium-sized blood vessels of the brain. Secondary intracerebral hemorrhage is associated with arteriovenous malformations (AVMs), intracranial aneurysms, intracranial neoplasms, or certain medications (eg, anticoagulants, amphetamines). The mortality rate has been reported to be as high as 48% at 30 days after an intracranial hemorrhage (Flaherty, Haverbusch, Sekar, et al., 2006). Patients who survive the acute phase of care usually have more severe deficits and a longer recovery phase compared to those with ischemic stroke.

Pathophysiology

The pathophysiology of hemorrhagic stroke depends on the cause and type of cerebrovascular disorder. Symptoms are produced when a primary hemorrhage, aneurysm, or AVM presses on nearby cranial nerves or brain tissue or, more dramatically, when an aneurysm or AVM ruptures, causing subarachnoid hemorrhage (hemorrhage into the cranial subarachnoid space). Normal brain metabolism is disrupted by the brain's exposure to blood; by an increase in ICP resulting from the sudden entry of blood into the subarachnoid space, which compresses and injures brain tissue; or by secondary ischemia of the brain resulting from the reduced perfusion pressure and vasospasm that frequently accompany subarachnoid hemorrhage.

Intracerebral Hemorrhage

An intracerebral hemorrhage, or bleeding into the brain tissue, is most common in patients with hypertension and cerebral atherosclerosis, because degenerative changes from these diseases cause rupture of the blood vessel. An intracerebral hemorrhage may also result from certain types of arterial pathology, brain tumors, and the use of medications (eg, oral anticoagulants, amphetamines, and illicit drug use).

Bleeding occurs most commonly in the cerebral lobes, basal ganglia, thalamus, brain stem (mostly the pons), and cerebellum (Hickey, 2009). Occasionally, the bleeding ruptures the wall of the lateral ventricle and causes intraventricular hemorrhage, which is frequently fatal.

Intracranial (Cerebral) Aneurysm

An intracranial (cerebral) aneurysm is a dilation of the walls of a cerebral artery that develops as a result of weakness in the arterial wall. The cause of aneurysms is unknown, although research is ongoing. An aneurysm may be due to atherosclerosis, which results in a defect in the vessel wall with subsequent weakness of the wall; a congenital defect of the vessel wall; hypertensive vascular disease; head trauma; or advancing age.

Any artery within the brain can be the site of a cerebral aneurysm, but these lesions usually occur at the bifurcations of the large arteries at the circle of Willis (Fig. 62-5). The cerebral arteries most commonly affected by an aneurysm are the internal carotid artery (ICA), anterior cerebral artery (ACA), anterior communicating artery (ACoA), posterior communicating artery (PCoA), posterior cerebral artery (PCA), and middle cerebral artery (MCA). Multiple cerebral aneurysms are not uncommon.

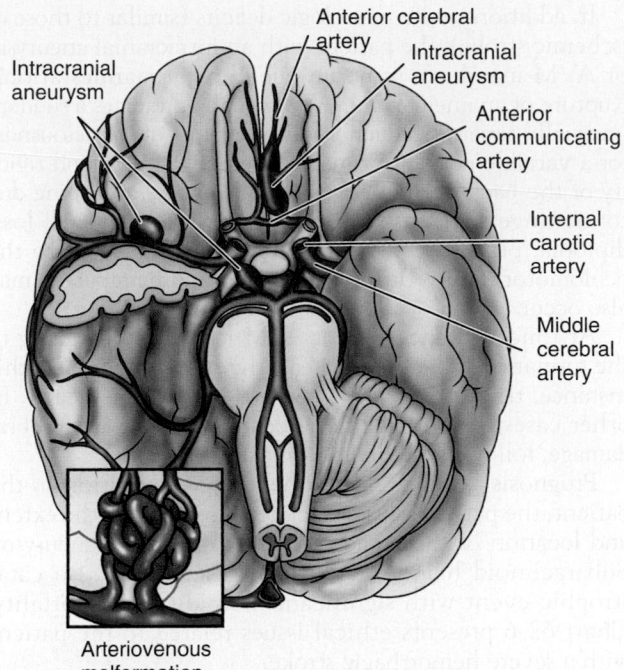

Figure 62-5 Common sites of intracranial aneurysms and an arteriovenous malformation.

Arteriovenous Malformations

Most AVMs are caused by an abnormality in embryonal development that leads to a tangle of arteries and veins in the brain that lacks a capillary bed (see Fig. 62-5). The absence of a capillary bed leads to dilation of the arteries and veins and eventual rupture. AVM is a common cause of hemorrhagic stroke in young people.

Subarachnoid Hemorrhage

A subarachnoid hemorrhage (hemorrhage into the subarachnoid space) may occur as a result of an AVM, intracranial aneurysm, trauma, or hypertension. The most common causes are a leaking aneurysm in the area of the circle of Willis and a congenital AVM of the brain.

Clinical Manifestations

The patient with a hemorrhagic stroke can present with a wide variety of neurologic deficits, similar to the patient with ischemic stroke. The conscious patient most commonly reports a severe headache. A comprehensive assessment reveals the extent of the neurologic deficits. Many of the same motor, sensory, cranial nerve, cognitive, and other functions that are disrupted after ischemic stroke are also altered after a hemorrhagic stroke. Table 62-2 reviews the neurologic deficits frequently seen in stroke patients. Table 62-3 compares the symptoms seen in right hemispheric stroke with those seen in left hemispheric stroke. Other symptoms that may be observed more frequently in patients with acute intracerebral hemorrhage (compared with ischemic stroke) are vomiting, an early sudden change in level of consciousness, and possibly focal seizures due to frequent brain stem involvement (Hickey, 2009).

In addition to the neurologic deficits (similar to those of ischemic stroke), the patient with an intracranial aneurysm or AVM may have some unique clinical manifestations. Rupture of an aneurysm or AVM usually produces a sudden, unusually severe headache and often loss of consciousness for a variable period of time. There may be pain and rigidity of the back of the neck (nuchal rigidity) and spine due to meningeal irritation. Visual disturbances (visual loss, diplopia, ptosis) occur if the aneurysm is adjacent to the oculomotor nerve. Tinnitus, dizziness, and hemiparesis may also occur.

At times, an aneurysm or AVM leaks blood, leading to the formation of a clot that seals the site of rupture. In this instance, the patient may show little neurologic deficit. In other cases, severe bleeding occurs, resulting in cerebral damage, followed rapidly by coma and death.

Prognosis depends on the neurologic condition of the patient, the patient's age, associated diseases, and the extent and location of the hemorrhage or intracranial aneurysm. Subarachnoid hemorrhage from an aneurysm is a catastrophic event with significant morbidity and mortality. Chart 62-6 presents ethical issues related to the patient with a severe hemorrhagic stroke.

Assessment and Diagnostic Findings

Any patient with suspected stroke should undergo a CT scan or MRI to determine the type of stroke, the size and location of the hematoma, and the presence or absence of ventricular blood and hydrocephalus. Cerebral angiography confirms the diagnosis of an intracranial aneurysm or AVM. These tests show the location and size of the lesion and provide information about the affected arteries, veins, adjoin-

ing vessels, and vascular branches. Lumbar puncture is performed if there is no evidence of increased ICP, the CT scan results are negative, and subarachnoid hemorrhage must be confirmed. Lumbar puncture in the presence of increased ICP could result in brain stem herniation or rebleeding. When diagnosing a hemorrhagic stroke in a patient younger than 40 years of age, some clinicians obtain a toxicology screen for illicit drug use.

Prevention

Primary prevention of hemorrhagic stroke is the best approach and includes managing hypertension and ameliorating other significant risk factors. Control of hypertension, especially in people older than 55 years of age, reduces the risk of hemorrhagic stroke (Luders, 2007). Additional risk factors are increased age, male gender, and excessive alcohol intake. Stroke risk screenings provide an ideal opportunity to lower hemorrhagic stroke risk by identifying high-risk individuals or groups and educating patients and the community about recognition and prevention.

Complications

Potential complications of hemorrhagic stroke include rebleeding or hematoma expansion; cerebral vasospasm resulting in cerebral ischemia; acute hydrocephalus, which results when free blood obstructs the reabsorption of cerebrospinal fluid (CSF) by the arachnoid villi; and seizures.

Cerebral Hypoxia and Decreased Blood Flow

Immediate complications of a hemorrhagic stroke include cerebral hypoxia, decreased cerebral blood flow, and extension of the area of injury. Providing adequate oxygenation of blood to the brain minimizes cerebral hypoxia. Brain function depends on delivery of oxygen to the tissues. Administering supplemental oxygen and maintaining the hemoglobin and hematocrit at acceptable levels will assist in maintaining tissue oxygenation.

Cerebral blood flow is dependent on the blood pressure, cardiac output, and integrity of cerebral blood vessels. Adequate hydration (IV fluids) must be ensured to reduce blood viscosity and improve cerebral blood flow. Extremes of hypertension or hypotension need to be avoided to prevent changes in cerebral blood flow and the potential for extending the area of injury.

A seizure can also compromise cerebral blood flow, resulting in further injury to the brain. Observing for seizure activity and initiating appropriate treatment are important components of care after a hemorrhagic stroke.

Vasospasm

The development of cerebral vasospasm (narrowing of the lumen of the involved cranial blood vessel) is a serious complication of subarachnoid hemorrhage and is the leading cause of morbidity and mortality in those who survive the initial subarachnoid hemorrhage (Kosty, 2005). The mechanism responsible for vasospasm is not clear, but it is associated with increasing amounts of blood in the subarachnoid cisterns and cerebral fissures, as visualized by CT scan. Monitoring for vasospasm may be performed through the use of bedside transcranial Doppler ultrasonography (TCD) or follow-up cerebral angiography.

CHART 62-6 *Ethics and Related Issues*

What Are the Ethical Issues Related to DNR Orders After Severe Stroke?

Situation

An 85-year-old patient is admitted with a large intracerebral hemorrhage, severe neurologic deficits, and a past medical history of coronary artery bypass graft surgery, hypertension, atrial fibrillation, and gout. The patient does not have an advanced directive. The attending physician suggests a do-not-resuscitate (DNR) order to the family.

Dilemma

The principle of autonomy for the patient (including death with dignity) conflicts with the principle of beneficence for the health care providers.

Discussion

1. What arguments would you pose in favor of the DNR order?
2. What arguments would you pose against the DNR order?
3. Does the family have the right to refuse?
4. Is a DNR order an example of "patient abandonment" by health care workers, or an attempt to limit treatment and avoid CPR in a patient with an anticipated poor outcome?

Vasospasm frequently occurs 3 to 14 days after initial hemorrhage, when the clot undergoes lysis (dissolution), and the chance of rebleeding is increased (Hickey, 2009). It leads to increased vascular resistance, which impedes cerebral blood flow and causes brain ischemia and infarction. The signs and symptoms reflect the areas of the brain involved. Vasospasm is often heralded by a worsening headache, a decrease in level of consciousness (confusion, lethargy, and disorientation), or a new focal neurologic deficit (aphasia, hemiparesis).

Management of vasospasm remains difficult and controversial. It is believed that early surgery to clip the aneurysm prevents rebleeding and that removal of blood from the basal cisterns around the major cerebral arteries may prevent vasospasm. Advances in technology have led to the introduction of interventional neuroradiology for the treatment of aneurysms. Endovascular techniques may be used in selected patients to occlude the artery supplying the aneurysm with a balloon, coils, or other techniques to occlude the aneurysm itself. As more studies on these techniques are completed, their use will increase.

Medication may be effective in the treatment of vasospasm. Based on one theory, that vasospasm is caused by an increased influx of calcium into the cell, medication therapy may be used to block or antagonize this action and prevent or reverse the action of vasospasm if already present. The most frequently used calcium channel blocker is nimodipine (Nimotop) (Devlin, 2008). Another therapy for vasospasm, referred to as "triple-H therapy," is aimed at minimizing the deleterious effects of the associated cerebral ischemia and includes (1) fluid volume expanders (hypervolemia), (2) induced arterial hypertension, and (3) hemodilution (Kosty, 2005).

Increased Intracranial Pressure

An increase in ICP can occur after either an ischemic or a hemorrhagic stroke but almost always follows a subarachnoid hemorrhage, usually because of disturbed circulation of CSF caused by blood in the basal cisterns. Neurologic assessments are performed frequently, and if there is evidence of deterioration from increased ICP (due to cerebral edema, herniation, hydrocephalus, or vasospasm), CSF drainage may be instituted by ventricular catheter drainage. Mannitol may be administered to reduce ICP. When mannitol is used as a long-term measure to control ICP, dehydration and disturbances in electrolyte balance (hyponatremia or hypernatremia; hypokalemia or hyperkalemia) may occur. Mannitol pulls water out of the brain tissue by osmosis and reduces total-body water through diuresis. The patient is monitored for signs of dehydration and for rebound elevation of ICP. Other interventions may include elevating the head of the bed, sedation, and hyperosmolar therapy (discussed in the vasospasm section) (Broderick, Connolly, Feldmann, et al., 2007; Presciutti, 2006).

Hypertension

Hypertension is the most common cause of intracerebral hemorrhage, and its treatment is critical. Specific goals for blood pressure management, which are individualized for each patient, remain controversial. Blood pressure goals may be dependent on the presence of increased ICP.

Clinical trials are currently ongoing to further investigate control of blood pressure in intracerebral hemorrhage (Broderick, et al., 2007). Systolic blood pressure may be lowered to prevent hematoma enlargement. If blood pressure is elevated, antihypertensive therapy (labetalol [Trandate], nicardipine [Cardene], nitroprusside [Nitropress], hydralazine [Apresoline]) may be prescribed. During the administration of antihypertensives, arterial hemodynamic monitoring is important to detect and avoid a precipitous drop in blood pressure, which can produce brain ischemia. Stool softeners are used to prevent straining, which can elevate the blood pressure.

Medical Management

The goals of medical treatment for hemorrhagic stroke are to allow the brain to recover from the initial insult (bleeding), to prevent or minimize the risk of rebleeding, and to prevent or treat complications. Management may consist of bed rest with sedation to prevent agitation and stress, management of vasospasm, and surgical or medical treatment to prevent rebleeding. If the bleeding is caused by anticoagulation with warfarin (Coumadin), the INR may be corrected with fresh-frozen plasma and vitamin K. Because seizures can occur after intracerebral hemorrhage, antiseizure agents are often administered prophylactically for a brief period of time. Analgesic agents may be prescribed for head and neck pain. The patient is fitted with sequential compression devices or anti-embolism stockings to prevent deep vein thrombosis (DVT). Fever should be treated. Hyperglycemia should also be treated (an IV insulin drip may be required to achieve control) (Broderick, et al., 2007; Presciutti, 2006). After discharge most patients will require antihypertensive medications to decrease their risk of another intracerebral hemorrhage.

Surgical Management

In many cases, a primary intracerebral hemorrhage is not treated surgically. However, if the diameter of the hematoma exceeds 3 cm and the Glasgow Coma Scale score decreases, surgical evacuation is strongly recommended for the patient with a cerebellar hemorrhage (Broderick, et al., 2007). Surgical evacuation is most frequently accomplished via a craniotomy (see Chapter 61).

The patient with an intracranial aneurysm is prepared for surgical intervention as soon as his or her condition is considered stable. Surgical treatment of the patient with an unruptured aneurysm is an option. The goal of surgery is to prevent bleeding in an unruptured aneurysm or further bleeding in an already ruptured aneurysm. This objective is accomplished by isolating the aneurysm from its circulation or by strengthening the arterial wall. An aneurysm may be excluded from the cerebral circulation by means of a ligature or a clip across its neck. If this is not anatomically possible, the aneurysm can be reinforced by wrapping it with some substance to provide support and induce scarring.

Less invasive endovascular treatments are now being used for aneurysms. These procedures are performed by neurosurgeons in neurointerventional radiology facilities. Two procedures include endovascular treatment (occlusion of the parent artery) and aneurysm coiling (obstruction of the aneurysm site with a coil). Although these techniques are associated with lower risks than intracranial surgery in general, secondary stroke and rupture of the aneurysm are still potential complications.

Postoperative complications include psychological symptoms (disorientation, amnesia, **Korsakoff's syndrome,** personality changes), intraoperative embolization, postoperative internal artery occlusion, fluid and electrolyte disturbances (from dysfunction of the neurohypophyseal system), and gastrointestinal bleeding.

NURSING PROCESS

THE PATIENT WITH A HEMORRHAGIC STROKE

Assessment

A complete neurologic assessment is performed initially and includes evaluation for the following:
- Altered level of consciousness
- Sluggish pupillary reaction
- Motor and sensory dysfunction
- Cranial nerve deficits (extraocular eye movements, facial droop, presence of ptosis)
- Speech difficulties and visual disturbance
- Headache and nuchal rigidity or other neurologic deficits

All patients should be monitored in the intensive care unit after an intracerebral or subarachnoid hemorrhage. Neurologic assessment findings are documented and reported as indicated. The frequency of these assessments varies depending on the patient's condition. Any changes in the patient's condition require reassessment and thorough documentation; changes should be reported immediately.

Alteration in level of consciousness often is the earliest sign of deterioration in a patient with a hemorrhagic stroke. Because nurses have the most frequent contact with patients, they are in the best position to detect subtle changes. Mild drowsiness and slight slurring of speech may be early signs that the level of consciousness is deteriorating.

Diagnosis

Nursing Diagnoses

Based on the assessment data, the patient's major nursing diagnoses may include the following:
- Ineffective tissue perfusion (cerebral) related to bleeding or vasospasm
- Disturbed sensory perception related to medically imposed restrictions (aneurysm precautions)
- Anxiety related to illness and/or medically imposed restrictions (aneurysm precautions)

Collaborative Problems/Potential Complications

Based on the assessment data, potential complications that may develop include the following:
- Vasospasm
- Seizures
- Hydrocephalus
- Rebleeding
- Hyponatremia

Planning and Goals

The goals for the patient may include improved cerebral tissue perfusion, relief of sensory and perceptual deprivation, relief of anxiety, and the absence of complications.

Nursing Interventions

Optimizing Cerebral Tissue Perfusion

The patient is closely monitored for neurologic deterioration resulting from recurrent bleeding, increasing ICP, or vasospasm. A neurologic flow record is maintained. The blood pressure, pulse, level of consciousness (an indicator of cerebral perfusion), pupillary responses, and motor function are checked hourly. Respiratory status is monitored, because a reduction in oxygen in areas of the brain with impaired autoregulation increases the chances of a cerebral infarction. Any changes are reported immediately.

IMPLEMENTING ANEURYSM PRECAUTIONS. Cerebral aneurysm precautions are implemented for the patient with a diagnosis of aneurysm to provide a nonstimulating environment, prevent increases in ICP, and prevent further bleeding. The patient is placed on immediate and absolute bed rest in a quiet, nonstressful environment, because activity, pain, and anxiety elevate the blood pressure, which increases the risk for bleeding. Visitors, except for family, are restricted.

The head of the bed is elevated 15 to 30 degrees to promote venous drainage and decrease ICP. Some neurologists, however, prefer that the patient remain flat to increase cerebral perfusion.

Any activity that suddenly increases the blood pressure or obstructs venous return is avoided. This includes the Valsalva maneuver, straining, forceful sneezing, pushing oneself up in bed, acute flexion or rotation of the head and neck (which compromises the jugular veins), and cigarette smoking. Any activity requiring exertion is contraindicated. The patient is instructed to exhale through the mouth during voiding or defecation to decrease strain. No enemas are permitted, but stool softeners and mild laxatives are prescribed. Both prevent constipation, which would cause an increase in ICP, as would enemas. Dim lighting is helpful, because photophobia (visual intolerance of light) is common. Coffee and tea, unless decaffeinated, are usually eliminated.

Anti-embolism stockings or sequential compression devices may be prescribed to decrease the incidence of DVT resulting from immobility. The legs are observed for signs and symptoms of DVT (tenderness, redness, swelling, warmth, and edema), and abnormal findings are reported.

The nurse administers all personal care. The patient is fed and bathed to prevent any exertion that might increase the blood pressure. External stimuli are kept to a minimum, including no television, no radio, and no reading. Visitors are restricted in an effort to keep the patient as quiet as possible. This precaution must be individualized based on the patient's condition and response to visitors. A sign indicating this restriction should be placed on the door of the room, and the restrictions should be discussed with both patient and family. The purpose of aneurysm precautions should be thoroughly explained to both the patient (if possible) and family.

Relieving Sensory Deprivation and Anxiety

Sensory stimulation is kept to a minimum for patients on aneurysm precautions. For patients who are awake, alert, and oriented, an explanation of the restrictions helps reduce the patient's sense of isolation. Reality orientation is provided to help maintain orientation.

Keeping the patient well informed of the plan of care provides reassurance and helps minimize anxiety. Appropriate reassurance also helps relieve the patient's fears and anxiety. The family also requires information and support.

Monitoring and Managing Potential Complications

VASOSPASM. The patient is assessed for signs of possible vasospasm: intensified headaches, a decrease in level of responsiveness (confusion, disorientation, lethargy), or evidence of aphasia or partial paralysis. These signs may develop several days after surgery or on the initiation of treatment and must be reported immediately. If vasospasm is diagnosed, calcium channel blockers or fluid volume expanders may be prescribed.

SEIZURES. Seizure precautions are maintained for every patient who may be at risk for seizure activity. Should a seizure occur, maintaining the airway and preventing injury are the primary goals. Medication therapy is initiated at this time, if not already prescribed. The medication of choice for many years has been phenytoin (Dilantin). Its use is being questioned based on the results of research including 527 patients that suggested that phenytoin may increase functional and cognitive disability after subarachnoid hemorrhage (Naidech, Kreiter, Janjua, et al., 2005).

HYDROCEPHALUS. Blood in the subarachnoid space or ventricles impedes the circulation of CSF, resulting in hydrocephalus. A CT scan that indicates dilated ventricles confirms the diagnosis. Hydrocephalus can occur within the first 24 hours (acute) after subarachnoid hemorrhage or several days (subacute) to several weeks (delayed) later. Symptoms vary according to the time of onset and may be nonspecific. Acute hydrocephalus is characterized by sudden onset of stupor or coma and is managed with a ventriculostomy drain to decrease ICP. Symptoms of subacute and delayed hydrocephalus include gradual onset of drowsiness, behavioral changes, and ataxic gait. A ventriculoperitoneal shunt is surgically placed to treat chronic hydrocephalus. Changes in patient responsiveness are reported immediately.

REBLEEDING. The rate of recurrent hemorrhage is approximately 2% after a primary intracerebral hemorrhage. Hypertension is the most serious risk factor, suggesting the importance of appropriate antihypertensive treatment.

Aneurysm rebleeding occurs most frequently during the first 2 weeks after the initial hemorrhage and is considered a major complication. Symptoms of rebleeding include sudden severe headache, nausea, vomiting, decreased level of consciousness, and neurologic deficit. Rebleeding is confirmed by CT scan. Blood pressure is carefully maintained with medications. The most effective preventive treatment is to secure the aneurysm if the patient is a candidate for surgery or endovascular treatment.

HYPONATREMIA. After subarachnoid hemorrhage, hyponatremia is found in up to 30% of patients (Naval, Stevens, Mirski, et al., 2006). Laboratory data must be checked frequently, and hyponatremia (defined as a serum sodium concentration of less than 135 mEq/L) must be identified as early as possible. The patient's primary health care provider needs to be notified of a low serum sodium level that has persisted for 24 hours or longer. The patient is then evaluated for syndrome of inappropriate antidiuretic hormone (SIADH) or cerebral salt-wasting syndrome. (SIADH is described in Chapter 14.) Cerebral salt-wasting syndrome occurs when the kidneys are unable to conserve sodium and volume depletion results. The treatment most often is the use of hypertonic 3% saline.

Promoting Home and Community-Based Care

TEACHING PATIENTS SELF-CARE. The patient and family are provided with information that will enable them to cooperate with the care and restrictions required during the acute phase of hemorrhagic stroke and to prepare them to return home. Patient and family teaching includes information about the causes of hemorrhagic stroke and its possible consequences. In addition, the patient and family are informed about the medical treatments that are implemented, including surgical intervention if warranted, and the importance of interventions taken to prevent and detect complications (ie, aneurysm precautions, close monitoring of the patient). Depending on the presence and severity of neurologic impairment and other complications resulting from the stroke, the patient may be transferred to a rehabilitation unit or center for additional patient and family teaching about strategies to regain self-care ability. Teaching addresses the use of assistive devices or modification of the home environment to help the patient live with the disability. Modifications of the home may be required to provide a safe environment.

CONTINUING CARE. The acute and rehabilitation phase of care focuses on obvious needs, issues, and deficits for the patient with a hemorrhagic stroke. The patient and family are reminded of the importance of following recommendations to prevent further hemorrhagic stroke and keeping follow-up appointments with health care providers for monitoring of risk factors. Referral for home care may be warranted to assess the home environment and the ability of the patient and to ensure that the patient and family are able to manage at home. Home visits provide opportunities to monitor the physical and psychological status of the patient and the ability of the family to cope with any alterations in the patient's status. In addition, the home care nurse reminds the patient and family of the importance of continuing health promotion and screening practices. Chart 62-7 lists teaching points for the patient recovering from a stroke.

Evaluation

Expected Patient Outcomes

Expected patient outcomes may include the following:

1. Demonstrates intact neurologic status and normal vital signs and respiratory patterns
   a. Is alert and oriented to time, place, and person

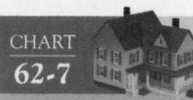

CHART 62-7 HOME CARE CHECKLIST
The Patient Recovering From a Stroke

At the completion of the home care instruction, the patient or caregiver will be able to:	PATIENT	CAREGIVER
• Discuss measures to prevent subsequent strokes.	✔	✔
• Identify signs and symptoms of specific complications.	✔	✔
• Identify potential complications and discuss measures to prevent them (blood clots, aspiration, pneumonia, urinary tract infection, fecal impaction, skin breakdown, contracture).	✔	✔
• Identify psychosocial consequences of stroke and appropriate interventions.	✔	✔
• Identify safety measures to prevent falls.	✔	✔
• State names, doses, indications, and side effects of medications.	✔	✔
• Demonstrate adaptive techniques for accomplishing ADLs.	✔	✔
• Demonstrate swallowing techniques (for patients with dysphagia).	✔	✔
• Demonstrate care of enteric feeding tube, if applicable.	✔	✔
• Demonstrate home exercises, use of splints or orthotics, proper positioning, and frequent repositioning.	✔	✔
• Describe procedures for maintaining skin integrity.	✔	✔
• Demonstrate indwelling catheter care, if applicable. Describe a bowel and bladder elimination program as appropriate.	✔	✔
• Identify appropriate recreational or diversional activities, support groups, and community resources.	✔	✔

b. Demonstrates normal speech patterns and intact cognitive processes
c. Demonstrates normal and equal strength, movement, and sensation of all four extremities
d. Exhibits normal deep tendon reflexes and pupillary responses
2. Demonstrates normal sensory perceptions
   a. States rationale for aneurysm precautions
   b. Exhibits clear thought processes
3. Exhibits reduced anxiety level
   a. Is less restless
   b. Exhibits absence of physiologic indicators of anxiety (eg, has normal vital signs; normal respiratory rate; absence of excessive, fast speech)
4. Is free of complications
   a. Exhibits absence of vasospasm
   b. Exhibits normal vital signs and neuromuscular activity without seizures
   c. Verbalizes understanding of seizure precautions
   d. Exhibits normal mental status and normal motor and sensory status
   e. Reports no visual changes

CRITICAL THINKING EXERCISES

1   A patient had symptoms of an ischemic stroke approximately 1 hour ago and is undergoing a CT scan. What are the time frames, criteria, and dosage for t-PA administration? What nursing assessments and actions would you take? What is your rationale for these assessments and actions?

2   A 58-year-old man is admitted with an ischemic stroke and has left-sided hemiplegia. He is concerned about how to resume sexual relations with his wife and the possibility of not being able to resume sexual intimacy. Identify possible causes of sexual dysfunction after a stroke. What interventions can the nurse implement to address his concerns?

3   A 50-year-old patient with a history of hypertension is expected to be discharged to home today after a 7-day stay for a stroke. She has residual right-sided weakness and a visual field deficit. What teaching would be indicated to prevent another stroke? What resources may be needed to enable her to go home as scheduled?

EBP   **4**   A patient is admitted to the hospital following a hemorrhagic stroke and is at high risk for vasospasm. What medical and nursing measures should be implemented to prevent vasospasm? Identify the evidence for and the criteria used to evaluate the strength of the evidence for the specific measures identified for prevention of vasospasm.

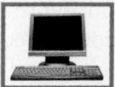

The Smeltzer suite offers these additional resources to enhance learning and facilitate understanding of this chapter:
• thePoint online resource, thepoint.lww.com/Smeltzer12E
• Student CD-ROM included with the book
• *Study Guide to Accompany Brunner & Suddarth's Textbook of Medical-Surgical Nursing*
• *Handbook for Brunner & Suddarth's Textbook of Medical-Surgical Nursing*

REFERENCES AND SELECTED READINGS

Asterisks indicate nursing research.
**Double asterisks indicate classic references.*

Books

American Association of Neuroscience Nurses. (2008). *Guide to the care of the hospitalized patient with ischemic stroke: AANN reference series for clinical practice*. Glenview, IL: Author.

Haines, D. (2006). *Fundamental neuroscience for basic and clinical application* (3rd ed.). Philadelphia: Churchill Livingston, Elsevier.

Hickey, J. V. (2009). *The clinical practice of neurological & neurosurgical nursing* (6th ed.). Philadelphia: Lippincott Williams & Wilkins.

Karch, A. (2008). *Lippincott's nursing drug guide*. Philadelphia: Lippincott Williams & Wilkins.

Porth, C. M. & Matfin, G. (2009). *Pathophysiology: Concepts of altered health states* (8th ed.). Philadelphia: Lippincott Williams & Wilkins.

Posner, J. B., Saper, C. B., Schiff, N. D., et al. (2007). *Plum and Posner's diagnosis of stupor and coma* (4th ed.). Oxford, UK: Oxford University Press.

Read, S. J. & Virley, D. (2005). *Stroke genomics: Methods and reviews*. Totowa, NJ: Humana Press.

Warlow, C.P., Dennis, M., van Gijn, J., et al. (2008). *Stroke: Practical management* (3rd ed.). Oxford, UK: Blackwell Science.

Journals and Electronic Documents

Adams, H. P., Zoppo, G., Alberts, M. J., et al. (2007). Guidelines for the early management of patients with ischemic stroke. A guideline from the American Heart Association/American Stroke Association Stroke Council, Clinical Cardiology Council, Cardiovascular Radiology and Intervention Council, and the Atherosclerotic Peripheral Vascular Disease and Quality of Care Outcomes in Research Interdisciplinary Working Groups. *Stroke, 38*(5), 1655–1711.

Berg, A., Palomäki, H., Lönnqvist, J., et al. (2005). Depression among caregivers of stroke survivors. *Stroke, 36*(3), 639–643.

Broderick, J., Connolly, S., Feldmann, E., et al. (2007). Guidelines for the management of spontaneous intracerebral hemorrhage in adults: 2007 update: A guideline from the American Heart Association/American Stroke Association Stroke Council, High Blood Pressure Research Council, and the Quality of Care and Outcomes in Research Interdisciplinary Working Group. *Stroke, 38*(6), 2001–2023.

Chae, J., Mascarenhas, D., Yu, D. T., et al. (2007). Poststroke shoulder pain: Its relationship to motor impairment, activity limitation, and quality of life. *Archives of Physical Medicine and Rehabilitation, 88*(3), 298–301.

Chaturvedi, S., Bruno, A., Feasby, T., et al. (2005). Carotid endarterectomy. An evidence-based review. *Neurology, 65*(6), 794–801.

Chiuve, S. E., Rexrode, K. M., Spiegelman, D., et al. (2008). Primary prevention of stroke by healthy lifestyle. *Circulation, 118*(8), 947–954.

*Coombs, U. (2007). Spousal caregiving for stroke survivors. *Journal of Neuroscience Nursing, 39*(2), 112–119.

Devlin, M. M. (2008). Nimodipine: Test your drug IQ. *Nursing, 38*(7), 56cc1–56cc2.

Duncan, P. W., Zorowitz, R., Bates, B., et al. (2005). Management of adult stroke rehabilitation care - A clinical practice guideline. *Stroke, 36*(9), e100–e143.

Elovic, E. P., Brashear, A., Kaelin, D., et al. (2008). Repeated treatments with botulinum toxin type A produce sustained decreases in the limitations associated with focal upper-limb poststroke spasticity for caregivers and patients. *Archives of Physical Medicine and Rehabilitation, 89*(5), 799–806.

Felton, R. P., Ogden, N. R. P., Pena, C., et al. (2005). The Food and Drug Administration medical device review process: Clearance of a clot retriever for use in ischemic stroke. *Stroke, 36*(2), 404–406.

Flaherty, M., Haverbusch, M., Sekar, P., et al. (2006). Long-term mortality after intracerebral hemorrhage. *Neurology, 66*(8), 1182–1186.

Fung, T. T., Chiuve, S. E., McCullough, M. L., et al. (2008). Adherence to a DASH-style diet and risk of coronary heart disease and stroke in women. *Archives of Internal Medicine, 168*(7), 713–720.

Gurm, H. S., Yadav, J. S., Fayad, P., et al., for the SAPPHIRE Investigators. (2008). Long-term results of carotid stenting versus endarterectomy in high-risk patients. *New England Journal of Medicine, 358*(15), 1572–1579.

*Harper, J. (2007). Emergency nurses' knowledge of evidence-based ischemic stroke care: A pilot study. *Journal of Emergency Nursing, 33*(3), 202–207.

Hinkle, J. L. & Guanci, M. (2007). Acute ischemic stroke review. *Journal of Neuroscience Nursing, 39*(5), 285–293, 310.

Johnson, J., Minarik, P., Nyström, K., et al. (2006). Poststroke depression incidence and risk factors: An integrative literature review. *Journal of Neuroscience Nursing, 38*(4), 316–327.

Kasner, S. E. (2006). Clinical interpretation and use of stroke scales. *Lancet Neurology, 5*(7), 603–612.

Kautz, D. (2007). Hope for love: Practical advice for intimacy and sex after stroke. *Rehabilitation Nursing, 32*(3), 95.

Kosty, T. (2005). Cerebral vasospasm after subarachnoid hemorrhage: An update. *Critical Care Nursing Quarterly, 28*(2), 122–134.

Kwakkel, G., Kollen, B. & Krebs, H. (2008). Effects of robot-assisted therapy on upper limb recovery after stroke: A systematic review. *Neurorehabilitation & Neural Repair, 22*(2), 111–121.

Lapchak, P. A. & Araujo, D. M. (2007). Advances in ischemic stroke treatment: Neuroprotective and combination therapies. *Expert Opinion on Emerging Drugs, 12*(1), 97–112.

Lewandowski, C. A., Rao, C. P. V. & Silver, B. (2008). Transient ischemic attack: Definitions and clinical presentations. *Annuals of Emergency Medicine, 52*(2), S7–S16.

*Lightbody, C., Auton, M., Baldwin, R., et al. (2007). The use of nurses' and carers' observations in the identification of poststroke depression. *Journal of Advanced Nursing, 60*(6), 595–604.

Luders, S. (2007). Drug therapy for the secondary prevention of stroke in hypertensive patients: Current issues and options. *Drugs, 67*(7), 955–963.

Naidech, A. M., Kreiter, K. T., Janjua, N., et al. (2005). Phenytoin exposure is associated with functional and cognitive disability after subarachnoid hemorrhage. *Stroke, 36*(3), 583–587.

Nassief, A. & Marsh, J. D. (2008). Statin therapy for stroke prevention. *Stroke, 39*(3), 1042–1048.

National Center for Health Statistics, Centers for Disease Control and Prevention. (2008). *Fast stats A to Z: Stroke*. Available at: www.cdc.gov/nchs/fastats/stroke.htm

**National Institute of Neurologic Disorders and Stroke (NINDS), rt-PA Stroke Study Group. (1995). Tissue plasminogen activator for acute ischemic stroke. *New England Journal of Medicine, 333*(24), 1581–1587.

Naval, N. S., Stevens, R. D., Mirski, M. A., et al. (2006). Controversies in the management of aneurysmal subarachnoid hemorrhage. *Critical Care Medicine, 34*(2), 511–524.

Presciutti, M. (2006). Nursing priorities in caring for patients with intracerebral hemorrhage. *Journal of Neuroscience Nursing, 38*(4), 296.

Ridker, P. M., Cook, N. R., Lee, I., et al. (2005). A randomized trial of low-dose aspirin in the primary prevention of cardiovascular disease in women. *New England Journal of Medicine, 353*(13), 1293–1304.

Rosamond, W., Flegal, K., Furie, K., et al., for the American Heart Association Statistics Committee and Stroke Statistics Subcommittee. (2008). Heart disease and stroke statistics—2008 update. A report from the American Heart Association Statistics Committee and Stroke Statistics Subcommittee. *Circulation, 117*, e25–e146.

Sacco, R. L., Adams, R., Albers, G., et al. (2006). Guidelines for prevention of stroke in patients with ischemic stroke or transient ischemic attack. A statement for healthcare professionals from the American Heart Association/American Stroke Association Council on Stroke. *Stroke, 37*(2), 577–617.

Saver, J. L. (2006). Time is brain quantified. *Stroke, 37*(1), 263–233.

U.S. Department of Health and Human Services. (2008). *Update to a public health action plan to prevent heart disease and stroke, celebrating our first five years*. Atlanta, GA: U.S. Department of Health and Human Services, Centers for Disease Control and Prevention. Available at: www.cdc.gov/dhdsp/library/action_plan/2008_update/pdfs/2008_Action_Plan_Update.pdf

Vranken, J. H., Dijkgraaf, M. G. W., Kruis, M. R., et al. (2008). Pregabalin in patients with central neuropathic pain: A randomized, double-blind, placebo-controlled trial of a flexible-dose regimen. *Pain, 136*(1–2), 150–157.

Wolf, S., Winstein, C., Miller, J., et al. (2006). Effect of constraint-induced movement therapy on upper extremity function 3 to 9 months after stroke: The EXCITE randomized clinical trial. *Journal of the American Medical Association, 296*(17), 2095–2104.

RESOURCES

American Association of Neuroscience Nurses, www.aann.org
American Stroke Association, a Division of the American Heart Association, www.strokeassociation.org
National Institute of Neurological Disorders and Stroke, www.ninds.nih.gov
National Stroke Association, www.stroke.org

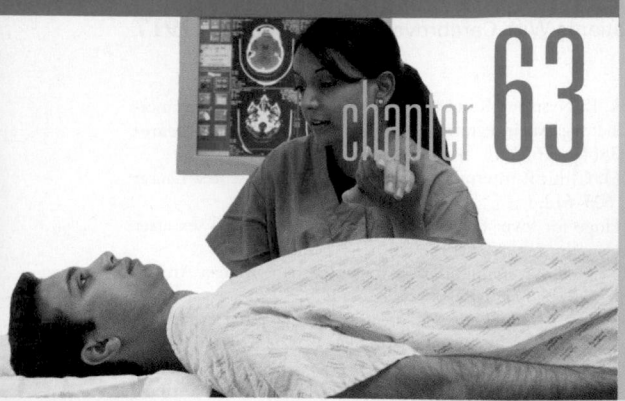

chapter 63

Management of Patients With Neurologic Trauma

Trauma involving the central nervous system can be life-threatening. Even if it is not life-threatening, brain and spinal cord injury may result in major physical and psychological dysfunction and can alter the patient's life completely. Neurologic trauma affects the patient, the family, the health care system, and society as a whole because of its major sequelae and the costs of acute and long-term care of patients with trauma to the brain and spinal cord.

Head Injuries

Head injury is a broad classification that includes injury to the scalp, skull, or brain. It is estimated that 1.4 million people sustain a head injury each year in the United States, and approximately 50,000 people die, 235,000 are hospitalized, and 1.1 million are treated and released from an emergency department (Langlois, Rutland-Brown & Thomas, 2006). A head injury may lead to conditions ranging from mild concussion to coma and death; the most serious form is known as a traumatic brain injury (TBI). The most common causes of TBIs are falls (28%), motor vehicle crashes (20%), being struck by objects (19%), and assaults (11%). People at highest risk for TBI are those in the 15- to 19-year age group. Males are twice as likely as females to sustain a TBI. Adults 75 years of age or older have the highest TBI-related hospitalization and death rates, and African Americans also have high mortality rates (Langlois, et al., 2006). An estimated 5.3 million Americans are currently living with a TBI-related disability (National Center for Injury Prevention and Control, 2007). The best approach to head injury is prevention (Chart 63-1).

Pathophysiology

Research suggests that not all brain damage occurs at the moment of impact. Damage to the brain from traumatic injury takes two forms: primary injury and secondary injury. **Primary injury** is the initial damage to the brain that results from the traumatic event. This may include contusions, lacerations, and torn blood vessels due to impact, acceleration/deceleration, or foreign object penetration. **Secondary injury** evolves over the ensuing hours and days after the initial injury and results from inadequate delivery of nutrients and oxygen to the cells (Littlejohns & Bader, 2005).

Physiology ■■■ Pathophysiology

Brain suffers traumatic injury

↓

Brain swelling or bleeding increases intracranial volume

↓

Rigid cranium allows no room for expansion of contents so intracranial pressure increases

↓

Pressure on blood vessels within the brain causes blood flow to the brain to slow

↓

Cerebral hypoxia and ischemia occur

↓

Intracranial pressure continues to rise. Brain may herniate

↓

Cerebral blood flow ceases

Figure 63-1 Pathophysiology of traumatic brain injury.

The cranial vault contains three main components: brain, blood, and cerebrospinal fluid (CSF). According to the Monro-Kellie doctrine, the cranial vault is a closed system, and if one of the three components increases in volume, at least one of the other two must decrease in volume, or the pressure increases. Any bleeding or swelling within the skull increases the volume of contents within the skull and therefore causes increased intracranial pressure (ICP) (see Chapter 61). If the pressure increases enough, it can cause displacement of the brain through or against the rigid structures of the skull. This causes restriction of blood flow to the brain, decreasing oxygen delivery and waste removal. Cells within the brain become anoxic and cannot metabolize properly, producing ischemia, infarction, irreversible brain damage, and, eventually, brain death (Fig. 63-1).

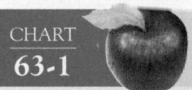

CHART 63-1

HEALTH PROMOTION
Preventing Head and Spinal Cord Injuries

- Advise drivers to obey traffic laws, and to avoid speeding or driving when under the influence of drugs or alcohol.
- Advise all drivers and passengers to wear seat belts and shoulder harnesses. Children younger than 12 years of age should be restrained in an age/size-appropriate system in the back seat.
- Caution passengers against riding in the back of pickup trucks.
- Advise motorcyclists, scooter riders, bicyclists, skateboarders, and roller skaters to wear helmets.

- Promote educational programs that are directed toward violence and suicide prevention in the community.
- Provide water safety instruction.
- Teach patients steps that can be taken to prevent falls, particularly in the elderly.
- Advise athletes to use protective devices. Recommend that coaches be educated in proper coaching techniques.
- Advise owners of firearms to keep them locked in a secure area where children cannot access them.

Scalp Injury

Isolated scalp trauma is generally classified as a minor injury. Because its many blood vessels constrict poorly, the scalp bleeds profusely when injured. Trauma may result in an abrasion (brush wound), contusion, laceration, or hematoma beneath the layers of tissue of the scalp (subgaleal hematoma). A large avulsion (tearing away) of the scalp may be potentially life-threatening and is a true emergency. Diagnosis of a scalp injury is based on physical examination, inspection, and palpation. Scalp wounds are potential portals of entry for organisms that cause intracranial infections. Therefore, the area is irrigated before the laceration is sutured, to remove foreign material and to reduce the risk for infection. Subgaleal hematomas (hematomas below the outer covering of the skull) usually reabsorb and do not require any specific treatment.

Skull Fractures

A skull fracture is a break in the continuity of the skull caused by forceful trauma. It may occur with or without damage to the brain. Skull fractures can be classified as simple, comminuted, depressed, or basilar. A simple (linear) fracture is a break in the continuity of the bone. A comminuted skull fracture refers to a splintered or multiple fracture line. Depressed skull fractures occur when the bones of the skull are forcefully displaced downward and can vary from a slight depression to bones of the skull being splintered and embedded within brain tissue. A fracture of the base of the skull is called a basilar skull fracture (Fig. 63-2) (Porth & Matfin, 2009). A fracture may be open, indicating a scalp laceration or tear in the dura (eg, from a bullet or an ice pick), or closed, in which case the dura is intact.

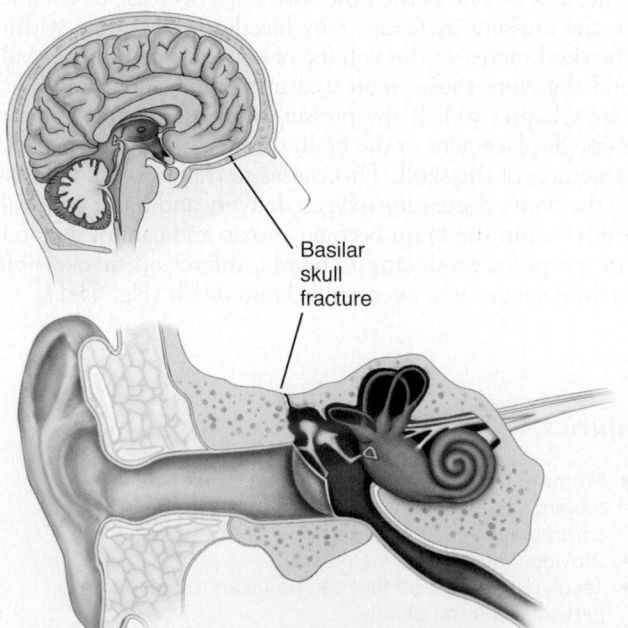

Figure 63-2 Basilar fractures allow cerebrospinal fluid to leak from the nose and ears. Adapted from Hickey, J. V. (2009). *The clinical practice of neurological and neurosurgical nursing* (6th ed.). Philadelphia: Lippincott Williams & Wilkins.

Basilar skull fracture

Clinical Manifestations

Symptoms, apart from those of the local injury, depend on the severity and the anatomic location of the underlying brain injury. Persistent, localized pain usually suggests that a fracture is present. Fractures of the cranial vault may or may not produce swelling in the region of the fracture; therefore, an x-ray is needed for diagnosis.

Fractures of the base of the skull tend to traverse the paranasal sinus of the frontal bone or the middle ear located in the temporal bone (see Fig. 63-2). Therefore, they frequently produce hemorrhage from the nose, pharynx, or ears, and blood may appear under the conjunctiva. An area of ecchymosis (bruising) may be seen over the mastoid (Battle's sign). Basilar skull fractures are suspected when CSF escapes from the ears (CSF otorrhea) and the nose (CSF rhinorrhea). Drainage of CSF is a serious problem, because meningeal infection can occur if organisms gain access to the cranial contents via the nose, ear, or sinus through a tear in the dura.

Assessment and Diagnostic Findings

X-rays confirm the presence and extent of a skull fracture (Porth & Matfin, 2009). A rapid physical examination and evaluation of neurologic status detects obvious brain injuries, and a computed tomography (CT) scan uses high-speed x-ray scanning to detect less apparent abnormalities. It is a fast, accurate, and safe diagnostic procedure that shows the presence, nature, location, and extent of acute lesions. It is also helpful in the ongoing management of head injury, because it can disclose cerebral edema, contusion, intracerebral or extracerebral hematoma, subarachnoid and intraventricular hemorrhage, and late changes (infarction, hydrocephalus) (Torpy, Lynm & Glass, 2005).

Magnetic resonance imaging (MRI) is used to evaluate patients with head injury when a more accurate picture of the anatomic nature of the injury is warranted and when the patient is stable enough to undergo this longer diagnostic procedure (Torpy, et al., 2005).

Cerebral angiography may also be used to identify supratentorial, extracerebral, and intracerebral hematomas and cerebral contusions. Lateral and anteroposterior views of the skull are obtained.

 Gerontologic Considerations

Elderly patients must be assessed carefully (Scheetz, 2005). Older patients with head injuries differ from those who are younger in terms of etiology of injury, higher mortality rates, and poorer functional outcomes (Flanagan, Hibbard & Gordon, 2005). The most common causes of injury in elderly patients are falls and motor vehicle crashes (Thompson & Bourbonniere, 2006). Physiologic changes related to aging may place the older adult at increased risk for injury, alter the type and severity of injury that occurs, or promote the development of complications. Two major factors place older adults at increased risk for hematomas. First, the dura becomes more adherent to the skull with increasing age. Second, many older adults take aspirin and anticoagulants as part of routine management of chronic conditions.

Medical Management

Nondepressed skull fractures generally do not require surgical treatment; however, close observation of the patient is essential. Nursing personnel may observe the patient in the hospital, but if no underlying brain injury is present, the patient may be allowed to return home. If the patient is discharged home, specific instructions must be given to the family (see later discussion of concussion).

Depressed skull fractures usually require surgery with elevation of the skull and débridement, usually within 24 hours of injury. Skull fractures can be a combination of open, compound, closed, or simple. Associated injuries include concurrent scalp laceration, dural tears, and brain injury directly below the fracture from compression of the tissue below the bony injury and from lacerations produced by the bony fragments (Hickey, 2009).

Brain Injury

The most important consideration in any head injury is whether the brain is injured. Even seemingly minor injury can cause significant brain damage secondary to obstructed blood flow and decreased tissue perfusion. The brain cannot store oxygen or glucose to any significant degree. Because the cerebral cells need an uninterrupted blood supply to obtain these nutrients, irreversible brain damage and cell death occur if the blood supply is interrupted for even a few minutes. Clinical manifestations of **brain injury** (injury to the brain that is severe enough to interfere with normal functioning) are listed in Chart 63-2. **Closed (blunt) brain injury** occurs when the head accelerates and then rapidly decelerates or collides with another object (eg, a wall, the dashboard of a car) and brain tissue is damaged but there is no opening through the skull and dura. **Open brain injury** occurs when an object penetrates the skull, enters the brain, and damages the soft brain tissue in its path (penetrating injury), or when blunt trauma to the head is so severe that it opens the scalp, skull, and dura to expose the brain.

CHART 63-2	*Assessing Traumatic Brain Injury*

Be alert for the following signs and symptoms:
- Altered level of consciousness
- Confusion
- Pupillary abnormalities (changes in shape, size, and response to light)
- Altered or absent gag reflex
- Absent corneal reflex
- Sudden onset of neurologic deficits
- Changes in vital signs (altered respiratory pattern, widened pulse pressure, bradycardia, tachycardia, hypothermia, or hyperthermia)
- Vision and hearing impairment
- Sensory dysfunction
- Headache
- Seizures

Types of Brain Injury

Concussion

A **concussion** after head injury is a temporary loss of neurologic function with no apparent structural damage. A concussion (also referred to as a mild TBI) may or may not produce a brief loss of consciousness. The mechanism of injury is usually blunt trauma from an acceleration-deceleration force, a direct blow, or a blast injury (Hoge, McGurk, Thomas, et al., 2008; Martin, Lu, Helmick, et al., 2008). If brain tissue in the frontal lobe is affected, the patient may exhibit bizarre irrational behavior, whereas involvement of the temporal lobe can produce temporary amnesia or disorientation.

There are two types of concussion: mild and classic. A mild concussion may lead to a period of observed or self-reported transient confusion, disorientation, or impaired consciousness. Commonly, there is a memory lapse at the time of injury and a loss of consciousness lasting less than 30 minutes. Other signs and symptoms of neurologic or neuropsychological dysfunction may include seizures, headache, dizziness, irritability, fatigue, or poor concentration (Hickey, 2009).

A classic concussion is an injury that results in a loss of consciousness; characteristically, this usually lasts less than 6 hours. This loss of consciousness is always accompanied by some degree of posttraumatic amnesia. Diagnostic studies may show no apparent structural sign of injury, but the duration of unconsciousness is an indicator of the severity of the concussion.

The patient may be hospitalized overnight for observation or discharged from the hospital in a relatively short time after a concussion. Monitoring includes observing the patient for headache, dizziness, lethargy, irritability, emotional lability, fatigue, poor concentration, decreased attention span, memory difficulties, and intellectual dysfunction that may occur from 1 week to 1 year after the initial injury (Hickey, 2009). The occurrence of these symptoms after injury is referred to as postconcussion syndrome. Recovery may appear complete, but long-term sequelae are possible. Problems at work and at home can result in interpersonal relationship problems or the loss of employment (Bay & McLean, 2007). The family is instructed to observe for the following signs and symptoms and to notify the physician or clinic (or bring the patient to the emergency department) if they occur: difficulty in awakening or speaking, confusion, severe headache, vomiting, and weakness of one side of the body.

Contusion

In cerebral **contusion,** a moderate to severe head injury, the brain is bruised and damaged in a specific area because of severe acceleration-deceleration force or blunt trauma. The impact of the brain against the skull leads to a contusion. Although a contusion may occur in any area of the brain, most are usually located in the anterior portions of the frontal and temporal lobes, around the sylvian fissure, at the orbital areas, and, less commonly, at the parietal and occipital areas.

Contusions are characterized by loss of consciousness associated with stupor and confusion. Other characteristics can include tissue alteration and neurologic deficit without hematoma formation, alteration in consciousness without localizing signs, and hemorrhage into the tissue that varies in size and is surrounded by edema. The effects of injury (hemorrhage and edema) peak after about 18 to 36 hours. Patient outcome depends on the area and severity of the injury. Temporal lobe contusions carry a greater risk of swelling, rapid deterioration, and brain herniation. Deep contusions are more often associated with hemorrhage and destruction of the reticular activating fibers altering arousal (Hickey, 2009).

Diffuse Axonal Injury

Diffuse axonal injury (DAI) results from widespread shearing and rotational forces that produce damage throughout the brain—to axons in the cerebral hemispheres, corpus callosum, and brain stem. The injured area may be diffuse, with no identifiable focal lesion. DAI is associated with prolonged traumatic coma; it is more serious and is associated with a poorer prognosis than a focal lesion or ischemia (Bay & McLean, 2007).

The patient with DAI in severe head trauma experiences no lucid interval, immediate coma, decorticate and decerebrate posturing (see Fig. 61-1 in Chapter 61), and global cerebral edema. Diagnosis is made by clinical signs in conjunction with a CT or MRI scan. Recovery depends on the severity of the axonal injury.

Intracranial Hemorrhage

Hematomas are collections of blood in the brain that may be epidural (above the dura), subdural (below the dura), or intracerebral (within the brain) (Fig. 63-3). Major symptoms are frequently delayed until the hematoma is large enough to cause distortion of the brain and increased ICP. The signs and symptoms of cerebral ischemia resulting from compression by a hematoma are variable and depend on the speed with which vital areas are affected and the area that is injured (American Association of Neuroscience Nurses [AANN], 2005). In general, a rapidly developing hematoma, even if small, may be fatal, whereas a larger but slowly developing one may allow compensation for increases in ICP.

Epidural Hematoma

After a head injury, blood may collect in the epidural (extradural) space between the skull and the dura mater. This can result from a skull fracture that causes a rupture or laceration of the middle meningeal artery, the artery that runs between the dura and the skull inferior to a thin portion of temporal bone. Hemorrhage from this artery causes rapid pressure on the brain (Vacca, 2007b).

Symptoms are caused by the expanding hematoma. Epidural hematomas are often characterized by a brief loss of consciousness followed by a lucid interval in which the patient is awake and conversant. During this lucid interval, compensation for the expanding hematoma takes place by rapid absorption of CSF and decreased intravascular volume, both of which help maintain a normal ICP. When these mechanisms can no longer compensate, even a small increase in the volume of the blood clot produces a marked elevation in ICP. The patient then becomes increasingly

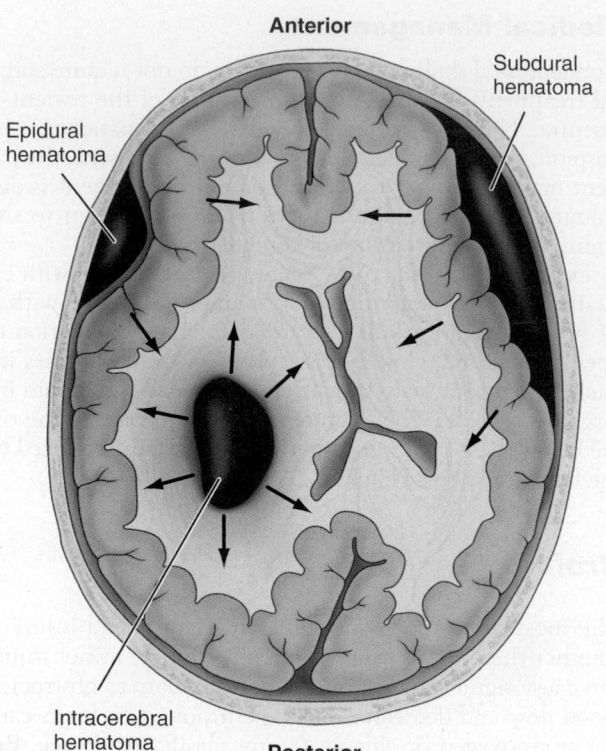

Figure 63-3 Location of epidural, subdural, and intracerebral hematomas.

restless, agitated, and confused as the condition progresses to coma. Then, often suddenly, signs of herniation appear (usually deterioration of consciousness and signs of focal neurologic deficits, such as dilation and fixation of a pupil or paralysis of an extremity), and the patient's condition deteriorates rapidly. The most common type of herniation syndrome associated with an epidural hematoma is uncal herniation (Vacca, 2007b).

An epidural hematoma is considered an extreme emergency; marked neurologic deficit or even respiratory arrest can occur within minutes. Treatment consists of making openings through the skull (burr holes) to decrease ICP emergently, remove the clot, and control the bleeding. A craniotomy may be required to remove the clot and control the bleeding. A drain is usually inserted after creation of burr holes or a craniotomy to prevent reaccumulation of blood.

Subdural Hematoma

A subdural hematoma is a collection of blood between the dura and the brain, a space normally occupied by a thin cushion of fluid. The most common cause of subdural hematoma is trauma, but it can also occur as a result of coagulopathies or rupture of an aneurysm. A subdural hemorrhage is more frequently venous in origin and is caused by the rupture of small vessels that bridge the subdural space (Vacca, 2007c). The subdural hematoma that results may be acute, subacute, or chronic, depending on the size of the involved vessel and the amount of bleeding.

Acute and Subacute Subdural Hematoma. Acute subdural hematomas are associated with major head injury involving contusion or laceration. Clinical symptoms develop over 24 to 48 hours. Signs and symptoms include changes in the level of consciousness (LOC), pupillary signs, and hemiparesis. There may be minor or even no symptoms with small collections of blood. Coma, increasing blood pressure, decreasing heart rate, and slowing respiratory rate are all signs of a rapidly expanding mass requiring immediate intervention. Subacute subdural hematomas are the result of less severe contusions and head trauma. Clinical manifestations usually appear between 48 hours and 2 weeks after the injury. Signs and symptoms are similar to those of an acute subdural hematoma.

If the patient can be transported rapidly to the hospital, an immediate craniotomy is performed to open the dura, allowing the subdural clot to be evacuated. Successful outcome also depends on the control of ICP and careful monitoring of respiratory function (see the discussion of intracranial surgery in Chapter 61). The mortality rate for patients with acute or subacute subdural hematoma is high because of associated brain damage.

Chronic Subdural Hematoma. Chronic subdural hematomas can develop from seemingly minor head injuries and are seen most frequently in the elderly. The elderly are prone to this type of head injury secondary to brain atrophy, which is a frequent consequence of the aging process. Seemingly minor head trauma may produce enough impact to shift the brain contents abnormally. The time between injury and onset of symptoms can be lengthy (eg, 3 weeks to months), so the actual injury may be forgotten.

A chronic subdural hematoma can resemble other conditions; for example, it may be mistaken for a stroke. The bleeding is less profuse, but compression of the intracranial contents still occurs. The blood within the brain changes in character in 2 to 4 days, becoming thicker and darker. In a few weeks, the clot breaks down and has the color and consistency of motor oil. Eventually, calcification or ossification of the clot takes place. The brain adapts to this foreign body invasion, and the clinical signs and symptoms fluctuate. Symptoms include severe headache, which tends to come and go; alternating focal neurologic signs; personality changes; mental deterioration; and focal seizures. The patient may be labeled neurotic or psychotic if the cause is overlooked.

The treatment of a chronic subdural hematoma consists of surgical evacuation of the clot. The procedure may be carried out through multiple burr holes, or a craniotomy may be performed for a sizable subdural mass that cannot be suctioned or drained through burr holes.

Intracerebral Hemorrhage and Hematoma

Intracerebral hemorrhage is bleeding into the substance of the brain. It is commonly seen in head injuries when force is exerted to the head over a small area (eg, missile injuries, bullet wounds, stab injuries). These hemorrhages within the brain may also result from the following:

- Systemic hypertension, which causes degeneration and rupture of a vessel
- Rupture of a saccular aneurysm
- Vascular anomalies
- Intracranial tumors

- Bleeding disorders such as leukemia, hemophilia, aplastic anemia, and thrombocytopenia
- Complications of anticoagulant therapy

Nontraumatic causes of intracerebral hemorrhage are discussed in Chapter 62.

The onset may be insidious, beginning with the development of neurologic deficits followed by headache. Management includes supportive care, control of ICP, and careful administration of fluids, electrolytes, and antihypertensive medications. Surgical intervention by craniotomy or craniectomy permits removal of the blood clot and control of hemorrhage but may not be possible because of the inaccessible location of the bleeding or the lack of a clearly circumscribed area of blood that can be removed.

Management of Brain Injuries

Assessment and diagnosis of the extent of injury are accomplished by the initial physical and neurologic examinations. CT and MRI scans are the primary neuroimaging diagnostic tools and are useful in evaluating the brain structure. Positron emission tomography (PET) is available in some trauma centers for assessing brain function. A flow chart developed by the Brain Trauma Foundation (2007) for the initial management of brain injury is presented in Figure 63-4.

Any patient with a head injury is presumed to have a cervical spine injury until proven otherwise. The patient is transported from the scene of the injury on a board with the head and neck maintained in alignment with the axis of the body. A cervical collar should be applied and maintained until cervical spine x-rays have been obtained and the absence of cervical spinal cord injury documented.

All therapy is directed toward preserving brain homeostasis and preventing secondary brain injury, which is injury to the brain that occurs after the original traumatic event (Littlejohns & Bader, 2005). Common causes of secondary injury are cerebral edema, hypotension, and respiratory depression that may lead to hypoxemia and electrolyte imbalance. Treatments to prevent secondary injury include stabilization of cardiovascular and respiratory function to maintain adequate cerebral perfusion, control of hemorrhage and hypovolemia, and maintenance of optimal blood gas values.

Treatment of Increased Intracranial Pressure

As the damaged brain swells with edema or as blood collects within the brain, an increase in ICP occurs; this requires aggressive treatment. See Chapter 61 for a discussion of the relationship of ICP to cerebral perfusion pressure (CPP). If the ICP remains elevated, it can decrease the CPP. Initial management is based on the principle of preventing secondary injury and maintaining adequate cerebral oxygenation (see Fig. 63-4).

Surgery is required for evacuation of blood clots, débridement and elevation of depressed fractures of the skull, and suture of severe scalp lacerations. ICP is monitored closely; if increased, it is managed by maintaining adequate oxygenation, elevating the head of the bed, and maintaining normal blood volume. Devices to monitor ICP or drain CSF can be inserted during surgery or at the bedside

Initial management

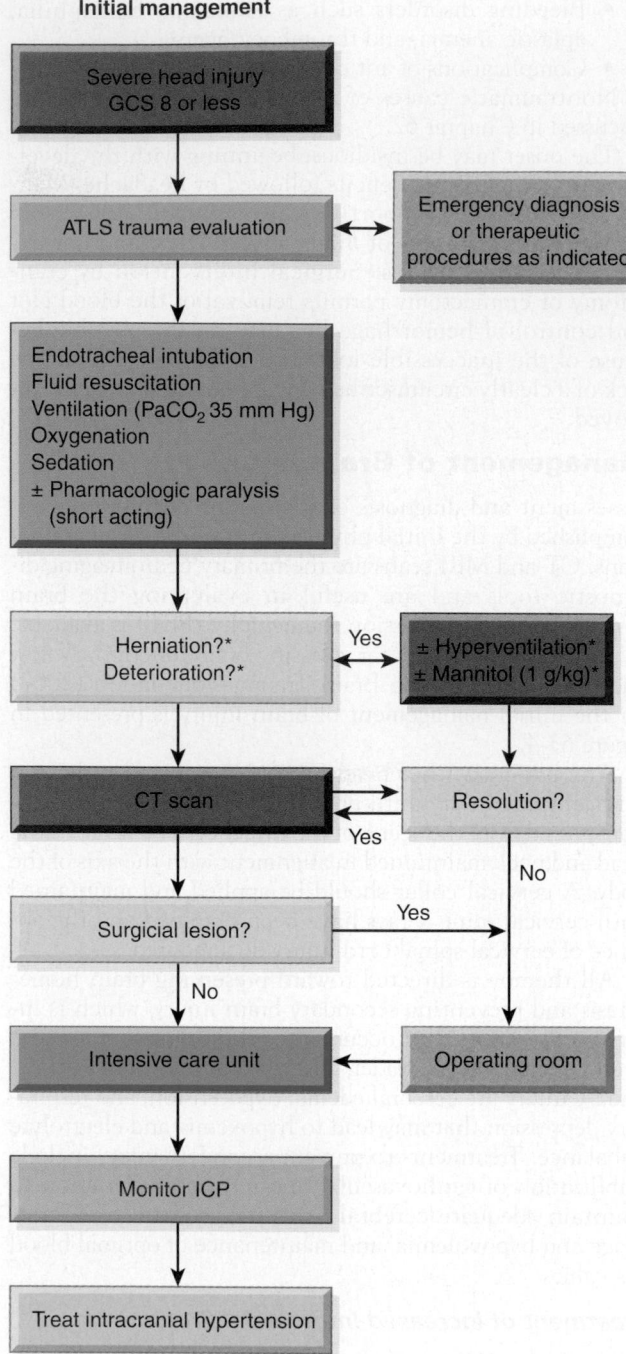

Figure 63-4 Initial management of the patient with traumatic brain injury (treatment option). Copyright © 2007 Brain Trauma Foundation. *Only in the presence of signs of herniation or progressive neurologic deterioration not attributable to extracranial factors. ATLS, Advanced Trauma Life Support; CT, computed tomography; GCS, Glasgow Coma Score; ICP, intracranial pressure.

using aseptic technique. The patient is cared for in the intensive care unit, where expert nursing care and medical treatment are readily available (AANN, 2005).

Supportive Measures

Treatment also includes ventilatory support, seizure prevention, fluid and electrolyte maintenance, nutritional support, and management of pain and anxiety. Comatose patients are intubated and mechanically ventilated to ensure adequate oxygenation and protect the airway.

Because seizures can occur after head injury and can cause secondary brain damage from hypoxia, antiseizure agents may be administered. If the patient is very agitated, benzodiazepines may be prescribed to calm the patient without decreasing LOC. These medications do not affect ICP or CPP, making them good choices for the patient with head injury. A nasogastric tube may be inserted, because reduced gastric motility and reverse peristalsis are associated with head injury, making regurgitation and aspiration common in the first few hours.

Brain Death

When a patient has sustained a severe head injury incompatible with life, the patient is a potential organ donor. The nurse may assist in the clinical examination for determination of brain death and in the process of organ procurement. All 50 states recognize the Uniform Determination of Brain Death Act that states death will be determined by accepted medical standards and indicates irreversible loss of all brain function, including the brain stem (Morton, Fontaine, Hudak, et al., 2010). The three cardinal signs of brain death on clinical examination are coma, the absence of brain stem reflexes, and apnea. Adjunctive tests, such as cerebral blood flow studies, electroencephalogram (EEG), transcranial Doppler, and brain stem auditory evoked potential, are often used to confirm brain death (Hickey, 2009). The health care team provides information to the family and assists them with the decision-making process about end-of-life care (Calvin, Kite-Powell & Hickey, 2007). For aspects of neuroscience-related end-of-life care, see Chart 63-3.

NURSING PROCESS

THE PATIENT WITH A TRAUMATIC BRAIN INJURY

Assessment

Depending on the patient's neurologic status, the nurse may elicit information from the patient, from the family, or from witnesses or emergency rescue personnel. Although all usual baseline data may not be collected initially, the immediate health history should include the following questions:

- When did the injury occur?
- What caused the injury? A high-velocity missile? An object striking the head? A fall?
- What was the direction and force of the blow?

A history of unconsciousness or amnesia after a head injury indicates a significant degree of brain damage, and changes that occur minutes to hours after the initial injury can reflect recovery or indicate the development of secondary brain damage. The nurse should determine if there was a loss of consciousness, the duration of the unconscious period, and if the patient could be aroused.

In addition to asking questions that establish the nature of the injury and the patient's condition immediately after

CHART 63-3
NURSING RESEARCH PROFILE
Perceptions About End-of-Life Care

Calvin, A. O., Kite-Powell, D. M. & Hickey, J. (2007). The neuroscience ICU nurse's perceptions about end-of-life care. *Journal of Neuroscience Nursing, 39*(3), 143–150.

Purpose

Little is known about palliative or end-of-life care in intensive care units. The purpose of this study was to explore nurses' perceptions of their roles in neuroscience intensive care units, especially their responsibilities in decision making during end-of-life care.

Design

Twelve registered nurses, all employed at the same hospital, volunteered to participate in this qualitative descriptive study. Researchers conducted moderately structured interviews using an interview guide that contained four questions for the first interview. During the second interview, participants were given an opportunity to read and react to a summary of the findings of their first interview. All interviews, which were audiotaped, were private and lasted approximately 1 hour.

Findings

Nurses described three major themes about end-of-life care. The first theme involved providing guidance to the patient and the family members during the end-of-life decision-making process. The second theme was being positioned at the "hub" of the communication process as they became intermediaries between the family members and physicians. The third theme was feeling emotions that covered a wide range from confusion, helplessness, and frustration to feeling emotionally drained, being overcome by very mixed feelings, and feeling privileged.

Nursing Implications

Little research has addressed the perceptions of nurses in neuroscience intensive care units about end-of-life care. This study shows that nurses working in such a unit have unique, central roles in the communication process surrounding the patient's end-of-life care and adds to the limited body of knowledge concerning critical care nurses' experiences with end-of-life care.

---

the injury, the nurse examines the patient thoroughly. This assessment includes determining the patient's LOC using the Glasgow Coma Scale (GCS) and assessing the patient's response to tactile stimuli (if unconscious), pupillary response to light, corneal and gag reflexes, and motor function. The GCS (Chart 63-4) is based on the three criteria of eye opening, verbal responses, and motor responses to verbal commands or painful stimuli. It is particularly useful for monitoring changes during the acute phase, the first few days after a head injury. It does not take the place of an in-depth neurologic assessment. Additional detailed assessments are made initially and at frequent intervals throughout the acute phase of care (Hickey, 2009). Baseline and ongoing assessments are critical in nursing assessment of the patient with brain injury, whose condition can worsen dramatically and irrevocably if subtle signs are overlooked. More information on assessment is provided in the following sections and in Figure 63-5 and Table 63-1.

Diagnosis

Nursing Diagnoses

Based on the assessment data, the patient's major nursing diagnoses may include the following:

- Ineffective airway clearance and impaired gas exchange related to brain injury
- Ineffective cerebral tissue perfusion related to increased ICP, decreased CPP, and possible seizures
- Deficient fluid volume related to decreased LOC and hormonal dysfunction
- Imbalanced nutrition, less than body requirements, related to increased metabolic demands, fluid restriction, and inadequate intake
- Risk for injury (self-directed and directed at others) related to seizures, disorientation, restlessness, or brain damage
- Risk for imbalanced body temperature related to damaged temperature-regulating mechanisms in the brain
- Risk for impaired skin integrity related to bed rest, hemiparesis, hemiplegia, immobility, or restlessness
- Disturbed thought processes (deficits in intellectual function, communication, memory, information processing) related to brain injury
- Disturbed sleep pattern related to brain injury and frequent neurologic checks
- Interrupted family processes related to unresponsiveness of patient, unpredictability of outcome, prolonged

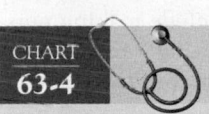

CHART 63-4
Assessment for Glasgow Coma Scale

The Glasgow Coma Scale is a tool for assessing a patient's response to stimuli. Scores range from 3 (deep coma) to 15 (normal).

Eye opening response	Spontaneous	4
	To voice	3
	To pain	2
	None	1
Best verbal response	Oriented	5
	Confused	4
	Inappropriate words	3
	Incomprehensible sounds	2
	None	1
Best motor response	Obeys command	6
	Localizes pain	5
	Withdraws	4
	Flexion	3
	Extension	2
	None	1
Total		3 to 15

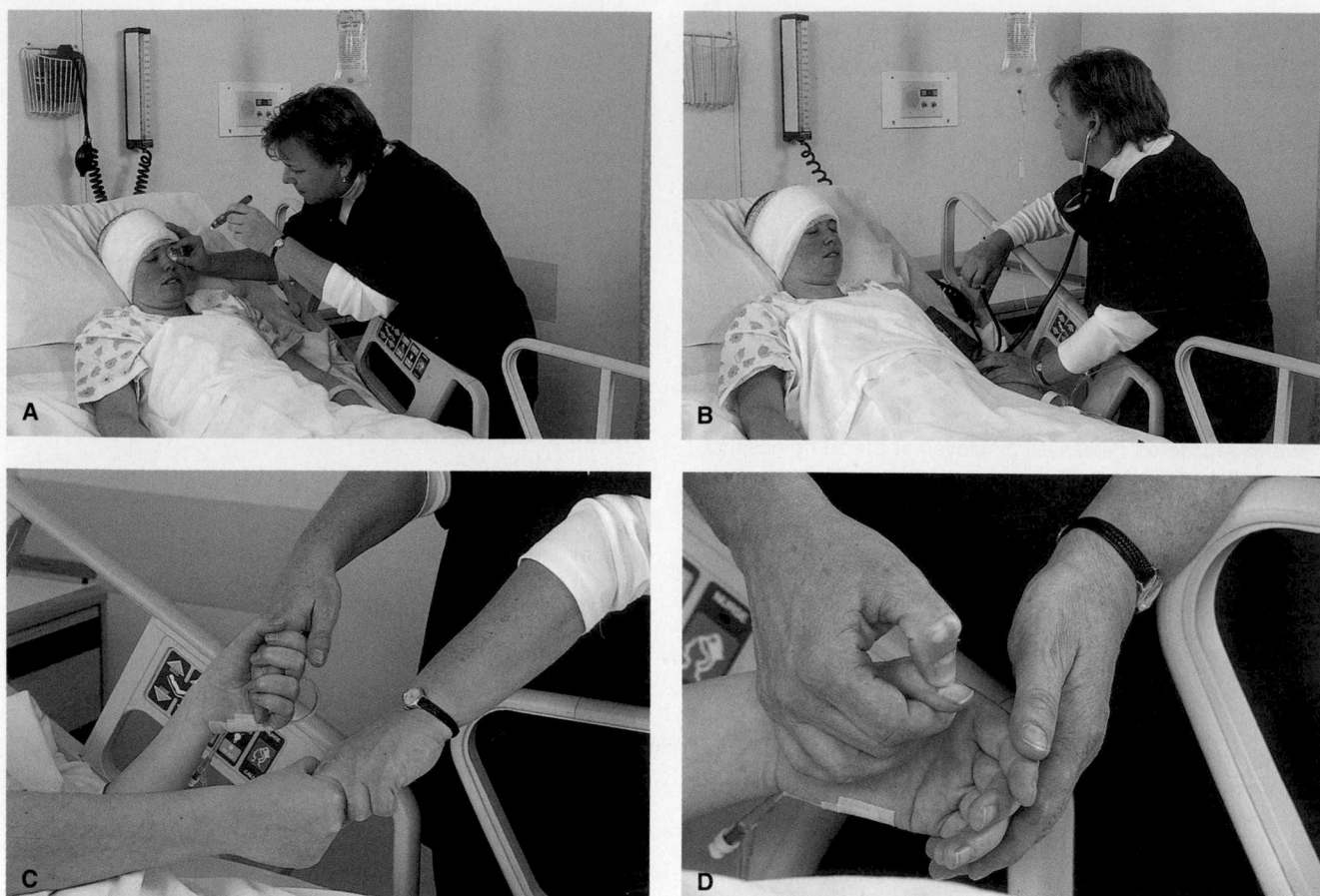

Figure 63-5 Assessment parameters for the patient with a head injury include **(A)** eye opening and responsiveness, **(B)** vital signs, and **(C, D)** motor response reflected in hand strength or response to painful stimulus. Photo © B. Proud.

recovery period, and the patient's residual physical disability and emotional deficit
- Deficient knowledge about brain injury, recovery, and the rehabilitation process

The nursing diagnoses for the unconscious patient and the patient with increased ICP also apply (see Chapter 61).

Collaborative Problems/Potential Complications

Based on all the assessment data, the major complications include the following:
- Decreased cerebral perfusion
- Cerebral edema and herniation
- Impaired oxygenation and ventilation
- Impaired fluid, electrolyte, and nutritional balance
- Risk of posttraumatic seizures

Planning and Goals

The goals for the patient may include maintenance of a patent airway, adequate CPP, fluid and electrolyte balance, adequate nutritional status, prevention of secondary injury, maintenance of normal body temperature, maintenance of skin integrity, improvement of cognitive function, prevention of sleep deprivation, effective family coping, increased knowledge about the rehabilitation process, and absence of complications.

Nursing Interventions

The nursing interventions for the patient with a head injury are extensive and diverse. They include making nursing assessments, setting priorities for nursing interventions, anticipating needs and complications, and initiating rehabilitation.

Monitoring Neurologic Function

The importance of ongoing assessment and monitoring of the patient with brain injury cannot be overstated. The following parameters are assessed initially and as frequently as the patient's condition requires. As soon as the initial assessment is made, the use of a neurologic flow chart is started and maintained.

LEVEL OF CONSCIOUSNESS. The GCS is used to assess LOC at regular intervals, because changes in the LOC precede all other changes in vital and neurologic signs. The patient's best responses to predetermined stimuli are recorded (see Chart 63-4). Each response is scored (the greater the number, the better the functioning), and the sum of these scores gives an indication of the severity of coma and a prediction of possible outcome. The lowest score is 3 (least responsive); the highest is 15 (most responsive). A GCS between 3 and 8 is generally accepted as indicating a severe head injury (Martin, et al., 2008).

Table 63-1	SUMMARY OF MULTISYSTEM ASSESSMENT MEASURES FOR THE PATIENT WITH TRAUMATIC BRAIN INJURY
System-Specific Considerations	**Assessment Data**

System-Specific Considerations	Assessment Data
Neurologic System • Severe head injury results in unconsciousness and alters many neurologic functions. • All body functions must be supported. • Increased ICP and herniation syndromes are life-threatening. • Measures are instituted to control elevated ICP.	• Assessment of neurologic signs • Assessment for signs and symptoms of ICP elevation • Calculation of cerebral perfusion pressure if ICP monitor is in place • Monitoring of antiseizure medication blood levels
Integumentary System (Skin and Mucous Membranes) • Immobility secondary to injury and unconsciousness contributes to the development of pressure areas and skin breakdown. • Intubation causes irritation of the mucous membrane.	• Assessment of skin integrity and character of the skin • Assessment of oral mucous membrane
Musculoskeletal System • Immobility contributes to musculoskeletal changes. • Decerebrate or decorticate posturing makes proper positioning difficult.	• Assessment of range of motion of joints and development of deformities or spasticity
Gastrointestinal System • Administration of corticosteroids places the patient at high risk for GI hemorrhage. • Injury to the GI tract can result in paralytic ileus. • Constipation can result from bed rest, NPO status, fluid restriction, and opioids given for pain control. • Bowel incontinence is related to the patient's unconscious state or altered mental state.	• Assessment of abdomen for bowel sounds and distention • Monitoring for decreased hemoglobin
Genitourinary System • Fluid restriction or use of diuretics can alter the amount of urinary output. • Urinary incontinence is related to the patient's unconscious state.	• Intake and output record
Metabolic (Nutritional) System • The patient receives all fluids IV for the first few days until the GI tract is functioning. • A nutritional consultation is initiated within the first 24–48 h; parenteral or enteral nutrition may be started.	• Assessment of fluid and electrolyte balance • Recording of weight, if possible • Hematocrit • Electrolyte studies
Respiratory System • Complete or partial airway obstruction will compromise the oxygen supply to the brain. • An altered respiratory pattern can result in cerebral hypoxia. • A short period of apnea at the moment of impact can result in spotty atelectasis. • Systemic disturbances from head injury can cause hypoxemia. • Brain injury can alter brain stem respiratory function. • Shunting of blood to the lungs as a result of a sympathetic discharge at the time of injury can cause neurogenic pulmonary edema.	• Assessment of respiratory function — Auscultate chest for breath sounds. — Note the respiratory pattern if possible (not possible if a ventilator is being used). — Note the respiratory rate. — Note whether the cough reflex is intact. • Arterial blood gas levels • Complete blood count • Chest x-ray studies • Sputum cultures • O_2 saturation using pulse oximetry
Cardiovascular System • The patient may develop cardiac dysrhythmias, tachycardia, or bradycardia. • The patient may develop hypotension or hypertension. • Because of immobility and unconsciousness, the patient is at high risk for deep vein thromboses and pulmonary emboli. • Fluid and electrolyte imbalance can be related to several problems, including alterations in antidiuretic hormone (ADH) secretion, the stress response, or fluid restriction. • Specific conditions may occur: — Diabetes insipidus (DI) — Syndrome of inappropriate secretion of ADH (SIADH) — Electrolyte imbalance — Hyperosmolar nonketotic hyperglycemia	• Assessment of vital signs • Monitoring for cardiac dysrhythmias • Assessment for deep vein thromboses of legs • Electrocardiogram • Electrolyte studies • Blood coagulation studies • I^{125} fibrinogen scan of legs • Blood glucose level • Blood acetone level • Blood osmolality • Urine specific gravity
Psychological/Emotional Response • The traumatic head-injured patient is unconscious. • The family needs emotional support to deal with the crisis.	• Collection of information about the family and the role of the head-injured person within the family • Assessment of the family to determine how functional it was before the injury occurred

VITAL SIGNS. Although a change in LOC is the most sensitive neurologic indication of deterioration of the patient's condition, vital signs also are monitored at frequent intervals to assess the intracranial status. Table 63-1 depicts the general assessment parameters for the patient with a head injury.

Signs of increasing ICP include slowing of the heart rate (bradycardia), increasing systolic blood pressure, and widening pulse pressure (Cushing's reflex). As brain compression increases, respirations become rapid, the blood pressure may decrease, and the pulse slows further. This is an ominous development, as is a rapid fluctuation of vital signs (Hickey, 2009). A rapid increase in body temperature is regarded as unfavorable because hyperthermia increases the metabolic demands of the brain and may indicate brain stem damage, a poor prognostic sign. The temperature is maintained at less than 38°C (100.4°F). Tachycardia and arterial hypotension may indicate that bleeding is occurring elsewhere in the body.

MOTOR FUNCTION. Motor function is assessed frequently by observing spontaneous movements, asking the patient to raise and lower the extremities, and comparing the strength and equality of the upper and lower extremities at periodic intervals. To assess upper extremity strength, the nurse instructs the patient to squeeze the examiner's fingers tightly. The nurse assesses lower extremity motor strength by placing the hands on the soles of the patient's feet and asking the patient to push down against the examiner's hands. Examination of the motor system is discussed in Chapter 60 in more detail. The presence or absence of spontaneous movement of each extremity is also noted, and speech and eye signs are assessed.

If the patient does not demonstrate spontaneous movement, responses to painful stimuli are assessed (Hickey, 2009). Motor response to pain is assessed by applying a central stimulus, such as pinching the pectoralis major muscle, to determine the patient's best response. Peripheral stimulation may provide inaccurate assessment data because it may result in a reflex movement rather than a voluntary motor response. Abnormal responses (lack of motor response; extension responses) are associated with a poorer prognosis.

OTHER NEUROLOGIC SIGNS. In addition to the patient's spontaneous eye opening, evaluated with the GCS, the size and equality of the pupils and their reaction to light are assessed. A unilaterally dilated and poorly responding pupil may indicate a developing hematoma, with subsequent pressure on the third cranial nerve due to shifting of the brain. If both pupils become fixed and dilated, this indicates overwhelming injury and intrinsic damage to the upper brain stem and is a poor prognostic sign (Adoni & McNett, 2007).

The patient with a head injury may develop deficits such as anosmia (lack of sense of smell), eye movement abnormalities, aphasia, memory deficits, and posttraumatic seizures or epilepsy. Patients may be left with residual psychological deficits (impulsiveness, emotional lability, or uninhibited, aggressive behaviors) and, as a consequence of the impairment, may lack insight into their emotional responses.

Maintaining the Airway

One of the most important nursing goals in the management of head injury is to establish and maintain an adequate airway. The brain is extremely sensitive to hypoxia, and a neurologic deficit can worsen if the patient is hypoxic. Therapy is directed toward maintaining optimal oxygenation to preserve cerebral function. An obstructed airway causes carbon dioxide retention and hypoventilation, which can produce cerebral vessel dilation and increased ICP.

Interventions to ensure an adequate exchange of air are discussed in Chapter 61 and include the following:

- Maintaining the unconscious patient in a position that facilitates drainage of oral secretions, with the head of the bed elevated about 30 degrees to decrease intracranial venous pressure (Bader, 2006b)
- Establishing effective suctioning procedures (pulmonary secretions produce coughing and straining, which increase ICP)
- Guarding against aspiration and respiratory insufficiency
- Closely monitoring arterial blood gas values to assess the adequacy of ventilation. The goal is to keep blood gas values within the normal range to ensure adequate cerebral blood flow.
- Monitoring the patient who is receiving mechanical ventilation for pulmonary complications such as acute respiratory distress syndrome (ARDS) and pneumonia (Hickey, 2009)

Monitoring Fluid and Electrolyte Balance

Brain damage can produce metabolic and hormonal dysfunctions. The monitoring of serum electrolyte levels is important, especially in patients receiving osmotic diuretics, those with syndrome of inappropriate antidiuretic hormone (SIADH) secretion, and those with posttraumatic diabetes insipidus.

Serial studies of blood and urine electrolytes and osmolality are carried out because head injuries may be accompanied by disorders of sodium regulation. Hyponatremia is common after head injury due to shifts in extracellular fluid, electrolytes, and volume. Hyperglycemia, for example, can cause an increase in extracellular fluid that lowers sodium. Hypernatremia may also occur as a result of sodium retention that may last several days, followed by sodium diuresis. Increasing lethargy, confusion, and seizures may be the result of electrolyte imbalance.

Endocrine function is evaluated by monitoring serum electrolytes, blood glucose values, and intake and output. Urine is tested regularly for acetone. A record of daily weights is maintained, especially if the patient has hypothalamic involvement and is at risk for the development of diabetes insipidus.

Promoting Adequate Nutrition

Head injury results in metabolic changes that increase calorie consumption and nitrogen excretion. Protein demand increases. Early initiation of nutritional therapy has been shown to improve outcomes in patients with head injury. Patients with brain injury are assumed to be catabolic and nutritional support consultation should be considered as soon as the patient is admitted. Parenteral nutrition via a central line or enteral feedings administered via a nasogastric or nasojejunal feeding tube should be considered (Hickey, 2009). If CSF rhinorrhea occurs, an oral feeding tube should be inserted instead of a nasal tube.

Laboratory values should be monitored closely in patients receiving parenteral nutrition. Elevating the head of the bed and aspirating the enteral tube for evidence of residual feeding before administering additional feedings can help prevent distention, regurgitation, and aspiration. A continuous-drip infusion or pump may be used to regulate the feeding. The principles and technique of enteral feedings are discussed in Chapter 36. Enteral or parenteral feedings are usually continued until the swallowing reflex returns and the patient can meet caloric requirements orally.

Preventing Injury

Often, as the patient emerges from coma, a period of lethargy and stupor is followed by a period of agitation. Each phase is variable and depends on the individual person, the location of the injury, the depth and duration of coma, and the patient's age. Restlessness may be caused by hypoxia, fever, pain, or a full bladder. It may indicate injury to the brain but may also be a sign that the patient is regaining consciousness. (Some restlessness may be beneficial because the lungs and extremities are exercised.) Agitation may also be the result of discomfort from catheters, intravenous (IV) lines, restraints, and repeated neurologic checks. Alternatives to restraints must be used whenever possible.

Strategies to prevent injury include the following:

- The patient is assessed to ensure that oxygenation is adequate and the bladder is not distended. Dressings and casts are checked for constriction.
- Padded side rails are used or the patient's hands are wrapped in mitts to protect the patient from self-injury and dislodging of tubes. Restraints are avoided, because straining against them can increase ICP or cause other injury. Enclosed or floor-level specialty beds may be indicated.
- Opioids are avoided as a means of controlling restlessness, because they depress respiration, constrict the pupils, and alter responsiveness.
- Environmental stimuli are reduced by keeping the room quiet, limiting visitors, speaking calmly, and providing frequent orientation information (eg, explaining where the patient is and what is being done).
- Adequate lighting is provided to prevent visual hallucinations.
- Efforts are made to minimize disruption of the patient's sleep–wake cycles.
- The patient's skin is lubricated with oil or emollient lotion to prevent irritation due to rubbing against the sheet.
- If incontinence occurs, an external sheath catheter may be used on a male patient. Because prolonged use of an indwelling catheter inevitably produces infection, the patient may be placed on an intermittent catheterization schedule.

Maintaining Body Temperature

Fever in the patient with a TBI can be the result of damage to the hypothalamus, cerebral irritation from hemorrhage, or infection. The nurse monitors the patient's temperature every 2 to 4 hours. If the temperature increases, efforts are made to identify the cause and to control it using acetaminophen and cooling blankets to maintain normothermia (Thompson, Kirkness & Mitchell, 2007). Cooling blankets should be used with caution so as not to induce shivering, which increases ICP. If infection is suspected, potential sites of infection are cultured and antibiotics are prescribed and administered.

Use of mild hypothermia to 34°C to 35°C (94°F to 96°F) has been tested in small randomized controlled trials for at least 12 hours versus normothermia (control) in patients with closed head injury. Early research showed improvement in patient outcomes but needs to be repeated in larger trials. Because hypothermia increases the risk of pneumonia and has other side effects, this treatment is not currently recommended outside of controlled clinical trials (Brain Trauma Foundation, 2007).

Maintaining Skin Integrity

Patients with TBI often require assistance in turning and positioning because of immobility or unconsciousness. Prolonged pressure on the tissues decreases circulation and leads to tissue necrosis. Potential areas of breakdown need to be identified early to avoid the development of pressure ulcers. Specific nursing measures include the following:

- Assessing all body surfaces and documenting skin integrity every 8 hours
- Turning and repositioning the patient every 2 hours
- Providing skin care every 4 hours
- Assisting the patient to get out of bed to a chair three times a day

Improving Cognitive Functioning

Although many patients with head injury survive because of resuscitative and supportive technology, they frequently have significant cognitive sequelae that may not be detected during the acute phase of injury. Cognitive impairment includes memory deficits, decreased ability to focus and sustain attention to a task (distractibility), reduced ability to process information, and slowness in thinking, perceiving, communicating, reading, and writing. Psychiatric, emotional, and relationship problems develop in many patients after head injury. Resulting psychosocial, behavioral, emotional, and cognitive impairments are devastating to the family as well as to the patient (Bay & Bergman, 2006; Jumisko, Lexell & Soderberg, 2005).

These problems require collaboration among many disciplines. A neuropsychologist (specialist in evaluating and treating cognitive problems) plans a program and initiates therapy or counseling to help the patient reach maximal potential. Cognitive rehabilitation activities help the patient to devise new problem-solving strategies. The retraining is carried out over an extended period and may include the use of sensory stimulation and reinforcement, behavior modification, reality orientation, computer training programs, and video games. Assistance from many disciplines is necessary during this phase of recovery. Even if intellectual ability does not improve, social and behavioral abilities may.

The patient recovering from a TBI may experience fluctuations in the level of cognitive function, with orientation, attention, and memory frequently affected. Many types of sensory stimulation programs have been tried, and research on these programs is ongoing (Hickey, 2009). When pushed to a level greater than the impaired cortical functioning allows, the patient may show symptoms of fatigue, anger, and stress (headache, dizziness). The Rancho Los Amigos Level of Cognitive Function scale is frequently used to assess cognitive function and evaluate ongoing recovery from head injury. Progress through the levels of cognitive function can vary widely for individual patients. Nursing management and a description of each level are included in Table 63-2.

Preventing Sleep Pattern Disturbance

Patients who require frequent monitoring of neurologic status may experience sleep deprivation as they are awakened hourly for assessment of LOC. To allow the patient longer times of uninterrupted sleep and rest, the nurse can group nursing care activities so that the patient is disturbed less frequently. Environmental noise is decreased, and the room lights are dimmed. Back rubs and other measures to increase comfort may promote sleep and rest.

Supporting Family Coping

Having a loved one sustain a TBI produces a great deal of stress in the family. This stress can result from the patient's physical and emotional deficits, the unpredictable outcome, and altered family relationships. Families report difficulties in coping with changes in the patient's temperament, behavior, and personality. Such changes are associated with disruption in family cohesion, loss of leisure pursuits, and loss of work capacity, as well as social isolation of the caretaker. The family may experience marital disruption, anger, grief, guilt, and denial in recurring cycles.

To promote effective coping, the nurse can ask the family how the patient is different now, what has been lost, and what is most difficult about coping with this situation. Helpful interventions include providing family members with accurate and honest information and encouraging them to continue to set well-defined short-term goals. Family counseling helps address the family members' overwhelming feelings of loss and helplessness and gives them guidance for the management of inappropriate behaviors. Support groups help the family members share problems, develop insight, gain information, network, and gain assistance in maintaining realistic expectations and hope.

The Brain Injury Association (see Resources) serves as a clearinghouse for information and resources for patients with head injuries and their families, including specific information on coma, rehabilitation, behavioral consequences of head injury, and family issues. This organization can provide names of facilities and professionals who work with patients with head injuries and can assist families in organizing local support groups.

Many patients with severe head injury die from their injuries, and many of those who survive experience long-term disabilities that prevent them from resuming their previous roles and functions. During the most acute phase of injury, family members need factual information and support from the health care team.

Many patients with severe head injuries that result in brain death are young and otherwise healthy and are therefore considered for organ donation. Family members of patients with such injuries need support during this extremely stressful time and assistance in making decisions to end life support and permit donation of organs. They need to know that the patient who is brain dead and whose respiratory and cardiovascular systems are maintained through life support is not going to survive and that the severe head injury, not the removal of the patient's organs or the removal of life support, is the cause of the patient's death. Bereavement counselors and members of the organ procurement team are often very helpful to family members in making decisions about organ donation and in helping them cope with stress.

Monitoring and Managing Potential Complications

DECREASED CEREBRAL PERFUSION PRESSURE. Maintenance of adequate CPP is important to prevent serious complications of head injury due to decreased cerebral perfusion. Adequate CPP is greater than 60 mm Hg. If CPP falls below a patient's threshold, a vasodilating cascade occurs, causing the volume of blood to increase inside the brain, causing ICP to increase. A decrease in CPP can impair cerebral perfusion and cause brain hypoxia and ischemia, leading to permanent brain damage. Once the threshold CPP is reached, vasoconstriction of the cerebral blood vessels occurs, causing ICP to decrease (Bader & Arbour, 2005). Therapy (eg, elevation of the head of the bed and increased IV fluids) is directed toward decreasing cerebral edema and increasing venous outflow from the brain. Systemic hypotension, which causes vasoconstriction and a significant decrease in CPP, is treated with increased IV fluids or vasopressors.

CEREBRAL EDEMA AND HERNIATION. The patient with a head injury is at risk for additional complications such as increased ICP and brain stem herniation. Cerebral edema is the most common cause of increased ICP in the patient with a head injury, with the swelling peaking approximately 48 to 72 hours after injury. Bleeding also may increase the volume of contents within the rigid, closed compartment of the skull, causing increased ICP and herniation of the brain stem and resulting in irreversible brain anoxia and brain death (Morton, et al., 2010). Measures to control ICP are discussed in Chapter 61 and listed in Chart 63-5.

IMPAIRED OXYGENATION AND VENTILATION. Impaired oxygen and ventilation may require mechanical ventilatory support. The patient must be monitored for a patent airway, altered breathing patterns, and hypoxemia and pneumonia. Interventions may include endotracheal intubation, mechanical ventilation, and positive end-expiratory pressure. These topics are discussed in further detail in Chapters 25 and 61.

Chart 63-5 • Controlling Intracranial Pressure in Patients With Severe Brain Injury

- Elevate the head of the bed as prescribed.
- Maintain the patient's head and neck in neutral alignment (no twisting or flexing the neck).
- Initiate measures to prevent the Valsalva maneuver (eg, stool softeners).
- Maintain normal body temperature.
- Administer O_2 to maintain PaO_2 >90 mm Hg.
- Maintain fluid balance with normal saline solution.
- Avoid noxious stimuli (eg, excessive suctioning, painful procedures).
- Administer sedation to reduce agitation.
- Maintain cerebral perfusion pressure >70 mm Hg.

Table 63-2 **RANCHO LOS AMIGOS SCALE: LEVELS OF COGNITIVE FUNCTION**

Cognitive Level	Description	Nursing Management
	For levels I–III, the key approach is to *provide stimulation.*	
I: No response	Completely unresponsive to all stimuli, including painful stimuli	Multiple modalities of sensory input should be used. Examples are listed here, but management should be individualized and expanded based on available materials and patient preferences (determined by obtaining information from the family).
II: Generalized response	Nonpurposeful response; responds to pain, but in a nonpurposeful manner	*Olfactory:* perfumes, flowers, shaving lotion *Visual:* family pictures, card, personal items
III: Localized response	Responses more focused: withdraws to pain; turns toward sound; follows moving objects that pass within visual field; pulls on sources of discomfort (eg, tubes, restraints); may follow simple commands but inconsistently and in a delayed manner	*Auditory:* radio, television, tapes of family voices or favorite recordings, talking to patient (nurse, family members). The nurse should tell patient what is going to be done, discuss the environment, provide encouragement. *Tactile:* touching of skin, rubbing various textures on skin *Movement:* range-of-motion exercises, turning, repositioning, use of water mattress
	For levels IV–VI, the key approach is to *provide structure.*	
IV: Confused, agitated response	Alert, hyperactive state in which patient responds to internal confusion/agitation; behavior nonpurposeful in relation to the environment; aggressive, bizarre behavior common	For level IV, which lasts 2–4 weeks, interventions are directed at decreasing agitation, increasing environmental awareness, and promoting safety. • Approach patient in a calm manner, and use a soft voice. • Screen patient from environmental stimuli (eg, sounds, sights); provide a quiet, controlled environment. • Remove devices that contribute to agitation (eg, tubes), if possible. • Functional goals cannot be set, because the patient is unable to cooperate.
V: Confused, inappropriate response	When agitation occurs, it is the result of external rather than internal stimuli; focused attention is difficult; memory is severely impaired; responses are fragmented and inappropriate to the situation; there is no carryover of learning from one situation to the other.	For levels V and VI, interventions are directed at decreasing confusion, improving cognitive function, and improving independence in performing ADLs. • Provide supervision. • Use repetition and cues to teach ADLs. Focus the patient's attention and help to increase his or her concentration.
VI: Confused, appropriate response	Follows simple directions consistently but is inconsistently oriented to time and place; short-term memory worse than long-term memory; can perform some ADLs	• Help the patient organize activity. • Clarify misinformation and reorient when confused. • Provide a consistent, predictable schedule (eg, post daily schedule on large poster board).
	For levels VII–X, the key approach is *integration into the community.*	
VII: Automatic, appropriate response	Appropriately responsive and oriented within the hospital setting; needs little supervision in ADLs; some carryover of learning; patient has superficial insight into disabilities; has decreased judgment and problem-solving abilities; lacks realistic planning for future	For levels VII–X, interventions are directed at increasing the patient's ability to function with minimal or no supervision in the community. • Reduce environmental structure. • Help the patient plan for adapting ADLs for self into the home environment. • Discuss and adapt home living skills (eg, cleaning, cooking) to patient's ability.
VIII: Purposeful, appropriate	Alert, oriented, intact memory; has realistic goals for the future. Able to complete familiar tasks for 1 h in a distracting environment; overestimates or underestimates abilities, argumentative, easily frustrated, self-centered; uncharacteristically dependent/independent	• Provide stand-by assistance as needed for ADLs and home living skills.
IX: Purposeful, appropriate	Independently shifts back and forth between tasks and completes them accurately for at least 2 consecutive hours; uses assistive memory devices to recall schedule and activities; aware of and acknowledges impairments and disabilities when they interfere with task completion; depression may continue; may be easily irritable and have a low frustration tolerance	• Provide assistance on request for adapting ADLs and home living skills.
X: Purposeful, appropriate	Able to handle multiple tasks simultaneously in all environments but may require periodic breaks; independently initiates and carries out familiar and unfamiliar tasks but may require more than usual amount of time and/or compensatory strategies to complete them; accurately estimates abilities and independently adjusts to task demands; periodic periods of depression may occur; irritability and low frustration tolerance when sick, fatigued, and/or under stress	• Monitor for signs and symptoms of depression. • Help the patient plan, anticipate concerns, and solve problems.

Used with permission from Los Amigos Research and Education Institute, Inc., Downey, CA 2002.

IMPAIRED FLUID, ELECTROLYTE, AND NUTRITIONAL BALANCE. Fluid, electrolyte, and nutritional imbalances are common in the patient with a head injury. Common imbalances include hyponatremia, which is often associated with SIADH (see Chapters 14 and 42), hypokalemia, and hyperglycemia. Modifications in fluid intake with tube feedings or IV fluids, including hypertonic saline, may be necessary to treat these imbalances (Hickey, 2009). Insulin administration may be prescribed to treat hyperglycemia.

Undernutrition is also a common problem in response to the increased metabolic needs associated with severe head injury. Decisions about early feeding should be individualized; options include IV hyperalimentation or placement of a feeding tube (jejunal or gastric). Caloric expenditure can increase up to 120% to 140% with TBI, requiring close monitoring of nutritional status. Feeding tubes should be placed 3 to 7 days after neurologic injury to replace energy and nitrogen losses, prevent increased mortality, and improve outcomes (Hickey, 2009).

POSTTRAUMATIC SEIZURES. Patients with head injury are at an increased risk for posttraumatic seizures. Posttraumatic seizures are classified as immediate (within 24 hours after injury), early (within 1 to 7 days after injury), or late (more than 7 days after injury) (Hickey, 2009). Seizure prophylaxis is the practice of administering antiseizure medications to patients with head injury to prevent seizures. It is important to prevent posttraumatic seizures, especially in the immediate and early phases of recovery, because seizures may increase ICP and decrease oxygenation. However, many antiseizure medications impair cognitive performance and can prolong the duration of rehabilitation. Therefore, it is important to weigh the overall benefit of these medications against their side effects. Research evidence supports the use of prophylactic antiseizure agents to prevent immediate and early seizures after head injury, but not for prevention of late seizures (Barker, 2008). The nursing management of seizures is addressed in Chapter 61.

Promoting Home and Community-Based Care

TEACHING PATIENTS SELF-CARE. Teaching early in the course of head injury often focuses on reinforcing information given to the family about the patient's condition and prognosis. As the patient's status and expected outcome change over time, family teaching may focus on interpretation and explanation of changes in the patient's physical and psychological responses.

If the patient's physical status allows discharge to home, the patient and family are instructed about limitations that can be expected and complications that may occur. The nurse explains to the patient and family, verbally and in writing, how to monitor for complications that merit contacting the neurosurgeon. Depending on the patient's prognosis and physical and cognitive status, the patient may be included in teaching about self-care management strategies.

If the patient is at risk for late posttraumatic seizures, antiseizure medications may be prescribed at discharge. The patient and family require instruction about the side effects of these medications and the importance of continuing to take them as prescribed.

CONTINUING CARE. The rehabilitation phase of care for the patient with a TBI begins at hospital admission. Admission to the rehabilitation unit is a milestone in a patient's recovery and requires intense work by the patient to complete the daily schedule of therapies. The goals of rehabilitation are to maximize the patient's ability to return to his or her highest level of functioning and to his or her home and the community, address concerns before discharge for a smooth transition to home or rehabilitation, and promote independence with adaptation to deficits (Hickey, 2009). The patient is encouraged to continue the rehabilitation program after discharge, because improvement in status may continue 3 or more years after injury. Changes in the patient with a TBI and the effects of long-term rehabilitation on the family and their coping abilities need ongoing assessment. Continued teaching and support of the patient and family are essential as their needs and the patient's status change. Teaching points to address with the family of the patient who is about to return home are described in Chart 63-6.

Depending on his or her status, the patient is encouraged to return to normal activities gradually. Referral to support

---

CHART 63-6	HOME CARE CHECKLIST *The Patient With a Traumatic Brain Injury*		
At the completion of the home care instruction, the patient or caregiver will be able to:		**PATIENT**	**CAREGIVER**
• Explain the need for monitoring for changes in neurologic status and for complications.		✔	✔
• Identify changes in neurologic status and signs and symptoms of complications that should be reported to the neurosurgeon or nurse.			✔
• Demonstrate safe techniques to assist patient with self-care, hygiene, and ambulation.			✔
• Demonstrate safe technique for eating, feeding patient, or assisting patient with eating.		✔	✔
• Explain rationale for taking medications as prescribed.		✔	✔
• Identify need for close monitoring of behavior due to changes in cognitive functioning.			✔
• Describe household modifications needed to ensure safe environment for the patient.			✔
• Describe strategies for reinforcing positive behaviors.			✔
• State importance of continuing follow-up by health care team.		✔	✔

groups and to the Brain Injury Association may be warranted.

During the acute and rehabilitation phases of care, the focus of teaching is on obvious needs, issues, deficits, and complications. Complications after TBI include infections (eg, pneumonia, urinary tract infection [UTI], septicemia, wound infection, osteomyelitis, meningitis, ventriculitis, brain abscess) and heterotrophic ossification (painful bone overgrowth in weight-bearing joints).

The nurse needs to remind the patient and family of the need for continuing health promotion and screening practices after the initial phase of care. Patients who have not been involved in these practices in the past are educated about their importance and are referred to appropriate health care providers.

Evaluation

Expected Patient Outcomes

Expected patient outcomes may include the following:

1. Attains or maintains effective airway clearance, ventilation, and brain oxygenation
   a. Achieves normal blood gas values and has normal breath sounds on auscultation
   b. Mobilizes and clears secretions
2. Achieves satisfactory fluid and electrolyte balance
   a. Demonstrates serum electrolytes within normal range
   b. Has no clinical signs of dehydration or overhydration
3. Attains adequate nutritional status
   a. Has less than 50 mL of aspirate in stomach before each tube feeding
   b. Is free of gastric distention and vomiting
   c. Shows minimal weight loss
4. Avoids injury
   a. Shows lessening agitation and restlessness
   b. Is oriented to time, place, and person
5. Maintains normal body temperature
   a. Absence of fever
   b. Absence of hypothermia
6. Demonstrates intact skin integrity
   a. Exhibits no redness or breaks in skin integrity
   b. Exhibits no pressure ulcers
7. Shows improvement in cognitive function and improved memory
8. Demonstrates normal sleep–wake cycle
9. Demonstrates absence of complications
   a. Exhibits normal vital signs and body temperature, and increasing orientation to time, place, and person
   b. Demonstrates normal or reduced ICP
10. Experiences no posttraumatic seizures
    a. Takes antiseizure medications as prescribed
    b. Identifies side effects/adverse effects of antiseizure medications
11. Family demonstrates adaptive family processes
    a. Joins support group
    b. Shares feelings with appropriate health care personnel
    c. Makes end-of-life decisions, if needed
12. Participates in rehabilitation process as indicated for patient and family members
    a. Takes active role in identifying rehabilitation goals and participating in recommended patient care activities
    b. Prepares for discharge

Spinal Cord Injury

Spinal cord injury (SCI) is a major health disorder. Almost 200,000 people in the United States live each day with a disability from SCI, and an estimated 11,000 new injuries occur each year (Hickey, 2009). SCI is primarily an injury of young adult males and 50% of those injured are between 16 and 30 years of age. Patients over the age of 60 years account for 10% of SCIs, and this figure has steadily risen over the past 25 years (Dawodu, 2007).

Motor vehicle crashes account for 48% of reported cases of SCI, with falls (23%), violence primarily from gunshot wounds (14%), recreational sporting activities (9%), and other events accounting for the remaining injuries. **Paraplegia** (paralysis of the lower body) and **tetraplegia** (formerly quadriplegia—paralysis of all four extremities) can occur, with incomplete tetraplegia (formerly quadriplegia) the largest category, followed by complete paraplegia, complete tetraplegia, and paraplegia.

The predominant risk factors for SCI include young age, male gender, and alcohol and drug use. The frequency with which these risk factors are associated with SCI serves to emphasize the importance of primary prevention. The same interventions suggested earlier in this chapter for head injury prevention serve to decrease the incidence of SCI as well (see Chart 63-1).

Most (80%) people who live with SCIs are men. The approximate ethnic distribution is 62% Caucasian, 22% African American, 13% Hispanic, and 3% other racial or ethnic groups (Dawodu, 2007). Life expectancy continues to increase for people with SCI because of improved health care but remains slightly lower than for those without SCI. The major causes of death are pneumonia, pulmonary emboli (PE), and septicemia (Dawodu, 2007; Hickey, 2009).

Pathophysiology

Damage in SCI ranges from transient concussion (from which the patient fully recovers), to contusion, laceration, and compression of the spinal cord substance (either alone or in combination), to complete **transection** (severing) of the spinal cord (which renders the patient paralyzed below the level of the injury). The vertebrae most frequently involved are the 5th, 6th, and 7th cervical vertebrae (C5 to C7), the 12th thoracic vertebra (T12), and the 1st lumbar vertebra (L1). These vertebrae are most susceptible because there is a greater range of mobility in the vertebral column in these areas (Sherwood, Crago, Spiro, et al., 2007).

SCIs can be separated into two categories: primary injuries and secondary injuries. Primary injuries are the result of the initial insult or trauma and are usually permanent. Secondary injuries are usually the result of a contusion or tear injury, in which the nerve fibers begin to swell and disintegrate. A secondary chain of events produces ischemia, hypoxia, edema, and hemorrhagic lesions, which in turn result in destruction of myelin and axons. The secondary injury is of primary concern for critical care nurses. Experts believe secondary injury is the principal cause of spinal cord degeneration at the level of injury and that it is reversible during the first 4 to 6 hours after injury. Methods of early treatment are essential to prevent partial damage from becoming total and permanent (Sherwood, et al., 2007).

Clinical Manifestations

Manifestations of SCI depend on the type and level of injury (Chart 63-7). The type of injury refers to the extent of injury to the spinal cord itself. **Incomplete spinal cord lesions** (the sensory or motor fibers, or both, are preserved below the lesion) are classified according to the area of spinal cord damage: central, lateral, anterior, or peripheral. The American Spinal Injury Association (ASIA) provides classification of SCI according to the degree of sensory and motor function present after injury (Chart 63-8). "Neurologic level" refers to the lowest level at which sensory and motor functions are normal. Below the neurologic level, there is total sensory and motor paralysis, loss of bladder and bowel control (usually with urinary retention and bladder distention), loss of sweating and vasomotor tone, and marked reduction of blood pressure from loss of peripheral vascular resistance. A **complete spinal cord lesion** (total loss of sensation and voluntary muscle control below the lesion) can result in paraplegia or tetraplegia.

If conscious, the patient usually complains of acute pain in the back or neck, which may radiate along the involved nerve. However, absence of pain does not rule out spinal injury, and a careful assessment of the spine should be conducted if there has been a significant force and mechanism of injury (ie, concomitant head injury). Often the patient speaks of fear that the neck or back is broken.

Respiratory dysfunction is related to the level of injury. The muscles contributing to respiration are the abdominals and intercostals (T1 to T11) and the diaphragm (C4). In high cervical cord injury, acute respiratory failure is the leading cause of death. Functional abilities by level of injury are described in Table 63-3.

Assessment and Diagnostic Findings

A detailed neurologic examination is performed. Diagnostic x-rays (lateral cervical spine x-rays) and CT scanning are usually performed initially. An MRI scan may be ordered as a further workup if a ligamentous injury is suspected, because significant spinal cord damage may exist even in the absence of bony injury (Hickey, 2009). If an MRI scan is contraindicated, a myelogram may be used to visualize the spinal axis. An assessment is made for other injuries, because spinal trauma often is accompanied by concomitant injuries, commonly to the head and chest. Continuous electrocardiographic monitoring may be indicated if a spinal cord injury is suspected, because bradycardia (slow heart rate) and asystole (cardiac standstill) are common in patients with acute spinal cord injuries.

Emergency Management

The immediate management at the scene of the injury is critical, because improper handling of the patient can cause further damage and loss of neurologic function. Any patient who is involved in a motor vehicle crash, a diving or contact sports injury, a fall, or any direct trauma to the head and neck must be considered to have SCI until such an injury is ruled out. Initial care must include a rapid assessment, immobilization, extrication, and stabilization or control of life-threatening injuries, and transportation to the most appropriate medical facility. Immediate transportation to a trauma center with the capacity to manage major neurologic trauma is then necessary (Hickey, 2009).

At the scene of the injury, the patient must be immobilized on a spinal (back) board, with the head and neck maintained in a neutral position, to prevent an incomplete injury from becoming complete. One member of the team must assume control of the patient's head to prevent flexion, rotation, or extension; this is done by placing the hands on both sides of the patient's head at about ear level to limit movement and maintain alignment while a spinal board or cervical immobilizing device is applied. If possible, at least four people should slide the patient carefully onto a board for transfer to the hospital. Any twisting movement may irreversibly damage the spinal cord by causing a bony fragment of the vertebra to cut into, crush, or sever the cord completely.

The standard of care is that the patient is referred to a regional spinal injury or trauma center because of the multidisciplinary personnel and support services required to counteract the destructive changes that occur in the first 24 hours after injury. However, no randomized controlled trials have been conducted to confirm that referral results in better outcomes for the patient with SCI (Jones & Bagnall, 2008). During treatment in the emergency and x-ray departments, the patient is kept on the transfer board. The patient must always be maintained in an extended position. No part of the body should be twisted or turned, and the patient is not allowed to sit up. Once the extent of the injury has been determined, the patient may be placed on a rotating specialty bed (Fig. 63-6) or in a cervical collar (Fig. 63-7). Later, if SCI and bone instability have been ruled out, the patient may be moved to a conventional bed or the collar may be removed without harm. If a specialty bed is needed but not available, the patient should be placed in a cervical collar and on a firm mattress.

Medical Management (Acute Phase)

The goals of management are to prevent secondary injury, to observe for symptoms of progressive neurologic deficits, and to prevent complications. The patient is resuscitated as necessary, and oxygenation and cardiovascular stability are maintained. SCI is a devastating event; new treatment methods and medications are continually being investigated for the acute and chronic phases of care (Fehlings & Baptiste, 2005).

Pharmacologic Therapy

Administration of high-dose IV corticosteroids or methylprednisolone sodium succinate in the first 24 or 48 hours is

Chart 63-7 • *Effects of Spinal Cord Injuries*

Central Cord Syndrome

- Characteristics: Motor deficits (in the upper extremities compared to the lower extremities; sensory loss varies but is more pronounced in the upper extremities); bowel/bladder dysfunction is variable, or function may be completely preserved.
- Cause: Injury or edema of the central cord, usually of the cervical area. May be caused by hyperextension injuries.

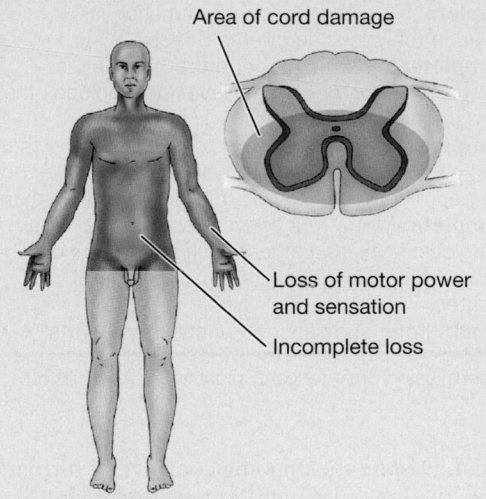

Area of cord damage

Loss of motor power and sensation

Incomplete loss

Central Cord Syndrome

Anterior Cord Syndrome

- Characteristics: Loss of pain, temperature, and motor function is noted below the level of the lesion; light touch, position, and vibration sensation remain intact.
- Cause: The syndrome may be caused by acute disk herniation or hyperflexion injuries associated with fracture-dislocation of vertebra. It also may occur as a result of injury to the anterior spinal artery, which supplies the anterior two thirds of the spinal cord.

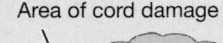

Area of cord damage

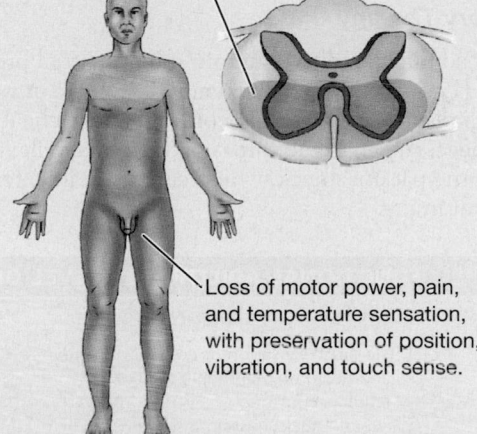

Loss of motor power, pain, and temperature sensation, with preservation of position, vibration, and touch sense.

Anterior Cord Syndrome

Brown-Séquard Syndrome (Lateral Cord Syndrome)

- Characteristics: Ipsilateral paralysis or paresis is noted, together with ipsilateral loss of touch, pressure, and vibration and contralateral loss of pain and temperature.
- Cause: The lesion is caused by a transverse hemisection of the cord (half of the cord is transected from north to south), usually as a result of a knife or missile injury, fracture-dislocation of a unilateral articular process, or possibly an acute ruptured disk.

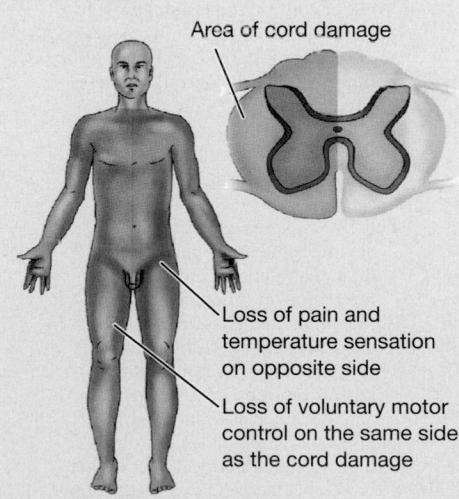

Area of cord damage

Loss of pain and temperature sensation on opposite side

Loss of voluntary motor control on the same side as the cord damage

Brown-Séquard Syndrome

Adapted from Hickey, L. (2009). *The clinical practice of neurological and neurosurgical nursing* (6th ed.). Philadelphia: Lippincott Williams & Wilkins.

Chart 63-8 • ASIA Impairment Scale

A = Complete: No motor or sensory function is preserved in the sacral segments S4–S5.

B = Incomplete: Sensory but not motor function is preserved below the neurologic level, and includes the sacral segments S4–S5.

C = Incomplete: Motor function is preserved below the neurologic level, and more than half of key muscles below the neurologic level have a muscle grade less than 3.

D = Incomplete: Motor function is preserved below the neurologic level, and at least half of key muscles below the neurologic level have a muscle grade of 3 or greater.

E = Normal: Motor and sensory function are normal.

Used with permission of American Spinal Injury Association.

controversial. Despite the ongoing controversy surrounding the practice, the use of IV high-dose methylprednisolone is accepted as standard therapy for SCI in many countries and remains an established clinical practice in most trauma centers in the United States (Hickey, 2009).

Respiratory Therapy

Oxygen is administered to maintain a high partial pressure of oxygen (PaO_2), because hypoxemia can create or worsen a neurologic deficit of the spinal cord. If endotracheal intubation is necessary, extreme care is taken to avoid flexing or extending the patient's neck, which can result in extension of a cervical injury.

In high cervical spine injuries, spinal cord innervation to the phrenic nerve, which stimulates the diaphragm, is lost. Diaphragmatic pacing (electrical stimulation of the phrenic nerve) attempts to stimulate the diaphragm to help the patient breathe (Sole, Klein & Moseley, 2009). Intramuscular diaphragmatic pacing is currently in the clinical trial phase for the patient with a high cervical injury. This is implanted via laparoscopic surgery, usually after the acute phase.

Skeletal Fracture Reduction and Traction

Management of SCI requires immobilization and reduction of dislocations (restoration of normal position) and stabilization of the vertebral column.

Cervical fractures are reduced, and the cervical spine is aligned with some form of skeletal traction, such as skeletal tongs or calipers, or with use of the halo device (Sole, et al., 2009). A variety of skeletal tongs are available, all of which involve fixation in the skull in some manner. The Gardner-Wells tongs require no predrilled holes in the skull. Crutchfield and Vinke tongs are inserted through holes made in the skull with a special drill under local anesthesia.

Traction is applied to the skeletal traction device by weights, the amount depending on the size of the patient and the degree of fracture displacement. The traction force is exerted along the longitudinal axis of the vertebral bodies, with the patient's neck in a neutral position. The traction is then gradually increased by adding more weights. As the amount of traction is increased, the spaces between the intervertebral disks widen and the vertebrae are given a chance to slip back into position. Reduction usually occurs after correct alignment has been restored. Once reduction is

Table 63-3	FUNCTIONAL ABILITIES BY LEVEL OF CORD INJURY			
Injury Level	**Segmental Sensorimotor Function**	**Dressing, Eating**	**Elimination**	**Mobility***
C1	Little or no sensation or control of head and neck; no diaphragm control; requires continuous ventilation	Dependent	Dependent	Limited. Voice or sip-n-puff controlled electric wheelchair
C2 to C3	Head and neck sensation; some neck control; independent of mechanical ventilation for short periods	Dependent	Dependent	Same as for C1
C4	Good head and neck sensation and motor control; some shoulder elevation; diaphragm movement	Dependent, may be able to eat with adaptive sling	Dependent	Limited to voice, mouth, head, chin, or shoulder-controlled electric wheelchair
C5	Full head and neck control; shoulder strength; elbow flexion	Independent with assistance	Maximal assistance	Electric or modified manual wheelchair, needs transfer assistance
C6	Fully innervated shoulder; wrist extension or dorsiflexion	Independent or with minimal assistance	Independent or with minimal assistance	Independent in transfers and wheelchair
C7 to C8	Full elbow extension; wrist plantar flexion; some finger control	Independent	Independent	Independent; manual wheelchair
T1 to T5	Full hand and finger control; use of intercostal and thoracic muscles	Independent	Independent	Independent; manual wheelchair
T6 to T10	Abdominal muscle control, partial to good balance with trunk muscles	Independent	Independent	Independent; manual wheelchair
T11 to L5	Hip flexors, hip abductors (L1–L3); knee extension (L2–L4); knee flexion and ankle dorsiflexion (L4–L5)	Independent	Independent	Short distance to full ambulation with assistance
S1 to S5	Full leg, foot, and ankle control; innervation of perineal muscles for bowel, bladder, and sexual function (S2–S4)	Independent	Normal to impaired bowel and bladder function	Ambulate independently with or without assistance

* Assistance refers to adaptive equipment, setup, or physical assistance.

From Porth, C. M. & Matfin, G. (2009). *Pathophysiology: Concepts of altered health states* (8th ed.). Philadelphia: Lippincott Williams & Wilkins.

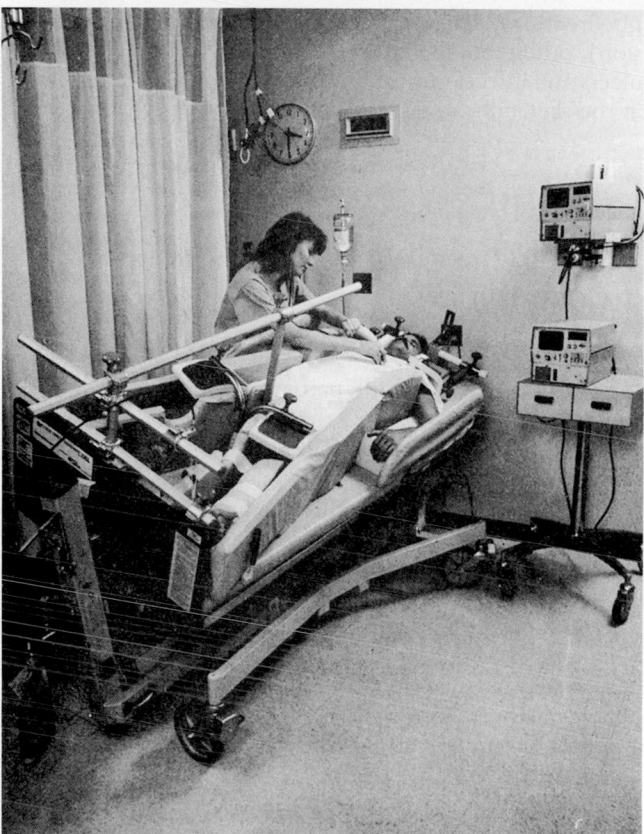

Figure 63-6 Roro Rest bed. Courtesy of Kinetic Concepts, San Antonio, TX.

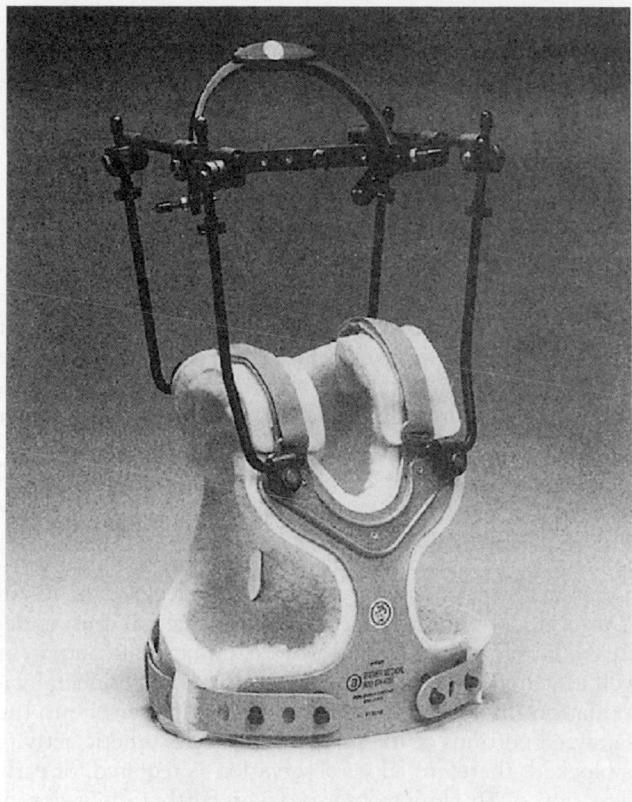

Figure 63-8 Halo and vest for cervical and thoracic injuries. Courtesy of Acromed Corp., Cleveland, OH.

achieved, as verified by cervical spine x-rays and neurologic examination, the weights are gradually removed until the amount of weight needed to maintain the alignment is identified. The weights should hang freely so as not to interfere with the traction. Traction is sometimes supplemented with manual manipulation of the neck by a surgeon to help achieve realignment of the vertebral bodies.

A halo device may be used initially with traction, or may be applied after removal of the tongs. It consists of a stainless steel halo ring that is fixed to the skull by four pins. The ring is attached to a removable **halo vest,** a device that

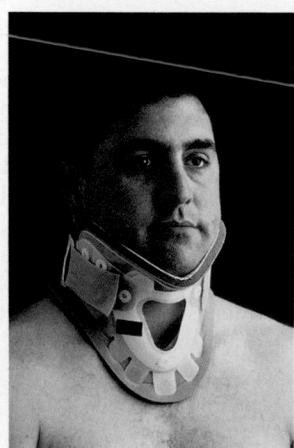

Figure 63-7 Cervical collar. Courtesy of Aspen Medical Products, Irvine, CA.

suspends the weight of the unit circumferentially around the chest. A metal frame connects the ring to the chest. Halo devices provide immobilization of the cervical spine while allowing early ambulation (Fig. 63-8).

Thoracic and lumbar injuries are usually treated with surgical intervention followed by immobilization with a fitted brace. Traction is not indicated either before or after surgery, due to the relative stability of the spine in these regions.

 NURSING ALERT

> The patient's vital organ functions and body defenses must be supported and maintained until spinal and neurogenic shock abates and the neurologic system has recovered from the traumatic insult; this can take up to 4 months (Hickey, 2009).

Surgical Management

Surgery is indicated in any of the following situations:
- Compression of the cord is evident.
- The injury results in a fragmented or unstable vertebral body.
- The injury involves a wound that penetrates the cord.
- Bony fragments are in the spinal canal.
- The patient's neurologic status is deteriorating.

Research indicates that early surgical stabilization improves the clinical outcome of patients compared to surgery performed later during the clinical course. The goals of surgical treatment are to preserve neurologic function by removing pressure from the spinal cord and to provide stability (Sherwood, et al., 2007).

Management of Acute Complications of Spinal Cord Injury

Spinal and Neurogenic Shock

The spinal shock associated with SCI reflects a sudden depression of reflex activity in the spinal cord (areflexia) below the level of injury. The muscles innervated by the part of the spinal cord segment below the level of the lesion are without sensation, paralyzed, and flaccid, and the reflexes are absent. In particular, the reflexes that initiate bladder and bowel function are affected. Bowel distention and paralytic ileus can be caused by depression of the reflexes and are treated with intestinal decompression by insertion of a nasogastric tube (Dawodu, 2007).

Neurogenic shock develops as a result of the loss of autonomic nervous system function below the level of the lesion (Dawodu, 2007). The vital organs are affected, causing decreases in blood pressure, heart rate, and cardiac output, as well as venous pooling in the extremities and peripheral vasodilation. In addition, the patient does not perspire in the paralyzed portions of the body, because sympathetic activity is blocked; therefore, close observation is required for early detection of an abrupt onset of fever. Further discussion of neurogenic shock can be found in Chapter 15.

With injuries to the cervical and upper thoracic spinal cord, innervation to the major accessory muscles of respiration is lost and respiratory problems develop. These include decreased vital capacity, retention of secretions, increased partial pressure of arterial carbon dioxide ($PaCO_2$) levels and decreased oxygen levels, respiratory failure, and pulmonary edema.

Deep Vein Thrombosis

Deep vein thrombosis (DVT) is a potential complication of immobility and is common in patients with SCI. Patients who develop DVT are at risk for PE, a life-threatening complication. Manifestations of PE include pleuritic chest pain, anxiety, shortness of breath, and abnormal blood gas values (increased $PaCO_2$ and decreased PaO_2). Low-dose anticoagulation therapy usually is initiated to prevent DVT and PE, along with the use of anti-embolism stockings or pneumatic compression devices. In some cases, permanent indwelling filters (see Chapter 23) may be placed prophylactically in the vena cava to prevent emboli (dislodged clots) from migrating to the lungs and causing a PE (Hickey, 2009).

 NURSING ALERT

The calves or thighs should never be massaged because of the danger of dislodging an undetected thromboemboli.

Other Complications

In addition to respiratory complications (respiratory failure, pneumonia) and **autonomic dysreflexia** (characterized by pounding headache, profuse sweating, nasal congestion, piloerection ["goose bumps"], bradycardia, and hypertension), other complications that may occur include pressure ulcers and infection (urinary, respiratory, and local infection at the skeletal traction pin sites) (Vacca, 2007a).

NURSING PROCESS

THE PATIENT WITH ACUTE SPINAL CORD INJURY

Assessment

The patient's breathing pattern and the strength of the cough are assessed, and the lungs are auscultated, because paralysis of abdominal and respiratory muscles diminishes coughing and makes clearing of bronchial and pharyngeal secretions difficult. Reduced excursion of the chest also results.

The patient is monitored closely for any changes in motor or sensory function and for symptoms of progressive neurologic damage. In the early stages of SCI, determining whether the cord has been severed may not be possible, because signs and symptoms of cord edema are indistinguishable from those of cord transection. Edema of the spinal cord may occur with any severe cord injury and may further compromise spinal cord function.

Motor and sensory functions are assessed through careful neurologic examination. These findings are recorded on a flow sheet so that changes in the baseline neurologic status can be monitored closely and accurately. The ASIA classification is commonly used to describe level of function for patients with SCI (see Chart 63-8). Chart 63-7 gives examples of the effects of altered spinal cord function. At the minimum:

- Motor ability is tested by asking the patient to spread the fingers, squeeze the examiner's hand, and move the toes or turn the feet.
- Sensation is evaluated by gently pinching the skin or touching it lightly with an object such as a tongue blade, starting at shoulder level and working down both sides of the extremities. The patient should have both eyes closed so that the examination reveals true findings, not what the patient hopes to feel. The patient is asked where the sensation is felt.
- Any decrease in neurologic function is reported immediately.

The patient is also assessed for spinal shock, a complete loss of all reflex, motor, sensory, and autonomic activity below the level of the lesion that causes bladder paralysis and distention. The lower abdomen is palpated for signs of urinary retention and overdistention of the bladder. Further assessment is made for gastric dilation and paralytic ileus caused by an atonic bowel, a result of autonomic disruption.

Temperature is monitored, because the patient may have periods of hyperthermia as a result of alteration in temperature control due to autonomic disruption.

Diagnosis

Nursing Diagnoses

Based on the assessment data, the patient's major nursing diagnoses may include the following:

- Ineffective breathing patterns related to weakness or paralysis of abdominal and intercostal muscles and inability to clear secretions
- Ineffective airway clearance related to weakness of intercostal muscles
- Impaired bed and physical mobility related to motor and sensory impairments
- Disturbed sensory perception related to motor and sensory impairment
- Risk for impaired skin integrity related to immobility and sensory loss
- Impaired urinary elimination related to inability to void spontaneously
- Constipation related to presence of atonic bowel as a result of autonomic disruption
- Acute pain and discomfort related to treatment and prolonged immobility

Collaborative Problems/Potential Complications

Based on the assessment data, potential complications that may develop include:
- DVT
- Orthostatic hypotension
- Autonomic dysreflexia

Planning and Goals

The goals for the patient may include improved breathing pattern and airway clearance, improved mobility, improved sensory and perceptual awareness, maintenance of skin integrity, relief of urinary retention, improved bowel function, promotion of comfort, and absence of complications.

Nursing Interventions

Promoting Adequate Breathing and Airway Clearance

Possible impending respiratory failure is detected by observing the patient, measuring vital capacity, monitoring oxygen saturation through pulse oximetry, and monitoring arterial blood gases. Early and vigorous attention to clearing bronchial and pharyngeal secretions can prevent retention of secretions and atelectasis. Suctioning may be indicated, but it should be used with caution to avoid stimulating the vagus nerve and producing bradycardia and cardiac arrest.

If the patient cannot cough effectively because of decreased inspiratory volume and inability to generate sufficient expiratory pressure, chest physical therapy and assisted coughing may be indicated. Specific breathing exercises are supervised by the nurse to increase the strength and endurance of the inspiratory muscles, particularly the diaphragm. Assisted coughing promotes clearing of secretions from the upper respiratory tract and is similar to the use of abdominal thrusts to clear an airway (see Chapter 25). Proper humidification and hydration are important to prevent secretions from becoming thick and difficult to remove even with coughing. The patient is assessed for signs of respiratory infection (eg, cough, fever, dyspnea).

Ascending edema of the spinal cord in the acute phase may cause respiratory difficulty that requires immediate intervention. Therefore, the patient's respiratory status must be monitored closely.

Improving Mobility

Proper body alignment is maintained at all times. The patient is repositioned frequently and is assisted out of bed as soon as the spinal column is stabilized. The feet are prone to footdrop; therefore, various types of splints are used to prevent footdrop. When used, the splints are removed and reapplied every 2 hours. Trochanter rolls, applied from the crest of the ilium to the midthigh of both legs, help prevent external rotation of the hip joints.

Patients with lesions above the midthoracic level have loss of sympathetic control of peripheral vasoconstrictor activity, leading to hypotension. These patients may tolerate changes in position poorly and require monitoring of blood pressure when positions are changed. If not on a rotating specialty bed, the patient should not be turned unless the spine is stable and the physician has indicated that it is safe to do so.

Contractures can develop rapidly with immobility and muscle paralysis. A joint that is immobilized too long becomes fixed as a result of contractures of the tendon and joint capsule. Atrophy of the extremities results from disuse. Contractures and other complications may be prevented by range-of-motion exercises that help preserve joint motion and stimulate circulation. Passive range-of-motion exercises should be implemented as soon as possible after injury. Toes, metatarsals, ankles, knees, and hips should be put through a full range of motion at least four, and ideally five, times daily.

For most patients who have a cervical fracture without neurologic deficit, reduction in traction followed by rigid immobilization for 6 to 8 weeks restores skeletal integrity. These patients are allowed to move gradually to an erect position. A neck brace or molded collar is applied when the patient is mobilized after traction is removed (see Fig. 63-7).

Promoting Adaptation to Sensory and Perceptual Alterations

The nurse assists the patient to compensate for sensory and perceptual alterations that occur with SCI. The intact senses above the level of the injury are stimulated through touch, aromas, flavorful food and beverages, conversation, and music. Additional strategies include the following:
- Providing prism glasses to enable the patient to see from the supine position
- Encouraging use of hearing aids, if indicated, to enable the patient to hear conversations and environmental sounds
- Providing emotional support to the patient
- Teaching the patient strategies to compensate for or cope with sensory deficits

Maintaining Skin Integrity

Pressure ulcers are a significant complication of SCI. The most common sites are over the ischial tuberosity, the greater trochanter, the sacrum, and the occiput (back of head). In the acute care setting, during the initial phase of hospitalization, it may be necessary to delay rehabilitation in 20% to 30% of patients because of pressure ulcers. Pressure ulcers may begin within hours of an acute SCI where pressure is continuous and where the peripheral circulation is inadequate as a result of spinal shock and a recumbent position. It is important to move the patient from the backboard as soon as possible and inspect the skin. In addition, patients who wear cervical collars for prolonged periods may develop breakdown from the pressure of the collar under the chin, on the shoulders, and at the occiput. In addition, pressure ulcers can add substantially to the personal and economic costs of living with a SCI. The prevalence of this complication ranges from 17% for people 2 months after injury to 33% for those living with an SCI.

The most effective approach to addressing this costly complication of SCI is prevention (King, Porter & Vertiz, 2008). The patient's position is changed at least every 2 hours. Turning not only assists in the prevention of pressure ulcers but also prevents pooling of blood and edema in the dependent areas. Careful inspection of the skin is made each time the patient is turned. The skin over the pressure points is assessed for redness or breaks; the perineum is checked for soilage, and the catheter is observed for adequate drainage. The patient's general body alignment and comfort are assessed. Special attention should be given to pressure areas in contact with the transfer board.

In addition, the patient's skin should be kept clean by washing with a mild soap, rinsing well, and blotting dry. Pressure-sensitive areas should be kept well lubricated and soft with hand cream or lotion. The patient is educated about the danger of pressure ulcers and is encouraged to take control and make decisions about appropriate skin care (King, et al., 2008). See Chapter 11 for other aspects of the prevention of pressure ulcers.

Maintaining Urinary Elimination

Immediately after SCI, the urinary bladder becomes atonic and cannot contract by reflex activity. Urinary retention is the immediate result. Because the patient has no sensation of bladder distention, overstretching of the bladder and detrusor muscle may occur, delaying the return of bladder function.

Intermittent catheterization is carried out to avoid overdistention of the bladder and UTI. If this is not feasible, an indwelling catheter is inserted temporarily. At an early stage, family members are shown how to carry out intermittent catheterization and are encouraged to participate in this facet of care, because they will be involved in long-term follow-up and must be able to recognize complications so that treatment can be instituted.

The patient is taught to record fluid intake, voiding pattern, amounts of residual urine after catheterization, characteristics of urine, and any unusual sensations that may occur. The management of a **neurogenic bladder** (bladder dysfunction that results from a disorder or dysfunction of the nervous system) is discussed in detail in Chapter 11.

Improving Bowel Function

Immediately after SCI, a paralytic ileus usually develops as a result of neurogenic paralysis of the bowel; therefore, a nasogastric tube is often required to relieve distention and to prevent vomiting and aspiration.

Bowel activity usually returns within the first week. As soon as bowel sounds are heard on auscultation, the patient is given a high-calorie, high-protein, high-fiber diet, with the amount of food gradually increased. The nurse administers prescribed stool softeners to counteract the effects of immobility and analgesic agents. A bowel program is instituted as early as possible.

Providing Comfort Measures: The Patient in Halo Traction

A patient who has had pins, tongs, or calipers placed for cervical stabilization may have a slight headache or discomfort for several days after the pins are inserted. Patients initially may be bothered by the rather startling appearance of these devices, but usually they readily adapt to it because the device provides comfort for the unstable neck (see Fig. 63-8). The patient may complain of being caged in and of noise created by any object coming in contact with the steel frame of a halo device, but he or she can be reassured that adaptation will occur.

The areas around the four pin sites of a halo device are cleaned daily and observed for redness, drainage, and pain. The pins are observed for loosening, which may contribute to infection. If one of the pins becomes detached, the head is stabilized in a neutral position by one person while another notifies the neurosurgeon. A torque screwdriver should be readily available in case the screws on the frame need tightening.

The skin under the halo vest is inspected for excessive perspiration, redness, and skin blistering, especially on the bony prominences. The vest is opened at the sides to allow the torso to be washed. The liner of the vest should not become wet, because dampness causes skin excoriation. Powder is not used inside the vest, because it may contribute to the development of pressure ulcers. The liner should be changed periodically to promote hygiene and good skin care. If the patient is to be discharged with the vest, detailed instructions must be given to the family, with time allowed for them to demonstrate the necessary skills of halo vest care (Chart 63-9).

Monitoring and Managing Potential Complications

THROMBOPHLEBITIS. Thrombophlebitis is a relatively common complication in patients after SCI. The patient must be assessed for symptoms of thrombophlebitis and PE. Chest pain, shortness of breath, and changes in arterial blood gas values must be reported promptly to the physician. The circumferences of the thighs and calves are measured and recorded daily; further diagnostic studies are performed if a significant increase is noted. Patients remain at high risk for thrombophlebitis for several months after the initial injury. Patients with paraplegia or tetraplegia are at increased risk for the rest of their lives. Immobilization and the associated venous stasis, as well as varying degrees of autonomic disruption, contribute to the high risk and susceptibility for DVT (Hickey, 2009).

Anticoagulation is initiated once head injury and other systemic injuries have been ruled out. Low-dose fractionated or unfractionated heparin may be followed by long-term oral anticoagulation (ie, warfarin) or subcutaneous fractionated heparin injections. Additional measures such as range-of-motion exercises, anti-embolism stockings, and adequate hydration are important preventive measures.

CHART 63-9	HOME CARE CHECKLIST *The Patient With a Halo Vest*		
At the completion of the home care instruction, the patient or caregiver will be able to:		**PATIENT**	**CAREGIVER**
• Describe the rationale for use of the halo vest.		✔	✔
• Demonstrate assessment of frame, traction, tongs, and pins.			✔
• Describe emergency measures if respiratory or other complications develop while patient is in halo vest or if frame becomes dislodged.			✔
• Demonstrate pin care using correct technique.			✔
• Identify signs and symptoms of infection.		✔	✔
• Assess the skin for reddened or irritated areas and breakdown.			✔
• Demonstrate care of skin.			✔
• Explain the reasons for and the method for changing the vest liner.		✔	✔
• Demonstrate safe techniques to assist patient with self-care, hygiene, and ambulation.			✔
• Identify signs and symptoms of complications (DVT, respiratory impairment, urinary tract infection).			✔

Pneumatic compression devices may also be used to reduce venous pooling and promote venous return. It is also important to avoid external pressure on the lower extremities that may result from flexion of the knees while the patient is in bed.

ORTHOSTATIC HYPOTENSION. For the first 2 weeks after SCI, the blood pressure tends to be unstable and quite low. It gradually returns to preinjury levels, but periodic episodes of severe orthostatic hypotension frequently interfere with efforts to mobilize the patient. Interruption in the reflex arcs that normally produce vasoconstriction in the upright position, coupled with vasodilation and pooling in abdominal and lower extremity vessels, can result in blood pressure readings of 40 mm Hg systolic and 0 mm Hg diastolic. Orthostatic hypotension is a particularly common problem for patients with lesions above T7. In some patients with tetraplegia, even slight elevations of the head can result in dramatic decreases in blood pressure.

A number of techniques can be used to reduce the frequency of hypotensive episodes. Close monitoring of vital signs before and during position changes is essential. Vasopressor medication can be used to treat the profound vasodilation. Anti-embolism stockings should be applied to improve venous return from the lower extremities. Abdominal binders may also be used to encourage venous return and provide diaphragmatic support when the patient is upright. Activity should be planned in advance, and adequate time should be allowed for a slow progression of position changes from recumbent to sitting and upright. Tilt tables frequently are helpful in assisting patients to make this transition.

AUTONOMIC DYSREFLEXIA. Autonomic dysreflexia (autonomic hyperreflexia) is an acute emergency that occurs as a result of exaggerated autonomic responses to stimuli that are harmless in normal people. It occurs only after spinal shock has resolved. This syndrome is characterized by a severe, pounding headache with paroxysmal hypertension, profuse diaphoresis (most often of the forehead), nausea, nasal congestion, and bradycardia. It occurs among patients with cord lesions above T6 (the sympathetic visceral outflow level) after spinal shock has subsided. The sudden increase in blood pressure may cause a rupture of one or more cerebral blood vessels or lead to increased ICP. A number of stimuli may trigger this reflex: distended bladder (the most common cause); distention or contraction of the visceral organs, especially the bowel (from constipation, impaction); or stimulation of the skin (tactile, pain, thermal stimuli, pressure ulcer). Because this is an emergency situation, the objectives are to remove the triggering stimulus and to avoid the possibly serious complications.

The following measures are carried out:

• The patient is placed immediately in a sitting position to lower blood pressure.
• Rapid assessment is performed to identify and alleviate the cause.
• The bladder is emptied immediately via a urinary catheter. If an indwelling catheter is not patent, it is irrigated or replaced with another catheter.
• The rectum is examined for a fecal mass. If one is present, a topical anesthetic agent is inserted 10 to 15 minutes before the mass is removed, because visceral distention or contraction can cause autonomic dysreflexia.
• The skin is examined for any areas of pressure, irritation, or broken skin.
• Any other stimulus that could be the triggering event, such as an object next to the skin or a draft of cold air, must be removed.
• If these measures do not relieve the hypertension and excruciating headache, a ganglionic blocking agent (hydralazine hydrochloride [Apresoline]) is prescribed and administered slowly by the IV route.
• The medical record or chart is labeled with a clearly visible note about the risk of autonomic dysreflexia.
• The patient is instructed about prevention and management measures.
• Any patient with a lesion above the T6 segment is informed that such an episode is possible and may occur even many years after the initial injury.

Promoting Home and Community-Based Care

TEACHING PATIENTS SELF-CARE. In most cases, patients with SCI (ie, patients with tetraplegia or paraplegia) need long-term rehabilitation. The process begins during hospitalization, as acute symptoms begin to subside or come under better control and the overall deficits and long-term effects of the injury become clear. The goals begin to shift from merely surviving the injury to learning strategies necessary to cope with the alterations that the injury imposes on activities of daily living (ADLs). The emphasis shifts from ensuring that the patient is stable and free of complications to specific assessment and planning designed to meet the patient's rehabilitation needs. Patient teaching may initially focus on the injury and its effects on mobility, dressing, and bowel, bladder, and sexual function. As the patient and family acknowledge the consequences of the injury and the resulting disability, the focus of teaching broadens to address issues necessary for carrying out the tasks of daily living and taking charge of their lives (Kinder, 2005). Teaching begins in the acute phase and continues throughout rehabilitation and throughout the patient's life as changes occur, the patient ages, and problems arise (Capoor & Stein, 2005).

Caring for the patient with SCI at home may at first seem a daunting task to the family. They will require dedicated nursing support to gradually assume full care of the patient. Although maintaining function and preventing complications will remain important, goals regarding self-care and preparation for discharge will assist in a smooth transition to rehabilitation and eventually to the community.

CONTINUING CARE. The goal of the rehabilitation process is independence. The nurse becomes a support to both the patient and the family, assisting them to assume responsibility for increasing aspects of patient care and management. Care for the patient with SCI involves members of all the health care disciplines, which may include nursing, medicine, rehabilitation, respiratory therapy, physical and occupational therapy, case management, and social services. The nurse often serves as coordinator of the management team and as a liaison with rehabilitation centers and home care agencies. The patient and family often require assistance in dealing with the psychological impact of the injury and its consequences; referral to a psychiatric clinical nurse specialist or other mental health care professional often is helpful.

The nurse should reassure female patients with SCI that pregnancy is not contraindicated and fertility is relatively unaffected, but that pregnant women with acute or chronic SCI pose unique management challenges. The normal physiologic changes of pregnancy may predispose women with SCI to many potentially life-threatening complications, including autonomic dysreflexia, pyelonephritis, respiratory insufficiency, thrombophlebitis, PE, and unattended delivery. Preconception assessment and counseling are strongly recommended to ensure that the woman is in optimal health and to increase the likelihood of an uneventful pregnancy and healthy outcomes (Smeltzer, 2007; Smeltzer & Wetzel-Effinger, 2009).

As more patients survive acute SCI, they face the changes associated with aging with a disability. Therefore, teaching in the home and community focuses on health promotion and addresses the need to minimize risk factors (eg, smoking, alcohol and drug abuse, obesity). Routine health screening and preventive services are needed for the older adult with SCI (Barker, 2008). Home care nurses and others who have contact with patients with SCI are in a position to teach patients about healthy lifestyles, remind them of the need for health screenings, and make referrals as appropriate. Assisting patients to identify accessible health care providers, clinical facilities, and imaging centers may increase the likelihood that they will participate in health screening.

Evaluation

Expected Patient Outcomes

Expected patient outcomes may include the following:

1. Demonstrates improvement in gas exchange and clearance of secretions, as evidenced by normal breath sounds on auscultation
   a. Breathes easily without shortness of breath
   b. Performs hourly deep-breathing exercises, coughs effectively, and clears pulmonary secretions
   c. Is free of respiratory infection (ie, has normal temperature, respiratory rate, and pulse; normal breath sounds; absence of purulent sputum)
2. Moves within limits of the dysfunction and demonstrates completion of exercises within functional limitations
3. Demonstrates adaptation to sensory and perceptual alterations
   a. Uses assistive devices (eg, prism glasses, hearing aids, computers) as indicated
   b. Describes sensory and perceptual alterations as a consequence of injury
4. Demonstrates optimal skin integrity
   a. Exhibits normal skin turgor; skin is free of reddened areas or breaks
   b. Participates in skin care and monitoring procedures within functional limitations
5. Regains urinary bladder function
   a. Exhibits no signs of UTI (ie, has normal temperature; voids clear, dilute urine)
   b. Has adequate fluid intake
   c. Participates in bladder training program within functional limitations
6. Regains bowel function
   a. Reports regular pattern of bowel movement
   b. Consumes adequate dietary fiber and oral fluids
   c. Participates in bowel training program within functional limitations
7. Reports absence of pain and discomfort
8. Is free of complications
   a. Demonstrates no signs of thrombophlebitis, DVT, or PE
   b. Maintains blood pressure within normal limits
   c. Reports no lightheadedness with position changes
   d. Exhibits no manifestations of autonomic dysreflexia (ie, absence of headache, diaphoresis, nasal congestion, bradycardia, or diaphoresis)

Medical Management of Long-Term Complications of Spinal Cord Injury

The patient faces a lifetime of disability, requiring ongoing follow-up and care. The expertise of a number of health professionals, including physicians (specifically a physiatrist), rehabilitation nurses, occupational therapists, physical therapists, psychologists, social workers, rehabilitation engineers, and vocational counselors, is necessary at different times as the need arises.

As people with SCI age, they have the same medical problems as other people. In addition, they face the threat of complications associated with their disability (Hickey, 2009). Usually, patients are encouraged to attend a spine clinic when complications and other issues arise. Lifetime care includes assessment of the urinary tract at prescribed intervals, because there is the likelihood of continuing alteration in detrusor and sphincter function, and the patient is prone to UTI.

Long-term problems and complications of SCI include premature aging, disuse syndrome, autonomic dysreflexia (discussed earlier), bladder and kidney infections, spasticity, and depression (Capoor & Stein, 2005). Pressure ulcers with potential complications of sepsis, osteomyelitis, and fistulas occur in about 10% of patients. Spasticity may be particularly disabling. Heterotopic ossification (overgrowth of bone) in the hips, knees, shoulders, and elbows occurs in many patients after SCI. Both of these complications are painful and can produce a loss of range of motion (Hickey, 2009). Management includes observing for and addressing any alteration in physiologic status and psychological outlook, as well as the prevention and treatment of long-term complications. The nursing role involves emphasizing the need for vigilance in self-assessment and care.

NURSING PROCESS

THE PATIENT WITH TETRAPLEGIA OR PARAPLEGIA

Assessment

Assessment focuses on the patient's general condition, complications, and how the patient is managing at that particular point in time. A head-to-toe assessment and review of systems should be part of the database, with emphasis on the areas that are prone to problems in this population. A thorough inspection of all areas of the skin for redness or breakdown is critical. The nurse reviews the established bowel and bladder program with the patient, because the program must continue uninterrupted. Patients with tetraplegia or paraplegia have varying degrees of loss of motor power, deep and superficial sensation, vasomotor control, bladder and bowel control, and sexual function. They are faced with potential complications related to immobility, skin breakdown and pressure ulcers, recurring UTIs, and contractures. Knowledge about these particular issues can further guide the assessment in any setting. Nurses in all settings, including home care, must be aware of these potential complications in the lifetime management of these patients.

An understanding of the emotional and psychological responses to tetraplegia or paraplegia is achieved by observing the responses and behaviors of the patient and family and by listening to their concerns. Documenting these assessments and reviewing the plan with the entire team on a regular basis provide insight into how both the patient and the family are coping with the changes in lifestyle and body functioning. Additional information frequently can be gathered from the social worker or psychiatric/mental health worker.

It takes time for the patient and family to comprehend the magnitude of the disability. They may go through stages of grief, including shock, disbelief, denial, anger, depression, and acceptance. During the acute phase of the injury, denial can be a protective mechanism to shield the patient from the overwhelming reality of what has happened. As the patient realizes the permanent nature of paraplegia or tetraplegia, the grieving process may be prolonged and all-encompassing because of the recognition that long-held plans and expectations are interrupted or permanently altered. A period of depression often follows as the patient experiences a loss of self-esteem in areas of self-identity, sexual functioning, and social and emotional roles. Exploration and assessment of these issues can assist in developing a meaningful plan of care.

Diagnosis

Nursing Diagnoses

Based on the assessment data, the major nursing diagnoses of the patient with tetraplegia or paraplegia may include the following:

- Impaired bed and physical mobility related to loss of motor function
- Risk for disuse syndrome
- Risk for impaired skin integrity related to permanent sensory loss and immobility
- Impaired urinary elimination related to level of injury
- Constipation related to effects of spinal cord disruption
- Sexual dysfunction related to neurologic dysfunction
- Ineffective coping related to impact of disability on daily living
- Deficient knowledge about requirements for long-term management

Collaborative Problems/Potential Complications

Based on all the assessment data, potential complications of tetraplegia or paraplegia that may develop include:

- Spasticity
- Infection and sepsis

Planning and Goals

The goals for the patient may include attainment of some form of mobility; maintenance of healthy, intact skin; achievement of bladder management without infection; achievement of bowel control; achievement of sexual expression; strengthening of coping mechanisms; and absence of complications.

Nursing Interventions

The patient requires extensive rehabilitation, which is less difficult if appropriate nursing management has been carried out during the acute phase of the injury or illness. Nursing care is one of the key factors determining the success of the rehabilitation program. The main objective is for the patient to live as independently as possible in the home and community.

Increasing Mobility

EXERCISE PROGRAMS. The unaffected parts of the body are built up to optimal strength to promote maximal self-care. The muscles of the hands, arms, shoulders, chest, spine, abdomen, and neck must be strengthened in the patient with paraplegia, because he or she must bear full weight on these muscles to ambulate. The triceps and the latissimus dorsi are important muscles used in crutch walking. The muscles of the abdomen and the back also are necessary for balance and for maintaining the upright position.

To strengthen these muscles, the patient can do push-ups when in a prone position and sit-ups when in a sitting position. Extending the arms while holding weights (traction weights can be used) also develops muscle strength. Squeezing rubber balls or crumbling newspaper promotes hand strength.

With encouragement from all members of the rehabilitation team, the patient with paraplegia can develop the increased exercise tolerance needed for gait training and ambulation activities. The importance of maintaining cardiovascular fitness is stressed to the patient. Alternative exercises to increase the heart rate to target levels must be designed within the patient's abilities.

MOBILIZATION. After the spine is stable enough to allow the patient to assume an upright posture, mobilization activities are initiated. A brace or vest may be used, depending on the level of the lesion. A patient whose paralysis is a result of complete transection of the cord can begin weight bearing early, because no further damage can be incurred. The sooner muscles are used, the less chance there is of disuse atrophy. The earlier the patient is brought to a standing position, the less opportunity there is for osteoporotic changes to take place in the long bones. Weight bearing also reduces the possibility of renal calculi and enhances many other metabolic processes.

Braces and crutches enable some patients with paraplegia to ambulate for short distances. Ambulation using crutches requires a high expenditure of energy. Motorized wheelchairs and specially equipped vans can provide greater independence and mobility for patients with high-level SCI or other lesions. Every effort should be made to encourage the patient to be as mobile and active as possible.

Preventing Disuse Syndrome

Patients are at high risk for development of contractures as a result of disuse syndrome due to the musculoskeletal system changes (atrophy) brought about by the loss of motor and sensory functions below the level of injury. Range-of-motion exercises must be provided at least four times a day, and care is taken to stretch the Achilles tendon with exercises. The patient is repositioned frequently and is maintained in proper body alignment whether in bed or in a wheelchair.

Contractures can complicate day-to-day care, increasing the difficulty of positioning and decreasing mobility. A number of surgical procedures have been tried with varying degrees of success. These techniques are used if more conservative approaches fail, but the best treatment is prevention.

Promoting Skin Integrity

Because these patients spend a great portion of their lives in wheelchairs, pressure ulcers are an ever-present threat. Contributing factors are permanent sensory loss over pressure areas; immobility, which makes relief of pressure difficult; trauma from bumps (against the wheelchair, toilet, furniture, and so forth) that cause unnoticed abrasions and wounds; loss of protective function of the skin from excoriation and maceration due to excessive perspiration and possible incontinence; and poor general health (anemia, edema, malnutrition), leading to poor tissue perfusion. The prevention and management of pressure ulcers are discussed in detail in Chapter 11.

The person with tetraplegia or paraplegia must take responsibility for monitoring (or directing monitoring) of his or her skin status. This involves relieving pressure and not remaining in any position for longer than 2 hours, in addition to ensuring that the skin receives meticulous attention and cleansing. The patient is taught that ulcers develop over bony prominences that are exposed to unrelieved pressure in the lying and sitting positions. The most vulnerable areas are identified. The patient with paraplegia is instructed to use mirrors, if possible, to inspect these areas morning and night, observing for redness, slight edema, or any abrasions. While in bed, the patient should turn at 2-hour intervals and then inspect the skin again for redness that does not fade on pressure. The bottom sheet should be checked for wetness and for creases. The patient with tetraplegia or paraplegia who cannot perform these activities is encouraged to direct others to check these areas and prevent ulcers from developing.

The patient is taught to relieve pressure while in the wheelchair by doing push-ups, leaning from side to side to relieve ischial pressure, and tilting forward while leaning on a table. The caregiver for the patient with tetraplegia will need to perform these activities if the patient cannot do so independently. A wheelchair cushion is prescribed to meet individual needs, which may change in time with changes in posture, weight, and skin tolerance. A referral can be made to a rehabilitation engineer, who can measure pressure levels while the patient is sitting and then tailor the cushion and other necessary aids and assistive devices to the patient's needs.

The diet for the patient with tetraplegia or paraplegia should be high in protein, vitamins, and calories to ensure minimal wasting of muscle and the maintenance of healthy skin, and high in fluids to maintain well-functioning kidneys. Excessive weight gain and obesity should be avoided, because they further limit mobility.

Improving Bladder Management

The effect of the spinal cord lesion on the bladder depends on the level of injury, the degree of cord damage, and the length of time after injury. A patient with tetraplegia or paraplegia usually has either a reflex or a nonreflex bladder (see Chapter 11). Both bladder types increase the risk of UTI.

The nurse emphasizes the importance of maintaining an adequate flow of urine by encouraging a fluid intake of about 2.5 L daily. The patient should empty the bladder frequently so that there is minimal residual urine and should pay attention to personal hygiene, because infection of the bladder and kidneys almost always occurs by the ascending route. The perineum must be kept clean and dry, and attention must be given to the perianal skin after defecation. Underwear should be cotton (which is more absorbent) and should be changed at least once a day.

If an external catheter (condom catheter) is used, the sheath is removed nightly; the penis is cleansed to remove urine and is dried carefully, because warm urine on the periurethral skin promotes the growth of bacteria. Attention also is given to the collection bag. The nurse emphasizes the importance of monitoring for signs of UTI: cloudy, foul-smelling urine or hematuria (blood in the urine); fever; or chills.

The female patient who cannot achieve reflex bladder control or self-catheterization may need to wear pads or waterproof undergarments. Surgical intervention may be indicated in some patients to create a urinary diversion.

Establishing Bowel Control

The objective of a bowel training program is to establish bowel evacuation through reflex conditioning, a technique described in Chapter 11. If the SCI occurs above the sacral segments or nerve roots and there is reflex activity, the anal sphincter may be massaged (digital stimulation) to stimulate defecation. If the cord lesion involves the sacral segment or nerve roots, anal massage is not performed, because the anus may be relaxed and lack tone. Massage is also contraindicated if there is spasticity of the anal sphincter. The anal sphincter is massaged by inserting a gloved finger (which has been adequately lubricated) 2.5 to 3.7 cm (1 to 1.5 inches) into the rectum and moving it in a circular motion or from side to side. It soon becomes apparent which area triggers the defecation response. This procedure should be performed at regular time intervals (usually every 48 hours), after a meal, and at a time that will be convenient for the patient at home. The patient also is taught the symptoms of impaction (frequent loose stools; constipation) and is cautioned to watch for hemorrhoids. A diet with sufficient fluids and fiber is essential to developing a successful bowel training program, avoiding constipation, and decreasing the risk of autonomic dysreflexia.

Counseling on Sexual Expression

Many patients with tetraplegia and paraplegia can have some form of meaningful sexual relationship, although modifications are necessary. The patient and partner benefit from counseling about the range of sexual expression possible, special techniques and positions, exploration of body sensations offering sensual feelings, and urinary and bowel hygiene as related to sexual activity. For men with erectile failure, penile prostheses enable them to have and sustain an erection, and impotence drugs may be helpful. Sildenafil (Viagra), vardenafil (Levitra), and tadalafil (Cialis), for example, are oral smooth muscle relaxants that cause blood to flow into the penis, resulting in an erection (see Chapter 49).

Sexual education and counseling services are included in the rehabilitation services at spinal centers. Small-group meetings in which patients can share their feelings, receive information, and discuss sexual concerns and practical aspects are helpful in producing effective attitudes and adjustments.

Enhancing Coping Mechanisms

The impact of the disability and loss becomes marked when the patient returns home. Each time something new enters the patient's life (eg, a new relationship, going to work), the patient is reminded anew of his or her limitations. Grief reactions and depression are common.

To work through this depression, the patient must have some hope for relief in the future. The nurse can encourage the patient to feel confident in his or her ability to achieve self-care and relative independence. The role of the nurse ranges from caretaker during the acute phase to teacher, counselor, and facilitator as the patient gains mobility and independence.

The patient's disability affects not only the patient but also the entire family. In many cases, family therapy is helpful in working through issues as they arise. Adjustment to the disability leads to the development of realistic goals for the future, making the best of the abilities that are left intact and reinvesting in other activities and relationships. Rejection of the disability causes self-destructive neglect and noncompliance with the therapeutic program, which leads to more frustration and depression. Crises for which interventions may be sought include social, psychological, marital, sexual, and psychiatric problems. The family usually requires counseling, social services, and other support systems to help them cope with the changes in their lifestyle and socioeconomic status.

A major goal of nursing management is to help the patient overcome his or her sense of futility and to encourage the patient in the emotional adjustment that must be made before he or she is willing to venture into the outside world. However, an excessively sympathetic attitude on the part of the nurse may cause the patient to develop an overdependence that defeats the purpose of the entire rehabilitation program. The patient is taught and assisted when necessary, but the nurse should avoid performing activities that the patient can do independently with a little effort. This approach to care more than repays itself in the satisfaction of seeing a completely demoralized and helpless patient become independent and find meaning in a newly emerging lifestyle.

Monitoring and Managing Potential Complications

SPASTICITY. Muscle spasticity is one of the most problematic complications of tetraplegia and paraplegia. These incapacitating flexor or extensor spasms, which occur below the level of the spinal cord lesion, interfere with both the rehabilitation process and ADLs. Spasticity results from an imbalance between the facilitatory and inhibitory effects on neurons that exist normally. The area of the cord distal to the site of injury or lesion becomes disconnected from the higher inhibitory centers located in the brain, so facilitatory impulses, which originate from muscles, skin, and ligaments, predominate.

Spasticity is defined as a condition of increased muscle tone in a muscle that is weak. Initial resistance to stretching is quickly followed by sudden relaxation. The stimulus that precipitates spasm can be obvious, such as movement or a position change, or subtle, such as a slight jarring of the wheelchair. Most patients with tetraplegia or paraplegia have some degree of spasticity. With SCI, the onset of spasticity usually occurs from a few weeks to 6 months after the injury. The same muscles that are flaccid during the period of spinal shock develop spasticity during recovery. The intensity of spasticity tends to peak approximately 2 years after the injury, after which the spasms tend to regress.

Management of spasticity is based on the severity of symptoms and the degree of incapacitation. The antispasmodic medication baclofen (Lioresal) is one of the most commonly used agents because it is available in an oral and an intrathecal form. Other medications such as diazepam (Valium) and dantrolene (Dantrium) are also effective in controlling spasm (Saulino & Jacobs, 2006). All of the antispasmodic medications cause drowsiness, weakness, and vertigo in some patients. Passive range-of-motion exercises and frequent turning and repositioning are helpful, because stiffness tends to increase spasticity. These activities also are essential in the prevention of contractures, pressure ulcers, and bowel and bladder dysfunction.

INFECTION AND SEPSIS. Patients with tetraplegia and paraplegia are at increased risk for infection and sepsis from a variety of sources: urinary tract, respiratory tract, and pressure ulcers. Sepsis remains a major cause of complications and death in these patients. Prevention of infection and sepsis is essential through maintenance of skin integrity, complete emptying of the bladder at regular intervals, and prevention of urinary and fecal incontinence. The risk for respiratory infection can be decreased by avoiding contact with people who have symptoms of respiratory infection, performing coughing and deep-breathing exercises to prevent pooling of respiratory secretions, receiving yearly influenza vaccines, and giving up smoking. A high-protein diet is important in maintaining an adequate immune system, as is avoiding factors that may reduce immune system function, such as excessive stress, drug abuse, and excessive alcohol intake.

If infection occurs, the patient requires thorough assessment and prompt treatment. Antibiotic therapy and adequate hydration, in addition to local measures (depending on the site of infection), are initiated immediately.

UTIs are minimized or prevented by aseptic technique in catheter management, adequate hydration, bladder training program, and prevention of overdistention of the bladder and urinary stasis.

Skin breakdown and infection are prevented by maintenance of a turning schedule; frequent back care; regular assessment of all skin areas; regular cleaning and lubrication of the skin; passive range-of-motion exercise to prevent contractures; pressure relief over broken skin areas, bony prominences, and heels; and wrinkle-free bed linen.

Pulmonary infections are managed and prevented by frequent coughing, turning, and deep-breathing exercises and chest physiotherapy; aggressive respiratory care and suctioning of the airway if a tracheostomy is present; assisted coughing as needed; and adequate hydration.

Infections of any kind can be life-threatening. Aggressive nursing interventions are key to prevention, detection, and early management.

Promoting Home and Community-Based Care

TEACHING PATIENTS SELF-CARE. Patients with tetraplegia or paraplegia are at risk for complications for the rest of their lives. Therefore, a major aspect of nursing care is teaching the patient and family about these complications and about strategies to minimize risks. UTIs, contractures, infected pressure ulcers, and sepsis may necessitate hospitalization. Other late complications that may occur include lower extremity edema, joint contractures, respiratory dysfunction, and pain. To avoid these and other complications, the patient and a family member are taught skin care, catheter care, range-of-motion exercises, breathing exercises, and other care techniques. Teaching is initiated as soon as possible and extends into the rehabilitation or long-term care facility and home. In all aspects of care, it is important for the nurse and patient to set mutual goals and discuss the tasks the patient is capable of doing independently and which tasks the patient needs assistance to complete. (See Chapter 11 for a more detailed discussion of rehabilitation.)

CONTINUING CARE. Referral for home care is often appropriate for assessment of the home setting, patient teaching, and evaluation of the patient's physical and emotional status. During visits by the home care nurse, teaching about strategies to prevent or minimize potential complications is reinforced. The home environment is assessed for adequacy for care and for safety. Environmental modifications are made, and specialized equipment is obtained, ideally before the patient goes home.

The home care nurse also assesses the patient's and the family's adherence to recommendations and their use of coping strategies. The use of inappropriate coping strategies (eg, drug and alcohol use) is assessed, and referrals to counseling are made for the patient and family. Appropriate and effective coping strategies are reinforced. The nurse reviews previous teaching and determines the need for further physical or psychological assistance. The patient's self-esteem and body image may be very poor at this time. Because people with high levels of social support often report feelings of well-being despite major physical disability, it is beneficial for the nurse to assess and promote further development of the support system and effective coping strategies for each patient.

The patient requires continuing, lifelong follow-up by the physician, physical therapist, and other rehabilitation team members, because the neurologic deficit is usually permanent and new deficits, complications, and secondary conditions can develop. These require prompt attention before they take their toll in additional physical impairment, time, morale, and financial costs. The local counselor for the Office of Vocational Rehabilitation works with the patient with respect to job placement or additional educational or vocational training.

The nurse is in a good position to remind patients and family members of the need for continuing health promotion and screening practices. Referral to accessible health care providers and imaging centers is important in health promotion and health screening. Chapter 10 has more information on chronic illness and disability.

Evaluation

Expected Patient Outcomes

Expected patient outcomes may include the following:

1. Attains some form of mobility
2. Contractures do not develop
3. Maintains healthy, intact skin
4. Achieves bladder control, absence of UTI
5. Achieves bowel control
6. Reports sexual satisfaction
7. Shows improved adaptation to environment and others
8. Exhibits reduction in spasticity
   a. Reports understanding of the precipitating factors
   b. Uses measures to reduce spasticity
9. Describes long-term management required
10. Exhibits absence of complications

CRITICAL THINKING EXERCISES

1 A 75-year-old man is brought to the emergency department by his family, who report that he fell approximately 2 weeks ago in the bathroom. The patient does not recall the event. His family states that he is sleeping more than usual and seems forgetful. The patient is prescribed warfarin (Coumadin) daily. What type of injury has he most likely sustained? What type of medical treatment might he undergo? What discharge instructions are warranted for this patient's family or caregiver?

2 A 19-year-old man with a spinal cord injury at the T6 level complains of a severe headache. He is diaphoretic and flushed above the level of injury. His blood pressure is 230/110 mm Hg. What do you suspect is happening? What are the possible causes of his condition, and how would you intervene? What is included in your teaching plan for the patient and family before discharge?

EBP **3** A 56-year-old man who is married and the father of two children was involved in a motor vehicle crash 2 days ago, and he sustained a C4 fracture with spinal cord injury. As a result, he has tetraplegia and is on a mechanical ventilator in a neurologic intensive care unit. What recommendations would you make for the care of this patient to prevent secondary injury? What is the evidence base for these recommendations? Identify the criteria used to evaluate the strength of the evidence for these practices.

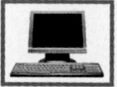

The Smeltzer suite offers these additional resources to enhance learning and facilitate understanding of this chapter:
• thePoint online resource, thepoint.lww.com/Smeltzer12E
• Student CD-ROM included with the book

• *Study Guide to Accompany Brunner & Suddarth's Textbook of Medical-Surgical Nursing*
• *Handbook for Brunner & Suddarth's Textbook of Medical-Surgical Nursing*

REFERENCES AND SELECTED READINGS

*Asterisk indicates nursing research.
**Double asterisk indicate classic reference.

Books

American Association of Neuroscience Nurses. (2005). *Guide to the care of the patient with intracranial pressure monitoring: AANN reference series for clinical practice.* Glenview, IL: Author.

Hickey, J. V. (2009). *The clinical practice of neurological & neurosurgical nursing* (6th ed.). Philadelphia: Lippincott Williams & Wilkins.

Langlois, J. A., Rutland-Brown, W. & Thomas, K. E. (2006). *Traumatic brain injury in the United States: Emergency department visits, hospitalizations and deaths.* Atlanta, GA: Centers for Disease Control and Prevention, National Center for Injury Prevention and Control.

Morton, P. G., Fontaine, D., Hudak, C., et al. (2010). *Critical care nursing a holistic approach* (9th ed.). Philadelphia: Lippincott Williams & Wilkins.

Porth, C. M. & Matfin, G. (2009). *Pathophysiology: Concepts of altered health status* (8th ed.). Philadelphia: Lippincott Williams & Wilkins.

Sole, M. L., Klein, D. G. & Moseley, M. J. (2009). *Introduction to critical care nursing* (5th ed.). St. Louis: Elsevier Saunders.

Journals and Electronic Documents

Head Injury

Adoni, A. & McNett, M. (2007). The pupillary response in traumatic brain injury: A guide for trauma nurses. *Journal of Trauma Nursing, 14*(4), 191–198.

Bader, M. K. (2006a). Gizmos and gadgets for the neuroscience intensive care unit. *Journal of Neuroscience Nursing, 38*(4), 248–260.

Bader, M. K. (2006b). Recognizing and treating ischemic insults to the brain: The role of brain tissue oxygen monitoring. *Critical Care Nursing Clinics of North America, 18*(2), 243–256.

Bader, M. K. & Arbour, R. (2005). Refractory increased intracranial pressure in severe traumatic brain injury: Barbiturate coma and bispectral index monitoring. *AACN Clinical Issues, 16*(4), 526–541.

*Bay, E. & Bergman, K. (2006). Symptom experience and emotional distress after traumatic brain injury. *Care Management Journal, 7*(1), 3–9.

Bay, E. & McLean, S. (2007). Mild traumatic brain injury: An update for advanced practice nurses. *Journal of Neuroscience Nursing, 39*(1), 43–51.

Brain Trauma Foundation. (2007). *Guidelines for the management of severe traumatic brain injury* (3rd ed.). Available at: www.braintrauma.org

*Calvin, A. O., Kite-Powell, D. M. & Hickey, J. (2007). The neuroscience ICU nurse's perceptions about end-of-life care. *Journal of Neuroscience Nursing, 39*(3), 143–150.

Flanagan, S. R., Hibbard, M. R. & Gordon, W. A. (2005). The impact of age on traumatic brain injury. *Physical Medicine and Rehabilitation Clinics of North America, 16*(1), 163–178.

**Hagen, C., Malkmus, D. & Durham, P. (1972). *Rancho Los Amigos Level of Cognitive Function scale.* Communication Disorders Service, Rancho Los Amigos Hospital, Downey, CA, 1972. Revised 11/15/74 by Danese Malkmus and Kathryn Stenderup.

Hoge, C. W., McGurk, D., Thomas, J. L., et al. (2008). Mild traumatic brain injury in U.S. soldiers returning from Iraq. *New England Journal of Medicine, 358*(5), 453–463.

*Jumisko, E., Lexell, J & Soderberg, S. (2005). The meaning of living with traumatic brain injury in people with moderate or severe traumatic brain injury. *Journal of Neuroscience Nursing, 37*(1), 42–50.

Kirkness, C. J., Burr, R. L., Cain, K. C., et al. (2006). Effect of continuous display of cerebral perfusion pressure on outcomes in patients with traumatic brain injury. *American Journal of Critical Care, 15*(6), 600–609.

Littlejohns, L. & Bader, M. K. (2005). Prevention of secondary brain injury: Targeting technology. *AACN Clinical Issues: Advanced Practice in Acute and Critical Care, 16*(4), 501–514.

Martin, E. M., Lu, W. C., Helmick, K., et al. (2008). Traumatic brain injuries sustained in the Afghanistan and Iraq wars. *American Journal of Nursing, 108*(4), 40–47.

McNett, M. (2007). A review of the predictive ability of Glasgow Coma Scale scores in head-injured patients. *Journal of Neuroscience Nursing, 39*(2), 68–75.

*Meeker, M., Du, R., Bacchetti, P., et al. (2005). Pupil examination: Validity and clinical utility of an automated pupillometer. *Journal of Neuroscience Nursing, 37*(1), 34–40.

National Center for Injury Prevention and Control, Centers for Disease Control and Prevention. (2007). *Traumatic brain injury, 2007.* Available at: www.cdc.gov/ncipc/factsheets/tbi.htm

Patterson, J., Bloom, S. A., Coyle, B., et al. (2005). Successful outcome in severe traumatic brain injury: A case study. *Journal of Neuroscience Nursing, 37*(5), 236–242.

*Scheetz, L. J. (2005). Relationship of age, injury severity, injury types, comorbid conditions, level of care, and survival among older motor vehicle trauma patients. *Research in Nursing and Health, 28*(3), 198–209.

Thompson, H. J. & Bourbonniere, M. (2006). Traumatic injury in the older adult from head to toe. *Critical Care Nursing Clinics of North America, 18*(3), 419–431.

Thompson, H. J., Kirkness, C. J. & Mitchell, P. H. (2007). Intensive care management of fever following traumatic brain injury. *Intensive & Critical Care Nursing, 23*(2), 91–96.

Torpy, J. M., Lynm, C. & Glass, R. M. (2005). Head injury. *Journal of the American Medical Association, 294*(12), 1580.

Vacca, V. M. (2007b). Epidural hemorrhage and hematoma. *Nursing, 37*(7), 72.

Vacca, V. M. (2007c). Subdural hematoma. *Nursing, 36*(3), 88.

Yanagawa, T., Bunn, F., Roberts, I., et al. (2005). Nutritional support for head-injured patients. *The Cochrane Database of Systematic Reviews, 3,* CD001530.

Spinal Cord Injury

Adams, M. G. & Pelter, M. M. (2005) Bedside monitoring of spinal cord injuries. *American Journal of Critical Care, 14*(1), 85–86.

Capoor, J. & Stein, A. B. (2005). Aging with spinal cord injury. *Physical Medicine and Rehabilitation Clinics of North America, 16*(1), 129–162.

Dawodu, S. T. (2007). *Spinal cord injury: Definition epidemiology pathophysiology.* Available at: www.emedicine.com/pmr/topic182.htm

Fehlings, M. G. & Baptiste, D. C. (2005). Current status of clinical trials for acute spinal cord injury. *Spinal Injury, 36*(suppl. 2), S113–S122.

Jones, L. & Bagnall, A. (2008). Spinal injuries centers (SCIs) for acute traumatic spinal cord injury. *The Cochrane Database of Systematic Reviews, 4,* CD004442.

*Kinder, R. A. (2005). Psychological hardiness in women with paraplegia. *Rehabilitation Nursing, 30*(2), 68–72.

*King, R. B., Porter, S. L. & Vertiz, K. B. (2008). Preventive skin care beliefs of people with spinal cord injury. *Rehabilitation Nursing, 33*(4), 154–162.

Saulino, M. & Jacobs, B. W. (2006). The pharmacological management of spasticity. *Journal of Neuroscience Nursing, 38*(6), 456–459.

Sherwood, P. R., Crago, E. A., Spiro, R. M., et al. (2007). Cervical spine injuries: Preserving function and improving outcomes. *American Nurse Today, 2*(9), 26–29.

Smeltzer, S. C. (2007). Pregnancy in women with physical disabilities. *Journal of Obstetric Gynecologic and Neonatal Nursing, 36*(1), 88–96.

Smeltzer, S. C. & Wetzel-Effinger, L. (2009). Pregnancy in women with spinal cord injury. *Topics in Spinal Cord Injury Rehabilitation, 15*(1), 29–42.

Smits, M., Dippel, D. W., Haan, H., et al. (2005). External validation of the Canadian CT head rule and the New Orleans criteria for CT scanning in patients with minor head injuries. *Journal of American Medical Association, 294*(12), 1519–1525.

Vacca, V. M. (2007a). Autonomic dysreflexia. *Nursing, 37*(9), 72.

RESOURCES

American Association of Neuroscience Nurses (AANN), www.aann.org
American Association of Spinal Cord Injury Nurses (AASCIN), www.aascin.org
Association of Rehabilitation Nurses, www.rehabnurse.org
Brain Trauma Foundation, www.braintrauma.org
Centers for Disease Control and Prevention, http://www.cdc.gov
Information Center for Individuals with Disabilities, www.disability.net
National Spinal Cord Injury Association, www.spinalcord.org
Paralyzed Veterans of America, www.pva.org
Waiting.com, www.waiting.com

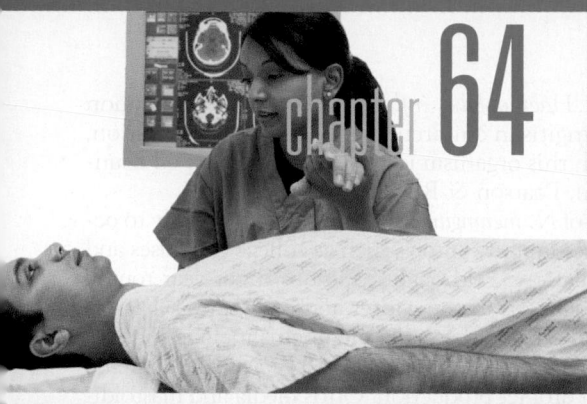

Management of Patients With Neurologic Infections, Autoimmune Disorders, and Neuropathies

LEARNING OBJECTIVES

On completion of this chapter, the learner will be able to:

1 Differentiate among the infectious disorders of the nervous system according to causes, manifestations, medical care, and nursing management.

2 Describe the pathophysiology, clinical manifestations, and medical and nursing management of multiple sclerosis, myasthenia gravis, and Guillain-Barré syndrome.

3 Use the nursing process as a framework for care of patients with multiple sclerosis and Guillain-Barré syndrome.

4 Describe disorders of the cranial nerves, their manifestations, and indicated nursing interventions.

5 Develop a plan of nursing care for the patient with a cranial nerve disorder.

GLOSSARY

ataxia: impaired coordination of movements

bulbar paralysis: immobility of muscles innervated by cranial nerves with their cell bodies in the lower portion of the brain stem

diplopia: double vision, or the awareness of two images of the same object occurring in one or both eyes

dyskinesia: impaired ability to execute voluntary movements

dysphagia: difficulty swallowing, causing the patient to be at risk for aspiration

dysphonia: voice impairment or altered voice production

neuropathy: general term indicating a disorder of the nervous system

paresthesia: a sensation of numbness or tingling or a "pins and needles" sensation

prion: a particle smaller than a virus that is resistant to standard sterilization procedures

spasticity: muscular hypertonicity with increased resistance to stretch often associated with weakness, increased deep tendon reflexes, and diminished superficial reflexes

spongiform: having the appearance or quality of a sponge

The diverse group of neurologic disorders that make up infectious and autoimmune disorders and cranial and peripheral neuropathies presents unique challenges for nursing care. The nurse who cares for patients with these disorders must have a clear understanding of the pathologic processes and the clinical outcomes. Some of the issues nurses must help patients and families confront include adaptation to the effects of the disease, potential changes in family dynamics, and, possibly, end-of-life issues.

INFECTIOUS NEUROLOGIC DISORDERS

The infectious disorders of the nervous system include meningitis, brain abscesses, various types of encephalitis, and Creutzfeldt-Jakob and variant Creutzfeldt-Jakob disease. The clinical manifestations, assessment, and diagnostic findings as well as the medical and nursing management are related to the specific infectious process.

Meningitis

Meningitis is an inflammation of the lining around the brain and spinal cord caused by bacteria or viruses (Iggulden, 2006). Meningitis can be the primary reason a patient is hospitalized or can develop during hospitalization and is classified as septic or aseptic. Septic meningitis is caused by bacteria. In aseptic meningitis, the cause is viral or secondary to lymphoma, leukemia, or human immunodeficiency virus (HIV). The bacteria *Streptococcus pneumoniae* and *Neisseria meningitides* are responsible for 80% of cases of meningitis in adults (van de Beek, de Gans, Tunkel,

et al., 2006). *Haemophilus influenzae* was once a common cause of meningitis in children, but, because of vaccination, infection with this organism is now rare in developed countries (Mazzoni, Pearson & Rowland, 2006).

Outbreaks of *N. meningitidis* infection are most likely to occur in dense community groups, such as college campuses and military installations. Although infections occur year round, the peak incidence is in the winter and early spring. Factors that increase the risk of bacterial meningitis include tobacco use and viral upper respiratory infection, because they increase the amount of droplet production. Otitis media and mastoiditis increase the risk of bacterial meningitis, because the bacteria can cross the epithelial membrane and enter the subarachnoid space. People with immune system deficiencies are also at greater risk for development of bacterial meningitis.

Pathophysiology

Meningeal infections generally originate in one of two ways: through the bloodstream as a consequence of other infections or by direct spread, such as might occur after a traumatic injury to the facial bones or secondary to invasive procedures.

N. meningitidis concentrates in the nasopharynx and is transmitted by secretion or aerosol contamination. Bacterial or meningococcal meningitis also occurs as an opportunistic infection in patients with acquired immunodeficiency syndrome (AIDS) and as a complication of Lyme disease (Chart 64-1).

Once the causative organism enters the bloodstream, it crosses the blood–brain barrier and proliferates in the cerebrospinal fluid (CSF). The host immune response stimulates the release of cell wall fragments and lipopolysaccharides, facilitating inflammation of the subarachnoid and pia mater. Because the cranial vault contains little room for

---

Chart 64-1• *Meningitis in Specific Populations*

Meningitis can occur as a complication of other diseases and is an opportunistic infection seen with greater frequency in patients who are immunocompromised.

Meningitis in Patients with Acquired Immunodeficiency Syndrome (AIDS)

- Aseptic, cryptococcal, and tuberculous forms of meningitis have been reported in patients with AIDS.
- Acute and chronic forms of aseptic meningitis may occur with AIDS; both are accompanied by headache, but signs of meningeal irritation usually occur with the acute form.
- Aseptic meningitis may be accompanied by cranial nerve palsies. The meningitis is thought to be related to direct infection of the central nervous system by human immunodeficiency virus (HIV) because it can be isolated from the cerebrospinal fluid (CSF).
- Cryptococcal meningitis is the most common fungal infection of the central nervous system in patients with AIDS. Patients may experience headache, nausea, vomiting, seizures, confusion, and lethargy. Treatment consists of IV administration of amphotericin B followed by fluconazole. Maintenance therapy with fluconazole may be necessary to prevent relapse.

- Some immunosuppressed patients develop few if any symptoms because of blunted inflammatory responses; others develop atypical features.

Meningitis in Patients with Lyme Disease

- Lyme disease is a multisystem inflammatory process caused by the tick-transmitted spirochete *Borrelia burgdorferi.*
- Neurologic abnormalities are seen in later stages (stages 2 or 3). Stage 2 occurs with the start of a characteristic rash or 1 to 6 months after the rash has disappeared.
- Neurologic abnormalities include aseptic meningitis, chronic lymphocytic meningitis, and encephalitis.
- Cranial nerve inflammation, including Bell's palsy and other peripheral neuropathies, is common.
- Stage 3 (the chronic form of the disease) begins years after the initial tick infection and is characterized by arthritis, skin lesions, and neurologic abnormalities.
- Most patients with stage 2 and 3 Lyme disease are treated with IV antibiotics, usually ceftriaxone or penicillin G.
- Meningeal and systemic symptoms begin to improve within days, although other symptoms, such as headache, may persist for weeks.

expansion, the inflammation may cause increased intracranial pressure (ICP). CSF circulates through the subarachnoid space, where inflammatory cellular materials from the affected meningeal tissue enter and accumulate.

The prognosis for bacterial meningitis depends on the causative organism, the severity of the infection and illness, and the timeliness of treatment. Acute fulminant presentation may include adrenal damage, circulatory collapse, and widespread hemorrhages (Waterhouse-Friderichsen syndrome). This syndrome is the result of endothelial damage and vascular necrosis caused by the bacteria. Complications include visual impairment, deafness, seizures, paralysis, hydrocephalus, and septic shock.

Clinical Manifestations

Headache and fever are frequently the initial symptoms. Fever tends to remain high throughout the course of the illness. The headache is usually either steady or throbbing and very severe as a result of meningeal irritation (Bickley, 2007). Meningeal irritation results in a number of other well-recognized signs common to all types of meningitis:

- Neck mobility: A stiff and painful neck (nuchal rigidity) can be an early sign and any attempts at flexion of the head are difficult because of spasms in the muscles of the neck. Normally the neck is supple, and the patient can easily bend the head and neck forward.
- Positive Kernig's sign: When the patient is lying with the thigh flexed on the abdomen, the leg cannot be completely extended (Fig. 64-1).
- Positive Brudzinski's sign: When the patient's neck is flexed (after ruling out cervical trauma or injury), flexion of the knees and hips is produced; when the lower extremity of one side is passively flexed, a similar movement is seen in the opposite extremity (see Fig. 64-1). Brudzinski's sign is a more sensitive indicator of meningeal irritation than Kernig's sign.
- Photophobia (extreme sensitivity to light): This finding is common, although the cause is unclear.

A rash can be a striking feature of *N. meningitidis* infection, occurring in about half of patients with this type of meningitis. Skin lesions develop, ranging from a petechial rash with purpuric lesions to large areas of ecchymosis.

Disorientation and memory impairment are common early in the course of the illness. The changes depend on the severity of the infection as well as the individual response to the physiologic processes. Behavioral manifestations are also common. As the illness progresses, lethargy, unresponsiveness, and coma may develop.

Seizures can occur and are the result of areas of irritability in the brain. ICP increases secondary to diffuse brain swelling or hydrocephalus (van de Beek, et al., 2006). The initial signs of increased ICP include decreased level of consciousness and focal motor deficits. If ICP is not controlled, the uncus of the temporal lobe may herniate through the tentorium, causing pressure on the brain stem. Brain stem herniation is a life-threatening event that causes cranial nerve dysfunction and depresses the centers of vital functions, such as the medulla. See Chapter 61 for discussion of the patient with a change in level of consciousness (LOC) or increased ICP.

An acute fulminant infection occurs in about 10% of patients with meningococcal meningitis, producing signs of overwhelming septicemia: an abrupt onset of high fever, extensive purpuric lesions (over the face and extremities), shock, and signs of disseminated intravascular coagulation (DIC). Death may occur within a few hours after onset of the infection.

Assessment and Diagnostic Findings

If the clinical presentation suggests meningitis, diagnostic testing is conducted to identify the causative organism. A computed tomography (CT) scan or magnetic resonance imaging (MRI) scan is used to detect a shift in brain contents (which may lead to herniation) prior to a lumbar puncture. Bacterial culture and Gram staining of CSF and blood are key diagnostic tests. CSF studies demonstrate low glucose, high protein levels, and high white blood cell count (Mazzoni, et al., 2006). Gram staining allows for rapid identification of the causative bacteria and initiation of appropriate antibiotic therapy (van de Beek, et al., 2006).

Researchers have developed a bedside risk score for use in adults with bacterial meningitis. Risks for an unfavorable outcome include older age, a heart rate of greater than 120 bpm, low Glasgow Coma score, cranial nerve palsies, and a positive Gram stain 1 hour after presentation to the hospital (Weisfelt, van de Beek, Spanjaard, et al., 2007).

Prevention

The Advisory Committee on Immunization Practices of the Centers for Disease Control and Prevention (CDC) (2008) recommends that the meningococcal conjugated vaccine be given to adolescents entering high school and to college freshmen living in dormitories. Freshmen living in dormitories have a three times greater risk of developing meningococcal meningitis as compared with the general population and students living off campus. Most states mandate education addressing meningococcal meningitis

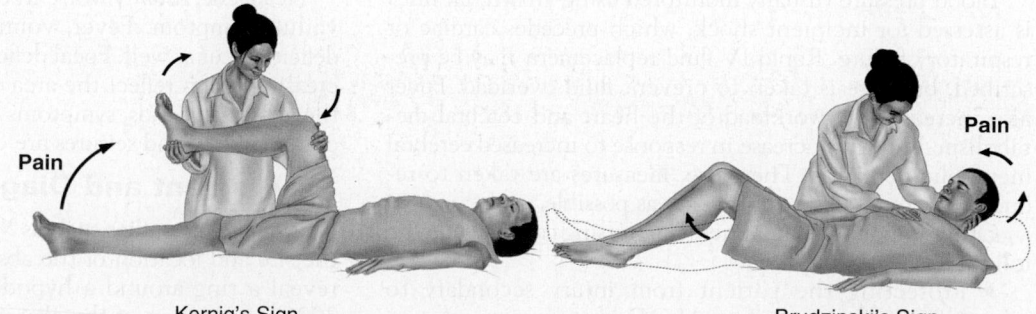

Figure 64-1 Testing for meningeal irritation. **A,** Kernig's sign. **B,** Brudzinski's sign.

Kernig's Sign

Brudzinski's Sign

and the availability of vaccination so that families can make informed decisions.

People in close contact with patients with meningococcal meningitis should be treated with antimicrobial chemoprophylaxis using rifampin (Rifadin), ciprofloxacin hydrochloride (Cipro), or ceftriaxone sodium (Rocephin). Therapy should be started within 24 hours after exposure because a delay in the initiation of therapy limits the effectiveness of the prophylaxis. Vaccination should also be considered as an adjunct to antibiotic chemoprophylaxis for anyone living with a person who develops meningococcal infection. Vaccination against *H. influenzae* and *S. pneumoniae* should be encouraged for children and at-risk adults (Matthews, Miller & Mott, 2007).

Medical Management

Successful outcomes depend on the early administration of an antibiotic that crosses the blood–brain barrier into the subarachnoid space in sufficient concentration to halt the multiplication of bacteria. Vancomycin hydrochloride in combination with one of the cephalosporins (eg, ceftriaxone sodium, cefotaxime sodium) is administered intravenously (IV) (van de Beek, et al., 2006).

Dexamethasone (Decadron) has been shown to be beneficial as adjunct therapy in the treatment of acute bacterial meningitis and in pneumococcal meningitis if it is administered 15 to 20 minutes before the first dose of antibiotic and every 6 hours for the next 4 days. Studies indicate that dexamethasone improves the outcome in adults and does not increase the risk of gastrointestinal bleeding (van de Beek, et al., 2006).

Dehydration and shock are treated with fluid volume expanders. Seizures, which may occur early in the course of the disease, are controlled with phenytoin (Dilantin). Increased ICP is treated as necessary (see Chapter 61).

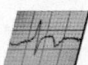 ## Nursing Management

The patient with meningitis is critically ill; therefore, many of the nursing interventions are collaborative with the physician, respiratory therapist, and other members of the health care team. The patient's safety and well-being depend on sound nursing judgment.

Neurologic status and vital signs are continually assessed. Pulse oximetry and arterial blood gas values are used to quickly identify the need for respiratory support if increasing ICP compromises the brain stem. Insertion of a cuffed endotracheal tube (or tracheotomy) and mechanical ventilation may be necessary to maintain adequate tissue oxygenation.

Blood pressure (usually monitored using an arterial line) is assessed for incipient shock, which precedes cardiac or respiratory failure. Rapid IV fluid replacement may be prescribed, but care is taken to prevent fluid overload. Fever also increases the workload of the heart and cerebral metabolism. ICP will increase in response to increased cerebral metabolic demands. Therefore, measures are taken to reduce body temperature as quickly as possible.

Other important components of nursing care include the following measures:

- Protecting the patient from injury secondary to seizure activity or altered LOC

- Monitoring daily body weight; serum electrolytes; and urine volume, specific gravity, and osmolality, especially if syndrome of inappropriate antidiuretic hormone (SIADH) is suspected
- Preventing complications associated with immobility, such as pressure ulcers and pneumonia
- Instituting infection control precautions until 24 hours after initiation of antibiotic therapy (oral and nasal discharge is considered infectious)

Any sudden, critical illness can be devastating to the family. Because the patient's condition is often critical and the prognosis guarded, the family needs to be informed about the patient's condition. Periodic family visits are essential to facilitate coping of the patient and family. An important aspect of the nurse's role is to support the family and assist them in identifying others who can be supportive to them during the crisis.

Brain Abscess

Brain abscesses account for less than 2% of space-occupying brain lesions in the United States and are more common in males during the first two decades of life (Mazzoni, et al., 2006). Brain abscesses are rare in immunocompetent people; they are more frequently diagnosed in people who are immunosuppressed as a result of an underlying disease or use of immunosuppressive mediations.

Pathophysiology

A brain abscess is a collection of infectious material within the tissue of the brain. Bacteria are the most common causative organisms. The most common predisposing conditions for abscesses among immunocompetent adults are otitis media and rhinosinusitis. An abscess can result from intracranial surgery, penetrating head injury, or tongue piercing. Organisms causing brain abscess may reach the brain by hematologic spread from the lungs, gums, tongue, or heart, or from a wound or intra-abdominal infection (Mazzoni, et al., 2006). Brain abscesses in immunocompromised people may result from various pathogens. To prevent brain abscess, otitis media, mastoiditis, rhinosinusitis, dental infections, and systemic infections should be treated promptly.

Clinical Manifestations

The clinical manifestations of a brain abscess result from alterations in intracranial dynamics (edema, brain shift), infection, or the location of the abscess (Chart 64-2).

Headache, usually worse in the morning, is the most prevailing symptom. Fever, vomiting, and focal neurologic deficits occur as well. Focal deficits such as weakness and decreasing vision reflect the area of brain that is involved. As the abscess expands, symptoms of increased ICP such as decreasing LOC and seizures are observed.

Assessment and Diagnostic Findings

Neuroimaging studies such as MRI or CT scanning identify the size and location of the abscess. The MRI or CT scans reveal a ring around a hypodense area (Mazzoni, et al., 2006). Aspiration of the abscess, guided by CT or MRI, is

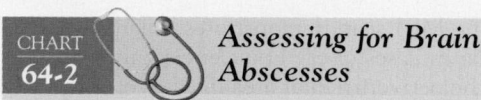

Assessing for Brain Abscesses

Be alert for the following signs and symptoms:

Frontal Lobe

Hemiparesis
Aphasia (expressive)
Seizures
Frontal headache

Temporal Lobe

Localized headache
Changes in vision
Facial weakness
Aphasia

Cerebellar Abscess

Occipital headache
Ataxia (inability to coordinate movements)
Nystagmus (rhythmic, involuntary movements of the eye)

the best method to culture and identify the infectious organism. Blood cultures are obtained if the abscess is believed to arise from a distant source. Chest x-ray is performed to rule out predisposing lung infections and an electroencephalogram (EEG) may help localize the lesion (Hickey, 2009).

Medical Management

Treatment is aimed at controlling increased ICP, draining the abscess, and providing antimicrobial therapy directed at the abscess and the primary source of infection. Large IV doses of antibiotics are administered to penetrate the blood–brain barrier and reach the abscess. The choice of the specific antibiotic medication is based on culture and sensitivity testing and directed at the causative organism. A stereotactic CT-guided aspiration may be used to drain the abscess and identify the causative organism. Corticosteroids may be prescribed to help reduce the inflammatory cerebral edema if the patient shows evidence of an increasing neurologic deficit. Antiseizure medications (phenytoin, phenobarbital) may be prescribed to prevent or treat seizures.

Nursing Management

Nursing care focuses on continuing to assess the neurologic status, administering medications, assessing the response to treatment, and providing supportive care.

Ongoing neurologic assessment alerts the nurse to changes in ICP, which may indicate a need for more aggressive intervention. The nurse also assesses and documents the responses to medications. Blood laboratory test results, specifically blood glucose and serum potassium levels, need to be closely monitored when corticosteroids are prescribed. Administration of insulin or electrolyte replacement may be required to return these values to normal or acceptable levels.

Patient safety is another key nursing responsibility. Injury may result from decreased LOC or falls related to motor weakness or seizures (Hughes, 2008).

The patient with a brain abscess is very ill, and neurologic deficits, such as hemiparesis, seizures, visual deficits, and cranial nerve palsies, may remain after treatment. Seizures are common sequelae. The nurse must assess the family's ability to express distress at the patient's condition, cope with the patient's illness and deficits, and obtain support.

Herpes Simplex Virus Encephalitis

Encephalitis is an acute inflammatory process of the brain tissue. Herpes simplex virus (HSV) is the most common cause of acute encephalitis in the United States (Mazzoni, et al., 2006). There are two herpes simplex viruses: HSV-1 and HSV-2. HSV-1 typically affects children and adults. HSV-2 most commonly affects neonates and is discussed in pediatric textbooks.

Pathophysiology

The pathology of encephalitis involves local necrotizing hemorrhage that becomes more generalized, followed by edema. There is also progressive deterioration of nerve cell bodies (Porth & Matfin, 2009).

Clinical Manifestations

The initial symptoms of HSV-1 encephalitis include fever, headache, and confusion. Focal neurologic symptoms reflect the areas of cerebral inflammation and necrosis and include fever, headache, behavioral changes, focal seizures, dysphasia, hemiparesis, and altered LOC (Porth & Matfin, 2009).

Assessment and Diagnostic Findings

Neuroimaging studies, such as EEG, and CSF examination are used to diagnose HSV encephalitis. MRI is the neuroimaging study of choice for detection of early changes caused by HSV-1; the study shows edema in the temporal lobe. The EEG shows diffuse slowing or focal changes in the temporal lobe in about 80% of patients (Mazzoni, et al., 2006). Lumbar puncture often reveals a high opening pressure and low glucose and high protein levels in CSF samples. Viral cultures are almost always negative. The polymerase chain reaction (PCR) is the standard test for early diagnosis of HSV-1 encephalitis. PCR identifies the DNA bands of HSV-1 in the CSF. The validity of PCR is very high between the 3rd and 10th days after symptom onset.

Medical Management

Acyclovir (Zovirax) or ganciclovir (Cytovene), antiviral agents, are the medications of choice in the treatment of HSV (Matthews, et al., 2007). Early administration of antiviral agents (usually well tolerated) improves the prognosis associated with HSV-1 encephalitis. The mode of action is inhibition of viral DNA replication. To prevent relapse, treatment should continue for up to 3 weeks. Slow IV administration over 1 hour prevents crystallization of the medication in the urine. The usual dose of acyclovir is decreased if the patient has a history of renal insufficiency. Studies are in progress to determine the effectiveness of an oral agent, valacyclovir hydrochloride (Valtrex), in the treatment of HSV-1 encephalitis.

Nursing Management

Assessment of neurologic function is key to monitoring the progression of disease. Comfort measures to reduce headache include dimming the lights, limiting noise and visitors, grouping nursing interventions, and administering analgesic agents (Matthews, et al., 2007). Opioid analgesic medications may mask neurologic symptoms; therefore, they are used cautiously. Seizures and altered LOC require care directed at injury prevention and safety. Nursing care addressing patient and family anxieties is ongoing throughout the illness. Monitoring of blood chemistry test results and urinary output alert the nurse to the presence of renal complications related to antiviral therapy.

Arthropod-Borne Virus Encephalitis

Arthropod vectors transmit several types of viruses that cause encephalitis. The primary vector in North America is the mosquito. In cases of West Nile virus, humans are the secondary host; birds are the primary host. Arbovirus infection (transmitted by arthropod vectors) occurs in specific geographic areas during the summer and fall. In the United States, West Nile and St. Louis are the most common types of arboviral encephalitis; both are members of the Japanese encephalitis serogroup. West Nile virus develops in 1 out of 150 cases of encephalitis (Matthews, et al., 2007; Mazzoni, et al., 2006).

Pathophysiology

Viral replication occurs at the site of the mosquito bite. The host immune response attempts to control viral replication. If the immune response is inadequate, viremia will ensue. The virus gains access to the central nervous system (CNS) via the cerebral capillaries, resulting in encephalitis. It spreads from neuron to neuron, predominantly affecting the cortical gray matter, the brain stem, and the thalamus. Meningeal exudates compound the clinical presentation by irritating the meninges and increasing ICP.

Clinical Manifestations

St. Louis and West Nile encephalitis most commonly affect adults. Climate, an environment conducive to arthropod proliferation, and human behavior contribute to the occurrence of St. Louis and West Nile encephalitis. An arboviral encephalitis begins with early flulike symptoms, but specific neurologic manifestations depend on the viral type. A unique clinical feature of St. Louis encephalitis is SIADH with hyponatremia. Signs and symptoms specific to West Nile encephalitis include a maculopapular or morbilliform rash on the neck, trunk, and arms; enlarged lymph nodes and legs; and flaccid paralysis (Matthews, et al., 2007). Both West Nile and St. Louis encephalitis can result in parkinsonianlike movements, reflecting inflammation of the basal ganglia. Seizures, a poor prognostic indicator, are present in both types of encephalitis but are more common in the St. Louis type.

Assessment and Diagnostic Findings

After a brief febrile prodrome, neurologic symptoms reflect the area of the brain that is involved. Neuroimaging and CSF evaluation are useful in the diagnosis of arboviral encephalitis. The MRI scan demonstrates inflammation of the basal ganglia in cases of St. Louis encephalitis and inflammation in the periventricular area in cases of West Nile encephalitis. Immunoglobulin M antibodies to West Nile virus are observed in serum and CSF. Serum cultures are not useful, because the viremia is brief. PCR evaluation of CSF may demonstrate viral ribonucleic acid (RNA).

Medical Management

No specific medication for arboviral encephalitis includes controlling the seizures and the increased ICP. Interferon may be useful in treating St. Louis encephalitis. Ribavirin and interferon alpha-2b show some effect against West Nile virus but have not been evaluated in controlled studies (Tunkel, Glaser, Block, et al., 2008). Neuropsychiatric complications, such as emotional outbursts and other behavior changes, occur frequently.

Nursing Management

If the patient is very ill, hospitalization may be required. The nurse carefully assesses neurologic status and identifies improvement or deterioration in the patient's condition. Injury prevention is key in light of the potential for falls or seizures. Arboviral encephalitis may result in death or lifelong residual health issues such as neurologic deficits and seizures (Mazzoni, et al., 2006). The family will need support and teaching to cope with these outcomes.

Public education addressing the prevention of arboviral encephalitis is a key nursing role. Clothing that provides coverage and insect repellents containing 25% to 30% diethyltoluamide (DEET) should be used on exposed clothing and skin in high-risk areas to decrease mosquito and tick bites. Screens should be in good repair in the home, and standing water should be removed. Blood donation centers screen all blood for West Nile virus. Cases of West Nile virus must be reported to the CDC.

Fungal Encephalitis

Fungal infections of the CNS occur rarely in healthy people. The presentation of fungal encephalitis is related to geographic area or to an immune system that is compromised due to disease or immunosuppressive medication. Causes of fungal infections include *Cryptococcus neoformans, Blastomyces dermatitidis, Histoplasma capsulatum, Aspergillus fumigatus, Candida,* and *Coccidioides immitis* (Mazzoni, et al., 2006). *C. immitis* is found mainly in California, Arizona, New Mexico, and Texas. *B. dermatitidis* exists in the southeastern United States and in the Ohio, St. Lawrence, and Mississippi River basins. It is a risk for coal miners, construction workers, and farmers. *C. neoformans* is associated with exposure to bird droppings and may be seen in bird handlers.

Pathophysiology

The fungal spores enter the body via inhalation. They initially infect the lungs, causing vague respiratory symptoms or pneumonitis. The fungi may enter the bloodstream, causing a fungemia. If the fungemia overwhelms the person's immune system, the fungus may spread to the CNS. The fungal invasion may cause meningitis, encephalitis, brain abscess, granuloma, or arterial thrombus (Mazzoni, et al., 2006).

Clinical Manifestations

The common symptoms of fungal encephalitis include fever, malaise, headache, meningeal signs, and change in LOC or cranial nerve dysfunction. Symptoms of increased ICP related to hydrocephalus often occur. C. *neoformans* and C. *immitis* are associated with specific skin lesions. H. *capsulatum* is associated with seizures, and A. *fumigatus* may cause ischemic or hemorrhagic strokes.

Assessment and Diagnostic Findings

A history of immunosuppression associated with AIDS or use of immunosuppressive medications may indicate fungal disease of the brain. Occupational and travel history may point to a fungal cause of CNS infection. Infections caused by H. *capsulatum* and C. *immitis* will demonstrate fungal antibodies in serologic tests. The CSF usually demonstrates elevated white cell and protein levels; glucose levels are decreased. C. *neoformans* is easily identified in CSF fungal cultures. *Candida* may be cultured from the blood or CSF. To identify B. *dermatitidis*, cisternal or ventricular cultures of CSF may need to be obtained. A. *fumigatus* is difficult to isolate in CSF and is diagnosed by lung biopsy. Neuroimaging is used to identify CNS changes related to fungal infection. MRI is the study of choice; it demonstrates areas of hemorrhage, abscess, or enhanced meninges indicating inflammation.

Medical Management

Medical management is directed at the causative fungus and the neurologic consequences of the infection. Seizures are controlled by standard antiseizure medications. Increased ICP is controlled by repeated lumbar punctures or shunting of CSF.

Antifungal agents are administered for a specific period to cure the infection in patients with competent immune systems. Patients with compromised immune systems receive antifungal therapy until the infection is controlled, after which they receive a maintenance dose of the medication for an indefinite period. Although the dose and duration of treatment depend on the causative fungi, amphotericin B is the standard antifungal agent used in treatment. Dosing depends on the causative organism, and it is usually administered by IV. The most common adverse reactions are fever, nausea and vomiting, anemia, uremia, and hypokalemia (Mazzoni, et al., 2006). Renal insufficiency is a serious reaction to amphotericin B that can occur. Fluconazole (Diflucan) or flucytosine (Ancobon) may be administered orally in conjunction with amphotericin B as maintenance therapy. Potential side effects of fluconazole include nausea, vomiting, and a transient increase in liver enzymes. The most common adverse reaction to flucytosine is bone marrow suppression. Therefore, patients receiving flucytosine should have leukocyte and platelet counts monitored regularly.

Nursing Management

The ICP will increase if hydrocephalus develops and the inflammatory response progresses. Nursing assessment aimed at early identification of increased ICP is necessary to ensure

early control and management. (See Chapter 61 for management of the patient with increased ICP.) Administering nonopioid analgesic agents, limiting environmental stimuli, and positioning may optimize patient comfort. Administering diphenhydramine (Benadryl) and acetaminophen (Tylenol) approximately 30 minutes before giving amphotericin B may prevent flulike side effects. If renal insufficiency develops, the dose may need to be reduced. Increasing levels of serum creatinine and blood urea nitrogen (BUN) may alert the nurse to the development of renal insufficiency and the need to address the patient's renal status.

Providing support assists the patient and family to cope with the illness. Workup of the patient for immunodeficiency diseases such as AIDS may put additional stress on the family. The nurse may need to mobilize community support systems for the patient and family, because the recovery may be long.

Creutzfeldt-Jakob and Variant Creutzfeldt-Jakob Disease

Creutzfeldt-Jakob disease (CJD) and variant Creutzfeldt-Jakob disease (vCJD) belong to a group of degenerative, infectious neurologic disorders called transmissible spongiform encephalopathies (TSE). CJD is very rare and has no identifiable cause. vCJD is the human variation of bovine spongiform encephalopathy (BSE); it results from the ingestion by humans of prions in infected beef. TSEs are caused by **prions,** proteinaceous particles that are smaller than a virus and are resistant to standard methods of sterilization. Although CJD and vCJD have distinct clinical features, one characteristic they share is a lack of CNS inflammation. CJD may lie dormant for decades before causing neurologic degeneration. The incubation period of vCJD seems to be shorter (less than 10 years). It is not known whether an increased number of cases will appear in the future. In both diseases, the symptoms are progressive, there is no definitive treatment, and the outcome is fatal.

About 150 cases of vCJD have been reported, almost all in the United Kingdom (Mazzoni, et al., 2006). The risk of vCJD in the United States is thought to be low, because cattle are fed primarily with soy-derived feed as opposed to feed containing animal parts.

Pathophysiology

The prion is a unique pathogen because it lacks nucleic acid, which enables the organism to withstand conventional means of sterilization. How the prion replicates in the absence of nucleic acid is unknown (Glatzel, Stoeck, Seeger, et al., 2005). In both CJD and vCJD, the prion crosses the blood–brain barrier and is deposited in brain tissue and causes degeneration of brain tissue. Cell death occurs, and spongy vacuoles are produced in the brain (**spongiform** changes). The spongiform vacuoles are surrounded by amyloid plaque.

Ninety percent of the cases of CJD appear sporadically; the incidence is 1 case per 1 million people. Although it is not transmittable by typical human contact, 5% of cases of sporadic CJD result from contaminated neurosurgical instruments, cadaver-derived growth factor, or corneal transplants. Ten percent of cases appear to be familial (Ward, Everington, Cousens, et al., 2007).

In 1996 the first case of vCJD was described. The mode of transmission was linked to the ingestion of beef contaminated with neurologic tissue. In 1998, additional concerns were raised about the safety of the blood supply in the United Kingdom. The prion exists in lymphoid tissue and blood in both vCJD and CJD. Both prion diseases are believed to be blood-borne. No method is available to screen blood for infectivity. The American Red Cross will not accept blood from anyone who has traveled to Europe in the past 6 months.

Clinical Manifestations

CJD and vCJD have several clinically distinct features. Psychiatric symptoms occur early in vCJD, whereas they are a late symptom in CJD. The mean age at onset of vCJD is 27 years, whereas the mean age for CJD onset is 50 years. The presenting symptoms of vCJD include affective symptoms (ie, behavioral changes), sensory disturbance, and limb pain. Muscle spasms and rigidity, dysarthria, incoordination, cognitive impairment, and sleep disturbances follow. Patients with sporadic CJD present with mental deterioration, ataxia, and visual disturbance. Memory loss, involuntary movement, paralysis, and mutism occur as the disease progresses. After clinical presentation, people with vCJD survive an average of 22 months; those with CJD survive for about 6 months (Mazzoni, et al., 2006).

Assessment and Diagnostic Findings

Historically, brain biopsy was used to diagnose CJD. The three diagnostic tests currently used in suspicious clinical presentations to support the diagnosis of CJD are immunologic assessment, electroencephalography, and MRI scanning. Immunologic assessment of CSF detects a protein kinase inhibitor called 14-3-3. The presence of this inhibitor indicates neuronal cell death, which is not specific to CJD but does support the diagnosis. The EEG reveals a characteristic pattern over the duration of the disease. After initial slowing, the EEG shows periodic activity. Later in the course of the disease, the EEG shows burst-suppressions characterized by periodic spikes alternating with slow periods. The MRI scan demonstrates symmetric or unilateral hyperintense signals arising from the basal ganglia.

Patients with vCJD do not demonstrate EEG or CSF changes, and the MRI scan shows bilateral hyperintensity of the posterior thalamus. The prion associated with vCJD has been shown to accumulate in the tonsils and other lymphoreticular tissues; therefore, tonsillar biopsy may be used in the diagnosis of vCJD.

Medical Management

After the onset of specific neurologic symptoms, progression of disease occurs quickly. There is no effective treatment for CJD or vCJD. The care of the patient is supportive and palliative. Goals of care include prevention of injury related to immobility and dementia, promotion of patient comfort, and provision of support and education for the family.

Nursing Management

The nursing care of patients is primarily supportive and palliative. Psychological and emotional support of the patient and family throughout the course of the illness is needed.

Care extends to providing for a dignified death and supporting the family through the processes of grief and loss. Hospice services are appropriate either at home or at an inpatient facility. See Chapter 17 for an in-depth discussion of end-of-life issues.

Prevention of disease transmission is an important part of nursing care. Although patient isolation is not necessary, use of standard precautions is important. Institutional protocols are followed for blood and body fluid exposure and decontamination of equipment. In the operating room, it is recommended that disposable instruments be used and then incinerated, because conventional methods of sterilization do not destroy the prion. The World Health Organization has guidelines that outline the stringent sterilization methods that must be used to destroy prions on surfaces.

AUTOIMMUNE PROCESSES

Autoimmune nervous system disorders include multiple sclerosis, myasthenia gravis, and Guillain-Barré syndrome.

Multiple Sclerosis

Multiple sclerosis (MS) is an immune-mediated, progressive demyelinating disease of the CNS. Demyelination refers to the destruction of myelin, the fatty and protein material that surrounds certain nerve fibers in the brain and spinal cord; it results in impaired transmission of nerve impulses (Fig. 64-2). MS may occur at any age but typically manifests in young adults between the ages of 20 and 40 years; it affects women more frequently than men (Porth & Matfin, 2009).

The cause of MS is an area of ongoing research (Costello & Sipe, 2008). Autoimmune activity results in demyelination, but the sensitized antigen has not been identified. Multiple factors play a role in the initiation of the immune process. Geographic prevalence is highest in Europe, New Zealand, southern Australia, the northern United States, and southern Canada (Olek, 2005). Researchers believe that some environmental exposure at a young age may play a role in the development of MS later in life.

Genetic predisposition is indicated by the presence of a specific cluster (haplotype) of human leukocyte antigens (HLAs) on the cell wall. Its presence may increase susceptibility to factors, such as viruses, that trigger the autoimmune response activated in MS. A specific virus capable of initiating the autoimmune response has not been identified. It is believed that deoxyribonucleic acid (DNA) on the virus mimics the amino acid sequence of myelin, resulting in an immune system cross-reaction in the presence of a defective immune system.

Pathophysiology

Sensitized T and B lymphocytes cross the blood–brain barrier; their function is to check the CNS for antigens and then leave. In MS, sensitized T cells remain in the CNS and promote the infiltration of other agents that damage the immune system. The immune system attack leads to inflammation that destroys myelin (which normally insulates the

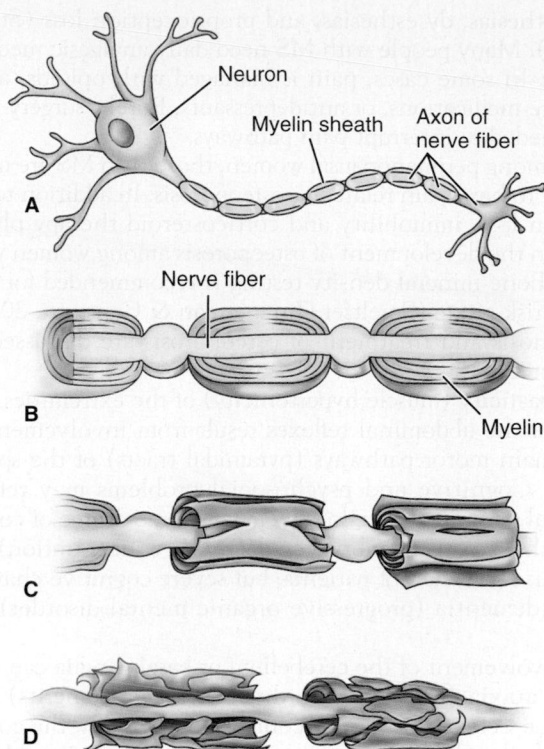

Figure 64-2 The process of demyelination. **A** and **B** depict a normal nerve cell and axon with myelin. **C** and **D** show the slow disintegration of myelin, resulting in a disruption in axon function.

axon and speeds the conduction of impulses along the axon) and the oligodendroglial cells that produce myelin in the CNS.

Demyelination interrupts the flow of nerve impulses and results in a variety of manifestations, depending on the nerves affected. Plaques appear on demyelinated axons, further interrupting the transmission of impulses. Demyelinated axons are scattered irregularly throughout the CNS (Fig. 64-3). The areas most frequently affected are the optic nerves, chiasm, and tracts; the cerebrum; the brain stem and cerebellum; and the spinal cord. The axons themselves begin to degenerate, resulting in permanent and irreversible damage (Costello & Sipe, 2008; Porth & Matfin, 2009).

Clinical Manifestations

The course of MS may assume many different patterns (Fig. 64-4) (Lublin & Reingold, 1996). In some patients, the disease follows a benign course, and symptoms are so mild that the patient does not seek health care or treatment. Between 80% and 85% of patients with MS have a relapsing-remitting (RR) course. With each relapse, recovery is usually complete; however, residual deficits may occur and accumulate over time, contributing to functional decline. Fifty percent of those with the RR course of MS progress to a secondary progressive course, in which disease progression occurs with or without relapses. Ten percent of patients have a primary progressive course, in which disabling symptoms steadily increase, with rare plateaus and temporary improvement. Primary progressive MS may result in quadriparesis, cognitive dysfunction,

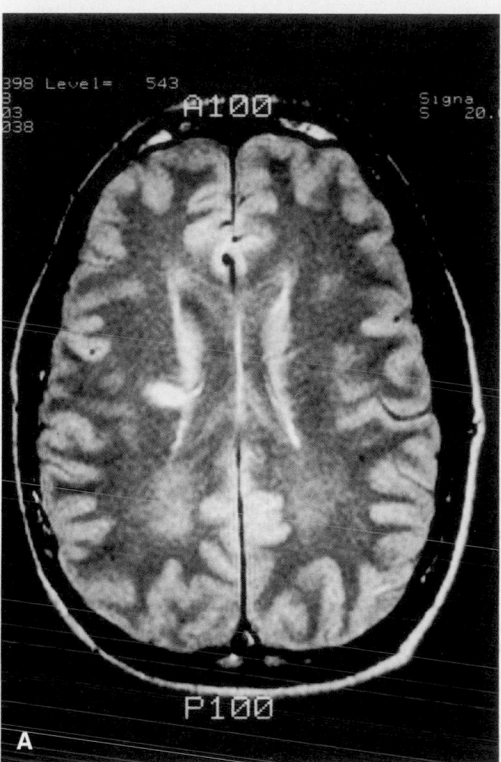

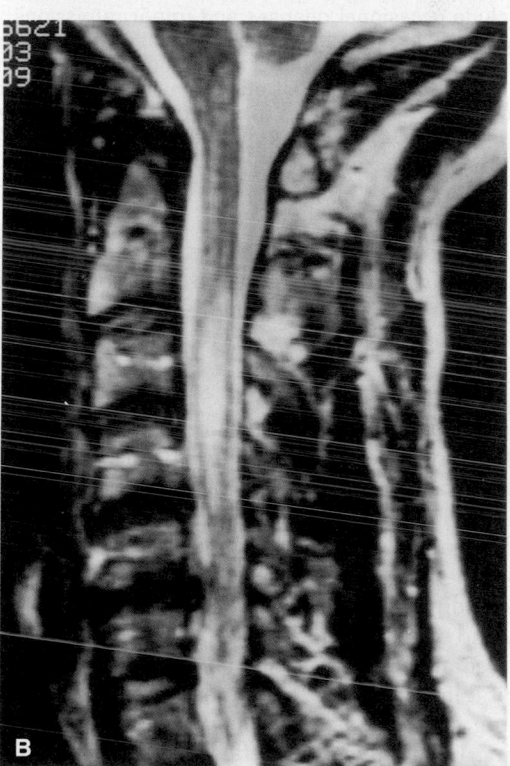

Figure 64-3 Multiple sclerosis. **A,** A computed tomography scan of brain demonstrates an area of demyelination in the periventricular white matter of the right frontal lobe. The plaque is perpendicular to the lateral ventricle, a typical finding in multiple sclerosis. **B,** A magnetic resonance image of the spinal cord in the same patient highlights another typical finding: a flame-shaped area of demyelination within the midcervical region of the spinal cord. Courtesy of the Danbury Hospital Department of Radiology.

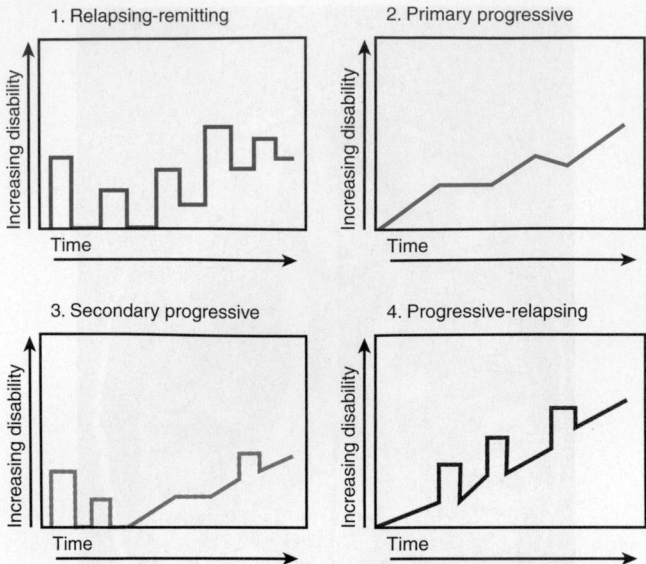

Figure 64-4 Types and courses of multiple sclerosis (MS). **1,** Relapsing-remitting (RR) MS is characterized by clearly acute attacks with full recovery or with sequelae and residual deficit upon recovery. Periods between disease relapses are characterized by lack of disease progression. **2,** Primary progressive (PP) MS is characterized by disease showing progression of disability from onset, without plateaus and temporary minor improvements. **3,** Secondary progressive (SP) MS begins with an initial RR course, followed by progression of variable rate, which may also include occasional relapses and minor remissions. **4,** Progressive-relapsing (PR) MS shows progression from onset but with clear acute relapses with or without recovery. From Lublin, F. D. & Reingold, S. C. (1996). Defining the clinical course of multiple sclerosis: Results of an international survey. *Neurology, 46*(64), 907–911. Used with permission from Lippincott Williams & Wilkins.

visual loss, and brain stem syndromes. The least common presentation (about 5% of cases) is the progressive relapsing course. It is characterized by relapses with continuous disabling progression between exacerbations (Mazzoni, et al., 2006).

The signs and symptoms of MS are varied and multiple, reflecting the location of the lesion (plaque) or combination of lesions. The primary symptoms most commonly reported are fatigue, depression, weakness, numbness, difficulty in coordination, loss of balance, and pain (Johnson, 2008; Newland, 2008). Visual disturbances due to lesions in the optic nerves or their connections may include blurring of vision, **diplopia** (double vision), patchy blindness (scotoma), and total blindness.

Fatigue affects most people with MS and is often the most disabling symptom. Heat, depression, anemia, deconditioning, and medication may contribute to fatigue. Avoiding hot temperatures, effective treatment of depression and anemia, and occupational and physical therapies may help control fatigue. Additional strategies include a balance of rest and activities, good nutrition, and a healthy lifestyle including avoidance of alcohol and cigarette smoking (Iggulden, 2006; Johnson, 2008).

Pain is another common symptom of MS that can contribute to social isolation. Lesions on the sensory pathways cause pain. Additional sensory manifestations include

paresthesias, dysesthesias, and proprioception loss (Stern, 2005). Many people with MS need daily analgesic medications. In some cases, pain is managed with opioids, antiseizure medications, or antidepressants. Rarely, surgery may be needed to interrupt pain pathways.

Among perimenopausal women, those with MS are more likely to have pain related to osteoporosis. In addition to estrogen loss, immobility and corticosteroid therapy play a role in the development of osteoporosis among women with MS. Bone mineral density testing is recommended for this high-risk group (Smeltzer, Zimmerman & Capriotti, 2005). Diagnosis and treatment of osteoporosis are discussed in Chapter 68.

Spasticity (muscle hypertonicity) of the extremities and loss of the abdominal reflexes result from involvement of the main motor pathways (pyramidal tracts) of the spinal cord. Cognitive and psychosocial problems may reflect frontal or parietal lobe involvement. Some degree of cognitive change (eg, memory loss, decreased concentration) occurs in about half of patients, but severe cognitive changes with dementia (progressive organic mental disorder) are rare.

Involvement of the cerebellum or basal ganglia can produce **ataxia** (impaired coordination of movements) and tremor. Loss of the control connections between the cortex and the basal ganglia may occur and cause emotional lability and euphoria. Bladder, bowel, and sexual dysfunctions are common.

Secondary complications of MS include urinary tract infections, constipation, pressure ulcers, contracture deformities, dependent pedal edema, pneumonia, reactive depression, and osteoporosis. Emotional, social, marital, economic, and vocational problems may also occur.

Exacerbations and remissions are characteristic of MS. During exacerbations, new symptoms appear and existing ones worsen; during remissions, symptoms decrease or disappear. Relapses may be associated with emotional and physical stress.

 Gerontologic Considerations

The life expectancy for patients with MS is not dramatically different from that of patients without MS; those diagnosed with secondary progressive disease live an average of 35 years after onset (Mazzoni, et al., 2006). Patients with MS who are elderly have specific physical and psychosocial challenges. They may have chronic health problems, for which they may be taking additional medications that could interact with medications prescribed for MS. The absorption, distribution, metabolism, and excretion of medications are altered in the elderly as a result of age-related changes in renal and liver functions. Therefore, elderly patients must be monitored closely for adverse and toxic effects of MS medications and for osteoporosis (particularly with frequent corticosteroid use that may be needed to treat exacerbations). The cost of medications may lead to poor adherence to the prescribed regimen in elderly patients on fixed incomes.

Elderly patients with MS are particularly concerned about increasing disability, family burden, marital concern, and the possible future need for nursing home care. Immobility resulting in fewer social opportunities contributes to loneliness and depression. Along with functional loss, spasticity, pain and bladder dysfunction, impaired sleep, and an increased need for assistance with self-care contribute to the physical challenges experienced by the elderly patient with MS (Stern, 2005).

Assessment and Diagnostic Findings

The diagnosis of MS is based on the presence of multiple plaques in the CNS observed with MRI (Mazzoni, et al., 2006). Electrophoresis of CSF identifies the presence of oligoclonal banding (several bands of immunoglobulin G bonded together, indicating an immune system abnormality). Evoked potential studies can help define the extent of the disease process and monitor changes. Underlying bladder dysfunction is diagnosed by urodynamic studies. Neuropsychological testing may be indicated to assess cognitive impairment. A sexual history helps identify changes in sexual function.

Medical Management

No cure exists for MS. An individual treatment program is indicated to relieve the patient's symptoms and provide continuing support, particularly for patients with cognitive changes, who may need more structure and support. The goals of treatment are to delay the progression of the disease, manage chronic symptoms, and treat acute exacerbations. Many patients with MS have a stable disease course and require only intermittent treatment, whereas others experience steady progression of their disease. Symptoms requiring intervention include spasticity, fatigue, bladder dysfunction, and ataxia. Management strategies target the various motor and sensory symptoms and effects of immobility that can occur.

Pharmacologic Therapy

Medications prescribed for MS include those for disease modification and those for symptom management. The disease-modifying therapies available to treat MS include immunomodulating therapies and immunosuppressive agents (Ross, Hackbarth, Rohl, et al., 2008).

Disease-Modifying Therapies

The disease-modifying medications reduce the frequency of relapse, the duration of relapse, and the number and size of plaques observed on MRI. All of the medications require injection.

Interferon beta-1a (Rebif) and interferon beta-1b (Betaseron) are administered subcutaneously. Another preparation of interferon beta-1a, Avonex, is administered intramuscularly once a week. Side effects of all the interferon-beta medications include flulike symptoms that can be managed with acetaminophen and ibuprofen and resolve after a few months. Additional side effects include potential liver damage, fetal abnormalities, and depression. For optimal control of disability, disease-modifying medications should be started early in the course of the disease (Ross, et al., 2008).

Glatiramer acetate (Copaxone) reduces the rate of relapse in the RR course of MS. It decreases the number of plaques noted on MRI and increases the time between relapses. Copaxone is administered subcutaneously daily. It

acts by increasing the antigen-specific suppressor T cells. Side effects are minimal and manageable (Miller & Jezewski, 2006). Copaxone is an option for those with an RR course; however, it may take 6 months for evidence of an immune response to appear.

IV methylprednisolone, the key agent in treating acute relapse in the RR course, shortens the duration of relapse. It exerts anti-inflammatory effects by acting on T cells and cytokines. One gram is administered IV daily for 3 days, followed by an oral taper of prednisone. Side effects include mood swings, weight gain, and electrolyte imbalances (Mazzoni, et al., 2006).

The medication mitoxantrone (Novantrone) is administered via IV infusion every 3 months. Novantrone can reduce the frequency of clinical relapses in patients with secondary-progressive or worsening relapsing-remitting MS. Patients must be very closely monitored for side effects, especially cardiac toxicity.

Symptom Management

Medications are also prescribed for management of specific symptoms. Baclofen (Lioresal), a gamma-aminobutyric acid (GABA) agonist, is the medication of choice for treating spasticity. It can be administered orally or by intrathecal injection for severe spasticity (Ridley & Rawlings, 2006). Benzodiazepines (Valium), tizanidine (Zanaflex), and dantrolene (Dantrium) may also be used to treat spasticity. Patients with disabling spasms and contractures may require nerve blocks or surgical intervention. Fatigue that interferes with activities of daily living (ADLs) may be treated with amantadine (Symmetrel), pemoline (Cylert), or fluoxetine (Prozac). Ataxia is a chronic problem most resistant to treatment. Medications used to treat ataxia include beta-adrenergic blockers (Inderal), antiseizure agents (Neurontin), and benzodiazepines (Klonopin).

Bladder and bowel problems are often among the most difficult ones for patients, and a variety of medications (anticholinergic agents, alpha-adrenergic blockers, antispasmodic agents) may be prescribed. Nonpharmacologic strategies also assist in establishing effective bowel and bladder elimination (see later discussion).

Urinary tract infection is often superimposed on the underlying neurologic dysfunction. Ascorbic acid (vitamin C) may be prescribed to acidify the urine, making bacterial growth less likely. Antibiotics are prescribed when appropriate.

NURSING PROCESS

THE PATIENT WITH MULTIPLE SCLEROSIS

Assessments

Nursing assessment addresses neurologic deficits, secondary complications, and the impact of the disease on the patient and family. The patient's mobility and balance are observed to determine whether there is risk of falling. Assessment of function is carried out both when the patient is well rested and when fatigued. The patient is assessed for weakness, spasticity, visual impairment, incontinence, and disorders of swallowing and speech. Additional areas of assessment include how MS has affected the patient's lifestyle, how the patient is coping, and what the patient would like to improve.

Diagnosis

Nursing Diagnoses

Based on the assessment data, the patient's major nursing diagnoses may include the following:

- Impaired bed and physical mobility related to weakness, muscle paresis, spasticity
- Risk for injury related to sensory and visual impairment
- Impaired urinary and bowel elimination (urgency, frequency, incontinence, constipation) related to nervous system dysfunction
- Impaired verbal communication and risk for aspiration related to cranial nerve involvement
- Disturbed thought processes (loss of memory, dementia, euphoria) related to cerebral dysfunction
- Ineffective individual coping related to uncertainty of course of MS
- Impaired home maintenance management related to physical, psychological, and social limits imposed by MS
- Potential for sexual dysfunction related to lesions or psychological reaction

Planning and Goals

The major goals for the patient may include promotion of physical mobility, avoidance of injury, achievement of bladder and bowel continence, promotion of speech and swallowing mechanisms, improvement of cognitive function, development of coping strengths, improved home maintenance management, and adaptation to sexual dysfunction.

Nursing Interventions

An individualized program of physical therapy, rehabilitation, and education is combined with emotional support. An educational plan of care is developed to enable the person with MS to deal with the physiologic, social, and psychological problems that accompany chronic disease. Research shows that depression, pain, fatigue, and walking difficulty all decrease physical activity (Motl, Snook & Schapiro, 2007). Assisting patients with management of these symptoms may help increase the level of physical activity and overall sense of well-being. (Chart 64-3).

Promoting Physical Mobility

Relaxation and coordination exercises promote muscle efficiency. Progressive resistive exercises are used to strengthen weak muscles, because diminishing muscle strength is often significant in MS.

EXERCISES. Walking improves the gait, particularly the problem of loss of position sense of the legs and feet. If certain muscle groups are irreversibly affected, other muscles can be trained to compensate. Instruction in the use of assistive devices may be needed to ensure their safe and correct use.

MINIMIZING SPASTICITY AND CONTRACTURES. Muscle spasticity is common and, in its later stages, is characterized by severe adductor spasm of the hips with flexor spasm of the hips and knees. Without relief, fibrous contractures of these joints occur. Warm packs may be beneficial, but hot baths should be avoided because of risk of burn injury secondary to sensory loss and increasing symptoms that may occur with elevation of the body temperature.

| CHART 64-3 | **NURSING RESEARCH PROFILE** *Physical Activity in People With Multiple Sclerosis* |

Motl, R. W., Snook, E. M. & Schapiro, R. T. (2007). Symptoms and physical activity behavior in individuals with multiple sclerosis. *Research in Nursing & Health, 31*(5), 466–475.

Purpose

Physical activity is a unique challenge for people with multiple sclerosis (MS). This study examined the relationships among overall and specific symptoms, such as difficulty walking and other physical activity issues in people with MS.

Design

In this cross-sectional descriptive study, 133 people (104 women and 78 men) with MS completed questionnaires measuring overall and specific symptoms (ie, depression, pain, and fatigue), difficulty walking, and physical activity. The purpose was to examine the relationships between overall and specific symptoms, difficulty walking, and physical activity. Participants in the study were recruited from local MS support groups over a 6-month time period.

Findings

The descriptive findings of the study showed that those with MS who have more intense overall symptoms had more difficulty walking and lower levels of physical activity. The path analysis suggested that higher levels of physical symptoms were directly and indirectly related to lower levels of physical activity. Another important finding was that the indirect pathway involved difficulty walking.

Nursing Implications

People with MS who have intense overall symptoms have a reduction in physical activity in comparison to those with MS and less intense overall symptoms. This study found that the reduction in physical activity can be partly explained by walking difficulty. The authors suggest that nursing interventions to promote physical activity in people with MS might need to include adaptive activities that do not require a lot of walking.

Daily exercises for muscle stretching are prescribed to minimize joint contractures. Special attention is given to the hamstrings, gastrocnemius muscles, hip adductors, biceps, and wrist and finger flexors. Muscle spasticity is common and interferes with normal function. A stretch–hold–relax routine is helpful for relaxing and treating muscle spasticity. Swimming and stationary bicycling are useful, and progressive weight bearing can relieve spasticity in the legs. The patient should not be hurried in any of these activities, because this often increases spasticity.

ACTIVITY AND REST. The patient is encouraged to work and exercise to a point just short of fatigue. Very strenuous physical exercise is not advisable, because it raises the body temperature and may aggravate symptoms. The patient is advised to take frequent short rest periods, preferably lying down. Extreme fatigue may contribute to the exacerbation of symptoms.

MINIMIZING EFFECTS OF IMMOBILITY. Because of the decrease in physical activity that often occurs with MS, complications associated with immobility, including pressure ulcers, expiratory muscle weakness, and accumulation of bronchial secretions, need to be considered and steps taken to prevent them. Measures to prevent such complications include assessing and maintaining skin integrity and having the patient perform coughing and deep-breathing exercises.

Preventing Injury

If motor dysfunction causes problems of incoordination and clumsiness, or if ataxia is apparent, the patient is at risk for falling. To overcome this disability, the patient is taught to walk with feet apart to widen the base of support and to increase walking stability. If loss of position sense occurs, the patient is taught to watch the feet while walking. Gait training may require assistive devices (walker, cane, braces, crutches, parallel bars) and instruction about their use by a physical therapist. If the gait remains inefficient, a wheelchair or motorized scooter may be the solution. The occupational therapist is a valuable resource person in suggesting and securing aids to promote independence. If incoordination is a problem and tremor of the upper extremities occurs when voluntary movement is attempted (intention tremor), weighted bracelets or wrist cuffs are helpful. The patient is trained in transfer and activities of daily living (ADLs).

Because sensory loss may occur in addition to motor loss, pressure ulcers are a continuing threat to skin integrity. The need to use a wheelchair continuously increases the risk. See Chapter 11 for a discussion of the prevention and treatment of pressure ulcers.

Enhancing Bladder and Bowel Control

Generally, bladder symptoms fall into the following categories: (1) inability to store urine (hyperreflexic, uninhibited); (2) inability to empty the bladder (hyporeflexic, hypotonic); and (3) a mixture of both types. The patient with urinary frequency, urgency, or incontinence requires special support. The sensation of the need to void must be heeded immediately, so the bedpan or urinal should be readily available. A voiding time schedule is set up (every 1.5 to 2 hours initially, with gradual lengthening of the interval).

The patient is instructed to drink a measured amount of fluid every 2 hours and then attempt to void 30 minutes after drinking. Use of a timer or wristwatch with an alarm may be helpful for the patient who does not have enough sensation to signal the need to empty the bladder. The nurse encourages the patient to take the prescribed medications to treat bladder spasticity, because this allows greater independence. Intermittent self-catheterization (see Chapter 11) has been successful in maintaining bladder control in patients with MS. If a female patient has permanent urinary incontinence, urinary diversion procedures may be considered. The male patient may wear a condom appliance for urine collection.

Bowel problems include constipation, fecal impaction, and incontinence. Adequate fluids, dietary fiber, and a bowel-training program are frequently effective in solving these problems. See Chapter 11 for a discussion of promoting bowel continence.

Enhancing Communication and Managing Swallowing Difficulties

If the cranial nerves that control the mechanisms of speech and swallowing are affected, dysarthrias (defects of articulation) marked by slurring, low volume of speech, and difficulties in phonation may occur. **Dysphagia** (difficulty swallowing) may also occur. A speech therapist evaluates speech and swallowing and instructs the patient, family, and health team members about strategies to compensate for speech and swallowing problems. The nurse reinforces this instruction and encourages the patient and family to adhere to the plan. Impaired swallowing increases the patient's risk of aspiration; therefore, strategies are needed to reduce that risk. Such strategies include having suction apparatus available, careful feeding, and proper positioning for eating.

Improving Sensory and Cognitive Function

Measures may be taken if visual defects or changes in cognitive status occur.

VISION. The cranial nerves affecting vision may be affected by MS. An eye patch or a covered eyeglass lens may be used to block the visual impulses of one eye if the patient has diplopia (double vision). Prism glasses may be helpful for patients who are confined to bed and have difficulty reading in the supine position. People who are unable to read regular-print materials are eligible for the free "talking book" services of the Library of Congress or may obtain large-print or audio books from local libraries.

COGNITION AND EMOTIONAL RESPONSES. Cognitive impairment and emotional lability occur early in MS in some patients and may impose numerous stresses on the patient and family. Some patients with MS are forgetful and easily distracted and may exhibit emotional lability.

Patients adapt to illness in a variety of ways, including denial, depression, withdrawal, and hostility. Emotional support assists patients and their families to adapt to the changes and uncertainties associated with MS and to cope with the disruption in their lives. The family should be made aware of the nature and degree of cognitive impairment. Patients with MS have identified that the support of family and friends is a primary need (Koopman, Benbow &

Vandervoort, 2006). The patient is assisted to set meaningful and realistic goals, to remain as active as possible, and to maintain interests and activities. Hobbies may help the patient's morale and provide satisfying interests if the disease progresses to the stage in which formerly enjoyed activities can no longer be pursued. The environment is kept structured, and lists and other memory aids are used to help the patient with cognitive changes maintain a daily routine. The occupational therapist can be helpful in formulating a structured daily routine.

STRENGTHENING COPING MECHANISMS. The diagnosis of MS is always distressing to the patient and family. They need to know that no two patients with MS have identical symptoms or courses of illness. Although some patients do experience significant disability early, others have a near-normal lifespan with minimal disability. Some families, however, face overwhelming frustrations and problems. MS affects people who are often in a productive stage of life and concerned about career and family responsibilities. Family conflict, disintegration, separation, and divorce are not uncommon. Often, very young family members assume the responsibility of caring for a parent with MS. Nursing interventions in this area include alleviating stress and making appropriate referrals for counseling and support to minimize the adverse effects of dealing with chronic illness.

The nurse, mindful of these complex problems, initiates home care and coordinates a network of services, including social services, speech therapy, physical therapy, and homemaker services. To strengthen the patient's coping skills, as much information as possible is provided. Patients need an updated list of available assistive devices, services, and resources.

Coping through problem solving involves helping the patient define the problem and develop alternatives for its management. Careful planning and maintaining flexibility and a hopeful attitude are useful for psychological and physical adaptation.

Improving Home Management

MS can affect every facet of daily living. Certain abilities are often impossible to regain after they are lost. Physical function may vary from day to day. Modifications that allow independence in home management should be implemented (eg, assistive eating devices, raised toilet seat, bathing aids, telephone modifications, long-handled comb, tongs, modified clothing). Exposure to heat increases fatigue and muscle weakness, so air conditioning is recommended in at least one room. Exposure to extreme cold may increase spasticity.

Promoting Sexual Functioning

Patients with MS and their partners face problems that interfere with sexual activity, both as a direct consequence of nerve damage and also from psychological reactions to the disease. Easy fatigability, conflicts arising from dependency and depression, emotional lability, and loss of self-esteem compound the problem. Erectile and ejaculatory disorders in men and orgasmic dysfunction and adductor spasms of the thigh muscles in women can make sexual intercourse difficult or impossible. Bladder and bowel incontinence and urinary tract infections add to the difficulties.

Collaboration between the patient, family, and health care provider is essential for supporting intimacy (Moore, 2007). A sexual counselor can help bring into focus the patient's or partner's sexual resources and suggest relevant information and supportive therapy. Sharing and communicating feelings, planning for sexual activity (to minimize the effects of fatigue), and exploring alternative methods of sexual expression may open up a wide range of sexual enjoyment and experiences.

Promoting Home and Community-Based Care

TEACHING PATIENTS SELF-CARE. As the disease progresses, the patient and family need to learn new strategies to maintain optimal independence. Teaching of new self-care techniques may be initiated in the hospital or clinic setting and reinforced in the home. Self-care education may address the use of assistive devices, self-catheterization, and administration of medications that affect the course of the disease or treat complications. A teaching plan that addresses intramuscular or subcutaneous administration of medications is developed for the patient and his or her family (Cox & Stone, 2006). One research study showed that use of a local anesthetic cream reduced pain and fear associated with intramuscular medication administration in 18 patients with MS (Buhse, 2006). Exercises that enable the patient to continue some form of activity or that maintain or improve swallowing, speech, or respiratory function may be taught to the patient and family (Chart 64-4).

CONTINUING CARE. After discharge, the home care nurse often provides teaching and reinforcement of new interventions in the patient's home. Nurses in the home setting assess for changes in the patient's physical and emotional status, provide physical care to the patient if required, coordinate outpatient services and resources, and encourage health promotion, appropriate health screenings, and adaptation. If changes in the disease or its course are noted, the home care nurse encourages the patient to contact the primary care provider, because treatment of an acute exacerbation or new problem may be indicated. Continuing health care and follow-up are recommended.

The patient with MS is encouraged to contact the local chapter of the National Multiple Sclerosis Society for services, publications, and contact with others who have MS (see Resources). Local chapters also provide direct services to patients. Through group participation, the patient has an opportunity to meet others with similar problems, share experiences, and learn self-help methods in a social environment.

Evaluation

Expected Patient Outcomes

Expected patient outcomes may include the following:

1. Improves physical mobility
   a. Participates in gait-training and rehabilitation program
   b. Establishes a balanced program of rest and exercise
   c. Uses assistive devices correctly and safely
2. Is free of injury
   a. Uses visual cues to compensate for decreased sense of touch or position
   b. Asks for assistance when necessary

CHART 64-4	HOME CARE CHECKLIST *The Patient With Multiple Sclerosis (MS)*		
At the completion of the home care instruction, the patient or caregiver will be able to:		**PATIENT**	**CAREGIVER**
• State how to access the local chapter of the National MS Society and available resources.		✔	✔
• Discuss the clinical course of MS.		✔	✔
• Identify strategies to manage symptoms (pain, cognitive responses, dysphagia, tremors, visual disturbances).		✔	✔
• State how to prevent complications (pressure ulcers, pneumonia, depression).		✔	✔
• Identify coping strategies.		✔	✔
• Identify ways to minimize fatigue.		✔	✔
• Explain how to prevent injury.		✔	✔
• State ways to adapt to sexual dysfunction.		✔	✔
• Discuss ways to control bowel and bladder function.		✔	✔
• Name benefits of exercise and physical activity.		✔	✔
• Identify ways to minimize immobility and spasticity.		✔	✔
• Describe medication regimen and potential adverse effects.		✔	✔
• Demonstrate correct techniques of administering injectable medications, if prescribed.		✔	✔

3. Attains or maintains control of bladder and bowel patterns
   a. Monitors self for urine retention and employs intermittent self-catheterization technique, if indicated
   b. Identifies the signs and symptoms of urinary tract infection
   c. Maintains adequate fluid and fiber intake
4. Participates in strategies to improve speech and swallowing
   a. Practices exercises recommended by speech therapist
   b. Maintains adequate nutritional intake without aspiration
5. Compensates for altered thought processes
   a. Uses lists and other aids to compensate for memory losses
   b. Discusses problems with trusted advisor or friend
   c. Substitutes new activities for those that are no longer possible
6. Demonstrates effective coping strategies
   a. Maintains sense of control
   b. Modifies lifestyle to fit goals and limitations
   c. Verbalizes desire to pursue goals and developmental tasks of adulthood
7. Adheres to plan for home maintenance management
   a. Uses appropriate techniques to maintain independence
   b. Engages in health promotion activities and health screenings as appropriate
8. Adapts to changes in sexual function
   a. Is able to discuss problem with partner and appropriate health professional
   b. Identifies alternative means of sexual expression

Myasthenia Gravis

Myasthenia gravis, an autoimmune disorder affecting the myoneural junction, is characterized by varying degrees of weakness of the voluntary muscles. Approximately 60,000 people have myasthenia gravis in the United States. Women are affected more frequently than men, and they tend to develop the disease at an earlier age (20 to 40 years of age, versus 60 to 70 years for men) (Mazzoni, et al., 2006).

Pathophysiology

Normally, a chemical impulse precipitates the release of acetylcholine from vesicles on the nerve terminal at the myoneural junction. The acetylcholine attaches to receptor sites on the motor endplate and stimulates muscle contraction. Continuous binding of acetylcholine to the receptor site is required for muscular contraction to be sustained.

In myasthenia gravis, antibodies directed at the acetylcholine receptor sites impair transmission of impulses across the myoneural junction. Therefore, fewer receptors are available for stimulation, resulting in voluntary muscle weakness that escalates with continued activity (Fig. 64-5). These antibodies are found in 80% to 90% of people with myasthenia gravis (Hickey, 2009). Eighty percent of people with myasthenia gravis have either thymic hyperplasia or a thymic tumor, and the thymus gland is believed to be the site of antibody production. In patients who are antibody negative, researchers believe that the offending antibody is directed at a portion of the receptor site rather than the whole complex.

Clinical Manifestations

The initial manifestation of myasthenia gravis in two thirds of patients involves the ocular muscles. Diplopia (double

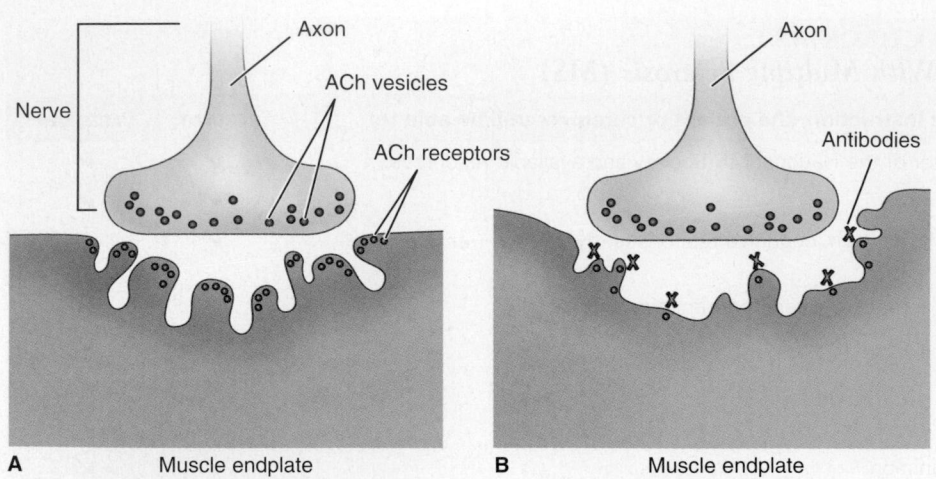

Figure 64-5 Myasthenia gravis. **A,** Normal acetylcholine (Ach) receptor site. **B,** ACh receptor site in myasthenia gravis.

vision) and ptosis (drooping of the eyelids) are common (Allen, 2006). Many patients also experience weakness of the muscles of the face and throat (bulbar symptoms) and generalized weakness. Weakness of the facial muscles results in a bland facial expression. Laryngeal involvement produces **dysphonia** (voice impairment) and increases the risk of choking and aspiration. Generalized weakness affects all the extremities and the intercostal muscles, resulting in decreasing vital capacity and respiratory failure. Myasthenia gravis is purely a motor disorder with no effect on sensation or coordination.

Assessment and Diagnostic Findings

An acetylcholinesterase inhibitor test is used to diagnose myasthenia gravis. The acetylcholinesterase inhibitor stops the breakdown of acetylcholine, thereby increasing availability at the neuromuscular junction. Edrophonium chloride (Tensilon), a fast-acting acetylcholinesterase inhibitor, is administered IV to diagnose myasthenia gravis. Thirty seconds after injection, facial muscle weakness and ptosis should resolve for about 5 minutes (Hickey, 2009). Immediate improvement in muscle strength after administration of this agent represents a positive test and usually confirms the diagnosis. Atropine should be available to control the side effects of edrophonium, which include bradycardia, sweating, and cramping.

The presence of acetylcholine receptor antibodies is identified in the serum (Mazzoni, et al., 2006). Repetitive muscle stimulation demonstrates a decrease in successive action potentials. The thymus gland, a site of acetylcholine receptor antibody production, may be enlarged in myasthenia gravis, and may be identified by MRI scan. A single-fiber electromyography (EMG) detects a delay or failure of neuromuscular transmission and is about 99% sensitive in confirming the diagnosis of myasthenia gravis (Hickey, 2009; Karpoff & Labus, 2008).

Medical Management

Management of myasthenia gravis is directed at improving function and reducing and removing circulating antibodies. Therapeutic modalities include administration of anticholinesterase medications and immunosuppressive therapy, plasmapheresis, and thymectomy. There is no cure for myasthenia gravis; treatments do not stop the production of the acetylcholine receptor antibodies.

Pharmacologic Therapy

Pyridostigmine bromide (Mestinon), an anticholinesterase medication, is the first line of therapy. It provides symptomatic relief by inhibiting the breakdown of acetylcholine and increasing the relative concentration of available acetylcholine at the neuromuscular junction. The dosage is gradually increased to a daily maximum and is administered in divided doses (usually four times a day). Adverse effects of anticholinesterase medications include fasciculations, abdominal pain, diarrhea, and increased oropharyngeal secretions (Allen, 2006). Pyridostigmine tends to have fewer side effects than other anticholinesterase medications (Chart 64-5).

If pyridostigmine bromide does not improve muscle strength and control fatigue, the next agents used are the immunomodulating drugs. The goal of immunosuppressive therapy is to reduce production of the antibody. Corticosteroids suppress the patient's immune response, decreasing the amount of antibody production, and this correlates with clinical improvement. An initial dose of prednisone is given daily; as symptoms improve, the medication is tapered and a maintenance dose may be given indefinitely (Mazzoni, et al., 2006). As the corticosteroid medications take effect the dosage of anticholinesterase medication can usually be lowered. Cytotoxic medications are used to treat myasthenia gravis if there is inadequate response to steroids. Azathioprine (Imuran) inhibits T lymphocytes and reduces acetylcholine receptor antibody levels. Therapeutic effects may not be evident for 3 to 12 months. Leukopenia and hepatotoxicity are serious adverse effects, so monthly evaluation of liver enzymes and white blood cell count is necessary.

Intravenous immune globulin (IVIG) is also used to treat exacerbations, and, in selected patients, it is used on a long-term adjunctive basis. IVIG treatment is easy to administer and involves the administration of pooled human gamma-globulin, and improvement occurs in a few days (Hickey, 2009).

A number of medications are contraindicated for patients with myasthenia gravis because they exacerbate the symptoms. The physician and the patient should weigh risks and benefits before any new medications are prescribed,

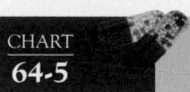

CHART
64-5

PHARMACOLOGY
Potential Adverse Effects of Anticholinesterase Medications

Central Nervous System

Irritability
Anxiety
Insomnia
Headache
Dysarthria
Syncope
Seizures
Coma
Diaphoresis

Respiratory

Bronchial relaxation
Increased bronchial secretions

Cardiovascular

Tachycardia
Hypotension

Gastrointestinal

Abdominal cramps
Nausea
Vomiting
Diarrhea
Anorexia
Increased salivation

Skeletal Muscles

Fasciculations
Spasms
Weakness

Genitourinary

Frequency
Urgency

Integumentary

Rash
Flushing

---

including antibiotics, cardiovascular medications, antiseizure and psychotropic medications, morphine, quinine and related agents, beta-blockers, and nonprescription medications (Allen, 2006). Procaine (Novocain) should be avoided, and the patient's dentist is informed of the diagnosis of myasthenia gravis.

Plasmapheresis

Plasmapheresis (plasma exchange) is a technique used to treat exacerbations. The patient's plasma and plasma components are removed through a centrally placed large-bore double-lumen catheter. The blood cells and antibody-containing plasma are separated, after which the cells and a plasma substitute are reinfused. Plasma exchange produces a temporary reduction in the level of circulating antibodies. The typical course of plasmapheresis consists of daily or alternate-day treatment, and the number of treatments is determined by the patient's response. Plasma exchange improves symptoms in 75% of patients; however, improvement lasts only a few weeks after treatment is completed (Hickey, 2009).

Surgical Management

Thymectomy (surgical removal of the thymus gland) can produce antigen-specific immunosuppression and result in clinical improvement. The procedure results in either partial or complete remission. A course of preoperative plasmapheresis decreases the time needed for postoperative mechanical ventilation. The entire gland must be removed for optimal clinical outcomes; therefore, surgeons prefer the transsternal surgical approach. After surgery, the patient is monitored in an intensive care unit, with special attention to respiratory function. The patient is weaned from mechanical ventilation after thorough respiratory assessment. After the thymus gland is removed, it may take up to 3 years

for the patient to benefit from the procedure, because of the long life of circulating T cells (Allen, 2006).

Complications

Respiratory Failure

A myasthenic crisis is an exacerbation of the disease process characterized by severe generalized muscle weakness and respiratory and bulbar weakness that may result in respiratory failure. Crisis may result from disease exacerbation or a specific precipitating event. The most common precipitator is respiratory infection; others include medication change, surgery, pregnancy, and medications that exacerbate myasthenia. A cholinergic crisis caused by overmedication with cholinesterase inhibitors is rare; atropine sulfate should be on hand to treat bradycardia or respiratory distress (Hickey, 2009).

Neuromuscular respiratory failure is the critical complication in myasthenic and cholinergic crises. Respiratory muscle and bulbar weakness combine to cause respiratory compromise. Weak respiratory muscles do not support inhalation. An inadequate cough and an impaired gag reflex, caused by bulbar weakness, result in poor airway clearance. A downward trend of two respiratory function tests, the negative inspiratory force and vital capacity, is the first clinical sign of respiratory compromise.

Endotracheal intubation and mechanical ventilation may be needed (see Chapter 25). Noninvasive positive-pressure ventilation uses an external device that provides respiratory support without endotracheal intubation. Cholinesterase inhibitors are stopped when respiratory failure occurs and gradually restarted after the patient demonstrates improvement with a course of plasmapheresis or IVIG. Nutritional support may be needed if the patient is intubated for a long period.

Nursing Management

Because myasthenia gravis is a chronic disease and most patients are seen on an outpatient basis, much of the nursing care focuses on patient and family teaching. Educational topics for outpatient self-care include medication management, energy conservation, strategies to help with ocular manifestations, and prevention and management of complications.

Medication management is a crucial component of ongoing care. Understanding the actions of the medications and taking them on schedule is emphasized, as are the consequences of delaying medication and the signs and symptoms of myasthenic and cholinergic crises. The patient can determine the best times for daily dosing by keeping a diary to determine fluctuation of symptoms and to learn when the medication is wearing off. The medication schedule can then be manipulated to maximize strength throughout the day.

► NURSING ALERT

Maintenance of stable blood levels of anticholinesterase medications is imperative to stabilize muscle strength. Therefore, the anticholinesterase medications must be administered on time. Any delay in administration of medications may exacerbate muscle weakness and make it impossible for the patient to take medications orally.

The patient is also taught strategies to conserve energy. To do this, the nurse helps the patient identify the optimal times for rest throughout the day. If the patient lives in a two-story home, the nurse can suggest that frequently used items (eg, hygiene products, cleaning products, snacks) be kept on each floor to minimize travel between floors. The patient is encouraged to apply for a handicapped license plate to minimize walking from parking spaces, and to schedule activities to coincide with peak energy and strength levels.

To minimize the risk of aspiration, mealtimes should coincide with the peak effects of anticholinesterase medication. In addition, rest before meals is encouraged to reduce muscle fatigue. The patient is advised to sit upright during meals, with the neck slightly flexed to facilitate swallowing. Soft foods in gravy or sauces can be swallowed more easily; if choking occurs frequently, the nurse can suggest puréed food with a puddinglike consistency. Suction should be available at home, with the patient and family instructed in its use. Supplemental feedings may be necessary in some patients to ensure adequate nutrition (Randell, Byars, Williams, et al., 2008).

Impaired vision results from ptosis of one or both eyelids, decreased eye movement, or double vision. To prevent corneal damage when the eyelids do not close completely, the patient is instructed to tape the eyes closed for short intervals and to regularly instill artificial tears. Patients who wear eyeglasses can have "crutches" attached to help lift the eyelids. Patching of one eye can help with double vision.

The patient is reminded of the importance of maintaining health promotion practices and of following health care screening recommendations. Factors that exacerbate symptoms and potentially cause crisis should be noted and avoided: emotional stress, infections (particularly respiratory infections), vigorous physical activity, some medications, and high environmental temperature. The Myasthenia Gravis Foundation of America provides support groups, services, and educational materials for patients, families, and health care providers (see Resources).

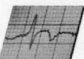

Myasthenic Crisis

Respiratory distress and varying degrees of dysphagia (difficulty swallowing), dysarthria (difficulty speaking), eyelid ptosis, diplopia, and prominent muscle weakness are symptoms of myasthenic crisis. The patient is placed in an intensive care unit for constant monitoring because of associated intense and sudden fluctuations in clinical condition.

Providing ventilatory assistance takes precedence in the immediate management of the patient with myasthenic crisis. Ongoing assessment for respiratory failure is essential. The nurse assesses the respiratory rate, depth, and breath sounds and monitors pulmonary function parameters (vital capacity and negative inspiratory force) to detect pulmonary problems before respiratory dysfunction progresses. Blood is drawn for arterial blood gas analysis. Endotracheal intubation and mechanical ventilation may be needed (see Chapter 25).

If the abdominal, intercostal, and pharyngeal muscles are severely weak, the patient cannot cough, take deep breaths, or clear secretions. Chest physical therapy, including postural drainage to mobilize secretions and suctioning to remove secretions, may have to be performed frequently. (Postural drainage should not be performed for 30 minutes after feeding.)

Assessment strategies and supportive measures include the following:

- Arterial blood gases, serum electrolytes, input and output, and daily weight are monitored.
- If the patient cannot swallow, nasogastric tube feedings may be prescribed.
- Sedatives and tranquilizers are avoided, because they aggravate hypoxia and hypercapnia and can cause respiratory and cardiac depression.

Guillain-Barré Syndrome

Guillain-Barré syndrome is an autoimmune attack on the peripheral nerve myelin. The result is acute, rapid segmental demyelination of peripheral nerves and some cranial nerves, producing ascending weakness with **dyskinesia** (inability to execute voluntary movements), hyporeflexia, and **paresthesias** (numbness). An antecedent event (most often a viral infection) precipitates clinical presentation (Palmieri, 2005). *Campylobacter jejuni*, cytomegalovirus, Epstein-Barr virus, *Mycoplasma pneumoniae*, *H. influenzae*, and HIV are the most common infectious agents that are associated with the development of Guillain-Barré syndrome.

The annual incidence of Guillain-Barré syndrome is 1 to 2 cases per 100,000, and it is more frequent in males between 16 and 25 years of age and between 45 and 60 years of age (Palmieri, 2005). Results of studies on recovery rates differ, but most indicate that 60% to 75% of patients recover completely. Residual deficits of varying degree occur in 20% to 25% of patients. Residual deficits are most likely in patients with rapid disease progression, those who require mechanical ventilation, and those 60 years of age or older. Death occurs in 5% of cases, resulting from respiratory failure, autonomic dysfunction, sepsis, or pulmonary emboli (Mazzoni, et al., 2006).

Pathophysiology

Myelin is a complex substance that covers nerves, providing insulation and speeding the conduction of impulses from the cell body to the dendrites. The cell that produces myelin in the peripheral nervous system is the Schwann cell. In Guillain-Barré syndrome, the Schwann cell is spared, allowing for remyelination in the recovery phase of the disease.

Guillain-Barré syndrome is the result of a cell-mediated and humoral immune attack on peripheral nerve myelin proteins that causes inflammatory demyelination. The best-accepted theory of cause is molecular mimicry, in which an infectious organism contains an amino acid that mimics the peripheral nerve myelin protein. The immune system cannot distinguish between the two proteins and attacks and destroys peripheral nerve myelin. The exact location of the immune attack within the peripheral nervous system is the ganglioside GM1b. With the autoimmune attack, there is an influx of macrophages and other immune-mediated agents that attack myelin and cause inflammation and destruction, interruption of nerve conduction, and axonal loss (Ho, Thakur, Gorson, et al., 2008; Palmieri, 2005).

Clinical Manifestations

Guillain-Barré syndrome typically begins with muscle weakness and diminished reflexes of the lower extremities. Hyporeflexia and weakness may progress to tetraplegia. Demyelination of the nerves that innervate the diaphragm and intercostal muscles results in neuromuscular respiratory failure. Sensory symptoms include paresthesias of the hands and feet and pain related to the demyelination of sensory fibers.

The antecedent event usually occurs 2 weeks before symptoms begin. Weakness usually begins in the legs and progresses upward. Maximum weakness, the plateau, varies in length but usually includes neuromuscular respiratory failure and bulbar weakness. The duration of the symptoms is variable; complete functional recovery may take up to 2 years. Any residual symptoms are permanent and reflect axonal damage from demyelination.

Cranial nerve demyelination can result in a variety of clinical manifestations. Optic nerve demyelination may result in blindness. Bulbar muscle weakness related to demyelination of the glossopharyngeal and vagus nerves results in the inability to swallow or clear secretions. Vagus nerve demyelination results in autonomic dysfunction, manifested by instability of the cardiovascular system. The presentation is variable and may include tachycardia, bradycardia, hypertension, or orthostatic hypotension. The symptoms of autonomic dysfunction occur and resolve rapidly. Guillain-Barré syndrome does not affect cognitive function or LOC.

Although the classic clinical features include areflexia and ascending weakness, variation in presentation occurs. There may be a sensory presentation, with progressive sensory symptoms; an atypical axonal destruction; or the Miller-Fisher variant, which includes paralysis of the ocular muscles, ataxia, and areflexia (Iggulden, 2006).

Assessment and Diagnostic Findings

The patient presents with symmetric weakness, diminished reflexes, and upward progression of motor weakness. A history of a viral illness in the previous few weeks suggests the diagnosis. Changes in vital capacity and negative inspiratory force are assessed to identify impending neuromuscular respiratory failure. Serum laboratory tests are not useful in the diagnosis. However, elevated protein levels are detected in CSF evaluation, without an increase in other cells. Evoked potential studies demonstrate a progressive loss of nerve conduction velocity.

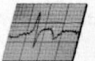

Medical Management

Because of the possibility of rapid progression and neuromuscular respiratory failure, Guillain-Barré syndrome is a medical emergency, requiring management in an intensive care unit. After baseline values are identified, assessment of changes in muscle strength and respiratory function alert the clinician to the physical and respiratory needs of the patient. Respiratory therapy or mechanical ventilation may be necessary to support pulmonary function and adequate oxygenation. Some clinicians recommend elective intubation before the onset of extreme respiratory muscle fatigue. Emergent intubation may result in autonomic dysfunction (Mazzoni, et al., 2006). Mechanical ventilation may be required for an extended period. The patient is weaned from mechanical ventilation after the respiratory muscles can again support spontaneous respiration and maintain adequate tissue oxygenation.

Other interventions are aimed at preventing the complications of immobility. These may include the use of anticoagulant agents and anti-embolism stockings or sequential compression boots to prevent thrombosis and pulmonary emboli.

Plasmapheresis and IVIG are used to directly affect the peripheral nerve myelin antibody level (Mazzoni, et al., 2006). Both therapies decrease circulating antibody levels and reduce the amount of time the patient is immobilized and dependent on mechanical ventilation. Studies indicate that IVIG and plasmapheresis are equally effective in treating Guillain-Barré syndrome; however, IVIG is the therapy of choice because it is associated with fewer side effects. The cardiovascular risks posed by autonomic dysfunction require continuous electrocardiographic (ECG) monitoring. Tachycardia and hypertension are treated with short-acting medications such as alpha-adrenergic blocking agents. The use of short-acting agents is important, because autonomic dysfunction is very labile. Hypotension is managed by increasing the amount of IV fluid administered.

NURSING PROCESS

THE PATIENT WITH GUILLAIN-BARRÉ SYNDROME

Assessment

Ongoing assessment for disease progression is critical. The patient is monitored for life-threatening complications (respiratory failure, cardiac dysrhythmias, deep vein thrombosis [DVT]), so that appropriate interventions can be initiated. Because of the threat to the patient in this sudden, potentially life-threatening disease, the nurse must assess the patient's and family's ability to cope and their use of coping strategies.

Diagnosis

Nursing Diagnoses

Based on the assessment data, the patient's major nursing diagnoses may include the following:

- Ineffective breathing pattern and impaired gas exchange related to rapidly progressive weakness and impending respiratory failure
- Impaired bed and physical mobility related to paralysis
- Imbalanced nutrition, less than body requirements, related to inability to swallow
- Impaired verbal communication related to cranial nerve dysfunction
- Fear and anxiety related to loss of control and paralysis

Collaborative Problems/Potential Complications

Based on the assessment data, potential complications that may develop include the following:

- Respiratory failure
- Autonomic dysfunction

Planning and Goals

The major goals for the patient may include improved respiratory function, increased mobility, improved nutritional status, effective communication, decreased fear and anxiety, and absence of complications.

Nursing Interventions

Maintaining Respiratory Function

Respiratory function can be maximized with incentive spirometry and chest physiotherapy. Monitoring for changes in vital capacity and negative inspiratory force is key to early intervention for neuromuscular respiratory failure. Mechanical ventilation is required if the vital capacity falls, making spontaneous breathing impossible and tissue oxygenation inadequate.

The potential need for mechanical ventilation should be discussed with the patient and family on admission to provide time for psychological preparation and decision making. Intubation and mechanical ventilation result in less anxiety if they are initiated on a nonemergency basis to a well-informed patient. The patient may require mechanical ventilation for a long period. Nursing management of the patient requiring mechanical ventilation is discussed in Chapter 25.

Bulbar weakness that impairs the ability to swallow and clear secretions is another factor in the development of res-

piratory failure in the patient with Guillain-Barré syndrome. Suctioning may be needed to maintain a clear airway.

The nurse assesses the blood pressure and heart rate frequently to identify autonomic dysfunction, so that interventions can be initiated quickly if needed. Medications are administered or a temporary pacemaker is placed for clinically significant bradycardia.

Enhancing Physical Mobility

Nursing interventions to enhance physical mobility and prevent the complications of immobility are key to the function and survival of patients. The paralyzed extremities are supported in functional positions, and passive range-of-motion exercises are performed at least twice daily. DVT and pulmonary embolism are threats to the paralyzed patient. Nursing interventions are aimed at preventing DVT. Range-of-motion exercises, position changes, anticoagulation, the use of anti-embolism stockings or sequential compression boots, and adequate hydration decrease the risk of DVT.

Padding may be placed over bony prominences, such as the elbows and heels, to reduce the risk of pressure ulcers (Igulden, 2006). The need for consistent position changes every 2 hours cannot be overemphasized. The nurse evaluates laboratory test results that may indicate malnutrition or dehydration, both of which increase the risk of pressure ulcers. The nurse collaborates with the physician and dietitian to develop a plan to meet the patient's nutritional and hydration needs.

Providing Adequate Nutrition

Paralytic ileus may result from insufficient parasympathetic activity. In this event, the nurse administers IV fluids and parenteral nutrition as a supplement and monitors for the return of bowel sounds. If the patient cannot swallow because of **bulbar paralysis** (immobility of muscles), a gastrostomy tube may be placed to administer nutrients. The nurse carefully assesses the return of the gag reflex and bowel sounds before resuming oral nutrition.

Improving Communication

Because of paralysis, the patient cannot talk, laugh, or cry and therefore has no method for communicating needs or expressing emotion. Establishing some form of communication with picture cards or an eye blink system provides a means of communication. Collaboration with the speech therapist may be helpful in developing a communication mechanism that is most effective for a specific patient.

Decreasing Fear and Anxiety

The patient and family are faced with a sudden, potentially life-threatening disease, and anxiety and fear are constant themes for them. The impact of disease on the family depends on the patient's role within the family. Referral to a support group may provide information and support to the patient and family.

The family may feel helpless in caring for the patient. Mechanical ventilation and monitoring devices may frighten and intimidate them. Family members often want to participate in physical care; with instruction and support by the nurse, they should be allowed and encouraged to do so.

In addition to fear, the patient may experience isolation, loneliness, and lack of control. Nursing interventions that increase the patient's sense of control include providing information about the condition, emphasizing a positive appraisal of coping resources, and teaching relaxation exercises and distraction techniques. The positive attitude and atmosphere of the multidisciplinary team are important to promote a sense of well-being.

Diversional activities are encouraged to decrease loneliness and isolation. Encouraging visitors, engaging visitors or volunteers to read to the patient, listening to music or books on tape, and watching television are ways to alleviate the patient's sense of isolation.

Monitoring and Managing Potential Complications

Thorough assessment of respiratory function at regular and frequent intervals is essential, because respiratory insufficiency and subsequent failure due to weakness or paralysis of the intercostal muscles and diaphragm may develop quickly. Respiratory failure is the major cause of mortality. In addition to the respiratory rate and the quality of respirations, vital capacity is monitored frequently and at regular intervals, so that respiratory insufficiency can be anticipated. Decreasing vital capacity with associated muscle weakness indicates impending respiratory failure. Signs and symptoms include breathlessness while speaking, shallow and irregular breathing, use of accessory muscles, tachycardia, weak cough, and changes in respiratory pattern.

Other complications include cardiac dysrhythmias, which necessitate ECG monitoring; transient hypertension; orthostatic hypotension; DVT; pulmonary embolism; urinary retention; and other threats to any immobilized and paralyzed patient. These require monitoring and attention to prevent them and prompt treatment if indicated.

Promoting Home and Community-Based Care

TEACHING PATIENTS SELF-CARE. Patients with Guillain-Barré syndrome and their families are usually frightened by the sudden onset of life-threatening symptoms and their severity. Therefore, teaching the patient and family about the disorder and its generally favorable prognosis is important (Chart 64-6).

During the acute phase of the illness, the patient and family are instructed about strategies they can implement to minimize the effects of immobility and other complications. As function begins to return, family members and other home care providers are instructed about care of the patient and their role in the rehabilitation process. Preparation for discharge is an interdisciplinary effort requiring family or caregiver education by all team members, including the nurse, physician, occupational and physical therapists, speech therapist, and respiratory therapist.

CONTINUING CARE. Most patients with Guillain-Barré syndrome experience complete recovery. Patients who have experienced total or prolonged paralysis require intensive rehabilitation; the extent depends on the patient's needs. Approaches include a comprehensive inpatient program if deficits are significant, an outpatient program if the patient can travel by car, or a home program of physical and occupational therapy. The recovery phase may be long and requires patience as well as involvement on the part of the patient and family.

During acute care, the focus is on immediate issues and deficits. The nurse needs to remind or instruct patients and family members of the need for continuing health promotion and screening practices after this initial phase of care.

Evaluation

Expected Patient Outcomes

Expected patient outcomes may include the following:

1. Maintains effective respirations and airway clearance
   a. Has normal breath sounds on auscultation
   b. Demonstrates gradual improvement in respiratory function

---

CHART 64-6 **HOME CARE CHECKLIST**
The Patient With Guillain-Barré Syndrome

At the completion of the home care instruction, the patient or caregiver will be able to:	PATIENT	CAREGIVER
• Describe the disease process of Guillain-Barré syndrome.	✔	✔
• Manage respiratory needs: tracheostomy care, suctioning.		✔
• Demonstrate proper body mechanics regarding lifting and transfers.		✔
• Practice gait training and strength endurance.	✔	✔
• Perform range-of-motion exercises.	✔	✔

• Perform activities of daily living and manage self-care:
  • Nutrition
  • Bowel and bladder management
  • Skin care
  • Adaptive equipment for bathing, hygiene, grooming, dressing
	✔
	✔
	✔
	✔
		✔
		✔
		✔
		✔

• Operate and explain function of medical equipment and mobility aids: walkers, wheelchairs, bedside commodes, tub transfer benches, adaptive devices.	✔	✔
• Use coping mechanisms and diversional activities appropriately.	✔	✔
• Implement safety measures in the home.	✔	✔
• Know how to contact and use community resources and the Guillain-Barré Syndrome Foundation International.	✔	✔

2. Shows increasing mobility
   a. Regains use of extremities
   b. Participates in rehabilitation program
   c. Demonstrates no contractures and minimal muscle atrophy
3. Receives adequate nutrition and hydration
   a. Consumes diet adequate to meet nutritional needs
   b. Swallows without aspiration
4. Demonstrates recovery of speech
   a. Communicates needs through alternative strategies
   b. Practices exercises recommended by the speech therapist
5. Shows lessening fear and anxiety
6. Has absence of complications
   a. Breathes spontaneously
   b. Has vital capacity within normal range
   c. Exhibits normal arterial blood gases and pulse oximetry

CRANIAL NERVE DISORDERS

Because the brain stem and cranial nerves involve vital motor, sensory, and autonomic functions of the body, these nerves may be affected by conditions arising primarily within these structures or in secondary extension from adjacent disease processes. The cranial nerves are examined separately and in sequence (see Chapter 60). Some cranial nerve deficits can be detected by observing the patient's face, eye movements, speech, and swallowing. EMG is used to investigate motor and sensory dysfunction. An MRI scan is used to obtain images of the cranial nerves and brain stem. An overview of disorders that may affect each of the cranial nerves, including clinical manifestations and nursing interventions, is presented in Table 64-1. The following discussion centers on the most common disorders of the cranial nerves: trigeminal neuralgia, a condition affecting the fifth cranial nerve, and Bell's palsy, caused by involvement of the seventh cranial nerve.

Trigeminal Neuralgia (Tic Douloureux)

Trigeminal neuralgia is a condition of the fifth cranial nerve that is characterized by paroxysms of pain in the area innervated by any of the three branches, but most commonly the second and third branches of the trigeminal nerve (Mazzoni, et al., 2006) (Fig. 64-6). The pain ends as abruptly as it starts and is described as a unilateral shooting and stabbing sensation. The unilateral nature of the pain is an important feature. Associated involuntary contraction of the facial muscles can cause sudden closing of the eye or twitching of the mouth, hence the former name *tic douloureux* (painful twitch). Although the cause is not certain, vascular compression and pressure are suggested causes. As the brain changes with age, a loop of a cerebral artery or vein may compress the nerve root entry point, and this can be identified on MRI scan (Gronseth, Cruccu, Alksne, et al., 2008).

Trigeminal neuralgia occurs most often before 35 years of age and is more common in women and in people with MS compared to the general population (Gronseth, et al., 2008; Mazzoni, et al., 2006). Pain-free intervals may be measured in terms of minutes, hours, days, or longer. With advancing years, the painful episodes tend to become more frequent and agonizing. The patient lives in constant fear of attacks.

Paroxysms can occur with any stimulation of the terminals of the affected nerve branches, such as washing the face, shaving, brushing the teeth, eating, and drinking. A draft of cold air or direct pressure against the nerve trunk may also cause pain. Certain areas are called trigger points because the slightest touch immediately starts a paroxysm or episode. To avoid stimulating these areas, patients with trigeminal neuralgia try not to touch or wash their faces, shave, chew, or do anything else that might cause an attack. These behaviors are a clue to the diagnosis.

Medical Management

Pharmacologic Therapy

Antiseizure agents, such as carbamazepine (Tegretol), relieve pain in most patients with trigeminal neuralgia by reducing the transmission of impulses at certain nerve terminals. Carbamazepine is taken with meals. Serum levels must be monitored to avoid toxicity in patients who require high doses to control the pain. Side effects include nausea, dizziness, drowsiness, and aplastic anemia. The patient is monitored for bone marrow depression during long-term therapy. Gabapentin (Neurontin) and baclofen (Lioresal) are also used for pain control. If pain control is still not achieved, phenytoin (Dilantin) may be used as adjunctive therapy.

Surgical Management

If pharmacologic management fails to relieve pain, a number of surgical options are available. Although these procedures may relieve facial pain for a few years, recurrence and complication rates are high (Hickey, 2009). The choice of procedure depends on the patient's preference and health status.

Microvascular Decompression of the Trigeminal Nerve

An intracranial approach is used to relieve the contact between the cerebral vessel and the trigeminal nerve root entry. With the aid of an operating microscope, the artery loop is lifted from the nerve to relieve the pressure, and a small prosthetic device is inserted to prevent recurrence of impingement on the nerve. The postoperative management is the same as for other intracranial surgeries (see Chapter 61).

Radiofrequency Thermal Coagulation

Percutaneous radiofrequency produces a thermal lesion on the trigeminal nerve. Although immediate pain relief is experienced, dysesthesia of the face and loss of the corneal reflex may occur. Use of stereotactic MRI for identification of the trigeminal nerve followed by gamma knife radiosurgery is being used at some medical centers.

Percutaneous Balloon Microcompression

Percutaneous balloon microcompression disrupts large myelinated fibers in all three branches of the trigeminal nerve. After its placement, the balloon is filled with a

Table 64-1 DISORDERS OF CRANIAL NERVES

Disorder	Clinical Manifestations	Nursing Interventions
Olfactory Nerve—I Head trauma Intracranial tumor Intracranial surgery	Unilateral or bilateral anosmia (temporary or persistent) Diminished taste for food	Assess sense of smell. Assess for cerebrospinal fluid rhinorrhea if patient has sustained head trauma.
Optic Nerve—II Optic neuritis Increased intracranial pressure Pituitary tumor	Lesions of optic tract producing homonymous hemianopsia	Assess visual acuity. Restructure environment to prevent injuries. Teach patient to accommodate for visual loss.
Oculomotor Nerve—III **Trochlear Nerve—IV** **Abducens Nerve—VI** Vascular Brain stem ischemia Hemorrhage and infarction Neoplasm Trauma Infection	Dilation of pupil with loss of light reflex on one side Impairment of ocular movement Diplopia Gaze palsies Ptosis of eyelid	Assess extraocular movement and for nonreactive pupil.
Trigeminal Nerve—V Trigeminal neuralgia Head trauma Cerebellopontine lesion Sinus tract tumor and metastatic disease Compression of trigeminal root by tumor	Pain in face Diminished or loss of corneal reflex Chewing dysfunction	Assess for pain and triggering mechanisms for pain. Assess for difficulty in chewing. Discuss trigger zones and pain precipitants with patient. Protect cornea from abrasion. Ensure good oral hygiene. Educate patient about medication regimen.
Facial Nerve—VII Bell's palsy Facial nerve tumor Intracranial lesion Herpes zoster	Facial dysfunction; weakness and paralysis Hemifacial spasm Diminished or absent taste Pain	Recognize facial paralysis as emergency; refer for treatment as soon as possible. Teach protective care for eyes. Select easily chewed foods; patient should eat and drink from unaffected side of mouth. Emphasize importance of oral hygiene. Provide emotional support for changed appearance of face.
Vestibulocochlear Nerve—VIII Tumors and acoustic neuroma Vascular compression of nerve Ménière's syndrome	Tinnitus Vertigo Hearing difficulties	Assess pattern of vertigo. Provide for safety measures to prevent falls. Ensure that patient can maintain balance before ambulating. Caution patient to change positions slowly. Assist with ambulation. Encourage use of assistive devices.
Glossopharyngeal Nerve—IX Glossopharyngeal neuralgia from neurovascular compression of cranial nerves IX and X Trauma Inflammatory conditions Tumor Vertebral artery aneurysms	Pain at base of tongue Difficulty in swallowing Loss of gag reflex Palatal, pharyngeal, and laryngeal paralysis	Assess for paroxysmal pain in throat, decreased or absent swallowing, and gag and cough reflexes. Monitor for dysphagia, aspiration, and nasal dysarthric speech. Position patient upright for eating or tube feeding.
Vagus Nerve—X Spastic palsy of larynx; bulbar paralysis; high vagal paralysis Guillain-Barré syndrome Vagal body tumors Nerve paralysis from malignancy, surgical trauma such as carotid endarterectomy	Voice changes (temporary or permanent hoarseness) Vocal paralysis Dysphagia	Assess for airway obstruction/provide airway management. Prevent aspiration. Support patient having voice reconstruction procedures.
Spinal Accessory Nerve—XI Spinal cord disorder Amyotrophic lateral sclerosis Trauma Guillain-Barré syndrome	Drooping of affected shoulder with limited shoulder movement Weakness or paralysis of head rotation, flexion, extension; shoulder elevation	Support patient undergoing diagnostic tests.
Hypoglossal Nerve—XII Medullary lesions Amyotrophic lateral sclerosis Polio and motor system disease, which may destroy hypoglossal nuclei Multiple sclerosis Trauma	Abnormal movements of tongue Weakness or paralysis of tongue muscles Difficulty in talking, chewing, and swallowing	Observe swallowing ability. Observe speech pattern. Be aware of swallowing or vocal difficulties. Prepare for alternate feeding methods (tube feeding) to maintain nutrition.

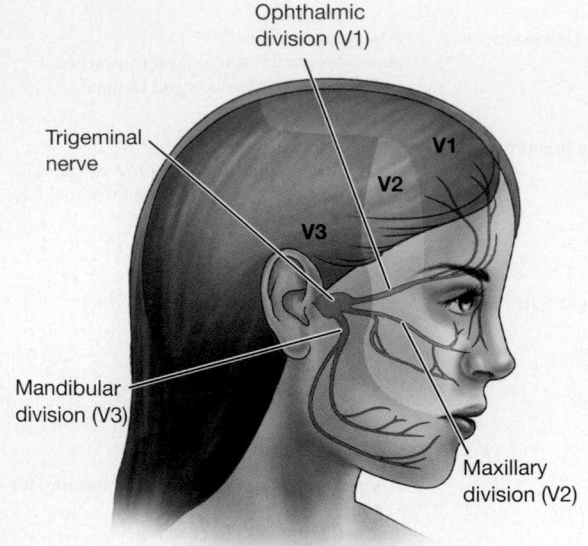

Figure 64-6 Distribution of trigeminal nerve branches.

contrast material for fluoroscopic identification. The balloon compresses the nerve root for 1 minute and provides microvascular decompression.

Nursing Management

Preventing Pain

Preoperative management of a patient with trigeminal neuralgia occurs mostly on an outpatient basis and includes recognizing factors that may aggravate excruciating facial pain, such as food that is too hot or too cold or jarring of the patient's bed or chair. Even washing the face, combing the hair, or brushing the teeth may produce acute pain. The nurse can assist the patient in preventing or reducing this pain by providing instructions about preventive strategies. Providing cotton pads and room temperature water for washing the face, instructing the patient to rinse with mouthwash after eating if tooth brushing causes pain, and performing personal hygiene during pain-free intervals are all effective strategies. The patient is instructed to take food and fluids at room temperature, to chew on the unaffected side, and to ingest soft foods. The nurse recognizes that anxiety, depression, and insomnia often accompany chronic painful conditions and uses appropriate interventions and referrals. See Chapter 13 for management of patients with chronic pain.

Providing Postoperative Care

Postoperative neurologic assessments are conducted to evaluate the patient for facial motor and sensory deficits in each of the three branches of the trigeminal nerve. If the surgery results in sensory deficits to the affected side of the face, the patient is instructed not to rub the eye because the pain of a resulting injury will not be detected. The eye is assessed for irritation or redness. Artificial tears may be prescribed to prevent dryness in the affected eye. The patient is cautioned not to chew on the affected side until numbness has diminished. The patient is observed carefully for any difficulty in eating or swallowing foods of different consistencies.

Bell's Palsy

Bell's palsy (facial paralysis) is caused by unilateral inflammation of the seventh cranial nerve, which results in weakness or paralysis of the facial muscles on the affected side (Fig. 64-7). Although the cause is unknown, theories about causes include vascular ischemia, viral disease (herpes simplex, herpes zoster), autoimmune disease, or a combination of all of these factors. Most adults with Bell's palsy are younger than 45 years of age (Carlson & Pfadt, 2005).

Bell's palsy may be a type of pressure paralysis. The inflamed, edematous nerve becomes compressed to the point of damage, or its blood supply is occluded, producing ischemic necrosis of the nerve. The face is distorted from paralysis of the facial muscles; increased lacrimation (tearing); and painful sensations in the face, behind the ear, and in the eye. The patient may experience speech difficulties and may be unable to eat on the affected side because of weakness or paralysis of the facial muscles. Most patients recover completely, and Bell's palsy rarely recurs (Carlson & Pfadt, 2005).

Medical Management

The objectives of treatment are to maintain the muscle tone of the face and to prevent or minimize denervation. The patient should be reassured that no stroke has occurred and that spontaneous recovery occurs within 3 to 5 weeks in most patients.

Corticosteroid therapy (prednisone) may be prescribed to reduce inflammation and edema; this reduces vascular compression and permits restoration of blood circulation to the nerve. Early administration of corticosteroid therapy appears to diminish the severity of the disease, relieve the pain, and prevent or minimize denervation (Carlson & Pfadt, 2005).

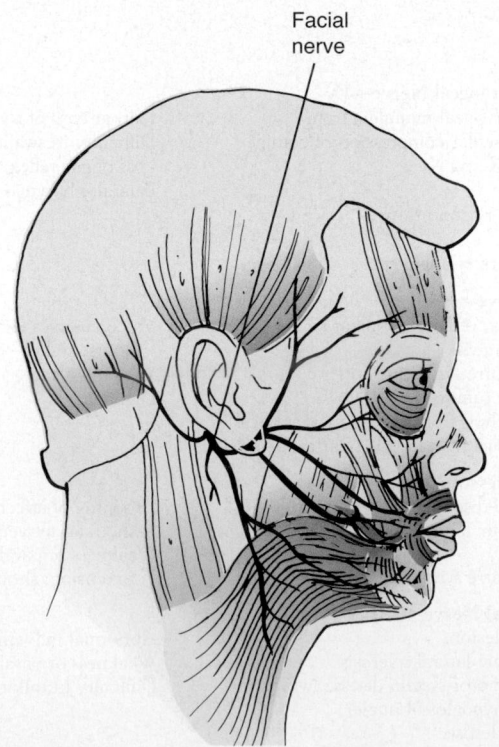

Figure 64-7 Distribution of the facial nerve.

Facial pain is controlled with analgesic agents. Heat may be applied to the involved side of the face to promote comfort and blood flow through the muscles. Electrical stimulation may be applied to the face to prevent muscle atrophy. Although most patients recover with conservative treatment, surgical exploration of the facial nerve may be indicated if a tumor is suspected, for surgical decompression of the facial nerve, or for surgical treatment of a paralyzed face.

Nursing Management

While the paralysis lasts, nursing care involves protection of the eye from injury. Frequently, the eye does not close completely and the blink reflex is diminished, so the eye is vulnerable to injury from dust and foreign particles. Corneal irritation and ulceration may occur. Distortion of the lower lid alters the proper drainage of tears. To prevent injury, the eye should be covered with a protective shield at night. The eye patch may abrade the cornea, however, because there is some difficulty in keeping the partially paralyzed eyelids closed. Moisturizing eye drops during the day and eye ointment at bedtime may help prevent injury (Carlson & Pfadt, 2005). The patient can be taught to close the paralyzed eyelid manually before going to sleep. Wrap-around sunglasses or goggles may be worn during the day to decrease normal evaporation from the eye.

After the sensitivity of the nerve to touch decreases and the patient can tolerate touching the face, the nurse can suggest massaging the face several times daily, using a gentle upward motion, to maintain muscle tone. Facial exercises, such as wrinkling the forehead, blowing out the cheeks, and whistling, may be performed with the aid of a mirror to prevent muscle atrophy. Exposure of the face to cold and drafts is avoided.

DISORDERS OF THE PERIPHERAL NERVOUS SYSTEM

Peripheral Neuropathies

A peripheral **neuropathy** (disorder of the nervous system) is a disorder affecting the peripheral motor and sensory nerves. Peripheral nerves connect the spinal cord and brain to all other organs. They transmit motor impulses from the brain and relay sensory impulses to the brain. Peripheral neuropathies are characterized by bilateral and symmetric disturbance of function, usually beginning in the feet and hands. The most common cause of peripheral neuropathy is diabetes with poor glycemic control (Tesfaye, Chaturvedi, Simon, et al., 2005). The major symptoms of peripheral nerve disorders are loss of sensation, muscle atrophy, weakness, diminished reflexes, pain, and paresthesia (numbness, tingling) of the extremities.

Peripheral nerve disorders are diagnosed by history, physical examination, and electrodiagnostic studies such as electroencephalography. The diagnosis of peripheral neuropathy in the geriatric population is challenging because many symptoms, such as decreased reflexes, can be associated with the normal aging process (Miller, 2009).

No specific treatment exists for peripheral neuropathy. Elimination or control of the cause may slow progression.

Patients with peripheral neuropathy are at risk for falls, thermal injuries, and skin breakdown. The plan of care includes inspection of the lower extremities for skin breakdown. Assistive devices such as a walker or cane may decrease the risk of falls. Bath water temperature is checked to avoid thermal injury. Footwear should be accurately sized. Driving may be limited or eliminated, thereby disrupting the patient's sense of independence.

Mononeuropathy

Mononeuropathy is limited to a single peripheral nerve and its branches. It arises when the trunk of the nerve is compressed or entrapped (as in carpal tunnel syndrome), traumatized (as when bruised by a blow), overstretched (as in joint dislocation), punctured by a needle used to inject a drug or damaged by the drugs thus injected, or inflamed because an adjacent infectious process extends to the nerve trunk. Mononeuropathy is frequently seen in patients with diabetes.

Pain is seldom a major symptom of mononeuropathy when the condition is due to trauma, but in patients with complicating inflammatory conditions such as arthritis, pain is prominent. Pain is increased with all body movements that tend to stretch, strain, or cause pressure on the injured nerve and sudden jarring of the body (eg, from coughing or sneezing). The skin in the areas supplied by nerves that are injured or diseased may become reddened and glossy, the subcutaneous tissue may become edematous, and the nails and hair in this area are altered. Chemical injuries to a nerve trunk, such as those caused by drugs injected into or near it, are often permanent.

The objective of treatment of mononeuropathy is to remove the cause, if possible (eg, freeing the compressed nerve). Local corticosteroid injections may reduce inflammation and the pressure on the nerve. Aspirin or codeine may be used to relieve pain.

Nursing care involves protection of the affected limb or area from injury, as well as appropriate patient teaching about mononeuropathy and its treatment.

CRITICAL THINKING EXERCISES

1 A 19-year-old college student is admitted with suspected meningitis. Identify two assessment parameters that indicate meningitis. What interventions would be included in your plan of care to protect the patient from injury? The patient's family has many questions about the disease and their risk of contracting meningitis. Develop a teaching plan that would describe meningitis and prophylactic therapy for the patient's family and close contacts.

2 Your patient has been prescribed a new medication for the treatment of MS that requires self-injection. She reports that she has a fear of self-injection. Identify additional assessment parameters that need to be used. Develop a teaching plan for self-injection. What resources may be needed to enable her to be successful?

EBP **3** Your 40-year-old patient is being investigated for trigeminal neuralgia. What is the current evidence base for diagnostic evaluation and treatment of trigeminal neuralgia? Identify the criteria used to evaluate the strength of the evidence for diagnostic evaluation and treatment of trigeminal neuralgia. How would you use this information in developing a nursing plan of care for this patient?

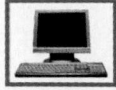 The Smeltzer suite offers these additional resources to enhance learning and facilitate understanding of this chapter:

- thePoint online resource, thepoint.lww.com/Smeltzer12E
- Student CD-ROM included with the book
- *Study Guide to Accompany Brunner & Suddarth's Textbook of Medical-Surgical Nursing*
- *Handbook for Brunner & Suddarth's Textbook of Medical-Surgical Nursing*

REFERENCES AND SELECTED READINGS

*Asterisk indicates nursing research.
**Double asterisk indicates classic reference.

Books

Bickley, L. S. (2007). *Bates' guide to physical examination and history taking* (9th ed.). Philadelphia: Lippincott Williams & Wilkins.

Hickey, J. V. (2009). *The clinical practice of neurological & neurosurgical nursing* (6th ed.). Philadelphia: Lippincott Williams & Wilkins.

Iggulden, H. (2006). *Care of the neurological patient.* Oxford: Blackwell Publishing.

Karch, A. (2008). *Lippincott's nursing drug guide.* Philadelphia: Lippincott Williams & Wilkins.

Karpoff, S. & Labus, D. M. (2008). *Portable diagnostic tests.* Philadelphia: Lippincott Williams & Wilkins.

Mazzoni, P., Pearson, T. S. & Rowland, L. P. (2006). *Merritt's neurology handbook.* Philadelphia: Lippincott Williams & Wilkins.

Miller, C. A. (2009). *Nursing for wellness in older adults* (5th ed.). Philadelphia: Lippincott Williams & Wilkins.

Olek, M. J. (2005). *Multiple sclerosis: Etiology, diagnosis and new treatment strategies.* Totowa, NJ: Humana Press.

Porth, C. M. & Matfin, C. (2009). *Pathophysiology: Concepts of altered health states* (8th ed.) Philadelphia: Lippincott Williams & Wilkins.

Posner, J. B., Saper, C. B., Schiff, N. D., et al. (2007). *Plum and Posner's diagnosis of stupor and coma* (4th ed.). Oxford: Oxford University Press.

Journals and Electronic Documents

General

Advisory Committee on Immunization Practices of the Centers for Disease Control and Prevention. (2008). *Recommended immunization schedule for persons aged 7–18 years—UNITED STATES 2008.* Available at: www.cispimmunize.org/

Hughes, R. G. (Ed.). (2008). *Patient safety and quality: An evidence-based handbook for nurses.* (AHRQ Publication No. 08-0043). Rockville, MD: Agency for Healthcare Research and Quality. www.ahrq.gov/qual/nurseshdbk/

CNS Infections

Matthews, C, Miller, L. & Mott, M. (2007). Getting ahead of acute meningitis and encephalitis. *Nursing, 37*(11), 37–42.

Tunkel, A. R., Glaser, C. A., Block, K. C., et al. (2008). The management of encephalitis: Clinical practice guidelines by the infectious diseases society of America. *Clinical Infectious Diseases, 47*(1), 303–327.

van de Beek, D., de Gans, J., Tunkel, A. R., et al. (2006). Community-acquired bacterial meningitis. *New England Journal of Medicine, 354*(1), 44–53.

Weisfelt, M., van de Beek, D., Spanjaard, L., et al. (2007). A risk score for unfavorable outcome in adults with bacterial meningitis. *Annals of Neurology, 63*(1), 90–97.

Creutzfeldt-Jakob Disease

Glatzel, M., Stoeck, K., Seeger, H., et al. (2005). Human prion diseases: Molecular and clinical aspects. *Archives of Neurology, 62*(4), 545–552.

Ward, H., Everington, D., Cousens, S. N., et al. (2007). Risk factors for sporadic Creutzfeldt-Jakob disease. *Annals of Neurology, 63*(3), 347–354.

Multiple Sclerosis

Buhse, M. (2006). Efficacy of EMLA cream to reduce fear and pain associated with interferon Beta-1a injection in patients with multiple sclerosis. *Journal of Neuroscience Nursing, 38*(4), 222–226.

Costello, K. & Sipe, J. C. (2008). Clabride tablets' potential in multiple sclerosis treatment. *Journal of Neuroscience Nursing, 40*(5), 275–280.

Cox, D. & Stone, J. (2006). Managing self-injection difficulties in patients with relapsing-remitting multiple sclerosis. *Journal of Neuroscience Nursing, 38*(3), 167–171.

Johnson, S. L. (2008). The concept of fatigue in multiple sclerosis. *Journal of Neuroscience Nursing, 40*(2), 72–77.

*Koopman, W. J., Benbow, C. & Vandervoort, M. (2006). Top 10 needs of people with multiple sclerosis and their significant others. *Journal of Neuroscience Nursing, 38*(5), 369–373.

**Lublin, F. D. & Reingold, S. C. (1996). Defining the clinical course of multiple sclerosis: Results of an international study. *Neurology, 46*(4), 907–911.

*Miller, C. E. & Jezewski, M. A. (2006). Relapsing MS patient's experiences with glatiramer acetate treatment: A phenomenological study. *Journal of Neuroscience Nursing, 38*(1), 37–41.

Moore, L. A. (2007). Intimacy and multiple sclerosis. *Nursing Clinics of North America, 42*(4), 606–620.

*Motl, R. W., Snook, E. M. & Schapiro, R. T. (2007). Symptoms and physical activity behavior in individuals with multiple sclerosis. *Research in Nursing & Health, 31*(5), 466–475.

*Newland, P. (2008). Pain in women with relapsing-remitting multiple sclerosis and in healthy women: A comparative study. *Journal of Neuroscience Nursing, 40*(5), 262–268.

Phillips, L. J. & Stuifbergen, A. K. (2009). Structural equation modeling of disability in women with fibromyalgia or Multiple Sclerosis. *Western Journal of Nurshing Research, 31*(1), 89–109.

Ridley, B. & Rawlings, P. K. (2006). Intrathecal Baclofen therapy: Ten steps toward best practice. *Journal of Neuroscience Nursing, 38*(2), 72–82.

Ross, A. P., Hackbarth, N., Rohl, C., et al. (2008). Effective multiple sclerosis management through improved patient assessment. *Journal of Neuroscience Nursing, 40*(3), 150–157.

*Smeltzer, S. C., Zimmerman, V. & Capriotti, T. (2005). Osteoporosis risk and bone mineral density in women with physical disabilities. *Archives of Physical Medicine and Rehabilitation, 86*(3), 582–586.

Stern, M. (2005). Aging with multiple sclerosis. *Physical Medicine and Rehabilitation Clinics of North America, 16*(1), 219–234.

Myasthenia Gravis and Guillain-Barré Syndrome

Allen, S. (2006). Management of myasthenia gravis. *Pharmaceutical Journal, 277*(19), 703–706.

Ho, D., Thakur, K., Gorson, K. C., et al. (2008). Influence of critical illness on axonal loss in Guillain-Barré syndrome. *Muscle & Nerve, 39*(1), 10–15.

Palmieri, R. L. (2005). Is it myasthenia gravis or Guillain-Barré Syndrome? *Nursing, 35*(12), 32hn1–32hn4.

Randell, D. J., Byars, A., Williams, F., et al. (2008). Glyconutrient supplementation in patients with myasthenia gravis. *Journal of Alternative and Complementary Medicine, 14*(9), 1–8.

Trigeminal Neuralgia and Neuropathies

Carlson, D. S. & Pfadt, E. (2005). When your patient has acute facial paralysis. *Nursing, 35*(4), 54–56.

Gronseth, G., Cruccu, G., Alksne, J., et al. (2008). Practice parameter: The diagnostic evaluation and treatment of trigeminal neuralgia. *Neurology, 71*(8), 1183–1190.

Tesfaye, S., Chaturvedi, N., Simon, E. M., et al. (2005). Vascular risk factors and diabetic neuropathy. *New England Journal of Medicine, 352*(4), 341–350.

RESOURCES

Guillain-Barré Syndrome Foundation International, http://gbs-cidp.org/
Myasthenia Gravis Foundation of America, www.myasthenia.org
National Multiple Sclerosis Society, www.nmss.org
The Neuropathy Association, Inc., www.neuropathy.org

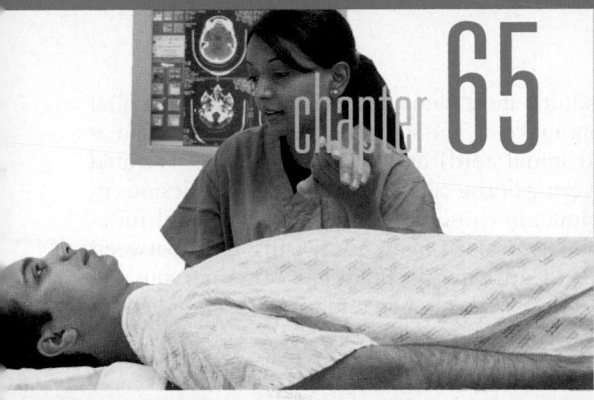

chapter 65

Management of Patients With Oncologic or Degenerative Neurologic Disorders

The occurrence of oncologic or degenerative disease processes in the neurologic system produces a unique set of nursing challenges. Oncologic disorders include brain and spinal cord tumors. Degenerative neurologic disorders include Parkinson's disease, Huntington disease, Alzheimer's disease, amyotrophic lateral sclerosis, muscular dystrophies, and degenerative disk disease. Postpolio syndrome is thought to be degenerative in nature and is included in this chapter.

ONCOLOGIC DISORDERS OF THE BRAIN AND SPINAL CORD

Oncologic disorders of the brain and spinal cord include several types of neoplasms, each with its own biology, prognosis, and treatment options. Because of the unique anatomy and physiology of the central nervous system (CNS), this collection of neoplasms is challenging to diagnose and treat.

Primary Brain Tumors

A brain tumor is a localized intracranial lesion that occupies space within the skull. A tumor usually grows as a spherical mass, but it also can grow diffusely and infiltrate tissue. The effects of neoplasms are caused by the compression and infiltration of tissue. A variety of physiologic changes result, causing any or all of the following pathophysiologic events:

- Increased intracranial pressure (ICP) and cerebral edema
- Seizure activity and focal neurologic signs
- Hydrocephalus
- Altered pituitary function

Primary brain tumors originate from cells and structures within the brain. Secondary, or metastatic, brain tumors develop from structures outside the brain and occur in 10% to 20% of patients with cancer. Brain tumors rarely metastasize outside the CNS (Arzbaecher, 2007). Metastatic lesions to the brain can occur from the lung, breast, lower gastrointestinal tract, pancreas, kidney, and skin (melanomas).

The cause of primary brain tumors is unknown. The strongest risk factor is exposure to ionizing radiation. Both glial and meningeal neoplasms have been linked to irradiation of the cranium, with a latency period of 10 to 20 years after exposure (American Brain Tumor Association [ABTA], 2007). Many additional risk factors have been investigated, but only rare genetic mutations, familial tendencies for astrocytoma, and epilepsy and seizures show strong evidence of an association. In the case of epilepsy and seizures, the relationship is unlikely to be causal (Pollock, 2006).

An estimated 21,810 new cases of malignant brain and other nervous system tumors are projected for the year 2008 (Jemal, Siegel, Ward, et al., 2008). Secondary tumors or metastases to the brain from a systemic primary cancer are even more common than new cases of malignant brain and other nervous system tumors. The highest incidence of brain tumors in adults occurs in the fifth, sixth, and seventh

decades. In adults, most brain tumors originate from glial cells (cells that make up the structure and support system of the brain and spinal cord) and are supratentorial (located above the covering of the cerebellum). Neoplastic lesions in the brain ultimately cause death by impairing vital functions, such as respiration, or by increasing ICP. Between 1990 and 2004, death rates for brain and other nervous system tumors declined in both men and women. The rates decreased by 12.6% for men and by 14.4% for women.

Types of Primary Brain Tumors

Brain tumors may be classified into several groups: those arising from the coverings of the brain (eg, dural meningioma), those developing in or on the cranial nerves (eg, acoustic neuroma), those originating within brain tissue (eg, glioma), and metastatic lesions originating elsewhere in the body. Tumors of the pituitary and pineal glands and of cerebral blood vessels are also types of brain tumors. Relevant clinical considerations include the location and the histologic character of the tumor. Tumors may be benign or malignant. A benign tumor, such as a colloid cyst, can occur in a vital area and can grow large enough to have serious effects (Richards & Ballard, 2008). See Chart 65-1 for the classification of brain tumors.

Gliomas

Glial tumors, the most common type of intracerebral brain neoplasm, are divided into many categories (Wen & Kesari, 2008). Astrocytomas are the most common type of glioma and are graded from I to IV, indicating the degree of malignancy (Arzbaecher, 2007). The grade is based on cellular density, cell mitosis, and appearance. Usually, these tumors spread by infiltrating into the surrounding neural connective tissue and therefore cannot be totally removed without causing considerable damage to vital structures.

Oligodendroglial tumors represent 20% of gliomas and are categorized as low grade or high grade (anaplastic) (ABTA, 2007). The histologic distinction between astrocy-

---

Chart 65-1 • *Classification of Brain Tumors in Adults*

I. **Intracerebral Tumors**
   A. Gliomas—infiltrate any portion of the brain; most common type of brain tumor
      1. Astrocytomas (grades I and II)
      2. Glioblastoma multiforme (astrocytoma grades III and IV)
      3. Oligodendrocytoma (low and high grades)
      4. Ependymoma (grades I to IV)
      5. Medulloblastoma
II. **Tumors Arising From Supporting Structures**
   A. Meningiomas
   B. Neuromas (acoustic neuroma, schwannoma)
   C. Pituitary adenomas
III. **Developmental Tumors**
   A. Angiomas
   B. Dermoid, epidermoid, teroma, craniopharyngioma
IV. **Metastatic Lesions**

tomas and oligodendrogliomas is difficult to make but important, because oligodendrogliomas are more sensitive than astrocytomas to chemotherapy.

Meningiomas

Meningiomas, which represent 15% of all primary brain tumors, are common benign encapsulated tumors of arachnoid cells on the meninges (Pollock, 2006). They are slow growing and occur most often in middle-aged adults (more often in women). Meningiomas most often occur in areas proximal to the venous sinuses. Manifestations depend on the area involved and are the result of compression rather than invasion of brain tissue. Preferred treatment for symptomatic lesions is surgery with complete removal or partial dissection.

Acoustic Neuromas

An acoustic neuroma is a tumor of the eighth cranial nerve, the cranial nerve most responsible for hearing and balance. It usually arises just within the internal auditory meatus, where it frequently expands before filling the cerebellopontine recess. An acoustic neuroma may grow slowly and attain considerable size before it is correctly diagnosed. The patient usually experiences loss of hearing, tinnitus, and episodes of vertigo and staggering gait. As the tumor becomes larger, painful sensations of the face may occur on the same side, as a result of the tumor's compression of the fifth cranial nerve. Many acoustic neuromas are benign and can be managed conservatively. Many that continue to grow can be surgically removed and have a good prognosis (see Chapter 59) (Pollock, 2006). Some acoustic neuromas may be suitable for stereotactic radiotherapy rather than open craniotomy. Stereotactic radiotherapy is discussed later in this chapter.

Pituitary Adenomas

Pituitary tumors represent about 10% to 15% of all brain tumors and cause symptoms as a result of pressure on adjacent structures or hormonal changes such as hyperfunction or hypofunction of the pituitary (Pollock, 2006).

Pressure Effects of Pituitary Adenomas

Pressure from a pituitary adenoma may be exerted on the optic nerves, optic chiasm, or optic tracts or on the hypothalamus or the third ventricle if the tumor invades the cavernous sinuses or expands into the sphenoid bone. These pressure effects produce headache, visual dysfunction, hypothalamic disorders (disorders of sleep, appetite, temperature, and emotions), increased ICP, and enlargement and erosion of the sella turcica.

Hormonal Effects of Pituitary Adenomas

Functioning pituitary tumors can produce one or more hormones normally produced by the anterior pituitary. There are prolactin-secreting pituitary adenomas (prolactinomas), growth hormone–secreting pituitary adenomas that produce acromegaly in adults, and adrenocorticotropic hormone (ACTH)–producing pituitary adenomas that result in Cushing's disease (Gordon, 2007). Adenomas that secrete thyroid-stimulating hormone or follicle-stimulating hormone and luteinizing hormone occur infrequently, whereas adenomas that produce both growth hormone and prolactin are relatively common.

The female patient whose pituitary gland is secreting excessive quantities of prolactin presents with amenorrhea or galactorrhea (excessive or spontaneous flow of milk). Male patients with prolactinomas may present with impotence and hypogonadism. Acromegaly, caused by excess growth hormone, produces enlargement of the hands and feet, distortion of the facial features, and pressure on peripheral nerves (entrapment syndromes). The clinical features of Cushing's disease, a condition associated with prolonged overproduction of cortisol, occur with excessive production of ACTH. Manifestations include a form of obesity with redistribution of fat to the facial, supraclavicular, and abdominal areas; hypertension; purple striae and ecchymoses; osteoporosis; elevated blood glucose levels; and emotional disorders. Endocrine disorders resulting from these tumors are discussed in Chapter 42.

Angiomas

Brain angiomas (masses composed largely of abnormal blood vessels) are found either in or on the surface of the brain. They occur in the cerebellum in 83% of cases. Some persist throughout life without causing symptoms; others cause symptoms of a brain tumor. Occasionally, the diagnosis is suggested by the presence of another angioma somewhere in the head or by a bruit (an abnormal sound) that is audible over the skull. Because the walls of the blood vessels in angiomas are thin, these patients are at risk for hemorrhagic stroke. In fact, cerebral hemorrhage in people younger than 40 years of age should suggest the possibility of an angioma.

 Gerontologic Considerations

The most frequent tumor types in the elderly are anaplastic astrocytoma, glioblastoma multiforme, and cerebral metastases from other sites. The incidence of primary brain tumors and the likelihood of malignancy increase with age. Intracranial tumors can produce personality changes, confusion, speech dysfunction, or disturbances of gait. In elderly patients, early signs and symptoms of intracranial tumors can be easily overlooked or incorrectly attributed to cognitive and neurologic changes associated with normal aging. Neurologic signs and symptoms in the elderly must be carefully evaluated, because 10% of brain metastases occur in patients with a history of prior cancer. Researchers are investigating patterns of care and clinical outcomes of elderly patients with primary brain tumors (Barnholtz-Sloan, Williams, Maldonado, et al., 2008).

Clinical Manifestations

Brain tumors can produce both focal or generalized neurologic signs and symptoms. Generalized symptoms reflect increased ICP, and the most common focal or specific signs and symptoms result from tumors that interfere with functions in specific brain regions. Figure 65-1 indicates common tumor sites in the brain.

Increased Intracranial Pressure

As discussed in Chapter 61, the skull is a rigid compartment containing essential noncompressible contents: brain matter,

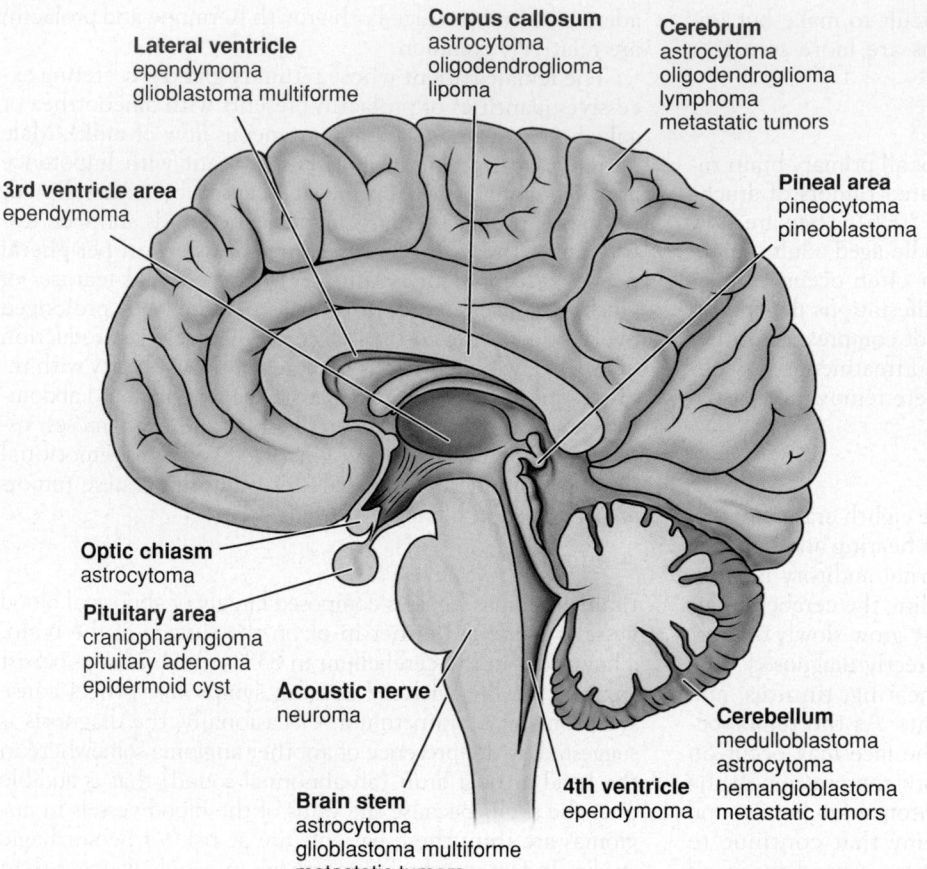

Lateral ventricle
ependymoma
glioblastoma multiforme

Corpus callosum
astrocytoma
oligodendroglioma
lipoma

Cerebrum
astrocytoma
oligodendroglioma
lymphoma
metastatic tumors

3rd ventricle area
ependymoma

Pineal area
pineocytoma
pineoblastoma

Optic chiasm
astrocytoma

Pituitary area
craniopharyngioma
pituitary adenoma
epidermoid cyst

Acoustic nerve
neuroma

Cerebellum
medulloblastoma
astrocytoma
hemangioblastoma
metastatic tumors

4th ventricle
ependymoma

Brain stem
astrocytoma
glioblastoma multiforme
metastatic tumors

Figure 65-1 Common brain tumor sites.

intravascular blood, and cerebrospinal fluid (CSF). According to the modified Monro-Kellie hypothesis, if any one of these skull components increases in volume, ICP increases unless one of the other components decreases in volume. Consequently, any change in volume occupied by the brain (as occurs with disorders such as brain tumor or cerebral edema) produces signs and symptoms of increased ICP.

Symptoms of increased ICP result from a gradual compression of the brain by the enlarging tumor. The effect is a disruption of the equilibrium that exists between the brain, the CSF, and the cerebral blood. As the tumor grows, compensatory adjustments may occur through compression of intracranial veins, reduction of CSF volume (by increased absorption or decreased production), a modest decrease in cerebral blood flow, or reduction of intracellular and extracellular brain tissue mass. When these compensatory mechanisms fail, the patient develops signs and symptoms of increased ICP, most often including headache, nausea with or without vomiting, and **papilledema** (edema of the optic disk) (Rowland, 2005). Personality changes and a variety of focal deficits, including motor, sensory, and cranial nerve dysfunction, are common.

Headache

Headache, although not always present, is most common in the early morning and is made worse by coughing, straining, or sudden movement. It is thought to be caused by the tumor's invading, compressing, or distorting the pain-sensitive structures or by edema that accompanies the tumor.

Headaches are usually described as deep or expanding or as dull but unrelenting. Frontal tumors usually produce a bilateral frontal headache; pituitary gland tumors produce pain radiating between the two temples (bitemporal); in cerebellar tumors, the headache may be located in the suboccipital region at the back of the head.

Vomiting

Vomiting, seldom related to food intake, is usually the result of irritation of the vagal centers in the medulla. Forceful vomiting is described as projectile vomiting.

Visual Disturbances

Papilledema is present in 70% to 75% of patients and is associated with visual disturbances such as decreased visual acuity, diplopia (double vision), and visual field deficits (Rowland, 2005).

Localized Symptoms

Common focal or localized symptoms are hemiparesis, seizures, and mental status changes (Rowland, 2005). When specific regions of the brain are affected, additional local signs and symptoms occur, such as sensory and motor abnormalities, visual alterations, alterations in cognition, and language disturbances (eg, aphasia). The progression of the signs and symptoms is important, because it indicates tumor growth and expansion. For example, a rapidly developing hemiparesis is more typical of a highly malignant glioma than of a low-grade tumor.

Although some tumors are not easily localized because they lie in so-called silent areas of the brain (ie, areas in which functions are not definitely determined), many tumors can be localized by correlating the signs and symptoms to specific areas in the brain, as follows:

- A motor cortex tumor produces seizurelike movements localized on one side of the body, called jacksonian seizures.
- An occipital lobe tumor produces visual manifestations: contralateral homonymous hemianopsia (visual loss in half of the visual field on the opposite side of the tumor) and visual hallucinations.
- A cerebellar tumor causes dizziness, an ataxic or staggering gait with a tendency to fall toward the side of the lesion, marked muscle incoordination, and nystagmus (involuntary rhythmic eye movements), usually in the horizontal direction.
- A frontal lobe tumor frequently produces personality disorders, changes in emotional state and behavior, and an apathetic mental attitude. The patient often becomes extremely untidy and careless and may use obscene language.
- A cerebellopontine angle tumor usually originates in the sheath of the acoustic nerve and gives rise to a characteristic sequence of symptoms. Tinnitus and vertigo appear first, soon followed by progressive nerve deafness (eighth cranial nerve dysfunction). Numbness and tingling of the face and tongue occur (due to involvement of the fifth cranial nerve). Later, weakness or paralysis of the face develops (seventh cranial nerve involvement). Finally, because the enlarging tumor presses on the cerebellum, abnormalities in motor function may be present.

Assessment and Diagnostic Findings

The history of the illness and the manner and time frame in which the symptoms evolved are key components in the diagnosis of brain tumors. A neurologic examination indicates the areas of the CNS that are involved. To assist in the precise localization of the lesion, a battery of tests is performed. Computed tomography (CT) scans, enhanced by a contrast agent, can give specific information concerning the number, size, and density of the lesions and the extent of secondary cerebral edema. CT scans can provide information about the ventricular system. A magnetic resonance imaging (MRI) scan is the most helpful diagnostic tool for detecting brain tumors, particularly smaller lesions, and tumors in the brain stem and pituitary regions, where bone is thick (Fig. 65-2). In a few instances, the appearance of a brain tumor on an MRI scan is so characteristic that a biopsy is unnecessary, especially when the tumor is located in a part of the brain that is difficult to biopsy (Rowland, 2005).

Positron emission tomography (PET) is used to supplement MRI scanning in centers where it is available. On PET scans, low-grade tumors are associated with hypometabolism and high-grade tumors show hypermetabolism. This information can be useful in making treatment decisions (ABTA, 2007). Computer-assisted stereotactic (three-dimensional) biopsy is used to diagnose deep-seated brain tumors and to provide a basis for treatment and prognosis.

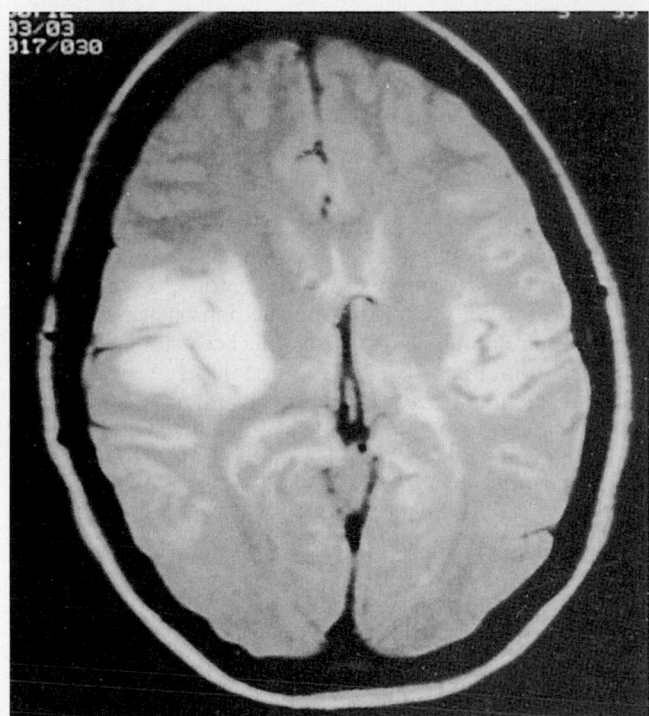

Figure 65-2 Low-grade glioma. Magnetic resonance image of the brain shows an abnormal density in the right temporal lobe. Courtesy of the Hospital of the University of Pennsylvania, Nuclear Medicine Section, Philadelphia, PA.

Cerebral angiography provides visualization of cerebral blood vessels and can localize most cerebral tumors.

An electroencephalogram (EEG) can detect an abnormal brain wave in regions occupied by tumor; it is used to evaluate temporal lobe seizures and to assist in ruling out other disorders. Cytologic studies of the CSF may be performed to detect malignant cells, because CNS tumors can shed cells into the CSF.

Medical Management

A variety of medical treatment modalities, including chemotherapy and external-beam radiation therapy, are used alone or in combination with surgical resection (Wen & Kesari, 2008). Radiation therapy, the cornerstone of treatment for many brain tumors, decreases the incidence of recurrence of incompletely resected tumors. Brachytherapy (the surgical implantation of radiation sources to deliver high doses at a short distance) has had promising results for primary malignancies. It is usually used as an adjunct to conventional radiation therapy or as a rescue measure for recurrent disease.

Intravenous (IV) autologous bone marrow transplantation is used in some patients who will receive chemotherapy or radiation therapy, because it can "rescue" the patient from the bone marrow toxicity associated with high doses of chemotherapy and radiation. A fraction of the patient's bone marrow is aspirated, usually from the iliac crest, and stored. The patient receives large doses of chemotherapy or radiation therapy to destroy large numbers of malignant cells. The marrow is then reinfused by IV after treatment is completed.

Gene transfer therapy uses retroviral vectors to carry genes to the tumor, reprogramming the tumor tissue for susceptibility to treatment. This approach is being tested (ABTA, 2007).

Surgical Management

The objective of surgical management is to remove or destroy the entire tumor without increasing the neurologic deficit (paralysis, blindness) or to relieve symptoms by partial removal (decompression). A variety of treatment modalities may be used; the specific approach depends on the type of tumor, its location, and its accessibility. In many patients, combinations of these modalities are used. Most pituitary adenomas are treated by transsphenoidal microsurgical removal (see Chapter 61), and the remainder of tumors that cannot be removed completely are treated by radiation (Pollock, 2006). An untreated brain tumor ultimately leads to death, either from increasing ICP or from the damage the tumor causes to brain tissue.

Conventional surgical approaches require a craniotomy (incision into the skull). See Chapter 61 for a discussion of care of the patient who has undergone a craniotomy. This approach is used in patients with meningiomas, acoustic neuromas, cystic astrocytomas of the cerebellum, colloid cysts of the third ventricle, congenital tumors such as dermoid cyst, and some of the granulomas. With improved imaging techniques and the availability of the operating microscope and microsurgical instrumentation, even large tumors can be removed through a relatively small craniotomy. For patients with malignant glioma, complete removal of the tumor and cure are not possible, but the rationale for resection includes relief of ICP, removal of any necrotic tissue, and reduction in the bulk of the tumor, which theoretically leaves behind fewer cells to become resistant to radiation or chemotherapy.

Stereotactic approaches involve the use of a three-dimensional frame that allows very precise localization of the tumor; a stereotactic frame and multiple imaging studies (x-rays, CT scans) are used to localize the tumor and verify its position (Fig. 65-3). New brain-mapping technology helps determine how close diseased areas of the brain are to structures essential for normal brain function. Lasers or radiation can be delivered with stereotactic approaches. Radioisotopes such as iodine 131 (^{131}I) can also be implanted directly into the tumor to deliver high doses of radiation to the tumor (brachytherapy) while minimizing effects on surrounding brain tissue.

Stereotactic procedures may be performed using a linear accelerator or gamma knife to perform radiosurgery. These procedures allow treatment of deep, inaccessible tumors, often in a single session. Precise localization of the tumor is accomplished by the stereotactic approach and by minute measurements and precise positioning of the patient. Multiple narrow beams then deliver a very high dose of radiation. An advantage of this method is that no surgical incision is needed; a disadvantage is the lag time between treatment and the desired result (Pollock, 2006; Swinson & Friedman, 2008).

Nursing Management

The patient with a brain tumor may be at increased risk for aspiration as a result of cranial nerve dysfunction. Preoperatively, the gag reflex and ability to swallow are evaluated. In

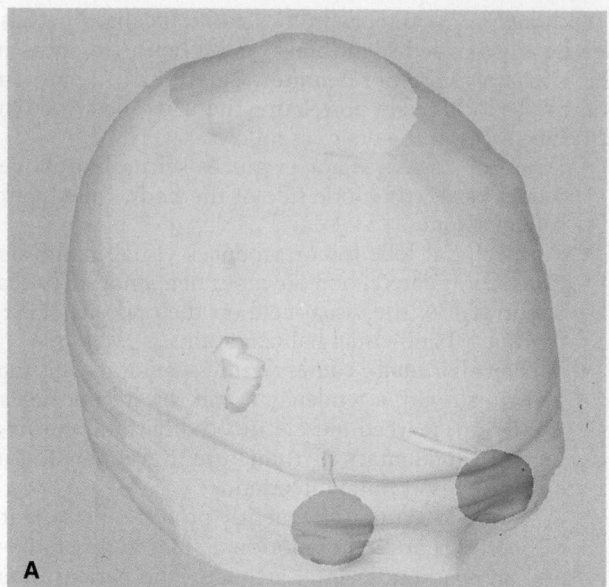

A

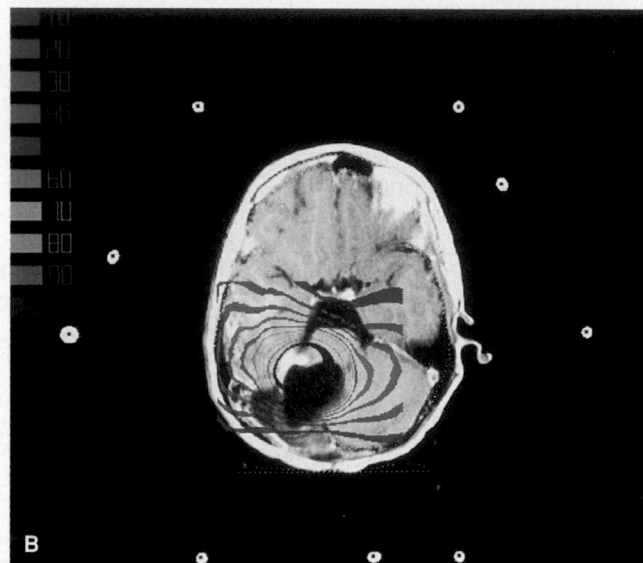

B

Figure 65-3 A, Using stereotactic or "brain-mapping" guided approach, a 3-D computer image fuses the computed tomography image and magnetic resonance image to pinpoint the exact location of the brain tumor. This low-grade astrocytoma is localized adjacent to the brain stem, is nonoperable, and is treated with radiation. Note the optic chasm and optic nerves. **B,** Computerized image of the prescribed radiation dose.

patients with diminished gag response, care includes teaching the patient to direct food and fluids toward the unaffected side, having the patient sit upright to eat, offering a semisoft diet, and having suction readily available. The effects of increased ICP caused by the tumor mass are reviewed in Chapter 61. The nurse performs neurologic checks, monitors vital signs, maintains a neurologic flow chart, spaces nursing interventions to prevent rapid increase in ICP, and reorients the patient when necessary to person, time, and place. Patients with changes in cognition caused by their lesion require frequent reorientation and the use of orienting devices (eg, personal possessions, photographs, lists, a clock), supervision of and assistance with self-care, and ongoing monitoring and intervention for prevention of injury. Patients with seizures are carefully monitored and protected from injury. Motor function is checked at intervals, because specific motor deficits may occur, depending on the tumor's location. Sensory disturbances are assessed. Speech is evaluated. Eye movement and pupillary size and reaction may be affected by cranial nerve involvement.

The psychosocial effects on family caregivers of a family member who has a primary malignant brain tumor may be significant (Schmer, Ward-Smith, Latham, et al., 2008) (Chart 65-2).

The nursing process for patients undergoing neurosurgery is discussed in Chapter 61. The patient's functional abilities should be reassessed postoperatively, because changes can occur.

Cerebral Metastases

A significant number of patients with cancer experience neurologic deficits caused by metastasis to the brain. Although metastatic lesions to the brain are the most common intracerebral tumor, their exact incidence is unknown (Raizer & Abrey, 2007). This high rate of occurrence is clinically important as more patients with all forms of cancer live longer because of improved therapies. Neurologic signs and symptoms include headache, gait disturbances, visual impairment, personality changes, altered mentation (memory loss and confusion), focal weakness, paralysis, aphasia, and seizures. These signs and symptoms can be devastating to both patient and family.

Medical Management

The treatment of metastatic brain cancer is palliative and involves eliminating or reducing serious symptoms. Even when palliation is the goal, distressing signs and symptoms can be relieved, thereby improving the quality of life for both patient and family. Patients with intracerebral metastases who are not treated have a steady downhill course with a limited survival time, whereas those who are treated may survive for slightly longer periods. The median survival time for patients with no treatment for brain metastases is 1 month; with corticosteroid treatment alone it is 2 months; radiation therapy extends the median survival time to 3 to 6 months.

The therapeutic approach includes radiation therapy (the foundation of treatment), surgery (usually for a single intracranial metastasis), and chemotherapy; more often, some combination of these treatments is the optimal method. Gamma knife radiosurgery is considered if three or fewer lesions are present.

Pharmacologic Therapy

Corticosteroids are useful in relieving headache and alterations in level of consciousness. Corticosteroids such as dexamethasone (Decadron) and prednisone are thought to reduce inflammation and edema around tumors (Karch, 2008). Other medications used include osmotic diuretics (eg, mannitol [Osmitrol]) to decrease the fluid content of the brain, which leads to a decrease in ICP. Antiseizure agents (eg, phenytoin [Dilantin]) are used to prevent and treat seizures (Rowland, 2005). The pharmacologic management of pituitary tumors is complex and usually carried

---

NURSING RESEARCH PROFILE
CHART 65-2 *The Caregiver Perspective When a Family Member Has a Malignant Brain Tumor*

Schmer, C., Ward-Smith, P., Latham, S., et al. (2008). When a family member has a malignant brain tumor: The caregiver perspective. *Journal of Neuroscience Nursing, 40*(2), 78–84.

Purpose

There have been no significant advances in the treatment of malignant brain tumors over the past 25 years, and care is performed primarily by family members. The purpose of this study was to explore the perspective of the caregiver for a patient receiving chemotherapy for initial treatment of a malignant brain tumor.

Design

This was a phenomenologic study that used interviews to explore caregiver perspectives. Ten family members (seven spouses, two daughters, and one son-in-law) provided data. Semi-structured interviews took place with the caregiver while the patient was receiving chemotherapy within the first 6 months of treatment for a primary malignant brain tumor. Data analysis was conducted using Colaizzi's method, a qualitative data analysis technique, to identify themes.

Findings

Data analysis uncovered three main themes. The first was that the diagnosis of a brain tumor is a shock; all participants used the work *shock* when explaining their feelings on hearing the diagnosis. The second was that immediate family role changes occur; diagnosis of a primary malignant brain tumor and subsequent treatment resulted in immediate family role changes for both the patient and caregiver. The final theme was that there are psychosocial effects for the caregiver, his or her family, and the person with the brain tumor. Participants did not perceive caring for the family member as a burden.

Nursing Implications

Little research has focused on the experience and changing roles of family members immediately after diagnosis or during the initial treatment phase of a terminal illness. This research provides beginning knowledge for health care professionals about the experience of a family caregiver of a patient with a primary brain tumor. During the first 6 months of treatment, there was a low physical need burden but significant psychosocial effects. Nurses working with patients and families should be prepared to address these psychosocial effects (eg, family role changes).

out on an outpatient basis (Gordon, 2007). Venous thromboembolic events, such as deep vein thrombosis (DVT) and pulmonary embolism (PE), occur in about 15% of patients and are associated with significant morbidity. Anticoagulants usually are not prescribed because of the risk of CNS hemorrhage; however, prophylactic therapy with low-molecular-weight heparin is under investigation.

Chemotherapy plays a small role in managing brain metastasis because of poor penetration across the blood–brain barrier. Drug penetration and sensitivity of brain cells are two factors that determine the responsiveness of metastatic brain tumors to chemotherapy. Research is being directed at multidrug regimens and drug resistance (ABTA, 2007). Encouraging results have been seen with chemotherapeutic agents such as carmustine (BCNU), lomustine (CCNU), and PCV (a triple-drug combination of procarbazine hydrochloride, lomustine, and vincristine). Promising results have been seen with the use of topotecan (Hycamtin), another chemotherapy agent.

Pain is managed by means of a stepped progression in the doses and type of analgesic agents needed for relief. If the patient has severe pain, morphine can be infused into the epidural or subarachnoid space through a spinal needle and a catheter placed as near as possible to the spinal segment where the pain is projected. Small doses of morphine are administered at prescribed intervals (see Chapter 13).

NURSING PROCESS

THE PATIENT WITH CEREBRAL METASTASES OR INCURABLE BRAIN TUMOR

Assessment

The nursing assessment includes a baseline neurologic examination and focuses on how the patient is functioning, moving, and walking; adapting to weakness or paralysis and to loss of vision and speech; and dealing with seizures. Assessment addresses symptoms that cause distress to the patient and affect the quality of life, including pain, respiratory problems, bowel and bladder disorders, sleep disturbances, and impairment of skin integrity, fluid balance, and temperature regulation (Arzbaecher, 2007). Tumor invasion, compression, or obstruction may cause these disorders.

Nutritional status is assessed, because cachexia (weak and emaciated condition) is common in patients with metastases. The nurse explores changes associated with poor nutritional status (anorexia, pain, weight loss, altered metabolism, muscle weakness, malabsorption, and diarrhea) and asks the patient about altered taste sensations that may be secondary to dysphagia, weakness, and depression and about distortions and impaired sense of smell (anosmia).

The nurse takes a dietary history to assess food intake, intolerance, and preferences. Calculation of body mass index can confirm the loss of subcutaneous fat and lean body mass (see Chapter 5). Biochemical measurements are reviewed to assess the degree of malnutrition, impaired cellular immunity, and electrolyte balance (see Appendix

A for normal laboratory values). A dietitian assists in determining the caloric needs of the patient.

The nurse works with other members of the health care team to assess the impact of the illness on the family in terms of home care, altered relationships, financial problems, time pressures, and family problems. This information is important in helping family members cope with the diagnosis and the changes associated with it.

Diagnosis

Nursing Diagnoses

Based on the assessment data, the patient's major nursing diagnoses may include the following:

- Self-care deficit (feeding, bathing, and toileting) related to loss or impairment of motor and sensory function and decreased cognitive abilities
- Imbalanced nutrition, less than body requirements, related to cachexia due to treatment and tumor effects, decreased nutritional intake, and malabsorption
- Anxiety related to fear of dying, uncertainty, change in appearance, or altered lifestyle
- Interrupted family processes related to anticipatory grief and the burdens imposed by the care of the person with a terminal illness

Other nursing diagnoses of the patient with cerebral metastases may include acute pain related to tumor compression; impaired gas exchange related to dyspnea; constipation related to decreased fluid and dietary intake and medications; impaired urinary elimination related to reduced fluid intake, vomiting, and side effects of medications; sleep pattern disturbances related to discomfort and fear of dying; impairment of skin integrity related to cachexia, poor tissue perfusion, and decreased mobility; deficient fluid volume related to fever, vomiting, and low fluid intake; and ineffective thermoregulation related to hypothalamic involvement, fever, and chills. See Chapter 16 for assessment and nursing interventions for the patient with cancer.

Planning and Goals

The goals for the patient may include compensating for self-care deficits, improving nutrition, reducing anxiety, enhancing family coping skills, and absence of complications.

Nursing Interventions

Compensating for Self-Care Deficits

The patient may have difficulty participating in goal setting as the tumor metastasizes and affects cognitive function. The nurse should encourage the family to keep the patient as independent as possible for as long as possible. Increasing assistance with self-care activities is required. Because the patient with cerebral metastasis and the family live with uncertainty, they are encouraged to plan for each day and to make the most of each day. The tasks and challenges are to assist the patient to find useful coping mechanisms, adaptations, and compensations for solving problems that arise. This helps patients maintain some sense of control. An individualized exercise program helps maintain strength, endurance, and range of motion. Eventually, referral for home or hospice care may be necessary (see Chapter 17).

Improving Nutrition

Patients with nausea, vomiting, diarrhea, breathlessness, and pain are rarely interested in eating. These symptoms are managed or controlled through assessment, planning, and care. The nurse teaches the family how to position the patient for comfort during meals. Meals are planned for times when the patient is rested and in less distress from pain or the effects of treatment.

The patient needs to be clean, comfortable, and free of pain for meals, in an environment that is as attractive as possible. Oral hygiene before meals helps to improve appetite. Offensive sights, sounds, and odors are eliminated. Creative strategies may be required to make food more palatable, provide enough fluids, and increase opportunities for socialization during meals. The family may be asked to keep a daily weight chart and to record the quantity of food eaten to determine the daily calorie count. Dietary supplements, if acceptable to the patient, can be provided to meet increased caloric needs. If the patient is not interested in most usual foods, those foods preferred by the patient should be offered. When the patient shows marked deterioration as a result of tumor growth and effects, some other form of nutritional support (eg, tube feeding, parenteral nutrition) may be indicated if consistent with the patient's end-of-life preferences (Dudek, 2006). Nursing interventions include assessing the patency of the central and IV lines or feeding tube, monitoring the insertion site for infection, checking the infusion rate, monitoring intake and output, and changing the IV tubing and dressing. Family members are instructed in these techniques if they will be providing care at home. Parenteral nutrition can be provided at home if indicated.

The patient's quality of life may guide the selection, initiation, maintenance, and discontinuation of nutritional support. The nurse and family should not place too much emphasis on eating or on discussions about food, because the patient may not desire aggressive nutritional intervention. The subsequent course of action must be congruent with the wishes and choices of the patient and family.

Relieving Anxiety

Patients with cerebral metastases may be restless, with changing moods that may include intense depression, euphoria, paranoia, and severe anxiety. The response of patients to terminal illness reflects their pattern of reaction to other crisis situations. Serious illness imposes additional strains that often bring other unresolved problems to light. The patient's own coping strategies can help deal with anxious and depressed feelings. Health care providers need to be sensitive to the patient's concerns and fears.

Patients need the opportunity to exercise some control over their situation. A sense of mastery can be gained as they learn to understand the disease and its treatment and how to deal with their feelings. The presence of family, friends, a spiritual advisor, and health professionals may be supportive. Support groups such as the Brain Tumor Support Group may provide a feeling of support and strength.

Spending time with patients allows them time to talk and to communicate their fears and concerns. Open communication and acknowledgment of fears are often therapeutic. Touch is also a form of communication. These patients need reassurance that continuing care will be provided and that they will not be abandoned. The situation becomes more endurable when others share in the experience of dying. If a patient's emotional reactions are very intense or prolonged, additional help from a spiritual advisor, social worker, or mental health professional may be indicated.

Enhancing Family Processes

The family needs to be reassured that their loved one is receiving optimal care and that attention will be paid to the patient's changing symptoms and concerns. When the patient can no longer carry out self-care, the family and additional support systems (social worker, home health aide, home care nurse, hospice nurse) may be needed. End-of-life care is provided with respect, and reassurance is provided by communicating the plan of care to the family (Fields, 2007).

Promoting Home and Community-Based Care

TEACHING PATIENTS SELF-CARE. The patient and family often have major responsibility for care at home. Therefore, teaching includes pain management strategies, prevention of complications related to treatment strategies, and methods to ensure adequate fluid and food intake (Chart 65-3). Teaching needs of the patient and family regarding care priorities are likely to change as the disease progresses. The nurse should assess the changing needs of the patient and the family and inform them about resources and services early, to assist them in dealing with changes in the patient's condition.

CONTINUING CARE. Home care nursing and hospice services are valuable resources that should be made available to the patient and the family early in the course of a terminal illness. Anticipating needs before they occur can assist in smooth initiation of services. Home care needs and interventions focus on four major areas: palliation of symptoms and pain control, assistance in self-care, control of treatment complications, and administration of specific forms of treatment, such as parenteral nutrition. The home care nurse assesses pain management, respiratory status, complications of the disorder and its treatment, and the patient's cognitive and emotional status. Additionally, the nurse assesses the family's ability to perform necessary care and notifies the physician about changing needs or complications if indicated.

The patient and family who elect to care for the patient at home as the disease progresses benefit from the care and support provided through hospice and palliative care services (Fields, 2007). Steps to initiate hospice care, including discussion of hospice care as an option, should not be postponed until death is imminent. Exploration of hospice care as an option should be initiated at a time when hospice services can provide support and care to the patient and family consistent with their end-of-life decisions and can assist in allowing death with dignity. End-of-life care is further described in Chapter 17.

Evaluation

Expected Patient Outcomes

Expected patient outcomes may include the following:

1. Engages in self-care activities as long as possible
   a. Uses assistive devices or accepts assistance as needed

HOME CARE CHECKLIST
The Patient With Cerebral Metastases

At the completion of the home care instruction, the patient or caregiver will be able to:	PATIENT	CAREGIVER
• State effects of the tumor according to its type and location in the brain.	✔	✔
• Describe side effects of treatment.	✔	✔
• Identify community resources, including:		
• Home health services	✔	✔
• Hospices	✔	✔
• Support groups	✔	✔
• American Brain Tumor Association	✔	✔
• Identify coping strategies, such as:		
• Taking control, setting daily goals, and staying positive	✔	✔
• Rehabilitation to improve self-care	✔	✔
• Relaxation techniques	✔	✔
• Family support		✔
• Verbalize an understanding of the treatment plan for:		
• Medications and pain control	✔	✔
• Nutritional needs	✔	✔
• Contacting the health care provider	✔	✔

    b. Schedules periodic rest periods to permit maximal participation in self-care

2. Maintains as optimal a nutritional status as possible

    a. Eats and accepts food within limits of condition and preferences

    b. Accepts alternative methods of providing nutrition if indicated

3. Reports being less anxious

    a. Is less restless and is sleeping better

    b. Verbalizes concerns and fears about death

    c. Participates in activities of personal importance as long as feasible

4. Family members seek help as needed

    a. Demonstrate ability to bathe, feed, and care for the patient and participate in pain management and prevention of complications

    b. Express feelings and concerns to appropriate health professionals

    c. Discuss and seek hospice care as an option

Spinal Cord Tumors

Tumors within the spine are classified according to their anatomic relation to the spinal cord. They include intramedullary lesions (within the spinal cord), extramedullary-intradural lesions (within or under the spinal dura), and extramedullary-extradural lesions (outside the dural membrane). Tumors that occur within the spinal cord or exert pressure on it cause symptoms ranging from localized or shooting pains and weakness and loss of reflexes above the tumor level to progressive loss of motor function and paralysis. Usually, sharp pain occurs in the area inner-vated by the spinal roots that arise from the cord in the region of the tumor. In addition, increasing sensory deficits develop below the level of the lesion.

Assessment and Diagnostic Findings

Neurologic examination and diagnostic studies are used to make the diagnosis. Neurologic examination includes assessment of pain, loss of reflexes, loss of sensation or motor function, and the presence of weakness and paralysis. Additional assessment findings usually include pain duration for longer than 1 month and an elevated erythrocyte sedimentation rate. Helpful diagnostic studies include x-rays, radionuclide bone scans, CT scans, MRI scans, and biopsy. The MRI scan is the most commonly used and the most sensitive diagnostic tool, and it is particularly helpful in detecting epidural spinal cord compression and metastases (Rowland, 2005).

Medical Management

Treatment of specific intraspinal tumors depends on the type and location of the tumor and the presenting symptoms and physical status of the patient. Surgical intervention is the primary treatment for most spinal cord tumors. Other treatment modalities include partial removal of the tumor, decompression of the spinal cord, chemotherapy, and radiation therapy, particularly for intramedullary tumors and metastatic lesions (Rowland, 2005).

Epidural spinal cord compression occurs in 5% to 7% of patients who die of cancer and is considered a neurologic emergency. For the patient with epidural spinal cord compression resulting from metastatic cancer (most commonly from breast, prostate, or lung), high-dose dexamethasone (Decadron) combined with radiation therapy is effective in relieving pain (Held-Warmkessel, 2005). See Chapter 16 for a discussion of care of the patient with spinal cord compression. Palliative care may be an option for the medical management of some patients.

Surgical Management

Tumor removal is desirable but not always possible. The goal is to remove as much tumor as possible while sparing uninvolved portions of the spinal cord. Microsurgical techniques have improved the prognosis for patients with intramedullary tumors. Prognosis is related to the degree of neurologic impairment at the time of surgery, the speed with which symptoms occurred, and the origin of the tumor. Patients with extensive neurologic deficits before surgery usually do not make significant functional recovery even after successful tumor removal.

Nursing Management

Providing Preoperative Care

The objectives of preoperative care include recognition of neurologic changes through ongoing assessments, pain control, and management of altered activities of daily living (ADLs) resulting from sensory and motor deficits and bowel and bladder dysfunction. The nurse assesses for weakness, muscle wasting, spasticity, sensory changes, bowel and bladder dysfunction, and potential respiratory problems, especially if a cervical tumor is present. The patient is also evaluated for coagulation deficiencies. A history of aspirin intake is obtained and reported, because the use of aspirin may impede hemostasis postoperatively. Breathing exercises are taught and demonstrated preoperatively. Postoperative pain management strategies are discussed with the patient before surgery.

Assessing the Patient After Surgery

The patient is monitored for deterioration in neurologic status. A sudden onset of neurologic deficit is an ominous sign and may be due to vertebral collapse associated with spinal cord infarction. Frequent neurologic checks are carried out, with emphasis on movement, strength, and sensation of the upper and lower extremities. Assessment of sensory function involves pinching the skin of the arms, legs, and trunk to determine if there is loss of feeling and, if so, at what level. Vital signs are monitored at regular intervals.

Managing Pain

The prescribed pain medication should be administered in adequate amounts and at appropriate intervals to relieve pain and prevent its recurrence. Pain is the hallmark of spinal metastasis. Patients with sensory root involvement or vertebral collapse may suffer excruciating pain, which requires effective pain management (Hickey, 2009).

The bed is usually kept flat initially. The nurse turns the patient as a unit, keeping shoulders and hips aligned and the back straight. The side-lying position is usually the most comfortable, because this position imposes the least pressure on the surgical site. Placement of a pillow between the knees of the patient in a side-lying position helps to prevent extreme knee flexion.

Monitoring and Managing Potential Complications

If the tumor was in the cervical area, respiratory compromise due to postoperative edema may occur. The nurse monitors the patient for asymmetric chest movement, abdominal breathing, and abnormal breath sounds. For a high cervical lesion, the endotracheal tube remains in place until adequate respiratory function is ensured. The patient is encouraged to perform deep-breathing and coughing exercises.

The area over the bladder is palpated or a bladder scan is performed to assess for urinary retention. The nurse also monitors for incontinence, because urinary dysfunction usually implies significant decompensation of spinal cord function. An intake and output record is maintained. Additionally, the abdomen is auscultated for bowel sounds.

Staining of the dressing may indicate leakage of CSF from the surgical site, which may lead to serious infection or to an inflammatory reaction in the surrounding tissues that can cause severe pain in the postoperative period.

Promoting Home and Community-Based Care

Teaching Patients Self-Care

In preparation for discharge, the patient is assessed for the ability to function independently in the home and for the availability of resources such as family members to assist in caregiving. Patients with residual sensory involvement are cautioned about the dangers of extremes in temperature. They should be alerted to the dangers of heating devices (eg, hot water bottles, heating pads, space heaters). The patient is taught to check skin integrity daily. Patients with impaired motor function related to motor weakness or paralysis may require training in ADLs and safe use of assistive devices, such as a cane, walker, or wheelchair.

The patient and family members are instructed about pain management strategies, bowel and bladder management, and assessment for signs and symptoms that should be reported promptly.

Continuing Care

Referral for inpatient or outpatient rehabilitation may be warranted to improve self-care abilities. A home care referral may be indicated and provides the home care nurse with the opportunity to assess the patient's physical and psychological status and the patient's and family's ability to adhere to recommended management strategies. During the home visit, the nurse determines whether changes in neurologic function have occurred. The patient's respiratory status and nutritional status are assessed. The adequacy of pain management is assessed, and modifications are made to ensure adequate pain relief. The need for hospice services or placement in an extended-care facility is discussed with the patient and family if warranted, and the patient is asked about preferences for end-of-life care. Additionally, social workers may be consulted to assist the patient and family members in identifying support groups and agencies that can provide help in coping with the disease process.

DEGENERATIVE DISORDERS

Disorders of the central and peripheral nervous system that are **neurodegenerative** (leading to deterioration of normal cells or function of the nervous system) are characterized by the slow onset of signs and symptoms. Patients are managed at home for as long as possible and are admitted to the acute care setting for exacerbations, treatments, and surgical interventions as needed.

Parkinson's Disease

Parkinson's disease is a slowly progressing neurologic movement disorder that eventually leads to disability. It is the fourth most common neurodegenerative disease, and 50,000 new cases are reported each year in the United States (Chen & Fernandez, 2007; Thomure, 2006). The disease affects men more often than women. Symptoms usually first appear in the fifth decade of life; however, cases have been diagnosed as early as 30 years of age.

The degenerative or idiopathic form of Parkinson's disease is the most common; there is also a secondary form with a known or suspected cause. Although the cause of most cases is unknown, research suggests several causative factors, including genetics, atherosclerosis, excessive accumulation of oxygen free radicals, viral infections, head trauma, chronic use of antipsychotic medications, and some environmental exposures.

Pathophysiology

Parkinson's disease is associated with decreased levels of dopamine resulting from destruction of pigmented neuronal cells in the substantia nigra in the basal ganglia region of the brain (Fig. 65-4). Fibers or neuronal pathways project from the substantia nigra to the corpus striatum, where neurotransmitters are key to the control of complex body movements. Through the neurotransmitters acetylcholine (excitatory) and dopamine (inhibitory), striatal neurons relay messages to the higher motor centers that control and refine motor movements. The loss of dopamine stores in this area of the brain results in more excitatory neurotransmitters than inhibitory neurotransmitters, leading to an imbalance that affects voluntary movement.

Clinical symptoms do not appear until 60% of the pigmented neurons are lost and the striatal dopamine level is decreased by 80%. Cellular degeneration impairs the extrapyramidal tracts that control semiautomatic functions and coordinated movements; motor cells of the motor cortex and the pyramidal tracts are not affected. Researchers are working on uncovering the exact mechanism of neurodegeneration; current theories suggest that it results from oxidative stress in a portion of the neuron known as Lewy bodies, protein aggregation, or a combination of the two mechanisms (Barker & Barasi, 2008).

Clinical Manifestations

Parkinson's disease has a gradual onset, and symptoms progress slowly over a chronic, prolonged course. The cardinal signs are tremor, rigidity, **bradykinesia** (abnormally slow movements), and postural instability (Chen & Fernandez, 2007; Thomure, 2006).

Tremor

Although symptoms are variable, a slow, unilateral resting tremor is present in the majority of patients at the time of diagnosis (Chen & Fernandez, 2007). Resting tremor

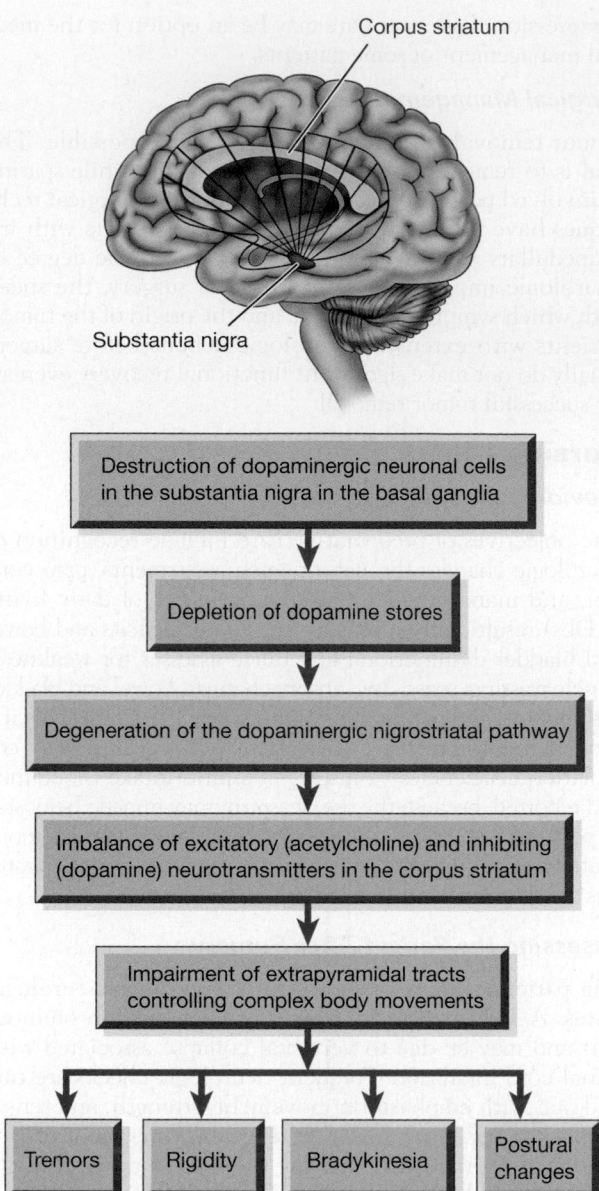

Figure 65-4 Pathophysiology of Parkinson's disease. The nuclei in the substantia nigra project fibers to the corpus striatum. The nerve fibers carry dopamine to the corpus striatum. The loss of dopamine nerve cells from the brain's substantia nigra is thought to be responsible for the symptoms of parkinsonism.

characteristically disappears with purposeful movement but is evident when the extremities are motionless. The tremor may manifest as a rhythmic, slow turning motion (pronation–supination) of the forearm and the hand and a motion of the thumb against the fingers as if rolling a pill between the fingers. Tremor is present while the patient is at rest; it increases when the patient is walking, concentrating, or feeling anxious.

Rigidity

Resistance to passive limb movement characterizes muscle rigidity. Passive movement of an extremity may cause the limb to move in jerky increments, referred to as lead-pipe or cog-wheel movements (Chen & Fernandez, 2007).

Involuntary stiffness of the passive extremity increases when another extremity is engaged in voluntary active movement. Stiffness of the arms, legs, face, and posture are common. Early in the disease, the patient may complain of shoulder pain due to rigidity.

Bradykinesia

One of the most common features of Parkinson's disease is bradykinesia, which refers to the overall slowing of active movement (Chen & Fernandez, 2007; Thomure, 2006). Patients may also take longer to complete activities and have difficulty initiating movement, such as rising from a sitting position or turning in bed.

Postural Instability

The patient commonly develops postural and gait problems. A loss of postural reflexes occurs, and the patient stands with the head bent forward and walks with a propulsive gait. The posture is caused by the forward flexion of the neck, hips, knees, and elbows. The patient may walk faster and faster, trying to move the feet forward under the body's center of gravity (shuffling gait). Difficulty in pivoting causes loss of balance (either forward or backward). Gait impairment and postural instability place the patient at increased risk for falls (Sadowski, Jones, Gordon, et al., 2007).

Other Manifestations

The effect of Parkinson's disease on the basal ganglia often produces autonomic symptoms that include excessive and uncontrolled sweating, paroxysmal flushing, orthostatic hypotension, gastric and urinary retention, constipation, and sexual dysfunction (Miller, 2009). Psychiatric changes include depression, **dementia** (progressive mental deterioration), delirium, and hallucinations. Depression is common; whether it is a reaction to the disorder or is related to a biochemical abnormality is uncertain. Mental changes may appear in the form of cognitive, perceptual, and memory deficits, although intellect is not usually affected. A number of psychiatric manifestations (personality changes, psychosis, dementia, and acute confusion) are common in elderly patients with Parkinson's disease. Dementia affects up to 75% of patients over the course of the disease (Weintraub & Hurtig, 2007). In addition, auditory and visual hallucinations have been reported in up to 40% of people with Parkinson's disease and may be associated with depression, dementia, lack of sleep, or adverse effects of medications.

Hypokinesia (abnormally diminished movement) is also common and may appear after the tremor. The freezing phenomenon refers to a transient inability to perform active movement and is thought to be an extreme form of bradykinesia. Additionally, the patient tends to shuffle and exhibits a decreased arm swing. As dexterity declines, **micrographia** (small handwriting) develops. The face becomes increasingly masklike and expressionless, and the frequency of blinking decreases. **Dysphonia** (soft, slurred, low-pitched, and less audible speech) may occur as a result of weakness and incoordination of the muscles responsible for speech. In many cases, the patient develops dysphagia, begins to drool, and is at risk for choking and aspiration.

Complications associated with Parkinson's disease are common and are typically related to disorders of movement.

As the disease progresses, patients are at risk for respiratory and urinary tract infection, skin breakdown, and injury from falls. The adverse effects of medications used to treat the symptoms are associated with numerous complications such as dyskinesia or orthostatic hypotension (Karch, 2008).

Assessment and Diagnostic Findings

Although laboratory tests and imaging studies are not helpful to the clinician in diagnosing Parkinson's disease, ongoing research with PET and single photon emission computed tomography (SPECT) scanning has been helpful in understanding the disease and advancing treatment. Currently, the disease is diagnosed clinically from the patient's history and the presence of two of the four cardinal manifestations: tremor, rigidity, bradykinesia, and postural changes.

Early diagnosis can be difficult because patients rarely are able to pinpoint when the symptoms started. Often, a family member notices a change such as stooped posture, a stiff arm, a slight limp, tremor, or slow, small handwriting. The medical history, presenting symptoms, neurologic examination, and response to pharmacologic management are carefully evaluated when making the diagnosis (Thomure, 2006).

Medical Management

Treatment is directed at controlling symptoms and maintaining functional independence, because no medical or surgical approaches in current use prevent disease progression. Care is individualized for each patient based on presenting symptoms and social, occupational, and emotional needs. Pharmacologic management is the mainstay of treatment, although advances in research have led to increased surgical options. Patients are usually cared for at home and are admitted to the hospital only for complications or to initiate new treatments.

Pharmacologic Therapy

Antiparkinsonian medications act by (1) increasing striatal dopaminergic activity; (2) reducing the excessive influence of excitatory cholinergic neurons on the extrapyramidal tract, thereby restoring a balance between dopaminergic and cholinergic activities; or (3) acting on neurotransmitter pathways other than the dopaminergic pathway.

Levodopa (Larodopa) is the most effective agent and the mainstay of treatment. Levodopa is converted to dopamine in the basal ganglia, producing symptom relief. Levodopa is available in three forms: immediate-release, orally disintegrating, and sustained-release tablets (Halkias, Haq, Huang, et al., 2007). The beneficial effects of levodopa are most pronounced in the first few years of treatment. Benefits begin to wane and adverse effects become more severe over time. Confusion, hallucinations, depression, and sleep alterations are associated with prolonged use.

Within 5 to 10 years, most patients develop a response to the medication characterized by **dyskinesia** (abnormal involuntary movements), including facial grimacing, rhythmic jerking movements of the hands, head bobbing, chewing and smacking movements, and involuntary movements of the trunk and extremities. The patient may experience an on–off syndrome in which sudden periods of near immobility ("off effect") are followed by a sudden return of effectiveness of the medication ("on effect"). Various adjunctive therapies are used to minimize dyskinesias (Chen & Fernandez, 2007). Another potential complication of long-term dopaminergic medication use is neuroleptic malignant syndrome, which is characterized by severe rigidity, stupor, and hyperthermia (Ward, 2005). Additional medications used to treat Parkinson's disease are described in Table 65-1.

Surgical Management

The limitations of levodopa therapy, improvements in stereotactic surgery, and new approaches in transplantation have renewed interest in the surgical treatment of Parkinson's disease. In patients with disabling tremor, rigidity, or severe levodopa-induced dyskinesia, surgery may be considered. Although surgery provides symptom relief in selected patients, it has not been shown to alter the course of the disease or to produce permanent improvement.

Stereotactic Procedures

Thalamotomy and pallidotomy are effective in relieving many of the symptoms of Parkinson's disease (Rowland, 2005). Patients eligible for these procedures are those who have had an inadequate response to medical therapy; they must meet strict criteria to be eligible. Candidates eligible for these procedures are patients with idiopathic Parkinson's disease who are taking maximum doses of antiparkinsonian medications. Patients with dementia and atypical Parkinson's disease are usually not considered for stereotactic procedures. Parkinson's disease rating scales and specific neurologic tests are used to identify eligible patients.

The intent of thalamotomy and pallidotomy is to interrupt the nerve pathways and thereby alleviate tremor or rigidity. During thalamotomy, a stereotactic electrical stimulator destroys part of the ventrolateral portion of the thalamus in an attempt to reduce tremor; the most common complications are ataxia and hemiparesis. Pallidotomy involves destruction of part of the ventral aspect of the medial globus

Table 65-1	SUMMARY OF MEDICATIONS USED TO TREAT PARKINSON'S DISEASE	
Medications	**Indications and Therapeutic Effects**	**Common Side Effects**
Anticholinergic Agents Trihexyphenidyl hydrochloride (Apo-Trihex) Benztropine mesylate (Cogentin)	Control of tremor and rigidity Counteract the action of acetylcholine	Blurred vision, flushing, rash, constipation, urinary retention, and acute confusional states Contraindicated in patients with narrow-angle glaucoma
Antiviral Agents Amantadine hydrochloride (Symmetrel)	Reduce rigidity, tremor, bradykinesia, and postural changes in early Parkinson's disease	Psychiatric disturbances (mood changes, confusion, depression, hallucinations), lower extremity edema, nausea, epigastric distress, urinary retention, headache, and visual impairment
Dopamine Agonists Bromocriptine mesylate (Parlodel) Pergolide (Permax)	Early Parkinson's disease as well as secondary drug therapy after carbidopa or levodopa loses effectiveness	Nausea, vomiting, diarrhea, lightheadedness, hypotension, impotence, and psychiatric effects
Nonergot Derivatives Ropinirole hydrochloride (Requip) Pramipexole (Mirapex)	Early stages of Parkinson's disease	May cause drowsiness or dizziness
Monoamine Oxidase Inhibitors Selegiline (Eldepryl) Rasagiline (Azilect)	Inhibit dopamine breakdown	Can cause hypertensive crisis
Catechol-O-Methyltransferase Inhibitors Entacapone (Comtan) Tolcapone (Tasmar)	Increase the duration of action of carbidopa or levodopa Reduce motor fluctuations in patients with advanced Parkinson's disease	
Antidepressants *Tricyclic Antidepressants* Amitriptyline hydrochloride (Elavil)	Anticholinergic and antidepressant	Hypertension, insomnia, dry mouth
Serotonin Reuptake Inhibitors Fluoxetine hydrochloride (Prozac) Bupropion hydrochloride (Wellbutrin)	Antidepressant	Clinical worsening and suicide risk
Antihistamines Diphenhydramine hydrochloride (Benadryl) Orphenadrine citrate (Banflex) Phenindamine hydrochloride (Neo-Synephrine)	May reduce tremors	Anticholinergic and sedative effects

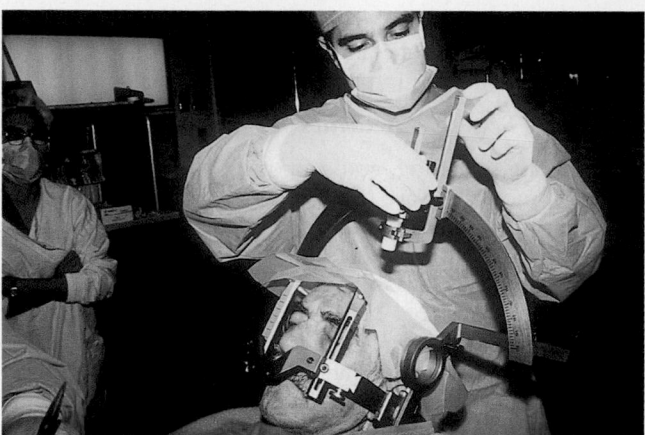

Figure 65-5 A stereotactic frame is applied to a patient's head in preparation for pallidotomy. The frame immobilizes the head.

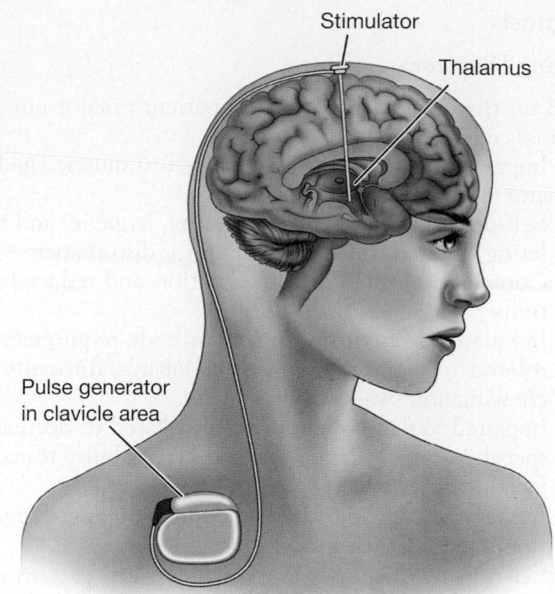

Figure 65-6 Deep brain stimulation is provided by a pulse generator surgically implanted in a pouch beneath the clavicle. The generator sends high-frequency electrical impulses to the thalamus, thereby blocking the nerve pathways associated with tremors in Parkinson's disease.

pallidus through electrical stimulation in patients with advanced disease. The procedure is effective in reducing rigidity, bradykinesia, and dyskinesia, thus improving motor function and ADLs in the immediate postoperative course. Potential complications include hemiparesis and stroke, as well as cognitive, speech, swallowing, and visual changes.

A CT scan, x-ray, MRI scan, or angiogram is used to localize the appropriate surgical site in the brain. Then the patient's head is positioned in a stereotactic frame (Fig. 65-5). After the surgeon makes an incision in the skin and a burr hole, an electrode is passed through to the target area in the thalamus or globus pallidum. The desired response of the patient to the electrical stimulation (ie, a decrease in rigidity) is the basis for the selection of the area of the brain to be destroyed. Stereotactic procedures are completed on one side of the brain at a time. If rigidity or tremor is bilateral, a 6-month interval is suggested between procedures.

Neural Transplantation

Ongoing research is exploring transplantation of porcine neuronal cells, human fetal cells, and stem cells (Rowland, 2005). Legal, ethical, and political concerns surrounding the use of fetal brain cells and stem cells have limited the implementation of these procedures.

Deep Brain Stimulation

Pacemakerlike brain implants are used to relieve tremors (Rowland, 2005). The stimulation can be bilateral or unilateral; bilateral stimulation of the subthalamic nucleus is thought to be of greater benefit to patients than results achieved with thalamotomy, pallidotomy, or fetal nigral transplantation. In deep brain stimulation, an electrode is placed in the thalamus and connected to a pulse generator that is implanted in a subcutaneous subclavicular or abdominal pouch. The battery-powered pulse generator sends high-frequency electrical impulses through a wire placed under the skin to a lead anchored to the skull (Fig. 65-6). The electrode blocks nerve pathways in the brain that cause tremors. These devices are not without complications that can result from both the surgical procedure needed for implantation and the device itself (eg, lead leakage) (Stewart, Desaloms & Sanghera, 2005).

NURSING PROCESS

THE PATIENT WITH PARKINSON'S DISEASE

Assessment

Assessment focuses on how the disease has affected the patient's ADLs and functional abilities. The patient is observed for degree of disability and functional changes that occur throughout the day, such as responses to medication. Almost every patient with a movement disorder has some functional alteration and may have some type of behavioral dysfunction. The following questions may be useful to assess alterations:

- Do you have leg or arm stiffness?
- Have you experienced any irregular jerking of your arms or legs?
- Have you ever been "frozen" or rooted to the spot and unable to move?
- Does your mouth water excessively? Have you (or others) noticed yourself grimacing or making faces or chewing movements?
- What specific activities do you have difficulty doing?

During this assessment, the nurse observes the patient for quality of speech, loss of facial expression, swallowing deficits (drooling, poor head control, coughing), tremors, slowness of movement, weakness, forward posture, rigidity, evidence of mental slowness, and confusion. Parkinson's disease symptoms, as well as side effects of medications, put these patients at high risk for falls; therefore, a fall risk assessment should be conducted (Sadowski, et al., 2007).

Diagnosis

Nursing Diagnoses

Based on the assessment data, the patient's major nursing diagnoses may include the following:

- Impaired physical mobility related to muscle rigidity and motor weakness
- Self-care deficits (feeding, dressing, hygiene, and toileting) related to tremor and motor disturbance
- Constipation related to medication and reduced activity
- Imbalanced nutrition, less than body requirements, related to tremor, slowness in eating, difficulty in chewing and swallowing
- Impaired verbal communication related to decreased speech volume, slowness of speech, inability to move facial muscles
- Ineffective coping related to depression and dysfunction due to disease progression

Other nursing diagnoses may include sleep pattern disturbances, deficient knowledge, risk for injury, risk for activity intolerance, disturbed thought processes, and compromised family coping.

Planning and Goals

The goals for the patient may include improving functional mobility, maintaining independence in ADLs, achieving adequate bowel elimination, attaining and maintaining acceptable nutritional status, achieving effective communication, and developing positive coping mechanisms.

Nursing Interventions

Improving Mobility

A progressive program of daily exercise will increase muscle strength, improve coordination and dexterity, reduce muscular rigidity, and prevent contractures that occur when muscles are not used. Walking, riding a stationary bicycle, swimming, and gardening are all exercises that help maintain joint mobility. Stretching (stretch–hold–relax) and range-of-motion exercises promote joint flexibility. Postural exercises are important to counter the tendency of the head and neck to be drawn forward and down. A physical therapist may be helpful in developing an individualized exercise program and can provide instruction to the patient and caregiver on exercising safely. Faithful adherence to an exercise and walking program helps delay the progress of the disease. Warm baths and massage, in addition to passive and active exercises, help relax muscles and relieve painful muscle spasms that accompany rigidity.

Balance may be adversely affected because of the rigidity of the arms (arm swinging is necessary in normal walking). Special walking techniques must be learned to offset the shuffling gait and the tendency to lean forward. The patient is taught to concentrate on walking erect, to watch the horizon, and to use a wide-based gait (ie, walking with the feet separated). A conscious effort must be made to swing the arms, raise the feet while walking, and use a heel–toe placement of the feet with long strides. The patient is advised to practice walking to marching music or to the sound of a ticking metronome, because this provides sensory rein-

forcement. Performing breathing exercises while walking helps move the rib cage and aerate parts of the lungs. Frequent rest periods aid in preventing frustration and fatigue.

Enhancing Self-Care Activities

Encouraging, teaching, and supporting the patient during ADLs promote self-care (Stewart, et al., 2005). See Chapter 11 for rehabilitation techniques.

Environmental modifications are necessary to compensate for functional disabilities. Patients may have severe mobility problems that make normal activities impossible. Adaptive or assistive devices may be useful. A hospital bed at home with bedside rails, an overbed frame with a trapeze, or a rope tied to the foot of the bed can provide assistance in pulling up without help. An occupational therapist can evaluate the patient's needs in the home, make recommendations regarding adaptive devices, and teach the patient and caregiver how to improvise.

Improving Bowel Elimination

The patient may have severe problems with constipation. Among the factors causing constipation are weakness of the muscles used in defecation, lack of exercise, inadequate fluid intake, and decreased autonomic nervous system activity. The medications used for the treatment of the disease also inhibit normal intestinal secretions. A regular bowel routine may be established by encouraging the patient to follow a regular time pattern, consciously increase fluid intake, and eat foods with moderate fiber content. Laxatives should be avoided. Psyllium (Metamucil), for example, decreases constipation but carries the risk of bowel obstruction (Karch, 2008). A raised toilet seat is useful, because the patient has difficulty in moving from a standing to a sitting position.

Improving Nutrition

Patients may have difficulty maintaining their weight. Eating becomes a very slow process, requiring concentration due to a dry mouth from medications and difficulty chewing and swallowing. These patients are at risk for aspiration because of impaired swallowing and the accumulation of saliva. They may be unaware that they are aspirating; subsequently, bronchopneumonia may develop.

Monitoring weight on a weekly basis indicates whether caloric intake is adequate. Supplemental feedings increase caloric intake. As the disease progresses, a nasogastric tube or percutaneous endoscopic gastroscopy may be necessary to maintain adequate nutrition. A dietitian can be consulted regarding nutritional needs.

Enhancing Swallowing

Swallowing difficulties and choking are common in Parkinson's disease (Chen & Fernandez, 2007). These can lead to problems with poor head control, tongue tremor, hesitancy in initiating swallowing, difficulty in shaping food into a bolus, and disturbances in pharyngeal motility. To offset these problems, the patient should sit in an upright position during mealtime. A semisolid diet with thick liquids is easier to swallow than solids; thin liquids should be avoided. Thinking through the swallowing sequence is helpful. The patient is taught to place the food on the tongue, close the lips and teeth, lift the tongue up and then back, and swallow. The patient is encouraged to chew first on one side of the mouth and then on the other. To control the buildup of saliva, the patient is reminded to hold the head upright and make a conscious effort to swallow. Massaging the facial and neck muscles before meals may be beneficial.

Encouraging the Use of Assistive Devices

An electric warming tray keeps food hot and allows the patient to rest during the prolonged time that it may take to eat. Special utensils also assist at mealtime. A plate that is stabilized, a nonspill cup, and eating utensils with built-up handles are useful self-help devices. The occupational therapist can assist in identifying appropriate adaptive devices.

Improving Communication

Speech disorders are present in most patients with Parkinson's disease. The low-pitched, monotonous, soft speech of patients requires that they make a conscious effort to speak slowly, with deliberate attention to what they are saying. The patient is reminded to face the listener, exaggerate the pronunciation of words, speak in short sentences, and take a few deep breaths before speaking. A speech therapist may be helpful in designing speech improvement exercises and assisting the family and health care personnel to develop and use a method of communication that meets the patient's needs. A small electronic amplifier is helpful if the patient has difficulty being heard.

Supporting Coping Abilities

Support can be given by encouraging the patient and pointing out that activities will be maintained through active participation. A combination of physiotherapy, psychotherapy, medication therapy, and support group participation may help reduce the depression that often occurs. Patients with Parkinson's disease can become withdrawn. It is best if patients are active participants in their therapeutic program, including social and recreational events. A planned program of activity throughout the day prevents too much daytime sleeping as well as disinterest and apathy.

Patients often feel embarrassed, apathetic, inadequate, bored, and lonely. In part, these feelings may result from physical slowness and the great effort that even small tasks require. The patient is assisted and encouraged to set achievable goals (eg, improvement of mobility). Every effort should be made to encourage patients to carry out the tasks involved in meeting their own daily needs and to remain independent. Doing things for the patient merely to save time undermines the basic goal of improving coping abilities and promoting a positive self-concept.

Promoting Home and Community-Based Care

TEACHING PATIENTS SELF-CARE. Patient and family education is important in the management of Parkinson's disease. Teaching needs depend on the severity of symptoms and the stage of the disease. Care must be taken not to overwhelm the patient and family with too much information early in the disease process. The patient's and family's need for information is ongoing as adaptations become necessary. The education plan should include a clear explanation of the disease and the goal of assisting the patient to remain functionally independent as long as possible. Every effort is made to explain the nature of the disease and its management to offset disabling anxieties and fears. The patient and family must be taught about the effects and side effects of medications and about the importance of reporting side effects to the physician (Chart 65-4).

CONTINUING CARE. In the early stages, the patient can be managed well at home. Family members often serve as caregivers, with home care or community services available to assist in meeting health care needs as the disease progresses. The family caregiver may be under considerable stress from living with and caring for a person with a significant disability. Providing information about treatment and care prevents many unnecessary problems. The caregiver is included in the plan and may be advised to learn stress reduction techniques, to include others in the caregiving process, to obtain periodic relief from responsibilities, and to have a yearly health assessment. Allowing family members to express feelings of frustration, anger, and guilt is often helpful to them.

The patient should be evaluated in the home for adaptation and safety needs and compliance with the plan of care. In the advanced stages, patients usually enter long-term care facilities if family support is absent. Periodically, admission to an acute care facility may be necessary for changes in medical management or treatment of complications. Nurses provide support, education, and monitoring of patients over the course of the illness.

The nurse involved in home and continuing care needs to remind the patient and family members of the importance of addressing health promotion needs such as screening for hypertension and stroke risk assessments in this predominantly elderly population. Patients are taught about the importance of these activities and are referred to appropriate health care providers. Informational booklets and a newsletter for patient education are published by the National Parkinson's Foundation, Inc., and the American Parkinson's Disease Association (see Resources).

Evaluation

Expected Patient Outcomes

Expected patient outcomes may include the following:

1. Strives toward improved mobility
   a. Participates in exercise program daily
   b. Walks with wide base of support; exaggerates arm swinging when walking
   c. Takes medications as prescribed
2. Progresses toward self-care
   a. Allows time for self-care activities
   b. Uses self-help devices
3. Maintains bowel function
   a. Consumes adequate fluid
   b. Increases dietary intake of fiber
   c. Reports regular pattern of bowel function
4. Attains improved nutritional status
   a. Swallows without aspiration
   b. Takes time while eating
5. Achieves a method of communication
   a. Communicates needs
   b. Practices speech exercises

CHART 65-4	HOME CARE CHECKLIST *The Patient With Parkinson's Disease*		
At the completion of the home care instruction, the patient or caregiver will be able to:		**PATIENT**	**CAREGIVER**
• Define Parkinson's disease and discuss its long-term effects.		✔	✔
• Identify the medication regimen and name adverse effects, and precautions.		✔	✔
• Discuss the risk for injury; prevent falls; implement adaptive measures in the home.		✔	✔
• Describe nutritional needs, dietary restrictions, dysphagia management, and ways to prevent aspiration.		✔	✔
• Manage constipation: fluid intake, bowel routine.		✔	✔
• Manage urinary problems: functional incontinence, retention (indwelling urinary catheter care, suprapubic catheter care).		✔	✔
• Explain effects of immobility and define preventive care: skin breakdown (frequent turning, pressure release, skin care), pneumonia (deep breathing, movement), contractures (range-of-motion exercises).		✔	✔
• Define benefits of daily exercise program.		✔	✔
• Walk and balance safely.		✔	
• Demonstrate speech and communication skills: speech exercises, communication techniques, breathing exercises.		✔	
• Name signs and symptoms of infection (urinary and respiratory) and state when health care provider should be notified.		✔	✔
• Describe strategies to promote self-care activities and independence.		✔	✔
• Identify resources: American Parkinson's Disease Association, National Parkinson's Disease Foundation, and local support groups.		✔	✔

6. Copes with effects of Parkinson's disease
   a. Sets realistic goals
   b. Demonstrates persistence in meaningful activities
   c. Verbalizes feelings to appropriate person

Huntington Disease

Huntington disease is a chronic, progressive, hereditary disease of the nervous system that results in progressive involuntary choreiform movement and dementia. The disease affects approximately 1 in 10,000 men or women of all races at midlife. It is transmitted as an autosomal dominant genetic disorder; therefore, each child of a parent with Huntington disease has a 50% risk of inheriting the disorder (Skirton, 2005).

A genetic marker for Huntington disease has been identified. Researchers can identify people who will develop this disease. However, genetic testing offers no hope of cure or even specific prediction of the timing of disease onset. Even though the gene was mapped in 1983 and presymptomatic testing has been offered since 1986, many patients choose not to be tested. For most people, the benefits of testing are unclear because of ethical issues and concerns about confidentiality. Genetic counseling is crucial after testing, and patients and their families may require long-term psychological counseling and emotional, financial, and legal support. People of childbearing age with a family history of Huntington disease often seek information about their risk of disease transmission.

Pathophysiology

The basic pathology involves premature death of cells in the striatum (caudate and putamen) of the basal ganglia, the region deep within the brain that is involved in the control of movement. Cells also are lost in the cortex, the region of the brain associated with thinking, memory, perception, and judgment, and in the cerebellum, the area that coordinates voluntary muscle activity. Why the protein destroys only certain brain cells is unknown, but several theories have been proposed to explain the phenomenon (Barker & Barasi, 2008; Skirton, 2005). One possible theory is that a building block for protein called glutamine abnormally collects in the cell nucleus, causing cell death (Walker, 2007).

Clinical Manifestations

The most prominent clinical features of the disease are **chorea** (abnormal involuntary movements), intellectual decline, and, often, emotional disturbance (Bickley, 2007; Walker, 2007). As the disease progresses, a constant writhing, twisting, uncontrollable movement may involve the entire body. These motions are devoid of purpose or rhythm, although patients may try to turn them into purposeful movement. All of the body musculature is involved. Facial movements produce tics and grimaces. Speech becomes slurred, hesitant, often explosive, and eventually unintelligible. Chewing and swallowing are difficult, and there is a constant danger of choking and aspiration. Choreiform movements persist during sleep but are diminished.

As with speech, the gait becomes disorganized to the point that ambulation eventually is impossible. Although independent ambulation should be encouraged for as long as possible, a wheelchair usually becomes necessary. Eventually, the patient is confined to bed when the chorea interferes with walking, sitting, and all other activities. Bladder and bowel control is lost. Cognitive function is usually affected, with dementia usually occurring. Initially, the patient is aware that the disease is responsible for the myriad dysfunctions that are occurring. The mental and emotional changes that occur may be more devastating to the patient and family than the abnormal movements. Personality changes may result in nervous, irritable, or impatient behaviors. In the early stages, patients are particularly subject to uncontrollable fits of anger; profound, often suicidal depression; apathy; anxiety; psychosis; or euphoria. Judgment and memory are impaired, and dementia eventually ensues. Hallucinations, delusions, and paranoid thinking may precede the appearance of disjointed movements. Emotional and cognitive symptoms often become less acute as the disease progresses (Walker, 2007).

Onset usually occurs between 35 and 45 years of age, although about 10% of patients are children. The disease progresses slowly. Despite a ravenous appetite, patients usually become emaciated and exhausted. Patients succumb in 10 to 20 years to heart failure, pneumonia, or infection, or as a result of a fall or choking.

Assessment and Diagnostic Findings

The diagnosis is made based on the clinical presentation of characteristic symptoms, a positive family history, the known presence of a genetic marker, and exclusion of other causes.

Management

Although no treatment halts or reverses the underlying process, medications may reduce chorea. Thiothixene hydrochloride (Navane) and haloperidol decanoate (Haldol), which predominantly block dopamine receptors, improve the chorea in many patients. Motor signs must be assessed and evaluated on an ongoing basis so that optimal therapeutic drug levels can be reached. **Akathisia** (motor restlessness) in the overmedicated patient is dangerous because it may be mistaken for the restless fidgeting of the illness and consequently may be overlooked. In certain types of the disease, hypokinetic motor impairment resembles Parkinson's disease. In patients who present with rigidity, some temporary benefit may be obtained from antiparkinson medications, such as levodopa (Larodopa).

Patients who have emotional disturbances, particularly depression, may be helped by antidepressant medications. The threat of suicide is present particularly early in the course of the disease (Walker, 2007). Psychotic symptoms usually respond to antipsychotic medications. Psychotherapy aimed at allaying anxiety and reducing stress may be beneficial. Nurses must look beyond the disease to focus on the patient's needs and capabilities (Chart 65-5). Chart 65-6 explores an ethical issue related to end-of-life care for a patient with Huntington disease.

Several new treatments, such as fetal tissue transplantation and the use of growth factor delivered to the basal ganglia region of the brain, are under investigation (Barker & Barasi, 2008; Skirton, 2005).

Promoting Home and Community-Based Care

Teaching Patients Self-Care

The needs of the patient and family for education depend on the nature and severity of the physical, cognitive, and psychological changes experienced by the patient. The patient and family members are taught about the medications prescribed and about signs indicating a need for change in medication or dosage. The teaching plan addresses strategies to manage symptoms such as chorea, swallowing problems, limitations in ambulation, and loss of bowel and bladder function. Consultation with a speech therapist may be indicated to assist in identifying alternative communication strategies if speech is affected.

Continuing Care

A program combining medical, nursing, psychological, social, occupational, speech, and physical rehabilitation services and palliative care is needed to help the patient and family cope with this severely disabling illness (Olson & Cristian, 2005). Huntington disease exacts enormous emotional, physical, social, and financial tolls on every member of the patient's family. The family needs supportive care as they adjust to the impact of the illness (Skirton, 2005; Walker, 2007). Regular follow-up visits help allay the fear of abandonment.

Home care assistance, day care centers, respite care, and eventually skilled long-term care can assist the patient and family in coping with the constant strain of the illness. Although the relentless progression of the disease cannot be halted, families can benefit from supportive care.

Voluntary organizations can be major aids to families and have been largely responsible for bringing the illness to national attention. The Huntington's Disease Foundation of America helps patients and families by providing information, referrals, family and public education, and support for research.

Alzheimer's Disease

Alzheimer's disease, or senile dementia of the Alzheimer's type, is a chronic, progressive, and degenerative brain disorder that is accompanied by profound effects on memory, cognition, and ability for self-care. Approximately 4.5 million people in the United States are affected (Ganzer, 2007). Alzheimer's disease is one of the most feared disorders of modern times because of its catastrophic consequences for the patient, family, and caregivers, who are faced with many crucial end-of-life decisions. Chapter 12 discusses the manifestations, management, and nursing care of the patient with Alzheimer's disease.

Amyotrophic Lateral Sclerosis

Amyotrophic lateral sclerosis (ALS) is a disease of unknown cause in which there is a loss of motor neurons (nerve cells controlling muscles) in the anterior horns of

Chart 65-5 • *Care of the Patient With Huntington Disease*

Nursing Diagnosis: Risk for injury from falls and possible skin breakdown (pressure ulcers, abrasions), resulting from constant movement

Nursing Interventions

Pad the sides and head of the bed; ensure that the patient can see over the sides of bed.
Use padded heel and elbow protectors.
Keep the skin meticulously clean.
Apply emollient cleansing agent and skin lotion as needed.
Use soft sheets and bedding.
Have patient wear football padding or other forms of padding.
Encourage ambulation with assistance to maintain muscle tone.
Secure the patient (only if necessary) in bed or chair with padded protective devices, making sure that they are loosened frequently.

Nursing Diagnosis: Imbalanced nutrition, less than body requirements, due to inadequate intake and dehydration resulting from swallowing or chewing disorders and danger of choking or aspirating food

Nursing Interventions

Administer phenothiazines as prescribed before meals (appears to calm some patients).
Talk to the patient before mealtime to promote relaxation; use mealtime for social interaction. Provide undivided attention and help the patient enjoy the mealtime experience.
Use a warming tray to keep food warm.
Learn the position that is best for *this* patient. Keep patient as close to upright as possible while feeding. Stabilize patient's head gently with one hand while feeding.
Show the food and explain what the foods are (eg, whether hot or cold).
Encircle the patient with one arm and get as close as possible to provide stability and support while feeding. Use pillows and wedges for additional support.
Do not interpret stiffness, turning away, or sudden turning of the head as rejection; these are uncontrollable choreiform movements.
For feeding, use a long-handled spoon (iced-tea spoon). Place spoon on middle of tongue and exert slight pressure.
Place bite-sized food between patient's teeth. Serve stews, casseroles, and thick liquids.
Disregard messiness and treat the person with dignity.

Wait for the patient to chew and swallow before introducing another spoonful. Make sure that bite-sized food is small.
Give between-meal feedings. Constant movement expends more calories. Patients often have voracious appetites, particularly for sweets.
Use blenderized meals if patient cannot chew; do not repeatedly give the same strained baby foods; gradually introduce increased textures and consistencies to the diet.
For swallowing difficulties:
Apply gentle deep pressure around the patient's mouth. Rub fingers in circles on the patient's cheeks and then down each side of the patient's throat.
Develop skill in Heimlich maneuver (to be used in the event of choking).

Nursing Diagnosis: Anxiety and impaired communication from excessive grimacing and unintelligible speech

Nursing Interventions

Read to the patient.
Employ biofeedback and relaxation therapy to reduce stress.
Consult with speech therapist to help maintain and prolong communication abilities.
Try to devise a communication system, perhaps using cards with words or pictures of familiar objects, before verbal communication becomes too difficult. Patients can indicate correct card by hitting it with hand, grunting, or blinking the eyes.
Learn how this particular patient expresses needs and wants—particularly nonverbal messages (widening of eyes, responses).
Patients can understand even if unable to speak. Do not isolate patients by ceasing to communicate with them.

Nursing Diagnosis: Disturbed thought processes and impaired social interaction

Nursing Interventions

Reorient the patient after awakening.
Have clock, calendar, and wall posters in view to assist in orientation.
Use every opportunity for one-to-one contact.
Use music for relaxation.
Have the patient wear a medical identification bracelet.
Keep the patient in the social mainstream.
Recruit and train volunteers for social interaction. Role-model appropriate and creative interactions.
Do not abandon a patient because the disease is eventually terminal. Patients are *living* until the end.

---

the spinal cord and the motor nuclei of the lower brain stem. It is often referred to as Lou Gehrig's disease after the famous baseball player who suffered from the disease. As motor neuron cells die, the muscle fibers that they supply undergo atrophic changes. Neuronal degeneration may occur in both the upper and lower motor neuron systems (see Chapter 60). The leading theory held by researchers is that overexcitation of nerve cells by the neurotransmitter glutamate results in cell injury and neuronal degeneration. Possible causes of ALS include autoimmune disease, free radical damage, and oxidative stress. In 5% to 10% of cases the cause is transmission of an autosomal dominant trait for familial ALS (Runge & Patterson, 2006; Tiwari, Xu &

Hayward, 2005). Several risk factors have been identified, but the exact cause is still unknown (Gal, Strom, Kilty, et al., 2007; Tiwari, et al., 2005).

Clinical Manifestations

Clinical manifestations depend on the location of the affected motor neurons, because specific neurons activate specific muscle fibers. The chief symptoms are fatigue, progressive muscle weakness, cramps, fasciculations (twitching), and incoordination. Loss of motor neurons in the anterior horns of the spinal cord results in progressive weakness and atrophy of the muscles of the arms, trunk, or legs. Spasticity usually is present, and the deep tendon stretch reflexes

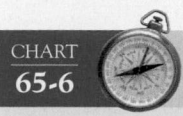

CHART 65-6 · *Ethics and Related Issues*

What Constitutes Assisted Suicide?

Situation

A 65-year-old man is admitted to the hospital with Huntington disease. He is in respiratory distress and near death and he is unable to communicate his wishes. The family state that they want no heroic measures, and the physician writes a "do not resuscitate" order on the chart.

Dilemma

The principle of beneficence and the nurse's duty to provide care conflict with the principle of respect for the person and the patient's right to death with dignity.

Discussion

1. Is the "do not resuscitate" order an act of assisted suicide?
2. Is it active or passive euthanasia? What is the nurse's role in caring for the patient if this action conflicts with his or her personal beliefs?
3. If no other nurse is available to provide care, does the nurse on duty have the right to refuse to provide care? Is this patient abandonment?

become brisk and overactive. Usually, the function of the anal and bladder sphincters remains intact, because the spinal nerves that control muscles of the rectum and urinary bladder are not affected.

In about 25% of patients, weakness starts in the muscles supplied by the cranial nerves, and difficulty in talking, swallowing, and ultimately breathing occurs. When the patient ingests liquids, soft palate and upper esophageal weakness causes the liquid to be regurgitated through the nose. Weakness of the posterior tongue and palate impairs the ability to laugh, cough, or even blow the nose. If bulbar muscles are impaired, speaking and swallowing are progressively difficult, and aspiration becomes a risk. The voice assumes a nasal sound, and articulation becomes so disrupted that speech is unintelligible. Some emotional liability may be present. It was traditionally believed that ALS spared cognitive function, but it is now recognized that some patients experience cognitive impairment.

The prognosis generally is based on the area of CNS involvement and the speed with which the disease progresses. Eventually, respiratory function is compromised. Death usually occurs as a result of infection, respiratory failure, or aspiration.

Assessment and Diagnostic Findings

ALS is diagnosed on the basis of the signs and symptoms, because no clinical or laboratory tests are specific for this disease. Electromyography and muscle biopsy studies of the affected muscles indicate reduction in the number of functioning motor units. An MRI scan may show high signal intensity in the corticospinal tracts; this differentiates ALS from a multifocal motor neuropathy. Neuropsychological testing can assist in assessment and diagnosis (Phukan, Pender & Hardiman, 2007).

Management

No specific therapy exists for ALS. The main focus of medical and nursing management is on interventions to maintain or improve function, well-being, and quality of life. The average survival time is 3 to 5 years with death due, most commonly, to respiratory insufficiency (Tiwari, et al., 2005).

The medication riluzole (Rilutek), a glutamate antagonist, is the only medication with U.S. Food and Drug Administration approval for treatment of ALS (Hickey, 2009). The action of riluzole is not clear, but its pharmacologic properties suggest that it may have a neuroprotective effect in the early stages of ALS. Symptomatic treatment and rehabilitative measures are used to support the patient and improve the quality of life. Baclofen (Lioresal), dantrolene sodium (Dantrium), or diazepam (Valium) may be useful for patients troubled by spasticity, which causes pain and interferes with self-care. Research evaluating the effect of ceftriaxone sodium (Rocephin) found that it slows the course of the disease in animals, but it has not yet been tested in humans (Brown, 2005).

Most patients with ALS are managed at home and in the community, with hospitalization for acute problems. The most common reasons for hospitalization are dehydration and malnutrition, pneumonia, and respiratory failure; recognizing these problems at an early stage in the illness allows for the development of preventive strategies. End-of-life issues include pain, dyspnea, and delirium (Olson & Cristian, 2005).

Mechanical ventilation (using negative-pressure ventilators) is an option if alveolar hypoventilation develops. Noninvasive positive-pressure ventilation is also an option. The use of noninvasive positive-pressure ventilation is particularly helpful at night and postpones the decision about whether to undergo a tracheotomy for long-term mechanical ventilation.

A patient experiencing aspiration and swallowing may require enteral feeding. A percutaneous endoscopic gastrostomy tube is inserted before the forced vital capacity drops below 50% of the predicted value. The tube can be safely placed in patients who are using noninvasive positive-pressure ventilation for ventilatory support (Hickey, 2009).

Decisions about life support measures are made by the patient and family and should be based on a thorough understanding of the disease, the prognosis, and the implications of initiating such therapy. Patients are encouraged to complete an advance directive or "living will" to preserve their autonomy in decision making. See Chapter 17 for additional discussion of end-of-life care.

The Amyotrophic Lateral Sclerosis Association has broad programs of research funding, patient and clinical services, patient information and support, and medical and public information. The *ALS Association Quarterly Newsletter* is a source of practical information (see Resources).

Muscular Dystrophies

The muscular dystrophies are a group of incurable muscle disorders characterized by progressive weakening and wasting of the skeletal or voluntary muscles. Most of these diseases are inherited. Duchenne muscular dystrophy, the most common type, occurs in 1 of every 3500 male births

(Rowland, 2005). The pathologic features include degeneration and loss of muscle fibers, variation in muscle fiber size, phagocytosis and regeneration, and replacement of muscle tissue by connective tissue. The common characteristics of these diseases include varying degrees of muscle wasting and weakness and abnormal elevation in serum levels of muscle enzymes (Barker & Barasi, 2008). Differences among these diseases center on the genetic pattern of inheritance, the muscles involved, the age at onset, and the rate of disease progression. The unique needs of these patients, who in the past did not live to adulthood, must be addressed as they live longer because of better supportive care.

Medical Management

Treatment of the muscular dystrophies focuses on supportive care and prevention of complications in the absence of a cure or specific pharmacologic interventions (Rowland, 2005). The goal of supportive management is to keep the patient active and functioning as normally as possible and to minimize functional deterioration. An individualized therapeutic exercise program is prescribed to prevent muscle tightness, contractures, and disuse atrophy. Night splints and stretching exercises are used to delay contractures of the joints, especially the ankles, knees, and hips. Braces may compensate for muscle weakness.

Spinal deformity is a severe problem. Weakness of trunk muscles and spinal collapse occur almost routinely in patients with severe neuromuscular disease. To help prevent spinal deformity, the patient is fitted with an orthotic jacket to improve sitting stability and reduce trunk deformity. This measure also supports cardiovascular status. In time, spinal fusion is performed to maintain spinal stability. Other procedures may be carried out to correct deformities.

Compromised pulmonary function may result either from progression of the disease or from deformity of the thorax secondary to severe scoliosis. Upper respiratory infections and fractures from falls must be vigorously treated in a way that minimizes immobilization because joint contractures become worse when the patient's activities are more restricted than usual.

Other difficulties may be manifested in relation to the underlying disease. Weakness of the facial muscles makes it difficult to attend to dental hygiene and to speak clearly. Gastrointestinal tract problems may include gastric dilation, rectal prolapse, and fecal impaction. Finally, cardiomyopathy appears to be a common complication in all forms of muscular dystrophy (Rowland, 2005).

Genetic counseling is advised for parents and siblings of the patient because of the genetic nature of this disease. The Muscular Dystrophy Association works to combat neuromuscular disease through research, programs of patient services and clinical care, and professional and public education (see Resources).

Nursing Management

The goals of the patient and the nurse are to maintain function at optimal levels and to enhance the quality of life. Therefore, the patient's physical requirements, which are considerable, are addressed without losing sight of emotional and developmental needs. The patient and family are actively involved in decision making, including end-of-life decisions.

During hospitalization for treatment of complications, the knowledge and expertise of the patient and family members responsible for caregiving in the home are assessed. Because the patient and family caregivers often have developed caregiving strategies that work effectively for them, these strategies need to be acknowledged and accepted, and provisions must be made to ensure that they are maintained during hospitalization.

Families of adolescents and young adults with muscular dystrophy need assistance to shift the focus of care from pediatric to adult care and to understand the usual disease course. Nursing goals include assisting the adolescent to make the transition to adult values and expectations while providing age-appropriate ongoing care. The nurse may need to help build the confidence of an older adolescent or adult patient by encouraging him or her to pursue job training to become economically independent. Other nursing interventions might include guidance in accessing adult health care and finding appropriate programs in sex education.

Promoting Home and Community-Based Care

Teaching Patients Self-Care

The management goals are addressed in special rehabilitation programs or in the patient's home and community. Therefore, the patient and family require information and instruction about the disorder, its anticipated course, and care and management strategies that will optimize the patient's growth and development and physical and psychological status. Members of a variety of health-related disciplines are involved in patient and family teaching; recommendations are communicated to all members of the health care team so that they may work toward common goals (Rowland, 2005).

Continuing Care

Both the neuromuscular disease and the associated deformities may progress in adolescence and adulthood. Self-help and assistive devices can aid in maintaining maximum independence. These devices, recommended by physical and occupational therapists, often become necessary as more muscle groups are affected.

The family is taught to monitor the patient for respiratory problems, because respiratory infection and cardiac failure are the most common causes of death (Rowland, 2005). As respiratory difficulties develop, patients and their families need information regarding respiratory support. Options currently exist that can provide ventilatory support (eg, negative-pressure devices, positive-pressure ventilators) while allowing mobility. Patients can remain relatively independent in a wheelchair, for example, while being maintained on a ventilator at home for many years.

The patient is encouraged to continue with range-of-motion exercises to prevent contractures, which are particularly disabling. Practical adaptations must be made, however, to cope with the effects of chronic neuromuscular disability. The patient at various stages of the disease may require a manual or an electric wheelchair, gait aids, upper and lower extremity and spinal orthoses, seating systems, bathroom equipment, lifts, ramps, and additional assistive devices, all of which require a team approach. The home care nurse assesses how the patient and family are managing, makes referrals, and coordinates the activities of the physical therapist, occupational therapist, and social services.

The patient is greatly concerned about issues surrounding the threat of increasing disability and dependence on others, accompanied by a significant deterioration in health-related quality of life. The patient is faced with a progressive loss of function, leading eventually to death. Feelings of helplessness and powerlessness are common. Each functional loss is accompanied by grief and mourning. The patient and family are assessed for depression, anger, or denial. The patient and family are assisted and encouraged to address decisions about end-of-life options before their need arises.

A psychiatric nurse clinician or other mental health professional may assist the patient to cope and adapt to the disease. By understanding and addressing the physical and psychological needs of the patient and family, the nurse provides a hopeful, supportive, and nurturing environment.

Degenerative Disk Disease

Low back pain is the second most common neurologic disorder in the United States. It is estimated that there were more than 450,000 lumbar spinal surgeries for herniated disks, stenosis, and degenerative changes in 2003 in the United States (Agency for Healthcare Research and Quality, 2008). There are significant economic costs to patients, their families, and society. Acute low back pain lasts less than 3 months, whereas chronic or degenerative disease has a duration of 3 months or longer. Most back problems are related to disk disease.

Pathophysiology

The intervertebral disk is a cartilaginous plate that forms a cushion between the vertebral bodies (Fig. 65-7A). This tough, fibrous material is incorporated in a capsule. A ball-like cushion in the center of the disk is called the nucleus

pulposus. In herniation of the intervertebral disk (ruptured disk), the nucleus of the disk protrudes into the annulus (the fibrous ring around the disk), with subsequent nerve compression. Protrusion or rupture of the nucleus pulposus usually is preceded by degenerative changes that occur with aging. Loss of protein polysaccharides in the disk decreases the water content of the nucleus pulposus. The development of radiating cracks in the annulus weakens resistance to nucleus herniation. After trauma (falls and repeated minor stresses such as lifting incorrectly), the cartilage may be injured.

For most patients, the immediate symptoms of trauma are short-lived, and those resulting from injury to the disk do not appear for months or years. Then, with degeneration in the disk, the capsule pushes back into the spinal canal, or it may rupture and allow the nucleus pulposus to be pushed back against the dural sac or against a spinal nerve as it emerges from the spinal column (see Fig. 65-7B). This sequence produces pain due to **radiculopathy** (pressure in the area of distribution of the involved nerve endings). Continued pressure may produce degenerative changes in the involved nerve, such as changes in sensation and deep tendon reflexes.

Clinical Manifestations

A herniated disk with accompanying pain may occur in any portion of the spine: cervical, thoracic (rare), or lumbar. The clinical manifestations depend on the location, the rate of development (acute or chronic), and the effect on the surrounding structures.

Assessment and Diagnostic Findings

A thorough health history and physical examination are important to rule out potentially serious conditions that may manifest as low back pain, including fracture, tumor, infection, or cauda equina syndrome (Hickey, 2009).

The MRI scan has become the diagnostic tool of choice for localizing even small disk protrusions, particularly for lumbar spine disease. If the clinical symptoms are not consistent with the pathology seen on MRI, CT scanning and

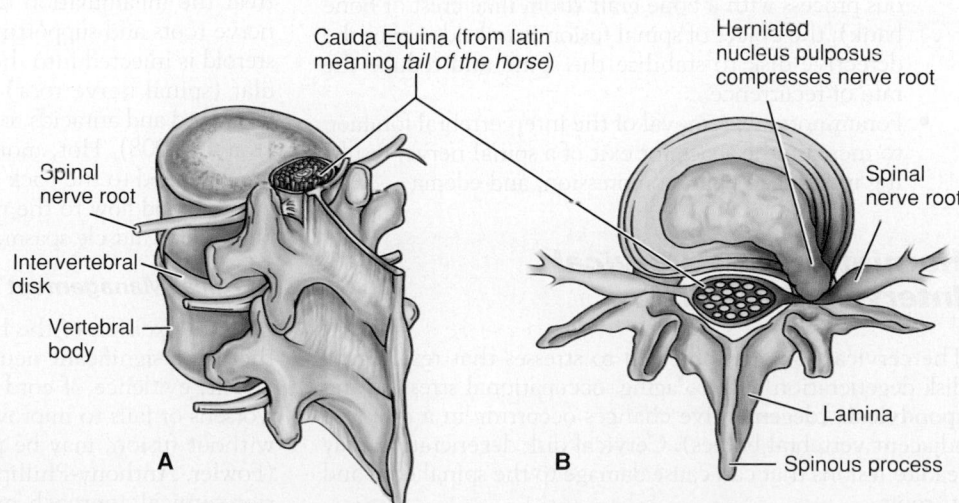

Cauda Equina (from latin meaning *tail of the horse*)

Herniated nucleus pulposus compresses nerve root

Spinal nerve root

Intervertebral disk

Vertebral body

Spinal nerve root

Lamina

Spinous process

A

B

Figure 65-7 A, Normal lumbar spine vertebrae, invertebral disks, and spinal nerve root. **B,** Ruptured vertebral disc.

myelography are performed. A neurologic examination is carried out to determine whether reflex, sensory, or motor impairment from root compression is present and to provide a baseline for future assessment. Electromyography may be used to localize the specific spinal nerve roots involved.

Medical Management

Herniations of the cervical and the lumbar disks occur most commonly and are usually managed conservatively with bed rest and medication (Hickey, 2009). Surgery is sometimes necessary.

Surgical Management

Surgical excision of a herniated disk is performed if there is evidence of a progressing neurologic deficit (muscle weakness and atrophy, loss of sensory and motor function, loss of sphincter control) and continuing pain or **sciatica** (leg pain resulting from sciatic nerve involvement) that are unresponsive to conservative management (Weber & Kelley, 2007). The goal of surgical treatment is to reduce the pressure on the nerve root to relieve pain and reverse neurologic deficits (Hickey, 2009). Microsurgical techniques make it possible to remove only the amount of tissue that is necessary, which preserves the integrity of normal tissue better and imposes less trauma on the body. During these procedures, spinal cord function can be monitored electrophysiologically.

To achieve the goal of pain relief, several surgical techniques are used, depending on the type and location of disk herniation, surgical morbidity, and results of previous surgery. Some of the surgical techniques available include:

- Microdiskectomy: removal of herniated or extruded fragments of intervertebral disk material
- Laminectomy: removal of the bone between the spinal process and facet pedicle junction to expose the neural elements in the spinal canal (Hickey, 2009); this allows the surgeon to inspect the spinal canal, identify and remove pathologic tissue, and relieve compression of the cord and roots
- Hemilaminectomy: removal of part of the lamina and part of the posterior arch of the vertebra
- Partial laminectomy or laminotomy: creation of a hole in the lamina of a vertebra
- Diskectomy with fusion: fusion of the vertebral spinous process with a bone graft (from iliac crest or bone bank); the object of spinal fusion is to bridge over the defective disk to stabilize the spine and reduce the rate of recurrence
- Foraminotomy: removal of the intervertebral foramen to increase the space for exit of a spinal nerve, resulting in reduced pain, compression, and edema

Herniation of a Cervical Intervertebral Disk

The cervical spine is subjected to stresses that result from disk degeneration (due to aging, occupational stresses) and **spondylosis** (degenerative changes occurring in a disk and adjacent vertebral bodies). Cervical disk degeneration may lead to lesions that can cause damage to the spinal cord and its roots.

Clinical Manifestations

A cervical disk herniation usually occurs at the C5–C6 or C6–C7 interspaces.

Pain and stiffness may occur in the neck, the top of the shoulders, and the region of the scapulae. Sometimes patients interpret these signs as symptoms of heart trouble or bursitis. Pain may also occur in the upper extremities and head, accompanied by **paresthesia** (tingling or a "pins and needles" sensation) and numbness of the upper extremities. Cervical MRI usually confirms the diagnosis.

Medical Management

The goals of treatment are to rest and immobilize the cervical spine to give the soft tissues time to heal and to reduce inflammation in the supporting tissues and the affected nerve roots in the cervical spine. Bed rest (usually 1 to 2 days) is important because it eliminates the stress of gravity and relieves the cervical spine of the need to support the head. It also reduces inflammation and edema in soft tissues around the disk, relieving pressure on the nerve roots. Proper positioning on a firm mattress may bring dramatic relief from pain.

The cervical spine may be rested and immobilized by a cervical collar, cervical traction, or a brace. A collar allows maximal opening of the intervertebral foramina and holds the head in a neutral or slightly flexed position. The patient may have to wear the collar 24 hours a day during the acute phase. The skin under the collar is inspected for irritation. After the patient is free of pain, cervical isometric exercises are started to strengthen the neck muscles.

Pharmacologic Therapy

Analgesic agents (nonsteroidal anti-inflammatory agents [NSAIDs], propoxyphene [Darvon], oxycodone [Tylox], or hydrocodone [Vicodin]) are prescribed during the acute phase to relieve pain, and sedatives may be administered to control the anxiety that is often associated with cervical disk disease. Muscle relaxants (cyclobenzaprine [Flexeril], methocarbamol [Robaxin], metaxalone [Skelaxin]) are administered to interrupt muscle spasm and to promote comfort. NSAIDs (aspirin, ibuprofen [Motrin, Advil], naproxen [Naprosyn, Anaprox]) or corticosteroids are prescribed to treat the inflammation that usually occurs in the affected nerve roots and supporting tissues. Occasionally, a corticosteroid is injected into the epidural space for relief of radicular (spinal nerve root) pain. NSAIDs are administered with food and antacids to prevent gastrointestinal irritation (Karch, 2008). Hot, moist compresses (for 10 to 20 minutes) applied to the back of the neck several times daily increase blood flow to the muscles and help relax the patient and reduce muscle spasm.

Surgical Management

Surgical excision of the herniated disk may be necessary if there is a significant neurologic deficit, progression of the deficit, evidence of cord compression, or pain that either worsens or fails to improve. A cervical diskectomy, with or without fusion, may be performed to alleviate symptoms (Fowler, Anthony-Phillips, Mehta, et al., 2005). An anterior surgical approach may be used through a transverse incision to remove disk material that has herniated into the spinal canal and foramina, or a posterior approach may be used at the appropriate level of the cervical spine. Potential complications with the anterior approach include carotid or vertebral artery injury, recurrent laryngeal nerve dysfunction, esophageal perforation, and airway obstruction. Complications of the posterior approach include damage to the nerve root or the spinal cord due to retraction or contusion of either of these structures, resulting in weakness of muscles supplied by the nerve root or cord.

Microsurgery, such as endoscopic microdiskectomy, may be performed in selected patients through a small incision, using magnification techniques. This usually results in less tissue trauma and pain, and patients consequently have a shorter hospital stay compared with those who have conventional surgery.

NURSING PROCESS

The Patient Undergoing a Cervical Diskectomy

Assessment

The patient is asked about past injuries to the neck (whiplash), because unresolved trauma can cause persistent discomfort, pain and tenderness, and symptoms of arthritis in the injured joint of the cervical spine. Assessment includes determining the onset, location, and radiation of pain and assessing for paresthesias, limited movement, and diminished function of the neck, shoulders, and upper extremities. It is important to determine whether the symptoms are bilateral; with large herniations, bilateral symptoms may be caused by cord compression. The area around the cervical spine is palpated to assess muscle tone and tenderness. Range of motion in the neck and shoulders is evaluated.

The patient is asked about any health issues that may influence the postoperative course and quality of life (Fowler, et al., 2005). It is also important to assess mood and stress levels (Starkweather, Witek-Janusek, Nockels, et al., 2006). The nurse determines the patient's need for information about the surgical procedure and reinforces what the physician has explained. Strategies for pain management are discussed with the patient.

Diagnosis

Nursing Diagnoses

Based on the assessment data, the patient's major nursing diagnoses may include the following:

- Acute pain related to the surgical procedure
- Impaired physical mobility related to the postoperative surgical regimen
- Deficient knowledge about the postoperative course and home care management

Other nursing diagnoses may include preoperative anxiety, postoperative constipation, urinary retention related to the surgical procedure, self-care deficits related to use of a neck orthosis, and sleep pattern disturbance related to disruption in lifestyle.

Collaborative Problems/Potential Complications

Based on all the assessment data, the potential complications may include the following:

- Hematoma at the surgical site, resulting in cord compression and neurologic deficit
- Recurrent or persistent pain after surgery

Planning and Goals

The goals for the patient may include relief of pain, improved mobility, increased knowledge and self-care ability, and prevention of complications.

Nursing Interventions

Relieving Pain

The patient may be kept flat in bed for 12 to 24 hours. If the patient has had a bone fusion with bone removed from the iliac crest, considerable pain may be experienced at the donor site. Interventions consist of monitoring the donor site for hematoma formation, administering the prescribed postoperative analgesic agent, positioning for comfort, and reassuring the patient that the pain can be relieved. If the patient experiences a sudden increase in pain, extrusion of the graft may have occurred, requiring reoperation. A sudden increase in pain should be promptly reported to the surgeon.

The patient may experience a sore throat, hoarseness, and dysphagia due to temporary edema. These symptoms are relieved by throat lozenges, voice rest, and humidification. A puréed diet may be given if the patient has dysphagia.

Improving Mobility

Postoperatively, a cervical collar (neck orthosis) is usually worn, which contributes to limited neck motion and altered mobility. The patient is instructed to turn the body instead of the neck when looking from side to side. The neck should be kept in a neutral (midline) position. The patient is assisted during position changes, to make sure that head, shoulders, and thorax are kept aligned. When assisting the patient to a sitting position, the nurse supports the patient's neck and shoulders. To increase stability, the patient should wear shoes when ambulating.

Monitoring and Managing Potential Complications

The patient is evaluated for bleeding and hematoma formation by assessing for excessive pressure in the neck or severe pain in the incision area. The dressing is inspected for serosanguineous drainage, which suggests a dural leak. If this occurs, meningitis is a threat. A complaint of headache requires careful evaluation. Neurologic checks are made for swallowing deficits and upper and lower extremity weakness, because cord compression may produce rapid or delayed onset of paralysis. The patient who has had an anterior cervical diskectomy is also assessed for a sudden return of radicular (spinal nerve root) pain, which may indicate instability of the spine.

Throughout the postoperative course, the patient is monitored frequently to detect any signs of respiratory difficulty, because retractors used during surgery may injure the recurrent laryngeal nerve, resulting in hoarseness and the inability to cough effectively and clear pulmonary secretions. In addition, the blood pressure and pulse are monitored to evaluate cardiovascular status.

Bleeding at the surgical site and subsequent hematoma formation may occur. Severe localized pain not relieved by analgesic agents should be reported to the surgeon. A change in neurologic status (motor or sensory function) should be reported promptly, because it suggests hematoma formation that may necessitate surgery to prevent irreversible motor and sensory deficits.

Promoting Home and Community-Based Care

TEACHING PATIENTS SELF-CARE. The patient's hospital stay is likely to be short; therefore, the patient and family should understand the care that is important for a smooth recovery. A cervical collar is usually worn for about 6 weeks. The patient is instructed in use and care of the cervical collar. The patient is instructed to alternate tasks that involve minimal body movement (eg, reading) with tasks that require greater body movement.

The patient is instructed about strategies for pain management and about signs and symptoms that may indicate complications that should be reported to the physician. The nurse assesses the patient's understanding of these management strategies, limitations, and recommendations. Additionally, the nurse assists the patient in identifying strategies to cope with ADLs (eg, self-care, childcare) and minimize risks to the surgical site (Chart 65-7). A discharge teaching plan is developed collaboratively by members of the health care team to decrease the risk of recurrent disk herniation. Topics include those previously discussed as well as proper body mechanics, maintenance of optimal weight, proper exercise techniques, and modifications in activity.

CONTINUING CARE. The patient is instructed to see the physician at prescribed intervals so that the physician can document the disappearance of old symptoms and assess the range of motion of the neck. Recurrent or persistent pain may occur despite removal of the offending disk or disk fragments. Patients who undergo discectomy usually have consented to surgery after prolonged pain; they have often

---

CHART 65-7

HOME CARE CHECKLIST
The Patient With Cervical Discectomy and Cervical Collar

At the completion of the home care instruction, the patient or caregiver will be able to:	PATIENT	CAREGIVER
• Care for the surgical incision site.		
• Keep staples or sutures clean and dry and cover with dry dressing.		✔
• Notify physician if any signs or symptoms of infection occur, such as fever, redness or irritation, drainage, increased pain.	✔	✔
• Demonstrate proper body mechanics and prescribed exercise techniques.	✔	
• Modify activity:		
• Avoid sitting or standing for more than 30 minutes.	✔	
• Avoid twisting, flexing, extending, or rotating the neck.	✔	
• Avoid long automobile rides.	✔	
• Avoid sleeping in a prone position or use of pillows, to minimize neck flexion in bed; keep head in a neutral position.	✔	
• Use adequate mattress and chair support.	✔	
• Wear low-heeled shoes.	✔	
• Follow physician's instructions regarding lifting, climbing stairs, driving a car, sexual activity, sports, exercise, and return to work.	✔	
• Practice stress reduction and relaxation techniques.	✔	
• Care of the cervical collar:		
• Wear the collar at all times until directed otherwise by the physician.	✔	
• Wash the neck twice a day with mild soap.	✔	✔
• Keep the neck still while the collar is open.	✔	
• With the assistance of a helper, wash the neck in steps:		
• Lie flat and supine.	✔	
• Open the Velcro tabs on each side of the collar and remove its front portion.		✔
• Gently wash and dry the neck.		✔
• Replace the front part of the collar and refasten the tabs.		✔
• Turn to one side with a thin pillow under the head.	✔	
• Open one tab.	✔	
• Gently wash and dry the back of the neck. Refasten the tab.		✔
• Turn to the other side and wash and dry this side. Refasten the tab.		✔
• Place a wrinkle-free silk scarf under the collar to increase comfort.	✔	✔
• **For men:** Shave without twisting or moving the neck. This may be done with help while lying flat or sitting. Remove only the front part of the collar for shaving.	✔	✔

undergone repeated courses of ineffective conservative management and previous surgeries to relieve the pain. Therefore, the recurrence or persistence of symptoms postoperatively, including pain and sensory deficits, is often discouraging for the patient and family. The patient who experiences recurrence of symptoms requires emotional support and understanding. Additionally, the patient is assisted in modifying activities and in considering options for subsequent treatment. The nurse reminds the patient and family members of the need to participate in health promotion and health screening practices.

Evaluation

Expected Patient Outcomes

Expected patient outcomes may include the following:

1. Reports decreasing frequency and severity of pain
2. Demonstrates improved mobility
   a. Demonstrates progressive participation in self-care activities
   b. Identifies prescribed activity limitations and restrictions
   c. Demonstrates proper body mechanics
3. Is knowledgeable about postoperative course, medications, and home care management
   a. Lists the signs and symptoms to be reported postoperatively
   b. Identifies dose, action, and potential side effects of medications
   c. Identifies appropriate home care management activities and any restrictions
4. Has absence of complications
   a. Reports no increase in incision pain or sensory symptoms
   b. Demonstrates normal findings on neurologic assessment

Herniation of a Lumbar Disk

Approximately 90% to 95% of lumbar disk herniations occur at the L5–S1 region (Hickey, 2009). A herniated lumbar disk produces low back pain accompanied by varying degrees of sensory and motor impairment.

Clinical Manifestations

The patient complains of low back pain with muscle spasms, followed by radiation of the pain into one hip and down into the leg (sciatica). Pain is aggravated by actions that increase intraspinal fluid pressure, such as bending, lifting, or straining (as in sneezing or coughing), and usually is relieved by bed rest. Usually there is some type of postural deformity, because pain causes an alteration of the normal spinal mechanics. If the patient lies on the back and attempts to raise a leg in a straight position, pain radiates into the leg; this maneuver, called the straight leg-raising test, stretches the sciatic nerve. Additional signs include muscle weakness, alterations in tendon reflexes, and sensory loss.

Assessment and Diagnostic Findings

The diagnosis of lumbar disk disease is based on the history and physical findings and the use of imaging techniques such as MRI, CT, and myelography.

Medical Management

The objectives of treatment are to relieve pain, slow disease progression, and increase the patient's functional ability. Bed rest, previously standard in treatment of back pain, is recommended for 2 days or less (Hickey, 2009).

Because muscle spasm is prominent during the acute phase, muscle relaxants are used. NSAIDs and systemic corticosteroids may be administered to counter the inflammation that usually occurs in the supporting tissues and the affected nerve roots. Moist heat and massage help relax muscles. Strategies for increasing the patient's functional ability include weight reduction, physical therapy, and biofeedback. Exercises, prescribed by physical therapists, can help strengthen back muscles and decrease pain (Hickey, 2009). Chapter 13 describes nursing interventions for the patient with pain.

Surgical Management

In the lumbar region, surgical treatment includes lumbar disk excision through a posterolateral laminotomy and the newer techniques of microdiskectomy and percutaneous diskectomy. In microdiskectomy, an operating microscope is used to visualize the offending disk and compressed nerve roots; it permits a small incision (2.5 cm [1 inch]) and minimal blood loss and takes about 30 minutes of operating time. Generally, the hospital stay is short, and the patient makes a rapid recovery. Several minimally invasive techniques in spinal surgery have led to improved patient outcomes and lower hospital costs, and research on these techniques is ongoing (Starkweather, Witek-Janusek, Nockels, et al., 2008). Research suggests that intraoperative wound infiltration with bupivacaine hydrochloride solution decreases pain and the need for opioids postoperatively (Ersayli, Gurget, Bekar, et al., 2006).

Complications of Disk Surgery

A patient undergoing a disk procedure at one level of the vertebral column may have a degenerative process at other levels. A herniation relapse may occur at the same level or elsewhere, so the patient may become a candidate for another disk procedure. Arachnoiditis (inflammation of the arachnoid membrane) may occur after surgery (and after myelography); it involves an insidious onset of diffuse, frequently burning pain in the lower back, radiating into the buttocks. Disk excision can leave adhesions and scarring around the spinal nerves and dura, which then produce inflammatory changes that create chronic neuritis and neurofibrosis. Disk surgery may relieve pressure on the spinal nerves, but it does not reverse the effects of neural injury and scarring and the pain that results. Failed disk syndrome (recurrence of sciatica after lumbar diskectomy) remains a cause of disability (Hickey, 2009).

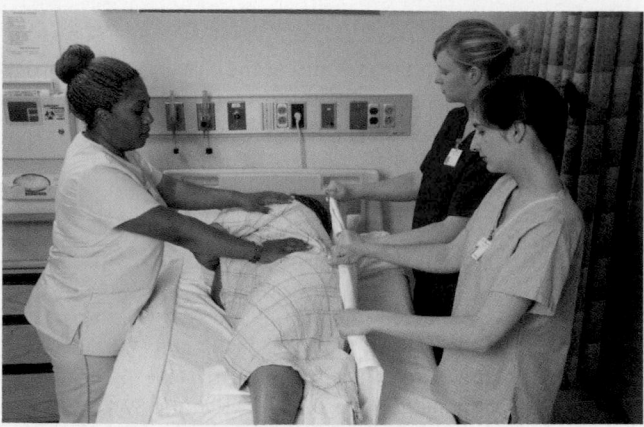

Figure 65-8 Before the patient undergoes laminectomy surgery, the logrolling technique that will be used for turning the patient should be demonstrated. The patient's arms will be crossed and the spine aligned. To avoid twisting the spine, the head, shoulders, knees, and hips are turned at the same time so that the patient rolls over like a log. When in a side-lying position, the patient's back, buttocks, and legs are supported with pillows.

Nursing Management

Providing Preoperative Care

Most patients fear surgery on any part of the spine and therefore need explanations about the surgery and reassurance that it will not weaken the back. When data are being collected for the health history, any reports of pain, paresthesia, or muscle spasm are recorded to provide a baseline for comparison after surgery. Health issues that may influence the postoperative course and quality of life (eg, fatigue, mood, stress, patient expectations) are important to assess (Saban & Penckofer, 2007; Starkweather, et al., 2008). Preoperative assessment also includes an evaluation of movement of the extremities as well as bladder and bowel function. To facilitate the postoperative turning procedure, the patient is taught to turn as a unit (called logrolling) as part of the preoperative preparation (see Fig. 65-8). Before surgery, the patient is also encouraged to take deep breaths, cough, and perform muscle-setting exercises to maintain muscle tone.

Assessing the Patient After Surgery

After lumbar disk excision, vital signs are checked frequently and the wound is inspected for hemorrhage, because vascular injury is a complication of disk surgery. Because postoperative neurologic deficits may occur from nerve root injury, the sensation and motor strength of the lower extremities are evaluated at specified intervals, along with the color and temperature of the legs and sensation of the toes. It is important to assess for urinary retention, another sign of neurologic deterioration.

In diskectomy with fusion, the patient has an additional surgical incision if bone fragments were taken from the iliac crest or fibula to serve as wedges in the spine. The recovery period is longer than for those patients who underwent diskectomy without spinal fusion, because bony union must take place.

Positioning the Patient

To position the patient, a pillow is placed under the head, and the knee rest is elevated slightly to relax the back muscles. When the patient is lying on one side, however, extreme knee flexion must be avoided. The patient is encouraged to move from side to side to relieve pressure and is reassured that no injury will result from moving. When the patient is ready to turn, the bed is placed in a flat position and a pillow is placed between the patient's legs. The patient turns as a unit (logrolls) without twisting the back.

To get out of bed, the patient lies on one side while pushing up to a sitting position. At the same time, the nurse or family member eases the patient's legs over the side of the bed. Coming to a sitting or standing posture is accomplished in one long, smooth motion. Most patients walk to the bathroom on the same day as the surgery. Sitting is discouraged except for defecation.

Promoting Home and Community-Based Care

Teaching Patients Self-Care

The patient is advised to increase activity gradually, as tolerated, because it takes up to 6 weeks for the ligaments to heal. Excessive activity may result in spasm of the paraspinal muscles.

Activities that produce flexion strain on the spine (eg, driving a car) should be avoided until healing has taken place. Heat may be applied to the back to relax muscle spasms. Scheduled rest periods are important, and the patient is advised to avoid heavy work for 2 to 3 months after surgery. Exercises are prescribed to strengthen the abdominal and erector spinal muscles. A back brace or corset may be necessary if back pain persists.

Continuing Care

Referral for inpatient or outpatient rehabilitation may be warranted to improve self-care abilities after medical or surgical treatment for herniation of a lumbar disk. A home care referral may be indicated and provides the home care nurse with the opportunity to assess the patient's physical and psychological status, as well as his or her ability to adhere to recommended management strategies. During the home visit, the nurse determines whether changes in neurologic function have occurred. The adequacy of pain management is assessed, and modifications are made to ensure adequate pain relief.

Postpolio Syndrome

People who survived the polio epidemic of the 1950s, many of whom are now elderly, are developing new symptoms of weakness, fatigue, and musculoskeletal pain. Researchers estimate that as many as 80% of the 1,000,000 polio survivors are experiencing the phenomenon known as postpolio syndrome. Men and women appear to be equally at risk for this condition (Bartels & Omura, 2005; Elrod, Jabben, Oswald, et al., 2005).

Pathophysiology

The exact cause of postpolio syndrome is not known, but researchers suspect that, with aging or muscle overuse, the neurons not destroyed by the poliovirus continue generating axon sprouts (Bartels & Omura, 2005). These new terminal axon sprouts reinnervate the affected muscles after the initial insult but may become more vulnerable as the body ages.

Assessment and Diagnostic Findings

No specific diagnostic test exists for postpolio syndrome. Clinical diagnosis is made on the basis of the history and physical examination and exclusion of other medical conditions that could be causing the new symptoms. Patients report a history of paralytic poliomyelitis followed by partial or complete recovery of function, with a plateau of function and then the recurrence of symptoms. Signs and symptoms may occur decades after the original onset of poliomyelitis (Elrod, et al., 2005).

Management

No specific medical or surgical treatment is available for this syndrome, and therefore nurses play a pivotal role in the team approach to assisting patients and families in dealing with the symptoms of progressive loss of muscle strength and significant fatigue. Other health care professionals who may assist in patient care include physical, occupational, speech, and respiratory therapists. Nursing interventions are aimed at maintaining the patient's strength as well as physical, psychological, and social well-being.

The patient needs to plan and coordinate activities to conserve energy and reduce fatigue. Rest periods should be planned and assistive devices used to reduce weakness and fatigue. Important activities should be planned for the morning, because fatigue often increases in the afternoon and evening (Bartels & Omura, 2005; Elrod, et al., 2005).

One study proposed an explanatory model of health promotion and quality of life in patients with postpolio syndrome (Stuifbergen, Seraphine, Harrison, et al., 2005). The results suggested that quality of life is the result of a complex interplay among contextual factors such as severity of impairment, antecedent variables, and health-promoting behaviors.

Pain in muscles and joints may be a problem. Nonpharmacologic techniques such as the application of heat and cold are most appropriate, because older patients may not tolerate or may have strong reactions to medications.

Maintaining a balance between adequate nutritional intake and avoiding excess calories that can lead to obesity in this sedentary group of patients is a challenge. Pulmonary hygiene and adequate fluid intake can help with airway management. Several interventions can improve sleep, including limiting caffeine intake before bedtime and assessing for nocturia. If nocturia is an issue, the patient needs to be evaluated for obstructive sleep apnea. Supportive ventilation may be appropriate, with continuous positive airway pressure if sleep apnea is a problem.

Bone density testing in patients with postpolio syndrome has revealed low bone mass and osteoporosis (Smeltzer, Zimmerman & Capriotti, 2005). Therefore, the importance of identifying risks, preventing falls, and treating osteoporosis must be discussed with patients and families. Families also need to be made aware of the possibility of changes in individual and family relationships due to the many symptoms of postpolio syndrome (Ward, 2008). The nurse also needs to remind patients and family members of the need for health promotion activities and health screening.

CRITICAL THINKING EXERCISES

1   A 48-year-old man is married with two young children and has been newly diagnosed with a metastatic spinal cord tumor. Assess and prioritize the patient's physiologic and psychosocial needs. Identify appropriate nursing interventions to alleviate the patient's and family's physiologic and emotional stressors. Address the patient's need for emotional support from both the nursing staff and the family.

2   A 75-year-old woman newly diagnosed with Parkinson's disease asks what type of medication she will be given. What are the possible medication regimens that may be used to treat her disease and the common side effects of each? How would your discharge teaching targeted toward medications be modified if the patient lives alone and is hearing impaired?

EBP **3**   A 45-year-old patient with Huntington disease has been referred for end-of-life care. What resources would you use to identify the current guidelines for end-of-life care? What is the current evidence base for end-of-life nursing care? Identify the criteria used to evaluate the strength of the evidence for end-of-life nursing care.

4   A 60-year-old patient with low back pain is seen in the clinic. What nursing interventions and actions would you suggest to assist in the management of low back pain? What strategies would you advise the patient to avoid? What is the rationale for your suggestions? State the types of health promotion activities you would recommend to this patient and the rationale for your recommendations.

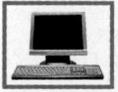

The Smeltzer suite offers these additional resources to enhance learning and facilitate understanding of this chapter:
- thePoint online resource, thepoint.lww.com/Smeltzer12E
- Student CD-ROM included with the book
- *Study Guide to Accompany Brunner & Suddarth's Textbook of Medical-Surgical Nursing*
- *Handbook for Brunner & Suddarth's Textbook of Medical-Surgical Nursing*

REFERENCES AND SELECTED READINGS

Asterisk indicates nursing research.

Books

Barker, R. A. & Barasi, S. (2008). *Neuroscience at a glance* (3rd ed.). Oxford: Blackwell Publishing.

Bickley, L. S. (2007). *Bates' guide to physical examination and history taking* (9th ed.). Philadelphia: Lippincott Williams & Wilkins.

Dudek, S. G. (2006). *Nutrition essentials for nursing practice* (5th ed.). Philadelphia: Lippincott Williams & Wilkins.

Hickey, J. V. (2009). *The clinical practice of neurological & neurosurgical nursing* (6th ed.). Philadelphia: Lippincott Williams & Wilkins.

Karch, A. M. (2008). *Lippincott's nursing drug guide*. Philadelphia: Lippincott Williams & Wilkins.

Koller, W. C. & Melamed, E. (2007). Parkinson's disease and related disorders (Part 1). In Minoff, M. J., Boller, F. & Swaab, D. F. *Handbook of clinical neurology* (Vol. 83). Philadelphia: Elsevier.

Miller, C. A. (2009). *Nursing for wellness in older adults* (5th ed.). Philadelphia: Lippincott Williams & Wilkins.

Pollock, B. E. (2006). *Guiding neurosurgery by evidence*. Basal: Karger.

Raizer, J. J. & Abrey, L. E. (Eds.). (2007) *Brain metastases*. New York: Springer.

Rice, J. N., Robichaux, C. & Leonard, A. (2005). Nervous system alterations. In Ropper, A. H., Gress, D., Diringer, M. N., et al. *Neurological and neurosurgical intensive care* (4th ed.). Philadelphia: Lippincott Williams & Wilkins.

Rowland, L. P. (2005). *Merritt's neurology* (11th ed.). Philadelphia: Lippincott Williams & Wilkins.

Runge, M. S. & Patterson, C. P. (2006). *Molecular medicine* (2nd ed.). Totowa, NJ: Humana Press.

Sole, M., Klein, D. G. & Moseley, M. J. (Eds.). (2009). *Introduction to critical care nursing* (5th ed.). St. Louis: Elsevier Saunders.

Weber, J. & Kelley, J. (2007). *Health assessment in nursing* (3rd ed.). Philadelphia: Lippincott Williams & Wilkins.

Wolfa, C. E. & Resnik, D. K. (2007). *Spine and peripheral nerves*. New York: Thieme.

Journals and Electronic Documents

General

Olson, E. & Cristian, A. (2005). The role of rehabilitation medicine and palliative care in the treatment of patients with end-stage disease. *Physical Medicine and Rehabilitation Clinics of North America, 16*(1), 285–305.

*Smeltzer, S. C., Zimmerman, V. & Capriotti, T. (2005). Osteoporosis risk and bone mineral density in women with physical disabilities. *Archives of Physical Medicine and Rehabilitation, 86*(3), 582–586.

Alzheimer's Disease

Cyr, N. R. (2007). Depression and older adults. *AORN Journal, 85*(2), 397–401.

Downey, D. (2008). Pharmacologic management of Alzheimer disease. *Journal of Neuroscience Nursing, 40*(1), 55–59.

Ganzer, C. A. (2007). Assessing Alzheimer's disease and dementia: Best practices in nursing care. *Geriatric Nursing, 28*(6), 358–365.

*Ward-Smith, P. & Forred, D. (2005). Participation in a dementia evaluation program: Perceptions of family members. *Journal of Neuroscience Nursing, 37*(2), 92–96.

Amyotrophic Lateral Sclerosis

Brown, R. H. (2005). Amyotrophic lateral sclerosis: A new role for old drugs. *New England Journal of Medicine, 352*(13), 1376–1378.

Gal, J., Strom, A., Kilty, R., et al. (2007). P62 accumulates and enhances aggregate formation in model systems of familial amyotrophic lateral sclerosis. *Journal of Biological Chemistry, 282*(15), 11068–11077.

Phukan, J., Pender, N. & Hardiman, O. (2007). Cognitive impairment in amyotrophic lateral sclerosis. *The Lancet Neurology, 6*(11), 994–1003.

Tiwari, A., Xu, Z. & Hayward, L. J. (2005). Aberrantly increased hydrophobicity shared by mutants of CU, Zn-superoxide dismutase in familial amyotrophic lateral sclerosis. *Journal of Biological Chemistry, 280*(33), 29771–29779.

Degenerative Disk Disease

Agency for Healthcare Research and Quality. (2008). Healthcare cost and utilization project. Available at: www.ahrq.gov/data/hcup/

Ersayli, D. T., Gurget, A., Bekar, A., et al. (2006). Effects of perioperatively administered bupivacaine and bupivacaine-methylprednisolone on pain after lumbar discectomy. *Spine, 31*(19), 2221–2226.

*Fowler, S., Anthony-Phillips, P., Mehta, D., et al. (2005). Health-related quality of life in patients undergoing anterior cervical discectomy. *Journal of Neuroscience Nursing, 37*(2), 97–100.

*Saban, K. L. & Penckofer, S. M. (2007). Patient expectations of quality of life following lumbar spinal surgery. *Journal of Neuroscience Nursing, 39*(3), 180–189.

*Starkweather, A. R., Witek-Janusek, L., Nockels, R. P., et al. (2006). The impact of psychological and immune factors in sciatic pain: A randomized controlled trial among herniated disc patients. *SCI Nursing, 23*(3), 1–11.

*Starkweather, A. R., Witek-Janusek, L., Nockels, R. P., et al. (2008). The multiple benefits of minimally invasive spinal surgery: Results comparing transforaminal lumbar interbody fusion and posterior lumbar fusion. *Journal of Neuroscience Nursing, 40*(1), 32–39.

Huntington Disease

Skirton, H. (2005). Huntington disease: A nursing perspective. *MedSurg Nursing, 14*(3), 167–173.

Walker, F. (2007). Huntington's disease. *Seminars in Neurology, 27*(2), 143–150.

Oncologic Disorders

American Brain Tumor Association (ABTA). (2007). *A primer of brain tumors: A patient's reference manual* (8th ed.). Available at: www.abta.org

American Caner Society (2009). *Caner facts & figures: 2009*. Available at: www.cancer.org

Arzbaecher, J. (2007). Spinal metastasis in glioblastoma multiforme: A case study. *Journal of Neuroscience Nursing, 39*(1), 21–25.

Barnholtz-Sloan, J. S., Williams, V. L., Maldonado, J. L., et al. (2008). Patterns of care and outcomes among elderly individuals with primary malignant astrocytoma. *Journal of Neurosurgery, 108*(4), 642–648.

Fields, L. (2007). DNR does not mean no care. *Journal of Neuroscience Nursing, 39*(5), 294–296.

Gordon, B. M. (2007). Pharmacological management of secreting pituitary tumors. *Journal of Neuroscience Nursing, 39*(1), 52–57.

Held-Warmkessel, J. (2005). Managing critical cancer complications. *Nursing, 35*(1), 58–63.

Jemal, A., Siegel, R., Ward, E., et al. (2008). Cancer statistics, 2008. *CA: A Cancer Journal for Clinicians, 58*(2), 71–97.

Richards, J. & Ballard, N. (2008). Colloid cyst: A case study. *Journal of Neuroscience Nursing, 40*(2), 103–105.

*Schmer, C., Ward-Smith, P., Latham, S., et al. (2008). When a family member has a malignant brain tumor: The caregiver perspective. *Journal of Neuroscience Nursing, 40*(2), 78–84.

Swinson, B. & Friedman, W. (2008). Linear accelerator stereotactic radiosurgery for metastatic brain tumors: Years of experience at the University of Florida. *Neurosurgery, 62*(5), 1018–1032.

Wen, P. Y. & Kesari, S. (2008). Malignant gliomas in adults. *New England Journal of Medicine, 359*(5), 492–507.

Parkinson's Disease

Chen, J. J. & Fernandez, H. H. (2007). Community and long-term care management of Parkinson's disease in the elderly. *Drugs & Aging, 24*(8), 663–680.

Halkias, I. A. C., Haq, I., Huang, Z., et al. (2007). When should Levodopa therapy be initiated in patients with Parkinson's disease? *Drugs & Aging, 24*(4), 261–273.

*Sadowski, C. A., Jones, C. A., Gordon, B., et al. (2007). Knowledge of risk factors for falling reported by patients with Parkinson disease. *Journal of Neuroscience Nursing, 39*(6), 336–341.

Stewart, R. M., Desaloms, J. M. & Sanghera, M. K. (2005). Stimulation of the subthalamic nucleus for the treatment of Parkinson's disease: Postoperative management programming and rehabilitation. *Journal of Neuroscience Nursing, 37*(2), 108–114.

Thomure, A. (2006). Helping your patient manage Parkinson's disease. *Nursing, 36*(8), 20.

Ward, C. (2005). Neuroleptic malignant syndrome in a patient with Parkinson's disease: A case study. *Journal of Neuroscience Nursing, 37*(3), 160–162.

Weintraub, D. & Hurtig, H. I. (2007). Presentation and management of psychosis in Parkinson's disease and dementia with Lewy bodies. *American Journal of Psychiatry, 164*(10), 1491–1498.

Postpolio Syndrome

Bartels, M. N. & Omura, A. (2005). Aging in polio. *Physical Medicine and Rehabilitation Clinics of North America, 16*(1), 197–218.

Elrod, L. M., Jabben, M., Oswald, G., et al. (2005). Vocational implications of post-polio syndrome. *Work, 25*(2), 155–161.

*Stuifbergen, A., Seraphine, A., Harrison, T., et al. (2005). An explanatory model of health promotion and quality of life for persons with post-polio syndrome. *Social Science and Medicine, 60*(2), 383–393.

Ward, S. (2008). Does anyone see me? Playing host to the uninvited guest of post-polio syndrome. *Qualitative Inquiry, 14*(3), 360–383.

RESOURCES

American Brain Tumor Association, www.abta.org

American Cancer Society, www.cancer.org

American Parkinson's Disease Association, www.apdaparkinson.org/userND/index.asp

The Michael J. Fox Foundation for Parkinson's Research, Church Street Station, www.michaeljfox.org

Amyotrophic Lateral Sclerosis Association, www.alsa.org

Huntington's Disease Society of America, www.hdsa.org

Muscular Dystrophy Association, www.mda.org

National Brain Tumor Foundation, www.braintumor.org

National Parkinson Foundation, Inc., www.parkinson.org

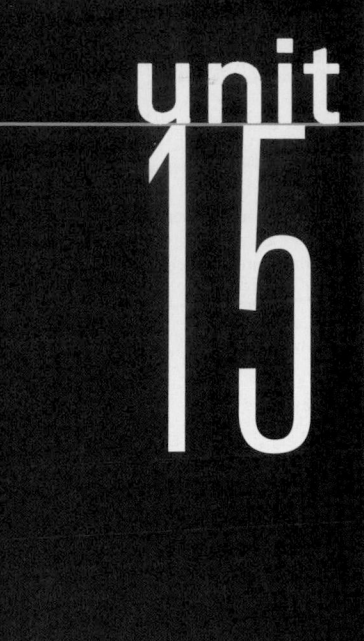

unit 15

Musculoskeletal Function

Case Study • Applying Concepts From NANDA, NIC, and NOC

A Patient With Musculoskeletal Limitations Complicated by a Medical Illness

Mrs. Waterman is a 70-year-old woman with severe osteoarthritis of the spine and a recent history of left total hip replacement. She has been attending outpatient physical therapy sessions three times a week and uses a rolling walker at home. She has been admitted to the hospital with a partial small bowel obstruction. The health care team anticipates that the obstruction will resolve with medical treatment, and her expected length of stay is 5 to 7 days. Currently she is allowed nothing by mouth, has a Salem sump tube in place, and is receiving peripheral parenteral nutrition. The nurse is concerned that Mrs. Waterman's already impaired physical mobility will decline further secondary to her illness and the medical treatments that make independent ambulation difficult.

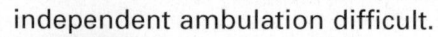

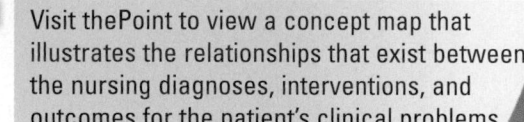

Visit thePoint to view a concept map that illustrates the relationships that exist between the nursing diagnoses, interventions, and outcomes for the patient's clinical problems.

Nursing Classifications and Languages

NANDA NURSING DIAGNOSES	NIC NURSING INTERVENTIONS	NOC NURSING OUTCOMES
		Return to functional baseline status, stabilization of, or improvement in:
IMPAIRED PHYSICAL MOBILITY— Limitation in independent, purposeful physical movement of the body or of one or more extremities	**EXERCISE PROMOTION—** Facilitation of regular physical exercise to maintain or advance a higher degree of fitness	**MOBILITY LEVEL—** Ability to move purposefully in own environment independently with or without assistive device
RISK FOR DISUSE SYNDROME— At risk for deterioration of body systems as the result of prescribed or unavoidable musculoskeletal inactivity	**EXERCISE PROMOTION: STRENGTH TRAINING—** Facilitating regular resistive muscle training to retain or increase muscle strength	**IMMOBILITY CONSEQUENCES: PHYSIOLOGICAL—** Severity of compromise in physiological functioning due to impaired physical mobility
	EMBOLUS PRECAUTIONS— Reduction of the risk of embolus in a patient with thrombi or at risk for developing thrombus formation	
	PRESSURE ULCER PREVENTION— Prevention of pressure ulcers for an individual at high risk for developing them	
	SURVEILLANCE— Purposeful and ongoing acquisition, interpretation, and synthesis of patient data for clinical decision-making	

Bulechek, G. M., Butcher, H. K., & Dochterman, J. M. (2008). *Nursing interventions classification (NIC)* (5th ed.). St. Louis: Mosby.
Johnson, M., Bulechek, G., Butcher, H. K., et al. (2006). *NANDA, NOC, and NIC linkages* (2nd ed.). St. Louis: Mosby.
Moorhead, S., Johnson, M., Mass, M. L., et al. (2008). *Nursing outcomes classification (NOC)* (4th ed.). St. Louis: Mosby.
NANDA International. (2007). *Nursing diagnoses: Definitions & classification 2007–2008*. Philadelphia: North American Nursing Diagnosis Association.

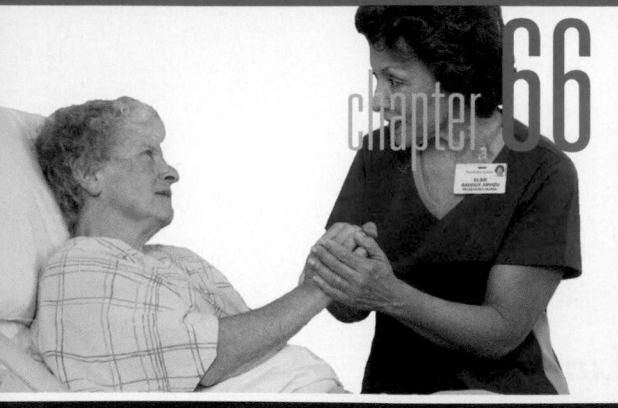

Assessment of Muscuskeletal

chapter 66

Assessment of Musculoskeletal Function

LEARNING OBJECTIVES

On completion of this chapter, the learner will be able to:

1 Describe the basic structure and function of the musculoskeletal system.

2 Discuss the significance of the health history to the assessment of musculoskeletal health.

3 Describe the significance of physical assessment to the diagnosis of musculoskeletal dysfunction.

4 Specify the diagnostic tests used for assessment of musculoskeletal function.

GLOSSARY

atonic: without tone; denervated muscle that atrophies

atrophy: shrinkagelike decrease in the size of a muscle

bursa: fluid-filled sac found in connective tissue, usually in the area of joints

callus: cartilaginous/fibrous tissue at fracture site

cancellous bone: latticelike bone structure; trabecular bone

cartilage: tough, elastic, avascular tissue at ends of bone

clonus: rhythmic contraction of muscle

contracture: abnormal shortening of muscle or joint, or both; fibrosis

cortical bone: compact bone

crepitus: grating or crackling sound or sensation; may occur with movement of ends of a broken bone or irregular joint surface

diaphysis: shaft of long bone

effusion: excess fluid in joint

endosteum: a thin, vascular membrane covering the marrow cavity of long bones and the spaces in cancellous bone

epiphysis: end of long bone

fascia (epimysium): fibrous tissue that covers, supports, and separates muscles

GLOSSARY *(Continued)*

fasciculation: involuntary twitch of muscle fibers

flaccid: limp; without muscle tone

hypertrophy: enlargement; increase in size of muscle

isometric contraction: muscle tension increased, length unchanged, no joint motion

isotonic contraction: muscle tension unchanged, muscle shortened, joint moved

joint: area where bone ends meet; provides for motion and flexibility

joint capsule: fibrous tissue that encloses bone ends and other joint surfaces

kyphosis: increase in the convex curvature of the spine

lamellae: mature compact bone structures that form concentric rings of bone matrix; lamellar bone

ligament: fibrous band connecting bones

lordosis: increase in lumbar curvature of the spine

ossification: process in which minerals (calcium) are deposited in bone matrix

osteoblast: bone-forming cell

osteoclast: bone resorption cell

osteocyte: mature bone cell

osteogenesis: bone formation

osteon: microscopic functional bone unit

paresthesia: abnormal sensation (eg, burning, tingling, numbness)

periosteum: fibrous connective tissue covering bone

remodeling: process that ensures bone maintenance through simultaneous bone resorption and formation

resorption: removal/destruction of tissue, such as bone

scoliosis: lateral curving of the spine

spastic: having greater-than-normal muscle tone

synovium: membrane in joint that secretes lubricating fluid

tendon: cord of fibrous tissue connecting muscle to bone

tone (tonus): normal tension (resistance to stretch) in resting muscle

trabeculae: latticelike bone structure; cancellous bone

The musculoskeletal system includes the bones, joints, muscles, tendons, ligaments, and bursae of the body. The functions of these components are highly integrated; therefore, disease in or injury to one component adversely affects the others. For instance, an infection in a joint (septic arthritis) causes degeneration of the articular surfaces of the bones within the joint and local muscle atrophy.

Diseases and injuries that involve the musculoskeletal system are commonly implicated in disability and death. For example, the leading cause of disability in the United States is arthritis (Centers for Disease Control and Prevention [CDC], 2005). Osteoporosis-related fractures account for more than 432,000 hospitalizations yearly in the United States (National Osteoporosis Foundation, 2008). Musculoskeletal diseases and injuries can significantly affect overall productivity, independence, and quality of life in people of all ages. Nurses in all practice areas encounter patients with malfunction in the musculoskeletal system.

Anatomic and Physiologic Overview

The musculoskeletal system provides protection for vital organs, including the brain, heart, and lungs; provides a sturdy framework to support body structures; and makes mobility possible. Muscles and tendons hold the bones together and joints allow the body to move. **Tendons** attach muscles to bones. They also move to produce heat that helps maintain body temperature. Movement facilitates the return of deoxygenated blood to the right side of the heart by massaging the venous vasculature. The musculoskeletal system serves as a reservoir for immature blood cells and essential minerals, including calcium, phosphorus, magnesium, and fluoride. More than 98% of total body calcium is present in bone.

Structure and Function of the Skeletal System

There are 206 bones in the human body, divided into four categories: long bones (eg, femur), short bones (eg, metacarpals), flat bones (eg, sternum), and irregular bones (eg, vertebrae). The shape and construction of a specific bone are determined by its function and the forces exerted on it. Bones are constructed of **cancellous** (trabecular) or **cortical** (compact) bone tissue. Long bones are shaped like rods or shafts with rounded ends (Fig. 66-1). The shaft, known as the **diaphysis,** is primarily cortical bone. The ends of the long bones, called **epiphyses,** are primarily cancellous bone. The epiphyseal plate separates the epiphyses from the diaphysis and is the center for longitudinal growth in children. It is calcified in adults. The ends of long bones are covered at the joints by articular **cartilage,** which is tough, elastic, avascular tissue. Long bones are designed for weight bearing and movement. Short bones consist of cancellous bone covered by a layer of compact bone. Flat bones are important sites of hematopoiesis and frequently protect vital organs. They are made of cancellous bone layered between compact bone. Irregular bones have unique shapes related to their function. Generally, irregular bone structure is similar to that of flat bones.

Bone is composed of cells, protein matrix, and mineral deposits. The cells are of three basic types—**osteoblasts,**

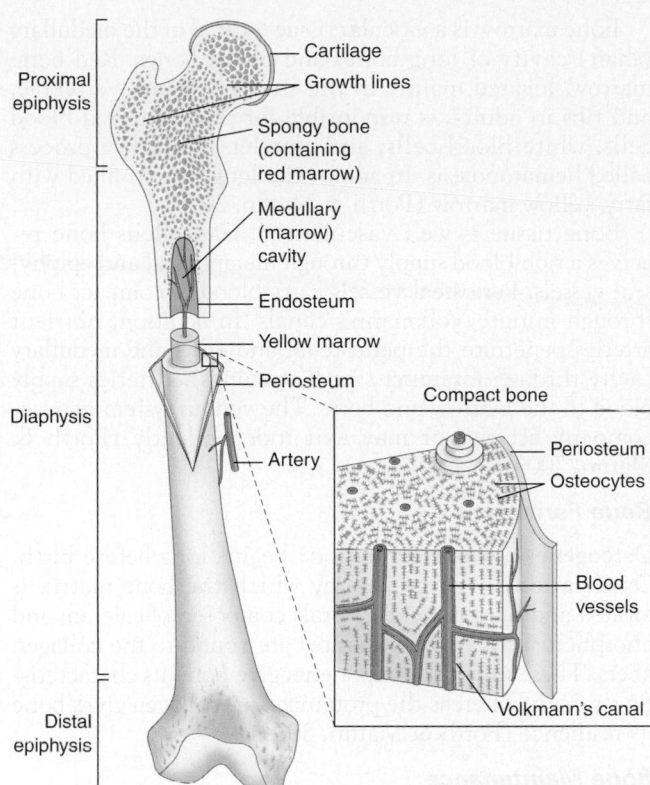

Figure 66-1 Structure of a long bone; composition of compact bone.

osteocytes, and **osteoclasts.** Osteoblasts function in bone formation by secreting bone matrix. The matrix consists of collagen and ground substances (glycoproteins and proteoglycans) that provide a framework in which inorganic mineral salts are deposited. These minerals are primarily composed of calcium and phosphorus. Osteocytes are mature bone cells involved in bone maintenance; they are located in lacunae (bone matrix units). Osteoclasts, located in shallow Howship's lacunae (small pits in bones), are multinuclear cells involved in dissolving and resorbing bone. The microscopic functioning unit of mature cortical bone is the **osteon** (Haversian system). The center of the osteon, the Haversian canal, contains a capillary. Around the capillary are circles of mineralized bone matrix called **lamellae.** Within the lamellae are lacunae that contain osteocytes. These are nourished through tiny structures, canaliculi (canals), which communicate with adjacent blood vessels within the Haversian system. Lacunae in cancellous bone are layered in an irregular lattice network **(trabeculae).** Red bone marrow fills the lattice network. Capillaries nourish the osteocytes located in the lacunae (Porth & Matfin, 2009).

Covering the bone is a dense, fibrous membrane known as the **periosteum.** This membranous structure nourishes bone and facilitates its growth. The periosteum contains nerves, blood vessels, and lymphatics. It also provides for the attachment of tendons and ligaments (Porth & Matfin, 2009).

The **endosteum** is a thin, vascular membrane that covers the marrow cavity of long bones and the spaces in cancellous bone. Osteoclasts, which dissolve bone matrix to maintain the marrow cavity, are located near the endosteum in Howship's lacunae (Porth & Matfin, 2009).

Bone marrow is a vascular tissue located in the medullary (shaft) cavity of long bones and in flat bones. Red bone marrow, located mainly in the sternum, ilium, vertebrae, and ribs in adults, is responsible for producing red blood cells, white blood cells, and platelets through a process called hematopoiesis. In adults, the long bone is filled with fatty, yellow marrow (Porth & Matfin, 2009).

Bone tissue is well vascularized. Cancellous bone receives a rich blood supply through metaphyseal and epiphyseal vessels. Periosteal vessels carry blood to compact bone through minute Volkmann's canals. In addition, nutrient arteries penetrate the periosteum and enter the medullary cavity through foramina (small openings). Arteries supply blood to the marrow and bone. The venous system may accompany arteries or may exit independently (Porth & Matfin, 2009).

Bone Formation

Osteogenesis (bone formation) begins long before birth. **Ossification** is the process by which the bone matrix is formed and hard mineral crystals composed of calcium and phosphorus (eg, hydroxyapatite) are bound to the collagen fibers. These mineral components give bone its characteristic strength, whereas the proteinaceous collagen gives bone its resilience (Porth & Matfin, 2009).

Bone Maintenance

Bone is a dynamic tissue in a constant state of turnover. During childhood, bones grow and form by a process called modeling. By early adulthood (ie, early 20s), **remodeling** is the primary process that occurs. Remodeling maintains bone structure and function through simultaneous **resorption** and osteogenesis, and as a result, complete skeletal turnover occurs every 10 years (U.S. Department of Health and Human Services [DHHS], 2004).

The balance between bone resorption and formation is influenced by the following factors: physical activity; dietary intake of certain nutrients, especially calcium; and several hormones, including calcitriol (ie, activated vitamin D), parathyroid hormone (PTH), calcitonin, thyroid hormone, cortisol, growth hormone, and the sex hormones estrogen and testosterone (DHHS, 2004).

Physical activity, particularly weight-bearing activity, acts to stimulate bone formation and remodeling. Bones subjected to continued weight bearing tend to be thick and strong. Conversely, people who are unable to engage in regular weight-bearing activities, such as those on prolonged bed rest or those with some physical disabilities, have increased bone resorption from calcium loss, and their bones become osteopenic and weak. These weakened bones may fracture easily.

Good dietary habits are integral to bone health. In particular, absorption of approximately 1000–1200 mg of calcium daily is essential to maintaining adult bone mass. This may be achieved through ingesting calcium-rich foods on a daily basis (eg, through drinking 16 to 24 ounces of milk daily).

Several hormones are vital in ensuring that calcium is properly absorbed and available for bone mineralization and matrix formation. Calcitriol functions to increase the amount of calcium in the blood by promoting absorption of calcium from the gastrointestinal tract. It also facilitates

mineralization of osteoid tissue. A deficiency of vitamin D results in bone mineralization deficit, deformity, and fracture (DHHS, 2004).

PTH and calcitonin are the major hormonal regulators of calcium homeostasis. PTH regulates the concentration of calcium in the blood, in part by promoting movement of calcium from the bone. In response to low calcium levels in the blood, increased levels of PTH prompt the mobilization of calcium, the demineralization of bone, and the formation of bone cysts. Calcitonin, secreted by the thyroid gland in response to elevated blood calcium levels, inhibits bone resorption and increases the deposit of calcium in bone (DHHS, 2004).

Both thyroid hormone and cortisol have multiple systemic effects with specific effects on bones. Excessive thyroid hormone production in adults (eg, Graves' disease) can result in increased bone resorption and decreased bone formation. Increased levels of cortisol have these same effects. Patients receiving long-term synthetic cortisol or corticosteroids (ie, prednisone) are at increased risk for steroid-induced osteopenia and fractures.

Growth hormone has direct and indirect effects on skeletal growth and remodeling. It stimulates the liver and to a lesser degree the bones to produce insulinlike growth factor-1 (IGF-I), which accelerates bone modeling in children and adolescents. Growth hormone also directly stimulates skeletal growth in children and adolescents. It is believed that the low levels of both growth hormone and IGF-I that occur with aging may be partly responsible for decreased bone formation and resultant osteopenia (DHHS, 2004).

The sex hormones testosterone and estrogen have important effects on bone remodeling. Estrogen stimulates osteoblasts and inhibits osteoclasts; therefore, bone formation is enhanced and resorption is inhibited. Testosterone has both direct and indirect effects on bone growth and formation. It directly causes skeletal growth in adolescence and has continued effects on skeletal muscle growth throughout the lifespan. Increased muscle mass results in greater weight-bearing stress on bones, resulting in increased bone formation. In addition, testosterone converts to estrogen in adipose tissue, providing an additional source of bone-preserving estrogen for aging men.

During the process of bone remodeling, osteoblasts produce a receptor for activated nuclear factor-kappa B ligand (RANKL) that binds to the receptor for activated nuclear factor-kappa B (RANK) present on the cell membranes of osteoclast precursors, causing them to differentiate and mature into osteoclasts, which causes bone resorption. Conversely, osteoblasts may produce osteoprogerin (OPG), which blocks the effects of RANKL, thereby turning off the process of bone resorption. T cells that may become activated as a result of the inflammatory process may also produce RANKL, overriding the effects of OPG and causing continued bone resorption during times of stress and injury, which can lead to loss of bone matrix and fractures. Research is currently focused on developing medications that block the effects of RANKL and on developing useful laboratory tests of RANKL levels that may guide therapy aimed at reducing the risk of fractures (McCormick, 2007).

Blood supply to the bone also affects bone formation. With diminished blood supply or hyperemia (congestion), osteogenesis and bone density decrease. Bone necrosis occurs when the bone is deprived of blood.

Bone Healing

Most fractures heal through a combination of intramembranous and endochondral ossification processes. When a bone is fractured, the bone fragments are not patched together with scar tissue. Instead, the bone regenerates itself.

Fracture healing occurs in the bone marrow, where endothelial cells rapidly differentiate into osteoblasts; in the bone cortex, where new osteons are formed; in the periosteum, where a hard **callus** (fibrous tissue) is formed through intramembranous ossification peripheral to the fracture, and where cartilage is formed through endochondral ossification adjacent to the fracture site; and in adjacent soft tissue, where a bridging callus forms that provides stability to the fractured bones.

The process of fracture healing occurs over three phases. These include the following:

Phase 1: Reactive phase: When a fracture occurs, the body's response is similar to that after injury elsewhere in the body. There is bleeding into the injured tissue and formation of a hematoma at the site of the fracture. Cytokines are released that initiate the fracture healing processes by causing the proliferation of fibroblasts and that cause angiogenesis to occur (ie, the growth of new blood vessels). Granulation tissue begins to form within the clot and becomes dense.

Phase II: Reparative phase: During this phase, the granulation tissue is initially replaced with a callus precursor, called procallus. Fibroblasts invade the procallus and produce a denser type of callus that is composed mostly of fibrocartilage. This fibrocartilaginous callus is replaced with denser bony callus within approximately 3 to 4 weeks postinjury. Lamellar bone then forms as the bony callus calcifies months postinjury.

Phase III: Remodeling phase: The final phase of fracture healing results in remodeling the new bone into its former structural arrangement. Remodeling may take months to years, depending on the extent of bone modification needed, the function of the bone, and the functional stresses on the bone.

Serial x-rays are used to monitor the progress of bone healing. The type of bone fractured, the adequacy of blood supply, the surface contact of the fragments, the immobility of the fracture site, and the age and general health of the person influence the rate of fracture healing. Adequate immobilization is essential until there is x-ray evidence of bone formation with ossification.

When fractures are treated with open rigid compression plate fixation techniques, the bony fragments can be placed in direct contact. Primary bone healing occurs through cortical bone (Haversian) remodeling. Little or no cartilaginous callus develops. Immature bone develops from the endosteum. There is an intensive regeneration of new osteons, which develop in the fracture line by a process similar to normal bone maintenance. Fracture strength is obtained when the new osteons have become established.

Structure and Function of the Articular System

The junction of two or more bones is called a **joint** (articulation). There are three basic kinds of joints: synarthrosis, amphiarthrosis, and diarthrosis joints. Synarthrosis joints are immovable (eg, the skull sutures). Amphiarthrosis joints (eg, the vertebral joints and the symphysis pubis) allow limited motion; the bones of amphiarthrosis joints are joined by fibrous cartilage. Diarthrosis joints are freely movable joints (Fig. 66-2).

There are several types of diarthrosis joints:
- *Ball-and-socket* joints (eg, the hip and the shoulder) permit full freedom of movement.
- *Hinge* joints permit bending in one direction only (eg, the elbow and the knee).
- *Saddle* joints allow movement in two planes at right angles to each other. The joint at the base of the thumb is a saddle, biaxial joint.
- *Pivot* joints are characterized by the articulation between the radius and the ulna. They permit rotation for such activities as turning a doorknob.
- *Gliding* joints allow for limited movement in all directions and are represented by the joints of the carpal bones in the wrist.

The ends of the articulating bones of a typical movable joint are covered with smooth hyaline cartilage. A tough, fibrous sheath called the **joint capsule** surrounds the articulating bones. The capsule is lined with a membrane, the **synovium,** which secretes the lubricating and shock-absorbing synovial fluid into the joint capsule. Therefore, the bone surfaces are not in direct contact. In some synovial joints (eg, the knee), fibrocartilage disks (eg, medial meniscus) are located between the articular cartilage surfaces. These disks provide shock absorption (Porth & Matfin, 2009).

Ligaments (fibrous connective tissue bands) bind the articulating bones together. Ligaments and muscle tendons, which pass over the joint, provide joint stability. In some joints, interosseous ligaments (eg, the cruciate ligaments of

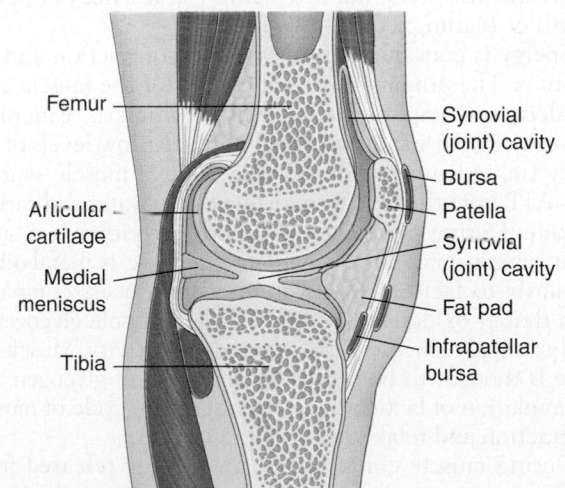

Figure 66-2 Hinge joint of the knee.

the knee) are found within the capsule and add anterior and posterior stability to the joint.

A **bursa** is a sac filled with synovial fluid that cushions the movement of tendons, ligaments, and bones at a point of friction. Bursae can be found in the joints of the elbow, shoulder, hip, and knee.

Structure and Function of the Skeletal Muscle System

Muscles are attached by tendons to bones, connective tissue, other muscles, soft tissue, or skin. The muscles of the body are composed of parallel groups of muscle cells (fasciculi) encased in fibrous tissue called **fascia** (epimysium). The more fasciculi contained in a muscle, the more precise the movements. Muscles vary in shape and size according to the activities for which they are responsible. Skeletal (striated) muscles are involved in body movement, posture, and heat-production functions. Muscles contract to bring the two points of attachment closer together, resulting in movement.

Skeletal Muscle Contraction

Each muscle cell (also referred to as a muscle fiber) contains myofibrils, which in turn are composed of a series of sarcomeres, the actual contractile units of skeletal muscle. Sarcomeres contain thick myosin and thin actin filaments.

Muscle cells contract in response to electrical stimulation delivered by an effector nerve cell at the motor end plate. When stimulated, the muscle cell depolarizes and generates an action potential in a manner similar to that described for nerve cells. These action potentials propagate along the muscle cell membrane and lead to the release of calcium ions that are stored in specialized organelles called sarcoplasmic reticula. When there is a local increase in calcium ion concentration, the myosin and actin filaments slide across one another. Shortly after the muscle cell membrane is depolarized, it recovers its resting membrane voltage. Calcium is rapidly removed from the sarcomeres by active reaccumulation in the sarcoplasmic reticulum. When the calcium concentration in the sarcomere decreases, the myosin and actin filaments cease to interact, and the sarcomere returns to its original resting length (relaxation). Actin and myosin do not interact in the absence of calcium (Porth & Matfin, 2009).

Energy is consumed during muscle contraction and relaxation. The primary source of energy for the muscle cells is adenosine triphosphate (ATP), which is generated through cellular oxidative metabolism. At low levels of activity (ie, sedentary activity), the skeletal muscle synthesizes ATP from the oxidation of glucose to water and carbon dioxide. During periods of strenuous activity, when sufficient oxygen may not be available, glucose is metabolized primarily to lactic acid, an inefficient process compared with that of oxidative pathways. Stored muscle glycogen is used to supply glucose during periods of activity. Muscle fatigue is thought to be caused by depletion of glycogen and accumulation of lactic acid. As a result, the cycle of muscle contraction and relaxation cannot continue.

During muscle contraction, the energy released from ATP is not completely used. The excess energy is dissipated in the form of heat. During isometric contraction, almost all of the energy is released in the form of heat; during isotonic contraction, some of the energy is expended in mechanical work. In some situations (eg, shivering), the need to generate heat is the primary stimulus for muscle contraction.

The contraction of muscle fibers can result in either isotonic or isometric contraction of the muscle. In **isometric contraction,** the length of the muscles remains constant but the force generated by the muscles is increased; an example of this is pushing against an immovable wall. **Isotonic contraction,** on the other hand, is characterized by shortening of the muscle with no increase in tension within the muscle; an example of this is flexing the forearm. In normal activities, many muscle movements are a combination of isometric and isotonic contraction. For example, during walking, isotonic contraction results in shortening of the leg, and isometric contraction causes the stiff leg to push against the floor.

The speed of the muscle contraction is variable. Myoglobulin is a hemoglobinlike protein pigment present in striated muscle cells that transports oxygen. Muscles containing large quantities of myoglobulin (red muscles) have been observed to contract slowly and powerfully (eg, respiratory and postural muscles). Muscles containing little myoglobulin (white muscles) contract quickly (eg, extraocular eye muscles). Most muscles contain both red and white muscle fibers (Porth & Matfin, 2009).

Muscle Tone

Relaxed muscles demonstrate a state of readiness to respond to contraction stimuli. This state of readiness, known as muscle **tone** (tonus), is produced by the maintenance of some of the muscle fibers in a contracted state. Muscle spindles, which are sense organs in the muscles, monitor muscle tone. Muscle tone is minimal during sleep and is increased when the person is anxious. A muscle that is limp and without tone is described as **flaccid;** a muscle with greater-than-normal tone is described as **spastic.** In conditions characterized by lower motor neuron destruction (eg, polio), denervated muscle becomes **atonic** (soft and flabby) and atrophies.

Muscle Actions

Muscles accomplish movement by contraction. Through the coordination of muscle groups, the body is able to perform a wide variety of movements (Fig. 66-3). The prime mover is the muscle that causes a particular motion. The muscles assisting the prime mover are known as synergists. The muscles causing movement opposite to that of the prime mover are known as antagonists. An antagonist must relax to allow the prime mover to contract, producing motion. For example, when contraction of the biceps causes flexion of the elbow joint, the biceps are the prime movers, and the triceps are the antagonists. A person with muscle paralysis (a loss of movement, possibly from nerve damage) may be able to retrain functioning muscles within the synergistic group to produce the needed movement. Muscles of the synergistic group then become the prime movers.

Exercise, Disuse, and Repair

Muscles need to be exercised to maintain function and strength. When a muscle repeatedly develops maximum or

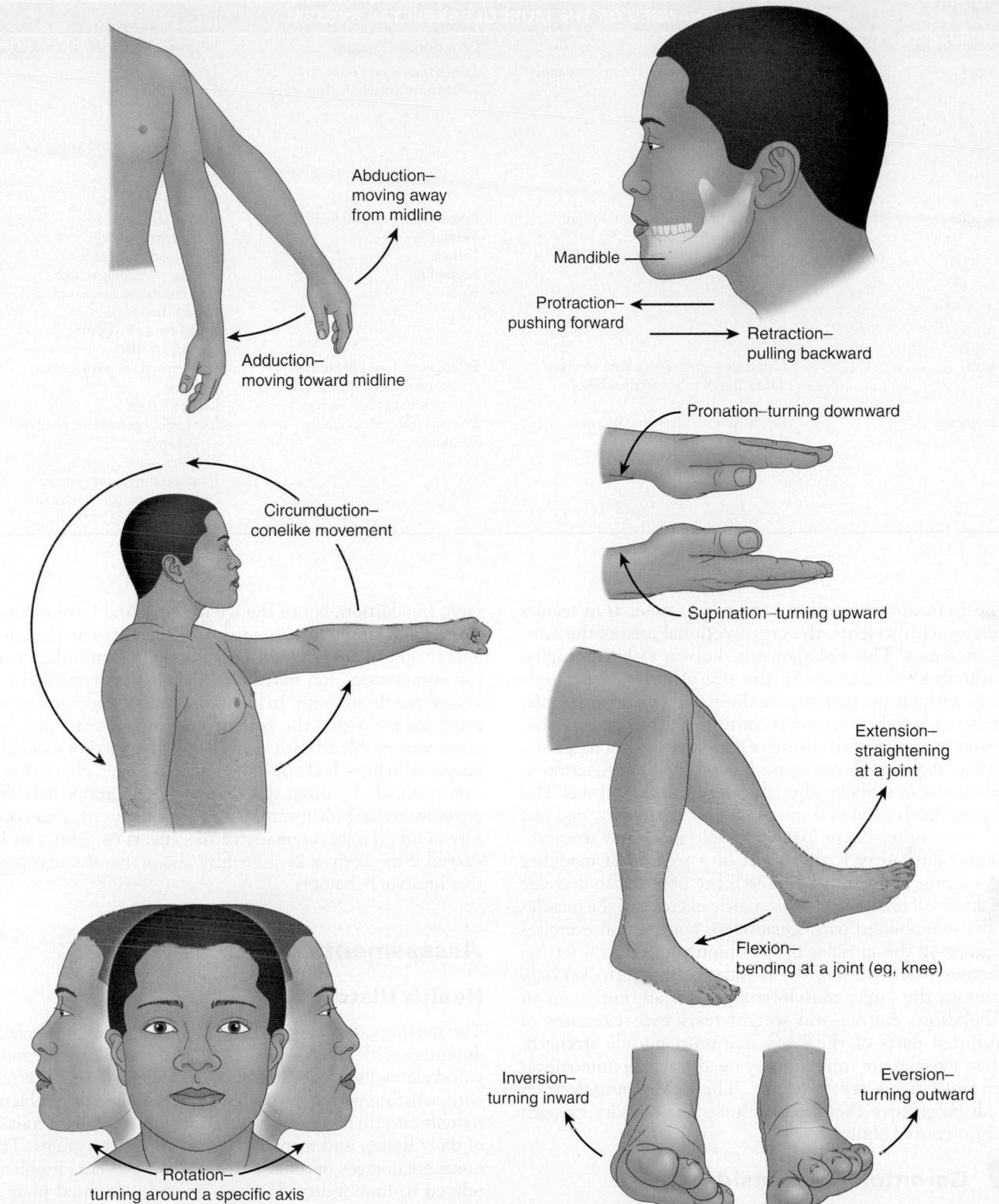

FIGURE 66-3 Body movements produced by muscle contraction.

Table 66-1	AGE-RELATED CHANGES OF THE MUSCULOSKELETAL SYSTEM		
Musculoskeletal System	**Structural Changes**	**Functional Changes**	**History and Physical Findings**
Bones	Gradual, progressive loss of bone mass after age 30 yr Vertebrae collapse	Bones fragile and prone to fracture: vertebrae, hip, wrist	Loss of height Posture changes Kyphosis Loss of flexibility Flexion of hips and knees Back pain Osteoporosis Fracture
Muscles	Increase in collagen and resultant fibrosis Muscles diminish in size (atrophy); wasting Tendons less elastic	Loss of strength and flexibility Weakness Fatigue Stumbling Falls	Loss of strength Diminished agility Decreased endurance Prolonged response time (diminished reaction time) Diminished tone Broad base of support History of falls
Joints	Cartilage—progressive deterioration Thinning of intervertebral disks	Stiffness, reduced flexibility, and pain interfere with activities of daily living	Diminished range of motion Stiffness Loss of height
Ligaments	Lax ligaments (less-than-normal strength; weakness)	Postural joint abnormality Weakness	Joint pain on motion; resolves with rest Crepitus Joint swelling/enlargement Osteoarthritis (degenerative joint disease)

close to maximum tension over a long time, as in regular exercise with weights, the cross-sectional area of the muscle increases. This enlargement, known as **hypertrophy**, results from an increase in the size of individual muscle fibers without an increase in their number. Hypertrophy persists only if the exercise is continued. The opposite phenomenon occurs with disuse of muscle over a long period of time. Age and disuse cause loss of muscular function as fibrotic tissue replaces the contractile muscle tissue. The decrease in the size of a muscle is called **atrophy.** Bed rest and immobility cause loss of muscle mass and strength. When immobility is the result of a treatment modality (eg, casting, traction, or bedrest), the patient can decrease the effects of immobility by isometric exercise of the muscles of the immobilized part. Quadriceps contraction exercises (tightening the muscles of the thigh) and gluteal setting exercises (tightening of the muscles of the buttocks) help maintain the larger muscle groups that are important in ambulation. Active and weight-resistance exercises of uninjured parts of the body maintain muscle strength. When muscles are injured, they need rest and immobilization until tissue repair occurs. The healed muscle then needs progressive exercise to resume its preinjury strength and functional ability.

Gerontologic Considerations

Multiple changes in the musculoskeletal system occur with aging (Table 66-1). There is a loss of height due to osteoporosis (abnormal excessive bone loss), kyphosis, thinned intervertebral disks, compressed vertebral bodies, and flexion of the knees and hips. Numerous metabolic changes, including menopausal withdrawal of estrogen and decreased activity, contribute to osteoporosis (DHHS, 2004; McCormick, 2007). Women lose more bone mass than

men. In addition, bones change in shape and have reduced strength. Fractures are common. Collagen structures are less able to absorb energy. Increased inactivity, diminished neuron stimulation, and nutritional deficiencies contribute to loss of muscle strength. In addition, remote musculoskeletal problems for which the patient has compensated may become new problems with age-related changes. For example, people who have had polio and who have been able to function normally by using synergistic muscle groups may discover increasing incapacity because of a reduced compensatory ability. However, many of the effects of aging can be slowed if the body is kept healthy and active through positive lifestyle behaviors.

Assessment

Health History

The nursing assessment of the patient with musculoskeletal dysfunction includes an evaluation of the effects of the musculoskeletal disorder on the patient. The nurse is concerned with assisting patients who have musculoskeletal problems to maintain their general health, accomplish their activities of daily living, and manage their treatment programs. The nurse encourages optimal nutrition and prevents problems related to immobility. Through an individualized plan of nursing care, the nurse helps the patient achieve maximum health.

Common Symptoms

During the interview and physical assessment, the patient with a musculoskeletal disorder may report pain, tenderness, tightness, and abnormal sensations. The nurse assesses and documents this information.

Pain

Most patients with diseases and traumatic conditions or disorders of the muscles, bones, and joints experience pain. Bone pain is characteristically described as a dull, deep ache that is "boring" in nature, whereas muscular pain is described as soreness or aching and is referred to as "muscle cramps." Fracture pain is sharp and piercing and is relieved by immobilization. Sharp pain may also result from bone infection with muscle spasm or pressure on a sensory nerve.

Rest relieves most musculoskeletal pain. Pain that increases with activity may indicate joint sprain, muscle strain, or compartment syndrome, whereas steadily increasing pain points to the progression of an infectious process (osteomyelitis), a malignant tumor, or neurovascular complications. Radiating pain occurs in conditions in which pressure is exerted on a nerve root. Pain is variable, and its assessment and nursing management must be individualized.

The nurse assesses the patient's pain as described in Chapter 13. Specific assessments that the nurse should make regarding the pain include the following:

- Is the body in proper alignment?
- Is there pressure from traction, bed linens, a cast, or other appliances?
- Is there tension on the skin at a pin site?

It is important that the patient's pain and discomfort be managed successfully. Not only is pain exhausting, but also, if prolonged, it can force the patient to become increasingly preoccupied and dependent (see Chapter 13).

Altered Sensations

Sensory disturbances are frequently associated with musculoskeletal problems. The patient may describe **paresthesias,** which are burning, tingling sensations or numbness. These sensations may be caused by pressure on nerves or by circulatory impairment. Soft tissue swelling or direct trauma to these structures can impair their function. The nurse assesses the neurovascular status of the involved musculoskeletal area.

Questions that the nurse should ask regarding altered sensations include the following:

- Is the patient experiencing any abnormal sensations or numbness?
- If the abnormal sensation or feeling of numbness involves an extremity, how does this feeling compare to sensation in the unaffected extremity?
- When did the condition begin? Is it getting worse?
- Does the patient also have pain? (If the patient has pain, then the questions and assessments for pain discussed previously should be followed.)

Assessments that the nurse should make regarding the altered sensations include the following:

- If the affected part is an extremity, how does its overall appearance compare to the unaffected extremity?
- Can the patient move the affected part? If an extremity is involved, does each toe/finger have normal sensation and motion (flexion and extension), and is the skin warm or cool?
- What is the color of the part distal to the affected area? Is it pale? Dusky? Mottled? Cyanotic?
- Does rapid capillary refill occur? (The nurse can gently squeeze a nail until it blanches, then release the pressure. The amount of time for the color under the nail to return to normal is noted. Color normally returns within 3 seconds. The return of color is evidence of capillary refill.)
- Is a pulse distal to the affected area palpable? If the affected area is an extremity, how does the pulse compare to the pulse of the unaffected extremity?
- Is edema present?
- Is any constrictive device or clothing causing nerve or vascular compression?
- Does elevating the affected part or modifying its position affect the symptoms?

Past Health, Social, and Family History

When assessing the musculoskeletal system, the nurse should gather pertinent data to include in the patient's health history, such as occupation (eg, does the patient's work require physical activity or heavy lifting?), exercise patterns, and dietary intake (eg, calcium and vitamin D). Concurrent health conditions (eg, diabetes, heart disease, chronic obstructive pulmonary disease, infection, preexisting disability) and related problems, such as familial or genetic abnormalities (Chart 66-1), also need to be considered when developing and implementing the plan of care.

Physical Assessment

An examination of the musculoskeletal system ranges from a basic assessment of functional capabilities to sophisticated physical examination maneuvers that facilitate diagnosis of specific bone, muscle, and joint disorders. The extent of assessment depends on the patient's physical complaints, health history, and physical clues that warrant further exploration. The nursing assessment is primarily a functional evaluation, focusing on the patient's ability to perform activities of daily living.

Techniques of inspection and palpation are used to evaluate the patient's posture, gait, bone integrity, joint function, and muscle strength and size. In addition, assessing the skin and neurovascular status is an important part of a complete musculoskeletal assessment. The nurse also should understand and be able to perform correct assessment techniques on patients with musculoskeletal trauma. When specific symptoms or physical findings of musculoskeletal dysfunction are apparent, the nurse carefully documents the examination findings and shares the information with the physician, who may decide that a more extensive examination and a diagnostic workup are necessary.

Posture

The normal curvature of the spine is convex through the thoracic portion and concave through the cervical and lumbar portions. Common deformities of the spine include **kyphosis,** an increased forward curvature of the thoracic spine; **lordosis,** or swayback, an exaggerated curvature of the lumbar spine; and **scoliosis,** a lateral curving deviation of the spine (Fig. 66-4). Kyphosis is frequently seen in elderly patients with osteoporosis and in some patients with neuromuscular diseases. Scoliosis may be congenital, idiopathic (without an identifiable cause), or the result of damage to the paraspinal muscles, as in polio. Lordosis

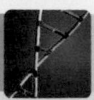

CHART 66-1

GENETICS IN NURSING PRACTICE
Musculoskeletal Disorders

When assessing a patient with musculoskeletal complaints, nurses must not overlook the possibility of a genetic component to the patient's problems.

Musculoskeletal Impairments Influenced by Genetic Factors

- Achondroplasia
- Congenital talipes equinovarus (clubfoot)
- Developmental dysplasia of the hip (DDH) (congenital hip dysplasia)
- Ehlers-Danlos syndrome
- Marfan syndrome
- Stickler syndrome
- Osteogenesis imperfecta
- Osteoporosis
- Scoliosis

Nursing Assessments

Family History

- Assess for other similarly affected family members.
- Assess for the presence of other related genetic conditions (eg, hematologic, cardiac, integumentary conditions).
- Determine the age at onset (eg, fractures present at birth as in osteogenesis imperfecta, hip dislocation present at birth in DDH, or early-onset osteoporosis).

Patient Assessment

- Assess stature for general screening purposes (unusually short stature may be related to achondroplasia; unusually tall stature may be related to Marfan syndrome).
- Assess for disease-specific skeletal findings (eg, pectus excavatum, scoliosis, long fingers [Marfan syndrome], osteoarthritis of the hip and waddling gait [DDH]).

- Assess for disease-specific skin findings (eg, velvety texture with unusual scarring and/or thin fragile skin [Ehlers-Danlos syndrome]).
- Assess for other common disease-specific findings (eg, vision impairment [Stickler syndrome, Marfan syndrome], blue/gray sclerae, opalescent dentin, hearing impairment [osteogenesis imperfecta]).

Management Issues Specific to Genetics

- Inquire whether DNA gene mutation or other genetic testing has been performed on affected family members.
- If indicated, refer patient for further genetic counseling and evaluation so that family members can discuss inheritance, risk to other family members, and the availability of genetic testing and gene-based interventions.
- Offer appropriate genetic information and resources.
- Assess patient's understanding of genetic information.
- Provide support to families with newly diagnosed genetic-related musculoskeletal disorders.
- Participate in management and coordination of care of patients with genetic conditions and people predisposed to develop or pass on a genetic condition.

Genetics Resources

Genetic Alliance—a directory of support groups for patients and families with genetic conditions; www.geneticalliance. org

Gene Clinics—a listing of common genetic disorders with up-to-date clinical summaries, genetic counseling and testing information; www. geneclinics.org

National Organization of Rare Disorders—a directory of support groups and information for patients and families with rare genetic disorders; www. rarediseases.org

OMIM: Online Mendelian Inheritance in Man—a complete listing of inherited genetic conditions; www.ncbi.nlm.nih.gov/entrez/query.fcgi?db=OMIM

---

is frequently seen during pregnancy as the woman adjusts her posture in response to changes in her center of gravity.

During inspection of the spine, the entire back, buttocks, and legs are exposed. The examiner inspects the spinal curves and trunk symmetry from posterior and lateral views. Standing behind the patient, the examiner notes any differences in the height of the shoulders or iliac crests. Shoulder and hip symmetry, as well as the line of the vertebral column, are inspected with the patient erect and with the patient bending forward (flexion). Scoliosis is evidenced by an abnormal lateral curve in the spine, shoulders that are not level, an asymmetric waistline, and a prominent scapula, accentuated by bending forward. Older adults experience a loss in height due to loss of vertebral cartilage and osteoporosis-related vertebral compression fractures. Therefore, an adult's height should be measured during health screenings.

Gait

Gait is assessed by having the patient walk away from the examiner for a short distance. The examiner observes the patient's gait for smoothness and rhythm. Any unsteadiness

or irregular movements (frequently noted in elderly patients) are considered abnormal. Limping motion is most frequently caused by painful weight bearing. In such instances, the patient can usually pinpoint the area of discomfort, thus guiding further examination. If one extremity is shorter than another, a limp may also be observed as the patient's pelvis drops downward on the affected side with each step. Limited joint motion may affect gait and a knee may be implicated. Evaluation of the knee involves the joints, bones, ligaments, tendons, and cartilage, and may include tests for the anterior and collateral ligaments, medial and lateral ligaments, and medical meniscus. In addition, a variety of neurologic conditions are associated with abnormal gaits, such as a spastic hemiparesis gait (stroke), steppage gait (lower motor neuron disease), and shuffling gait (Parkinson's disease).

Bone Integrity

The bony skeleton is assessed for deformities and alignment. Symmetric parts of the body, such as extremities, are compared. Abnormal bony growths due to bone tumors may be

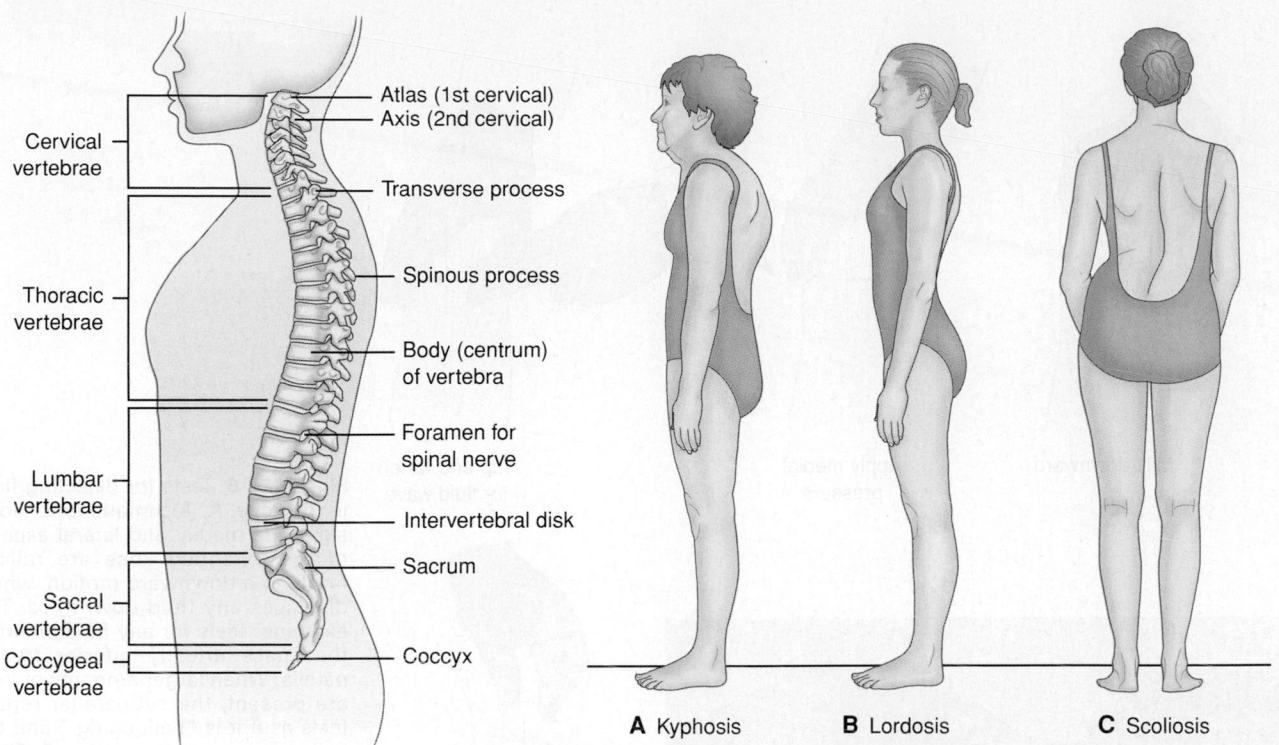

Cervical vertebrae
— Atlas (1st cervical)
— Axis (2nd cervical)
— Transverse process
— Spinous process

Thoracic vertebrae
— Body (centrum) of vertebra

Lumbar vertebrae
— Foramen for spinal nerve
— Intervertebral disk
— Sacrum

Sacral vertebrae
— Coccyx

Coccygeal vertebrae

A Kyphosis   **B** Lordosis   **C** Scoliosis

Figure 66-4 A normal spine and three abnormalities. **A,** Kyphosis: an increased convexity or roundness of the spine's thoracic curve. **B,** Lordosis: swayback; exaggeration of the lumbar spine curve. **C,** Scoliosis: a lateral curvature of the spine.

observed. Shortened extremities, amputations, and body parts that are not in anatomic alignment are noted. Fracture findings may include abnormal angulation of long bones, motion at points other than joints, and **crepitus** (a grating sound) at the point of abnormal motion. Movement of fracture fragments must be minimized to avoid additional injury.

Joint Function

The articular system is evaluated by noting range of motion, deformity, stability, and nodular formation. Range of motion is evaluated both actively (the joint is moved by the muscles surrounding the joint) and passively (the joint is moved by the examiner). The examiner is familiar with the normal range of motion of major joints (see Chapter 11). Precise measurement of range of motion can be made by a goniometer (a protractor designed for evaluating joint motion). Limited range of motion may be the result of skeletal deformity, joint pathology, or **contracture** (shortening of surrounding joint structures) of the surrounding muscles, tendons, and joint capsule. In elderly patients, limitations of range of motion associated with osteoarthritis may reduce their ability to perform activities of daily living.

If joint motion is compromised or the joint is painful, the joint is examined for **effusion** (excessive fluid within the capsule), swelling, and increased temperature that may reflect active inflammation. An effusion is suspected if the joint is swollen and the normal bony landmarks are obscured. The most common site for joint effusion is the knee. If large amounts of fluid are present in the joint spaces beneath the patella, it may be identified by assessing for the balloon sign and for ballottement of the knee (Fig. 66-5). If

inflammation or fluid is suspected in a joint, consultation with a physician is indicated.

Joint deformity may be caused by contracture, dislocation (complete separation of joint surfaces), subluxation (partial separation of articular surfaces), or disruption of structures surrounding the joint. Weakness or disruption of joint-supporting structures may result in a weak joint that requires an external supporting appliance (eg, brace).

Palpation of the joint while it is passively moved provides information about the integrity of the joint. Normally, the joint moves smoothly. A snap or crack may indicate that a ligament is slipping over a bony prominence. Slightly roughened surfaces, as in arthritic conditions, result in crepitus (grating, crackling sound or sensation) as the irregular joint surfaces move across one another.

The tissues surrounding joints are examined for nodule formation. Rheumatoid arthritis, gout, and osteoarthritis may produce characteristic nodules. The subcutaneous nodules of rheumatoid arthritis are soft and occur within and along tendons that provide extensor function to the joints. The nodules of gout are hard and lie within and immediately adjacent to the joint capsule itself. They may rupture, exuding white uric acid crystals onto the skin surface. Osteoarthritic nodules are hard and painless and represent bony overgrowth that has resulted from destruction of the cartilaginous surface of bone within the joint capsule. They are frequently seen in older adults.

Often, the size of the joint is exaggerated by atrophy of the muscles proximal and distal to that joint. This is seen in rheumatoid arthritis of the knees, in which the quadriceps muscle may atrophy dramatically. In rheumatoid arthritis,

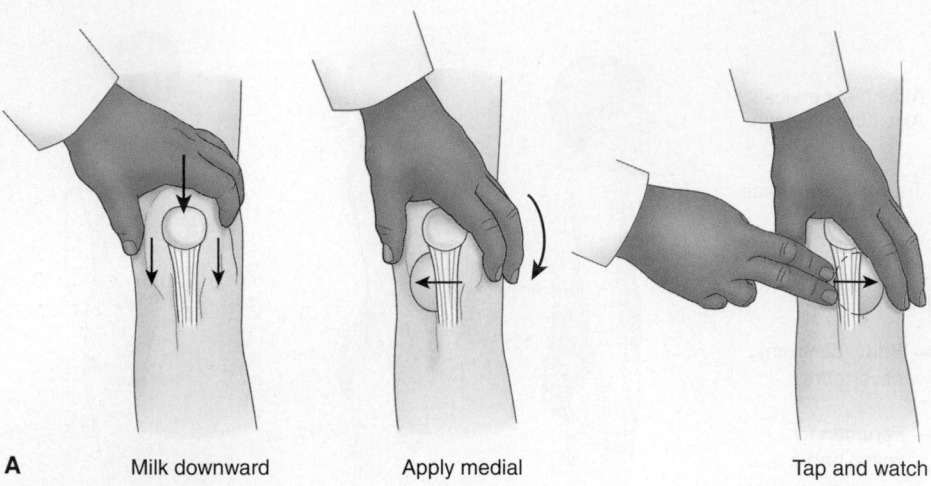

A   Milk downward   Apply medial pressure   Tap and watch for fluid wave

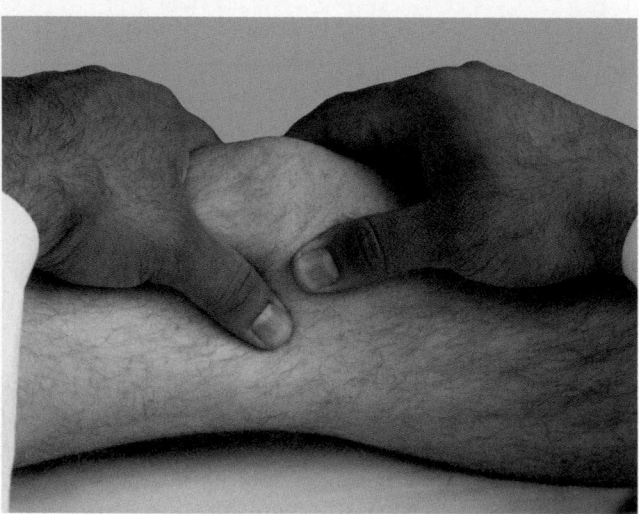

B

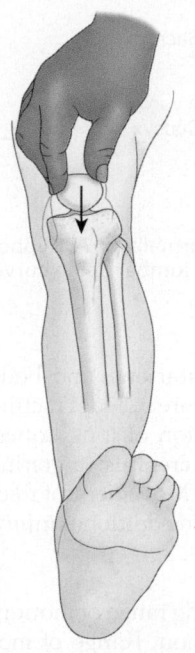

Figure 66-5 Tests for detecting fluid in the knee. **A,** Technique for balloon sign. The medial and lateral aspects of the extended knee are milked firmly in a downward motion, which displaces any fluid downward. The examiner feels for any fluid entering the space directly inferior to the patella. When larger amounts of fluid are present, the subpatellar region feels as if it is "ballooning," and the balloon sign test is positive. **B,** Technique for ballottement sign. The medial and lateral aspects of the extended knee are milked firmly in a downward motion. The examiner pushes the patella toward the femur and observes for fluid return to the region superior to the patella. When larger amounts of fluid are present, the patella elevates, there is visible return of fluid to the region directly superior to the patella, and the ballottement test is positive. Photograph used with permission from Bickley, L. S. (2007). *Bates' guide to physical examination and history taking* (9th ed.). Philadelphia: Lippincott Williams & Wilkins.

joint involvement assumes a symmetric pattern (Fig. 66-6). (See Chapter 54 for further information about rheumatoid arthritis.)

Muscle Strength and Size

The muscular system is assessed by noting muscular strength and coordination, the size of individual muscles, and the patient's ability to change position. Weakness of a group of muscles might indicate a variety of conditions, such as polyneuropathy, electrolyte disturbances (particularly potassium and calcium), myasthenia gravis, poliomyelitis, and muscular dystrophy. By palpating the muscle while passively moving the relaxed extremity, the nurse can determine the muscle tone. The nurse assesses muscle strength by having the patient perform certain maneuvers with and without added resistance. For example, when the biceps are tested, the patient is asked to extend the arm fully and then

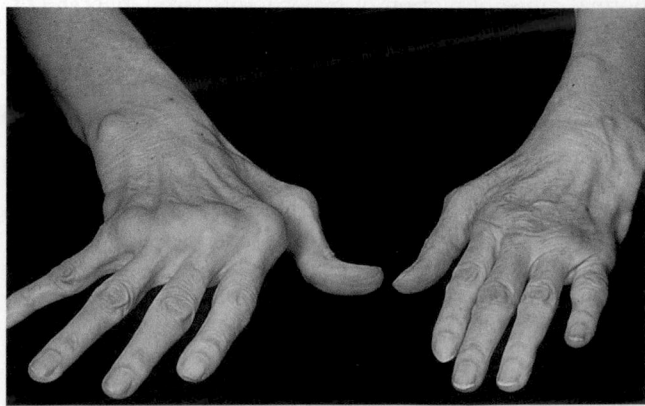

Figure 66-6 Rheumatoid arthritis joint deformity with ulnar deviation of fingers and "swan neck" deformity of fingers (ie, hyperextension of proximal interphalangeal joints with flexion of distal interphalangeal joints).

to flex it against resistance applied by the nurse. A simple handshake may provide an indication of grasp strength.

The nurse may elicit muscle **clonus** (rhythmic contractions of a muscle) in the ankle or wrist by sudden, forceful, sustained dorsiflexion of the foot or extension of the wrist. **Fasciculation** (involuntary twitching of muscle fiber groups) may be observed.

The nurse measures the girth of an extremity to monitor increased size due to exercise, edema, or bleeding into the muscle. Girth may decrease due to muscle atrophy. The unaffected extremity is measured and used as the reference standard for the affected extremity. Measurements are taken at the maximum circumference of the extremity. It is important that the measurements be taken at the same location on the extremity, and with the extremity in the same position, with the muscle at rest. Distance from a specific anatomic landmark (eg, 10 cm below the medial aspect of the knee for measurement of the calf muscle) should be indicated in the patient's record so that subsequent measurements can be made at the same point. For ease of serial assessment, the nurse may indicate the point of measurement by marking the skin. Variations in size greater than 1 cm are considered significant.

Skin

In addition to assessing the musculoskeletal system, the nurse inspects the skin for edema, temperature, and color. Palpation of the skin can reveal whether any areas are warmer, suggesting increased perfusion or inflammation, or cooler, suggesting decreased perfusion, and whether edema is present. Cuts, bruises, skin color, and evidence of decreased circulation or inflammation can influence nursing management of musculoskeletal conditions.

Neurovascular Status

It is important for the nurse to perform frequent neurovascular assessments of patients with musculoskeletal disorders (especially of those with fractures) because of the risk for tissue and nerve damage. Chart 66-2 describes tests of peripheral nerve function that the nurse may perform. One complication that the nurse needs to be alert for when assessing the patient is compartment syndrome, which is described in detail later in this unit. This major neurovascular problem is caused by pressure within a muscle compartment that increases to such an extent that microcirculation diminishes, leading to nerve and muscle anoxia and necrosis. Function can be permanently lost if the anoxic situation continues for longer than 6 hours. Assessment of neurovascular status (Chart 66-3) is frequently referred to as assessment of CMS (circulation, motion, and sensation).

Diagnostic Evaluation

Imaging Procedures

X-Ray Studies

X-ray studies are important in evaluating patients with musculoskeletal disorders. Bone x-rays determine bone density, texture, erosion, and changes in bone relationships. X-ray study of the cortex of the bone reveals any widening,

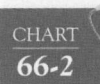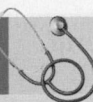

CHART 66-2

Assessing for Peripheral Nerve Function

Assessment of peripheral nerve function has two key elements: evaluation of sensation and evaluation of motion. The nurse may perform one or all of the following during a musculoskeletal assessment.

Nerve	Test of Sensation	Test of Movement
Peroneal nerve	Prick the skin midway between the great and second toe. 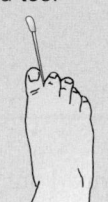	Ask the patient to dorsiflex the foot and extend the toes. 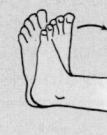
Tibial nerve	Prick the medial and lateral surface of the sole. 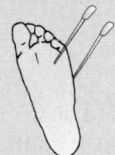	Ask the patient to plantar flex toes and foot. 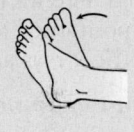
Radial nerve	Prick the skin midway between the thumb and second finger. 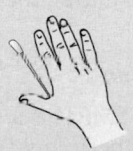	Ask the patient to stretch out the thumb, then the wrist, and then the fingers at the metacarpal joints. 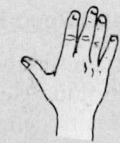
Ulnar nerve	Prick the distal fat pad of the small finger. 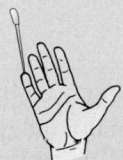	Ask the patient to abduct all fingers. 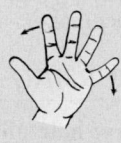
Median nerve	Prick the top or distal surface of the index finger. 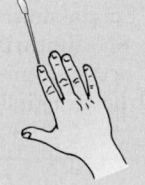	Ask the patient to touch the thumb to the little finger. Also observe whether the patient can flex the wrist. 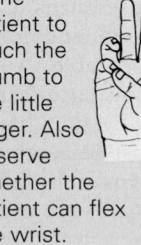

Chart 66-3 • *Indicators of Peripheral Neurovascular Dysfunction*

Circulation

Color: Pale, cyanotic, or mottled
Temperature: Cool
Capillary refill: More than 3 seconds

Motion

Weakness
Paralysis

Sensation

Paresthesia
Unrelenting pain
Pain on passive stretch
Absence of feeling

narrowing, or signs of irregularity. Joint x-rays reveal fluid, irregularity, spur formation, narrowing, and changes in the joint structure. Multiple x-rays, with multiple views (eg, anterior-posterior, lateral), are needed for full assessment of the structure being examined. Serial x-rays may be indicated to determine the status of the healing process. After being positioned for the study, the patient must remain still while the x-rays are obtained.

Computed Tomography

A computed tomography (CT) scan, which may be performed with or without the use of contrast agents, shows in detail a specific plane of involved bone and can reveal tumors of the soft tissue or injuries to the ligaments or tendons. It is used to identify the location and extent of fractures in areas that are difficult to evaluate (eg, acetabulum). The patient must remain still during the procedure (Goodhart & Page, 2007).

Magnetic Resonance Imaging

Magnetic resonance imaging (MRI) is a noninvasive imaging technique that uses magnetic fields, radiowaves, and computers to demonstrate abnormalities (ie, tumors or narrowing of tissue pathways through bone) of soft tissues such as muscle, tendon, cartilage, nerve, and fat. Because an electromagnet is used, patients with any metal implants, clips, or pacemakers are not candidates for MRI.

> ▶ **NURSING ALERT**
>
> Jewelry, hair clips, hearing aids, credit cards with magnetic strips, and other metal-containing objects must be removed before the MRI is performed; otherwise, they can become dangerous projectile objects or cause burns. Credit cards with magnetic strips may be erased, and nonremovable cochlear devices can become inoperable. Also, transdermal patches (eg, NicoDerm, Transderm-Nitro, Transderm Scopolamine, Catapres-TTS) that have a thin layer of aluminized backing must be removed before MRI because they can cause burns. The physician should be notified before the patches are removed.

To enhance visualization of anatomic structures, intravenous (IV) contrast agent may be used. During the MRI, the patient must lie still and will hear a rhythmic knocking sound. Patients who experience claustrophobia may be unable to tolerate the confinement of closed MRI equipment without sedation. Open MRI systems are available, but they use lower-intensity magnetic fields, which produce lower-quality images. Advantages of open MRI include increased patient comfort, reduced problems with claustrophobic reactions, and reduced noise.

Arthrography

Arthrography is useful in identifying acute or chronic tears of the joint capsule or supporting ligaments of the knee, shoulder, ankle, hip, or wrist. A radiopaque contrast agent or air is injected into the joint cavity to visualize irregular surfaces. The joint is put through its range of motion to distribute the contrast agent while a series of x-rays is obtained. If a tear is present, the contrast agent leaks out of the joint and is evident on the x-ray image.

After an arthrogram, a compression elastic bandage is applied as prescribed and the joint is usually rested for 12 hours. The nurse provides additional comfort measures (mild analgesia, ice) as appropriate and explains to the patient that it is normal to experience clicking or crackling in the joint for a day or two after the procedure, until the contrast agent or air is absorbed.

Nursing Interventions for Imaging Studies

Before the patient undergoes an imaging study, the nurse assesses for conditions that may require special consideration during the study or that may be contraindications to the study (eg, pregnancy; claustrophobia; inability to tolerate required positioning due to age, debility, or disability; metal implants). If contrast agents will be used for CT scan, MRI, or arthrography, the patient is assessed for possible allergies (Goodhart & Page, 2007).

Bone Densitometry

Bone densitometry is used to estimate bone mineral density (BMD). This can be performed through the use of x-rays or ultrasound. The most common modalities used include dual-energy x-ray absorptiometry (DXA or DEXA), quantitative computed tomography (QCT), and quantitative ultrasound (QUS). DXA BMD measures of the hip and spine are very accurate in estimating the extent of osteoporosis and monitoring a patient's response to treatment for osteoporosis. Peripheral DXA (pDXA) may be an alternative test that measures BMD of the forearm, finger, or heel, though its ability to project hip or spine fracture risk is less accurate than DXA. While the BMD of the heel can be used to diagnose and monitor osteoporosis, predicting hip fracture risk related to osteoporosis is best achieved through DXA of the hip; hence, it is the most commonly prescribed diagnostic test for determining BMD (Bonnick, 2005; National Osteoporosis Foundation, 2008). (See Chapter 68 for a further discussion of osteoporosis risks.)

Bone Scan

A bone scan is performed to detect metastatic and primary bone tumors, osteomyelitis, some fractures, and aseptic necrosis. A bone-seeking radioisotope is injected

IV. The scan is performed 2 to 3 hours after the injection. At this point, distribution and concentration of the isotope in the bone are measured. The degree of nuclide uptake is related to the metabolism of the bone. An increased uptake of isotope is seen in primary skeletal disease (osteosarcoma), metastatic bone disease, inflammatory skeletal disease (osteomyelitis), and fractures that do not heal as expected.

Nursing Interventions

Before the patient undergoes a bone scan, the nurse inquires about possible allergies to the radioisotope and assesses for any condition that would contraindicate performing the procedure (eg, pregnancy). In addition, the patient is encouraged to drink plenty of fluids to help distribute and eliminate the isotope. Before the scan, the nurse asks the patient to empty the bladder, because a full bladder interferes with accurate scanning of the pelvic bones.

Arthroscopy

Arthroscopy is a procedure that allows direct visualization of a joint to diagnose joint disorders. Treatment of tears, defects, and disease processes may be performed through the arthroscope. The procedure is performed in the operating room under sterile conditions; injection of a local anesthetic agent into the joint or general anesthesia is used. A large-bore needle is inserted, and the joint is distended with saline. The arthroscope is introduced, and joint structures, synovium, and articular surfaces are visualized. After the procedure, the puncture wound is closed with adhesive strips or sutures and covered with a sterile dressing. Complications are rare but may include infection, hemarthrosis, neurovascular compromise, thrombophlebitis, stiffness, effusion, adhesions, and delayed wound healing.

Nursing Interventions

After the arthroscopic procedure, the joint is wrapped with a compression dressing to control swelling. In addition, ice may be applied to control edema and enhance comfort. Frequently, the joint is kept extended and elevated to reduce swelling. It is important to monitor and document the neurovascular status. Analgesic agents are administered as needed. The patient is instructed about activities and exercises that may be performed. The patient and family are informed of the symptoms (eg, swelling, numbness, cool skin) to watch for in order to determine whether complications are occurring and of the importance of notifying the physician of these observations.

Arthrocentesis

Arthrocentesis (joint aspiration) is carried out to obtain synovial fluid for purposes of examination or to relieve pain due to effusion. Examination of synovial fluid is helpful in the diagnosis of septic arthritis and other inflammatory arthropathies and reveals the presence of hemarthrosis (bleeding into the joint cavity), which suggests trauma or a bleeding disorder. Normally, synovial fluid is clear, pale, straw colored, and scanty in volume. Using aseptic technique, the physician inserts a needle into the joint and aspirates fluid. Anti-inflammatory medications may be injected into the joint. A sterile dressing is applied after aspiration. There is a risk of infection after this procedure.

Electromyography

Electromyography (EMG) provides information about the electrical potential of the muscles and the nerves leading to them. The test is performed to evaluate muscle weakness, pain, and disability. The purpose of the procedure is to determine any abnormality of function and to differentiate muscle and nerve problems. Needle electrodes are inserted into selected muscles, and responses to electrical stimuli are recorded on an oscilloscope. Warm compresses may relieve residual discomfort after the study.

Biopsy

Biopsy may be performed to determine the structure and composition of bone marrow, bone, muscle, or synovium to help diagnose specific diseases. The nurse teaches the patient about the procedure and assures the patient that analgesic agents will be provided. The nurse monitors the biopsy site for edema, bleeding, pain, and infection. Ice is applied as prescribed to control bleeding and edema. In addition, analgesic agents are administered as prescribed for comfort.

Laboratory Studies

Examination of the patient's blood and urine can provide information about a primary musculoskeletal problem (eg, Paget's disease of the bone), a developing complication (eg, infection), the baseline for instituting therapy (eg, anticoagulant therapy), or the response to therapy. Before surgery, coagulation studies are performed to detect bleeding tendencies (because bone is vascular tissue).

Serum calcium levels are altered in patients with osteomalacia, parathyroid dysfunction, Paget's disease, metastatic bone tumors, or prolonged immobilization. Serum phosphorus levels are inversely related to calcium levels and are diminished in osteomalacia associated with malabsorption syndrome. Acid phosphatase is elevated in Paget's disease and metastatic cancer. Alkaline phosphatase is elevated during early fracture healing and in diseases with increased osteoblastic activity (eg, metastatic bone tumors). Bone metabolism may be evaluated through thyroid studies and determination of calcitonin, PTH, and vitamin D levels. Serum enzyme levels of creatine kinase and aspartate aminotransferase become elevated with muscle damage. Serum osteocalcin (bone GLA protein) indicates the rate of bone turnover. Urine calcium levels increase with bone destruction (eg, parathyroid dysfunction, metastatic bone tumors, multiple myeloma) (McCormick, 2007).

Specific urine and serum biochemical markers can be used to provide information about bone formation. These include urinary N-telopeptide of type 1 collagen (N-Tx) and deoxypyridinoline (Dpd), both of which reflect increased osteoclast activity and increased bone resorption. Conversely, elevated serum levels of bone-specific alkaline phosphatase (ALP), osteocalcin, and intact *N*-terminal propeptide of type 1 collagen (P1NP) reflect increased activity of osteoblasts and enhanced bone remodeling activity (McCormick, 2007).

CRITICAL THINKING EXERCISES

EBP **1** A 72-year-old Caucasian woman arrives at the emergency department where you are the triage nurse. She is complaining of severe pain in her right groin area and has some discomfort when she puts weight on or moves her right hip. She stated that she did not fall or injure the extremity; she just was walking down the steps and felt a "force" on her right leg. There are no deformities noted. What are the first evaluation assessments that you would perform? What is the evidence base that indicates that this woman may be at increased risk for osteoporosis-related fractures? What recommendations might be made for appropriate testing in this patient? What are the most important medical history questions you would ask her?

2 A 15-year-old high school football player came into the orthopedic office after sustaining a "direct blow" to the left knee last night during a game. He has slight edema and complains of pain with movement and weight bearing. What is your first physical assessment activity? How would you assess the stability of his left knee? What diagnostic tests are most likely indicated?

EBP **3** You are a parish nurse teaching a class to senior citizens in your parish centered on age-associated changes in the musculoskeletal system. The participants have experienced many of the changes you identify and ask you what they can do about them. What is the evidence base that supports the strategies that these elderly citizens might implement to minimize these changes and maximize musculoskeletal health? What is the strength of the evidence of the effectiveness of these strategies? Focus your teaching strategies on prevention of falls and on prevention of osteoporosis.

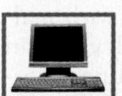

The Smeltzer suite offers these additional resources to enhance learning and facilitate understanding of this chapter:
• thePoint online resource, thepoint.lww.com/Smeltzer12E

• Student CD-ROM included with the book
• *Study Guide to Accompany Brunner & Suddarth's Text-book of Medical-Surgical Nursing*

REFERENCES AND SELECTED READINGS

Books

Argur, A. & Dalley, A. (2005). *Grants atlas of anatomy*. Philadelphia: Lippincott Williams & Wilkins.

Bickley, L. S. (2007). *Bates' guide to physical examination and history taking* (9th ed.). Philadelphia: Lippincott Williams & Wilkins.

Fischbach, F. T. & Dunning, M. B. (2008). *A manual of laboratory and diagnostic tests* (8th ed.). Philadelphia: Lippincott Williams & Wilkins.

National Association of Orthopaedic Nurses. (2007). *Core curriculum for orthopaedic nursing* (6th ed.). Boston: Pearson Custom Publishing.

National Osteoporosis Foundation. (2008). *Clinician's guide to prevention and treatment of osteoporosis*. Washington, DC: Author.

Porth, C. M. & Matfin, G. (2009). *Pathophysiology: Concepts of altered health states* (8th ed.). Philadelphia: Lippincott Williams & Wilkins.

Reider, B. (2005). *The orthopaedic physical examination* (2nd ed.). St. Louis: Elsevier.

U.S. Department of Health and Human Services. (2004). *Bone health and osteoporosis: A report of the Surgeon General*. Rockville, MD: U.S. Department of Health and Human Services/Public Health Service, Office of the Surgeon General.

Journals and Electronic Documents

Bonnick, S. L. (2005). Bone mass measurement techniques in clinical practice: Methods, applications, and interpretation. *Topics in Geriatric Rehabilitation, 21*(1), 30–41.

Centers for Disease Control and Prevention. (2005). *Arthritis: Data and statistics*. www.cdc.gov/arthritis/data_statistics/index.htm

Goodhart, J. & Page, J. (2007). Radiology nursing. *Orthopaedic Nursing, 26*(1), 36–39.

McCormick, R. K. (2007). Osteoporosis: Biomarkers and other diagnostic correlates into the management of bone fragility. *Alternative Medicine Review, 12*(2), 113–145.

National Association of Orthopedic Nurses. (2005). Palliative care: Improving the quality of care for patients with chronic, incurable musculoskeletal conditions: Consensus document. *Orthopaedic Nursing, 24*(1), 8–11.

RESOURCES

American College of Sports Medicine, www.acsm.org
National Association of Orthopaedic Nurses (NAON), www.orthonurse.org
National Institute of Arthritis and Musculoskeletal and Skin Diseases, www.niams.nih.gov
National Osteoporosis Foundation, www.nof.org

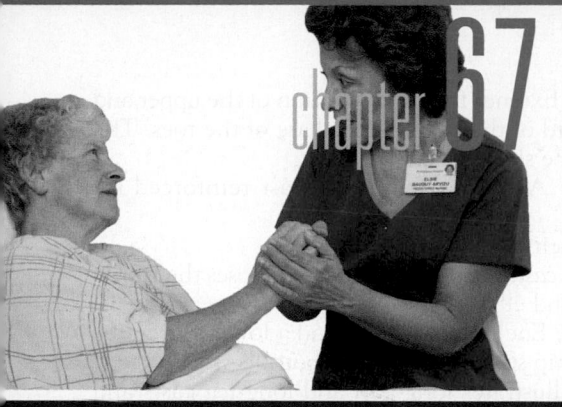

chapter 67

Musculoskeletal Care Modalities

LEARNING OBJECTIVES

On completion of this chapter, the learner will be able to:

1 Identify the preventive and health teaching needs of the patient with a cast, brace, or splint.

2 Describe the nursing management of the patient with a cast, brace, or splint.

3 Describe the various types of traction and the principles of effective traction.

4 Identify the preventive nursing care needs of the patient in traction.

5 Describe the nursing management of the patient in traction.

6 Compare the nursing needs of the patient undergoing total hip replacement with those of the patient undergoing total knee replacement.

7 Use the nursing process as a framework for care of the patient undergoing orthopedic surgery.

GLOSSARY

abduction: movement away from the center or median line of the body

adduction: movement toward the center or median line of the body

avascular necrosis: death of tissue due to insufficient blood supply

brace: externally applied device to support the body or a body part, control movement, and prevent injury

cast: rigid external immobilizing device molded to contours of body part

cast syndrome: psychological (claustrophobic reaction) or physiologic (superior mesenteric artery syndrome) responses to confinement in body cast

continuous passive motion (CPM) device: a device that promotes range of motion, circulation, and healing

edema: soft tissue swelling due to fluid accumulation

external fixator: external metal frame attached to bone fragments to stabilize them

fracture: a break in the continuity of the bone

heterotopic ossification: misplaced formation of bone

neurovascular status: neurologic (motor and sensory components) and circulatory functioning of a body part

open reduction with internal fixation (ORIF): open surgical procedure to repair and stabilize a fracture

osteomyelitis: infection of the bone

osteotomy: surgical cutting of bone

sling: bandage used to support an arm

splint: device designed specifically to support and immobilize a body part in a desired position

traction: application of a pulling force to a part of the body

trapeze: overhead assistive device to promote patient mobility in bed

The management of musculoskeletal injuries and disorders frequently includes the use of casts, braces, splints, traction, surgery, or a combination of these. Patient education is essential for optimal outcomes. The nurse prepares the patient for immobilization with casts or traction, and for surgery, when indicated. Nursing care is planned to maximize the effectiveness of these treatment modalities and to prevent potential complications associated with each of the interventions. The patient is taught to manage care at home and how to safely resume activities.

The Patient in a Cast, Splint, or Brace

Casts

A **cast** is a rigid external immobilizing device that is molded to the contours of the body. A cast is used specifically to immobilize a reduced **fracture,** to correct a deformity, to apply uniform pressure to underlying soft tissue, or to support and stabilize weakened joints (Altizer, 2004). Generally, casts permit mobilization of the patient while restricting movement of a body part.

The condition being treated influences the type and thickness of the cast applied. Generally, the joints proximal and distal to the area to be immobilized are included in the cast. However, with some fractures, cast construction and molding may allow movement of a joint while immobilizing a fracture (eg, three-point fixation in a patellar tendon weight-bearing cast). Various types of casts include the following:

Short-arm cast: Extends from below the elbow to the palmar crease, secured around the base of the thumb. If the thumb is included, it is known as a *thumb spica* or *gauntlet* cast.

Long-arm cast: Extends from the axillary fold to the proximal palmar crease. The elbow usually is immobilized at a right angle.

Short-leg cast: Extends from below the knee to the base of the toes. The foot is flexed at a right angle in a neutral position.

Long-leg cast: Extends from the junction of the upper and middle third of the thigh to the base of the toes. The knee may be slightly flexed.

Walking cast: A short- or long-leg cast reinforced for strength.

Body cast: Encircles the trunk.

Shoulder spica cast: A body jacket that encloses the trunk, shoulder, and elbow.

Hip spica cast: Encloses the trunk and a lower extremity. A double hip spica cast includes both legs.

Figure 67-1 illustrates long-arm and long-leg casts and areas in which pressure problems commonly occur with these casts.

Fiberglass Casts

Fiberglass casts are composed of water-activated polyurethane materials that have the versatility of plaster (see later discussion) but are lighter in weight, stronger, and more durable than plaster. In addition, they are water resistant (Altizer, 2004). They consist of an open-weave, nonabsorbent fabric impregnated with cool water–activated hardeners that bond and reach full rigid strength in minutes. Heat is given off (an exothermic reaction) while the cast is applied. Therefore, a newly applied fiberglass cast should not be placed on a plastic surface. The heat given off during this reaction can be uncomfortable, and the nurse should prepare the patient for the sensation of increasing warmth so that the patient does not become alarmed. While the cast is setting, it can be dented. Therefore, it must be handled with the palms of the hands and not allowed to rest on hard surfaces or sharp edges. Cast dents may press on the skin, causing irritation and skin breakdown.

Some fiberglass casts use a waterproof lining (Gore-Tex), which permits the patient to shower, swim, or engage in hydrotherapy (use of water for treatment). When the cast is wet, the patient is instructed to shake or drain water out of it; thorough drying is important to prevent skin breakdown. The best results are achieved with casts that can easily drain, such as short-arm casts. Heels and elbows encased in wet casts may become macerated from the trapped water and therefore are associated with more skin breakdown.

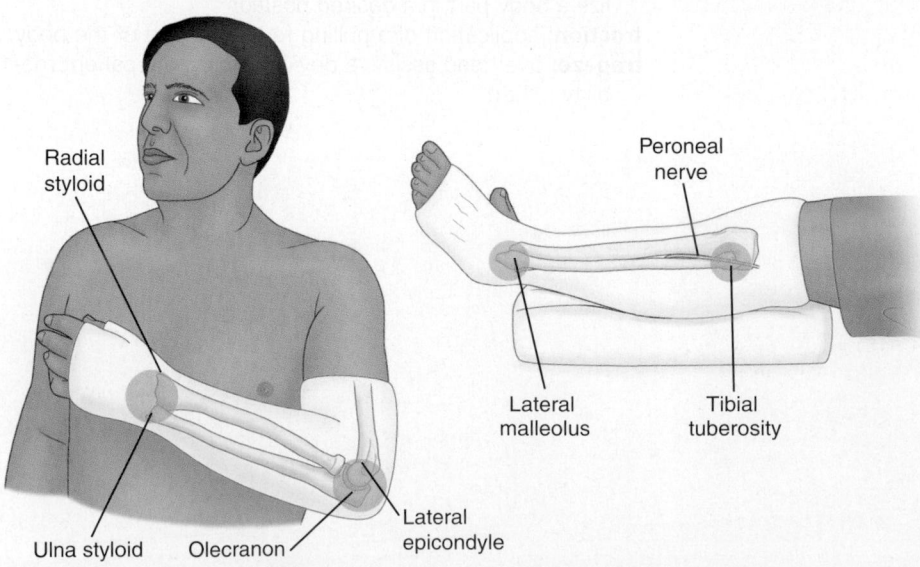

Figure 67-1 Pressure areas in common types of casts. **Left,** Long-arm cast. **Right,** Short-leg cast.

Radial styloid

Peroneal nerve

Lateral malleolus

Tibial tuberosity

Ulna styloid Olecranon Lateral epicondyle

Plaster Casts

Casts made of plaster are less costly and achieve a better mold than fiberglass casts; however, they are not as durable and take longer to dry. Rolls of plaster of Paris-impregnated bandages are wet in cool water and applied smoothly to the body. These will also cause an exothermic reaction, similar to that seen with fiberglass casts. The crystallization process produces a rigid dressing in 15 to 20 minutes. After the plaster sets, the cast remains wet and somewhat soft. It does not have its full strength until it is dry. The plaster cast requires 24 to 72 hours to dry completely, depending on its thickness and the environmental drying conditions. A freshly applied cast should be exposed to circulating air to dry and should not be covered with clothing or bed linens or placed on plastic-coated mats or bedding. A wet plaster cast appears dull and gray, sounds dull on percussion, feels damp, and smells musty. A dry plaster cast is white and shiny, resonant to percussion, odorless, and firm.

Splints and Braces

Many injuries that were previously treated with casts may now be treated with other immobilization devices (eg, braces, splints) (Nash, Mickan, Del Mar, et al., 2005).

Contoured **splints** of plaster or pliable thermoplastic materials may be used for conditions that do not require rigid immobilization, for those in which swelling may be anticipated, and for those that require special skin care. Splints made of thermoplastics are warmed and molded to fit the patient (eg, hand splints and thoracolumbosacral orthotics [TLSOs], clamshell-type back braces). The splint needs to immobilize and support the body part in a functional position and it must be well padded to prevent pressure, skin abrasion, and skin breakdown. The splint is overwrapped with an elastic bandage applied in a spiral fashion and with pressure uniformly distributed so that circulation is not restricted. Splints are generally indicated for short-term use (Gravlee & Van Durme, 2007).

Braces (ie, orthoses) are used to provide support, control movement, and prevent additional injury. They are custom fitted to various parts of the body. The orthotist adjusts the brace for fit, positioning, and motion so that movement is enhanced, any deformities are corrected, and discomfort is minimized. Braces are generally indicated for longer use than splints (Gravlee & Van Durme, 2007).

Many splints and braces are prefabricated. They may be made of plastic and other materials such as cloth, leather, metal, elastic and Velcro. Knee immobilizers, ankle stirrups, and cock-up wrist splints are types of prefabricated splints and braces.

General Nursing Management of a Patient in a Cast, Splint, or Brace

Before the cast, brace, or splint is applied, the nurse completes an assessment of the patient's general health, presenting signs and symptoms, emotional status, understanding of the need for the device, and condition of the body part to be immobilized. Physical assessment of the part to be immobilized must include assessment of the **neurovascular status** (ie, neurologic and circulatory functioning) of the body part and degree and location of swelling, bruising, and skin abrasions. In addition, the nurse gives the patient information about the underlying pathologic condition and the purpose and expectations of the prescribed treatment regimen. This knowledge promotes the patient's active participation in and compliance with the treatment program. It is important to prepare the patient for the application of the cast, brace, or splint by describing the anticipated sights, sounds, and sensations (eg, heat from the hardening reaction of the fiberglass or plaster). The patient needs to know what to expect during application and the reason the body part must be immobilized (Chart 67-1).

The nurse must carefully evaluate pain associated with the musculoskeletal condition, asking the patient to indicate the exact site and to describe the character and intensity of the pain to help determine its cause. Most pain can be relieved by elevating the involved part, applying cold packs, and administering analgesic agents as prescribed.

 NURSING ALERT

A patient's unrelieved pain must be immediately reported to the physician to avoid possible paralysis and necrosis.

Pain associated with the underlying condition (eg, fracture) is frequently controlled by immobilization. Pain due to **edema** that is associated with trauma, surgery, or bleeding into the tissues can frequently be controlled by elevation and, if prescribed, intermittent application of cold packs. Ice bags (one-third to one-half full) or cold application devices are placed on each side of the cast, if prescribed, making sure not to indent or wet the cast.

Pain may be indicative of complications. Pain associated with compartment syndrome (see Chapter 69 and later in this chapter) is relentless and is not controlled by modalities such as elevation, application of cold if prescribed, and usual dosages of analgesic agents. Severe burning pain over bony prominences, especially the heels, anterior ankles, and elbows, warns of an impending pressure ulcer. These may also occur from too-tight ace wraps used to hold splints in place. Pain decreases when ulceration occurs. Discomfort due to pressure on the skin may be relieved by elevation that controls edema or by positioning that alters pressure. It may be necessary to modify the dressing, ace wrap, or cast, or to apply a new cast.

 NURSING ALERT

The nurse must never ignore complaints of pain from the patient in a cast because of the possibility of problems, such as impaired tissue perfusion or pressure ulcer formation.

Every joint that is not immobilized should be exercised and moved through its range of motion to maintain function. If the patient has a leg cast, brace, or splint, the nurse encourages toe exercises. If the patient has an arm immobilized, the nurse encourages finger exercises.

To promote healing, it is important to treat any skin lacerations and abrasions that may have occurred as a result of the trauma that caused the fracture before the cast, brace, or

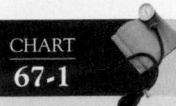

CHART 67-1 Guidelines for Applying a Cast

Equipment

- Drape for patient
- Knitted material (eg, stockinette)
- Nonwoven roll padding
- Casting material
- Water and basin
- Cast knife or cutter

Implementation

Procedure	Rationale
1. Support extremity or body part to be casted.	1. Minimizes movement; maintains reduction and alignment; increases comfort
2. Position and maintain part to be casted in position indicated by physician during casting procedure.	2. Facilitates casting; reduces incidence of complications (eg, malunion, nonunion, contracture)
3. Drape patient.	3. Avoids undue exposure; protects other body parts from contact with casting materials
4. Wash and dry part to be casted.	4. Reduces incidence of skin breakdown
5. Place at least three layers of knitted material* (eg, stockinette) over part to be casted. • Apply in smooth and nonconstrictive manner. • Allow additional material.	5. Protects skin from casting materials Protects skin from pressure Folds over edges of cast when finishing application; creates smooth, padded edge; protects skin from abrasion
6. Wrap soft, nonwoven roll padding* smoothly and evenly around part. • Use additional padding around bony prominences to protect superficial nerves (eg, head of fibula, olecranon process).	6. Protects skin from pressure of cast Protects skin at bony prominences Protects superficial nerves
7. Apply plaster or fiberglass casting material evenly on body part. • Choose appropriate-width bandage. • Overlap preceding turn by half the width of the bandage. • Use continuous motion, maintaining constant contact with body part. • Use additional casting material (splints) at joints and at points of anticipated cast stress.	7. Creates smooth, solid, well-contoured cast Facilitates smooth application Creates smooth, solid, immobilizing cast Shapes cast properly for adequate support Strengthens cast
8. "Finish" cast. • Smooth edges. • Trim and reshape with cast knife or cutter.	8. Protects skin from abrasion Allows full range of motion of adjacent joints
9. Remove particles of casting materials from skin.	9. Prevents particles from loosening and sliding underneath cast
10. Support cast during hardening. • Handle hardening casts with palms of hands. • Support cast on firm, smooth surface. • Do not rest cast on hard surfaces or on sharp edges. • Avoid pressure on cast.	10. Casting materials begin to harden in minutes. Maximum hardness of nonplaster cast occurs in minutes. Maximum hardness of plaster cast occurs with drying (24 to 72 hours, depending on environment and thickness of cast). Avoids denting of cast and development of pressure areas
11. Promote drying of cast. • Leave cast uncovered and exposed to air. • Turn patient every 2 hours, supporting major joints. • Fans may be used to increase air flow and speed drying.	11. Facilitates drying

*Nonabsorbent materials are used with nonplaster casts.

---

splint is applied. The nurse thoroughly cleans the skin and treats it as prescribed. The patient may require a tetanus booster if the wound is dirty and if the last known booster was administered more than 5 years ago. Sterile dressings are used to cover the injured skin. If the skin wounds are extensive, an alternative method (eg, external fixator) may be chosen to immobilize the body part. While the cast is on, the nurse observes the patient for systemic signs of infection; odors from the cast, brace, or splint; and purulent

drainage staining the cast. It is important to notify the physician if any of these occur.

The nurse monitors circulation, motion, and sensation of the affected extremity, assessing the fingers or toes of the affected extremity and comparing them with those of the opposite extremity. Normal findings include minimal edema, minimal discomfort, pink color, warm to touch, rapid capillary refill response, normal sensations, and ability to exercise fingers or toes (Konstantakos, Dalstrom, Nelles,

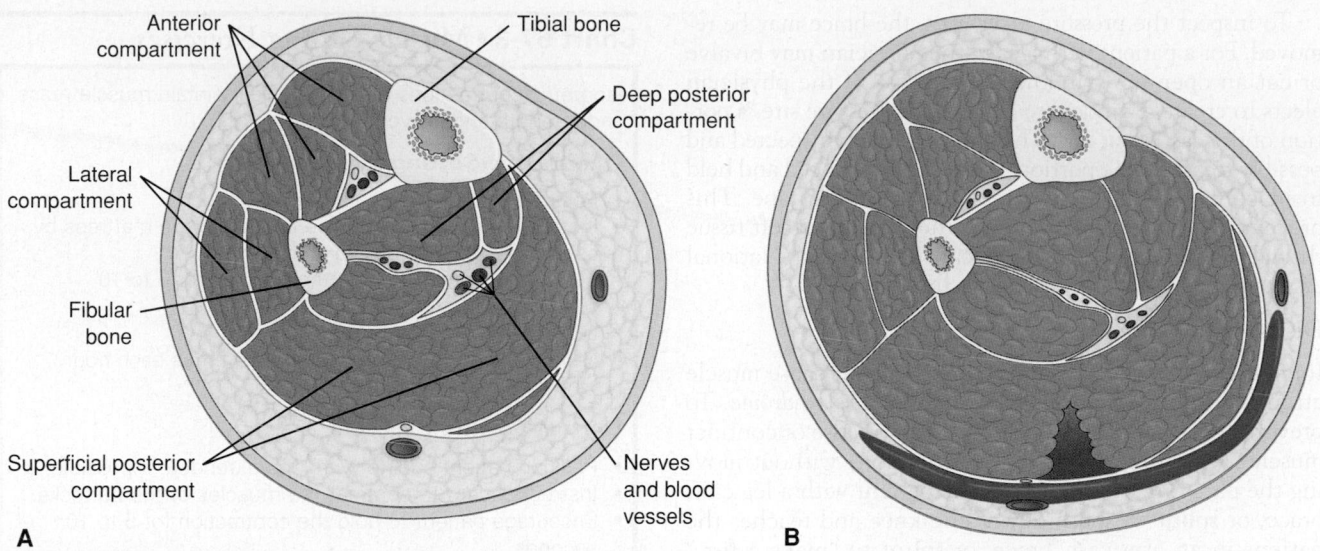

Figure 67-2 A, Cross-section of normal lower leg with muscle compartments. **B,** Cross-section of lower leg with compartment syndrome. Swelling of muscles causes compression of nerves and blood vessels.

Labels in figure A: Anterior compartment, Tibial bone, Deep posterior compartment, Lateral compartment, Fibular bone, Superficial posterior compartment, Nerves and blood vessels

et al., 2007). The nurse encourages the patient to move all fingers or toes hourly when awake to stimulate circulation.

It is important to perform frequent, regular assessments of neurovascular status. The "five P's" that require assessment are symptoms of neurovascular compromise: *p*ain, *p*allor, *p*ulselessness, *p*aresthesia, and *p*aralysis. Early recognition of diminished circulation and nerve function is essential to prevent loss of function. The nurse adjusts the extremity so that it is no higher than heart level to enhance arterial perfusion and control edema and notifies the physician at once if signs of compromised neurovascular status are present.

Monitoring and Managing Potential Complications

Potential complications related to casts, braces, and splints include compartment syndrome, pressure ulcer formation, and disuse syndrome. These most commonly occur when a cast is applied, because the cast is not easily removable, and are least commonly associated with use of a splint, because splints tend to be used for the short term.

Compartment Syndrome

Edema is a natural response of the tissue to trauma. The patient may complain that the cast, brace, or splint is too tight. Vascular insufficiency and nerve compression due to unrelieved swelling can result in compartment syndrome (Fig. 67-2). Compartment syndrome occurs when there is increased tissue pressure within a limited space (eg, cast, muscle compartment) that compromises the circulation and the function of the tissue within the confined area. To relieve the pressure, the cast must be bivalved (cut in half longitudinally) while maintaining alignment, and the extremity must be elevated no higher than heart level to ensure arterial perfusion (Chart 67-2). If pressure is not relieved and circulation is not restored, a fasciotomy may be necessary to relieve the pressure within the muscle compartment. The nurse closely monitors the patient's response to conservative and surgical management of compartment syndrome (Konstantakos, et al., 2007). The nurse records

neurovascular responses and promptly reports changes to the physician. (See Chapter 69 for further discussion of compartment syndrome.)

Pressure Ulcers

Pressure of a cast or an inappropriately applied brace on soft tissues may cause tissue anoxia and pressure ulcers. Lower extremity sites most susceptible to pressure ulcers are the heel, malleoli, dorsum of the foot, head of the fibula, and anterior surface of the patella. The main pressure sites on the upper extremity are located at the medial epicondyle of the humerus and the ulnar styloid (see Fig. 67-1).

Usually, the patient with a pressure ulcer reports pain and tightness in the area. A warm area on the cast or brace suggests underlying tissue erythema. Skin breakdown may occur. The drainage may stain the cast or brace and emit an odor. Even if discomfort does not occur with skin breakdown and tissue necrosis, there may still be extensive loss of tissue. The nurse must monitor the patient with a cast or brace for pressure ulcer development and report findings to the physician.

Chart 67-2 • *Procedure for Bivalving a Cast*

The following procedure is followed when a cast is bivalved.
1. With a cast cutter, a longitudinal cut is made to divide the cast in half.
2. The underpadding is cut with scissors.
3. The cast is spread apart with cast spreaders to relieve pressure and to inspect and treat the skin without interrupting the reduction and alignment of the bone.
4. After the pressure is relieved, the anterior and posterior parts of the cast are secured together with an elastic compression bandage to maintain immobilization.
5. To control swelling and promote circulation, the extremity is elevated (but no higher than heart level, to minimize the effect of gravity on perfusion of the tissues).

To inspect the pressure ulcer area, the brace may be removed. For a patient with a cast, the physician may bivalve or cut an opening (window) in the cast. If the physician elects to create a window to inspect the pressure site, a portion of the cast is cut out. The affected area is inspected and possibly treated. The portion of the cast is replaced and held in place by an elastic compression dressing or tape. This prevents window edema, which is the swelling of soft tissue through the area unopposed by casting material (National Association of Orthopedic Nurses [NAON], 2007).

Disuse Syndrome

Immobilization in a cast, brace, or splint can cause muscle atrophy and loss of strength, known as *disuse syndrome*. To prevent this, the patient needs to learn to tense or contract muscles (eg, isometric muscle contraction) without moving the part. The nurse teaches the patient with a leg cast, brace, or splint to "push down" the knee and teaches the patient in an arm cast, brace, or splint to "make a fist." Muscle-setting exercises (eg, quadriceps-setting and gluteal-setting exercises) are important in maintaining muscles essential for walking (Chart 67-3). Isometric exercises should be performed hourly while the patient is awake.

Promoting Home and Community-Based Care

Teaching the Patient Self-Care

Self-care deficits occur when a portion of the body is immobilized. The nurse encourages the patient to participate actively in personal care and to use assistive devices safely. The nurse must assist the patient in identifying areas of self-

care deficit and in developing strategies to achieve independence in activities of daily living (ADLs) (Chart 67-4). The patient's participation in planning and accomplishing ADLs is an important aspect of self-care, independence, maintaining control, and avoiding untoward psychological reactions, such as depression. Patient and caregiver education is also described in Chart 67-4.

Chart 67-3 • *Muscle-Setting Exercises*

Isometric contractions of the muscle maintain muscle mass and strength and prevent atrophy.

Quadriceps-Setting Exercise

- Position patient supine with leg extended.
- Instruct patient to push knee back onto the mattress by contracting the anterior thigh muscles.
- Encourage patient to hold the position for 5 to 10 seconds.
- Let patient relax.
- Have patient repeat the exercise 10 times each hour when awake.

Gluteal-Setting Exercise

- Position patient supine with legs extended, if possible.
- Instruct patient to contract the muscles of the buttocks.
- Encourage patient to hold the contraction for 5 to 10 seconds.
- Let the patient relax.
- Have patient repeat the exercise 10 times each hour when awake.

CHART 67-4 HOME CARE CHECKLIST
The Patient With a Cast, Splint, or Brace

At the completion of the home care instruction, the patient or caregiver will be able to:	PATIENT	CAREGIVER
• Describe techniques to promote cast drying (eg, do not cover, leave exposed to circulating air, handle damp plaster cast with palms of hands and do not rest the cast on hard surfaces or sharp edges that can dent soft cast).	✔	✔
• Describe approaches to controlling swelling and pain (eg, elevate immobilized extremity to heart level, apply intermittent ice bag if prescribed, take analgesic agents as prescribed).	✔	✔
• Report pain uncontrolled by elevating the immobilized limb and by analgesic agents (may be an indicator of impaired tissue perfusion—compartment syndrome or pressure ulcer).	✔	
• Demonstrate ability to transfer (eg, from a bed to a chair).	✔	
• Use mobility aids safely.	✔	
• Avoid excessive use of injured extremity; observe prescribed weight-bearing limits.	✔	
• Manage minor skin irritations (eg, for skin irritation from edge of cast, splint, or brace; pad rough edges with tape; to relieve itching, blow cool air from hair dryer; do not insert objects inside the cast, splint, or brace).	✔	✔
• Demonstrate exercises to promote circulation and minimize disuse syndrome.	✔	
• State indicators of complications to report promptly to physician (eg, uncontrolled swelling and pain; cool, pale fingers or toes; paresthesia; paralysis; purulent drainage staining cast; signs of systemic infection; cast, splint, or brace breaks).	✔	✔
• Describe care of extremity following cast, splint, or brace removal (eg, skin care; gradual resumption of normal activities to protect limb from undue stresses; management of swelling).	✔	✔

Continuing Care

For the patient with a cast that is ready for removal, the nurse should prepare the patient by explaining what to expect. The cast is cut with a cast cutter, which vibrates. The patient can feel the vibration and pressure during its use. The cutter does not penetrate deeply enough to injure the patient's skin. The cast padding is cut with scissors.

After removal of a splint, and especially after removal of a brace or cast, both of which are typically applied for longer periods of time, the formerly immobilized body part is weak from disuse, is stiff, and may appear atrophied. There may be extreme stiffness even after only a few weeks of immobilization. Therefore, support is needed when the cast, brace, or splint is removed. The skin, which is usually dry and scaly from accumulated dead skin, is vulnerable to injury from scratching. The skin needs to be washed gently and lubricated with an emollient lotion.

The nurse and physical therapist teach the patient to resume activities gradually within the prescribed therapeutic regimen. Exercises prescribed to help the patient regain joint motion are explained and demonstrated. Because the muscles are weak from disuse, the body part that has been immobilized cannot withstand normal stresses immediately. In addition, the nurse teaches the patient with noticeable swelling of the affected extremity after removal of the immobilizing device (eg, cast, brace, or splint) to continue to elevate the extremity to control swelling until normal muscle tone and use are reestablished.

Nursing Management of the Patient With an Immobilized Upper Extremity

The patient whose arm is immobilized must readjust to many routine tasks. The unaffected arm must assume all the upper extremity activities. The nurse, in consultation with an occupational therapist, suggests devices designed to aid one-handed activities. The patient may experience fatigue due to modified activities and the weight of the cast, brace, or splint. Frequent rest periods are necessary.

To control swelling, the immobilized arm is elevated. When the patient is lying down, the arm is elevated so that each joint is positioned higher than the preceding proximal joint (eg, elbow higher than the shoulder, hand higher than the elbow).

A **sling** may be used when the patient ambulates. To prevent pressure on the cervical spinal nerves, the sling should distribute the supported weight over a large area and not on the back of the neck. The nurse encourages the patient to remove the arm from the sling and elevate it frequently.

Circulatory disturbances in the hand may become apparent with signs of cyanosis, swelling, and an inability to move the fingers. One serious effect of impaired circulation in the arm is Volkmann's contracture, a specific type of compartment syndrome. Contracture of the fingers and wrist occurs as the result of obstructed arterial blood flow to the forearm and hand. The patient is unable to extend the fingers, describes abnormal sensation (eg, unrelenting pain, pain on passive stretch), and exhibits signs of diminished circulation to the hand. Permanent damage develops

within a few hours if action is not taken (see Chapter 69). This serious complication can be prevented with nursing surveillance and proper care.

Neurovascular checks must be done frequently (see Chapter 66). If a cast is used for immobility, compartment syndrome is managed in part by bivalving (cutting) the cast and releasing the constricting cast and dressings. A fasciotomy may be necessary to improve vascular status.

Nursing Management of the Patient With an Immobilized Lower Extremity

The application of a leg cast, brace, or splint imposes a degree of immobility on the patient. Casts may include short-leg casts, extending to the knees, or long-leg casts, extending to the groin. Hinged knee braces and immobilizers typically extend from ankle to groin.

The patient's leg must be supported on pillows to heart level to control swelling, and ice packs should be applied as prescribed over the fracture site for 1 or 2 days. The patient is taught to elevate the immobilized leg when seated. The patient should also assume a recumbent position several times a day with the immobilized leg elevated to promote venous return and control swelling.

The nurse assesses circulation by observing the color, temperature, and capillary refill of the exposed toes. Nerve function is assessed by observing the patient's ability to move the toes and by asking about the sensations in the foot. Numbness, tingling, and burning may be caused by peroneal nerve injury from pressure at the head of the fibula.

 NURSING ALERT

> Injury to the peroneal nerve as a result of pressure is a cause of footdrop (the inability to maintain the foot in a normally flexed position). Consequently, the patient drags the foot when ambulating.

The nurse and physical therapist teach the patient how to transfer and ambulate safely with assistive devices (eg, crutches, walker) (see Chapter 11). The gait to be used depends on whether the patient is permitted to bear weight. If weight bearing is allowed, the cast, splint, or brace is reinforced to withstand the body weight. A cast boot, worn over the casted foot, provides a broad, nonskid walking surface.

Nursing Management of the Patient With a Body or Spica Cast

Casts that encase the trunk (body cast) and portions of one or two extremities (spica cast) require special nursing strategies. Body casts are used to immobilize the spine. Hip spica casts are used for some femoral fractures and after some hip joint surgeries, and shoulder spica casts are used for some humeral neck fractures.

Nursing responsibilities include preparing and positioning the patient, assisting with skin care and hygiene, and monitoring for **cast syndrome,** (see discussion on next page) (NAON, 2007). Explaining the casting procedure helps reduce the patient's apprehension about being encased in a large cast. The nurse reassures the patient that several people will provide care during the application, support for the injured area will be adequate, and care providers will be as gentle as possible. Medications for pain relief and relaxation administered before the procedure enable the patient to cooperate during application of the cast.

The nurse turns the patient as a unit toward the uninjured side every 2 hours to relieve pressure and to allow the cast to dry. It is important to avoid twisting the patient's body within the cast. Sufficient personnel (at least three people) or mechanical assistive devices are needed when the patient is turned because of the added weight of the cast. The nurse encourages the patient to assist in the repositioning, if not contraindicated, by use of the **trapeze** or bed rail. A stabilizing abduction bar incorporated into a spica cast should never be used as a turning device. The nurse adjusts the pillows to provide support without creating areas of pressure.

The nurse turns the patient to a prone position, twice daily if tolerated, to provide postural drainage of the bronchial tree and to relieve pressure on the back. A small pillow under the abdomen enhances comfort. The nurse can either place a pillow lengthwise under the dorsa of the feet or allow the toes to hang over the edge of the bed to prevent the toes from being forced into the mattress.

The nurse inspects the skin around the edges of the cast frequently for signs of irritation. The nurse can inspect some of the skin under the cast by pulling the skin taut and using a flashlight. The skin can be bathed and massaged by reaching under the cast edges with the fingers.

The perineal opening must be large enough for hygienic care. To protect the cast from soiling, Gore-Tex liners are used prior to hip spica casting. If the cast is not Gore-Tex lined, the nurse can insert clean dry plastic sheeting under the dry cast and over the cast edge before elimination by the patient. Usually, fracture bedpans are easier to use than regular bedpans for patients with a hip spica cast.

Patients immobilized in large casts may develop cast syndrome that may include psychological or physiologic manifestations. The psychological component is similar to a claustrophobic reaction. The patient exhibits an acute anxiety reaction characterized by behavioral changes and autonomic responses (eg, increased respiratory rate, diaphoresis, dilated pupils, increased heart rate, elevated blood pressure). The nurse needs to recognize the anxiety reaction and provide an environment in which the patient feels secure.

Physiologic cast syndrome responses (eg, superior mesenteric artery syndrome) are associated with immobility in a body cast. With decreased physical activity, gastrointestinal motility decreases, intestinal gases accumulate, intestinal pressure increases, and ileus may occur. The patient exhibits abdominal distention, abdominal discomfort, nausea, and vomiting. As with other instances of adynamic ileus, the patient is treated conservatively with decompression (nasogastric intubation connected to suction) and intravenous (IV) fluid therapy until gastrointestinal motility is restored (Adams, Hawkins, Ferdinand, et al., 2007). If the cast restricts the abdomen, the abdominal window must be enlarged. After the ileus resolves and bowel sounds resume, the patient gradually resumes an oral diet. Rarely, the distention places traction on the superior mesenteric artery,

reducing the blood supply to the bowel, which can result in gangrenous bowel. The descending aorta may also sustain pressure as it may be compressed between the spine and pressure of abdominal distention, which results in ischemia. If the descending aorta becomes ischemic, its rupture could cause exsanguination and death.

NURSING ALERT

The nurse monitors the patient in a large body cast for potential cast syndrome, noting bowel sounds every 4 to 8 hours, and reports distention, nausea, and vomiting to the physician.

The patient with a body or spica cast is often cared for at home. The nurse teaches family members how to care for the patient, which includes providing hygienic and skin care, ensuring proper positioning, preventing complications, and recognizing symptoms that should be reported to the health care provider.

The Patient With an External Fixator

External fixators are used to manage open fractures with soft tissue damage. They provide stable support for severe comminuted (crushed or splintered) fractures while permitting active treatment of damaged soft tissues (Fig. 67-3). Complicated fractures of the humerus, forearm, femur, tibia, and pelvis are managed with external skeletal fixators. The fracture is reduced, aligned, and immobilized by a series of pins inserted in the bone. Pin position is maintained through attachment to a portable frame. The fixator facilitates patient comfort, early mobility, and active exercise of adjacent uninvolved joints; thus, complications due to disuse and immobility are minimized (Holmes & Brown, 2005).

Nursing Management

It is important to prepare the patient psychologically for application of the external fixator. The apparatus looks clumsy and foreign. Reassurance that the discomfort associated with the device is minimal and that early mobility is anticipated promotes acceptance of the device.

After the external fixator is applied, the extremity is elevated to reduce swelling. If there are sharp points on the fixator or pins, they are covered with caps to prevent device-induced injuries. The nurse monitors the neurovascular status of the extremity every 2 to 4 hours and assesses each pin site for redness, drainage, tenderness, pain, and loosening of the pin. Some serous drainage from the pin sites is to be expected. The nurse must be alert for potential problems caused by pressure from the device on the skin, nerves, or blood vessels and for the development of compartment syndrome (see Chapter 69). The nurse carries out pin care as prescribed to prevent pin tract infection. This typically includes cleaning each pin site separately one or two times a day with cotton-tipped applicators soaked in chlorhexidine solution (Holmes & Brown, 2005). If signs of infection are present or if the pins or clamps seem loose, the nurse notifies the physician.

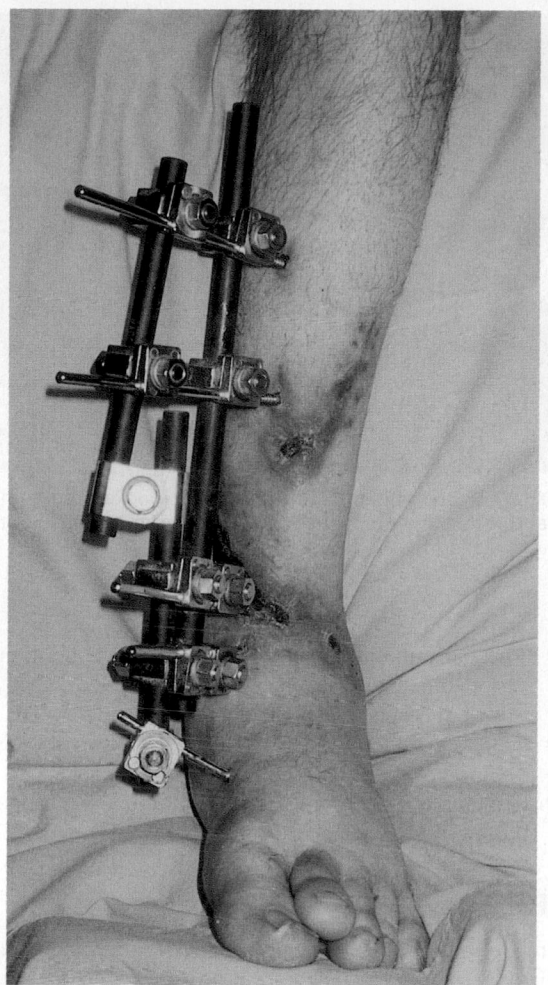

Figure 67-3 External fixation device. Pins are inserted into bone. The fracture is reduced and aligned and then stabilized by attaching the pins to a rigid portable frame. The device facilitates treatment of soft tissue damaged in complex fractures.

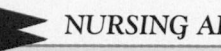 **NURSING ALERT**

The nurse never adjusts the clamps on the external fixator frame. It is the physician's responsibility to do so.

The nurse encourages isometric and active exercises as tolerated. When the swelling subsides, the nurse helps the patient become mobile within the prescribed weight-bearing limits (non–weight bearing to full weight bearing). Adherence to weight-bearing instructions minimizes the chance of loosening of the pins when stress is applied to the bone–pin interface. The fixator is removed after the soft tissue heals. The fracture may require additional stabilization by a cast or molded orthosis while healing.

The Ilizarov external fixator is a special device used to correct angulation and rotational defects, to treat nonunion (failure of bone fragments to heal), and to lengthen limbs. Tension wires are attached to fixator rings, which are joined by telescoping rods. Bone formation is stimulated by prescribed daily adjustment of the telescoping rods. It is important to teach the patient how to adjust the telescoping rods and how to perform skin care. Generally, the nurse can encourage weight bearing. After the desired correction has been achieved, no additional adjustments are made, and the fixator is left in place until the bone heals.

The nurse teaches the patient to perform pin site care according to the prescribed protocol (clean technique can be used at home [Holmes & Brown, 2005]) and to report promptly any signs of pin site infection: redness, tenderness, increased or purulent pin site drainage, or fever. The nurse also instructs the patient and family to monitor neurovascular status and report any changes promptly. The nurse teaches the patient or family member to check the integrity of the fixator frame daily and to report loose pins or clamps. A physical therapy referral is helpful in teaching the patient how to transfer, use ambulatory aids safely, and adjust to weight-bearing limits and altered gait patterns (Chart 67-5).

CHART 67-5 HOME CARE CHECKLIST
The Patient With an External Fixator

At the completion of the home care instruction, the patient or caregiver will be able to:	PATIENT	CAREGIVER
• Demonstrate prescribed pin site care.	✔	✔
• State signs of pin site infection (eg, redness, tenderness, increased or purulent pin site drainage) to be reported promptly.	✔	✔
• Describe approaches to controlling swelling and pain (eg, elevate extremity to heart level, take analgesic agents as prescribed).	✔	✔
• Report pain uncontrolled by elevation and analgesic agents (may be an indicator of impaired tissue perfusion, compartment syndrome, or pin tract infection).	✔	
• Demonstrate ability to transfer.	✔	
• Use mobility aids safely.	✔	
• Avoid excessive use of injured extremity; observe prescribed weight-bearing limits.	✔	
• State indicators of complications to report promptly to physician (eg, uncontrolled swelling and pain; cool, pale fingers or toes; paresthesia; paralysis; purulent drainage; signs of systemic infection; loose fixator pins or clamps).	✔	✔
• Describe care of extremity after fixator removal (eg, gradual resumption of normal activities to protect limb from undue stresses).	✔	✔

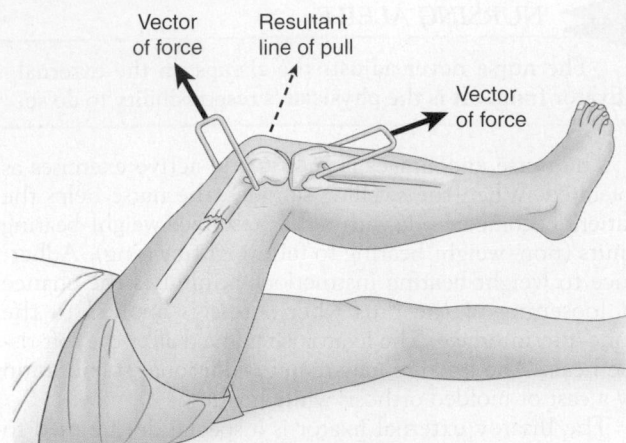

Figure 67-4 Traction may be applied in different directions to achieve the desired therapeutic line of pull. Adjustments in applied forces may be prescribed over the course of treatment.

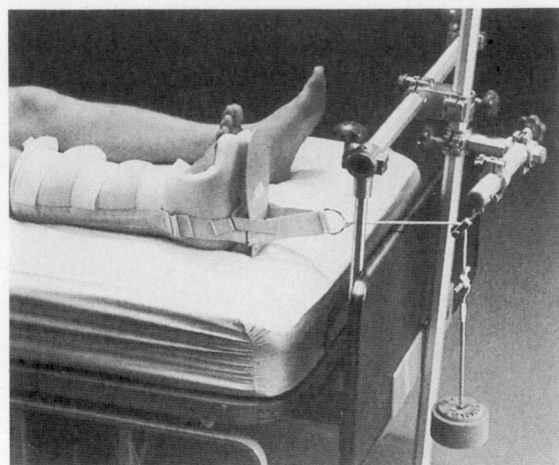

Figure 67-5 Buck's extension traction. Lower extremity in unilateral Buck's extension traction is aligned in a foam boot and traction applied by the free-hanging weight.

The Patient in Traction

Traction is the application of a pulling force to a part of the body. Traction is used to minimize muscle spasms; to reduce, align, and immobilize fractures; to reduce deformity; and to increase space between opposing surfaces. Traction must be applied in the correct direction and magnitude to obtain its therapeutic effects. As muscle and soft tissues relax, the amount of weight used may be changed to obtain the desired effect (NAON, 2007).

At times, traction needs to be applied in more than one direction to achieve the desired line of pull. When this is done, one of the lines of pull counteracts the other. These lines of pull are known as the vectors of force. The actual resultant pulling force is somewhere between the two lines of pull (Fig. 67-4). The effects of traction are evaluated with x-ray studies, and adjustments are made if necessary.

Traction is used primarily as a short-term intervention until other modalities, such as external or internal fixation, are possible. These modalities reduce the risk of disuse syndrome and minimize the length of hospitalization, often allowing the patient to be cared for in the home setting (NAON, 2007).

PRINCIPLES OF EFFECTIVE TRACTION

Whenever traction is applied, countertraction must be used to achieve effective traction. Countertraction is the force acting in the opposite direction. Usually, the patient's body weight and bed position adjustments supply the needed countertraction.

The following are additional principles to follow when caring for the patient in traction:
- Traction must be continuous to be effective in reducing and immobilizing fractures.
- Skeletal traction is *never* interrupted.
- Weights are not removed unless intermittent traction is prescribed.
- Any factor that might reduce the effective pull or alter its resultant line of pull must be eliminated:

- The patient must be in good body alignment in the center of the bed when traction is applied.
- Ropes must be unobstructed.
- Weights must hang freely and not rest on the bed or floor.
- Knots in the rope or the footplate must not touch the pulley or the foot of the bed.

TYPES OF TRACTION

There are several types of traction. *Straight* or *running traction* applies the pulling force in a straight line with the body part resting on the bed. Buck's extension traction (Fig. 67-5) is an example of straight traction. *Balanced suspension traction* (Fig. 67-6) supports the affected extremity off the bed and allows for some patient movement without disruption of the line of pull.

Traction may be applied to the skin (*skin traction*) or directly to the bony skeleton (*skeletal traction*). The mode of application is determined by the purpose of the traction. Traction can be applied with the hands (*manual traction*). This is temporary traction that may be used when applying a cast, giving skin care under a Buck's extension foam boot, or adjusting the traction apparatus.

Skin Traction

Skin traction is used to control muscle spasms and to immobilize an area before surgery. Skin traction is accomplished by using a weight to pull on traction tape or on a foam boot attached to the skin. The amount of weight applied must not exceed the tolerance of the skin. No more than 2 to 3.5 kg (4.5 to 8 lb) of traction can be used on an extremity. Pelvic traction is usually 4.5 to 9 kg (10 to 20 lb), depending on the weight of the patient.

Types of skin traction used for adults include Buck's extension traction (applied to the lower leg) (described below), the cervical head halter (occasionally used to treat neck pain), and the pelvic belt (sometimes used to treat back pain).

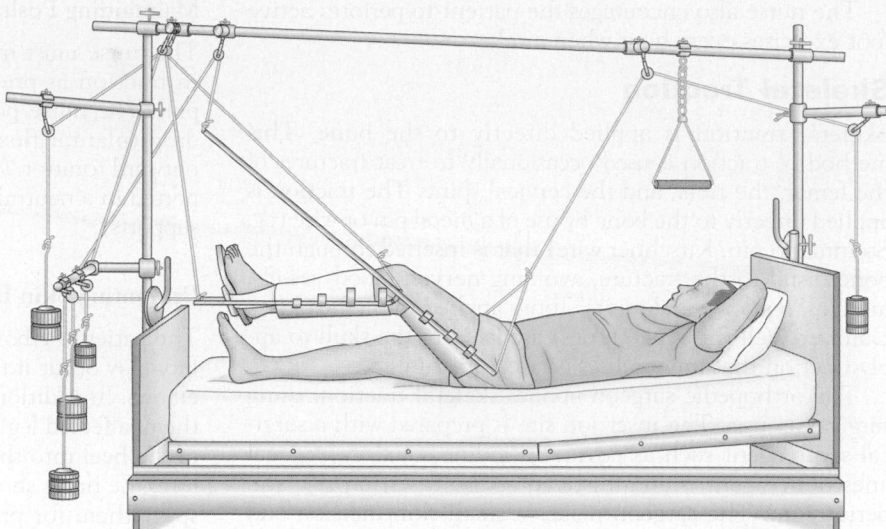

Figure 67-6 Balanced suspension skeletal traction with Thomas leg splint. The patient can move vertically as long as the resultant line of pull is maintained.

Buck's Extension Traction

Buck's extension traction (unilateral or bilateral) is skin traction to the lower leg. The pull is exerted in one plane when partial or temporary immobilization is desired (see Fig. 67-5). It is used to immobilize fractures of the proximal femur before surgical fixation.

Before the traction is applied, the nurse inspects the skin for abrasions and circulatory disturbances. The skin and circulation must be in healthy condition to tolerate the traction. The extremity should be clean and dry before the foam boot or traction tape is applied.

To apply Buck's traction, one nurse elevates and supports the extremity under the patient's heel and knee while another nurse places the foam boot under the leg, with the patient's heel in the heel of the boot. Next, the nurse secures Velcro straps around the leg. Traction tape overwrapped with elastic bandage in a spiral fashion may be used instead of the boot. Excessive pressure is avoided over the malleolus and proximal fibula during application to prevent pressure ulcers and nerve damage. The nurse then passes the rope affixed to the spreader or footplate over a pulley fastened to the end of the bed and attaches the prescribed weight—usually 5 to 8 pounds—to the rope.

Nursing Interventions

Ensuring Effective Traction

To ensure effective skin traction, it is important to avoid wrinkling and slipping of the traction bandage and to maintain countertraction. Proper positioning must be maintained to keep the leg in a neutral position. To prevent bony fragments from moving against one another, the patient should not turn from side to side; however, the patient may shift position slightly with assistance.

Monitoring and Managing Potential Complications

Skin Breakdown. During the initial assessment, the nurse identifies sensitive, fragile skin (common in older adults). The nurse also closely monitors the status of the skin in

contact with tape or foam to ensure that shearing forces are avoided. The nurse performs the following procedures to monitor and prevent skin breakdown:

- Removes the foam boots to inspect the skin, the ankle, and the Achilles tendon three times a day. A second nurse is needed to support the extremity during the inspection and skin care.
- Palpates the area of the traction tapes daily to detect underlying tenderness.
- Provides back care at least every 2 hours to prevent pressure ulcers. The patient who must remain in a supine position is at increased risk for development of a pressure ulcer.
- Uses special mattress overlays (eg, air-filled, high-density foam) to prevent pressure ulcers.

Nerve Damage. Skin traction can place pressure on peripheral nerves. When traction is applied to the lower extremity, care must be taken to avoid pressure on the peroneal nerve at the point at which it passes around the neck of the fibula just below the knee. Pressure at this point can cause footdrop. The nurse regularly questions the patient about sensation and asks the patient to move the toes and foot. The nurse should immediately investigate any complaint of a burning sensation under the traction bandage or boot. Dorsiflexion of the foot demonstrates function of the peroneal nerve. Weakness of dorsiflexion or foot movement and inversion of the foot might indicate pressure on the common peroneal nerve. Plantar flexion demonstrates function of the tibial nerve. In addition, the nurse should promptly report altered sensation or impaired motor function.

Circulatory Impairment. After skin traction is applied, the nurse assesses circulation of the foot within 15 to 30 minutes and then every 1 to 2 hours. Circulatory assessment consists of the following:

- Peripheral pulses, color, capillary refill, and temperature of the fingers or toes
- Indicators of deep vein thrombosis (DVT), including unilateral calf tenderness, warmth, redness, and swelling

The nurse also encourages the patient to perform active foot exercises every hour when awake.

Skeletal Traction

Skeletal traction is applied directly to the bone. This method of traction is used occasionally to treat fractures of the femur, the tibia, and the cervical spine. The traction is applied directly to the bone by use of a metal pin or wire (eg, Steinmann pin, Kirschner wire) that is inserted through the bone distal to the fracture, avoiding nerves, blood vessels, muscles, tendons, and joints. Tongs applied to the head (eg, Gardner-Wells or Vinke tongs) are fixed to the skull to apply traction that immobilizes cervical fractures.

The orthopedic surgeon applies skeletal traction, using surgical asepsis. The insertion site is prepared with a surgical scrub agent such as povidone–iodine solution. A local anesthetic agent is administered at the insertion site and periosteum. The surgeon makes a small skin incision and drills the sterile pin or wire through the bone. The patient feels pressure during this procedure and possibly some pain when the periosteum is penetrated.

After insertion, the pin or wire is attached to the traction bow or caliper. The ends of the pin or wire are covered with caps to prevent injury to the patient or caregivers. The weights are attached to the pin or wire bow by a rope-and-pulley system that exerts the appropriate amount and direction of pull for effective traction. Skeletal traction frequently uses 7 to 12 kg (15 to 25 lb) to achieve the therapeutic effect. The weights applied initially must overcome the shortening spasms of the affected muscles. As the muscles relax, the traction weight is reduced to prevent fracture dislocation and to promote healing.

Often, skeletal traction is balanced traction, which supports the affected extremity, allows for some patient movement, and facilitates patient independence and nursing care while maintaining effective traction. The Thomas splint with a Pearson attachment is frequently used with skeletal traction for fractures of the femur (see Fig. 67-6). Because upward traction is required, an overbed frame is used.

When skeletal traction is discontinued, the extremity is gently supported while the weights are removed. The pin is cut close to the skin and removed by the physician. Internal fixation, casts, or splints are then used to immobilize and support the healing bone.

Nursing Interventions

Maintaining Effective Traction

When skeletal traction is used, the nurse checks the traction apparatus to see that the ropes are in the wheel grooves of the pulleys, that the ropes are not frayed, that the weights hang freely, and that the knots in the rope are tied securely. The nurse also evaluates the patient's position, because slipping down in bed results in ineffective traction.

 NURSING ALERT

The nurse must never remove weights from skeletal traction unless a life-threatening situation occurs. Removal of the weights completely defeats their purpose and may result in injury to the patient.

Maintaining Positioning

The nurse must maintain alignment of the patient's body in traction as prescribed to promote an effective line of pull. The nurse positions the patient's foot to avoid footdrop (plantar flexion), inward rotation (inversion), and outward rotation (eversion). The patient's foot may be supported in a neutral position by orthopedic devices (eg, foot supports).

Preventing Skin Breakdown

The patient's elbows frequently become sore, and nerve injury may occur if the patient repositions by pushing on the elbows. In addition, patients frequently push on the heel of the unaffected leg when they raise themselves. This digging of the heel into the mattress may injure the tissues. Therefore, the nurse should protect the elbows and heels and inspect them for pressure ulcers. To encourage movement without using the elbows or heel, a trapeze can be suspended overhead within easy reach of the patient. The trapeze helps the patient move about in bed and move on and off the bedpan.

Specific pressure points are assessed for redness and skin breakdown. Areas that are particularly vulnerable to pressure caused by a traction apparatus applied to the lower extremity include the ischial tuberosity, popliteal space, Achilles tendon, and heel. If the patient is not permitted to turn on one side or the other, the nurse must make a special effort to provide back care and to keep the bed dry and free of crumbs and wrinkles. The patient can assist by holding the overhead trapeze and raising the hips off the bed. If the patient cannot do this, the nurse can push down on the mattress with one hand to relieve pressure on the back and bony prominences and to provide for some shifting of weight. A pressure-relieving air-filled or high-density foam mattress overlay may reduce the risk of pressure ulcer.

For change of bed linens, the patient raises the torso while nurses on both sides of the bed roll down and replace the upper mattress sheet. Then, as the patient raises the buttocks off the mattress, the nurses slide the sheets under the buttocks. Finally, the nurses replace the lower section of the bed linens while the patient rests on the back. Sheets and blankets are placed over the patient in such a way that the traction is not disrupted.

Monitoring Neurovascular Status

The nurse assesses the neurovascular status of the immobilized extremity at least every hour initially and then every 4 hours. The nurse instructs the patient to report any changes in sensation or movement immediately so that they can be promptly evaluated. DVT is a significant risk for the immobilized patient. The nurse encourages the patient to do active flexion–extension ankle exercises and isometric contraction of the calf muscles (calf-pumping exercises) 10 times an hour while awake to decrease venous stasis. In addition, anti-embolism stockings, compression devices, and anticoagulant therapy may be prescribed to help prevent thrombus formation.

> ### NURSING ALERT
>
> The nurse must promptly investigate every report of discomfort expressed by the patient in traction. Prompt recognition of a developing neurovascular problem is essential so that corrective measures can be instituted promptly.

Providing Pin Site Care. The wound at the pin insertion site requires attention. The goal is to avoid infection and development of **osteomyelitis.** For the first 48 hours after insertion, the site is covered with a sterile absorbent nonstick dressing and a rolled gauze or Ace-type bandage. After this time, a loose cover dressing or no dressing is recommended. (A bandage is necessary if the patient is exposed to airborne dust.) Pin site care is performed initially one or two times a day. The frequency of pin care needs to be increased if mechanical looseness of pins or early signs of infection are present (eg, edema, purulent drainage, erythema, tenderness). Chlorhexidine solution is recommended as the most effective cleansing solution; however, water and saline are alternate choices (Holmes & Brown, 2005). Although hydrogen peroxide and Betadine solutions have been used, they are believed to be cytotoxic to osteoblasts and may actually damage healthy tissue (Lethaby, Temple & Santy, 2008).

The nurse must inspect the pin sites every 8 hours for reaction (ie, normal changes that occur at the pin site after insertion) and infection. Signs of reaction may include redness, warmth, and serous or slightly sanguinous drainage at the site. These signs subside after 72 hours. Signs of infection may mirror those of reaction but also include the presence of purulent drainage, pin loosening, and odor. Minor infections may be readily treated with antibiotics, whereas infections that result in systemic manifestations may additionally warrant pin removal until the infection resolves (Holmes & Brown, 2005). When pins are mechanically stable (after 48 to 72 hours), weekly pin site care is recommended.

> ### NURSING ALERT
>
> The nurse must inspect the pin site at least every 8 hours for signs of inflammation and evidence of infection.

Due to a lack of evidence-based research findings, controversy remains about management of crusts that may form at the pin insertion site, frequency of pin care and showering, and use of massage to release skin adherence to pins (Holmes & Brown, 2005). The patient should be taught to perform any prescribed pin site care prior to discharge from the hospital and should be provided with written follow-up instructions that include the signs and symptoms of infection. Patients permitted to take showers within 5 to 10 days of pin insertion are encouraged to leave the pins exposed to water flow. The sites are dried with a clean towel and left open to air, or dressings are applied as prescribed.

Promoting Exercise. Patient exercises, within the therapeutic limits of the traction, assist in maintaining muscle strength and tone and in promoting circulation. Active exercises include pulling up on the trapeze, flexing and extending the feet, and range-of-motion and weight-resistance exercises for noninvolved joints. Isometric exercises of the immobilized extremity (quadriceps-setting and gluteal-setting exercises) are important for maintaining strength in major ambulatory muscles (see Chart 67-3). Without exercise, the patient will lose muscle mass and strength, and rehabilitation will be greatly prolonged.

Nursing Management

Assessing Anxiety

The nurse must consider the psychological and physiologic impact of the musculoskeletal problem, traction device, and immobility. Traction restricts mobility and independence. The equipment often looks threatening, and its application can be frightening. Confusion, disorientation, and behavioral problems may develop in patients who are confined in a limited space for an extended time. Therefore, the nurse must assess and monitor the patient's anxiety level and psychological responses to traction.

Assisting With Self-Care

Initially, the patient may require assistance with self-care activities. The nurse helps the patient eat, bathe, dress, and toilet. Convenient arrangement of items such as the telephone, tissues, water, and assistive devices (eg, reachers, overbed trapeze) may facilitate self-care. With resumption of self-care activities, the patient feels less dependent and less frustrated and experiences improved self-esteem. Because some assistance is required throughout the period of immobility, the nurse and the patient can creatively develop routines that maximize the patient's independence.

It is important to evaluate the body part to be placed in traction and its neurovascular status (ie, color, temperature, capillary refill, edema, pulses, ability to move, and sensations) and compare it to the unaffected extremity. The nurse also assesses skin integrity along with body system functioning for baseline data. Ongoing assessment is indicated for the patient in traction.

Monitoring and Managing Potential Complications

Immobility-related complications may include pressure ulcers, atelectasis, pneumonia, constipation, loss of appetite, urinary stasis, urinary tract infections, and venous thromboemboli formation. Early identification of preexisting or developing conditions facilitates prompt interventions to resolve them.

Atelectasis and Pneumonia

The nurse auscultates the patient's lungs every 4 to 8 hours to assess respiratory status and teaches the patient deep-breathing and coughing exercises to aid in fully expanding the lungs and clearing pulmonary secretions. If the patient history and baseline assessment indicate that the patient is at risk for development of respiratory complications, specific therapies (eg, use of incentive spirometer) may be indicated. If a respiratory complication develops, prompt institution of prescribed therapy is needed.

Constipation and Anorexia

Reduced gastrointestinal motility results in constipation and anorexia. A diet high in fiber and fluids may help stimulate gastric motility. If constipation develops, therapeutic measures may include stool softeners, laxatives, suppositories, and enemas. To improve the patient's appetite, the patient's food preferences are included, as appropriate, within the prescribed therapeutic diet.

Urinary Stasis and Infection

Incomplete emptying of the bladder related to positioning in bed can result in urinary stasis and infection. In addition, the patient may find use of the bedpan uncomfortable and may limit fluids to minimize the frequency of urination. The nurse monitors the fluid intake and the character of the urine. The nurse teaches the patient to consume adequate amounts of fluid and to void every 3 to 4 hours. If the patient exhibits signs or symptoms of urinary tract infection, the nurse notifies the physician.

Venous Thromboembolism

Venous stasis that predisposes the patient to venous thromboembolism occurs with immobility. The nurse teaches the patient to perform ankle and foot exercises within the limits of the traction therapy every 1 to 2 hours when awake to prevent DVT. The patient is encouraged to drink fluids to prevent dehydration and associated hemoconcentration, which contribute to stasis. The nurse monitors the patient for signs of DVT, including unilateral calf tenderness, warmth, redness, and swelling (increased calf circumference). The nurse promptly reports findings to the physician for definitive evaluation and therapy.

During traction therapy, the nurse encourages the patient to exercise muscles and joints that are not in traction to prevent deterioration, deconditioning, and venous stasis. The physical therapist can design bed exercises that minimize loss of muscle strength. During the patient's exercise, the nurse ensures that traction forces are maintained and that the patient is properly positioned to prevent complications resulting from poor alignment.

The Patient Undergoing Orthopedic Surgery

Many patients with musculoskeletal dysfunction undergo surgery to correct the condition. Conditions that may be corrected by surgery include unstabilized fracture, deformity, joint disease, necrotic or infected tissue, and tumors. Frequent surgical procedures include **open reduction with internal fixation (ORIF)** and closed reduction with internal fixation (fracture fragments are not surgically exposed) for fractures; arthroplasty, meniscectomy, and joint replacement for joint conditions; amputation for severe extremity conditions (eg, gangrene, massive trauma); bone graft for joint stabilization, defect filling, or stimulation of bone healing; and tendon transfer for improving motion. The goals include improving function by restoring motion and stability and relieving pain and disability. Chart 67-6 describes common orthopedic surgeries.

Indications for a surgical procedure are based on the patient's age, underlying orthopedic condition, and general physical health and the impact of joint disability on daily activities. Timing of these procedures is important to ensure

Chart 67-6 • *Common Orthopedic Surgical Procedures*

Open reduction: the correction and alignment of the fracture after surgical dissection and exposure of the fracture

Internal fixation: the stabilization of the reduced fracture by the use of metal screws, plates, wires, nails, and pins

Arthroplasty: the repair of joint problems through the operating arthroscope (an instrument that allows the surgeon to operate within a joint without a large incision) or through open joint surgery

Hemiarthroplasty: the replacement of one of the articular surfaces (eg, in a hip hemiarthroplasty, the femoral head and neck are replaced with a femoral prosthesis—the acetabulum is not replaced)

Joint arthroplasty or replacement: the replacement of joint surfaces with metal or synthetic materials

Total joint arthroplasty or replacement: the replacement of both articular surfaces within a joint with metal or synthetic materials

Meniscectomy: the excision of damaged joint fibrocartilage

Amputation: the removal of a body part

Bone graft: the placement of bone tissue (autologous or homologous grafts) to promote healing, to stabilize, or to replace diseased bone

Tendon transfer: the insertion of tendon to improve function

Fasciotomy: the incision and diversion of the muscle fascia to relieve muscle constriction, as in compartment syndrome, or to reduce fascia contracture

maximum function. In general, surgery should be performed before surrounding muscles become contracted and atrophied and serious structural abnormalities occur.

Because most of these are elective procedures, many patients donate their own blood during the weeks preceding their surgery. This blood is used to replace blood lost during surgery. Autologous blood transfusions eliminate many of the risks of transfusion therapy (see Chapter 33).

Blood is conserved during surgery to minimize loss. During orthopedic surgery on a limb (eg, total knee replacement [TKR]), a pneumatic tourniquet may be applied to produce a "bloodless field." This technique has the advantages of keeping the surgical field dry, minimizing blood loss, and providing some additional limb anesthesia (O'Connor & Murphy, 2007). Intraoperative blood salvage with reinfusion is used when a large volume of blood loss is anticipated. Postoperative blood salvage with intermittent autotransfusion also reduces the need for blood transfusion.

JOINT REPLACEMENT

Patients with severe joint pain and disability may undergo joint replacement. Conditions contributing to joint degeneration include osteoarthritis, rheumatoid arthritis, trauma, and congenital deformity. Some fractures (eg, femoral neck fracture) may cause disruption of the blood supply and subsequent **avascular necrosis;** management with joint replacement may be elected over ORIF. Joints frequently replaced include the hip, knee (Fig. 67-7), and finger joints.

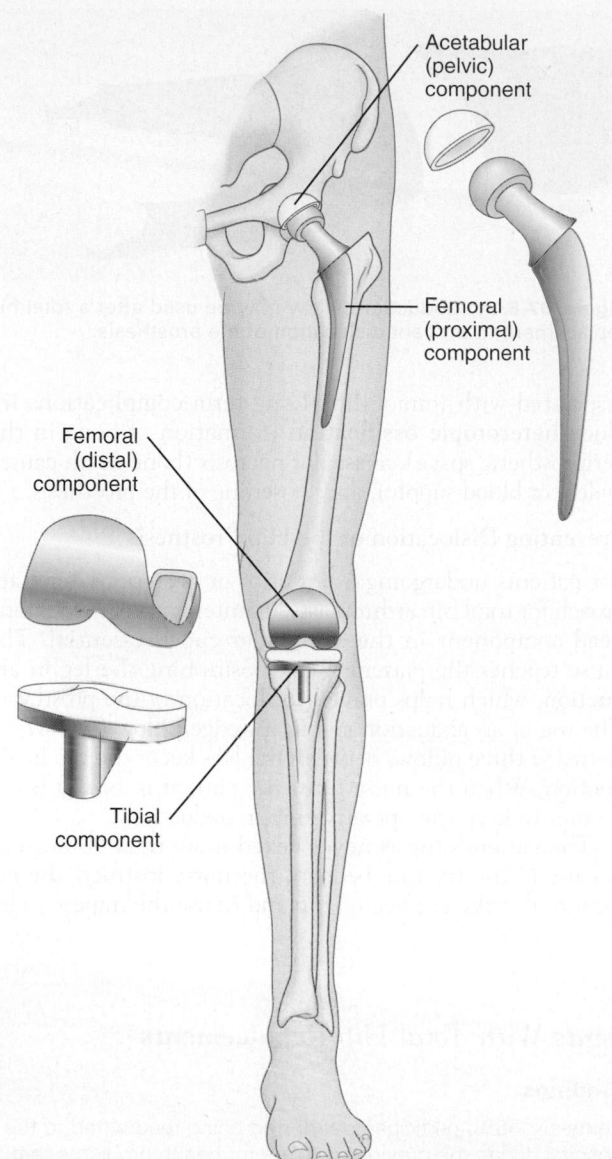

Acetabular (pelvic) component

Femoral (proximal) component

Femoral (distal) component

Tibial component

Figure 67-7 Examples of hip and knee replacement.

Less frequently, more complex joints (shoulder, elbow, wrist, ankle) are replaced.

Most joint replacements consist of metal (eg, cobalt-chromium, titanium) and high-density polyethylene components. The joint implants may be cemented in the prepared bone with polymethylmethacrylate (PMMA), a bone-bonding agent that has properties similar to bone. Loosening of the prosthesis due to cement–bone interface failure is a common cause of prosthesis failure. Press-fit, ingrowth prostheses (porous-coated, cementless artificial joint components) that allow the patient's bone to grow into and securely fix the prosthesis in the bone are alternatives to cemented prostheses. Accurate fitting and the presence of healthy bone with adequate blood supply are important in the use of cementless components (Lucas, 2008a). Much progress has been made in reducing prosthesis failure rates through improved techniques, improved materials, and use of bone grafts.

With joint replacement, excellent pain relief is obtained in most patients. Return of motion and function depends on preoperative soft tissue condition, soft tissue reactions, and general muscle strength. Early failure of joint replacement is associated with excessive activity and preoperative joint and bone pathology.

Nursing Interventions

Assessment of the patient and preoperative management are aimed at having the patient in optimal health at the time of surgery. Preoperatively, it is important to evaluate cardiovascular, respiratory, renal, and hepatic functions. Age, obesity, preoperative leg edema, a history of any venous thromboemboli, and varicose veins increase the risk for postoperative DVT and pulmonary embolism.

Preoperatively, it is important to assess the neurovascular status of the extremity undergoing joint replacement (Lucas, 2008a). Postoperative assessment data are compared with preoperative assessment data to identify changes and deficits. For example, an absent pulse postoperatively is of concern unless the pulse was also absent preoperatively. Nerve palsy could occur as a result of surgery.

Preventing Infection

Preoperative assessment of the patient for infections, including urinary tract infection, is necessary because of the risk for postoperative infection. Any infection 2 to 4 weeks before planned surgery may result in postponement of surgery. Preoperative skin preparation frequently begins 1 or 2 days before the surgery. Airborne bacteria that contaminate the wound at the time of surgery cause most deep infections. Therefore, as with any surgery, there is strict adherence to aseptic principles, and the operating area is made as bacteria free as possible (Lucas, 2008a).

Research findings suggest that prophylactic antibiotics given 60 minutes prior to incision are effective in preventing postoperative infection (Hawn, Gray, Vick, et al., 2006). Culture of the joint during surgery may be important in identifying and treating subsequent infections.

If osteomyelitis develops, it is difficult to treat. Persistent infection at the site of the prosthesis usually requires removal of the implant and joint revision. It is not always possible to achieve a functional joint when the reconstruction procedure has to be repeated.

Promoting Ambulation

Patients with total hip or total knee replacement begin ambulation with a walker or crutches within a day after surgery. The nurse and the physical therapist assist the patient in achieving the goal of independent ambulation. At first, the patient may be able to stand for only a brief period because of orthostatic hypotension. Specific weight-bearing limits on the prosthesis are based on the patient's condition, the procedure, and the fixation method. Usually, patients with cemented prostheses can proceed to weight bearing as tolerated. If the patient has a press-fit, cementless, ingrowth prosthesis, weight bearing immediately after surgery may be limited to minimize micromotion of the prosthesis in the bone (Lucas, 2008b). As the patient is able to tolerate more activity, the nurse encourages transferring to a chair several times a day for short periods and walking for progressively greater distances.

Total Hip Replacement

Total hip replacement is the replacement of a severely damaged hip with an artificial joint. Indications for this surgery include osteoarthritis, rheumatoid arthritis, femoral neck fractures, failure of previous reconstructive surgeries (failed prosthesis, **osteotomy**), and conditions resulting from developmental dysplasia or Legg-Calve-Perthes (avascular necrosis of the hip in childhood). A variety of total hip prostheses are available. Most consist of a metal femoral component topped by a spherical ball, of metal, ceramic, or plastic, fitted into a plastic or metal acetabular socket (see Fig. 67-7).

The surgeon selects the prosthesis that is best suited to the individual patient, considering various factors, including skeletal structure and activity level. The patient has irreversibly damaged hip joints, and the potential benefits, including improved quality of life (Chart 67-7), outweigh the surgical risks. With the advent of improved prosthetic materials and operative techniques, the life of the prosthesis has been extended, and today younger patients with severely damaged and painful hip joints are undergoing total hip replacement.

Nursing Interventions

The nurse must be aware of and monitor for specific potential complications associated with total hip replacement. Complications that may occur include dislocation of the hip prosthesis, excessive wound drainage, thromboembolism, infection, and heel pressure ulcer (Chart 67-8). Other complications for which the nurse must monitor include those

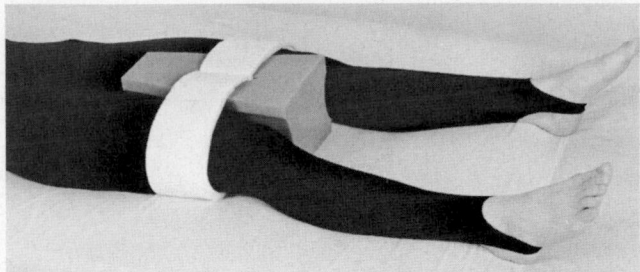

Figure 67-8 An abduction pillow may be used after a total hip replacement to prevent dislocation of the prosthesis.

associated with immobility. Long-term complications include **heterotopic ossification** (formation of bone in the periprosthetic space), avascular necrosis (bone death caused by loss of blood supply), and loosening of the prosthesis.

Preventing Dislocation of the Hip Prosthesis

For patients undergoing a posterior or posterior-lateral approach for total hip arthroplasty, maintenance of the femoral head component in the acetabular cup is essential. The nurse teaches the patient about positioning the leg in **abduction**, which helps prevent dislocation of the prosthesis. The use of an abduction splint, a wedge pillow (Fig. 67-8), or two or three pillows between the legs keeps the hip in abduction. When the nurse turns the patient in bed, it is important to keep the operative hip in abduction.

The patient's hip is never flexed more than 90 degrees. For use of the fracture bedpan, the nurse instructs the patient to flex the unaffected hip and to use the trapeze to lift

---

CHART	
67-7	**NURSING RESEARCH PROFILE**
	Quality of Life Over the Long-Term for Patients With Total Hip Replacements

McMurray, A., Grant, S., Griffiths, S., et al. (2005). Mapping recovery after total hip replacement surgery: Health-related quality of life after three years. *Australian Journal of Advanced Nursing, 22*(4), 20–25.

Purpose

Total hip replacement (THR) surgery is generally considered a cost-effective and successful surgical intervention that results in improved mobility and quality of life. While many studies have examined quality-of-life outcomes among patients who have had THR, few have measured quality-of-life outcomes beyond a few weeks or months during the postoperative period. This study compared quality-of-life outcomes among patients who had THR at 12 weeks and at 3 years after hospital discharge postsurgery.

Design

Patients who had participated in a previous study of postoperative patients who had THR were called and invited to participate in this study. Of the original cohort of 95 participants, 62 agreed to participate in this study. Thirty-two (52%) of these patients were female, and 37 (60%) were over 75 years of age. These participants were asked to respond to items from the Short Form health survey (SF-36), which they had previously completed at 1, 2, 4, 8, and 12 weeks post–hospital discharge.

Findings

Thirty-six (58%) participants reported being readmitted to the hospital during the previous 3 years for health problems that were not related to their THR. Approximately half (*n* = 33) reported unmet health needs that were mostly related to non–hip-related problems. There were no significant changes found on any SF-36 scores from 12 weeks to 3 years post–hospital discharge for THR. However, the overall physical functioning scores for women were less than population-based norms, while the physical function scores among men were higher than population-based norms. Twenty-six (42%) participants reported an increase in participation of social activities from the preoperative period.

Nursing Implications

Many patients who have had hip replacement surgery report greater mobility and less pain that improves their ability to resume social activities postoperatively. Findings from this study suggest that gains made in engagement in social activities after THR may continue for several years postoperatively among patients with THR. Gains in other quality-of-life indicators may also persist for at least 3 years postoperatively. While men who have had THR may enjoy long-term improvements in physical function, this may not be the case for women who have had THR. Women who have had THR may require more vigilant long-term follow-up.

CHART
67-8

PLAN OF NURSING CARE
The Patient With a Total Hip Replacement

NURSING DIAGNOSIS: Pain related to total hip replacement
GOAL: Relief of pain

Nursing Interventions	Rationale	Expected Outcomes
1. Assess patient for pain using a standard pain intensity scale.	1. Pain is expected after a surgical procedure because of the surgical trauma and tissue response. Muscle spasms occur after total hip replacements. Immobility causes discomfort at pressure points.	• Describes discomfort • Expresses confidence in efforts to control pain • States pain is reduced; pain intensity scores are decreasing • Appears comfortable and relaxed • Uses physical, psychological, and pharmacologic measures to reduce pain and discomfort
2. Ask patient to describe discomfort.	2. Pain characteristics may help to determine the cause of discomfort. Pain may be due to complications (hematoma, infection, dislocation). Pain is an individual experience—it means different things to different people.	
3. Acknowledge existence of pain; inform patient of available analgesic agents or muscle relaxants.	3. The nurse can reduce the stress experienced by patient by communicating concern and availability of assistance to help the patient deal with the pain.	

4. Use pain-modifying techniques.
  a. Administer analgesic agents as prescribed.
 	
  b. Change position within prescribed limits.
 	
  c. Modify environment.
 	
  d. Notify surgeon about persistent pain.
	4.
	  a. Patient will require parenteral opioids during the first 24–48 hours, and then will progress to oral analgesic agents.
	  b. Use of pillows to provide adequate support and relief of pressure on bony prominences assists in minimizing pain.
	  c. Interactions with others, distractions, and sensory overload or deprivation may affect pain experience.
	  d. Surgical intervention may be necessary if pain is due to hematoma or excessive edema.	

5. Evaluate and record discomfort and effectiveness of pain-modifying techniques.	5. Effectiveness of action is based on experience; data provide a baseline about pain experiences, management, and pain relief.	

NURSING DIAGNOSIS: Impaired physical mobility related to positioning, weight-bearing, and activity restrictions after hip replacement
GOAL: Achieves pain-free, functional, stable hip joint

Nursing Interventions	Rationale	Expected Outcomes
1. Maintain proper positioning of hip joint (abduction, neutral rotation, limited flexion).	1. Prevents dislocation of hip prosthesis	• Maintains prescribed position • No heel pressure • Assists in position changes • Shows increased independence in transfers • Exercises hourly • Participates in progressive ambulation program • Actively participates in exercise regimen • Uses ambulatory aids correctly and safely
2. Keep pressure off heel.	2. Prevents pressure ulcer on heel	
3. Instruct and assist in position changes and transfers.	3. Encourages patient's active participation while preventing dislocation	
4. Instruct and supervise isometric quadriceps- and gluteal-setting exercises.	4. Strengthens muscles needed for walking	
5. In consultation with physical therapist, instruct and supervise progressive safe ambulation within limitations of weight-bearing prescription.	5. Amount of weight-bearing depends on patient's condition and prosthesis; ambulatory aids are used to assist the patient with non–weight-bearing and partial weight-bearing ambulation.	

Continued on following page

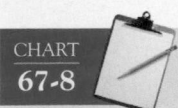

CHART 67-8

PLAN OF NURSING CARE
The Patient With a Total Hip Replacement (Continued)

Nursing Interventions	Rationale	Expected Outcomes
6. Offer encouragement and support exercise regimen.	6. Reconditioning exercises can be uncomfortable and fatiguing; encouragement helps patient comply with exercise program.	
7. Instruct and supervise safe use of ambulatory aids.	7. Prevents injury from unsafe use and prevents falls	

COLLABORATIVE PROBLEMS: Hemorrhage; neurovascular compromise; dislocation of prosthesis; deep vein thrombosis; infection related to surgery
GOAL: Absence of complications

Nursing Interventions	Rationale	Expected Outcomes
Hemorrhage		
1. Monitor vital signs, observing for shock.	1. Changes in pulse, blood pressure, and respirations may indicate development of shock. Blood loss and stress of surgery may contribute to development of shock.	• Vital signs stabilize within normal limits. • Amount of drainage decreases. • No bright red bloody drainage. • Hematology values are within normal limits.
2. Note character and amount of drainage.	2. Within 48 hours, bloody drainage collected in portable suction device should decrease to 25–30 mL per 8 hours. Excessive drainage (more than 250 mL in first 8 hours after surgery) and bright red drainage may indicate active bleeding.	
3. Notify surgeon if patient develops shock or excessive bleeding and prepare for administration of fluids, blood component therapy, and medications.	3. Corrective measures need to be instituted.	
4. Monitor hemoglobin and hematocrit values.	4. Anemia due to blood loss may develop. Blood replacement or iron supplementation may be needed.	
Neurovascular Dysfunction		
1. Assess affected extremity for color and temperature.	1. The skin becomes pale and feels cool with decreased tissue perfusion. Venous congestion may produce cyanosis.	• Color normal • Extremity warm • Normal capillary refill • Moderate edema and swelling; tissue not palpably tense • Pain controllable • No pain with passive dorsiflexion • Normal sensations • No paresthesia • Normal motor abilities • No paresis or paralysis • Pulses strong and equal
2. Assess toes for capillary refill response.	2. After compression of the nail, rapid return of pink color indicates good capillary perfusion.	
3. Assess extremity for edema and swelling. Report patient complaints of leg tightness.	3. The trauma of surgery will cause edema. Excessive swelling and hematoma formation can compromise circulation and function.	
4. Elevate extremity (keep leg lower than hip when in chair).	4. Minimizes dependent edema	
5. Assess for deep, throbbing, unrelenting pain.	5. Surgical pain can be controlled; pain due to neurovascular compromise is not relieved by treatment.	
6. Assess for pain on passive flexion of foot.	6. With nerve ischemia, there will be pain on passive stretch. Additionally, pain or tenderness may indicate deep vein thrombosis.	
7. Assess for change in sensations and numbness.	7. Diminished pain and sensory function may indicate nerve damage. Sensation in web between great and second toe—peroneal nerve; sensation on sole of foot—tibial nerve	

Continued

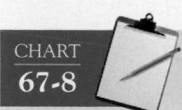

CHART
67-8

PLAN OF NURSING CARE
The Patient With a Total Hip Replacement (Continued)

Nursing Interventions	Rationale	Expected Outcomes
8. Assess ability to move foot and toes.	8. Dorsiflexion of ankle and extension of toes indicate function of peroneal nerve. Plantar flexion of ankle and flexion of toes indicate function of tibial nerve.	
9. Assess pedal pulses in both feet.	9. Indicator of extremity circulation	
10. Notify surgeon if altered neurovascular status is noted.	10. Function of extremity needs to be preserved.	

Dislocation of Prosthesis

Nursing Interventions	Rationale	Expected Outcomes
1. Position patient as prescribed.	1. Hip component positioning (femoral component in acetabular component) needs to be maintained.	• Prosthesis not dislocated • Adheres to recommendations to prevent dislocation
2. Use abductor splint or pillows to maintain position and to support extremity.	2. Keeps hip in abduction and in a neutral rotation to prevent dislocation	
3. Support leg and place pillows between legs when patient is turning and side-lying; turn to the unaffected side.	3–5. Prevent dislocation	
4. Avoid acute flexion of hip (head of bed at 60 degrees or less).		
5. Avoid crossing legs.		
6. Assess for dislocation of prosthesis (extremity shortens, internally or externally rotated, severe hip pain, patient unable to move extremity)	6. Findings may indicate dislocation of prosthesis.	
7. Notify surgeon of possible dislocation.	7. Joint dislocations compromise neurovascular status and future function of extremity.	

Deep Vein Thrombosis

Nursing Interventions	Rationale	Expected Outcomes
1. Use anti-embolism stocking or sequential compression device as prescribed.	1. Aids in venous blood return and prevents stasis	• Wears anti-embolism stockings; uses compression device • No skin breakdown • Pulses equal and strong • Skin temperature normal • No calf pain or tenderness • Changes position with assistance and supervision • Participates in exercise regimen • Well hydrated • No chest pain; lungs clear to auscultation; no evidence of pulmonary emboli
2. Remove stocking for 20 minutes twice a day and provide skin care.	2. Skin care is necessary to avoid breakdown. Extended removal of stockings defeats purpose of stockings.	
3. Assess popliteal, dorsalis pedis, and posterior tibial pulses.	3. Pulses indicate arterial perfusion of extremity.	
4. Assess skin temperature of legs.	4. Local inflammation will increase local skin temperature.	
5. Assess for unilateral calf pain or tenderness every 8 hours.	5. Pain or tenderness may indicate deep vein thrombosis.	
6. Avoid pressure on popliteal blood vessels from equipment (eg, abductor splint straps, sequential compression stockings) or pillows.	6. Compression of blood vessels diminishes blood flow.	
7. Change position and increase activity as prescribed.	7. Activity promotes circulation and diminishes venous stasis.	
8. Supervise ankle exercises hourly.	8. Muscle exercise promotes circulation.	
9. Monitor body temperature.	9. Body temperature increases with inflammation.	
10. Encourage fluids.	10. Dehydration increases blood viscosity.	

Infection

Nursing Interventions	Rationale	Expected Outcomes
1. Monitor vital signs.	1. Temperature, pulse, and respirations increase in response to infection. (Magnitude of response may be minimal in an elderly patient.)	• Vital signs normal • Well-approximated incision without drainage or excessive inflammatory response

Continued on following page

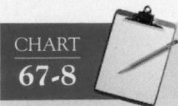

CHART 67-8

PLAN OF NURSING CARE
The Patient With a Total Hip Replacement (Continued)

Nursing Interventions	Rationale	Expected Outcomes
2. Use aseptic technique for dressing changes and emptying of portable drainage.	2. Avoids introducing organisms	• Minimal discomfort; no hematoma • Tolerates antibiotics
3. Assess wound appearance and character of drainage.	3. Red, swollen, draining incision is indicative of infection.	
4. Assess complaints of pain.	4. Pain may be due to wound hematoma—a possible locus of infection—that needs to be surgically evacuated.	
5. Administer prophylactic antibiotics if prescribed, and observe for side effects.	5. Infected prosthesis is avoided.	

NURSING DIAGNOSIS: Risk for ineffective health maintenance related to total hip replacement
GOAL: Cares for self at home

Nursing Interventions	Rationale	Expected Outcomes
1. Assess home environment for discharge planning.	1. Physical barriers (especially stairs, bathrooms) may limit patient's ability to ambulate and care for self at home.	• Home is accessible for patient at time of discharge • Appears relaxed and develops strategies to deal with identified problems • Personal assistance is available • Demonstrates ability to provide necessary assistance within therapeutic prescription • Complies with home care program • Keeps follow-up health care appointments
2. Encourage patient to express concerns about care at home; explore together possible solutions to the problem.	2. Patient may have special problems that need to be identified and resolved.	
3. Assess availability of physical assistance for health care activities.	3. Because of limitation of mobility and limited hip range of motion, patient may require some assistance in routine health care.	
4. Teach home health care regimen to caregiver.	4. Understanding of rehabilitative regimen is necessary for compliance.	

5. Instruct patient on posthospital care:
  a. Activity limitations (hip precautions, weight-bearing limits)
  b. Exercise instructions
  c. Safe use of ambulatory aids
  d. Wound care
  e. Measures to promote healing
  f. Medications, if any
  g. Potential problems
  h. Continuing health care supervision and management
	5. Lack of knowledge and poor preparation for care at home contribute to patient anxiety, insecurity, and nonadherence to therapeutic regimen.	

the pelvis onto the pan. The patient is also reminded not to flex the affected hip.

Limited flexion is maintained during transfers and when sitting. When the patient is initially assisted out of bed, an abduction splint or pillows are kept between the legs. The nurse encourages the patient to keep the affected hip in extension, instructing the patient to pivot on the unaffected leg with assistance by the nurse, who protects the affected hip from **adduction,** flexion, internal or external rotation, and excessive weight bearing.

High-seat (orthopedic) chairs, semireclining wheelchairs, and raised toilet seats are used to minimize hip joint flexion. When sitting, the patient's hips should be higher than the knees. The patient's affected leg should not be elevated when sitting. The patient may flex the knee.

The nurse teaches the patient protective positioning, which includes maintaining abduction and avoiding inter-

nal and external rotation, hyperextension, and acute flexion. A cradle boot may be used to prevent leg rotation and to support the heel off the bed, preventing development of a pressure ulcer. The patient should use pillows between the legs when in a supine or side-lying position and when turning. Generally, the nurse instructs the patient not to sleep on the side on which the surgery was performed. At no time should the patient cross his or her legs. The patient should not bend at the waist to put on shoes and socks. Occupational therapists can provide the patient with devices to assist with dressing below the waist (Lucas, 2008b). Hip precautions should be enforced for 4 or more months after surgery (Chart 67-9). A patient who has had an anterior surgical approach may not need these precautions.

Dislocation may occur with positioning that exceeds the limits of the prosthesis. The nurse must recognize dislocation of the prosthesis. Indicators are as follows:

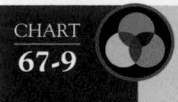

CHART 67-9

PATIENT EDUCATION
Avoiding Hip Dislocation After Replacement Surgery With Posterior or Posterolateral Approach

Until the hip prosthesis stabilizes after hip replacement surgery, it is necessary to follow instructions for proper positioning so that the prosthesis remains in place. Dislocation of the hip is a serious complication of surgery that causes pain and loss of function and necessitates reduction under anesthesia to correct the dislocation. Desirable positions include abduction, neutral rotation, and flexion of less than 90 degrees. When you are seated, the knees should be lower than the hip.

Methods for avoiding displacement include the following:
- Keep the knees apart at all times.
- Put a pillow between the legs when sleeping.
- Never cross the legs when seated.
- Avoid bending forward when seated in a chair.
- Avoid bending forward to pick up an object on the floor.
- Use a high-seated chair and a raised toilet seat.
- Do not flex the hip to put on clothing such as pants, stockings, socks, or shoes. Positions to avoid after total hip replacement are illustrated below.

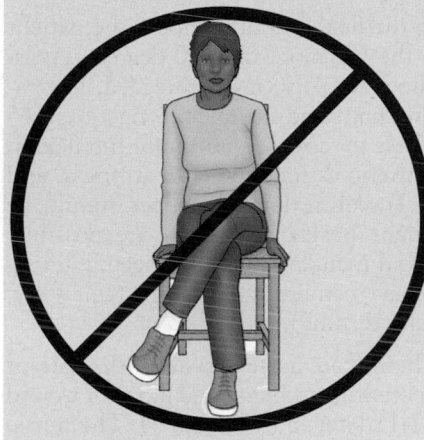
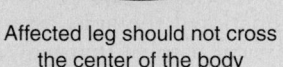

Affected leg should not cross the center of the body

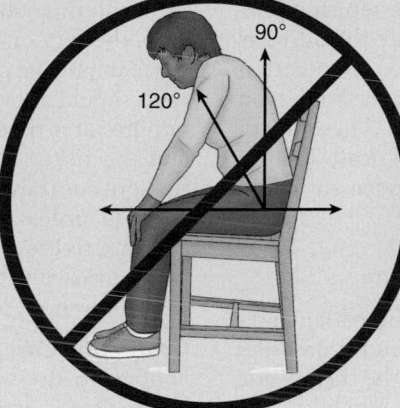

Hip should not bend more than 90 degrees

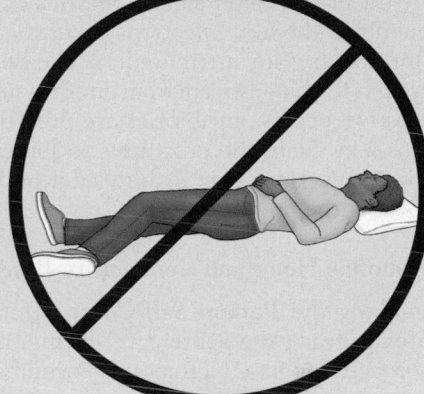

Affected leg should not turn inward

- Increased pain at the surgical site, swelling, and immobilization
- Acute groin pain in the affected hip or increased discomfort
- Shortening of the leg
- Abnormal external or internal rotation
- Restricted ability or inability to move the leg
- Reported "popping" sensation in the hip

If a prosthesis becomes dislocated, the nurse (or the patient, if at home) immediately notifies the surgeon, because the hip must be reduced and stabilized promptly so that the leg does not sustain circulatory and nerve damage. After closed reduction, the hip may be stabilized with Buck's traction or a brace to prevent recurrent dislocation. As the muscles and joint capsule heal, the chance of dislocation diminishes. Stresses to the new hip joint should be avoided for the first 8 to 12 weeks, when the risk of dislocation is greatest (Lucas, 2008b).

Monitoring Wound Drainage

Fluid and blood accumulating at the surgical site are usually drained with a portable suction device. This prevents accumulation of fluid, which could contribute to discomfort and provide a site for infection. Drainage of 200 to 500 mL in the first 24 hours is expected; by 48 hours postoperatively, the total drainage in 8 hours usually decreases to 30 mL or less, and the suction device is then removed. The nurse promptly notifies the physician of any drainage volumes greater than anticipated.

If extensive blood loss is anticipated after total joint replacement surgery, an autotransfusion drainage system (in which the drained blood is filtered and reinfused into the patient during the immediate postoperative period) may be used to decrease the need for homologous blood transfusions.

Preventing Deep Vein Thrombosis

The risk of venous thromboembolism (VTE) is particularly great after reconstructive hip surgery. The incidence of DVT is 48% for patients who have not had any type of VTE preventive measures instituted, which includes mechanical prophylaxis (eg, anti-embolism stockings) and pharmacologic prophylaxis (eg, antithrombotic medications) (Haas, Barrack, Westrich, et al., 2008). DVT formation can lead to pulmonary embolism (PE), which can be fatal. Therefore, the nurse must institute preventive measures and monitor the patient closely for the development of DVT and PE. Signs of DVT include calf pain, swelling, and tenderness. Medications that include fondaparinux (Arixtra) or low-molecular-weight heparin (eg, enoxaparin [Lovenox], dalteparin [Fragmin]) are indicated as prophylaxis for VTE after hip replacement surgery (Hirsh, Guyatt, Albers, et al., 2008).

Preventing Infection

Infection, a serious complication of total hip replacement, may necessitate removal of the prosthesis. Patients who are elderly, are obese, are poorly nourished, smoke cigarettes, or use corticosteroid medications (eg, prednisone) and patients who have diabetes, rheumatoid arthritis, concurrent infections (eg, urinary tract infection, dental abscess), or hematomas are at high risk for infection (Doherty & Way, 2006).

Potential sources of infection are avoided. If indwelling urinary catheters or portable wound suction devices are used, they are removed as soon as possible to avoid infection. Prophylactic antibiotics are prescribed if the patient needs any future surgical or invasive procedures, such as tooth extraction or cystoscopic examination.

Acute infections may occur within 3 months after surgery and are associated with progressive superficial infections or hematomas. Delayed surgical infections may appear 4 to 24 months after surgery and may cause return of discomfort in the hip. Infections occurring more than 2 years after surgery are attributed to the spread of infection through the bloodstream from another site in the body. If an infection occurs, antibiotics are prescribed. These infections may cause the prosthesis to loosen (Lucas, 2008b). Severe infections may require surgical débridement or removal of the prosthesis.

Promoting Home and Community-Based Care

Teaching the Patient Self-Care. Before the patient prepares to leave the acute care setting, the nurse provides thorough teaching to promote continuity of the therapeutic regimen and active participation in the rehabilitation process (Chart 67-10). The nurse advises the patient of the importance of the daily exercise program in maintaining the functional motion of the hip joint and strengthening the abductor muscles of the hip, and reminds the patient that it will take time to strengthen and retrain the muscles.

Assistive devices (crutches, walker, or cane) are used for a time. After sufficient muscle tone has developed to permit a normal gait without discomfort, these devices are not necessary. In general, by 3 months, the patient can resume routine ADLs. Stair climbing is permitted as prescribed but is kept to a minimum for 3 to 6 months. Frequent walks, swimming, and use of a high rocking chair are excellent for hip exercises. Sexual intercourse should be carried out with the patient in the dependent position (flat on the back) for 3 to 6 months to avoid excessive adduction and flexion of the new hip.

At no time during the first 4 months should the patient cross the legs or flex the hip more than 90 degrees. Assistance in putting on shoes and socks may be needed. The patient should avoid low chairs and sitting for longer than 45 minutes at a time. These precautions minimize hip flexion and the risks of prosthetic dislocation, hip stiffness, and flexion contracture. Traveling long distances should be avoided unless frequent position changes are possible. Other activities to avoid include tub baths, jogging, lifting heavy loads, and excessive bending and twisting (eg, lifting, shoveling snow, forceful turning).

Continuing Care. A home care nurse may assess the patient at home to assess for potential problems and monitor wound healing (see Chart 67-11 later in this chapter). The nurse, physical therapist, or occupational therapist assesses the home environment for physical barriers that may impede

---

Chart 67-10 • *Providing Home Care After Hip Replacement*

Considerations

- Pain management
- Wound care
- Mobility
- Self-care (activities of daily living)
- Potential complications

Nursing Interventions

Discuss with patient methods to reduce pain:
- Periodic rest
- Distraction and relaxation techniques
- Medication therapy (eg, nonsteroidal anti-inflammatory drugs, opioid analgesic agents): actions of medications, administration, schedule, side effects

Instruct patient in the following:
- Keeping incision clean and dry
- Taking care of the wound and changing the dressing
- Recognizing signs of wound infection (eg, pain, swelling, drainage, fever)

Explain that sutures or staples will be removed 10 to 14 days after surgery.

Teach patient about the following:
- Safe use of assistive devices
- Weight-bearing limits
- How to change positions frequently
- Limitations on hip flexion and adduction (eg, avoid acute flexion and crossing legs)

- How to stand without flexing hip acutely
- Avoidance of low-seated chairs
- Sleeping with pillow between legs to prevent adduction
- Gradual increase in activities and participation in prescribed exercise regimen
- Use of important medications such as warfarin (Coumadin) and aspirin

Assess home environment for physical barriers.

Instruct patient to use elevated toilet seat and to use reachers to aid in dressing.

Encourage patient to accept assistance with activities of daily living during early convalescence until mobility and strength improve.

Arrange services and accommodations to address the patient's disability or illness, as appropriate.

Assess patient for development of potential problems, and instruct patient to report signs of potential complications:
- Dislocation of prosthesis (eg, increased pain, shortening of leg, inability to move leg, popping sensation in hip, abnormal rotation)
- Deep vein thrombosis (eg, calf pain, swelling)
- Wound infection (eg, swelling, purulent drainage, pain, fever)
- Pulmonary emboli (eg, sudden dyspnea, tachypnea, pleuritic chest pain)

Discuss with patient the need to continue regular health care (routine physical examinations) and screenings.

the patient's rehabilitation. In addition, the nurse or therapist may need to assist the patient in acquiring devices such as reachers or long-handled tongs to help with dressing, or toilet seat extenders to elevate the toilet.

After successful surgery and rehabilitation, the patient can expect a hip joint that is free or almost free of pain, has good motion, is stable, and permits normal or near-normal ambulation.

Total Knee Replacement

Total knee replacement surgery is considered for patients who have severe pain and functional disabilities related to destruction of joint surfaces by osteoarthritis or rheumatoid arthritis. Metal and acrylic prostheses designed to provide the patient with a functional, painless, stable joint may be used. If the patient's ligaments have weakened, a fully constrained (hinged) or semiconstrained prosthesis may be used to provide joint stability. A nonconstrained prosthesis depends on the patient's ligaments for joint stability.

Nursing Interventions

Postoperatively, the knee is dressed with a compression bandage. Ice may be applied to control edema and bleeding. The nurse assesses the neurovascular status of the leg. It is important to encourage active flexion of the foot every hour when the patient is awake. Efforts are directed at preventing complications (thromboembolism, peroneal nerve palsy, infection, limited range of motion) (Lucas, 2008b).

A wound suction drain removes fluid accumulating in the joint. Drainage ranges from 200 to 400 mL during the first 24 hours after surgery and diminishes to less than 25 mL by 48 hours, at which time the surgeon removes the drains. If extensive bleeding is anticipated, an autotransfusion drainage system may be used during the immediate postoperative period. The color, type, and amount of drainage are documented, and any excessive drainage or change in characteristics of the drainage is promptly reported to the physician.

Use of a **continuous passive motion (CPM) device** in conjunction with physical therapy is associated with decreased hospital length of stay as well as improved patient postoperative knee mobility and decreased use of analgesic agents (Milne, Brosseau, Robinson, et al., 2008). The patient's leg is placed in this device, which increases circulation and range of motion of the knee joint. The rate and amount of extension and flexion are prescribed. Usually, 10 degrees of extension and 50 degrees of flexion are prescribed initially, increasing to 90 degrees of flexion with full extension (0 degrees) by discharge (Fig. 67-9).

The nurse encourages the patient to use the CPM device. The physical therapist supervises exercises for strength and range of motion. If satisfactory flexion is not achieved, gentle manipulation of the knee joint under general anesthesia may be necessary about 2 weeks after surgery.

The nurse assists the patient to get out of bed on the evening or the day after surgery. The knee is usually protected with a knee immobilizer (eg, cast, brace, splint) and is elevated when the patient sits in a chair. The physician prescribes weight-bearing limits. Progressive ambulation, using assistive devices and within the prescribed weight-bearing limits, begins on the day after surgery.

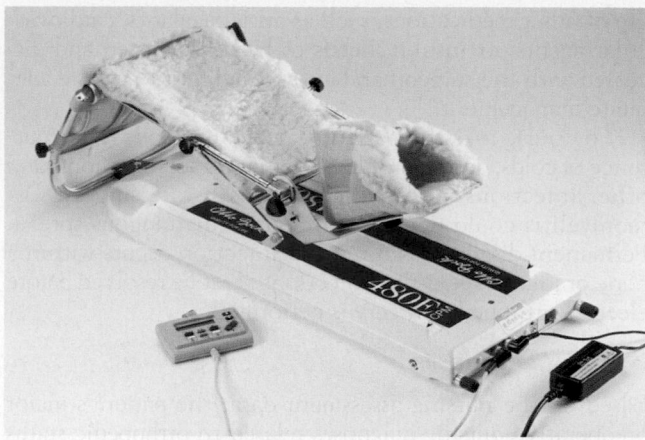

Figure 67-9 Lower-limb continuous passive motion (CPM) device. The Otto Bock 480E Knee CPM is 11 kg (24 lb) and combines durable construction with portability and ease of operation. CPM is best applied immediately after surgery and continued, uninterrupted, for up to 6 weeks as prescribed by the physician. Photo courtesy of Otto Bock Healthcare, Minneapolis, MN.

After discharge from the hospital, the patient may continue to use the CPM device at home and may undergo physical therapy on an outpatient basis. Late complications that may occur include infection and loosening of prosthetic components (Lucas, 2008b). Patients usually can achieve a pain-free, functional joint and participate more fully in life activities than before the surgery (Marx, Jones, Atwan, et al., 2005; Rasanen, Paavoalinen, Sintonen, et al., 2007).

NURSING PROCESS

PREOPERATIVE CARE OF THE PATIENT UNDERGOING ORTHOPEDIC SURGERY

Assessment

Assessment of the patient is focused on hydration status, current medication history, and possible infection. Adequate hydration is an important goal for orthopedic patients. Immobilization and bed rest contribute to the following complications: DVT, PE, urinary stasis and associated bladder infections, and kidney stone formation. Adequate hydration decreases blood viscosity and venous stasis and ensures adequate urine flow. To determine preoperative hydration status, the nurse assesses the skin and mucous membranes, vital signs, urinary output, and laboratory values.

The medication history provides information for perioperative management. The patient with chronic illness (eg, adrenal insufficiency, rheumatoid arthritis, chronic pulmonary disease, multiple sclerosis) or with a transplanted organ frequently has received long-term administration of corticosteroid medications to control disease symptoms or prevent rejection. The corticosteroid should be administered preoperatively, intraoperatively, and postoperatively as prescribed to prevent the occurrence of acute adrenal insufficiency from suppressed adrenal function. The patient's use of other medications, such as anticoagulants, cardiovascular agents, or insulin, needs to be documented and discussed with the surgeon and anesthesiologist to ensure adequate management.

The nurse asks the patient specifically about the occurrence of colds, dental problems, urinary tract infections, and other infections within the 2 weeks before surgery. Osteomyelitis could develop through hematologous spread. Permanent disability can result if infection occurs within a bone or joint. Preexisting infections must be resolved before elective orthopedic surgery is performed.

Nursing Diagnoses

Based on the nursing assessment data, the patient's major preoperative nursing diagnoses related to orthopedic status may include the following:

- Acute pain related to fracture, joint degeneration, swelling, or inflammation
- Risk for peripheral neurovascular dysfunction related to swelling, constricting devices, or impaired venous return
- Risk for ineffective therapeutic regimen management related to insufficient knowledge or lack of available support and resources
- Impaired physical mobility related to pain, swelling, and possible presence of an immobilization device
- Risk for situational low self-esteem and/or disturbed body image related to impact of musculoskeletal disorder

Planning and Goals

The major goals for the patient before orthopedic surgery may include relief of pain, adequate neurovascular function, health promotion, improved mobility, and positive self-esteem.

Nursing Interventions

Relieving Pain

Discomfort is decreased with immobilization of a fractured bone or an injured, inflamed joint. Elevation of an edematous extremity promotes venous return and reduces associated discomfort. Ice, if prescribed, relieves swelling and reduces discomfort by diminishing nerve stimulation.

Analgesic agents are frequently prescribed to control the acute pain of musculoskeletal injury or surgery and associated muscle spasm. During the immediate postoperative period, the nurse needs to discuss and coordinate the administration of effective analgesic medications (eg, opioids, nonsteroidal anti-inflammatory drugs) with the anesthesia provider and surgeon. (See Chapter 13 for a further discussion of assessment and management of pain.)

Maintaining Adequate Neurovascular Function

Trauma, edema, or immobilization devices may interrupt tissue perfusion. The nurse must frequently assess neurovascular status (ie, color, temperature, capillary refill, pulses, edema, pain, sensation, motion) of the extremity and document the findings. If circulation is compromised, the nurse institutes measures to restore adequate circulation. These include promptly notifying the physician, elevating the extremity, and releasing constricting wraps or assisting with bivalving constrictive casts as prescribed.

Promoting Health

The nurse assists the patient in performing activities that promote health during the perioperative period. The nurse assesses nutritional status and hydration. The nurse monitors fluid intake, urinary output, and urinalysis findings. At times, patients may intentionally limit their fluid intake to minimize the use of a bedpan. A small fracture bedpan may be more comfortable for the patient to use. An indwelling catheter should be used only when necessary to minimize the risk of urinary tract infection. A preexisting urinary tract infection must be effectively treated prior to surgery.

If the surgery is elective, the orthopedic surgeon may instruct the patient to shower with a germicidal soap at home prior to surgery. The patient may also be asked to mark the operative site prior to surgery to minimize the risk that the wrong site is selected in the operating room.

The nurse discusses with the patient and the family the need for assistance with ADLs and the therapeutic regimen during convalescence so that adequate support is available when the patient is discharged. Modification of the home environment may be necessary to accommodate the altered mobility of the patient after surgery. Referral to a social worker and case manager may be needed to ensure a smooth transition to home care.

Improving Mobility

Preoperatively, the patient's mobility may be impaired by pain, swelling, and immobilizing devices (eg, splints, casts, traction). The nurse should elevate and adequately support edematous extremities with pillows. It is important to control pain before an injured part is moved by administering analgesic medication in time for it to take effect. The injured part is supported when it is moved. The nurse encourages movement within the limits of therapeutic immobility. The patient should perform active range-of-motion exercises of uninvolved joints, and, unless contraindicated, the nurse teaches gluteal-setting and quadriceps-setting isometric exercises to maintain the muscles needed for ambulation (see Chart 67-3). The patient who will be using assistive devices postoperatively may exercise to strengthen the upper extremities and shoulders. If the use of assistive devices (eg, crutches, walker, wheelchair) is anticipated, the nurse encourages the patient to practice with them preoperatively to facilitate their safe use and to promote earlier independent mobility.

Helping the Patient Maintain Self-Esteem

Preoperatively, orthopedic patients may need assistance in accepting changes in body image, diminished self-esteem, or inability to perform their roles and responsibilities. The degree of assistance required in this area varies greatly, depending on the events preceding hospitalization, the surgery and rehabilitation planned, and the temporary or permanent nature of the problems. The nurse promotes a trusting relationship so that the patient feels comfortable expressing concerns and anxieties, and helps the patient examine his or her feelings about changes in self-concept. The nurse clarifies any misconceptions the patient may have and helps the patient work through modifications needed to adapt to alterations in physical capacity and to reestablish positive self-esteem.

Evaluation

Expected Patient Outcomes

Expected patient outcomes may include:

1. Reports relief of pain
   a. Uses multiple approaches to reduce pain
   b. States that medication is effective in relieving pain
   c. Moves with increasing comfort
2. Exhibits adequate neurovascular function
   a. Exhibits normal skin color
   b. Has warm skin
   c. Has normal capillary refill response
   d. Reports normal sensation and demonstrates joint motion
   e. Demonstrates reduced swelling
3. Promotes health
   a. Consumes diet appropriate to meet nutritional needs
   b. Maintains adequate hydration
   c. Abstains from smoking
   d. Practices respiratory exercises
   e. Repositions self to relieve skin pressure
   f. Engages in strengthening and preventive exercises
   g. Plans for assistance during convalescence at home
4. Maximizes mobility within therapeutic limits
   a. Requests assistance when moving
   b. Elevates edematous extremity after transfer
   c. Uses immobilizing devices and assistive devices safely as prescribed
5. Expresses positive self-esteem
   a. Acknowledges temporary or permanent changes in body image
   b. Discusses role performance changes
   c. Participates in decisions about care

NURSING PROCESS

POSTOPERATIVE CARE OF THE PATIENT UNDERGOING ORTHOPEDIC SURGERY

Assessment

After orthopedic surgery, the nurse continues the preoperative care plan, modifying it to match the patient's current postoperative status. The nurse reassesses the patient's needs related to pain, neurovascular status, health promotion, mobility, and self-esteem. Skeletal trauma and surgery performed on bones, muscles, or joints can produce significant pain, especially during the first 1 or 2 postoperative days. Tissue perfusion must be monitored closely, because edema and bleeding into the tissues can compromise circulation and result in compartment syndrome. Inactivity contributes to venous stasis and the development of venous thromboemboli that may include DVTs or PEs. General anesthesia, analgesia, and immobility can result in altered functioning of the respiratory, gastrointestinal, and urinary systems.

The nurse notes the prescribed limits on mobility and assesses the patient's understanding of the mobility restrictions. The nurse discusses the plan of care with the patient and encourages his or her active participation in the plan.

Frequent assessment of vital signs including pain, level of consciousness, neurovascular status, wound drainage, breath sounds, bowel sounds, and fluid balance provides the nurse with data that may suggest the possible development of complications. The nurse reports abnormal findings to the physician promptly.

With major orthopedic surgery, there is a risk for hypovolemic shock because of blood loss. Muscle dissection frequently produces wounds in which hemostasis is poor. Wounds that are closed under tourniquet control may bleed during the postoperative period. The nurse must be alert for signs of hypovolemic shock.

Changes in the patient's pulse rate, respiratory rate, or color of the skin or mucous membranes may indicate pulmonary or cardiovascular complications. Atelectasis and pneumonia are common and may be related to preexisting pulmonary disease, deep anesthesia, decreased activity, and reduced respiratory reserve due to advanced age or an underlying musculoskeletal disorder (eg, restrictive lung expansion secondary to kyphosis, rheumatoid arthritis, or osteoporosis).

Voiding in unnatural positions may contribute to urinary retention. In addition, elderly men usually have some degree of prostate enlargement and may already have difficulty voiding. Therefore, it is important to monitor urinary output.

Temperature elevations within the first 48 hours are frequently related to atelectasis or other respiratory problems. Temperature elevations during the next few days are frequently associated with urinary tract infections. Superficial wound infections take 4 to 6 days to develop. Fever from phlebitis usually occurs during the end of the first week through the second week.

Venous thromboembolus (see discussions of DVT in Chapter 31 and PE in Chapter 23) is one of the most common and most dangerous of all complications occurring in the postoperative orthopedic patient. Advanced age, venous stasis, lower extremity orthopedic surgery, and immobilization are significant risk factors. The nurse assesses the patient daily for unilateral calf swelling, tenderness, warmth, and redness. The nurse promptly reports abnormal findings to the physician.

In addition, fat emboli syndrome (FES) (see Chapter 69) may occur with orthopedic surgery. The nurse must be alert to any signs and symptoms that may suggest the development of FES. These may include respiratory distress; onset of delirium or any acute change in level of consciousness; and development of unusual skin rashes, especially a papular rash on the upper torso.

Diagnosis

Nursing Diagnoses

Based on all assessment data, the patient's major nursing diagnoses after orthopedic surgery may include the following:

- Acute pain related to the surgical procedure, swelling, and immobilization
- Risk for peripheral neurovascular dysfunction related to swelling, constricting devices, or impaired circulation
- Risk for ineffective therapeutic regimen management related to insufficient knowledge or available support and resources
- Impaired physical mobility related to pain, edema, or the presence of an immobilizing device (eg, splint, cast, or brace)
- Risk for situational low self-esteem, disturbed body image, or ineffective role performance related to impact of the musculoskeletal disorder

Collaborative Problems/Potential Complications

Based on the assessment data, potential complications may include the following:

- Hypovolemic shock
- Atelectasis; pneumonia
- Urinary retention
- Infection
- Venous thromboembolism, including DVT or PE
- Constipation and fecal impaction

Planning and Goals

The major goals for the patient after orthopedic surgery may include relief of pain, adequate neurovascular function, health promotion, improved mobility, positive self-esteem, and absence of complications.

Nursing Interventions

Relieving Pain

After orthopedic surgery, pain can be intense. Edema, hematomas, and muscle spasms contribute to the pain. Some patients report that the pain is less than that experienced preoperatively, and only moderate amounts of analgesic agents are needed. The nurse assesses the patient's level of pain, evaluates the patient's response to therapeutic measures, and makes every effort to relieve the pain and discomfort. Pain assessment must occur on an ongoing basis and take place at least as often as vital signs are assessed.

Multiple pharmacologic approaches to pain management exist. Patient-controlled analgesia (PCA) and epidural analgesia may be prescribed to relieve the pain. If the patient is receiving preemptive analgesia on an ongoing basis via a PCA IV pump, the nurse ensures that the patient receives boluses of the analgesic agent prior to performing planned physical activities. If intramuscular and oral analgesic agents are prescribed on an as-needed basis (PRN), the nurse should administer medications on a preventive basis within the prescribed intervals if the onset of pain can be predicted (eg, 30 minutes before planned activity such as transfer or exercise). The nurse should offer the medication at set intervals.

In addition to pharmacologic approaches to controlling pain, elevation of the operative extremity and application of cold packs, if prescribed, help control edema and pain. Surgical drains inserted in the wound decrease fluid accumulation and hematoma formation. The nurse may find

that repositioning, relaxation, distraction, and guided imagery help in reducing the patient's pain.

The nurse should report increasing and uncontrollable pain to the orthopedic surgeon for evaluation. Pain should diminish rapidly after the initial postoperative period. After 2 to 3 days, most patients require only occasional oral analgesia for residual muscle soreness and spasm.

Maintaining Adequate Neurovascular Function

The nurse monitors the neurovascular status of the involved body part and notifies the physician promptly of any indications of diminished tissue perfusion. The patient is reminded to perform muscle-setting, ankle, and calf-pumping exercises hourly while awake to enhance circulation.

Maintaining Health

It is important to encourage the patient to participate in the postoperative treatment regimen. A diet that includes adequate protein and vitamins is essential for wound healing. The patient progresses to a regular diet as soon as possible.

The nurse assesses the patient for early manifestations of pressure ulcers (eg, redness over bony prominences), which are a threat to any patient who must spend an extended time in bed or who is elderly, malnourished, or unable to move without assistance. Turning the patient frequently at preset intervals (eg, at least every 2 hours), washing and drying the skin, and minimizing pressure over bony prominences are necessary to avoid skin breakdown.

Improving Physical Mobility

Patients are frequently reluctant to move after orthopedic surgery. Preoperative education about the planned postoperative treatment regimen promotes patient adherence to an optimal rehabilitation regimen. Patients often increase their mobility once they have been reassured that movement within therapeutic limits is beneficial, that the nurse will provide assistance, and that discomfort can be controlled.

Metal pins, screws, rods, and plates used for internal fixation are designed to maintain the position of the bone until ossification occurs. They are not designed to support the body's weight, and they can bend, loosen, or break if stressed. The estimated strength of the bone, the stability of the fracture, reduction and fixation, and the amount of bone healing are important considerations in determining weight-bearing limits. Although the incision may appear healed, the underlying bone requires more time to repair and regain normal strength. Some orthopedic procedures require weight-bearing restrictions. The orthopedic surgeon will prescribe the weight-bearing limits and the use of protective devices (orthoses), if necessary, after surgery.

The physical therapist tailors the rehabilitation program to each patient's needs. The goal is the patient's return to the highest level of function in the shortest time possible. Rehabilitation involves progressive increases in the patient's activities and exercises. Assistive devices (crutches, walker) may be used for postoperative mobility. Preoperative practice with assistive devices helps the patient use them appropriately postoperatively. The nurse makes sure that the patient uses these devices safely (see discussions of crutch walking and use of a walker in Chapter 11).

Maintaining Self-Esteem

The nurse and the patient set realistic goals. Increased ability to perform self-care activities within the limits of the therapeutic regimen and resumption of roles facilitate the patient's recognition of abilities and promote self-esteem, personal identity, and role performance. Acceptance of altered body image is facilitated by support provided by the nurse, family, and others.

Monitoring and Managing Potential Complications

HYPOVOLEMIC SHOCK. Excessive loss of blood during or after surgery can result in shock. The nurse monitors the patient for signs and symptoms of hypovolemic shock: increased pulse rate (eg, greater than 100 bpm), decreased blood pressure (eg, less than 90/60 mm Hg), narrowed pulse pressure (eg, less than 20 mm Hg), urine output less than 30 mL/h, restlessness, change in mentation, thirst, and decreased hemoglobin and hematocrit. The nurse reports these findings to the orthopedic surgeon and assists in appropriate management. (See Chapter 15 for a discussion of managing shock.)

ATELECTASIS AND PNEUMONIA. The nurse monitors the patient's breath sounds and encourages deep-breathing and coughing exercises. Full expansion of the lungs prevents the accumulation of pulmonary secretions and the development of atelectasis and pneumonia. Incentive spirometry use is encouraged. If signs of respiratory problems develop (eg, increased respiratory rate, productive cough, diminished or adventitious breath sounds, fever), the nurse reports the findings to the surgeon.

URINARY RETENTION. The nurse closely monitors the patient's urinary output after surgery. The nurse encourages the patient to void every 3 to 4 hours to prevent urinary retention and bladder distention. It is important to provide privacy during toileting. Because the patient may need to void in an unusual position, the nurse assists the patient with positioning. Fracture bedpans may be more comfortable to use than other bedpans. Voiding in the side-lying position may be helpful to the male patient. Some male patients can void only if standing, and clarification with the surgeon of the activity prescription may be needed before the patient is assisted to a standing position.

If the patient cannot void, intermittent catheterizations may be prescribed until the patient can void independently. Indwelling urinary catheters should be used only when necessary and should be removed as soon as possible. The patient may follow a catheterization protocol that incorporates the use of a bladder scanner to estimate the amount of urine in the bladder, thereby determining if catheterization is necessary. Catheterization protocol use has decreased the number of nosocomial urinary tract infections associated with unnecessary catheterizations (Wald, Ma, Bratzler, et al., 2008).

INFECTION. Infection is a risk after any surgery, but it is of particular concern for the postoperative orthopedic patient because of the risk of osteomyelitis. Osteomyelitis often requires prolonged courses of IV antibiotics. At times, the infected bone and prosthesis or internal fixation device must be surgically removed. Therefore, prophylactic systemic antibiotics are usually prescribed during the perioperative and immediate postoperative periods. The nurse assesses the patient's response to these antibiotics. When changing dressings and emptying wound drainage devices, aseptic technique is essential. The nurse monitors the patient's vital signs, incision, and drainage. The nurse monitors the patient for signs of urinary tract infection. Prompt assessment for and treatment of infection are essential.

VENOUS THROMBOEMBOLISM AND DEEP VEIN THROMBOSIS. Prevention of DVT requires use of ankle and calf-pumping exercises, anti-embolism stockings, and sequential compression devices. Adequate hydration and early mobilization are equally important. Prophylactic fondaparinux, low-molecular-weight heparin (eg, enoxaparin, dalteparin), warfarin (Coumadin), or low-dose unfractionated heparin may be prescribed in the immediate postoperative period. Typically, fondaparinux, a low-molecular-weight heparin, or warfarin is prescribed during the later rehabilitation period for DVT prophylaxis (Hirsh, et al., 2008). The nurse monitors the patient for signs of DVT and promptly reports findings to the physician for management.

CONSTIPATION. Constipation is a frequently overlooked complication, because patients are discharged to a rehabilitation or home setting in 3 or 4 days. Constipation occurs because of decreased mobility and hydration, coupled with the use of opioids. Prevention of constipation requires continual monitoring of bowel function. Adequate hydration, early mobilization, and stool softeners may be prescribed to prevent fecal impaction (see Chapter 38).

Promoting Home and Community-Based Care

TEACHING THE PATIENT SELF-CARE. Because the length of stay in the hospital after orthopedic surgery is usually 3 or 4 days, most convalescence and rehabilitation take place at home or in a nonacute care setting. The nurse teaches the patient and the family to recognize complications that must be reported promptly to the orthopedic surgeon. The patient must understand the prescribed medication regimen. The nurse should demonstrate proper wound care. The patient gradually resumes physical activities and adheres to weight-bearing limits. The patient must be able to perform transfers and to use mobility aids safely. If the patient has a cast or other immobilizing device, family members are instructed about how to assist the patient in a way that is safe for the patient and for the family member (eg, using proper body mechanics when assisting the patient). Specific exercises need to be taught and practiced before discharge. The nurse discusses recovery and health promotion, emphasizing a healthy lifestyle and diet (Chart 67-11).

CONTINUING CARE. If special equipment or home modifications are needed for safe care at home, they must be in place before the patient is discharged home. Discharge planning begins immediately after surgery. The nurse, physical therapist, and social worker can assist the patient and family in identifying their needs and in getting ready to care for the patient at home.

Frequently, home health nursing and home physical therapy are part of the discharge plan of care. These referrals provide resources and help the patient and the family

CHART
67-11

HOME CARE CHECKLIST
The Patient Who Has Had Orthopedic Surgery

At the completion of the home care instruction, the patient or caregiver will be able to:	PATIENT	CAREGIVER
• Describe wound care.	✔	✔
• State indicators of wound infections (eg, redness, swelling, tenderness, purulent drainage, fever).	✔	✔
• Consume a healthy diet to promote wound and bone healing.	✔	
• Participate in prescribed exercise regimen to promote circulation and mobility.	✔	
• Use mobility aids safely.	✔	
• Observe prescribed weight-bearing and activity limits.	✔	
• Take prescribed therapeutic and prophylactic medications (eg, antibiotics, anticoagulants, analgesic agents).	✔	
• State indicators of complications to report promptly to physician (eg, uncontrolled swelling and pain; cool, pale fingers or toes; paresthesia; paralysis; purulent drainage; signs of systemic infection; signs of deep vein thrombosis or pulmonary embolism).	✔	✔
• Identify modifications of home environment to promote safe environment and independence during recovery and rehabilitation.	✔	✔

cope with the demands of care during recovery and rehabilitation. The nurse assesses the patient's progress and monitors for possible complications. Regular medical follow-up care after discharge needs to be arranged. The nurse reminds the patient and family about the importance of continuing health promotion and screening practices.

Evaluation

Expected Patient Outcomes

Expected patient outcomes may include:

1. Reports decreased level of pain
   a. Uses multiple approaches to reduce pain
   b. Uses oral analgesic medication as needed to control discomfort
   c. Elevates extremity to control edema and discomfort
   d. Moves with greater comfort
2. Exhibits adequate neurovascular function
   a. Exhibits normal color and temperature of skin
   b. Has warm skin
   c. Has normal capillary refill response
   d. Demonstrates intact sensory and motor function
   e. Demonstrates reduced swelling
3. Promotes health
   a. Eats diet appropriate for nutritional needs
   b. Maintains adequate hydration
   c. Abstains from smoking
   d. Practices respiratory exercises
   e. Repositions self to relieve pressure on skin
   f. Engages in strengthening and preventive exercises
4. Maximizes mobility within the therapeutic limits
   a. Requests assistance when moving
   b. Elevates edematous extremity after transfer
   c. Uses immobilizing devices as prescribed
   d. Complies with prescribed weight-bearing limitation

5. Expresses positive self-esteem
   a. Discusses temporary or permanent changes in body image
   b. Discusses role performance
   c. Views self as capable of assuming responsibilities
   d. Actively participates in planning care and in the therapeutic regimen
6. Exhibits absence of complications
   a. Does not experience shock
   b. Maintains normal vital signs and blood pressure
   c. Has clear lung sounds
   d. Demonstrates wound healing without signs of infection
   e. Does not experience urinary retention
   f. Voids clear urine
   g. Exhibits no signs of DVT or PE
   h. Does not experience constipation

CRITICAL THINKING EXERCISES

EBP **1** A 64-year-old man has had a right total knee replacement for osteoarthritis. On his second postoperative day, he complains to you that he would rather not use his CPM device, and wonders why his participation in physical therapy alone is not sufficient. How would you respond to him? Why is CPM indicated for patients who have had knee replacement surgery? What is the strength of the evidence that supports the use of CPM either singly or in tandem with physical therapy postoperatively in this patient population?

2 A 50-year-old woman has had a repair of a fracture of her right tibia. She has a plaster cast over her right leg, with a window placed over her incision. During the evening of her second postoperative day, she complains of increasing pain and slight paresthesias of her right toes. Opioid analgesic agents have only moderately relieved her pain. The night-shift nurse documents her findings and asks you, as the oncoming day-shift nurse, to report these findings to the orthopedic surgeon when he makes his rounds. You assess the patient after report and find that she now describes her right lower leg as "feeling tight" and that she has sensations of "pins and needles." Capillary refill of her right toes is longer than 3 seconds, and they feel much cooler than the left toes. What additional assessments might you make at this time? What is your priority nursing diagnosis and intervention?

EBP **3** You are an experienced perioperative nurse. You note that different orthopedic surgical groups have different preoperative hygiene protocols for patients undergoing total knee replacement surgery who come to the surgical center where you work. One surgical group tells its patients to shower with Betadine solution once daily for 2 days prior to surgery; another tells its patients to shower with chlorhexidine solution the morning of surgery; while another does not give any specific preoperative hygiene instructions. What is the strength of the evidence that identifies which preoperative hygiene protocol is most effective for patients scheduled to have total knee replacement surgery?

4 A 70-year-old woman with a long-standing history of osteoarthritis has had a right total hip replacement. On the second postoperative day, a physical therapy assistant helps the patient get out of bed. She has been sitting out of bed for approximately an hour when she requests to be placed back in bed. What is the best way to accomplish this transfer from chair to bed? What specific precautions might you follow?

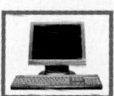

The Smeltzer suite offers these additional resources to enhance learning and facilitate understanding of this chapter:
- thePoint online resource, thepoint.lww.com/Smeltzer12E
- Student CD-ROM included with the book
- *Study Guide to Accompany Brunner & Suddarth's Textbook of Medical-Surgical Nursing*

REFERENCES AND SELECTED READINGS

Asterisk indicates nursing research.

Books

Doherty, G. M. & Way, L. W. (2006). *Current surgical diagnosis and treatment.* New York: Lange Medical Books.

Kneale, J. (2005). *Orthopaedic nursing* (2nd ed.). Philadelphia: Elsevier.

National Association of Orthopedic Nurses. (2007). *Core curriculum for orthopaedic nursing* (6th ed.). Boston: Pearson.

Journals and Electronic Documents

Adams, J. B., Hawkins, M. L., Ferdinand, C. H., et al. (2007). Superior mesenteric artery syndrome in the modern trauma patient. *American Surgeon*, 73(8), 803–806.

Altizer, L. (2004). Casting for immobilization. *Orthopaedic Nursing*, 23(2), 136–141.

Barrett, J., Losina, E., Baron, J. A., et al. (2005). Survival following total hip replacement. *Journal of Bone and Joint Surgery*, 87(9), 1965–1971.

Gravlee, J. R. & Van Durme, D. J. (2007). Braces and splints for musculoskeletal conditions. *American Family Physician*, 75(3), 342–348.

Haas, S. B., Barrack, R. L., Westrich, G., et al. (2008). Venous thromboembolic disease after total hip and knee arthroplasty. *Journal of Bone and Joint Surgery*, 90(12), 2763–2780.

Hawn, M. T., Gray, S. H., Vick, C. C., et al. (2006). Timely administration of prophylactic antibiotics for major surgical procedures. *Journal of the American College of Surgeons*, 203(6), 803–811.

Hessmann, M., Ingelfinger, P. & Rommens, P. M. (2007). Compartment syndrome of the lower extremity. *European Journal of Trauma and Emergency Surgery*, 33(6), 589–599.

Hirsh, J., Guyatt, G., Albers, G. W., et al. (2008). ACCP guidelines: Antithrombotic and thrombolytic therapy. *Chest*, 133(6), 71S–105S.

Holmes, S. B. & Brown, S. J. (2005). Skeletal pin site care: National Association of Orthopaedic Nurses guidelines for orthopaedic nursing. *Orthopaedic Nursing*, 24(2), 99–107.

Iyengar, K. P., Ivanovic, N. & Mahale, A. (2007). Targeted early rehabilitation at home after total hip and knee joint replacement: Does it work? *Disability and Rehabilitation*, 29(6), 495–502.

Janzing, H. M. (2007). Epidemiology, etiology, pathophysiology and diagnosis of the acute compartment syndrome of the extremity. *European Journal of Trauma & Emergency Surgery*, 33(6), 576–583.

Kearon, C., Kahn, S. R., Agnelli, G., et al. (2008). Antithrombotic therapy for venous thromboembolic disease. American College of Chest Physicians evidence-based clinical practice guidelines. *Chest*, 133(Suppl. 6), 454S–545S.

Khan, R. J., Carey-Smith, R. L., Alakeson, R., et al. (2006). Operative and nonoperative treatment options for dislocation of the hip following total hip arthroplasty: A perioperative pain experience. *Cochrane Database of Systematic Reviews*, CD005320.

Konstantakos, E. K., Dalstrom, D. J., Nelles, M. E., et al. (2007). Diagnosis and management of extremity compartment syndromes: An orthopaedic perspective. *American Surgeon*, 73(12), 1199–1209.

Lethaby, A., Temple, J. & Santy, J. (2008). Pin site care for preventing infections associated with external bone fixators and pins. *Cochrane Database of Systematic Reviews*, CD004551.

Lucas, B. (2008a). Total hip and total knee replacement: Preoperative nursing management. *British Journal of Nursing*, 17(21), 1346–1351.

Lucas, B. (2008b). Total hip and total knee replacement: Postoperative nursing management. *British Journal of Nursing*, 17(22), 1410–1414.

Marx, R. G., Jones, E. C., Atwan, N. C., et al. (2005). Measuring improvement following total hip and knee arthroplasty using patient-based measures of outcome. *Journal of Bone and Joint Surgery*, 87(9), 1999–2005.

* McMurray, A., Grant, S., Griffiths, S., et al. (2005). Mapping recovery after total hip replacement surgery: Health-related quality of life after three years. *Australian Journal of Advanced Nursing*, 22(4), 20–25.

Milne, S., Brosseau, L., Robinson, V., et al. (2008). Continuous passive motion following total knee arthroplasty. *Cochrane Database of Systematic Reviews*, CD004260.

Nash, C. E., Mickan, S. M., Del Mar, C. B., et al. (2005). Injured limbs recover better with early mobilization and function bracing than cast immobilization. *The Journal of Bone and Joint Surgery*, 87(5), 1167.

O'Connor, C. & Murphy, S. (2007). Pneumatic tourniquet use in the perioperative environment. *Journal of Perioperative Practice*, 17(8), 391–397.

Rasanen, P., Paavolainen, P., Sintonen, H., et al. (2007). Effectiveness of hip or knee replacement surgery in terms of quality-adjusted life years and costs. *Acta Orthopaedica*, 78(1), 108–115.

Sanchez-Sotelo, J., Haidukewych, G. J. & Boberg, C. J. (2006). Hospital cost of dislocation after primary total hip arthroplasty. *Journal of Bone and Joint Surgery*, 88(2), 290–294.

*Stomberg, M. W. & Oman, U. (2006). Patients undergoing total hip arthroplasty: A perioperative pain experience. *Journal of Clinical Nursing*, 15(4), 451–458.

Wald, H. L., Ma, A., Bratzler, D. W., et al. (2008). Indwelling urinary catheter use in the postoperative period: Analysis of the national surgical infection prevention project data. *Archives of Surgery*, 143(6), 551–557.

RESOURCES

National Association of Orthopaedic Nurses (NAON), www.orthonurse.org

National Institute of Arthritis and Musculoskeletal and Skin Diseases, National Institutes of Health, www.niams.nih.gov

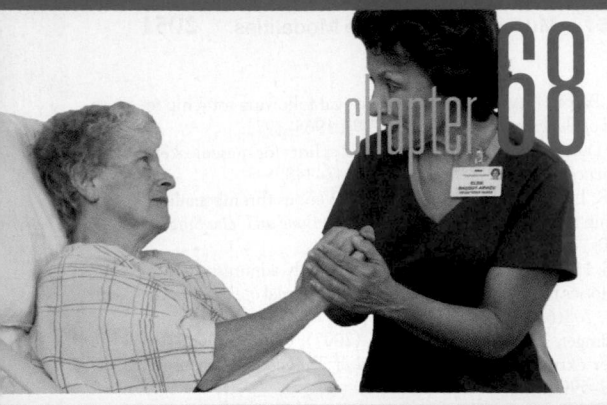

Chapter 68

Management of Patients With Musculoskeletal Disorders

LEARNING OBJECTIVES

On completion of this chapter, the learner will be able to:

1 Describe the nursing management, rehabilitation, and health education needs of the patient with low back pain.

2 Identify common conditions of the hand or wrist and nursing care of the patient undergoing surgery of the hand or wrist.

3 Describe common conditions of the foot and nursing care of the patient undergoing foot surgery.

4 Explain the pathophysiology, pathogenesis, prevention, and management of osteoporosis.

5 Use the nursing process as a framework for care of the patient with osteoporosis.

6 Identify the causes and related medical management of osteomalacia.

7 Identify medication modalities for the patient with Paget's disease.

8 Use the nursing process as a framework for care of the patient with osteomyelitis.

9 Describe the nursing management of the patient with a bone tumor.

GLOSSARY

bursitis: inflammation of a fluid-filled sac in a joint

contracture: abnormal shortening of muscle or fibrosis of joint structures

involucrum: new bone growth around a sequestrum

radiculopathy: disease of a nerve root

sciatica: sciatic nerve pain; pain travels down back of thigh into foot

sequestrum: dead bone in abscess cavity

tendinitis: inflammation of muscle tendons

Musculoskeletal disorders, particularly impairment of the back and spine, are leading health problems and causes of disability. The functional and psychological limitations imposed on the patient may be severe. The economic costs, in terms of loss of productivity, medical expenses, and other costs that are not compensated, are estimated to exceed $100 billion in direct and indirect costs in North America yearly (Sahar, Cohen, Matan, et al., 2008).

Low Back Pain

The number of visits to primary care providers resulting from low back pain is second only to the number of visits for upper respiratory illnesses (Sahar, et al., 2008). Most low back pain is caused by one of many musculoskeletal problems, including acute lumbosacral strain, unstable lumbosacral ligaments and weak muscles, osteoarthritis of the spine, spinal stenosis, intervertebral disk problems, and unequal leg length. Obesity, stress, and occasionally depression may contribute to low back pain. Back pain due to musculoskeletal disorders usually is aggravated by activity, whereas pain due to other conditions is not.

Older patients may experience back pain associated with osteoporotic vertebral fractures, osteoarthritis of the spine and spinal stenosis (Weiner, Sakamoto, Perera, et al., 2006). Other causes include kidney disorders, pelvic problems, retroperitoneal tumors, and abdominal aortic aneurysms.

Pathophysiology

The spinal column can be considered an elastic rod constructed of rigid units (vertebrae) and flexible units (intervertebral disks) held together by complex facet joints, multiple ligaments, and paravertebral muscles. Its unique construction allows for flexibility while providing maximum protection for the spinal cord. The spinal curves absorb vertical shocks from running and jumping. The trunk muscles help stabilize the spine. The abdominal and thoracic muscles are important in lifting activities, working together to minimize stress on the spinal units. Disuse weakens these supporting muscular structures. Obesity, postural problems, structural problems, and overstretching of the spinal supports may result in back pain (Porth & Matfin, 2009).

The intervertebral disks change in character as a person ages. A young person's disks are mainly fibrocartilage with a gelatinous matrix. As a person ages, the fibrocartilage becomes dense and irregularly shaped. Disk degeneration is a common cause of back pain. The lower lumbar disks, L4–L5 and L5–S1, are subject to the greatest mechanical stress and the greatest degenerative changes. Disk protrusion (herniated nucleus pulposus) or facet joint changes can cause pressure on nerve roots as they leave the spinal canal, which results in pain that radiates along the nerve (Porth & Matfin, 2009). Management of intervertebral disk disease is discussed in Chapter 65.

Clinical Manifestations

The typical patient reports either acute back pain (lasting less than 3 months) or chronic back pain (lasting more than 3 months without improvement) and fatigue. The patient

may report pain radiating down the leg, which is known as **radiculopathy** or **sciatica;** presence of this symptom suggests nerve root involvement. The patient's gait, spinal mobility, reflexes, leg length, leg motor strength, and sensory perception may be affected. Physical examination may disclose paravertebral muscle spasm (greatly increased muscle tone of the back postural muscles) with a loss of the normal lumbar curve and possible spinal deformity.

Assessment and Diagnostic Findings

The initial evaluation of acute low back pain includes a focused history and physical examination, including general observation of the patient, back examination, and neurologic testing (reflexes, sensory impairment, straight-leg raising, muscle strength, and muscle atrophy). The findings suggest either nonspecific back symptoms or potentially serious problems, such as sciatica, spine fracture, cancer, infection, or rapidly progressing neurologic deficit. If the initial examination does not suggest a serious condition, no additional testing is performed during the first 4 weeks of symptoms.

The diagnostic procedures described in Chart 68-1 may be indicated for the patient with potentially serious or prolonged low back pain. The nurse prepares the patient for these studies, provides the necessary support during the testing period, and monitors the patient for any adverse responses to the procedures.

Medical Management

Most back pain is self-limited and resolves within 4 weeks with analgesic agents, rest, and relaxation. Based on initial assessment findings, the patient is reassured that the assessment indicates that the back pain is not due to a serious condition. Management focuses on relief of pain and discomfort, activity modification, and patient education.

Nonprescription analgesic agents such as acetaminophen (Tylenol) and nonsteroidal anti-inflammatory drugs (NSAIDs) (eg, ibuprofen [Motrin]) and prescription muscle

---

Chart 68-1 • *Diagnostic Procedures for Low Back Pain*

X-ray of the spine—may demonstrate a fracture, dislocation, infection, osteoarthritis, or scoliosis

Bone scan and blood studies—may disclose infections, tumors, and bone marrow abnormalities

Computed tomography (CT)—useful in identifying underlying problems, such as obscure soft tissue lesions adjacent to the vertebral column and problems of vertebral disks

Magnetic resonance imaging (MRI)—permits visualization of the nature and location of spinal pathology

Electromyogram (EMG) and nerve conduction studies—used to evaluate spinal nerve root disorders (radiculopathies)

Myelogram—permits visualization of segments of the spinal cord that may have herniated or may be compressed

Ultrasound—useful in detecting tears in ligaments, muscles, tendons, and soft tissues in the back

relaxants (eg, cyclobenzaprine [Flexeril]) are effective in relieving acute low back pain, while tricyclic antidepressants (eg, amitriptyline [Elavil) are effective in relieving chronic low back pain. Other medications, including opioids (eg, morphine), tramadol (Ultram), benzodiazepines (eg, diazepam [Valium]), and gabapentin (Neurontin) (ie, prescribed for pain from radiculopathy) are also effective, though the evidence of their effectiveness is not as strong as that for the previously noted medications. Systemic corticosteroids are generally not considered effective in alleviating low back pain (Chou & Huffman, 2007b).

Effective nonpharmacologic interventions for acute low back pain include the application of superficial heat and spinal manipulation (eg, chiropractic therapy). Cognitive-behavioral therapy (eg, biofeedback), exercise regimens, spinal manipulation, physical therapy, acupuncture, massage, and yoga are all effective nonpharmacologic interventions for treating chronic low back pain but not acute low back pain (Chou & Huffman, 2007a).

Most patients need to alter their activity patterns to avoid aggravating the pain. They should avoid twisting, bending, lifting, and reaching, all of which stress the back. The patient is taught to change position frequently. Sitting should be limited to 20 to 50 minutes based on level of comfort. Bed rest is recommended for 1 to 2 days, for a maximum of 4 days and *only* if pain is severe. A gradual return to activities and a program of low-stress aerobic exercise are recommended. Conditioning exercises for the trunk muscles are begun after about 2 weeks.

If there is no improvement within 1 month, additional assessments for physiologic abnormalities are performed. Management is based on findings.

Nursing Assessment

The nurse asks the patient with low back pain to describe the discomfort (eg, location, severity, duration, characteristics, radiation, associated weakness in the legs). Descriptions of how the pain occurred—with a specific action (eg, opening a garage door) or with an activity in which weak muscles were overused (eg, weekend gardening)—and how the patient has dealt with the pain often suggest areas for intervention and patient teaching.

If back pain is a recurrent problem, information about previous successful pain control methods helps in planning current management. The nurse also asks how the back pain affects the patient's lifestyle. Information about work and recreational activities helps identify areas for back health education. Because stress and anxiety can evoke muscle spasms and pain, the nurse assesses environmental variables, work situations, and family relationships. In addition, the nurse assesses the effect of chronic pain on the emotional well-being of the patient. Referral to a mental health professional (eg, psychiatric advanced practice nurse) for assessment and management of stressors contributing to the low back pain and related depression may be appropriate.

During the interview, the nurse observes the patient's posture, position changes, and gait. Often, the patient's movements are guarded, with the back kept as still as possible. The patient often selects a chair of standard seat height with arms for support. The patient may sit and stand in an unusual position, leaning away from the most painful side, and may ask for assistance when undressing for the physical examination.

On physical examination, the nurse assesses the spinal curve, any leg length discrepancy, and pelvic crest and shoulder symmetry. The nurse palpates the paraspinal muscles and notes spasm and tenderness. When the patient is in a prone position, the paraspinal muscles relax, and any deformity caused by spasm subsides. The nurse asks the patient to bend forward and then laterally and notes any discomfort or limitations in movement. It is important to determine the effect of these limitations in movement on activities of daily living (ADLs). The nurse evaluates nerve involvement by assessing deep tendon reflexes, sensations (eg, paresthesia), and muscle strength. Back and leg pain on straight-leg raising (with the patient supine, the patient's leg is lifted upward with the knee extended) suggest nerve root involvement. Obesity can contribute to low back pain. If the patient is obese, the nurse completes a nutritional assessment (see Chapter 5) (Bickley, 2007).

Nursing Management

The major nursing goals for the patient may include relief of pain, improved physical mobility, use of back-conserving techniques of body mechanics, improved self-esteem, and weight reduction (as necessary) (Chart 68-2).

The nurse assesses the patient's response to analgesic agents. As the acute pain subsides, medication dosages are reduced. The nurse evaluates and notes the patient's response to various pain management modalities. (Other generic interventions that may relieve pain are discussed in Chapter 13.)

The nurse instructs the patient with severe pain to limit activities for 1 to 2 days. Extended periods of inactivity are not effective and result in deconditioning. A firm, nonsagging mattress (a bed board may be used) is recommended. Lumbar flexion is increased by elevating the head and thorax 30 degrees using pillows or a foam wedge and slightly flexing the knees supported on a pillow. Alternatively, the patient can assume a lateral position with knees and hips flexed (curled position) with a pillow between the knees and legs and a pillow supporting the head (Fig. 68-1). A prone position should be avoided because it accentuates lordosis. The nurse instructs the patient to get out of bed by rolling to one side and placing the legs down while pushing the torso up, keeping the back straight (National Institute of Neurological Disorders and Stroke [NINDS], 2009).

As the patient achieves comfort, activities are gradually resumed, and an exercise program is initiated. Initially, low-stress aerobic exercises, such as short walks or swimming, are suggested. After 2 weeks, conditioning exercises for the abdominal and trunk muscles are started. The physical therapist designs an exercise program for the individual patient to reduce lordosis, increase flexibility, and reduce strain on the back. It may include hyperextension exercises to strengthen the paravertebral muscles, flexion exercises to increase back movement and strength, and isometric flexion exercises to strengthen trunk muscles. Each exercise period begins with relaxation. Exercise begins gradually and increases as the patient recovers.

PATIENT EDUCATION
Strategies for Treating and Preventing Acute Low Back Pain

Treatment

- Limit bed rest; keep your knees flexed to decrease strain on your back.
- Try nonpharmacologic approaches such as application of superficial heat or chiropractic therapy.
- Pharmacologic approaches: Take nonsteroidal anti-inflammatory drugs, acetaminophen (Tylenol), and muscle relaxants as prescribed.
- Weight reduction as needed: Modify diet to achieve ideal body weight.

Prevention

Exercise

- Stretch to enhance flexibility. Do strengthening exercises.
- Perform prescribed back exercises to increase function, gradually increasing time and repetitions.

Body Mechanics

- Practice good posture.
- Avoid twisting your body.
- Push objects rather than pull them.
- Keep load close to your body when lifting.
- Bend your knees and tighten abdominal muscles when lifting.
- Avoid overreaching.
- Use a wide base of support.

Work Modifications

- Adjust work area to avoid stress on back.
- Adjust height of chair or work table.
- Use lumbar support in chair.
- Avoid prolonged standing and repetitive tasks.
- Avoid bending, twisting, and lifting heavy objects.
- Avoid work involving continuous vibrations.

The nurse encourages the patient to adhere to the prescribed exercise program. The patient should exercise 30 minutes daily using low-impact activities that may include speed walking, swimming, stationary bike riding, or yoga. Some patients may find it difficult to adhere to a program of prescribed exercises for a long period; in these instances, alternating activities may help facilitate compliance (NINDS, 2009). Patients are encouraged to improve their posture and use good body mechanics on a regular basis. Activities should not cause excessive lumbar strain, twisting, or discomfort; for example, activities such as horseback riding and weight lifting should be avoided.

Good body mechanics and posture are essential to avoid recurrence of back pain. The patient must be taught how to stand, sit, lie, and lift properly (Fig. 68-2). Providing the patient with a list of suggestions helps in making these long-term changes (Chart 68-3). The patient who wears high heels is encouraged to change to low heels with good arch support. The patient who is required to stand for long periods should shift weight frequently and should rest one foot on a low stool, which decreases lumbar lordosis. Patients who stand in place for a long period of time (eg, cashiers)

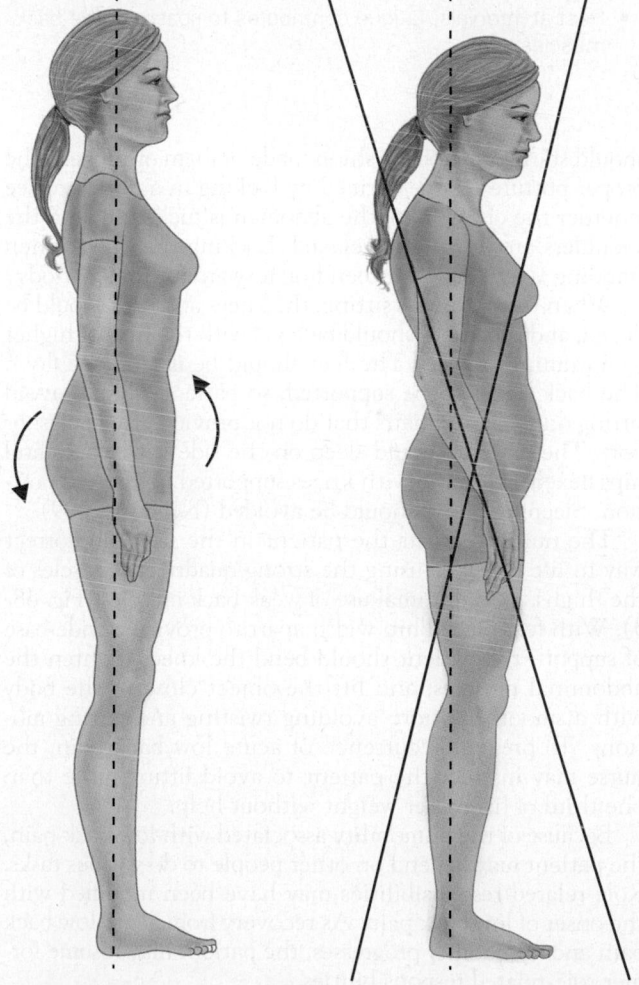

Figure 68-2 Proper and improper standing postures. **Left,** Abdominal muscles contracted, giving a feeling of upward pull, and gluteal muscles contracted, giving a downward pull. **Right,** Slouch position, showing abdominal muscles relaxed and body out of proper alignment.

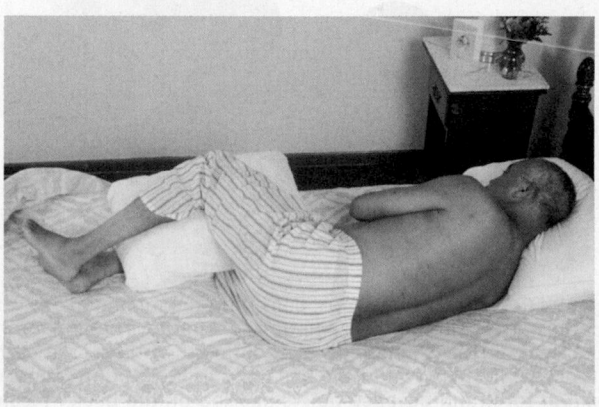

Figure 68-1 Positioning to promote lumbar flexion. © B. Proud.

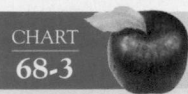

HEALTH PROMOTION
Activities to Promote a Healthy Back

CHART 68-3

Standing. Advise the patient to adhere to the following guidelines:
- Avoid prolonged standing and walking.
- When standing for any length of time, rest one foot on a small stool or box to relieve lumbar lordosis.
- Avoid forward flexion work positions.
- Avoid high heels.

Sitting. Discuss the following strategies with the patient:
- Avoid sitting for prolonged periods.
- Sit in a straight-back chair with back well supported and arm rests to support some of the body weight; use a footstool to position knees higher than hips if necessary.
- Eradicate the hollow of the back by sitting with the buttocks "tucked under."
- Maintain back support; use a soft support at the small of the back.
- Avoid knee and hip extension. When driving a car, have the seat pushed forward as far as possible for comfort.
- Guard against extension strains—reaching, pushing, sitting with legs straight out.
- Alternate periods of sitting with walking.

Lying. Encourage the patient to do the following:
- Rest at intervals; fatigue contributes to spasm of the back muscles.

- Place a firm bed board under the mattress.
- Avoid sleeping in a prone position.
- When lying on the side, place a pillow under the head and one between the legs, with the legs flexed at the hips and knees.
- When supine, use a pillow under the knees to decrease lordosis.

Lifting. Emphasize the importance of the following strategies:
- When lifting, keep the back straight and hold the load as close to the body as possible.
- Lift with the large leg muscles, not the back muscles.
- Use trunk muscles to stabilize the spine.
- Squat while keeping the back straight when it is necessary to pick something off the floor.
- Avoid twisting the trunk of the body, lifting above waist level, and reaching up for any length of time.

Exercising. Daily exercise is important in the prevention of back problems.
- Walk daily and gradually increase the distance and pace of walking.
- Perform prescribed back exercises twice daily, increasing exercise gradually.
- Avoid jumping and jarring activities.

should stand on a foot cushion made of foam or rubber. The proper posture can be verified by looking in a mirror to see whether the chest is up, the abdomen is tucked in, and the shoulders are down and relaxed. Locking the knees when standing is avoided, as is bending forward for long periods.

When the patient is sitting, the knees and hips should be flexed, and the knees should be level with the hips or higher to minimize lordosis. The feet should be flat on the floor. The back needs to be supported, so patients should avoid sitting on stools or chairs that do not provide firm back support. The patient should sleep on the side with knees and hips flexed, or supine with knees supported in a flexed position. Sleeping prone should be avoided (NINDS, 2009).

The nurse instructs the patient in the safe and correct way to lift objects—using the strong quadriceps muscles of the thighs, with minimal use of weak back muscles (Fig. 68-3). With feet placed hip-width apart to provide a wide base of support, the patient should bend the knees, tighten the abdominal muscles, and lift the object close to the body with a smooth motion, avoiding twisting and jarring motions. To prevent recurrence of acute low back pain, the nurse may instruct the patient to avoid lifting more than one third of his or her weight without help.

Because of the immobility associated with low back pain, the patient may depend on other people to do various tasks. Role-related responsibilities may have been modified with the onset of low back pain. As recovery from acute low back pain and immobility progresses, the patient may resume former role-related responsibilities.

However, if these activities contributed to the development of low back pain, it may be difficult to resume them without the development of chronic low back pain, with associated disability and depression. If the patient experi-

ences secondary gains associated with low back disability (eg, worker's compensation, easier lifestyle or workload, increased emotional support), a "low back neurosis" may develop. The patient may need help in coping with specific stressors and in learning how to control stressful situations. Psychotherapy or counseling may be needed to assist the person in resuming a full, productive life. Back clinics use multidisciplinary approaches to help the patient with pain and with resumption of role-related responsibilities.

Obesity contributes to back strain by stressing the relatively weak back muscles. Exercises are less effective and more difficult to perform when the patient is overweight. Weight reduction through diet modification may prevent

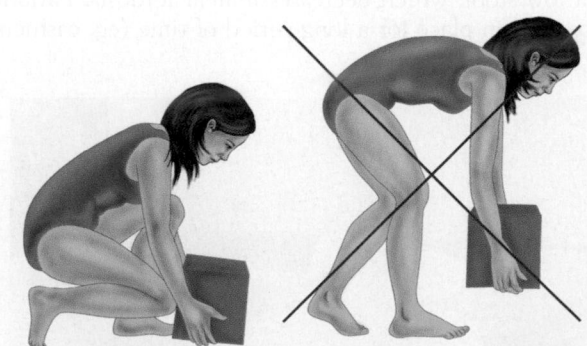

Figure 68-3 Proper and improper lifting techniques. **Left,** Correct position for lifting. This person is using the long and strong muscles of the arms and legs and holding the object so that the line of gravity falls within the base of support. **Right,** Incorrect position for lifting because pull is exerted on the back muscles and leaning causes the line of gravity to fall outside the base.

recurrence of back pain. Weight reduction is based on a sound nutritional plan that includes a change in eating habits to maintain desirable weight. Monitoring weight reduction, noting achievement, and providing encouragement and positive reinforcement facilitate adherence. Frequently, back problems resolve as optimal weight is achieved (NINDS, 2009).

Common Upper Extremity Problems

The structures in the upper extremities are frequently the sites of painful syndromes. The structures most frequently affected are the shoulder, wrist, and hand.

BURSITIS AND TENDINITIS

Bursitis and **tendinitis** are inflammatory conditions that commonly occur in the shoulder. Bursae are fluid-filled sacs that prevent friction between joint structures during joint activity. When inflamed, they are painful. Similarly, muscle tendon sheaths become inflamed with repetitive stretching. The inflammation causes proliferation of synovial membrane and pannus formation, which restricts joint movement. Traditional conservative treatment includes rest of the extremity, intermittent ice and heat to the joint, and NSAIDs to control the inflammation and pain. Newer therapies that include extracorporeal shock wave therapy (ie, use of focused high-intensity acoustic radiation), pulsed magnetic field therapy, laser phototherapy, and radiofrequency coblation therapy (ie, use of focused radiowaves) may accelerate tendon healing, although further research is needed to determine their overall effectiveness (Sharma & Maffulli, 2005). Arthroscopic synovectomy may be considered if shoulder pain and weakness persist.

LOOSE BODIES

Loose bodies may occur in a joint as a result of articular cartilage wear and bone erosion. These fragments interfere with joint movement, locking the joint, resulting in painful movement. Loose bodies are removed by arthroscopic surgery.

IMPINGEMENT SYNDROME

Impingement syndrome is a general term that describes all lesions that involve the rotator cuff of the shoulder (Trampas & Kitsios, 2006). Impingement usually occurs from repetitive overhead movement of the arm or from acute trauma (Trojian, Stevenson & Agrawal, 2005), resulting in irritation and eventual inflammation of the rotator cuff tendons or the subacromial bursa as they grate against the coracoacromial arch. Stage I impingement syndrome is characterized by edema and hemorrhage of the rotator cuff tendons or subacromial bursa (Trampas & Kitsios, 2006). The patient experiences pain, shoulder tenderness, limited movement, muscle spasm, and eventual atrophy. The process may progress to a partial or complete rotator cuff tear (referred to as Stage II or Stage III impingement syndrome, respectively (Trojian, et al., 2005) (see Chapter 69 for a discussion of rotator cuff tears).

Medications used to treat Stage I impingement syndrome include oral NSAIDs (eg, ibuprofen) or intra-articular (ie, subacromial) injections of corticosteroids (eg, triamcinolone [Aristocort]). Treatment with corticosteroids generally results in speedier symptomatic improvement than that with NSAIDs, though the use of both medications concomitantly does not appear to confer any additional improvements (Trojian, et al., 2005). Application of superficial cold or heat does not improve patients' symptoms, but a therapeutic exercise program (eg, physical therapy) does reduce pain and improve shoulder function (Trampas & Kitsios, 2006) (Chart 68-4).

CARPAL TUNNEL SYNDROME

Carpal tunnel syndrome is an entrapment neuropathy that occurs when the median nerve at the wrist is compressed by a thickened flexor tendon sheath, skeletal encroachment, edema, or a soft tissue mass. It most commonly occurs in women between 30 and 60 years of age. It is commonly caused by repetitive hand and wrist movements, but it may also be associated with arthritis, diabetes, tumors, or trauma (Schoen, 2005). Patients who perform repetitive movements or those whose hands are repeatedly exposed to cold temperatures, vibrations, or extreme direct pressure are at an increased risk for carpal tunnel syndrome. The patient experiences pain, numbness, paresthesia, and possibly weakness along the median nerve (thumb, index, and middle fingers). Tinel's sign may be used to help identify carpal tunnel syndrome (Fig. 68-4). Night pain is common.

Treatment of carpal tunnel syndrome is based on the cause of the condition. Research findings suggest that intra-articular injections of corticosteroids (eg, methylprednisolone [Medrol]) or oral corticosteroids (eg, prednisone) are very effective at relieving symptoms. Application of wrist splints to prevent hyperextension and prolonged

---

CHART **68-4** PATIENT EDUCATION
Measures to Promote Shoulder Healing of Impingement Syndrome

- Rest the joint in a position that minimizes stress on the joint structures to prevent further damage and the development of adhesions.
- Support the affected arm on pillows while sleeping to keep from turning onto the shoulder.
- Gradually resume motion and use of the joint. Assistance with dressing and other activities of daily living may be needed.

- Avoid working and lifting above shoulder level or pushing an object against a "locked" shoulder.
- Perform the prescribed daily range-of-motion and strengthening exercises.

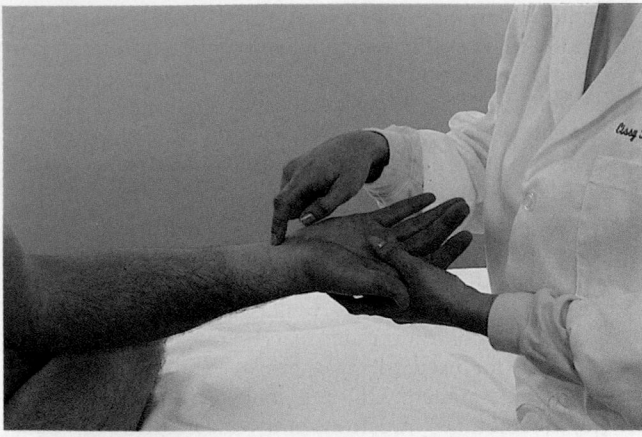

Figure 68-4 Tinel's sign may be elicited in patients with carpal tunnel syndrome by percussing lightly over the median nerve, located on the inner aspect of the wrist. If the patient reports tingling, numbness, and pain, the test for Tinel's sign is considered positive. From Weber, J. W. & Kelley, J. (2006). *Health assessment in nursing* (3rd ed.). Philadelphia: Lippincott Williams & Wilkins. © B. Proud.

flexion of the wrist are also effective interventions. However, yoga, laser therapy, and ultrasound therapy are ineffective therapies, as are the use of NSAIDs, diuretics, and vitamin B_6 (Piazzini, Aprile, Ferrara, et al., 2007).

Traditional open nerve release or endoscopic laser surgery are the two most common surgical management options for treatment of carpal tunnel syndrome. Both of these procedures are performed under local anesthesia and involve making small incisions into the affected wrist, cutting the carpal ligament so that the carpal tunnel is widened. Smaller incisions are made with the endoscopic laser procedure, and there is less scar formation and a shorter recovery time than with the open method. Following either of these procedures, the patient wears a hand splint and limits hand use during healing. The patient may need assistance with personal care and ADLs. Full recovery of motor and sensory function after either type of nerve release surgery may take several weeks or months.

GANGLION

A ganglion, a collection of gelatinous material near the tendon sheaths and joints, appears as a round, firm, cystic swelling, usually on the dorsum of the wrist. It most frequently occurs in women younger than 50 years. The ganglion is locally tender and may cause an aching pain. When a tendon sheath is involved, weakness of the finger occurs. Treatment may include aspiration, corticosteroid injection, or surgical excision. After treatment, a compression dressing and immobilization splint are used.

DUPUYTREN'S DISEASE

Dupuytren's disease results in a slowly progressive **contracture** of the palmar fascia, called Dupuytren's contracture, which causes flexion of the fourth and fifth fingers, and frequently the middle finger. This renders the fingers more or less useless (Fig. 68-5). It is caused by an inherited autosomal dominant trait and occurs most frequently in men who

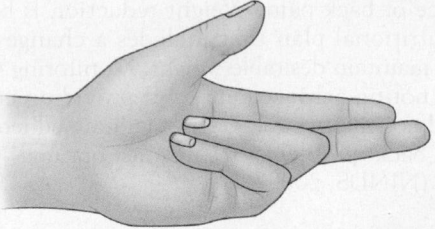

Figure 68-5 Dupuytren's contracture, a flexion deformity caused by an inherited trait, is a slowly progressive contracture of the palmar fascia, which severely impairs the function of the fourth, fifth, and, sometimes, middle finger.

are older than 50 years and who are of Scandinavian or Celtic origin. It is also associated with arthritis, diabetes, gout, cigarette smoking, and alcoholism (Childs, 2005). It starts as a nodule of the palmar fascia. The nodule may not change, or it may progress so that the fibrous thickening extends to involve the skin in the distal palm and produces a contracture of the fingers. The patient may experience dull aching discomfort, morning numbness, cramping, and stiffness in the affected fingers. This condition starts in one hand, but eventually both hands are affected. Finger-stretching exercises or intranodular injections of corticosteroids (eg, triamcinolone) may prevent contractures (Trojian & Chu, 2007). With contracture development, palmar and digital fasciectomies are performed to improve function. Finger exercises are begun on postoperative day 1 or 2.

NURSING MANAGEMENT OF THE PATIENT UNDERGOING SURGERY OF THE HAND OR WRIST

Surgery of the hand or wrist, unless related to major trauma, is generally an ambulatory procedure. Before surgery, the nurse assesses the patient's level and type of discomfort and limitations in function caused by the ganglion, carpal tunnel syndrome, Dupuytren's contracture, or other condition of the hand.

Neurovascular assessment of the exposed fingers every hour for the first 24 hours following surgery is essential for monitoring function of the nerves and perfusion of the hand. The nurse instructs the patient and any family caregivers on these parameters for periodic neurovascular assessment and gives instructions on when to notify the physician. The nurse compares the affected hand with the unaffected hand and the postoperative status with the documented preoperative status. The patient describes sensations in the hands and demonstrates finger mobility. With tendon repairs and nerve, vascular, or skin grafts, motor function is tested as necessary. The temperature of the affected hand is assessed. Dressings provide support but are nonconstrictive. Pain uncontrolled by analgesic agents suggests compromised neurovascular functioning.

Pain may be related to surgery, edema, hematoma formation, or restrictive bandages. To control swelling that may increase the patient's pain and discomfort, the nurse instructs the patient to elevate the hand to heart level with pillows. If the patient is ambulatory, the arm is elevated in a conventional sling with the hand at heart level.

CHART 68-5	HOME CARE CHECKLIST *Hand Surgery*		
At the completion of the home care instruction, the patient or caregiver will be able to:		**PATIENT**	**CAREGIVER**
• Demonstrate how to assess neurovascular status.		✔	✔
• State abnormal findings (eg, unrelenting pain; paralysis; paresthesia; cool, nonblanching fingers) to report to physician promptly.		✔	✔
• Demonstrate control of edema by elevating hand above elbow and applying ice intermittently if prescribed.		✔	✔
• Identify signs and symptoms of infection (eg, elevated temperature, purulent drainage).		✔	✔
• Demonstrate finger exercises to promote circulation, unless contraindicated.		✔	
• Describe methods to prevent wound infection (eg, keeping hand dressing clean and dry during activities of daily living).		✔	✔
• Describe use of prescribed medications.		✔	✔
• Demonstrate use of assistive devices, if appropriate.		✔	

Intermittent use of ice packs to the surgical area during the first 24 to 48 hours may be prescribed to control edema. Unless contraindicated, active extension and flexion of the fingers to promote circulation are encouraged, even though movement is limited by the bulky dressing.

Generally, the pain and discomfort can be controlled by oral analgesic agents. If the patient is hospitalized, the nurse evaluates the patient's response to analgesic agents and to other pain control measures. Patient education concerning analgesic agents is important.

During the first few days after surgery, the patient needs assistance with ADLs because one hand is bandaged and independent self-care is impaired. The patient may need to arrange for assistance with feeding, bathing and hygiene, dressing, grooming, and toileting. Within a few days, the patient develops skills in one-handed ADLs and is usually able to function with minimal assistance and use of assistive devices. The nurse encourages the patient to use the involved hand, unless contraindicated, within the limits of discomfort. As rehabilitation progresses, the patient resumes use of the injured hand. Physical or occupational therapy–directed exercises may be prescribed. The nurse emphasizes compliance with the therapeutic regimen.

As with all surgery, there is a risk of infection. The nurse teaches the patient to monitor temperature and signs and symptoms that suggest an infection. It also is important to instruct the patient to keep the dressing clean and dry and to report any drainage, foul odor, or increased pain and swelling. Patient education includes aseptic wound care as well as education related to prescribed prophylactic antibiotics.

Promoting Home and Community-Based Care

Teaching Patients Self-Care

After the patient has undergone hand surgery, the nurse teaches the patient how to monitor neurovascular status and the signs of complications that need to be reported to the surgeon (eg, paresthesia, paralysis, uncontrolled pain, coolness of fingers, extreme swelling, excessive bleeding, purulent drainage, fever). The nurse discusses prescribed medications with the patient. In addition, the nurse teaches the

patient to elevate the hand above the elbow and to apply ice (if prescribed) to control swelling. Unless contraindicated, the nurse encourages extension and flexion exercises of the fingers to promote circulation. The use of assistive devices is encouraged if they would be helpful in promoting accomplishment of ADLs. For bathing, the nurse instructs the patient to keep the dressing dry by covering it with a secured plastic bag. Generally, the wound is not redressed until the patient's follow-up visit with the surgeon (Chart 68-5).

Common Foot Problems

Disorders of the foot may be caused by poorly fitting shoes, which distort normal anatomy while inducing deformity and pain. Dermatologic problems commonly affect the feet in the form of fungal infections and plantar warts. Several systemic diseases affect the feet. Patients with diabetes are prone to develop corns and peripheral neuropathies with diminished sensation, leading to ulcers at pressure points of the foot. Patients with peripheral vascular disease and arteriosclerosis complain of burning and itching feet, resulting in scratching and skin breakdown. Foot deformities may occur with rheumatoid arthritis. Obesity can cause a host of foot anomalies, including plantar fasciitis (Cole, Seto & Gazewood, 2005).

The discomforts of foot strain are treated with rest, elevation, physiotherapy, supportive strappings, and orthotic devices. The patient must inspect the foot and skin under pads and orthotic devices for pressure and skin breakdown daily. If a "window" is cut into shoes to relieve pressure over a bony deformity, the skin must be monitored daily for breakdown from pressure exerted at the "window" area. Active foot exercises promote circulation and help strengthen the feet. Walking in properly fitting shoes is considered the ideal exercise.

PLANTAR FASCIITIS

Plantar fasciitis, an inflammation of the foot-supporting fascia, presents as an acute onset of heel pain experienced with the first steps in the morning. The pain is localized to the anterior medial aspect of the heel and diminishes with gentle stretching of the foot and Achilles tendon. Management includes stretching exercises, wearing shoes with support and cushioning to relieve pain, orthotic devices (eg, heel cups, arch supports, night splints), and corticosteroid injections (Cole, et al., 2005). Unresolved plantar fasciitis may progress to fascial tears at the heel and eventual development of heel spurs.

CORN

A corn is an area of hyperkeratosis (overgrowth of a horny layer of epidermis) produced by internal pressure (the underlying bone is prominent because of a congenital or acquired abnormality, commonly arthritis) or external pressure (ill-fitting shoes). The fifth toe is most frequently involved, but any toe may be involved.

Corns are treated by a podiatrist by soaking and scraping off the horny layer, by application of a protective shield or pad, or by surgical modification of the underlying offending osseous structure. Soft corns are located between the toes and are kept soft by moisture. Treatment consists of drying the affected spaces and separating the affected toes with lamb's wool or gauze. A wider shoe may be helpful. Usually, a podiatrist is consulted to treat the underlying cause.

CALLUS

A callus is a discretely thickened area of the skin that has been exposed to persistent pressure or friction. Faulty foot mechanics usually precede the formation of a callus. Treatment consists of eliminating the underlying causes and having the callus treated by a podiatrist if it is painful. A keratolytic ointment may be applied and a thin plastic cup worn over the heel if the callus is on this area. Felt padding with an adhesive backing is also used to prevent and relieve pressure. Orthotic devices can be made to remove the pressure from bony protuberances, or the protuberance may be excised.

INGROWN TOENAIL

An ingrown toenail (onychocryptosis) is a condition in which the free edge of a nail plate penetrates the surrounding skin, either laterally or anteriorly. A secondary infection or granulation tissue may develop. This painful condition is caused by improper self-treatment, external pressure (tight shoes or stockings), internal pressure (deformed toes, growth under the nail), trauma, or infection. Trimming the nails properly (clipping them straight across and filing the corners consistent with the contour of the toe) can prevent this problem. Active treatment consists of washing the foot twice a day, followed by the application of a local antibiotic ointment, and relieving the pain by decreasing the pressure of the nail plate on the surrounding soft tissue. Warm, wet soaks help drain an infection. A toenail may need to be excised by the podiatrist if there is severe infection.

HAMMER TOE

Hammer toe is a flexion deformity of the interphalangeal joint, which may involve several toes (Fig. 68-6A). The condition is usually an acquired deformity. Tight socks or shoes may push an overlying toe back into the line of the

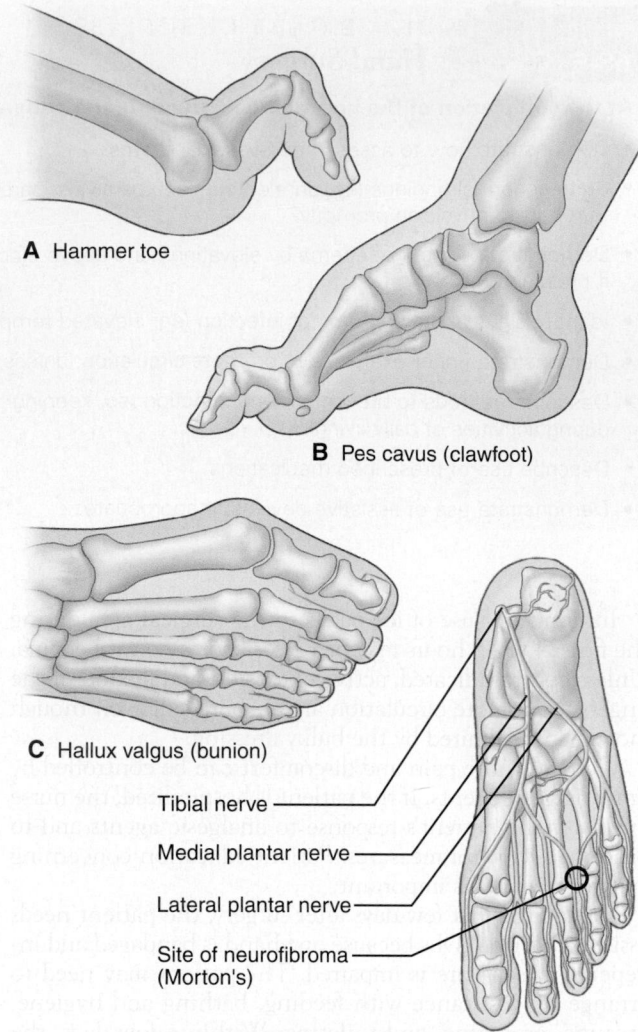

A Hammer toe

B Pes cavus (clawfoot)

C Hallux valgus (bunion)

Tibial nerve
Medial plantar nerve
Lateral plantar nerve
Site of neurofibroma (Morton's)

D Neurofibroma (Morton's neuroma)

Figure 68-6 Common foot deformities.

other toes. The toes usually are pulled upward, forcing the metatarsal joints (ball of the foot) downward. Corns develop on top of the toes, and tender calluses develop under the metatarsal area. The treatment consists of conservative measures: wearing open-toed sandals or shoes that conform to the shape of the foot, carrying out manipulative exercises, and protecting the protruding joints with pads. Surgery (osteotomy) may be used to correct a resulting deformity. There is little evidence to support treatment of hammer toe when the patient does not report pain or other symptoms (Badlissi, Dunn, Link, et al., 2005).

HALLUX VALGUS

Hallux valgus (commonly called a bunion) is a deformity in which the great toe deviates laterally (see Fig. 68-6C). Associated with this is a marked prominence of the medial aspect of the first metatarsophalangeal joint. There is also osseous enlargement (exostosis) of the medial side of the first metatarsal head, over which a bursa may form (secondary to pressure and inflammation). Acute bursitis symptoms include a reddened area, edema, and tenderness.

Factors contributing to bunion formation include heredity, ill-fitting shoes, and gradual lengthening and widening of the foot associated with aging. Osteoarthritis is frequently associated with hallux valgus. Treatment depends on the patient's age, the degree of deformity, and the severity of symptoms. If a bunion deformity is uncomplicated, wearing a shoe that conforms to the shape of the foot or that is molded to the foot to prevent pressure on the protruding portions may be the only treatment needed. Corticosteroid injections control acute inflammation. Surgical removal of the bunion (exostosis) and osteotomies to realign the toe may be required to improve function, appearance, and symptoms (Badlissi, et al., 2005). Complications related to bunionectomy include limited range of motion, paresthesias, tendon injury, and recurrence of deformity.

Postoperatively, the patient may have intense throbbing pain at the operative site, requiring opioid analgesia (eg, morphine). The foot is elevated to the level of the heart to decrease edema and pain. The neurovascular status of the toes is assessed. The duration of immobility and initiation of ambulation depend on the procedure used. Toe flexion and extension exercises are initiated to facilitate walking. Shoes that fit the shape and size of the foot are recommended.

PES CAVUS

Pes cavus (clawfoot) refers to a foot with an abnormally high arch and a fixed equinus deformity of the forefoot (see Fig. 68-6B). The shortening of the foot and increased pressure produce calluses on the metatarsal area and on the dorsum of the foot. Charcot-Marie-Tooth disease (a peripheral neuromuscular disease associated with a familial degenerative disorder), diabetes mellitus, and tertiary syphilis are common causes of pes cavus. Exercises are prescribed to manipulate the forefoot into dorsiflexion and relax the toes. Orthotic devices alleviate pain and can protect the foot (Burns, Landorf, Ryan, et al., 2008). In severe cases, arthrodesis (fusion) is performed to reshape and stabilize the foot.

MORTON'S NEUROMA

Morton's neuroma (plantar digital neuroma, neurofibroma) is a swelling of the third (lateral) branch of the median plantar nerve (see Fig. 68-6D). The third digital nerve, which is located in the third intermetatarsal (web) space, is most commonly involved. Microscopically, digital artery changes cause an ischemia of the nerve.

The result is a throbbing, burning pain in the foot that is usually relieved when the patient rests. Conservative treatment consists of inserting innersoles and metatarsal pads designed to spread the metatarsal heads and balance the foot posture. Local injections of a corticosteroid (eg, hydrocortisone [Acticort]) and a local anesthetic agent may provide relief. If these fail, surgical excision of the neuroma is necessary. Pain relief and loss of sensation are immediate and permanent.

FLATFOOT

Flatfoot (pes planus) is a common disorder in which the longitudinal arch of the foot is diminished. It may be caused by congenital abnormalities or associated with bone or ligament injury, muscle and posture imbalances, excessive weight, muscle fatigue, poorly fitting shoes, or arthritis. Signs and symptoms include a burning sensation, fatigue, clumsy gait, edema, and pain.

Exercises to strengthen the muscles and to improve posture and walking habits are helpful. A number of foot orthoses are available to give the foot additional support.

NURSING MANAGEMENT OF THE PATIENT UNDERGOING FOOT SURGERY

Surgery of the foot may be necessary because of various conditions, including neuromas and foot deformities (bunion, hammer toe, clawfoot). Generally, foot surgery is performed on an outpatient basis. Before surgery, the nurse assesses the patient's ambulatory ability and balance and the neurovascular status of the foot. Additionally, the nurse considers the availability of assistance at home and the structural characteristics of the home in planning for care during the first few days after surgery.

After surgery, neurovascular assessment of the exposed toes every 1 to 2 hours for the first 24 hours is essential to monitor the function of the nerves and the perfusion of the tissues. If the patient is discharged within several hours after the surgery, the nurse teaches the patient and family how to assess for edema and neurovascular status (circulation, motion, sensation). Compromised neurovascular function can increase the patient's pain (see Chart 66-3 in Chapter 66).

Pain experienced by patients who undergo foot surgery is related to inflammation and edema. Formation of a hematoma may contribute to the discomfort. To control the edema, the foot should be elevated on several pillows when the patient is sitting or lying. Ice packs applied intermittently to the surgical area during the first 24 to 48 hours may be prescribed to control edema and provide some pain relief. As activity increases, the patient may find that dependent positioning of the foot is uncomfortable. Simply elevating the foot often relieves the discomfort. Oral analgesic agents may be used to control the pain. The nurse instructs the patient and family about appropriate use of these medications.

After surgery, the patient will have a bulky dressing on the foot, protected by a light cast or a special protective boot. Limits for weight bearing on the foot will be prescribed by the surgeon. Some patients are allowed to walk on the heel and progress to weight bearing as tolerated; other patients are restricted to non–weight-bearing activities. Assistive devices (eg, crutches, walker) may be needed. The choice of the devices depends on the patient's general condition and balance and on the weight-bearing prescription. Safe use of the assistive devices must be ensured through adequate patient education and practice before discharge. Strategies to move around the house safely while using assistive devices are discussed with the patient. As healing progresses, the patient gradually resumes ambulation within prescribed limits. The nurse emphasizes compliance with the therapeutic regimen.

Any surgery carries a risk of infection. In addition, percutaneous pins may be used to hold bones in position, and these pins serve as potential sites for infection. Care must be taken

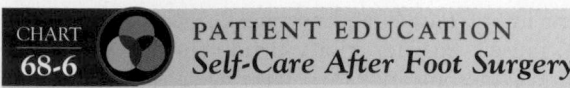

CHART 68-6

PATIENT EDUCATION
Self-Care After Foot Surgery

Neurovascular Status

The following signs and symptoms indicate impaired circulation and should be reported to your health care provider right away:

- Change in sensation
- Inability to move toes
- Toes or foot cool to touch
- Color changes

Pain Management

Methods to reduce pain include the following:

- Elevate foot to heart level.
- Apply ice as prescribed.
- Use analgesic agents as prescribed.
- Report pain that is not relieved.

Mobility

- Use assistive devices safely.
- Comply with prescribed weight-bearing limits.
- Wear special protective shoe over the dressing.

Wound Care

- Keep the dressing or cast clean and dry.
- Report signs of wound infection (eg, pain, drainage, fever) immediately.
- Follow the prescribed antibiotic regimen.
- Keep your appointment with the surgeon for the initial dressing change.

to protect the surgical wound from dirt and moisture. When bathing, the patient can secure a plastic bag over the dressing to prevent it from getting wet. Patient instructions concerning aseptic wound care and pin care may be necessary.

The nurse teaches the patient to monitor for temperature changes and infection. Drainage on the dressing, a foul odor, or increased pain and swelling could indicate infection. The nurse instructs the patient to promptly report any of these findings to the physician. If prophylactic antibiotics are prescribed, the nurse provides instruction about their correct use. The nurse plans patient teaching for home care, focusing on neurovascular status, pain management, mobility, and wound care (Chart 68-6).

Metabolic Bone Disorders

OSTEOPOROSIS

Osteoporosis is the most prevalent bone disease in the world. More than 10 million Americans have osteoporosis and an additional 33.6 million have osteopenia, the precursor to osteoporosis. The consequence of osteoporosis is bone fracture. It is projected that one of every two Caucasian women and one of every five men will have an osteoporosis-related fracture at some point in their lives (National Osteoporosis Foundation [NOF], 2008). The costs incurred from treating osteoporosis-related fractures in the United States are estimated at $20 billion annually (Sambrook & Cooper, 2006).

Prevention

Peak adult bone mass is achieved between the ages of 18 and 25 years in both females and males and is affected by genetic factors. Bone mass during these years is affected by nutrition, physical activity, medications, endocrine status, and general health (NOF, 2008). Risk factors for osteoporosis and their effects on bone remodeling and maintenance are noted in Figure 68-7.

Primary osteoporosis occurs in women after menopause (usually between the ages of 45 and 55 years) and in men later in life, but it is not merely a consequence of aging. Failure to develop optimal peak bone mass during childhood, adolescence, and young adulthood contributes to the development of osteoporosis. Early identification of at-risk

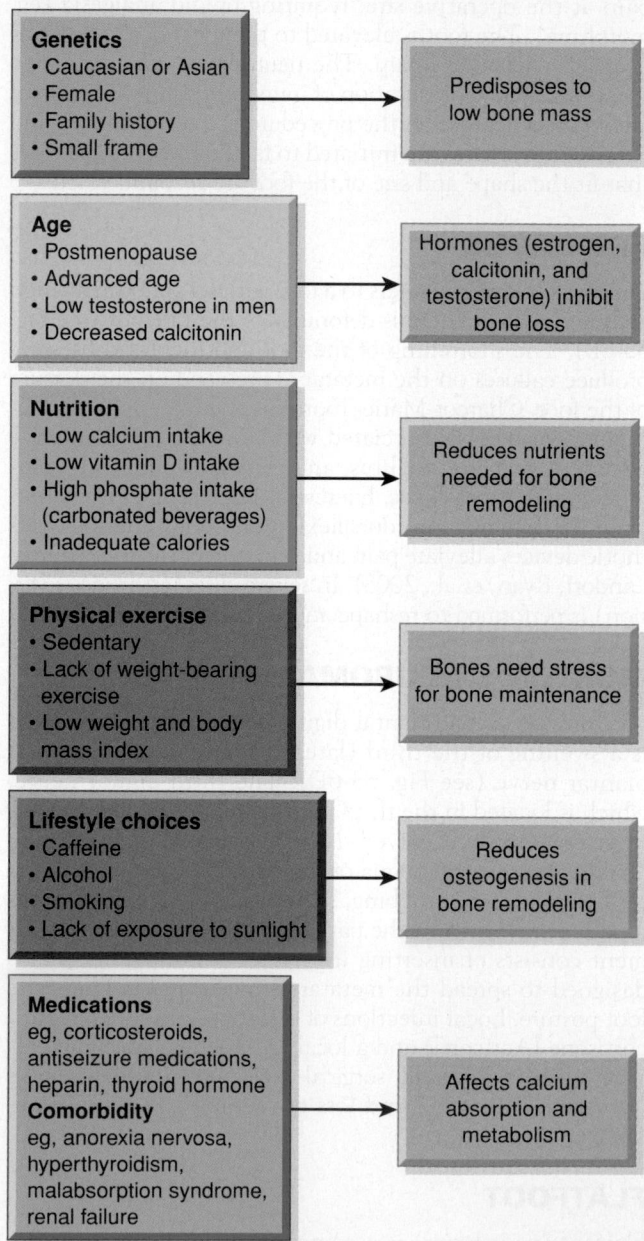

FIGURE 68-7 Risk factors for osteoporosis, and the effects of these factors on bone.

teenagers and young adults, increased calcium intake, participation in regular weight-bearing exercise, and modification of lifestyle (eg, reduced use of caffeine, cigarettes, carbonated soft drinks, and alcohol) are interventions that decrease the risk of osteoporosis, fractures, and associated disability later in life (NOF, 2008).

Secondary osteoporosis is the result of medications or other conditions and diseases that affect bone metabolism. Specific disease states (eg, celiac disease, hypogonadism) and medications (eg, corticosteroids, antiseizure medications) that place patients at risk need to be identified and therapies instituted to reverse the development of osteoporosis (NOF, 2008). The degree of osteoporosis is related to the duration of medication therapy. When the therapy is discontinued or the metabolic problem is corrected, the progression of osteoporosis is halted, but restoration of lost bone mass usually does not occur.

 Gerontologic Considerations

The prevalence of osteoporosis in women older than 80 years is 50%. The average 75-year-old woman has lost 25% of her cortical bone and 40% of her trabecular bone. With the aging of the population, the incidence of fractures (more than 1.5 million osteoporotic fractures per year), pain, and disability associated with osteoporosis is increasing. Most residents of long-term care facilities have a low bone mineral density (BMD) and are at risk for bone fracture. It is estimated that the number of hip fractures and their associated costs will at least double by the year 2040 because of the projected aging of the U.S. population (NOF, 2008).

Asymptomatic osteoporotic-related vertebral fractures are associated with loss of height, respiratory dysfunction, increased risk of mortality, and increased risk of subsequent fractures. Elderly men are also at heightened risk for osteoporosis and fractures. One third of all hip fractures occur among men and these tend to be more lethal than those seen in women. Men are more likely than women to have secondary causes of osteoporosis that may lead to fractures, including use of corticosteroids (eg, prednisone) and excessive alcohol intake (Ebeling, 2008).

Elderly people absorb dietary calcium less efficiently and excrete it more readily through their kidneys; therefore, postmenopausal women and the elderly need to consume approximately 1200 mg of daily calcium; quantities larger than this may place patients at heightened risk for renal calculi (ie, kidney stones) or cardiovascular disease (NOF, 2008).

Pathophysiology

Osteoporosis is characterized by reduced bone mass, deterioration of bone matrix, and diminished bone architectural strength. Normal homeostatic bone turnover is altered; the rate of bone resorption that is maintained by osteoclasts is greater than the rate of bone formation that is maintained by osteoblasts, resulting in a reduced total bone mass. The bones become progressively porous, brittle, and fragile; they fracture easily under stresses that would not break normal bone. These increase susceptibility to fracture, which occur most commonly as compression fractures (Fig. 68-8) of the

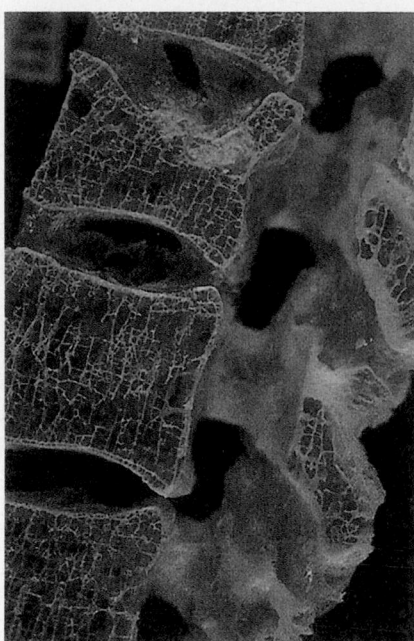

Figure 68-8 Progressive osteoporotic bone loss and compression fractures. From Rubin, E., Gorstein, F., Schwarting, R., et al. (2004). *Pathology* (4th ed.). Philadelphia: Lippincott Williams & Wilkins.

thoracic and lumbar spine, hip fractures, and Colles' fractures of the wrist. These fractures may be the first clinical manifestation of osteoporosis (NOF, 2008).

The gradual collapse of a vertebra may be asymptomatic; it is observed as progressive kyphosis. With the development of kyphosis (ie, "dowager's hump"), there is an associated loss of height (Fig. 68-9). The postural changes result in relaxation of the abdominal muscles and a protruding abdomen. The deformity may also produce pulmonary insufficiency.

Age-related loss begins soon after the peak bone mass is achieved (ie, in the fourth decade). Calcitonin, which inhibits bone resorption and promotes bone formation, is decreased. Estrogen, which inhibits bone breakdown, decreases with aging. On the other hand, parathyroid hormone (PTH) increases with aging, increasing bone turnover and resorption. The consequence of these changes is net loss of bone mass over time.

The withdrawal of estrogens at menopause or with oophorectomy causes an accelerated bone resorption that continues during the postmenopausal years. Women develop osteoporosis more frequently and more extensively than men because of lower peak bone mass and the effect of estrogen loss during menopause. More than half of all women older than 50 years show evidence of osteopenia.

Risk Factors

Small-framed, nonobese Caucasian women are at greatest risk for osteoporosis (see Fig. 68-7). Also, Asian women of slight build are at risk for low peak BMD. African American women, who have a greater bone mass than Caucasian women, are less susceptible to osteoporosis. Men have a greater peak bone mass and do not experience sudden

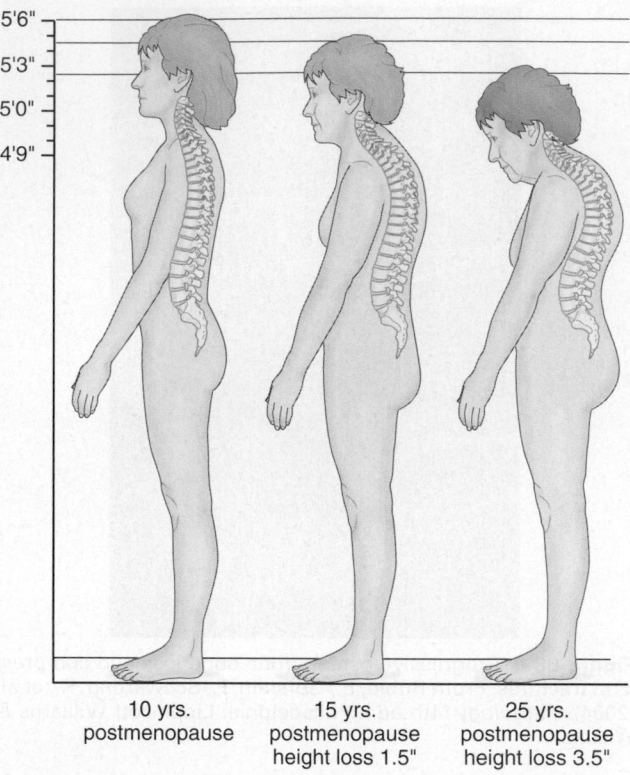

5'6"
5'3"
5'0"
4'9"

10 yrs.
postmenopause

15 yrs.
postmenopause
height loss 1.5"

25 yrs.
postmenopause
height loss 3.5"

Figure 68-9 Typical loss of height associated with osteoporosis and aging.

estrogen reduction. As a result, osteoporosis occurs in men at a lower rate and at an older age (about one decade later). It is believed that testosterone and estrogen are important in achieving and maintaining bone mass in men. Risk for osteoporosis increases with increasing age (Chart 68-7).

Nutritional factors contribute to the development of osteoporosis. A diet that includes adequate calories and nutrients needed to maintain bone, calcium, and vitamin D must be consumed. Vitamin D is necessary for calcium absorption and for normal bone mineralization. Dietary calcium and vitamin D must be adequate to maintain bone remodeling and body functions. The best source of calcium and vitamin D is fortified milk. A cup of milk or calcium-fortified orange juice contains about 300 mg of calcium. The recommended adequate intake (RAI) level of calcium for all individuals is 1000 to 1200 mg daily (NOF, 2008). The recommended vitamin D intake for adults 50 years of age and older is 800 to 1000 international units (IU) daily (NOF, 2008). Patients who have had bariatric surgery are at increased risk for osteoporosis as the duodenum is bypassed, which is the primary site for absorption of calcium (Hogan, 2005), as are patients who have gastrointestinal diseases that cause malabsorption (eg, celiac disease).

Bone formation is enhanced by the stress of weight and muscle activity. Resistance and impact exercises are most beneficial in developing and maintaining bone mass. Immobility contributes to the development of osteoporosis. When immobilized by casts, general inactivity, paralysis, or

---

CHART 68-7

NURSING RESEARCH PROFILE
Beliefs of Osteoporosis Risks in Men and Women 50 Years of Age and Older

Doheny, M. O., Sedlak, C. A., Estok, P. J., et al. (2007). Osteoporosis knowledge, health beliefs, and DXA T-scores in men and women 50 years of age and older. *Orthopaedic Nursing, 26*(4), 243–250.

Purpose

Osteoporosis is prevalent among older adults, particularly women older than 65 years of age. Although older men and postmenopausal women are at lesser risk for osteoporosis than elderly women, these populations of adults are nonetheless at risk. Yet, contemporary society seems to identify that osteoporosis is a disease of elderly women. The threefold purposes of this study were to determine if there was a difference in knowledge about osteoporosis, a difference in health beliefs related to osteoporosis, and a difference in bone density scores between men older than 50 years of age and women between 50 and 65 years of age.

Design

This study utilized a secondary analysis of data from a prior study of 218 healthy community-based women who were between 50 and 65 years of age and 226 healthy community-based men who were at least 50 years of age. These study participants responded to the 24-item Osteoporosis Knowledge Test (OKT), the 42-item Osteoporosis Health Belief Scale (OHBS), and the 12-item Osteoporosis Self-Efficacy

Scale (OSES). In addition, they had dual-energy x-ray absorptiometry (DXA) scans performed that yielded T-scores.

Findings

Neither the women nor men in the sample were knowledgeable about osteoporosis, although the women's mean OKT scores were higher than the men's scores. Men believed that they were less susceptible to osteoporosis, thought that it was less serious, had less faith in the efficacy of calcium in preventing and treating osteoporosis, and felt that there were fewer barriers to exercise to prevent osteoporosis than the sampled women. Less than half of the sampled men and women had normal DXA T-scores. Less than half of each group had T-scores that were consistent with osteopenia; approximately 10% of each sample had T-scores consistent with osteoporosis.

Nursing Implications

Both men and women are at risk for osteoporosis by the time they reach the age of 50, yet few of these adults believe that they are at risk. Results from this study suggest that as many as 10% of healthy men who are at least 50 years of age and healthy women who are between 50 and 65 years of age may already have osteoporosis. Nurses are in ideal positions to educate these adults about their risks and provide them with education aimed at preserving bone matrix and preventing fractures associated with osteoporosis.

other disability, the bone is resorbed faster than it is formed, and osteoporosis results (Porth & Matfin, 2009).

Assessment and Diagnostic Findings

Osteoporosis may be undetectable on routine x-rays until there has been 25% to 40% demineralization, resulting in radiolucency of the bones. When the vertebrae collapse, the thoracic vertebrae become wedge shaped and the lumbar vertebrae become biconcave. Osteoporosis is diagnosed by dual-energy x-ray absorptiometry (DXA), which provides information about BMD at the spine and hip (see Chapter 66 for further discussion of tests for BMD). The DXA scan data are analyzed and reported as T-scores (the number of standard deviations [SDs] above or below the average BMD value for a young, healthy Caucasian woman).

BMD testing is recommended for all women older than 65 years of age, for all men older than 70 years of age, for postmenopausal women and men older than 50 years of age with osteoporosis risk factors, and for all people who have had a fracture thought to occur as a consequence of osteoporosis (Bonnick, 2005; NOF, 2008). BMD studies are useful in identifying osteopenic and osteoporotic bone and in assessing response to therapy. Through early screening (using both assessment of risk factors and BMD scans), promotion of adequate dietary intake of calcium and vitamin D, encouragement of lifestyle changes, and early institution of preventive medications, bone loss and osteoporosis can be reduced, resulting in a reduced incidence of fracture.

Laboratory studies (eg, serum calcium, serum phosphate, serum alkaline phosphatase, urine calcium excretion, urinary hydroxyproline excretion, hematocrit, erythrocyte sedimentation rate [ESR]) and x-ray studies are used to exclude other possible disorders (eg, multiple myeloma, osteomalacia, hyperparathyroidism, malignancy) that contribute to bone loss.

Medical Management

A diet rich in calcium and vitamin D throughout life, with an increased calcium intake during adolescence, young adulthood, and the middle years, protects against skeletal demineralization. Such a diet includes three glasses of skim or whole vitamin D–enriched milk or other foods high in calcium (eg, cheese and other dairy products, steamed broccoli, canned salmon with bones) daily.

Regular weight-bearing exercise promotes bone formation. From 20 to 30 minutes of aerobic exercise (eg, walking), 3 days or more a week, is recommended. Weight training stimulates an increase in BMD. In addition, exercise improves balance, reducing the incidence of falls and fractures (Chart 68-8).

Pharmacologic Therapy

The first-line medications used to treat and prevent osteoporosis include calcium and vitamin D supplements and bisphosphonates. To ensure adequate calcium intake, a calcium supplement (eg, Caltrate, Citracal) with vitamin D may be prescribed and taken with meals or with a beverage high in vitamin C to promote absorption. The recommended daily dose should be split and not taken as a single dose. Common side effects of calcium supplements are

abdominal distention and constipation. Other medications that might be prescribed after these medications are tried include calcitonin, selective estrogen receptor modulators, and anabolic agents (Johnson, Clifford & Smith, 2008).

Bisphosphonates that include daily or weekly oral preparations of alendronate (Fosamax) or risedronate (Actonel), monthly oral preparations of ibandronate (Boniva), or yearly intravenous (IV) infusions of zoledronic acid (Reclast) increase bone mass and decrease bone loss by inhibiting osteoclast function (Johnson, et al., 2008). These medications have demonstrated cost-effectiveness in preventing osteoporotic-related fractures in women 65 years of age and older (Pfister, Welch, Lester, et al., 2006). In particular, alendronate is very effective therapy in preventing fractures in postmenopausal women with osteoporosis (Wells, Cranney, Peterson, et al., 2008).

Adequate calcium and vitamin D intake is needed for maximum effect, but these supplements should not be taken at the same time of day as bisphosphonates. Side effects of bisphosphonates include gastrointestinal symptoms (eg, dyspepsia, nausea, flatulence, diarrhea, constipation). Some patients may develop esophageal ulcers, gastric ulcers, or osteonecrosis of the jaw related to bisphosphonate use (Johnson, et al., 2008). Patients who take oral bisphosphonates must take these medications on an empty stomach on arising in the morning with a full glass of water and must sit upright for 30 to 60 minutes after their administration.

Calcitonin (Miacalcin) directly inhibits osteoclasts, thereby reducing bone loss and increasing BMD. Calcitonin is administered by nasal spray or by subcutaneous or intramuscular injection. Side effects include nasal irritation, flushing, gastrointestinal disturbances, and urinary frequency. It should not be prescribed for patients with seafood allergies (Johnson, et al., 2008).

Selective estrogen receptor modulators (SERMs), such as raloxifene (Evista), reduce the risk of osteoporosis by preserving BMD without estrogenic effects on the uterus. They are indicated for both prevention and treatment of osteoporosis. They are contraindicated in women with a history of venous thromboembolism (Johnson, et al., 2008).

Teriparatide (Forteo) is a subcutaneously administered anabolic agent that is administered once daily. As a recombinant PTH, it stimulates osteoblasts to build bone matrix and facilitates overall calcium absorption (Johnson, et al., 2008).

Fracture Management

Fractures of the hip that occur as a consequence of osteoporosis are managed surgically by joint replacement or by closed or open reduction with internal fixation (eg, hip pinning) as described in Chapters 67 and 69, respectively. Management of Colles' fractures is also described in Chapter 69. Patients need to be evaluated for osteoporosis and treated, as indicated, in order to prevent additional fractures.

Osteoporotic compression fractures of the vertebrae are managed conservatively. Additional vertebral fractures and progressive kyphosis are common. Pharmacologic and dietary treatments are aimed at increasing vertebral bone density. Most patients who experience these fractures are asymptomatic and do not require acute care management;

CHART 68-8	HOME CARE CHECKLIST *Osteoporosis*		
At the completion of the home care instruction, the patient or caregiver will be able to:		**PATIENT**	**CAREGIVER**
Adolescents and Young Adults			
• List risk factors for osteoporosis.		✔	✔
• Identify calcium- and vitamin D–rich foods.		✔	
• Consume diet with adequate calcium (1000–1200 mg/day) and vitamin D.		✔	
• Engage in weight-bearing exercise daily.		✔	
• Modify lifestyle choices—avoid smoking, alcohol, caffeine, and carbonated beverages.		✔	
Menopausal and Postmenopausal Women			
• List risk factors for osteoporosis.		✔	✔
• Identify calcium- and vitamin D–rich foods.		✔	
• Consume diet with adequate calcium (1000–1200 mg/day) and vitamin D.		✔	
• Discuss calcium supplements.		✔	
• Engage in weight-bearing exercise at least three times weekly.		✔	
• Engage in exercise that improves balance to reduce the incidence of falls.		✔	
• Demonstrate good body mechanics.		✔	
• Modify lifestyle choices—avoid smoking, alcohol, caffeine, and carbonated beverages.		✔	
• Discuss pharmacologic agents to maintain and enhance bone mass.		✔	
• Review concurrent medical conditions and medications with health care provider to identify factors that contribute to bone mass loss.		✔	✔
• Assess home environment for hazards contributing to falls.		✔	✔
Men			
• List risk factors associated with osteoporosis in men, including medications (eg, corticosteroids, antiseizure medications, aluminum-containing antacids); chronic diseases (eg, kidney, lung, gastrointestinal); and undiagnosed low testosterone levels.		✔	✔
• Modify lifestyle choices—avoid smoking, alcohol, caffeine, and carbonated beverages.		✔	
• Engage in weight-bearing exercise daily, such as walking, weight lifting, and resistance exercise.		✔	
• Consume diet with adequate calcium (1000–1200 mg/day) and vitamin D.		✔	
• Participate in screening for osteoporosis.		✔	
• Talk with health care provider about use of medications (eg, alendronate) to enhance bone mass or to correct testosterone deficiency.		✔	
• Assess home environment for hazards contributing to falls.		✔	✔

for those who experience pain, acute care management is indicated as outlined in the following Nursing Process section. Percutaneous vertebroplasty or kyphoplasty (injection of polymethylmethacrylate bone cement into the fractured vertebra, followed by inflation of a pressurized balloon to restore the shape of the affected vertebra) can provide rapid relief of acute pain and improve quality of life (NOF, 2008). Patients who have not responded to first-line approaches to the treatment of vertebral compression fracture can be considered for the procedure. It is contraindicated in the presence of infection, old fractures, and certain coagulopathies.

NURSING PROCESS

THE PATIENT WITH A SPONTANEOUS VERTEBRAL FRACTURE RELATED TO OSTEOPOROSIS

Assessment

Health promotion, identification of people at risk for osteoporosis, and recognition of problems associated with osteoporosis form the basis for nursing assessment. The health history includes questions concerning the occurrence of osteopenia and osteoporosis and focuses on family history, previous fractures, dietary consumption of calcium, exercise patterns, onset of menopause, and use of corticosteroids as well as alcohol, smoking, and caffeine intake. Any symptoms the patient is experiencing, such as back pain, constipation, or altered body image, are explored.

Physical examination may disclose a fracture, kyphosis of the thoracic spine, or shortened stature. Problems in mobility and breathing may exist as a result of changes in posture and weakened muscles.

Nursing Diagnoses

Based on the assessment data, the major nursing diagnoses for the patient who experiences a spontaneous vertebral fracture related to osteoporosis may include the following:
- Deficient knowledge about the osteoporotic process and treatment regimen
- Acute pain related to fracture and muscle spasm
- Risk for constipation related to immobility or development of ileus (intestinal obstruction)
- Risk for injury: additional fractures related to osteoporosis

Planning and Goals

The major goals for the patient may include knowledge about osteoporosis and the treatment regimen, relief of pain, improved bowel elimination, and absence of additional fractures.

Nursing Interventions

Promoting Understanding of Osteoporosis and the Treatment Regimen

Patient teaching focuses on factors influencing the development of osteoporosis, interventions to arrest or slow the process, and measures to relieve symptoms. It is emphasized that all people continue to need sufficient calcium, vitamin D, and weight-bearing exercise to slow the progression of osteoporosis. Patient teaching related to medication therapy as described previously is important.

Relieving Pain

Relief of back pain resulting from compression fracture may be accomplished by resting in bed in a supine or side-lying position several times a day. The mattress should be firm and nonsagging. Knee flexion increases comfort by relaxing back muscles. Intermittent local heat and back rubs promote muscle relaxation. The nurse instructs the patient to move the trunk as a unit and to avoid twisting. The nurse encourages good posture and teaches body mechanics. When the patient is assisted out of bed, a trunk orthosis (eg, lumbosacral corset) may be worn for temporary support and immobilization, although such a device is frequently uncomfortable and is poorly tolerated by many elderly patients (NOF, 2008). The patient gradually resumes activities as pain diminishes.

Improving Bowel Elimination

Constipation is a problem related to immobility and medications. Early institution of a high-fiber diet, increased fluids, and the use of prescribed stool softeners help prevent or minimize constipation. If the vertebral collapse involves the T10–L2 vertebrae, the patient may develop a paralytic ileus. The nurse therefore monitors the patient's intake, bowel sounds, and bowel activity.

Preventing Injury

Physical activity is essential to strengthen muscles, improve balance, prevent disuse atrophy, and retard progressive bone demineralization. Isometric exercises can strengthen trunk muscles. The nurse encourages walking, good body mechanics, and good posture. Daily weight-bearing activity, preferably outdoors in the sunshine to enhance the body's ability to produce vitamin D, is encouraged. Sudden bending, jarring, and strenuous lifting are avoided.

GERONTOLOGIC CONSIDERATIONS. Elderly people fall frequently as a result of environmental hazards, neuromuscular disorders, diminished senses and cardiovascular responses, and responses to medications. The patient and family need to be included in planning for care and preventive management regimens. For example, the home environment should be assessed for safety and elimination of potential hazards (eg, scatter rugs, cluttered rooms and stairwells, toys on the floor, pets underfoot). A safe environment can then be created (eg, well-lighted staircases with secure hand rails, grab bars in the bathroom, properly fitting footwear).

Evaluation

Expected Patient Outcomes

Expected patient outcomes may include:

1. Acquires knowledge about osteoporosis and the treatment regimen
   a. States relationship of calcium and vitamin D intake and exercise to bone mass
   b. Consumes adequate dietary calcium and vitamin D
   c. Increases level of exercise
   d. Takes prescribed medications, following instructions for administration
   e. Adheres to prescribed screening and monitoring procedures
2. Achieves pain relief
   a. Experiences pain relief at rest
   b. Experiences minimal discomfort during ADLs
   c. Demonstrates diminished tenderness at fracture site
3. Demonstrates normal bowel elimination
   a. Has active bowel sounds
   b. Reports regular pattern of bowel movements
4. Experiences no new fractures
   a. Maintains good posture
   b. Uses good body mechanics
   c. Consumes a diet high in calcium and vitamin D
   d. Engages in weight-bearing exercises (walks daily)
   e. Rests by lying down several times a day
   f. Participates in outdoor activities
   g. Creates a safe home environment
   h. Accepts assistance and supervision as needed

OSTEOMALACIA

Osteomalacia is a metabolic bone disease characterized by inadequate mineralization of bone. As a result of faulty mineralization, there is softening and weakening of the skeleton, causing pain, tenderness to touch, bowing of the bones, and pathologic fractures. On physical examination, skeletal deformities (spinal kyphosis and bowed legs) give patients an unusual appearance and a waddling or limping gait. These patients may be uncomfortable with their appearance. As a result of calcium deficiency, muscle weakness, and unsteadiness, there is an increased risk for falls and fractures, particularly pathologic fractures of the distal radius and the proximal femur (Porth & Matfin, 2009).

Pathophysiology

The primary defect in osteomalacia is a deficiency of activated vitamin D (calcitriol), which promotes calcium absorption from the gastrointestinal tract and facilitates mineralization of bone. The supply of calcium and phosphate in the extracellular fluid is low. Without adequate vitamin D, calcium and phosphate are not moved to calcification sites in bones.

Osteomalacia may result from failed calcium absorption (eg, malabsorption syndrome) or from excessive loss of calcium from the body. Gastrointestinal disorders (eg, celiac disease, chronic biliary tract obstruction, chronic pancreatitis, small bowel resection) in which fats are inadequately absorbed are likely to produce osteomalacia through loss of vitamin D (along with other fat-soluble vitamins) and calcium, the latter being excreted in the feces with fatty acids. In addition, liver and kidney diseases can produce a lack of vitamin D because these are the organs that convert vitamin D to its active form.

Severe renal insufficiency results in acidosis. The body uses available calcium to combat the acidosis, and PTH stimulates the release of skeletal calcium in an attempt to reestablish a physiologic pH. During this continual drain of skeletal calcium, bony fibrosis occurs, and bony cysts form. Chronic glomerulonephritis, obstructive uropathies, and heavy metal poisoning result in a reduced serum phosphate level and demineralization of bone.

Hyperparathyroidism leads to skeletal decalcification and thus to osteomalacia by increasing phosphate excretion in the urine. Prolonged use of antiseizure medication (eg, phenytoin [Dilantin], phenobarbital) poses a risk of osteomalacia, as does insufficient vitamin D (dietary, sunlight).

Osteomalacia that results from malnutrition (deficiency in vitamin D often associated with poor intake of calcium) is a result of poverty, poor dietary habits, and lack of knowledge about nutrition. It occurs most frequently in parts of the world where vitamin D is not added to food, where dietary deficiencies exist, and where sunlight is rare (Porth & Matfin, 2009).

 Gerontologic Considerations

A nutritious diet is particularly important in elderly people. Adequate intake of calcium and vitamin D is promoted. Because sunlight is necessary for synthesizing vitamin D, people should be encouraged to spend some time in the sun. Prevention, identification, and management of osteomalacia in the elderly are essential to reduce the incidence of fractures. When osteomalacia is combined with osteoporosis, the incidence of fracture increases.

Assessment and Diagnostic Findings

On x-ray studies, generalized demineralization of bone is evident. Studies of the vertebrae may show a compression fracture with indistinct vertebral endplates. Laboratory studies show low serum calcium and phosphorus levels and a moderately elevated alkaline phosphatase concentration. Urine excretion of calcium and creatinine is low. Bone biopsy demonstrates an increased amount of osteoid, a demineralized, cartilaginous bone matrix that is sometimes referred to as "prebone."

Medical Management

Physical, psychological, and pharmaceutical measures are used to reduce the patient's discomfort and pain. When assisting the patient to change positions, the nurse handles the patient gently, and pillows are used to support the body. As the patient responds to therapy, the skeletal discomfort diminishes.

If possible, the underlying cause of osteomalacia is corrected. Frequently, skeletal problems associated with osteomalacia resolve themselves when the underlying nutritional deficiency or pathologic process is adequately treated.

If osteomalacia is caused by malabsorption, increased doses of vitamin D, along with supplemental calcium, are usually prescribed (Lyman, 2005). Exposure to sunlight may be recommended; ultraviolet radiation transforms a cholesterol substance (7-dehydrocholesterol) present in the skin into vitamin D.

If osteomalacia is dietary in origin, a diet with adequate protein and increased calcium and vitamin D is provided. The patient is instructed about dietary sources of calcium and vitamin D (eg, fortified milk and cereals, eggs, chicken livers). The safe use of supplements is reviewed. Because high doses of vitamin D are toxic and increase the risk for hypercalcemia, the importance of monitoring serum calcium levels is stressed. Vitamin D raises the concentrations of calcium and phosphorus in the extracellular fluid and thus makes these ions available for mineralization of bone.

Long-term monitoring of the patient is appropriate to ensure stabilization or reversal of osteomalacia. Some persistent orthopedic deformities may need to be treated with braces or surgery (eg, osteotomy may be performed to correct long bone deformity).

PAGET'S DISEASE OF THE BONE

Paget's disease (osteitis deformans) is a disorder of localized rapid bone turnover, most commonly affecting the skull, femur, tibia, pelvic bones, and vertebrae. The disease occurs in about 2% to 3% of the population older than 50 years. The incidence is slightly greater in men than in women and increases with aging. A family history has been noted, with siblings often developing the disease. The cause of Paget's disease is not known (Josse, Hanley, Kendler, et al., 2007).

Pathophysiology

In Paget's disease, there is a primary proliferation of osteoclasts, which induce bone resorption. This is followed by a compensatory increase in osteoblastic activity that replaces the bone. As bone turnover continues, a classic mosaic (disorganized) pattern of bone develops. Because the diseased bone is highly vascularized and structurally weak, pathologic fractures occur. Structural bowing of the legs causes malalignment of the hip, knee, and ankle joints, which contributes to the development of arthritis and back and joint pain (Josse, et al., 2007).

Clinical Manifestations

Paget's disease is insidious; most patients never experience symptoms. Some patients do not experience symptoms but have skeletal deformity; a few patients have symptomatic deformity and pain. The condition is most frequently identified on x-ray studies performed during a routine physical examination or during a workup for another problem. Sclerotic changes, skeletal deformities (eg, bowing of the femur and tibia, enlargement of the skull, deformity of pelvic bones), and cortical thickening of the long bones occur.

In most patients, skeletal deformity involves the skull or long bones. The skull may thicken, and the patient may report that a hat no longer fits. In some cases, the cranium, but not the face, is enlarged. This gives the face a small, triangular appearance. Most patients with skull involvement have impaired hearing from cranial nerve compression and dysfunction. Other cranial nerves may also be compressed.

The femurs and tibiae tend to bow, producing a waddling gait. The spine is bent forward and is rigid; the chin rests on the chest. The thorax is compressed and immobile on respiration. The trunk is flexed on the legs to maintain balance and the arms are bent outward and forward and appear long in relation to the shortened trunk (Porth & Matfin, 2009).

Pain, tenderness, and warmth over the bones may be noted. The pain is mild to moderate, deep, and aching; it increases with weight bearing if the lower extremities are involved. Pain and discomfort may precede skeletal deformities of Paget's disease by years and are often wrongly attributed by the patient to old age or arthritis.

The temperature of the skin overlying the affected bone increases because of increased bone vascularity. Patients with large, highly vascular lesions may develop high-output cardiac failure because of the increased vascular bed and metabolic demands.

Assessment and Diagnostic Findings

Elevated serum alkaline phosphatase concentration and urinary hydroxyproline excretion reflect increased osteoblastic activity. Higher values suggest more active disease. Patients with Paget's disease have normal blood calcium levels. X-rays confirm the diagnosis of Paget's disease. Local areas of demineralization and bone overgrowth produce characteristic mosaic patterns and irregularities. Bone scans demonstrate the extent of the disease. Bone biopsy may aid in the differential diagnosis (Porth & Matfin, 2009).

Medical Management

Pain usually responds to NSAIDs. Gait problems from bowing of the legs are managed with walking aids, shoe lifts, and physical therapy. Weight is controlled to reduce stress on weakened bones and malaligned joints. Asymptomatic patients may be managed with diets adequate in calcium and vitamin D and periodic monitoring.

Fractures, arthritis, and hearing loss are complications of Paget's disease. Fractures are managed according to location. Healing occurs if fracture reduction, immobilization,

and stability are adequate. Severe degenerative arthritis may require total joint replacement. Loss of hearing is managed with hearing aids and communication techniques used with hearing-impaired people (eg, speech reading, body language) (see Chapter 59).

Pharmacologic Therapy

Patients with moderate to severe disease may benefit from specific antiosteoclastic therapy. Several medications reduce bone turnover, reverse the course of the disease, relieve pain, and improve mobility.

Calcitonin, a polypeptide hormone, retards bone resorption by decreasing the number and availability of osteoclasts. Calcitonin therapy facilitates remodeling of abnormal bone into normal lamellar bone, relieves bone pain, and helps alleviate neurologic and biochemical signs and symptoms. Calcitonin is administered subcutaneously or by nasal inhalation. Side effects include flushing of the face and nausea. The effect of calcitonin therapy is evident in 3 to 6 months through reduction of bone loss and pain.

Bisphosphonates produce rapid reduction in bone turnover and relief of pain (Keating & Scott, 2007). They also reduce serum alkaline phosphatase and urinary hydroxyproline levels. Food inhibits absorption of these medications. Adequate daily intake of calcium and vitamin D is required during therapy.

Plicamycin (Mithracin), a cytotoxic antibiotic, may be used to control the disease. This medication is reserved for severely affected patients with neurologic compromise and for those whose disease is resistant to other therapy. This medication has dramatic effects on pain reduction and on serum calcium, alkaline phosphatase, and urinary hydroxyproline levels. It is administered by IV infusion; hepatic, renal, and bone marrow function must be monitored during therapy. Clinical remissions may continue for months after the medication is discontinued.

 Gerontologic Considerations

Because Paget's disease tends to affect elderly people, careful assessment of a patient's pain and discomfort is necessary. Patient teaching helps the patient understand the treatment regimen, the need for a diet with adequate calcium and vitamin D, and how to compensate for altered musculoskeletal functioning. The home environment is assessed for safety to prevent falls and to reduce the risk of fracture. Strategies for coping with a chronic health problem and its effect on quality of life need to be developed.

Musculoskeletal Infections

OSTEOMYELITIS

Osteomyelitis is an infection of the bone that results in inflammation, necrosis, and formation of new bone (Davis, 2005). Osteomyelitis is classified as:

- Hematogenous osteomyelitis (ie, due to bloodborne spread of infection)
- Contiguous-focus osteomyelitis, from contamination from bone surgery, open fracture, or traumatic injury (eg, gunshot wound)

- Osteomyelitis with vascular insufficiency, seen most commonly among patients with diabetes and peripheral vascular disease, most commonly affecting the feet (Davis, 2005)

Patients who are at high risk for osteomyelitis include those who are poorly nourished, elderly, or obese. Other patients at risk include those with impaired immune systems, those with chronic illnesses (eg, diabetes, rheumatoid arthritis), and those receiving long-term corticosteroid therapy or other immunosuppressive agents.

Postoperative surgical wound infections occur within 30 days after surgery. They are classified as incisional (superficial, located above the deep fascia layer) or deep (involving tissue beneath the deep fascia). If an implant has been used, deep postoperative infections may occur within a year. Deep sepsis after arthroplasty may be classified as follows:

- Stage 1, acute fulminating: occurring during the first 3 months after orthopedic surgery; frequently associated with hematoma, drainage, or superficial infection
- Stage 2, delayed onset: occurring between 4 and 24 months after surgery
- Stage 3, late onset: occurring 2 or more years after surgery, usually as a result of hematogenous spread

Bone infections are more difficult to eradicate than soft tissue infections because the infected bone is mostly avascular and not accessible to the body's natural immune response. Also, there is decreased penetration by antibiotics. Osteomyelitis may become chronic and may affect the patient's quality of life.

Pathophysiology

Over 50% of bone infections are caused by *Staphylococcus aureus*. Other pathogens that are frequently found in osteomyelitis include gram-positive organisms that include streptococci and enterococci, followed by gram-negative bacteria that include *Pseudomonas* species (Venugopalan & Martin, 2007).

The initial response to infection is inflammation, increased vascularity, and edema. After 2 or 3 days, thrombosis of the local blood vessels occurs, resulting in ischemia with bone necrosis. The infection extends into the medullary cavity and under the periosteum and may spread into adjacent soft tissues and joints. Unless the infective process is treated promptly, a bone abscess forms. The resulting abscess cavity contains dead bone tissue (the **sequestrum**), which does not easily liquefy and drain. Therefore, the cavity cannot collapse and heal, as it does in soft tissue abscesses. New bone growth (the **involucrum**) forms and surrounds the sequestrum. Although healing appears to take place, a chronically infected sequestrum remains and produces recurring abscesses throughout the patient's life. This is referred to as chronic osteomyelitis.

Clinical Manifestations

When the infection is bloodborne, the onset is usually sudden, occurring often with the clinical and laboratory manifestations of sepsis (eg, chills, high fever, rapid pulse, general malaise). The systemic symptoms at first may overshadow the local signs. As the infection extends through the cortex of the bone, it involves the periosteum and the soft tissues. The infected area becomes painful, swollen, and extremely tender. The patient may describe a constant, pulsating pain that intensifies with movement as a result of the pressure of the collecting purulent material (ie, pus). When osteomyelitis occurs from spread of adjacent infection or from direct contamination, there are no symptoms of sepsis. The area is swollen, warm, painful, and tender to touch (Davis, 2005; Forman, Forman & Rose, 2005).

The patient with chronic osteomyelitis presents with a nonhealing ulcer that overlies the infected bone with a connecting sinus that will intermittently and spontaneously drain pus (Davis, 2005).

Assessment and Diagnostic Findings

In acute osteomyelitis, early x-ray findings demonstrate soft tissue edema. In about 2 to 3 weeks, areas of periosteal elevation and bone necrosis are evident. Radioisotope bone scans, particularly the isotope-labeled white blood cell (WBC) scan, and magnetic resonance imaging (MRI) help with early definitive diagnosis. Blood studies reveal leukocytosis and an elevated ESR. Wound and blood culture studies are performed, although they are only positive in 50% of cases. Therefore, treatment with antibiotics may be prescribed without definitively isolating the offending organism (Davis, 2005).

With chronic osteomyelitis, large, irregular cavities; raised periosteum; sequestra; or dense bone formations are seen on x-ray. Bone scans may be performed to identify areas of infection. The ESR and the WBC count are usually normal. Anemia, associated with chronic infection, may be evident. Cultures of blood specimens and drainage from the sinus tract are frequently unreliable; antibiotic therapy is many times prescribed presumptively without isolating the offending pathogen (Davis, 2005).

Prevention

Prevention of osteomyelitis is the goal. Elective orthopedic surgery should be postponed if the patient has a current infection (eg, urinary tract infection, sore throat) or a recent history of infection. During orthopedic surgery, careful attention is paid to the surgical environment and to techniques to decrease direct bone contamination. Prophylactic antibiotics, administered to achieve adequate tissue levels at the time of surgery and for 24 hours after surgery, are helpful. Urinary catheters and drains are removed as soon as possible to decrease the incidence of hematogenous spread of infection.

Treatment of focal infections diminishes hematogenous spread. Aseptic postoperative wound care reduces the incidence of superficial infections and osteomyelitis. Prompt management of soft tissue infections reduces extension of infection to the bone. When patients who have had joint replacement surgery undergo dental procedures or other invasive procedures (eg, cystoscopy), prophylactic antibiotics are frequently recommended.

Medical Management

The initial goal of therapy is to control and halt the infective process. Antibiotic therapy depends on the results of blood and wound cultures. General supportive measures (eg, hydration, diet high in vitamins and protein, correction of anemia) should be instituted. The area affected with osteomyelitis is immobilized to decrease discomfort and to prevent pathologic fracture of the weakened bone (Sheff, 2005).

Pharmacologic Therapy

As soon as the culture specimens are obtained, IV antibiotic therapy begins, based on the assumption that infection results from a staphylococcal organism that is sensitive to a penicillin or cephalosporin. The aim is to control the infection before the blood supply to the area diminishes as a result of thrombosis. Around-the-clock dosing is necessary to maintain a high therapeutic blood level of the antibiotic. After results of the culture and sensitivity studies are known, an antibiotic to which the causative organism is sensitive is prescribed. IV antibiotic therapy continues for 3 to 6 weeks. After the infection appears to be controlled, the antibiotic may be administered orally for up to 3 months. To enhance absorption of the orally administered medication, antibiotics should not be administered with food (Davis, 2005; Sheff, 2005).

Surgical Management

If the infection is chronic and does not respond to antibiotic therapy, surgical débridement is indicated. The infected bone is surgically exposed, the purulent and necrotic material is removed, and the area is irrigated with sterile saline solution. Antibiotic-impregnated beads may be placed in the wound for direct application of antibiotics for 2 to 4 weeks (Kent, Rapp & Smith, 2006). IV antibiotic therapy is continued.

In chronic osteomyelitis, antibiotics are adjunctive therapy to surgical débridement. A sequestrectomy (removal of enough involucrum to enable the surgeon to remove the sequestrum) is performed. In many cases, sufficient bone is removed to convert a deep cavity into a shallow saucer (saucerization). All dead, infected bone and cartilage must be removed before permanent healing can occur. A closed suction irrigation system may be used to remove debris. Wound irrigation using sterile physiologic saline solution may be performed for 7 to 8 days.

The wound is either closed tightly to obliterate the dead space or packed and closed later by granulation or possibly by grafting. The débrided cavity may be packed with cancellous bone graft to stimulate healing. With a large defect, the cavity may be filled with a vascularized bone transfer or muscle flap (in which a muscle is moved from an adjacent area with blood supply intact). These microsurgery techniques enhance the blood supply. The improved blood supply facilitates bone healing and eradication of the infection. These surgical procedures may be staged over time to ensure healing. Because surgical débridement weakens the bone, internal fixation or external supportive devices may be needed to stabilize or support the bone to prevent pathologic fracture (Davis, 2005).

NURSING PROCESS

THE PATIENT WITH OSTEOMYELITIS

Assessment

The patient reports an acute onset of signs and symptoms (eg, localized pain, edema, erythema, fever) or recurrent drainage of an infected sinus with associated pain, edema, and low-grade fever. The nurse assesses the patient for risk factors (eg, older age, diabetes, long-term corticosteroid therapy) and for a history of previous injury, infection, or orthopedic surgery. The patient avoids pressure and movement of the area. In acute hematogenous osteomyelitis, the patient exhibits generalized weakness due to the systemic reaction to the infection.

Physical examination reveals an inflamed, markedly edematous, warm area that is tender. Purulent drainage may be noted. The patient has an elevated temperature. With chronic osteomyelitis, the temperature elevation may be minimal, occurring in the afternoon or evening.

Nursing Diagnoses

Based on the nursing assessment data, nursing diagnoses for the patient with osteomyelitis may include the following:
- Acute pain related to inflammation and edema
- Impaired physical mobility related to pain, use of immobilization devices, and weight-bearing limitations
- Risk for extension of infection: bone abscess formation
- Deficient knowledge related to the treatment regimen

Planning and Goals

The patient's goals may include relief of pain, improved physical mobility within therapeutic limitations, control and eradication of infection, and knowledge of the treatment regimen.

Nursing Interventions

Relieving Pain

The affected part may be immobilized with a splint to decrease pain and muscle spasm. The nurse monitors the neurovascular status of the affected extremity. The wounds are frequently very painful, and the extremity must be handled with great care and gentleness. Elevation reduces swelling and associated discomfort. Pain is controlled with prescribed analgesic agents and other pain-reducing techniques.

Improving Physical Mobility

Treatment regimens restrict activity. The bone is weakened by the infective process and must be protected by immobilization devices and by avoidance of stress on the bone. The patient must understand the rationale for the activity restrictions. The joints above and below the affected part should be gently moved through their range of motion. The nurse encourages full participation in ADLs within the physical limitations to promote general well-being.

Controlling the Infectious Process

The nurse monitors the patient's response to antibiotic therapy and observes the IV access site for evidence of phlebitis, infection, or infiltration. With long-term, intensive antibiotic therapy, the nurse monitors the patient for signs of superinfection (eg, oral or vaginal candidiasis, loose or foul-smelling stools).

If surgery is necessary, the nurse takes measures to ensure adequate circulation to the affected area (wound suction to prevent fluid accumulation, elevation of the area to promote venous drainage, avoidance of pressure on the grafted area), to maintain needed immobility, and to ensure the

CHART 68-9	HOME CARE CHECKLIST *Osteomyelitis*		
At the completion of the home care instruction, the patient or caregiver will be able to:		**PATIENT**	**CAREGIVER**
• Describe osteomyelitis.		✔	✔
• Relieve pain with pharmacologic and nonpharmacologic interventions.		✔	
• State weight-bearing and activity restrictions.		✔	✔
• Demonstrate safe use of ambulatory aids and assistive devices.		✔	
• Describe use of prescribed medications.		✔	✔
• Comply with antibiotic regimen.		✔	
• Promote healing through aseptic dressing changes.		✔	✔
• Demonstrate proper wound care.		✔	✔
• Report signs and symptoms of continuing infection or superinfection.		✔	✔

patient's adherence to weight-bearing restrictions. The nurse changes dressings using aseptic technique to promote healing and to prevent cross-contamination.

The nurse continues to monitor the general health and nutrition of the patient. A diet high in protein promotes a positive nitrogen balance and healing. The nurse encourages adequate hydration as well.

Promoting Home and Community-Based Care

TEACHING PATIENTS SELF-CARE. The patient and family are taught about the importance of strictly adhering to the therapeutic regimen of antibiotics and preventing falls or other injuries that could result in bone fracture. They need to learn to maintain and manage the IV access and IV administration equipment in the home. Teaching includes medication name, dosage, frequency, administration rate, safe storage and handling, adverse reactions, and necessary laboratory monitoring. In addition, aseptic dressing and warm compress techniques are taught.

The nurse carefully monitors the patient for the development of additional sites that are painful or sudden increases in body temperature. The nurse instructs the patient and family to observe for and report elevated temperature, drainage, odor, signs of increased inflammation, adverse reactions, and signs of superinfection.

CONTINUING CARE. Management of osteomyelitis, including wound care and IV antibiotic therapy, is usually performed at home. The patient must be medically stable and physically able and motivated to adhere strictly to the therapeutic regimen of antibiotic therapy. The home care environment needs to be conducive to the promotion of health and to the requirements of the therapeutic regimen.

If warranted, the nurse completes a home assessment to determine the patient's and family's abilities regarding continuation of the therapeutic regimen. If the patient's support system is questionable or if the patient lives alone, a home care nurse may be needed to assist with IV administration of the antibiotics. The nurse monitors the patient for response to the treatment, signs and symptoms of superinfections, and adverse drug reactions. The nurse stresses the importance of

follow-up health care appointments and recommends age-appropriate health screening (Chart 68-9).

Evaluation

Expected Patient Outcomes

Expected patient outcomes may include:

1. Experiences pain relief
   a. Reports decreased pain
   b. Experiences no tenderness at site of previous infection
   c. Experiences no discomfort with movement
2. Increases physical mobility
   a. Participates in self-care activities
   b. Maintains full function of unimpaired extremities
   c. Demonstrates safe use of immobilizing and assistive devices
   d. Modifies environment to promote safety and to avoid falls
3. Shows absence of infection
   a. Takes antibiotic as prescribed
   b. Reports normal temperature
   c. Exhibits no edema
   d. Reports absence of drainage
   e. Laboratory results indicate normal white blood cell count and erythrocyte sedimentation rate
   f. Wound cultures are negative
4. Adheres to therapeutic plan
   a. Takes medications as prescribed
   b. Protects weakened bones
   c. Demonstrates proper wound care
   d. Reports signs and symptoms of complications promptly
   e. Consumes a diet high in protein
   f. Keeps follow-up health care appointments
   g. Reports increased strength
   h. Reports no elevation of temperature or recurrence of pain, edema, or other symptoms at the site

SEPTIC (INFECTIOUS) ARTHRITIS

Joints can become infected through spread of infection from other parts of the body (hematogenous spread) or directly through trauma or surgical instrumentation. Previous trauma to joints, joint replacement, coexisting arthritis, and diminished host resistance contribute to the development of an infected joint. *S. aureus* causes at least 50% of all joint infections, and 80% of cases of septic arthritis in patients with rheumatoid arthritis and diabetes. The knee is the joint that is most commonly infected (50% of cases), followed by the hip and the shoulder, respectively (Davis, 2005). Prompt recognition and treatment of an infected joint are important because accumulating purulent material results in chondrolysis (destruction of hyaline cartilage).

Clinical Manifestations

The patient with acute septic arthritis usually presents with a warm, painful, swollen joint with decreased range of motion. Systemic chills, fever, and leukocytosis are present. Risk factors include advanced age, diabetes, rheumatoid arthritis, and preexisting joint disease or joint replacement. Elderly patients and patients taking corticosteroids or immunosuppressive medications are at heightened risk; yet, these patients may not exhibit typical clinical manifestations of infection. Therefore, they require ongoing assessment to detect infection as early as possible in the infectious process (Gavet, Tournadre, Soubrier, et al., 2005).

Assessment and Diagnostic Findings

An assessment for the source and cause of infection is performed. Diagnostic studies include aspiration, examination, and culture of the synovial fluid. Computed tomography (CT) and MRI may reveal damage to the joint lining. Radioisotope scanning may be useful in localizing the infectious process.

Medical Management

Prompt treatment is essential and may save a prosthesis for patients who have had joint replacement surgery. Broad-spectrum IV antibiotics are started promptly and then changed to organism-specific antibiotics after culture results are available. The IV antibiotics are continued until symptoms resolve. The synovial fluid is aspirated and analyzed periodically for sterility and decrease in WBCs.

In addition to prescribing antibiotics, the physician may aspirate the joint with a needle to remove excessive joint fluid, exudate, and debris. This promotes comfort and decreases joint destruction caused by the action of proteolytic enzymes in the purulent fluid. Occasionally, arthrotomy or arthroscopy is used to drain the joint and remove dead tissue (Davis, 2005).

The inflamed joint is supported and immobilized in a functional position by a splint that increases the patient's comfort. Analgesic agents, such as codeine, may be prescribed to relieve pain. After the infection has responded to antibiotic therapy, NSAIDs may be prescribed to limit joint damage. The patient's nutrition and fluid status is monitored. Progressive range-of-motion exercises are prescribed as soon as the patient can begin movement without exacerbating symptoms of acute pain (Davis, 2005).

If septic joints are treated promptly, recovery of normal function is expected. The patient is assessed periodically for recurrence. If the articular cartilage was damaged during the inflammatory reaction, joint fibrosis and diminished function may result.

Nursing Management

The nurse describes the septic arthritis physiologic process to the patient and teaches the patient how to relieve pain using pharmacologic and nonpharmacologic interventions. The nurse also explains the importance of supporting the affected joint, adhering to the prescribed antibiotic regimen, and observing weight-bearing and activity restrictions. Additionally, the nurse demonstrates and encourages the patient to practice safe use of ambulatory aids and assistive devices.

The nurse teaches the patient strategies to promote healing through aseptic dressing changes and proper wound care. The patient is then encouraged to perform range-of-motion exercises after the infection subsides.

Bone Tumors

Neoplasms of the musculoskeletal system are of various types, including osteogenic, chondrogenic, fibrogenic, muscle (rhabdomyogenic), and marrow (reticulum) cell tumors as well as nerve, vascular, and fatty cell tumors. They may be primary tumors or metastatic tumors from primary cancers elsewhere in the body (eg, breast, lung, prostate, kidney). Metastatic bone tumors are more common than primary bone tumors (Weber, 2005).

Types

Benign Bone Tumors

Benign tumors of the bone and soft tissue are more common than malignant primary bone tumors. Benign bone tumors generally are slow growing, well circumscribed, and encapsulated; present few symptoms; and are not a cause of death.

Benign primary neoplasms of the musculoskeletal system include osteochondroma, enchondroma, bone cyst (eg, aneurysmal bone cyst), osteoid osteoma, rhabdomyoma, and fibroma. Some benign tumors, such as giant cell tumors, have the potential to become malignant.

Osteochondroma is the most common benign bone tumor. It usually occurs as a large projection of bone at the end of long bones (at the knee or shoulder). It develops during growth and then becomes a static bony mass. In fewer than 1% of patients, the cartilage cap of the osteochondroma may undergo malignant transformation after trauma, and a chondrosarcoma or osteosarcoma may develop.

Enchondroma is a common tumor of the hyaline cartilage that develops in the hand, femur, tibia, or humerus. Usually, the only symptom is a mild ache. Pathologic fractures may occur.

Bone cysts are expanding lesions within the bone. Aneurysmal (widening) bone cysts are seen in young adults, who present with a painful, palpable mass of the long bones, vertebrae, or flat bone. Unicameral (single cavity) bone cysts occur in children and cause mild discomfort and possible pathologic fractures of the upper humerus and femur, which may heal spontaneously.

Osteoid osteoma is a painful tumor that occurs in children and young adults. The neoplastic tissue is surrounded by reactive bone formation that can be identified by x-ray.

Giant cell tumors (osteoclastomas) are benign for long periods but may invade local tissue and cause destruction. They occur in young adults and are soft and hemorrhagic. Eventually, giant cell tumors may undergo malignant transformation and metastasize (Porth & Matfin, 2009).

Malignant Bone Tumors

Primary malignant musculoskeletal tumors are relatively rare and arise from connective and supportive tissue cells (sarcomas) or bone marrow elements (multiple myeloma; see Chapter 33). Malignant primary musculoskeletal tumors include osteosarcoma, chondrosarcoma, Ewing's sarcoma, and fibrosarcoma. Soft tissue sarcomas include liposarcoma, fibrosarcoma of soft tissue, and rhabdomyosarcoma. Bone tumor metastasis to the lungs is common.

Osteosarcoma (ie, osteogenic sarcoma) is the most common and most often fatal primary malignant bone tumor. Prognosis depends on whether the tumor has metastasized to the lungs at the time the patient seeks health care. Osteosarcoma appears most frequently in children, adolescents and young adults (in bones that grow rapidly), in older people with Paget's disease of the bone, and in people with a prior history of radiation exposure. Clinical manifestations typically include localized bone pain that may be accompanied by a tender, palpable soft tissue mass. The primary lesion may involve any bone, but the most common sites are the distal femur, the proximal tibia, and the proximal humerus (Skubitz & D'Adamo, 2007).

Malignant tumors of the hyaline cartilage are called chondrosarcomas. These tumors are the second most common primary malignant bone tumor. They are large, bulky, tumors that may grow and metastasize slowly or very fast, depending on the characteristics of the tumor cells involved (ie, grade). Patients with low-grade chondrosarcomas tend to have a much better prognosis than those with high-grade chondrosarcomas (see Chapter 16 for a discussion of tumor grades). The usual tumor sites include the pelvis, femur, humerus, spine, scapula, and tibia. Metastasis to the lungs occurs in less than half of patients. When these tumors are well differentiated, large bloc excision or amputation of the affected extremity results in increased survival rates. These tumors may recur, however (Skubitz & D'Adamo, 2007).

Metastatic Bone Disease

Metastatic bone disease (secondary bone tumor) is more common than primary bone tumors. Tumors arising from tissues elsewhere in the body may invade the bone and produce localized bone destruction (lytic lesions) or bone overgrowth (blastic lesions). The most common primary sites of tumors that metastasize to bone are the kidney, prostate, lung, breast, ovary, and thyroid. Metastatic tumors most frequently attack the skull, spine, pelvis, femur, and humerus and often involve more than one bone (polyostotic) (Porth & Matfin, 2009).

Pathophysiology

A tumor in the bone causes the normal bone tissue to react by osteolytic response (bone destruction) or osteoblastic response (bone formation). Primary tumors cause bone destruction, which weakens the bone, resulting in bone fractures. Adjacent normal bone responds to the tumor by altering its normal pattern of remodeling. The bone's surface changes and the contours enlarge in the tumor area.

Malignant bone tumors invade and destroy adjacent bone tissue. Benign bone tumors, in contrast, have a symmetric, controlled growth pattern and place pressure on adjacent bone tissue. Malignant bone tumors invade and weaken the structure of the bone until it can no longer withstand the stress of ordinary use; pathologic fracture commonly results.

Clinical Manifestations

Patients with metastatic bone tumor may have a wide range of associated clinical manifestations. They may be symptom-free or have pain that ranges from mild and occasional to constant and severe, varying degrees of disability, and, at times, obvious bone growth. Weight loss, malaise, and fever may be present. The tumor may be diagnosed only after pathologic fracture has occurred.

With spinal metastasis, spinal cord compression may occur. It can progress rapidly or slowly. Neurologic deficits (eg, progressive pain, weakness, gait abnormality, paresthesia, paraplegia, urinary retention, loss of bowel or bladder control) must be identified early and treated with decompressive laminectomy to prevent permanent spinal cord injury.

Assessment and Diagnostic Findings

The differential diagnosis is based on the history, physical examination, and diagnostic studies, including CT, bone scans, myelography, arteriography, MRI, biopsy, and biochemical assays of the blood and urine. Serum alkaline phosphatase levels are frequently elevated with osteogenic sarcoma. With metastatic carcinoma of the prostate, serum acid phosphatase levels are elevated. Hypercalcemia is present with bone metastases from breast, lung, or kidney cancer. Symptoms of hypercalcemia include muscle weakness, fatigue, anorexia, nausea, vomiting, polyuria, cardiac dysrhythmias, seizures, and coma. Hypercalcemia must be identified and treated promptly.

A surgical biopsy is performed for histologic identification. Extreme care is taken during the biopsy to prevent seeding and resultant recurrence after excision of the tumor.

Chest x-rays are performed to determine the presence of lung metastasis. Surgical staging of musculoskeletal tumors is based on tumor grade and site (intracompartmental or extracompartmental), as well as on metastasis. Staging is used for planning treatment.

During the diagnostic period, the nurse explains the diagnostic tests and provides psychological and emotional support to the patient and family. The nurse assesses coping behaviors and encourages use of support systems.

Medical Management

Primary Bone Tumors

The goal of primary bone tumor treatment is to destroy or remove the tumor. This may be accomplished by surgical excision (ranging from local excision to amputation and disarticulation), radiation therapy if the tumor is radiosensitive, and chemotherapy (preoperative, intraoperative [neoadjuvant], postoperative, and adjunctive for possible micrometastases). Chemotherapy may be delivered intra-arterially for patients with osteosarcoma; this mode of delivery is associated with improved limb preservation (Matthews, Snell & Coats, 2006). Major gains are being made in the use of wide bloc excision with restorative grafting technique (Muscolo, Ayerza, Aponte-Tinao, et al., 2005). Survival and quality of life are important considerations in procedures that attempt to save the involved extremity.

Limb-sparing (salvage) procedures are used to remove the tumor and adjacent tissue. A customized prosthesis, total joint arthroplasty, or bone tissue from the patient (autograft) or from a cadaver donor (allograft) replaces the resected tissue. Soft tissue and blood vessels may need grafting because of the extent of the excision. Complications may include infection, loosening or dislocation of the prosthesis, allograft nonunion, fracture, devitalization of the skin and soft tissues, joint fibrosis, and recurrence of the tumor. Function and rehabilitation after limb salvage depend on positive encouragement and reducing the risk of complications.

Surgical removal of the tumor may require amputation of the affected extremity, with the amputation extending well above the tumor to achieve local control of the primary lesion (see Nursing Process: The Patient Undergoing an Amputation in Chapter 69).

Because of the danger of metastasis with malignant bone tumors, chemotherapy is started before and continued after surgery in an effort to eradicate micrometastatic lesions. The goal of combined chemotherapy is greater therapeutic effect at a lower toxicity rate with reduced resistance to the medications. There is an improved long-term survival rate when a localized osteosarcoma is removed and chemotherapy is initiated. Soft tissue sarcomas are treated with radiation, limb-sparing excision, and adjuvant chemotherapy (see Chapter 16).

Secondary Bone Tumors

The treatment of metastatic bone cancer is palliative. The therapeutic goal is to relieve the patient's pain and discomfort while promoting quality of life.

If metastatic disease weakens the bone, structural support and stabilization are needed to prevent pathologic fracture. At times, large bones with metastatic lesions are strengthened by prophylactic internal fixation. Internal fixation of pathologic fractures, arthroplasty, or methylmethacrylate (bone cement) reconstruction minimizes associated disability and pain. Patients with metastatic disease are at higher risk than other patients for postoperative pulmonary congestion, hypoxemia, deep vein thrombosis (DVT), and hemorrhage.

Hypercalcemia results from breakdown of bone. It needs to be recognized promptly. Treatment includes hydration with IV administration of normal saline solution; diuresis; mobilization; and medications such as bisphosphonates, (eg, pamidronate [Aredia]) and calcitonin. Because inactivity leads to loss of bone mass and increased calcium in the blood, the nurse assists the patient to increase activity and ambulation.

Hematopoiesis is frequently disrupted by tumor invasion of the bone marrow or by treatment (chemotherapy or radiation). Blood component therapy restores hematologic factors. Pain can result from multiple factors, including the osseous metastasis, surgery, chemotherapy or radiation side effects, and arthritis. Pain must be assessed accurately and managed with adequate and appropriate opioid, nonopioid, and nonpharmaceutical interventions. External beam radiation to involved metastatic sites may be used. Patients with multiple bony metastases may achieve pain control with systemically administered "bone-seeking" isotopes (eg, strontium 89). See Chapter 13 for more information about pain management.

Additional therapies are used to treat the original cancer. Radiation and hormonal therapy may be effective in promoting healing of osteolytic lesions. Chemotherapy is used to control the primary disease (see Chapter 16).

Nursing Management

The nurse asks the patient about the onset and course of symptoms. During the interview, the nurse assesses the patient's understanding of the disease process, how the patient and the family have been coping, and how the patient has managed the pain. On physical examination, the nurse gently palpates the mass and notes its size and associated soft tissue swelling, pain, and tenderness. Assessment of the neurovascular status and range of motion of the extremity provides baseline data for future comparisons. The nurse evaluates the patient's mobility and ability to perform ADLs.

The nursing care of a patient who has undergone excision of a bone tumor is similar in many respects to that of other patients who have had skeletal surgery. Vital signs are monitored; blood loss is assessed; and observations are made to assess for the development of complications such as DVT, pulmonary embolism, infection, contracture, and disuse atrophy. The affected part is elevated to reduce edema, and the neurovascular status of the extremity is assessed.

Patient and family teaching about the disease process and diagnostic and management regimens is essential. Explanation of diagnostic tests, treatments (eg, wound care), and expected results (eg, decreased range of motion, numbness, change of body contours) helps the patient deal with the procedures and changes and comply with the therapeutic regimen. The nurse can most effectively reinforce and clarify information provided by the physician by being present during these discussions.

Accurate pain assessment and use of pharmacologic and nonpharmacologic pain management techniques are used to relieve pain and increase the patient's comfort level. The nurse works with the patient in designing the most effective pain management regimen, thereby increasing the patient's control over the pain. The nurse prepares the patient and gives support during painful procedures. Prescribed IV or epidural analgesic medications are used during the early postoperative period. Later, oral or transdermal opioid or nonopioid analgesic agents are indicated to alleviate pain. In addition, external radiation or systemic radioisotopes (eg, strontium 89) may be prescribed to control pain (see Chapter 13 for further discussion of nursing management for patients in pain).

Bone tumors weaken the bone to a point at which normal activities or even position changes can result in fracture. During nursing care, the affected extremities must be supported and handled gently. External supports (eg, splints) may be used for additional protection. At times, the patient may elect to have surgery (eg, open reduction with internal fixation, joint replacement) in an attempt to prevent pathologic fracture. Prescribed weight-bearing restrictions must be followed. The nurse and physical therapist teach the patient how to use assistive devices safely and how to strengthen unaffected extremities.

The nurse encourages the patient and family to verbalize their fears, concerns, and feelings. They need to be supported as they deal with the impact of the malignant bone tumor. Feelings of shock, despair, and grief are expected. Referral to a psychiatric advanced practice nurse, psychologist, counselor, or spiritual advisor may be indicated for specific psychological help and emotional support.

Independence versus dependence is an issue for the patient who has a malignancy. Lifestyle is dramatically changed, at least temporarily. It is important to support the family in working through the adjustments that must be made. The nurse assists the patient in dealing with changes in body image due to surgery and possible amputation (see Chapter 69 for nursing management of a patient with an amputation). It is helpful to provide realistic reassurance about the future and resumption of role-related activities and to encourage self-care and socialization. The patient participates in planning daily activities. The nurse encourages the patient to be as independent as possible. Involvement of the patient and family throughout treatment encourages confidence, restoration of self-concept, and a sense of being in control of one's life.

Monitoring and Managing Potential Complications

Delayed Wound Healing

Wound healing may be delayed because of tissue trauma from surgery, previous radiation therapy, inadequate nutrition, or infection. The nurse minimizes pressure on the wound site to promote circulation to the tissues. An aseptic, nontraumatic wound dressing promotes healing. Monitoring and reporting of laboratory findings facilitate initiation of interventions to promote homeostasis and wound healing.

Repositioning the patient at frequent intervals reduces the incidence of skin breakdown and pressure ulcers. Special therapeutic beds or mattresses may be needed to prevent skin breakdown and to promote wound healing after extensive surgical reconstruction and skin grafting.

Inadequate Nutrition

Because loss of appetite, nausea, and vomiting are frequent side effects of chemotherapy and radiation therapy, it is necessary to provide adequate nutrition for healing and health promotion. Antiemetics and relaxation techniques reduce the adverse gastrointestinal effects of chemotherapy. Stomatitis is controlled with anesthetic or antifungal mouthwash (see Chapter 16). Adequate hydration is essential. Nutritional supplements or parenteral nutrition may be prescribed to achieve adequate nutrition.

Osteomyelitis and Wound Infections

Prophylactic antibiotics and strict aseptic dressing techniques are used to diminish the occurrence of osteomyelitis and wound infections. During healing, other infections (eg, upper respiratory infections) need to be prevented so that hematogenous spread does not result in osteomyelitis. If the patient is receiving chemotherapy, it is important to monitor the WBC count and to instruct the patient to avoid contact with people who have colds or other infections.

Hypercalcemia

Hypercalcemia is a dangerous complication of bone cancer. The symptoms must be recognized and treatment initiated promptly. Symptoms include muscular weakness, incoordination, anorexia, nausea and vomiting, constipation, electrocardiographic changes (eg, shortened QT interval and ST segment, bradycardia, heart blocks), and altered mental states (eg, confusion, lethargy, psychotic behavior). See Chapter 14 for a discussion of hypercalcemia and its management.

Promoting Home and Community-Based Care

Teaching Patients Self-Care

Preparation for and coordination of continuing health care are begun early as a multidisciplinary effort. Patient teaching addresses medication, dressing changes, treatment regimens, and the importance of physical and occupational therapy programs. The nurse teaches weight-bearing limitations and special handling to prevent pathologic fractures. It is important that the patient and family know the signs and symptoms of possible complications as well as resources available for continuing care (Chart 68-10).

Continuing Care

Frequently, arrangements are made with a home health care agency for home care supervision and follow-up. The home care nurse assesses the patient's and family's abilities to meet the patient's needs and determines whether the services of other agencies are needed. The nurse advises the patient to have readily available the telephone numbers of people to contact in case concerns arise.

The nurse emphasizes the need for long-term health supervision to ensure cure or to detect tumor recurrence or metastasis and the need for recommended health screening. If the patient has metastatic disease, end-of-life issues may need to be explored. Referral for hospice care is made if appropriate.

CHART
68-10

HOME CARE CHECKLIST
Bone Tumor

At the completion of the home care instruction, the patient or caregiver will be able to:	PATIENT	CAREGIVER
• Describe tumor growth process.	✔	✔
• Control pain with pharmacologic and nonpharmacologic interventions.	✔	✔
• Support affected musculoskeletal area.	✔	
• Describe use of prescribed medications.	✔	✔
• Comply with medication regimen.	✔	
• Consume diet to promote healing and health.	✔	
• State weight-bearing and activity restrictions.	✔	✔
• Demonstrate safe use of ambulatory aids and assistive devices.	✔	
• Protect affected bone from pathologic fracture.	✔	✔
• Identify complications of tumor and therapy.	✔	✔
• Report signs and symptoms of complications promptly.	✔	✔
• Use effective coping strategies.	✔	
• Maintain role performance.	✔	

CRITICAL THINKING EXERCISES

EBP **1**   You are a staff nurse employed at a family practice clinic. A 52-year-old mechanic has been seeking treatment at the clinic for low back pain of 2 weeks' duration. He has been prescribed a muscle relaxant and told to take over-the-counter NSAIDs. He is not reporting significant relief from his symptoms, though he reports taking his prescribed medications diligently. You note that this patient is obese. The patient tells you that he is getting frustrated that he continues to have significant low back pain that interferes with his ability to work. Identify other therapies or interventions that might be reasonable alternatives or adjuncts that might relieve this patient's low back pain. What is the strength of the evidence for each of these potential therapies or interventions?

2   Your 30-year-old cousin tells you that she was diagnosed 3 months ago with impingement syndrome of her right shoulder. She was treated with intra-articular corticosteroids and physical therapy and has had a very good response to these interventions. She is a flight attendant and is concerned whether she is likely to have recurrent episodes or whether she is at risk for worse shoulder injuries. What is the likelihood that she may have either recurrence of her symptoms or worse rotator cuff injuries? What advice might you share with her so that she might continue her career as a flight attendant?

EBP **3**   On the general medical unit where you are a staff nurse, a 74-year-old man is admitted with pneumonia and a history of chronic obstructive pulmonary disease (COPD). He also has a history of heavy cigarette smoking and alcohol consumption. You note during his screening process that he has lost 1 inch in height over the past year, and he has notable kyphosis of his lumbar vertebrae. What musculoskeletal condition is he at risk of developing? What specific questions would you ask him to determine the status of his bone health? Discuss the strength of the evidence that supports any risk factor reduction strategies you consider implementing.

EBP **4**   At the orthopedic clinic where you work as a nurse, a 20-year-old college athlete presents for a workup because of persistent right shoulder pain with point tenderness at his proximal humerus and a palpable soft tissue mass. An extensive workup confirms an osteosarcoma. He is stunned with the diagnosis and tells you that he would rather die than have his right arm amputated (he is right-sided dominant and is his football team's quarterback). What is the evidence that supports limb salvage over amputation in patients with osteosarcoma of an extremity? What can he expect in terms of quality of life after an amputation versus more conservative limb salvage interventions? What support systems would you mobilize for this patient?

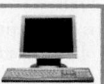

The Smeltzer suite offers these additional resources to enhance learning and facilitate understanding of this chapter:
- thePoint online resource, thepoint.lww.com/Smeltzer12E
- Student CD-ROM included with the book
- *Study Guide to Accompany Brunner & Suddarth's Textbook of Medical-Surgical Nursing*
- *Handbook for Brunner & Suddarth's Textbook of Medical-Surgical Nursing*

REFERENCES AND SELECTED READINGS

Asterisk indicates nursing research.

Books

Bickley, L. S. (2007). *Bates' guide to physical examination and history taking* (9th ed.). Philadelphia: Lippincott Williams & Wilkins.

National Association of Orthopaedic Nurses. (2007). *Core curriculum for orthopaedic nursing* (6th ed.). Boston: Pearson Custom Publishing.

National Osteoporosis Foundation (NOF). (2008). *Clinician's guide to prevention and treatment of osteoporosis.* Washington, DC: Author.

Porth, C. M. & Matfin, G. (2009). *Pathophysiology: Concepts of altered health states* (8th ed.). Philadelphia: Lippincott Williams & Wilkins.

U.S. Department of Health and Human Services. (2004). *Bone health and osteoporosis: A report of the Surgeon General.* Rockville, MD: U.S. Department of Health and Human Services/Public Health Service, Office of the Surgeon General.

World Health Organization. (2003). *Prevention and management of osteoporosis.* Geneva, Switzerland: World Health Organization.

Journals and Electronic Documents

Anders, M., Turner, L. & Wallace, L. S. (2007). Use of decision rules for osteoporosis prevention and treatment: Implications for nurse practitioners. *Journal of the American Academy of Nurse Practitioners, 19*(6), 299–305.

Badlissi, F., Dunn, J. E., Link, C. L., et al. (2005). Foot musculoskeletal disorders, pain, and foot-related functional limitation in older persons. *Journal of the American Geriatrics Society, 53*(6), 1029–1033.

Bonnick, S. L. (2005). Bone mass measurement techniques in clinical practice: Methods, applications, and interpretation. *Topics in Geriatric Rehabilitation, 21*(1), 30–41.

Burns, J., Landorf, K. B., Ryan, M. M., et al. (2008). Interventions for the prevention and treatment of pes cavus (review). *Cochrane Database of Systematic Reviews, 4,* CD006154.

Carne, K. (2009). Osteoporosis: Maintaining bone health and preventing fractures. *Journal of Community Nursing, 23*(1), 11–13.

Childs, S. G. (2005). Dupuytren's disease. *Orthopaedic Nursing, 24*(2), 160–165.

Chou, R. & Huffman, L. H. (2007a). Nonpharmacologic therapies for acute and chronic low back pain: A review of the evidence for an American Pain Society/American College of Physicians clinical practice guideline. *Annals of Internal Medicine, 147*(7), 492–504.

Chou, R. & Huffman, L. H. (2007b). Medications for acute and chronic low back pain: A review of the evidence for an American Pain Society/American College of Physicians clinical practice guideline. *Annals of Internal Medicine, 147*(7), 505–514.

Cole, C., Seto, C. & Gazewood, J. (2005). Plantar fasciitis: Evidence-based review of diagnosis and therapy. *American Family Physician, 72*(11), 2237–2242.

*Davis, G. C., White, T. L. & Yang, A. (2006). A bone health intervention for older adults living in residential settings. *Research in Nursing and Health, 29*(6), 566–575.

Davis, J. S. (2005). Management of bone and joint infections due to *Staphylococcus aureus. Internal Medicine Journal, 35*(suppl. 2), S79–S96.

*Doheny, M. O., Sedlak, C. A., Estok, P. J., et al. (2007). Osteoporosis knowledge, health beliefs, and DXA T-scores in men and women 50 years of age and older. *Orthopaedic Nursing, 26*(4), 243–250.

Donaldson, A. D., Jalaludin, B. B. & Chan, R. C. (2007). Patient perceptions of osteomyelitis, septic arthritis and prosthetic joint infection: The psychological influence of methicillin-resistant *Staphylococcus aureus. Internal Medicine Journal, 37*(8), 536–542.

Ebeling, P. R. (2008). Osteoporosis in men. *New England Journal of Medicine, 358*(14), 1474–1482.

Ferreira, A. (2006). Development of renal bone disease. *European Journal of Clinical Investigation, 26*(S2), 2–12.

Forman, T. A., Forman, S. K. & Rose, N. E. (2005). A clinical approach to diagnosing wrist pain. *American Family Physician, 72*(9), 1753–1758.

Gavet, F., Tournadre, A., Soubrier, M., et al. (2005). Septic arthritis in patients aged 80 and older: A comparison with younger adults. *Journal of the American Geriatrics Society, 53*(7), 1210–1213.

Hogan, S. L. (2005). The effects of weight loss on calcium and bone. *Critical Care Nursing Quarterly, 28*(3), 269–275.

Holick, M. F. (2007). Review article: Optimal vitamin D status for the prevention and treatment of osteoporosis. *Drugs and Aging, 24*(12), 1017–1029.

Hurwitz, E. L., Morganstern, H. & Chiao, C. (2005). Effects of recreational physical activity and back exercises on low back pain and psychological distress: Findings from the UCLA Low Back Pain Study. *American Journal of Public Health, 95*(10), 1817–1824.

Jeon, I. H., Choi, C. H., Seo, J. S., et al. (2006). Arthroscopic management of septic arthritis of the shoulder joint. *Journal of Bone and Joint Surgery, 88*(8), 1802–1806.

Johnson, N., K., Clifford, T. & Smith, K. M. (2008). Treatment of risk factors, screening, and treatment of postmenopausal osteoporosis. *Orthopedics, 31*(7), 676–680.

Josse, R. G., Hanley, D. A., Kendler, D., et al. (2007). Position paper: Diagnosis and treatment of Paget's disease of bone. *Clinical Investigative Medicine, 30*(5), E210–E233.

Keating, G., M. & Scott, L. J. (2007). Zoledronic acid: A review of its use in treatment of Paget's disease of bone. *Drugs, 67*(5), 793–804.

Kent, M. E., Rapp, R. P. & Smith, K. M. (2006). Antibiotic beads and osteomyelitis: Here today, what's coming tomorrow? *Orthopedics, 29*(7), 599–603.

Kern, L. M., Rowe, N. R., Levine, M. A., et al. (2005). Association between screening for osteoporosis and the incidence of hip fracture. *Annals of Internal Medicine, 142*(3), 173–181.

Landis, D. M. (2005). Fracture risk in postmenopausal women. *Nurse Practitioner, 30*(11), 48, 53–58.

Liberman, U. A. (2006). Long-term safety of bisphosphonate therapy for osteoporosis. *Drugs and Aging, 23*(4), 289–298.

Licata, A. A. (2007). Update on therapy for osteoporosis. *Orthopaedic Nursing, 26*(3), 162–166.

Lyman, D. (2005). Undiagnosed vitamin D deficiency in the hospitalized patient. *American Family Physician, 71*(2), 299–304.

Matthews, E., Snell, K. & Coats, H. (2006). Intra-arterial chemotherapy for limb preservation in patients with osteosarcoma: Nursing implications. *Clinical Journal of Oncology Nursing, 10*(5), 581–589.

Migues, A., Campaner, G., Slullitel, G., et al. (2007). Minimally invasive surgery in hallux valgus and digital deformities. *Orthopedics, 30*(7), 523–526.

Muscolo, D. L., Ayerza, M. A., Aponte-Tinao, L. A., et al. (2005). Use of distal femoral osteoarticular allografts in limb salvage surgery. *Journal of Bone and Joint Surgery, 87A*(11), 2449–2455.

National Institute of Neurological Disorders and Stroke (NINDS). (2009). Low back pain fact sheet. Available at: www.ninds.nih.gov/disorders/backpain/detail_backpain.htm

Piazzini, D. B., Aprile, I., Ferrara, P. E., et al. (2007). A systematic review of conservative treatment of carpal tunnel syndrome. *Clinical Rehabilitation, 21*(4), 299–314.

Pfister, A. K., Welch, C. A., Lester, M. D., et al. (2006). Cost-effectiveness strategies to treat osteoporosis. *Southern Medical Journal, 99*(2), 123–131.

Resnik, L. & Dobrykowski, E. (2005). Outcomes measurement for patients with low back pain. *Orthopaedic Nursing, 24*(1), 14–24.

Sadler, C. & Huff, M. (2007). African-American women: Health beliefs, lifestyle, and osteoporosis. *Orthopaedic Nursing, 26*(2), 96–103.

Sahar, T., Cohen, M. J., Matan, J., et al. (2008). Insoles for prevention and treatment of back pain. *Cochrane Database of Systematic Reviews, 4,* CD005275.

Sambrook, P. & Cooper, C. (2006). Osteoporosis. *Lancet, 367*(9527), 2010–2018.

Schoen, D. C. (2005). Injuries of the wrist. *Orthopaedic Nursing, 24*(4), 304–307.

Schousboe, J. T., Ensrud, K. E., Nyman, J. A., et al. (2005). Universal bone densitometry screening combined with alendronate therapy for those diagnosed with osteoporosis is highly cost-effective for elderly women. *Journal of the American Geriatrics Society, 53*(10), 1697–1704.

*Sedlak, C. A., Doheny, M. O., Estok, P. J., et al. (2005). Tailored interventions to enhance osteoporosis prevention in women. *Orthopaedic Nursing, 24*(4), 270–278.

Sharma, P. & Maffulli, N. (2005). Tendon injury and tendinopathy: Healing and repair. *Journal of Bone & Joint Surgery, 87*(1), 187–202.

Sheff, E. K. (2005). Solving the mystery of osteomyelitis. *Nursing, 35*(7), 32hn1–32hn3.

Sim, M. F., Stone, M. D., Phillips, C. J., et al. (2005). Cost effectiveness analysis of using quantitative ultrasound as a selective pre-screen for bone densitometry. *Technology and Health Care, 13*(2), 75–85.

Skubitz, K. M. & D'Adamo, D. R. (2007). Sarcoma. *Mayo Clinic Proceedings, 82*(11), 1409–1432.

*Smeltzer, S. C. & Zimmerman, V. L. (2005). Usefulness of the SCORE index as a predictor of osteoporosis in women with disabilities. *Orthopaedic Nursing, 24*(1), 33–39.

Solomon, D. H., Morris, C., Cheng, H., et al. (2005). Medication use patterns for osteoporosis: An assessment of guidelines, treatment rates, and quality improvement interventions. *Mayo Clinic Proceedings, 80*(2), 194–202.

Termaat, M. F., Raijmakers, P. G., Scholten, H. J., et al. (2005). The accuracy of diagnostic imaging for the assessment of chronic osteomyelitis: A systematic review and meta-analysis. *Journal of Bone & Joint Surgery, 87*(11), 2464–2471.

Trampas, A. & Kitsios, A. (2006). Exercise and manual therapy for the treatment of impingement syndrome of the shoulder: A systematic review. *Physical Therapy Reviews, 11,* 125–142.

Trojian, T. H. & Chu, S. M. (2007). Dupuytren's disease: Diagnosis and treatment. *American Family Physician, 76*(1), 86–89, 90.

Trojian, T., Stevenson, J. H. & Agrawal, N. (2005). What can we expect from nonoperative treatment options for shoulder pain? *Journal of Family Practice, 54*(3), 216–223.

Venugopalan, V. & Martin, C. A. (2007). Selecting anti-infective agents for the treatment of bone infections: New anti-infective agents and chronic suppressive therapy. *Orthopedics, 30*(1), 832–834.

Weber, K. L. (2005). What's new in musculoskeletal oncology. *Journal of Bone and Joint Surgery, 87*(6), 1400–1410.

Weiner, D. K., Sakamoto, S., Perera, S., et al. (2006). Chronic low back pain in older adults: Prevalence, reliability, and validity of physical examination findings. *Journal of the American Geriatrics Society, 54*(1), 11–20.

Wells, G. A., Cranney, A., Peterson, J., et al. (2008). Alendronate for the primary and secondary prevention of osteoporotic fractures in postmenopausal women. *Cochrane Database of Systematic Reviews, 1,* CD001155.

RESOURCES

National Institute of Arthritis and Musculoskeletal and Skin Diseases, www.niams.nih.gov

National Osteoporosis Foundation, www.nof.org

The Paget Foundation, www.paget.org

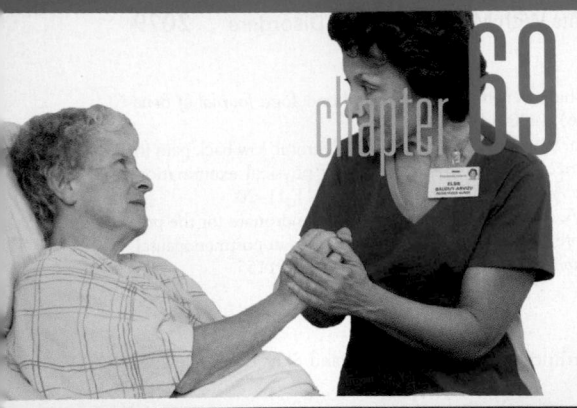

Management of Patients With Musculoskeletal Trauma

LEARNING OBJECTIVES

On completion of this chapter, the learner will be able to:

1 Differentiate between contusions, strains, sprains, dislocations, and subluxations.

2 Identify sport and occupational injuries and their signs, symptoms, and treatments.

3 Identify the signs and symptoms of an acute fracture.

4 Describe the treatment procedures of fracture reduction, fracture immobilization, and management of open and intra-articular fractures.

5 Describe the prevention and management of immediate and delayed complications of fractures.

6 Describe the rehabilitation needs of patients with fractures of the upper and lower extremities, pelvis, and hips.

7 Describe nursing management of the elderly patient with a fracture of the hip.

8 Describe the rehabilitation and health education needs of the patient who has had an amputation.

9 Use the nursing process as a framework for care of the patient with an amputation.

GLOSSARY

allograft: tissue harvested from a donor for use in another person

amputation: removal of a body part, usually a limb or part of a limb

arthroscope: surgical scope injected into the joint to examine or repair

autograft: tissue harvested from one area of the body and used for transplantation to another area of the same body

avascular necrosis: death of tissue secondary to a decrease or lack of perfusion

contusion: blunt force injury to soft tissue

crepitus: a grating sound or sensation by rubbing bony fragments together

débridement: surgical removal of contaminated and devitalized tissues and foreign material

delayed union: prolongation of expected healing time for a fracture

disarticulation: amputation through a joint

dislocation: complete separation of joint surfaces

fracture: a break in the continuity of a bone

fracture reduction: restoration of fracture fragments into anatomic alignment

malunion: healing of a fractured bone in a malaligned position

nonunion: failure of fractured bones to heal together

phantom limb pain: pain perceived in an amputated section

RICE: acronym for *r*est, *i*ce, *c*ompression, *e*levation

sprain: an injury to ligaments and muscles and other soft tissues at a joint

strain: a musculotendinous stress injury

subluxation: partial separation of joint surfaces

Injury to one part of the musculoskeletal system results in malfunction of adjacent muscles, joints, and tendons. The type and severity of injury affects the mobility of the injured area. Treatment of injury to the musculoskeletal system involves providing support to the injured part until healing is complete. Some injuries or situations require traction to be applied to maintain proper anatomical alignment of the extremity. Pain assessment and management are essential. After the immediate painful effects of the injury have decreased, treatment efforts are focused on proper exercise and mobility, with assistance if needed.

Contusions, Strains, and Sprains

A **contusion** is a soft tissue injury produced by blunt force, such as a blow, kick, or fall, causing small blood vessels to rupture and bleed into soft tissues (ecchymosis, or bruising). A hematoma develops from bleeding at the site of impact. Local symptoms (pain, swelling, and discoloration) are controlled with intermittent application of cold packs applied with pressure to the site and elevation of the extremity above the heart level. Most contusions resolve in 1 to 2 weeks.

A **strain,** or a "pulled muscle or tendon," is an injury caused by overuse, overstretching, or excessive stress. Strains are graded along a continuum based on postinjury symptoms and loss of function and reflect the degree of injury. Three types of strain are recognized:

- A first-degree strain is mild stretching of the muscle or tendon. Signs and symptoms may include minor edema, tenderness, and mild muscle spasm, without noticeable loss of function.
- A second-degree strain involves partial tearing of the muscle or tendon. Signs and symptoms include loss of load-bearing strength with accompanying edema, tenderness, muscle spasm, and ecchymosis.
- A third-degree strain is severe muscle or tendon stretching with rupturing and tearing of the involved tissue. Signs and symptoms include significant pain, muscle spasm, ecchymosis, edema, and loss of function. An x-ray should be obtained to rule out bone injury, because an avulsion fracture (in which a bone fragment is pulled away from the bone by a tendon) may be associated with a third-degree strain. Magnetic resonance imaging (MRI) will reveal a third-degree strain, but x-rays do not reveal injuries to soft tissue or muscles, tendons, or ligaments.

A **sprain** is an injury to the ligaments and tendons that surround a joint. It is caused by a twisting motion or hyperextension (forcible) of a joint. The function of a ligament is to stabilize a joint while permitting mobility. A torn ligament causes a joint to become unstable. Blood vessels rupture and edema occurs; the joint is tender, and movement of the joint becomes painful. The degree of disability and pain increases during the first 2 to 3 hours after the injury because of the associated swelling and bleeding, especially if treatment is delayed. Sprains are graded in a manner similar to the grading system used for strains:

- A first-degree sprain is caused by stretching the ligamentous fibers, resulting in minimum damage. It is manifested by mild edema, local tenderness, and pain that is elicited when the joint is moved.
- A second-degree sprain involves partial tearing of the ligament. It results in increased edema, tenderness, pain with motion, joint instability, and partial loss of normal joint function.
- A third-degree sprain occurs when a ligament is completely torn or ruptured. A third-degree sprain may also cause an avulsion of the bone. Symptoms include severe pain, tenderness, increased edema, and abnormal joint motion.

Nursing Management

Treatment of contusions, strains, and sprains consists of resting and elevating the affected part, applying cold, and using a compression bandage. (The acronym **RICE**—*rest, ice, compression, elevation*—is helpful for remembering treatment interventions.) Rest prevents additional injury and promotes healing. Intermittent application of moist or dry cold packs for 20 to 30 minutes during the first 24 to 48 hours after injury produces vasoconstriction, which decreases bleeding, edema, and discomfort. Care must be taken to avoid skin and tissue damage from excessive cold. An elastic compression bandage controls bleeding, reduces edema, and provides support for the injured tissues. Elevation controls the swelling. If the sprain or strain is third degree, surgical repair or immobilization by a splint, brace, or cast may be necessary so that the joint will not lose its stability. The neurovascular status (circulation, motion, sensation) of the injured extremity is monitored every 15 minutes for the first 1 to 2 hours after injury; then, every 30 minutes until stable. Decreases in sensation or motion and increases in pain level should be documented and reported to the physician immediately so that compartment syndrome can be prevented (see later discussion).

After the acute inflammatory stage (eg, 24 to 48 hours after injury), heat may be applied intermittently (for 15 to 30 minutes four times a day) to relieve muscle spasm and to promote vasodilation, absorption, and repair. Depending on the severity of injury, progressive passive and active exercises may begin in 2 to 5 days. Severe sprains and strains may require 1 to 3 weeks of immobilization before exercises are initiated. Excessive exercise early in the course of treatment delays recovery. Strains and sprains take weeks or months to heal because ligaments and tendons have minimal blood supply. Splinting may be used to maintain stability at the injury site.

Joint Dislocations

A **dislocation** of a joint is a condition in which the articular surfaces of the distal and proximal bones that form the joint are no longer in anatomic alignment. A **subluxation** is a partial dislocation and does not cause as much deformity as a complete dislocation. In complete dislocation, the bones are literally "out of joint." Traumatic dislocations are orthopedic emergencies because the associated joint structures, blood supply, and nerves are displaced and may be entrapped with extensive pressure on them. If a dislocation or subluxation is not reduced immediately, **avascular necrosis** (AVN) may develop. AVN of bone is caused by ischemia, which leads to necrosis or death of the bone cells.

Signs and symptoms of a traumatic dislocation include acute pain, change in positioning of the joint, shortening of the extremity, deformity, and decreased mobility. X-rays confirm the diagnosis and reveal any associated fracture.

Medical Management

The affected joint needs to be immobilized at the scene and during transport to the hospital. The dislocation is promptly reduced and displaced parts are placed back in proper anatomic position to preserve joint function. Analgesia, muscle relaxants, and possibly anesthesia are used to facilitate closed reduction. The joint is immobilized by splints, casts, or traction and is maintained in a stable position. Neurovascular status is assessed at a minimum of every 15 minutes until stable. After reduction, if the joint is stable, gentle, progressive, active and passive movement is begun to preserve range of motion (ROM) and restore strength. The joint is supported between exercise sessions.

Nursing Management

Nursing attention is geared to frequent assessment and evaluation of the injury including complete neurovascular assessment with proper documentation and communication with the physician. The patient and supportive family members are educated regarding proper exercises and activities as well as danger signs and symptoms to look for, such as increasing pain (even with analgesics), "numbness or tingling," and increased edema in the extremity. These signs and symptoms may indicate compartment syndrome, and if this is not identified and communicated to the treating physician, the patient may lose the extremity (see later discussion).

Injuries to the Tendons, Ligaments, and Menisci

ROTATOR CUFF TEARS

A rotator cuff tear is a tear in a tendon that connects one of the rotator muscles to the humeral head. The rotator cuff stabilizes the humeral head and is composed of four muscles and their tendons that include the supraspinatous, infraspinatous, teres minor, and subscapularis.

Rotator cuff tears may result from an acute injury or from chronic joint stresses. Patients complain of pain, limited ROM, and some joint dysfunction, including muscle weakness. In many cases, patients with a rotator cuff tear experience night pain and cannot sleep on the involved side. Patients cannot perform over-the-head activities. The acromioclavicular joint is tender. X-rays are helpful in evaluating the joint. Arthrography and MRI or ultrasound are used to determine soft tissue pathology and the extent of the rotator cuff tear.

Initial conservative management includes use of nonsteroidal anti-inflammatory drugs (NSAIDs), rest with modification of activities, injection of a corticosteroid into the shoulder joint, and progressive stretching, ROM, and lengthening exercises (Trojian, Stevenson & Agrawal, 2005). Some rotator cuff tears require arthroscopic **débridement** (removal of devitalized tissue) or arthroscopic or open acromioplasty with tendon repair. Postoperatively, the shoulder is immobilized for several days to 4 weeks. Physical

therapy with shoulder exercises is begun as prescribed, and the patient is instructed in how to perform the exercises at home. Full recovery is expected in 6 to 12 months.

EPICONDYLITIS

Epicondylitis is a chronic, painful condition that is caused by excessive, repetitive extension, flexion, pronation, and supination motions of the forearm. These motions result in inflammation (tendinitis) and minor tears in the tendons at the origin of the muscles on the lateral or medial epicondyles. Lateral epicondylitis (ie, tennis elbow) is frequently identified in someone who repeatedly extends the wrist or frequently pronates and supinates the forearm. Pain develops over the lateral epicondyle and in the extensor muscles. If action is continued, pain continues to increase (Clinton & Murthi, 2008). Medial epicondylitis (ie, golfer's or pitcher's elbow) is consistent with repetitive wrist flexion. Extreme tenderness occurs at the medial epicondyle. Pain greatly increases with wrist flexion against resistance.

Application of ice and administration of NSAIDs usually relieve the pain. In some instances, the arm is immobilized in a molded splint or cast. Because of its degenerative effects on tendons, local injection of a corticosteroid is reserved for patients with severe pain who do not respond to NSAIDs and immobilization. After pain subsides, rehabilitation exercises include gentle and gradual increased stretching of the tendons (Clinton & Murthi, 2008). A tennis elbow counterforce strap that limits extension of the elbow may be prescribed when activity is resumed.

LATERAL AND MEDIAL COLLATERAL LIGAMENT INJURY

Lateral and medial collateral ligaments of the knee (Fig. 69-1) provide stability lateral and medial to the knee. Injury to these ligaments occurs when the foot is firmly planted and the knee is struck—either medially, causing stretching and tearing injury to the lateral collateral ligament, or laterally, causing stretching and tearing injury to the medial collateral ligament. The patient experiences an acute onset of pain, point tenderness, joint instability, and inability to walk without assistance.

Medical Management

Early management includes RICE. The joint is evaluated for fracture. Hemarthrosis (bleeding into the joint) may develop, contributing to the pain. The joint fluid may be aspirated to relieve pressure.

Treatment depends on the severity of the injury. Conservative management includes limited weight bearing and use of a protective brace. As pain subsides, ROM exercise is encouraged. The patient's return to full activities, including sports, depends on return of motion, functional stability of the joint, and muscle strength.

If needed, surgical reconstruction may be performed immediately or it may be delayed. The leg is immobilized for approximately 6 to 8 weeks. A progressive rehabilitation program helps restore the function and strength of the knee. Rehabilitation occurs over many months, and the patient may need to wear a derotational brace while engaging in sports to prevent reinjury.

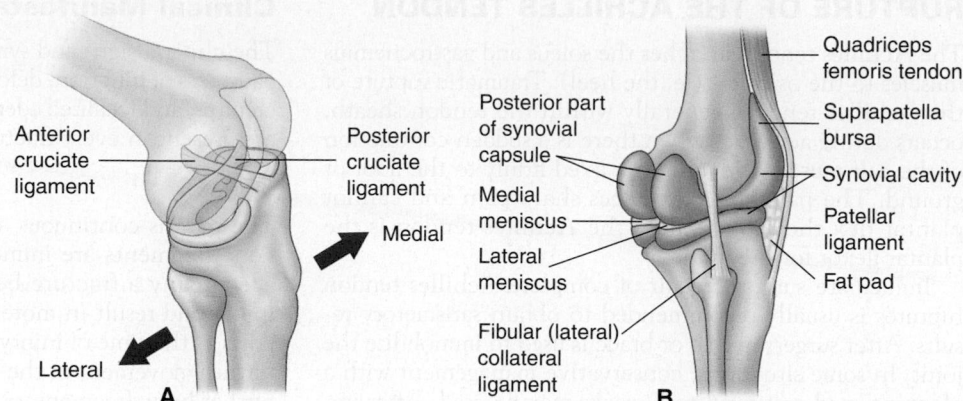

Figure 69-1 Knee ligaments, tendons, and menisci. **A,** Anterolateral view. **B,** Posterolateral view.

Nursing Management

The nurse instructs the patient about proper use of ambulatory devices, the healing process, and activity limitation to promote healing. Education addresses pain management, analgesic use, antibiotic use, brace use, wound care, signs and symptoms of possible complications (eg, altered neurovascular status, infection, skin breakdown), and self-care.

CRUCIATE LIGAMENT INJURY

The anterior cruciate ligament (ACL) and the posterior cruciate ligament (PCL) of the knee stabilize anterior and posterior motion of the tibia articulating with the femur (see Fig. 69-1). These ligaments cross each other in the center of the knee. Injury occurs when the foot is firmly planted and the leg sustains direct force, forward or backward. If the force is forward, the ACL suffers the impact from the force; whereas, backward force places force on the PCL. The injured person may report feeling and hearing a "pop" in the knee with this injury. If the patient exhibits significant swelling of the joint within 2 hours after the injury, the ACL or PCL may be torn. A torn cruciate ligament produces pain, joint instability, and pain with weight bearing. Immediate postinjury management includes RICE and stabilization of the joint until it is evaluated for a fracture. Severe joint effusion and hemarthrosis may require joint aspiration and wrapping with an elastic compression dressing.

Treatment depends on the severity of the injury and the effect of the injury on daily activities. Early treatment involves application of a brace and physical therapy. Surgical ACL or PCL reconstruction may be scheduled after near-normal joint ROM is achieved and includes tendon repair with grafting. This is typically performed as ambulatory arthroscopic surgery, a procedure in which the surgeon uses an **arthroscope** to visualize and repair the damage. The best surgical candidates include patients who are young and physically active. Older and less active patients, particularly with concomitant osteoarthritis, tend to benefit from non-surgical therapy (Alford & Bach, 2004). After surgery, the patient is taught to control pain with oral analgesics and cryotherapy (a cooling pad incorporated in a dressing). The patient and family are taught about monitoring the neurovascular status of the leg, wound care, and signs of complications

that need to be reported promptly to the surgeon. Exercises (ankle pumps, quadriceps sets, and hamstring sets) are encouraged during the early postoperative period. The patient must protect the graft by complying with exercise restrictions. The physical therapist supervises progressive ROM and weight bearing (as permitted). Continuous passive motion may be helpful in restoring full ROM.

MENISCAL INJURIES

Two crescent-shaped (semilunar) cartilages in the knee, called menisci, are located on the right and left side of the proximal tibia, between the tibia and the femur (see Fig. 69-1). These structures act as shock absorbers in the knee. Normally, little twisting movement is permitted in the knee joint. Twisting of the knee or repetitive squatting and impact may result in either tearing or detachment of the cartilage from its attachment to the head of the tibia. The peripheral third of the menisci have a small amount of blood flow, which allows that portion to heal if torn.

These injuries leave loose cartilage in the knee joint that may slip between the femur and the tibia, preventing full extension of the leg. If this happens during walking or running, the patient often describes the leg as "giving way." The patient may hear or feel a click in the knee when walking, especially when extending the leg that is bearing weight. When the cartilage is attached to the front and back of the knee but torn loose laterally (bucket-handle tear), it may slide between the bones to lie between the condyles and prevent full flexion or extension. As a result, the knee "locks."

When a meniscus is torn, the synovial membrane secretes additional synovial fluid due to the irritation and the knee becomes very edematous. Initial conservative treatment includes immobilization of the knee, use of crutches, anti-inflammatory agents, analgesics, and modification of activities to avoid those that cause the symptoms. An MRI is the diagnostic tool used to detect a torn meniscus. Damaged cartilage is surgically removed (meniscectomy) arthroscopically. After surgery, a pressure dressing is applied. The most common complication is an effusion into the knee joint, which produces pain. The patient is instructed to continue quadriceps-setting and ROM exercises.

RUPTURE OF THE ACHILLES TENDON

The Achilles tendon attaches the soleus and gastrocnemius muscles to the os calcis (ie, the heel). Traumatic rupture of the Achilles tendon, generally within the tendon sheath, occurs during activities when there is a sudden contraction of the calf muscle with the foot fixed firmly to the floor or ground. The patient experiences sharp pain and cannot plantar flex the foot because the Achilles tendon is the plantar flexor for the ankle.

Immediate surgical repair of complete Achilles tendon ruptures is usually recommended to obtain satisfactory results. After surgery, a cast or brace is used to immobilize the joint. In some situations, conservative management with a plantar-flexed cast for 6 to 8 weeks may be used. After immobilization, a heel lift is worn and progressive physical therapy to promote ankle ROM and strength is begun.

Fractures

A **fracture** is a complete or incomplete disruption in the continuity of bone structure and is defined according to its type and extent. Fractures occur when the bone is subjected to stress greater than it can absorb. Fractures may be caused by direct blows, crushing forces, sudden twisting motions, and extreme muscle contractions. When the bone is broken, adjacent structures are also affected, resulting in soft tissue edema, hemorrhage into the muscles and joints, joint dislocations, ruptured tendons, severed nerves, and damaged blood vessels. Body organs may be injured by the force that caused the fracture or by fracture fragments.

Types of Fractures

A *complete fracture* involves a break across the entire cross-section of the bone and is frequently displaced (removed from its normal position). An *incomplete fracture* (eg, greenstick fracture) involves a break through only part of the cross-section of the bone. A *comminuted* fracture is one that produces several bone fragments. A *closed fracture* (simple fracture) is one that does not cause a break in the skin. An *open fracture* (compound, or complex, fracture) is one in which the skin or mucous membrane wound extends to the fractured bone (Whiteing, 2008). Open fractures are graded according to the following criteria:

- Grade I is a clean wound less than 1 cm long.
- Grade II is a larger wound without extensive soft tissue damage.
- Grade III is highly contaminated, has extensive soft tissue damage, and is the most severe.

Fractures may also be described according to the anatomic placement of fragments. Specific types of fractures are reviewed in Figure 69-2.

An intra-articular fracture extends into the joint surface of a bone. Because each end of a long bone is cartilaginous, if the fracture is nondisplaced, x-rays will not always reveal the fracture because cartilage is nonradiopaque. An MRI or arthroscopy will identify the fracture and confirm the diagnosis. The joint is stabilized and immobilized with a splint or cast and no weight bearing is allowed until the fracture has healed. Intra-articular fractures often lead to posttraumatic arthritis.

Clinical Manifestations

The clinical signs and symptoms of a fracture include acute pain, loss of function, deformity, shortening of the extremity, crepitus, and localized edema and ecchymosis. Not all of these are present in every fracture (Whiteing, 2008).

Pain

The pain is continuous and increases in severity until the bone fragments are immobilized. The muscle spasms that accompany a fracture begin within 20 minutes after the injury and result in more intense pain than the patient reports at the time of injury. The muscle spasms can minimize further movement of the fracture fragments or can result in further bony fragmentation or malalignment.

Loss of Function

After a fracture, the extremity cannot function properly because normal function of the muscles depends on the integrity of the bones to which they are attached. Pain contributes to the loss of function. In addition, abnormal movement (false motion) may be present.

Deformity

Displacement, angulation, or rotation of the fragments in a fracture of the arm or leg causes a deformity that is detectable when the limb is compared with the uninjured extremity.

Shortening

In fractures of long bones, there is actual shortening of the extremity because of the compression of the fractured bone. Sometimes muscle spasms can cause the distal and proximal site of the fracture to overlap, causing the extremity to shorten.

Crepitus

When the extremity is gently palpated, a crumbling sensation, called **crepitus,** can be felt. It is caused by the rubbing of the bone fragments against each other.

 NURSING ALERT

Testing for crepitus can produce further tissue damage and should be minimized as much as possible.

Localized Edema and Ecchymosis

Localized edema and ecchymosis occur after a fracture as a result of trauma and bleeding into the tissues. These signs may not develop for several hours after the injury or may develop within an hour, depending on the severity of the fracture.

Emergency Management

Immediately after injury, if a fracture is suspected, it is important to immobilize the body part before the patient is moved. Adequate splinting is essential. Joints proximal and distal to the fracture must be immobilized to prevent movement of fracture fragments. Immobilization of the long bones of the lower extremities may be accomplished by bandaging the legs together, with the unaffected extremity

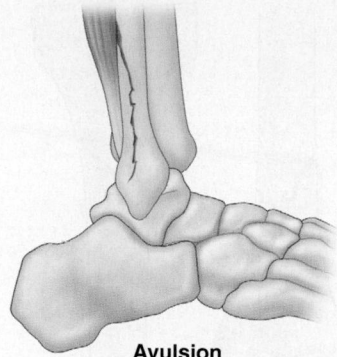

Avulsion
A fracture in which a fragment of bone has been pulled away by a tendon and its attachment

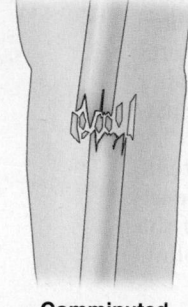

Comminuted
A fracture in which bone has splintered into several fragments

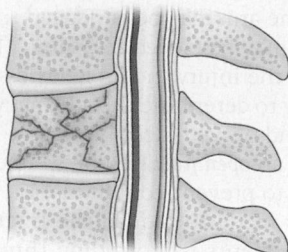

Compression
A fracture in which bone has been compressed (seen in vertebral fractures)

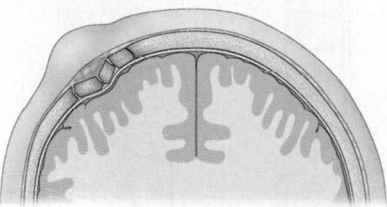

Depressed
A fracture in which fragments are driven inward (seen frequently in fractures of skull and facial bones)

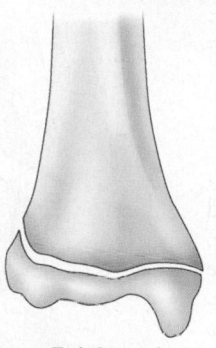

Epiphyseal
A fracture through the epiphysis

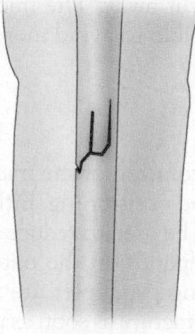

Greenstick
A fracture in which one side of a bone is broken and the other side is bent

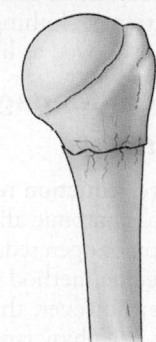

Impacted
A fracture in which a bone fragment is driven into another bone fragment

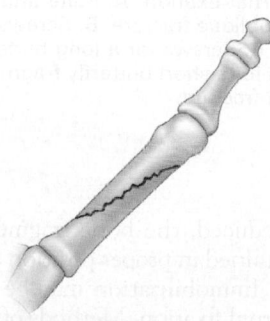

Oblique
A fracture occurring at an angle across the bone (less stable than a transverse fracture)

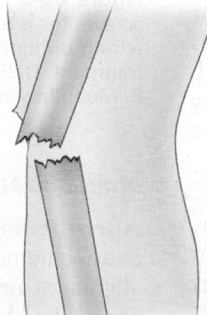

Open
A fracture in which damage also involves the skin or mucous membranes, also called a compound fracture

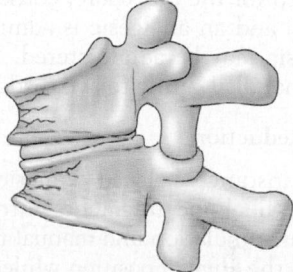

Pathologic
A fracture that occurs through an area of diseased bone (eg, osteoporosis, bone cyst, Paget's disease, bony metastasis, tumor); can occur without trauma or fall

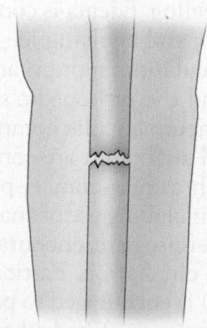

Simple
A fracture that remains contained, with no disruption of the skin integrity

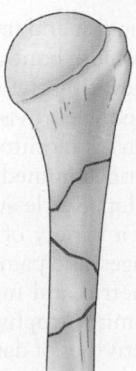

Spiral
A fracture that twists around the shaft of the bone

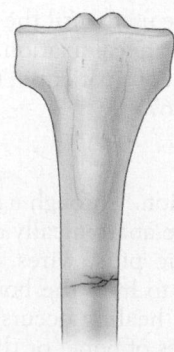

Stress
A fracture that results from repeated loading of bone and muscle

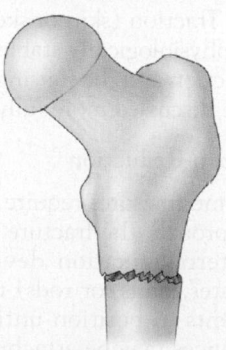

Transverse
A fracture that is straight across the bone shaft

Figure 69-2 Specific types of fractures.

serving as a splint for the injured one. In an upper extremity injury, the arm may be bandaged to the chest, or an injured forearm may be placed in a sling. The neurovascular status distal to the injury should be assessed both before and after splinting to determine the adequacy of peripheral tissue perfusion and nerve function.

With an *open fracture*, the wound is covered with a sterile dressing to prevent contamination of deeper tissues. No attempt is made to reduce the fracture, even if one of the bone fragments is protruding through the wound. Splints are applied for immobilization.

In the emergency department, the patient is evaluated completely. The clothes are gently removed, first from the uninjured side of the body and then from the injured side. The patient's clothing may be cut away. The fractured extremity is moved as little as possible to avoid more damage.

Medical Management

Reduction

Fracture reduction refers to restoration of the fracture fragments to anatomic alignment and positioning. Either closed reduction or open reduction may be used to reduce a fracture. The specific method selected depends on the nature of the fracture; however, the underlying principles are the same. Usually, the physician reduces a fracture as soon as possible to prevent loss of elasticity from the tissues through infiltration by edema or hemorrhage. In most cases, fracture reduction becomes more difficult as the injury begins to heal.

Before fracture reduction and immobilization, the patient is prepared for the procedure; consent for the procedure is obtained, and an analgesic is administered as prescribed. Anesthesia may be administered. The injured extremity must be handled gently to avoid additional damage.

Closed Reduction

In most instances, closed reduction is accomplished by bringing the bone fragments into anatomic alignment through manipulation and manual traction. The extremity is held in the aligned position while the physician applies a cast, splint, or other device. Reduction under anesthesia with percutaneous pinning may also be used. The immobilizing device maintains the reduction and stabilizes the extremity for bone healing. X-rays are obtained to verify that the bone fragments are correctly aligned.

Traction (skin or skeletal) may be used until the patient is physiologically stable to undergo surgical fixation. Use of traction and the nursing management of a patient in traction are discussed more fully in Chapter 67.

Open Reduction

Some fractures require open reduction. Through a surgical approach, the fracture fragments are anatomically aligned. Internal fixation devices (metallic pins, wires, screws, plates, nails, or rods) may be used to hold the bone fragments in position until solid bone healing occurs. These devices may be attached to the sides of bone, or they may be inserted through the bony fragments or directly into the medullary cavity of the bone (Fig. 69-3). Internal fixation devices ensure firm approximation and fixation of the bony fragments.

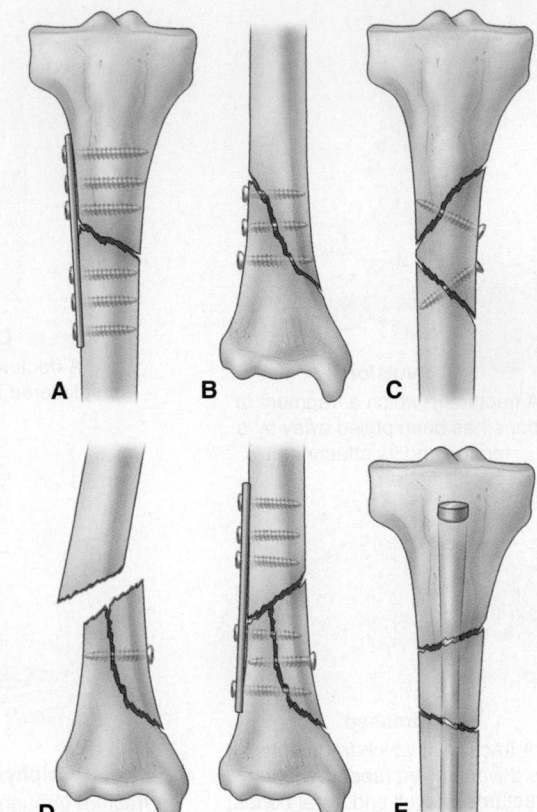

Figure 69-3 Techniques of internal fixation. **A,** Plate and six screws for a transverse or short oblique fracture. **B,** Screws for a long oblique or spiral fracture. **C,** Screws for a long butterfly fragment. **D,** Plate and six screws for a short butterfly fragment. **E,** Medullary nail for a segmental fracture.

Immobilization

After the fracture has been reduced, the bone fragments must be immobilized and maintained in proper position and alignment until union occurs. Immobilization may be accomplished by external or internal fixation. Methods of external fixation include bandages, casts, splints, continuous traction, and external fixators.

Maintaining and Restoring Function

Reduction and immobilization are maintained as prescribed to promote bone and soft tissue healing. Edema is controlled by elevating the injured extremity and applying ice as prescribed. Neurovascular status (circulation, motion and sensation) is monitored routinely, and the orthopedic surgeon is notified immediately if signs of neurovascular compromise develop. Restlessness, anxiety, and discomfort are controlled with a variety of approaches, such as reassurance, position changes, and pain relief strategies, including use of analgesics. Isometric and muscle-setting exercises are encouraged to minimize atrophy and to promote circulation. Participation in activities of daily living (ADLs) is encouraged to promote independent functioning and self-esteem. Gradual resumption of activities is promoted within the therapeutic prescription. With internal fixation, the surgeon determines the amount of movement and weight-bearing stress the extremity can sustain and prescribes the level of activity.

(See Nursing Process sections in Chapter 67 for more information about caring for patients who have a cast, are in traction, or are undergoing orthopedic surgery.)

Nursing Management

Patients With Closed Fractures

The patient with a closed fracture has no opening in the skin at the fracture site. The fractured bones may be nondisplaced or slightly displaced, but the skin is intact. The nurse instructs the patient regarding the proper methods to control edema and pain (Chart 69-1). It is important to teach exercises to maintain the health of unaffected muscles and to increase the strength of muscles needed for transferring and for using assistive devices such as crutches, walkers, and special utensils. The patient is also taught how to use assistive devices safely. Plans are made to help patients modify the home environment as needed and to ensure safety, such as removing floor rugs or anything that obstructs walking paths throughout the house. Patient teaching includes self-care, medication information, monitoring for potential complications, and the need for continuing health care supervision. Fracture healing and restoration of strength and mobility may take an average maximum of 6 to 8 weeks, depending on the quality of the patient's bone tissue.

Patients With Open Fractures

In an open fracture, there is a risk for osteomyelitis, tetanus, and gas gangrene. The objectives of management are to prevent infection of the wound, soft tissue, and bone and to promote healing of bone and soft tissue. Intravenous (IV) antibiotics are administered immediately upon the patient's arrival in the hospital along with tetanus toxoid if needed.

Wound irrigation and débridement are initiated in the operating room as soon as possible. The wound is cultured and bone grafting may be performed to fill in areas of bone defects. The fracture is carefully reduced and stabilized by external fixation and the wound is usually left open for 5 to 7 days for intermittent irrigation and cleansing (see Chapter 67). If there is any damage to blood vessels, soft tissue, muscles, nerves, or tendons, appropriate treatment is implemented.

With open fractures, primary wound closure is usually delayed. Heavily contaminated wounds are left unsutured and dressed with sterile gauze to permit edema and wound drainage. Wound irrigation and débridement may be repeated, removing infected and devitalized tissue and increasing vascularity in the region.

The extremity is elevated to minimize edema. It is important to assess neurovascular status frequently. Temperature is monitored at regular intervals and the patient is monitored for signs of infection. In 4 to 8 weeks, bone grafting may be necessary to bridge bone defects and to stimulate bone healing.

Fracture Healing and Complications

Weeks to months are required for most fractures to heal. Many factors influence the time frame of the healing process (Chart 69-2). With a comminuted fracture, fragments must be properly aligned to attain the best healing possible. It is essential for the fractured bone to have blood supply to the area to facilitate the healing process. In general, fractures of flat bones (pelvis, sternum, and scapula) heal rapidly. A complex, comminuted fracture may heal slower. Fractures at the ends of long bones, where the bone is more vascular and cancellous, heal more quickly than do fractures in areas where the bone is dense and less vascular (midshaft). Weight bearing stimulates healing of stabilized fractures of the long bones in the lower extremities.

CHART 69-1

HOME CARE CHECKLIST
Closed Fracture

At the completion of the home instruction, the patient or caregiver will be able to:	PATIENT	CAREGIVER
• Describe approaches to control swelling and pain (eg, elevate extremity to heart level; take analgesics as prescribed).	✔	✔
• Report pain uncontrolled by elevation and analgesics (may be an indicator of impaired tissue perfusion or compartment syndrome).	✔	✔
• Describe management of immobilizing device or care of incision.	✔	✔
• Consume diet to promote bone healing.	✔	
• Demonstrate ability to transfer.	✔	
• Use mobility aids and assistive devices safely.	✔	
• Avoid excessive use of injured extremity; observe prescribed weight-bearing limits.	✔	
• State indicators of complications to report promptly to physician (eg, uncontrolled swelling and pain; cool, pale fingers or toes; paresthesia; paralysis; signs of local and systemic infection; signs of venous thromboembolism; problems with immobilization device).	✔	✔
• State possible delayed complications of fractures (ie, delayed union; nonunion; avascular necrosis; reaction to internal fixation device; complex regional pain syndrome [CRPS], formally called reflex sympathetic dystrophy syndrome; heterotopic ossification).	✔	✔
• Describe gradual resumption of normal activities when medically cleared, and discuss how to protect fracture site from undue stresses.	✔	✔

Chart 69-2 • *Factors That Affect or Inhibit Fracture Healing*

Factors That Enhance Fracture Healing

- Immobilization of fracture fragments
- Maximum bone fragment contact
- Sufficient blood supply
- Proper nutrition
- Exercise: weight bearing for long bones
- Hormones: growth hormone, thyroid, calcitonin, vitamin D, anabolic steroids
- Electric potential across fracture

Factors That Inhibit Fracture Healing

- Extensive local trauma
- Bone loss
- Weight bearing prior to approval
- Malalignment of the fracture fragments
- Inadequate immobilization
- Space or tissue between bone fragments
- Infection
- Local malignancy
- Metabolic bone disease (eg, Paget's disease of the bone)
- Irradiated bone (radiation necrosis)
- Avascular necrosis
- Intra-articular fracture (synovial fluid contains fibrolysins, which lyse the initial clot and retard clot formation)
- Age (elderly persons heal more slowly)
- Corticosteroids (inhibit the repair rate)

If fracture healing is disrupted, bone union may be delayed or stopped completely. Factors that can impair fracture healing include inadequate fracture immobilization, inadequate blood supply to the fracture site or adjacent tissue, extensive space between bone fragments, interposition of soft tissue between bone ends, displacement of fracture fragments or ends, infection, and metabolic problems.

Complications of fractures may be either acute or chronic. Early complications include shock, fat embolism, compartment syndrome, and venous thromboemboli (deep vein thrombosis [DVT], pulmonary embolism [PE]). Delayed complications include delayed union, malunion, nonunion, AVN of bone, reaction to internal fixation devices, complex regional pain syndrome (CRPS, formerly called reflex sympathetic dystrophy [RSD]), and heterotopic ossification.

Early Complications

Shock

Hypovolemic shock resulting from hemorrhage is more frequently noted in trauma patients with pelvic fractures and in patients with a displaced or open femoral fracture in which the femoral artery is torn by bone fragments. Treatment of shock consists of stabilizing the fracture to prevent further hemorrhage, restoring blood volume and circulation, relieving the patient's pain, providing proper immobilization, and protecting the patient from further injury and other complications. (See Chapter 15 for a discussion of shock.)

Fat Embolism Syndrome

After fracture of long bones or pelvic bones, or crush injuries, fat emboli may develop. Fat embolism syndrome (FES) occurs most frequently in adults younger than 40 years of age and in men. It is also more common in patients with multiple fractures (Stein, Yaekoub, Matta, et al., 2008). At the time of fracture, fat globules may diffuse from the marrow into the vascular compartment. The fat globules (ie, emboli) may occlude the small blood vessels that supply the lungs, brain, kidneys, and other organs. The onset of symptoms is rapid, typically within 12 to 48 hours of injury (Harvey, 2006), but may occur up to 10 days after injury (Whiteing, 2008).

Clinical Manifestations. Presenting features include hypoxia, tachypnea, tachycardia, and pyrexia. The respiratory distress response includes tachypnea, dyspnea, crackles, wheezes, precordial chest pain, cough, large amounts of thick white sputum, and tachycardia. Occlusion of a large number of small vessels causes the pulmonary pressure to rise. Edema and hemorrhages in the alveoli impair oxygen transport, leading to hypoxia. Arterial blood gas values show the partial pressure of oxygen (PaO_2) to be less than 60 mm Hg, with an early respiratory alkalosis and later respiratory acidosis. The chest x-ray shows a typical "snowstorm" infiltrate. Without prompt, definitive treatment, acute pulmonary edema, acute respiratory distress syndrome (ARDS), and heart failure may develop. Cerebral disturbances (due to hypoxia and the lodging of fat emboli in the brain) are manifested by mental status changes varying from headache and mild agitation to delirium and coma.

> ### NURSING ALERT
>
> **Subtle personality changes, restlessness, irritability, or confusion in a patient who has sustained a fracture are indications for immediate arterial blood gas studies.**

With systemic embolization, the patient appears pale. Petechiae, possibly due to a transient thrombocytopenia, are noted in the buccal membranes and conjunctival sacs, on the hard palate, and over the chest and anterior axillary folds. The patient develops a fever greater than 39.5°C (103°F). Free fat may be found in the urine if emboli are filtered by the renal tubules. Acute tubular necrosis and renal failure may develop (Harvey, 2006).

Prevention and Management. Immediate immobilization of fractures including early surgical fixation, minimal fracture manipulation, and adequate support for fractured bones during turning and positioning, and maintenance of fluid and electrolyte balance are measures that may reduce the incidence of fat emboli.

Prompt initiation of respiratory support, assessment, and monitoring is essential. The objectives of management are to support the respiratory system, to prevent respiratory failure, and to correct homeostatic disturbances. Acute pulmonary edema and ARDS are the most common causes of death. Respiratory support is provided with high-flow oxygen. Controlled-volume ventilation with positive end-expiratory pressure (PEEP) may be used to prevent or treat pulmonary edema. Corticosteroids may be administered IV to treat the inflammatory lung reaction and to control cerebral edema (Harvey, 2006) (see Chapter 23 for the nursing management of respiratory failure and Chapter 25 for care of the patient on a ventilator). Vasopressor medications to support cardiovascular function are administered IV to prevent and treat hypotension, shock, and interstitial pulmonary edema. Accurate fluid intake and output records facilitate adequate fluid replacement therapy.

Compartment Syndrome

An anatomic compartment is an area of the body encased by bone or fascia (eg, the fibrous membrane that covers and separates muscles) that contains muscles, nerves, and blood vessels. The human body has 46 anatomic compartments, and 36 of these are located in the extremities (Fig. 69-4). Compartment syndrome in an extremity is a limb-threatening condition that occurs when perfusion pressure falls below tissue pressure within a closed anatomic compartment.

Acute compartment syndrome involves a sudden and severe decrease in blood flow to the tissues distal to an area of injury that results in ischemic necrosis if prompt, decisive intervention does not occur. The patient complains of deep, throbbing, unrelenting pain, which continues to increase despite the administration of opioids and seems out of proportion to the injury. A hallmark sign is pain that occurs or intensifies with passive ROM (eg, pain intensifies with dorsiflexion of the wrist of the affected extremity). This pain can be caused by (1) a reduction in the size of the muscle

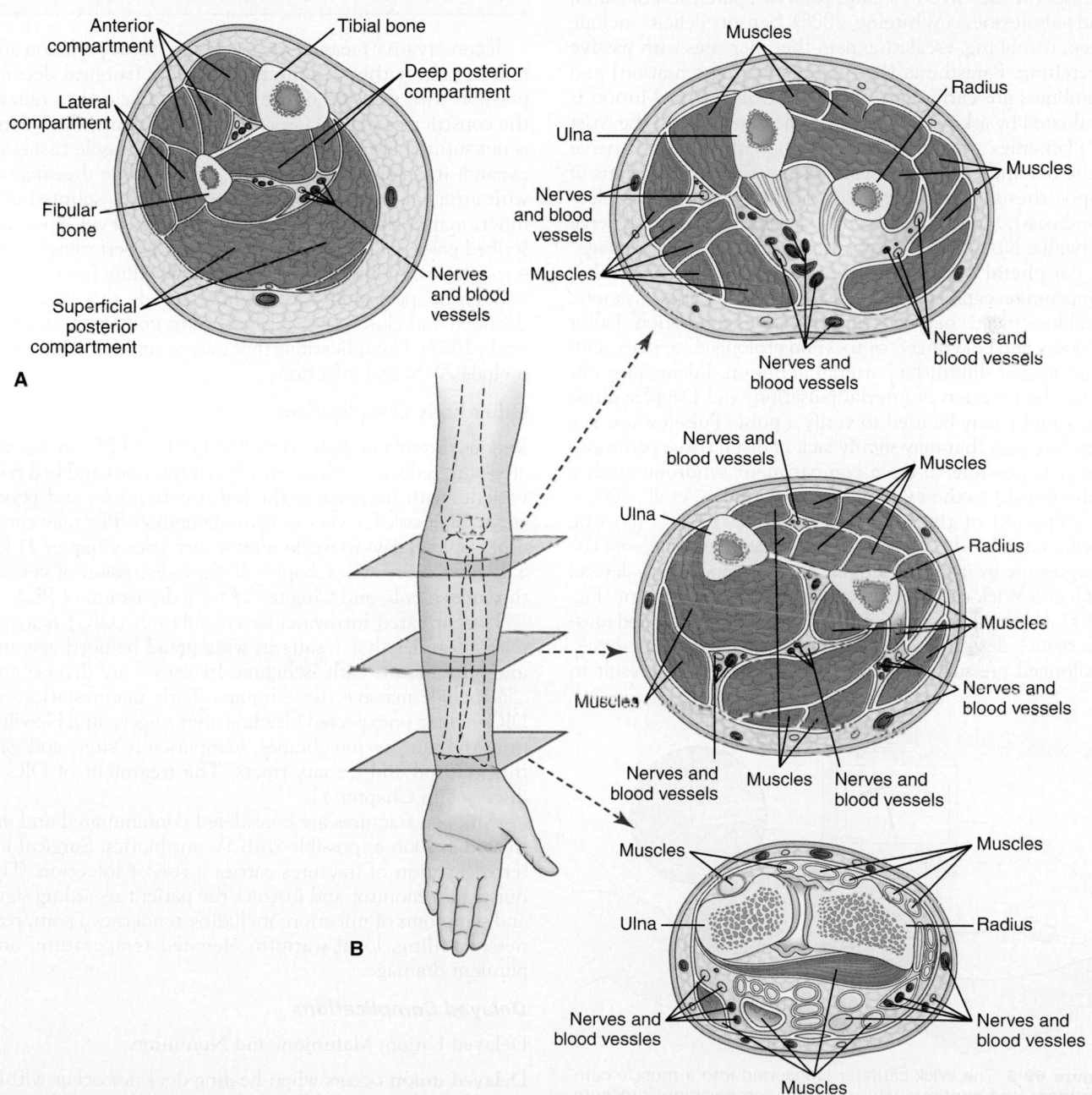

Figure 69-4 Cross-sections of anatomic compartments. **A,** Compartments of the left lower leg. **B,** Compartments of the left forearm. From Chapman, M. W., Szabo, R. M. & Marder, R. A. (2000). *Chapman's orthopaedic surgery* (3rd ed., pp. 395–396). Philadelphia: Lippincott Williams & Wilkins.

compartment because the enclosing muscle fascia is too tight or a cast or dressing is constrictive or (2) an increase in compartment contents because of edema or hemorrhage from the fracture site. The lower leg is most frequently involved, but the forearm is also at risk (see figure 67-2 for an illustration of compartment syndrome of the lower leg). The pressure within a muscle compartment may increase to such an extent that microcirculation diminishes, causing nerve and muscle anoxia and necrosis (Konstantakos, Dalstrom, Nelles, et al., 2007). Permanent function can be lost if the anoxic situation continues for longer than 6 hours (Harvey, 2006).

Assessment and Diagnostic Findings. Frequent assessment of neurovascular function after a fracture is essential and focuses on the "five Ps": *p*ain, *p*aralysis, *p*aresthesias, *p*allor, and *p*ulselessness (Whiteing, 2008). Sensory deficits include deep, throbbing, escalating pain that increases with passive stretching. Paresthesia (burning or tingling sensation) and numbness are early signs of nerve involvement. Motion is evaluated by asking the patient to flex and extend the wrist or plantarflex and dorsiflex the foot. With continued nerve ischemia and edema, the patient experiences sensations of hypoesthesia (diminished sensation followed by complete numbness). Motor weakness may occur as a late sign of nerve ischemia. No movement (paralysis) indicates nerve damage.

Peripheral circulation is evaluated by assessing color, temperature, capillary refill time, edema, and pulses. Cyanotic (ie, blue-tinged) nail beds suggest venous congestion. Pallor or dusky and cold fingers or toes and prolonged capillary refill time suggest diminished arterial perfusion. Edema may obscure the function of arterial pulsation, and Doppler ultrasonography may be used to verify a pulse. Pulselessness is a very late sign that may signify lack of distal tissue perfusion, but it is possible to have compartment syndrome with a pulse (weak) to the extremity (Konstantakos, et al., 2007).

Palpation of the muscle, if possible, reveals it to be swollen and hard. The orthopedic surgeon may measure tissue pressure by inserting a tissue pressure–monitoring device, such as a Wick catheter, into the muscle compartment (Fig. 69-5). (Normal pressure is 8 mm Hg or less.) Nerve and muscle tissues deteriorate as compartment pressure increases. Prolonged pressure of more than 30 mm Hg can result in

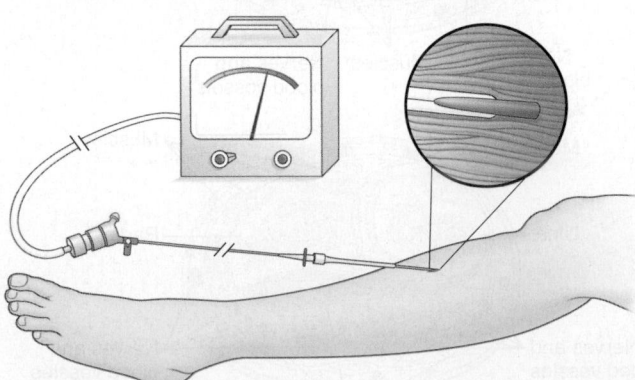

Figure 69-5 The Wick catheter is inserted into a muscle compartment and continuously monitors compartment pressure. From Chapman, M. W., Szabo, R. M. & Marder, R. A. (2000). *Chapman's orthopaedic surgery* (3rd ed., p. 401). Philadelphia: Lippincott Williams & Wilkins.

compromised microcirculation (Hessmann, Ingelfinger & Rommens, 2007).

Medical Management. Prompt management of acute compartment syndrome is essential. The surgeon needs to be notified immediately if neurovascular compromise is suspected. Delay in treatment may result in permanent nerve and muscle damage or even necrosis and amputation.

 NURSING ALERT

Compartment syndrome is managed by maintaining the extremity at the heart level (*not above heart level*), and opening and bivalving the cast (see Chart 67-2) or opening the splint, if one or the other are present.

If conservative measures do not restore tissue perfusion and relieve pain within 1 hour, a fasciotomy (surgical decompression with excision of the fascia) is indicated to relieve the constrictive muscle fascia. After fasciotomy, the wound is not sutured but is left open to allow the muscle tissues to expand; it is covered with moist, sterile saline dressings or with artificial skin. The affected arm or leg is splinted in a functional position and elevated to heart level, and prescribed passive ROM exercises are usually performed every 4 to 6 hours. In 3 to 5 days, when the swelling has resolved and tissue perfusion has been restored, the wound is débrided and closed (possibly with skin grafts) (Hessmann, et al., 2007). Complications that may occur after fasciotomy include AVN and infection.

Other Early Complications

Venous thromboemboli, including DVT and PE, are associated with reduced skeletal muscle contractions and bed rest. Patients with fractures of the lower extremities and pelvis are at high risk for venous thromboemboli. PEs may cause death several days to weeks after injury. (See Chapter 31 for a discussion of DVT; Chapter 30 for a discussion of venous thromboemboli; and Chapter 23 for a discussion of PE.)

Disseminated intravascular coagulation (DIC) is a systemic disorder that results in widespread hemorrhage and microthrombosis with ischemia. Its causes are diverse and can include massive tissue trauma. Early manifestations of DIC include unexpected bleeding after surgery, and bleeding from the mucous membranes, venipuncture sites, and gastrointestinal and urinary tracts. The treatment of DIC is discussed in Chapter 33.

All open fractures are considered contaminated and are treated as soon as possible with IV antibiotics. Surgical internal fixation of fractures carries a risk of infection. The nurse must monitor and instruct the patient regarding signs and symptoms of infection, including tenderness, pain, redness, swelling, local warmth, elevated temperature, and purulent drainage.

Delayed Complications

Delayed Union, Malunion, and Nonunion

Delayed union occurs when healing does not occur within the expected time frame for the location and type of fracture. Delayed union may be associated with distraction (pulling apart) of bone fragments, systemic or local infection, poor nutrition, or comorbidity (eg, diabetes mellitus, autoimmune disease). The healing time is prolonged; but the fracture eventually heals (Whiteing, 2008).

Nonunion results from failure of the ends of a fractured bone to unite, whereas **malunion** results from failure of the ends of a fractured bone to unite in normal alignment. In both of these instances, the patient complains of persistent discomfort and abnormal movement at the fracture site. Factors contributing to nonunion and malunion include infection at the fracture site, interposition of tissue between the bone ends, inadequate immobilization or manipulation that disrupts callus formation, excessive space between bone fragments, limited bone contact, and impaired blood supply resulting in AVN. In nonunion, fibrocartilage or fibrous tissue exists between the bone fragments; no bone salts have been deposited. A false joint (pseudarthrosis) often develops at the site of the fracture (Whiteing, 2008).

Medical Management. The physician treats nonunion with internal fixation, bone grafting, electrical bone stimulation, or a combination of these therapies. Internal fixation stabilizes the bone fragments and ensures bone contact.

Bone grafts promote osteogenesis, osteoconduction, and osteoinduction. *Osteogenesis* (bone formation) occurs after transplantation of bone because the graft contains osteoblasts, which build bony matrix. Building of this structural bony matrix promotes *osteoconduction*, the growth of blood vessels and osteoblasts within the matrix. *Osteoinduction* is the stimulation of host stem cells to differentiate into osteoblasts by several growth factors, including bone morphogenetic proteins (BMPs), particularly BMP-2, BMP-6, and BMP-9 (Boden, 2005).

Grafted bone undergoes a reconstructive process that results in a gradual replacement of the graft with new bone. During surgery the bone fragments are débrided and aligned, infection (if present) is removed, and a bone graft is placed in the bony defect. The bone graft may be an **autograft** (tissue, frequently from the iliac crest, harvested from the patient for his or her own use) or an **allograft** (tissue harvested from a donor). The bone graft fills the bone gap and provides a lattice structure for invasion by bone cells and actively promotes bone growth. The type of bone selected for grafting depends on function: cortical bone is used for structural strength, cancellous bone for osteogenesis, and corticocancellous bone for strength and rapid incorporation. Free vascularized bone autografts are grafted with their own blood supply, allowing for primary fracture healing.

After grafting, immobilization and non–weight-bearing exercises are required while the bone graft becomes incorporated and the fracture or defect heals. Depending on the type of bone grafted and the age of the patient, healing may take from 6 to 12 months or longer. Bone grafting complications include wound or graft infection, fracture of the graft, and nonunion (Boden, 2005). Specific problems associated with autografts include a limited quantity of bone available for harvest and harvest site pain that may persist for up to 2 years after harvest (Boden, 2005). Infrequent specific allograft complications include partial acceptance (lack of host and donor histocompatibility, which retards graft incorporation), graft rejection (rapid and complete resorption of the graft), and transmission of disease (rare).

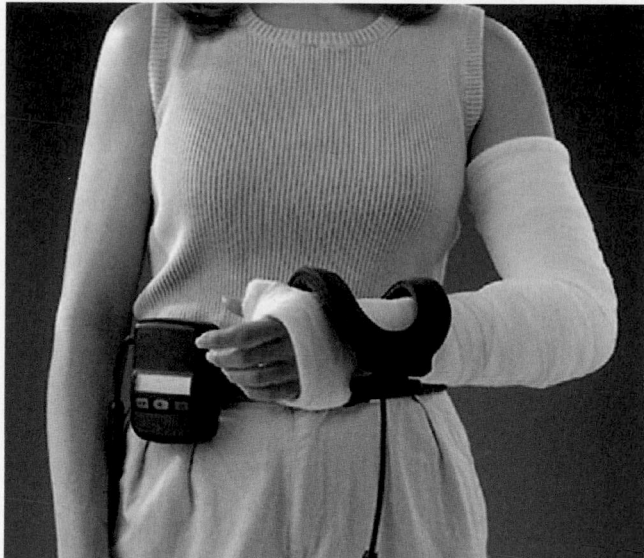

Figure 69-6 Bone healing stimulator applied to the arm. Courtesy of EBI Medical Systems, Parsippany, NJ.

Osteogenesis may be stimulated by electrical impulses; the effectiveness is similar to that of bone grafting. Use of electrical impulses is not effective with large bone gaps. The electrical stimulation modifies the tissue environment, making it electronegative, which enhances mineral deposition and bone formation that promotes bone growth. In some situations, pins that act as cathodes are inserted percutaneously, directly into the fracture site, and electrical impulses are directed to the fracture continuously. This method cannot be used when infection is present.

Another method for stimulating osteogenesis is noninvasive inductive coupling. Pulsing electromagnetic fields are delivered to the fracture for approximately 10 hours each day by an electromagnetic coil over the nonunion site (Fig. 69-6). During the electrical stimulation treatment period, which takes 3 to 6 months or longer, rigid fracture fixation with adequate support is needed.

Nursing Management. The patient with a nonunion has experienced an extended time in fracture treatment and frequently becomes frustrated with prolonged therapy. The nurse provides emotional support and encouragement to the patient and encourages compliance with the treatment regimen. The orthopedic surgeon evaluates the progression of bone healing with periodic x-rays.

Nursing care for the patient with a bone graft includes pain management and monitoring the patient for possible complications. The nurse needs to reinforce educational information concerning the objectives of the bone graft, immobilization, non–weight-bearing exercises, wound care, monitoring for signs of infection, and the importance of follow-up care with the orthopedic surgeon.

Nursing care for the patient with electrical bone stimulation focuses on patient education that addresses immobilization, weight-bearing restrictions, and correct daily use of the stimulator as prescribed.

Avascular Necrosis of Bone

AVN occurs when the bone loses its blood supply and dies. It may occur after a fracture with disruption of the blood supply to the distal area. It is also seen with dislocations, bone transplantation, prolonged high-dose corticosteroid therapy, chronic renal disease, sickle cell anemia, and other diseases. The devitalized bone may collapse or reabsorb. The patient develops pain and experiences limited movement. X-rays reveal loss of mineralized matrix and structural collapse. Treatment generally consists of attempts to revitalize the bone with bone grafts, prosthetic replacement, or arthrodesis (joint fusion).

Reaction to Internal Fixation Devices

Internal fixation devices may be removed after bony union has taken place. However, in most patients, the device is not removed unless it produces symptoms. Pain and decreased function are the prime indications that a problem has developed. Problems may include mechanical failure (inadequate insertion and stabilization); material failure (faulty or damaged device); corrosion of the device, causing local inflammation; allergic response to the metallic alloy used; and osteoporotic remodeling adjacent to the fixation site (Bucholz, Heckman, Court-Brown, et al., 2005). If the device is removed, the bone needs to be protected from refracture related to osteoporosis, altered bone structure, and trauma.

Complex Regional Pain Syndrome

CRPS is a painful sympathetic nervous system problem. It occurs infrequently; but when it does occur, it is most often in an upper extremity after trauma and is seen more frequently in women. Clinical manifestations of CRPS include severe burning pain, local edema, hyperesthesia, stiffness, discoloration, vasomotor skin changes (ie, fluctuating warm, red, dry and cold, sweaty, cyanotic), and trophic changes that may include glossy, shiny skin and increased hair and nail growth. This syndrome is frequently chronic, with extension of symptoms to adjacent areas of the body. Disuse muscle atrophy and bone deossification (osteoporosis) may occur with persistent CRPS.

Nursing Management. Prevention may include elevation of the extremity after injury or surgery and selection of an immobilization device (eg, external fixator) that allows for the greatest ROM and functional use of the rest of the extremity. Early effective pain relief is the focus of management. Pain may need to be controlled with analgesics. NSAIDs, corticosteroids, and muscle relaxants also may be used. The nurse helps the patient to cope with CRPS manifestations and explores multiple ways to control pain (see Chapter 13).

NURSING ALERT

The nurse avoids using the affected extremity for blood pressure measurements and venipuncture in the patient with CRPS.

Heterotopic Ossification

Heterotopic ossification (myositis ossificans) is the abnormal formation of bone, near bones or in muscle, in response to soft tissue trauma or fracture after blunt trauma or total joint replacement. The muscle is painful, and normal muscular contraction and movement are limited. Early mobilization may prevent its occurrence. Usually the bone lesion resorbs over time, but the abnormal bone eventually may need to be excised if symptoms persist.

Fractures of Specific Sites

CLAVICLE

Fracture of the clavicle (collar bone) is a common injury that results from a fall or a direct blow to the shoulder. The clavicle helps maintain the shoulder in the upward, outward, and backward position from the thorax. Therefore, when the clavicle is fractured, the patient assumes a protective position, slumping the shoulders and immobilizing the arm to prevent shoulder movements. The treatment goal is to align the shoulder in its normal position by means of closed reduction and immobilization.

Most of these fractures occur in the middle third of the clavicle. A clavicular strap, also called a *figure-eight bandage* (Fig. 69-7), may be used to pull the shoulders back, reducing and immobilizing the fracture. The nurse monitors the circulation and nerve function of the affected arm and compares it with the unaffected arm to determine variations, which may indicate disturbances in neurovascular status. A sling

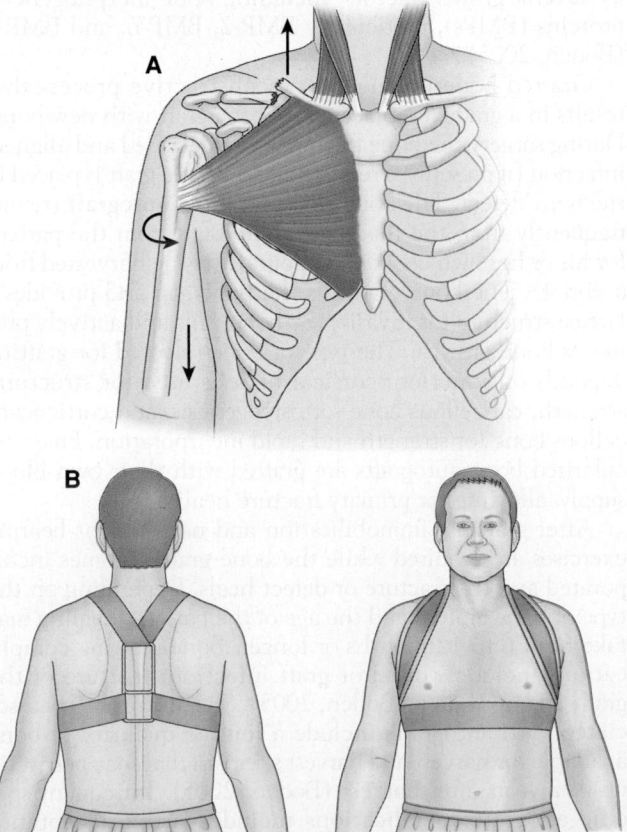

Figure 69-7 Fracture of the clavicle. **A,** Anteroposterior view shows typical displacement in midclavicular fracture. **B,** Immobilization is accomplished with a clavicular strap.

may be used to support the arm and relieve pain. The patient may be permitted to use the arm for light activities within the range of comfort.

Fracture of the distal third of the clavicle, without displacement and ligament disruption, is treated with a sling and restricted motion of the arm. When a fracture in the distal third is accompanied by a disruption of the coracoclavicular ligament that connects the coracoid process of the scapula and the inferior surface of the clavicle, the bony fragments are frequently displaced. This type of injury may be treated by open reduction with internal fixation (ORIF) (see Chapter 67 for discussion of ORIF).

The nurse cautions the patient not to elevate the arm above shoulder level until the fracture has healed (about 6 weeks) but encourages the patient to exercise the elbow, wrist, and fingers as soon as possible. When prescribed, shoulder exercises are performed to obtain full shoulder motion (Fig. 69-8). Vigorous activity is limited for approximately 3 months.

Complications of clavicular fractures include trauma to the nerves of the brachial plexus, injury to the subclavian vein or artery from a bony fragment, and malunion.

HUMERAL NECK

Fractures of the proximal humerus may occur through the neck of the humerus. Impacted fractures of the surgical neck of the humerus are seen most frequently in older women after a fall on an outstretched arm. Active middle-aged patients who are injured in a fall may suffer severely displaced humeral neck fractures with associated rotator cuff damage.

The patient presents with the affected arm hanging limp at the side or supported by the uninjured hand. Neurovascular

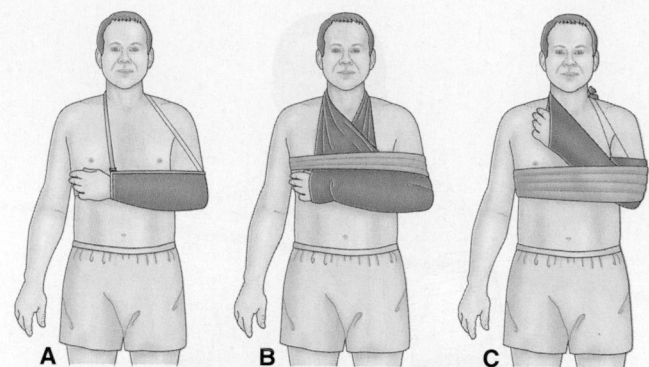

Figure 69-9 Immobilizers for proximal humeral fractures. **A,** Commercial sling with immobilizing strap permits easy removal for hygiene and is comfortable on the neck. **B,** Conventional sling and swathe. **C,** Stockinette Velpeau and swathe are used when there is an unstable surgical neck component. This position relaxes the pectoralis major.

assessment of the extremity is essential to evaluate the full extent of injury and the possible involvement of the nerves and blood vessels of the arm.

Many impacted fractures of the surgical neck of the humerus are not displaced and do not require reduction. The arm is supported and immobilized by a sling and swathe that secure the supported arm to the trunk (Fig. 69-9). Limitation of motion and stiffness of the shoulder occur with disuse. Therefore, pendulum exercises begin as soon as tolerated by the patient. In pendulum or circumduction exercises, the physical therapist instructs the patient to lean forward and allow the affected arm to hang in abduction and rotate. These fractures require approximately 6 to 10 weeks to heal, and the patient should avoid vigorous arm activity for an additional 4 weeks. Residual stiffness, aching, and some limitation of ROM may persist for 6 months or longer.

When a humeral neck fracture is displaced, treatment consists of closed reduction, ORIF, or a total shoulder replacement. Exercises are begun after an adequate period of immobilization.

HUMERAL SHAFT

Fractures of the shaft of the humerus are most frequently caused by (1) direct trauma that results in a transverse, oblique, or comminuted fracture or (2) an indirect twisting force that results in a spiral fracture. The nerves and brachial blood vessels may be injured with these fractures, so neurovascular assessment is essential to monitor the status of the nerve or blood vessels. Damage to either requires immediate attention.

Well-padded splints are used to initially immobilize the upper arm and to support the arm in 90 degrees of flexion at the elbow. A sling or collar and cuff support the forearm. The weight of the hanging arm and splints puts traction on the fracture site. External fixators are used to treat open fractures of the humeral shaft (see Chapter 67). ORIF of a fracture of the humerus is necessary with nerve palsy, blood vessel damage, comminuted fracture, or displaced fracture.

Functional bracing is another form of treatment used for these fractures. A contoured thermoplastic sleeve is secured in place with interlocking fabric (Velcro) closures around

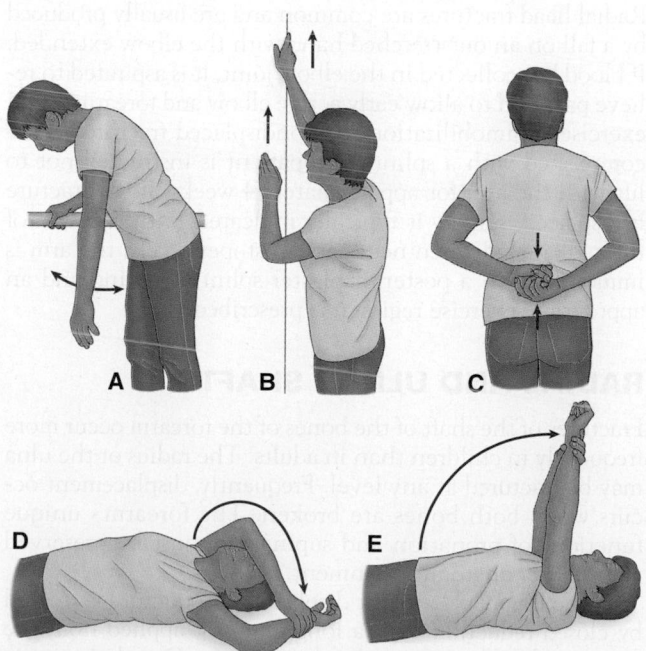

Figure 69-8 Exercises that promote shoulder range of motion include **(A)** pendulum exercise and **(B)** wall climbing. The unaffected arm is used to assist with **(C)** internal rotation, **(D)** external rotation, and **(E)** elevation. In C, D, and E, the unaffected arm is used for power.

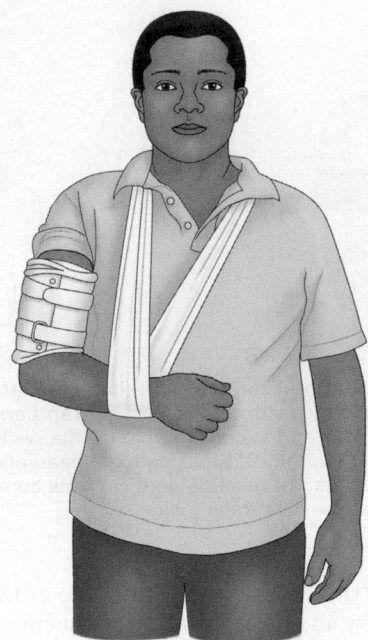

Figure 69-10 Functional humeral brace with collar and cuff sling.

the upper arm, immobilizing the reduced fracture. As swelling decreases, the sleeve is tightened, and uniform pressure and stability are applied to the fracture. The forearm is supported with a collar and cuff sling (Fig. 69-10). Functional bracing allows active use of muscles, shoulder and elbow motion, and good approximation of fracture fragments. Pendulum shoulder exercises are performed as prescribed to provide active movement of the shoulder, thereby preventing a "frozen shoulder." Isometric exercises may be prescribed to prevent muscle atrophy. The callus that develops is substantial, and the sleeve can be discontinued in about 8 weeks. Complications that are seen with humeral shaft fractures include delayed union and nonunion because of decreased blood supply in that area.

ELBOW

Fractures of the distal humerus result from motor vehicle crashes, falls on the elbow (in the extended or flexed position), or a direct blow. These fractures may result in injury to the median, radial, or ulnar nerves.

The patient is evaluated for paresthesia and signs of compromised circulation in the forearm and hand. The most serious complication of a supracondylar fracture of the humerus is Volkmann's contracture (an acute compartment syndrome), which results from antecubital swelling or damage to the brachial artery (Chart 69-3). The nurse needs to monitor the patient regularly for compromised neurovascular status and signs and symptoms of acute compartment syndrome. Other potential complications are damage to the joint articular surfaces and hemarthrosis (ie, blood in the joint), which may be treated by needle aspiration by the physician to relieve the pressure and pain.

The goal of therapy is prompt reduction and stabilization of the distal humeral fracture, followed by controlled active motion after swelling has subsided and healing has begun. If

the fracture is not displaced, the arm is immobilized in a cast or posterior splint with the elbow at 45 to 90 degrees of flexion and placed in a sling. A thermoplastic splint is used to support the fracture.

Usually a displaced fracture is treated with ORIF. Excision of bone fragments may be necessary. Additional external support with a splint is then applied. Active finger exercises are encouraged. Gentle ROM exercise of the injured joint is begun about 1 week after internal fixation. Motion promotes healing of injured joints by producing movement of synovial fluid into the articular cartilage. Active exercise to prevent residual limitation of motion is performed as prescribed.

RADIAL HEAD

Radial head fractures are common and are usually produced by a fall on an outstretched hand with the elbow extended. If blood has collected in the elbow joint, it is aspirated to relieve pain and to allow early active elbow and forearm ROM exercises. Immobilization for nondisplaced fractures is accomplished with a splint. The patient is instructed not to lift with the arm for approximately 4 weeks. If the fracture is displaced, surgery is typically indicated, with excision of the radial head when necessary. Postoperatively, the arm is immobilized in a posterior plaster splint and sling and an appropriate exercise regimen is prescribed.

RADIAL AND ULNAR SHAFTS

Fractures of the shaft of the bones of the forearm occur more frequently in children than in adults. The radius or the ulna may be fractured at any level. Frequently, displacement occurs when both bones are broken. The forearm's unique functions of pronation and supination must be preserved with proper anatomic alignment.

If the fragments are not displaced, the fracture is treated by closed reduction with a long-arm cast applied from the upper arm to the proximal palmar crease. Circulation, motion, and sensation of the hand are assessed before and after the cast is applied. The arm is elevated to control edema. Frequent finger flexion and extension are encouraged to reduce edema. Active motion of the involved shoulder is essential. The reduction and alignment are monitored closely by x-rays to ensure proper alignment. The fracture is immobilized for about 12 weeks; during the last 6 weeks, the arm may be in a functional forearm brace that allows exercise of the wrist and elbow. Lifting and twisting are avoided.

Displaced fractures are managed by ORIF, using a compression plate with screws, intramedullary nails, or rods. The arm is usually immobilized in a plaster splint or cast. Open and displaced fractures may be managed with external fixation devices. The arm is elevated to control swelling. Neurovascular status is assessed and documented. Elbow, wrist, and hand exercises are begun when prescribed by the physician.

WRIST

Fractures of the distal radius (Colles fracture) are common and are usually the result of a fall on an open, dorsiflexed hand. This fracture is frequently seen in elderly women with osteoporotic bones and weak soft tissues that do not dissipate the energy of the fall. The patient presents with a deformed wrist, pain, swelling, weakness, limited finger ROM, and complaints of "tingling" in the affected hand.

Treatment usually consists of closed reduction and immobilization with a short-arm cast. For fractures with extensive comminution, ORIF, arthroscopic percutaneous pinning, or external fixation is used to achieve and maintain reduction. The wrist and forearm are elevated for 48 hours after reduction to control swelling.

Active motion of the fingers and shoulder should begin promptly. The patient is taught to perform the following exercises to reduce swelling and prevent stiffness:

- Hold the hand at the level of the heart.
- Move the fingers from full extension to flexion. Hold and release. (Repeat at least 10 times every hour when awake.)
- Use the hand in functional activities.
- Actively exercise the shoulder and elbow, including complete ROM exercises of both joints.

The fingers may swell due to diminished venous and lymphatic return. The nurse assesses the sensory function of the median nerve by pricking the distal aspect of the index finger. The motor function is assessed by the patient's ability to touch the thumb to the little finger. Diminished circulation and nerve function must be treated promptly (see previous discussion of Compartment Syndrome).

HAND

Trauma to the hand often requires extensive reconstructive surgery. The objective of treatment is always to regain maximum function of the hand.

For a nondisplaced fracture of the phalanx (finger bone), the finger is splinted for 3 to 4 weeks to relieve pain and to protect the finger from further trauma. Displaced fractures and open fractures may require ORIF, using wires or pins.

The neurovascular status of the injured hand is evaluated and documented. Swelling is controlled by elevation of the hand. Functional use of the uninvolved portion of the hand is encouraged. Assistive devices might be recommended to aid the patient in performing ADLs until the hand has healed and functional status returns.

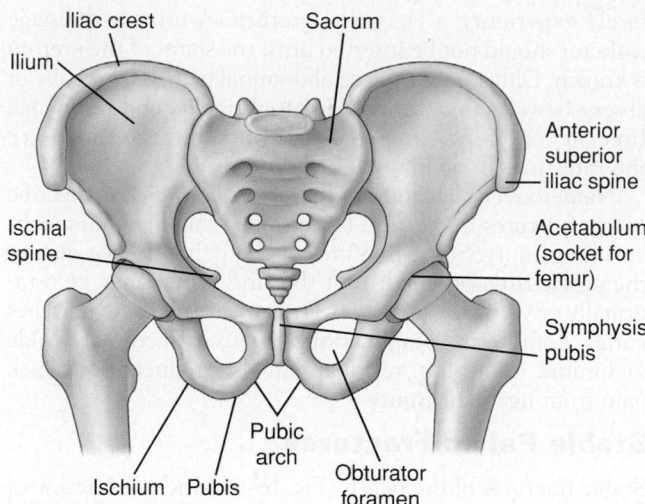

Figure 69-11 Pelvic bones.

PELVIS

The sacrum, ilium, pubis, and ischium bones form the pelvic bone, a fused, stable, bony ring in adults (Fig. 69-11). Falls, motor vehicle crashes, and crush injuries can cause pelvic fractures. Pelvic fractures are serious because at least two thirds of affected patients have significant and multiple injuries. Management of severe, life-threatening pelvic fractures is coordinated with the trauma team. Hemorrhage and thoracic, intra-abdominal, and cranial injuries have priority over treatment of fractures. There is a high mortality rate associated with pelvic fractures, related to hemorrhage, pulmonary complications, fat emboli, thromboembolic complications, and infection.

Signs and symptoms of pelvic fracture include ecchymosis; tenderness over the symphysis pubis, anterior iliac spines, iliac crest, sacrum, or coccyx; local edema; numbness or tingling of the pubis, genitals, and proximal thighs; and inability to bear weight without discomfort. Computed tomography (CT) of the pelvis helps determine the extent of injury by demonstrating sacroiliac joint disruption, soft tissue trauma, pelvic hematoma, and fractures. Neurovascular assessment of the lower extremities is completed to detect any injury to pelvic blood vessels and nerves (Kobziff, 2006).

Hemorrhage and shock are two of the most serious consequences that may occur. Bleeding arises mainly from the laceration of veins and arteries by bone fragments and possibly from a torn iliac artery. The peripheral pulses, especially the dorsalis pedis pulses of both lower extremities, are palpated; absence of a pulse may indicate a tear in the iliac artery or one of its branches. Peritoneal lavage or abdominal CT may be performed to detect intra-abdominal hemorrhage. The patient is handled gently to minimize further bleeding and shock (Bucholz, et al., 2005).

The nurse assesses for injuries to the bladder, rectum, intestines, other abdominal organs, and pelvic vessels and nerves. To assess for urinary tract injury, the patient's urine is analyzed for blood. A voiding cystourethrogram and an IV urogram may be performed. Laceration of the urethra is suspected in males with anterior fracture of the pelvis and blood at the urethral meatus (Bucholz, et al., 2005). Females rarely experience a lacerated urethra. A urinary drainage catheter should not be inserted until the status of the urethra is known. Diffuse and intense abdominal pain, hyperactive or absent bowel sounds, and abdominal rigidity and resonance (free air) or dullness to percussion (blood) suggest injury to the intestines or abdominal bleeding.

Numerous classification systems have been used to describe pelvic fractures in relation to anatomy, stability, and mechanism of injury. Some fractures of the pelvis do not disrupt the pelvic ring; others disrupt the ring, which may be rotationally or vertically unstable. The severity of pelvic fractures varies. Long-term complications of pelvic fractures include malunion, nonunion, residual gait disturbances, and back pain from ligament injury.

Stable Pelvic Fractures

Stable fractures of the pelvis (Fig. 69-12) include fracture of a single pubic or ischial ramus, fracture of ipsilateral pubic and ischial rami, fracture of the pelvic wing of the ilium (Duverney fracture), and fracture of the sacrum or coccyx. If injury results in only a slight widening of the pubic symphysis or the anterior sacroiliac joint and the pelvic ligaments are intact, the disrupted pubic symphysis is likely to heal spontaneously with conservative management. Most fractures of the pelvis heal rapidly because the pelvic bones are mostly cancellous bone, which has a rich blood supply.

Stable pelvic fractures are treated with a few days of bed rest and symptom management until discomfort is controlled. Fluids, dietary fiber, ankle and leg exercises, anti-embolism stockings to aid venous return, logrolling, deep breathing, and skin care reduce the risk of complications and increase the patient's comfort. The patient with a fractured sacrum is at risk for paralytic ileus; therefore, bowel sounds should be monitored.

The patient with a fracture of the coccyx experiences pain when sitting and when defecating. Sitz baths may be prescribed to relieve pain, and stool softeners may be given to ease defecation. As pain resolves, activity is gradually resumed with the use of assistive mobility devices. Early mobilization reduces problems related to immobility.

Unstable Pelvic Fractures

Unstable fractures of the pelvis (Fig. 69-13) may result in rotational instability (eg, the "open book" type, in which a separation occurs at the symphysis pubis with sacroiliac

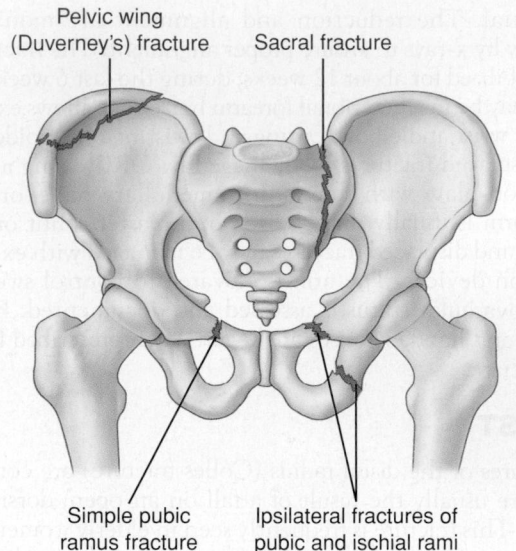

Figure 69-12 Stable pelvic fractures.

ligament disruption), vertical instability, or a combination of both. Lateral or anterior–posterior compression of the pelvis produces rotationally unstable pelvic fractures. Vertically unstable pelvic fractures occur when force is exerted on the pelvis vertically, as may occur when the patient falls onto extended legs or is struck from above by a falling object. Vertical shear pelvic fractures involve the anterior and posterior pelvic ring with vertical displacement, usually through the sacroiliac joint. There is generally complete disruption of the posterior sacroiliac, sacrospinous, and sacrotuberous ligaments.

Immediate treatment in the emergency department of a patient with an unstable pelvic fracture includes stabilizing the pelvic bones and compressing bleeding vessels with a pelvic girdle, an external binding and stabilizing device. If major vessels are lacerated, the bleeding may be stopped through embolization using interventional radiology techniques prior to surgery. Approximately 20% of patients with unstable pelvic fractures bleed excessively, requiring more than 15 units of blood products within the first 24 hours after injury (Bongiovanni, Bradley & Kelley, 2005). These patients are at risk for hemorrhagic shock (see Chapter 15 for nursing management of the patient in shock). When the

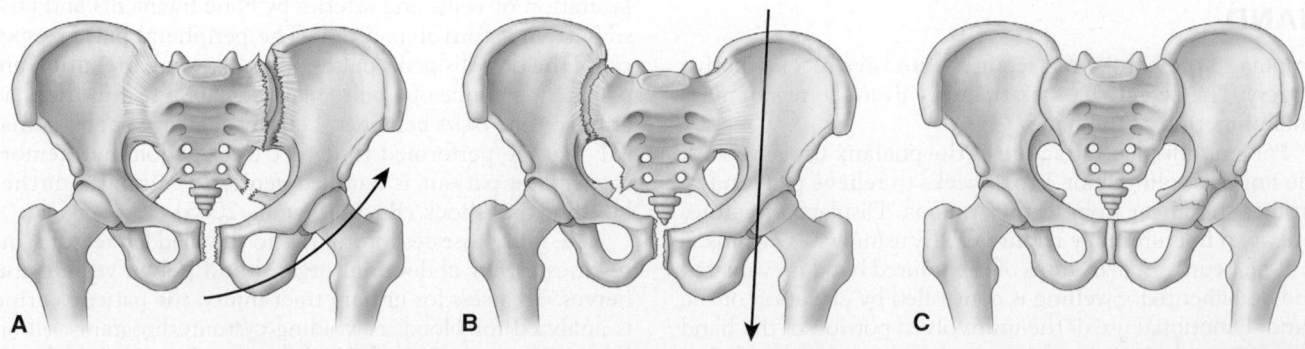

Figure 69-13 Unstable pelvic fracture. **A,** Rotationally unstable fracture. The symphysis pubis is separated and the anterior sacroiliac, sacrotuberous, and sacrospinous ligaments are disrupted. **B,** Vertically unstable fracture. The hemipelvis is displaced anteriorly and posteriorly through the symphysis pubis, and the sacroiliac joint ligaments are disrupted. **C,** Undisplaced fracture of the acetabulum.

patient is hemodynamically stable, treatment generally involves external fixation or ORIF. These measures promote hemostasis, hemodynamic stability, comfort, and early mobilization.

Acetabulum

Drivers and passengers sitting in the right front seat in motor vehicle crashes may forcibly propel their knees into the dashboard, injuring the knee-thigh-hip complex (Rupp & Schneider, 2004). The acetabulum is particularly vulnerable to fracture with injuries. Treatment depends on the pattern of fracture. Stable, nondisplaced fractures may be managed with traction and protective weight bearing so that the affected foot is only placed on the floor for balance. Displaced and unstable acetabular fractures are treated with open reduction, joint débridement, and internal fixation or arthroplasty. Internal fixation permits early non–weight-bearing ambulation and ROM exercise. Complications seen with acetabular fractures include nerve palsy, heterotopic ossification, and posttraumatic arthritis.

HIP

Elderly people (particularly women) who have low bone density from osteoporosis and who tend to fall frequently have a high incidence of hip fracture. Weak quadriceps muscles, general frailty due to age, and conditions that produce decreased cerebral arterial perfusion (transient ischemic attacks, anemia, emboli, cardiovascular disease, effects of medications) contribute to the incidence of falls. Mortality rates 1 year post–hip fracture range between 12% and 32% (Schoen, 2006).

There are two major types of hip fracture. *Intracapsular fractures* are fractures of the neck of the femur. *Extracapsular fractures* are fractures of the trochanteric region (between the base of the neck and the lesser trochanter of the femur) and of the subtrochanteric region (Fig. 69-14). Fractures of the neck of the femur may damage the vascular system that supplies blood to the head and the neck of the femur, and the bone may become ischemic. For this reason, AVN is common in patients with femoral neck fractures.

Extracapsular intertrochanteric fractures have an excellent blood supply and heal more rapidly. However, extensive soft

tissue damage may occur at the time of injury. It is not uncommon for the fracture to be comminuted and unstable. The elderly are particularly vulnerable to intertrochanteric fractures and do not have a prognosis as favorable as younger patients.

Clinical Manifestations

With fractures of the femoral neck, the leg is shortened, adducted, and externally rotated. The patient reports pain in the hip and groin or in the medial side of the knee. With most fractures of the femoral neck, the patient cannot move the leg without a significant increase in pain. The patient is most comfortable with the leg slightly flexed in external rotation. Impacted intracapsular femoral neck fractures cause moderate discomfort (even with movement), may allow the patient to bear weight, and may not demonstrate obvious shortening or rotational changes. With extracapsular femoral fractures of the trochanteric or subtrochanteric regions, the extremity is significantly shortened, externally rotated to a greater degree than intracapsular fractures, exhibits muscle spasm that resists positioning of the extremity in a neutral position, and has an associated area of ecchymosis. The diagnosis is confirmed by x-ray.

 Gerontologic Considerations

Hip fractures cause more than 340,000 hospitalizations annually among adults 65 years of age and older (Schoen, 2006). They are frequent contributors to physical disability and institutionalization among the elderly (Schoen, 2006). Stress and immobility related to the trauma predispose the older adult to atelectasis, pneumonia, sepsis, venous thromboemboli, pressure ulcers, and reduced ability to cope with other health problems. Many elderly people hospitalized with hip fractures exhibit delirium as a result of the stress of the trauma, unfamiliar surroundings, sleep deprivation, and medications. In addition, delirium that develops in some elderly patients may be caused by mild cerebral ischemia or mild hypoxemia. Other factors associated with delirium include responses to medications and anesthesia, malnutrition, dehydration, infectious processes, mood disturbances, and blood loss (see Chapter 12).

To prevent complications, the nurse must assess the elderly patient for chronic conditions that require close monitoring. Examination of the legs may reveal edema due to heart failure or absence of peripheral pulses from peripheral vascular disease. Similarly, chronic respiratory problems may be present and may contribute to the possible development of atelectasis or pneumonia. Coughing and deep-breathing exercises are encouraged. Frequently, elderly people take cardiac, antihypertensive, or respiratory medications that need to be continued. The patient's responses to these medications should be monitored.

Dehydration and poor nutrition may be present. At times, elderly people who live alone cannot call for help at the time of injury. A day or two may pass before assistance is provided, and as a result dehydration occurs. Dehydration contributes to hemoconcentration and predisposes the patient to the development of venous thromboemboli. Dehydration, inadequate nutritional intake, and immobility contribute to the development of pressure ulcers. Therefore, the patient needs

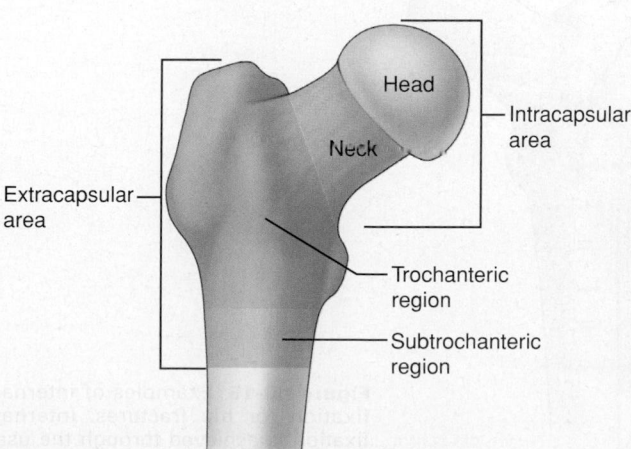

Figure 69-14 Regions of the proximal femur.

to be encouraged to consume adequate fluids and a healthy diet.

Muscle weakness may have initially contributed to the fall and fracture. Bed rest and immobility cause an additional loss of muscle strength unless the nurse encourages the patient to move all joints except the involved hip and knee. Patients are encouraged to use their arms and the overhead trapeze to reposition themselves. This strengthens the arms and shoulders, which facilitates walking with assistive devices.

Medical Management

Buck's extension traction, a type of temporary skin traction, may be applied to reduce muscle spasm, to immobilize the extremity, and to relieve pain, although its efficacy has not been demonstrated in clinical trials (Parker & Handoll, 2006). The goal of surgical treatment of hip fractures is to obtain a satisfactory fixation so that the patient can be mobilized quickly and avoid secondary medical complications. Surgical treatment consists of (1) open or closed reduction of the fracture and internal fixation, (2) replacement of the femoral head with a prosthesis (hemiarthroplasty), or (3) closed reduction with percutaneous stabilization for an intracapsular fracture. Surgical intervention is carried out as soon as possible after injury. The preoperative objective is to ensure that the patient is in as favorable a condition as possible for the surgery. Displaced femoral neck fractures are treated as emergencies, with reduction and internal fixation performed within 12 to 24 hours after fracture. The femoral head is often replaced with a prosthesis if there is complete disruption of blood flow to the femoral head, which may cause AVN.

After general or spinal anesthesia, the hip fracture is reduced under x-ray visualization. A stable fracture is usually fixed with nails, a nail-and-plate combination, multiple pins, or compression screw devices (Fig. 69-15). The orthopedic surgeon determines the specific fixation device based on the fracture site or sites. Adequate reduction is important for fracture healing: the better the reduction, the better the healing.

Total hip replacement (see Chapter 67) may be used in selected patients with acetabular defects.

Nursing Management

The immediate postoperative care for a patient with a hip fracture is similar to that for other patients undergoing major surgery (see Chapters 20 and 67). Attention is given to pain management, prevention of secondary medical problems, and early mobilization of the patient so that independent functioning can be restored (Chart 69-4).

During the first 24 to 48 hours, relief of pain and prevention of complications are important, and continuous neurovascular assessment is essential. The nurse encourages deep breathing and dorsiflexion and plantar flexion exercises every 1 to 2 hours. Thigh-high anti-embolism stockings or pneumatic compression devices are used, and anticoagulants are administered as prescribed to prevent the formation of venous thromboemboli. The nurse administers prescribed prophylactic IV antibiotics and monitors the patient's hydration, nutritional status, and urine output. A pillow placed between the legs is essential to maintain abduction and alignment and provide needed support when turning the patient.

Repositioning the Patient

The most comfortable and safest way to turn the patient is to turn to the uninjured side. The standard method involves placing a pillow between the patient's legs to keep the affected leg in an abducted position. Proper alignment and supported abduction are maintained while turning.

Promoting Exercise

The patient is encouraged to exercise as much as possible by means of the overbed trapeze. This device helps strengthen the arms and shoulders in preparation for protected ambulation (eg, toe touch, partial weight bearing). On the first postoperative day, the patient transfers to a chair with assistance and begins assisted ambulation. The amount of weight bearing that can be permitted depends on the stability of the fracture reduction. The physician prescribes the degree of weight bearing. In general, hip flexion and internal rotation restrictions apply only if the patient has had a hemiarthroplasty or total arthroplasty (see Chapter 67). Physical therapists

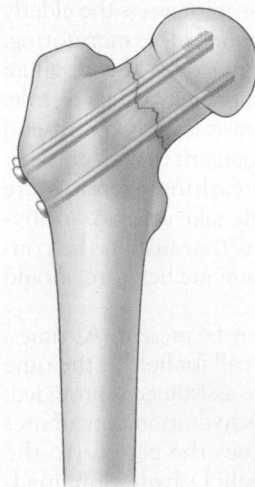

Cannulated screw
fixation

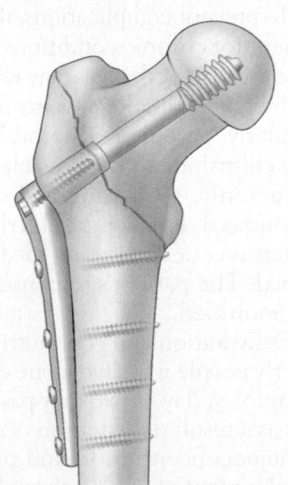

Compression hip screw
and side plate

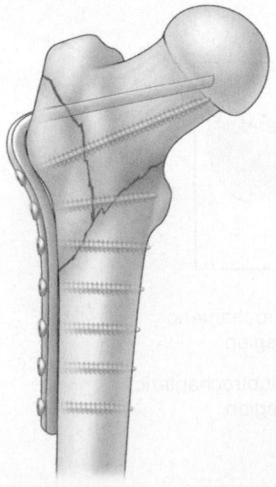

Blade plate
fixation

Figure 69-15 Examples of internal fixation for hip fractures. Internal fixation is achieved through the use of screws and plates specifically designed for stability and fixation.

CHART 69-4

NURSING RESEARCH PROFILE
Functional Recovery After Hip Fracture Surgery

Folden, S. & Tappen, R. (2007). Factors influencing function and recovery following hip repair surgery. *Orthopaedic Nursing, 26*(4), 234–241.

Purpose

The incidence of hip fractures will rise with the projected aging of the American population. Most hip fractures are repaired surgically and incur high rates of morbidity and mortality. Although prior research identifies factors associated with functional recovery following hip repair surgery for patients with hip fractures, these studies utilized data gathered close to the time of surgery. There is sparse research targeted at identifying factors that influence functional recovery following hip repair surgery more than 1 month postoperatively. Therefore, the purpose of this study was to identify factors that are associated with improved functional recovery 3 months post–hip repair surgery.

Design

Seventy-three patients who had hip repair surgery post–hip fracture and who were enrolled in a study on the effects of a postoperative educational intervention provided data for this study, which used secondary analysis of data from a previous study. The mean age of this sample was 73.93 years (SD = 8.40) and most participants were Caucasian (98.4%) and female (66.7%). All participants had hip repair surgery, were admitted to rehabilitation units posthospital discharge, and were planning to return to their communities postrehabilitation. Participants had to be able to read and write English and had to demonstrate satisfactory mental status by achieving a minimum score on the Mini-Mental Status Exam (MMSE) in order to be able to participate in the original study (and therefore also to provide data for this secondary analysis).

A variety of factors that affect functional recovery were assessed on these participants using self-report measures. These included fatigue, measured with the Fatigue Severity Scale (FSS); depression, measured with the Center for Epidemiologic Studies–Depression Scale (CES-D); fear of falling, measured with the Fall Efficacy Scale (FES); cognitive status, measured with the MMSE; pain, measured with a visual analog scale (VAS); performance of activities of daily living (ie, functional level), measured with the Functional Life Scale (FLS); and balance, measured with the Berg Balance Scale. Functional recovery was calculated by subtracting participants' FLS scores at 3 months from the FLS scores they reported preoperatively.

Findings

Cognitive status and balance were the best predictors of functional recovery 3 months postdischarge among sampled patients who had hip repair surgery. In addition, men had higher functional levels 3 months postdischarge and had a greater likelihood of returning to their preoperative functional level.

Nursing Implications

Results from this study suggest that the best predictors of functional recovery among patients who have hip repair surgery are improved balance and cognitive status. Women may be at higher risk of not achieving functional recovery. Nurses are in ideal positions to educate postoperative hip repair patients of the potential benefits of engaging in exercise regimens that improve balance, including resistance exercises, yoga, and tai chi.

---

work with the patient on transfers, ambulation, and the safe use of assistive devices.

The patient can anticipate discharge to home or to an extended care facility with the use of assistive devices (see Chapter 11). Some modifications in the home may be needed, such as installation of elevated toilet seats and grab bars.

Monitoring and Managing Potential Complications

Elderly people with hip fractures are prone to complications that may require more vigorous treatment. Achievement of homeostasis after injury and after surgery is accomplished through careful monitoring and collaborative management.

Neurovascular complications may occur from direct injury or edema in the area that causes compression of nerves and blood vessels. With hip fracture, bleeding into the tissues and edema are expected. Monitoring and documenting the neurovascular status of the affected leg are vital.

To prevent DVT, the nurse encourages intake of fluids and ankle and foot exercises. Anti-embolism stockings, pneumatic compression devices, and prophylactic anticoagulant therapy may be prescribed. Assessment of the patient's legs every 2 to 4 hours for signs of DVT, which may include unilateral calf tenderness, warmth, redness, and swelling, is indicated.

Pulmonary complications (eg, atelectasis, pneumonia) are a threat to elderly patients undergoing hip surgery. Coughing and deep-breathing exercises, a change of position at least every 2 hours, and the use of an incentive spirometer may help prevent respiratory complications. Pain must be treated with analgesic agents, typically opioids; otherwise, the patient may not be able to cough, deep breathe, or engage in prescribed activities. The nurse assesses breath sounds at least every 2 to 4 hours to detect adventitious or diminished sounds.

Skin breakdown is often seen in elderly patients with hip fracture. Blisters caused by tape are related to the tension of soft tissue edema under the nonelastic tape. An elastic hip wrap dressing or elastic tape applied in a vertical fashion may reduce the incidence of tape blisters. In addition, patients with hip fractures tend to remain in one position and may develop pressure ulcers. Proper skin care, especially on the bony prominences, helps to relieve pressure. High-density foam mattress overlays may provide protection by distributing pressure evenly.

Loss of bladder control (incontinence or retention) may occur. In general, the routine use of an indwelling catheter is avoided because of the high risk for urinary tract infection. If a catheter is inserted at the time of surgery, it usually is removed on the first postoperative day. Because urinary retention is common after surgery, the nurse must assess the patient's voiding patterns. To ensure proper urinary tract function, the nurse encourages liberal fluid intake if the patient has no preexisting cardiac disease.

Delayed complications of hip fractures include infection, nonunion, AVN of the femoral head (particularly with femoral neck fractures), and fixation device problems (eg, protrusion of the fixation device through the acetabulum, loosening of hardware). Infection is suspected if the patient complains of constant pain in the hip and has an elevated erythrocyte sedimentation rate.

The nursing management of the elderly patient with a hip fracture is summarized in the Plan of Nursing Care (Chart 69-5).

Health Promotion

Osteoporosis screening of patients who have experienced hip fracture is important for prevention of future fractures. With dual-energy x-ray absorptiometry (DXA) scan testing, the risk for additional fracture can be predicted. Specific patient education regarding dietary requirements, lifestyle changes, and weight-bearing exercise to promote bone health is needed. Specific therapeutic interventions need to be initiated to slow bone loss and to build bone mineral density (see Chapter 68). Prevention of falls is also important and may be achieved through exercises to improve muscle tone and balance and through the elimination of environmental hazards.

FEMORAL SHAFT

Considerable force is required to break the shaft of a femur in adults. Most femoral fractures occur in young adults who have been involved in a motor vehicle crash or who have fallen from a high place. Frequently, these patients have associated multiple injuries.

The patient presents with an edematous, deformed, painful thigh and cannot move the hip or the knee. The fracture may be transverse, oblique, spiral, or comminuted. Frequently the patient develops shock, because the loss of 2 to 3 units of blood into the tissues is common with these fractures. The diameter of the thigh should be closely monitored because expansion may indicate continued bleeding. Types of femoral fractures are illustrated in Figure 69-16A.

Assessment and Diagnostic Findings

Assessment includes checking the neurovascular status of the extremity, especially circulatory perfusion of the lower leg and foot (popliteal, posterior tibial, and pedal pulses and toe capillary refill time). A Doppler ultrasound may be indicated to assess blood flow. Dislocation of the hip and knee may accompany these fractures. Knee effusion suggests ligament damage and possible instability of the knee joint.

Medical Management

Continued neurovascular monitoring and documentation are important. The fracture is immobilized so that additional soft tissue damage does not occur. Generally, skeletal traction (Fig. 69-16B,C) or splinting is used to immobilize fracture fragments until the patient is physiologically stable and ready for ORIF procedures.

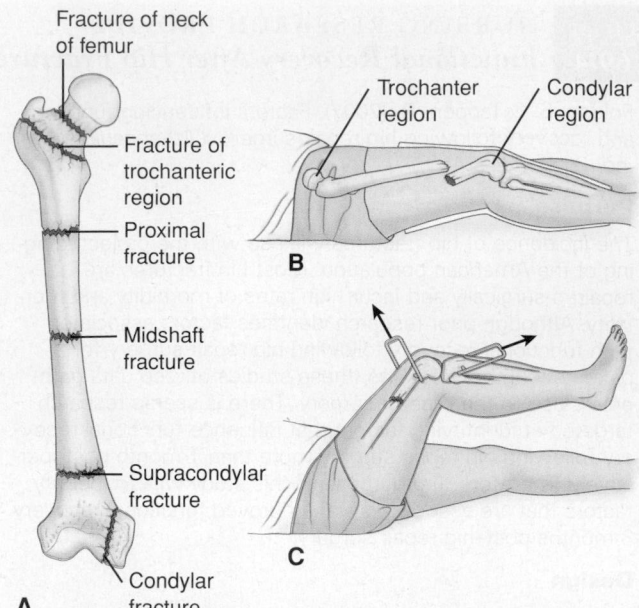

Figure 69-16 A, Types of femoral fractures. **B,** Example of deformity on admission to hospital. **C,** Adequate reduction is achieved when additional wire is inserted in the lower femoral fragment and vertical lift is secured.

Internal fixation usually is carried out within 24 hours after injury (Scalea, 2008). Intramedullary locking nail devices are used for midshaft (diaphyseal) fractures. Depending on the supracondylar fracture pattern, intramedullary nailing or screw plate fixation may be used. Internal fixation permits early mobilization. A thigh cuff orthosis may be used for external support. To preserve muscle strength, the patient is instructed to exercise the hip and the lower leg, foot, and toes on a regular basis. Active muscle movement enhances healing by increasing blood supply and electrical potentials at the fracture site. Prescribed weight-bearing limits are based on the type and location of the fracture and treatment approach. Physical therapy includes ROM and strengthening exercises, safe use of assistive devices, and gait training. Ambulation stimulates fracture healing in approximately 4 to 6 months.

Compression plates and intramedullary nails are sometimes removed after 12 to 18 months due to loosening. After the plates are removed, a thigh cuff orthosis is used for several months to provide support while bone remodeling takes place.

Infrequently because of patient risk associated with anesthesia and surgery, middle shaft and distal fractures may be managed with skeletal traction. Between 2 and 4 weeks after injury, when pain and swelling have subsided, skeletal traction is removed and the patient is placed in a cast brace. The cast brace is a total contact device (ie, encircles the limb) and holds the reduced fracture. The muscle, through hydrodynamic compression, stabilizes the bone and stimulates healing. Minimal partial weight bearing is begun and is progressed to full weight bearing as tolerated. The cast brace is worn for 12 to 14 weeks.

An external fixator may be used if the patient has experienced an open fracture, has extensive soft tissue trauma, has lost bone, has an infection, or has hip and tibial fractures.

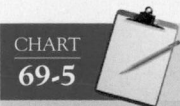

**CHART
69-5**

PLAN OF NURSING CARE
Care of the Elderly Patient With a Fractured Hip

NURSING DIAGNOSIS: Acute pain related to fracture, soft tissue damage, muscle spasm, and surgery
GOAL: Relief of pain

Nursing Interventions	Rationale	Expected Outcomes
1. Assess type and location of patient's pain whenever vital signs are obtained and as needed.	1. Pain is expected after fracture; soft tissue damage and muscle spasm contribute to discomfort; pain is subjective and is best evaluated on a pain scale of 0 to 10 and through description of characteristics and location, which are important for identifying cause of discomfort and for proposing interventions. Continuing pain may indicate development of neurovascular problems. Pain must be assessed periodically to gauge effectiveness of continuing analgesic therapy.	• Patient describes and rates pain on scale of 0 to 10 • Expresses confidence in efforts to control pain • Expresses comfort with position changes • Expresses comfort when leg is positioned and immobilized • Minimizes movement of extremity before reduction and fixation • Uses physical, psychological, and pharmacologic measures to reduce discomfort • Describes a decrease in pain in 24 to 48 hours after surgery • Requests pain medications and uses pain relief measures early in pain cycle • States that positioning provides comfort • Appears comfortable and relaxed • Moves with increasing comfort as healing progresses
2. Acknowledge existence of pain; inform patient of available analgesics; record patient's baseline discomfort.	2. Reduces stress experienced by the patient by communicating concern and availability of help in dealing with pain. Documentation provides baseline data.	
3. Handle the affected extremity gently, supporting it with hands or pillow.	3. Movement of bone fragments is painful; muscle spasms occur with movement; adequate support diminishes soft tissue tension.	
4. Apply Buck's traction if prescribed. Use trochanter roll.	4. Immobilizes fracture to decrease pain, muscle spasm, and external rotation of hip.	
5. Use pain-modifying strategies.	5. Pain perception can be diminished by distraction and refocusing of attention.	
a. Modify the environment.	a. Interaction with others, distraction, and environmental stimuli may modify pain experiences.	
b. Administer prescribed analgesics as needed.	b. Analgesics reduce the pain; muscle relaxants may be prescribed to decrease discomfort associated with muscle spasm.	
c. Encourage patient to use pain relief measures to relieve pain.	c. Mild pain is easier to control than severe pain.	
d. Evaluate patient's response to medications and other pain-reduction techniques.	d. Assessment of effectiveness of measures provides basis for future management interventions; early identification of adverse reactions is necessary for corrective measures and care plan modifications.	
e. Consult with physician if relief of pain is not obtained.	e. Change in treatment plan may be necessary.	
6. Position for comfort and function.	6. Alignment of body facilitates comfort; positioning for function diminishes stress on musculoskeletal system.	
7. Assist with frequent changes in position.	7. Change of position relieves pressure and associated discomfort.	

Continued on following page

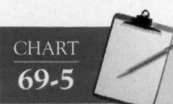

CHART 69-5

PLAN OF NURSING CARE
Care of the Elderly Patient With a Fractured Hip (*Continued*)

NURSING DIAGNOSIS: Impaired physical mobility related to fractured hip
GOAL: Achieves pain-free, functional, stable hip

Nursing Interventions	Rationale	Expected Outcomes
1. Maintain neutral positioning of hip.	1. Prevents stress at the site of fixation.	• Patient engages in therapeutic positioning
2. Use trochanter roll; roll to uninjured side.	2. Minimizes external rotation.	• Uses pillow between legs when turning
3. Place pillow between legs when turning.	3. Supports leg; prevents adduction.	• Assists in position changes; shows increased independence in transfers
4. Instruct and assist in position changes and transfers.	4. Encourages patient's active participation while preventing stress on hip fixation.	• Exercises every 2 hours while awake
5. Instruct in and supervise isometric, quadriceps-setting, and gluteal-setting exercises.	5. Strengthens muscles needed for walking.	• Uses trapeze • Participates in progressive ambulation program
6. Encourage use of trapeze.	6. Strengthens shoulder and arm muscles necessary for use of ambulatory aids.	• Actively participates in exercise regimen
7. In consultation with physical therapist, instruct in and supervise progressive safe ambulation within limitations of weight-bearing prescription.	7. Amount of weight bearing depends on the patient's condition, fracture stability, and fixation device; ambulatory aids are used to assist the patient with non–weight-bearing and partial-weight-bearing ambulation.	• Uses ambulatory aids correctly and safely
8. Offer encouragement and support exercise regimen.	8. Reconditioning exercises can be uncomfortable and fatiguing; encouragement helps patient comply with the program.	
9. Instruct in and supervise safe use of ambulatory aids.	9. Prevents injury from unsafe use.	

NURSING DIAGNOSIS: Risk for infection related to surgical incision
GOAL: Maintains asepsis

Nursing Interventions	Rationale	Expected Outcomes
1. Monitor vital signs.	1. Temperature, pulse, and respiration increase in response to infection. (Magnitude of response may be minimal in elderly patients.)	• Patient maintains vital signs within normal range
2. Perform aseptic dressing changes.	2. Avoids introducing infectious organisms.	• Exhibits well-approximated incision without drainage or excessive inflammatory response
3. Assess wound appearance and character of drainage.	3. Red, swollen, draining incision is indicative of infection.	• Relates minimal discomfort; demonstrates no hematoma
4. Assess report of pain.	4. Pain may be due to wound hematoma, a possible locus of infection, which needs to be surgically evacuated.	• Tolerates antibiotics; exhibits no evidence of osteomyelitis
5. Administer prophylactic antibiotic if prescribed, and observe for side effects.	5. Antibiotics reduce the risk for infection.	

NURSING DIAGNOSIS: Readiness for enhanced urinary elimination related to immobility
GOAL: Maintains normal urinary elimination patterns

Nursing Interventions	Rationale	Expected Outcomes
1. Monitor intake and output.	1. Adequate fluid intake ensures hydration; adequate urinary output minimizes urinary stasis.	• Intake and output are adequate; patient exhibits normal voiding patterns
2. Avoid/minimize use of indwelling catheter.	2. Source of bladder infection.	• Demonstrates no evidence of urinary tract infection
3. Perform intermittent catheterization for urinary retention.	3. Empties bladder; reduces urinary tract infections.	

Continued

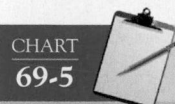

CHART
69-5

PLAN OF NURSING CARE
Care of the Elderly Patient With a Fractured Hip (Continued)

NURSING DIAGNOSIS: Readiness for enhanced coping related to injury, anticipated surgery, and dependence
GOAL: Uses effective coping mechanisms to modify stress

Nursing Interventions	Rationale	Expected Outcomes
1. Encourage patient to express concerns and to discuss the possible impact of fractured hip.	1. Verbalization helps patient deal with problems and feelings. Clarification of thoughts and feelings promotes problem solving.	• Patient describes feelings concerning fractured hip and implications for lifestyle
2. Support use of coping mechanisms. Involve significant others and support services as needed.	2. Coping mechanisms modify disabling effects of stress; sharing concerns lessens the burden and facilitates necessary modification.	• Uses available resources and coping mechanisms; develops health promotion strategies
3. Contact social services, if needed.	3. Anxiety may be related to financial or social problems; facilitates management of problems associated with continuing care.	• Uses community resources as needed • Participates in development of health care plan
4. Explain anticipated treatment regimen and routines to facilitate positive attitude in relation to rehabilitation.	4. Understanding of plan of care helps to diminish fears of the unknown.	
5. Encourage patient to participate in planning.	5. Participating in care provides for some control of self and environment.	

NURSING DIAGNOSIS: Risk for disturbed thought process related to age, stress of trauma, unfamiliar surroundings, and medication therapy
GOAL: Remains oriented and participates in decision making

Nursing Interventions	Rationale	Expected Outcomes
1. Assess orientation status.	1. Evaluate presenting orientation of patient; confusion may result from stress of fracture, unfamiliar surroundings, coexisting systemic disease, cerebral ischemia, hypoxemia, or other factors. Baseline data are important for determining change.	• Patient establishes effective communication
2. Interview family regarding patient's orientation and cognitive abilities before injury.	2. Provides data for evaluation of current findings.	• Demonstrates orientation to time, place, and person
3. Assess patient for auditory and visual deficits.	3. Diminished vision and auditory acuity frequently occur with aging; glasses and hearing aid may increase patient's ability to interact with environment.	• Participates in self-care activities • Remains mentally alert • Avoids episodes of confusion
a. Assist patient with use of sensory aids (eg, glasses, hearing aid) b. Control environmental distractors	a. Aids must be in good working order and available for use. b. Facilitates communication.	
4. Orient to and stabilize environment. a. Use orientation activities and aids (eg, clock, calendar, pictures, Introduction of self). b. Minimize number of staff working with patient.	4. a. Short-term memory may be faulty in the elderly; frequent reorientation helps. b. Consistency of caregivers promotes trust.	
5. Give simple explanations of procedures and plan of care.	5. Promotes understanding and active participation.	
6. Encourage participation in hygiene and nutritional activities.	6. Participation in routine activities promotes orientation, increases awareness of self.	
7. Provide for safety. a. Keep light on at night. b. Have call bell available. c. Provide prompt response to requests for assistance.	7. Mechanism for securing assistance is available to patient; independent activities based on faulty judgment may result in injury.	

Continued on following page

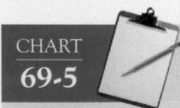

CHART 69-5

PLAN OF NURSING CARE
Care of the Elderly Patient With a Fractured Hip (*Continued*)

Nursing Interventions	Rationale	Expected Outcomes
8. Assess mental responses to medications, especially sedatives and analgesics.	8. Elderly people tend to be more sensitive to medications; abnormal responses (eg, hallucinations, depression) may occur.	

COLLABORATIVE PROBLEMS: Hemorrhage; pulmonary complications; peripheral neurovascular dysfunction; deep vein thrombosis; pressure ulcers related to surgery and immobility
GOAL: Absence of complications

Nursing Interventions	Rationale	Expected Outcomes
Hemorrhage		
1. Monitor vital signs, observing for shock.	1. Changes in pulse, blood pressure, and respirations may indicate development of shock; blood loss and stress may contribute to development of shock.	• Vital signs are stabilized within normal limits • Experiences no excessive or bright red drainage • Exhibits stable postoperative hemoglobin and hematocrit values • Patient has clear breath sounds • Breath sounds present in all fields • Exhibits no shortness of breath, chest pain, or elevated temperature
2. Consider preinjury blood pressure values and management of coexisting hypertension, if present.	2. Necessary for interpretation of current blood pressure determinations.	
3. Note character and amount of drainage.	3. Excessive drainage and bright red drainage may indicate active bleeding.	
4. Notify surgeon if patient develops shock or excessive bleeding.	4. Corrective measures need to be instituted.	
5. Note hemoglobin and hematocrit values, and report decreases in values.	5. Anemia due to blood loss may develop; bleeding into tissues after hip fracture may be extensive; blood replacement may be needed.	
Pulmonary Complications		
1. Assess respiratory status: respiratory rate, depth, and duration, breath sounds, sputum. Monitor temperature.	1. Anesthesia and bed rest diminish respiratory effort and cause pooling of respiratory secretions. Adventitious breath sounds, pain on respiration, shortness of breath, blood tinged sputum, cough, etc., indicate pulmonary dysfunction.	• Vital signs are stabilized within normal limits • Patient has clear breath sounds • Breath sounds present in all fields • Exhibits no shortness of breath, chest pain, or elevated temperature • PaO_2 on room air within normal limits • Performs respiratory exercises; uses incentive spirometer as instructed • Changes position frequently • Consumes adequate fluids
2. Report adventitious and diminished breath sounds and elevated temperature.	2. Elevated temperature in the early postoperative period may be due to atelectasis or pneumonia.	
3. Supervise deep breathing and coughing exercises. Encourage use of incentive spirometer if prescribed.	3. Promote optimal ventilation. Coexisting respiratory conditions diminish lung expansion.	
4. Administer oxygen as prescribed.	4. Reduced ventilatory efforts may diminish PaO_2 when patient is breathing room air.	
5. Turn and reposition patient at least every 2 hours. Mobilize patient (assist patient out of bed) as soon as possible.	5. Promotes optimal ventilation. Diminishes pooling of respiratory secretions.	
6. Ensure adequate hydration.	6. Liquefies respiratory secretions. Facilitates expectoration.	
Peripheral Neurovascular Dysfunction		
1. Assess affected extremity for color and temperature.	1. The skin becomes pale and feels cool with decreased tissue perfusion. Venous congestion may cause cyanosis.	• Patient has normal color and the extremity is warm • Demonstrates normal capillary refill response • Exhibits moderate swelling; tissue not palpably tense • States pain is tolerable
2. Assess toes for capillary refill response.	2. After compression of the nail, rapid return of pink color indicates good capillary perfusion.	

Continued

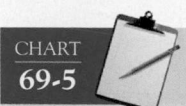

Nursing Interventions	Rationale	Expected Outcomes
3. Assess affected extremity for edema and swelling.	3. The trauma of surgery will cause swelling; excessive swelling and hematoma formation can compromise circulation and function; edema may be due to coexisting cardiovascular disease.	• Reports no pain with passive dorsiflexion • Reports normal sensations and no paresthesia • Demonstrates normal motor abilities and no paresis or paralysis • Has strong and equal pulses
4. Elevate affected extremity.	4. Minimizes dependent edema.	
5. Assess for deep, throbbing, unrelenting pain.	5. Surgical pain can be controlled; pain due to neurovascular compromise is refractory to treatment with analgesics.	
6. Assess for pain on passive flexion of foot.	6. With nerve ischemia, there will be pain on passive stretch.	
7. Assess for sensations and numbness.	7. Diminished pain and paresthesia may indicate nerve damage. Sensation in web between great and second toe-peroneal nerve; sensation on sole of foot-tibial nerve.	
8. Assess ability to move foot and toes.	8. Dorsiflexion of ankle and extension of toes indicate function of peroneal nerve. Plantar flexion of ankle and flexion of toes indicate functioning of tibial nerve.	
9. Assess pedal pulses in both feet.	9. Indicates circulatory status of extremities.	
10. Notify surgeon if diminished neurovascular status occurs.	10. Function of extremity needs to be preserved.	

Deep Vein Thrombosis

Nursing Interventions	Rationale	Expected Outcomes
1. Apply thigh-high anti-embolism stockings and/or sequential compression device as prescribed.	1. Compression aids venous blood return and prevents stasis.	• Wears thigh-high anti-embolism stockings • Uses sequential compression device • Experiences no more warmth than usual in skin areas • Exhibits no increase in calf circumference • Demonstrates no evidence of calf tenderness, warmth, redness, or swelling • Changes position with assistance and supervision • Participates in exercise regimen • Experiences no chest pain; has lungs clear to auscultation; presents no evidence of pulmonary emboli • Exhibits no signs of dehydration; has normal hematocrit • Maintains normal body temperature
2. Remove stockings for 20 minutes twice a day, and provide skin care.	2. Skin care is necessary to avoid skin breakdown. Extended removal of stocking or device defeats purpose.	
3. Assess popliteal, dorsalis pedis, and posterior tibial pulses.	3. Pulses indicate arterial perfusion of extremity. With coexisting arteriosclerotic vascular disease, pulses may be diminished or absent.	
4. Assess skin temperature of legs.	4. Local inflammation increases local skin temperature.	
5. Assess calf every 4 hours for tenderness, warmth, redness, and swelling.	5. Unilateral calf tenderness, warmth, redness, and swelling may indicate deep vein thrombosis.	
6. Measure calf circumference twice daily.	6. Increased calf circumference indicates edema or altered perfusion.	
7. Avoid pressure on popliteal blood vessels from appliances or pillows.	7. Compression of blood vessels diminishes blood flow.	
8. Change patient's position and increase activity as prescribed.	8. Activity promotes circulation and diminishes venous stasis.	
9. Supervise ankle exercises hourly while patient is awake.	9. Muscle exercise promotes circulation.	
10. Ensure adequate hydration.	10. Elderly people may become dehydrated because of low fluid intake, resulting in hemoconcentration.	
11. Monitor body temperature.	11. Body temperature increases with inflammation (magnitude of response minimal in elderly people).	

Continued on following page

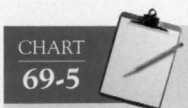

PLAN OF NURSING CARE
Care of the Elderly Patient With a Fractured Hip (Continued)

CHART 69-5

Nursing Interventions	Rationale	Expected Outcomes
Pressure Ulcers 1. Monitor condition of skin at pressure points (eg, heels, sacrum, shoulders); inspect heels at least twice a day. 2. Reposition patient at least every 2 hours. Avoid skin shearing. 3. Administer skin care, especially to pressure points. 4. Use special care mattress and other protective devices (eg, heel protectors); support heel off the mattress. 5. Institute care according to protocol at first indication of potential skin breakdown.	1. Elderly patients are subject to skin breakdown at points of pressure because of diminished subcutaneous tissue. 2. Avoids prolonged pressure and trauma to the skin. 3. Immobility causes pressure at bony prominences; position changes relieve pressure. 4. Devices minimize pressure on skin at bony prominences. 5. Early interventions prevent tissue destruction and prolonged rehabilitation.	• Patient exhibits no signs of skin breakdown • Skin remains intact • Repositions self frequently • Uses protective devices

NURSING DIAGNOSIS: Risk for ineffective health maintenance related to fractured hip and impaired mobility
GOAL: Exhibits health maintenance/promotion behaviors

Nursing Interventions	Rationale	Expected Outcomes
1. Assess home environment for discharge planning. 2. Encourage patient to express concerns about care at home; explore with patient possible solutions to problems. 3. Assess availability of physical assistance for ADLs and health care activities. 4. Teach caregiver the home health care regimen. 5. Instruct patient in posthospital care: a. Activity limitations. b. Reinforce exercise instructions. c. Safe use of ambulatory aids. d. Wound care. e. Measures to promote healing (nutrition, wound care). f. Medications. g. Potential problems. h. Continuing health care supervision.	1. Physical barriers (especially stairs, bathrooms) may limit patient's ability to ambulate and care for self at home. 2. Patient may have special problems that need to be identified so that solutions might be identified. 3. Because of limitation of mobility, patient requires some assistance in ADLs and routine health care. 4. Understanding of rehabilitative regimen is necessary for compliance. 5. Lack of knowledge and poor preparation for care at home contribute to patient anxiety, insecurity, and nonadherence to therapeutic regimen.	• Home is accessible for patient at time of discharge • Patient appears relaxed and develops strategies to deal with identified problems • Has personal assistance available • Demonstrates ability to use necessary assistive devices within therapeutic prescription • Complies with home care program; keeps follow-up health care appointments

A common complication after fracture of the femoral shaft is restriction of knee motion. Active and passive knee exercises begin as soon as possible, depending on the stability of the fracture and knee ligaments. Other complications include malunion, delayed union or nonunion, pudendal nerve palsy, and infection.

KNEE

Fracture to the most distal portion of the femur, the patella (kneecap), and fracture to the most proximal portion of the tibia, may be defined as fractures of the knee. These fractures may be caused by motor vehicle crashes, direct blows to the knee from contact sports or intentionally inflicted trauma,

or falls. The patient typically presents with acute pain to the affected knee and cannot ambulate or bear weight on the affected extremity. The affected knee is notably edematous.

Assessment and Diagnostic Findings

If a patient presents with acute knee pain that occurs as a result of an injury (such as a fall or direct blow to the knee), a CT scan may be indicated to determine the extent of injury. Not all knee injuries are evident on x-ray. An MRI or CT scan can define the details of the injury of bone, cartilage, tendons, and ligaments. If the bones of the knee area are fractured, there is usually limited ROM and sometimes crepitus with motion.

Medical Management

Patients with significant joint effusions may benefit from arthrocentesis to provide relief of intra-articular pressure. Anti-inflammatory and analgesic effects of NSAIDs such as ibuprofen (Motrin, Advil) may be prescribed. Other treatments that may be prescribed depend on the knee bone that is fractured and the extent of the injury, including whether the fracture is displaced or nondisplaced. Nondisplaced fractures may be effectively treated with 6 weeks of immobilization and gradual increases in weight bearing, while displaced fractures typically require ORIF surgical procedures.

TIBIA AND FIBULA

The most common fractures below the knee are tibia and fibula fractures. Fractures of the tibia and fibula often occur in association with each other and tend to result from a direct blow, falls with the foot in a flexed position, or a violent twisting motion. The patient presents with pain, deformity, obvious hematoma, and considerable edema. Frequently, these fractures are open and involve severe soft tissue damage because there is little subcutaneous tissue in the area.

Assessment and Diagnostic Findings

The peroneal nerve is assessed and if damaged, the patient cannot dorsiflex the great toe and has diminished sensation in the first web space. The tibial artery is assessed for damage by evaluating pulses, skin temperature, and color and by testing the capillary refill response. Hemiarthrosis or ligament damage may occur with a fracture near the joint.

The patient is monitored for an anterior acute compartment syndrome. Signs and symptoms include pain that is not relieved by analgesics, pain that increases with plantar flexion, complaints of paresthesias, and sometimes a weak or absent pulse.

Medical Management

Most closed tibial fractures are treated with closed reduction and initial immobilization in a long-leg walking cast or a patellar tendon–bearing cast. As with other lower extremity fractures, the leg is elevated to control edema. Partial weight bearing is usually prescribed after 7 to 10 days, depending on the type of fracture. Activity decreases edema and increases circulation. The cast is changed to a short-leg cast or brace in 3 to 4 weeks, which allows for knee motion. Fracture healing takes 6 to 10 weeks. Percutaneous pins may be placed in the bone and held in position by an external fixator.

Comminuted fractures may be treated with skeletal traction, internal fixation with intramedullary nails or plates and screws, or external fixation. External support may be used with internal fixation. Hip, foot, and knee exercises are encouraged within the limits of the immobilizing device. Partial weight bearing is begun when prescribed and is progressed as the fracture heals in 4 to 8 weeks.

Open fractures are treated with external fixation. Distal fractures with extensive soft tissue damage heal slowly and may require bone grafting.

Continued neurovascular evaluation is important. The development of acute compartment syndrome requires prompt recognition and communication to the orthopedic surgeon. Other complications include delayed union, infection, impaired wound edge healing due to limited soft tissue, and loosening of the internal fixation hardware.

RIB

Uncomplicated fractures of the lower ribs occur frequently in adults and usually result in no impairment of function. Because these fractures cause pain with respiratory effort, the patient tends to decrease respiratory excursions and refrains from coughing. As a result, tracheobronchial secretions are not mobilized, aeration of the lung is diminished, and a predisposition to atelectasis and pneumonia results. To help the patient cough and take deep breaths, the nurse may splint the chest with his or her hands. Occasionally, an anesthesia care provider administers intercostal nerve blocks to relieve pain and to permit productive coughing.

Chest strapping to immobilize the rib fracture is not used because decreased chest expansion may result in atelectasis and pneumonia. The pain associated with rib fracture diminishes significantly in 3 or 4 days, and the fracture heals within 6 weeks. In addition to atelectasis and pneumonia, complications may include a flail chest, pneumothorax, and hemothorax. The assessment and management of patients with these conditions are discussed in Chapter 23.

THORACOLUMBAR SPINE

Fractures of the thoracolumbar spine may involve (1) the vertebral body, (2) the laminae and articulating processes, and (3) the spinous processes or transverse processes. The T12 to L2 area of the spine is most vulnerable to fracture. Fractures generally result from indirect trauma caused by excessive loading, sudden muscle contraction, or excessive motion beyond physiologic limits. Osteoporosis contributes to vertebral body collapse (compression fracture) (Bucholz, et al., 2005).

Stable spinal fractures are caused by flexion, extension, lateral bending, or vertical loading. The anterior structural column (vertebral bodies and disks) or the posterior structural column (neural arch, articular processes, ligaments) are disrupted. Unstable fractures occur with fracture dislocations and involve disruption of both anterior and posterior structural columns. There is always the potential for neural damage (eg, spinal cord injury).

The patient with a spinal fracture presents with acute tenderness, swelling, paravertebral muscle spasm, and change in the normal curves or in the gap between spinous processes. Pain is greater with moving, coughing, or weight bearing. Immobilization is essential until initial assessments have determined if there is any spinal cord injury and whether the fracture is stable or unstable (see Chapter 63). If spinal cord injury with neurologic deficit does occur, it usually requires immediate surgery (laminectomy with spinal fusion) to decompress the spinal cord.

Stable spinal fractures are treated conservatively with limited bed rest. The head of the bed is elevated less than 30 degrees until the acute pain subsides (several days). Analgesics are prescribed for pain relief. The patient is monitored for a transient paralytic ileus caused by associated retroperitoneal hemorrhage. Sitting is avoided until the pain subsides. A spinal brace or plastic thoracolumbar orthosis may be applied for support during progressive ambulation and resumption of activities.

The patient with an unstable fracture is treated with bed rest, possibly with the use of a special turning device or bed to maintain spinal alignment. Within 24 hours after fracture, open reduction, decompression, and fixation with spinal fusion and instrument stabilization are usually accomplished. Neurologic status is monitored closely during the preoperative and postoperative periods. Postoperatively, the patient may be cared for on the turning device or in a bed with a firm mattress. Progressive ambulation is begun a few days after surgery, with the patient using a body brace orthosis. Patient teaching emphasizes good posture, good body mechanics, and, after healing is sufficient, back-strengthening exercises. (Spinal cord injury is discussed in Chapter 63.)

Sports-Related Injuries

Sport activities are very common, and, unfortunately, sports-related injuries are also common consequences. Table 69-1 displays common sports injuries, their mechanisms of injury, assessment findings, and acute care management.

Management

Patients who have experienced sports-related injuries are often highly motivated to return to their previous level of activity. Compliance with restriction of activities and gradual resumption of activities need to be reinforced. Injured athletes are at risk for reinjury and require follow-up and monitoring. With recurrence of symptoms, athletes need to diminish their level and intensity of activity to a comfortable level. The time required to recover from a sports-related injury can be as short as a few days or considerably longer than 6 weeks, depending on the severity of the injury. Increasing activities gradually to acclimate the muscles, tendons, and joints to the sport motions will assist in recovery and rehabilitation.

Prevention

Sports-related injuries can often be prevented by using proper equipment (eg, running shoes for joggers, wrist guards for skaters) and by effectively training and conditioning the body. Specific training needs to be tailored to the person and the sport. Stretching prior to engaging in sports or exercise had long been recommended; however, studies suggest that stretching may not prevent injury (Hart, 2005).

Occupation-Related Injuries

According to the U.S. Department of Labor, occupation-related musculoskeletal disorders are injuries or illnesses of the muscles, nerves, tendons, joints, cartilage, and bones that occur because of exposure to work-related risks. In 2005, more than 4.2 million cases of nonfatal musculoskeletal injuries and illnesses occurred in the workplace in the private sector (eg, not including the military or government agencies); of these, 1.4 million injuries resulted in lost work days (U.S. Department of Labor, Bureau of Labor Statistics, 2005).

The most frequent types of single injuries that occurred were sprains, strains, and tears (40.8%), cuts, lacerations,

and punctures (9.6%), bruises and contusions (8.7%), fractures, (7.8%), soreness and pain (5.3%), multiple injuries (4.1%), and back pain (2.9%) (U.S. Department of Labor, 2005). Management of sprains, strains, and fractures is described earlier in this chapter; management of low back pain is described in Chapter 68.

Amputation

Amputation is the removal of a body part, often an extremity. Amputation of a lower extremity is often necessary because of progressive peripheral vascular disease (often a sequela of diabetes mellitus), fulminating gas gangrene, trauma (crushing injuries, burns, frostbite, electrical burns, explosions, ballistic injuries), congenital deformities, chronic osteomyelitis, or malignant tumor. Of all these causes, peripheral vascular disease accounts for most amputations of lower extremities (see Chapter 31). Amputation of an upper extremity occurs less frequently than a lower extremity and is most often necessary because of either traumatic injury or a malignant tumor. It is estimated that 1.7 million Americans has had some type of an amputation (National Lower Limb Information Center, 2006).

Amputation is used to relieve symptoms, to improve function, and, most important, to save or improve the patient's quality of life. If the health care team communicates a positive attitude, the patient adjusts to the amputation more readily and actively participates in the rehabilitative plan, learning how to modify activities and how to use assistive devices for ADLs and mobility.

Levels of Amputation

Amputation is performed at the most distal point that will heal successfully. The site of amputation is determined by two factors: circulation in the part and functional usefulness (ie, meets the requirements for the use of a prosthesis).

The circulatory status of the extremity is evaluated through physical examination and diagnostic studies. Muscle and skin perfusion is important for healing. Doppler flow studies with duplex ultrasound, segmental blood pressure determinations, and transcutaneous PaO_2 of the extremity are valuable diagnostic aids. Angiography is performed if revascularization is considered an option.

The objective of surgery is to conserve as much extremity length as needed to preserve function and possibly to achieve a good prosthetic fit. Preservation of knee and elbow joints is desirable. Figure 69-17 shows the levels at which an extremity may be amputated. Most amputations involving extremities can be eventually fitted with a prosthesis.

The amputation of toes and portions of the foot can cause changes in gait and balance. A Syme amputation (modified ankle **disarticulation** amputation) is performed most frequently for extensive foot trauma and aims to produce a durable extremity end that can withstand full weight bearing. Below-knee amputation (BKA) is preferred to above-knee amputation (AKA) because of the importance of the knee joint and the energy requirements for walking. Knee disarticulations are most successful with young, active patients who can develop precise control of the prosthesis. When AKAs are performed, all possible length is preserved,

Table 69-1	COMMON SPORTS INJURIES			
Anatomic Area	**Mechanism of Injury**	**Assessment Findings**	**Sports Activity**	**Acute Management**
Clavicle fracture	Fall on shoulder or outstretched arm Direct blow to the clavicle	Crepitus Holds arm closely to body Unable to raise affected arm above head Can feel movement of both ends of clavicle	Football Rugby Hockey Wrestling Gymnastics	Sling or shoulder immobilizer Ice NSAIDs
Dislocated shoulder	*Anterior:* Some combination of hyperextension, external rotation, and abduction Anterior blow to shoulder *Posterior:* Fall on flexed and adducted arm Direct axial load to humerus	Pain Lack of motion May feel empty shoulder socket Uneven posture in comparison to other shoulder Affected arm appears longer Abduction limited	Rugby Hockey Wrestling Skiing	Closed reduction Immobilizer Pendulum exercises
Dislocated elbow	Falling on a hand with a flexed elbow Elbow overextended	Intense pain Edema Limited motion Deformity Ecchymosis	Football Gymnastics Squash Wrestling Cycling Skiing	Immobilization Ice ROM exercises
Wrist sprain or fracture	Falling on an outstretched arm	Pain Edema Ecchymosis Deformity Limited motion	Skating Hockey Wrestling Skiing Soccer Handball Horseback riding	Ice Elevation Immobilization Gentle ROM for 4 to 6 weeks (for sprain only)
Knee sprain	Twisting injury that produces incomplete tear of ligaments and capsule around the joint	Pain Limited motion Edema Ecchymosis Tenderness over joint Joint appears stable	Basketball Football High jump	Ice Elevation Compression wrap Active ROM exercises Isometric exercises May immobilize
Knee strain	Sudden forced motion causing muscle to be stretched beyond normal capacity	Pain Limited motion Pain aggravated by activity	Soccer Swimming Skiing	Ice Elevation Rest Gradual return to activities
Meniscal tears of knee	Sharp, sudden pivot Direct blow to knee Forced internal rotation Wear from repetitive squatting or climbing Torsional weight-bearing force	Edema *Medial tear:* Pain occurs with hyperflexion, hyperextension, and turning in of knee with knee flexed *Lateral tear:* Pain occurs with hyperflexion and hyperextension and internal rotation of foot with knee flexed *Displaced fragment:* Inability to extend knee; "locked" Positive McMurray's sign*	Hockey Basketball Football	*Conservative:* RICE Exercising of quadriceps and hamstrings Resistive exercising NSAIDs Physical therapy *Surgical:* Arthroscopy
Ankle sprain	Foot is twisted, causing stretching or tearing of ligaments	Pain Edema Limited motion Ecchymosis	Tennis Basketball Football Skating	Immobilization in cast or brace Ice Elevation Rest
Ankle strain	Sudden forced motion, stretching muscles beyond normal capacity	*Acute:* Severe pain *Chronic:* Achy pain	Running All ball sports	Immobilization in cast or brace Ice Elevation Rest

Continued on following page

Table 69-1	COMMON SPORTS INJURIES (Continued)			
Anatomic Area	**Mechanism of Injury**	**Assessment Findings**	**Sports Activity**	**Acute Management**
Ankle fracture	Inward turning on sole of foot and front of foot Supination with internal rotation Pronation with external rotation	Pain Edema Deformity Inability to bear weight	Contact sports Tennis Basketball	Ice Elevation Cast (4 to 6 weeks) Surgery if fracture is displaced or unstable
Metatarsal stress fracture	Occurs with repeated loading of bone; often in an unconditioned extremity	Forefoot pain that progressively worsens with activity Minimal or no forefoot swelling	Running Dance Skating	Rest Stop sports-related activity for 6 weeks Ice Weight-bearing as indicated

NSAIDs, nonsteroidal anti-inflammatory drugs; ROM, range of motion; RICE, rest, ice, compression, elevation.
*McMurray's sign—manipulation of tibia while knee flexed produces audible "click".
Reprinted with permission from National Association of Orthopedic Nurses. (2007). *Core curriculum for orthopaedic nursing* (6th ed.). Boston: Pearson.

muscles are stabilized and shaped, and hip contractures are prevented to maximize ambulatory potential. Most people who have a hip disarticulation amputation must rely on a wheelchair for mobility.

Upper extremity amputations are performed with the goal of preserving maximal functional length. The prosthesis is fitted early to ensure maximum function.

A *staged amputation* may be used when gangrene and infection exist. Initially, a guillotine amputation (eg, nonclosed residual limb) is performed to remove the necrotic and infected tissue. The wound is débrided and allowed to drain. Sepsis is treated with systemic antibiotics. In a few days,

after the infection has been controlled and the patient's condition has stabilized, a definitive amputation with skin closure is performed.

Complications

Complications that may occur with amputation include hemorrhage, infection, skin breakdown, phantom limb pain, and joint contracture. Because major blood vessels have been severed, massive bleeding may occur. Infection is a risk with all surgical procedures. The risk of infection increases with contaminated wounds after traumatic amputation. Skin irritation caused by the prosthesis may result in

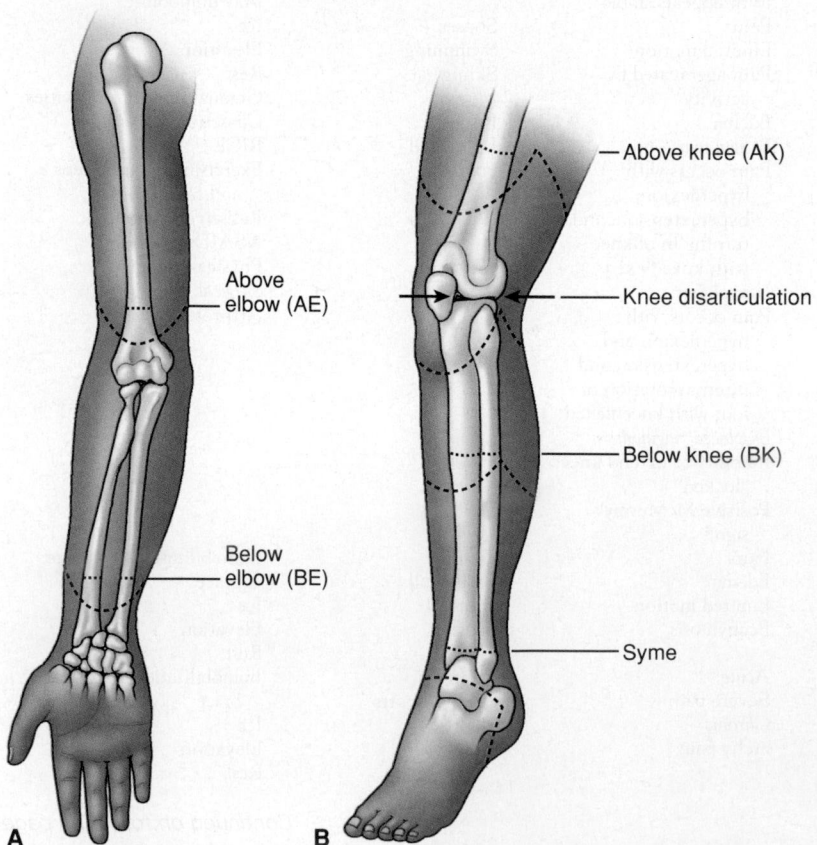

— Above knee (AK)

Above elbow (AE)

Knee disarticulation

Below knee (BK)

Below elbow (BE)

Syme

A

B

Figure 69-17 Levels of amputation are determined by circulatory adequacy, type of prosthesis, function of the part, and muscle balance. **A**, Levels of amputation of upper extremity. **B**, Levels of amputation of lower extremity.

skin breakdown. **Phantom limb pain** is caused by the severing of peripheral nerves. Joint contracture is caused by positioning and a protective flexion withdrawal pattern associated with pain and muscle imbalance.

Medical Management

The objective of treatment is to achieve healing of the amputation wound, the result being a nontender residual limb with healthy skin for prosthetic use. Healing is enhanced by gentle handling of the residual limb, control of residual limb edema through rigid or soft compression dressings, and use of aseptic technique in wound care to avoid infection.

A closed rigid cast dressing or an elastic residual limb shrinker that covers the residual limb may be used to provide uniform compression, to support soft tissues, to control pain, and to prevent joint contractures. Immediately after surgery, a sterilized residual limb sock is applied to the residual limb. Padding is placed over pressure-sensitive areas.

For the patient with a lower extremity amputation, the cast may be equipped to attach a temporary prosthetic extension (pylon) and an artificial foot. This rigid dressing technique is used as a means of creating a socket for immediate postoperative prosthetic fitting. The length of the prosthesis is tailored to the individual patient. Early minimal weight bearing on the residual limb with a rigid cast dressing and a pylon attached produces little discomfort. The cast is changed in about 10 to 14 days. A fever, severe pain, or a loose-fitting cast may necessitate earlier replacement.

A removable rigid dressing may be placed over a soft dressing to control edema, to prevent joint flexion contracture, and to protect the residual limb from unintentional trauma during transfer activities. This rigid dressing is removed several days after surgery for wound inspection and is then replaced to control edema. The dressing facilitates residual limb shaping.

A soft dressing with or without compression may be used if there is significant wound drainage and frequent inspection of the residual limb is required. An immobilizing splint may be incorporated in the dressing. Residual limb wound hematomas are controlled with wound drainage devices to minimize infection.

Rehabilitation

The multidisciplinary rehabilitation team (patient, nurse, physician, social worker, physical therapist, occupational therapist, psychologist, prosthetist, vocational rehabilitation worker) helps the patient achieve the highest possible level of function and participation in life activities (Fig. 69-18). Prosthetic clinics and amputee support groups facilitate this rehabilitation process (Marzen-Groller & Bartman, 2005).

Patients who undergo amputation need support as they grieve the loss and change in body image. Their reactions can include anger, bitterness, and hostility. Psychological issues (eg, denial, withdrawal) may be influenced by the type of support the patient receives from the rehabilitation team and by how quickly ADLs and use of the prosthesis are learned. Knowing the full options and capabilities available with the various prosthetic devices can give the patient a sense of control over the resulting disability (Kelly & Dowling, 2008).

Patients who require amputation because of severe trauma are usually, but not always, young and healthy, heal

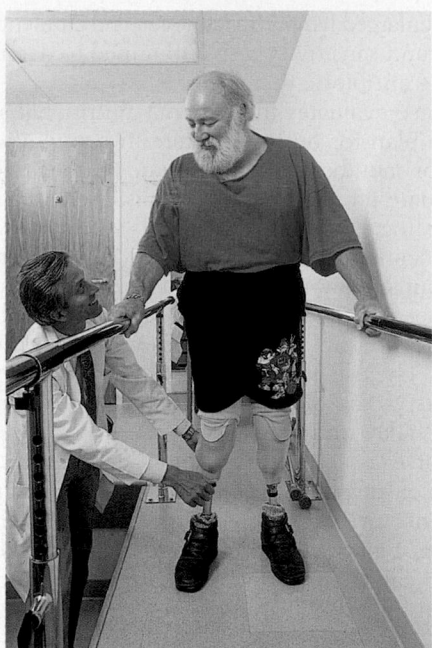

Figure 69-18 Many patients with amputations receive prostheses soon after surgery and begin learning how to use them with the help and support of the rehabilitation team, which includes nurses, physicians, physical therapists, and others.

rapidly, and are physically able to participate in a vigorous rehabilitation program. Because the amputation is the result of an injury, the patient needs psychological support in accepting the sudden change in body image and in dealing with the stresses of hospitalization, long-term rehabilitation, and modification of lifestyle.

Within the past decade, numerous U.S. soldiers have lost limbs because of ballistic injuries received while fighting in Iraq and Afghanistan. In order to best meet the complex needs of these young, previously healthy men and women, the U.S. Army instituted both a specialized treatment center for patients with amputations at Walter Reed Army Hospital in Washington, D.C., and a database registry to facilitate their long-term treatment and management. Treatment for these injured soldiers addresses not only their physical rehabilitation needs but also their emotional needs. Behavioral health services are considered key components to their therapy (Peake, 2005).

NURSING PROCESS

THE PATIENT UNDERGOING AN AMPUTATION

Assessment

Before surgery, the nurse must evaluate the neurovascular and functional status of the extremity through history and physical assessment. If the patient has experienced a traumatic amputation, the nurse assesses the function and condition of the residual limb. The nurse also assesses the circulatory status and function of the unaffected extremity. If infection or gangrene develops, the patient may have associated enlarged lymph nodes, fever, and purulent drainage. A culture and sensitivity test is obtained to determine the appropriate antibiotic therapy.

The nurse evaluates the patient's nutritional status and develops a plan for nutritional care in consultation with a dietitian or metabolic support team, if indicated. A diet with adequate protein and vitamins is essential to promote wound healing.

Any concurrent health problems (eg, dehydration, anemia, cardiac insufficiency, chronic respiratory problems, diabetes mellitus) need to be identified and treated so that the patient is in the best possible condition to withstand the surgical procedure. The use of corticosteroids, anticoagulants, vasoconstrictors, or vasodilators may influence management and prolong or delay wound healing.

The nurse assesses the patient's psychological status. Evaluation of the patient's emotional reaction to amputation is important. Grief responses to permanent alterations in body image, function, and mobility are likely. Professional counseling can help the patient cope in the aftermath of amputation surgery.

Diagnosis

Nursing Diagnoses

Based on the assessment data, the patient's major nursing diagnoses may include the following:

- Acute pain related to amputation
- Disturbed sensory perception: phantom limb pain related to amputation
- Impaired skin integrity related to surgical amputation
- Disturbed body image related to amputation of body part
- Grieving and/or risk for complicated grieving related to loss of body part and resulting disability
- Self-care deficit: feeding, bathing/hygiene, dressing/grooming, or toileting, related to loss of extremity
- Impaired physical mobility related to loss of extremity

Collaborative Problems/Potential Complications

Based on the assessment data, potential complications that may develop include the following:

- Postoperative hemorrhage
- Infection
- Skin breakdown

Planning and Goals

The major goals of the patient may include relief of pain, absence of altered sensory perceptions, wound healing, acceptance of altered body image, resolution of the grieving process, independence in self-care, restoration of physical mobility, and absence of complications.

Nursing Interventions

Relieving Pain

Pain may be incisional or may be caused by inflammation, infection, pressure on a bony prominence, or hematoma. Muscle spasms may add to the patient's discomfort. Surgical pain can be effectively controlled with opioid analgesics that may be accompanied with evacuation of a hematoma or accumulated fluid. Changing the patient's position or

placing a light sandbag on the residual limb to counteract the muscle spasm may improve the patient's level of comfort. Evaluation of the patient's pain and responses to interventions is an important component of pain management. The pain may be an expression of grief and alteration of body image.

Minimizing Altered Sensory Perceptions

A person who has had an amputation may begin to experience phantom limb pain soon after surgery or 2 to 3 months after amputation. It occurs more frequently in patients who have had AKAs. The patient describes pain or unusual sensations, such as numbness, tingling, or muscle cramps, as well as a feeling that the extremity is present, crushed, cramped, or twisted in an abnormal position. When a patient describes phantom pains or sensations, the nurse acknowledges these feelings as real and encourages the patient to verbalize when in pain so that effective treatment may be given. Although phantom sensations diminish over time for many patients, they do not occur in all patients with amputations (Ebrahimzadeh, Fattahi & Nejad, 2006).

The pathogenesis of the phantom limb phenomenon is unknown. Keeping the patient active helps decrease the occurrence of phantom limb pain. Early intensive rehabilitation and residual limb desensitization with kneading massage bring relief. Distraction techniques and activity are helpful. In addition to the nursing interventions, transcutaneous electrical nerve stimulation (TENS), ultrasound, or local anesthetics may provide relief for some patients. In addition, beta-blockers may relieve dull, burning discomfort; antiseizure medications control stabbing and cramping pain; and tricyclic antidepressants may not only alleviate phantom pain, they may also be prescribed to improve mood and coping ability.

Promoting Wound Healing

The residual limb must be handled gently. Whenever the dressing is changed, aseptic technique is required to prevent wound infection and possible osteomyelitis.

> ▶ **NURSING ALERT**
>
> If the cast or elastic dressing inadvertently comes off, the nurse must immediately wrap the residual limb with an elastic compression bandage. If this is not done, excessive edema will develop in a short time, resulting in a delay in rehabilitation. The nurse notifies the surgeon if a cast dressing comes off, so that another cast can be applied promptly.

Residual limb shaping is important for prosthesis fitting. The nurse instructs the patient and family to apply elastic wraps on the residual limb. Using ace wraps on the residual limb is discouraged because they may apply inconsistent pressure on the residual limb, causing problems with shaping it to fit a prosthetic. After the incision is healed, the patient is instructed how to care for the residual limb.

Enhancing Body Image

Amputation is a procedure that alters the patient's body image. The nurse who has established a trusting relationship with the patient is better able to communicate acceptance of the patient who has experienced an amputation. The nurse encourages the patient to look at, feel, and care for the residual limb. It is important to identify the patient's strengths and resources to facilitate rehabilitation. The nurse helps the patient regain the previous level of independent functioning. The patient who is accepted as a whole person is more readily able to resume responsibility for self-care; self-concept improves, and body-image changes are accepted. Even with highly motivated patients, this process may take months.

Helping the Patient to Resolve Grieving

The loss of an extremity (or part of one) may come as a shock even if the patient was prepared preoperatively. The patient's behavior (eg, crying, withdrawal, apathy, anger) and expressed feelings (eg, depression, fear, helplessness) reveal how the patient is coping with the loss and working through the grieving process.

The nurse creates an accepting and supportive atmosphere in which the patient and family are encouraged to express and share their feelings and work through the grief process. The support from family and friends promotes the patient's acceptance of the loss. The nurse helps the patient deal with immediate needs and become oriented to realistic rehabilitation goals and future independent functioning. Mental health and support group referrals may be appropriate (Marzen-Groller & Bartman, 2005).

Promoting Independent Self-Care

Amputation of an extremity affects the patient's ability to provide adequate self-care. The patient is encouraged to be an active participant in self-care. The patient needs time to accomplish these tasks and must not be rushed. Practicing an activity with consistent, supportive supervision in a relaxed environment enables the patient to learn self-care skills. The patient and the nurse need to maintain positive attitudes and to minimize fatigue and frustration during the learning process.

Independence in dressing, toileting, and bathing depends on balance, transfer abilities, and physiologic tolerance of the activities. The nurse works with the physical therapist and occupational therapist to teach and supervise the patient in these self-care activities.

The patient with an upper extremity amputation has self-care deficits in feeding, bathing, and dressing. Assistance is provided only as needed; the nurse encourages the patient to learn to do these tasks, using assistive feeding and dressing aids when needed. The nurse, therapists, and prosthetist work with the patient to achieve maximum independence.

Helping the Patient to Achieve Physical Mobility

Proper positioning prevents the development of hip or knee joint contracture in the patient with a lower extremity amputation. Abduction, external rotation, and flexion of the lower extremity are avoided. The residual limb may be placed in an extended position or elevated for a brief period after surgery.

 NURSING ALERT

The residual limb should not be placed on a pillow because a flexion contracture of the hip may result.

The nurse encourages the patient to turn from side to side and to assume a prone position, if possible, to stretch the flexor muscles and to prevent flexion contracture of the hip. The patient is encouraged not to sit for long periods of time to prevent flexion contracture. The legs should remain close together to prevent an abduction deformity. The nurse encourages the patient to use assistive devices to more readily perform self-care activities and to identify what home modifications, if any, should be made to perform these activities in the home environment.

Postoperative ROM exercises are started early because contracture deformities develop rapidly. ROM exercises include hip and knee exercises for patients with BKAs and hip exercises for patients with AKAs. It is important that the patient understand the importance of exercising the residual limb.

The upper extremities, trunk, and abdominal muscles are exercised and strengthened. The extensor muscles in the arm and the depressor muscles in the shoulder play an important part in crutch walking. The patient uses an overbed trapeze to change position and strengthen the biceps. The patient may flex and extend the arms while holding weights. Doing push-ups while seated strengthens the triceps muscles. Exercises (such as hyperextension of the residual limb), conducted under the supervision of the physical therapist, also aid in strengthening muscles as well as increasing circulation, reducing edema, and preventing atrophy.

Because a patient who has had an upper extremity amputated uses both shoulders to operate the prosthesis, the muscles of both shoulders are exercised. A patient with an above-the-elbow amputation or shoulder disarticulation is likely to develop a postural abnormality caused by loss of the weight of the amputated extremity. Postural exercises are helpful.

Strength and endurance are assessed, and activities are increased gradually to prevent fatigue. As the patient progresses to independent use of the wheelchair, use of ambulatory aids, or ambulation with a prosthesis, the nurse emphasizes safety considerations. Environmental barriers (eg, steps, inclines, doors, throw rugs, wet surfaces) are identified, and methods of managing them are implemented. It is important to anticipate, identify, and manage problems associated with the use of the mobility aids. Proper instructions in using assistive devices will help prevent these problems.

Amputation of the leg changes the center of gravity; therefore, the patient may need to practice position changes (eg, standing from sitting, standing on one foot). The patient is taught transfer techniques early and is reminded to maintain good posture when getting out of bed. A well-fitting shoe with a nonskid sole should be worn. During position changes, the patient should be guarded and stabilized with a transfer belt at the waist to prevent falling.

As soon as possible, the patient with a lower extremity amputation is assisted to stand between parallel bars to allow extension of the temporary prosthesis to the floor with minimal weight bearing. How soon after surgery the patient is allowed to bear full body weight on the prosthesis depends on the patient's physical status and wound healing. As endurance increases and balance is achieved, ambulation is started with the use of parallel bars or crutches. The patient learns to use a normal gait, with the residual limb moving back and forth while walking with the crutches. To prevent a permanent flexion deformity from occurring, the residual limb should *not* be held up in a flexed position.

The patient with an upper extremity amputation is taught how to carry out ADLs with one arm. The patient is started on one-handed self-care activities as soon as possible. The use of a temporary prosthesis is encouraged. The patient who learns to use the prosthesis soon after the amputation is less dependent on one-handed self-care activities.

The patient with an upper extremity amputation may wear a cotton T-shirt to prevent contact between the skin and shoulder harness and to promote absorption of perspiration. The prosthetist advises about cleaning the washable portions of the harness. Periodically, the prosthesis is inspected for potential problems.

The residual limb must be conditioned and shaped into a conical form to permit accurate fit, maximum comfort, and function of the prosthetic device. Elastic bandages, an elastic residual limb shrinker, or an air splint is used to condition and shape the residual limb. The nurse teaches the patient or a member of the family the correct method of bandaging.

Bandaging supports the soft tissue and minimizes the formation of edema while the residual limb is in a dependent position. The bandage is applied in such a manner that the remaining muscles required to operate the prosthesis are as firm as possible. An improperly applied elastic bandage contributes to circulatory problems and a poorly shaped residual limb.

Effective preprosthetic care is important to ensure proper fitting of the prosthesis. The major problems that can delay prosthetic fitting during this period are (1) flexion deformities, (2) nonshrinkage of the residual limb, and (3) abduction deformities of the hip.

The physician usually prescribes activities to condition or "toughen" the residual limb in preparation for a prosthesis. The patient begins by pushing the residual limb into a soft pillow, then into a firmer pillow, and finally against a hard surface. The patient is taught to massage the residual limb to mobilize the surgical incision site, decrease tenderness, and improve vascularity. Massage is usually started once healing has occurred and is first performed by the physical therapist. Skin inspection and preventive care are taught.

The prosthesis socket is custom molded to the residual limb by the prosthetist. Prostheses are designed for specific activity levels and patient abilities. Types of prostheses include hydraulic, pneumatic, biofeedback-controlled, myoelectrically controlled, and synchronized prostheses. Adjustments of the prosthetic socket are made by the prosthetist to accommodate the residual limb changes that occur during the first 6 months to 1 year after surgery.

Some patients are not candidates for a prosthesis and are thus nonambulatory patients with amputations. If use of a prosthesis is not possible, the patient is instructed in the safe use of a wheelchair to achieve independence. A special wheelchair designed for patients who have had amputations is recommended. Because of the decreased weight in the front, a regular wheelchair may tip backward when the patient sits in it. In wheelchairs designed for patients who have had amputations, the rear axle is set back about 5 cm (2 in) to compensate for the change in weight distribution.

Monitoring and Managing Potential Complications

After any surgery, efforts are made to reestablish homeostasis and to prevent complications related to surgery, anesthesia, and immobility. The nurse assesses body systems (eg, respiratory, hematological, gastrointestinal, genitourinary, skin) for problems associated with immobility (eg, atelectasis, pneumonia, DVT, PE, anorexia, constipation, urinary stasis, pressure ulcers).

Massive hemorrhage due to a loosened suture is the most threatening problem. The nurse monitors the patient for any signs or symptoms of bleeding and monitors the patient's vital signs and suction drainage.

 NURSING ALERT

Immediate postoperative bleeding may develop slowly or may take the form of massive hemorrhage resulting from a loosened suture. A large tourniquet should be in plain sight at the patient's bedside so that, if severe bleeding occurs, it can be applied to the residual limb to control the hemorrhage. The nurse immediately notifies the surgeon in the event of excessive bleeding.

Infection is a common complication of amputation. Patients who have undergone traumatic amputation have contaminated wounds. The nurse administers antibiotics as prescribed. It is important to monitor the incision, dressing, and drainage for indications of infection (eg, change in color, odor, or consistency of drainage; increasing discomfort). The nurse also assesses for systemic indicators of infection (eg, elevated temperature, leukocytosis with an increase of more than 10% bands on the differential) and promptly reports indications of infection to the surgeon.

Skin breakdown may result from immobilization or from pressure from various sources. The prosthesis may cause pressure areas to develop. The nurse and the patient assess for breaks in the skin. Careful skin hygiene is essential to prevent skin irritation, infection, and breakdown. The healed residual limb is washed and dried (gently) at least twice daily. The skin is inspected for pressure areas, dermatitis, and blisters. If they are present, they must be treated before further skin breakdown occurs. Usually a residual limb sock is worn to absorb perspiration and to prevent direct contact between the skin and the prosthetic socket. The sock is changed daily and must fit smoothly to prevent irritation caused by wrinkles. The socket of the prosthesis is washed with a mild detergent, rinsed, and dried thoroughly with a clean cloth. It must be thoroughly dry before the prosthesis is applied.

Promoting Home and Community-Based Care

TEACHING THE PATIENT TO MANAGE SELF-CARE. Before the patient is discharged to the home or to a rehabilitation facility, the patient and family are encouraged to become active participants in care. They participate in care of the skin, residual limb, and prosthesis as appropriate. The patient receives ongoing instructions and practice sessions to learn to transfer and to use mobility aids and other assistive devices safely. The nurse explains the signs and symptoms of complications that must be reported to the physician (Chart 69-6).

CONTINUING CARE IN THE HOME AND COMMUNITY. After the patient has achieved physiologic homeostasis and has demonstrated achievement of major health care goals, rehabilitation continues either in a rehabilitation facility or at home. Continued support and evaluation by the home care nurse are essential.

The patient's home environment should be assessed prior to discharge. Modifications are made to ensure the patient's continuing care, safety, and mobility. An overnight or weekend experience at home may be tried to identify problems that were not identified on the assessment visit. Physical therapy and occupational therapy may continue in the home or on an outpatient basis. Transportation to continuing health care appointments must be arranged. The social service department of the hospital or the home health agency may be of great assistance in securing personal assistance and transportation services.

During follow-up health visits, the nurse evaluates the patient's physical and psychosocial adjustment. Periodic preventive health assessments are necessary. An elderly spouse may not be able to provide the assistance required if needed at home. Modifications in the plan of care are made on the basis of such findings. Often, the patient and family find involvement in a post-amputation support group to be of value; here they can share problems, solutions, and resources. Talking with those who have successfully dealt with a similar problem may help the patient develop a satisfactory solution.

Because patients and their family members and health care providers tend to focus on the most obvious needs and issues, the nurse reminds the patient and family about the importance of continuing health promotion and screening practices, such as regular physical examinations and diagnostic screening tests. Accessible facilities for screening, health care, and exercise are identified. Patients are instructed about their importance and are referred to appropriate health care providers.

Evaluation

Expected Patient Outcomes

Expected patient outcomes may include:

1. Experiences no pain
   a. Appears relaxed
   b. Verbalizes comfort
   c. Uses measures to increase comfort
   d. Participates in self-care and rehabilitative activities
2. Experiences no phantom limb pain
   a. Reports diminished phantom sensations
   b. Uses distraction techniques
   c. Performs residual limb desensitization massage
3. Achieves wound healing
   a. Controls residual limb edema
   b. Exhibits healed, nontender, nonadherent scar
   c. Demonstrates residual limb care

CHART 69-6 HOME CARE CHECKLIST
Amputation

At the completion of the home instruction, the patient or caregiver will be able to:	PATIENT	CAREGIVER
• Describe approaches to controlling pain (eg, take analgesics as prescribed; use nonpharmacologic interventions).	✔	✔
• Report pain that is uncontrolled by analgesics and other pain management techniques.	✔	
• Describe care of residual limb and conditioning for prosthesis.	✔	✔
• Consume healthy diet to promote wound healing.	✔	
• Demonstrate ability to transfer.	✔	
• Use mobility and activity aids safely.	✔	
• Participate in rehabilitation program to regain functional independence.	✔	
• State indicators of complications to report promptly to physician (eg, uncontrolled pain; signs of local or systemic infection; residual limb skin breakdown).	✔	✔
• Identify professionals and community agencies to help with transition to home.	✔	✔
• Identify support group to facilitate rehabilitation.	✔	✔
• Describe effects of amputation on self-image.	✔	
• Acknowledge grieving as part of coping process.	✔	✔
• Identify modifications of home environment to promote safe environment and independence during rehabilitation.	✔	✔
• Identify the importance of keeping follow-up appointments and participating in health screening and health promotion activities, including exercises.	✔	✔

4. Demonstrates improved body image and effective coping
   a. Acknowledges change in body image
   b. Participates in self-care activities
   c. Demonstrates increasing independence
   d. Projects self as a whole person
   e. Resumes role-related responsibilities
   f. Reestablishes social contacts
   g. Demonstrates confidence in abilities
5. Exhibits resolution of grieving
   a. Expresses grief
   b. Works through feelings with family and friends
   c. Focuses on future functioning
   d. Participates in support group
6. Achieves independent self-care
   a. Asks for assistance when needed
   b. Uses aids and assistive devices to facilitate self-care
   c. Verbalizes satisfaction with abilities to perform ADLs
7. Achieves maximum independent mobility
   a. Avoids positions contributing to contracture development
   b. Demonstrates full active ROM
   c. Maintains balance when sitting and transferring
   d. Increases strength and endurance
   e. Demonstrates safe transferring technique
   f. Achieves functional use of prosthesis
   g. Overcomes environmental barriers to mobility
   h. Uses community services and resources as needed
8. Exhibits absence of complications of hemorrhage, infection, or skin breakdown
   a. Does not experience excessive bleeding
   b. Maintains normal blood values
   c. Is free of local or systemic signs of infection
   d. Repositions self frequently
   e. Is free of pressure-related problems
   f. Reports any skin discomfort and irritations promptly

Prevention of Injuries in Nursing Personnel

Nursing is consistently ranked among the top ten occupations that are most involved in occupation-related injuries and lost work days. The types of injuries that are most common include back, neck, shoulder, wrist, and knee injuries (de Castro, 2006). Most of these injuries have occurred during patient handling and movement activities. Traditional methods to prevent musculoskeletal injuries among nursing personnel during patient handling and moving have revolved around training sessions on proper body mechanics and "safe" lifting of patients and use of back belts, yet there is no research-based evidence that suggests that these methods reduce caregiver injuries (Nelson & Baptiste, 2006). The American Nurses Association (ANA) launched a "Handle with Care" campaign aimed at reducing occupational musculoskeletal work-related injuries among nurses (de Castro, 2006). In particular, the ANA advocates include that:

- Hospitals, long-term care facilities, and other health care organizations should purchase patient handling equipment (eg, inflatable lateral-assist devices to transfer patients) and train nursing personnel in their appropriate use.
- Health care organizations should institute "no lift" policies for individual nursing personnel. Rather, patient lift teams should be organized.
- Health care organizations should devise methods to assess their patient care ergonomic risks and develop algorithms for patient handling and movement that include patient transfer and movement activities.

CRITICAL THINKING EXERCISES

1 You are a staff nurse in the emergency department, and a patient is brought in with an open tibia/fibula fracture. He is not in respiratory distress, with an SaO_2 of 99%, and is communicating appropriately with you, but complains of pain. What assessments will you gather first, second, and third on this patient? Explain your rationale for the priority order of your assessments.

EBP **2** You are the nurse manager of an orthopedic unit. In the past 3 months, four of the staff members have sustained back injuries when lifting or turning patients. What is your plan to prevent similar staff injuries in the future? Are there any evidence-based guidelines that you might follow to help you prevent recurrence of these injuries?

EBP **3** You are a staff nurse on an orthopedic unit and receive a patient from surgery who had ACL repair after sustaining a "knee injury." Upon arrival to the unit, the patient appeared comfortable. His left leg was in a compression wrap and a belted brace. About 4 hours after arrival on the floor, he began to ask for pain medication. Morphine was administered as prescribed, yet 40 minutes after administration his pain level actually increased from 7 to 9 on the numeric pain scale. What assessment would you perform immediately on this patient? What should you do with the findings of the assessment? What actions do you anticipate you may initiate with this patient? What evidenced-based information supports your actions?

4 You are a home health nurse and are assigned a new patient to your caseload, a National Guard veteran who was released from duty after having amputations of both legs after stepping on a land mine. His right leg had a below-the-knee amputation and his left leg had an above-the-knee amputation 2 months ago. Identify this patient's unique nursing, medical, physical therapy, occupational therapy, social, and emotional needs. Devise a nursing plan of care that addresses these needs.

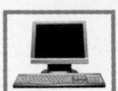 The Smeltzer suite offers these additional resources to enhance learning and facilitate understanding of this chapter:

- thePoint online resource, thepoint.lww.com/Smeltzer12E
- Student CD-ROM included with the book
- *Study Guide to Accompany Brunner & Suddarth's Textbook of Medical-Surgical Nursing*
- *Handbook for Brunner & Suddarth's Textbook of Medical-Surgical Nursing*

REFERENCES AND SELECTED READINGS

*Asterisk indicates nursing research.

Books

Bickley, L. S. (2007). *Bates' guide to physical assessment* (9th ed.). Philadelphia: Lippincott Williams & Wilkins.

Bucholz, R. W., Heckman, J. D., Court-Brown, C., et al. (2005). *Rockwood and Green's fractures in adults* (6th ed.). Philadelphia: Lippincott Williams & Wilkins.

National Association of Orthopedic Nurses. (2007). *Core curriculum for orthopaedic nursing* (6th ed.). Boston: Pearson.

Porth, C. M. & Matfin, G. (2009). *Pathophysiology: Concepts of altered health states* (8th ed.). Philadelphia: Lippincott Williams & Wilkins.

Wiegand, D. L. M. & Carlson, K. (2005). *AACN procedure manual for critical care* (5th ed.). St. Louis: Elsevier-Saunders.

Journals and Electronic Documents

Alford, J. W. & Bach, B. B. (2004). Managing ACL tears: When to treat, when to refer. *Journal of Musculoskeletal Medicine, 21*(1), 520–526.

Altizer, L. (2004). Compartment syndrome. *Orthopaedic Nursing, 23*(6), 391–396.

Boden, S. D. (2005). The ABCs of BMPs. *Orthopaedic Nursing, 24*(1), 49–52.

Bongiovanni, M. S., Bradley, S. L. & Kelley, D. M. (2005). Orthopaedic trauma: Critical care nursing issues. *Critical Care Nursing Quarterly, 28*(1), 60–71.

Clinton, R. E. & Murthi, A. M. (2008). Lateral epicondylitis. *Current Orthopaedic Practice, 19*(6), 612–615.

Cole, P. A., Miclau, T., Ly, T. V., et al. (2008). What's new in orthopaedic trauma. *Journal of Bone and Joint Surgery, 90*(12), 2804–2822.

de Castro, A. B. (2006). Handle with care: The American Nurses Association's campaign to address work-related musculoskeletal disorders. *Orthopaedic Nursing, 25*(6), 356–365.

Ebrahimzadeh, M. H., Fattahi, A. S. & Nejad, B. A. (2006). Long-term follow-up of Iranian veteran upper extremity amputees from the Iran-Iraq war (1980–1988). *Journal of Trauma, 61*(4), 886–888.

*Folden, S. & Tappan, R. (2007). Factors influencing function and recovery following hip repair surgery. *Orthopaedic Nursing, 26*(4), 234–240.

Gerden, A. C., Hogan, M. V. & Miller, M. D. (2009). What's new in sports medicine. *The Journal of Bone and Joint Surgery, 91*(1), 241–256.

Hart, L. (2005). Effect of stretching on sport injury risk: A review. *Clinical Journal of Sports Medicine, 15*(2), 113.

Harvey, C. V. (2006). Complications. *Orthopaedic Nursing, 25*(6), 410–411.

Hessman, M. H., Ingelfinger, P. & Rommens, P. M. (2007). Compartment syndrome of the lower extremity. *European Journal of Trauma and Emergency Surgery, 33*(6), 589–599.

Kelly, M. & Dowling, M. (2008). Patient rehabilitation following lower limb amputation. *Nursing Standard, 22*(49), 35–40.

Kobziff, L. (2006). Traumatic pelvic fractures. *Orthopaedic Nursing, 25*(4), 235–241.

Konstantakos, E. K., Dalstrom, D. J., Nelles, M. E., et al. (2007). Diagnosis and management of extremity compartment syndromes: An orthopaedic perspective. *American Surgeon, 73*, 1199–1209.

Marzen-Groller, K. D. & Bartman, K. (2005). Building a successful support group for post-amputation patients. *Journal of Vascular Nursing, 23*(2), 42–45.

*Marzen-Groller, K. D., Tremblay, S. M., Kaszuba, J., et al. (2008). Testing the effectiveness of the Amputee Mobility Protocol: A pilot study. *Journal of Vascular Nursing, 26*(3), 74–81.

National Lower Limb Information Center. (2006). Fact sheet: Amputation statistics by cause: Limb loss in the United States. Available at: www.amputee coalition.org/fact_sheets/amp_stats_cause.html

*Nelson, A. & Baptiste, A. (2006). Evidence-based practices for safe patient handling and movement. *Orthopaedic Nursing, 25*(6), 367–379.

Parker, M. J. & Handoll, H. H. (2006). Preoperative traction for fractures of the proximal femur in adults. *Cochrane Database of Systematic Reviews, 3,* CD000168.

Peake, J. B. (2005). Beyond the Purple Heart: Continuity of care for the wounded in Iraq. *New England Journal of Medicine, 352*(3), 219–222.

*Pellino, T. A., Owen, B., Knapp, L., et al. (2006). The evaluation of mechanical devices for lateral transfers on perceived exertion and patient comfort. *Orthopaedic Nursing, 25*(1), 4–10.

Rupp, J. D. & Schneider, L. W. (2004). Injuries to the hip joint in frontal motor-vehicle crashes: Biomechanical and real-world perspectives. *Orthopaedic Clinics of North America, 35*(4), 493–504.

Scalea, T. M. (2008). Optimal timing of fracture fixation: Have we learned anything in the past 20 years? *Journal of Trauma, 65*(2), 253–260.

Schoen, D. C. (2006). Hip fractures. *Orthopaedic Nursing, 25*(2), 148–152.

Silvis, M. L., Clinch, C., Randall, D. O., et al. (2008). What is the best way to evaluate an acute traumatic knee injury? *Journal of Family Practice, 57*(2), 116–118.

Stein, P. D., Yaekoub, A. Y., Matta, F., et al. (2008). Fat embolism syndrome. *American Journal of the Medical Sciences, 336*(6), 472–477.

Trojian, T., Stevenson, J. H. & Agrawal, N. (2005). What can we expect from nonoperative treatment options for shoulder pain? *Journal of Family Practice, 54*(3), 216–223.

U.S. Department of Labor, Bureau of Labor Statistics. (2005). Workplace injuries and illnesses. Available at: www.bls.gov/iif/oshwc/osh/os/osnr0025. pdf

Whiteing, N. L. (2008). Fractures: Pathophysiology, treatment and nursing care. *Nursing Standard, 23*(2), 49–57.

RESOURCES

American College of Sports Medicine, www.acsm.org

Amputee Resource Foundation of America, Inc., www.amputeeresource.org

National Amputation Foundation, www.nationalamputation.org

National Association of Orthopaedic Nurses (NAON), www.orthonurse.com

National Institute for Occupational Safety and Health, www.cdc.gov.niosh. html

National Institute of Arthritis and Musculoskeletal and Skin Diseases, www. niams.nih.gov

U.S. Department of Labor, Occupational Safety and Health Administration, www.osha.gov

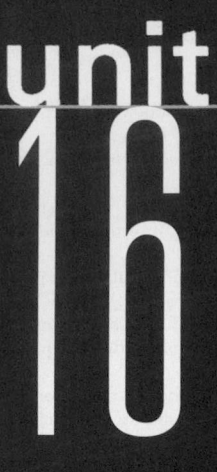

unit 16

Other Acute Problems

Case Study • Applying Concepts From NANDA, NIC, and NOC

A Patient With Multiple Trauma Resulting in Hemorrhage and Risk for Shock

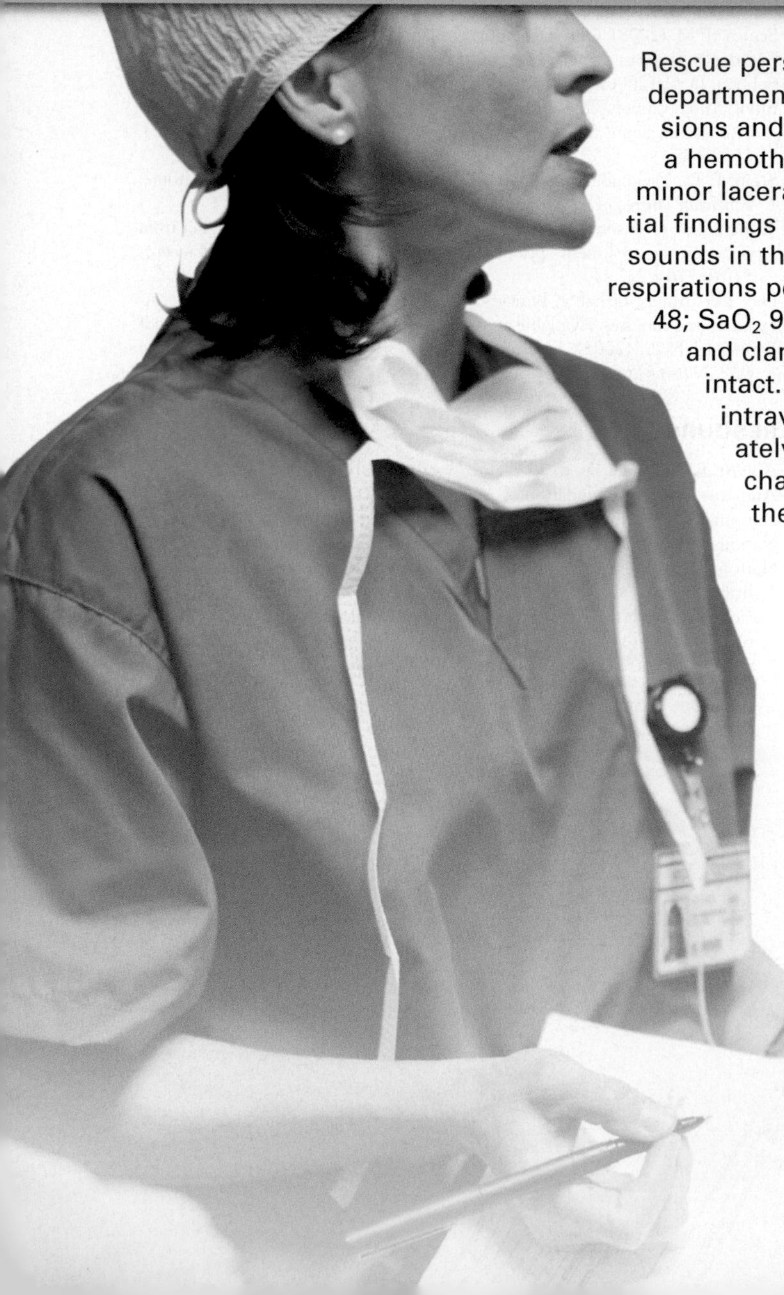

Rescue personnel bring 19-year-old **Anna Woo** to the emergency department (ED) after a motorcycle crash. She has facial contusions and lacerations, a fractured sternum, three fractured ribs, a hemothorax, a dislocated hip, a fractured pelvis, and multiple minor lacerations. She is moaning but responds to her name. Initial findings include an unobstructed airway with absent breath sounds in the right basilar lung field, tachypnea with 32 shallow respirations per minute, and ABG values as follows: pH 7.29; pCO_2 48; SaO_2 90%; HCO_3^- 24. Blood pressure is 94/70; skin is cool and clammy; heart rate is 100; and peripheral pulses are intact. After a preliminary survey and placement of intravenous access lines, a chest tube is inserted. Immediately, 300 mL of bloody fluid drains into the collection chamber. Grossly bloody fluid continues to drain from the chest tube at a rate of 20 mL every 15 minutes.

Visit thePoint to view a concept map that illustrates the relationships that exist between the nursing diagnoses, interventions, and outcomes for the patient's clinical problems.

Nursing Classifications and Languages

NANDA NURSING DIAGNOSES	NIC NURSING INTERVENTIONS	NOC NURSING OUTCOMES
		Return to functional baseline status, stabilization of, or improvement in:
INEFFECTIVE BREATHING PATTERN—Inspiration and/or expiration that does not provide adequate ventilation	**AIRWAY MANAGEMENT**—Facilitation of patency of air passages	**RESPIRATORY STATUS: AIRWAY PATENCY**—Open, clear tracheobronchial passages for air exchange
IMPAIRED GAS EXCHANGE—Excess or deficit in oxygenation and/or carbon dioxide elimination at the alveolar–capillary membrane	**RESPIRATORY MONITORING**—Collection and analysis of patient data to ensure airway patency and adequate gas exchange	**RESPIRATORY STATUS: VENTILATION**—Movement of air in and out of the lungs
DEFICIENT FLUID VOLUME—Decreased intravascular, interstitial, and/or intracellular fluid	**OXYGEN THERAPY**—Administration of oxygen and monitoring of its effectiveness	**RESPIRATORY STATUS: GAS EXCHANGE**—Alveolar exchange of carbon dioxide and oxygen to maintain arterial blood gas concentrations
DECREASED CARDIAC OUTPUT—Inadequate blood pumped by the heart to meet metabolic demands of the body	**ACID–BASE MANAGEMENT**—Promotion of acid–base balance and prevention of complications resulting from acid–base imbalance	**ELECTROLYTE AND ACID/BASE BALANCE**—Balance of electrolytes and nonelectrolytes in the intracellular and extracellular compartments of the body
	HEMORRHAGE CONTROL—Reduction or elimination of rapid and excessive blood loss	**CIRCULATION STATUS**—Unobstructed, unidirectional blood flow at an appropriate pressure through large vessels of the systemic and pulmonary circuits
	IV INSERTION—Insertion of a needle into a peripheral or central vein for the purpose of administering fluids, blood, or medications	**VITAL SIGNS**—Extent to which temperature, pulse, respiration, and blood pressure are within normal range for the individual
	HYPOVOLEMIA MANAGEMENT—Expansion of intravascular fluid volume in a patient who is volume-depleted	**CARDIAC PUMP EFFECTIVENESS**—Adequacy of blood volume ejected from the left ventricle to support systolic perfusion pressure
	BLOOD PRODUCTS ADMINISTRATION—Administration of blood or blood products and monitoring of patient's response	
	VITAL SIGNS MONITORING—Collection and analysis of cardiovascular, respiratory, and body temperature data to determine and prevent complications	
	SHOCK PREVENTION—Detecting and treating a patient at risk for impending shock	
	SHOCK MANAGEMENT—Facilitation of the delivery of oxygen and nutrients to systemic tissue with removal of cellular waste products in a patient with severely altered tissue perfusion	

Bulechek, G. M., Butcher, H. K., & Dochterman, J. M. (2008). *Nursing interventions classification (NIC)* (5th ed.). St. Louis: Mosby.
Johnson, M., Bulechek, G., Butcher, H. K., et al. (2006). *NANDA, NOC, and NIC linkages* (2nd ed.). St. Louis: Mosby.
Moorhead, S., Johnson, M., Mass, M. L., et al. (2008). *Nursing outcomes classification (NOC)* (4th ed.). St. Louis: Mosby.
NANDA International. (2007). *Nursing diagnoses: Definitions & classification 2007–2008.* Philadelphia: North American Nursing Diagnosis Association.

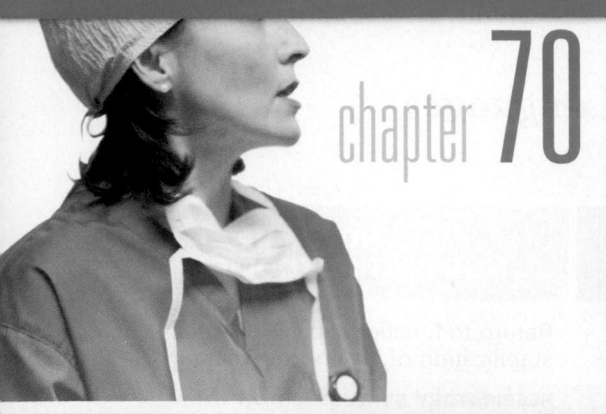

chapter 70

Management of Patients With Infectious Diseases

LEARNING OBJECTIVES

On completion of this chapter, the learner will be able to:

1 Differentiate between colonization, infection, and disease.

2 Identify federal and local resources available to the nurse seeking information about infectious diseases.

3 Identify the benefits of vaccines recommended for health care workers.

4 Identify the reasons for Standard and Transmission-Based Precautions and discuss the elements of these standards.

5 Describe the concept of emerging infectious diseases and factors that led to the development of these diseases.

6 Use the nursing process as a framework for care of patients with sexually transmitted disease.

7 Describe home health care measures that reduce the risk of infection.

8 Use the nursing process as a framework for care of patients with infectious diseases.

GLOSSARY

bacteremia: laboratory-proven presence of bacteria in the bloodstream

community-associated methicillin-resistant *Staphylococcus aureus* (CA-MRSA): a strain of MRSA infecting persons who have not been treated in a health care setting

carrier: person who has an organism without apparent signs and symptoms; one who is able to transmit an infection to others

colonization: microorganisms present in or on a host, without host interference or interaction and without eliciting symptoms in the host

emerging infectious diseases: human infectious diseases with incidence increased within the past two decades or potential increase in the near future

fungemia: a bloodstream infection caused by a fungal organism

health care–associated infection (HAI): an infection not present or incubating at the time of admission to the health care setting; this term is replacing the term "nosocomial infection," which refers only to those infections acquired in a hospital

GLOSSARY *(Continued)*

host: an organism that provides living conditions to support a microorganism

immune: person with protection from a previous infection or immunization who resists reinfection when re-exposed to the same agent

incubation period: time between contact and onset of signs and symptoms

infection: condition in which the host interacts physiologically and immunologically with a microorganism

infectious disease: the consequences that result from invasion of the body by microorganisms that can produce harm to the body and potentially death

latency: time interval after primary infection when a microorganism lives within the host without producing clinical evidence

methicillin-resistant Staphylococcus aureus (MRSA): *Staphylococcus aureus* bacterium that is not susceptible to extended-penicillin antibiotic formulas, such as methicillin, oxacillin, or nafcillin; MRSA may occur in a health care or in a community setting

normal flora: persistent nonpathogenic organisms colonizing a host

reservoir: any person, plant, animal, substance, or location that provides living conditions for microorganisms and that enables further dispersal of the organism

Standard Precautions: strategy of assuming all patients may carry infectious agents and using appropriate barrier precautions for all health care worker–patient interactions

susceptible: not possessing immunity to a particular pathogen

transient flora: organisms that have been recently acquired and are likely to be shed in a relatively short period

Transmission-Based Precautions: precautions used in addition to Standard Precautions when contagious or epidemiologically significant organisms are recognized; the three types of Transmission-Based Precautions are Airborne, Droplet, and Contact Precautions

vancomycin-resistant *Enterococcus* (VRE): *Enterococcus* bacterium that is resistant to the antibiotic vancomycin

vancomycin-resistant *Staphylococcus aureus* (VRSA): *Staphylococcus aureus* bacterium that is not susceptible to vancomycin

virulence: degree of pathogenicity of an organism

An infectious disease is any disease caused by the growth of pathogenic microbes in the body. It may or may not be communicable (ie, contagious). Modern science has controlled, eradicated, or decreased the incidence of many infectious diseases. However, increases in other infections, such as those caused by antibiotic-resistant organisms and emerging infectious diseases, are of great and growing concern. Examples of these infectious diseases are presented in this chapter. Other infectious diseases are discussed in the appropriate chapters (for example, see Chapter 23 for information on tuberculosis [TB]). It is important to understand infectious causes and the treatment of contagious, serious, and common infections. Table 70-1 presents an overview of many infectious diseases, their causative organisms, mode of transmission, and usual **incubation periods** (time between contact and development of the first signs and symptoms).

The nurse plays an important role in infection control and prevention. Educating patients may decrease their risk of becoming infected or may decrease the sequelae of infection. Using appropriate barrier precautions, observing prudent hand hygiene, and ensuring aseptic care of intravenous

(IV) catheters and other invasive equipment also assists in reducing infections.

The Infectious Process

The Chain of Infection

A complete chain of events is necessary for infection to occur. Figure 70-1 illustrates the elements of the chain and identifies points where health care workers can intervene to interrupt the chain. Six elements are necessary for infection to occur. These essentials are (1) a causative organism, (2) a reservoir of available organisms, (3) a portal or mode of exit from the reservoir, (4) a mode of transmission from reservoir to host, (5) a susceptible host, and (6) a mode of entry to the host.

Causative Organism

The types of microorganisms that cause infections are bacteria, rickettsiae, viruses, protozoa, fungi, and helminths.

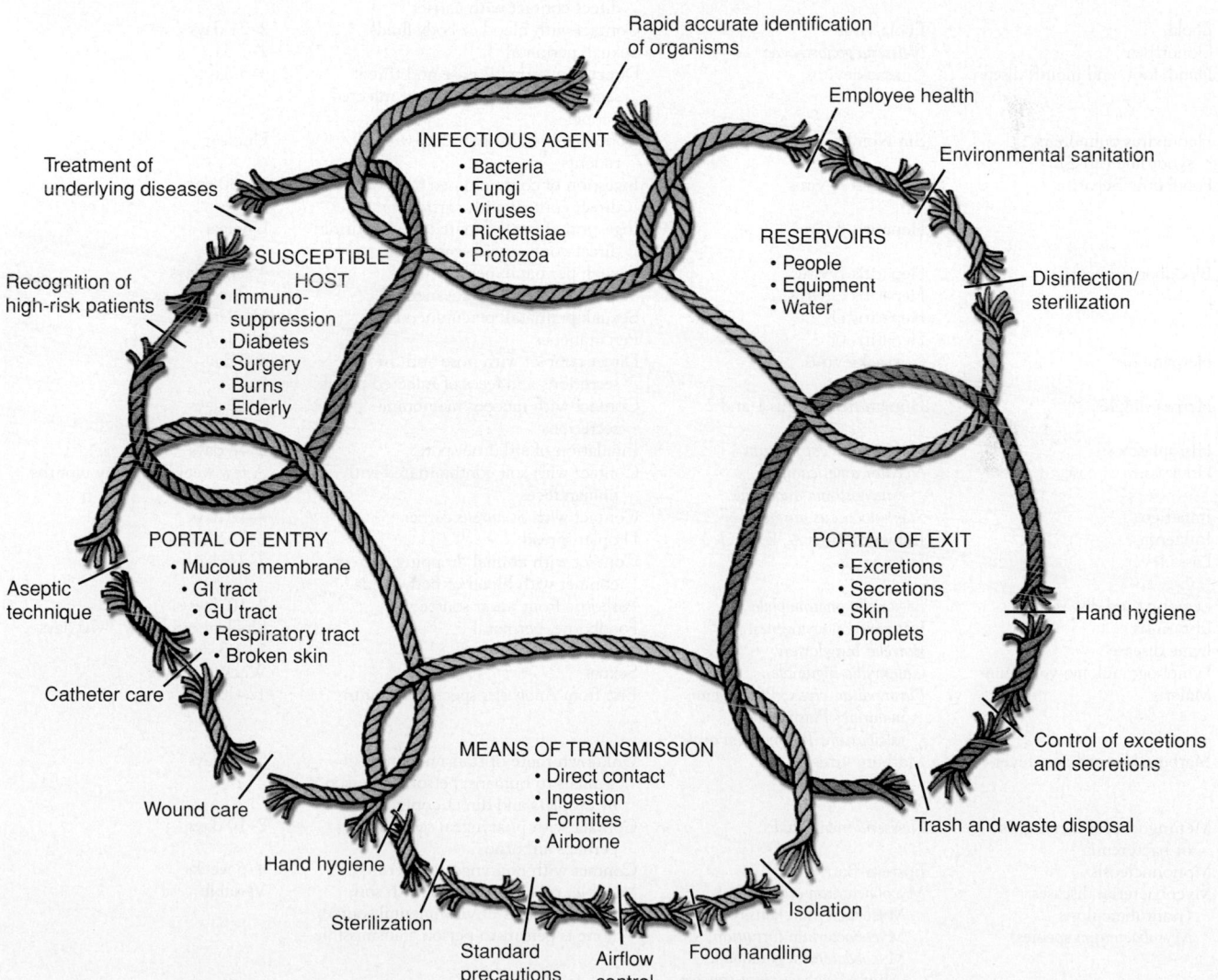

Figure 70-1 Health care workers' interventions used to break the chain of infection transmission.

Table 70-1 INFECTIOUS DISEASES, CAUSATIVE ORGANISMS, MODES OF TRANSMISSION, AND USUAL INCUBATION PERIODS

Disease or Condition	Organism	Usual Mode of Transmission	Usual Incubation Period (Infection to First Symptom)
Acquired immunodeficiency syndrome (AIDS)	Human immunodeficiency virus (HIV)	Sexual; percutaneous; perinatal	Median of 10 years
Amebiasis	*Entamoeba histolytica*	Contaminated water	2–4 weeks
Anthrax	*Bacillus anthracis*	Airborne or contact	2–60 days
Chancroid	*Haemophilus ducreyi*	Sexual	3–5 days
Chickenpox	Varicella zoster	Airborne or contact	About 14 days
Cholera	*Vibrio cholerae*	Ingestion of water contaminated with human waste	A few hours to 5 days
Cryptococcosis	*Cryptococcus neoformans*	Probably by inhalation	Unknown
Cryptosporidiosis	*Cryptosporidium* species	Ingestion of contaminated water; direct contact with carrier	Probably 1–12 days
Cytomegalovirus (CMV) infection	Cytomegalovirus	Transfusion and transplantation; sexual; perinatal	Highly variable: 3–8 weeks after transfusion, 3–12 weeks after delivery of newborn
Diarrheal disease (common causes)	*Campylobacter* species	Ingestion of contaminated food	3–5 days
	Clostridium difficile	Fecal–oral	Variable; in part related to the influence of antibiotics 12–36 hours
	Salmonella species	Ingestion of contaminated food or drink	1–3 days
	Shigella species	Ingestion of contaminated food or drink; direct contact with carrier	1–3 days
	Yersinia species	Ingestion of contaminated food or drink; direct contact with carrier	
Ebola	Ebola virus	Contact with blood or body fluids	2–21 days
Gonorrhea	*Neisseria gonorrhoeae*	Sexual; perinatal	2–7 days
Hand, foot, and mouth disease	Coxsackievirus	Direct contact with nose and throat secretions and with feces of infected people	3–5 days
Hantavirus pulmonary syndrome (HPS)	Sin Nombre virus	Contact (direct or indirect) with rodents	Unclear
Foodborne hepatitis	Hepatitis A virus	Ingestion of contaminated food or drink; direct contact with carrier	15–50 days
	Hepatitis E virus	Ingestion of contaminated food or drink; direct contact with carrier	Unclear
Bloodborne hepatitis	Hepatitis B virus	Sexual; perinatal; percutaneous	45–160 days
	Hepatitis C virus	Sexual; perinatal; percutaneous	6–9 months
	Hepatitis D	Sexual; perinatal; percutaneous	Unclear
	Hepatitis G	Percutaneous	Unclear
Herpangina	Coxsackievirus	Direct contact with nose and throat secretions and feces of infected people	3–5 days
Herpes simplex	Human herpesvirus 1 and 2	Contact with mucous membrane secretions	2–12 days
Histoplasmosis	*Histoplasma capsulatum*	Inhalation of airborne spores	5–18 days
Hookworm disease	*Necator americanus; Ancylostoma duodenale*	Contact with soil contaminated with human feces	A few weeks to many months
Impetigo	*Staphylococcus aureus*	Contact with *S. aureus* carrier	4–10 days
Influenza	Influenza virus A, B, or C	Droplet spread	24–72 hours
Lassa fever	Lassa virus	Contact with animal droppings; direct contact with blood or body fluids	7–21 days
Legionnaires' disease	*Legionella pneumophila*	Airborne from water source	2–10 days
Listeriosis	*Listeria monocytogenes*	Foodborne; perinatal	Unclear; probably 3–70 days
Lyme disease	*Borrelia burgdorferi*	Tick bite	14–23 days
Lymphogranuloma venereum	*Chlamydia inguinale*	Sexual	Weeks to years
Malaria	*Plasmodium vivax; Plasmodium malariae; Plasmodium falciparum; Plasmodium ovale*	Bite from *Anopheles* species mosquito	12–30 days
Marburg hemorrhagic fever	Marburg virus	Unknown route of transmission from animals to humans; person-to-person by droplets and direct contact	5–10 days
Meningococcal meningitis or bacteremia	*Neisseria meningitidis*	Contact with pharyngeal secretions; perhaps airborne	2–10 days
Mononucleosis	Epstein-Barr virus	Contact with pharyngeal secretions	4–6 weeks
Mycobacterial diseases (nontuberculosis *Mycobacterium* species)	*Mycobacterium avium; Mycobacterium kansasii; Mycobacterium fortuitum; Mycobacterium gordonae;* other *Mycobacterium* species	Variable; probably contact with soil, water, or other environmental source; none is person-to-person transmissible	Variable
Mycoplasmal pneumonia	*Mycoplasma pneumoniae*	Droplet inhalation	14–21 days

Continued

Table 70-1 INFECTIOUS DISEASES, CAUSATIVE ORGANISMS, MODES OF TRANSMISSION, AND USUAL INCUBATION PERIODS (Continued)

Disease or Condition	Organism	Usual Mode of Transmission	Usual Incubation Period (Infection to First Symptom)
Norovirus	Norovirus	Fecal–oral by food or water or by person-to-person spread	24–48 hours
Pediculosis	Pediculus humanus capitis (head louse); Phthirus pubis (crab louse)	Direct contact	1–2 weeks
Pertussis (whooping cough)	Bordetella pertussis	Contact with respiratory droplets	7–10 days
Pinworm disease	Enterobius vermicularis	Direct contact with egg-contaminated articles	4- to 6-week life cycle; often takes months of infection before recognition
Pneumocystis jiroveci pneumonia	Pneumocystis jiroveci	Unknown; not transmitted person-to-person	Infants: 1–2 months; adults: unclear
Pneumococcal pneumonia	Streptococcus pneumoniae	Droplet spread	Probably 1–3 days
Rabies	Rabies virus	Bite from rabid animal	2–8 weeks
Respiratory syncytial disease	Respiratory syncytial virus	Self-inoculation by mouth or nose after contact with infectious respiratory secretions	3–7 days
Ringworm	Microsporum species; Trichophyton species	Direct and indirect contact with lesions	4–10 days
Rocky mountain spotted fever	Rickettsia rickettsii	Bite from infected tick	3–14 days
Roseola infantum	Human herpes virus 6	Saliva	10–15 days
Rotavirus gastroenteritis	Rotavirus	Fecal–oral route	About 48 hours
Rubella	Rubella virus	Droplet spread; direct contact	14–21 days
Scabies	Sarcoptes scabei	Direct skin contact	2–6 weeks
Severe acute respiratory syndrome (SARS)	SARS-associated coronavirus (SARS-CoV)	Droplet; direct contact; occasionally airborne	2–10 days
Smallpox	Variola major	Airborne and contact	7–14 days
Syphilis	Treponema pallidum	Sexual; perinatal	10 days to 10 weeks
Tetanus	Clostridium tetani	Puncture wound	4–21 days
Trichinosis	Trichinella spiralis	Ingestion of insufficiently cooked foods, especially pork and beef	10–14 days
Tuberculosis	Mycobacterium tuberculosis	Airborne	4–12 weeks to the formation of primary lesion
West Nile virus	West Nile virus	Bite of infected mosquitoes; from transfusions and transplants; perinatal	3–14 days

Reservoir

Reservoir is the term used for any person, plant, animal, substance, or location that provides nourishment for microorganisms and enables further dispersal of the organism. Infections may be prevented by eliminating the causative organisms from the reservoir.

Mode of Exit

The organism must have a mode of exit from a reservoir. An infected host must shed organisms to another or to the environment for transmission to occur. Organisms exit through the respiratory tract, the gastrointestinal tract, the genitourinary tract, or the blood.

Route of Transmission

A route of transmission is necessary to connect the infectious source with its new host. Organisms may be transmitted through sexual contact, skin-to-skin contact, percutaneous injection, or infectious particles carried in the air. A person who carries or transmits an organism but does not have apparent signs and symptoms of infection is called a **carrier.**

Specific organisms require specific routes of transmission for infection to occur. For example, *Mycobacterium tuberculosis* is almost always transmitted by the airborne route. Health care providers do not "carry" M. *tuberculosis* bacteria on their hands or clothing. In contrast, bacteria such as *Staphylococcus aureus* are easily transmitted from patient to patient on the hands of health care providers.

When appropriate, the nurse should explain routes of disease transmission to patients. For example, a nurse may explain that sharing a room with a patient who is infected with human immunodeficiency virus (HIV) does not pose a risk because intimate contact (ie, sexual or parenteral) is necessary for transmission to occur.

Susceptible Host

For infection to occur, the **host** must be **susceptible** (not possessing immunity to a particular pathogen). Previous infection or vaccine administration may render the host **immune** (not susceptible) to further infection with an agent. Although exposure to potentially infectious microorganisms occurs essentially on a constant basis, people have elaborate immune systems that generally prevent infection from occurring. A person who is immunosuppressed has much greater susceptibility to infection than a healthy person.

Portal of Entry

A portal of entry is needed for the organism to gain access to the host. Again, specific organisms may require specific portals of entry for infection to occur. For example, airborne M. *tuberculosis* does not cause disease when it settles on the skin of an exposed host; the only entry route for M. *tuberculosis* is through the respiratory tract.

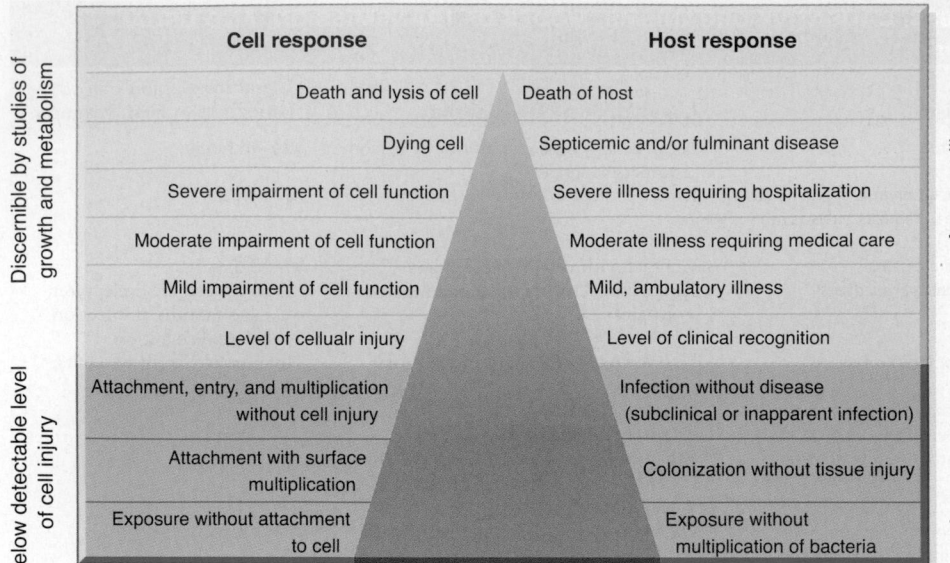

Cell response	Host response
Death and lysis of cell	Death of host
Dying cell	Septicemic and/or fulminant disease
Severe impairment of cell function	Severe illness requiring hospitalization
Moderate impairment of cell function	Moderate illness requiring medical care
Mild impairment of cell function	Mild, ambulatory illness
Level of cellualr injury	Level of clinical recognition
Attachment, entry, and multiplication without cell injury	Infection without disease (subclinical or inapparent infection)
Attachment with surface multiplication	Colonization without tissue injury
Exposure without attachment to cell	Exposure without multiplication of bacteria

Discernible by studies of growth and metabolism

Below detectable level of cell injury

Apparent illness

Inapparent

Figure 70-2 Biologic spectrum of response to bacterial infection at the cellular level (*left*) and of the intact host (*right*). Redrawn from Evans, A. S. & Brachman, P. S. (1998). *Bacterial infections in humans.* New York: Plenum.

Colonization, Infection, and Infectious Disease

Relatively few anatomic sites (eg, brain, blood, bone, heart, vascular system) are sterile. Bacteria found throughout the body usually provide beneficial **normal flora** to compete with potential pathogens, to facilitate digestion, or to work in other ways symbiotically with the host.

Colonization

The term **colonization** is used to describe microorganisms present without host interference or interaction. Organisms reported in microbiology test results often reflect colonization rather than infection. The patient's health care team must interpret microbiology test results accurately to ensure appropriate treatment.

Infection

Infection indicates a host interaction with an organism. A patient colonized with S. *aureus* may have staphylococci on the skin without any skin interruption or irritation. However, if the patient has an incision, S. *aureus* could enter the wound, resulting in an immune system reaction of local inflammation and migration of white cells to the site. Clinical evidence of redness, heat, and pain and laboratory evidence of white blood cells on the wound specimen smear suggest infection. In this situation, the host identifies the staphylococci as *foreign*. Infection is recognized by the host reaction (manifested by signs and symptoms) and by laboratory-based evidence of white blood cell reaction and microbiologic organism identification.

Infectious Disease

It is important to recognize the difference between infection and infectious disease. **Infectious disease** is the state in which the infected host displays a decline in wellness due to the infection. When the host interacts immunologically with an organism but remains symptom free, the definition of infectious disease has not been met. For example, when a person is first infected with M. *tuberculosis*, infection can be detected by a positive tuberculin skin test, which demonstrates immunologic recognition. Most people who are infected with M. *tuberculosis* have latent infection, but few people (approximately 10%) actually become ill and demonstrate symptoms of TB (fever, weight loss, and advancing pneumonia). Figure 70-2 depicts response to bacterial infection at the cellular level and at the host level.

The primary source of information about most bacterial infections is the microbiology laboratory report, which should be viewed as a tool to be used along with clinical indicators to determine if a patient is colonized, infected, or diseased. Microbiology reports from clinical specimens usually show three components: the smear and stain, the culture and organism identification, and the antimicrobial susceptibility (ie, sensitivity). As a marker for the likelihood of infection, the smear and stain generally provide the most helpful information because they describe the mix of cells present at the anatomic site at the time of specimen collection. Culture and sensitivity results specify which organisms are recognized and which antibiotics actively affect the bacteria.

Infection Control and Prevention

The World Health Organization (WHO) and the Centers for Disease Control and Prevention (CDC) are the principal agencies involved in setting guidelines about infection prevention. In recent years, attention to **health care–associated infections (HAIs)** has grown with increased input from the Joint Commission, the Institute for Healthcare Improvement (IHI), and Medicare.

The impact of infectious diseases changes over time as microorganisms mutate, as human behavior patterns shift, or as therapeutic options change. The CDC provides timely recommendations about many of the situations that a nurse may face when caring for or teaching a patient with an infectious disease. The CDC routinely publishes recommendations, guidelines, and summaries. Through its Internet site and its weekly journal, the *Morbidity and Mortality Weekly Report* (*MMWR*), the CDC reports significant cases,

Table 70-2	SELECTED IMPORTANT CENTERS FOR DISEASE CONTROL WEB SITES
Web Site	**Features**
www.cdc.gov	CDC home page
	Entry point to other sites; information about current situations in infectious diseases
www.cdc.gov/flu	Information about influenza and links to information, data, recommendations, and updates
www.cdc.gov/STD	Sexually transmitted diseases information, statistics, treatment guidelines, and laboratory guidelines
www.bt.cdc.gov/Agent/Agentlist.asp	Bioterrorism history, bioterrorism agents, updates, situations, and recommendations
www.cdc.gov/vaccines/vpd-vac/default.htm	Menu-driven overview of vaccine-preventable diseases
www.cdc.gov/drugresistance/	Overview of antibiotic/antimicrobial resistance, educational resources, laboratory information, and fact sheets
www.cdc.gov/ncidod/dhqp/index.html	Issues in health care settings, including infection control guidelines for isolation, surgical site infections, pneumonia, intravascular catheter–related infections, urinary tract infections, and infection control in long-term care facilities
www.cdc.gov/hiv/	Information about the epidemiology of HIV/AIDS, including fact sheets, slide sets, and statistics

outbreaks, environmental hazards, or other public health problems. Examples of important CDC guidelines and summaries are *Guidelines for Preventing the Transmission of Tuberculosis in Health Care Facilities* (2005g), *Updated US Public Health Service Guidelines for the Management of Occupation as Exposure to HIV and Recommendations for Post Exposure Prophylaxis* (2005e), *Sexually Transmitted Diseases Treatment Guidelines* (2006b), and *Recommended Immunization Schedules for Persons Aged 0 Through 18 years United States, 2009* (2009d).

This chapter summarizes several aspects of infectious diseases. However, the field of infection control and prevention changes rapidly. Health care workers should seek the most current information when they address patient care concerns or develop infection control policies. Table 70-2 presents an overview of selected CDC Web sites.

Preventing Infection in the Hospital

Isolation Precautions

Isolation precautions are guidelines created to prevent transmission of microorganisms in hospitals. The Hospital Infection Control Practices Advisory Committee (HICPAC) of the CDC recommends two tiers of isolation precautions. The first tier, called Standard Precautions, is designed for the care of *all* patients in the hospital and is the primary strategy for preventing HAIs. The second tier, called Transmission-Based Precautions, is designed for care of patients with known or suspected infectious diseases spread by airborne, droplet, or contact routes.

Standard Precautions

The premise of **Standard Precautions** is that all patients are colonized or infected with microorganisms, whether or not there are signs or symptoms, and that a uniform level of caution should be used in the care of all patients. The health care worker should use additional barriers in the form of personal protective equipment (PPE), including masks, eye protection, and cover gowns, depending on the degree of expected exposure to patient excretions or secretions. The

elements of Standard Precautions include hand hygiene, use of PPE, proper handling of patient care equipment and linen, environmental control, prevention of injury from sharps devices, and patients' room assignments within health care facilities. Hand hygiene, glove use, needlestick prevention, and avoidance of splash or spray of body fluids are discussed in the following sections. Chart 52-4 in Chapter 52 describes the Standard Precautions in detail.

Hand Hygiene. The most frequent cause of infection outbreaks in health care institutions is spread of microorganisms by the hands of health care workers. Hands should be washed or decontaminated frequently during patient care.

Chart 70-1 • *Hand-Hygiene Methods*

Hand Decontamination With Alcohol-Based Product

- After contact with body fluids, excretions, mucous membranes, nonintact skin, or wound dressings as long as hands are not visibly soiled
- After contact with a patient's intact skin (as after taking pulse or blood pressure or lifting a patient)
- In patient care, when moving from a contaminated body site to a clean body site
- After contact with inanimate objects in the patient's immediate vicinity
- Before caring for patients with severe neutropenia or other forms of severe immune suppression
- Before donning sterile gloves when inserting central catheters
- Before inserting urinary catheters or other devices that do not require a surgical procedure
- After removing gloves

Handwashing

- When hands are visibly dirty or contaminated with biologic material from patient care
- When health care workers do not tolerate waterless alcohol product

Chart 70-1 describes the recommended hand-hygiene methods.

When hands are visibly dirty or contaminated with biologic material from patient care, hands should be washed with soap and water. In intensive care units and other locations in which virulent or resistant organisms are likely to be present, antimicrobial agents (eg, chlorhexidine gluconate, iodophor, chloroxylenol, and triclosan) may be used. Effective handwashing requires at least *15 seconds of vigorous scrubbing*, with special attention to the area around nail beds and between fingers, where there is a high bacterial load. Hands should be thoroughly rinsed after washing.

If hands are not visibly soiled, health care providers are strongly encouraged to use alcohol-based, waterless antiseptic agents (eg, Avagard or Endure) for routine hand decontamination. These solutions are superior to soap or antimicrobial handwashing agents in their speed of action and effectiveness against microorganisms. Because they are formulated with emollients, they are usually better tolerated than other agents, and because they can be used without sinks and towels, health care workers have been found to be more compliant with their use. Nurses working in home health care or other settings where they are relatively mobile should carry pocket-size containers of alcohol-based solutions (Rhinehart & McGoldrick, 2005).

Normal skin flora usually consist of coagulase-negative staphylococci or diphtheroids. In the health care setting, workers may temporarily carry other bacteria (ie, **transient flora**) such as *S. aureus, Pseudomonas aeruginosa,* or other organisms with increased pathogenic potential. Generally, transient flora are superficially attached and are shed with hand hygiene and skin regeneration.

Hand hygiene reduces the bacterial load and decreases the risk of transfer to other patients. The Joint Commission has included hand hygiene as one of the national patient safety goals and focuses on this behavior in all surveys of health care facilities. All health care settings should have mechanisms to evaluate compliance with hand hygiene by all personnel who care for patients.

When providing patient care, nurses should not wear artificial fingernails or nail extenders because they have been epidemiologically linked to several significant outbreaks of infections. Natural nails should be kept less than 0.25 inches (0.6 cm) long, and nail polish should be removed when chipped because it can support increased bacterial growth (CDC, 2002a).

Glove Use. Gloves provide an effective barrier for hands from the microflora associated with patient care. Gloves should be worn when a health care worker has contact with any patient secretions or excretions and must be discarded after each patient care contact. Because microbial organisms colonizing health care workers' hands can proliferate in the warm, moist environment provided by gloves, hands must be washed or disinfected after gloves are removed. As patient advocates, nurses have an important role in promoting hand hygiene and glove use by other hospital workers, such as laboratory personnel, technicians, and others who have contact with patients.

Compared with vinyl gloves, latex or nitrile gloves are preferred because they resist puncture better and provide greater comfort and fit. Latex gloves have been improved to reduce the incidence of latex hypersensitivity, but some workers continue to experience local skin irritation or more severe reactions, including generalized dermatitis, conjunctivitis, asthma, angioedema, and anaphylaxis (see Chapter 53). The nurse who experiences irritation or an allergic reaction associated with exposure to latex should report symptoms to an occupational health specialist or a physician.

Needlestick Prevention. The most important aspect of reducing the risk of bloodborne infection is avoidance of percutaneous injury. Extreme care is essential in all situations in which needles, scalpels, and other sharp objects are handled. Used needles should not be recapped. Instead, they are placed directly into puncture-resistant containers near the place where they are used. If a situation dictates that a needle must be recapped, the nurse must use a mechanical device to hold the cap or use a one-handed approach to decrease the likelihood of skin puncture. Since 2001, the Occupational Safety and Health Administration (OSHA) has required use of needleless devices and other instruments designed to prevent injury from sharps when appropriate.

Avoidance of Splash and Spray. When the health care provider is involved in an activity in which body fluids may be sprayed or splashed, appropriate barriers must be used. If a splash to the face may occur, goggles and a face mask are warranted. If the health care worker is involved in a procedure in which clothing may be contaminated with biologic material, a cover gown should be worn.

Transmission-Based Precautions

Some microbes are so contagious or epidemiologically significant that precautions in addition to the Standard Precautions should be used when such organisms have been identified. The CDC recommends a second tier of precautions, called **Transmission-Based Precautions.** The isolation categories are Airborne, Droplet, and Contact Precautions (Siegel, Rhinehart, Jackson, et al., 2007).

Airborne Precautions are required for patients with presumed or proven pulmonary TB, chickenpox, or other airborne pathogen. Airborne Precautions would also be advised if a patient were infected with smallpox (eg, as a result of a bioterrorist attack). When hospitalized, patients should be in airborne infection isolation rooms (AIIR), engineered to provide negative air pressure, rapid turnover of air, and air either highly filtered or exhausted directly to the outside. Health care providers should wear an N-95 respirator (ie, protective mask) at all times while in the patient's room.

Droplet Precautions are used for organisms such as influenza or meningococcus that can be transmitted by close respiratory or mucous membrane contact with respiratory secretions. While taking care of a patient requiring Droplet Precautions, the nurse should wear a face mask, but because the risk of transmission is limited to close contact, the door may remain open.

Contact Precautions are used for organisms that are spread by skin-to-skin contact, such as antibiotic-resistant organisms or *Clostridium difficile.* Contact Precautions are designed to emphasize cautious technique and the use of barriers for organisms that have serious epidemiologic consequences or those easily transmitted by contact between health care

Chart 70-2 • *Summary of Types of Precautions and Patients Requiring the Precautions*

Standard Precautions

Use Standard Precautions for the care of all patients.

Airborne Precautions

In addition to Standard Precautions, use Airborne Precautions for patients known or suspected to have serious illnesses transmitted by airborne droplet nuclei. Examples of such illnesses include the following:
- Measles
- Varicella (including disseminated zoster)*
- Tuberculosis

Droplet Precautions

In addition to Standard Precautions, use Droplet Precautions for patients known or suspected to have serious illnesses transmitted by large particle droplets. Examples of such illnesses include:
- Invasive *Haemophilus influenzae* type b disease, including meningitis, pneumonia, epiglottitis, and sepsis
- Invasive *Neisseria meningitidis* disease, including meningitis, pneumonia, and sepsis
- Other serious bacterial respiratory infections spread by droplet transmission, including:
- Diphtheria (pharyngeal)
- Primary atypical pneumonia (*Mycoplasma pneumoniae*)
- Pertussis
- Pneumonic plague
- Streptococcal (group A) pharyngitis, pneumonia, or scarlet fever in infants and young children
- Serious viral infections spread by droplet transmission, including:
- Adenovirus*
- Influenza
- Mumps
- Parvovirus B19
- Rubella

Contact Precautions

In addition to Standard Precautions, use Contact Precautions for patients known or suspected to have serious illnesses easily transmitted by direct patient contact or by contact with items in the patient's environment. Examples of such illnesses include:
- Gastrointestinal, respiratory, skin, or wound infections or colonization with multidrug-resistant bacteria judged by the infection control program, based on current state, regional, or national recommendations, to be of special clinical and epidemiologic significance
- Enteric infections with a low infectious dose or prolonged environmental survival, including:
  - *Clostridium difficile*
  - For diapered or incontinent patients: enterohemorrhagic *Escherichia coli* O157:H7, *Shigella* species, hepatitis A, or rotavirus
- Respiratory syncytial virus, parainfluenza virus, or enteroviral infections in infants and young children
- Skin infections that are highly contagious or that may occur on dry skin, including:
- Diphtheria (cutaneous)
- Herpes simplex virus (neonatal or mucocutaneous)
- Impetigo
- Major (noncontained) abscesses, cellulitis, or pressure ulcers
- Pediculosis
- Scabies
- Staphylococcal furunculosis in infants and young children
- Zoster (disseminated or in the immunocompromised host)*
- Viral and hemorrhagic conjunctivitis
- Viral hemorrhagic infections (Ebola, Lassa, or Marburg)

*Certain infections require more than one type of precaution.
From Centers for Disease Control and Prevention, Atlanta, GA, 2007.

worker and patient. When possible, the patient requiring contact isolation is placed in a private room to facilitate hand hygiene and decreased environmental contamination. Masks are not needed, and doors do not need to be closed (Chart 70-2).

Specific Organisms with Health Care–Associated Infection Potential

Clostridium Difficile

This spore-forming bacterium has significant HAI potential. A more virulent strain has affected health care facilities throughout North America in the past several years, and rates of C. *difficile* infection increased significantly in the United States since 2000 (McDonald, 2007). Infection is usually preceded by antibiotics that disrupt normal intestinal flora and allow the antibiotic-resistant C. *difficile* spores to proliferate within the intestine. The organism causes pathology by releasing toxins into the lumen of the bowel. In pseudomembranous colitis, the most extreme form of C. *difficile* infection, debris from the injured lumen of the bowel and from white blood cells, accumulates in the form of pseudomembranes or studded areas of the colon. The destruction of such a large anatomic area can produce profound sepsis.

Because antibiotics are used so extensively in health care settings, many patients are at risk for infection with C. *difficile*. The potential for health care–associated acquisition is increased because the spore is relatively resistant to disinfectants and can be spread on the hands of health care providers after contact with equipment previously contaminated with C. *difficile*. Control is best achieved by using Contact Precautions for infected patients, with use of gowns and gloves for all patient contact. Because the spores are resistant to alcohol, waterless hand products are not as effective as handwashing with soap and water for use in hand hygiene. Bleach-based solutions and cleaning products are preferred over other hospital disinfectants for environmental cleaning. Frequently touched equipment (such as the overbed table and side rails) should be cleaned daily and whenever visibly soiled. IV poles and other peripheral items should be cleaned when the patient is discharged.

Methicillin-Resistant Staphylococcus Aureus

Methicillin-resistant Staphylococcus aureus (MRSA), a common human pathogen, refers to *S. aureus* that is resistant to methicillin or its comparable pharmaceutic agents, oxacillin and nafcillin. Soon after penicillin was discovered in the 1940s, *S. aureus* became all but universally penicillin resistant. Alternative therapies in the form of cephalosporins and synthetic penicillin solutions such as methicillin were introduced. However, since the late 1970s, MRSA became increasingly more prevalent, and transmission within hospitals and nursing homes is well documented. In the past 10 years, MRSA has also been found in otherwise healthy people who have not been in health care settings (CDC, 2006a).

Health Care–Associated MRSA. Health care providers transmit MRSA to patients easily because *S. aureus* has an affinity for skin colonization. The patient who is colonized with MRSA has an increased probability of developing health care–associated MRSA (HA-MRSA), especially when invasive procedures, such as IV therapy, respiratory therapy, or surgery are performed. The colonized patient also serves as a reservoir of MRSA that can be transmitted to others. HA-MRSA may persist as normal flora in the patient for an extended time. From the early 1990s to 2003, the proportion of MRSA in *S. aureus* samples grew from approximately 20% to approximately 60% (CDC, 2006a).

Community-Associated MRSA. MRSA is not limited to health care facilities, and in recent years there has been a significant increase in the incidence of MRSA infections in children, members of sports teams, prison inmates, and in other people who have no apparent health care exposure. These **community-associated MRSA** (CA-MRSA) infections are typically caused by strains of *S. aureus* that are molecularly distinct from HA-MRSA. The CA-MRSA strains typically produce more toxins than HA-MRSA, and localized skin symptoms can lead to necrotizing fasciitis or bacteremia (Weber, 2005). Often, skin symptoms are initially mistaken for spider or bug bites. CA-MRSA infections have resulted in serious skin and soft tissue infections, pneumonia, and, in rare cases, death. Once introduced into a health care facility, the virulent CA-MRSA strains can be transmitted to other patients in a manner typically associated with HA-MRSA (Gonzalez, Rueda, Shelburne, et al., 2006).

Control of MRSA in Health Care Facilities. The CDC recommends Contact Precautions for patients with MRSA colonization or infection. In recent years, there has been a growing debate about the benefits of active surveillance cultures to determine unrecognized carriers. In active surveillance, asymptomatic patients are cultured routinely (on admission or on a regular basis) to determine unrecognized carriers. Although the epidemiologic evidence does not clearly indicate whether this strategy reduces patient risk, a growing number of states have mandated this approach (Milstone & Perl, 2008). Nurses who participate in active surveillance programs must be prepared to educate patients and their families about the definitions of colonization and infection and the reason for the vigorous isolation efforts.

Vancomycin (Vancocin) and linezolid (Zyvox) are typically the preferred treatments for serious MRSA infection. However, there is concern that MRSA will eventually become resistant to even these medications because they are used so commonly. Since 2002, a very small but disturbing number of patients have been diagnosed with *S. aureus* infections that are completely resistant to vancomycin (ie, **vancomycin-resistant Staphylococcus aureus [VRSA]**). Researchers have also noted decreased efficacy of vancomycin both in the laboratory and in clinical settings (Wang, Hindler, Ward, et al., 2006). The threat of VRSA is considered a very serious public health concern because of the commonality and pathogenicity of *S. aureus*. Without effective antibiotics, many patients with *S. aureus* infections would have a poor outcome (CDC, 2002b). Control of MRSA is an important goal, and it may also make the emergence of VRSA strains less likely.

Vancomycin-Resistant Enterococcus

Vancomycin-resistant Enterococcus (VRE) is the second most frequently isolated source of HAIs in the United States. This gram-positive bacterium, which is part of the normal flora of the gastrointestinal tract, can produce significant disease when it infects blood, wounds, or the urinary tract.

Enterococcus has several traits that make it an easily transmittable HAI organism. It is a normal part of the gastrointestinal flora of the host; it is bile resistant and able to withstand harsh anatomic sites, such as the intestine; and it persists well on the hands of health care providers and on environmental objects.

As a relatively resistant organism at baseline, therapy for *Enterococcus* is limited to penicillin formulations (eg, ampicillin), vancomycin in combination with an aminoglycoside (eg, gentamicin), or linezolid (Zyvox). Between 1994 and 2003, the CDC recorded an increase of more than 62% in the number of cases of VRE infections in patients in intensive care units (CDC, 2004b). This rapid increase has serious implications. Because many strains of VRE are resistant to all other antimicrobial therapies, clinicians are left with few choices for effective therapy. Equally important, VRE colonization and infection may serve as a reservoir of vancomycin-resistant coded genes that may be transferred to the more virulent *S. aureus* (CDC, 2002b).

Multidrug-Resistant Gram-Negative Organisms

During the past several decades, the incidence of infections caused by multidrug-resistant gram-negative organisms has also increased significantly. Extensive use of antibiotics induces resistance. The bacteria that most commonly develop resistance include *P. aeruginosa* (resistant to fluoroquinolone antibiotics and/or carbapenems), *Acinetobacter* species (resistant to many antibiotics, including carbapenems), and both *Klebsiella pneumoniae* and *Escherichia coli* (resistant to extended-spectrum beta-lactam antibiotics). These pathogens are also associated with outbreaks in health care facilities. Transmission has been associated with contamination of equipment and with transfer via the hands of health care workers (CDC, 2002b).

Preventing Health Care-Associated Bloodstream Infections (Bacteremia and Fungemia)

Reducing the risk of health care–associated bloodstream infections requires preventive activities in addition to the Standard Precautions. If a health care–associated

Chart 70-3 • *Conditions That Suggest the Presence of Health Care–Associated Vascular Access Device-Related Bacteremia or Fungemia*

- The patient has catheter in place, appears septic, but has no obvious reason to suggest predisposition to sepsis.
- There is no infection at another body site to indicate probable source of sepsis.
- The site of vascular line insertion is red, swollen, or draining (especially purulent drainage).
- The patient has a central vascular line in place at the onset of sepsis.
- The bloodstream infection is caused by *Candida* species or by common skin organisms such as coagulase-negative staphylococci, *Bacillus* species, or *Corynebacterium* species.
- The patient remains septic after appropriate therapy without removal of the vascular access device.

bloodstream infection occurs, early diagnosis is important to prevent complications, such as endocarditis and brain abscess. Mortality rates associated with infection by some organisms are estimated to average 18%. The estimated cost attributed to catheter-related bloodstream infections ranges from $12,000 to $54,000 per case (Pronovost, Needham, Berenholtz, et al., 2006).

Bacteremia is defined as the laboratory-confirmed presence of bacteria in the bloodstream. **Fungemia** is a bloodstream infection caused by a fungal organism. Any vascular access device (VAD) can serve as the source for a bloodstream infection. Most hospitalized patients receive VADs, and increasingly, long-term central catheters are used to provide IV therapy to outpatients in clinic or home settings. In all instances, the nurse must use appropriate care to reduce the risk of bacteremia and to be alert for signs of bacteremia. Chart 70-3 identifies conditions that suggest the presence of health care–associated VAD-related bacteremia or fungemia.

Hand hygiene and strict attention to aseptic technique are essential during the insertion of all VADs. Health care personnel who insert central catheters should use surgical technique, including sterile gloves, sterile gowns with long sleeves, masks, and a large drape over the patient.

Disinfecting Skin

The patient's own flora, traversing the exterior of a peripherally inserted catheter or contaminating the central catheter hub, is the most common bacterial source of catheter-related bacteremia (CDC, 2002b). Rarely, IV fluid itself can become contaminated and serve as a source of infection. The preferred solution for disinfection of the insertion site is chlorhexidine gluconate (CHG, Hibiclens). Alternative solutions are povidone-iodine (Betadine) or alcohol.

There is no apparent difference in risk or benefit when comparing transparent polyurethane dressings and gauze dressings. However, if blood is oozing from the catheter insertion site, a gauze dressing should be used. Most importantly, the dressing should be applied using aseptic technique and should be sealed along its entire perimeter. A highly absorbent CHG-impregnated dressing (Biopatch

Antimicrobial Dressing), which releases disinfectant for up to 7 days, may be used to reduce risk in patients older than 2 months of age (Marschall, Mermel, Classen, et al., 2008).

Changing Infusion Sets, Caps, and Solutions

Infusion sets and stopcock caps should be changed no more frequently than every 3 days, unless an infusion set is used for the delivery of blood or lipid solutions. Infusion sets and tubing for blood, blood products, or lipid emulsions should be changed within 24 hours of initiating the infusion. Blood infusions should finish within 4 hours of hanging the blood; lipid solutions should be completed within 24 hours of hanging. There are no guidelines for the appropriate intervals for the hang time of other solutions. Injection ports should be cleaned with 70% alcohol or iodophor before accessing the system (CDC, 2002b).

Preventing Infection in the Community

The CDC and state and local public health departments share responsibility for prevention and control of infection in the community. Methods of infection prevention include sanitation techniques (eg, water purification, disposal of sewage and other potentially infectious materials), regulated health practices (eg, the handling, storage, packaging, and preparation of food by institutions), and immunization programs. In the United States, immunization programs have markedly decreased the incidence of infectious diseases.

Vaccination Programs

The goal of vaccination programs is to use wide-scale efforts to prevent specific infectious diseases from occurring in a population. Public health decisions about vaccination efforts are complex. Risks and benefits for the person and the community must be evaluated in terms of morbidity, mortality, and financial cost and benefit. The most successful vaccine programs have been ones for the prevention of smallpox, measles, mumps, rubella, polio, diphtheria, pertussis, and tetanus. Table 70-3 demonstrates this success.

More than 25 vaccines are currently licensed in the United States. Vaccines are suspensions of antigen preparations, intended to produce a human immune response to protect the host from future encounters with the organism. Because no vaccine is completely safe for all recipients, contraindications on package inserts of a vaccine must be heeded. These guidelines provide details about studied experiences with allergy and other complications and provide crucial information about refrigeration, storage, dosage, and administration. The most common adverse effects are allergic reaction to the antigen or carrier solution and the occurrence of the actual disease (often in modified form) when live vaccine is used.

The standard recommended immunization schedules for adults as developed by the CDC can be found at the CDC Web site (2009b). The schedule is revised as epidemiologic evidence warrants; nurses should consult the CDC to determine the most recent schedule. Variations to the recommended immunization schedule should be made on a case-by-case basis, depending on the patient's risk factors. The recommended vaccines for adults are designed to protect those with underlying diseases that increase infection risk, those with potential for occupational exposure, and those

Table 70-3   IMPACT OF VACCINES IN THE TWENTIETH AND TWENTY-FIRST CENTURIES

Disease	20th-Century Annual Morbidity	2006 Total	% Decrease
Smallpox	48,164	0	100
Diphtheria	175,885	0	100
Pertussis	147,271	15,632	89
Tetanus	1314	41	97
Polio (paralytic)	16,316	0	100
Measles	503,282	55	>99.9
Mumps	152,209	6,584	96
Rubella	47,745	11	>99.9
Congenital rubella	823	1	88.8
Haemophilus influenzae (<5 years)	20,000 (EST)	208 (serotype b or unknown)	99

Centers for Disease Control and Prevention. (2008). Atkinson, W., Hamborsky, J., McIntyre, L., et al. (Eds.). *Epidemiology and prevention of vaccine-preventable diseases* (10th ed. 2nd printing). Washington DC: Public Health Foundation.

who may be exposed to infectious agents during travel. Immunosuppressed adults (including those who have had a splenectomy) should be vaccinated for pneumococcus (*Streptococcus pneumoniae*) and meningococcus (*Neisseria meningitidis*). Health care workers should be immune to measles, mumps, rubella, pertussis, tetanus, hepatitis B, and varicella. An annual influenza vaccine is recommended for people with chronic conditions such as immune suppression, asthma, and cardiac or respiratory diseases, as well as for *all* health care workers and for people 65 years of age and older.

The CDC (2009a) gives information about individual vaccines and vaccine-preventable diseases. It also provides a 24-hour telephone hotline (see Resources below) for routine pediatric or adult vaccine advice. Advice about optimal vaccinations for travelers is also available at the CDC (2006d) Web site and by phone (see Resources).

The incidence of vaccine-preventable diseases, such as measles, mumps, rubella, and diphtheria, is affected by immigration from developing countries. Vaccine campaigns in developing countries are often financially and logistically constrained, and immigrants from such areas may be more likely than U.S. residents to be unprotected. Individual risk and epidemic risk are reduced when vaccination campaigns reach all communities, including those with a high proportion of immigrants.

Common Vaccines

Measles, Mumps, and Rubella Vaccine. Since the measles, mumps, and rubella (MMR) vaccines were licensed, endemic rubella has been eliminated in the United States (CDC, 2005a), and mumps and rubella have decreased by more than 99%. To maintain this effective public health strategy, routine MMR vaccination should be administered to children at 12 to 15 months of age, with repeat dosing at 4 to 6 years of age (CDC, 2007a).

Patients should be advised that fever, transient lymphadenopathy, or hypersensitivity reaction might occur following an MMR vaccination. The risk of side effects is greater in vaccine recipients who have not previously received the vaccine than in those who have received repeat doses. Antipyretics may be used to decrease the risk of fever.

Varicella (Chickenpox) Vaccine and Zoster (Shingles) Vaccine. Varicella zoster is the virus that causes chicken-

pox and herpes zoster. In its natural state, the varicella virus often attacks children, causing disseminated disease in the form of chickenpox. Although the incidence of varicella is lower in adults, the severity of chickenpox and possible sequelae, including death, is substantially greater (CDC, 2007a). Transmission occurs by the airborne and contact routes. With rare exception, varicella infects a person only once. The incubation period is about 2 weeks (range, 10 to 21 days). During a prodrome of general malaise (often noticed about 2 days before the rash develops), the newly infected host is capable of transmitting the virus to other susceptible contacts. Typically, the vesicular, pustular rash spreads rapidly from few too many lesions in a matter of hours. New lesions continue to form for 2 to 3 days and appear at different stages throughout this time. By the fourth symptomatic day, the lesions begin to dry, and new lesions usually do not develop. Fever is common during the 4 to 6 days of rash progression. When the lesions have crusted, the patient is no longer contagious.

Between 1995, when the varicella vaccine was first licensed in the United States, and 2004, the incidence of chickenpox decreased by 83% to 93%. The vaccine is effective in preventing chickenpox in approximately 70% to 90% of people who receive vaccinations, and it is 90% to 100% effective in preventing severe varicella (CDC, 2007a). The vaccine should not be given to those who have depressed immune function, are pregnant, have received blood products in the past 6 months, or have demonstrated allergy to varicella vaccine.

Herpes zoster, also known as shingles, is a painful, localized rash caused by recurrent varicella. Vesicles are restricted to areas supplied by single associated nerve groups. Varicella may be transmitted from the rash of those with shingles to people who are susceptible to varicella; the new varicella infections are manifested as chickenpox. It is estimated that more than 50% of unvaccinated people who live to at least 85 years of age will develop shingles.

In 2006, the Food and Drug Administration approved Zostavax, a vaccine to reduce the risk of shingles. The vaccine is recommended for people older than 60 years of age because it reduces the risk of shingles by approximately 50% in those people (CDC, 2007a).

Influenza Vaccine. Influenza is an acute viral respiratory disease that predictably and periodically causes worldwide epidemics known as pandemics. Epidemics occur every 2 to 3 years, with a highly variable degree of severity. An estimated 36,000 deaths per year are attributed to influenza or its sequelae (ie, pneumonia, cardiopulmonary collapse). Elderly people are more susceptible to influenza, and the incidence of the disease in the United States is increasing as the proportion of the elderly increases (CDC, 2007a).

Each year a new vaccine is composed of the three virus strains (two type A influenza strains and one type B influenza strain) considered most likely to occur in the coming season. If the correct influenza agents have been included in that year's vaccine, the vaccine offers approximately 70% to 90% protection for healthy children and adults younger than 65 years of age. Although less effective in preventing disease in the elderly, it decreases the severity of illness in those who become infected. In extended care facilities, the vaccine is approximately 80% effective in preventing death and 50% to 60% effective in preventing hospitalization (CDC, 2007a). The vaccine is administered as an injection with inactivated virus or as a nasal spray with live attenuated virus.

The Advisory Committee for Immunization Practices of the Public Health Service recommends annual influenza vaccinations for the following groups: people older than 50 years of age, children 6 to 59 months of age, pregnant women, residents of extended care facilities, and those with chronic medical diseases or disabilities. In addition, health care providers and household members of those in high-risk groups should receive the vaccine to reduce the risk of transmission to people vulnerable to influenza sequelae. Vaccine campaigns in health care workers and patients should be intensified when there is evidence of community influenza.

Reporting Problems With Vaccines

Nurses should ask parents or adult vaccine recipients to provide information about any problems encountered after vaccination. As mandated by law, a Vaccine Adverse Event Reporting System (VAERS) form must be completed with the following information: type of vaccine received, timing of vaccination, onset of the adverse event, current illnesses or medication, history of adverse events after vaccination, and demographic information about the recipient. Forms are obtained by telephone or via the Internet (see Resources section) and can be submitted online.

Contraindications to Vaccines

Patients who have developed encephalopathy within 7 days of a previous diphtheria, tetanus, and pertussis dose and those who have developed anaphylaxis or other moderate or severe sequelae after a previous dose should not receive further doses. Diphtheria, tetanus, and acellular pertussis (DTap) is often deferred for the child who previously developed a fever higher than 40.5°C (105°F) within 48 hours of vaccination or who had a seizure or developed a shocklike state within 3 days of previous vaccination. Some live vaccines (eg, varicella, MMR, yellow fever) are contraindicated for people who are severely immunosuppressed or who are pregnant. All decisions about vaccination should be made by the patient's primary health care provider after careful review of vaccine-specific contraindications.

Planning for an Influenza Pandemic

A pandemic is a global outbreak of a disease. For example, influenza caused three pandemics in the 20th century. In the United States, the pandemic influenza caused more than 500,000 deaths in the 1918 "Spanish flu" pandemic, about 70,000 deaths in 1957 in the "Asian flu" pandemic, and about 34,000 deaths in 1968 in the "Hong Kong flu" pandemic. In June 2009, the WHO announced that a novel influenza virus, H1N1 had reached pandemic proportion. At the time of this printing, the extent of the H1N1 pandemic cannot be characterized, but its rapid dissemination worldwide with sustained human to human transmission in many locations was well recognized.

Subtypes of influenza viruses have pandemic potential because they constantly change within animals and secondarily within humans. As a result of these changes, essentially new viruses can "emerge" and can expose entire populations who are immunologically unprotected.

Influenza pandemics are likely to be more catastrophic than other anticipated public health problems because they last longer than other emergency events, they often occur in "waves," they deplete the available health care workforce, and they reduce the supply of medical equipment because of their widespread nature. The frequency and severity of pandemics cannot be accurately predicted, but models suggest that a medium-intensity pandemic could cause more than 200,000 deaths in the United States and quickly overwhelm the existing health care infrastructure. The CDC encourages all health care institutions to have a pandemic plan and to test the components of the plan regularly. A tool to help estimate the number of hospitalizations that will occur, the need for intensive care unit beds, and the need for ventilators can be found at http://www.cdc.gov/flu/flusurge.htm.

Avian Influenza Pandemic

Avian influenza (bird flu) is an infection caused by influenza viruses that chiefly infect birds and poultry. The H5N1 strain (named for the characteristics of the viral surface proteins hemagglutinin and neuraminidase) is of particular concern. It has caused a number of outbreaks in poultry since 2003, and the problem is ongoing; flocks of migratory birds have rapidly disseminated the virus throughout much of the world. Although many avian influenza viruses are natural and nonpathogenic in birds, H5N1 is unusual because of its high mortality rate in birds and because it has shown a limited ability to be transmitted from a bird source to mammals, including humans. The human mortality rate from H5N1 avian influenza has been more than 60% (WHO, 2008a). The majority of human cases of H5N1 are attributed to direct contact with poultry, but there are rare instances that suggest occasional human-to-human transmission.

Scientists are especially concerned that avian influenza H5N1 may change, either through mutation or reassortment, to become easily transmitted from human to human. If H5N1 were easily transmissible to humans, it would be likely to cause a severe pandemic because the human population has no immunity to the virus and because development of an appropriate vaccine would take too long to effectively stop the pandemic (U.S. Department of Health and Human Services [USDHHS], 2008).

The symptoms associated with H5N1 avian influenza in humans have ranged from the symptoms typically seen with seasonal influenza (cough, fever, and muscle aches) to severe pneumonia and multiorgan failure. Influenza antiviral therapy (ie, oseltamivir [Tamiflu] and zanamivir [Relenza]) is stockpiled as part of a national strategy, with hopes that they would be effective in treating humans infected with the pandemic strain of H5N1. Simple infection control strategies using careful hand hygiene and masks will be especially important in an avian influenza pandemic. Health departments throughout the country are also planning how to implement isolation programs to keep symptomatic people away from schools and work places (USDHHS, 2008).

Home-Based Care of the Patient With an Infectious Disease

The nurse who cares for the patient with an infectious disease in the home should provide information about infection risk prevention to the patient, the family, and the caregiver (Chart 70-4). Recognizing that a health history may not identify all active or latent infections, the caregiver should carefully follow Standard Precautions in the home. The nurse should establish a work environment that facilitates hand hygiene and aseptic technique.

Family caregivers should receive an annual influenza vaccine. This is especially true if the caregiver or the patient is older than 50 years of age, has underlying cardiac or pulmonary disease, or has underlying immunosuppression.

Patients requiring home care are often people with immunosuppression from underlying conditions, such as HIV infection or cancer, or those who have treatment-induced immunosuppression, as occurs with many antineoplastic agents. Careful assessment for signs of infection is important.

Reducing Risk to the Patient

Equipment Care

All caregivers must pay careful attention to disinfection and aseptic technique while using medical equipment. Catheter-related sepsis should be suspected in a patient who has unexplained fever, redness, swelling, and drainage around a vascular catheter insertion site. Indwelling urinary catheters should be discontinued whenever possible, because each day of use increases the risk of infection. The nurse should promptly report signs of urinary tract infection or of generalized sepsis to the patient's physician.

Patient Teaching

When assessing the risk of the immunosuppressed patient in the home environment for infection, it is important to realize that intrinsic colonizing bacteria and latent viral infections present a greater risk than do extrinsic environmental contaminants. The nurse should reassure the patient and family that their home needs to be clean but not sterile. Common-sense approaches to cleanliness and risk reduction are helpful.

For patients with neutropenia or T-cell dysfunction (eg, patients with acquired immunodeficiency syndrome [AIDS]), it is wise to restrict visits of people with potentially contagious illnesses. The patient who is severely neutropenic should not eat uncooked fruits and vegetables. The immunosuppressed patient is vulnerable to acquiring bacterial infection with enteric pathogens from food; therefore, family members should be reminded about the need to follow recommendations for hygiene and safe cooking times and temperatures.

Reducing Risk to Household Members

Establishing reasonable barriers to infection transmission in the household is an important part of home care. The route of transmission of the organism in question must first be determined. The nurse can then teach household members strategies to reduce their risk of becoming infected. If the patient has active pulmonary TB, the public health department should be contacted to provide screening and treatment for family members. If the patient has shingles (herpes zoster), family members who have had varicella vaccine or who have previously had chickenpox are considered immune and need no precautions. However, if a family member is immunosuppressed or otherwise susceptible to varicella, maintaining physical separation may be an important strategy during the time when the patient has draining

---

CHART
70-4
HOME CARE CHECKLIST
Prevention of Infection in the Home Care Setting

At the completion of the home care instruction, the patient or caregiver will be able to:	PATIENT	CAREGIVER
• Demonstrate aseptic technique in the care of technical equipment such as intravenous catheter and indwelling urinary catheter.	✔	✔
• Demonstrate thorough hand hygiene after patient care. (Use alcohol-based disinfectant *or* handwashing.)	✔	✔
• Complies with antibiotic regimen (patient) or with completion of vaccination series (patient and caregiver).	✔	✔
• State the rationale for thoroughly cooking all foods and storing meat products separate from other food groups.	✔	✔
• Use separate eating utensils and towels.	✔	✔
• Avoid contact with someone who has a known infectious disease.	✔	✔

lesions. When the patient is infected with *Shigella*, *Salmonella*, *C. difficile*, hepatitis A, or other enteric organisms, the family should be reassured that common household disinfectants are effective in controlling environmental contamination.

Family members who assist in the care of a patient with a bloodborne infection such as HIV or hepatitis C can prevent transmission by carefully handling any sharp objects that are contaminated with blood. Family teaching may include discussion about the need for caution when shaving the patient; performing dressing changes; or administering any IV, intramuscular, or subcutaneous medication. To collect and dispose of used needles, syringes, and vascular access equipment, the family should use containers designed for sharps disposal. With the exception of TB, the opportunistic infections associated with AIDS do not usually pose a risk to the healthy family member. Family members should be reassured that dishes are safe to use after being washed with hot water and that linens and clothing are safe to use after being washed in a hot-water cycle.

Nursing Management

Assessment

The health history and physical examination and the use of diagnostic tests are important for determining the presence of infection and infectious diseases. Symptoms of infectious diseases vary significantly between and within diseases. For some infections, visible symptoms such as rash, redness, or swelling provide early warnings of infection. In other infections, such as TB and HIV, asymptomatic latency is prolonged, and infection must be determined through diagnostic procedures.

The history is obtained to establish the likelihood and probable source of infection as well as the degree of associated pathology and symptoms. The patient's previous medical record is reviewed when possible. In obtaining a health history, the following questions may be asked:

- Does the patient have a history of previous or recurrent infections?
- Has there been fever? How high has the patient's temperature been? Is the temperature constant, or does it rise and fall? Has fever been associated with chills? Has the patient taken any medication to relieve fever?
- Is there cough? Is the cough chronic or acute? Is it associated with shortness of breath? Does the cough produce sputum? Is the sputum bloody? Has the patient had a tuberculin skin test (TST) recently? If so, what were the results? Has the patient been given isoniazid (INH) prophylaxis for TB infection? Has the patient been treated for TB in the past?
- Is there pain? Where is the pain? What is the nature of the pain? Does the patient have a sore throat, headache, myalgias, or arthralgias? Is there pain on urination or other activity?
- Is there edema? Is there drainage associated with the edema? Is the edematous area warm to touch?
- Is there a draining lesion? Is the drainage associated with trauma or a previous procedure? Is the drainage purulent or clear?
- Does the patient have diarrhea, vomiting, or abdominal pain?

- Is there a rash? What is the nature of the rash—is it flat, raised, red, crusted, purulent, or lacelike? Has the patient taken medications that could induce rash? Has there been exposure to another person who has an identified infectious disease or rash?
- What is the patient's vaccination history?
- Has there been an insect or animal bite? Has there been an animal scratch or other exposure to pets, farm animals, or experimental animals?
- What medications are used? Have antibiotics been taken recently or long term? Is the patient being treated with corticosteroids, immunosuppressive agents, or chemotherapy?
- Has the patient been treated in the past for other infectious diseases? Has the patient been hospitalized for infectious diseases?
- If sexual history is pertinent, has there been sexual exposure to another person with a known sexually transmitted disease (STD)? Has the patient been treated for STDs in the past? Is the patient pregnant, or has she recently been pregnant? Has the patient been tested for HIV?
- Has the patient traveled abroad, including developing countries? What was the immunization or antimicrobial prophylaxis used for protection while traveling?
- What is the patient's occupation? What are the patient's recreational activities? Hobbies?

Because infection may occur in any body system, physical examination may reveal signs of infection at any body site. Generalized signs of chronic infection may include significant weight loss or pallor associated with anemia of chronic diseases. Acute infection may manifest with fever, chills, lymphadenopathy, or rash. Localized signs vary by source of infection. Purulent drainage, pain, edema, and redness are strongly associated with localized infection. Cough and shortness of breath may be caused by influenza, pneumonia, or TB, as well as many noninfectious causes.

Nursing Interventions

Preventing Infection Transmission

Preventing the spread of infection requires an understanding of the usual routes of transmission of the organism. The hospitalized patient may pose a contagious risk to others if the disease is easily spread (such as *C. difficile*) or is spread through an airborne route (such as TB). In these situations, strict adherence to isolation measures is important in reducing the opportunity for spread. Preventing transmission of organisms from patient to patient requires participation of the health care team. Transmission of organisms on the hands and gloves of health care workers remains a common source of cross-infection in the hospital or clinic setting.

Nurses serve an important role in preventing the transfer of organisms in two ways. First, as the health professionals who spend the most time with patients, nurses have a greater opportunity for spreading organisms. It is imperative that nurses disinfect their hands before and after contact with patients and after performing a potentially hand-contaminating activity. Hands must be disinfected each time gloves are removed. For example, the nurse who has performed endotracheal suctioning should remove the gloves, wash the hands, and put on a new pair of gloves before performing wound care on the same patient. Second, nurses can reduce hand-to-hand spread of organisms by serving as patient advocates. To the degree feasible, the nurse should observe the hand-hygiene activities of other professionals and discuss with them any lapses in technique that are observed.

Teaching About the Infectious Process

Interruption of transmission requires diagnosis and patient compliance with the treatment regimen. The nurse's role is to educate the patient and, in some situations, to report the case to public health officials for contact tracing and verification of follow-up.

The nurse must stress the importance of immunization to parents of young children and to others for whom vaccines are recommended, such as patients who are elderly, are immunosuppressed, or have chronic illnesses or disabilities. Nurses should recognize their personal responsibility to receive the hepatitis B vaccine and an annual influenza vaccine to reduce potential transmission to themselves and vulnerable patient groups.

Infectious diseases often seem mysterious and frequently are socially stigmatizing. Patient teaching efforts require empathy and sensitivity. For example, in the past, TB was a stigmatizing disease. The nurse may need to provide basic information to the patient who needs INH prophylaxis to promote understanding and allay anxiety that the patient may feel.

Controlling Fever and Accompanying Discomforts

Fever must always be investigated to determine whether infection is the source. Evidence indicates that fever, mediated by the hypothalamus, may potentiate beneficial functions in the syndrome of reactions known as *acute-phase reaction*. These reactions include changes in liver protein synthesis; alterations in serum metals, such as iron; and increased production of certain classes of white blood cells and other cells of the immune system. Most fevers are physiologically controlled so that the temperature remains below 41°C (105.8°F). However, severe fever, as occurs with meningococcal meningitis, may cause heat stroke and other complications. Even milder fevers accompanied by fatigue, chills, and diaphoresis are often uncomfortable for the patient. Whether fever is treated or untreated, adequate fluid intake is important during febrile episodes.

> ◣ **NURSING ALERT**
>
> Because fever offers clues about infection severity and the success of antibiotic therapy, outpatients with fever should be taught to obtain accurate temperature readings. Frequently, family caregivers know that a patient has warm skin but do not disturb the patient by taking a temperature reading. Body temperature information can be very helpful in adjusting therapy or in reevaluating a preliminary diagnosis.

Monitoring and Managing Potential Complications

The patient with a rapidly progressive infectious disease should have vital signs and level of consciousness closely monitored. X-ray findings and microbiologic, immunologic, hematologic, cytologic, and parasitologic laboratory values must be interpreted in the context of other clinical findings to assess the course of the infectious disease.

Antibiotic therapy is frequently complex, and modifications are necessary because of sensitivity test results and disease progression. To ensure therapeutic blood levels rapidly, antibiotic therapy should be initiated as soon as it is prescribed rather than waiting until routine medication scheduling times. The Plan of Nursing Care in Chart 70-5 describes nursing interventions for specific complications of infection.

Diarrheal Diseases

Diarrheal diseases, which are especially prevalent in the developing world, cause significant morbidity and mortality. It is estimated that diarrheal diseases kill more than 6,000 children per day in Asia, Africa, and Latin America. The most important cause of death associated with these diseases is dehydration, and the most important treatment that decreases death rates is rehydration therapy (Guerrant & Steiner, 2005).

In the United States, the epidemiology of diarrheal diseases is changing constantly. Water disinfection, pasteurization, and appropriate food packaging have decreased the incidence of diseases such as typhoid and cholera. However, importation of foreign foods, environmental and ecological changes, and changes in diagnostic test modalities have led to recognition of important new trends and outbreaks.

Transmission

The portal of entry of all diarrheal pathogens is oral ingestion. Although food is far from sterile, the high acidity of the stomach and the antibody-producing cells of the small bowel generally serve to decrease the potential of pathogens. Infection can occur when the infectious dose is high enough or if the food neutralizes the acidic environment. Decreased gastric acidity with disruption of normal bowel flora (as occurs after surgery), use of antimicrobial agents, and the immune dysfunction of AIDS all decrease intestinal defenses.

Causes

There are many bacterial, viral, and parasitic causes of diarrheal diseases. Common causes of bacterial infection include *E. coli* and *Salmonella*, *Shigella*, *Campylobacter*, and *Yersinia* species. The most significant viral causes of diarrhea are *Rotavirus*, which commonly results in diarrhea in young children, and *Calicivirus* (often called *Norovirus*), a virus associated with outbreaks in long-term care facilities and cruise ships. Parasitic infections of importance include *Giardia* and *Cryptosporidium* species and *Entamoeba histolytica*.

Campylobacter Infections

Campylobacter species are the most frequent cause of diarrheal disease worldwide. The bacterium, which is abundant in animal foods, is especially common in poultry but can also be found in beef and pork. Direct person-to-person transmission appears to be less common than it is for other enteric pathogens, such as *Shigella*. Guillain-Barré syndrome, a serious neurologic disorder characterized by

CHART
70-5

PLAN OF NURSING CARE
Care of the Patient With an Infectious Disease

NURSING DIAGNOSIS: Risk for infection transmission
GOAL: Prevention of transmission of infectious agents

Nursing Interventions	Rationale	Expected Outcomes
1. Prevent patient-to-patient infection spread.	1. Organisms that are spread through an airborne route or are very contagious through direct contact can be transmitted in a health care setting.	• No evidence of patient-to-patient transmission of infection • No evidence of transmission via health care workers • No occupationally acquired infections in nurses and other health care workers • No evidence of transmission due to contaminated equipment • Absence of bacteremia, septicemia, and sepsis • Absence of urinary tract infections • Absence of pneumonia
a. Provide isolation according to CDC guidelines and Standard Precautions.	a. CDC isolation strategies are developed to reduce the likelihood of transmission from patient to patient.	

b. Ensure that patients with airborne infections remain in private rooms during hospital stay. If they must leave their rooms, arrangements should be made to decrease the likelihood of contact with other patients. Rooms should be ventilated according to CDC criteria. Personal protective equipment in the form of N95 respirators should be worn as indicated.
   The N95 respirator is the minimal level of personal protection for tuberculosis control. The "N" indicates the filter resistance to oil aerosols; and the "95" indicates that the respirator has 95% effectiveness in filtering test particles.
   In any care setting where patients may have increased risk for the sequelae of influenza, annual influenza vaccination should be encouraged for personnel and patients.
	b. Engineering controls are important in the prevention of airborne diseases. Influenza vaccine safely reduces risk of illness associated with this highly communicable, and frequently virulent, condition.	

c. Ensure that patients with highly transmissible, nonairborne organisms such as *Clostridium difficile* and *Shigella* species are physically separated from other patients if hygiene or institutional policy dictates.	c. Increased prevention strategies are needed when the organism has high epidemic potential.	
2. Prevent health care workers' transfer of organisms from patient to patient.	2. Transfer of organisms on the hands of health care workers is a common route of transmission. Hospital organisms colonizing the hands of health care workers may be virulent.	
a. Perform hand hygiene (by hand washing or by use of alcohol-based solution) consistently and thoroughly, disinfecting hands before and after each patient contact, and after procedures that offer contamination risk while caring for an individual patient.	a. Hand hygiene is important in reducing transient flora on outer epidermal layers of skin. Alcohol-based hand disinfectants are effective methods to reduce transient flora.	
b. Use gloves when handling any body fluid from any patient. Change gloves between patient care activities, and disinfect hands after gloves are removed.	b. Gloves provide effective barrier protection. Gloves quickly become contaminated and then become a potential vehicle for the transfer of organisms between patients. Microflora on hands are likely to proliferate while gloves are worn.	

Continued on following page

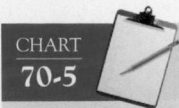

CHART 70-5

PLAN OF NURSING CARE
Care of the Patient With an Infectious Disease (Continued)

Nursing Interventions	Rationale	Expected Outcomes
c. Avoid wearing artificial fingernails or extenders when providing patient care. Keep natural nails less than ¼ inch long.	c. Artificial fingernails and extenders harbor microorganisms.	
d. Monitor the hand hygiene and glove use behaviors of health care professionals caring for the patient.	d. Poor compliance with hand hygiene among health care workers has been well documented and should be anticipated. It is important for the nurse as the patient's advocate to communicate protective behavior.	
3. Prevent patient-to-health care worker transmission of infection.	3. Health care workers may acquire infections occupationally due to close contact with patients.	
a. Avoid risk of infection with tuberculosis.	a. The most important element in the reduction of tuberculosis is early identification. Many of the symptoms of tuberculosis are subtle, and may be first observed by the nurse who has prolonged contact with the patient.	
(1) Participate in the early identification of patients with active disease. Patients will be asked about risk factors, symptoms, previous exposure, and tuberculin skin test (TST) status.	(1) Identification of patients at risk can help to prevent exposure.	
(2) Expedite diagnostic work-up with chest x-ray, sputum analysis for organisms, and TST administration as appropriate.	(2) Confirmation of diagnosis facilitates development of an appropriate treatment plan, including prevention of spread of infection.	
(3) Maintain engineering controls. Keep the patient in a private room with a closed door.	(3) Confining airflow to the immediate vicinity of the patient and exhausting air to the outside reduce the likelihood of transmission to health care workers in areas outside of the patient room.	
(4) Use protection in isolation room or when participating in procedures that are likely to generate cough, such as suctioning, intubation, or administering nebulized medications.	(4) N95 respirators are designed to reduce health care workers' risk.	
b. Avoid risk of transmission of blood-borne diseases such as hepatitis B, hepatitis C, and the human immunodeficiency virus.	b. Health care workers can contract blood-borne diseases via percutaneous injury such as needlestick or by contact with blood or body fluids to mucous membranes, such as eyes and mouth.	
(1) Get hepatitis B vaccination.	(1) Hepatitis B vaccine should be administered to reduce risk from this contagious blood-borne virus.	

Continued

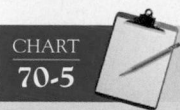

CHART
70-5

PLAN OF NURSING CARE
Care of the Patient With an Infectious Disease (Continued)

Nursing Interventions	Rationale	Expected Outcomes
(2) Use Standard Precautions as defined by the CDC.	(2) Standard Precautions are based on the recognition that most patients are not identified as infected by physical assessment or history taking. Health care workers must assume that all patients may be infected with bloodborne or other infection and must use barrier precautions appropriately for *all* patients.	
(3) Use "needleless" syringes and other injury-preventing devices.	(3) Use of injury-preventing devices decreases risk of transmission of blood-borne diseases.	
c. Avoid risk of airborne diseases. (1) Receive influenza vaccination annually. (2) Get vaccinated or produce proof of immunity to measles, mumps, rubella, and varicella.	c. Influenza vaccine is recommended for health care workers to reduce the likelihood of transmission in health care settings where immunocompromised patients can be exposed.	
4. Prevent patient exposure to contaminated medical equipment.	4. Technologic advances offer increased opportunity for invasive procedures. Equipment may be complex and difficult to clean.	
a. Ensure that equipment that is inserted through intact skin is sterilized between patient uses.	a. Sterilization renders equipment free of all microorganisms.	
b. Ensure that equipment that has contact with mucous membranes is sterilized or receives "high-level disinfection" between patient uses.	b. High-level disinfection renders an object free of all microorganisms with the possible exception of spore-producing organisms.	
c. Ensure that equipment used against intact skin is thoroughly cleaned and receives "low-level disinfection" between patient uses.	c. The disinfection goal for low-level disinfection is to reduce the load of microorganisms to a level that is not threatening to the host with intact skin.	
5. Follow established guidelines for the routine removal and replacement of intravenous devices.	5. Indwelling intravenous devices can serve as a conduit for organisms to migrate into the bloodstream.	
6. Remove urinary catheters at the earliest time possible.	6. The risk of urinary tract infections is directly proportional to the length of time that a urinary catheter remains in place.	
7. Remove endotracheal and nasogastric tubes as soon as possible.	7. The risk for pneumonia is increased as the use of indwelling equipment increases.	

NURSING DIAGNOSIS: Deficient knowledge about disease, cause of infection, and preventive measures
GOAL: Acquisition of knowledge about the infectious process

Nursing Interventions	Rationale	Expected Outcomes
1. Listen carefully to what the patient says about illness and previous treatment.	1. Listening facilitates detection of misunderstanding and misinformation and provides opportunity for education.	• Patient actively participates in treatment • Patient complies with infection control measures
2. Provide pertinent explanations about: a. Organism and route of transmission b. Treatment goals c. Follow-up schedule d. Prevention of transmission to others	2. Knowledge about specific diagnoses and treatments may increase compliance.	
3. Allow opportunities for questions and discussions.	3. The patient's questions indicate issues that need clarification.	

Continued on following page

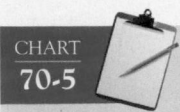

CHART
70-5

PLAN OF NURSING CARE
Care of the Patient With an Infectious Disease (Continued)

Nursing Interventions	Rationale	Expected Outcomes

4. Teach the patient and family about:
  a. Prophylaxis or immunization, if recommended
  b. Community resources, if necessary
  c. Means of preventing transmission within the home
	4. Understanding of the risks and precautions associated with an infectious disease may reduce the opportunity for further spread.	

NURSING DIAGNOSIS: Risk for imbalanced body temperature (fever) related to the presence of infection
GOAL: Patient comfort and return of normal temperature

Nursing Interventions	Rationale	Expected Outcomes
1. Monitor temperature, pulse, and respirations at regular intervals. 2. Administer antipyretics as prescribed.	1. Graph fever curve to help evaluate when fever occurs, how long it lasts, and whether it responds to therapy. 2. Prompt treatment will improve outcomes.	• Body temperature within normal limits • Maintenance of fluid and electrolyte balance • Patient comfortable

COLLABORATIVE PROBLEMS: Among potential complications are septicemia, bacteremia, or sepsis, septic shock, dehydration, abscess formation, endocarditis, infectious disease–related cancers, and infertility
GOAL: Absence of complications

Nursing Interventions	Rationale	Expected Outcomes
Septicemia, Bacteremia, Sepsis 1. Monitor patient for evidence of infection at any location. 2. Assess treatment effectiveness of all identified infections. 3. Administer antibiotics as prescribed with first dose given at the earliest time possible.	1. Vigilance for bacterial or fungal infection at any site promotes early recognition and treatment and reduces the likelihood of secondary infections. 2. The natural course of some infections may be rapid unless antibiotics are administered promptly. 3. Prompt treatment will improve outcomes.	• No episode of infection • Effective treatment of identified bacterial and fungal infections without progression to bloodstream infection • Early improvement in septic course

Septic Shock
1. Routinely, and as warranted, monitor vital signs for patients with recognized infections and severely immunosuppressed patients at risk for shock. In particular, be alert for signs of:
  a. Fever
  b. Tachycardia (more than 90 bpm)
  c. Tachypnea (more than 20 breaths/min)
  d. Evidence of decreased perfusion or dysfunction of vital organs in the form of
    (1) Change of mental status
    (2) Hypoxemia as measured by arterial blood gases
    (3) Elevated lactate levels
    (4) Urine output (less than 30 mL/h)
2. Administer antibiotics, fluid replacement, vasopressors, and oxygen as prescribed.
	1. Early recognition of the signs and prompt treatment of impending shock may reduce the associated severity or mortality.
	
	2. Therapeutic maintenance of hemodynamic and respiratory status is necessary until infection is effectively treated with antimicrobial regimen.
		• Absence of symptoms of septic shock
		• Hemodynamic and respiratory status within normal range

Dehydration 1. Assess for dehydration (thirst, dryness of mucous membranes, loss of skin turgor, reduced peripheral pulses, urine output less than 30 mL/h). 2. Monitor weight.	1. Signs of dehydration provide a basis for fluid replacement and suggest possible further complications of circulatory collapse. 2. Rapid changes in weight indicate fluid volume changes.	• Attains fluid balance (output approximates intake: body weight unchanged) • Mucous membranes appear moist; normal skin turgor • Serum electrolytes are within normal limits

Continued

CHART
70-5

PLAN OF NURSING CARE
Care of the Patient With an Infectious Disease (Continued)

Nursing Interventions	Rationale	Expected Outcomes
3. Monitor intake and output and serum electrolyte levels.	3. Dehydration produces a deficit in some electrolytes. Decreased urine production may indicate hypovolemia and decreased renal perfusion.	
4. Replace fluids as needed. If the patient can tolerate oral fluids, offer fluids every 2–4 hours. Administer intravenous fluids as prescribed.	4. When possible, oral hydration is preferable because the patient can select the beverage, control the rate and interval of replacement, and care for self at home. Additionally, the risks associated with vascular devices are avoided. If intravenous fluid is required, intravenous solutions are selected to facilitate intestinal reabsorption of fluid and electrolytes.	

Abscess Formation

1. Assess vascular access sites, wound sites, pressure ulcers, and other appropriate sites for apparent collections of purulent material.	1. Collections of purulent material often require drainage before antimicrobial therapy is effective.	• Absence of abscess • Takes antibiotics as prescribed
2. Assess the patient who has had abdominal surgery or trauma to abdominal area for localized signs of intra-abdominal abscess. These signs include: a. Low-grade fever b. Elevated peripheral white blood cell count c. Localized pain d. Abdominal tenderness e. Visible or palpable mass f. Postoperative diarrhea g. GI bleeding	2. Intra-abdominal abscess formation is most common following traumatic or surgical disruption of the GI tract. Signs are often initially subtle.	
3. Assess patient who has had percutaneous abscess drainage to determine whether drainage has been successful. Be alert for all of the above signs and symptoms.	3. After percutaneous drainage, recurrent or persistent signs of abscess may indicate the need for surgical treatment.	
4. Administer antibiotics as prescribed.	4. Antibiotics, along with drainage, are the most important elements of intra-abdominal abscess management.	

Endocarditis
Prevention

1. Teach patients with the following conditions about the importance of antibiotic prophylaxis for events and procedures that may introduce the risk of endocarditis: a. Valvular disease b. Congenital heart disease c. Intracardiac prosthesis d. Previous endocarditis	1. Patients with underlying valvular disease and other cardiac abnormalities are at increased risk for "seeding" of the cardiac valves during procedures that can cause bacteremia.	• Informs health care professionals of cardiac conditions that require antibiotic prophylaxis before invasive procedures • Takes prophylactic antibiotics as prescribed

Management

1. Obtain blood cultures as prescribed; carefully record results. Note persistent bloodstream infections with a particular organism.	1. A definitive diagnosis of endocarditis requires blood culture confirmation.	• Endocarditis is diagnosed, treated, and cured
2. Obtain a detailed history about the duration of fever in the absence of well-recognized cause.	2. Endocarditis should be suspected in patients who report an unexplained fever of more than 1 week's duration	

Continued on following page

CHART
70-5

PLAN OF NURSING CARE
Care of the Patient With an Infectious Disease (Continued)

Nursing Interventions	Rationale	Expected Outcomes
3. Administer intravenous antibiotic therapy at prescribed time schedule.	3. Intravenous therapy is usually required for cure. The goal of therapy is complete eradication of all organisms. Careful adherence to following the scheduled administration is therefore essential.	

Infectious Disease-Related Cancers and Infertility

These potential complications of infectious diseases are prevented by primary avoidance of infection. Management of them is directed toward treating each of them as a noninfectious entity. For example, the management of cancer secondary to hepatitis B is handled as an oncology issue, not as an infectious disease issue.

temporary paralysis, is a complication of approximately 1 of 1000 cases of *Campylobacter* infection.

Cooking and storing food at appropriate temperatures protects against *Campylobacter*. It is important that kitchen utensils used in meat preparation be kept away from other food to prevent *Campylobacter* transmission.

After a person is infected, the bacterium directly attacks the lumen of the intestine and may cause disease through enterotoxin release. Symptoms can range from mild abdominal cramping and minimal diarrhea to severe disease with profuse watery bloody diarrhea and debilitating abdominal cramping. Antimicrobial therapy is recommended only for patients who are seriously ill (CDC, 2005d).

Salmonella Infection

Salmonella is a gram-negative bacillus with many species, including the very pathogenic *Salmonella typhi* (ie, typhoid fever). Of the nontyphi species, most organisms are prevalent in animal food sources. *Salmonella* species contaminate over 30% of commercially available chicken products and are frequently found in eggs (intact and with broken shells), in turkeys, and occasionally in beef (U.S. Department of Agriculture [USDA], 2008). Most of the deaths caused by *Salmonella* enteritis occur in elderly nursing home residents because of their weakened immune systems (CDC, 2005d).

Variable symptoms are associated with *Salmonella* species infection, including an asymptomatic carrier state, gastroenteritis, and systemic infection. Diarrhea with gastroenteritis is common. Disseminated disease and bacteremia, sometimes accompanied by diarrhea, occur less often.

The person with *Salmonella*-caused diarrhea can on rare occasions be a source for transmission to others. The importance of good hygiene should be emphasized, and health care workers should use special care when handling bedpans, stool specimens, or other objects that may be contaminated with feces. Hand hygiene is imperative after any contact with a person with *Salmonella* diarrhea. Although patients with systemic salmonellosis require antimicrobial therapy, those with gastroenteritis only are not usually treated, because antibiotic use may increase the period of time that the patient carries the bacteria while not improving the clinical outcome.

Shigella Infection

The *Shigella* species is a gram-negative organism that invades the lumen of the intestine and causes disease and severe watery (possibly bloody) diarrhea. *Shigella* species are spread through the fecal–oral route, with easy transmission from one person to another. *Shigella* exhibits high levels of **virulence** (degree of pathogenicity of an organism); infection with a very small number of organisms can cause disease. Because transmission occurs easily with improper hygiene, it is not surprising that *Shigella* organisms disproportionately affect pediatric populations. Disease in the very young may infrequently be complicated by pulmonary or neurologic symptoms.

Antimicrobial therapy should be instituted early. Frequently, initial therapy choices must be altered when final microbiologic testing reveals the organism's sensitivity.

Escherichia coli

E. coli is the most common aerobic organism colonizing the large bowel. When *E. coli* bacteria are cultured from fecal specimens, the results usually reflect normal flora. However, certain strains of *E. coli* with increased virulence have been responsible for significant outbreaks of diarrheal disease in recent years. These stronger pathologic strains are subgrouped as enterotoxigenic *E. coli* (ETEC) because of their production of enterotoxins. ETEC strains often cause cholera-like disease, with rapid, severe dehydration and an increased risk of death.

Several outbreaks of an *E. coli* species, 0157:H7, have been linked to the ingestion of undercooked beef and to vegetables that have been contaminated by animal waste water. This bacterium lives in the intestines of cattle and can be introduced into meat at the time of slaughter. Prevention of disease from *E. coli* 0157:H7 is aimed at teaching the public to cook ground beef thoroughly (ie, until the meat is no longer pink and the juices run clear). During an important outbreak of *E. coli* 0157:H7 that resulted from contaminated spinach in 2006, spinach from an implicated packager was recalled. Consumers were advised to boil or fry fresh spinach if there was a concern that it might be from the contaminated area (CDC, 2006c).

Calicivirus (Norwalk-like Virus; Norovirus)

Calicivirus, which is often referred to as the Norwalk-like virus or the *Norovirus*, is a very common cause of foodborne illness. This agent has been associated with important diarrheal outbreaks in long-term care facilities, hospitals, and cruise ships. Onset of illness is usually acute, with vomiting and watery diarrhea that generally last for approximately 2 days. Dehydration is the most common complication.

Calicivirus is transmitted easily from person to person by direct contact and by ingesting contaminated food. Waterborne outbreaks have been associated with sewage-contaminated wells and contaminated swimming pools. Although people with *Calicivirus* infection typically recover within 2 to 3 days, they may continue to transmit the virus to others for approximately 2 more weeks.

Caliciviruses can withstand environmental extremes of heat or cold and are resistant to chemical disinfection, which are significant reasons for their epidemic potential. Control of *Calicivirus* in health care facilities requires a co-ordinated program with decisions about isolation, environmental disinfection, diagnosis, and coordination with public health officials. Contact Precautions should be used when caring for patients with incontinence and during outbreaks of the virus. Workers should wear masks if they are cleaning heavily soiled areas or caring for a patient who is actively vomiting. No Environmental Protection Agency (EPA)–approved disinfectants have specific claims about effectiveness for *Calicivirus*. Therefore, the CDC recommends that surface disinfection be accomplished with a freshly prepared solution of 1 part bleach to 50 parts water or with the peroxygen compound Virkon-S, which has been approved for feline *Calicivirus* and may be similarly effective for human viruses (CDC, 2005d).

Giardia Lamblia

Transmission of the protozoan *Giardia lamblia* occurs when food or drink is contaminated with viable cysts of the organism. People often become infected while traveling to endemic areas or by drinking contaminated water from mountain streams within the United States. The organism can be transmitted by close contact, such as occurs in day care settings. Transmission by sexual contact has also been documented.

Frequently, the infection goes unnoticed. Infection is often recognized more easily in children than in adults. In extreme cases, the patient may experience abdominal pain and chronic diarrhea, usually described as containing mucus and fat but not blood. Microscopic examination of stool specimens reveals the trophozoite or cyst stages of the parasitic life cycle.

Metronidazole (Flagyl) is commonly used to treat *Giardia*, but success rates for this and alternative therapies are inconsistent. Patients with *Giardia* infections should be instructed that the organism can be easily transmitted in family or group settings. Personal hygiene measures should be reinforced, and those who travel or camp where water is not treated and filtered should be advised to avoid local water supplies unless water is purified before drinking or using it in cooking.

Vibrio Cholerae

Although reported cases of cholera have been rare in the United States in recent decades, no discussion of infectious diarrhea is complete without mention of this very serious infectious disease. Historically, epidemics of cholera have influenced all aspects of life—from medical to political—and infection rates have been significant enough to destroy governments and armies. Cholera is always a concern when wars or natural disasters result in inadequately processed waste water. *Vibrio cholerae* also may be found naturally in brackish rivers and coastal waters.

V. cholerae is a gram-negative organism with several different serotypes. The type usually associated with epidemics is toxigenic *V. cholerae* 01. The organism is transmitted by contaminated food or water. Most recent cases in the United States have been from contaminated shellfish found in the Gulf of Mexico or from contaminated shellfish brought into the United States by visitors. However, even though the incidence in other *Vibrio* species increased in the aftermath of Hurricane Katrina, in 2005, there were no cases of toxigenic *V. cholerae* 01 reported (CDC, 2005f).

Cholera causes disease with a very rapid onset of copious diarrhea in which up to 1 L of fluid per hour can be lost. Dehydration, with subsequent cardiopulmonary collapse, may cause rapid progression from onset of signs and symptoms to death. Rehydration efforts should be vigorous and sustained. If oral rehydration cannot be accomplished, the patient needs IV therapy.

In the United States, cholera should be suspected in patients who have watery diarrhea after eating shellfish harvested from the Gulf of Mexico. Confirmation of the causative organism can be made by stool culture. It is imperative that all cases are reported to local and state public health authorities. People traveling to areas where cholera occurs regularly should remember the simple rule of thumb: "boil it, cook it, peel it, or forget it."

NURSING PROCESS

THE PATIENT WITH INFECTIOUS DIARRHEA

Assessment

The most important element of assessment in the patient with diarrhea is to determine hydration status. The goal of rehydration is to correct the dehydration. Assessment includes evaluation for thirst, dryness of oral mucous membranes, sunken eyes, a weakened pulse, and loss of skin turgor. Careful observation for these signs is especially important in cases of rapidly dehydrating diseases (most notably cholera) and in younger children.

Intake and output measurements are crucial in determining fluid balance. Liquid stool should be measured and recorded, along with the frequency of stools. It is important to note the consistency and appearance of stool as key indicators of the type and severity of the diarrheal disease. The presence of mucus or blood should also be documented.

When conducting a health history, the nurse asks if the patient has recently traveled, if the patient is being treated with antibiotics, if the patient has been in contact with anyone who has recently had diarrheal disease, and what the patient has recently eaten. Frequently, patients attribute the most recent meal eaten as the cause of symptoms. However, the incubation period for most diarrheal conditions is longer than the time interval between meals, and the nurse needs to get detailed information about the meal preceding the illness and about all food intake in the previous 3 to 4 days. When eliciting this kind of history, it is helpful to ask the patient to list every food tasted. The nurse also asks the patient if he or she is employed in a food preparation service, because the local public health departments should be notified about any person with infectious diarrhea who works in the food industry.

Diagnosis

Nursing Diagnoses

Based on the assessment data, the patient's major nursing diagnoses may include the following:

- Deficient fluid volume related to fluid lost through diarrhea
- Deficient knowledge about the infection and the risk of transmission to others

Collaborative Problems/Potential Complications

Based on the assessment data, potential complications that may develop include the following:

- Bacteremia
- Hypovolemic shock

Planning and Goals

The most important goals are maintenance of fluid and electrolyte balance, increased knowledge about the disease and risk of transmission, and absence of complications.

Nursing Interventions

Correcting Dehydration Associated With Diarrhea

The patient is assessed to determine the degree of dehydration and the amount and route of rehydration needed. Oral rehydration therapy is a strategy used to reduce the severe complications of diarrheal disease regardless of causative agent. It is inexpensive and effective for most patients, but it is often underused because of cultural beliefs discouraging oral intake during episodes of diarrhea. The World Health Organization (WHO) and the United Nations International Children's Emergency Fund (UNICEF) recommend an oral rehydration solution (ORS) for the treatment of children and adults with dehydration and electrolyte imbalance associated with cholera and other forms of diarrheal disease. It contains (in millimoles per liter) sodium, 90; potassium, 20; chloride, 80; citrate, 10; and glucose, 111.

MILD DEHYDRATION. The patient exhibits dry oral mucous membranes of the mouth and increased thirst. The rehydration goal at this level of dehydration is to deliver about 50 mL of ORS per 1 kg of weight over a 4-hour interval.

MODERATE DEHYDRATION. Common findings are sunken eyes, loss of skin turgor, increased thirst, and dry oral mucous membranes. The rehydration goal at this level of dehydration is to deliver about 100 mL/kg of ORS over 4 hours.

SEVERE DEHYDRATION. The patient with severe dehydration shows signs of shock (ie, rapid thready pulse, cyanosis, cold extremities, rapid breathing, lethargy, or coma) and should receive IV replacement until hemodynamic and

mental status return to normal. When improvement is evident, the patient can be treated with ORS.

Administering Rehydration Therapy

Because diarrheal episodes are often accompanied by vomiting, rehydration and refeeding can be difficult. Oral rehydration therapy should be delivered frequently in small amounts. When patients are persistently vomiting, they often require frequent administration of fluids by spoonfuls. IV therapy is necessary for the patient who is severely dehydrated or in shock.

It is important for children and adults with acute diarrheal symptoms to maintain caloric intake. As soon as dehydration has been corrected, an age-appropriate, unrestricted diet is allowed. Recommended foods include starches, cereals, yogurt, fruits, and vegetables. Foods that are high in simple sugars, such as undiluted apple juice or gelatin, should be avoided.

 NURSING ALERT

Sports drinks do not replace fluid losses correctly and should not be used.

Increasing Knowledge and Preventing Spread of Infection

Public health nurses, school nurses, and others who are involved in patient teaching should emphasize principles of safe food preparation, with special attention to meat preparation and cooking. Ground beef should be cooked until no longer pink, and all meat should be maintained at temperatures below 40°F or above 140°F. In planning events for groups of people, adequate provision for storage and reheating to temperature thresholds is important. When preparing food, it is important to use different surfaces, knives, and other equipment for meat and nonmeat items.

Diarrheal diseases discussed in this section must be reported to local or state health departments. The goal of reporting is to provide information for determining incidence trends and promptly identifying any restaurants or other food preparation establishments that have served contaminated food.

The need for rehydration and refeeding should be taught to parents of children with diarrheal disease. Beliefs about illness and food patterns may have a traditional or cultural basis, and any teaching of health facts requires cultural sensitivity.

In both homes and health care delivery settings, good hygiene and principles of Standard Precautions should be emphasized.

Monitoring and Managing Potential Complications

BACTEREMIA. E. coli, Salmonella, and Shigella are organisms that can enter the bloodstream and disseminate to other organs. Blood cultures are necessary in the acutely febrile patient with diarrhea. If initial smear results reveal gram-negative organisms, antibiotic therapy is instituted.

HYPOVOLEMIC SHOCK. Shock associated with diarrheal diseases demands accurate intake and output assessment and vigorous fluid replacement. In rare instances, patients with severe fluid imbalance require intensive care nursing support with aggressive hemodynamic monitoring. For further information, see Chapter 15.

Evaluation

Expected Patient Outcomes

Expected patient outcomes may include the following:

1. Attains fluid balance
   a. Output approximates intake
   b. Mucous membranes appear moist
   c. Skin turgor is normal
   d. Adequate amounts of fluids and calories ingested
   e. Absence of vomiting
   f. Stools are of normal color and consistency
2. Acquires knowledge and understanding about infectious diarrhea and transmission potential
   a. Takes proper precautions to prevent spread of infection to others
   b. Describes principles and techniques of safe food storage, preparation, and cooking
3. Absence of complications
   a. Temperature is within normal range
   b. Blood culture reports are negative
   c. Fluid balance is achieved

Sexually Transmitted Diseases

An STD (also known as a sexually transmitted infection [STI]) is a disease acquired through sexual contact with an infected person. Table 70-4 identifies diseases that can be classified as STDs. Infections caused by organisms not generally considered STDs can also be transmitted during sexual contact; for example, G. lamblia, usually associated with contaminated water, can be transmitted through sexual exposure.

STDs are the most common infectious diseases in the United States and are epidemic in most parts of the world. Portals of entry of STD-causing microorganisms and sites of

Table 70-4 CONDITIONS CLASSIFIED AS SEXUALLY TRANSMITTED DISEASES (STDS) AND THEIR ROUTES OF TRANSMISSION

Disease	Route(s) of Transmission
Chancroid, *Lymphogranuloma venereum*, and *Granuloma inguinale*	Sexual
Chlamydia	Sexual
Cytomegalovirus (CMV)	Sexual, less intimate contact
Gonorrhea	Sexual, perinatal
Hepatitis B (HBV)	Sexual, percutaneous, perinatal
Hepatitis C (HCV)	Percutaneous, probably sexual, probably perinatal
Herpes simplex	Sexual
HIV infection/AIDS	Sexual, percutaneous, perinatal
Human papillomavirus (HPV)	Sexual
Syphilis	Sexual, perinatal

infection include the skin and mucosal linings of the urethra, cervix, vagina, rectum, and oropharynx.

Approximately 19 million Americans become infected with STDs annually. STDs have severe health consequences. In addition, they represent a financial burden estimated to be as high as $15.3 billion per year (CDC, 2009e). To determine the most effective methods for communicating information about STDs to people between 25 and 45 years of age (those who are most at risk for STDS), the CDC sought the help of focus groups. These groups proposed that using straightforward language and personal testimonials, developing materials for targeted audiences (eg, people who want information about protecting themselves), and conducting presentations in trusted establishments (eg, churches, health care facilities) might be effective. These suggestions could serve as a resource to all health care personnel who specialize in the prevention of STDs (CDC, 2004c).

Education about prevention of STDs includes information about risk factors and behaviors that can lead to infection. Included in this education is information about the relative value of condoms in reducing risk of infection. The use of condoms to provide a protective barrier from transmission of STD-related organisms has been broadly promoted, especially since the recognition of HIV/AIDS. At first referred to as a method to ensure *safe sex*, the use of condoms has been shown to reduce but not eliminate the risk of transmission of HIV and other STDs. Thus, the term *safer sex* more appropriately connotes the public health message to be used when promoting the use of condoms.

STDs provide a unique set of challenges for nurses, physicians, and public health officials. Because of perceived stigma and possible threat to emotional relationships, people with symptoms of STDs are often reluctant to seek health care in a timely fashion. STDs may progress without symptoms and a delay in diagnosis and treatment is potentially harmful because the risk of complications for the infected person and the risk of transmission to others increase over time.

Infection with one STD suggests the possibility of infection with other diseases as well. After one STD is identified, diagnostic evaluation for others should be conducted. The possibility of HIV infection should be pursued when any STD is diagnosed.

HUMAN IMMUNODEFICIENCY VIRUS

HIV is the causative agent of AIDS. The definition of AIDS, as determined by the CDC, sets a point in the continuum of HIV pathogenesis in which the host has clinically demonstrated profound immune dysfunction. Since 1993, the AIDS definition has also included a CD4-positive (CD4+) cell count of less than 200 cells/mm^3 as a threshold criterion. CD4+ cells are a subset of lymphocytes and one of the targets of HIV infection. Many opportunistic infections and neoplasms occur with severe immunosuppression.

HIV is transmitted through sexual contact or percutaneous injection of contaminated blood or from infected mother to fetus. Most people infected by the percutaneous route are IV or injecting drug users who share contaminated needles, but transmission is also remotely possible through contaminated blood transfusion. Since 1985, all blood transfusions have been screened, and transfusion-related transmission of HIV is now extremely unlikely. Additional information about HIV is provided in Chapter 52.

Risk to Health Care Workers

Health care workers can be infected through the percutaneous route if needlestick or other injury from a sharp object introduces contaminated blood. Prospective studies of this risk demonstrate that less than 1% of occupational exposures in which the source patient is infected with HIV lead to transmission (CDC, 2005e). Despite the rarity of transmission, health care workers are advised to use extreme care to avoid needlestick or mucous membrane exposure to blood from all patients.

In health care facilities, employers are required to provide devices designed to reduce the risk of needlestick and other injuries. Health care workers should understand the need to report a needlestick or other percutaneous exposure immediately. Since 1996, the CDC has recommended postexposure prophylaxis (PEP) for significant occupational exposures to HIV (further discussion of PEP is provided in Chapter 52). Counseling about the advisability of prophylaxis, appropriate combination of drugs, and dosing is made on a case-by-case basis.

SYPHILIS

Syphilis is an acute and chronic infectious disease caused by the spirochete *Treponema pallidum*. It is acquired through sexual contact or may be congenital in origin.

Stages of Syphilis

In the untreated person, the course of syphilis can be divided into three stages: primary, secondary, and tertiary. These stages reflect the time from infection and the clinical manifestations observed in that period and are the basis for treatment decisions.

Primary syphilis occurs 2 to 3 weeks after initial inoculation with the organism. A painless lesion at the site of infection is called a *chancre*. Untreated, these lesions usually resolve spontaneously within about 2 months.

Secondary syphilis occurs when the hematogenous spread of organisms from the original chancre leads to generalized infection. The rash of secondary syphilis occurs about 2 to 8 weeks after the chancre and involves the trunk and the extremities, including the palms of the hands and the soles of the feet. Transmission of the organism can occur through contact with these lesions. Generalized signs of infection may include lymphadenopathy, arthritis, meningitis, hair loss, fever, malaise, and weight loss.

After the secondary stage, there is a period of **latency,** when the infected person has no signs or symptoms of syphilis. Latency can be interrupted by a recurrence of secondary syphilis symptoms.

Tertiary syphilis is the final stage in the natural history of the disease. It is estimated that between 20% and 40% of those infected do not exhibit signs and symptoms in this final stage. Tertiary syphilis presents as a slowly progressive inflammatory disease with the potential to affect multiple organs. The most common manifestations at this level are aortitis and neurosyphilis, as evidenced by dementia, psychosis, paresis, stroke, or meningitis.

Assessment and Diagnostic Findings

Because syphilis shares symptoms with many diseases, clinical history and laboratory evaluation are important. The conclusive diagnosis of syphilis can be made by direct identification of the spirochete obtained from the chancre lesions of primary syphilis. Serologic tests used in the diagnosis of secondary and tertiary syphilis require clinical correlation in interpretation. The serologic tests are summarized as follows:

- *Nontreponemal* or *reagin tests*, such as the Venereal Disease Research Laboratory (VDRL) or the rapid plasma reagin circle card test (RPR-CT), are generally used for screening and diagnosis. After adequate therapy, the test result is expected to decrease quantitatively until it is read as negative, usually about 2 years after therapy is completed.
- *Treponemal tests*, such as the fluorescent treponemal antibody absorption test (FTA-ABS) and the microhemagglutination test (MHA-TP), are used to verify that the screening test did not represent a false-positive result. Positive results usually are positive for life and therefore are not appropriate to determine therapeutic effectiveness.

Medical Management

Treatment of all stages of syphilis is administration of antibiotics. Penicillin G benzathine is the medication of choice for early syphilis or early latent syphilis of less than 1 year's duration. It is administered by intramuscular injection at a single session. Patients with late latent or latent syphilis of unknown duration should receive three injections at 1-week intervals. Patients who are allergic to penicillin are usually treated with doxycycline (Adoxa). The patient treated with penicillin is monitored for 30 minutes after the injection to observe for a possible allergic reaction.

Treatment guidelines established by the CDC are updated on a regular basis. Recommendations provide special guidelines for treatment in the setting of pregnancy, allergy, HIV infection, pediatric infection, congenital infection, and neurosyphilis (CDC, 2006b).

Nursing Management

Syphilis is a reportable communicable disease. In any health care facility, a mechanism must be in place to ensure that all diagnosed patients are reported to the state or local public health department to ensure community follow-up. The public health department is responsible for identification of sexual contacts, contact notification, and contact screening.

Lesions of primary and secondary syphilis may be highly infective. Gloves are worn when direct contact with lesions is likely, and hand hygiene is performed after gloves are removed. Isolation in a private room is not required (Chart 70-6).

CHLAMYDIA TRACHOMATIS AND NEISSERIA GONORRHOEAE INFECTIONS

Chlamydia trachomatis and *Neisseria gonorrhoeae* are the most commonly reported infectious diseases in the United States. Coinfection with *C. trachomatis* often occurs in patients infected with *N. gonorrhoeae*. The greatest risk of *C. trachomatis* infection occurs in young women between 15 and 19 years of age (CDC, 2007b).

Clinical Manifestations

Women

Both *C. trachomatis* and *N. gonorrhoeae* infections frequently do not cause symptoms in women. When symptoms are present, mucopurulent cervicitis with exudates in the endocervical canal is the most frequent finding. Women with gonorrhea can also present with symptoms of urinary tract infection or vaginitis.

Men

Although men are more likely than women to have symptoms when infected, infection with *N. gonorrhoeae* or *C. trachomatis* can be asymptomatic. When symptoms are present, they may include burning during urination and penile discharge. Patients with *N. gonorrhoeae* infection may also report painful, swollen testicles.

Complications

In women, pelvic inflammatory disease (PID), ectopic pregnancy, endometritis, and infertility are possible complications of either *N. gonorrhoeae* or *C. trachomatis* infection. In men, epididymitis, a painful disease that may lead to infertility, may result from infection with either bacterium. In people of either gender, arthritis or bloodstream infection may be caused by *N. gonorrhoeae*.

Assessment and Diagnostic Findings

The patient is assessed for fever, discharge (urethral, vaginal, or rectal), and signs of arthritis. Diagnostic methods used in *N. gonorrhoeae* infection include Gram stain (appropriate only for male urethral samples), culture, and nucleic acid amplification tests (NAATs). Gram stain and the direct fluorescent antibody test can be used in chlamydia. NAATs are also available for *C. trachomatis* but demand strict attention to laboratory procedures to ensure test reliability. In the female patient, samples are obtained from the endocervix, anal canal, and pharynx. In the male patient, specimens are obtained from the urethra, anal canal, and pharynx. Because *N. gonorrhoeae* organisms are susceptible to environmental changes, specimens for culture must be delivered to the laboratory immediately after they are obtained.

Because as many as 70% of chlamydial infections are asymptomatic, the CDC recommends annual *Chlamydia* testing for all pregnant women, sexually active women younger than 25 years of age, and older women with a new sexual partner or multiple partners (CDC, 2006b).

Medical Management

Because patients are often coinfected with both gonorrhea and chlamydia, the CDC recommends dual therapy even if only gonorrhea has been laboratory proven. The CDC-recommended treatment for chlamydia is either doxycycline or azithromycin (Zithromax) and one of the following for gonorrhea: ceftriaxone (Rocephin), cefixime (Suprax), or ciprofloxacin (Cipro). These antibiotics are not recommended during pregnancy. CDC guidelines should be used to determine alternative therapy for the patient who is pregnant or allergic or who has a complicated chlamydial infection.

Patients with uncomplicated gonorrhea who are treated with CDC-recommended therapy do not routinely need to return for a proof-of-cure visit. If the patient reports a new episode of symptoms or tests are positive for gonorrhea again, the most likely explanation is reinfection rather than treatment failure. Serologic testing for syphilis and HIV should be offered to patients with gonorrhea or chlamydia, because any STD increases the risk of other STD infections.

Nursing Management

Gonorrhea and chlamydia are reportable communicable diseases. In any health care facility, a mechanism should be in place to ensure that all diagnosed patients are reported to the local public health department to ensure follow-up of the patient. The public health department also is responsible for interviewing the patient to identify sexual contacts, so that contact notification and screening can be initiated.

The target group for preventive patient teaching about gonorrhea and chlamydia is the adolescent and young adult population. Along with reinforcing the importance of abstinence, when appropriate, education should address postponing the age of initial sexual exposure, limiting the number of sexual partners, and using condoms for barrier protection. Young women and pregnant women should also be instructed about the importance of routine screening for chlamydia.

NURSING PROCESS

THE PATIENT WITH A SEXUALLY TRANSMITTED DISEASE

Assessment

The patient should be asked to describe the onset and progression of symptoms and to characterize any lesions by location and by describing drainage, if present. Brief explanations of why the information is needed are often helpful. Clarification of terms may be necessary if either the patient or nurse uses words that are unfamiliar to the other.

Protecting confidentiality is important when discussing sexual issues. When a detailed sexual history is necessary, it is important to respect the patient's right to privacy. When obtaining a sexual history, the CDC recommends the following systematic interview of key areas, the five Ps: partners, prevention of pregnancy, protection from STDs, practices, past history of STDs (CDC, 2006b).

Asking specific information about sexual contacts usually should be done only when the nurse is part of a team that will conduct partner notification. The nurse should describe to the patient the public health notification process and resources that are available to assist sexual partners or infants and children.

During the physical examination, the examiner looks for rashes, lesions, drainage, discharge, or swelling. Inguinal nodes are palpated to elicit tenderness and to assess swelling. Women are examined for abdominal or uterine tenderness. The mouth and throat are examined for signs of inflammation or exudate. The nurse wears gloves while examining the mucous membranes, and gloves are changed and replaced after vaginal or rectal examination.

Diagnosis

Nursing Diagnoses

Based on assessment data, the patient's major nursing diagnoses may include the following:

- Deficient knowledge about the disease and risk for spread of infection and reinfection
- Anxiety related to anticipated stigmatization and to prognosis and complications
- Noncompliance with treatment

Collaborative Problems/Potential Complications

Based on assessment data, potential complications that may develop include the following:
- Increased risk for ectopic pregnancy
- Infertility
- Transmission of infection to fetus, resulting in congenital abnormalities and other outcomes
- Neurosyphilis
- Gonococcal meningitis
- Gonococcal arthritis
- Syphilitic aortitis
- HIV-related complications

Planning and Goals

Major goals are increased patient understanding of the natural history and treatment of the infection, reduction in anxiety, increased compliance with therapeutic and preventive goals, and absence of complications.

Nursing Interventions

Increasing Knowledge and Preventing Spread of Disease

Education about STDs and prevention of the spread to others is often accomplished simultaneously. The infected patient should be told what the causative organism is and

should receive an explanation of the usual course of the infection (including the interval of potential communicability to others) and possible complications. The nurse should stress the importance of following therapy as prescribed and the need to report any side effects or symptom progression.

Discussion should emphasize that the same behaviors that led to infection with one STD increase the risk for any other STD, including HIV. Methods used to contact sexual partners should be discussed. The patient should understand that until the partner has been treated, continued sexual exposure to the same person may lead to reinfection. The relative value of condoms in reducing the risk for infection with STDs should be addressed. When appropriate, the patient should be encouraged to discuss any reasons for resistance to condom use to promote thoughtful decision making about this preventive method.

Reducing Anxiety

When appropriate, the patient is encouraged to discuss anxieties and fear associated with the diagnosis, treatment, or prognosis. By individualizing teaching efforts, factual information applied to specific needs may offer reassurance. Patients may need help in planning discussion with partners. If the patient is especially apprehensive about this aspect, referral to a social worker or other specialist may be appropriate. For example, such support is especially important when the patient has newly diagnosed HIV infection. Patients with HIV may benefit from programs that combine support, education, counseling, and therapeutic goals. Such programs are designed to offer coordinated care throughout the course of disease progression.

Increasing Compliance

In group settings (eg, an outpatient obstetric setting) or in a one-to-one setting, open discussion about STD information facilitates patient teaching. Discomfort can be reduced by factual explanation of causes, consequences, treatments, prevention, and responsibilities. Because most communities have expanded STD prevention resources, referrals to appropriate agencies can complement individual educational efforts and ensure that later questions or uncertainties can be addressed by experts. Patients can obtain more information by accessing the CDC Web site (2009c).

Monitoring and Managing Potential Complications

INFERTILITY AND INCREASED RISK OF ECTOPIC PREGNANCY. STDs may lead to PID and, with it, increased risk of ectopic pregnancy and infertility. For additional information, see Chapters 46 and 47.

CONGENITAL INFECTIONS. All STDs can be transmitted to infants in utero or at the time of birth. Complications of congenital infection can range from localized infection (eg, throat infection with N. gonorrhoeae), to congenital abnormalities (eg, stunting of growth or deafness from congenital syphilis), to life-threatening disease (eg, congenital herpes simplex virus).

NEUROSYPHILIS, GONOCOCCAL MENINGITIS, GONOCOCCAL ARTHRITIS, AND SYPHILITIC AORTITIS. STDs can cause disseminated infection. The central nervous system may be infected, as seen in cases of neurosyphilis or gonococcal meningitis. Gonorrhea that infects the skeletal system may result in gonococcal arthritis. Syphilis can infect the cardiovascular system by forming vegetative lesions on the mitral or aortic valves.

HUMAN IMMUNODEFICIENCY VIRUS–RELATED COMPLICATIONS. HIV infection leads to the profound immunosuppression characteristic of AIDS. Complications of HIV infection include many opportunistic infections, including those due to *Pneumocystis jiroveci*, *Cryptococcus neoformans*, cytomegalovirus, and *Mycobacterium avium* (see Chapter 52).

Evaluation

Expected Patient Outcomes

Expected patient outcomes may include the following:

1. Exhibits knowledge about STDs and their transmission
2. Demonstrates a less anxious demeanor
   a. Discusses anxieties and goals for treatment
   b. Inspects self for lesions, rashes, and discharge
   c. Accepts support, education, and counseling when indicated
   d. Assists with sharing information about infection with sexual partners
   e. Discusses risk-reduction behaviors and safer sex practices
3. Complies with treatment
4. Achieves effective treatment
5. Reports for follow-up examinations if necessary
6. Absence of complications

Emerging Infectious Diseases

As defined by the CDC, **emerging infectious diseases** are human diseases of infectious origin that have increased within the past two decades or that are likely to increase in the near future. Examples of emerging infectious diseases presented here include West Nile virus, Legionnaires' disease, pertussis, hantavirus pulmonary syndrome, and viral hemorrhagic fevers. Some multiple resistant strains of common bacteria such as CA-MRSA and gram-negative organisms that are resistant to extended-spectrum beta-lactam antibiotics or carbapenem-based antibiotics are also often considered causes of emerging diseases. This is especially true of CA-MRSA, because its presentation in people without underlying disease and its aggressive nature in skin and soft tissue infections are different from those seen with HA-MRSA. Table 70-1 provides an overview of infectious diseases, including emerging infectious diseases.

Many factors contribute to newly emerging or re-emerging infectious diseases. These include travel, globalization of food supply and central processing of food, population growth, increased urban crowding, population movements (eg, those that result from war, famine, or man-made or natural disasters), ecologic changes, human behavior (eg, risky sexual behavior, IV/injection drug use), antimicrobial resistance, and breakdown in public health measures.

These diseases are important from an epidemiologic standpoint because their incidence has not yet stabilized. When the pattern of disease in a community is not well understood in the medical-scientific community, patients, families, and others in the community often become alarmed about these diseases. During times of increased concern about bioterrorism, whether triggered by actual events or by hoaxes, nurses have responsibility to rationally separate facts from fears. In discussions with patients and other caregivers, it is important to keep the focus on what is known and to clarify the plan for diagnosis, treatment, and containment.

WEST NILE VIRUS

The West Nile virus was first recognized in the 1930s in Africa and was first seen in humans in the United States in 1999. Although most human infections are mild or asymptomatic, a range of presentations is possible. Approximately 20% of infected people have a mild disease called West Nile fever. These patients usually experience headache, fever, and a persistent fatigue that may continue for several months. In these patients, fewer than 1 in 150 infections develop into more serious disease, which is characterized by severe neuroinvasive illness, meningitis, encephalitis, and paralysis or poliomyelitis. The mortality rate for people with the milder West Nile fever and meningitis is less than 1%, but this rate increases to approximately 20% for those with encephalitis and as high as 50% for those with paralysis (Sejvar, 2007). Although age-related factors do not appear to affect a person's chances of acquiring West Nile virus, the risk of neuroinvasive disease is greater in those older than 64 years of age (Hayes, Komar, Nasci, et al., 2005).

The incubation period (ie, from mosquito bite to onset of symptoms) is between 3 and 14 days. Currently, there is no treatment for West Nile virus infection. Medical and nursing management consists of fluid replacement, airway management, and supportive nursing care when meningitis or symptoms are present.

Birds are the natural reservoir for the virus, and since 1999, the population of infected birds in the eastern United States has increased steadily. Mosquitoes become infected when feeding on birds and can transmit the virus to animals and humans. Although human-to-human transmission of West Nile virus is very rare, transmission has occurred as the result of occupational exposure in laboratory workers, infant exposure transplacentally and from breastfeeding, and blood transfusion or organ transplant from infected donors (CDC, 2004a).

LEGIONNAIRES' DISEASE

Legionnaires' disease is a multisystem illness that usually includes pneumonia and is caused by the gram-negative bacterium *Legionella pneumophila*. Named after an outbreak among people attending a convention of the American Legion in 1976, its potential to cause outbreaks has been demonstrated repeatedly in hospitals and other settings. It continues to be considered an emerging infectious disease because there are new patterns in recent years. There has been an approximate 70% increase in new cases since 2003 compared with earlier time periods, and a disproportionate increase in the eastern United States (Neil & Berkeman, 2008).

Legionella organisms are found in many man-made and naturally occurring water sources. Although the organisms may initially be introduced to the plumbing system in low numbers, growth is enhanced by water storage, sediment, temperatures ranging from 25°C to 42°C (77°F to 107°F), and certain amoebae frequently present in water that can support intracellular growth of legionellae. As incidence appears to increase in the summer and autumn months, vacation-related exposure to hotel or cruise ship plumbing and air conditioning systems, whirlpool spas, and decorative fountains may be the causative risk.

Pathophysiology

L. pneumophila is transmitted by the aerosolized route from an environmental source to a person's respiratory tract. It is not transmitted from person to person. In hospitals, patients may be exposed to aerosols created by cooling towers, water exposure from in-room plumbing, and respiratory therapy equipment. Because underlying medical conditions can increase host susceptibility and subsequent severity of disease and because hospital plumbing systems are often very complex, outbreaks occur in hospitals more frequently than at other centers within the community. The mortality rate for Legionnaires' disease may be as high as 40% in some populations (CDC, 2008a).

Risk Factors

Risk factors for *Legionella* infection include diseases that lead to severe immunosuppression, such as AIDS, hematologic malignancy, end-stage renal disease, or use of immunosuppressive agents. Other factors associated with increased risk include diabetes, smoking, exposure to whirlpool spas, and recent travel.

Clinical Manifestations

The lungs are the principal organs of infection; however, other organs may also be involved. The incubation period ranges from 2 to 10 days. Early symptoms may include malaise, myalgias, headache, and dry cough. The patient develops increasing pulmonary symptoms, including productive cough, dyspnea, and chest pain. Patients are usually febrile, and body temperatures may reach or exceed 39.4°C (103°F). Diarrhea and other gastrointestinal symptoms are common. In severe cases, multiorgan involvement and failure may follow.

Assessment and Diagnostic Findings

The diagnostic approach generally involves accumulation of information obtained from the history, physical examination, x-rays, laboratory findings, and assessment of therapeutic effectiveness. Chest x-ray abnormalities may vary in severity and in location within the lungs. Laboratory tests available for the diagnosis of *Legionella* include culture or tests that detect either antigen or antibody. The most frequently used test is the urinary antigen. The greatest limitation of the test is that it detects only one subgroup of one of the several species of *Legionella*. The CDC recommends using multiple tests when Legionnaires' disease is suspected because none of the tests is completely accurate.

Medical Management

The antibiotics of choice are azithromycin or a fluoroquinolone such as moxifloxacin (Avelox) (Mandell, Wunderink, Anzueto, et al., 2007). The antibiotic doxycycline may also be used.

Nursing Management

The nursing management described for the patient with any pneumonia (see Chapter 23) should form the basis of care for the patient with *Legionella* pneumonia. Isolation is not required because *Legionella* is not transmitted between humans. When the patient has acquired the infection in a health care facility, water cultures should be performed to determine if the water supply is contaminated.

PERTUSSIS

Pertussis, also known as whooping cough, a common childhood disease in the prevaccine era, is an example of a disease that has reemerged. Incidence rates declined until the 1980s, when rates for all age groups began to increase steadily for the next two decades. In the short period from 2001 to 2003, the incidence of cases in adolescents and adults more than doubled compared with the period from 1990 to 1993 (CDC, 2008b) (Fig. 70-3).

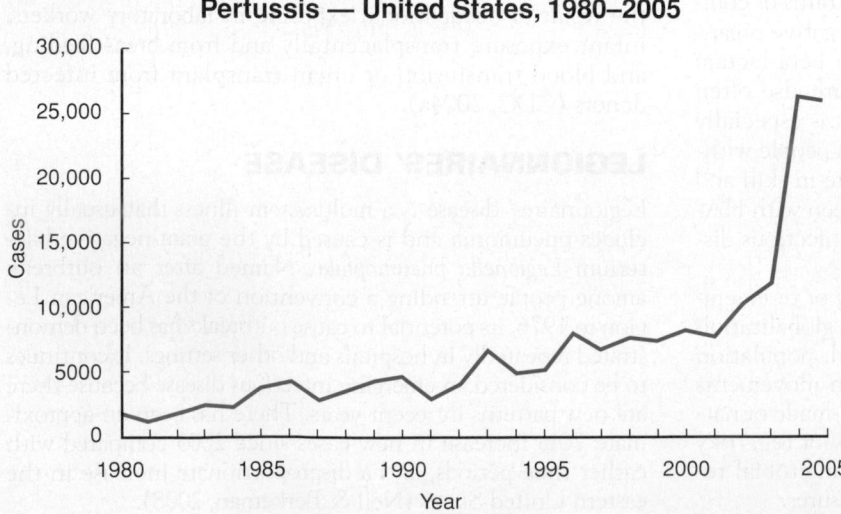

Pertussis — United States, 1980–2005

Figure 70-3 Graph showing increased incidence of pertussis in the United States, 1980–2005. From Centers of Disease Control and Prevention. (2007). Epidemiology and prevention of vaccine preventable diseases broadcasts: Slide sets. (10th ed.). Available at: www.cdc.gov/vaccines/ed/epivac07/epivac07-slides.htm

Pertussis is highly contagious, and patients usually present to health care professionals with a sudden (paroxysmal) cough that is accompanied by a characteristic whoop, a high-pitched noise heard when inhaling. Whooping cough is caused by the bacterium *Bordetella pertussis*.

Pathophysiology

B. pertussis is transmitted by droplets. The bacteria easily attach to pharyngeal epithelial cells, where they release a number of antigens, toxins, and other substances that trigger the immune system. Because most of the disease manifestations are caused by this immune reaction, patients are usually contagious only early in the disease (when the bacteria are still present) and not during the protracted period of cough (when the immune reaction is causing the pathology).

Clinical Manifestations

Pertussis causes a range of respiratory symptoms, with cough being the most frequent. It is generally most severe for infants who have not yet been vaccinated. Pneumonia is the most common consequence of infection, but the disease can also lead to seizures, encephalopathy, and rarely death. People who have been vaccinated seldom have severe disease.

Assessment and Diagnostic Findings

Most diagnoses of pertussis are made, at least initially, without laboratory confirmation. The clinical case definition, unless there is a preexisting condition to explain the symptoms, is a new cough lasting at least 2 weeks with inspiratory whoop or vomiting after cough. Laboratory confirmation can be made by clinical culture or by polymerase chain reaction (PCR) assay for *B. pertussis*. Serologic testing, although less reliable, can also strengthen the diagnostic suspicion. The best source for a culture is a nasopharyngeal specimen.

Medical Management

The antibiotics of choice are azithromycin, erythromycin (Erythrocin), or clarithromycin (Biaxin). The antibiotic trimethoprim sulfate (Bactrim) may also be used (Mandell, et al., 2007). Close contacts of a patient with proven or suspected pertussis should receive prophylaxis with one of these agents to reduce the risk of disease.

Nursing Management

Hospitalized patients with pertussis should be isolated in Droplet Precautions until they have received 5 days of appropriate therapy. Household members should receive antimicrobial prophylaxis and should be advised to report any symptoms of an upper respiratory infection.

HANTAVIRUS PULMONARY SYNDROME

Hantavirus pulmonary syndrome is caused by a member of the Hantavirus family of viruses. In the United States, the Sin Nombre hantavirus causes severe cardiopulmonary illness, with a case mortality rate of approximately 50%. It occurs most frequently in the western United States, but the rodents known to carry the virus are found throughout the country (Vaheri & Calisher, 2002).

The diagnosis of hantavirus pulmonary syndrome should be suspected in patients who live in rural areas; who may have had exposure to rodents; and who report fever, aching muscles, and nausea. Thrombocytopenia and hemoconcentration are also common.

No specific treatment for hantavirus pulmonary syndrome has been approved. Early identification, assessment, and maintenance of respiratory status are the most important aspects of care for patients with the disease. Intake and output should be monitored closely because overhydration is possible, with resultant cardiopulmonary compromise.

Prevention requires strategies to reduce human contact with rodents and their droppings. Public health programs and clinics in rural areas should regularly teach people to eliminate rodent food sources that are in areas close to humans. Openings in walls or cabinets should be sealed. Traps should be used in areas such as sheds and barns in which humans work and rodents may enter. Gloves should be worn when removing an animal from a trap, and the trap should be disinfected with a 1:10 bleach solution. People entering such areas should be taught to avoid stirring up dust or breathing potentially contaminated dust. Brooms and vacuum cleaners should be used with caution; areas that may emit dust while being cleaned should be first dampened with a bleach solution to reduce viral contaminants and the potential for dust dispersion.

VIRAL HEMORRHAGIC FEVERS

Viral hemorrhagic fevers are a group of illnesses caused by several families of viruses (the arenaviruses, filoviruses, bunyaviruses, and flaviviruses). These viruses cause a syndrome characterized by multisystem involvement, resulting in a damaged vascular system. Although most cases of hemorrhagic fever are severe, some cases are less acute. The viruses as a whole can be found throughout the world; however, each virus usually causes disease only in its own limited geographic area.

The Ebola and Marburg viruses, both belonging to the filovirus family, are the best-known viral hemorrhagic fever viruses. Since the 1960s, they have been the source of an irregular pattern of sporadic outbreaks. The clinical course differs among patients but often includes fever, hemorrhage, vomiting, diarrhea, cough, and jaundice. Symptoms usually occur rapidly, and the course of the illness often progresses rapidly to profound hemorrhage, organ destruction, and shock. The mortality rate ranges from 25% to 80%. When patients survive, the recovery period is often prolonged, and weakness, malaise, and cachexia are common (Heymann, 2004).

Nonhuman animals or insects appear to be the natural reservoirs of the viruses. Humans usually become infected when exposed to the natural reservoir (eg, after exposure to an unrecognized host or an insect bite). However, human-to-human transmission occurs occasionally; it involves close contact and usually occurs via the bloodborne route after exposure to blood or other body fluid. Percutaneous exposure requires only a very low inoculum of contaminated blood for transmission to occur. Mucous membrane exposure is another method of transmission. Although airborne transmission does not appear to be likely, the possibility has not been entirely eliminated.

A diagnosis of Ebola or Marburg should be considered in a patient who has a febrile, hemorrhagic illness after traveling to Asia or Africa or who has handled animals or animal carcasses from those parts of the world. The CDC should be contacted immediately when Ebola and Marburg viruses are suspected because hospital and local public health laboratories would not be able to confirm a diagnosis. Because no cases of Ebola or Marburg have been diagnosed in the United States to date, more likely diagnoses should also be considered whenever one of these diseases is a diagnostic possibility.

All health care workers who are involved in caring for patients with filoviruses must adhere to strict infection control measures. Systems must be set up to have objective observers ensure that each worker wears complete protective equipment in the form of cap, goggles, mask, gown, gloves, and shoe covers.

Treatment is largely supportive maintenance of the circulatory system and respiratory systems. It is likely that the infected patient will need ventilator and dialysis support during the acute phases of illness (CDC, 2005b). Supportive care for a patient with such a devastating disease requires psychological support for the patient and family. The patient, family, health care workers, and others in the community need substantial, coordinated education about the known elements and approach. Intervention may be required from those trained to provide psychological support for national emergencies or crises.

Travel and Immigration

Travel, trade, migration, and wars have led to many epidemics throughout history. The potential for epidemics is greatest when travelers and immigrants introduce microorganisms to which the host population has little or no immunity. Examples of important epidemics in the Western Hemisphere have included yellow fever, malaria, hookworm, leprosy, smallpox, measles, mumps, and syphilis. The HIV epidemic demonstrates the way that travel and immigration allow a disease to spread undetected worldwide. The 2003 severe acute respiratory syndrome (SARS) outbreak demonstrates how global travel contributes to a rapidly occurring epidemic involving an unrecognized pathogen.

In the United States, an infrastructure with enforced vaccination, clean water, and insect and rodent control decreases the risk that epidemics will progress even when travel may introduce exotic microorganisms. However, the recent experience with West Nile virus has reinforced knowledge that insect transmission can lead to significant human outbreaks. Thus, the concern grows that vector-borne diseases such as dengue and malaria may increase in the United States as mosquitoes can transmit disease locally when a reservoir of infected humans is established. The CDC maintains an active surveillance system to monitor and halt the incidence of many diseases prospectively.

Immigration and Acquired Immunodeficiency Disease Syndrome

The fact that AIDS reached pandemic proportions less than a decade after its recognition attests to the efficiency of world travel in spreading disease. Such rapid transmission rates are especially dramatic because HIV essentially requires intimate contact between two people through sexual activity or sharing blood through needles.

HIV/AIDS is now an international health disaster. Since the start of the epidemic, more than 67 million people have become infected with HIV and more than 27 million have died of AIDS. Control of the epidemic anywhere in the world requires control everywhere. More than 95% of the current burden is felt in economically depressed countries, which means that the control of the disease, using antiretroviral therapy and public health education, requires investment from nations, corporations, and people throughout the world, especially the wealthy nations (UNAIDS, 2008).

Immigration and Tuberculosis

Although there are substantive efforts to eliminate TB in the United States, TB remains a growing epidemic in developing nations. Approximately one third of the world's population is currently infected with TB. Between 5% and 10% of those infected eventually develop disease; therefore, approximately 9 million people per year become ill with TB (WHO, 2008b). Immigration has always been an important influence in the dynamic epidemiology of TB in the United States. In 2007, the incidence of TB in the United States was 9.7 times greater in foreign-born people than in native-born people (CDC, 2008b).

The association between immigration and transmission risk is greatest in urban areas because these locations are frequently heavily populated and frequently visited by foreign-born people. These locales are also often the epicenter of the HIV epidemic. Because HIV infection depletes T cells, which are necessary for TB protection, the geographic closeness of these two microorganisms potentiates increased rates of both infections.

A positive tuberculin skin test (TST) establishes that TB infection has occurred at some time in a person's life but does not provide information about current infectivity. The reliability of TST interpretation is decreased among foreign-born people because the bacille Calmette-Guérin (BCG) vaccine is used in many countries. After receiving BCG, people often have some degree of TST reactivity for a prolonged time.

Immigration and Vector-Borne Diseases

Malaria and dengue are diseases that cause significant morbidity and mortality throughout the developing world. These diseases may be "imported" to the United States via travel, immigration, or commerce. They are caused by microorganisms that can be spread to humans by mosquitoes in the United States that thrive in tropical zones and breed in stagnant water sources. Although malaria was eradicated in the United States in the 1950s, limited local outbreaks have occurred regularly when mosquitoes acquire the bacteria from a person recently traveling from an area in which malaria is endemic and transmit it to a small number of people. Similarly, an increase of dengue virus in the Caribbean has caused concern that outbreaks may occur in the United States.

CRITICAL THINKING EXERCISES

1 Several elderly patients in your community have developed skin infections caused by MRSA. What should nurses in different roles in the community do to reduce the risk of new infections and to reduce people's anxiety? What strategies are used to control MRSA in health care facilities?

2 Several patients in your long-term care facility have developed fever and diarrhea. What steps should be taken to reduce the risk of further outbreaks?

EBP 3 Audits of hand hygiene in your health care facility demonstrate poor compliance with recommended methods of hand hygiene. What methods of hand hygiene should be used? What strategies should be used to improve compliance and to sustain appropriate behavior once acceptable rates are achieved? What is the evidence base for these practices?

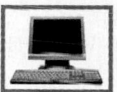 The Smeltzer suite offers these additional resources to enhance learning and facilitate understanding of this chapter:
- thePoint online resource, thepoint.lww.com/Smeltzer12E
- Student CD-ROM included with the book
- *Study Guide to Accompany Brunner & Suddarth's Textbook of Medical-Surgical Nursing*

REFERENCES AND SELECTED READINGS

Books

Centers for Disease Control and Prevention (CDC). (2007a). *Epidemiology and prevention of vaccine-preventable diseases.* Washington DC: Public Health Foundation.

Guerrant, R. L. & Steiner, T. S. (2005). Principles and syndromes of enteric infection. In Mandell, G. L., Bennett, R. D., Dolin, R. (Eds.). *Mandell, Douglas and Bennett's principles and practice of infectious diseases* (6th ed.). Philadelphia: Elsevier.

Heymann, D. L. (Ed.). (2004). *Control of communicable disease manual* (18th ed.). Washington, DC: American Public Health Association.

Rhinehart, E. & McGoldrick, M. (2005). *Infection control in home care and hospice* (2nd ed.). Boston: Jones and Bartlett.

Journals and Electronic Sources

Centers for Disease Control and Prevention (CDC). (2002a). Guideline for hand hygiene in health care settings. MMWR: *Morbidity and Mortality Weekly Report, 51*(RR-16), 1–56.

Centers for Disease Control and Prevention (CDC). (2002b). *Staphylococcus aureus* resistant to vancomycin—United States, 2002. MMWR: *Morbidity and Mortality Weekly Report, 51*(26), 565–567.

Centers for Disease Control and Prevention (CDC). (2004a). Information and guidance for clinicians: West Nile virus: Epidemiologic information for clinicians. Available at: www.cdc.gov/ncidod/dvbid/westnile/clinicians/pdf/wnv-epidemiology-clinguidance.pdf

Centers for Disease Control and Prevention (CDC). (2004b). National nosocomial infections surveillance system report: Data summary, from January 1992–June 2004, issued October 2004. *American Journal of Infection Control, 32*(8), 470–485.

Centers for Disease Control and Prevention (CDC). (2004c). STD communications database. General public focus group findings. February 2004. Available at: www.cdc.gov/std/HealthComm/ExecSumHPVGenPub2004.pdf

Centers for Disease Control and Prevention (CDC). (2005a). Achievements in public health: Elimination of rubella and congenital rubella syndrome—United States, 1969–2004. MMWR: *Morbidity and Mortality Weekly Report, 54*(11), 279–282.

Centers for Disease Control and Prevention (CDC). (2005b). Brief report: Outbreak of Marburg virus hemorrhagic fever—Angola, October 1, 2004–March 29, 2005. MMWR: *Morbidity and Mortality Weekly Report, 54*(Dispatch), 1–2.

Centers for Disease Control and Prevention (CDC). (2005c). Norovirus in healthcare facilities. Available at: www.cdc.gov/ncidod/dhqp/id_norovirusfs.html

Centers for Disease Control and Prevention (CDC). (2005d). *Salmonella enteritis.* Available at: www.cdc.gov/ncidod/dbmd/diseaseinfo/salment_g.htm

Centers for Disease Control and Prevention (CDC). (2005e) Updated U.S. Public Health Service Guidelines for the management of occupational exposures to HIV and recommendations for postexposure prophylaxis. Available at: www.cdc.gov/mmwr/preview/mmwrhtml/rr5409a1.htm

Centers for Disease Control and Prevention (CDC). (2005f). Vibrio illnesses after Hurricane Katrina—Multiple states, August–September 2005. Available at: www.cdc.gov/MMWR/preview/mmwrhtml/mm5437a5.htm

Centers for Disease Control and Prevention (CDC). (2005g). Guidelines for preventing the transmission of mycobacterium tuberculosis in health-care settings, 2005. Available at www.cdc.gov/mmwr/preview/mmwrhtml/rr5417q.1. htm?s_cid=5417a1_e.

Centers for Disease Control and Prevention (CDC). (2006a). Management of multidrug-resistant organisms in healthcare settings, 2006. Available at: www.cdc.gov/ncidod/dhqp/pdf/ar/mdroguideline2006.pdf

Centers for Disease Control and Prevention (CDC). (2006b). Sexually transmitted diseases treatment guidelines, 2006. MMWR: *Morbidity and Mortality Weekly Report, 55*(RR11), 1–94.

Centers for Disease Control and Prevention (CDC). (2006c). Update on multistate outbreak of *E. coli* 157:H7 infections from fresh spinach, October 6, 2006. Available at: www.cdc.gov/ecoli/2006/september/updates/100606.htm

Centers for Disease Control and Prevention (CDC). (2006d). Travelers health: Vaccinations. Available at: wwwn.cdc.gov/travel/contentVaccinations.aspx

Centers for Disease Control and Prevention (CDC). (2006e). Pandemic influenza resources. FluSurge 2.0. Available at: www.cdc.gov/flu/flusurge.htm

Centers for Disease Control and Prevention (CDC). (2008a). Legionellosis resource site. Top 10 things every clinician needs to know about legionellosis. Available at: www.cdc.gov/legionella/top10.htm

Centers for Disease Control and Prevention (CDC). (2008b). Vaccine preventable diseases surveillance manual. Available at: www.cdc.gov/vaccines/Pubs/surv-manual/chpt10-pertussis.pdf

Centers for Disease Control and Prevention (CDC). (2008c). Prevention and control of influenza: Recommendations of the Advisory Committee on Immunization Practices. MMWR: *Morbidity and Mortality Weekly Report: CDC Surveillance Summaries, 57*(Early release), 1–60.

Centers for Disease Control and Prevention (CDC). (2008d). Trends in tuberculosis—2007. MMWR: *Morbidity and Mortality Weekly Review, 57*(11), 281–285.

Centers for Disease Control and Prevention (CDC). (2009a). MMWR Quick Guide. Recommended adult immunization schedule. United States 2009. Available at: www.cdc.gov/mmwr/pdf/wk/mm5753-Immunization.pdf

Centers for Disease Control and Prevention (CDC). (2009b). Vaccines and recommendations: ACIP recommendations. Available at: www.cdc.gov/vaccines/pubs/ACIP-list.htm

Centers for Disease Control and Prevention (CDC). (2009c). Sexually transmitted diseases. General information. Available at: www.cdc.gov/std/general/

Centers for Disease Control and Prevention (CDC). (2009d). Recommended immunization schedules for persons aged 0 though 18 years-United States, 2009. Available at www.cdc.gov/mmwr/preview/mmwrhtml/mm5751a5.htm?s_cid=mm5751a5_e.

Centers for Disease Control and Prevention (CDC). (2009e). Trends in reportable sexually transmitted diseases in the United States, 2007. National surveillance data for chlamydia, gonorrhea, and syphilis. Available at: www.cdc.gov/std/stats07/trends.pdf

Davey, V. J. (2007). Questions and answers on pandemic influenza. *American Journal of Nursing, 107*(7), 50–56.

Gonzalez, B. E., Rueda A. M., Shelburne, S. A., et al. (2006). Community-associated strains of methicillin-resistant *Staphylococcus aureus* as the cause of healthcare-associated infection. *Infection Control and Hospital Epidemiology, 27*(10), 1051–1056.

Hayes, E. B., Komar, N., Nasci, R. S., et al. (2005). Epidemiology and transmission dynamics of West Nile virus disease. Emerging infectious diseases. Available at: www.cdc.gov/ncidod/EID/vol11no08/05-0289a.htm

Joint Commission. (2008). *2009 National patient safety goals.* Available at: www.jointcommission.org/PatientSafety/NationalPatientSafetyGoals/

Mandell, L. A., Wunderink, R. G., Anzueto, A., et al. (2007). Infectious Disease Society of America/American Thoracic Society consensus guidelines on the management of community-acquired pneumonia in adults. *Clinical Infectious Diseases, 44*(S2), S27–S72.

Marschall, J., Mermel, L. A., Classen, D., et al. (2008). Strategies to prevent central line-associated bloodstream infections in acute care hospitals. *Infection Control and Hospital Epidemiology, 29*(Suppl 1), S22–S30.

McDonald, L. C. (2007). Confronting *Clostridium difficile* in inpatient health care facilities. *Clinical Infectious Diseases, 45*(10), 1274–1276.

Milstone, A. M. & Perl, T. M. (2008). Fact, fiction, or no data: What does surveillance for methicillin-resistant *Staphylococcus aureus* prevent in the intensive care unit? *Clinical Infectious Diseases, 46*(11), 1726–1728.

Neil, K. & Berkeman, R. (2008). Increasing incidence of legionellosis in the United States, 1990–2005: Changing epidemiologic trends. *Clinical Infectious Diseases, 47*(5), 591–599.

Pronovost, P., Needham, D., Berenholtz, S., et al. (2006). An intervention to decrease catheter-related bloodstream infections in the ICU. *New England Journal of Medicine, 355*(26), 2725–2732.

Sejvar, J. (2007). The long-term outcomes of human West Nile virus infection. *Clinical Infectious Diseases, 44*(12), 1617–1624.

Siegel, J. D., Rhinehart, E., Jackson, M., et al. (2007). Guideline for isolation precautions: preventing transmission of infectious agents in healthcare settings, June 2007. Available at: www.cdc.gov/ncidod/dhqp/gl_isolation.html

UNAIDS. (2008). Global AIDS report 2008. Available at: www.unaids.org/en/KnowledgeCentre/HIVData/GlobalReport/2008/2008_Global_report.asp

U.S. Department of Agriculture (USDA). (2008). Quarterly progress report on *Salmonella* testing of selected raw meat and poultry products: Preliminary results, January–March 2008. Available at: www.fsis.usda.gov/Science/Q1_2008_Salmonella_Testing_Tables/Index.asp#table1

U.S. Department of Health and Human Services (USDHH). (2008). Pandemic influenza. Available at: www.pandemicflu.gov

Vaheri, A. & Calisher, C. (2002). Conference summary: The fifth international conference on hemorrhagic fever with renal syndrome, hantavirus pulmonary syndrome, and hantaviruses. *Emerging Infectious Diseases, 8*(1), 109.

Wang, G., Hindler, J. F., Ward, K. W., et al. (2006). Increased Vancomycin MICs for *Staphylococcus aureus* clinical isolates from a university hospital during a 5-year period. *Journal of Clinical Microbiology, 44*(11), 3883–3886.

Weber, J. T. (2005). Community-associated methicillin-resistant *Staphylococcus aureus*. *Clinical Infectious Diseases, 41*(Suppl 4), S269–S272.

World Health Organization (WHO). (2008a). Avian influenza update number 142. Available at: www.wpro.who.int/NR/rdonlyres/FA932417-F88C-4DC2-B24F-E8FC6A679C76/0/AIWeekly142WPRO8_4_08.pdf

World Health Organization (WHO). (2008b). Global tuberculosis control: Surveillance, planning and financing. Available at: www.who.int/tb/publications/global_report/en/index.html

Writing Committee of the World Health Organization (WHO). (2005). Consultation on human influenza A/H5. Avian influenza A (H5N1) infection in humans. *New England Journal of Medicine, 353*(13), 1374–1385.

RESOURCES

American Lung Association, www.lungusa.org
American Public Health Association (APHA), www.apha.org
Association for Professionals in Infection Control and Epidemiology (APIC), Inc., www.apic.org
Centers for Disease Control and Prevention (CDC), www.cdc.gov
Centers for Disease Control and Prevention (CDC), adult or pediatric vaccine advice hotline, 800 232-4636
Centers for Disease Control and Prevention (CDC), traveler's vaccination advice, 877-FYI-TRIP or 877 394-8747
Department of Infectious and Parasitic Disease Pathology, Armed Forces Institute of Pathology (AFIP), www.afip.org
Infectious Diseases Society of America (IDSA), www.idsociety.org
National Foundation for Infectious Diseases (NFID), www.nfid.org
National Institute of Allergy and Infectious Diseases (NIAID), www.niaid.nih.gov/default.htm
Occupational Safety and Health Administration (OSHA), www.osha.gov
Society for Healthcare Epidemiology of America (SHEA), www.shea-online.org
Vaccine Adverse Event Reporting System, 800 822-7967, www.vaers.hhs.gov
World Health Organization (WHO), www.who.int/home-page

chapter 71

Emergency Nursing

LEARNING OBJECTIVES

On completion of this chapter, the learner will be able to:

1 Describe emergency care as a collaborative, holistic approach that includes the patient, the family, and significant others.

2 Discuss priority emergency measures instituted for the patient with an emergency condition.

3 Describe the emergency management of patients with intra-abdominal injuries.

4 Identify the priorities of care for the patient with multiple injuries.

5 Compare and contrast the emergency management of patients with heat stroke, frostbite, and hypothermia.

6 Specify the similarities and differences of the emergency management of patients with swallowed or inhaled poisons, skin contamination, and food poisoning.

7 Discuss the emergency management of patients with drug overdose and with acute alcohol intoxication.

8 Describe the significance of crisis intervention in the care of rape victims.

9 Differentiate between the emergency care of patients who are overactive, those who are violent, those who are depressed, and those who are suicidal.

GLOSSARY

antivenin: antitoxin manufactured from venom of poisonous snakes to assist the patient's immune system response to an envenomation

carboxyhemoglobin: hemoglobin that is bound to carbon monoxide and therefore is unable to bind with oxygen, resulting in hypoxemia

corrosive poison: alkaline or acidic agent; causes tissue destruction after contact

cricothyroidotomy: surgical opening of the cricothyroid membrane to obtain an airway that is maintained with a tracheostomy or endotracheal tube

diagnostic peritoneal lavage: instillation of lactated Ringer's or normal saline solution into the abdominal cavity to detect red blood cells, white blood cells, bile, bacteria, amylase, or gastrointestinal contents indicative of abdominal injury

emergent: triage category signifying potentially life-threatening injuries or illnesses requiring immediate treatment

envenomation: injection of a poisonous material by sting, spine, bite, or other means

fasciotomy: surgical incision of the extremity to the level of the fascia to relieve pressure and restore neurovascular function to the extremity

Hare traction: portable in-line traction applied to the lower extremity to manage femur or hip fractures or dislocations

minor: triage category signifying non–life-threatening injuries or illnesses that can be routinely managed in a clinic or physician's office or that require no medical care

nonurgent: triage category signifying episodic or minor injury or illness in which treatment may be delayed several hours or longer without increased morbidity

resuscitation: triage category signifying life-threatening injuries or illnesses requiring immediate intervention

triage: process of assessing patients to determine management priorities

urgent: triage category signifying serious illness or injury that is not immediately life-threatening

The term *emergency management* traditionally refers to care given to patients with urgent and critical needs. However, because many people lack access to health care, the emergency department (ED) is increasingly used for nonurgent problems. Therefore, the philosophy of emergency management has broadened to include the concept that an emergency is whatever the patient or the family considers it to be.

Large numbers of people seek emergency care for serious life-threatening conditions, such as cardiac dysrhythmias, acute coronary syndrome (ACS), acute heart failure, pulmonary edema, and stroke. Priorities for managing these cardiac and other conditions are discussed in Chapters 27, 28, 30, and 62. Emergency management of trauma and conditions not found elsewhere in this book are discussed in this chapter. It is assumed that care and treatment are provided under the direction of a physician or emergency nurse practitioner. Facts about ED visits in the United States are presented in Chart 71-1.

SCOPE AND PRACTICE OF EMERGENCY NURSING

The emergency nurse has had specialized education, training, experience, and expertise in assessing and identifying patients' health care problems in crisis situations. In addition, the emergency nurse establishes priorities, monitors and continuously assesses acutely ill and injured patients, supports and attends to families, supervises allied health personnel, and teaches patients and families within a time-limited, high-pressured care environment. Nursing interventions are accomplished interdependently, in consultation with or under the direction of a physician or nurse practitioner. The roles of nursing and medicine are complementary in an emergency situation. Appropriate nursing and medical interventions are anticipated based on assessment data. The emergency health care staff members work as a team in performing the highly technical, hands-on skills required to care for patients in emergency situations.

The nursing process provides a logical framework for problem solving in this environment. Patients in the ED have a wide variety of actual or potential problems, and their condition may change. Therefore, nursing assessment must be continuous, and nursing diagnoses change with the patient's condition. Although a patient may have several diagnoses at a given time, the focus is on the most life-threatening ones; often, both independent and interdependent nursing interventions are required.

Issues in Emergency Nursing Care

Emergency nursing is demanding because of the diversity of conditions and situations that present unique challenges. These challenges include legal issues, occupational health and safety risks for ED staff, and the challenge of providing holistic care in the context of a fast-paced, technology-driven environment in which serious illness and death are encountered on a daily basis. Another dimension of emergency nursing is nursing in disasters. With the increasing use of weapons of terror and mass destruction, the emergency nurse must recognize and treat patients exposed to biologic and other weapons and anticipate nursing care in the event of a mass casualty incident (see Chapter 72).

Chart 71-1 • *Facts About Emergency Department Visits*

In 2005, there were 115.3 million visits to emergency departments (EDs), a 31% increase from 1995. This was accompanied by a 10% decrease in the number of EDs and an increased utilization by 7%.

- The highest rate of ED visits in people 65 years of age and older were from long-term care facilities.
- More than 15.5% of patients arrived at the ED by ambulance.
- Patients with Medicaid used EDs more often than patients with private health insurance, Medicare, or self-pay.
- Injuries accounted for 41.9% of all ED visits.
- The leading causes of injuries, including falls and motor vehicle crashes, accounted for 31% of injury-related ED visits. For those injured, 36.9% were transported to designated trauma centers.
- The average ED waiting time before being seen by a health care provider for definitive treatment was 2.4 hours, with 7 of 10 patients spending less than 4 hours in the ED.

Source: National Hospital Ambulatory Medical Care Survey. (2005). *2005 Emergency department summary.* Available at: www.cdc.gov/nchs/data/ad/ad386.pdf and www.cdc.gov/nchs/data/hus/hus07.pdf#091

Documentation of Consent and Privacy

Consent to examine and treat the patient is part of the ED record. The patient must consent to invasive procedures (eg, angiography, lumbar puncture) unless he or she is unconscious or in critical condition and unable to make decisions. If the patient is unconscious and brought to the ED without family or friends, this fact must be documented. Monitoring of the patient's condition, as well as all instituted treatments and the times at which they were performed, must be documented. After treatment, a notation is made on the record about the patient's condition, response to the treatment, and condition at discharge or transfer and about instructions given to the patient and family for follow-up care.

The patient is also provided with a statement of the privacy policy of the health care agency, according to federal law. Patients involved in violent events are often provided with an alias, and access to the medical record, both paper and electronic, is limited to protect the privacy of the patient. A patient may also request extra privacy by limiting access to his or her room and by choosing not to receive phone calls, mail, flowers, other gifts, or certain visitors. These practices relate to the federally mandated privacy policy stipulated in the Health Insurance Portability and Accountability Act (HIPAA).

Limiting Exposure to Health Risks

Because of the increasing numbers of people infected with hepatitis B and C, with human immunodeficiency virus (HIV), and other infectious diseases, health care providers are at an increased risk for exposure to communicable diseases through blood, respiratory droplets, or other body fluids. This risk is further compounded in the ED because of the common use of invasive treatments in patients who may have a wide range of conditions and who frequently cannot provide a comprehensive medical history. All emergency health care providers must adhere strictly to standard precautions for minimizing exposure.

The reemergence of tuberculosis as a major health problem is complicated by multi–drug-resistant tuberculosis and by tuberculosis concomitant with HIV infection. Early identification and adherence to transmission-based precautions for patients who are potentially infectious are crucial. Nurses in the ED are usually fitted with personal high-efficiency particulate air (HEPA) filter masks to use when treating patients with airborne diseases.

The potential for exposure to highly contagious organisms, hazardous chemicals or gases, and radiation related to acts of terrorism or natural or manmade disasters presents additional risks to ED staff (see Chapter 72 for information about decontamination procedures).

Violence in the Emergency Department

Not only do ED staff members encounter patients who may be violent because of the effects of substance abuse, injury, or other emergencies, but they may also encounter other violent situations. Frequently, patients and families waiting for assistance are emotionally volatile. Often, waiting rooms are the sites where feelings of dissatisfaction, fear, and anger are channeled violently. Some EDs assign security officers to the area and have installed silent alarm systems or metal detectors to identify weapons in order to protect patients, families, and staff. Safety is the first priority.

It is not unusual for a patient or family member to come to the ED armed. To avoid angry confrontations, members of gangs and feuding families need to be separated in the ED, in the waiting room, and later in the inpatient nursing unit. Nurses and other personnel must be prepared to deal with these circumstances. The ED should be locked against entry if security is questionable.

Patients from prison and those who are under guard need to be handcuffed to the bed and appropriately assessed to ensure the safety of hospital staff and other patients. The following precautions are taken:

- The hand or ankle restraint (handcuff) is never released.
- A guard is always present in the room.
- The patient is placed face down on the stretcher to avoid injury from head-butting, spitting, or biting.
- Restraints are used on any violent patient as needed.
- Medication is administered as necessary to control violent behavior until definitive treatment can be obtained.

In the case of gunfire in the ED, self-protection is a priority. There is no advantage to protecting others if medical caregivers are injured. Security officers and police must gain control of the situation first, and then care is provided to the injured.

Providing Holistic Care

Patients and families experiencing sudden injury or illness are often overwhelmed by anxiety because they have not had time to adapt to the crisis. They experience real and terrifying fear of death, mutilation, immobilization, and other assaults on their personal identity and body integrity. When confronted with trauma, severe disfigurement, severe illness, or sudden death, the family experiences several stages of crisis. The stages begin with anxiety and progress through denial, remorse and guilt, anger, grief, and reconciliation. The initial goal for the patient and family is anxiety reduction, a prerequisite to effective and appropriate coping. During this stressful time, safety is of prime importance. Close observation and preplanning are essential and security personnel are stationed nearby in the event that a patient or family member responds to stress with physical violence.

Assessment of the patient and family's psychological function includes evaluating emotional expression, degree of anxiety, and cognitive functioning. Possible nursing diagnoses include:

- General anxiety or death anxiety related to uncertain potential outcomes of the illness or trauma
- Ineffective coping related to acute situational crisis

Possible nursing diagnoses for the family include:

- Grieving
- Interrupted family processes
- Compromised or disabled family coping related to acute situational crises

Patient-Focused Interventions

Clinicians caring for the patient should act confidently and competently to relieve anxiety and promote a sense of security. Explanations should be given that the patient can understand. Human contact and reassuring words reduce the panic of the severely injured or ill person and aid in dispelling fear of the unknown.

The unconscious patient should be treated as if conscious; that is, the patient should be touched, called by name, and given an explanation of every procedure that is performed. As the patient regains consciousness, the nurse should orient the patient by stating his or her name, the date, and the location. This basic information should be provided repeatedly, as needed, in a reassuring way.

Family-Focused Interventions

The family is kept informed about where the patient is, how he or she is doing, and the care that is being given. Allowing family members to stay with the patient, when possible, also helps allay their anxieties. In many facilities, family presence during resuscitation is permitted to assist the family to cope through this difficult time. Many family members respond very well to this approach, and it provides some answers to the question "Was everything done?" (Walker, 2008). Additional interventions are based on the assessment of the stage of crisis that the family is experiencing. Measures to help family members cope with sudden death are presented in Chart 71-2.

Anxiety and Denial. During these crises, family members are encouraged to recognize and talk about their feelings of anxiety. Asking questions is encouraged. Honest answers given at the level of the family's understanding must be provided. Although denial is an ego-defense mechanism that protects one from recognizing

Chart 71-2 • *Helping Family Members Cope With Sudden Death*

- Take the family to a private place.
- Talk to the family together, so that they can grieve together.
- Reassure the family that everything possible was done; inform them of the treatment rendered.
- Avoid using euphemisms such as "passed on." Show the family that you care by touching, offering coffee, water, and the services of a chaplain.
- Encourage family members to support each other and to express emotions freely (grief, loss, anger, helplessness, tears, disbelief).
- Avoid giving sedation to family members; this may mask or delay the grieving process, which is necessary to achieve emotional equilibrium and to prevent prolonged depression.
- Encourage the family to view the body if they wish; this action helps to integrate the loss. Cover disfigured and injured areas before the family sees the body. Go with the family to see the body. Show acceptance by touching the body to give the family "permission" to touch.
- Spend time with the family, listening to them and identifying any needs that they may have for which the nursing staff can be helpful.
- Allow family members to talk about the deceased and what he or she meant to them; this permits ventilation of feelings of loss. Encourage the family to talk about events preceding admission to the emergency department. Do not challenge initial feelings of anger or denial.
- Avoid volunteering unnecessary information (eg, the patient was drinking).

painful and disturbing aspects of reality, prolonged denial is not encouraged or supported. The family must be prepared for the reality of what has happened and what may come.

Remorse and Guilt. Expressions of remorse and guilt are common, with family members accusing themselves (or each other) of negligence or minor omissions. Family members are urged to verbalize their feelings to help them cope appropriately.

Anger. Expressions of anger, common in crisis situations, are a way of handling anxiety and fear. Anger is frequently directed by the family at the patient, but it is also often expressed toward the physician, the nurse, or admitting personnel. The therapeutic approach is to allow the anger to be expressed and to assist the family members to identify their feelings of frustration.

Grief. Grief is a complex emotional response to anticipated or actual loss. The key nursing intervention is to help family members work through their grief and to support their coping mechanisms, letting them know that it is normal and acceptable for them to cry, feel pain, and express loss. The hospital chaplain and social services staff serve as invaluable members of the team when assisting families to work through their grief.

Caring for Emergency Personnel

Concerted efforts have been made to focus on the needs of the ED staff, especially after serious and stressful events (Emergency Nurses Association [ENA], 2007). Events can range from a local trauma case involving children; to treating someone known to the emergency worker, such as a colleague or family member; to a more complex natural disaster or multicasualty situation. It is important to remember that all staff members may not necessarily respond in the same way; an event that is stressful for one person may not be as stressful for another. In addition, because stress is a daily occurrence in the ED, the staff may not recognize the personal effect of any one event. The availability of nonjudgmental counseling is essential to promoting a healthy staff. After serious events, critical incident stress debriefing necessary to critique individual and group performance. In addition, personal and group stress debriefing is also essential.

Emergency Nursing and the Continuum of Care

A key principle underlying emergency care is that the patient is rapidly assessed, treated, and referred to the appropriate setting for ongoing care. This makes the ED a temporary point on the continuum of care. Most patients who receive emergency care are discharged directly from the ED to their homes, and emergency nurses must plan and facilitate the patient's safe discharge and follow-up care in the home and the community.

Discharge Planning

Before discharge, verbal and written instructions for continuing care are given to the patient and the family or significant others. Many EDs have preprinted standard instruction sheets for the more common conditions, which can then be individualized. Discharge instructions should be available in a variety of languages. A language interpreter should be used as necessary to provide both written and verbal instructions.

Instructions should include information about prescribed medications, treatments, diet, activity, and when to contact a health care provider or schedule follow-up appointments. It is imperative that instructions are written legibly, use simple language, and are clear in their teaching. When providing discharge instructions, the nurse also considers any special needs the patient may have related to hearing or visual impairments. Alternate formats of instruction (eg, large print, Braille, audiotape) should be available to meet the needs of patients with hearing or visual impairments.

Community Services

Before discharge, some patients require the services of a social worker to help them meet continuing health care needs. Home care resources may be contacted before discharge to arrange services. This is particularly important for patients who are elderly or disabled and who need assistance. Identifying continuing health care needs and making arrangements for meeting these needs can prevent return visits to the ED or readmission to the hospital.

For patients who are returning to long-term care facilities and for those who already rely on community agencies for continuing health care, communication about the patient's condition and any changes in health care needs that have occurred must be provided to the appropriate facilities or agencies. This communication is essential to promote continuity of care and to ensure ongoing care to meet the patient's changing health care needs.

 Gerontologic Considerations

The ED is a common point of entry into the health care system for patients 65 years and older. In fact, patients in this age group account for more than 41% of the admissions to the hospital from the ED. Of the 115 million ED visits in the United States in 2005, 2.2 million of these were patients from long-term care facilities (National Hospital Ambulatory Medical Care Survey, 2005) (see Chart 71-1). Elderly patients typically arrive with one or more presenting conditions. Nonspecific symptoms, such as weakness and fatigue, episodes of falling, incontinence, and change in mental status, may be manifestations of acute, potentially life-threatening illness in the elderly person. Emergencies in this age group may be more difficult to manage because elderly patients may have an atypical presentation, an altered response to treatment, a greater risk of developing complications, or a combination of these factors.

The elderly patient may perceive the emergency as a crisis signaling the end of an independent lifestyle or even resulting in death. The nurse should give attention to the patient's feelings of anxiety and fear.

The older patient may have limited sources of social and financial support during these times of crises. The nurse should assess the psychosocial resources of the patient (and of the caregiver, if necessary) and anticipate discharge needs. Referrals for support services (eg, to the social service department or a gerontologic nurse specialist) may be necessary.

PRINCIPLES OF EMERGENCY CARE

By definition, emergency care is care that must be rendered without delay. In an ED, several patients with diverse health problems—some life-threatening, some not—may present to the ED simultaneously. One of the first principles of emergency care is triage.

Triage

The word **triage** comes from the French word *trier*, meaning "to sort." In the daily routine of the ED, triage is used to sort patients into groups based on the severity of their health problems and the immediacy with which these problems must be treated.

A basic and widely used triage system that has been in use for many years has three categories: emergent, urgent, and nonurgent (Berner, 2005). **Emergent** patients have the highest priority—their conditions are life-threatening and they must be seen immediately. **Urgent** patients have serious health problems but not immediately life-threatening ones; they must be seen within 1 hour. **Nonurgent** patients have

episodic illnesses that can be addressed within 24 hours without increased morbidity (Berner, 2005). A fourth category that is increasingly used is "fast-track." These patients require simple first aid or basic primary care and may be treated in the ED or safely referred to a clinic or physician's office.

A more refined comprehensive triage system, which recognizes that EDs are used for both emergency and routine health care, has been implemented. This system has five levels: resuscitation, emergent, urgent, nonurgent, and minor (Tanabe, Gimbel, Yarnold, et al., 2004). The increased number of triage levels assists the triage nurse to more precisely determine the needs of the patient and the urgency for treatment. This five-level triage system is currently used throughout the United States, Australia, the United Kingdom, and Canada.

In the five-level system, patients in the emergent category identified in the previously used three-level system have been divided into two distinct groupings, resuscitation and emergent. Patients in the **resuscitation** category need treatment immediately to prevent death. Patients in the emergent category may deteriorate rapidly and develop a major life-threatening situation or require time-sensitive treatment. Patients in the urgent category have non–life-threatening conditions but require two or more resources (defined below) to provide their care. If these patients' vital signs deviate significantly from their baseline, they may require "up-triaging" to the emergent category. Patients in the nonurgent category have non–life-threatening conditions and likely need only one resource to provide for their needs. Patients in the **minor** category have no life-threatening conditions and likely require no resources to provide their evaluation and management.

Resources include imaging studies, medications administered by intravenous (IV) or intramuscular (IM) routes, and invasive procedures. Insertion of an indwelling catheter is an example of a one-resource procedure. Use of moderate sedation is a two-resource procedure because it requires frequent monitoring and IV medications.

Triage is an advanced skill. Emergency nurses spend many hours learning to classify different illnesses and injuries to ensure that patients most in need of care do not needlessly wait. Protocols may be followed to initiate laboratory or x-ray studies while the patient is in the triage area. Collaborative protocols are developed and used by the triage nurse based on his or her level of experience. Nurses in the triage area collect additional crucial baseline data: full vital signs including pain assessment, history of the current event and past medical history, neurologic assessment findings, weight, allergies (especially to latex and medications), domestic violence screening, and necessary diagnostic data. Some facilities collect these data in a computerized system, which helps guide the nurse through assessment and documentation. The following questions reflect the minimum information that should be obtained from the patient or from the person who accompanied the patient to the ED and then are documented.

- What were the circumstances, precipitating events, location, and time of the injury or illness?
- When did the symptoms appear?
- Was the patient unconscious after the injury or onset of illness?

- How did the patient get to the ED?
- What was the health status of the patient before the injury or illness?
- Is there a history of medical illness or previous surgeries? A history of admissions to the hospital?
- Is the patient currently taking any medications, especially hormones, insulin, digitalis, or anticoagulants? Is the patient using any complementary or alternative therapies such as herbology, naturopathy, reiki, massage, or acupuncture?
- Does the patient have any allergies, especially to latex, medications, eggs, or nuts?
- Does the patient smoke or use recreational drugs? How frequently? What type? When was the last time they were used?
- Does the patient have any fears? Does the patient feel that he or she is in danger or in an unsafe situation?
- When was the last meal eaten? (This is important if general anesthesia is to be given or if the patient is unconscious.)
- When was the last menstrual period?
- Is the patient under a physician's care? What are the name and contact information for the physician?
- What was the date of the patient's most recent tetanus immunization?

In addition to the collection of initial vital signs and medical history, triage consists of providing basic first aid, which may include application of ice, bleeding control, and basic wound care, as well as initiating protocol-based orders (eg, x-rays, administering antipyretics or mild analgesics, obtaining an electrocardiogram [ECG] or urinalysis, removing sutures). The triage nurse also is responsible for and monitors the waiting area, maintains a safe environment, reassesses waiting patients, and is the initial liaison to the families of patients.

Routine ED triage protocols differ significantly from the triage protocols used in disasters and mass casualty incidents (field triage). Routine triage directs all available resources to the patients who are most critically ill, regardless of potential outcome. In field triage (or hospital triage during a disaster), scarce resources must be used to benefit the most people possible. This distinction affects triage decisions (see Chapter 72).

Assess and Intervene

For the patient assigned to a resuscitation, emergent, or urgent triage category, stabilization, provision of critical treatments, and prompt transfer to the appropriate setting (intensive care unit, operating room, general care unit) are the priorities of emergency care. Although treatment is initiated in the ED, ongoing definitive treatment of the underlying problem is provided in other settings, and the sooner the patient is stabilized and moved to that area, the better the outcome.

A systematic approach to effectively establishing and treating health priorities is the primary survey/secondary survey approach. The primary survey focuses on stabilizing life-threatening conditions. The ED staff work collaboratively and follow the ABCD (airway, breathing, circulation, disability) method:

- Establish a patent airway.
- Provide adequate ventilation, employing resuscitation measures when necessary. (Trauma patients must have the cervical spine protected and chest injuries assessed first, immediately after the airway is established.)
- Evaluate and restore cardiac output by controlling hemorrhage, preventing and treating shock, and maintaining or restoring effective circulation. This includes the prevention and management of hypothermia. In addition, peripheral pulses are examined, and any immediate closed reductions of fractures or dislocations are performed if an extremity is pulseless.
- Determine neurologic disability by assessing neurologic function using the Glasgow Coma Scale and a motor and sensory evaluation of the spine (see Chapter 60).

After these priorities have been addressed, the ED team proceeds with the secondary survey. This includes the following:

- A complete health history and head-to-toe assessment (includes a reassessment of airway and breathing parameters)
- Diagnostic and laboratory testing
- Insertion or application of monitoring devices such as ECG electrodes, arterial lines, or urinary catheters
- Splinting of suspected fractures
- Cleansing, closure, and dressing of wounds
- Performance of other necessary interventions based on the patient's condition

Once the patient has been assessed, stabilized, and tested, appropriate medical and nursing diagnoses are formulated, initial important treatment is started, and plans for the proper disposition of the patient are made. Many emergent and urgent conditions and priority emergency interventions are discussed in detail in the remaining sections of this chapter.

In addition to the management of the illness or injury, the ED nurse must also focus on providing comfort and emotional support to the patient and family. Included in this is pain management. Effective pain management must be instituted early and should include rapid-acting agents that result in minimal sedation so that the patient can continue to interact with the staff for continued assessment. Moderate sedation can help facilitate short procedures in the ED; the patient will not remember the procedure later. The patient is closely monitored during the procedure and then rapidly awakens when it is complete (see Chapter 19).

It is essential that family crisis intervention services are available for families of ED patients. Even if a patient's condition is not emergent, the situation may be perceived as such by the family. Every family needs attention and support. The chaplain and social worker may be available to assist with interventions.

AIRWAY OBSTRUCTION

Acute upper airway obstruction is a life-threatening medical emergency.

Pathophysiology

The airway may be partially or completely occluded. Partial obstruction of the airway can lead to progressive hypoxia, hypercarbia, and respiratory and cardiac arrest. If the airway is completely obstructed, permanent brain injury or death will occur within 3 to 5 minutes secondary to hypoxia. Air movement is absent in the presence of complete airway obstruction. Oxygen saturation of the blood decreases rapidly because obstruction of the airway prevents entry of air into the lungs. Oxygen deficit occurs in the brain, resulting in unconsciousness, with death following rapidly.

Upper airway obstruction has a number of causes, including aspiration of foreign bodies, anaphylaxis, viral or bacterial infection, trauma, and inhalation or chemical burns. For elderly patients, especially those in extended-care facilities, sedatives and hypnotic medications, diseases affecting motor coordination (eg, Parkinson's disease), and mental dysfunction (eg, dementia, mental retardation) are risk factors for asphyxiation by food. In adults, aspiration of a bolus of meat is the most common cause of airway obstruction. Peritonsillar abscesses, epiglottitis, and other acute infectious processes of the posterior pharynx can also result in airway obstruction (Marx, 2006).

Clinical Manifestations

Typically, a person with a foreign body airway obstruction cannot speak, breathe, or cough. The patient may clutch the neck between the thumb and fingers (ie, universal distress signal). Other common signs and symptoms include choking, apprehensive appearance, refusing to lie flat, inspiratory and expiratory stridor, labored breathing, use of accessory muscles (suprasternal and intercostal retraction), flaring nostrils, increasing anxiety, restlessness, and confusion. Cyanosis and loss of consciousness develop as hypoxia worsens. Cyanosis and loss of consciousness are late signs. Action must be taken before these manifestations develop, if possible, or immediately if the patient has already exhibited these signs.

Assessment and Diagnostic Findings

Assessment of the patient who has a foreign object occluding the airway may involve simply asking the person whether he or she is choking and requires help. If the person is unconscious, inspection of the oropharynx may reveal the offending object. X-rays, laryngoscopy, or bronchoscopy also may be performed.

Management

If the patient can breathe and cough spontaneously, a partial obstruction should be suspected. The victim is encouraged to cough forcefully and to persist with spontaneous coughing and breathing efforts as long as good air exchange exists. There may be some wheezing between coughs. If the patient demonstrates a weak, ineffective cough, high-pitched noise while inhaling, increased respiratory difficulty, or cyanosis, the patient should be managed as if there were complete airway obstruction.

After the obstruction is removed, rescue breathing is initiated. If the patient has no pulse, cardiac compressions are instituted. These measures provide oxygen to the brain, heart, and other vital organs until definitive medical treatment can restore and support normal heart and ventilatory activity.

Establishing an Airway

Establishing an airway may be as simple as repositioning the patient's head to prevent the tongue from obstructing the pharynx. Alternatively, other maneuvers, such as abdominal thrusts, the head-tilt–chin-lift maneuver, the jaw-thrust maneuver, or insertion of specialized equipment, may be needed to open the airway, remove a foreign body, or maintain the airway. In all maneuvers, the cervical spine must be protected from injury. After these maneuvers are performed, the patient is assessed for breathing by watching for chest movement and listening and feeling for air movement. In such a case, nursing diagnoses would include ineffective airway clearance related to obstruction of the airway by the tongue, an object, or fluids (blood, saliva) and ineffective breathing pattern related to airway obstruction or injury.

Abdominal Thrusts

The terms *subdiaphragmatic abdominal thrusts, abdominal thrusts,* and *Heimlich maneuver* are used interchangeably. This maneuver causes elevation of the diaphragm, forcing air from the lungs to create an artificial cough that can move and expel an obstructing foreign body from the airway. Chart 71-3 describes how to manage a foreign body obstruction using abdominal or chest thrusts.

Head-Tilt–Chin-Lift Maneuver

The patient is placed supine on a firm, flat surface. If the patient is lying face down, the body is turned as a unit so that the head, shoulders, and torso move simultaneously with no twisting (ie, logroll). Next, the airway is opened using either the head-tilt–chin-lift maneuver or the jaw-thrust maneuver. In the head-tilt–chin-lift maneuver, one hand is placed on the victim's forehead, and firm backward pressure is applied with the palm to tilt the head back. The fingers of the other hand are placed under the bony part of the lower jaw near the chin and lifted up. The chin and the teeth are brought forward almost to occlusion to support the jaw.

 NURSING ALERT

The head-tilt–chin-lift maneuver, which helps tilt the head back, should be used only if it is determined that the patient's cervical spine is not injured.

Jaw-Thrust Maneuver

After one hand is placed on each side of the patient's jaw, the angles of the patient's lower jaw are grasped and lifted, displacing the mandible forward. This is a safe approach to opening the airway of a patient with suspected spinal cord injury because it can be accomplished without extending the neck.

Oropharyngeal Airway Insertion

An oropharyngeal airway is a semicircular tube or tubelike plastic device that is inserted over the back of the tongue into the lower posterior pharynx in a patient who is breathing spontaneously but who is unconscious (Chart 71-4). This type of airway prevents the tongue from falling back

Chart 71-3 • *Managing a Foreign Body Airway Obstruction*

Assess for Indications of Airway Obstruction

- Person may clutch the neck between thumb and fingers
- Weak, ineffective cough; high-pitched noises on inspiration
- Increased respiratory distress
- Inability to speak, breathe, or cough
- Collapse

Heimlich Maneuver (Subdiaphragmatic Abdominal Thrusts)

For Standing or Sitting Conscious Patient

Stand behind the patient, wrap your arms around the patient's waist, and proceed as follows:

1. Make a fist with one hand, placing the thumb side of the fist against the patient's abdomen, in the midline slightly above the umbilicus and well below the xiphoid process. Grasp the fist with the other hand.
2. Press your fist into the patient's abdomen with a quick inward and upward thrust. Each new thrust should be a separate and distinct maneuver. All thrusts should be in rapid sequence.

For Patient Lying Down (Unconscious)

1. Position patient on the back.
2. Kneel astride the patient's thighs, facing the head.
3. Place the heel of one hand against the patient's abdomen, in the midline slightly above the umbilicus and well below the tip of the xiphoid; place the second hand directly on top of the first.
4. Press into the abdomen with a quick upward thrust. All thrusts should be in rapid sequence.

Finger Sweep

1. Open the adult patient's mouth by grasping both the tongue and lower jaw between the thumb and fingers and lifting the mandible (tongue-jaw lift). This maneuver is to be used *only in the unconscious adult patient*. This action

draws the tongue away from the back of the throat and away from the foreign body that may be lodged there.
2. If a foreign body is visible in the mouth, insert the index finger of the other hand down along the inside of the cheek and scrape across the back of the throat.
3. Use a hooking action to dislodge the foreign body and maneuver it into the mouth for removal. Care is used to avoid forcing the object deeper into the throat.

Chest Thrusts With Conscious Patient Standing or Sitting

This technique is to be used *only in the patient in advanced stages of pregnancy or in the markedly obese person.*

1. Stand behind the patient with your arms under the patient's axillae to encircle the patient's chest.
2. Place the thumb side of your fist on the middle of the patient's sternum, taking care to avoid the xiphoid process and the margins of the rib cage.
3. Grasp your fist with the other hand and perform backward thrusts until the foreign body is expelled or the patient becomes unconscious. Each thrust should be administered with the intent of relieving the obstruction. All thrusts should be in rapid sequence.

Chest Thrust With Patient Lying (Unconscious)

This maneuver is *used only in the patient in advanced stages of pregnancy or when the rescuer cannot apply the Heimlich maneuver effectively to the unconscious, markedly obese person.*

1. Place the patient on the back and kneel close to the side of the patient's body.
2. Place the heel of your hand on the lower half of the sternum.
3. Deliver each chest thrust slowly and distinctly with the intent of relieving the obstruction.

Adapted from American Heart Association. (2005). BLS for healthcare providers. Available at: www.americanheart.org.

against the posterior pharynx and obstructing the airway. It also allows health care providers to suction secretions.

Endotracheal Intubation

The purpose of endotracheal intubation is to establish and maintain the airway in patients with respiratory insufficiency or hypoxia. Endotracheal intubation is indicated to establish an airway for a patient who cannot be adequately ventilated with an oropharyngeal airway, bypass an upper airway obstruction, prevent aspiration, permit connection of the patient to a resuscitation bag or mechanical ventilator, or facilitate the removal of tracheobronchial secretions (Fig. 71-1). Because the procedure requires skill, endotracheal intubation is performed only by those who have had extensive training. These may include physicians, nurse anesthetists, respiratory therapists, flight nurses, and nurse practitioners. However, the emergency nurse is commonly called on to assist with intubation.

Rapid sequence intubation may be indicated, which provides management of the patient in a situation similar to that in the operating room. Medications used to facilitate

rapid sequence intubation include a sedative, an analgesic, and a neuromuscular blockade agent; these are usually administered by the practitioner performing the intubation.

Intubation With a Combitube or Laryngeal Mask Airway

If the patient is not hospitalized and cannot be intubated in the field, emergency medical personnel may insert a Combitube, which rapidly provides pharyngeal ventilation. When the tube is inserted into the trachea, it functions like an endotracheal tube (Fig. 71-2).

The two balloons that surround the tube are inflated after the tube is inserted. One balloon is large (100 mL) and occludes the oropharynx. This permits ventilation by forcing air through the larynx. The smaller balloon is inflated with 15 mL of air and is supposed to anchor the device in the esophagus at a site distal to the glottis; however, it can occlude the trachea if it is inadvertently placed there. Breath sounds are auscultated after balloon inflation to make sure that the oropharyngeal balloon (or cuff) does not obstruct the glottis. The patient can be ventilated through either one of the two ports (eg, tracheal or esophageal) of

Chart 71-4 • *Inserting an Oropharyngeal Airway*

1. Measure the oral airway alongside the head. The airway should reach from lip to ear.
2. Extend the patient's head by placing one hand under the bony chin (*only if the cervical spine is uninjured*). With the other hand, tilt the head backward by applying pressure to the forehead while simultaneously lifting the chin forward.
3. Open the patient's mouth.

4. **(A)** Insert the oropharyngeal airway with the tip facing up toward the roof of the mouth until it passes the uvula. **(B)** Rotate the tip 180 degrees so that the tip is pointed down toward the pharynx. This displaces the tongue anteriorly, and the patient then breathes through and around the airway.
5. The distal end of the oropharyngeal airway is in the hypopharynx, and the flange is approximately at the patient's lips. Make sure that the tongue has not been pushed into the airway.

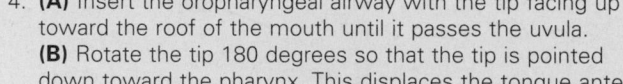

A   B

the tube, depending on whether the tube is placed in the trachea or esophagus.

If it is difficult to establish an airway, a laryngeal mask airway (LMA) may be inserted as an interim airway device. The design of the LMA provides a "mask" in the subglottic airway with a cuff inflated within the esophagus. It allows easy insertion for rapid airway control until a more definitive airway can be placed. Some LMAs also permit removal of secretions from the esophagus (see Chapter 19).

Cricothyroidotomy (Cricothyroid Membrane Puncture)

Cricothyroidotomy is the opening of the cricothyroid membrane to establish an airway. This procedure is used in emergency situations in which endotracheal intubation is

either not possible or contraindicated, as in airway obstruction from extensive maxillofacial trauma, cervical spine injuries, laryngospasm, laryngeal edema (after an allergic reaction or extubation), hemorrhage into neck tissue, or obstruction of the larynx. A cricothyroidotomy is replaced with a formal tracheostomy when the patient is able to tolerate this procedure.

Maintaining Ventilation

Only a few conditions, such as an obstructed airway or a sucking wound of the chest, take precedence over the immediate control of hemorrhage. After the airway is determined to be unobstructed, the nurse must ensure that ventilation is adequate by checking for equal bilateral breath sounds. Satisfactory management of ventilations may prevent hypoxia and hypercapnia. The nurse must quickly assess for absent or diminished breath sounds, open chest wounds, and difficulty delivering artificial breaths for the patient. The nurse should monitor pulse oximetry, capnography, and arterial blood gases if the patient requires airway or ventilatory assistance. A tension pneumothorax can mimic hypovolemia, so ventilatory assessment precedes assessment for hemorrhage. A pneumothorax (both simple and tension) or sucking (open) chest wound is managed with a chest tube; immediate relief of increasing positive intrathoracic pressure and maintenance of adequate ventilation should occur immediately.

HEMORRHAGE

Stopping bleeding is essential to the care and survival of patients in an emergency or disaster situation. Hemorrhage that results in the reduction of circulating blood

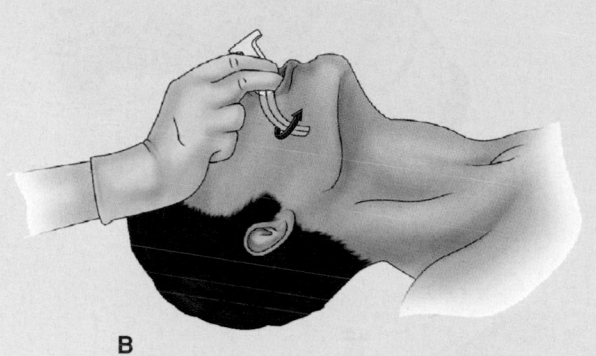

Laryngoscope
Tongue
Tongue
Epiglottis
Vocal cords
Trachea
Arytenoid muscle

A   B

Figure 71-1 Endotracheal intubation in a patient without a cervical spine injury. **A,** The primary glottic landmarks for tracheal intubation as visualized with proper placement of the laryngoscope. **B,** Positioning the endotracheal tube.

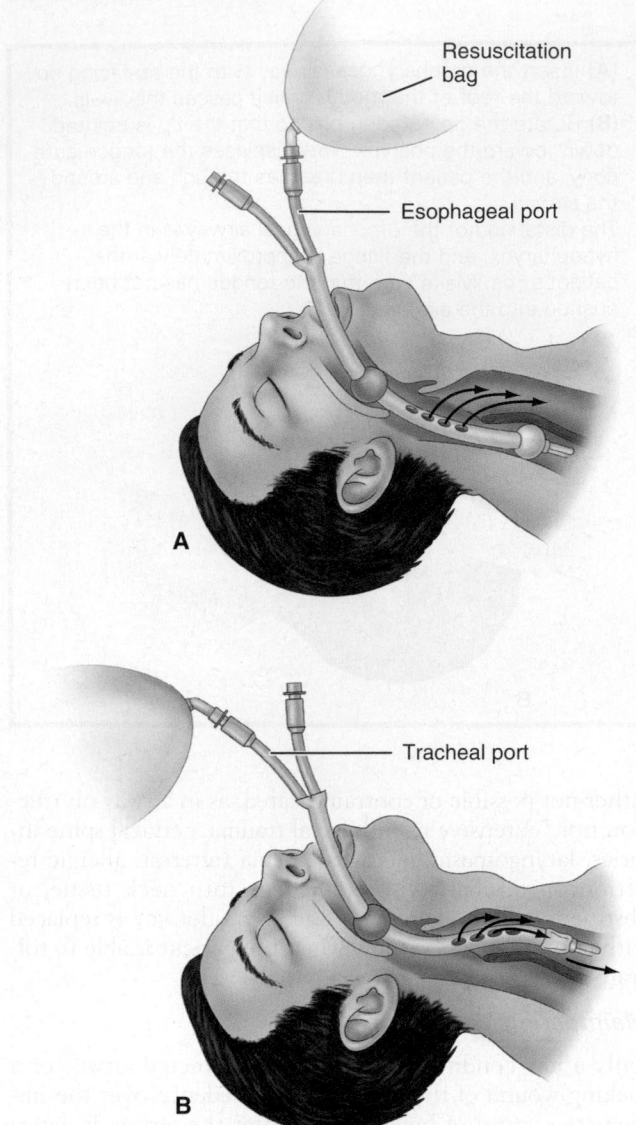

Resuscitation bag

Esophageal port

A

Tracheal port

B

Figure 71-2 A, Combitude in esophageal position. **B,** Combitude tracheal position.

volume is a primary cause of shock. Minor bleeding, which is usually venous, generally stops spontaneously unless the patient has a bleeding disorder or has been taking anticoagulants.

The patient is assessed for signs and symptoms of shock: cool, moist skin (resulting from poor peripheral perfusion), decreasing blood pressure, increasing heart rate, delayed capillary refill, and decreasing urine volume (see Chapter 15). The goals of emergency management are to control the bleeding, maintain adequate circulating blood volume for tissue oxygenation, and prevent shock. Patients who hemorrhage are at risk for cardiac arrest caused by hypovolemia with secondary anoxia. Nursing interventions are carried out collaboratively with other members of the emergency health care team.

Management

Fluid Replacement

Whenever a patient is hemorrhaging—whether externally or internally—a loss of circulating blood results in a fluid volume deficit and decreased cardiac output. Therefore, fluid replacement is imperative to maintain circulation. Typically, two large-gauge IV catheters are inserted to provide a means for fluid and blood replacement, and blood samples are obtained for analysis, typing, and cross-matching. Replacement fluids are administered as prescribed, depending on clinical estimates of the type and volume of fluid lost. Replacement fluids may include isotonic electrolyte solutions (eg, lactated Ringer's, normal saline), colloids, and blood component therapy.

Packed red blood cells are infused when there is massive blood loss, which may also necessitate transfusion of other blood components, including platelets and clotting factors. (See Chapter 33 for full discussion of blood component therapy indications and treatment.)

> ⚑ **NURSING ALERT**
>
> The infusion rate is determined by the severity of the blood loss and the clinical evidence of hypovolemia. If massive blood replacement is necessary, the blood must be warmed in a commercial blood warmer, because administration of large amounts of blood that has been refrigerated has a core cooling effect that may lead to cardiac arrest and coagulopathy.

Control of External Hemorrhage

If a patient is hemorrhaging externally (eg, from a wound), a rapid physical assessment is performed as the patient's clothing is cut away in an attempt to identify the area of hemorrhage. Direct, firm pressure is applied over the bleeding area or the involved artery at a site that is proximal to the wound (Fig. 71-3). Most bleeding can be stopped or at least controlled by application of direct pressure. Otherwise, unchecked arterial bleeding results in death. A firm pressure dressing is applied, and the injured part is elevated to stop venous and capillary bleeding if possible. If the injured area is an extremity, the extremity is immobilized to control blood loss.

A tourniquet is applied to an extremity only as a *last resort* when the external hemorrhage cannot be controlled in any other way and immediate surgery is not feasible. Care must be taken when applying a tourniquet because of the risk of loss of the extremity. The tourniquet is applied just proximal to the wound and tied tightly enough to control arterial blood flow. The patient is tagged with a skin-marking pencil or on adhesive tape on the forehead with a "T," stating the location of the tourniquet and the time applied (Lakstein, Blumenfeld, Sokolov, et al., 2003). If there is no arterial bleeding, the tourniquet is removed and a pressure dressing is applied. If the patient has suffered a traumatic amputation with uncontrollable hemorrhage, the tourniquet remains in place until the patient is in the operating room.

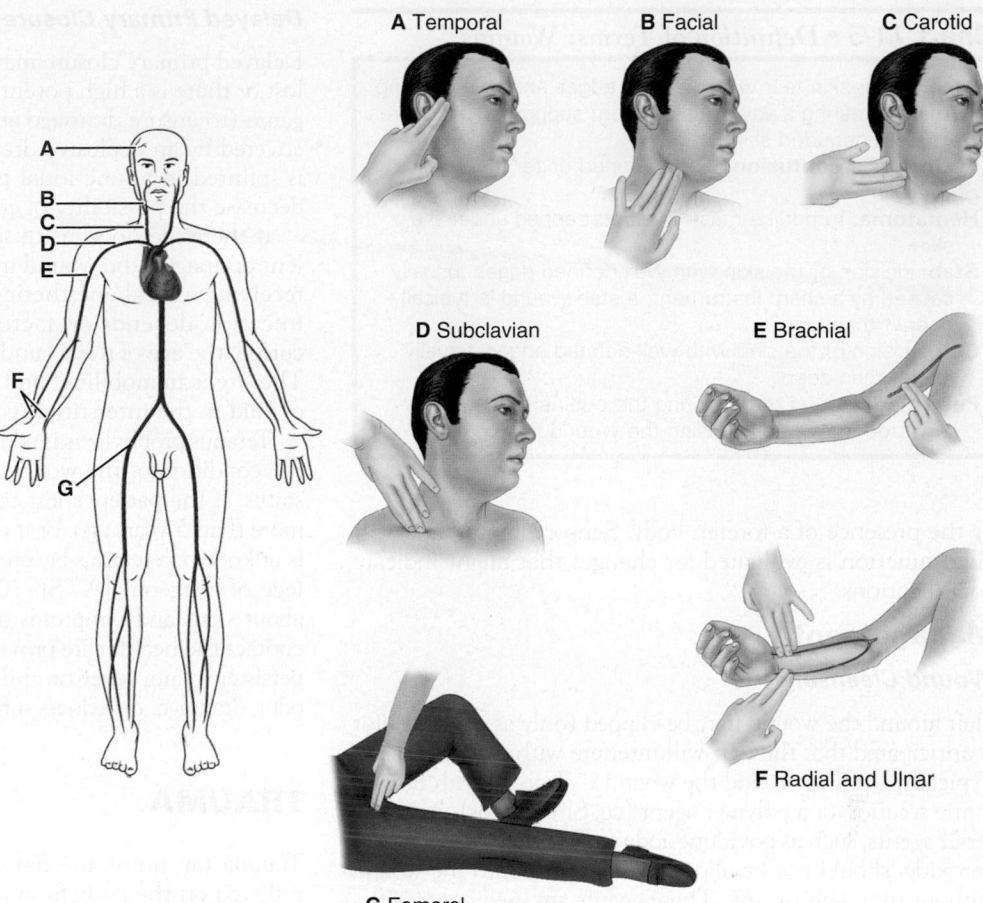

A Temporal **B** Facial **C** Carotid

D Subclavian **E** Brachial

F Radial and Ulnar

G Femoral

Figure 71-3 Pressure points for control of hemorrhage.

Control of Internal Bleeding

If the patient shows no external signs of bleeding but exhibits tachycardia, falling blood pressure, thirst, apprehension, cool and moist skin, or delayed capillary refill, internal hemorrhage is suspected. Typically, packed red blood cells are administered at a rapid rate, and the patient is prepared for more definitive treatment (eg, surgery, pharmacologic therapy). In addition, arterial blood gas specimens are obtained to evaluate pulmonary function and tissue perfusion and to establish baseline hemodynamic parameters, which are then used as an index for determining the amount of fluid replacement the patient can tolerate and the response to therapy. The patient is maintained in the supine position and monitored closely until hemodynamic or circulatory parameters improve, or until he or she is transported to the operating room or intensive care unit.

HYPOVOLEMIC SHOCK

Shock is a condition in which there is loss of effective circulating blood volume. Inadequate organ and tissue perfusion follows, ultimately resulting in cellular metabolic derangements. In any emergency situation, the onset of shock should be anticipated by assessing all injured people immediately. The underlying cause of shock (hypovolemic, cardiogenic, neurogenic, anaphylactic or septic) must be determined. Of these, hypovolemia is the most common cause (see Chapter 15 for further discussion of management of hypovolemic shock).

WOUNDS

Wounds involving injury to soft tissues can vary from minor tears to severe crushing injuries. The types of wounds that may occur are defined in Chart 71-5. The primary goal of treatment is to restore the physical integrity and function of the injured tissue while minimizing scarring and preventing infection. Proper documentation of the characteristics of the wound, using precise descriptions and correct terminology, is essential. Such information may be needed in the future for forensic evidence. Photographs are helpful because they provide an accurate, visible depiction of the wound. Photographs also become important for exigent wounds (ie, wounds that will eventually heal). Patients involved in domestic violence or trauma may need the photographs later to visually describe the extent of injury.

Determining *when* and *how* the wound occurred is important because a treatment delay increases infection risk. Using aseptic technique, the clinician inspects the wound to determine the extent of damage to underlying structures

Chart 71-5 • *Definition of Terms: Wounds*

Laceration: skin tear with irregular edges and vein bridging

Avulsion: tearing away of tissue from supporting structures

Abrasion: denuded skin

Ecchymosis/contusion: blood trapped under the surface of the skin

Hematoma: tumorlike mass of blood trapped under the skin

Stab: incision of the skin with well-defined edges, usually caused by a sharp instrument; a stab wound is typically deeper than long

Cut: incision of the skin with well-defined edges, usually longer than deep

Patterned: wound representing the outline of the object (eg, steering wheel) causing the wound

or the presence of a foreign body. Sensory, motor, and vascular function is evaluated for changes that might indicate complications.

Management

Wound Cleansing

Hair around the wound may be clipped (only as directed) if it is anticipated that the hair will interfere with wound closure. Typically, the area around the wound is cleansed with normal saline solution or a polymer agent (eg, Shur-Clens). Antibacterial agents, such as povidone-iodine (Betadine) or hydrogen peroxide, should not be allowed to get deep into the wound without thorough rinsing. These agents are used only for the initial cleansing because they injure exposed and healthy tissue, resulting in further tissue damage.

If indicated, the area is infiltrated with a local intradermal anesthetic through the wound margins or by regional block. Patients with soft tissue injuries usually have localized pain at the site of injury. The nurse then assists with cleaning and débriding the wound. The wound is irrigated gently and copiously with sterile isotonic saline solution to remove surface dirt. Devitalized tissue and foreign matter are removed because they impede healing and may promote infection. Any small bleeding vessels are clamped, tied, or cauterized. After wound treatment, a nonadherent dressing is applied to protect the wound and to serve as a splint and as a reminder to the patient that the area is injured.

Primary Closure

The decision to suture a wound depends on the nature of the wound, the time since the injury was sustained, the degree of contamination, and the vascularity of tissues. If primary closure is indicated, the wound is sutured or stapled, usually by the physician, with the patient receiving either local anesthesia or moderate sedation (see Chapter 19). Wound closure begins when subcutaneous fat is brought together loosely with a few sutures to close off the dead space. The subcuticular layer is then closed, and finally the epidermis is closed. Sutures are placed near the wound edge, with the skin edges leveled carefully to promote optimal healing. Instead of sutures, sterile strips of reinforced microporous tape or a bonding agent (skin glue) may be used to close clean, superficial wounds.

Delayed Primary Closure

Delayed primary closure may be indicated if tissue has been lost or there is a high potential for infection. A thin layer of gauze (to ensure drainage and prevent pooling of exudate), covered by an occlusive dressing, may be used. The wound is splinted in a functional position to prevent motion and decrease the possibility of contracture.

If there are no signs of suppuration (formation of purulent drainage), the wound may be sutured (with the patient receiving a local anesthetic). Use of antibiotics to prevent infection depends on factors such as how the injury occurred, the age of the wound, and the risk of contamination. The site is immobilized and elevated to limit accumulation of fluid in the interstitial spaces of the wound.

Tetanus prophylaxis is administered as prescribed, based on the condition of the wound and the patient's immunization status. If the patient's last tetanus booster was administered more than 5 years ago, or if the patient's immunization status is unknown, a tetanus booster must be given (American College of Surgeons [ACS], 2008). The patient is instructed about signs and symptoms of infection and is instructed to contact the health care provider or clinic if there is sudden or persistent pain, fever or chills, bleeding, rapid swelling, foul odor, drainage, or redness surrounding the wound.

TRAUMA

Trauma (an unintentional or intentional wound or injury inflicted on the body from a mechanism against which the body cannot protect itself) is the fourth leading cause of death in the United States. Trauma is the leading cause of death in children and in adults younger than 44 years of age. The incidence is increasing in adults older than 44 years of age. Alcohol and drug abuse are often implicated as factors in both blunt and penetrating trauma (McQuillan, VonReuden, Hartsock, et al., 2008).

Collection of Forensic Evidence

In assessing and managing any patient with an emergency condition, but especially the patient experiencing trauma, meticulous documentation is essential. Included in documentation are descriptions of all wounds, mechanism of injury, time of events, and collection of evidence. In trauma care, the nurse must be exceedingly careful with all potential evidence, handling and documenting it properly.

The basics of care management for patients with traumatic injury include an understanding that trauma in any patient (living or dead) has potential legal or forensic implications if criminal activity is suspected. Hence, proper management from both a medical and forensic perspective is essential.

When clothing is removed from the patient who has experienced trauma, the nurse must be careful not to cut through or disrupt any tears, holes, blood stains, or dirt present on the clothing if criminal activity is suspected. Each piece of clothing should be placed in an individual paper bag. If the clothing is wet, it should be hung to dry. Clothing should not be given to families. Valuables should be inventoried and either placed in the hospital safe or it should be clearly documented to which family member they were given. If a police officer is present to collect clothing or any other items from the patient, each item is labeled. The transfer of custody to the officer, the officer's name, the date, and the time are documented.

If suicide or homicide is suspected in a deceased trauma patient, the medical examiner examines the body on site or has the body moved to the coroner's office for autopsy. All tubes and lines must remain in place. The patient's hands must be covered with paper bags to protect evidence on the hands or under the fingernails. In the surviving patient, tissue specimens may be swabbed from the hands and nails as potential evidence. Photographs of wounds or clothing are essential and should include a reference ruler in one photo and one without the ruler.

Documentation should also include any statements made by the patient in the patient's own words and surrounded by quotation marks. A chain of evidence is essential. If the patient's case is reviewed in a court of law in the future, clear documentation assists the judicial process and helps to identify the activities that occurred in the ED.

Injury Prevention

Any discussion of trauma management must address injury prevention. A component of the emergency nurse's daily role is to provide injury prevention information to every patient with whom there is contact, including patients admitted for reasons other than injury. The only way to reduce the incidence of trauma is through prevention.

There are three components of injury prevention. The first is education. Providing information and materials to help prevent violence and to maintain safety at home and in vehicles is important. Involvement in local injury prevention organizations, nursing organizations, and health fairs promotes wellness and safety. In practice, nursing and other health care professionals should avoid using the word "accident," because trauma events are *preventable* and should be viewed as such rather than as "fate" or "happenstance." Responsibility and accountability must be assigned to traumatic incidents, particularly because of the high rate of trauma recidivism (repeated trauma). People who are at risk for trauma and trauma recidivism should be identified and provided with education and counseling directed toward altering risky behaviors and preventing further trauma (ENA, 2007).

The second component of injury prevention is legislation. Nurses should be actively involved in safety legislation at the local, state, and federal levels. Such legislation is meant to provide universal safety measures, not to infringe on rights.

The third component is automatic protection. Airbags and automotive design are included in this category. These mechanisms provide for safety without requiring personal intervention.

Multiple Trauma

Multiple trauma is caused by a single catastrophic event that causes life-threatening injuries to at least two distinct organs or organ systems. Patients with single-system trauma still receive full assessment, because even single-system injuries can be life-threatening or more severe than they initially appear. Mortality in patients with multiple trauma is related to the severity of the injuries and the number of systems and organs involved. Immediately after injury, the body is hypermetabolic, hypercoagulable, and severely stressed.

Care of the patient with multiple injuries requires a team approach, with one person responsible for coordinating the treatment. The nursing staff assumes responsibility for assessing and monitoring the patient, ensuring airway and IV access, administering prescribed medications, collecting laboratory specimens, and documenting activities and the patient's subsequent responses.

Assessment and Diagnostic Findings

Evidence of trauma may be sparse or absent. Patients with multiple trauma should be assumed to have a spinal cord injury until it is proven otherwise. The injury regarded as the least significant in appearance may be the most lethal. For example, the pelvic fracture not identified until an x-ray is obtained may cause rapid and massive hemorrhage into the pelvic cavity, but an obvious amputation of the arm may have already stopped bleeding from the body's normal response of vasoconstriction.

Management

The goals of treatment are to determine the extent of injuries and to establish priorities of treatment. Any injury interfering with a vital physiologic function (eg, airway, breathing, circulation) is an immediate threat to life and has the highest priority for immediate treatment. Essential life-saving procedures are performed simultaneously by the emergency team. As soon as the patient is resuscitated, clothes are removed or cut off and a rapid physical assessment is performed. Transfer from field management to the ED must be orderly and controlled, with attention given to the verbal report from emergency medical services. Treatment in a trauma center is appropriate for patients experiencing major trauma. Treatment priorities are presented in Chart 71-6.

Intra-Abdominal Injuries

Intra-abdominal injuries are categorized as penetrating or blunt trauma. *Penetrating* abdominal injuries (ie, gunshot wounds, stab wounds) are serious and usually require surgery. Penetrating abdominal trauma results in a high incidence of injury to hollow organs, particularly the small bowel. The liver is the most frequently injured solid organ. In gunshot wounds, the most important prognostic factor is the velocity at which the missile enters the body. High-velocity missiles (bullets) produce extensive tissue damage. All abdominal gunshot wounds that cross the peritoneum or are associated with peritoneal signs require surgical exploration. On the other hand, some stab wounds may be managed nonoperatively due to low velocity and less penetration of the implement (ie, weapon).

Blunt trauma to the abdomen may result from motor vehicle crashes, falls, blows, or explosions. Blunt trauma is commonly associated with extra-abdominal injuries to the chest, head, or extremities. Patients with blunt trauma are a

Chart 71-6 • *Priority Management in Patients with Multiple Injuries*

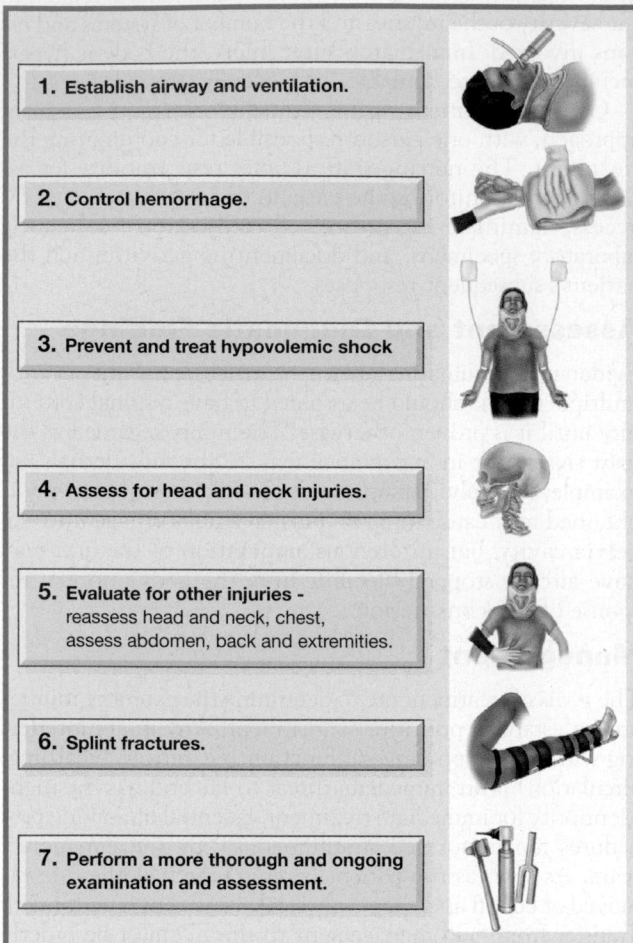

1. **Establish airway and ventilation.**

2. **Control hemorrhage.**

3. **Prevent and treat hypovolemic shock**

4. **Assess for head and neck injuries.**

5. **Evaluate for other injuries -**
   reassess head and neck, chest,
   assess abdomen, back and extremities.

6. **Splint fractures.**

7. **Perform a more thorough and ongoing
   examination and assessment.**

challenge because injuries may be difficult to detect. The incidence of delayed and trauma-related complications is greater than for penetrating injuries. This is especially true of blunt injuries involving the liver, kidneys, spleen, or blood vessels, which can lead to massive blood loss into the peritoneal cavity.

Assessment and Diagnostic Findings

As the history of the traumatic event is obtained, the abdomen is inspected as a part of the secondary survey for obvious signs of injury, including penetrating injuries, bruises, and abrasions. Abdominal assessment continues with auscultation of bowel sounds to provide baseline data from which changes can be noted. Absence of bowel sounds may be an early sign of intraperitoneal involvement, although stress can also decrease or halt peristalsis and bowel sounds. Further abdominal assessment may reveal progressive abdominal distention, involuntary guarding, tenderness, pain, muscular rigidity, or rebound tenderness along with changes in bowel sounds, all of which are signs of peritoneal irritation. Hypotension and signs and symptoms of shock may also be noted. Additionally, the chest and other body systems are assessed for injuries that frequently accompany intra-abdominal injuries.

Laboratory studies that aid in assessment include the following:

- Urinalysis to detect hematuria (indicative of a urinary tract injury)
- Serial hemoglobin and hematocrit levels to evaluate trends reflecting the presence or absence of bleeding
- White blood cell (WBC) count to detect elevation (generally associated with trauma)
- Serum amylase analysis to detect increasing levels, which suggest pancreatic injury or perforation of the gastrointestinal tract

Internal Bleeding

Hemorrhage frequently accompanies abdominal injury, especially if the liver or spleen has been traumatized. Therefore, the patient is assessed continuously for signs and symptoms of external and internal bleeding. The front of the body, flanks, and back are inspected for bluish discoloration, asymmetry, abrasion, and contusion. Abdominal computed tomography (CT) scans permit detailed evaluation of abdominal contents and retroperitoneal examination. Abdominal ultrasounds can rapidly assess hemodynamically unstable patients to detect intraperitoneal bleeding. This is referred to as the focused assessment sonography for trauma (FAST) examination (Kirkpatrick, Sirois, Laupland, et al., 2005). Pain in the left shoulder is common in a patient with bleeding from a ruptured spleen, whereas pain in the right shoulder can result from laceration of the liver. During the resuscitation period, pain is managed using administration of small dosages of opioids (ACS, 2008).

Intraperitoneal Injury

The abdomen is assessed for tenderness, rebound tenderness, guarding, rigidity, spasm, increasing distention, and pain. Referred pain is a significant finding because it suggests intraperitoneal injury. To determine if there is intraperitoneal injury and bleeding, the patient is usually prepared for diagnostic procedures, such as peritoneal lavage, abdominal ultrasonography, or abdominal CT scanning. **Diagnostic peritoneal lavage** (DPL), although no longer the standard diagnostic study used to evaluate a traumatized abdomen, remains a backup procedure that is easily performed and is very useful during mass casualty situations when CT scanners may not be readily available. DPL involves the instillation of 1 L of warmed lactated Ringer's or normal saline solution into the abdominal cavity. After a minimum of 400 mL has been returned, a fluid specimen is sent to the laboratory for analysis. Positive laboratory findings include a red blood cell count greater than $100,000/mm^3$; a WBC count greater than $500/mm^3$; or the presence of bile, feces, or food.

In patients with stab wounds, sinography may be performed to detect peritoneal penetration; a purse-string suture is placed around the wound and a small catheter is introduced through the wound. A contrast agent is then introduced through the catheter, and x-rays are taken to identify any peritoneal penetration.

Genitourinary Injury

A focused genitourinary examination, which typically includes a rectal and/or vaginal examination, is performed to determine any injury to the pelvis, bladder, urethra, or intestinal wall. To decompress the bladder and monitor urine output, an indwelling catheter is inserted after a rectal examination has been completed (not before). In the male patient, a high-riding prostate gland (abnormal position) discovered during a rectal examination indicates a potential urethral injury.

 NURSING ALERT

Urethral catheter insertion with a possible urethral injury is contraindicated; a urology consultation and further evaluation of the urethra are required.

Management

As indicated by the patient's condition, resuscitation procedures (restoration of airway, breathing, and circulation) are initiated as previously described.

With blunt trauma, the patient is kept on a stretcher to immobilize the spine. A backboard may be used for transporting the patient to the x-ray department, to the operating room, or to the intensive care unit. Cervical spine immobilization is maintained until cervical x-rays have been obtained and cervical spine injury has been ruled out. Likewise, once the patient has arrived at the definitive destination, the backboard is removed, and logrolling can be used to protect the spine until x-rays are obtained and confirm there is no evidence of injuries.

Knowing the mechanism of injury (eg, penetrating force from a gunshot or knife, blunt force from a blow) is essential to determining the type of management needed. All wounds are located, counted, and documented. If abdominal viscera protrude, the area is covered with sterile, moist saline dressings to keep the viscera from drying.

Typically, oral fluids are withheld in anticipation of surgery, and the stomach contents are aspirated with a nasogastric tube to reduce the risk of aspiration and to decompress the stomach in preparation for diagnostic procedures.

Trauma predisposes the patient to infection by disruption of mechanical barriers, exposure to exogenous bacteria from the environment at the time of injury, aspiration of vomitus, and diagnostic and therapeutic procedures (hospital-acquired infection). Tetanus prophylaxis and broad-spectrum antibiotics are administered as prescribed.

Throughout the stay in the ED, the patient's condition is continuously monitored for changes. If there is continuing evidence of shock, blood loss, free air under the diaphragm, evisceration, hematuria, severe head injury, or suspected or known abdominal injury, the patient is rapidly transported to surgery. In most cases, blunt liver and spleen injuries are managed nonsurgically.

Crush Injuries

Crush injuries occur when a person is caught between opposing forces (eg, run over by a moving vehicle, crushed between two cars, crushed under a collapsed building).

Assessment and Diagnostic Findings

The patient is observed for the following:

- Hypovolemic shock resulting from extravasation of blood and plasma into injured tissues after compression has been released

- Paralysis of a body part
- Erythema and blistering of skin
- Damaged body part (usually an extremity) appearing swollen, tense, and hard
- Renal dysfunction (prolonged hypotension causes kidney damage and acute renal insufficiency; myoglobinuria secondary to muscle damage can cause acute tubular necrosis and acute renal failure)

Management

In conjunction with maintaining the airway, breathing, and circulation, the patient is observed for acute renal insufficiency. Injury to the back can cause kidney damage. Severe muscular damage may cause rhabdomyolysis, which signifies a release of myoglobin from ischemic skeletal muscle, resulting in acute tubular necrosis. In addition, major soft tissue injuries are splinted promptly to control bleeding and pain. The serum lactic acid level is monitored; a decrease to less than 2.5 mmol/L is an indication of successful resuscitation (Blow, Magliore, Claridge, et al., 1999).

If an extremity is injured, it is elevated to relieve swelling and pressure. If compartment syndrome develops, the physician may perform a **fasciotomy** (ie, surgical incision to the level of the fascia) to restore neurovascular function (see Chapter 69). Medications for pain and anxiety are then administered as prescribed, and the patient is quickly transported to the operating suite for wound débridement and fracture repair. A hyperbaric oxygen chamber (if available) may be used to hyperoxygenate crushed tissue, if indicated.

Fractures

Immediate appropriate management of a fracture may determine the patient's eventual outcome and may mean the difference between recovery and disability. When the patient is being examined for fracture, the body part is handled gently and as little as possible. Clothing is cut off to visualize the affected body part. Assessment is conducted for pain over or near a bone, swelling (from blood, lymph, and exudate infiltrating the tissue), and circulatory disturbance. The patient is assessed for ecchymosis, tenderness, and crepitation (see Chapter 69). The nurse must remember that the patient may have multiple fractures accompanied by head, chest, spine, or abdominal injuries.

Management

Immediate attention is given to the patient's general condition. Assessment of airway, breathing, and circulation (which includes pulses in the extremities) is conducted. The patient is also evaluated for neurologic or abdominal injuries before the extremity is treated, unless a pulseless extremity is detected.

If a pulseless extremity is identified, repositioning of the extremity to proper alignment is required. If the pulseless extremity involves a fractured hip or femur, **Hare traction** (a portable in-line traction device) may be applied to assist with alignment. If repositioning is ineffective in restoring the pulse, a rapid total-body assessment must be completed, followed by transfer of the patient to the operating room for arteriography and possible arterial repair.

After the initial evaluation has been completed, all injuries identified are evaluated and treated. The fractured body part is inspected. Using a systematic head-to-toe approach, the nurse inspects the entire body, observing for lacerations, swelling, and deformities, including angulation (bending), shortening, rotation, and asymmetry. All peripheral pulses, especially those distal to the fractured extremity, are palpated. The extremity is also assessed for coolness, blanching, and decreased sensation and motor function, which are indicative of injury to the extremity's neurovascular supply.

A splint is applied before the patient is moved. Splinting immobilizes the joint at a site distal and proximal to the fracture, relieves pain, restores or improves circulation, prevents further tissue injury, and prevents a closed fracture from becoming an open one. To splint an extremity, one hand is placed distal to the fracture and some traction is applied while the other hand is placed beneath the fracture for support. The splints should extend beyond the joints adjacent to the fracture. Upper extremities must be splinted in a functional position. If the fracture is open, a moist, sterile dressing is applied.

After splinting, the vascular status of the extremity is checked by assessing color, temperature, pulse, and blanching of the nail bed. In addition, the patient is assessed for neurovascular compromise if pain or pressure is reported. (See Chapter 69 for a complete description of fracture management.)

ENVIRONMENTAL EMERGENCIES

Heat Stroke

Heat stroke is an acute medical emergency caused by failure of the heat-regulating mechanisms of the body. The most common cause of heat stroke is prolonged exposure to an environmental temperature of greater than 39.2°C (102.5°F). It usually occurs during extended heat waves, especially when they are accompanied by high humidity.

People at risk for heat stroke are those not acclimatized to heat, those who are elderly or very young, those unable to care for themselves, those with chronic and debilitating diseases, and those taking certain medications (eg, major tranquilizers, anticholinergics, diuretics, beta-blockers). Exertional heat stroke occurs in healthy individuals during sports or work activities (eg, exercising in extreme heat and humidity). Hyperthermia results because of inadequate heat loss. This type of heat stroke can also cause death. Strategies used to prevent heat stroke are reviewed in Chart 71-7.

Another form of heat stroke is heat exhaustion in which the patient's temperature may be normal to 40°C (104°F). The patient demonstrates weakness, hypotension, increased heart rate, and increased thirst.

Gerontologic Considerations

Most heat-related deaths occur in the elderly because their circulatory systems are unable to compensate for stress imposed by heat. Elderly people have a decreased ability to perspire as well as a decreased ability to vasodilate and vasoconstrict. They have less subcutaneous tissue, a decreased thirst mechanism, and a diminished ability to concentrate

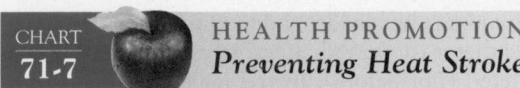

urine to compensate for heat. Many elderly people do not drink adequate amounts of fluid, partly because of fear of incontinence, and thus have a greater risk of heat stroke. In addition, many elderly people fear being victims of crime, so they tend to keep windows closed, even when the temperature and humidity levels are high.

Assessment and Diagnostic Findings

Heat stroke causes thermal injury at the cellular level, resulting in coagulopathies and widespread damage to the heart, liver, and kidneys. Recent patient history reveals exposure to elevated ambient temperature or excessive exercise during extreme heat. When assessing the patient, the nurse notes the following symptoms: profound central nervous system (CNS) dysfunction (manifested by confusion, delirium, bizarre behavior, coma); elevated body temperature (40.6°C [105°F] or higher); hot, dry skin; and usually anhidrosis (absence of sweating), tachypnea, hypotension, and tachycardia.

Management

The primary goal is to reduce the high body temperature as quickly as possible, because mortality is directly related to the duration of hyperthermia. Simultaneous treatment focuses on stabilizing oxygenation using the ABCs (airway, breathing, and circulation) of basic life support. This includes establishing IV access for fluid administration.

After the patient's clothing is removed, the core (internal) temperature is reduced to 39°C (102°F) as rapidly as possible, preferably within 1 hour (Hoyt & Selfridge-Thomas, 2007). One or more of the following methods may be used as prescribed:

- Cool sheets and towels or continuous sponging with cool water
- Ice applied to the neck, groin, chest, and axillae while spraying with tepid water
- Cooling blankets
- Immersion of the patient in a cold water bath (if possible) (Auerbach, 2007)

During cooling procedures, an electric fan is positioned so that it blows on the patient to augment heat dissipation by convection and evaporation. The patient's temperature is constantly monitored with a thermistor placed in the rectum, bladder, or esophagus to evaluate core temperature. Caution is used to avoid hypothermia and to prevent hyperthermia, which may recur spontaneously within 3 to 4 hours. The cooling process should stop at 38.8°C (102°F) in order to avoid iatrogenic hypothermia (Hoyt & Selfridge-Thomas, 2007).

Throughout treatment, the patient's status is monitored carefully, including vital signs, ECG findings (for possible myocardial ischemia, myocardial infarction, and dysrhythmias), central venous pressure (CVP), and level of responsiveness, all of which may change with rapid alterations in body temperature. A seizure may be followed by recurrence of hyperthermia. To meet tissue needs exaggerated by the hypermetabolic condition, 100% oxygen is administered. Endotracheal intubation and mechanical ventilation to support failing cardiopulmonary systems may be required.

IV infusion therapy of normal saline or lactated Ringer's solution is initiated as directed to replace fluid losses and maintain adequate circulation. Fluids are administered carefully because of the dangers of myocardial injury from high body temperature and poor renal function. Cooling redistributes fluid volume from the periphery to the core.

Urine output is also measured frequently, because acute tubular necrosis may occur as a complication of heat stroke from rhabdomyolysis (myoglobin in the urine). Blood specimens are obtained for serial testing to detect bleeding disorders, such as disseminated intravascular coagulation (DIC), and for serial enzyme studies to estimate thermal hypoxic injury to the liver, heart, and muscle tissue. Permanent liver, cardiac, and CNS damage may occur.

Additional supportive care may include dialysis for renal failure, antiseizure medications to control seizures, potassium for hypokalemia, and sodium bicarbonate to correct metabolic acidosis. Benzodiazepines (eg, diazepam [Valium]) or chlorpromazine (Thorazine) may be prescribed to suppress seizure activity. Patient education regarding the prevention of heat stroke (see Chart 71-7) is also important to prevent a recurrence.

Frostbite

Frostbite is trauma from exposure to freezing temperatures and freezing of the intracellular fluid and fluids in the intercellular spaces. It results in cellular and vascular damage. Frostbite can result in venous stasis and thrombosis. Body parts most frequently affected by frostbite include the feet, hands, nose, and ears. Frostbite ranges from first degree (redness and erythema) to fourth degree (full-depth tissue destruction).

Assessment and Diagnostic Findings

A frozen extremity may be hard, cold, and insensitive to touch and may appear white or mottled blue-white. The extent of injury from exposure to cold is not always initially known. The patient history should include environmental temperature, duration of exposure, humidity, and the presence of wet conditions.

Management

The goal of management is to restore normal body temperature. Constrictive clothing and jewelry that could impair circulation are removed. Wet clothing is removed as rapidly as possible. If the lower extremities are involved, the patient should not be allowed to ambulate.

Controlled yet rapid rewarming is instituted. Frozen extremities are usually placed in a 37°C to 40°C (98.6°F to 104°F) circulating bath for 30- to 40-minute spans. This treatment is repeated until circulation is effectively restored. Early rewarming appears to decrease the amount of ultimate tissue loss. During rewarming, an analgesic for pain is administered as prescribed, because the rewarming process may be very painful. To avoid further mechanical injury, the body part is not handled. Massage is contraindicated.

Once rewarmed, the part is protected from further injury and is elevated to help control swelling. Sterile gauze or cotton is placed between affected fingers or toes to prevent maceration, and a bulky dressing is placed on the extremity. A foot cradle may be used to prevent contact with bedclothes if the feet are involved. Hemorrhagic blebs, which may develop 1 hour to a few days after rewarming, are left intact and not ruptured. Nonhemorrhagic blisters are débrided to decrease the inflammatory mediators found in the blister fluid.

A physical assessment is conducted with rewarming to observe for concomitant injury, such as soft tissue injury, dehydration, alcohol coma, or fat embolism. Problems such as hyperkalemia (eg, from release of potassium in the damaged cells) and hypovolemia, which occur frequently in people with frostbite, are corrected. Risk of infection is also great; therefore, strict aseptic technique is used during dressing changes, and tetanus prophylaxis is administered as indicated. Nonsteroidal anti-inflammatory medication is prescribed for its anti-inflammatory effects and to control pain.

Additional measures that may be carried out when appropriate include the following:

- Whirlpool bath for the affected body parts to aid circulation and débridement of necrotic tissue to help prevent infection
- Escharotomy (incision through the eschar) to prevent further tissue damage, to allow for normal circulation, and to permit joint motion
- Fasciotomy to treat compartment syndrome

After rewarming, hourly active motion of any affected digits is encouraged to promote maximal restoration of function and to prevent contractures. Discharge instructions also include encouraging the patient to avoid tobacco, alcohol, and caffeine because of their vasoconstrictive effects, which further reduce the already deficient blood supply to injured tissues.

Hypothermia

Hypothermia is a condition in which the core (internal) temperature is 35°C (95°F) or less as a result of exposure to cold or an inability to maintain body temperature in the absence of low ambient temperatures. Urban hypothermia (extreme exposure to cold in an urban setting) is associated with a high mortality rate; elderly people, infants, people with concurrent illnesses, and the homeless are particularly susceptible. Alcohol ingestion increases susceptibility because it causes systemic vasodilation. Some medications (eg, phenothiazines) or medical conditions (eg, hypothyroidism, spinal cord injury) decrease the ability to shiver, hampering the body's innate ability to generate body heat. Trauma victims are also at risk for hypothermia resulting from treatment with cold fluids, unwarmed oxygen, and exposure during examination. The patient may also have frostbite, but hypothermia takes precedence in treatment.

Assessment and Diagnostic Findings

Hypothermia leads to physiologic changes in all organ systems. There is progressive deterioration, with apathy, poor judgment, ataxia, dysarthria, drowsiness, pulmonary edema, acid–base abnormalities, coagulopathy, and eventual coma. Shivering may be suppressed at a temperature of less than 32.2°C (90°F), because the body's self-warming mechanisms become ineffective. The heartbeat and blood pressure may be so weak that peripheral pulses become undetectable. Cardiac dysrhythmias may also occur. Other physiologic abnormalities include hypoxemia and acidosis.

Management

Management consists of removal of wet clothing, continuous monitoring, rewarming, and supportive care.

Monitoring

The ABCs of basic life support are a priority. The patient's vital signs, CVP, urine output, arterial blood gas levels, blood chemistry determinations (blood urea nitrogen, creatinine, glucose, electrolytes), and chest x-rays are evaluated frequently. Body temperature is monitored with an esophageal, bladder, or rectal thermistor. Continuous ECG monitoring is performed, because cold-induced myocardial irritability leads to conduction disturbances, especially ventricular fibrillation. An arterial line is inserted and maintained to record blood pressure and to facilitate blood sampling.

Rewarming

Rewarming methods include active internal (core) rewarming and passive or active external (spontaneous) rewarming.

Active internal (core) rewarming methods are used for moderate to severe hypothermia (less than 28°C to 32.2°C [82.5°F to 90°F]) and include cardiopulmonary bypass, warm fluid administration, warm humidified oxygen by ventilator, and warmed peritoneal lavage. Monitoring for ventricular fibrillation as the patient's temperature increases from 31°C to 32°C (88°F to 90°F) is essential.

Passive or active external rewarming is used for mild hypothermia (32.2°C to 35°C [90°F to 95°F]). Passive active rewarming uses over-the-bed heaters to the extremities and increases blood flow to the acidotic, anaerobic extremities. The cold blood from peripheral tissues has high lactic acid levels. As this blood returns to the core, it causes a significant drop in the core temperature (ie, core temperature

afterdrop) and can potentially cause cardiac dysrhythmias and electrolyte disturbances. Active external rewarming uses forced air warm blankets. Care must be taken to prevent extremity burn from these devices, because the patient may not have effective sensation to feel the burn.

Supportive Care

Supportive care during rewarming includes the following as directed:

- External cardiac compression (typically performed only as directed in patients with temperatures higher than 31°C [88°F]).
- Defibrillation of ventricular fibrillation. A patient whose temperature is less than 32°C [90°F] experiences spontaneous ventricular fibrillation if moved or touched. Defibrillation is ineffective in patients with temperatures lower than 31°C (88°F); therefore, the patient must be rewarmed first.
- Mechanical ventilation with positive end-expiratory pressure (PEEP) and heated humidified oxygen to maintain tissue oxygenation.
- Administration of warmed IV fluids to correct hypotension and to maintain urine output and core rewarming, as described previously.
- Administration of sodium bicarbonate to correct metabolic acidosis if necessary.
- Administration of antiarrhythmic medications.
- Insertion of an indwelling urinary catheter to monitor urinary output and renal function.

Near Drowning

Near drowning is defined as survival for at least 24 hours after submersion that caused a respiratory arrest. The most common consequence is hypoxemia. Drowning is the second most common cause of unintentional death in children younger than 14 years. An estimated 8000 drownings and 90,000 near drownings occur yearly in the United States (Hoyt & Selfridge-Thomas, 2007).

Factors associated with drowning and near drowning include alcohol ingestion, inability to swim, diving injuries, hypothermia, and exhaustion. The majority of drowning events occur in pools, lakes, and bathtubs. Suicide by drowning rarely occurs in pools and rarely involves alcohol (Auerbach, 2007).

Efforts to save the patient should not be abandoned prematurely. Successful resuscitation with full neurologic recovery has occurred in near-drowning patients after prolonged submersion in cold water. This is possible because of a decrease in metabolic demands and/or the diving reflex. The near-drowning process involves the onset of hypoxia, hypercapnia, bradycardia, and dysrhythmias. If there is a violent struggle associated with the near-drowning episode, exercise-induced acidosis and tachypnea can result in aspiration. Hypoxia and acidosis cause eventual apnea and loss of consciousness. When the victim loses consciousness and makes a final effort to breathe, the terminal gasp occurs. Water then moves passively into the airways prior to death.

After resuscitation, hypoxia and acidosis are the primary complications experienced by a person who has nearly drowned; immediate intervention in the ED is essential. Resultant pathophysiologic changes and pulmonary injury depend on the type of fluid (fresh or salt water) and the volume aspirated. Fresh water aspiration results in a loss of surfactant and, therefore, an inability to expand the lungs. Salt water aspiration leads to pulmonary edema from the osmotic effects of the salt within the lungs. If a person survives submersion, acute respiratory distress syndrome (ARDS), resulting in hypoxia, hypercarbia, and respiratory or metabolic acidosis, can occur.

Management

Therapeutic goals include maintaining cerebral perfusion and adequate oxygenation to prevent further damage to vital organs. Immediate cardiopulmonary resuscitation is the factor with the greatest influence on survival. The most important priority in resuscitation is to manage the hypoxia, acidosis, and hypothermia. Prevention and management of hypoxia are accomplished by ensuring an adequate airway and respiration, thus improving ventilation (which helps correct respiratory acidosis) and oxygenation. Arterial blood gases are monitored to evaluate oxygen, carbon dioxide, bicarbonate levels, and pH. These parameters determine the type of ventilatory support needed. Use of endotracheal intubation with PEEP improves oxygenation, prevents aspiration, and corrects intrapulmonary shunting and ventilation–perfusion abnormalities (caused by aspiration of water). If the patient is breathing spontaneously, supplemental oxygen may be administered by mask. However, an endotracheal tube is necessary if the patient does not breathe spontaneously.

Because of submersion, the patient is usually hypothermic. A rectal probe is used to determine the degree of hypothermia. Prescribed rewarming procedures (eg, extracorporeal warming, warmed peritoneal dialysis, inhalation of warm aerosolized oxygen, torso warming) are started during resuscitation. The choice of warming method is determined by the severity and duration of hypothermia and available resources. Intravascular volume expansion and inotropic agents are used to treat hypotension and impaired tissue perfusion. ECG monitoring is initiated, because dysrhythmias frequently occur. An indwelling urinary catheter is inserted to measure urine output. Hypothermia and accompanying metabolic acidosis may compromise renal function. Nasogastric intubation is used to decompress the stomach and to prevent the patient from aspirating gastric contents.

Even if the patient appears healthy, close monitoring continues with serial vital signs, serial arterial blood gas values, ECG monitoring, intracranial pressure assessments, serum electrolyte levels, intake and output, and serial chest x-rays. After a near-drowning, the patient is at risk for complications such as hypoxic or ischemic cerebral injury, ARDS, pulmonary damage secondary to aspiration, and life-threatening cardiac arrest.

Decompression Sickness

Decompression sickness, also called "the bends," occurs in patients who have engaged in diving (lake, as well as ocean, diving), high-altitude flying, or flying in commercial aircraft within 24 hours after diving. It occurs relatively infrequently in the United States, but its effects can be hazardous. Being aware of decompression sickness and assessing the patient properly ensures proper management and results in the least morbidity possible.

Decompression sickness results from formation of nitrogen bubbles that occur with rapid changes in atmospheric pressure. They may occur in joint or muscle spaces, resulting in musculoskeletal pain, numbness, or hypesthesia. More significantly, nitrogen bubbles can become air emboli in the bloodstream and thereby produce stroke, paralysis, or death. Taking a rapid history about the events preceding the symptoms is essential. Recompression is necessary as soon as possible and may necessitate a low-altitude flight to the nearest hyperbaric chamber.

Assessment and Diagnostic Findings

To identify decompression sickness, a detailed history is obtained from the patient or diving partner. Evidence of rapid ascent, loss of air in the tank, buddy breathing, recent alcohol intake or lack of sleep, or a flight within 24 hours after diving suggests possible decompression sickness. Some patients describe a perfect dive yet still have the signs and symptoms of decompression sickness, and they must receive treatment for the condition.

Signs and symptoms include joint or extremity pain, numbness, hypesthesia, and loss of range of motion. Neurologic symptoms mimicking those of a stroke or spinal cord injury can indicate an air embolus. Cardiopulmonary arrest can also occur in severe cases and is usually fatal. Any neurologic symptoms should be rapidly assessed. All patients with decompression sickness need rapid transfer to a hyperbaric chamber.

Management

A patent airway and adequate ventilation are established, as described previously, and 100% oxygen is administered throughout treatment and transport. A chest x-ray is obtained to identify aspiration, and at least one IV line is started with lactated Ringer's or normal saline solution.

The cardiopulmonary and neurologic systems are supported as needed. If an air embolus is suspected, the head of the bed should be lowered. The patient's wet clothing is removed, and the patient is kept warm. Transfer to the closest hyperbaric chamber for treatment is initiated. If air transport is necessary, low-altitude flight (below 1000 feet) is required. However, the patient who is awake and alert without central neurologic deficits may be able to travel by ground ambulance or by automobile, depending on the severity of symptoms. Throughout treatment, the patient is continually assessed, and changes are documented. If aspiration is suspected, antibiotics and other treatment may be prescribed.

Anaphylactic Reaction

An anaphylactic reaction is an acute systemic hypersensitivity reaction that occurs within seconds or minutes after exposure to certain foreign substances, such as medications (eg, penicillin, iodinated contrast material), and other agents, such as latex, insect stings (eg, bee, wasp, yellow jacket, hornet), or foods (eg, eggs, peanuts). Repeated administration

Chart 71-8 • *Nursing Interventions for Preventing Anaphylactic Reactions*

- Be aware of the danger of anaphylactic reactions and the early signs of anaphylaxis.
- Ask the patient about previous allergies to medications, foods, stings, latex, pollen, peanuts, nuts from trees, eggs, and so on.
- Before giving a foreign serum or other type of antigenic agent, ask the patient or caregiver whether the agent was received at some earlier time.
- Avoid giving medications to patients with hay fever, asthma, or other allergic disorders unless necessary.
- Avoid giving parenteral medications unless absolutely necessary, because anaphylactic reactions are more likely to occur when the agent is given parenterally.
- Perform a skin test before administration of certain materials known to produce anaphylactic reactions (eg, horse serum). Remember that negative skin test results do not always indicate safety and that skin testing can precipitate anaphylaxis in highly sensitive patients. Have epinephrine, intravenous infusions, and intubation and tracheostomy equipment available as precautionary measures.
- If the patient is an outpatient, keep him or her in the office, hospital, or clinic for at least 30 minutes after injection of any agent. Caution the patient to return if symptoms develop.
- Caution patients who are highly sensitive (eg, to insect bites and stings) to carry kits equipped to treat insect stings (epinephrine). Instruct the patient, family, and significant others in the use of the emergency supplies.
- Encourage patients with allergies to wear medical identification tags or bracelets.

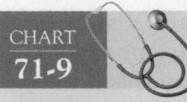

CHART 71-9 — *Assessing for Anaphylaxis*

Be alert for the following signs and symptoms:

Respiratory Signs

- Nasal congestion
- Itching
- Sneezing and coughing
- Possible respiratory distress that progresses rapidly (caused by bronchospasm or edema of the larynx)
- Chest tightness
- Other respiratory difficulties, such as wheezing, dyspnea, and cyanosis

Skin Manifestations

- Flushing with a sense of warmth and diffuse erythema
- Generalized itching over the entire body (indicates developing general systemic reaction)
- Urticaria (hives)
- Massive facial angioedema possible with accompanying upper respiratory edema

Cardiovascular Manifestations

- Tachycardia or bradycardia
- Peripheral vascular collapse as indicated by
  - Pallor
  - Imperceptible pulse
  - Decreasing blood pressure
  - Circulatory failure, leading to coma and death

Gastrointestinal Problems

- Nausea
- Vomiting
- Colicky abdominal pains
- Diarrhea

of parenteral or oral therapeutic agents (eg, repeated exposures to penicillin) may also precipitate an anaphylactic reaction when initially only a mild allergic response occurred. Anaphylaxis prevention strategies are given in Chart 71-8.

An anaphylactic reaction is the result of an antigen–antibody interaction in a sensitized person who, as a consequence of previous exposure, has developed a special type of antibody (immunoglobulin) that is specific for that particular allergen. Immunoglobulin E (IgE) is responsible for most of the immediate types of human allergic responses. A second exposure to the same antigen results in a more severe and more rapid response (see Chapter 53).

An anaphylactic reaction produces a wide range of clinical manifestations, especially respiratory symptoms (difficulty breathing and stridor secondary to laryngeal edema), fainting, itching, swelling of mucous membranes, and a sudden decrease in blood pressure secondary to massive vasodilation that may progress to shock (Chart 71-9). (See Chapters 15 and 53 for additional discussion and management of anaphylactic reactions.)

Insect Stings

A person may have an extreme sensitivity to the venoms of insects in the order Hymenoptera (bees, hornets, yellow jackets, fire ants, and wasps). Venom allergy is thought to be an IgE-mediated reaction, and it constitutes an acute emergency. Although stings in any area of the body can trigger anaphylaxis, stings of the head and neck or multiple stings are especially serious.

Clinical manifestations range from generalized urticaria, itching, malaise, and anxiety due to laryngeal edema to severe bronchospasm, shock, and death. Generally, the shorter the time between the sting and the onset of severe symptoms, the worse the prognosis.

Management includes stinger removal if the sting is from a bee because the venom is associated with sacs around the barb of the stinger itself. The stinger is removed with one quick scrape of a fingernail over the site. Wound care with soap and water is sufficient for stings. Scratching is avoided because it results in a histamine response. Ice application reduces swelling and also decreases venom absorption. An oral antihistamine and analgesic will decrease the itching and pain.

In the case of an anaphylactic or severe allergic response, the patient is treated as discussed previously in Chapter 53. Desensitization therapy should be given to people who have had systemic or significant local reactions. Patient and family education is an important measure in preventing exposure to stinging insects (Chart 71-10).

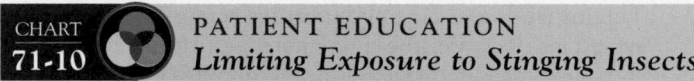

CHART 71-10

PATIENT EDUCATION
Limiting Exposure to Stinging Insects

To Minimize Your Chances of Being Stung:
- Avoid places where stinging insects congregate, such as camp and picnic sites, and insect feeding areas, such as flower beds, ripe fruit orchards, garbage, and fields of clover.
- Wear covering on the feet, and avoid going barefoot outdoors, because yellow jackets nest and pollinate on the ground.
- Avoid perfumes, scented soaps, and bright colors, which attract bees.
- Keep car windows closed.
- Spray garbage cans with quick-acting insecticide.
- Secure a professional exterminator to dispose of wasp and hornet nests or beehives in the home area.

- Remain motionless if an insect is buzzing around. Motion, especially running, increases the likelihood of being stung.
- If allergic, carry a self-treatment kit containing injectable (EpiPen) and inhalant forms of epinephrine, an oral antihistamine, and written instructions. Carry it with you at all times.

If You are Stung, Do the Following:
1. Inject self immediately with epinephrine if allergy is known or allergic response occurs.
2. Remove the stinger with one quick scrape of the fingernail. *Do not* squeeze the venom sac because this may cause injection of additional venom.
3. Clean the area with soapy water, and apply ice.
4. Report to the nearest health care facility for further examination if allergic response or allergy is suspected.

Animal and Human Bites

Bites are a common reason for visits to the ED. Dog bites constitute 90% of these bites and are responsible for the majority of deaths from bites by a nonvenomous animal. Cat bites have a high risk of infection because of the presence of *Pasteurella* in their saliva. All animal bites must be reported to public health authorities, which must provide follow-up screening of the offending animal for rabies. If the animal cannot be located and rabies vaccination verified, rabies prophylaxis for the person who has been bitten must be instituted.

Human bites are frequently associated with rapes, sexual assaults, or other forms of battery. The human mouth contains more bacteria than that of most other animals, so a high risk of bite-related infection exists. Depending on the circumstances surrounding the event, the victim may delay seeking treatment. The ED nurse should inspect any bitten tissue for pus, erythema, or necrosis. A health care provider should take photographs, which can be used as evidence in criminal and legal proceedings. Cleansing with soap and water is then necessary, followed by the administration of antibiotics and tetanus toxoid as prescribed.

Snake Bites

Venomous (poisonous) snakes cause 7000 to 8000 bites in the United States each year and result in 10 to 15 deaths (Hoyt & Selfridge-Thomas, 2007). Children between 1 and 9 years of age are the most likely victims. The greatest number of bites occurs during the daylight hours and early evening of the summer months. The most frequent poisonous snake bite occurs from pit vipers (Crotalidae). The most common site is the upper extremity. Of these bites, only 20% to 25% result in **envenomation** (injection of a poisonous material by sting, spine, bite, or other means). Venomous snake bites are medical emergencies (Daley & Barbee, 2008).

Nineteen different species of venomous snakes are found in various regions within the United States. Nurses should be familiar with the types of snakes common to the geographic region in which they practice.

Clinical Manifestations

Snake venom consists primarily of proteins and has a broad range of physiologic effects. It may affect multiple organ systems, especially the neurologic, cardiovascular, and respiratory systems.

Classic clinical signs of envenomation are edema, ecchymosis, and hemorrhagic bullae, leading to necrosis at the site of envenomation. Symptoms include lymph node tenderness, nausea, vomiting, numbness, and a metallic taste in the mouth. Without decisive treatment, these clinical manifestations may progress to include fasciculations, hypotension, paresthesias, seizures, and coma (Daley & Barbee, 2008).

Management

Initial first aid at the site of the snake bite includes having the person lie down, removing constrictive items such as rings, providing warmth, cleansing the wound, covering the wound with a light sterile dressing, and immobilizing the injured body part below the level of the heart. Airway, breathing, and circulation are the priorities of care. Ice or a tourniquet is *not* applied. Initial evaluation in the ED is performed quickly and includes information about the following:

- Whether the snake was venomous or nonvenomous; if the snake is dead, it should be transported to the ED with the patient for identification. However, caution should be taken when handling the transported snake. Frequently, the patient and family transport the snake in a stunned, not dead, state.
- Where and when the bite occurred and the circumstances of the bite
- Sequence of events, signs and symptoms (fang punctures, pain, edema, and erythema of the bite and nearby tissues)
- Severity of poisonous effects
- Vital signs
- Circumference of the bitten extremity or area at several points; the circumference of the extremity that was bitten is compared with the circumference of the opposite extremity

• Laboratory data (complete blood count, urinalysis, and coagulation studies)

The course and prognosis of snake bite injuries depend on the kind and amount of venom injected, where on the body the bite occurred, and the general health, age, and size of the patient. There is no one specific protocol for treatment of snake bites. Generally, ice, tourniquets, heparin, and corticosteroids are not used during the acute stage. Corticosteroids are contraindicated in the first 6 to 8 hours after the bite because they may depress antibody production and hinder the action of **antivenin** (antitoxin manufactured from the snake venom and used to treat snake bites).

Parenteral fluids may be used to treat hypotension. If vasopressors are used to treat hypotension, their use should be short term. Surgical exploration of the bite is rarely indicated. Typically, the patient is observed closely for at least 6 hours. The patient is *never* left unattended.

Administration of Antivenin (Antitoxin)

Although envenomation is rare, it can occur with snake bites. An assessment of progressive signs and symptoms is essential before considering administration of antivenin, which is most effective if administered within 4 hours and no greater than 12 hours after the snake bite. Two antivenins are available: Antivenin Polyvalent (ACP) and Crotalidae Polyvalent Immune Fab Antivenin (FabAV) (Auerbach, 2007). The dose depends on the type of snake and the estimated severity of the bite. Indications for antivenin depend on the progression of symptoms, including coagulopathy and systemic reaction. Children may require more antivenin than adults because their smaller bodies are more susceptible to the toxic effects of venom.

A skin or eye test should be performed before the initial dose to detect allergy to the antivenin, because as many as 33% of patients who are given ACP (horse serum–derived antivenin) develop hypersensitivity reactions to it. Because even the skin test can cause an anaphylactic reaction, patients should not be tested unless antivenin will be given. If the dose exceeds 10 vials, serum sickness will most likely occur. Serum sickness is a type of hypersensitivity response that results in fever, arthralgias, pruritus, lymphadenopathy, and proteinuria and can progress to neuropathies.

FabAV is more potent than ACP, with less associated hypersensitivity and serum sickness (Auerbach, 2007). However, FabAV must be administered cautiously to patients receiving anticoagulation therapy. Administration of FabAV may result in a recurring coagulopathy. The dosage and administration of FabAV are different from ACP and should be reviewed carefully before the medication is given.

Before administering antivenin and every 15 minutes thereafter, the circumference of the affected part is measured. Premedication with diphenhydramine (Benadryl) or cimetidine (Tagamet) is indicated because these antihistamines may decrease the allergic response to antivenin. Antivenin is administered as an IV infusion whenever possible, although IM administration can be used.

Depending on the severity of the snake bite, the antivenin is diluted in 500 to 1000 mL of normal saline solution. The infusion is started slowly, and the rate is increased after 10 minutes if there is no reaction. The total dose should be infused during the first 4 to 6 hours after the bite.

The initial dose is repeated until symptoms decrease. After symptoms decrease, the circumference of the affected part should be measured every 30 to 60 minutes for the next 48 hours to detect symptoms of compartment syndrome (swelling, loss of pulse, increased pain, and paresthesias).

The most common cause of allergic reaction to the antivenin is too-rapid infusion, although about 3% of patients with negative skin test results develop reactions unrelated to infusion rate. Reactions may consist of a feeling of fullness in the face, urticaria, pruritus, malaise, and apprehension. These symptoms may be followed by tachycardia, shortness of breath, hypotension, and shock. In this situation, the infusion should be stopped immediately and IV diphenhydramine administered. Vasopressors are used for patients in shock, and resuscitation equipment must be on standby while antivenin is infusing.

Spider Bites

There are two venomous spiders found in the United States that typically interact with humans: the brown recluse and the black widow. Both are usually found in dark places such as closets, woodpiles, and attics, as well as in shoes.

Brown recluse spider bites are painless. Systemic effects such as fever and chills, nausea and vomiting, malaise, and joint pain develop within 24 to 72 hours. The site of the bite may appear reddish to purple in color within 2 to 8 hours after the bite. Necrosis occurs in the next 2 to 4 days in approximately 10% of cases. The center of the bite may become necrotic, and surgical débridement may be necessary. Wound care consists of cleansing with soap and water, and hyperbaric oxygen treatments may be helpful. Most wounds heal within 2 to 3 months.

Black widow spider bites feel like pinpricks. Systemic effects usually occur within 30 minutes—much more rapidly than with brown recluse spider bites. Signs and symptoms include abdominal rigidity, nausea and vomiting, hypertension, tachycardia, and paresthesias. Severe pain also develops within 60 minutes and increases over 1 to 2 days. Treatment involves application of ice to the site to decrease systemic toxin delivery. Cardiopulmonary monitoring is essential. Antivenin is effective for black widow spider bites. This antivenin is horse serum–based; therefore, testing for sensitivity must be performed prior to administration (Auerbach, 2007).

Tick Bites

Tick bites are common in many areas of the United States, and they usually occur in grassy or wooded areas. It is important to learn the place where the bite occurred as well as the location of the bite on the body. The patient may demonstrate weakness; joint pain; skin rash, especially on the palms and soles of feet; headache; and fever. Ticks can carry diseases such as Rocky Mountain spotted fever, tularemia, and Lyme disease. The tick bite itself is not usually the problem; rather, it is the pathogen transmitted by the tick that can cause serious disease. The tick should be removed, and the patient should be informed of the signs and symptoms of diseases carried by ticks, especially if the patient lives in an area endemic for tick-related diseases (eg, Lyme disease).

Lyme disease has three stages. Stage I presents with a "bull's eye" rash (ie, erythema migrans) that typically can be found in the axilla, groin, or thigh area and that appears within 4 weeks after the tick bite, with a peak manifestation time of 7 days after the bite. Classically, this rash is at least 5 cm in diameter with bright red borders. It is accompanied by flulike signs and symptoms that may include chills, fever, myalgia, fatigue, and headache. Without treatment, the rash subsides within 3 to 4 weeks. However, the rash and flulike manifestations can be significantly reduced within days if prompt treatment with antibiotics is initiated. If antibiotics are not administered, stage II Lyme disease may present within 4 to 10 weeks following the tick bite and may manifest with joint pain, memory loss, poor motor coordination, and meningitis. Stage III can begin anywhere from weeks to more than a year after the bite and has serious long-term chronic sequelae, including arthritis, neuropathy, myalgia, and myocarditis.

POISONING

A poison is any substance that, when ingested, inhaled, absorbed, applied to the skin, or produced within the body in relatively small amounts, injures the body by its chemical action. Poisoning from inhalation and ingestion of toxic materials, both intentional and unintentional, constitutes a major health hazard and an emergency situation. Emergency treatment is initiated with the following goals:

- To remove or inactivate the poison before it is absorbed
- To provide supportive care in maintaining vital organ function
- To administer a specific antidote to neutralize a specific poison
- To implement treatment that hastens the elimination of the absorbed poison

Ingested (Swallowed) Poisons

Swallowed poisons may be corrosive. **Corrosive poisons** include alkaline and acid agents that can cause tissue destruction after coming in contact with mucous membranes. Alkaline products include lye, drain cleaners, toilet bowl cleaners, bleach, nonphosphate detergents, oven cleaners, and button batteries (batteries used to power watches, calculators, or cameras). Acid products include toilet bowl cleaners, pool cleaners, metal cleaners, rust removers, and battery acid.

Control of the airway, ventilation, and oxygenation are essential. In the absence of cerebral or renal damage, the patient's prognosis depends largely on successful management of respiration and circulation. Measures are instituted to stabilize cardiovascular and other body functions. ECG, vital signs, and neurologic status are monitored closely for changes. Shock may result from the cardiodepressant action of the substance ingested, from venous pooling in the lower extremities, or from reduced circulating blood volume resulting from increased capillary permeability. An indwelling urinary catheter is inserted to monitor renal function. Blood specimens are obtained to determine the concentration of drug or poison.

Efforts are made to determine what substance was ingested; the amount; the time since ingestion; signs and symptoms, such as pain or burning sensations, any evidence of redness or burn in the mouth or throat, pain on swallowing or an inability to swallow, vomiting, or drooling; age and weight of the patient; and pertinent health history.

 NURSING ALERT

The local poison control center should be called if an unknown toxic agent has been taken or if it is necessary to identify an antidote for a known toxic agent.

Measures are instituted to remove the toxin or decrease its absorption. The patient who has ingested a corrosive poison, which can be a strong acid or alkaline substance, is given water or milk to drink for dilution. However, dilution is not attempted if the patient has acute airway edema or obstruction or if there is clinical evidence of esophageal, gastric, or intestinal burn or perforation. The following gastric emptying procedures may be used as prescribed:

- Syrup of ipecac to induce vomiting in the alert patient (*never* use with corrosive poisons)
- Gastric lavage for the obtunded patient (Chart 71-11); gastric aspirate is saved and sent to the laboratory for testing (toxicology screens)
- Activated charcoal administration if the poison is one that is absorbed by charcoal
- Cathartic, when appropriate

NURSING ALERT

Vomiting is never induced after ingestion of caustic substances (acid or alkaline) or petroleum distillates.

If there is a specific chemical or physiologic antagonist (antidote), it is administered as early as possible to reverse or diminish the effects of the toxin. If this measure is ineffective, procedures may be initiated to remove the ingested substance. These procedures include administration of multiple doses of charcoal, diuresis (for substances excreted by the kidneys), dialysis, or hemoperfusion. Hemoperfusion involves detoxification of the blood by processing it through an extracorporeal circuit and an adsorbent cartridge containing charcoal or resin, after which the cleansed blood is returned to the patient.

Throughout detoxification, the patient's vital signs, CVP, and fluid and electrolyte balance are monitored closely. Hypotension and cardiac dysrhythmias are possible. Seizures are also possible because of CNS stimulation from the poison or from oxygen deprivation. If the patient complains of pain, analgesics are administered cautiously. Severe pain causes vasomotor collapse and reflex inhibition of normal physiologic functions.

After the patient's condition has stabilized and discharge is imminent, written material should be given to the patient

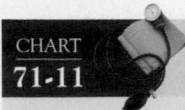

CHART 71-11   *Guidelines for Assisting With Gastric Lavage*

Gastric lavage is the aspiration of stomach contents and washing out of the stomach by means of a large-bore gastric tube. Gastric lavage is contraindicated after acid or alkali ingestion, in the presence of seizures, or after ingestion of hydrocarbons or petroleum distillates. It is particularly dangerous after ingestion of strong corrosive agents.

Purposes:
- For urgent removal of ingested substance to decrease systemic absorption
- To empty the stomach before endoscopic procedures
- To diagnose gastric hemorrhage and to arrest hemorrhage

Equipment:
Large-bore Levin tubes or large-bore Ewald tube
Large irrigating syringe with adapter
Large plastic funnel with adapter to fit tube
Water-soluble lubricant
Tap water or appropriate antidote (milk, saline solution, sodium bicarbonate solution, fruit juice, activated charcoal)
Container for aspirate; suction apparatus
Nasotracheal or endotracheal tubes with inflatable cuffs
Containers for specimens

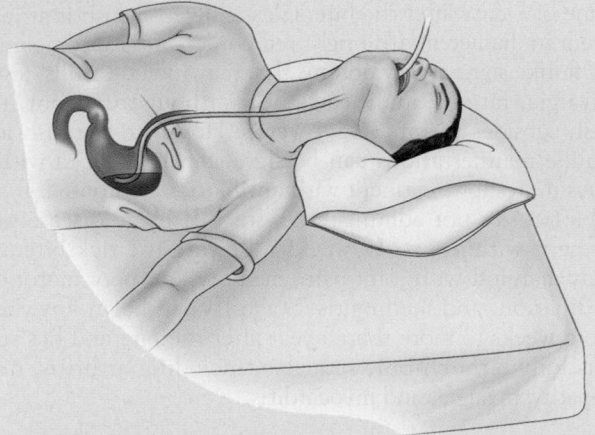

During gastric lavage, the patient is positioned on the left side, which allows the gastic contents to pool and decreases the passage of fluid into the duodenum.

Action	Rationale
1. Remove dentures and inspect the oral cavity for loose teeth.	1. This will prevent aspiration of teeth.
2. Measure the distance between the bridge of the nose and the xiphoid process. Mark the tube with indelible pencil or tape.	2. This distance is a rule-of-thumb measurement of the distance the tube must be passed to reach the stomach. This avoids curling and kinking of excess tubing in the stomach.
3. Lubricate the tube with water-soluble lubricant.	3. Lubrication eases insertion of the tube.
4. If comatose, the patient is intubated with a cuffed nasotracheal or endotracheal tube before placement of the nasogastric tube.	4. A cuffed nasotracheal or endotracheal tube decreases the risk of aspiration of gastric contents.
5. Place the patient in a left lateral position with the head lowered about 15 degrees.	5. This position decreases passage of gastric contents into the duodenum during lavage.
6. Pass the tube orally while keeping the patient's head in a neutral position. Pass the tube to the adhesive marking or about 50 cm (20 in). Encourage patient to swallow to assist with passage of the tube. Then lower the head of the stretcher or bed. Have standby suction available.	6. The depth of insertion of the tube varies according to the size of the patient. If the tube enters the trachea instead of the esophagus, the patient will experience coughing, dyspnea, stridor, and cyanosis. Positive confirmation of tube placement is accomplished by x-ray.
7. Aspirate the stomach contents with the syringe attached to the tube before instilling water or an antidote. Save the specimen for analysis. Ensure correct placement before installation.	7. Aspiration is carried out to determine that the tube is in the stomach and to remove the stomach contents. Positive confirmation of tube placement is accomplished by x-ray.
8. Remove the syringe. Attach the funnel to the end of the tube, or use a 50-mL syringe to instill solution in the gastric tube. The volume of fluid placed in the stomach should be small.	8. Overfilling of the stomach may cause regurgitation and aspiration or force the stomach contents through the pylorus.
9. Elevate the funnel above the patient's head and pour 150 to 200 mL of solution into the funnel.	9. Gravity allows the solution to flow into the tube.
10. Lower the funnel and siphon the gastric contents into the container or connect to suction.	10. The fluid should flow in freely and drain by gravity.
11. Save samples of the first two washings.	11. Keep the first washing sample isolated from other washings for toxicologic analysis.
12. Repeat the lavage procedure until the returns are relatively clear and no particulate matter is seen.	12. This usually requires a total volume of at least 2 L; some clinicians advocate the use of 5 to 20 L.

Continued

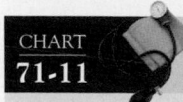

CHART 71-11 *Guidelines for Assisting With Gastric Lavage (Continued)*

Action	Rationale

13. At the completion of lavage:
  a. The stomach may be left empty.
 	
  b. An adsorbent (powder form of activated charcoal mixed with water to form a liquid the consistency of thick soup) may be instilled in the tube and allowed to remain in the stomach.
  c. A saline cathartic may be instilled in the tube.
	13.
	  a. The stomach is kept empty if no further medications are required.
	  b. Activated charcoal reduces absorption by adsorbing (attaching to its surface) a wide range of substances; it renders the poison inaccessible to the circulation, thereby reducing its toxicity.
	  c. A cathartic may be given to hasten the elimination of remaining ingested material.

14. Pinch off the tube during removal or maintain suction while the tube is being withdrawn. Keep the patient's head lower than the body. 15. Warn the patient that his stools will turn black from the charcoal.	14. Pinching off the tube prevents aspiration and the initiation of the gag reflex. Keeping the patient's head lower than the body also helps to prevent initiation of the gag reflex. 15. Patient teaching is important to reduce anxiety.

indicating the signs and symptoms of potential problems related to the poison ingested and signs or symptoms requiring evaluation by a physician. If poisoning was determined to be a suicide or self-harm attempt, a psychiatric consultation should be requested before the patient is discharged. In cases of inadvertent poison ingestion, poison prevention and home poison-proofing instructions should be provided to the patient and family.

Carbon Monoxide Poisoning

Carbon monoxide poisoning may occur as a result of industrial or household incidents or attempted suicide. It is implicated in more deaths than any other toxin except alcohol. Carbon monoxide exerts its toxic effect by binding to circulating hemoglobin and thereby reducing the oxygen-carrying capacity of the blood. Hemoglobin absorbs carbon monoxide 200 times more readily than it absorbs oxygen. Carbon monoxide–bound hemoglobin, called **carboxyhemoglobin,** does not transport oxygen.

Clinical Manifestations

Because the CNS has a critical need for oxygen, CNS symptoms predominate with carbon monoxide toxicity. A person with carbon monoxide poisoning may appear intoxicated (from cerebral hypoxia). Other signs and symptoms include headache, muscular weakness, palpitation, dizziness, and confusion, which can progress rapidly to coma. Skin color, which can range from pink or cherry-red to cyanotic and pale, is not a reliable sign. Pulse oximetry is also not valid, because the hemoglobin is well saturated. It is not saturated with oxygen, but the pulse oximeter indicates only if the hemoglobin is saturated; in this case, it is saturated with carbon monoxide rather than with oxygen.

Management

Exposure to carbon monoxide requires immediate treatment. Goals of management are to reverse cerebral and myocardial hypoxia and to hasten elimination of carbon

monoxide. Whenever a patient inhales a poison, the following general measures apply:

- Carry the patient to fresh air immediately; open all doors and windows.
- Loosen all tight clothing.
- Initiate cardiopulmonary resuscitation if required; administer 100% oxygen.
- Prevent chilling; wrap the patient in blankets.
- Keep the patient as quiet as possible.
- Do not give alcohol in any form or permit the patient to smoke.

In addition, for the patient with carbon monoxide poisoning, carboxyhemoglobin levels are analyzed on arrival at the ED and before treatment with oxygen if possible. One hundred percent oxygen is administered at atmospheric or preferably hyperbaric pressures to reverse hypoxia and accelerate the elimination of carbon monoxide. Oxygen is administered until the carboxyhemoglobin level is less than 5%. The patient is monitored continuously. Psychoses, spastic paralysis, ataxia, visual disturbances, and deterioration of mental status and behavior may persist after resuscitation and may be symptoms of permanent brain damage.

When unintentional carbon monoxide poisoning occurs, the health department should be contacted so that the dwelling or building in question can be inspected. A psychiatric consultation is warranted if poisoning was determined to be a suicide attempt.

Skin Contamination Poisoning (Chemical Burns)

Skin contamination injuries from exposure to chemicals are challenging because of the large number of possible offending agents with diverse actions and metabolic effects. The severity of a chemical burn is determined by the mechanism of action, the penetrating strength and concentration, and the amount and duration of exposure of the skin to the chemical.

The skin should be drenched immediately with running water from a shower, hose, or faucet, except in the case of lye and white phosphorus, which should be brushed off the skin, dry.

NURSING ALERT

Water should not be applied to burns from lye or white phosphorus because of the potential for an explosion or for deepening of the burn. All evidence of these chemicals should be brushed off the patient before any flushing occurs.

The skin should be flushed with a constant stream of water as the patient's clothing is removed. The skin of health care personnel assisting the patient should be appropriately protected if the burn is extensive or if the agent is significantly toxic or is still present. Prolonged lavage with generous amounts of tepid water is important.

Attempts to determine the identity and characteristics of the chemical agent are necessary in order to specify future treatment. The standard burn treatment appropriate for the size and location of the wound (antimicrobial treatment, débridement, tetanus prophylaxis, antidote administration as prescribed) is instituted. (see Chapter 57) The patient may require plastic surgery for further wound management. The patient is instructed to have the affected area reexamined at 24 and 72 hours and in 7 days because of the risk of underestimating the extent and depth of these types of injuries.

Food Poisoning

Food poisoning is a sudden illness that occurs after ingestion of contaminated food or drink. Botulism is a serious form of food poisoning that requires continual surveillance (see Chapter 72). Assessment questions for patients with food poisoning are discussed in Chart 71-12.

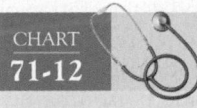

| CHART 71-12 | Assessment for Food Poisoning |

Use the following questions to elicit information about the circumstances surrounding the possibility of food poisoning:

• How soon after eating did the symptoms occur? (Immediate onset suggests chemical, plant, or animal poisoning.)
• What was eaten in the previous meal? Did the food have an unusual odor or taste? (Most foods causing bacterial poisoning *do not* have unusual odor or taste.)
• Did anyone else become ill from eating the same food?
• Did vomiting occur? What was the appearance of the vomitus?
• Did diarrhea occur? (Diarrhea is usually absent with botulism and with shellfish or other fish poisoning.)
• Are any neurologic symptoms present? (These occur in botulism and in chemical, plant, and animal poisoning.)
• Does the patient have a fever? (Fever is characteristic in salmonella, ingestion of fava beans, and some fish poisoning.)

The key to treatment is determining the source and type of food poisoning. If possible, the suspected food should be brought to the medical facility and a history obtained from the patient or family.

Food, gastric contents, vomitus, serum, and feces are collected for examination. The patient's respirations, blood pressure, level of consciousness, central venous pressure (CVP) (if indicated), and muscular activity are monitored closely. Measures are instituted to support the respiratory system. Death from respiratory paralysis can occur with botulism, fish poisoning, and some other food poisonings.

Because large volumes of electrolytes and water are lost by vomiting and diarrhea, fluid and electrolyte status should be assessed. Severe vomiting produces alkalosis, and severe diarrhea produces acidosis. Hypovolemic shock may also occur from severe fluid and electrolyte losses. The patient is assessed for signs and symptoms of fluid and electrolyte imbalances, including lethargy, rapid pulse rate, fever, oliguria, anuria, hypotension, and delirium. Weight and serum electrolyte levels are obtained for future comparisons.

Measures to control nausea are also important to prevent vomiting, which could exacerbate fluid and electrolyte imbalances. An antiemetic medication is administered parenterally as prescribed if the patient cannot tolerate fluids or medications by mouth. For mild nausea, the patient is encouraged to take sips of weak tea, carbonated drinks, or tap water. After nausea and vomiting subside, clear liquids are usually prescribed for 12 to 24 hours, and the diet is gradually progressed to a low-residue, bland diet.

SUBSTANCE ABUSE

Substance abuse is the misuse of specific substances, such as drugs or alcohol, to alter mood or behavior. Drug abuse is the use of drugs for other than legitimate medical purposes. People who abuse drugs often take a variety of drugs simultaneously (such as alcohol, barbiturates, opioids, and tranquilizers), and the combination may have additive and addictive effects. "Rave" parties are large-scale parties attended by hundreds of teenagers involved in drug use. At these events, one of the most commonly used drugs is 3,4-methylenedioxymethamphetamine (MDMA), or Ecstasy, a methamphetamine-based drug that users believe produces a "harmless high." ED nurses should be aware of "rave" parties in their geographic area so they can prepare for a potential influx of patients who abuse this drug. Others may combine Ecstasy with sildenafil (Viagra); this drug combination is nicknamed "sextasy." People who abuse IV/injection drugs are at increased risk for HIV infection, acquired immunodeficiency syndrome (AIDS), hepatitis B and C, and tetanus.

Clinical manifestations vary with the substance used, but the underlying principles of management are essentially the same. Table 71-1 identifies commonly abused drugs, listing their clinical manifestations and therapeutic management. Treatment goals for a patient with a drug overdose are to support the respiratory and cardiovascular functions, to enhance clearance of the agent, and to provide for safety of the patient and staff.

Table 71-1 EMERGENCY MANAGEMENT OF PATIENTS WITH DRUG OVERDOSE

Drug	Clinical Manifestations	Therapeutic Management

Stimulants
Cocaine
  Intranasally ("snorting"): inhaled into nostrils through straws
  By smoking ("freebasing"): cocaine hydrochloride dissolved in ether to yield a pure cocaine alkaloid base (called "crack," "rocks"); smoking in a small pipe delivers large quantities of cocaine to lungs
  Intravenously
  Polysubstance (cocaine and heroin)
	Cocaine is a central nervous system (CNS) stimulant that can increase heart rate and blood pressure and cause hyperpyrexia, seizures, increased energy, agitation, aggression, and ventricular dysrhythmias. It produces intense euphoria, then anxiety, sadness, insomnia, and sexual indifference; cocaine hallucinations with delusions; psychosis with extreme paranoia and ideas of persecution; and hypervigilance. Chronic psychotic symptoms may persist.
	Overall psychotic symptoms are short-lived compared to methamphetamines
		1. Maintain airway and provide respiratory support
		2. Control seizures.
		3. Monitor cardiovascular effects; have lidocaine and defibrillator available.
		4. Treat for hyperthermia.
		5. If cocaine was ingested, evacuate stomach contents and use activated charcoal to treat. Whole bowel irrigation may be necessary to treat body packers ("mules").
		6. Refer for psychiatric evaluation and treatment in an inpatient unit that eliminates access to the drug. Include drug rehabilitation counseling.

Opioids Heroin Opium or paregoric Morphine, codeine, semisynthetic derivatives: oxycodone (OxyContin), methadone, meperidine (Demerol), propoxyphene (Darvon), tramadol (Ultram), fentanyl (Sublimaze)	Acute intoxication (overdose) Pinpoint pupils (may be dilated with severe hypoxia); decreased blood pressure Marked respiratory depression/ arrest Pulmonary edema Stupor → coma Seizures Fresh needle marks along course of any superficial vein; skin abscesses	1. Support respiratory and cardiovascular functions. 2. Establish an intravenous (IV) line; obtain blood for chemical and toxicologic analysis. Patient may be given bolus of glucose to eliminate possibility of hypoglycemia. 3. Give narcotic antagonist (naloxone hydrochloride IV, IM [Narcan]) as prescribed to reverse severe respiratory depression and coma. 4. Continue to monitor level of responsiveness and respirations, pulse, and blood pressure. Duration of action of naloxone hydrochloride is shorter than that of heroin; repeated dosages may be necessary. 5. Send urine for analysis; opioids can be detected in urine. 6. Obtain an electrocardiogram. 7. Do not leave patient unattended; he or she may lapse back into coma rapidly. Clinical status may change from minute to minute. Hemodialysis may be indicated for severe drug intoxication. Activated charcoal may be considered if opioids were taken orally and if the patient is alert. 8. Monitor for pulmonary edema, which is frequently seen in patients who abuse/overdose on narcotics. 9. Refer patient for psychiatric and drug rehabilitation evaluation before discharge.

Barbiturates
Pentobarbital (Nembutal), secobarbital (Seconal), amobarbital (Amytal), gamma-hydroxybutyrate (GHB, "liquid Ecstasy")
	Acute intoxication (may mimic alcohol intoxication):
	• Respiratory depression
	• Flushed face
	• Decreased pulse rate; decreased blood pressure
	• Increasing nystagmus
	• Depressed deep tendon reflexes
	• Decreasing mental alertness
	• Difficulty in speaking
	• Poor motor coordination
	• Coma, death
	GHB:
	• Sexual disinhibition
	• Amnesia, myoclonus, agitation
	• Overdoses when mixed with alcohol
		1. Maintain airway and provide respiratory support.
		2. Endotracheal intubation or tracheostomy is considered if there is any doubt about the adequacy of airway exchange.
		  a. Check airway frequently.
		  b. Perform suctioning as necessary.
		3. Support cardiovascular and respiratory functions; most deaths result from respiratory depression or shock.
		4. Start infusion through large-gauge needle or IV catheter to support blood pressure; coma and dehydration result in hypotension and respond to infusion of intravenous fluids with elevation of blood pressure. Sodium bicarbonate may be prescribed to alkalinize urine; it promotes excretion of barbiturates.
		5. Evacuate stomach contents or lavage as soon as possible to prevent absorption; repeated doses of activated charcoal may be administered.

Continued on following page

Table 71-1	EMERGENCY MANAGEMENT OF PATIENTS WITH DRUG OVERDOSE (Continued)

Drug	Clinical Manifestations	Therapeutic Management
		6. Assist with hemodialysis for severely overdosed patient. 7. Maintain neurologic and vital sign flow sheet. 8. Patient awakening from overdose may demonstrate combative behavior. 9. Refer for psychiatric and drug rehabilitation consultation to evaluate suicide potential and drug abuse.
Inhalants Amyl nitrate Freon Propane Trichloroethylene Gasoline Perchloroethylene Toluene (metallic paint spray)	Effects mimic those of alcohol, with dizziness and imbalance Euphoria, headache, altered level of consciousness to coma Renal, hepatic, and cardiac toxicity Aplastic anemia Fetal growth retardation Respiratory depression Vasodilation Nosebleeding Circumoral red spots	1. Provide airway support, ventilation, and oxygen. 2. Treat cardiac dysrhythmias and hypotension. 3. Provide advanced cardiac life support (ACLS) as needed. 4. Monitor for profound hypotension when amyl nitrate is combined with MDMA and sildenafil.
Amphetamine-Type Drugs (pep pills, "uppers," "speed," "crystal meth") Amphetamine (Benzedrine) Dextroamphetamine (Dexedrine) Methamphetamine (Desoxyn, "speed") 3,4-Methylenedioxymethamphetamine (MDMA) ("Ecstasy," "Adam")* 3,4-Methylenedioxymethamphetamine (MDEA) ("Eve") 3,4-Methylenedioxyamphetamine (MDA) methylphenidate (Ritalin) "ice," "rocks," "crystal meth"	Nausea, vomiting, anorexia, palpitations, tachycardia, increased blood pressure, tachypnea, anxiety, nervousness, diaphoresis, mydriasis Repetitive or stereotyped behavior Irritability, insomnia, agitation Visual misperceptions, auditory hallucinations Fearfulness, anxiety, depression, hostility, paranoia Hyperactivity, rapid speech, euphoria, hyperalertness Decreased inhibition Seizures, coma, hyperthermia, cardiovascular collapse, rhabdomyolysis MDMA is both a hallucinogenic and stimulant	1. Provide airway support, ventilation, cardiac monitoring; insert IV line. 2. Use gastrointestinal (GI) evacuation in cases of oral overdose; activated charcoal, gastric lavage. 3. Keep in calm, cool, quiet environment; elevated temperature potentiates amphetamine toxicity. Maintain normothermia cooling the patient as necessary. 4. Use small doses of diazepam (Valium) (IV) or haloperidol (Haldol) as prescribed for CNS and muscular hyperactivity. 5. Administer appropriate pharmacologic therapy as prescribed for severe hypertension and ventricular dysrhythmias. 6. Treat seizures with benzodiazepines (eg, diazepam) as prescribed. 7. Treat sympathetic stimulation with beta-blocker agents as prescribed. 8. Try to communicate with patient if delusions or hallucinations are present. 9. Place in a protective environment (preferably psychiatric security room with video monitoring) to observe for suicide attempt. 10. Refer for psychiatric and drug rehabilitation evaluation.

Hallucinogens or Psychedelic-Type Drugs
Lysergic acid diethylamide (LSD)
Phencyclidine HCl (PCP, "angel dust")
Mescaline, psilocybin
Cannabinoids (marijuana)
Ketamine ("special K")
	Nystagmus
	Mild hypertension
	Marked confusion bordering on panic
	Incoherence, hyperactivity
	Withdrawn
	Combative behavior; delirium, mania, self-injury (lasts 6 to 12 hours)
	Hallucinations, body image distortion
	Hypertension, hyperthermia, renal failure
	Flashback: recurrence of LSD-like state without having taken the drug; may occur weeks or months after drug was taken
	Ketamine: "out-of-body" experience; increased aggressiveness
		1. Evaluate and maintain patient's airway, breathing, and circulation.
		2. Determine by urine or serum drug screen whether the patient has ingested hallucinogenic drug or has a toxic psychosis.
		3. Try to communicate with and reassure the patient.
		  a. "Talking down" involves understanding the process through which the patient is proceeding and helping him overcome his fears while establishing contact with reality.
		  b. Remind the patient that fear is common with this problem.

Continued

Table 71-1 EMERGENCY MANAGEMENT OF PATIENTS WITH DRUG OVERDOSE (Continued)

Drug	Clinical Manifestations	Therapeutic Management

		c. Reassure the patient that he is not losing his mind but is experiencing the effect of drugs and that this will wear off.
		 d. Instruct the patient to keep the eyes open; this reduces the intensity of reaction.
		 e. Reduce sensory stimuli: minimize noise, lights, movement, tactile stimulation.
		 4. Sedate the patient as prescribed if hyperactivity cannot be controlled; diazepam (Valium) or a barbiturate may be prescribed.
		 5. Search for evidence of trauma; hallucinogen users have a tendency to "act out" their hallucinations.
		 6. Manage seizures with benzodiazepines (eg, diazepam) as necessary.
		 7. Observe patient closely; patient's behavior may become hazardous. Have safety officers stationed near the patient's room.
		 8. Monitor for hypertensive crisis if patient has prolonged psychosis due to drug ingestion.
		 9. Place patient in a protected environment under proper medical supervision to prevent self-inflicted bodily harm.
		
		 Management for Phencyclidine Abusers
		 1. Place patient in a calm, supportive environment to minimize stimuli; protect from self-injury.
		 2. Avoid talking down.
		 3. Do not leave patient unobserved. Treat symptoms as they occur.
		   a. Drug effects are unpredictable and prolonged.
		   b. Symptoms are likely to exacerbate; patient becomes out of control.
		 4. Refer all patients in this category for psychiatric and drug evaluation/rehabilitation.

Drugs Producing Sedation, Intoxication, or Psychological and Physical Dependence (nonbarbiturate sedatives)		

Diazepam (Valium)
 Chlordiazepoxide (Librium)
 Oxazepam (Serax)
 Lorazepam (Ativan)
 Midazolam (Versed)
 Flunitrazepam (Rohypnol, "roofies," "date rape drug")*
	Seizures, coma, circulatory collapse, death
	 Acute intoxication:
	 • Respiratory depression
	 • Decreasing mental alertness
	 • Confusion
	 • Slurred speech, decreased blood pressure
	 • Ataxia
	 • Pulmonary edema
	 • Coma, death
	
	 Flunitrazepam:
	 • Disinhibition with antegrade amnesia
	 • Weakness and unsteadiness with impaired judgment
	 • Powerlessness
		1. Endotracheal tube is inserted as a precaution; use assisted ventilation to stabilize and correct respiratory depression. Observe for sudden apnea and laryngeal spasm.
		 2. Assess for hypotension
		   a. Insert indwelling urinary catheter for comatose patient; decreased urinary volume is an index of reduced renal flow associated with reduced intravascular volume or vascular collapse.
		   b. Start volume expansion with saline or dextrose as prescribed.
		 3. Evacuate stomach contents; emesis; lavage; activated charcoal; cathartic.
		 4. Start ECG monitoring. Observe for dysrhythmias.
		 5. Administer flumazenil (Romazicon), a benzodiazepine antagonist (reversal agent).
		 6. Refer patient for psychiatric evaluation (potential suicide intent).

Continued on following page

Table 71-1   EMERGENCY MANAGEMENT OF PATIENTS WITH DRUG OVERDOSE (Continued)

Drug	Clinical Manifestations	Therapeutic Management
Salicylate Poisoning Aspirin (present in compound analgesic tablets) Toxic levels (150–200 mg/kg body weight) Chronic toxicity (occurs in elderly due to decreased renal function) Long-term intoxication (>100 mg/kg/day for more than 2 days)	Restlessness, tinnitus, deafness, blurring of vision Hyperpnea, hyperpyrexia, sweating Epigastric pain, vomiting, dehydration Respiratory alkalosis and metabolic acidosis Disorientation, coma, cardiovascular collapse Coagulopathy	1. Treat respiratory depression. 2. Induce gastric emptying by lavage. 3. Give activated charcoal to adsorb aspirin; a cathartic may be administered with charcoal to help ensure intestinal cleansing. 4. Support patient with IV infusions as prescribed to establish hydration and correct electrolyte imbalances, including administration of sodium bicarbonate. 5. Enhance elimination of salicylates as directed by forced diuresis, alkalinization of urine, peritoneal dialysis, or hemodialysis, according to severity of intoxication. 6. Monitor serum salicylate level for efficacy of treatment. 7. Administer specific prescribed pharmacologic agent for bleeding and other problems. 8. Concretions formed in the gut may result in prolonged exposure as they are digested. 9. Refer patient for psychiatric evaluation (potential suicide intent).
Acetaminophen (present in prescription and nonprescription analgesics, antipyretics, and cold remedies)	Lethargy to encephalopathy and death GI upset, diaphoresis Right upper quadrant pain Abnormal liver function tests, prolonged prothrombin time, increased bilirubin, disseminated intravascular coagulation Hepatomegaly leading to liver failure Metabolic acidosis Hypoglycemia	1. Maintain airway. 2. Obtain acetaminophen level. Levels ≥140 mg/kg are toxic. 3. Laboratory studies—liver function tests, prothrombin time/partial thromboplastin time, complete blood count, blood urea nitrogen, creatinine. 4. Administer syrup of ipecac and follow emesis with activated charcoal. 5. Prepare for possible hemodialysis, which clears acetaminophen but does not halt liver damage. 6. Administer N-acetylcysteine (NAC, Mucomyst) as soon as possible. NAC replenishes essential liver enzymes and requires a total of 18 doses every 4 hours. Charcoal absorbs NAC; do not administer together. Repeat NAC dose if patient vomits. 7. Refer patient for psychiatric evaluation (potential suicide intent).
Tricyclic Antidepressants (TCAs) Amitriptyline (Elavil) Doxepin (Sinequan) Nortriptyline (Aventyl) Imipramine (Tofranil)	Dysrhythmia: ventricular fibrillation/ tachycardia, tachycardia Hypotension Pulmonary edema, hypoxemia, acidosis Confusion, agitation, coma Visual hallucinations Clonus, tremors, hyperactive reflexes, nystagmus, myoclonic jerking Seizures Blurred vision, flushing, hyperthermia	1. Provide airway support, ventilation, cardiac monitoring; insert IV line with normal saline solution. 2. If within 1–2 hours after overdose, insert a nasogastric tube and instill activated charcoal with sorbitol every 4 hours × 3. 3. Administer a sodium bicarbonate drip to decrease dysrhythmias; the alkaline environment increases the protein binding of the metabolite. 4. Administer vasopressors. 5. Use only Class IB antiarrhythmics (eg, lidocaine), as some other types of antiarrhythmics have the same effect as TCA. 6. Manage seizure activity with benzodiazepines (eg, diazepam) as necessary. 7. Refer patient for psychiatric evaluation for potential suicide intent and evaluation of medication regimen for effectiveness.

Continued

Table 71-1	EMERGENCY MANAGEMENT OF PATIENTS WITH DRUG OVERDOSE (Continued)	
Drug	**Clinical Manifestations**	**Therapeutic Management**
Selective Serotonin Reuptake Inhibitors (SSRIs) and Other Antidepressants Trazodone (Desyrel) Fluoxetine (Prozac) Paroxetine (Paxil) Sertraline (Zoloft) Venlafaxine (Effexor) Escitalopram (Lexapro) Bupropion (Wellbutrin)	Decreased level of consciousness, confusion Respiratory depression Increased heart rate **Serotonin syndrome:** Agitation, seizures Hyperthermia, diaphoresis Hypertension	1. Administer activated charcoal with possibly whole-bowel irrigation if a sustained-release medication was taken. 2. Use seizure precautions and administer benzodiazepines (eg, diazepam) as ordered. 3. Serotonin syndrome may occur if the SSRI was taken in conjunction with dextromethorphan or meperidine.

*Polydrug use at "rave clubs" frequently involves MDMA, alcohol, amphetamines, LSD, and sometimes dextromethorphan. Terms such as "Ecstasy" may refer to flunitrazepam (Rohypnol), GHB, ephedrine, and/or caffeine, in addition to MDMA. The Web site www.clubdrugs.gov provides more information about possible drug abuse and how it may relate to emergency nursing care.

Acute Alcohol Intoxication

Alcohol is a psychotropic drug that affects mood, judgment, behavior, concentration, and consciousness. Many heavy drinkers are young adults or people older than 60 years of age. There is a high prevalence of alcoholism among ED patients. Because patients who abuse alcohol return frequently to the ED, they often frustrate and tax the patience of the health care professionals who care for them. Their management requires patience and thoughtful, accurate, long-term treatment (Thompson, Lande & Kalapatapu, 2008).

Alcohol, or ethanol, is a multisystem toxin and CNS depressant that causes drowsiness, impaired coordination, slurring of speech, sudden mood changes, aggression, belligerence, grandiosity, and uninhibited behavior. In excess, it can also cause stupor, coma, and death. Increasingly, underage minors and college students arrive at the ED with alcohol poisoning from binge drinking. All too frequently, the result is death.

In the ED, the patient is assessed for head injury, hypoglycemia (which mimics intoxication), and other health problems. Possible nursing diagnoses include ineffective breathing pattern related to CNS depression and risk for violence (self-directed or other-directed) related to severe intoxication from alcohol.

Treatment involves detoxification of the acute poisoning, recovery, and rehabilitation. Commonly, the patient uses mechanisms of denial and defensiveness. The nurse should approach the patient in a nonjudgmental manner, using a firm, consistent, accepting, and reasonable attitude. Speaking in a calm and slow manner is helpful because alcohol interferes with thought processes. If the patient appears intoxicated, hypoxia, hypovolemia, and neurologic impairment must be ruled out before it is assumed that the patient is intoxicated. Typically, a blood specimen is obtained for analysis of the blood alcohol level.

If drowsy, the patient should be allowed to sleep off the state of alcoholic intoxication. During this time, maintenance of a patent airway and observation for symptoms of CNS depression are essential. The patient should be undressed and kept warm with blankets. On the other hand, if the patient is noisy or belligerent, sedation may be necessary. If sedation is used, the patient should be monitored carefully for hypotension and decreased level of consciousness.

In addition, the patient is examined for alcohol withdrawal delirium and also for injuries and organic disease (such as head injury, seizures, pulmonary infections, hypoglycemia, and nutritional deficiencies) that may be masked by alcoholic intoxication. People with alcoholism suffer more injuries than the general population. Also, acute alcohol intoxication is the cause of trauma for many nonalcoholic patients. Pulmonary infections are also more common in patients with alcoholism, resulting from respiratory depression, an impaired defense system, and a tendency toward aspiration of gastric contents. The patient may show little increase in temperature or WBC count. The patient may be hospitalized or admitted to a detoxification center in an effort to examine problems underlying the substance abuse.

Alcohol Withdrawal Syndrome/Delirium Tremens

Alcohol withdrawal syndrome is an acute toxic state that occurs as a result of sudden cessation of alcohol intake after a bout of heavy drinking or, more typically, after prolonged intake of alcohol. Severity of symptoms depends on how much alcohol was ingested and for how long. Delirium tremens may be precipitated by acute injury or infection (pneumonia, pancreatitis, hepatitis) and is the most severe form of alcohol withdrawal syndrome (Larson, 2008).

Patients with alcohol withdrawal syndrome show signs of anxiety, uncontrollable fear, tremor, irritability, agitation, insomnia, and incontinence. They are talkative and preoccupied and experience visual, tactile, olfactory, and auditory hallucinations that often are terrifying. Autonomic overactivity occurs and is evidenced by tachycardia, dilated pupils, and profuse perspiration. Usually, all vital signs are elevated in the alcoholic toxic state. Delirium tremens is a life-threatening condition and carries a high mortality rate.

The goals of management are to give adequate sedation and support to allow the patient to rest and recover without danger of injury or peripheral vascular collapse. A physical examination is performed to identify preexisting or contributing illnesses or injuries (eg, head injury, pneumonia).

A drug history is obtained to elicit information that may facilitate adjustment of any sedative requirements. Baseline blood pressure is determined, because the patient's subsequent treatment may depend on blood pressure changes.

Usually, the patient is sedated as directed with a sufficient dosage of benzodiazepines to establish and maintain sedation, which reduces agitation, prevents exhaustion, prevents seizures, and promotes sleep. The patient should be calm, able to respond, and able to maintain an airway safely on his or her own. A variety of medications and combinations of medications are used (eg, chlordiazepoxide [Librium], lorazepam [Ativan], and clonidine [Catapres]). Haloperidol (Haldol) or droperidol (Inapsine) may be administered for severe acute alcohol withdrawal syndrome. Dosages are adjusted according to the patient's symptoms (agitation, anxiety) and blood pressure response.

The patient is placed in a calm, nonstressful environment (usually a private room) and observed closely. The room remains lighted to minimize the potential for illusions (visual misrepresentations) and hallucinations. Homicidal or suicidal responses may result from hallucinations. Closet and bathroom doors are closed to eliminate shadows. Someone is designated to stay with the patient as much as possible. The presence of another person has a reassuring and calming effect, which helps the patient maintain contact with reality. To orient the patient to reality, any illusions are explained.

◤ NURSING ALERT

Restraints are used as prescribed, if necessary, if the client is aggressive or violent, but only when other alternatives have been unsuccessful. The least restrictive device that will prevent the patient from injuring self or others is used. Caution is taken to ensure that restraints are applied properly and that they are not impairing circulation to any part of the body or interfering with respirations. Restraints should be used in tandem with verbal intervention to calm the patient and promote compliance. Restraints must be released according to protocol. Physical observation (eg, skin integrity, circulatory status, respiratory status) is ongoing, and the patient's response is documented.

Fluid losses may result from gastrointestinal losses (vomiting), profuse perspiration, and hyperventilation. In addition, the patient may be dehydrated as a result of alcohol's effect of decreasing antidiuretic hormone. The oral or IV route is used to restore fluid and electrolyte balance.

Temperature, pulse, respiration, and blood pressure are recorded frequently (every 30 minutes in severe forms of delirium) to monitor for peripheral circulatory collapse or hyperthermia (the two most serious complications). Phenytoin (Dilantin) or other antiseizure medications may be prescribed to prevent repeated withdrawal seizures.

Frequently seen complications include infections (eg, pneumonia), trauma, hepatic failure, hypoglycemia, and cardiovascular problems. Hypoglycemia may accompany alcohol withdrawal, because alcohol depletes liver glycogen stores and impairs gluconeogenesis; many patients with alcoholism also are malnourished. Parenteral dextrose may be prescribed if the liver glycogen level is depleted. Orange juice, Gatorade, or other sources of carbohydrates are given to stabilize the blood glucose level and counteract tremulousness. Supplemental vitamin therapy and a high-protein diet are provided as prescribed to counteract nutritional deficits. The patient should be referred to an alcoholic treatment center for follow-up care and rehabilitation.

VIOLENCE, ABUSE, AND NEGLECT

Family Violence, Abuse, and Neglect

EDs are often the first place where victims of family violence, abuse, or neglect go to seek help. Each year in the United States, there are 4.8 million women and 2.9 million men who experience physical assaults involving their intimate partners. Intimate partner violence (IPV) caused 1544 deaths in 2004; of these victims, 75% were females and 25% were male. Costs related to IPV are estimated to exceed $8.3 billion annually (Centers for Disease Control and Prevention [CDC], 2006a).

It is estimated that up to one third of all patients in the ED have experienced IPV at some point in their lives. Research studies suggest that as many as 44% of all women murdered by a partner had visited an ED within the 2 years prior to death. Researchers believe that most persons who have experienced IPV are willing to disclose their causes of injury, but as few as 4% to 10% of cases are accurately identified in EDs (Daugherty & Houry, 2008). ED nurses must be vigilant in their assessments of both women and men who present with injuries that may be consistent with IPV. In addition, ED nurses must be aware that men and women with disabilities are at higher risk of domestic violence and abuse than nondisabled people and should include questions to that effect in their evaluations.

It is estimated that between 700,000 and 1.2 million elders are abused or neglected annually (American Geriatrics Society, 2005). Elder abuse takes many forms, including physical, emotional, and verbal abuse; neglect; violation of personal rights; and financial abuse (see Chapters 5 and 46).

Clinical Manifestations

When people who have been abused seek treatment, they may present with physical injuries or with health problems such as anxiety, insomnia, or gastrointestinal symptoms that are related to stress. The possibility of abuse should be investigated whenever a person presents with multiple injuries that are in various stages of healing, when injuries are unexplained, and when the explanation does not fit the physical picture (Chart 71-13). The possibility of neglect should be investigated whenever a dependent person shows evidence of inattention to hygiene, to nutrition, or to known medical needs (eg, unfilled medication prescriptions, missed appointments with health care providers). In the ED, the most common physical injuries seen are unexplained bruises, lacerations, abrasions, head injuries, or fractures. The most common clinical manifestations of neglect are malnutrition and dehydration.

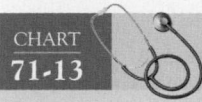

CHART 71-13

Assessing for Abuse, Maltreatment, and Neglect

The following questions may be helpful when assessing a patient for abuse, maltreatment, and neglect:

- I noticed that you have a number of bruises. Can you tell me how they happened? Has anyone hurt you?
- You seem frightened. Has anyone ever hurt you?
- Sometimes patients tell me that they have been hurt by someone at home or at work. Could this be happening to you?
- Are you afraid of anyone at home or work, or of anyone with whom you come in contact?
- Has anyone failed to help you to take care of yourself when you needed help?
- Has anyone prevented you from seeing friends or other people whom you wish to see?
- Have you signed any papers that you did not understand or did not wish to sign?
- Has anyone forced you to sign papers against your will?
- Has anyone forced you to engage in sexual activities within the past year?
- Has anyone prevented you from using an assistive device (eg, wheelchair, walker) within the past year?
- Has anyone you depend on refused to help you take your medicine, bathe, groom, or eat within the past year?

Assessment and Diagnostic Findings

Nurses in EDs are in an ideal position to provide early detection and interventions for victims of IPV. This requires an acute awareness of the signs of possible abuse, maltreatment, and neglect. Nurses must be skilled in interviewing techniques that are likely to elicit accurate information. A careful history is crucial in the screening process. Asking questions in private—away from others—may be helpful in eliciting information about abuse, maltreatment, and neglect.

Whenever evidence leads one to suspect abuse or neglect, an evaluation with careful documentation of descriptions of events and drawings or photographs of injuries is important, because the medical record may be used as part of a legal proceeding. Assessment of the patient's general appearance and interactions with significant others, an examination of the entire surface area of the body, and a mental status examination are crucial.

Management

Whenever abuse, maltreatment, or neglect is suspected, the health care provider's primary concern should be the safety and welfare of the patient. Treatment focuses on the consequences of the abuse, violence, or neglect and on prevention of further injury. Protocols of most EDs require that a multidisciplinary approach be used. Nurses, physicians, social workers, and community agencies work collaboratively to develop and implement a plan for meeting the patient's needs.

If the patient is in immediate danger, he or she should be separated from the abusing or neglecting person whenever possible. Referral to a shelter may be the most appropriate action, but many shelters are inaccessible to people with mobility limitations.

When abuse or neglect is the result of stress experienced by a caregiver who is no longer able to cope with the burden of caring for an elderly person or a person with chronic disease or a disability, respite services may be necessary. Support groups may be helpful to these caregivers. When mental illness of the abuser or neglecter is responsible for the situation, alternative living arrangements may be required.

Nurses must be mindful that competent adults are free to accept or refuse the help that is offered to them. Some patients insist on remaining in the home environment where the abuse or neglect is occurring. The wishes of patients who are competent and not cognitively impaired should be respected. However, all possible alternatives, available resources, and safety plans should be explored with the patient.

Mandatory reporting laws in most states require health care workers to report *suspected* child or elder abuse to an official agency, usually Adult (or Child) Protective Services. All that is required for reporting is the suspicion of abuse; the health care worker is not required to prove abuse or neglect. Likewise, health care workers who report suspected abuse are immune from civil or criminal liability if the report is made in good faith. Subsequent home visits resulting from the report of suspected abuse are a part of gathering information about the patient in the home environment. In addition, many states have resource hotlines for use by health care workers and by patients who seek answers to questions about abuse and neglect.

Sexual Assault

The definition of *rape* is forced sexual acts, especially if these acts involve vaginal or anal penetration. Perpetrators and victims may be either male or female. Society is focused on the rights and care of people who have been sexually assaulted, and law enforcement agencies are increasingly sensitive and aggressive in managing these crimes. Rape crisis centers offer support and education and help people who have been sexually assaulted through the subsequent police investigation and courtroom experience.

The manner in which the patient is received and treated in the ED is important to his or her future psychological well-being. Crisis intervention should begin when the patient enters the health care facility. The patient should be seen immediately. Most hospitals have a written protocol that addresses the patient's physical and emotional needs as well as collection of forensic evidence.

In many states, the emergency nurse has the opportunity to become trained as a sexual assault nurse examiner (SANE). Preparing for this role requires specific training in forensic evidence collection, history taking, documentation, and ways to approach the patient and family. Specialized training also includes learning proper photographic methods and the use of colposcopy. Colposcopy facilitates assessment by magnifying tissues and looking for evidence of microtrauma. Evidence is collected through photography, videography, and analysis of specimens. Another tool useful to the SANE is the light-staining microscope, which enables the examiner to identify motile and nonmotile sperm and infectious organisms. This tool saves time and also enhances assessment. The SANE complements the ED staff and they can spend more time with both the patient and police officers investigating the incident (Lynch, 2006).

Assessment and Diagnostic Findings

The patient's reaction to rape has been termed *rape trauma syndrome* and is seen as an acute stress reaction to a life-threatening situation. The nurse performing the assessment is aware that the patient may go through several phases of psychological reactions (Lynch, 2006), which have been described as follows:

- An acute disorganization phase, which may manifest as an expressed state in which shock, disbelief, fear, guilt, humiliation, anger, and other such emotions are encountered or as a controlled state in which feelings are masked or hidden and the victim appears composed
- A phase of denial and unwillingness to talk about the incident, followed by a phase of heightened anxiety, fear, flashbacks, sleep disturbances, hyperalertness, and psychosomatic reactions that is consistent with posttraumatic stress disorder (PTSD) (see Chapter 7 for further discussion of PTSD)
- A phase of reorganization, in which the incident is put into perspective; some victims never fully recover and go on to develop chronic stress disorders and phobias

Management

The goals of management are to provide support, to reduce the patient's emotional trauma, and to gather available evidence for possible legal proceedings. All of the interventions are aimed at encouraging the patient to gain a sense of control over his or her life.

Throughout the patient's stay in the ED, the patient's privacy and sensitivity must be respected. The patient may exhibit a wide range of emotional reactions, such as hysteria, stoicism, or feelings of being overwhelmed. Support and caring are crucial. The patient should be reassured that anxiety is natural and asked whether a support person may be called. Appropriate support is available from professional and community resources. The Rape Victim Companion Program, if available in the community, can be contacted, and the services of a volunteer can be requested. The patient should never be left alone.

Physical Examination

A written, witnessed informed consent must be obtained from the patient (or parent or guardian if the patient is a minor) for examination, for taking of photographs, and for release of findings to police. A history is obtained only if the patient has not already talked to a police officer, social worker, or crisis intervention worker. The patient should not be asked to repeat the history. Any history of the event that is obtained should be recorded in the patient's own words. The patient is asked whether he or she has bathed, douched, brushed his or her teeth, changed clothes, urinated, or defecated since the attack, because these actions may alter interpretation of subsequent findings. The time of admission, time of examination, date and time of the alleged rape, and the patient's emotional state and general appearance (including any evidence of trauma, such as discoloration, bruises, lacerations, secretions, or torn and bloody clothing) are documented.

For the physical examination, the patient is helped to undress and is draped properly. Each item of clothing is placed in a separate paper bag. Plastic bags are not used because they retain moisture; moisture may promote mold and mildew formation, which can destroy evidence. The bags are labeled and given to appropriate law enforcement authorities.

The patient is examined (from head to toe) for injuries, especially injuries to the head, neck, breasts, thighs, back, and buttocks. Body diagrams and photographs aid in documenting the evidence of trauma. The physical examination focuses on the following:

- External evidence of trauma (bruises, contusions, lacerations, stab wounds)
- Dried semen stains (appearing as crusted, flaking areas) on the patient's body or clothes
- Broken fingernails and body tissue and foreign materials under nails (if found, samples are taken)
- Oral examination, including a specimen of saliva and cultures of gum and tooth areas

Pelvic and rectal examinations are also performed. The perineum and other areas are examined with a Wood lamp or other filtered ultraviolet light. Areas that appear fluorescent may indicate semen stains. The color and consistency of any discharge present is noted. A water-moistened rather than a lubricated vaginal speculum is used for the examination. Lubricant contains chemicals that may interfere with later forensic testing of specimens and acid phosphatase determinations. The rectum is examined for signs of trauma, blood, and semen. During the examination, the patient should be advised of the nature and necessity of each procedure and given the rationale for each question asked.

Specimen Collection

During the physical examination, numerous laboratory specimens may be collected, including the following:

- Vaginal aspirate, examined for presence or absence of motile and nonmotile sperm
- Secretions (obtained with a sterile swab) from the vaginal pool for acid phosphatase, blood group antigen of semen, and precipitin test against human sperm and blood
- Separate smears from the oral, vaginal, and anal areas
- Culture of body orifices for gonorrhea
- Blood serum for syphilis and HIV testing and DNA analysis; a sample of serum for syphilis may be frozen and saved for future testing
- Pregnancy test if there is a possibility that the patient may be pregnant
- Any foreign material (leaves, grass, dirt), which is placed in a clean envelope
- Pubic hair samples obtained by combing or trimming. Several pubic hairs with follicles are placed in separate containers and identified as the patient's hair

To preserve the chain of evidence, each specimen is labeled with the name of the patient, the date and time of collection, the body area from which the specimen was obtained, and the names of personnel collecting specimens. Then the specimens are given to a designated person (eg, crime laboratory technician), and an itemized receipt is obtained.

Treating Potential Consequences of Rape

After the initial physical examination is completed and specimens have been obtained, any associated injuries are treated as indicated. The patient is given the option of prophylaxis against sexually transmitted disease (STD) (also referred to as sexually transmitted infection [STI]). Ceftriaxone (Rocephin), administered intramuscularly with 1% lidocaine (Xylocaine), may be prescribed as prophylaxis for gonorrhea. In addition, a single oral dose of metronidazole (Flagyl) and either a single oral dose of azithromycin (Zithromax) or a 7-day oral regimen of doxycycline (Vibramycin) may be prescribed as prophylaxis for syphilis and chlamydia (CDC, 2006b).

Antipregnancy measures may be considered if the patient is of childbearing age (CDC, 2006b). A postcoital contraceptive medication, such as an oral contraceptive medication that contains levonorgestrel and ethinyl estradiol (Alesse, Seasonique), may be prescribed after a pregnancy test. To promote effectiveness, the contraceptive medication should be administered within 12 to 24 hours and no later than 72 hours after intercourse. The 21-day package rather than the 28-day package is prescribed so that the patient does not take the inert tablets by mistake. An antiemetic may be administered as prescribed to decrease discomfort from side effects. A cleansing douche, mouthwash, and fresh clothing are usually offered (Lynch, 2006).

Follow-Up Care

The patient is informed of counseling services to prevent long-term psychological effects. Counseling services should be made available to both the patient and the family. A referral is made to the Rape Victim Companion Program, if available. Appointments for follow-up surveillance for pregnancy and for STD and HIV testing also are made (CDC, 2006b).

The patient is encouraged to return to his or her previous level of functioning as soon as possible. When leaving the health care facility, the patient should be accompanied by a family member or friend.

PSYCHIATRIC EMERGENCIES

A psychiatric emergency is an urgent, serious disturbance of behavior, affect, or thought that makes the patient unable to cope with life situations and interpersonal relationships. A patient presenting with a psychiatric emergency may display overactive or violent, underactive or depressed, or suicidal behaviors.

The most important concern of the ED personnel is determining whether the patient is at risk for injuring self or others. The aim is to try to maintain the patient's self-esteem (and life, if necessary) while providing care. Determining whether the patient is currently under psychiatric care is important so that contact can be made with the therapist or physician who works with the patient.

Overactive Patients

Patients who display disturbed, uncooperative, and paranoid behavior and those who feel anxious and panicky may be prone to assaultive and destructive impulses and abnormal social behavior. Intense nervousness, depression, and crying are evident in some patients. Disturbed and noisy behavior may be exacerbated or compounded by alcohol or drug intoxication.

A reliable source for obtaining an accurate history is needed to identify events leading to the crisis. Past mental illness, hospitalizations, injuries, serious illnesses, use of alcohol or drugs, crises in interpersonal relationships, or intrapsychic conflicts are explored. Because abnormal thoughts and behavior may be manifestations of an underlying physical disorder, such as hypoglycemia, drug or alcohol toxicity, a stroke, a seizure disorder, or head injury, a physical assessment is also performed.

The immediate goal is to gain control of the situation. If the patient is potentially violent, security or local police should be nearby. Restraints are used as a *last* resort and only as prescribed. Approaching the patient with a calm, confident, and firm manner is therapeutic and has a calming effect. Helpful interventions include the following:

- Introduce yourself by name.
- Tell the patient, "I am here to help you."
- Repeat the patient's name from time to time.
- Speak in one-thought sentences and be consistent.
- Give the patient space and time to slow down.
- Show interest in, listen to, and encourage the patient to talk about personal thoughts and feelings.
- Offer appropriate and honest explanations.

A psychotropic agent (eg, one that exerts an effect on the mind) may be prescribed for emergency management of functional psychosis. However, a patient with a personality disorder should not be treated with psychotropic medications, and psychotropic medications should not be used if the patient's behavior results from the use of hallucinogens (eg, lysergic acid diethylamide [LSD]).

Agents such as chlorpromazine and haloperidol act specifically against psychotic symptoms of thought fragmentation and perceptual and behavioral aberrations. The initial dose depends on the patient's body weight and the severity of the symptoms. After administration of the initial dose, the patient is observed closely to determine the degree of change in psychotic behavior. Subsequent doses depend on the patient's response. Typically, after stabilization, the patient is transferred to an inpatient psychiatric unit or psychiatric outpatient treatment is arranged.

Violent Behavior

Violent and aggressive behavior, usually episodic, is a means of expressing feelings of anger, fear, or hopelessness about a situation. Usually, the patient has a history of outbursts of rage, temper tantrums, or impulsive behavior. People with a tendency for violence frequently lose control when intoxicated with alcohol or drugs. Family members are the most frequent victims of their aggression. Patients with a propensity for violence include those intoxicated by drugs or alcohol; those going through drug or alcohol withdrawal; and those diagnosed with acute paranoid schizophrenic state, acute organic brain syndrome, acute psychosis, paranoid character, borderline personality, or antisocial personality disorders.

The goal of treatment is to bring the violence under control. A specially designated room with at least two exits should be used for the interview. The door of the room should be kept open, and the nurse should remain in clear view of the staff, *staying between the patient and the door*. However, the patient's exit to the door must not be blocked, because the patient may feel trapped and threatened. No objects that could be used as weapons should be in sight, in the room, or carried in with health care personnel. If the interviewer feels anxious or uneasy about the patient's response, security staff, a family member, or another health care worker should be asked to remain in the hall nearby in the event that additional help is needed. The patient should never be left alone, because this may be interpreted as rejection or provide an opportunity for self-harm.

To bring the violence under control, it is crucial to use a calm, noncritical approach while remaining in control of the situation. Sudden movements are avoided. If the patient is carrying a weapon, the emergency health care provider should ask that it be surrendered. If the patient is unwilling to surrender the weapon, the security staff is called. If necessary, the security staff may seek further assistance from the local police department.

The patient's violent behavior is a crisis situation for the patient and the ED. Crisis intervention, achieved by talking and listening to the patient, is best accomplished by expressing an interest in the patient's well-being while attempting to tune in to the patient and remain firm. The patient's agitated state is acknowledged by statements such as, "I want to work with you to relieve your distress."

The patient is allowed the opportunity to express anger verbally. If the patient is delusional, challenging the patient is avoided. Trying to hear what the patient is saying, conveying an expectation of appropriate behavior, and making the patient aware that help is available are key. The patient should be informed that violent behavior may be frightening to others and that violence is not acceptable. Help that is available in crisis situations (from a clinic or mental health facility) should be described and offered. Often, the offer of protection by hospitalization is welcomed by the patient, who fears losing control or harming self or others. If the patient does not calm down, security personnel or police intervention may be necessary.

If these measures fail to alleviate the patient's tension, medication may be prescribed (rapid sedation with haloperidol, diazepam, or chlorpromazine) to reduce tension, anxiety, and hyperactivity. Soft restraints must be prescribed by a physician only if other measures to calm the patient have failed (Hoyt & Selfridge-Thomas, 2007). After combativeness, agitation, and fear have decreased, the patient is referred for further mental health treatment.

Posttraumatic Stress Disorder

PTSD is the development of characteristic symptoms after a psychologically stressful event that is considered outside the range of normal human experience (eg, rape, combat, motor vehicle crash, natural catastrophe, terrorist attack). Symptoms of this disorder include intrusive thoughts and dreams, phobic avoidance reaction (avoidance of activities that arouse recollection of the traumatic event), heightened vigilance, exaggerated startle reaction, generalized anxiety, and societal withdrawal. PTSD may be acute, chronic, or delayed. PTSD often presents as multiple readmissions to the ED for minor or recurring complaints without evidence of injury. Refer to Chapter 7 for further discussion of assessment, diagnostic findings, and management of patients with PTSD.

Underactive or Depressed Patients

In the ED, depression may be seen as the primary condition bringing the patient to the health care facility or it may be masked by anxiety and somatic complaints. The depressed person has a mood disturbance.

Any patient who is depressed may be at risk of suicide. Attempts are made to find out whether the patient has thought about or attempted suicide. Questions such as, "Have you ever thought about taking your own life?" may be helpful. Generally, the patient is relieved to have an opportunity to discuss personal feelings. If the patient is seriously depressed, relatives should be notified. The patient should never be left alone, because suicide is usually committed in solitude. See Chapter 7 for further discussion of assessment, diagnostic findings, and management of patients with depression.

Suicidal Patients

Attempted suicide is an act that stems from depression (eg, loss of a loved one, loss of body integrity or status, poor self-image) and can be viewed as a cry for help and intervention. Males are at greater risk than females. Others at risk are elderly people; young adults; people who are enduring unusual loss or stress; those who are unemployed, divorced, widowed, or living alone; those showing signs of significant depression (eg, weight loss, sleep disturbances, somatic complaints, suicidal preoccupation); and those with a history of a previous suicide attempt, suicide in the family, or psychiatric illness.

Being aware of people at risk and assessing for specific factors that predispose a person to suicide are key management strategies. Specific signs and symptoms of potential suicide include the following:

- Communication of *suicidal intent,* such as preoccupation with death or talking of someone else's suicide (eg, "I'm tired of living. I've put my affairs in order. I'm better off dead. I'm a burden to my family.")
- History of a previous suicide attempt (the risk is much greater in these cases)

- Family history of suicide
- Loss of a parent at an early age
- Specific plan for suicide
- A means to carry out the plan

Emergency management focuses on treating the consequences of the suicide attempt (eg, gunshot wound, drug overdose) and preventing further self-injury. A patient who has made a suicidal attempt may do so again. Crisis intervention is used to determine suicidal potential, to discover areas of depression and conflict, to find out about the patient's support system, and to determine whether hospitalization or psychiatric referral is necessary. Depending on the patient's potential for suicide, the patient may be admitted to the intensive care unit, referred for follow-up care, or admitted to the psychiatric unit.

CRITICAL THINKING EXERCISES

1 An elderly man arrives at the ED by ambulance after a car crash. He is immobilized on a backboard with a cervical collar and an oxygen mask is in place. There is a bruise across his abdomen where the seat belt was applied. He is groaning loudly and seems confused; he cannot tell you what has happened, where he is at present, nor what day of the week it is, although he can tell you his full name. You note a shallow, rapid breathing pattern of 26 breaths per minute. How would you prioritize the patient's needs? Develop an assessment strategy, identify diagnostic studies that will benefit the patient, and describe the patient's priority treatment needs.

EBP **2** Two men choose to go ice fishing for the first time of the season. They chose to wear light clothing, expecting the cabin to be warm, but neglected to take into account the 4 inches of snow on the ground and the high humidity. They spent the day fishing on the ice without moving much. One man now presents to the ED for treatment of frostbite of his feet. His friend has been massaging them en route to the ED, and the patient insists that this makes his feet feel better. You tell them to cease massage. Describe the explanation you would give to this patient and the evidence base that guides your response. Tell how you would proceed with managing this patient's care. Describe the treatment dilemmas for this type of injury.

3 The following four patients present to the triage desk of the ED within minutes of each other. How would you prioritize and categorize each of these patients? Which ones need immediate attention? What initial care would you provide at triage? Which patient could wait or be sent to the clinic for management?
a. A college-student with a history of exercise-induced asthma and known noncompliance to prescribed medications presents with rapid, shallow respirations and wheezing after jogging 5 miles. His girlfriend is very anxious. He has been this way for about 15 minutes.
b. An attorney who has had a cold for 3 days says she has no primary care physician and must be seen right now because she cannot breathe. Her respirations are normal, pulse oxygenation saturations are 100%, and she has complaints of sinus drainage and a headache.
c. A middle-age woman experienced sudden dyspnea and chest tightness while making dinner. Instead of calling 911, her husband drove her to the ED. She is complaining of left scapular pain and tingling in her left arm, her skin appears ashen, and she is diaphoretic.
d. An elderly woman with a known history of diabetes presents with complaints of 24 hours of vomiting. Her vital signs are normal, but she is diaphoretic and appears weak.

4 A patient arrives to the triage area of the ED complaining of flulike symptoms. He has developed a rash that seems to be primarily located on the soles of his feet and palms of his hands. He cannot remember touching anything that he knows he is allergic to, and he has not been walking barefoot. He does like to hunt, and only a week ago was in his deer stand for most of the weekend. What potential disease symptoms are being exhibited by this patient? What other questions would you ask? What will you focus on when you examine his skin?

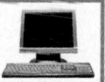 The Smeltzer suite offers these additional resources to enhance learning and facilitate understanding of this chapter:
- thePoint online resource, thepoint.lww.com/Smeltzer12E
- Student CD-ROM included with the book
- *Study Guide to Accompany Brunner & Suddarth's Textbook of Medical-Surgical Nursing*

REFERENCES AND SELECTED READINGS

**Double asterisk indicates classic reference.*

Books

American College of Surgeons (ACS). (2008). *Advanced trauma life support* (8th ed.). Chicago: Author.

Auerbach, P. S. (2007). *Wilderness medicine* (5th ed.). St. Louis, MO: Elsevier-Mosby.

Berner, A. R. (2005). Triage. In Harwood-Nuss, A. (Ed.). *The clinical practice of emergency medicine* (4th ed.). Philadelphia: Lippincott Williams & Wilkins.

Emergency Nurses Association (ENA). (2007). *Trauma nurse core course provider manual* (6th ed.). Chicago: Author.

Emergency Nurses Association (ENA) & Newberry, L. (2006). *Sheehy's emergency nursing* (6th ed.). St. Louis, MO: Mosby.

Hoyt, K. S. & Selfridge-Thomas, J. (2007). *Emergency nursing core curriculum* (6th ed.). St Louis, MO: Saunders.

Lynch, V. (2006). *Forensic nursing.* St. Louis, MO: C. V. Mosby.

Marx, J. (2006). *Rosen's emergency medicine: Concepts and clinical practice* (6th ed.). Philadelphia: Mosby Elsevier.

McQuillan, K., VonReuden, K., Hartsock, R., et al. (2008). *Trauma nursing: Resuscitation through rehabilitation* (4th ed.). Philadelphia: Saunders.

Nayduch, D. (2009). *Nurse to nurse trauma care:* New York: McGraw Hill.

Journals and Electronic Documents

American Geriatrics Society. (2005). Aging in the know: Elder mistreatment. Available at: www.healthinaging.org/agingintheknow/chapters_ch_trial.asp?ch=9

American Heart Association. (2005). Guidelines for cardiopulmonary resuscitation and emergency cardiovascular care. *Circulation, 112*(24 Supp), 1–203.

**Blow, O., Magliore, L., Claridge, J. A., et al. (1999). The golden hour and the silver day: Detection and correction of occult hypoperfusion within 24 hours improves outcome from major trauma. *Journal of Trauma, 47*(5), 964–969.

Centers for Disease Control and Prevention (CDC). (2006a). Factsheet: Understanding intimate partner violence. Available at: www.cdc.gov/ncipc/dvp/ipv_factsheet.pdf

Centers for Disease Control and Prevention (CDC). (2006b). Sexually transmitted diseases' treatment guidelines. *Morbidity and Mortality Weekly Reports*, 55(RR-11), 1–100.

Daley, B. J. & Barbee, J (2008). Snakebite. Available at: www.emedicine.com/article/168828-overview

Daugherty, J. D. & Houry, D. E. (2008). Intimate partner violence screening in the emergency department. *Journal of Postgraduate Medicine*, 54(4), 301–305.

Kirkpatrick, A. W., Sirois, M., Laupland, K. B., et al. (2005). Prospective evaluation of hand-held focused abdominal sonography for trauma (FAST) in blunt and abdominal trauma. *Canadian Journal of Surgery*, 48(6), 453–460.

Lakstein, D., Blumenfeld, A., Sokolov, T., et al. (2003). Tourniquets for hemorrhage control on the battlefield: A 4-year accumulated experience. *Journal of Trauma*, 154(5), 5221–5225.

Larson, M. (2008). Alcohol-related psychosis. Available at: http://emedicine.medscape.com/article/289848-overview

National Hospital Ambulatory Medical Care Survey. (2005). 2005. Emergency department summary. Available at: www.cdc.gov/nchs/data/ad/ad386.pdf

Shepard, S. M., Martin, J. & Shoff, W. H. (2008). Drowning. Available at: http://emedicine.medscape.com/article/772753-overview

Tanabe, P., Gimbel, R., Yarnold, P. R., et al. (2004). The Emergency Severity Index (version 3) 5-level triage systems scores predict ED resource consumption. *Journal of Emergency Nursing*, 30(1), 22–29.

Thompson, W., Lande, R. G. & Kalapatapu, R. K. (2008). Alcoholism. Available at: http://emedicine.medscape.com/article/285913-overview

Walker, W. (2008). Accident and emergency staff opinion on the effects of family presence during adult resuscitation: Critical literature review. *Journal of Advanced Nursing*, 61(4), 348–362.

Zeglin, D. (2005). Brown recluse spider bites. *American Journal of Nursing*, 105(2), 64–68.

RESOURCES

American College of Surgeons, Committee on Trauma, www.facs.org
American Heart Association, www.americanheart.org
American Trauma Society, www.amtrauma.org
Centers for Disease Control and Prevention, www.cdc.gov
Divers Alert Network, www.diversalertnetwork.org
Emergency Nurses Association, www.ena.org
National Safety Council, www.nsc.org
Society of Trauma Nurses, http://traumanursesoc.org

chapter 72

Terrorism, Mass Casualty, and Disaster Nursing

LEARNING OBJECTIVES

On completion of this chapter, the learner will be able to:

1 Identify the necessary components of an emergency operations plan.

2 Discuss how triage in a disaster differs from triage in an emergency.

3 Develop a plan of care for a patient experiencing short-term or long-term psychological effects after a disaster.

4 Evaluate the different levels of personal protection and decontamination procedures that may be necessary during an event involving mass casualties or weapons of mass destruction (WMD).

5 Identify physical injuries that may occur after blast events.

6 Describe isolation precautions necessary for bioterrorism agents.

7 Identify the differences among the various chemical agents used in terrorist events, their effects, and the decontamination and treatment procedures that are necessary.

8 Determine the injuries associated with varying levels of radiation or chemical exposure and the associated decontamination processes.

GLOSSARY

biological warfare: use of a biological agent, such as anthrax, as a WMD

chemical warfare: use of a chemical agent, such as chlorine, as a WMD

decontamination: process of removing, or rendering harmless, contaminants that have accumulated on personnel, patients, and equipment

mass casualty incident (MCI): situation in which the number of casualties exceeds the number of resources

material safety data sheet (MSDS): provides information to employees and health care providers regarding specific chemical agents; includes chemical name, physical data, chemical ingredients, fire and explosive hazard data, health and reactive data, spill or leak procedures, special protection information, and special precautions; also known as the Worker's Right to Know

nuclear warfare: use of nuclear contamination as a WMD

personal protective equipment (PPE): equipment beyond standard precautions; may include level A, B, C, and D equipment

terrorism: unlawful use of violence or threats of violence against people in order to coerce or intimidate

weapons of mass destruction (WMD): weapons used to cause widespread death and destruction

The possibility and reality of mass casualties associated with disasters, terrorism, and biologic warfare are not new to human history; nor is the concept of using **weapons of mass destruction (WMD)**. In fact, the use of WMD dates as far back as the 6th century BCE for biological weapons and the year 436 BCE for chemical weapons (U.S. Army Medical Research Institute of Chemical Defense, 1999). However, geopolitical forces and interests and the availability of destructive technology have brought the possibility of more terrorist events to our doorstep. **Terrorism** systematically involves using violence to create feelings of fear. Examples include the 1993 bombing of the World Trade Center in New York City; the 1995 Oklahoma City bombing of the Murrah Federal Building; the total destruction of the World Trade Center towers and the damage to the Pentagon on September 11, 2001; and the London subway bombing of 2005. Terrorists have become increasingly sophisticated, organized, and therefore effective. It is no longer a question of *whether* a terrorist event will again lead to mass casualties, but *when* such an event will occur.

In 1999, the National Domestic Preparedness Organization, a federal agency, was developed to coordinate preparedness in the event of a terrorist attack. The Department of Homeland Security was created after the attacks of September 11, 2001, to coordinate federal and state efforts to combat terrorist activity. Every facility receiving preparedness funds must have a plan that adheres to guidelines devised by the National Incident Management System (NIMS), directed by the Federal Emergency Management Agency (FEMA).

Warfare and terrorism are just two of the reasons that health care providers need to plan for mass casualties. Airplane crashes, train crashes, toxic substance spills, and infectious disease outbreaks are other disasters that can result in casualties and tax the resources of health care facilities and their communities. In addition, natural phenomena such as floods, tornadoes, hurricanes (eg, Hurricane Katrina, the category 5 storm that struck New Orleans, Louisiana, and Biloxi, Mississippi, in 2006), fires, and earthquakes, kill and injure hundreds of thousands of people worldwide each year. Acute care facilities must be prepared for any and all of these disasters. This chapter focuses on disaster preparedness, especially providing information about possible terrorist-related injuries and illnesses that can occur after biologic, chemical, and nuclear or radiation attacks. Information about the process of responding to these emergencies is applicable to other types of mass disasters as well.

Federal, State, and Local Responses to Emergencies

Many resources are available at the federal, state, and local levels to assist in the management of **mass casualty incidents (MCIs),** disasters, and emergencies. An MCI is defined as any incident that results in more patients than daily resources can handle (Emergency Nurses Association, 2007). Local communities must be prepared to act in isolation and provide competent care for up to 5 days before federal or other state resources become available (Hoyt &

Chart 72-1 • *Disaster Levels*

Disasters are often classified by the resultant anticipated necessary response:

Level I: Local emergency response personnel and organizations can contain and effectively manage the disaster and its aftermath.

Level II: Regional efforts and aid from surrounding communities are sufficient to manage the effects of the disaster.

Level III: Local and regional assets are overwhelmed; statewide or federal assistance is required.

Selfridge-Thomas, 2007). Initiating the request for federal assistance should not be delayed, however, so that resources do not become exhausted.

Disasters are often categorized by level to indicate the anticipated level of response (Chart 72-1). A list of local resources with specific instructions about how and when to contact these agencies or organizations should be readily available to local disaster planning committees and frequently reviewed by those committees for needed updates.

A disaster response strategy cannot succeed without appropriate physical assets and a staff trained and prepared to carry out the plan. Assets such as increased security; stockpiles of equipment and medications; and planning, drills, and training are essential (Lusby, 2006). Hazard vulnerability assessments should be performed to identify potential and actual threats that involve a particular facility and community. Mutual aid agreements among various communities must take these vulnerabilities into account. Successful execution of a response plan is based on knowledge, confidence, and readiness.

Federal Agencies

State authorities must request federal assistance with resources through appropriate government channels. A request for federal resources generally is made when local resources have become or are expected to become depleted.

Federal agencies that may provide resources in response to an MCI or a disaster include the Department of Health and Human Services (DHHS), the Department of Justice, Department of Defense, and the Department of Homeland Security. Each of these federal departments oversees hundreds of agencies that may respond to MCIs. For example, personnel from the Federal Bureau of Investigation (FBI) (structured under the Department of Justice) may be used for scene control and collection of forensic evidence. FEMA, which is overseen by the Department of Homeland Security, can activate teams such as the Urban Search and Rescue Teams (USRTs). The DHHS administers the Centers for Disease Control and Prevention (CDC) and the National Disaster Medical System. The National Disaster Medical System has many medical support teams, such as Disaster Medical Assistance Teams (DMATs), Disaster Mortuary Response Teams (DMORTs), Veterinary Medical Assistance Teams (VMATs), and National Medical Response Teams for Weapons of Mass Destruction (NMRTs).

The DMAT organizes voluntary medical personnel who can set up and staff a field hospital; DMATs are located across the country. There are four NMRTs: the

Table 72-1 DEPARTMENT OF HOMELAND SECURITY THREAT LEVELS	
Level of Security Threat	**Actions**
Red: severe, usually site is specified	Lockdown for security Prevention of parking close to the site Activation of the Emergency Operation Plan and Incident Command System
Orange: high, risk of attack but a specific site may not yet be identified	Increased security and screenings Activation of the Incident Command System
Yellow: elevated, possible risk but no defined site	Increased awareness and monitoring of activities Continued training for the Emergency Operations Plan
Blue: guarded, general risk but no specific risks identified	Ensure readiness with drill practice
Green: low, little or no risk perceived or known	Continued preparedness with drill practice

U.S. Department of Homeland Security, 2003.

mobile California, North Carolina, and Colorado teams and the Washington, D.C., team, which is stationary. These specialty teams were developed to respond to situations involving WMD. They consist of specially trained medical and technical personnel. The National Guard Civil Strike Teams are specially trained units that may respond to MCIs or disasters. In addition, the Department of Homeland Security designates a level of security threat that is intended to alert the country to credible threats (Table 72-1).

Additional federal resources that may be activated include the teams from the CDC. This is the main federal agency for disease prevention, and it controls activities and provides backup support to state and local health departments. Additional support is available from the American Red Cross, which provides many support systems and shelter as needed.

State and Local Agencies

Some state and local agencies may be branches of the same agencies already listed (eg, local CDC and FBI). Other state and local resources may include the American Red Cross, poison control centers, and other local volunteer organizations. The Metro Medical Response Teams Systems are local teams of health care providers that are located in cities considered possible terrorist targets and are funded for specialty response to WMD. Many state and federal task forces have been developed to assist in the development and improvement of civilian medical response to chemical and biologic terrorism.

Most cities and all states have an Office of Emergency Management (OEM) or Office of Emergency Services (OES). The OEM/OES coordinates the disaster relief efforts at the state and local levels. The OEM/OES is responsible for providing interagency coordination during an emergency. It maintains a corps of emergency management personnel, including a leader, responders, planners, and administrative and support staff.

The Incident Command System

The Incident Command System (ICS) is a federally mandated command structure that coordinates personnel, facilities, equipment, and communication in any emergency situation. The ICS is the center of operations for organization, planning, and transport of patients in the event of a specific local MCI. Successful incident management requires equip-

ment compatibility, effective communication, adequate distribution of resources, and clear differentiation of members' roles. The ICS ensures that any hazardous substances used during an MCI are identified promptly and that appropriate personal protection equipment is distributed. In addition to all of these responsibilities, the ICS is also responsible for determining when an MCI has ended.

The hospital incident command system (HICS) is a modification of the ICS that is used by both hospitals and law enforcement agencies. The HICS incident commander is the hospital emergency preparedness coordinator who oversees and coordinates all efforts surrounding the event. The HICS team includes a safety officer, public information officer, liaison officer, operations chief, logistics chief, planning chief, and finance chief. Each team member has a specific responsibility and communicates directly back to the incident commander (Dara, Ashton, Farmer, et al., 2005).

Hospital Emergency Preparedness Plans

Health care facilities are required by the Joint Commission to create a plan for emergency preparedness and to practice this plan at least twice a year (Joint Commission, 2006). Generally, these plans are developed by the facility's safety committee and are overseen by an administrative liaison.

Before the basic emergency operations plan (EOP) can be developed, the planning committee of the health care facility first evaluates characteristics of the community to identify the likely types of natural and man-made disasters that might occur. This hazard vulnerability analysis process is the responsibility of the local health care facility and its safety committee, safety officer, or emergency department (ED) manager. This information can be gathered by questioning local law enforcement, fire departments, and emergency medical systems and assessing the patterns of local train traffic, automobile traffic, and flood, earthquake, tornado, or hurricane activity. Consideration is also given to possible mass casualties that could arise because of the community's proximity to chemical plants, nuclear facilities, or military bases. Federal, judicial, or financial buildings, schools, and any places where large groups of people gather can be considered high-risk areas.

The emergency preparedness planning committee must have a realistic understanding of its resources. It must determine, for example, whether the facility has or needs a pharmaceutical stockpile available to treat specific chemical or biological agents (Hoyt & Selfridge-Thomas, 2007). Another scenario that might be anticipated may include the dispersal of a pulmonary intoxicant or choking agent, which would require that emergency operations planners determine how many ventilators are available within the facility and throughout the greater community. The committee might also outline how staff would triage and assign priority to patients when the number of ventilators is limited. Multiple factors influence a facility's ability to respond effectively to a sudden influx of injured patients, and the committee must anticipate various scenarios to improve its preparedness.

Components of the Emergency Operations Plan

The principles of emergency management must be a part of the EOP design and include a comprehensive plan for tackling all potential and actual hazards. The primary goal is protection of the community. The EOP should be integrated with local, state, and federal government plans and coordinated with the private sector and volunteers. It must be coordinated in advance to achieve a single common purpose, yet the plan must be flexible enough to adapt to any likely situation at hand. Predetermined organization is essential to minimize confusion, ensure that all key operations are directed, and promote a well-coordinated response. Essential components of the EOP include the following:

- An *activation response:* The EOP activation response of a health care facility defines where, how, and when the response is initiated.
- An *internal/external communication plan:* Communication is critical for all parties involved, including communication to and from the prehospital arena (Dara, et al., 2005).
- A *plan for coordinated patient care:* A response is planned for coordinated patient care into and out of the facility, including transfers to other facilities. The site of the disaster can determine where the greater number of patients may self-refer.
- *Security plans:* A coordinated security plan involving facility and community agencies is key to the control of an otherwise chaotic situation.
- *Identification of external resources:* External resources are identified, including local, state, and federal resources and information about how to activate these resources.
- A *plan for people management and traffic flow:* "People management" includes strategies to manage the patients, the public, the media, and personnel. Specific areas are assigned, and a designated person is delegated to manage each of these groups (Dara, et al., 2005).
- A *data management strategy:* A data management plan for every aspect of the disaster will save time at every step. A backup system for charting, tracking, and staffing is developed if the facility has a computer system.
- *Demobilization response:* Deactivation of the response is as important as activation; resources should not be unnecessarily exhausted. The person who decides when the facility resumes daily activities is clearly identified. Any possible residual effects of a disaster must be considered before this decision is made.
- An *after-action report or corrective plan:* Facilities often see increased volumes of patients 3 months or more after an incident. Postincident response must include a critique and a debriefing for all parties involved, immediately and again at a later date.
- A *plan for practice drills:* Practice drills that include community participation allow for troubleshooting any issues before a real-life incident occurs.
- *Anticipated resources:* Food and water must be available for staff, families, and others who may be at the facility for an extended period.
- *MCI planning:* MCI planning includes such issues as planning for mass fatalities and morgue readiness.
- An *education plan for all of the above:* A strong education plan for all personnel regarding each step of the plan allows for improved readiness and additional input for fine-tuning of the EOP (Dara, et al., 2005).

Initiating the Emergency Operations Plan

Notification of a disaster situation to a health care facility varies with each situation. Generally, the notification to the facility comes from outside sources unless the initial incident occurred at the facility. The disaster activation plan should clearly state how the EOP is to be initiated. If communication is functioning, field incident command will give notice of the approximate number of arriving patients, although the number of self-referring patients will not be known.

Identifying Patients and Documenting Patient Information

Patient tracking is a critical component of casualty management. Disaster tags, which are numbered and include triage priority, name, address, age, location and description of injuries, and treatments or medications given, are used to communicate patient information. The tag should be securely placed on the patient and remain with the patient at all times. The tag number and the patient's name, if known, are recorded in a disaster log. The log is used by the command center to track patients, assign beds, and provide families with information.

Triage

Triage is the sorting of patients to determine the priority of their health care needs and the proper site for treatment. In nondisaster situations, health care workers assign a high priority and allocate the most resources to those who are the most critically ill. For example, a young adult who has a chest injury and is in full cardiac arrest would receive advanced cardiopulmonary resuscitation, including medications, chest tubes, intravenous (IV) fluids, blood, and possibly emergency surgery in an effort to restore life. However, in a disaster, when health care providers are faced with a large number of casualties, the fundamental principle

Table 72-2	TRIAGE CATEGORIES DURING A MASS CASUALTY INCIDENT (MCI)			
Triage Category		**Priority**	**Color**	**Typical Conditions**
Immediate: Injuries are life-threatening but survivable with minimal intervention. Individuals in this group can progress rapidly to expectant if treatment is delayed.		1	Red	Sucking chest wound, airway obstruction secondary to mechanical cause, shock, hemothorax, tension pneumothorax, asphyxia, unstable chest and abdominal wounds, incomplete amputations, open fractures of long bones, and 2nd/3rd degree burns of 15%–40% total body surface area.
Delayed: Injuries are significant and require medical care, but can wait hours without threat to life or limb. Individuals in this group receive treatment only after immediate casualties are treated.		2	Yellow	Stable abdominal wounds without evidence of significant hemorrhage; soft tissue injuries; maxillofacial wounds without airway compromise; vascular injuries with adequate collateral circulation; genitourinary tract disruption; fractures requiring open reduction, débridement, and external fixation; most eye and CNS injuries.
Minimal: Injuries are minor and treatment can be delayed hours to days. Individuals in this group should be moved away from the main triage area.		3	Green	Upper extremity fractures, minor burns, sprains, small lacerations without significant bleeding, behavioral disorders or psychological disturbances.
Expectant: Injuries are extensive and chances of survival are unlikely even with definitive care. Persons in this group should be separated from other casualties, but not abandoned. Comfort measures should be provided when possible.		4	Black	Unresponsive patients with penetrating head wounds, high spinal cord injuries, wounds involving multiple anatomical sites and organs, 2nd/3rd degree burns in excess of 60% of body surface area, seizures or vomiting within 24 hours after radiation exposure, profound shock with multiple injuries, agonal respirations; no pulse, no blood pressure, pupils fixed and dilated.

guiding resource allocation is to do the greatest good for the greatest number of people. Decisions are based on the likelihood of survival and consumption of available resources. Therefore, this same patient, and others with conditions associated with a high mortality rate, would be assigned a low triage priority in a disaster situation, even if the person is conscious. Although this may sound uncaring, from an ethical standpoint the expenditure of limited resources on people with a low chance of survival, and denial of those resources to others with serious but treatable conditions, cannot be justified.

The triage officer rapidly assesses those injured at the disaster scene. Patients are immediately tagged and transported or given life-saving interventions. One person performs the initial triage while other emergency medical services (EMS) personnel perform life-saving measures (eg, intubation) and transport patients. Although EMS personnel carry out initial field triage, secondary and continuous triage at all subsequent levels of care is essential.

Staff should control all entrances to the acute care facility so that incoming patients are directed to the triage area first. The triage area may be outside the entry or just at the door of the ED. This facilitates the triage of all patients, including those arriving by medical transport and those who walk into the ED. Some patients who have already been seen in the field may be reclassified in the triage area, based on their current presentation.

Triage categories separate patients according to severity of injury. A special color-coded tagging system is used during an MCI so that the triage category is immediately obvious. There are several triage systems in use across the country, and every nurse should be aware of the system used by his or her facility and community. The North Atlantic Treaty Organization (NATO) triage system is one that is widely used. It consists of four colors—red, yellow,

green, and black. Each color signifies a different level of priority. Table 72-2 describes each category and gives examples of how different injuries would be classified. (See Chapter 71 for discussion of triage in non-MCI situations.)

Managing Internal Problems

Each facility must determine its supply lists based on its own needs assessment. The Red Cross has developed a basic survival/shelter resource kit. The EOP committee should determine the top 10 critical medications used during normal day-to-day operations and then anticipate which other medications may be required in a disaster or an MCI. For example, the health care facility might plan to have available a stockpile of antidotes (eg, cyanide kits) or antibiotics used in treating biologic agents. Information should be available about stocking or restocking any of the basic and special supplies, how those supplies are requested, and the time required to receive those supplies.

Communicating With the Media and Family

Communication is a key component of disaster management. Communication within the vast team of disaster responders is paramount; however, effective, informative communication with the media and worried family members is also crucial.

Managing Media Requests for Information

Although the media have an obligation to report the news and can play a significant positive role in communication, the number of reporters and newscasters and their support teams can be overwhelming, possibly compromising operations and patient confidentiality. A clearly defined process for managing media requests that includes a designated spokesperson, the public information officer, a site for the

Chart 72-2 • *Cultural Considerations*

Any disaster or mass casualty incident can be expected to involve members of diverse religious, ethnic, and cultural groups or may be targeted at and predominately affect a specific religious or ethnic group. Health care providers likewise include members of all religious, ethnic, and cultural backgrounds and should bear in mind that victims may have:
- Language difficulties that increase fears and frustrations
- Specific religious practices related to medical treatment, hygiene, or diet
- Specific places/times for prayer
- Rituals about handling the dead
- Timing of funeral services

Some religious communities have plans for emergencies and disasters, and local hospitals should integrate these plans to the extent possible into their emergency operations plans.

dissemination of information (away from patient care areas), and a regular schedule for providing updates should be part of the disaster plan.

The EOP helps prevent the release of contradictory or inaccurate information. Initial statements should focus on current efforts and what is being done to better understand the scope and impact of the situation. Information about casualties should not be released. Security staff should not allow media personnel access to patient care areas.

Caring for Families

Friends and family members converging on the scene must be cared for by the facility. The public information officer's role is to provide direction for the families and provide them with information as it becomes available. They may be feeling intense anxiety, shock, or grief and should be provided with information and updates about their loved ones as soon as possible and regularly thereafter. They should not be in the triage or treatment areas but in a designated area staffed by available social workers, counselors, therapists, or clergy. Access to this area should be controlled to prevent families from being disturbed. Chart 72-2 discusses cultural variables to consider when coping with disaster-related injuries and death.

The Nurse's Role in Disaster Response Plans

The role of the nurse during a disaster varies. Nurses may be asked to perform duties outside their areas of expertise and may take on responsibilities normally held by physicians or advanced practice nurses. For example, a critical care nurse may intubate a patient or even insert a chest tube. A nurse may perform wound débridement or suturing. A nurse may serve as the triage officer.

Although the exact role of a nurse in disaster management depends on the specific needs of the facility at the time, it should be clear which nurse or physician is in charge of a given patient care area and which procedures each individual nurse may or may not perform. Assistance can be obtained through the HICS, and nonmedical personnel can provide services where possible. For example, family members can provide nonskilled interventions for

their loved ones. Nurses should remember that nursing care in a disaster focuses on essential care from a perspective of what is best for all patients.

New settings and atypical roles for nurses arise during a disaster; for example, the nurse may provide shelter care in a temporary housing area or bereavement support and assistance with identification of deceased loved ones. People may require crisis intervention, or the nurse may participate in counseling other staff members and in Critical Incident Stress Management. Special care may be warranted for at-risk populations during a disaster (Chart 72-3).

Considering Ethical Conflicts

Disasters can present a disparity between the resources of the health care agency and the needs of the victims. This generates ethical dilemmas for nurses and other health care providers. Issues include conflicts related to the following:
- Rationing care
- Futile therapy
- Consent
- Duty
- Confidentiality
- Resuscitation
- Assisted suicide

Nurses may find it difficult to not provide care to the dying or to withhold information to avoid spreading fear and panic. Clinical scenarios that are unimaginable in normal circumstances confront the nurse in extreme instances. Other ethical dilemmas may arise out of health care providers' instincts for self-protection and protection of their families. For example, what should a pregnant nurse do when incoming disaster victims have been exposed to radiation yet too few nurses are available?

Nurses can plan for the ethical dilemmas they will face during disasters by establishing a framework for evaluating

Chart 72-3 • *Caring for People With Disabilities During a Disaster*

When a disaster occurs, the multiple agencies involved attempt to provide food, water, and shelter to all those affected. People with disabilities have specific needs that require attention. It is recommended that people with disabilities have a personal support network to check on them after a disaster and to provide needed assistance. They should also have a back-up system and an evacuation plan. Agencies need to be aware that service animals are also affected during a disaster and may be brought to shelters with their companions.

Evacuation assistance is imperative for people with disabilities. Directions to personal equipment (eg, communication aids, medications, oxygen) should be available to rescue personnel. In a rapid evacuation, mobility devices, oxygen, suction, and medications will be needed at the shelters. Special efforts to keep those with vision or hearing impairment informed should be implemented. People skilled in sign language are also valuable resources during a disaster. On its Web site, the American Red Cross provides a handbook for disaster preparedness for people with disabilities: www.redcross.org/services/disaster/ beprepared/ disability/html

ethical questions before they arise and by identifying and exploring possible responses to difficult clinical situations. They can consider how the fundamental ethical principles of utilitarianism, beneficence, and justice will influence their decisions and care in disaster response (see Chapter 3).

Managing Behavioral Issues

Although most people pull together and function well during a disaster, both people and communities suffer immediate and sometimes long-term psychological trauma. Common responses to disaster include the following:

- Depression
- Anxiety
- Somatization (fatigue, general malaise, headaches, gastrointestinal disturbances, skin rashes)
- Posttraumatic stress disorder (PTSD)
- Substance abuse
- Interpersonal conflicts
- Impaired performance

Factors that influence a person's response to disaster include the degree and nature of the exposure to the disaster, loss of friends and loved ones, existing coping strategies, available resources and support, and the personal meaning attached to the event. Other factors, such as loss of home and valued possessions, extended exposure to danger, and exposure to toxic contamination, also influence response and increase the risk of adjustment problems. Those exposed to the dead and injured, those endangered by the event, the elderly, children, emergency first responders, and health care personnel caring for victims are considered to be at higher risk for emotional sequelae.

Nurses can assist disaster victims through active listening and providing emotional support, giving information, and referring patients to therapists or social workers. Health care workers must refer people to mental health care services because experience has shown that few disaster victims seek these services, and early intervention minimizes psychological consequences. Nurses can also discourage victims from subjecting themselves to repeated exposure to the event through media replays and news articles, and encourage them to return to normal activities and social roles when appropriate.

Critical Incident Stress Management

Critical Incident Stress Management (CISM) is an approach to preventing and treating the emotional trauma that can affect emergency responders as a consequence of their jobs and that can also occur to anyone involved in a disaster or MCI. CISM is handled by its own teams, which are available to the OEM. There are 350 such teams in the United States. All branches of emergency services have CISM teams, as do the military and many industries (eg, airline industry).

Components of a management plan include education before an incident occurs about critical incident stress and coping strategies; field support (ensuring that staff get adequate rest, food, and fluids, and rotating work loads) during an incident; and defusings, debriefings, demobilization, and follow-up care after the incident.

Defusing is a process by which the person receives education about recognition of stress reactions and management strategies for handling stress. Debriefing is a more complicated intervention; it involves a 2- to 3-hour process during which participants are asked about their emotional reactions to the incident, what symptoms they may be experiencing (eg, flashbacks, difficulty sleeping, intrusive thoughts), and other psychological ramifications. In follow-up, members of the CISM team contact the participants of a debriefing and schedule a follow-up meeting if necessary. People with ongoing stress reactions are referred to mental health specialists.

Preparedness and Response

Recognition and Awareness

Preparedness for terrorism and other disasters includes awareness of the potential for covert use of WMD, self-protection, and early detection, containment, or decontamination of substances and agents that may affect others by secondary exposure. The strength of many toxins, mobility of many members of society, and long incubation periods for some organisms and diseases can result in an epidemic that can quickly and silently spread across the entire country. For example, a formerly healthy person with a rapid onset of flulike symptoms can have an ominous illness, such as anthrax or severe acute respiratory syndrome (SARS), both of which are discussed in more detail later in the chapter.

Nurses should have a heightened awareness of trends that may suggest deliberate dispersal of toxic or infectious agents, including the following:

- An unusual increase in the number of people seeking care for fever, respiratory, or gastrointestinal symptoms
- Clusters of patients who present with the same unusual illness from a single location. For example, clusters can be from a specific geographic location, such as a city, or from a single sporting or entertainment event.
- A large number of rapidly fatal cases, especially when death occurs within 72 hours after hospital admission.
- Any increase in disease incidence in a normally healthy population. These cases should be reported to the state health department and to the CDC.

If any of these trends are noted, an extensive patient history is taken in an attempt to identify the possible agent involved. This history includes an occupational, work, and environmental assessment, in addition to the regular admission history. An exposure history contains, at a minimum, information about current and past exposures to possible hazards and an assessment of the patient's typical day and any deviations in routines. The work history includes, at a minimum, a description of all previous jobs, including short-term, seasonal, and part-time employment and any military service. The environmental history includes assessment of present and previous home locations, water supply, and any hobbies, to name a few factors. The admission history should include such information as recent travel and contact with others who have been ill or have recently died of a fatal illness. This is just a brief review of the extensive history that may need to be obtained to identify an exposure agent (Agency for Toxic Substances and Disease Registry, 2009).

Suspicions or findings are reported to the appropriate resources in the facility and to proper authorities in the community. Resources can include the infection control department, **material safety data sheets (MSDS)** or the Chemtrac database, the state health department, the CDC, the local poison control center, and many Internet sites (Dara, et al., 2005). Reporting furnishes data elements to those agencies responsible for epidemiology and response. Reporting also allows for sharing of information among facilities and jurisdictions and can help determine the source of infections or exposure and prevent further exposures and even deaths.

Personal Protective Equipment

Another component of preparedness and response involves the protection of the health care provider by additional **personal protective equipment (PPE).** Chemical or biologic agents and radiation are silent killers and are generally colorless and odorless. The purpose of PPE is to shield health care workers from the chemical, physical, biologic, and radiologic hazards that may exist when caring for contaminated patients. The U.S. Environmental Protection Agency (EPA) has divided protective clothing and respiratory protection into the following four categories, levels A through D:

- Level A protection is worn when the highest level of respiratory, skin, eye, and mucous membrane protection is required. This includes a self-contained breathing apparatus (SCBA) and a fully encapsulating, vapor-tight, chemical-resistant suit with chemical-resistant gloves and boots.
- Level B protection requires the highest level of respiratory protection but a lesser level of skin and eye protection than with level A situations. This level of protection includes the SCBA and a chemical-resistant suit, but the suit is not vapor tight (Hoyt & Selfridge-Thomas, 2007).
- Level C protection requires the air-purified respirator, which uses filters or sorbent materials to remove harmful substances from the air. A chemical-resistant coverall with splash hood, chemical-resistant gloves, and boots are included in level C protection.
- Level D protection is the typical work uniform.

Levels C and D PPE are the levels most often used in hospital facilities (Hoyt & Selfridge-Thomas, 2007).

Protective equipment must be donned before contact with a contaminated patient. The acute care facility's standard precaution PPE (level D) generally is not adequate for protection from a chemically, biologically, or radiologically contaminated patient. Level C PPE is adequate for the average patient exposure. The health care provider must use equipment that is capable of providing protection against the agent involved. This may mean using a splash suit along with a full-face positive-pressure or negative-pressure respirator (a filter-type gas mask) or even an SCBA for medical personnel in the field.

No single PPE is capable of protecting against all hazards. Under no circumstances should responders wear any PPE without proper training, practice, and fit testing of respirator masks as necessary.

Decontamination

Decontamination, the process of removing accumulated contaminants, is critical to the health and safety of health care providers by preventing secondary contamination. The decontamination plan should establish procedures and educate employees about decontamination procedures, identify the equipment needed and methods to be used, and establish methods for disposal of contaminated materials (Dara, et al., 2005).

Although many principles and theories surround decontamination of a patient, authorities agree that, to be effective, decontamination must include a minimum of two steps. The first step is removal of the patient's clothing and jewelry and then rinsing the patient with water. Depending on the type of exposure, this step alone can remove a large amount of the contamination and decrease secondary contamination. The second step consists of a thorough soap-and-water wash and rinse. When patients arrive at the facility after being assessed and treated by a prehospital provider, it should not be assumed that they have been thoroughly decontaminated. The hospital must be prepared to perform additional decontamination prior to entry into the facility. The hospital personnel may also treat "walking wounded" who did not receive any decontamination at the scene.

Natural Disasters

Natural disasters may result in mass casualties. Natural disasters can occur anywhere at any time and include events such as tornadoes, hurricanes, floods, avalanches, tidal waves (eg, tsunamis), earthquakes, and volcanic eruptions. In the event of a natural disaster, loss of communications, potable water, and electricity is usually the greatest obstacle to a well-coordinated emergency response, and preparatory planning is essential. Even wireless technology (eg, cellular phones, computers, other communication devices) may not be functional.

The majority of the immediate casualties are trauma related. These mass casualties tax the trauma system to its limits to provide triage, transport of patients (in poor weather and road conditions), and management within the trauma centers. The majority of patients usually begin arriving within an hour of the event. However, the "walking wounded" may not seek care for 5 days to 2 weeks after the event or may seek care for injuries received during clean-up activities. Casualties arrive at hospitals in three waves. The first wave consists of minimally (generally) injured people who arrive of their own accord. The second wave consists of severely injured patients. The third wave consists of injured patients who arrive after they are discovered by rescuers. For example, in the event of earthquakes, buildings collapse and cause the majority of fatalities from injuries that primarily involve the head and chest (Kano, 2005). The majority of the patients usually begin arriving within an hour of the event; the "walking wounded" may not seek care for 5 days to 2 weeks after the event or may seek care for injuries inflicted during the clean-up activities.

Excessive exposure to the natural elements and the need for food and water (by both patients and emergency responders) are critical issues. Without cover (eg, buildings may be unsafe or destroyed) or potable water (eg, water may be either contaminated or unavailable), injuries from exposure to heat, cold, or contaminated food or water can occur. Safety equipment that protects rescue workers from injury, exposure, and potentially dangerous animals (eg, snakes, alligators, spiders) must be readily available. Rescue workers may also injure themselves in the process of extrication or cleanup (eg, chain saws, building collapse). Hypothermia can occur rapidly in workers who are exposed to water at temperatures of 23.9°C (75°F) or less. As is true during all disasters, mental health workers and shelters are needed throughout the community. Veterinary assistance is also essential because pets are frequently abandoned and injured. In addition, emergency response workers must be prepared to treat the most common ailments experienced after exposure to a specific natural disaster. For instance, pulmonary problems peak with earthquakes and volcanic eruptions because of the increased particulate matter in the air. Most volcano-related deaths are from suffocation. After floods or water disasters, waterborne transmission of agents such as *Escherichia coli,* salmonella, shigella, typhoid, leptospirosis, malaria, and tularemia are common and cause widespread disease. In addition, other waterborne hazards can include human exposure to poisonous snakes and alligators in the flood waters.

In some instances, early warning systems have assisted in decreasing the number of deaths from tornadoes and hurricanes. However, even with the advent of early warning systems, some people are unable or unwilling to leave prior to the occurrence of the natural disaster. When buildings collapse, rapid response to identify and remove trapped victims is the only means of improving survivability. There is a direct relationship between time trapped and survival; fewer than 50 percent of people survive if they are trapped more than 2 to 6 hours. Water-damaged buildings are not safe and require extensive examination before experts can ensure safe occupancy. Larger-scale issues that can cause significant later morbidity and mortality include the absence of water purification, waste removal, removal of human and animal remains, and vector control. Removal or disposal of biologic, chemical, and nuclear agents must also be considered.

Weapons of Terror

Although biologic, chemical, and radiologic events are not everyday events, they can occur at any facility, and every nurse needs to know the basics of caring for affected patients. An explosion may spread the dangerous material. Therefore, treatment of blast injuries must be anticipated and planned.

Blast Injury

Examples of recent highly publicized bombings that have caused significant injuries or loss of lives include those in a disco in Tel Aviv in 2001, in the London subway system in 2005, and on the Mumbai (India) commuter trains in 2006. Terrorist bombings occur frequently throughout the Middle East today, particularly in Iraq and Afghanistan. Several types of bombs are typically used, resulting in various injuries.

Types of Explosive Devices

Commonly used bombs include pipe bombs, Molotov cocktails, fertilizer bombs, and "dirty" bombs (so-called because they spread radiation). The most commonly utilized bomb is the pipe bomb, which consists of relatively low-velocity explosives and may also contain nails or other implements that cause more damage when the explosive ignites. Another type of commonly used explosive device is the Molotov cocktail, which uses a common flammable liquid such as gasoline in a glass bottle and a source of ignition, such as a rag. This forms a simple yet effective incendiary device. Other common explosive devices include fertilizer bombs, which were used in the Oklahoma City bombing in 1995, and dirty bombs, which include a radioactive source that spreads radiation after the initial blast. Common hazards following a bombing include secondary devices (set to explode at a predetermined time, typically after the arrival of rescue personnel), building collapse, contamination from biological, chemical, or radiological weapons, and the presence of terrorists among the patients and bystanders. The entire scene of the bombing is a crime scene and is treated as such. Triage of patients involved in a bombing is the same as for all disasters, with a heightened awareness that serious internal injuries from the blast wave may not be evident.

Physical Injuries

The actual blast that occurs during the initial seconds of the bombing causes a pressure wave or primary blast wave. Injuries can result from the impact of the explosion, the primary blast wave, or shrapnel within the bomb. The majority of injuries are caused by the primary blast wave (CDC, 2006). A blast wave has four effects. These include spalling, which refers to the pressure wave; implosion, which refers to rupture of organs from entrapped gases; shearing, which refers to the blast response of different body tissues dependent on their density; and irreversible work, which refers to the presence of forces that exceed the tensile strength of an organ or tissue.

Different phases of the blast may result in common injuries that include blast lung, tympanic membrane rupture, and head and abdominal injuries (Table 72-3). Although approximately 50% to 70% of deaths result from head injuries, the majority of head injuries are not life-threatening (CDC, 2006). Bombings that occur in enclosed spaces amplify the blast wave, resulting in more pressure wave injuries. Distance from the blast, whether the blast space was enclosed, composition of the explosive, whether a building collapsed, and the efficiency of medical resources available after the blast all affect patient outcomes after a blast injury.

Blast Lung

Blast lung results from the blast wave as it passes through air-filled lungs. The result is hemorrhage and tearing of the lung, ventilation-perfusion mismatch, and possible air emboli. Typical signs and symptoms include dyspnea, hypoxia, tachypnea or apnea (depending on severity), cough, chest pain, and hemodynamic instability. Management involves providing respiratory support that includes administration of supplemental oxygen, but may also require intubation and mechanical ventilation. If a hemothorax or pneumothorax is present, a chest tube must be inserted to re-expand the lung. In the event of an air embolus, the patient should be immediately placed in the prone left lateral position to

Table 72-3 PHASES OF BLASTS AND ASSOCIATED COMMON INJURIES	
Phase of Blast Injury	**Common Injuries**
Primary: results from pressure wave	Pulmonary barotraumas, including pulmonary contusions Head injuries, including concussion, other severe brain injuries Tympanic membrane rupture, middle ear injury Abdominal hollow organ perforation, hemorrhage
Secondary: results from debris or shrapnel within the bomb or from the scene	Penetrating trunk, skin, and soft tissue injuries Fractures, traumatic amputations
Tertiary: results from pressure wave that causes the victim to be thrown, resulting in traumatic injury	Head injuries Fractures, including skull
Quaternary: results from preexisting conditions exacerbated by the force of the blast or by postblast injury complications	Severe injuries with complex injury patterns: burns, crush injuries, head injuries Common preexisting conditions that become exacerbated: COPD, asthma, cardiac conditions, diabetes, and hypertension
Quinary: thought to result from a hyperinflammatory state commonly seen in bystanders near to the blast and due to toxic substances or uncommon explosives	Hyperpyrexia Diaphoresis

COPD, chronic obstructive pulmonary disease
Kluger, Y., Nimrod, A., Biderman, P., et al. (2006). The quinary pattern of blast injury. *Journal of Emergency Management*, 4(1), 51–55.

prevent migration of the embolus and will require emergent treatment in a hyperbaric chamber. Complications following blast lung can include respiratory failure as well as acute respiratory distress syndrome (ARDS) (see Chapter 23 for further discussion).

Tympanic Membrane Rupture

The tympanic membrane (TM) is the most frequent injury after subjection to a pressure wave because it is the body's most sensitive organ to pressure. There is an increased incidence of TM rupture when a blast occurs in close proximity to the patient and when it occurs in an enclosed space. Signs and symptoms include hearing loss, tinnitus, pain, dizziness, and otorrhea. The majority of TM ruptures heal spontaneously. Approximately 5% of patients with TM rupture from a blast will require hearing aids, whereas the majority will suffer only mild high-frequency hearing loss (Ritenour, Wickley, Ritenour, et al., 2008). Other ear injuries may include ossicular disruption and impaction of foreign bodies.

Abdominal and Head Injuries

Blast abdomen may be evidenced by abdominal hemorrhage and internal organ injury. The typical signs and symptoms of internal abdominal injury can include pain, guarding, rebound tenderness, rectal bleeding, nausea, and vomiting (see Chapter 71 for further discussion of abdominal trauma) (CDC, 2006).

Head injuries are typically minor but those that are severe result in the majority of postblast deaths. These injuries can occur without a direct blow to the head and may result from the blast itself, building collapse, or flying debris. Concussions commonly occur postblast and the usual follow-up evaluation and treatment for postconcussive syndrome is indicated (see Chapter 62 for further discussion of head injuries) (CDC, 2006).

Special Populations

Special populations may have different blast-associated risks. For instance, the elderly are particularly susceptible to bone fractures because they tend to have decreased bone density. They also tend to have more preexisting morbid conditions that may be exacerbated by the explosion. Pregnant patients' abdomens are particularly susceptible to placental shear forces that may result in abruptio placentae. People with mobility disabilities may have difficulty extricating themselves from the site of the blast (CDC, 2006).

Biologic Weapons

Biologic weapons are weapons that spread disease among the general population or the military.

Effects of Biologic Weapons

Biologic warfare is a covert method of effecting terrorist objectives. Biologic weapons are easily obtained and easily disseminated and can result in significant mortality and morbidity. The potential use of biologic agents calls for continuous increased surveillance by health departments and an increased index of suspicion by clinicians. Many biologic weapons result in signs and symptoms similar to those of common disease processes. Appropriate management of a biologic threat includes rapid recognition of the potential agent; use of proper PPE; decontamination, isolation or quarantine of infected patients when appropriate; and the administration of appropriate vaccinations, antidotes, or medications to people at risk.

Biologic agents are delivered in either a liquid or dry state, applied to foods or water, or vaporized for inhalation or direct contact. Vaporization may be accomplished through spray or explosives loaded with the agent. Because of increases in business and pleasure travel by people in industrialized nations, an agent could be released in one city and affect people in other cities thousands of miles away. The vector can be an insect, animal, or person, or there may be direct contact with the agent itself.

The following is a discussion of two of the agents most likely to be used or weaponized. Table 72-4 describes other easily weaponized biologic agents.

Table 72-4	**EXAMPLES OF BIOLOGIC AGENTS THAT CAN BE USED AS WEAPONS**			
Agent/Organism	**Contagion**	**Decontamination and Protective Equipment**	**Signs and Symptoms**	**Treatment (Mortality Rate)**
Tularemia— *Francisella tularensis*: gram-negative coccobacillus, one of the most infectious bacteria known	Direct contact with infected animals or aerosolized as a bioterror weapon; bites Not contagious through human-to-human contact	Standard barrier precautions Clothing and linens should be laundered under the usual hospital protocol	*Initial:* Abrupt onset of fever, fatigue, chills, headache, lower backache, malaise, rigor, coryza, dry cough, and sore throat without adenopathy. Nausea and vomiting or diarrhea possible. *As disease progresses:* Sweating, fever, progressive weakness, anorexia, and weight loss demonstrate continued illness. *Mortality secondary to:* pneumonitis (if inhalation is the source) with copious watery or purulent sputum, hemoptysis, respiratory insufficiency, sepsis, and shock.	Streptomycin or gentamicin/aminoglycoside for 10–14 days. Inhalation tularemia must be treated within 48 hours of onset. In mass casualty situations, doxycycline or ciprofloxacin is recommended. For persons exposed to tularemia, tetracycline or doxycycline is recommended for 14 days. (Mortality rate = 2%)
Botulism— Clostridium botulinum: Botulinum blocks acetylcholine-containing vesicles from fusing with the terminal membranes of the motor-neuron endplate, resulting in a flaccid paralysis.	Direct contact Not contagious through human-to-human contact	Any skin exposure to the botulism toxin can be treated with soap and water or a 0.1% hypochlorite solution Standard precautions are used when treating patients with botulism	*Gastrointestinal botulism:* abdominal cramps, nausea, vomiting, and diarrhea. *Inhalation botulism:* fever; symmetric descending flaccid paralysis with multiple cranial nerve palsies. Classic signs and symptoms include diplopia, dysphagia, dry mouth, lack of fever, and alert mental status. Other possible symptoms include ptosis of the eyelids, blurred vision, enlarged sluggish pupils, dysarthria, and dysphonia. *Mortality secondary to:* airway obstruction and inadequate tidal volume.	Supportive ventilatory therapy is necessary if respiratory infection occurs. Aminoglycosides and clindamycin are contraindicated because they exacerbate neuromuscular blockage. Equine antitoxin is used to minimize subsequent nerve damage. There is a 2% rate of anaphylaxis to the antitoxin; therefore, diphenhydramine (Benadryl) and epinephrine must be immediately available for use. Supportive care—mechanical ventilation, nutrition, fluids, prevention of complications (Mortality rate = 5%)
Plague—*Yersinia pestis:* nonsporulating gram-negative coccobacillus. The bacterium causes destruction and necrosis of the lymph nodes.	Contagious *Bubonic plague:* transmitted through flea bites with no person-to-person transmission *Pneumonic plague:* transmitted through respiratory droplet contact	Isolation barrier precautions with full face respirators; the patient should wear a mask Rooms should receive a terminal cleaning Clothing and linens with body fluids on them should be cleaned with the usual disinfectant Routine precautions should be used in the case of death	*Bubonic plague:* Sudden fever and chills, weakness, a swollen and tender lymph node (bubo) in the groin, axilla, or cervical area. The resultant bacteremia progresses to septicemia from the endotoxin and, finally, shock and death. *Primary septicemic plague:* Disseminated intravascular coagulation (DIC), necrosis of small vessels, purpura, and gangrene of the digits and nose (black death). *Pneumonic plague:* Severe bronchospasm, chest pain, dyspnea, cough, and hemoptysis. There is a 100% mortality associated with pneumonic plague if not treated within the first 24 hours.	Streptomycin or gentamicin for 10–14 days. Tetracycline or doxycycline is an acceptable alternative if an aminoglycoside cannot be given. People with close contact exposure (<2 m) require prophylaxis with doxycycline for 7 days. (Mortality rate = 50%)

Types of Biologic Agents

Anthrax

Anthrax is recognized as the most likely weaponized biologic agent available and has been recognized as a highly debilitating agent for centuries. *Bacillus anthracis* is a naturally occurring gram-positive, encapsulated rod that lives in the soil in the spore state throughout the world. The bacterium sporulates (ie, is liberated) when exposed to air and is infective only in the spore form. Contact with infected animal products (raw meat) or inhalation of the spores results in infection. Cattle and other herbivores are vaccinated against anthrax to prevent transmission through contaminated meat.

It is believed that approximately 8000 to 50,000 spores must be inhaled to put a person at risk (Tasota, Henker & Hoffman, 2002). As an aerosol, anthrax is odorless and invisible and can travel a great distance before disseminating;

hence, the site of release and the site of infection can be miles apart.

Clinical Manifestations. Anthrax is caused by replicating bacteria that release toxin, resulting in hemorrhage, edema, and necrosis. The incubation period is 1 to 6 days. There are three primary methods of infection: skin contact, inhalation, and gastrointestinal ingestion. Skin lesions (the most common infection) cause edema with pruritus and macule or papule formation, resulting in ulceration with 1- to 3-mm vesicles. A painless eschar develops, which falls off in 1 to 2 weeks.

Ingestion of anthrax results in fever, nausea and vomiting, abdominal pain, bloody diarrhea, and occasionally ascites. If severe diarrhea develops, decreased intravascular volume becomes the primary treatment concern. The bacterium targets the terminal ileum and cecum. Sepsis can occur.

Inhaling anthrax results in the most severe clinical manifestations. Its symptoms mimic those of the flu, and usually treatment is sought only when the second stage of severe respiratory distress occurs. Current antibiotic therapy does not halt the progress of the disease. Inhaled anthrax can incubate for up to 60 days, making it difficult to identify its source. Initial signs and symptoms include cough, headache, fever, vomiting, chills, weakness, mild chest discomfort, dyspnea, and syncope, without rhinorrhea or nasal congestion. Most patients have a brief recovery period followed by the second stage within 1 to 3 days, characterized by fever, severe respiratory distress, stridor, hypoxia, cyanosis, diaphoresis, hypotension, and shock. These patients require optimization of oxygenation, correction of electrolyte imbalances, and ventilatory and hemodynamic support. More than 50% of these patients have hemorrhagic mediastinitis on a chest x-ray (a hallmark sign) (Auerbach, 2007). The disease can also progress to include meningitis with subarachnoid hemorrhage. Death results approximately 24 to 36 hours after the onset of severe respiratory distress. The mortality rate approaches 100%.

Treatment. At present, anthrax is penicillin sensitive; however, strains of penicillin-resistant anthrax are thought to exist. Recommended treatment includes penicillin (Penicillin V), erythromycin (E-mycin, Erythrocin), gentamicin (Garamycin), or doxycycline (Vibramycin). If antibiotic treatment begins within 24 hours after exposure, death can be prevented. In a mass casualty situation, treatment with ciprofloxacin (Cipro) or doxycycline is recommended. Treatment is continued for 60 days. For patients who have been directly exposed to anthrax but have no signs and symptoms of disease, ciprofloxacin or doxycycline is used for prophylaxis for 60 days.

Standard precautions are the only ones indicated to protect the caregiver exposed to a patient infected with anthrax. The patient is not contagious, and the disease cannot spread from person to person. Equipment should be cleaned using standard hospital disinfectant. After death, cremation is recommended because the spores can survive for decades and represent a threat to morticians and forensic medicine personnel.

There is a vaccine for anthrax that has been used in the military; however, it is not yet widely used because it requires multiple time-interval–sensitive boosters and has up to a 48% systemic reaction rate. The federal government is investigating the potential for development of a community-wide vaccine that has fewer side effects and that requires fewer boosters.

Smallpox

Smallpox (variola) is classified as a DNA virus. It has an incubation period of approximately 12 days. It is extremely contagious and is spread by direct contact, by contact with clothing or linens, or by droplets from person to person only after the fever has decreased and the rash phase has begun (Karwa, Currie & Kvetan, 2005). There is an associated 30% case-fatality rate (ie, the likelihood of fatality per case diagnosed). Aerosolization of the virus would result in widespread dissemination.

The World Health Organization declared smallpox eradicated in 1977 and stopped worldwide vaccination in 1980. In the United States, the last child was vaccinated in 1972. Therefore, a large portion of the current population has no immunity to the virus. A smallpox vaccination plan introduced in 2003 proposed that a designated number of ED staff receive the first vaccinations to ensure that ED staff would be immunized in the event of a smallpox outbreak. The government estimated that 0.1% of those people receiving the vaccine would have serious side effects. Of these, approximately 4% would have life-threatening complications, and 0.1% would die. Plans for any type of select or mass vaccinations for smallpox are not under current consideration, given the risks associated with vaccination.

Clinical Manifestations. Signs and symptoms of smallpox infection include high fever, malaise, headache, backache, and prostration. After 1 to 2 days, a maculopapular rash appears, evolving at the same rate, beginning on the face, mouth, pharynx, and forearms (Fig. 72-1). Only then does the rash progress to the trunk and also become vesicular to pustular (Hoyt & Selfridge-Thomas, 2007). There is a large amount of the virus in the saliva and pustules. Smallpox is contagious only after the appearance of the rash. There are two forms of smallpox, variola major and variola minor. Variola major is more common, results in a higher fever and more extensive rash, and has a 30% case-fatality rate. Hemorrhagic smallpox, a subtype of variola major, includes all of the above signs and symptoms plus a dusky erythema and petechiae leading to frank hemorrhage of the skin and mucous membranes, and it results in death by day 5 or 6.

Treatment. Treatment includes supportive care with antibiotics for any additional infection. The patient must be isolated with the use of transmission precautions. Laundry and biologic wastes should be autoclaved before being washed with hot water and bleach. Standard decontamination of the room is effective. All people who have household or face-to-face contact with the patient after the fever begins should be vaccinated within 4 days to prevent infection and death. A patient with a temperature of 38°C (101°F) or higher within 17 days after exposure must be placed in isolation. Cremation is preferred for all deaths because the virus can survive in scabs for up to 13 years.

Severe Acute Respiratory Syndrome

Not all mass casualty biologic events are terrorist based. The SARS outbreak in 2003 is a prime example of a

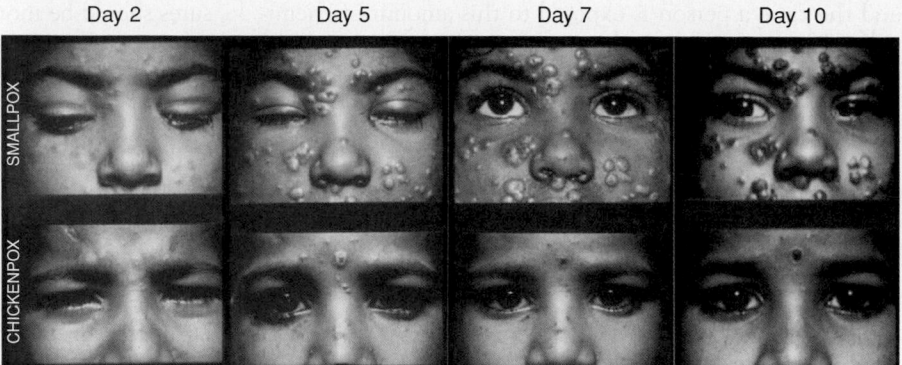

Figure 72-1 Comparison of progression of smallpox rash and chicken pox rash. From World Health Organization. (2001). WHO slide set on the diagnosis of smallpox. Reproduced by permission of the World Health Organization. Available at: www.who.int/emc/diseases/smallpox/slideset/index.htm

non–terrorist-based mass casualty biologic event. The disease started as "atypical" pneumonia in China in February and spread to 29 countries throughout the world by July. Air travel and worldwide trade have increased the possibility that any contagious disease may spread rapidly.

SARS is caused by a virus, officially named SARS-CoV. Its incubation period is 2 to 10 days. People at risk include health care workers who have had unprotected exposure to SARS-CoV. See Chapter 23 for further discussion of SARS.

Chemical Weapons

Agents that may be used in **chemical warfare** or for terrorist purposes are overt agents in that the effects are more apparent and occur more quickly than those caused by biologic weapons Refer to Table 72-5 for an overview of common chemical agents.

Characteristics of Chemicals

Volatility

Volatility is the tendency for a chemical to become a vapor. The most common volatile agents are phosgene and cyanide. Most chemicals are heavier than air, except for hydrogen cyanide. Therefore, in the presence of most chemicals, people should stand up to avoid heavy exposure (because the chemical will sink toward the floor or ground).

Persistence

Persistence means that the chemical is less likely to vaporize and disperse. More volatile chemicals do not evaporate very quickly. Most industrial chemicals (eg, cyanide) are not very persistent. Weaponized agents (chemicals developed as weapons by the military or terrorists [eg, mustard gas]) are more likely than industrial chemicals to penetrate skin and mucous membranes and also cause secondary exposure.

Toxicity

Toxicity is the potential of an agent to cause injury to the body. The median lethal dose (LD_{50}) is the amount of the chemical that will cause death in 50% of those who are exposed. The median effective dose (ED_{50}) is the amount of the chemical that will cause signs and symptoms in 50% of those who are exposed. The concentration time (CT) is the concentration released multiplied by the time exposed (mg/min). For example, if 1000 mg of a chemical is released

Agent	Action	Signs and Symptoms	Decontamination and Treatment
TABLE 72-5	**COMMON CHEMICAL AGENTS**		
Nerve Agents Sarin Soman organophosphates	Inhibition of cholinesterase	Increased secretions, gastrointestinal motility, diarrhea, bronchospasm.	Soap and water Supportive care Benzodiazepine Pralidoxime Atropine
Blood Agent Cyanide	Inhibition of aerobic metabolism	Inhalation—tachypnea, tachycardia, coma, seizures. Can progress to respiratory arrest, respiratory failure, cardiac arrest, death.	Sodium nitrite Sodium thiocyanate Amyl nitrate Hydroxocobalamin
Vesicant Agents Lewisite Sulfur mustard Nitrogen mustard Phosgene	Blistering agents	Superficial to partial-thickness burn with vesicles that coalesce.	Soap and water Blot; do not rub dry
Pulmonary Agents Phosgene Chlorine	Separation of alveoli from capillary bed	Pulmonary edema, bronchospasm.	Airway management Ventilatory support Bronchoscopy

and the time a person is exposed to this amount of chemical is 10 minutes, then the concentration time would be 10,000 mg/min.

Latency

Latency is the time from absorption to the appearance of signs and symptoms. Sulfur mustards and pulmonary agents have the longest latency, whereas other vesicants, nerve agents, and cyanide produce signs and symptoms within seconds.

Limiting Exposure

Evacuation is essential, as is removal of the person's clothing and decontamination as close to the scene as possible and before transport of the exposed person. Soap and water are effective means of decontamination in most cases. Staff involved in decontamination efforts must wear PPE and contain and dispose of the runoff after decontamination procedures.

Types of Chemicals

Vesicants

Vesicants are chemicals that cause blistering and result in burning, conjunctivitis, bronchitis, pneumonia, hematopoietic suppression, and death. Examples of vesicants include lewisite, phosgene, nitrogen mustard, and sulfur mustard. In World War I and in the Iran–Iraq conflict of 1980 to 1988, vesicants were used to disable opponents. Vesicants were the primary incapacitating agents, resulting in minimal (less than 5%) death but large numbers of injuries (Dara, et al., 2005). Liquid sulfur mustard was the most frequently used vesicant in these conflicts.

Clinical Manifestations. The initial presentation after exposure to a vesicant is similar to that of a large superficial to partial-thickness burn in the warm and moist areas of the body (ie, perineum, axillae, antecubital spaces). There is stinging and erythema for approximately 24 hours, followed by pruritus, painful burning, and small vesicle formation after 2 to 18 hours. These vesicles can coalesce into large, fluid-filled bullae. Lewisite and phosgene result in immediate pain after exposure. Tissue damage occurs within minutes.

If the eye is exposed, there is pain, photophobia, lacrimation, and decreased vision. This progresses to conjunctivitis, blepharospasm, corneal ulcer, and corneal edema.

Respiratory effects are more serious and often are the cause of mortality with vesicant exposure. Purulent fibrinous pseudomembrane discharge may cause obstruction of the airways. Gastrointestinal exposure may cause nausea and vomiting, leukopenia, and upper gastrointestinal bleeding.

Treatment. Appropriate decontamination includes soap and water. Scrubbing and the use of hypochlorite solutions should be avoided because they increase penetration. Once the substance has penetrated, it cannot be removed. Eye exposure requires copious irrigation. For respiratory exposure, intubation and bronchoscopy to remove necrotic tissue are essential. With lewisite exposure, dimercaprol (BAL in oil) is administered intravenously for systemic toxicity and topically for skin lesions. All persons with sulfur mustard expo-

sures should be monitored for 24 hours for delayed (latent) effects.

Nerve Agents

The most toxic agents in existence are the nerve agents such as sarin, soman, tabun, VX, and organophosphates (pesticides). They are inexpensive, effective in small quantities, and easily dispersed. In the liquid form, nerve agents evaporate into a colorless, odorless vapor. Organophosphates are similar in nature to the nerve agents used in warfare and are readily available. Nerve agents can be inhaled or absorbed percutaneously or subcutaneously. These agents bond with acetylcholinesterase, so that acetylcholine is not inactivated; the adverse result is continuous stimulation (hyperstimulation) of the nerve endings. Carbamates, which are insecticides originally extracted from the Calabar bean, are derivatives of carbamic acid; they are nerve agents that specifically inhibit acetylcholinesterase for several hours and then spontaneously become unbound from the acetylcholinesterase. However, organophosphates require the formation of new enzyme (acetylcholinesterase) before nervous system function can be restored.

A very small drop of a nerve agent is enough to result in sweating and twitching at the site of exposure. A larger amount results in more systemic symptoms. Effects can begin anywhere from 30 minutes up to 18 hours after exposure. The more common organophosphates and carbamates (eg, sevin and malathion) that are used in agriculture result in less severe symptoms than do those used in warfare or in terrorist attacks. In an ordinary situation (eg, nonwarfare, nonterrorist attack situation), a patient could arrive at the ED having been unintentionally or intentionally exposed to organophosphates in a suicidal attempt.

Clinical Manifestations. Signs and symptoms of nerve gas exposure are those of cholinergic crisis and include bilateral miosis, visual disturbances, increased gastrointestinal motility, nausea and vomiting, diarrhea, substernal spasm, indigestion, bradycardia and atrioventricular block, bronchoconstriction, laryngeal spasm, weakness, fasciculations, and incontinence. The patient must be examined in a dark area to truly identify miosis. Neurologic responses include insomnia, forgetfulness, impaired judgment, depression, and irritability. A lethal dose results in loss of consciousness, seizures, copious secretions, fasciculations, flaccid muscles, and apnea.

Treatment. Decontamination with copious amounts of soap and water or saline solution for 8 to 20 minutes is essential. The water is blotted off, not wiped off, the skin. Fresh 0.5% hypochlorite solution (bleach) can also be used. The airway is maintained, and suctioning is frequently required. Plastic airway equipment should not be used because plastic will absorb sarin gas and may result in continued exposure to the agent.

Atropine 2 to 4 mg is administered by IV, followed by 2 mg every 3 to 8 minutes for up to 24 hours of treatment. Alternatively, IV atropine 1 to 2 mg/h may be administered until clear signs of anticholinergic activity have returned (decreased secretions, tachycardia, and decreased gastrointestinal motility). Another medication that may serve as an antidote is pralidoxime (Protopam), which allows cholinesterase to become active against acetylcholine. Pralidoxime 1 to 2 g in 100 to 150 mL of normal saline solution is administered over 15 to 30 minutes. Pralidoxime has no effect on secretions and may have any of the following side effects: hypertension, tachycardia, weakness, dizziness, blurred vision, and diplopia. Diazepam (Valium) or other benzodiazepines are used to control seizures, to decrease fasciculations, and to alleviate apprehension and agitation.

Military personnel believed to be at risk for chemical attack are provided with Mark I automatic injectors, which contain 2 mg atropine and 600 mg pralidoxime chloride. Diazepam may be administered by a partner.

Blood Agents

Blood agents such as hydrogen cyanide and cyanogen chloride have a direct effect on cellular metabolism, resulting in asphyxiation through alterations in hemoglobin. Cyanide is an agent that has profound systemic effects. It is commonly used in the mining of gold and silver and in the plastics and dye industries. In 1984, the Union Carbide pesticide plant in Bhopal, India, inadvertently released large amounts of cyanide in an industrial disaster and hundreds of deaths occurred.

A cyanide release is often associated with the odor of bitter almonds. In house fires, cyanide is released during the combustion of plastics, rugs, silk, furniture, and other construction materials. There is a significant correlation between blood cyanide and carbon monoxide levels in patients who survive fires, and in many cases, the cause of death is cyanide poisoning.

Clinical Manifestations. Cyanide can be ingested, inhaled, or absorbed through the skin and mucous membranes. Cyanide is protein bound and inhibits aerobic metabolism, leading to respiratory muscle failure, respiratory arrest, cardiac arrest, and death. Its inhalation results in flushing, tachypnea, tachycardia, nonspecific neurologic symptoms, stupor, coma, and seizure preceding respiratory arrest.

Treatment. Rapid administration of amyl nitrate, sodium nitrite, and sodium thiosulfate is essential to the successful management of cyanide exposure. First, the patient is intubated and placed on a ventilator. Next, amyl nitrate pearls are crushed and placed in the ventilator reservoir to induce methemoglobinemia. Cyanide has a 20% to 25% higher affinity for methemoglobin than it does for hemoglobin; it binds methemoglobin to form either cyanomethemoglobin or sulfmethemoglobin. The cyanomethemoglobin is then detoxified in the liver by the enzyme rhodanese. Next, IV sodium nitrite is administered to induce the rapid formation of methemoglobin. IV sodium thiosulfate is then administered; it has a higher affinity for cyanide than methemoglobin does and stimulates the conversion of cyanide to sodium thiocyanate, which can be excreted by the kidneys. Although they may be life-saving, these emergency medications do have side effects: sodium nitrite can result in severe hypotension, and thiocyanate can cause vomiting, psychosis, arthralgia, and myalgia.

The production of methemoglobin is contraindicated in patients with smoke inhalation, because they already have decreased oxygen-carrying capacity secondary to the carboxyhemoglobin produced by smoke inhalation. In facilities where a hyperbaric chamber is available, it may be used to provide oxygenation while the previously discussed therapies are initiated. An alternative suggested treatment for cyanide poisoning is hydroxocobalamin (vitamin $B_{12}a$). Hydroxocobalamin binds cyanide to form cyanocobalamin (vitamin B_{12}). It must be administered by IV in large doses. Administration of vitamin $B_{12}a$ can result in a transient pink discoloration of mucous membranes, skin, and urine. In high doses, tachycardia and hypertension can occur, but they usually resolve within 48 hours.

Pulmonary Agents

Pulmonary agents such as phosgene and chlorine destroy the pulmonary membrane that separates the alveolus from the capillary bed, disrupting alveolar–capillary oxygen transport mechanisms. Capillary leakage results in fluid-filled alveoli. Phosgene and chlorine both vaporize, rapidly causing this pulmonary injury. Phosgene has the odor of fresh-mown hay.

Signs and symptoms include pulmonary edema with shortness of breath, especially during exertion. An initial hacking cough is followed by frothy sputum production. A particulate air-filter mask is the only protection required to protect health care personnel. Phosgene does not injure the eyes.

Nuclear Radiation Exposure

The threat of **nuclear warfare** or radiation exposure is very real with the availability of nuclear material and easily concealed simple devices, such as the so-called dirty bomb, for dispersal. A dirty bomb is a conventional explosive (eg, dynamite) that is packaged with radioactive material that scatters when the bomb is detonated. It disperses radioactive material and may be called a radiologic weapon, but is not a nuclear weapon, which uses a complex nuclear fission reaction that is thousands of times more devastating than the dirty bomb.

Sources of radioactive material include not only nuclear weapons but also reactors and simple radioactive samples, such as weapons-grade plutonium or uranium, freshly spent nuclear fuel, or medical supplies (eg, radium, certain cesium isotopes) used in cancer treatments and radiology. Exposure of a large number of people can be accomplished by placing a radioactive sample in a public place. Thousands may be exposed this way; some may be immediately affected, and others may require health monitoring for many years to assess long-term effects. The effectiveness of these weapons was demonstrated in the devastating results of the bombings of Hiroshima and Nagasaki in World War II.

Nuclear reactor incidents have occurred in the Chernobyl (1986) and Three Mile Island (1979) nuclear facilities. There were 31 official deaths on the day of the Chernobyl incident, which involved a core meltdown and explosion, releasing radiation throughout the community. The long-term effects of this incident, including increased incidence of thyroid cancers and leukemia, continue to be evaluated.

Any terrorist-sponsored or unintentional radiation release can be sizable and may require the entire hospital and prehospital staff to be prepared, recognize signs and symptoms of exposure, and rapidly treat victims without contamination of personnel, visitors, patients, or the facility itself.

Types of Radiation

Atoms consist of protons, neutrons, and electrons. The protons and neutrons are in balance in the nucleus. The protons repel each other because they are all positively charged. The number of protons is specific for each element in the periodic table. There is a specific ratio of protons and neutrons for each different atom, and the result is element stability. When an element is radioactive, there is an imbalance in the nucleus, resulting from an excess of neutrons.

To achieve stability, a radioactive nuclide can eject particles until the most stable number (an even number) of protons and neutrons exists. A proton can become a neutron by ejecting a positron; conversely, a neutron can become a proton by ejecting a negative electron. An alpha particle is released when two protons and two electrons are ejected.

Alpha particles cannot penetrate the skin. A thin layer of paper or clothing is all that is necessary to protect the skin from alpha radiation. However, this low-level radiation can enter the body through inhalation, ingestion, or injection (open wound). Only localized damage occurs.

Beta particles have the ability to moderately penetrate the skin to the layer in which skin cells are being produced. This high-energy radiation can cause skin damage if the skin is exposed for a prolonged period and can cause injury if beta particles penetrate the skin.

Gamma radiation is a short-wavelength electromagnetic energy that is emitted when there is excess core nucleus energy. Gamma particles are penetrating. Therefore, it is difficult to shield against gamma radiation. X-rays are an example of gamma radiation. Gamma radiation often accompanies both alpha particle and beta particle emission.

Measurement and Detection

Radiation is measured in several different units. The *rad* is the basic unit of measurement. A rad is equivalent to 0.01 J of energy per kilogram of tissue. To determine the damaging effect of the rad, a conversion to the *rem* (roentgen equivalents human) is necessary. The rem reflects the type of radiation absorbed and the potential for damage. For example, 200,000 mrem results in mild radiation sickness (1 rem = 1000 mrem) (Dara, et al., 2005). Typical natural yearly exposure for a person is 360 mrem. Another important concept is *half-life*. The half-life of a radioactive product is the time it takes to lose half of its radioactivity.

The only way to detect radiation is through a device that determines the exposure per minute. There are various devices for this purpose. The Geiger counter (or Geiger-Mueller survey meter) can measure background radiation quickly through detection of gamma radiation and some beta radiation. With high-level radiation, the Geiger counter may underestimate exposure. Other devices include the ionization chamber survey meter, alpha monitors, and dose-rate meters. Personal dosimeters are simple tools that identify radiation exposure and are worn by radiology personnel.

Exposure

Exposure is affected by time, distance, and shielding. The longer a person is within the radiation area, the higher the exposure. Also, the larger the amount of radioactive material in the area, the greater the exposure. The farther away the person is from the radiation source, the lower the exposure. Shielding from the radiation source also decreases exposure.

Three types of radiation-induced injury can occur: external irradiation, contamination with radioactive materials, and incorporation of radioactive material into body cells, tissues, or organs:

- *External irradiation* exposure occurs when all or part of the body is exposed to radiation that penetrates or passes completely through the body. In this type of exposure, the person is not radioactive and does not require special isolation or decontamination measures. Irradiation does not necessarily constitute a medical emergency.
- *Contamination* occurs when the body is exposed to radioactive gases, liquids, or solids either externally or internally. If internal, the contaminant can be deposited within the body. Contamination requires immediate medical management to prevent incorporation.
- *Incorporation* is the actual uptake of radioactive material into the cells, tissues, and susceptible organs. The organs involved are usually the kidneys, bones, liver, and thyroid.

Sequelae of contamination and incorporation can occur days to years later. The thyroid gland can be largely protected from radiation exposure by administration of stable iodine (potassium iodide, or KI) before or promptly after the intake of radioactive iodine (Dara, et al., 2005).

Priorities in the treatment of any type of radiation exposure are always treatment of life-threatening injuries and illnesses first, followed by measures to limit exposure, contamination control, and finally decontamination.

Decontamination

Hospital and community disaster plans should be in effect when managing a radiation disaster. Access restriction is essential to prevent contamination of other areas of the hospital. Triage outside the hospital is the most effective means of preventing contamination of the facility itself. Floors are covered to prevent tracking of contaminants throughout the treatment areas. Strict isolation precautions should be in effect. All air ducts and vents must be sealed to prevent spread. Waste is controlled through double-bagging and the use of plastic-lined containers outside of the facility. All radiation-contaminated waste must be disposed in appropriate color-coded yellow and magenta canisters.

Staff are required to wear protective clothing, such as water-resistant gowns, two pairs of gloves, masks, caps, goggles, and booties. Dosimetry devices should be worn by all staff members participating in patient care. The radiation safety officer in the hospital should be notified immediately to assist with surveys (using a radiation survey meter) of the incoming patients and to provide dosimeters to all staff personnel involved in direct care of exposed patients. There is minimal risk to staff if the patients are properly surveyed and decontaminated. The majority of patients can be safely decontaminated with soap and water.

Each patient arriving at the hospital should first be surveyed with the radiation survey meter for external contamination and then directed toward the decontamination area as needed. Decontamination occurs outside of the ED with a shower, collection pool, tarp, and collection containers for patient belongings, as well as soap, towels, and disposable paper gowns for patients. Water runoff needs to be contained. Patients who are uninjured can perform self-decontamination with handheld showers. After the patient has showered, a resurvey is conducted to determine whether the radioactive contaminants have been removed. Additional washings should occur until the patient is free of contamination. It is important to ensure that during showers previously clean areas are not contaminated with runoff from the washed contaminated areas (eg, hair should be washed in a position that protects the body from contamination). Wounds are irrigated and then covered with a water-resistant dressing prior to total body decontamination.

Internal contamination or incorporation requires decontamination through catharsis, gastric lavage with chelating agents (agents that bind with radioactive substances and are then excreted), or both. Samples of urine, feces, and vomitus are surveyed to determine internal contamination levels. Biologic samples are taken through nasal and throat swabs, and a complete blood count with differential is obtained.

Acute Radiation Syndrome

Acute radiation syndrome (ARS) can occur after exposure to radiation. It is the dose, rather than the source, that determines whether ARS develops. Factors that determine whether the patient's response to exposure will result in ARS include a high dose (minimum 100 rad) and rate of radiation with total body exposure and penetrating-type radiation. Age, medical history, and genetics also affect the outcome after exposure. The course is predictable. Table 72-6 identifies the phases of ARS.

Each body system is affected differently in ARS. Systems with cells that rapidly reproduce are most commonly affected. The effects on the hematopoietic system include decreased numbers of lymphocytes, granulocytes, thrombocytes, and reticulocytes. It is the first system affected and serves as an indicator of the severity of radiation exposure (Dara, et al., 2005). A predictor of outcome is the absolute lymphocyte count at 48 hours after exposure. A significant exposure would be indicated by blood lymphocyte counts of 300 to 1200/mm³. Barrier precautions should be implemented to protect the patient from infection. Neutrophils decrease within 1 week, platelets decrease within 2 weeks, and red blood cells decrease within 3 weeks. Hemorrhagic complications, fever, and sepsis are common.

The gastrointestinal system, with its rapidly reproducing cells, is also readily affected by radiation. Doses of radiation required to produce symptoms are approximately 600 rad or higher. The gastrointestinal symptoms usually occur at the same time as the changes in the hematopoietic system. Nausea and vomiting occur within 2 hours after exposure. Sepsis, fluid and electrolyte imbalance, and opportunistic infections can occur as complications. An ominous sign is the presence of high fever and bloody diarrhea; these typically appear on day 10 after exposure.

The central nervous system is affected when the dose exceeds 1000 rad (Dara, et al., 2005). The symptoms occur when damage to the blood vessels of the brain results in fluid leakage. Signs and symptoms include cerebral edema, nausea, vomiting, headache, and increased intracranial pressure (ICP). Increased ICP heralds a poor outcome and imminent death. Central nervous system injury with this amount of exposure is irreversible and occurs before hematopoietic or gastrointestinal system symptoms appear. Cardiovascular collapse is usually seen in conjunction with these injuries.

Skin effects can also indicate the dose of radiation exposure. With exposure of 600 to 1000 rad, erythema occurs; it can disappear within hours, and then reappear. The exposed patient must be evaluated hourly for the presence of erythema. With exposures greater than 1000 rad, desquamation (radiation dermatitis) of the skin occurs. Necrosis becomes evident within a few days to months at doses greater than 5000 rad.

Secondary injury can occur when the radiation exposure occurs during a traumatic event such as a blast or burn. Trauma in addition to radiation exposure increases patient mortality. Attention must first be directed toward the primary assessment for trauma. Airway, breathing, circulation, and fracture reduction require immediate attention. All definitive treatments must occur within the first 48 hours. Thereafter, all surgical procedures should be delayed for 2 to 3 months because of the potential for delayed wound healing and the possible development of opportunistic infections several weeks after exposure.

Survival

There are three categories of predicted survival after radiation exposure: probable, possible, and improbable. Triage of victims at the scene, after decontamination, is conducted using the routine system for disaster triage. Presenting signs

TABLE 72-6	PHASES OF EFFECTS OF RADIATION EXPOSURE	
Phase	**Time of Occurrence**	**Signs and Symptoms**
Prodromal phase (presenting symptoms)	48–72 h after exposure	Nausea, vomiting, loss of appetite, diarrhea, fatigue High-dose radiation: fever, respiratory distress, and increased excitability
Latent phase (a symptom-free period)	After resolution of prodromal phase; can last up to 3 wk With high-dose radiation, latent period is shorter	Decreasing lymphocytes, leukocytes, thrombocytes, red blood cells
Illness phase	After latent period phase	Infection, fluid and electrolyte imbalance, bleeding, diarrhea, shock, and altered level of consciousness
Recovery phase OR	After illness phase	Can take weeks to months for full recovery
Death	After illness phase	Increased intracranial pressure is a sign of impending death

and symptoms determine the potential for survival and therefore the category of predicted survival during triage.

Probable survivors have either no initial symptoms or only minimal symptoms (eg, nausea and vomiting), or these symptoms resolve within a few hours. These patients should have a complete blood count drawn and may be discharged with instructions to return if any symptoms recur.

Possible survivors present with nausea and vomiting that persist for 24 to 48 hours. They experience a latent period, during which leukopenia, thrombocytopenia, and lymphocytopenia occur. Barrier precautions and protective isolation are implemented if the patient's lymphocyte count is less than 1200/mm³. Supportive treatment includes administration of blood products, prevention of infection, and provision of enhanced nutrition.

Improbable survivors have received more than 800 rad of total body penetrating irradiation. People in this group demonstrate an acute onset of vomiting, bloody diarrhea, and shock. Any neurologic symptoms suggest a lethal dose of radiation (CDC, 2005). These patients still require decontamination to prevent further contamination of the area and of others. Personal protection is essential, because it is virtually impossible to fully decontaminate these patients; all of their internal organs have been irradiated. The survival time is variable; however, death usually occurs swiftly due to shock. If there are no neurologic symptoms, patients may be alert and oriented, similar to a patient with extensive burns. In a mass casualty situation, these patients would be triaged into the black category, where they will receive comfort measures and emotional support. If it is not a mass casualty situation, aggressive fluid and electrolyte therapies are essential.

CRITICAL THINKING EXERCISES

1 You are the triage nurse at the receiving facility for casualties after a tornado. As you prepare to set up a triage station, "walking wounded" begin to arrive on their own. Among them is a hysterical adult woman with a facial abrasion who is otherwise apparently unharmed, carrying a 7-year-old child who has a Glasgow Coma Scale (GCS) score of 6 and is apneic. A 20-year-old man believes he has broken his arm; if fractured, it appears to be a closed fracture and the arm is warm with good pulses. As you quickly assess these patients, an ambulance arrives with an 80-year-old man with a sucking chest wound who is apneic and with a pulse barely palpable only at the carotids. The emergency medical services (EMS) personnel were unable to intubate him. In addition, a 15-year-old girl arrives with a cold pulseless foot from an obvious ankle fracture dislocation. How would you initially tag and triage these patients to provide optimal use of resources, remembering that this is only the first wave of injuries from multiple building collapses? Family members, members of the press, and city officials also begin arriving at the hospital in large numbers. How should the family members be managed? How should the other people be managed?

2 A patient arrives at the triage desk of the emergency department complaining of a sudden onset of a high fever and respiratory flulike symptoms. He has recently returned from a trip to Asia. At this point, there are no skin signs that suggest disease. What signs and symptoms should you identify if you suspect a biologic warfare agent or contagious process? Which agents cause pneumonia-like signs and symptoms? What precautions should be taken to protect staff and patients? What type of isolation would be typical if you suspected a contagion that is transmitted by the respiratory tract? Would you consider the patient's recent travel to Asia an important piece of information?

3 You are a member of the safety committee at your hospital. The committee is charged with updating the hospital's emergency operations plan (EOP). What types of disasters may occur in and around your facility? How do you determine the hazards and vulnerability of your facility? How does your facility plan comply with the National Incident Management System requirements? What plan for triage will be included in the EOP? What types of personal protective equipment (PPE) will you recommend?

4 Your facility is closest to a bombing event on the mass transit system. You initiate the hospital emergency plan. What special considerations should you address, including possible use of chemical and biological weapons? What types of blast injuries do you expect? How many phases of injury are involved with a blast effect?

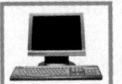 The Smeltzer suite offers these additional resources to enhance learning and facilitate understanding of this chapter:
- thePoint online resource, thepoint.lww.com/Smeltzer12E
- Student CD-ROM included with the book
- *Study Guide to Accompany Brunner & Suddarth's Textbook of Medical-Surgical Nursing*

REFERENCES AND SELECTED READINGS

Books

Auerbach, P. S. (2007). *Wilderness medicine* (5th ed). St. Louis, MO: Mosby.

Emergency Management Institute, National Emergency Training Center. (2002). *Mass fatalities incident response course*. Emmitsburg, MD: Federal Emergency Management Agency.

Emergency Nurses Association. (2007). *Trauma nurse core course provider manual* (6th ed). Chicago: Author.

Hoyt, K. S & Selfridge-Thomas, J. (2007). *Emergency nursing core curriculum* (6th ed.). St Louis: Saunders Elsevier.

Nayduch, D. (2009). *Nurse to nurse trauma care*. New York: McGraw Hill.

U.S. Army Medical Research Institute of Chemical Defense. (1999). *Medical management of chemical casualties handbook*. Fort Detrick, MD: Aberdeen Proving Ground.

U.S. Department of Homeland Security. (2003). *Homeland security exercise and evaluation program*, vol. 1. Washington, DC: U.S. Department of Homeland Security Office for Domestic Preparedness.

Journals and Electronic Documents

Agency for Toxic Substances and Disease Registry. (2009). Medical management guidelines. Available at: www.atsdr.cdc.gov/mtfmi/mmg.html

American Red Cross Disaster Services. (2001). Disaster preparedness for people with disabilities. Available at: www.redcross.org/www-files/Documents/Preparing/A4497.pdf

Centers for Disease Control and Prevention (CDC). (2004). Severe acute respiratory syndrome (SARS). Available at: www.cdc.gov/ncidod/sars

Centers for Disease Control and Prevention (CDC). (2005). Acute radiation syndrome: A fact sheet for physicians. Available at: www.bt.cdc.gov/radiation/arsphysicianfactsheet.asp

Centers for Disease Control and Prevention (CDC). (2006). Bombings: Injury patterns and care. Available at: http://emergency.cdc.gov/masscasualties/bombings_injurycare.asp

Cox, E. & Briggs, S. (2004). Disaster nursing: New frontiers for critical care. *Critical Care Nurse, 24*(3), 16–22.

Dara, S. I., Ashton, R. W., Farmer, J. C., et al. (2005). Worldwide disaster medical response. *Critical Care Medicine, 33*(Suppl 1), S2–S6.

Joint Commission. (2006). Hospital accreditation standards for emergency management planning. Available at: www.jcrinc.com/common/PDFs/fpdfs/pubs/pdfs/JCReqs/JCP-06-08-51.pdf

Karwa, M., Currie, B. & Kvetan, V. (2005). Bioterrorism: Preparing for the impossible or the improbable. *Critical Care Medicine, 33*(Suppl 1), S75–S95.

Kano, M. (2005). Characteristics of earthquake-related injuries treated in emergency departments following the 2001 Nisqually earthquake in Washington. *Journal of Emergency Management, 3*(1), 33–45.

Kapucu, N. (2006). Emergency logistics planning and disaster preparedness. *Journal of Emergency Management, 4*(6), 21–24.

Kluger, Y., Nimrod, A., Biderman, P., et al. (2006). The quinary pattern of blast injury. *Journal of Emergency Management, 4*(1), 51–55.

Lusby, L. G. (2006). Are you ready to execute your facility's emergency management plans? *Journal of Trauma Nursing, 13*(2), 74–77.

Nicholson, W. C. (2006). The role of the incident command system. *Journal of Emergency Management, 4*(1), 19–21.

Ritenour, A. E., Wickley, A., Ritenour, J. S., et al. (2008). Tympanic membrane perforation and hearing loss from blast overpressure in Operation Enduring Freedom and Operation Iraqi Freedom wounded. *Journal of Trauma, 64*(2), S174–S178.

Stambler, K. (2004). Psychological and social characteristics of a terrorist and their application in society and emergency management. *Journal of Emergency Management, 2*(4), 20–23.

Tasota, F. J., Henker, R. A. & Hoffman, L. A. (2002). Anthrax as a biological weapon: An old disease that poses a new threat. *Critical Care Nurse, 22*(5), 21–34.

Waugh, W. L. (2007). The principles of emergency management. *Journal of Emergency Management, 5*(3), 15–16.

RESOURCES

Agency for Toxic Substances and Disease Registry, www.atsdr.cdc.gov
American Red Cross, http://redcross.org/services/disaster/beprepared
Centers for Disease Control and Prevention, www.cdc.gov
U.S. Department of Homeland Security, www.dhs.gov/training.fema.gov

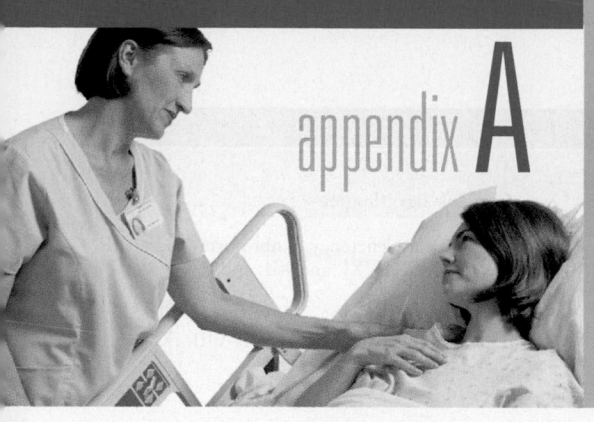

Diagnostic Studies and Interpretation

Test Value Studied

- Reference Ranges—Hematology
- Reference Ranges—Serum, Plasma and Whole Blood Chemistries
- Reference Ranges—Immunodiagnostic Tests
- Reference Ranges—Urine Chemistry
- Reference Ranges—Cerebrospinal Fluid (CSF)
- Miscellaneous Values

Selected Abbreviations Used in Reference Ranges

Conventional Units

kg = kilogram
gm = gram
mg = milligram
μg = microgram
μμg = micromicrogram
ng = nanogram
pg = picogram
dL = 100 milliliters
mL = milliliter
gm = gram
mm³ = cubic millimeter

fL = femtoliter
mM = millimole
nM = nanomole
mOsm = milliosmole
mm = millimeter
μm = micron or micrometer
mm Hg = millimeters of mercury
U = unit
mU = milliunit
μU = microunit
mEq = milliequivalent
IU = International Unit
mIU = milliInternational Unit

SI Units

g = gram
L = liter
d = day
h = hour
mol = mole
mmol = millimole
μmol = micromole
nmol = nanomole
pmol = picomole

Table A-1 REFERENCE RANGES—HEMATOLOGY*

Determination	Reference Range		Clinical Significance
	Conventional Units	SI Units	
A₂ hemoglobin	2.0%–3.2% of total hemoglobin	Mass fraction: 0.015–0.035 of total hemoglobin	Increased in certain types of thalassemia
Bleeding time	1.5–9.5 min	1.5–9.5 min	Prolonged in thrombocytopenia, defective platelet function, and aspirin therapy
Factor V assay (pro-accelerin factor)	60%–140%		
Factor VIII assay (antihemophiliac factor)	60%–140%		Deficient in classical hemophilia
Factor IX assay (plasma thromboplastin component)	60%–140%		Deficient in Christmas disease (pseudohemophilia)
Factor X (Stuart factor)	60%–140%		Deficient in Stuart clotting defect
Fibrinogen	200–400 mg/dL	2–4 g/dL	Increased in pregnancy, infections accompanied by leukocytosis, nephrosis Decreased in severe liver disease, abruptio placentae
Fibrin split (degradation) products	<5 μg/mL	<5 μg/mL	Increased in disseminated intravascular coagulation
Fibrinolysins (whole blood clot lysis time)	No lysis in 24 h		Increased activity associated with massive hemorrhage, extensive surgery, transfusion reactions

Continued on following page

Table A-1 REFERENCE RANGES—HEMATOLOGY* (Continued)

Determination	Reference Range		Clinical Significance
	Conventional Units	SI Units	
Partial thrombo-plastin time (activated)	Lower limit of normal: 20–25 sec; Upper limit of normal: 32–39 sec		Prolonged in deficiency of fibrinogen, factors II, V, VIII, IX, X, XI, and XII, and in heparin therapy
Prothrombin consumption	Lower limit of normal: 10 sec Lower limit of normal: 14 sec		Impaired in deficiency of factors VIII, IX, and X
Prothrombin time INR	9.5–12 sec 1.0 2–3 for therapy in atrial fibrillation, deep vein thrombosis, and pulmonary enbolism 2.5–3.5 for therapy in prosthetic heart valves		Prolonged by deficiency of factors I, II, V, VII, and X, fat malabsorption, severe liver disease, coumarin anticoagulant therapy INR used to standardize the prothrombin time and anticoagulation therapy
Erythrocyte count	Males: 4,600,000– 6,200,000/cu mm Females: 4,200,000– 5,400,000/cu mm	$4.6–6.2 \times 10^{12}$/L $4.2–5.4 \times 10^{12}$/L	Increased in severe diarrhea and dehydration, polycythemia, acute poisoning, pulmonary fibrosis Decreased in all anemias, in leukemia, and after hemorrhage when blood volume has been restored
Erythrocyte indices			
Mean corpuscular volume (MCV)	84–96 cu μm	84–96 fL	Increased in macrocytic anemias; decreased in microcytic anemia
Mean corpuscular hemoglobin (MCH)	28–33 μμg/cell	28–33 pg	Increased in macrocytic anemias; decreased in microcytic anemia
Mean corpuscular hemoglobin concentration (MCHC)	33%–35%	Concentration fraction: 0.33–0.35	Decreased in severe hypochromic anemia
Reticulocytes	0.5%–1.5% of red cells	Number fraction: 0.005–0.015	Increased with any condition stimulating increase in bone marrow activity (ie, infection, blood loss [acute and chronically following iron therapy in iron deficiency anemia], polycythemia rubra vera) Decreased with any condition depressing bone marrow activity, acute leukemia, late stage of severe anemias
Erythrocyte sedimentation rate (ESR)—Westergren method	Males under 50 yr: <15 mm/h Males over 50 yr: <20 mm/h Females under 50 yr: <25 mm/h Females over 50 yr: <30 mm/h	<15 mm/h <20 mm/h <25 mm/h <30 mm/h	Increased in tissue destruction, whether inflammatory or degenerative; during menstruation and pregnancy; and in acute febrile diseases
Erythrocyte sedimentation ratio—Zeta centrifuge	<50 yr: <55% 50–80 yr: 40%–60%	Volume fraction: <0.55 0.40–0.60	Significance similar to ESR
Hematocrit	Males: 42%–52% Females: 35%–47%	Volume fraction: 0.42–0.52 Volume fraction: 0.35–0.47	Decreased in severe anemias, anemia of pregnancy, acute massive blood loss Increased in erythrocytosis of any cause, and in dehydration or hemoconcentration associated with shock
Hemoglobin	Males: 13–18 gm/dL Females: 12–16 gm/dL	2.02–2.79 mmol/L 1.86–2.48 mmol/L	Decreased in various anemias, pregnancy, severe or prolonged hemorrhage, and with excessive fluid intake Increased in polycythemia, chronic obstructive pulmonary disease, failure of oxygenation because of congestive heart failure, and normally in people living at high altitudes
Hemoglobin F	Less than 2% of total hemoglobin	Mass fraction: <0.02	Increased in infants and children, and in thalassemia and many anemias

Continued

Table A-1 REFERENCE RANGES—HEMATOLOGY* (Continued)

Determination	Reference Range		Clinical Significance
	Conventional Units	SI Units	
Leukocyte alkaline phosphatase	Score of 15–130 (varies among labs)		Increased in polycythemia vera, myelofibrosis, and infections. Decreased in chronic granulocytic leukemia, paroxysmal nocturnal hemoglobinuria, hypoplastic marrow, and viral infections, particularly infectious mononucleosis
Leukocyte count	Total: 4,500–11,000/cu mm	4.5–11 × 10⁹/L	
Neutrophils	45%–73%	Number fraction: 0.45–0.73	Neutrophils increased with acute infections, trauma or surgery, leukemia, malignant disease, necrosis; decreased with viral infections, bone marrow suppression, primary bone marrow disease
Eosinophils	0%–4%	Number fraction: 0.00–0.04	Eosinophils increased in allergy, parasitic disease, collagen disease, subacute infections; decreased with stress, use of some medications (ACTH, epinephrine, thyroxine)
Basophils	0%–1%	Number fraction: 0.00–0.01	Basophils increased with acute leukemia and following surgery or trauma; decreased with allergic reactions, stress, allergy, parasitic disease, use of corticosteroids
Lymphocytes	20%–40%	Number fraction: 0.2–0.4	Lymphocytes increased with infectious mononucleosis, viral and some bacterial infections, hepatitis; decreased with aplastic anemia, SLE, immunodeficiency including AIDS
Monocytes	2%–8%	Number fraction: 0.02–0.08	Monocytes increased with viral infections, parasitic disease, collagen and hemolytic disorders; decreased with use of corticosteroids, RA, HIV infection
Platelet count	150,000–450,000/cu mm	0.15–0.45 × 10¹²/L	Increased in malignancy, myeloproliferative disease, rheumatoid arthritis, and postoperatively; about 50% of patients with unexpected increase of platelet count will be found to have a malignancy. Decreased in thrombocytopenic purpura, acute leukemia, aplastic anemia, and during cancer chemotherapy

*Laboratory values may vary according to the techniques used in different laboratories.

Table A-2 REFERENCE RANGES—SERUM, PLASMA, AND WHOLE BLOOD CHEMISTRIES

Determination	Normal Adult Reference Range		Clinical Significance	
	Conventional Units	SI Units	Increased	Decreased
Acetoacetate	0.2–1.0 mg/dL	19.6–98 μmol/L	Diabetic ketoacidosis Fasting	
Acetone	0.3–2.0 mg/dL	51.6–344.0/μmol/L	Diabetic ketoacidosis Toxemia of pregnancy Carbohydrate-free diet High-fat diet	
Acid, total phosphatase	Males: 2–12 UL Females: 0.3–9.2 UL	Males: 2–12 UL Females: 0.3–9.2 UL	Carcinoma of prostate Advanced Paget's disease Hyperparathyroidism Gaucher's disease	
Acid, phosphatase, prostatic—RIA	2.5–3.37 ng/mL	2.5–3.37 μg/L	Carcinoma of prostate	
Alkaline phosphatase	Adults: 50–120 UL	50–120 UL	Conditions reflecting increased osteoblastic activity of bone Rickets Hyperparathyroidism Hepatic disease Bone disease	

Continued on following page

Table A-2 REFERENCE RANGES—SERUM, PLASMA, AND WHOLE BLOOD CHEMISTRIES (Continued)

Determination	Normal Adult Reference Range — Conventional Units	SI Units	Clinical Significance — Increased	Decreased
Alkaline phosphatase, thermostable fraction	Hepatic: >25% Combined: 10%–25% Skeletal: <10%			
Adrenocorticotropic hormone (ACTH) (plasma)—RIA*	<50 pg/mL	<50 ng/L	Pituitary-dependent Cushing's syndrome Ectopic ACTH syndrome Primary adrenal atrophy	Adrenocortical tumor Adrenal insufficiency secondary to hypopituitarism
Aldolase	3–8 Sibley-Lehninger U/dL at 37°C	22–59 mU/L at 37°C	Hepatic necrosis Granulocytic leukemia Myocardial infarction Skeletal muscle disease	
Aldosterone (plasma)—RIA	Supine: 3–10 ng/dL Upright: 5–30 ng/dL Adrenal vein: 200–800 ng/dL	0.08–0.30 nmol/L 0.14–0.90 nmol/L 5.54–22.16 nmol/L	Primary aldosteronism Secondary aldosteronism	Addison's disease
Alpha-1-antitrypsin	110–140 mg/dL	1.1–1.4 g/L		Certain forms of chronic lung and liver disease in young adults
Alpha-1-fetoprotein	<15 ng/mL	<15 μg/L	Hepatocarcinoma Metastatic carcinoma of liver Germinal cell carcinoma of the testicle or ovary Fetal neural tube defects— elevation in maternal serum	
Alpha-hydroxybutyric dehydrogenase	<140 U/L	<140 U/L	Myocardial infarction Granulocytic leukemia Hemolytic anemias Muscular dystrophy	
Ammonia (plasma)	15–45 μg/dL (varies with method)	11–32/μmol/L	Severe liver disease Hepatic decompensation	
Amylase	60–160 Somogyi U/dL	111–296 U/L	Acute pancreatitis Mumps Duodenal ulcer Carcinoma of head of pancreas Prolonged elevation with pseudocyst of pancreas Increased by medications that constrict pancreatic duct sphincters: morphine, codeine, cholinergics	Chronic pancreatitis Pancreatic fibrosis and atrophy Cirrhosis of liver Pregnancy (2nd and 3rd trimesters)
Arsenic	<70 μg/dL; poisoning: 100–150 μg/dL	<0.93–2.6 μmol/L; poisoning: 133–6.65 μmol/L	Intentional or unintentional poisoning Excessive occupational exposure	
Ascorbic acid (vitamin C)	0.4–1.5 mg/dL	23–85 μmol/L	Large doses of ascorbic acid as a prophylactic against the common cold	
ALT (alanine aminotransferase), formerly SGPT	Males: 10–40 U/mL Females: 8–35 U/mL	Males: 0.17–0.68 μkat/L Females: 0.14–0.60 μkat/L	Same conditions as AST (SGOT), but increase is more marked in liver disease than AST (SGOT)	
AST (aspartate aminotransferase), formerly SGOT	Males: 10–40 U/L Females: 15–30 U/L	Males: 0.34–0.68 μkat/L Females: 0.25–0.51 μkat/L	Myocardial infarction Skeletal muscle disease Liver disease	
Bilirubin	Total: 0.3–1.0 mg/dL Direct: 0.1–0.4 mg/dL Indirect: 0.1–0.4 mg/dL	5–17 μmol/L 1.7–3.7 μmol/L 3.4–11.2 μmol/L	Hemolytic anemia (indirect) Biliary obstruction and disease Hepatocellular damage (hepatitis) Pernicious anemia Hemolytic disease of newborn	
Blood gases Oxygen, arterial (whole blood): Partial pressure (PaO$_2$)	85–95 mm Hg	10.64–12.64 kPa	Polycythemia	Anemia Cardiac or pulmonary disease

Continued

Table A-2   REFERENCE RANGES—SERUM, PLASMA, AND WHOLE BLOOD CHEMISTRIES (Continued)

Determination	Normal Adult Reference Range		Clinical Significance	
	Conventional Units	SI Units	Increased	Decreased
Saturation (SaO$_2$)	95%–99%	Volume fraction: 0.95–0.99		Cardiac decompensation Chronic obstructive lung disease
Carbon dioxide, arterial (whole blood) partial pressure (PaCO$_2$)	35–45 mm Hg	4.66–5.99 kPa	Respiratory acidosis Metabolic alkalosis	Respiratory alkalosis Metabolic acidosis
pH (whole blood, arterial)	7.35–7.45	7.35–7.45	Vomiting Hyperventilation Fever Intestinal obstruction	Uremia Diabetic ketoacidosis Hemorrhage Nephritis
Brain (B-type) natriuretic peptide (BNP)	<100 pg/mL	100 ng/L	Heart failure Cardiac volume overload	
Calcitonin	Basal: <19 pg/mL Stimulation test Males: <350 pg/mL Females: <100 pg/mL	19 ng/L <350 ng/L <100 ng/L	Medullary carcinoma of the thyroid Some nonthyroid tumors Zollinger-Ellison syndrome	
Calcium	8.6–10.2 mg/dL	2.15–2.55 mmol/L	Tumor or hyperplasia of parathyroid Hypervitaminosis D Multiple myeloma Nephritis with uremia Malignant tumors Sarcoidosis Hypoparathyroidism Skeletal immobilization Excess calcium intake: milk alkali syndrome	Hyperthyroidism Diarrhea Celiac disease Vitamin D deficiency Acute pancreatitis Nephrosis After parathyroidectomy
CO$_2$, venous	Adults: 24–32 mEq/L Infants: 18–24 mEq/L	24–32 mmol/L 18–24 mmol/L	Tetany Respiratory disease Intestinal obstruction Vomiting	Acidosis Nephritis Eclampsia Diarrhea Anesthesia
Catecholamines (plasma)—RIA	Epinephrine: <100 pg/mL Norepinephrine: <400 pg/mL Dopamine: <143 pg/mL	<540 pmol/L <2360 pmol/L <935 pmol/L	Pheochromocytoma	
Ceruloplasmin	20–40 mg/dL	1.26–2.52 μmol/L		Wilson's disease (hepatolenticular degeneration)
Chloride	97–107 mEq/L	97–107 mmol/L	Nephrosis Nephritis Urinary obstruction Cardiac decompensation Anemia	Diabetes mellitus Diarrhea Vomiting Pneumonia Heavy metal poisoning Cushing's syndrome Intestinal obstruction Febrile conditions
Cholesterol	150–200 mg/dL	3.9–5.2 mmol/L	Lipemia Obstructive jaundice Diabetes Hyperthyroidism	Pernicious anemia Hemolytic anemia Hypothyroidism Severe infection Terminal states of debilitating disease
Cholesterol esters	60%–70% of total	Fraction of total cholesterol: 0.6–0.7		The esterified fraction decreases in liver diseases
Cholinesterase	Serum: 0.6–1.6 delta pH Red cells: 0.6–1 delta pH	0.6–1.6 U 0.6–1 U	Nephrosis Exercise	Nerve gas exposure (greater effect on red cell activity) Insecticide poisoning
Chorionic gonadotropin, beta subunit	0–5 IU/L	0–5 IU/L	Pregnancy Hydatidiform mole Choriocarcinoma	Threatened abortion Ectopic pregnancy

Continued on following page

Table A-2   REFERENCE RANGES—SERUM, PLASMA, AND WHOLE BLOOD CHEMISTRIES (Continued)

Determination	Normal Adult Reference Range		Clinical Significance	
	Conventional Units	SI Units	Increased	Decreased
Complement, C_3	80–170 mg/dL	0.8–1.7 g/L	Some inflammatory diseases, acute myocardial infarction, cancer	Acute glomerulonephritis Disseminated lupus erythematosus with renal involvement
Complement, C_4	18–51 mg/dL	180–510 mg/L	Some inflammatory diseases, acute myocardial infarction, cancer	Often decreased in immunologic disease, especially with active systemic lupus erythematosus Hereditary angioneurotic edema
Complement, total (hemolytic)	90%–94% complement	25–70 U/mL	Some inflammatory diseases	Acute glomerulonephritis Epidemic meningitis Subacute bacterial endocarditis
Copper	70–150 μg/dL	11–24 μmol/L	Cirrhosis of liver Pregnancy	Wilson's disease
Cortisol-RIA	8 AM: 5–25/μg/dL 4 PM: 3–16 μg/dL	138–690 nmol/L 83–442 nmol/L	Stress: infectious disease, surgery, burns, etc. Pregnancy Cushing's syndrome Pancreatitis Eclampsia	Addison's disease Anterior pituitary hypofunction
C-peptide reactivity	0.9–4.0 ng/mL	0.9–4.0 μg/L	Insulinoma	Diabetes mellitus
Creatine	0.2–0.8 mg/mL	15.3–61 μmol/L	Pregnancy Skeletal muscle necrosis or atrophy Starvation Hyperthyroidism	
Creatine phosphokinase (CPK)	Males: 50–325 mU/mL Females: 50–250 mU/mL	50–325 U/L 50–250 U/L	Myocardial infarction Skeletal muscle diseases Intramuscular injections Crush syndrome Hypothyroidism Alcohol withdrawal delirium Alcoholic myopathy Cerebrovascular disease	
Creatine kinase (CK) isoenzymes	MM band present (skeletal muscle)- MB band absent (heart muscle)		MB band increased in myocardial infarction, ischemia	
Creatinine	0.7–1.4 mg/dL	62–124 μmol/L	Nephritis Chronic renal disease	
Creatinine clearance	Males: 85–125 mL/min Females: 75–115 mL/min	1.42–2.08 mL/s 1.25–1.92 mL/s		Kidney diseases Kidney diseases
Cryoglobulins, qualitative	Negative		Multiple myeloma Chronic lymphocytic leukemia Lymphosarcoma Systemic lupus erythematosus Rheumatoid arthritis Infective subacute endocarditis Some malignancies Scleroderma	
11-Deoxycortisol	1 μg/dL	<0.029 μmol/L	Hypertensive form of virilizing adrenal hyperplasia due to an 11-β-hydroxylase defect	
Dibucaine number	Normal: 70%–85% inhibition Heterozygote: 50%–65% inhibition Homozygote: 16%–25% inhibition			Important in detecting carriers of abnormal cholinesterase activity who are susceptible to succinylcholine anesthetic shock

Continued

Table A-2   REFERENCE RANGES—SERUM, PLASMA, AND WHOLE BLOOD CHEMISTRIES (Continued)

Determination	Normal Adult Reference Range		Clinical Significance	
	Conventional Units	SI Units	Increased	Decreased
Dihydrotestosterone	Males: 50–210 ng/dL Females: none detectable	1.72–7.22 nmol/L		Testicular feminization syndrome
Estradiol—RIA	Females: Follicular: 10–90 pg/mL Midcycle: 100–500 pg/mL Luteal: 50–240 pg/mL Follicular phase: 2–20 ng/dL Midcycle: 12–40 ng/dL Luteal phase: 10–30 ng/dL Postmenopausal: 1–5 ng/dL Males: 0.5–5 ng/dL	37–370 pmol/L 367–1835 pmol/L 184–881 pmol/L	Pregnancy, ovarian tumor	Ovarian failure

Estriol—RIA	Nonpregnant females:
	  <0.5 ng/mL
	Pregnant females:
	  1st trimester: up to 1 ng/mL
	  2nd trimester: 0.8–7 ng/mL
	  3rd trimester: 5–25 ng/mL
		<1.75 nmol/L
		
		Up to 3.5 nmol/L
		2.8–24.3 nmol/L
		17.4–86.8 nmol/L
			Pregnancy	Ovarian failure

Estrogens, total—RIA	Females: cycle days:
	  Day 1–10: 61–394 pg/mL
	  Day 11–20: 122–437 pg/mL
	  Day 21–30: 156–350 pg/mL
	  Males: 40–115 pg/mL
		61–394 ng/L
		122–437 ng/L
		156–350 ng/L
		40–115 ng/L
			Pregnancy
			Measured on a daily basis, can be used to evaluate response of hypogonadotrophic, hypoestrogenic women to human menopausal or pituitary gonadotropin
				Fetal distress
				Ovarian failure

Estrone—RIA	Females:
	  Day 1–10:4.3–18 ng/dL
	  Day 11–20:7.5–19.6 ng/dL
	  Day 21–30: 13–20 ng/dL
	  Males: 2.5–7.5 ng/dL
		15.9–66.6 pmol/L
		27.8–72.5 pmol/L
		48.1–74 pmol/L
		9.3–27.8 pmol/L
			Pregnancy	Ovarian failure

Ferritin—RIA	Males: 20–250 ng/mL Females: 12–250 ng/mL	20–250 µg/L 12–250 µg/L	Nephritis Hemochromatosis Certain neoplastic diseases Acute myelogenous leukemia Multiple myeloma	Iron deficiency
Folic acid—RIA	2.5–20 ng/mL	6–46 nmol/L		Megaloblastic anemias of infancy and pregnancy Inadequate diet Liver disease Malabsorption syndrome Severe hemolytic anemia

Follicle stimulating hormone (FSH)—RIA	Males: 2–10 mIU/mL
	Females:
	  Follicular phase:
	    5–20 mIU/mL
	  Peak of middle cycle:
	    12–30 mIU/mL
	  Luteinic phase:
	    5–15 mIU/mL
	  Menopausal females:
	    40–200 mIU/mL
		
		5–20 IU/L
		
		12–30 IU/L
		
		5–15 IU/L
		
		40–200 IU/L
			Menopause and primary ovarian failure	Pituitary failure

Galactose	<5 mg/dL	<0.28 mmol/L		Galactosemia
Gamma glutamyl transpeptidase	Males: 20–30 U/L Females: 1–24 U/L	0.03–0.5/µkat/L 0.02–0.4/µkat/L	Hepatobiliary disease Drug toxicity Myocardial infarction Renal infarction Zollinger-Ellison syndrome	
Gastrin—RIA	Fasting: 50–155 pg/mL Postprandial: 80–170 pg/mL	50–155 ng/L 80–170 ng/L	Peptic ulceration of the duodenum Pernicious anemia	

Continued on following page

Table A-2 REFERENCE RANGES—SERUM, PLASMA, AND WHOLE BLOOD CHEMISTRIES (Continued)				
	Normal Adult Reference Range		**Clinical Significance**	
Determination	**Conventional Units**	**SI Units**	**Increased**	**Decreased**
Glucose	Fasting: 60–110 mg/dL Postprandial (2 h): 65–140 mg/dL	3.3–6.05 mmol/L 3.58–7.7 mmol/L	Diabetes mellitus Nephritis Hypothyroidism Early hyperpituitarism Cerebral lesions Infections Pregnancy Uremia	Hyperinsulinism Hyperthyroidism Late hyperpituitarism Pernicious vomiting Addison's disease Extensive hepatic damage

Glucose tolerance (oral)	Features of a normal
	  response:
	1. Normal fasting
	  between 60–110 mg/dL
	2. No sugar in urine
	3. Upper limits of normal:
	  Fasting = 125
	  1 hour = 190
	  2 hours = 140
	  3 hours = 125
		
		3.3–6.05 mmol/L
		
		6.88 mmol/L
		10.45 mmol/L
		7.70 mmol/L
		6.88 mmol/L
			Two-hour value >200 mg/dL
			  (11.1 mmol/L) is
			  diagnostic for diabetes
			  mellitus
				Decreased 2- and 3-hour
				  values may occur with
				  hypoglycemia in
				  diabetes mellitus

Glucose-6-phosphate
  dehydrogenase (red cells)
	Screening:
	  Decolorization in
	  20–100 min
	  Quantitative: 1.86–2.5
	  IU/mL RBC
		
		1860–2500 U/L
				Drug-induced hemolytic
				  anemia
				Hemolytic disease of
				  newborn

Glycoprotein (alpha-1-acid)	50–120 mg/dL	0.5–1.2 g/L	Neoplasm
			Tuberculosis
			Diabetes mellitus
			  complicated by
			  degenerative vascular
			  disease
			Pregnancy
			Rheumatoid arthritis
			Rheumatic fever
			Infectious liver disease
			Lupus erythematosus	

Growth hormone—RIA	Males: 0–4 ng/mL Females: 0–18 ng/mL	0.4 μg/L 0–18 μg/L	Acromegaly	Hypopituitarism

Haptoglobin	30–200 mg/dL	0.3–2.0 g/L	Pregnancy
			Estrogen therapy
			Chronic infections
			Various inflammatory
			  conditions
				Hemolytic anemia
				Hemolytic blood
				  transfusion reaction

Hemoglobin (plasma)	0.5–5 mg/dL	5–50 mg/L	Transfusion reactions
			Paroxysmal nocturnal
			  hemoglobinuria
			Intravascular hemolysis
			Suboptimal glucose control
				Anemia, pregnancy,
				  chronic renal failure

Glycohemoglobin (GHB,
  hemoglobin A1c,
  hemoglobin A1)
	Nondiabetics and diabetics
	  with good control:
	  4.4%–6.4%			

Hexosaminidase, total	Controls: 333–375
	  nM/mL/h
		333–375 μmol/L/h	Sandhoff's disease	Tay-Sachs disease and
				  heterozygotes

Hexosaminidase A	Controls: 49%–68%
	  of total
	Heterozygotes: 26%–45%
	  of total
	Tay-Sachs disease:
	  0%–4% of total
	Diabetics: 39%–59%
	  of total
		Fraction of total:
		  0.49–0.68
		0.26–0.45
		
		0–0.04
		0.39–0.59		

High-density lipoprotein
  cholesterol (HDL
  cholesterol)
	Males: 35–70 mg/dL
	Females: 35–85 mg/dL
		0.91–1.81 mmol/L
		0.91–2.20 mmol/L
				HDL cholesterol is lower
				  in patients with increased
				  risk for coronary heart
				  disease

17 Hydroxy-
  progesterone—RIA
	Males: 0.5–2.0 ng/mL
	Females: 0.2–3.0 ng/mL
	Children: <1.0 ng/mL
		1.5–6.0 nmol/L
		0.6–9.0 nmol/L
		<3.0 nmol/L
			Congenital adrenal
			  hyperplasia
			Pregnancy
			Some cases of adrenal or
			  ovarian adenomas	

Continued

Table A-2	**REFERENCE RANGES—SERUM, PLASMA, AND WHOLE BLOOD CHEMISTRIES** (Continued)			
	Normal Adult Reference Range		**Clinical Significance**	
Determination	**Conventional Units**	**SI Units**	**Increased**	**Decreased**
Immunoglobulin A	Adults: 80–400 mg/dL	0.8–4.0 g/L	Gamma A myeloma Wiskott-Aldrich syndrome Autoimmune disease Hepatic cirrhosis	Ataxia telangiectasis Agammaglobulinemia Hypogamma-globulinemia, transient Dysgammaglobulinemia Protein-losing enteropathies
Immunoglobulin D	0.5–12.0 mg/dL	5–120 mg/L	IgD multiple myeloma Some patients with chronic infectious diseases	
Immunoglobulin E	<1.0 mg/mL	<10 mg/L	Allergic patients and those with parasitic infections	
Immunoglobulin G	Adults: 600–1800 mg/dL	6.0–18.0 g/L	IgG myeloma Following hyperimmunization Autoimmune disease states Chronic infections	Congenital and acquired hypogam-maglobu-linemia IgA myelomas, Waldenström's (IgM) macroglobulinemia Some malabsorption syndromes Extensive protein loss
Immunoglobulin M	Adults: 55–250 mg/dL	0.55–2.5 g/L	Waldenström's macroglobulinemia Parasitic infections Hepatitis	Agammaglobulinemias Some IgG and IgA myelomas Chronic lymphatic leukemia
Insulin—RIA	5–25 μU/mL	0.2–1 μg/L	Insulinoma Acromegaly	Diabetes mellitus
Iron	50–160/μg/dL	9–29 μmol/L	Pernicious anemia Aplastic anemia Hemolytic anemia Hepatitis Hemochromatosis	Iron deficiency anemia
Iron-binding capacity	IBC: 250–350 μg/dL TIBC: 250–475 μg/dL % Saturation: 20–50	45–63 μmol/L 45–85 μmol/L Fraction of total iron-binding capacity: 0.2–0.5	Iron deficiency anemia Acute and chronic blood loss Hepatitis	Chronic infectious diseases Cirrhosis
Isocitric dehydrogenase	50–180 U	0.83–3 UIL	Hepatitis, cirrhosis Obstructive jaundice Metastatic carcinoma of the liver Megaloblastic anemia	
Lactic acid (whole blood)	Venous: 5–15 mg/dL Arterial: 3–11 mg/dL	0.5–1.7 mmol/L 0.36–1.25 mmol/L	Increased muscular activity Congestive heart failure Hemorrhage Shock Lactic acidosis Some febrile infections May be increased in severe liver disease	
Lactic dehydrogenase (LDH)	90–176 mU/mL	90–176 U/L	Untreated pernicious anemia Myocardial infarction Pulmonary infarction Liver disease	
*Lactic dehydrogenase isoenzymes Total lactic dehy-drogenase	90–176 mU/mL	90–176 U/L Fraction of total LDH:	LDH-1 and LDH-2 are increased in myocardial infarction, megaloblastic anemia, and hemolytic anemia LDH-4 and LDH-5 are increased in pulmonary infarction, congestive heart failure, and liver disease	
LDH-1 LDH-2 LDH-3 LDH-4 LDH-5	22%–36% 35%–46% 13%–26% 3%–10% 2%–12%	0.2–0.36 0.35–0.46 0.13–0.26 0.03–0.10 0.02–0.12		
Lead (whole blood)	Up to 40 μg/dL	Up to 2 μmol/L	Lead poisoning	
Leucine aminopeptidase	80–200 U/mL	19.2–48 U/L	Liver or biliary tract diseases Pancreatic disease Metastatic carcinoma of liver and pancreas Biliary obstruction	

Continued on following page

Table A-2   REFERENCE RANGES—SERUM, PLASMA, AND WHOLE BLOOD CHEMISTRIES (Continued)

Determination	Normal Adult Reference Range		Clinical Significance	
	Conventional Units	SI Units	Increased	Decreased
†Lipase	<200 U/mL	<200 U/L	Acute and chronic pancreatitis Biliary obstruction Cirrhosis Hepatitis Peptic ulcer	
Lipids, total	400–800 mg/dL	4–8 g/L	Hypothyroidism Diabetes mellitus Nephrosis Glomerulonephritis Hyperlipoproteinemias	Hyperthyroidism
Low-density lipoprotein cholesterol (LDL cholesterol)	mg/dL desirable levels: <160 if no coronary artery disease (CAD) and <2 risk factors <130 if no CAD and 2 or more risk factors <100 if CAD present		LDL cholesterol is higher in patients with increased risk for coronary heart disease	

Luteinizing hormone—RIA	Males: 1.5–9.3 mU/mL
	Females:
	  Follicular phase:
	  1.9–12.5 mU/mL
	  Midcycle: 8.7–76.3 mU/mL
		1.5–9.3 U/L
		
		1.9–12.5 U/L
		8.7–76.3 U/L
			Pituitary tumor
			Ovarian failure
				Pituitary failure

Lysozyme (muramidase)	4.0–15.6 µg/mL	0.28–1.10 µmol/L	Certain types of leukemia (acute monocytic leukemia) Inflammatory states and infections	Acute lymphocytic leukemia
Magnesium	1.3–2.3 mg/dL	0.62–0.95 mmol/L	Excess ingestion of magnesium-containing antacids	Chronic alcoholism Severe renal disease Diarrhea Defective growth
Mercury	<10 µg/L	<50 µmol/L	Mercury poisoning	
Myoglobin	5–70 ng/mL	5–70 µg/mL	Myocardial infarction Myocardial ischemia Rhabdomyolysis Malignant hyperthermia	Rheumatoid arthritis Myasthenia gravis
5' Nucleotidase	3.2–11.6 IU/L	3.2–11.6 U/L	Hepatobiliary disease	
Osmolality	275–300 mOsm/kg	275–300 mmol/L	Diabetes insipidus, osmotic diuresis	Inappropriate secretion of ADH Addison's disease
Parathyroid hormone	10–65 pg/mL	10–65 ng/L	Hyperparathyroidism, chronic renal failure	Hypoparathyroidism
Phenylalanine	1.2–3.5 mg/dL 1st week 0.7–3.5 mg/dL thereafter	0.07–0.21 mmol/L 0.04–0.21 mmol/L	Phenylketonuria	
Phosphohexose isomerase	20–90 IU/L	20–90 U/L	Malignancy Disease of heart, liver, and skeletal muscles	
Phospholipids	125–300 mg/dL	1.25–3 g/L	Diabetes mellitus Nephritis	
Phosphorus, inorganic	2.5–4.5 mg/dL	0.8–1.45 mmol/L	Chronic nephritis Hypoparathyroidism	
Potassium	3.5–5 mEq/L	3.5–5 mmol/L	Renal Failure Acidosis Cell lysis Tissue breakdown or hemolysis	Hyperparathyroidism Vitamin D deficiency GI losses Diuretic administration
Prealbumin	16.0–35.0 mg/dL	160–350 mg/L	Malnutrition Severe or chronic illness Liver disease	

Continued

Table A-2	REFERENCE RANGES—SERUM, PLASMA, AND WHOLE BLOOD CHEMISTRIES (Continued)			
	Normal Adult Reference Range		**Clinical Significance**	
Determination	**Conventional Units**	**SI Units**	**Increased**	**Decreased**
Progesterone—RIA	Follicular phase: up to 0.8 ng/mL	2.5 nmol/L	Useful in evaluation of menstrual disorders and infertility and in the evaluation of placental function during pregnancies complicated by toxemia, diabetes mellitus, or threatened miscarriage	
	Luteal phase: 10–20 ng/mL	31.8–63.6 nmol/L		
	End of cycle: <1 ng/mL	<3 nmol/L		
	Pregnant: up to 50 ng/mL in 20th week	Up to 160 nmol/L		
Prolactin—RIA	4–30 ng/mL	4–30 µg/L	Pregnancy Functional or structural disorders of the hypothalamus Pituitary stalk section Pituitary tumors	
Prostate-specific antigen	<4 ng/mL		Prostatic cancer, benign prostatic hyperplasia, prostatitis	
Protein, total	6–8 gm/dL	60–80 g/L	Hemoconcentration	Malnutrition
Albumin	3.5–5.5 g/dL	40–55 g/L	Shock	Hemorrhage
Globulin	1.7–3.3 g/dL	17–33 g/L	Globulin fraction increased in multiple myeloma, chronic infection, liver disease	Loss of plasma from burns Proteinuria
Protein Electrophoresis		35–50 g/L		
Albumin	3.5–5.5 g/dL	40–55 g/L		
Alpha-1 globulin	0.15–0.25 g/dL	1.5–2.5 g/L		
Alpha-2 globulin	0.43–0.75 g/dL	4.3–7.5 g/L		
Beta globulin	0.5–1.0 g/dL	5–10 g/L		
Gamma globulin	0.6–1.3 g/dL	6–13 g/L		
Protoporphyrin erythrocyte (whole blood)	Males: 11–45 µg/dL	0.20–0.80 µmol/L	Lead toxicity	
	Females: 19–52 µg/dL	0.34–0.92 µmol/L	Erythropoietic porphyria	
Pyridoxine	5–30 ng/mL	20–1.21 nmol/L		A wide spectrum of clinical conditions, such as mental depression, peripheral neuropathy, anemia, neonatal seizures, and reactions to certain drug therapies
Pyruvic acid (whole blood)	0.3–0.9 mg/dL	34–102 µmol/L	Diabetes mellitus Severe thiamine deficiency Acute phase of some infections, possibly secondary to increased glycogenolysis and glycolysis	
Renin (plasma)—RLA	Normal diet:		Renovascular hypertension	Frank primary aldosteronism
	Supine: 0.3–1.9 ng/mL/h	0.08–0.52 ng/L/S	Malignant hypertension	
	Upright: 0.6–3.6 ng/mL/h	0.16–1.00 µg/L/S	Untreated Addison's disease	Increased salt intake
	Low salt diet:		Primary salt-losing nephropathy	Salt–retaining steroid therapy
	Supine: 0.9–4.5 ng/mL/h	0.25–1.25 µg/L/S		
	Upright: 4.1–9.1 ng/mL/h	1.13–2.53 µg/L/S	Low-salt diet Diuretic therapy Hemorrhage	Antidiuretic hormone therapy Blood transfusion
Sodium	135–145 mEq/L	135–145 mmol/L	Hemoconcentration Nephritis Pyloric obstruction	Alkali deficit Addison's disease Myxedema
Sulfate (inorganic)	0.5–1.5 mg/dL	0.05–0.15 mmol/L	Nephritis Nitrogen retention	

Continued on following page

Table A-2   REFERENCE RANGES—SERUM, PLASMA, AND WHOLE BLOOD CHEMISTRIES (Continued)

| Determination | Normal Adult Reference Range | | Clinical Significance | |
	Conventional Units	SI Units	Increased	Decreased

Testosterone—RIA	Females: 20–80 ng/dL
	Males: 240–1200 ng/dL
		0.7–2.8 nmol/L
		18.3–41.8 nmol/L
			Females:
			Polycystic ovary
			Virilizing tumors
				Males:
				Orchidectomy for
				  neoplastic disease
				  of the prostate
				  or breast
				Estrogen therapy
				Klinefelter's syndrome
				Hypopituitarism
				Hypogonadism
				Hepatic cirrhosis

T₃ (triiodothyronine)
  uptake
	24%–34%	Relative uptake
		  fraction: 0.24–0.34
			Hyperthyroidism
			Thyroxine-binding globulin
			  (TBG) deficiency
			Androgens and anabolic
			  steroids
				Hypothyroidism
				Pregnancy
				TBG excess
				Estrogens and
				  antiovulatory drugs

T₃ total circulating—RIA	70–204 ng/dL	1.08–3.14 nmol/L	Pregnancy Hyperthyroidism	Hypothyroidism

T₄ (thyroxine)—RIA	5–11 μg/dL	65–138 nmol/L	Hyperthyroidism
			Thyroiditis
			Elevated thyroxine-binding
			  proteins caused by oral
			  contraceptives
			Pregnancy
				Primary and pituitary
				  hypothyroidism
				Idiopathic involvement
				Cases of diminished
				  thyroxine-binding
				  proteins caused by
				  androgenic and anabolic
				  steroids
				Hypoproteinemia
				Nephrotic syndrome

T₄, free	0.8–2.7 ng/dL	10.3–35 pmol/L	Euthyroid patients with
			  normal free thyroxine
			  levels may have abnormal
			  T3 and T4 levels caused
			  by drug preparations	

Thyroid-stimulating hormone (TSH)—RIA		0.4–4.2 mIU/L	Hypothyroidism	Hyperthyroidism

Thyroid-binding globulin	10–26 μg/dL	100–260/μg/L	Hypothyroidism
			Pregnancy
			Estrogen therapy
			Oral contraceptive use
			Genetic and idiopathic
			  liver disease
				Use of androgens and
				  anabolic steroids
				Nephrotic syndrome
				Marked hypoproteinemia

Transferrin	200–380 mg/dL	2.3–3.2 g/L	Pregnancy
			Iron deficiency anemia
			  due to hemorrhaging
			Acute hepatitis
			Polycythemia
			Oral contraceptive use
				Pernicious anemia in
				  relapse
				Thalassemic and sickle
				  cell anemia
				Chromatosis
				Neoplastic and hepatic
				  diseases
				Malnutrition

Triglycerides	100–200 mg/dL	1.13–3.8 mmol/L	Increased risk for atherosclerosis	

Troponin
  Troponin I
  Troponin T
	<0.35 ng/mL
	<0.2 ng/mL
		<0.35 μg/L
		<0.2 μg/L
			Myocardial infarction
			Rhabdomyolysis
			Severe crushing injuries	

Tryptophan	1.4–3 mg/dL	68.6–147 nmol/L	Tyrosinosis	Tryptophan-specific malabsorption syndrome
Tyrosine	0.5–4 mg/dL	27.6–220.8 mmol/L	Acute glomerulonephritis	Severe hepatic failure
Urea nitrogen (BUN)	10–20 mg/dL	3.6–7.2 mmol/L	Obstructive uropathy Mercury poisoning Nephrotic syndrome	Pregnancy

Uric acid	2.5–8 mg/dL	0.15–0.5 mmol/L	Gouty arthritis
			Acute leukemia
			Lymphomas treated by
			  chemotherapy
			Toxemia of pregnancy
				Defective tubular
				  reabsorption

Viscosity	1.4–1.8 relative to water
	  at 37°C (98.6°F)
			Patients with marked
			  increases of the gamma
			  globulins
			Hypervitaminosis A	

Continued

Table A-2 REFERENCE RANGES—SERUM, PLASMA, AND WHOLE BLOOD CHEMISTRIES (Continued)

Determination	Normal Adult Reference Range		Clinical Significance	
	Conventional Units	SI Units	Increased	Decreased
Vitamin A	30–120 μg/dL	1.05–4.20 μmol/L		Vitamin A deficiency
				Celiac disease
				Sprue
				Obstructive jaundice
				Giardiasis
				Parenchymal hepatic disease
Vitamin B₁ (thiamine)	1.6–4 μg/dL	47.4–135.7 nmol/L		Anorexia
				Beriberi
				Polyneuropathy
				Cardiomyopathies
Vitamin B₆ (pyridoxal phosphate)	5–30 ng/mL	20–121 nmol/L		Chronic alcoholism
				Malnutrition
				Uremia
				Neonatal seizures
				Malabsorption, such as celiac syndrome
Vitamin B₁₂—RIA	200–900 pg/mL	148–666 pmol/L	Hepatic cell damage and in association with the myeloproliferative disorders (the highest levels are encountered in myeloid leukemia)	Strict vegetarianism
				Alcoholism
				Pernicious anemia
				Total or partial gastrectomy
				Ileal resection
				Sprue and celiac disease
				Fish tapeworm infestation
Vitamin E	0.5–1.8 mg/dL	12–42 μmol/L		Vitamin E deficiency
Xylose absorption test	2 hr, 30–50 mg/dL	2–3.35 mmol/L		Malabsorption syndrome
Zinc	55–150 μg/dL	7.65–22.95 μmol/L	Coronary artery disease	Metastatic liver disease
			Arteriosclerosis	Tuberculosis
			Industrial exposure	Sprue

*By radioimmunoassay.
†Varies among methods.

Table A-3 REFERENCE RANGES—IMMUNODIAGNOSTIC TEST

Determination	Normal Value	Clinical Significance
Acetylcholine receptor binding antibody	Negative or <0.03 nmol/L	Considered to be diagnostic for myasthenia gravis in patients with symptoms.
Anti-ds-DNA antibody	<70 U by enzyme-linked immunosorbent assay (ELISA) <1:20 by indirect fluorescence	Valuable in supporting diagnosis or monitoring disease activity and prognosis of systemic lupus erythematosus (SLE).
Antiglomerular basement membrane antibody	Negative or less than 5εUL	Primarily used in the differential diagnosis of glomerular nephritis induced by antiglomerular basement membrane antibodies from other types of glomerular nephritis.
Anti-insulin antibody	<3% binding of labeled beef and pork insulin by patient's serum; or <9 mIU/L	Helpful in determining the best therapeutic agent in diabetics and the cause of allergic manifestations. Also used to identify insulin resistance.
Antinuclear antibody	Negative, <1:40	Increased in SLE, chronic hepatitis, scleroderma, leukemia, and mononucleosis.
Anti-parietal cell antibody	Negative	Helpful in diagnosing chronic gastric disease and differentiating autoimmune pernicious anemia from other megaloblastic anemias.
Antiribonucleoprotein antibody	Negative	Helpful in differential diagnosis of systemic rheumatic disease.
Antiscleroderma antibody	Negative	Highly diagnostic for scleroderma.
Anti-Smith antibody	Negative	Highly diagnostic of SLE.
Anti-SS-A/anti-SS-B antibody	Negative	SS-A antibodies are found in Sjögren's syndrome alone or associated with lupus. SS-B antibodies are associated with primary Sjögren's syndrome.
Antithyroglobulin and antimicrosomal antibodies	<1:100 titer by gelatin or hemagglutination	Presence and concentration is important in evaluation and treatment of various thyroid disorders, such as Hashimoto's thyroiditis and Graves' disease. May indicate previous antoimmune disorders.
CA 15-3 tumor marker	<30 IU/mL	Increased in metastatic breast cancer.
CA 19-9 tumor marker	<37 IU/mL	Increased in pancreatic, hepatobiliary, gastric, and colorectal cancer, gallstones.

Continued on following page

Table A-3   REFERENCE RANGES—IMMUNODIAGNOSTIC TEST (Continued)

Determination	Normal Value	Clinical Significance
CA 125	0–35 IU/mL	Increased in colon, upper gastrointestinal (GI), ovarian, and other gynecologic cancers: pregnancy, peritonitis.
Carcinoembryonic antigen (CEA)—RLK	0–2.5 μg/L (nonsmoker) 0–5/μg/L (smoker)	The repeatedly high incidence of this antigen in cancers of the colon, rectum, pancreas, and stomach suggests that CEA levels may be useful in the therapeutic monitoring of these conditions, but it is not a screening test.
Cold agglutinins	Negative or <1:32	Increased in mycoplasma pneumonia, viral illness, mononucleosis, multiple myeloma, scleroderma.
C-reactive protein	<1mg/dL (<10 mg/L)	Increase indicates active inflammation.
High sensitivity assay for C-reactive protein (hs-CRP)	0.2–8.0 mg/L	Cardiovascular disease risk.
Cytomegalovirus antibodies (CMV IgG)	Negative: <0.9 units/mL	Positive >1:0 unit/mL if exposed to CMV at any time. Acute and convalescent specimens can help identify acute infection.
Cytomegalovirus antibodies (CMV IgM)	Negative: <0:79 Equivocal: 0:80–1.20	Positive >1:20 usually indicates acute infection. Repeat specimen in 1–2 weeks for equivocal result.
Epstein-Barr virus serology (viral capsid antigen IgG and IgM, early antigen IgG, and nuclear antigen IgG)	Negative: <1:20 or <1:20 for each individual test	Differentiation of acute from chronic or old infection by interpretation of table below.

EBV Interpretation

	VCA-IgG	VCA-IgM	EA-IgG	EBV-NA
Susceptible	−	−	−	−
Acute infection	+	+	±	−
Convalescent phase	+	±	±	+
Chronic or reactivated	+	−	+	±
Old infection	±	−	−	+

Antibody present: +
Antibody absent: −
VCA, viral capsid antigen; EA, early antigen; EBV-NA, Epstein Barr virus-nuclear antigen

Hepatitis A virus antibodies, IgM (HAV-Ab/IgM)	Negative	Positive in acute-stage hepatitis A; develops early in disease.
Hepatitis A virus antibodies, IgG (HAV-Ab/IgG)	Negative	Positive if previous exposure and immunity to hepatitis A.
Hepatitis B surface antigen (HBsAg)	Negative	Positive in acute-stage hepatitis B.
Hepatitis B surface antibody (HBsAb)	Negative	Positive if previous exposure and immunity to hepatitis B.
Hepatitis C virus antibodies	Negative	Positive in exposure to hepatitis C virus; may indicate acute, chronic, or cleared infection.
Hepatitis C virus RNA	Negative	Positive in hepatitis C infection, can be quantitative
Homocysteine	0.54–2.30 mg/L (4–17 μmol/L)	Cardiovascular disease risk Folic acid deficiency Vitamin B_{12} deficiency
Infectious mononucleosis tests (monospot, monotest, heterophile antigen test, Epstein-Barr virus [EBV], antiviral capsid antigen IgM and IgG)	Negative	Positive monospot and monotest are presumptive, positive EBV IgM and IgG indicate acute and recent or past infection, respectively.
Lyme disease titer	Negative, <1:256 by indirect fluorescent antibody method; nonreactive by ELISA	Positive results help diagnose Lyme disease. False positive may occur with high rheumatoid factor titers or syphilis. Positive ELISA confirmed by Western blot test.
Pyroglobulin test	Negative	These abnormal proteins may be associated with myeloma, lymphoma, polycythemia vera, and SLE.
Rheumatoid factor	Negative or less than 40 IU/mL	Elevated in rheumatoid arthritis, lupus endocarditis, tuberculosis, syphilis, sarcoidosis, cancer.
T and B cell lymphocyte surface markers T-helper/T-suppressor ratio	T and B cell lymphocyte surface markers: Percent T cells (CD2) 60–88% Percent helper cells (CD4) 34–67% Percent suppressor cells (CD8) 10–42% Percent B cells (CD19) 3–21% Absolute counts: Lymphocytes 0.66–4.60 thou/mL T cells 644–2201 cells/mL Helper cells 493–1191 cells/mL Suppressor T cells 182–785 cells/mL B cells 92–392 cells/mL Lymphocyte ratio: T_H/T_S ratio >1	Used to evaluate immune system by identifying the specific cells involved in the immune response. Valuable in diagnosis of lymphocytic leukemia, lymphoma, and immunodeficiency diseases including acquired immunodeficiency syndrome, and in the assessment of patient response to chemotherapy and radiation.

Table A-4   REFERENCE RANGES—URINE CHEMISTRY

	Normal Adult Reference Range		Clinical Significance	
Determination	Conventional Units	SI Units	Increased	Decreased
Acetone and acetoacetate	Zero		Diabetic ketoacidosis Starvation	
Aldosterone	With normal salt diet: Normal: 4–20 µg/24 h Renovascular: 10–40 µg/24 h Tumor: 20–100 µg/24 h	11.1–55.5 nmol/24h 27.7–111 nmol/24 h 55.4–277 nmol/24 h	Primary aldosteronism (adrenocortical tumor) Secondary aldosteronism Salt depletion Potassium loading ACTH in large doses Cardiac failure Cirrhosis with ascites formation Nephrosis Pregnancy	
Alpha amino nitrogen	50–200 mg/24 h	3.6–14.3 nmol/24 h	Leukemia Phenylketonuria Other metabolic diseases	
Amylase	35–260 units excreted per h	6.5–48.1 U/h	Acute pancreatitis	
Arylsulfatase A	>2.4 U/mL			
Bence-Jones protein	None detected		Myeloma	Metachromatic leukodystrophy
Calcium	100–250 mg/24 h	2.5–6.2 mmol/24 h	Hyperparathyroidism Vitamin D intoxication Fanconi's syndrome	Hypoparathyroidism
Catecholamines	Total: 0–275 µg/24 h Epinephrine: 10%–40% Norepinephrine: 60%–90%	0–275 µg/24 h Fraction total: 0.10–8.4 Fraction total: 0.60–0.90	Pheochromocytoma Neuroblastoma	Vitamin D deficiency
Chorionic gonadotrophin, qualitative (pregnancy test)	Negative		Pregnancy Chorionepithelioma Hydatidiform mole	
Copper	15–60 µg/24 h	0.22–0.9 µmol/24 h	Wilson's diseases Cirrhosis Nephrosis	
Coproporphyrin	50–300 µg/24 h	0.075–0.45 µmol/24 h	Poliomyelitis Lead poisoning Porphyria	
Cortisol, free	20–90 µg/24 h	55.2–248.4 nmol/d	Cushing's syndrome	
Creatinine	Males: 1–2 g/24 h Females: 0.8–1.8 g/24 h	8.8–17.7 mmol/24 h 7.1–15.9 mmol/24 h	Muscular dystrophy Fever Carcinoma of liver Pregnancy Hyperthyroidism Myositis	
Creatine	0–270 mg/24 h	0–2.05 mmol/24 h	Typhoid fever Salmonella infections Tetanus	Muscular atrophy Anemia Advanced degeneration of kidneys Leukemia
Creatinine clearance	Males: 85–125 mL/min Females: 75–115 mL/min	1.42–2.08 mL/s 1.25–1.92 mL/s		Renal diseases
Cystine and cysteine	10–100 mg/24 h	0.08–0.83 mmol/24 h	Cystinuria	
Delta aminolevulinic acid	0–0.54 mg/dL	0–40/µmol/L	Lead poisoning Porphyria hepatica Hepatitis Hepatic carcinoma	
11-Desoxycortisol	20–100 µg/24 h	0.6–2.9/µmol/d	Hypertensive form of virilizing adrenal hyperplasia due to an 11-beta hydroxylase defect	
Estriol (placental)	Weeks of pregnancy 12 16 20 24 28 32 36 40	µm/24 h <1 2–7 4–9 6–13 8–22 12–43 14–45 19–46	mmol/24 h <3.5 7–24.5 14–32 21–45.5 28–77 42–150 49–158 66.5–160	Decreased values occur with fetal distress of many conditions, including preeclampsia, placental insufficiency, and poorly controlled diabetes mellitus

Continued on following page

Table A-4   REFERENCE RANGES—URINE CHEMISTRY   (Continued)

Determination	Normal Adult Reference Range		Clinical Significance	
	Conventional Units	SI Units	Increased	Decreased
Estrogens, total (fluorometric)	Females: Onset of menstruation: 4–25 μg/24 h	4–25 μg/24 h	Hyperestrogenism due to gonadal or adrenal neoplasm	Primary or secondary amenorrhea
	Ovulation peak: 28–100 μg/24 h	28–100 μg/24 h		
	Luteal peak: 22–105 μg/24 h	22–105 μg/24 h		
	Menopausal: 1.4–19.6 μg/24 h	1.4–19.6 μg/24 h		
	Males: 5–18 μg/24 h	5–18 μg/24 h		
Etiocholanolone	Males: 1.9–6 mg/24 h	6.5–20.6 μmol/24 h	Adrenogenital syndrome	
	Females: 0.5–4 mg/24 h	1.7–13.8 μmol/24 h	Idiopathic hirsutism	
Follicle-stimulating hormone—RIA	Females: Follicular: 5–20 IU/24 h	5–20 IU/d	Menopause and primary ovarian failure	Pituitary failure
	Luteal: 5–15 IU/24 h	5–15 IU/d		
	Midcycle: 15–60 IU/24 h	15–60 IU/d		
	Menopausal: 50–100 IU/24 h	50–100 IU/d		
	Males: 5–25 IU/24 h	5–25 IU/d		
Glucose	Negative		Diabetes mellitus	
			Pituitary disorders	
			Increased ICP	
			Lesion in floor of 4th ventricle	
Hemoglobin and myoglobin	Negative		Extensive burns	
			Transfusion of incompatible blood	
			Myoglobin increased in severe crushing injuries to muscles	
Homovanillic acid		5.5–27.5 μmol/d	Neuroblastoma	Addison's disease
17-hydroxycortic-osteroids	8 mg/24 h 2–10 mg/24 h	5.5–27.5 μmol/d	Cushing's disease	Anterior pituitary hypofunction
5-Hydroxyindoleacetic acid, qualitative	Negative		Malignant carcinoid tumors	
17-ketosteroids, total	Males: 10–22 mg/24 h	35–76 μmol/24h	Interstitial cell tumor of testes	Thyrotoxicosis
	Females: 6–16 mg/24 h	21–55 μmol/24h	Simple hirsutism, occasionally	Female hypogonadism
				Diabetes mellitus
			Adrenal hyperplasia	Hypertension
			Cushing's syndrome	Debilitating disease of mild to moderate severity
			Adrenal cancer, virilism	Eunuchoidism
			Adrenoblastoma	Addison's disease
				Panhypopituitarism
				Myxedema
				Nephrosis
Lead	<125 μg/24 h	<60 μmol/24 h	Lead poisoning	
Luteinizing hormone	Males: 5–18 IU/24 h		Pituitary tumor	Failure of pituitary or hypothalamus
	Females:		Ovarian failure	Anorexia nervosa
	Follicular phase: 2–25 IU/24 h	2–25 IU/d		
	Ovulatory peak: 30–95 IU/24 h	30–95 IU/d		
	Luteal phase: 2–20 IU/24 h	2–20 IU/d		
	Postmenopausal: 40–110 IU/24 h	40–110 IU/d		
Metanephrines, total	<1.4 mg/24 h	<7 μmol/24h	Pheochromocytoma; a few patients with pheochromocytoma may have elevated urinary metanephrines but normal catecholamines and vanillylmandelic acid (VMA)	
Osmolality	250–900 mOsm/kg	250–900 mmol/kg	Useful in the study of electrolyte and water balance	

Continued

Table A-4   REFERENCE RANGES—URINE CHEMISTRY (Continued)

| Determination | Normal Adult Reference Range | | Clinical Significance | |
	Conventional Units	SI Units	Increased	Decreased
Oxalate	Up to 45 mg/24 h	Up to 500/μmol/24 h	Primary hyperoxaluria	
Phenylpyruvic acid qualitative	Negative		Phenylketonuria	
Phosphorus, inorganic	0.9–1.3 g/24 h	29–42 mmol/24 h	Hypoparathyroidism Vitamin D intoxication Paget's disease Metastatic neoplasm to bone	Hypoparathyroidism Vitamin D deficiency
Porphobilinogen, qualitative	Negative		Chronic lead poisoning Acute porphyria Liver disease	
Porphobilinogen quantitative	0–1 mg/24 h	0–4.4 μmol/24 h	Acute porphyria Liver disease	
Porphyrins, qualitative	Negative		See porphyrins, quantitative	
Porphyrins, quantitative (coproporphyrin and uroporphyrin)	Coproporphyrin: 50–160 μg/24 h Uroporphyrin: up to 50 μg/24 h	0.075–0.24 μmol/24h Up to 0.06 μmol/24 h	Porphyria Lead poisoning (only coproporphyrin increased)	
Potassium	26–123 mEq/24 h	26–123 mmol/24 h	Hemolysis Chronic renal failure Acidosis Cushing's disease Corpus luteum cysts	Diarrhea Adrenocortical insufficiency
Pregnanediol	Females: Proliferative phase: 0.5–1.5 mg/24 h Luteal phase: 2–7 mg/24 h Menopause: 0.2–1 mg/24 h	1.6–4.8 μmol/24 h 6–22 μmol/24 h 0.6–3.1 μmol/24 h	When placental tissue remains in the uterus following parturition Some cases of adrenocortical tumors	Placental dysfunction Threatened abortion Intrauterine death
Pregnancy: Weeks of gestation 10–12 12–18 18–24 24–28 28–32	mg/24 h 5–15 5–25 15–33 20–42 27–47	μmol/24 h 15.6–47 15.6–78.0 47.0–103.0 62.4–131.0 84.2–146.6		
Pregnanetriol	Females: 0.1–2.2 mg/24 h Males: 0.4–2.5 mg/24 h	0.3–6.5 μmol/24 h 1.2–7.5 μmol/24 h	Congenital adrenal androgenic hyperplasia	
Protein	<150 mg/24 h	<150 mg/24 h	Nephritis Cardiac failure Mercury poisoning Bence-Jones protein in multiple myeloma Febrile states Hematuria	
Sodium	75–200 mEq/24 h	75–200 mmol/24 h	Useful in detecting gross changes in water and salt balance	
Titratable acidity	20–40 mEq/24 h	20–40 mmol/24 h	Metabolic acidosis	Metabolic alkalosis
Urea nitrogen	9–16 gm/24 h	0.32–0.57 mol/L	Excessive protein catabolism	Impaired kidney function
Uric acid	250–750 mg/24 h	1.48–4.43 mmol/24 h	Gout	Nephritis
Urobilinogen	Random urine: <0.25 mg/dL 24-hour urine: up to 4 mg/24 h	<0.42 mol/24 h Up to 6.76 μmol/24 h	Liver and biliary tract disease Hemolytic anemias	Complete or nearly complete biliary obstruction Diarrhea
Vanillylmandelic acid (VMA)	0.7–6.8 mg/24 h	3.5–34.3 μmol/24 h	Pheochromocytoma Neuroblastoma Ingestion of coffee, tea, aspirin, bananas, and several different drugs	Renal insufficiency
Xylose absorption test (5-hour)	16%–33% of ingested xylose	Fraction absorbed: 0.16–0.33		
Zinc	0.15–1.2 mg/24 h	2.3–18.4 μmol/24h		Malabsorption syndromes

TABLE A-5 REFERENCE RANGES—CEREBROSPINAL FLUID (CSF)

Determination	Normal Adult Reference Range		Clinical Significance	
	Conventional Units	SI Units	Increased	Decreased
Albumin	15–30 mg/dL	150–300 mg/L	Certain neurologic disorders Lesion in the choroid plexus or blockage of the flow of CSF Damage to the blood–brain barrier	
Cell count (white blood cells)	0–5 cells per cu mm	$0–5 \times 10^6$/L	Bacterial meningitis Neurosyphilis Anterior poliomyelitis Encephalitis lethargica	
Chloride	120–130 mEq/L	120–130 mmol/L	Uremia	Acute generalized meningitis Tuberculous meningitis
Glucose	40–80 mg/dL; 50%–80% of blood glucose value	2.75–4.13 mmol/L	Diabetes mellitus Diabetic coma Epidemic encephalitis Uremia	Acute meningitis Tuberculous meningitis Insulin shock Subarachnoid hemorrhage
Glutamine	6–15 mg/dL	0.41–1 mmol/L	Hepatic encephalopathies, including Reye's syndrome Hepatic coma Cirrhosis	
IgG	<5 mg/dL	<50 mg/L	Damage to the blood– brain barrier Multiple sclerosis Neurosyphilis Subacute sclerosing panencephalitis Chronic phases of CNS infections	
Lactic acid	4.5–28.8 mg/dL	0.5–3.2 mmol/L	Bacterial meningitis Hypocapnia Hydrocephalus Brain abscesses Cerebral ischemia Fungal meningitis	
Lactate dehydrogenase	1/10 that of serum level	Activity fraction: 0.1 of serum	CNS disease Acute meningitis	
Protein	16–45 mg/dL	150–450 mg/L	Tubercular meningitis Neurosyphilis Poliomyelitis Guillain-Barré syndrome Subdural hematoma Brain tumor Multiple sclerosis	

TABLE A-6   MISCELLANEOUS VALUES

Determination	Normal Values	Clinical Significance	
		Conventional Units	**SI Units**
Acetaminophen	Zero	Therapeutic level = 10–30 µg/mL	10–30 mg/L
Aminophylline (theophylline)	Zero	Therapeutic level = 10–20/µg/mL	10–20 mg/L
Bromide	Zero	Therapeutic level = 5–50 mg/dL	50–500 mg/L
Carbamazepine	Zero	Therapeutic level = 4–12 µg/mL	34–51 µmol/L
Carbon monoxide	0%–2%	Symptoms with 10%–30% saturation	
Chlordiazepoxide	Zero	Therapeutic level = 0.7–1.0 µg/mL	0.7–1.0 mg/L
Diazepam	Zero	Therapeutic level = 0.2–1.0 µg/mL	0.2–1.0 mg/L
Digitoxin	Zero	Therapeutic level = 18–35 ng/mL	18–35 µg/L
Digoxin	Zero	Therapeutic level = 0.8–2 ng/mL	0.8–2/µg/L
Ethanol	0%–0.01%	Legal intoxication level = 0.1% or above	
		0.3%–0.4% = marked intoxication	
		0.4%–0.5% = alcoholic stupor	
Fosphenytoin	Zero	10–20 mg/L	
Gentamicin	Zero	Therapeutic level = 4–10 µg/mL	4–10 mg/L
Lithium	Zero	Therapeutic level = 0.6–1.2 mEq/L	0.6–1.2 mmol/L
Methanol	Zero	May be fatal in concentration as low as 10 mg/dL	100 mg/L
Phenobarbital	Zero	Therapeutic level = 15–40 µg/mL	15–40 mg/L
Phenytoin	Zero	Therapeutic level = 10–20 µg/mL	10–20 mg/L
Primidone	Zero	Therapeutic level = 5–12 µg/mL	5–12 mg/L
Quinidine	Zero	Therapeutic level = 0.2–0.5 mg/dL	2–5 mg/L
Salicylate	Zero	Therapeutic level = 2–25 mg/dL	20–250 mg/L
		Toxic level = >30 mg/dL	300 mg/L
Vancomycin	Zero	Therapeutic peak 20–40 µg/mL	
Amitriptyline	Zero	Therapeutic trough 5–10 µg/mL	
		Therapeutic level 80–200 ng/mL	289–722 nmol/L
Doxepin	Zero	Therapeutic level 150–250 ng/mL (includes metabolites)	540–900 nmol/L
Imipramine	Zero	Therapeutic level 100–300 ng/mL (includes metabolites)	360–1070 nmol/L
Lidocaine	Zero	Therapeutic level 1.5–5 µg/mL	6.4–21.4 µmol/L
Methotrexate	Zero	Toxic (48 h after high dose) 454 mg/mL	1000 mmol/L
Propranolol	Zero	Therapeutic level 50–100 ng/mL	193–386 nmol/L
Valproic acid	Zero	Therapeutic level 50–100 ng/mL	347–693 µmol/L

REFERENCES

1. *Jacobs and Demott's Laboratory Test Handbook.* 5th ed. Lexi-Comp. Inc. Hudson (OH), 2001.

2. Traub SL. *Basic Skills in Interpreting Laboratory Data.* 2nd ed. American Society of Health-Systems Pharmacy, Bethesda, 1996.

3. www.bioscientia.de

4. http://www.gpnotebook.co.uk/simplepage.cfm?ID=429195241&linkID=8734

5. www.bloodbook.com/ranges.html

6. http://www.buymedicals.com/MedicalInfo/2-urine.asp

7. http://thailabonline.com/lab-normalrange1.htm

8. Directory of Services and Interpretive Guide. LabCorp. 2001.

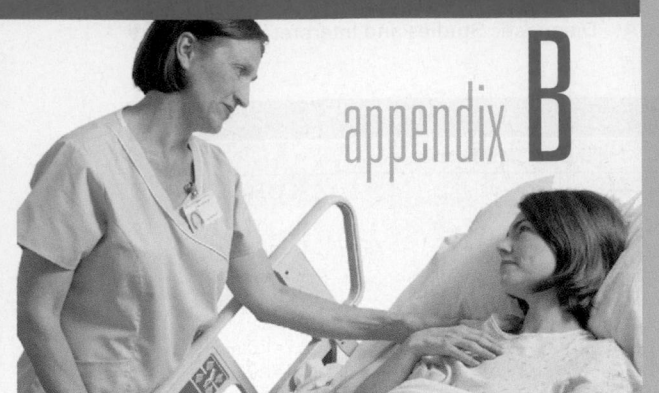

Understanding Clinical Pathways

Clinical pathways (also called critical pathways) are care plans developed collaboratively by physicians, nurses, physical and occupational therapists, technicians, pharmacists, speech therapists, case managers, and other staff members involved in patient care. Nurses are instrumental in ensuring the successful use of clinical pathways and can best contribute by gaining a thorough understanding of why and how pathways are used.

Understanding and Using Clinical Pathways in Patient Care

Clinical pathways grew out of financial upheaval in the health care industry. They represent a significant change in how patient care is managed. In the past (and currently for many patients), each health care discipline developed its own plan of care and used the patient's medical record as the primary communication tool. Each care provider needed to read the notes of health care providers of other disciplines to get a complete picture of the plan of care and the patient's progress. Although there was probably general agreement about how patient progress would be facilitated and measured, individual steps in the processes of care and outcomes to be achieved were often not identified and communicated. The physician managed the case and most patients remained in the hospital until they required very little care or could be discharged home or transferred to a convalescent center. A hospital stay of 2 to 3 weeks in an acute care facility was not unusual.

Cost and Effects

Although this system worked for decades, it was expensive. The federal government and insurance companies balked at paying these costs when highly skilled care was no longer needed. As a result, the number of days of hospitalization that a patient with a specific diagnosis required was determined. Then insured parties were paid only for that number of days. Decreasing the length of stay was seen as one way to decrease costs and save money. Patients were discharged to home or rehabilitation centers much sooner than before. They were weaker, had relatively fresh incisions, or often could not independently perform even minimal self-care. As hospital stays became shorter, nurses, physicians, consumers, and regulatory agencies expressed concerns about the quality of care. These concerns compelled hospital administrators and clinicians to develop new ways to measure and manage costs, quality, and outcomes. Assessment of how patient care was provided exposed inefficiencies, including lack of face-to-face communication among disciplines. Case management was developed and widely adopted to provide more cost-effective care while saving hundreds of thousands of dollars yearly.

Case Management

Using the case management model, care is planned collaboratively so that important events, such as initiation of physical therapy, home care consultation, or discontinuation of invasive treatments, occur on a schedule that clinicians, through research or experience, have identified as optimum for enhancing recovery. Care is mapped out by day or by other pivotal time intervals, and goals or desired outcomes are specified for each time frame. When the patient has met all the goals, he or she is ready for discharge to home or to the next level of care. Responsibility for monitoring the patient's progress and tracking variance or deviation from the pathway is given to the case manager, who usually (but not always) is a nurse. The tool on which all this information is contained is the clinical pathway. The purposes of a clinical pathway are to
- Promote quality care and improve clinical outcomes
- Standardize important aspects of care
- Reduce unnecessary delays in care
- Reduce costs

Elements of a Clinical Pathway

Clinical pathways are now used in a variety of settings and cover diverse diagnoses and conditions. They are often developed by individual organizations and, although the format varies from institution to institution, clinical pathways have major features in common.

Patient Population

The first important element of the clinical pathway is the patient population (Fig. B-1A). Each pathway clearly specifies those patients who are appropriate for inclusion on the pathway. Pathways tend to cover patient groups in which the treatment and recovery are relatively predictable. Diagnosis-related groups (DRGs) are usually used to identify patients for a specific pathway, but qualifiers may be added. For example, a pathway for community-acquired pneumonia may exclude patients with *Pneumocystis* pneumonia or underlying obstructive pulmonary disease because those patients require highly individualized treatment plans and may not respond as quickly to intervention as patients without these underlying disorders.

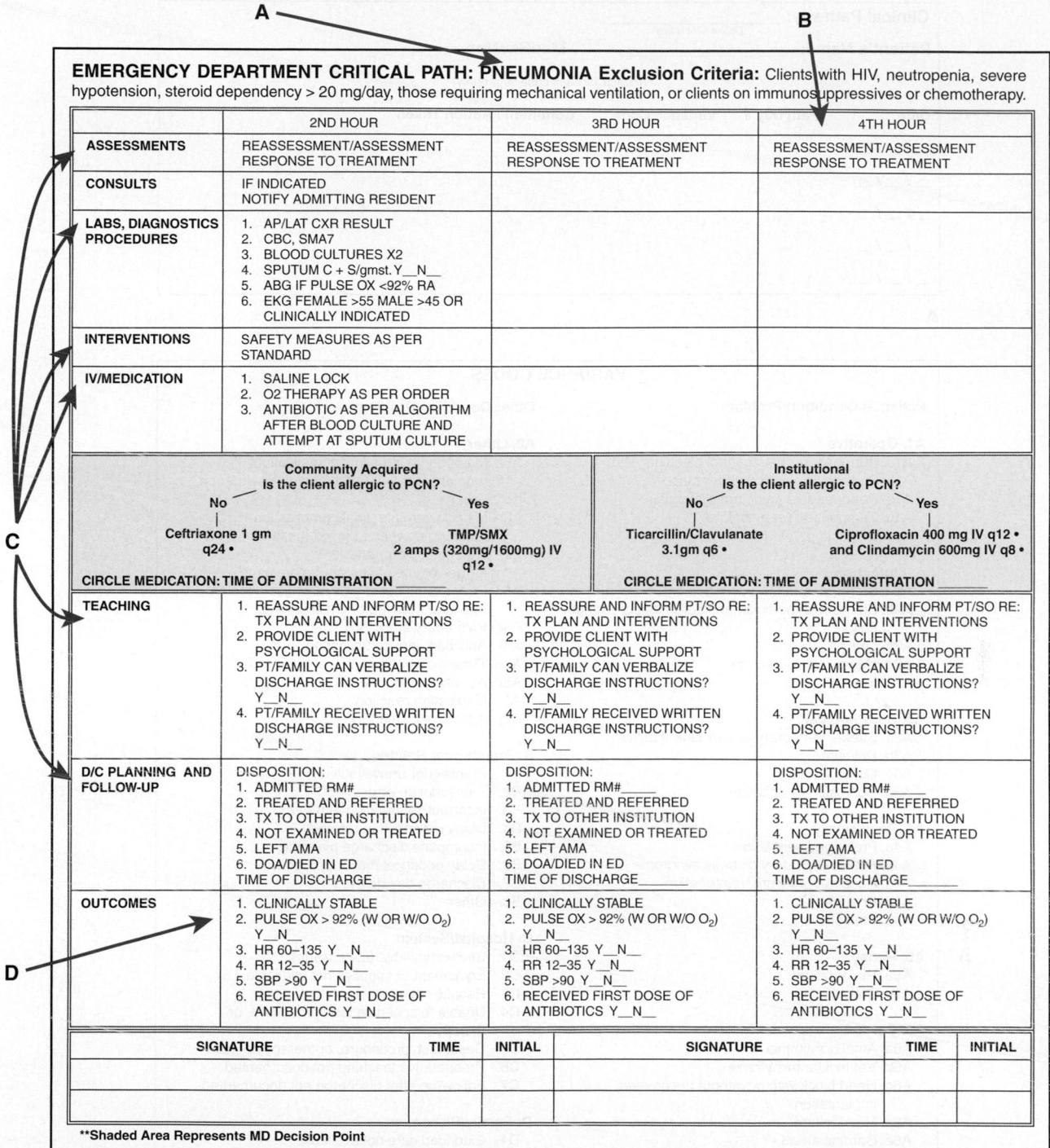

EMERGENCY DEPARTMENT CRITICAL PATH: PNEUMONIA Exclusion Criteria: Clients with HIV, neutropenia, severe hypotension, steroid dependency > 20 mg/day, those requiring mechanical ventilation, or clients on immunosuppressives or chemotherapy.

	2ND HOUR	3RD HOUR	4TH HOUR
ASSESSMENTS	REASSESSMENT/ASSESSMENT RESPONSE TO TREATMENT	REASSESSMENT/ASSESSMENT RESPONSE TO TREATMENT	REASSESSMENT/ASSESSMENT RESPONSE TO TREATMENT
CONSULTS	IF INDICATED NOTIFY ADMITTING RESIDENT		
LABS, DIAGNOSTICS PROCEDURES	1. AP/LAT CXR RESULT 2. CBC, SMA7 3. BLOOD CULTURES X2 4. SPUTUM C + S/gmst. Y__N__ 5. ABG IF PULSE OX <92% RA 6. EKG FEMALE >55 MALE >45 OR CLINICALLY INDICATED		
INTERVENTIONS	SAFETY MEASURES AS PER STANDARD		
IV/MEDICATION	1. SALINE LOCK 2. O2 THERAPY AS PER ORDER 3. ANTIBIOTIC AS PER ALGORITHM AFTER BLOOD CULTURE AND ATTEMPT AT SPUTUM CULTURE		

Community Acquired Is the client allergic to PCN?		**Institutional** Is the client allergic to PCN?	
No — Ceftriaxone 1 gm q24 •	Yes — TMP/SMX 2 amps (320mg/1600mg) IV q12 •	No — Ticarcillin/Clavulanate 3.1gm q6 •	Yes — Ciprofloxacin 400 mg IV q12 • and Clindamycin 600mg IV q8 •
CIRCLE MEDICATION: TIME OF ADMINISTRATION _____		CIRCLE MEDICATION: TIME OF ADMINISTRATION _____	

TEACHING	1. REASSURE AND INFORM PT/SO RE: TX PLAN AND INTERVENTIONS 2. PROVIDE CLIENT WITH PSYCHOLOGICAL SUPPORT 3. PT/FAMILY CAN VERBALIZE DISCHARGE INSTRUCTIONS? Y__N__ 4. PT/FAMILY RECEIVED WRITTEN DISCHARGE INSTRUCTIONS? Y__N__	1. REASSURE AND INFORM PT/SO RE: TX PLAN AND INTERVENTIONS 2. PROVIDE CLIENT WITH PSYCHOLOGICAL SUPPORT 3. PT/FAMILY CAN VERBALIZE DISCHARGE INSTRUCTIONS? Y__N__ 4. PT/FAMILY RECEIVED WRITTEN DISCHARGE INSTRUCTIONS? Y__N__	1. REASSURE AND INFORM PT/SO RE: TX PLAN AND INTERVENTIONS 2. PROVIDE CLIENT WITH PSYCHOLOGICAL SUPPORT 3. PT/FAMILY CAN VERBALIZE DISCHARGE INSTRUCTIONS? Y__N__ 4. PT/FAMILY RECEIVED WRITTEN DISCHARGE INSTRUCTIONS? Y__N__
D/C PLANNING AND FOLLOW-UP	DISPOSITION: 1. ADMITTED RM#____ 2. TREATED AND REFERRED 3. TX TO OTHER INSTITUTION 4. NOT EXAMINED OR TREATED 5. LEFT AMA 6. DOA/DIED IN ED TIME OF DISCHARGE_____	DISPOSITION: 1. ADMITTED RM#____ 2. TREATED AND REFERRED 3. TX TO OTHER INSTITUTION 4. NOT EXAMINED OR TREATED 5. LEFT AMA 6. DOA/DIED IN ED TIME OF DISCHARGE_____	DISPOSITION: 1. ADMITTED RM#____ 2. TREATED AND REFERRED 3. TX TO OTHER INSTITUTION 4. NOT EXAMINED OR TREATED 5. LEFT AMA 6. DOA/DIED IN ED TIME OF DISCHARGE_____
OUTCOMES	1. CLINICALLY STABLE 2. PULSE OX > 92% (W OR W/O O2) Y__N__ 3. HR 60–135 Y__N__ 4. RR 12–35 Y__N__ 5. SBP >90 Y__N__ 6. RECEIVED FIRST DOSE OF ANTIBIOTICS Y__N__	1. CLINICALLY STABLE 2. PULSE OX > 92% (W OR W/O O2) Y__N__ 3. HR 60–135 Y__N__ 4. RR 12–35 Y__N__ 5. SBP >90 Y__N__ 6. RECEIVED FIRST DOSE OF ANTIBIOTICS Y__N__	1. CLINICALLY STABLE 2. PULSE OX > 92% (W OR W/O O2) Y__N__ 3. HR 60–135 Y__N__ 4. RR 12–35 Y__N__ 5. SBP >90 Y__N__ 6. RECEIVED FIRST DOSE OF ANTIBIOTICS Y__N__

SIGNATURE	TIME	INITIAL	SIGNATURE	TIME	INITIAL

**Shaded Area Represents MD Decision Point

Figure B-1 Key elements of a clinical pathway. (**A**) Patient population clearly defined. (**B**) Clinically meaningful time frames. (**C**) Interventional categories. (**D**) Outcomes for each time frame should be specific and measurable. Reproduced with permission from Graduate Hospital, Philadelphia, Pennsylvania.

Time Frames

All pathways are divided into useful time frames, for example, minutes, hours, days, weeks, or phases (Fig. B-1B). Conditions requiring emergency treatment (eg, myocardial infarction, head injury, stroke) might be divided into 15-minute intervals, whereas conditions requiring chronic care (eg, chronic pain, spinal cord injury rehabilitation) may be divided into weekly or monthly intervals. An example of interventions by phases might be seen in postanesthesia care pathways.

Clinical Pathway: _____
(Department Name)

Patient's Name: _____   **MedRecNo:** _ _ _ _ _ _

(Please list each code separately)

Date	Path Day #	Variance Code	Comment / Action Taken
__/__/__			
__/__/__			
__/__/__			
__/__/__			
__/__/__			

A

VARIANCE CODES

Patient's Condition/Problem

A1. Operative
A1a. Further surgery to control bleeding
A1b. Further surgery for other reason
A1c. Perioperative myocardial infarction
A1d. Tamponade (early or late)
A1e. Dissection

A2. Infection
A2a. Sternum, requiring debridement
A2b. Sternum, superficial (antibiotics and dressings only)
A2c. Leg
A2d. Urinary tract infection
A2e. Sepsis

A3. Neurological
A3a. Stroke, temporary or permanent deficit
A3b. Delirium
A3c. Coma
A3d. Confusion or agitation

A4. Respiratory
A4a. Prolonged ventilation
A4b. Acute respiratory distress syndrome
A4c. Respiratory failure, reintubation
A4d. Pneumonia
A4e. Atelectasis

A5. Renal
A5a. Renal failure
A5b. Dialysis

A6. Cardiac
A6a. Atrial arrhythmia
A6b. Ventricular arrhythmia
A6c. Heart block with or without pacemaker implantation
A6d. Heart failure
A6e. Cardiac arrest
A6f. Hemodynamic instability
A6g. Unable to wean off inotropic agents

A7. Vascular
A7a. Deep vein thrombosis
A7b. Limb ischemia

Other Condition/Problem

A8. Other
A8a. Major gastrointestinal complication requiring surgery (eg, bleeding, perforation, ileus)
A8b. Minor gastrointestinal complication requiring bowel rest (eg, ileus, nausea, high nasogastric output)
A8c. Large volume of chest-tube drainage
A8d. Poor wound healing (ie, significant sterile drainage from leg or chest wound)
A8e. Pulmonary embolism
A8f. Anticoagulant complication
A8g. Thromboembolism
A8h. Activity intolerance
A8i. Medication reaction
A8j. Altered skin integrity

B: Practitioner Related
B1. Practitioner unavailability
B2. Transcription error
B3. Incorrect sequencing of therapy
B4. Delay in consult or referral
B5. Incomplete discharge planning
B6. Delay or cancel test or procedure
B7. Discharge day delay
B8. Other

C: Hospital/System
C1. Bed unavailable (state issue)
C2. Equipment or supplies not available
C3. Results not available
C4. Unable to schedule test, procedure, or therapy
C5. Case, test, procedure, or therapy delayed
C6. Preoperative teaching not documented
C7. Follow-up after discharge not documented

D: Family/Placement
D1. Extended care not available
D2. Homecare not available
D3. Patient or family delaying discharge planning
D4. Financial issues
D5. Other

Form used at Westchester County Medical Center for tracking variances from clinical pathway for cardiac surgery (CABG).

B

Figure B-2 Variance record. (**A**) Blank pages for recording variance. (**B**) Variance codes. Reproduced with permission from *Critical Care Nurse, 17*(16), December 1997, pp. 29–30.

Acute Ischemic Stroke Critical Pathway Card

	Admission Day Day 0-1 (1st 24 hrs) ER to ASU/NICU (or direct to ASU) / /	Day 2 ASU / /	Day 3 ASU/General Floor / /
Goals/Outcomes	Identify acute ischemic stroke patient Document time of symptom onset Evaluate for appropriate treatment options and/or clinical trial Avoid Aspiration **NIH Stroke Scale (NIHSS)** _____ **Barthel Index** _____	Neuro status stabilized/improved Avoid medical complications (Aspiration, Fever, Infection) Initial Diagnostic tests results documented Rehab therapies initiated as appropriate **t-PA pts. transferred from NICU to ASU**	Neuro status stabilized/improved Avoid medical complications Diagnostic tests documented Rehab therapies continued as appropriate Pt/Family understands disease process **Transfer from ASU→Floor** Discharge if appropriate **NIHSS** _____ **Barthel Index** _____ (upon dischrg)

**Laboratory/
Diagnostic Tests**
	STAT CT brain CBC, PT/PTT
	  without contrast SMA-7
	EKG SMA-12
	CXR ESR
	Carotid Dopplers RPR
	Echocardiogram UA (if febrile)
	  To Consider: **To Consider:**
	   • MRI/MRA • ACLA, LA
	   • CTA • ANA, RF
	   • TCD • Fibrinogen level
	    • Protein C & S, AT III
	     (if age <55; venous infarct)
		Fasting Lipid profile
		Fasting Homocysteine level
		Follow up on abnormal tests as needed
		PTT daily if on heparin
		PT/INR daily if on warfarin
		If patient received t-PA:
		   CT brain without contrast
		To Consider:
		   • **MRI/MRA**
		   • CTA
		   • TCD (if VB circulation)
		   • TEE
			PTT if on heparin
			PT/INR if on warfarin
			Follow-up abnormal tests
			
			To Consider:
			   • Modified Barum Swallow
			   • SPECT
			   • Angiogram

**Assessments/RN
Interventions**
	VS as per Unit/t-PA protocol
	Neuro check as per Unit/t-PA protocol
	Cardiac monitoring
	Continuous Pulse Ox, and titrate O$_2$ to keep
	    SpO$_2$ > 95%
	Bowel/Bladder/Skin assessment
	Avoid foley cath
	Compression boots (unless anticoagulated)
	HOB up 30°/Aspiration Precautions
	Institute Falls Risk Precautions
	Barthel Index completed and documented
		VS and Neuro checks per Unit protocol
		Cardiac monitoring
		Continuous Pulse Ox, and titrate O$_2$ to keep
		    SpO$_2$ > 95%
		Bowel/Bladder/Skin assessment
		Avoid foley cath
		Compression boots (unless anticoagulated)
		HOB up 30°/Aspiration Precautions
		Pulmonary toilet
		Turn q2h if pt on bed rest
		ROM as per Rehab if paralysis exists
		Hand/foot splint as per Rehab as needed
			VS and Neuro checks per Unit protocol
			Cardiac monitoring (ASU)
			Continuous Pulse Ox, and titrate O$_2$ to keep
			    SpO$_2$ > 95%
			Bowel/Bladder/Skin assessment
			Avoid foley cath
			Compression boots (unless anticoagulated)
			HOB up 30°/Aspiration Precautions
			Pulmonary toilet
			Turn q2h if pt on bed rest
			ROM as per Rehab, if paralysis exists
			Hand/foot splint as per Rehab as needed
			
			To Consider:
			   • D/C cardiace monitor & Pulse Ox & transfer to floor
			    -or-
			   • D/C to home

**Medications/
Treatments**
	IV NSS
	Evaluate admission medications
	BP meds w/parameters as needed
	Acetaminophen 650 mg p.o./PR q 4° prn temp > 100°
	Sliding Scale Insulin as needed
	Bowel regimen prn
	
	To Consider:
	   • Antiplatelet treament
	   • IV heparin
	   • t-PA (No ASA, Heparin or Warfarin for 24
	    hrs.–Refer to t-PA protocol)
	   • Investigational drug (refer to Protocol)
		Renew IVF or IV to heplock
		Reassess BP meds w/parameters as needed
		Acetaminophen 650 mg p.o./PR q 4° prn temp > 100°
		Sliding Scale Insulin as needed
		Bowel regimen prn
		Continue from Day One as needed
		   Antiplatelet Therapy
		   IV Heparin
		
		To Consider:
		   • Warfarin if indicated
		   • If pt recieved t-PA, begin antiplatelet treatment
		    or heparin as appropriate
		   • Investigational drug, follow Protocol
			Renew IVF, IV to hep lock, or D/C IV
			Reassess BP meds w/parameters as needed
			Acetaminophen 650 mg p.o./PR q 4° prn temp > 100°
			Sliding Scale Insulin and restart diabetic regimen if
			   appropriate
			Bowel regimen prn
			
			Continue as appropriate
			   -Antiplatelet Therapy
			   -IV Heparin → Warfarin
			
			If investigational Drug, follow Protocol

Consults	**Notify Case Manager on Admission**
	Notify Social Work on Admission
	Consult as Needed:
	   • Physical Medicine & Rehabilitation (PM&R)
	   • Speech Therapy
	   • Primary MD
	   • Cardiology
		Completion of consults ordered Day 1
		Consult as Needed:
		   • Home Health
		   • Rehab Coordinator
		   • Neuropsych
		   • Neurosurgery
		   • Vascular Surgery
			Completion of Consults ordered Day 2
			GI if feeding tube needed

Activity	Bed rest (HOB up 30°)
	    -or-
	Increase activity as tolerated
	To Consider:
	   • Pt may come off monitor for testing or traveling
	    to Rehab Dept.
		Bed rest (HOB up 30°)
		Increase activity as tolerated
		    -or-
		Increase activity per PM&R
			Increase activity as tolerated
			    -or-
			Pt. seen by PT/OT
			Increase activity per PM&R

Nutrition	Nutrition Screen
	NPO/Aspiration Precautions
	    -or-
	Diet as recommended by Speech
		NPO/Aspiration Precautions
		Advance diet or per Speech/Dietitian recommendations
		
		To Consider:
		   • Temporary Feeding tube
			NPO/Aspiration Precautions
			Tube feeding per Dietitian recommendations
			    -or-
			Advance diet per Speech/Dietitian Guidelines

Patient/Family Education D/C Planning	Orient to unit routine Educate about disease process Educate about diagnostic tests and meds Discharge Planning Assessment Initiated	Educate about diagnostic tests and meds Discuss discharge care options	Ongoing Stroke Education Start Warfarin teaching as needed **Finalize disp. plans (Home, Rehab, SNF)** **Discharge if appropriate**
Comments			

Figure B-3   Clinical pathway for acute ischemic stroke. Courtesy of Thomas Jefferson University Hospital, Philadelphia, PA. Available at www.stroke-site.org

Acute Ischemic Stroke Critical Pathway Card

	Day 4 / / ASU/General Floor	Day 5-7 / / ASU/General Floor	Post Discharge Care/Home Health

Goals/Outcomes	Neuro status stabilized/improved
	Pt transferred to floor
	Rehab therapies continued as appropriate
	NIHSS and Barthel Index documented, if patient discharged
	Discharge if appropriate
	
	NIHSS _____ Barthel Imdex _____ (upon discharge)
		Neuro status stabilized/improved
		Special diagnostic tests documented
		Rehab therapies continued as appropriate
		NIHSS and Barthel Index documented,
		  if patient discharged
		Discharge if appropriate
		
		NIHSS _____ Barthel Imdex _____ (upon discharge)
			Maintain compliance with meds, diet and risk
			  factor reduction
			Follow-up with Primary MD/Neurology
			Absence of recurrent symptoms
			Return to baseline activity level
			Recognise Signs & Symptoms and when to call Physician
			Advance diet accordingly

Laboratory/
Diagnostic Tests
	PTT if on heparin
	PT/INR if on warfarin
	Follow-up abnormal tests
	
	To Consider:
	• Modified Barium Swallow
		PTT if on heparin
		PT/INR if on warfarin
			Labs per MD order
			  -PT/INR if on warfarin
			  -CBC q2 weeks x 3 months if on Ticlopidine

Assessments/RN
Interventions
	VS and Neuro Checks per Unit Protocol
	Cardiac monitoring (ASU)
	Continuous Pulse Ox, and titrate O2 to keep
	  SpO2 > 95%
	Bowel/Bladder/Skin Assessment
	Avoid foley cath
	Compresssion boots (unless anticoagulated)
	HOB up 30°/Aspiration Precautions
	Turn q2h if pt on bed rest
	ROM as per Rehab, if paralysis exists
	Hand/foot splint as per Rehab as needed
	
	To Consider:
	• D'C cardiac monitoring & Pulse Ox & transfer to floor
	  -or-
	• D'C to home
		VS and Neuro checks per Unit Protocol
		Cardiac monitoring as needed
		Continuous Pulse Ox as needed
		Bowel/Bladder/Skin Assessment
		Avoid foley cath
		Compresssion boots (unless anticoagulated)
		HOB up 30°/Aspiration Precautions
		Turn q2h if pt on bed rest
		ROM as per Rehab, if paralysis exists
		Hand/foot splint as per Rehab as needed
			Vital Signs
			Assess for and educate about recurrent signs
			  and stmptoms of TIA/Stroke
			Complete Oasis Tool
			Asses PT/OT/Speech and swallow needs
			Assess feeding tube functioning
			Evaluate support systems
			Bowel/Bladder Training

Medications/
Treatments
	IV to hep lock or D'C IV
	Reassess BP meds and parameters as needed
	Consider antihypertensive regimen
	Acetaminophen 650mg p.o./PR q4 prn temp. > 100
	Diabetic regimen if appropriate
	Bowel regimen prn
	
	Continue as appropriate
	  -Antiplatelet therapy
	  -IV Heparin Æ Warfarin (D'C heparin when INR 2-3)
	
	If Investigational Drug, follow Protocol
		IV to hep lock or D'C IV
		Adjust antihypertensive regimen as needed
		Adjust diabetic regimen as needed
		
		Continue as appropriate
		  -Antiplatelet Therapy
		  -IV Heparin → Warfarin (D'C heparin when INR 2-3)
		
		If Investigational Drug, follow Protocol
			Review medications
			Set up med schedule via mediplan or calendar

Consults		Feeding tube placement if needed	Home Health Aid as needed Home PT/OT/Speech as needed Social Work /Registered Dietician if needed Case Management telephone follow-up
Activity	Increase activity as tolerated -or- Increase activity per PM&R	Increase activity as tolerated/as per Rehab guidelines	Encourage increase in activity as tolerated Exercise/Therapy protocols as per PT/OT

Nutrition	Increase tube feedings as tolerated as per
	  Dietitian Guidelines
	  -or-
	Advance diet as tolerated/as per
	  Speech/Dietitian recommendations
		NPO for feeding tube placement
		  -or-
		Advance diet as tolerated per
		  Speech/Dietitian recommendations
			Reinforce prescribed diet
			Refer as necessary to Out-Patient Dietitian X5077
			Consider Swallow re-eval for removal of feeding tube

Patient/Family
Education D/C
Planning
	Ongoing Stroke Education
	Warfarin teaching as needed
	
	Finalize disp. plans (Home, Rehab, SNF)
	Discharge if appropriate
		Ongoing Stroke Education
		Warfarin teaching as needed
		
		D'C instructions based on disposition plans
		Discharge if appropriate
			Reinforce signs/symptoms of stroke and need for
			  urgent intervention
			Reinforce importance of risk factor reduction and
			  med compliance
			Reinforce need to stay on meds
			Encourage pt/family that rehab process continues
			  long after hospital stay and to continue to work
			  towards improvement
			Advise on the availability of community/ financial/
			  transportation resources
			Warfarin teaching as needed

Comments			

Figure B-3 (Continued).

UNIT NO.

NAME

ADDRESS

BIRTH DATE:

VISIT NUMBER:

(if handwritten, record name, unit no., birth date, and visit no.)

PERMANENT PART OF MEDICAL RECORD

YALE NEW HAVEN HOSPITAL
CLINICAL PATHWAY

ACUTE CORONARY SYNDROME WITH OR WITHOUT PERCUTANEOUS CORONARY INTERVENTION [F-5021]

DIAGNOSIS: ❑ **RO/MI** ❑ **UNSTABLE ANGINA (USA)** ❑ **NON ST ELEVATION MI** ❑ **ST ELEVATION MI (STEMI)**

***EXPECTED OUTCOMES - PATIENT IS FREE FROM:**

DATE:	DATE:	DATE:	DATE:	DATE:
Patient Problem	**Patient Problem**	**Patient Problem**	**Patient Problem**	**Patient Problem**
• Myocardial ischemia (angina, ST/T-wave ECG changes, SOB) • Dysrhythmias • Hypotension / hypertension • Bleeding / hematoma • Hypoxemia (by SpO_2, ABG's) • Heart Failure • Maladaptive coping mechanisms • Education barriers (language, impaired vision or hearing, dementia, developmentally delayed) • Inability to verbalize understanding of: - reportable conditions (CP, etc) - activity limitations - plan of care • Self-care deficit-unable to return home/previous residence	• Myocardial ischemia • Dysrhythmias • Hypotension / hypertension • Bleeding / hematoma • Hypoxemia • Heart Failure • Maladaptive coping mechanisms • Education barriers (language, impaired vision or hearing, dementia, developmentally delayed) • Inability to verbalize understanding of: - reportable conditions - activity limitations - plan of care • Self-care deficit-unable to return home/previous residence	• Myocardial ischemia • Dysrhythmias • Hypotension / hypertension • Bleeding / hematoma • Hypoxemia • Heart Failure • Maladaptive coping mechanisms • Education barriers (language, impaired vision or hearing, dementia, developmentally delayed) • Inability to verbalize understanding of: - reportable conditions - activity limitations - plan of care • Self-care deficit-unable to return home/previous residence	• Myocardial ischemia • Dysrhythmias • Hypotension / hypertension • Bleeding / hematoma • Hypoxemia • Heart Failure • Maladaptive coping mechanisms • Education barriers (language, impaired vision or hearing, dementia, developmentally delayed) • Inability to verbalize understanding of: - reportable conditions - activity limitations - plan of care • Self-care deficit-unable to return home/previous residence	• Myocardial ischemia • Dysrhythmias • Hypotension / hypertension • Bleeding / hematoma • Hypoxemia • Heart Failure • Maladaptive coping mechanisms • Education barriers (language, impaired vision or hearing, dementia, developmentally delayed) • Inability to verbalize understanding of: - reportable conditions - activity limitations - plan of care • Self-care deficit-unable to return home/previous residence
AMI Quality Indicators				
• Aspirin • Beta Blocker • If STEM - Primary PTCA within 90 minutes	• Aspirin • Beta Blocker	• Aspirin • Beta Blocker	• Aspirin • Beta Blocker	• If LDL > 100 mg/dl - D/C on statin • Discharged on ASA, beta blocker • EF ≤40%– D/C on ACEI • Complete D/C instructions provided • Smoking cessation advice

* Variance reporting - circle variance, write History and Progress note, individualize Clinical Pathway - If problem cannot be resolved within 8-12 hour shift, add problem to IPOC/NPOC

Figure B-4 Clinical pathway for acute coronary syndrome with or without percutaneous coronary intervention. Courtesy of Yale New Haven Hospital, New Haven, CT.

PERMANENT PART OF MEDICAL RECORD
YALE NEW HAVEN HOSPITAL
CLINICAL PATHWAY

ACUTE CORONARY SYNDROME
WITH OR WITHOUT PERCUTANEOUS
CORONARY INTERVENTION   [F-5021]

UNIT NO.

NAME

ADDRESS

BIRTH DATE:

VISIT NUMBER:

(if handwritten, record name, unit no., birth date, and visit no.)

INTERVENTIONS

PATIENT/FAMILY EDUCATION	DATE: ___ UNIT: ___ Initiate GPE: YATAP /SCALES			DATE: ___ UNIT: ___ Initiate GPE: YATAP /SCALES			DATE: ___ UNIT: ___ Initiate GPE: YATAP /SCALES			DATE: ___ UNIT: ___ Initiate GPE: YATAP /SCALES		
	Method	*Response*	*Initials*	*Method*	*Response*	*Initials*	*Method*	*Response*	*Initials*	*Method*	*Response*	*Initials*
Key Patient Teaching Method Response	ventilator			ventilator			ventilator			ventilator		
G=Good V=Verbal	Monitoring equipment			Monitoring equipment			Monitoring equipment			Monitoring equipment		
F=Fair W=Written	other:			other:			other:			other:		
P=Poor TV= Video	symptoms to report			symptoms to report			symptoms to report			symptoms to report		
R=Refused	plan of care / priority problems			plan of care / priority problems			plan of care / priority problems			plan of care / priority problems		
G = complete understanding/ independent in performing skill	diet			diet			diet			diet		
F = limited understanding requires reminders/ multiple cues to demonstrate skill	activity			activity			activity			activity		
	smoking cessation			smoking cessation			smoking cessation			smoking cessation		
	medications			medications			medications			medications		
P = no understanding/ unable to demonstrate skill	weigh / monitor for HF symptoms daily			weigh / monitor for HF symptoms daily			weigh / monitor for HF symptoms daily			weigh / monitor for HF symptoms daily		
	emotions/coping with illness			emotions/coping with illness			emotions/coping with illness			emotions/coping with illness		
Booklets Distributed: ❑ Coumadin	risk factors			risk factors			risk factors			risk factors		
❑ Heart Failure ❑ Patient Pathway	tests/procedures			tests/procedures			tests/procedures			tests/procedures		
❑ Take Care ❑ Stent ❑ Stepping Toward Control ❑ Straight from the Heart ❑ Quit Smoking for Life ❑ Women's Heart Advantage ❑ Other:	other:			other:			other:			other:		

Figure B-4 *(Continued).*

UNIT NO.

NAME

ADDRESS

BIRTH DATE:

VISIT NUMBER:

(if handwritten, record name, unit no., birth date, and visit no.)

PERMANENT PART OF MEDICAL RECORD
YALE NEW HAVEN HOSPITAL
CLINICAL PATHWAY

ACUTE CORONARY SYNDROME
WITH OR WITHOUT PERCUTANEOUS
CORONARY INTERVENTION   [F-5021]

INTERVENTIONS

	DATE: UNIT:	DATE: UNIT:	DATE: UNIT:	DATE: UNIT:
ASSESSMENT	Cardiac risk factors: ☐ premature family history ☐ tobacco use within year ☐ diabetes ☐ hypertension ☐ hypercholesterolemia ☐ obesity ☐ sedentary Signs and symptoms of: angina/angina equivalent hypoxemia decreased perfusion bleeding maladaptive coping Cardiac rate/rhythm per CMP: Continuous ECG monitoring Hemodynamic parameter, T, RR, lung sound, SpO2 Other: _____ ☐ PA catheter per NOPM ☐ ABP per NOPM ☐ EF 40% or HF present – I&O weight per SCALES Program ☐ DM - finger sticks ac & hs or as ordered Follow diagnostic and lab data	Cardiac risk factors: ☐ premature family history ☐ tobacco use within year ☐ diabetes ☐ hypertension ☐ hypercholesterolemia ☐ obesity ☐ sedentary Signs and symptoms of: angina/angina equivalent hypoxemia decreased perfusion bleeding maladaptive coping Cardiac rate/rhythm per CMP Hemodynamic parameter, T, RR, lung sound, SpO2 Other: _____ ☐ EF 40% or HF present – I&O weight per SCALES Program ☐ DM - finger sticks ac & hs or as ordered Follow diagnostic and lab data If discharge-dependent labs drawn, label specimens with special sticker	Signs and symptoms of: angina/angina equivalent hypoxemia decreased perfusion bleeding maladaptive coping Cardiac rate/rhythm per CMP Hemodynamic parameter, T, RR, lung sound, SpO2 Other: _____ ☐ EF 40% or HF present – I&O weight per SCALES Program ☐ DM - finger sticks ac & hs or as ordered Follow diagnostic and lab data If discharge-dependent labs drawn, label specimens with special sticker	Signs and symptoms of: angina/angina equivalent hypoxemia decreased perfusion bleeding maladaptive coping mechanisms D/C continuous ECG monitoring ☐ EF 40% or HF present – I&O weight per SCALES Program ☐ DM - finger sticks ac & hs or as ordered If discharge-dependent labs drawn, label specimens with special sticker
MEDICATIONS	*SAAB (Statin, ASA, ACEI, Beta Blocker) if indicated Consider: IV GP IIB / IIIA platelet inhibitor, clopidogrel, anticoagulant, nitrate, nicotine replacement tx/bupropion, if tobacco user O2 via N/C @2L/min IV fluids or IID as ordered	*SAAB if indicated Consider: IV GP IIB / IIIA platelet inhibitor, clopidogrel, anticoagulant, nitrate, nicotine replacement tx/bupropion, if tobacco user Consider discontinuing O2 via N/C @ 2L/min if SPO2 95% IV fluids or IID as ordered	*SAAB if indicated Consider: IV GP IIB / IIIA platelet inhibitor, anticoagulant, nitrate, clopidogrel IV fluids or IID as ordered	*SAAB if indicated If EF 40% discharge on ACE I; if not prescribed, document rationale IV fluids or IID as ordered
PAIN Ischemic pain	Assess for pain with vital signs & within one hour of an intervention for pain Interventions - CMP: Anginal Symptoms	Assess for pain with vital signs & within 1 hour of an intervention for pain Interventions - CMP: Anginal Symptoms	Assess for pain with vital signs & within 1 hour of an intervention for pain Interventions - CMP: Anginal Symptoms	Assess for pain with vital signs & within 1 hour of an intervention for pain Interventions - CMP: Anginal Symptoms
Other pain source	Add on to IPOC/NPOC	Add onto IPOC/NPOC	Add onto IPOC/NPOC	Add on to IPOC/NPOC

Figure B-4 (*Continued*).

PERMANENT PART OF MEDICAL RECORD

YALE NEW HAVEN HOSPITAL
CLINICAL PATHWAY

ACUTE CORONARY SYNDROME WITH OR WITHOUT PERCUTANEOUS CORONARY INTERVENTION [F-5021]

UNIT NO.

NAME

ADDRESS

BIRTH DATE:

VISIT NUMBER:

(if handwritten, record name, unit no., birth date, and visit no.)

INTERVENTIONS

	DATE: ___ UNIT: ___	DATE: ___ UNIT: ___	DATE: ___ UNIT: ___	DATE: ___ UNIT: ___	DATE: ___ UNIT: ___
TESTS / PROCEDURES	Labs: *** Lipid profile,** troponin - draw at: CK, CK/MB every 8 hrs X 3 – draw at: CBC, platelets, lytes, bun/CR, LFTs, PT/PTT CXR, ECG (with RV leads if IWMI) □ stress test with imaging □ cardiac echo - EF ___ % □ other: **REFER TO PAGE 5 OF INTERVENTIONS** □ cardiac catheterization □ PTCA /stent: ___ □ brachytherapy	□ stress test with imaging □ cardiac echo - EF ___ % □ other: **REFER TO PAGE 5 OF INTERVENTIONS** □ cardiac catheterization □ PTCA /stent: □ brachytherapy	□ stress test with imaging □ cardiac echo - EF ___ % □ other: **REFER TO PAGE 5 OF INTERVENTIONS** □ cardiac catheterization □ PTCA /stent: □ brachytherapy	□ stress test with imaging □ cardiac echo - EF ___ % □ other: **REFER TO PAGE 5 OF INTERVENTIONS** □ cardiac catheterization □ PTCA /stent: □ brachytherapy	□ stress test with imaging □ cardiac echo - EF ___ % □ other: **REFER TO PAGE 5 OF INTERVENTIONS** □ cardiac catheterization □ PTCA /stent: □ brachytherapy
ACTIVITY	□ Bed rest □ Bed rest with bedside commode □ Bed rest - OOB to bathroom	□ USA: Advance as tolerated □ AMI: Out of bed to chair tid; Ambulate 50 ft, bathroom privileges □ Other:	□ USA: Advance as tolerated □ AMI: Out of bed to chair as tolerated; Ambulate 100 - 300 ft; Shower sitting - with supervision □ Other:	□ USA: Advance as tolerated □ AMI: Out of bed to chair as tolerated; Ambulate 100 - 300 ft; Shower sitting - with supervision □ Other:	□ USA: Advance as tolerated □ AMI: Ambulates 300-400 ft tid/qid □ Other:
DISCHARGE PROCESS	Identify key contact person and current home care services	Determine self-management needs (home care services, transportation, care provider) If Discharge Day: complete W-10, CR Referral and Written Instructions in CCSS. If AMI, assure quality indicators are addressed	Determine self-management needs If Discharge Day: complete W-10, CR Referral and Written Instructions in CCSS. If AMI, assure quality indicators are addressed	Determine self-management needs If Discharge Day: complete W-10, CR Referral and Written Instructions in CCSS. If AMI, assure quality indicators are addressed	If Discharge Day: complete W-10, CR Referral and Written Instructions in CCSS. If AMI, assure quality indicators are addressed
SIGN OFF PRINT NAME SIGN SHIFT					

Figure B-4 (Continued).

UNIT NO.
NAME
ADDRESS
BIRTH DATE:
VISIT NUMBER:

(if handwritten, record name, unit no., birth date, and visit no.)

PERMANENT PART OF MEDICAL RECORD
YALE NEW HAVEN HOSPITAL
CLINICAL PATHWAY
ACUTE CORONARY SYNDROME
WITH OR WITHOUT PERCUTANEOUS
CORONARY INTERVENTION   [F-5021]

INTERVENTIONS

	PRE-PROCEDURE	POST-PROCEDURE
MEDICATIONS	**DATE:** If allergy to contrast dye, consider prophylactic therapy Consider hydration If creatinine ≥ 1.3 mg/dl, consider acetylcystein 20%- 600 mg bidor 2 days Diabetes: give 1/2 NPH dose, cover with sliding scale; Hold Metformin for 48 hours Hold warfarin ASA PO platelet inhibitor if stent anticipated Discontinue heparin on-call to CV Lab as prescribed	**DATE:** Offer pain medication and sedatives PRN IV hydration Hold Metformin If on warfarin pre-procedure, consider restarting ASA If stent placed - p.o. platelet inhibitor Ensure order written to continue/discontinue heparin; If prescribed begin infusion 4-6 hours after sheath is removed.
TESTS / PROCEDURES		PTCA only: ECG, I&O, CK with MB in AM ☐ Femostop per CCSS orders - Remove @ _____ ☐ ACT prior to sheath removal @ _____ Pull sheaths when ACT ≤ 175 If receiving IIBIIIA platelet inhibitor, draw platelets 4 hours after bolus/infusion initiated - Draw @ _____
ASSESSMENT	Establish baseline lower extremity circulation, movement, sensation (CMS) bilaterally Comfort level or pain with vital signs	Vital signs every 30 minutes X 6, then as needed Monitor CMS of affected extremity and catheter insertion site for bleeding, hematoma every 15 min X 4, every 30 min X2, then every 1 hr Comfort level/pain with vital signs
ACTIVITY		Post cardiac catheterization: Right-sided catheterization - bed rest 4 hours OOB @ _____ Left-sided catheterization - bed rest 6 hours OOB @ _____ Immobilize affected extremity, head of bed <30° If vascular closure device used: ambulate after 1-2 hrs of bed rest or when puncture site stable: OOB @ _____ Post PTCA: bed rest while arterial sheaths in place maintain bed rest 6-8 hours after sheaths removed - OOB @ _____ head of bed <30° If vascular closure devise used: Bed rest x 4hrs then ambulate (see CMP) If IIB IIIA inhibitor infusing - bed rest untill infusion completed

PATIENT / FAMILY EDUCATION

Method	Response	Initials
pre-procedure teaching – sensations/experiences		
other:		

Method	Response	Initials
activity restrictions post-procedure		
hold pressure on groin to cough or sneeze		
call nurse for loss of sensation in extremity below puncture site or bleeding		

Key

Patient response	Teaching Method
G = good	V = Verbal
F = fair	W = Written
P = poor	TV = Video

DIET

If afternoon procedure scheduled - light breakfast, then NPO

Resume diet - encourage PO fluids unless contraindicated

Figure B-4 (Continued).

Interventional Categories

Interventional categories consist of the groups of activities that make up a comprehensive treatment plan and are shown in the left-hand column of the pathway (Fig. B-1C). Although the order in which they are listed varies, these categories typically include

- Tests
- Treatments and nursing interventions
- Consultations
- Medications
- Diet
- Activity
- Patient and family education
- Discharge planning

Outcomes

Defined outcomes provide the focus for patient care activities for the various disciplines. Pathways include outcomes identified for each time interval (Fig. B-1D). They should be realistic, reflect incremental progress, and be achievable by 90% of the population. Pathway outcomes include physiologic, psychological, social, and educational outcomes.

Variance Record

The variance record (Fig. B-2) is an extremely important part of the pathway and represents the mechanism through which improvements in patient care can be accomplished. Variance is defined as any deviation from the pathway. Because all events on the pathway are critical to recovery, deviations can negatively affect outcomes. If the pathway calls for a specific test or treatment on day 2 and it is not carried out on day 2, a variance has occurred. If the patient is to ambulate 3 times a day and ambulates only once, a variance has occurred. The variance and the causes are recorded. Some variance records require a written note; others use code numbers or electronic systems to record variance (see Fig. B-2).

Case managers collect and analyze the variance data to identify trends in patient care and outcomes. For example, a pneumonia pathway may specify that the first dose of antibiotics be given within 3 hours of admission to the hospital (delays in administration of the first dose of an antibiotic are associated with increased morbidity and mortality). The case manager reviews the variance records and determines that only 40% of pneumonia patients are receiving the antibiotic in the specified time frame. Assessment of the issue reveals that delays are a result of the length of time it takes for the medication order to be taken off the chart and delivered to the pharmacy and the length of time it takes for the medication to be delivered. The pneumonia pathway team discusses this issue and determines that the first dose of medication should be given in the emergency department since the emergency department stocks these medications. The pathway is then revised to reflect this change in care. At the next review, the case manager reports that 92% of pneumonia patients on the clinical pathway received their antibiotics within 1 to 2 hours of admission. This ex-ample illustrates how pathway use and variance data collection provide the forum for assessing an issue, determining a plan of action, implementing the plan, and evaluating the effectiveness of the plan.

The Nurse's Role

Nurses have a key role in all aspects of clinical pathway use. Participating in the development of the pathway is the first step. Because nurses begin and end the chain of staff involved in delivering care, they have a unique perspective in how health care systems work to enhance or impede the delivery of care. In the above example about antibiotic administration, staff nurses were able to identify the issue quickly and suggest solutions. Staff from other disciplines, being single links in the chain, cannot supply this global view of the problem.

Nurses are also responsible for initiating the pathway for appropriate patients and ensuring that the various events occur as planned. In some care settings or conditions, case managers who are advanced practice nurses closely follow pathway patients; in others, staff nurses or community-based nurses function as case managers. In any setting, enhancing and monitoring outcome achievement is a nursing activity. Patients may be given a printed copy of the patient pathway for reference. The pathway describes the care plan in simple language and pictures. The nurse discusses the pathway with the patient and focuses on achieving specific outcomes.

Nurses are also responsible for completing required documentation. Well-designed pathways strive for simplicity and should not duplicate documentation required elsewhere. For example, a separate nursing plan of care is not necessary when using a clinical pathway. The outcome section of the pathway usually requires documentation; other areas may need to be checked off or initialed so that other providers can readily see what has been accomplished. Documenting variance and initiating steps to address the variance are equally important, as is participating in redesigning care practices to promote the highest quality of cost-effective care.

Pathways in Practice

Several pathways are provided in the following pages to demonstrate the variety of formats the nurse may encounter. Figure B-3 is a pathway used at Thomas Jefferson University Hospital for patients with acute ischemic stroke. The pathway provides clear expected outcomes as well as a variety of checklists identifying all significant and sequential aspects of patient care. Figure B-4 is a pathway used at Yale New Haven Hospital for a patient with acute coronary syndrome with or without percutaneous coronary intervention.

Whatever format is used or condition treated, clinical pathways are documents in transition; they will change as research suggests better treatment strategies and as variance data are analyzed. Nurses' participation in these processes is essential for the successful implementation of clinical pathways and, ultimately, the opportunity to improve patient care.

INDEX

Page numbers followed by c indicate charts; those followed by f indicate figures; those followed by t indicate tables.